Congenital Heart Disease

A Clinical, Pathological, Embryological, *and* Segmental Analysis

Congenital Heart Disease

A Clinical, Pathological, Embryological, *and* Segmental Analysis

Richard Van Praagh, MD
Professor of Pathology Emeritus
Harvard Medical School
Director of the Cardiac Registry Lab Emeritus
Research Associate in Cardiac Surgery Emeritus
Emeritus Member of the Departments of Cardiology,
Pathology, and Cardiac Surgery
Boston Children's Hospital
Boston, Massachusetts

ELSEVIER

Elsevier
1600 John F. Kennedy Blvd.
Ste 1800
Philadelphia, PA 19103-2899

CONGENITAL HEART DISEASE: A CLINICAL, PATHOLOGICAL, EMBRYOLOGICAL, AND SEGMENTAL ANALYSIS

ISBN: 978-1-56053-368-9

Notice

Senior Content Strategist: Charlotta Kryhl
Senior Content Development Manager: Laura Schmidt
Publishing Services Manager: Catherine Jackson
Senior Project Manager: Daniel Fitzgerald
Designer: Amy Buxton

Printed in India.

Last digit is the print number: 9 8 7 6 5 4 3 2 1

This book is dedicated to all patients with congenital heart disease and to their physicians, surgeons, nurses, and other health care providers.

ACKNOWLEDGMENTS

To understand the bridge that exists between the genome and the operating room, one should study all the stages that make up this bridge. My postgraduate training (1954 to 1965) represents my attempt to do that. **The following are some of the outstanding individuals who have helped to guide and to contribute to my studies.** Also indicated are the names of my training positions and where and when this postgraduate work was done.

Dr. Laurence Chute and his staff at the Hospital for Sick Children in Toronto, Canada, introduced me to clinical pediatrics. I served as a Junior Assistant Resident in Pediatrics from 1955 to 1956.

Dr. Charles A. Janeway and his staff at the Children's Hospital Medical Center in Boston, Massachusetts, from 1957 to 1958. This position was known as a Senior Assistant Residency in Pediatrics.

Dr. John Craig, who masterfully directed my basic science year in general pediatric pathology at the Children's Hospital Medical Center in Boston, Massachusetts, from 1956 to 1957. This position was known as an Assistant Residency in Pathology.

Dr. MacDonald introduced me to adult internal medicine at Sunnybrook Hospital in Toronto, Canada, from 1958 to 1959. During this year I also finished a paper on the causes of death in hemolytic disease in a newborn—my first scientific paper. This position was known as an Assistant Residency in Internal Medicine.

Dr. Helen B. Taussig and Dr. Catherine Neill taught me during my first year of clinical pediatric cardiology at Johns Hopkins Hospital in Baltimore, Massachusetts, from 1959 to 1960. This position was known as a Fellowship in Pediatric Cardiology.

Dr. Jeremy Swan, Dr. Owings Kincaid, and Dr. Alberto Barcia (a visiting radiologist from Uruguay), and **Dr. Jesse Edwards** (a great pathologist) introduced me to cardiac catheterization and angiocardiography at the Mayo Clinic in Rochester, Minnesota, from 1959-1961—one whole year spent in this laboratory as a Fellow in Cardiopulmonary Physiology.

Dr. John D. Keith, Dr. Richard Rowe, Dr. Peter Vlad, and Dr. Stella Zacharioudaki (my future wife and a pediatric cardiologist) at the Hospital for Sick Children in Toronto, Canada, from 1961 to 1963. I was a Senior Fellow in Cardiology.

Dr. Maurice Lev at the Congenital Heart Disease Research and Training Center in Chicago, Illinois, from 1963 to 1965, where I became an Assistant Professor of Pathology concentrating on congenital cardiac morphology.

Dr. Robert DeHaan of the Carnegie Institute of Washington, where I did experimental and observational embryology, from January 1 to June 30, 1966. My title was Visiting Scientist.

Dr. Alexander Nadas, Chief of the Department of Cardiology, **Dr. Robert E. Gross**, Chief of the Department of Surgery, and **Dr. Sidney Farber,** Chief of the Department of Pathology—all three invited me to become a member of the staff of Children's Hospital Medical Center in Boston, Massachusetts. **Dr. Stella Van Praagh,** by then my wife, was included in this invitation.

The unfailing expert assistance of **Elsevier** was greatly appreciated.

Dr. Maurice Lev's morphologic method in cardiac chamber identification has been an inspiration. **Dr. Jesse Edwards'** clinicopathologic correlation has been exemplary.

Dr. Richard Van Praagh founded the Cardiac Registry, where he did many of the lectures for the medical fellows and staff, including some for only the nurses, and he also did most of the cardiac dissections. He became Professor of Pathology at Harvard Medical School, Boston, Massachusetts, in 1974.

Dr. Stella Van Praagh was the Assistant Director of the Cardiac Registry, and her assistance was enormously appreciated. She had the very important task of teaching our cardiac surgical residents.

Drs. Richard and Stella Van Praagh retired in 2002. **Dr. Stella Van Praagh** died in 2006. **Dr. Richard Van Praagh** did a "working retirement." It is now 2021. In the last 19 years, he has written 38 scientific papers and this book, *Congenital Heart Disease*. Following a Cardiac Surgery Meeting in Kraków, Poland, he was invited to write a paper for his Polish colleagues that resulted in the development of 15 new cardiovascular equations. These equations constitute a new approach to the understanding of congenital heart disease.

CONTENTS

SECTION I

Historical Perspective

1

Brief History of the Cardiovascular System

Who really discovered the circulation of the blood? Although much has been written,[1-223] the correct answer to this fundamental question remains largely unknown. The early history of the development of understanding of the cardiovascular system may be summarized chronologically as follows:

In 2625 BCE, the Chinese emperor **Huang Ti** *(Nei Ching)* realized that the heartbeat and the pulse go together. He may have had some understanding of the circulation of the blood, but evidence of this is lacking.

In 1550 BCE, the **ancient Egyptians** knew that the heart is the center of the vascular system. But they did not distinguish between arteries and veins. Regarding the pulse as the "voice" of the heart, they developed an extensive pulse lore.

In 330 BCE, **Praxagoras of Cos** first distinguished between arteries and veins. This distinction was further developed by his student, Herophilus of Alexandria, Egypt, about 300 BCE.

In approximately 330 BCE, **Aristotle** (Aristoteles) (Fig. 1.1) discovered the cardiovascular *system*. Aristotle, the tutor and friend of Alexander the Great, was the first to realize that the heart sits at the center of a system of arteries and veins. Aristotle understood that both the arteries and the veins arise from the heart. Prior to that time, the veins were thought to originate from the liver. Aristotle said that the heart normally has three cavities (ventricles), apparently because he did not regard the right atrium as a cardiac chamber. Instead, he interpreted the right atrium as a dilatation of the great vein—our superior and inferior venae cavae.[1]

In 300 BCE, **Herophilus** and **Erasistratus** of Alexandria saw chyliferous vessels in the mesentery of sheep. Erasistratus discovered that the heart is a pump. He was also the first to describe and name the tricuspid and bicuspid (mitral) valves. However, Erasistratus thought that the arteries contain air (which they do at autopsy, because the blood tends to drain into the more distensible veins). This erroneous concept impeded the discovery of the circulation of the blood.

In 25 CE, **Rufus of Ephesus** named what we call the base of the heart the "head" of the heart. He observed that on each side of the head of the heart there are soft, hollow, wing-like things that pulsate; he called them the "ears" of the heart because they were on both sides of the head of the heart. "Ears" in Latin is "auriculae," which became auricles in medical English. So Rufus realized that the right atrium is indeed part of the heart because it beats, and he was the first to distinguish between auricles and ventricles.[1]

In about 190 CE, **Claudius Galen** (Fig. 1.2) of Pergamos in Asia Minor showed that arteries contain blood, not air, as had been previously thought. Galen believed that arterial blood is admixed with air, resulting in aerated (spirituous) blood, as opposed to venous blood. Galen contended that venous blood passes from the right ventricle into the left ventricle via invisible pores in the interventricular septum. He also thought that a small amount of blood passes from the right ventricle via the pulmonary artery and lungs into the left heart. So Galen had a partial understanding of the pulmonary (or lesser) circulation.

In about 1250 CE, **Ibn al-Nafis** deduced the existence of the pulmonary (lesser) circulation.[2,3] He thought that the pulmonary trunk is too large to be there only for the nutrition of the lungs, and hence he deduced that the blood of the right heart must flow to the left heart via the large pulmonary trunk and the lungs.

In 1505, **Leonardo da Vinci** (Fig. 1.3) concluded that the human heart has "lower ventricles" (chambers) and "upper ventricles" (chambers) and that the upper chambers have "ears" (auricles). Hence the concept of Rufus of Ephesus concerning the auricles, which the influential Galen had opposed, was finally accepted after a lapse of some 1500 years.

In 1543, **Andreas Vesalius** (Fig. 1.4) of Brussels, Belgium, in his epochal *De Humani Corporis Fabrica*, described no openings in the interventricular septum but did not flatly contradict Galen's dogma of invisible pores.

In 1547, **Giambattista Canano of Ferrara** described a few of the valves in the azygos vein.

In 1553, **Michael Servetus** (Serveto) rediscovered the pulmonary (lesser) circulation, apparently unaware of the prior work of Ibn al-Nafis. Servetus also denied the permeability of the ventricular septum. At the insistence of Calvin, Servetus was burned at the stake in Geneva, Switzerland, on October 27, 1553, because of his unorthodox views on the Christian Holy Trinity. All but two copies of his 1553 book, *Christianismi Restituto (The Restitution of Christianity),* were also burned. Calvin is thought to have strongly disapproved of an earlier work of Servetus, *De Trinitatis Erroribus libri septum* (*On the Errors of the Trinity,* in seven books), published in 1531.

In 1555, Andreas Vesalius, in the second edition of his *Fabrica,* stated that he could not understand how any blood could pass through the ventricular septum. But he deduced no further conclusions from this observation. We (R.V.P. and S.V.P.)[a] translated much of Book VI of the *Fabrica* in order to

[a]S.V.P. was my dear departed wife, Dr. Stella Van Praagh. She was born in Crete, Greece, and was an expert in ancient Greek. I am an old Latin scholar; we worked together on the translation.

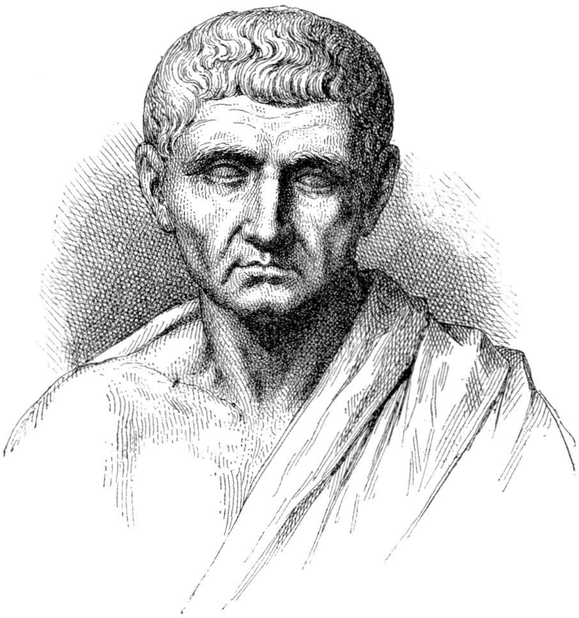

Fig. 1.1 Aristotle (384–322 BCE) discovered the cardiovascular system about 330 BCE. Born in Stagira, Macedonia, he studied under Plato at the Academy (367–347 BCE), tutored Alexander the Great at the Macedonian court (342–339 BCE), and opened his own school, the Lyceum, in Athens (335 BCE). His was also called the Peripatetic school because of his practice of lecturing in the Lyceum's covered portico or walking place *(peripatos)*. Aristotle was a one-man university for the Athenians, the Arabs, the Jews, and later for the medieval Europeans.

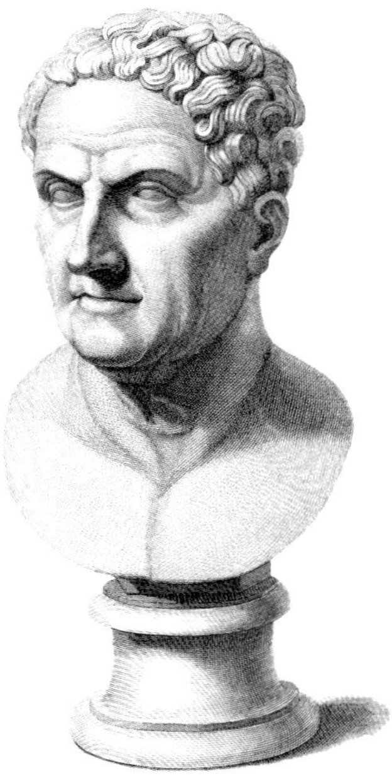

Fig. 1.2 Claudius Galen (c 130–201 CE) demonstrated that the arteries contain blood, not air as had previously been thought. *Artery* means air-containing in Greek (Greek *arteria*, from *aer*, air + *terein*, to keep or contain). Galen was a Greek from Pergamos in Asia Minor. After studying in Asia Minor, Greece, and Alexandria, he returned to Pergamos as physician to the gladiators—where no doubt he witnessed spurting arteries. From c 162 CE onward, he resided chiefly in Rome, where he became physician to Emperor Marcus Aurelius and wrote approximately 500 publications. Galen remained the pre-eminent medical authority until the publication by Andreas Vesalius (1514–1564) of *De Humani Corporis Fabrica (The Construction of the Human Body)* in 1543.

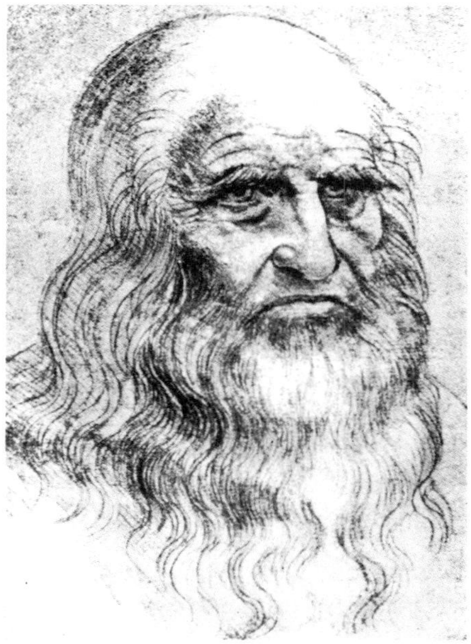

Fig. 1.3 Leonardo da Vinci (1452–1519), Italian painter, sculptor, architect, musician, engineer, and scientist. In 1505, he confirmed the distinction between the upper cardiac chambers ("ventricles") that have auricles (ears), and the lower cardiac chambers ("ventricles") that do not have auricles. This distinction between auricles and ventricles had first been made by Rufus of Ephesus in about 25 CE but had been effectively opposed by Galen. (Reproduced from Hemmeter JC. The history of the circulation of the blood. In Hemmeter JC: *Master Minds in Medicine*. New York: Medical Life Press; 1927:226.)

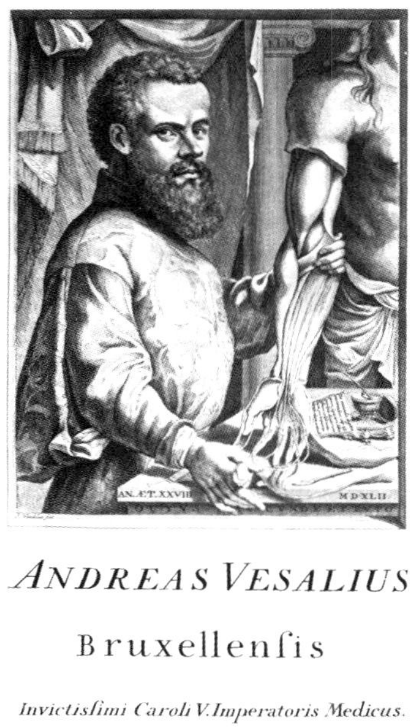

Fig. 1.4 Andreas Vesalius (1514–1564), Flemish anatomist from Brussels working in Padua, described no openings in the interventricular septum in his monumental work, *De Humani Corporis Fabrica* (1543). However, he did not flatly contradict Galen's erroneous dogma of invisible pores in the interventricular septum. Although Vesalius is now widely regarded as the father of modern anatomy and modern medicine, he did not understand the circulation of the blood. (Reproduced with permission from Van Praagh R, Van Praagh S. Aristotle's "triventricular" heart and the relevant early history of the cardiovascular system. *Chest* 1983;84:462.)

see if Vesalius understood that the blood circulates, that is, flows in a circle. No evidence was found that he did.

In 1559, **Matteo Realdo Columbo** described the pulmonary circulation and the impermeability of the ventricular septum, claiming both as his discoveries.

In 1564, Bartholomaeus **Eustacheus** discovered the thoracic duct in the horse.

In 1571, **Andreas Cesalpinus** (Andrea Cesalpino in Italian), the physician and philosopher of Arezzo, first described the circulation of the blood in his *Peripateticarum Quaestionum libri quinque* (*Of Peripatetic Questions* in five books).[4] Regarding the title of his work, it should be recalled that the school of Aristotle (see Fig. 1.1) was known as the Peripatetic school. Hence peripatetic questions are scientific and philosophic matters considered in the Aristotelian way.

Cesalpino stated that the blood is in constant transition from arteries to veins in all parts of the body by means of tiny anastomoses that he defined as *"vasa in capillamenta resoluta"* (vessels resolved into hairlike vessels). This is where our term *capillary* comes from; *capillus* means hair (Latin).

Cesalpino coined the term *circulatio,* by which he meant that the blood flowed in a *circle:* from the veins to the right heart, then to the lungs, thence to the left heart, and then to the arteries.

Cesalpino also realized that the pulmonary artery is an artery (not a vein, as Galen had said) and that the pulmonary vein is a vein (not an artery, as Galen had stated).

In 1583, Andrea Cesalpino published *De Plantis* (Of Plants), in which he confirmed his theory that the blood circulates.[4]

In 1593, Andrea Cesalpino published *Questionum Medicarum libri II* (*Medical Questions* in two books) in which he gave experimental proof of the circulation of the blood. These were the same two experiments later used by Harvey[4]:

1. Cesalpino observed that when a vein is first divided, dark venous blood comes out, which then becomes lighter and lighter in color, which favored the theory that the blood is circulating.
2. Cesalpino also observed that when veins are occluded, they always swell between the ligature and the capillaries, not between the ligature and the heart—as they should if Galen's concept of centrifugal venous blood flow were correct.

Consequently, as the American physician, linguist, and historian John C. Hemmeter[4] wrote in 1927, to Andrea Cesalpino of Arezzo "belongs the fame of being the first to have recognized and demonstrated the general circulation of the blood." In 1583, in his outstanding work *De Plantis,* Cesalpino stated: the blood is led through the veins to the heart, and is distributed by the arteries to the entire body (... *sanguiinem per venas duci ad cor, et per arterias in universum corpus distribui*). Cesalpino discovered the circulation of the blood without knowing about the valves in the veins.

In 1598, **Carlo Ruini** of Bologna published a book on the anatomy and diseases of the horse, in which it is clear that he understood the function of the valves of the heart.

In 1603, **Hieronymus Fabricius ab Aquapendente** (Fabrizio in Italian) described valves in the entire venous system in his work *De Venarum Ostiolis,* but he did not understand their function correctly. Fabricius was the tutor of William Harvey at Padua (1598–1602).

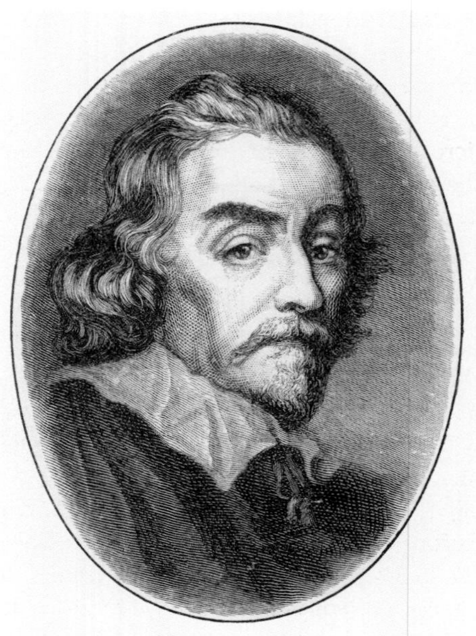

Fig. 1.5 William Harvey of Folkestone, Kent, England, was the third "discoverer" of the circulation (in 1628), after Cesalpino (1571, 1583, 1593) and Sarpi (1623). Harvey deserves the credit for having persuaded the medical world, despite considerable opposition, that the blood does indeed circulate.

In Milan in 1622, **Gaspare Aselli** observed chyliferous vessels in the mesentery of the dog and called them lactiferous vessels.

In 1623, **Paolo Sarpi**, the famous theologian and canonist of the republic of Venice, as well as a student and friend of Fabricius, described the function of the venous valves correctly. From this understanding, he deduced the circulation of the blood. Unfortunately, however, the manuscripts of Sarpi in the library of the Servitians at Venice were destroyed in a monastery fire in September 1769. Hence, Paolo Sarpi may be regarded as the second "discoverer" (or first rediscoverer after Caesalpinus) of the circulation of the blood.

In 1628, **William Harvey** (Fig. 1.5) of Folkestone, Kent, England, described the circulation of the blood in a 72-page book titled *Exercitatio Anatomica de Motu Cordis et Sanguinis in Animalibus (Anatomic Experience Concerning the Motion of the Heart and Blood in Animals),* and he demonstrated the circulation experimentally. After the publication of his little book at Frankfurt, Harvey was accused of plagiarism by many of his contemporaries (Micanzio, Vesling, Walaens, Riolan, Bartholin, and others). Harvey is now considered to have been the third "discoverer" (or the second rediscoverer, after Sarpi) of the circulation of the blood.[4] Harvey deserves the credit not for discovering the circulation of the blood but for eventually persuading the scientific world, over considerable opposition, that the blood does indeed circulate.

In 1648, while a student in Paris, **Jean Pecquet** discovered the thoracic duct in humans and realized that the lactiferous vessels do not return to the liver but to the thoracic duct and thence to the left subclavian vein.

In 1650, **Olaf Rudbeck** was a student at Uppsala University when he discovered the lymphatics of the liver and found that they too drained into the thoracic duct.

In 1661, at the University of Bologna, **Marcello Malpighi,** using a microscope, was the first to observe the motion of the blood in the capillaries of the lung in frogs. Malpighi had discovered the postulated capillaries of Caesalpinus.

In 1771, **Lazzaro Spallanzani,** again with the aid of a microscope, saw blood flowing in the umbilical vessels of the chick embryo. This was the first direct observation of the circulation of the blood in a warm-blooded animal.

Thus, the *normal* circulation of the blood and lymph was discovered and documented over approximately 4,400 years from 2625 BCE (Huang Ti; *Nei Ching*) to 1771 CE (Lazzaro Spallanzani).

The story of the discovery and documentation of the *abnormal* circulation of the blood in infants and children is much more recent, being little more than 330 years old. Very largely, this is the history of congenital (as opposed to acquired) heart disease in infants and children.

For example:

The anomaly now known as the **tetralogy of Fallot** was first described by the Danish physician/priest **Niels Stensen** (1648–86) in 1671,[6] the patient being a macerated stillborn fetus with cervical ectopia cordis.

The malformation now known as **transposition of the great arteries** was discovered and described by **Matthew Baillie** (1761–1823) of London, England, in 1797.[7] However, by the dawn of the 19th century, congenital heart disease remained mostly unknown. **Single left ventricle** (LV) with absence of the right ventricular sinus and double-inlet LV was not discovered and reported until 1824 by **Andrew F. Holmes** (1797–1860) of Montreal, Canada.[8]

Corrected transposition of the great arteries was not discovered and reported until 1875 by **Carl von Rokitansky** (1804–78) of Vienna.[9]

Thus, the seeds of the understanding of congenital heart disease were sown in the 19th century by Thomas B. Peacock,[10] Carl von Rokitansky,[9] E. Théremin,[11] and others. It was in the 20th century that these seeds came to fruition. Many **books** appeared dealing with different aspects of heart in infants and children—cardiology, radiology, echocardiography, epidemiology, surgery, pathology, embryology, and etiology. Some of these books are listed alphabetically in Box 1.1.

"Are there any good books on congenital heart disease?" I am often asked. My answer to this important question is yes. But a list of "good" books on congenital heart disease is surprisingly hard to find, hence Box 1.1. I hope that this box of "old friends," which is by no means complete, will serve as a helpful reference list for students and investigators.

The history of the development of our understanding of congenital heart disease in the 20th century is clearly indicated—concerning any subject—by studying these books *chronologically* (see Box 1.1).

I would like to salute the investigators cited in Box 1.1, many of whom are friends. They and their colleagues are largely responsible for the remarkable progress that has occurred in pediatric cardiology and cardiac surgery during the 20th century.

In addition to the books referred to in Box 1.1 that are concerned *in part* with the history of heart disease in infants and children, there are also many fascinating books that focus *mainly* on history. Some of my favorites include the works of Garrison,[5] Majno,[220] Lyons and Petrucelli,[221] East,[222] and Harris.[223]

Is an understanding of history important to the comprehension of congenital heart disease? The brief answer is yes. Consequently, history is often an integral part of the presentation concerning many types of congenital heart disease.

BOX 1.1 Some of the Books Concerning Heart Disease in Infants and Children That Have Appeared During the 20th Century

Authors and References

Abbott ME[12,13]
Adams FH, Emmanouilides GC[14]
Adams FH, Emmanouilides GC, Riemenschneider TA[15]
Albou E, Lanfranchi J, Piton J-L, LeGoubey J[16]
Allwork SP[17]
Anderson RH, Shinebourne EA[20]
Anderson WAD[18,19]
Ando M[21,22]
Anselmi G, Munoz H, Espino Vela J, Arguello C[23]
Arey LB[24]
Aziz KU[25]
Bailey FR, Miller AM[26]
Bankl[27,28]
Barratt-Boyes BG, Neutze JM, Harris EA[29]
Barth LG[30]
Becker AE, Anderson RH[31]
Behrman RE, Kliegman RM, Nelson WE, Vaughan VC III[32]
Bergsma D, McKusick VA, Neill C, Rowe R, Lindstrom J, Jackson C, Rogers J[33]
Berri GG[34]
Beuren AJ[35]
Bharati S, Lev M[36,37]
Bharati S, Lev M, Kirklin JW[38]
Bianchi T, Invernizzi G, Parenzan L[39]
Bourne GH[40]
Boyd W[41]
Braunwald E[42]
Bremer JL[43]
Bucharin VA, Podzolkov VP[44]
Burakovsky VI, Bukharin VA, Bockeria LA[45]
Cassells DE[46]
Castañeda AR, Jonas RA, Mayer JE, Hanley FL[47]
Castellanos y Gonzalez[48]
Christidès C, Cabrol C[49]
Clark EB, Markwald RR, Takao A[50]
Clark EB, Takao A[51]
Cooley DA, Hallman GL[52]
Corone P[53]
Cotran RS, Kumar V, Robbins SL[54]
Crupi G, Parenzan L, Anderson RH[55]
Davies MJ, Anderson RH, Becker AE[56]
Davis JA, Dobbing J[57]

Continued

BOX 1.1 Some of the Books Concerning Heart Disease in Infants and Children That Have Appeared During the 20th Century—cont'd

Davila JC[58]
DeHaan RL, Ursprung H[59]
De la Cruz y Toyos, Munoz Castellanos L, Espino Vela J, Attie Cury F[60]
De Medeiros Sobrinho JH[61]
De Vivie ER, Hellberg K, Ruschewski W[62]
Donzelot E, D'Allaines F[63]
Dordevic BS, Kanjuh VI, Saradnici I[64]
Doyle EF, Engle MA, Gersony WM, Rashkind WJ, Talner NS[65]
Dupuis C, Kachaner J, Freedom RM, Payot M, Davignon A[66]
Edwards JE, Carey LLS, Neufeld HN, Lester RG[67]
Edwards JE, Lev M, Abell MR[68]
Eldredge WJ, Goldberg H, Lemole GM[69]
Elliott LP, Schiebler GL[70]
Emmanouilides GC, Riemenschneider TA, Allen HD, Gutgesell HP[71]
Engle MA[72]
Fawcett DW[73]
Feigenbaum H[74]
Feldt RH[75]
Fenoglio JJ[76]
Ferencz C, Rubin JD, Loffredo CA, Magee CA[77]
Fitzgerald MJT[78]
Fontana RS, Edwards JE[79]
Fraser FC, Nora JJ[80]
Freedom RM, Benson LN, Smallhorn JF[81]
Freedom RM, Culham JAG, Moes CAF[82]
Friedman WF, Lesch M, Sonnenblick EH[83]
Fyler DC[84]
Garson A, Bricker JT, McNamara DG[85]
Gasser RF[86]
Gasul BM, Arcilla RA, Lev M[87]
Giuliani ER, Gersh BJ, McGoon MD, Hayes DL, Schaff HV[88]
Godman MJ[89]
Goodwin JF[90]
Goor DA, Lillehei CW[91]
Gould SE[92]
Grant JCB[93,94]
Gray H[95]
Gross RE[96,97]
Hallman GL, Cooley DA[98]
Ham AW, Leeson TS[99]
Hamilton HL[100]
Hamilton WJ, Mossman HW[101]
Harris P, Heath D[102]
Hernández Rodríguez M[103]
Hamburger V[104]
Hudson REB[105]
Hyman LH[106]
Jones KL[107]
Kahn DR, Strang RH, Wilson WS[108]
Keck EW[109]
Keibel F, Mall FP[110]
Keith JD, Rowe RD, Vlad P[111]
Kidd BSL, Keith JD[112]
Kidd BSL, Rowe RD[113]
Kirklin JW[114]
Kirklin JW, Barratt-Boyes BG[115]
Kirklin JW, Karp RB[116]
Kissane JM[117]
Kjellberg SR, Mannheimer G, Rudhe U, Jonsson B[118]
Kreutzer EA[119,120]
Krovetz LJ, Gessner IH, Schiebler GL[121]
Langman J[122]
Lansing AI[123]
Lev M[124]
Lewis T[125]
Lieberman M, Sano T[126]
Litwin SB[127]
Lock JE, Keane JF, Fellows KE[128]
Long WA[129]
Lozsádi K[130]
Lue H-C, Takao A[131]
Macartney FJ[132]
Marino B, Dallapiccola B, Mastroiacovo P[133]
Marino B, Thiene G[134]
Markowitz M, Gordis L[135]
Mavroudis C, Backer CL[136]
McKusick VA[137,138]
Meszaros WT[139]
Miller SW[140]
Minot CS[141]
Moller JH[142,143]
Moss AJ, Adams FH[144]
Moss AJ, Adams FH, Emmanouilides GC[145]
Moulaert AJMG[146]
Nadas AS[147]
Nadas AS, Fyler DC[148]
Nebesar RA, Kornblith PL, Pollard JJ, Michels NA[149]
Neill CA, Clark EB, Clark C[150]
Netter FH[151,152]
Neufeld HN, Schneeweiss A[153]
Nichols DG, Cameron DE, Greeley WJ, Lappe DG, Ungerleider RM, Wetzel RC[154]
Nishimura H, Okamoto N[155]
Nora JJ, Fraser FC[156]
Nora JJ, Takao A[157]
Norman JC[158]
Okamoto N[159]
Olsen EGJ[160]
Ongley PA, Sprague HB, Rappaport MB, Nadas AS[161]
Parenzan L, Carcassonne M[162]
Patten BM[163]
Pearson AA, Sauter RW[164]
Perloff JK[165]
Pexieder T[166,167]
Pierson RN, Kriss JP, Jones RH, Macintyre WJ[168]
Pomerance A, Davies MJ[169]
Pongpanich B, Sueblinvong V, Vongprateep C[170]
Potter EL[171]
Potter EL, Craig JM[172]
Pugh L[173]
Quero Jiménez M, Arteaga Martínez M[174]
Rashkind WJ[175]
Ravitch MM[176]
Robb GP[177]
Robb JS[178]
Robbins SL[179]
Romanoff AL[180]

BOX 1.1 Some of the Books Concerning Heart Disease in Infants and Children That Have Appeared During the 20th Century—cont'd

Rosenquist GC, Bergsma D[181]
Rowe RD, Freedom RM, Mehrizi A, Bloom KR[182]
Rowe RD, Mehrizi A[183]
Roberts WC[184]
Rudolph AM[185]
Rushmer RF[186]
Sabiston DC, Spencer FC[187]
Sade RM, Cosgrove DM, Castaneda AR[188]
Shaher RM[189]
Simeunovic SD[190]
Smith CA[191]
Spitzer A[192]
Squarcia U[193]
Stark J, de Leval M[194]
Starling EH[195]
Stewart JR, Kincaid OW, Edwards JE[196]
Smith DW[197]
Takahashi M, Wells WJ, Lindesmith GC[198]
Taran LM[199]
Taussig HB[200]
Thiene G, Frescura C[201]
Tucker BL, Lindesmith GC[202]
Tucker BL, Lindesmith GC, Takahashi M[203]
Van Mierop LHS, Oppenheimer-Dekker A, Bruins CLDC[204]
Van Praagh R, Takao A,[205]
Van Praagh R, Van Praagh S[206]
Venables AW[207]
Vince DJ[208]
Vlodaver Z, Neufeld HN, Edwards JE[209]
Wagenvoort CA, Heath D, Edwards JE[210]
Walmsley R, Watson H[211]
Watson H[212]
Wenink ACG, Oppenheimer-Dekker A, Moulaert AJ[213]
White PD[214]
Williams RG, Bierman FZ, Sanders SP[215]
Williams RG, Tucker C[216]
Wolstenholme GEW, O'Connor M[217]
Wood P[218]
Zimmerman HA[219]

REFERENCES

1. Van Praagh R, Van Praagh S. Aristotle's "triventricular" heart and the relevant early history of the cardiovascular system. *Chest.* 1983;84:462.
2. Myerhof M. Ibn An-Nafis (XIIIth cent.) and his theory of the lesser circulation. *Isis.* 1935;23:100.
3. Bittar EE. The influence of Ibn Nafis: a linkage in medical history. *Hamdard Med Dig.* 1960;4:9.
4. Hemmeter JC. The history of the circulation of the blood. In: Hemmeter JC, ed. *Master Minds in Medicine.* New York: Medical Life Press; 1927:226.
5. Garrison FH. *An Introduction to the History of Medicine, with Medical Chronology, Suggestions for Study and Bibliographic Data.* Philadelphia: WB Saunders Co; 1967.
6. Stensen N. Translated and quoted by Goldstein D. *Bull Hist Med* 1948;29:526.
7. Baillie M. *Morbid Anatomy of Some of the Most Important Parts of the Human Body, London*; 1793:38. J. Johnson and G. Nicol.
8. Holmes AF. Case of malformation of the heart. *Trans Med-Chir Soc Edinb.* 1824:252.
9. von Rokitansky CF. *Die Defecte der Scheidewande des Herzens.* Vienna, W: Braumüller; 1875:83.
10. Peacock TB. *On Malformations, etc., of the Human Heart.* London: John Churchill; 1858.
11. Théremin E. *Études Sur Les Affections Congenital Du Coeur.* Paris: Asselin et Houzeau; 1895.
12. Abbott ME. Congenital cardiac disease. *Osler & McCrae's Modern Medicine.* 2nd ed. Vol. IV. Philadelphia and New York: Lea & Febiger; 1915:323.
13. Abbott ME. *Atlas of Congenital Cardiac Disease.* New York: American Heart Association; 1936.
14. Adams FH, Emmanouilides GC, eds. *Moss' Heart Disease in Infants, Children, and Adolescents.* 3rd ed. Baltimore: Williams & Wilkins; 1983.
15. Adams FH, Emmanouilides GC, Riemenschneider TA, eds. *Moss' Heart Disease in Infants, Children, and Adolescents.* 4th ed. Baltimore: Williams & Wilkins; 1989.
16. Albou E, Lanfranchi J, Piton J-L, LeGoubey J. *Atlas D'Angiocardiographie Des Cardiopathies Congenitales.* Paris: Geigy Laboratories; 1971.
17. Allwork SP. *Pathological Correlation after Cardiac Surgery.* Oxford: Butterworth-Heinemann Ltd; 1991.
18. Anderson WAD. *Pathology.* St. Louis: CV Mosby; 1961.
19. Anderson WAD. *Synopsis of Pathology.* St. Louis: CV Mosby; 1952.
20. Anderson RH, Shinebourne EA, eds. *Paediatric Cardiology 1977.* Edinburgh: Churchill Livingstone; 1978.
21. Ando M. *Necropsied Cases of Japanese Patients with Congenital Heart Disease, Tokyo*; 1984. Unpublished data.
22. Ando M. *Cardiac Registry, Tokyo*; 1984. Unpublished data.
23. Anselmi G, Munoz H, Espino Vela J, Arguello C. *Side by Side Great Arteries.* Mexico: Francisco Mendez Oteo; 1984.
24. Arey LB. *Developmental Anatomy, A Textbook and Laboratory Manual of Embryology.* Philadelphia: WB Saunders Co; 1965.
25. Aziz KU. *Heart Disease in Children.* Karachi: Shakoor Sons Printers; 1991.
26. Bailey FR, Miller AM. *Text-Book of Embryology.* New York: William Wood and Co; 1921.
27. Bankl H. *Missbildungen des arteriellen Herzendes.* Munich: Urban & Schwarzenberg; 1971.
28. Bankl H. *Congenital Malformations of the Heart and Great Vessels.* Baltimore and Munich: Urban & Schwarzenberg; 1977.
29. Barratt-Boyes BG, Neutze JM, Harris EA. *Heart Disease in Infancy, Diagnosis and Surgical Treatment.* Edinburgh and London: Churchill Livingstone; 1973.
30. Barth LG. *Embryology.* New York: Dryden Press, Inc; 1953.
31. Becker AE, Anderson RH. *Pathology of Congenital Heart Disease.* London: Butterworths; 1981.
32. Behrman RE, Kliegman RM, Nelson WE, Vaughan III VC. *Nelson Textbook of Pediatrics.* Philadelphia: WB Saunders Co; 1992.

33. Bergsma D, McKusick VA, Neill C, eds.*The Fourth Conference on the Clinical Delineation of Birth Defects, Part XV the Cardiovascular System*. Vol. 8. Baltimore: Williams and Wilkins Co.; 1972. Birth Defects: Original Article Series.
34. Berri GG. *Dextrocardias Y Levocardias*. Buenos Aires: Hector Macchi; 1958.
35. Beuren AJ. *Die Angiokardiographische Darstellung Kongenitaler Herzfehler, Ein Atlas*. Berlin: Walter De Gruyter & Co; 1966.
36. Bharati S, Lev M. *The Cardiac Conduction System in Unexplained Sudden Death*. Mount Kisco, NY: Futura Publishing Company, Inc; 1990.
37. Bharati S, Lev M. *The Pathology of Congenital Heart Disease, a Personal Experience with More than 6,300 Congenitally Malformed Hearts*. Armonk, NY: Futura Publishing Company Inc; 1996.
38. Bharati S, Lev M, Kirklin JW. *Cardiac Surgery and the Conduction System*. Mount Kisco, NY: Futura Publishing Company, Inc; 1992.
39. Bianchi T, Invernizzi G, Parenzan L, eds. *20 Anni Di Cardiochirurgia*. Bergamo: Carrara; 1988.
40. Bourne GH, ed. *Heart and Heart-like Organs*. Vol. 1. New York: Comparative Anatomy and Development; 1980 (Academic Press).
41. Boyd W. *A Text-Book of Pathology, an Introduction to Medicine*. Philadelphia: Lea & Febiger; 1953.
42. Braunwald E, ed. *Heart Disease, A Textbook of Cardiovascular Medicine*. Philadelphia: W.B. Saunders Co; 1992.
43. Bremer JL. *Congenital Anomalies of the Viscera, Their Embryological Basis*. Cambridge, Massachusetts: Harvard University Press; 1957.
44. Bucharin VA, Podzolkov VP. *Anomalies of Intrathoracic Cardiac Position*. Moscow: Meditsina; 1979.
45. Burakovsky VI, Bukharin VA, Bockeria LA, eds. *Second Joint USSR-USA Symposium on Congenital Heart Disease*. Moscow: Mir Publishers; 1976.
46. Cassels DE, ed. *The Heart and Circulation in the Newborn and Infant*. New York: Grune & Stratton; 1966.
47. Castañeda AR, Jonas RA, Mayer JE, Hanley FL. *Cardiac Surgery of the Neonate and Infant*. Philadelphia: W.B. Saunders Co; 1994.
48. Castellanos y Gonzalez A. *Cardiopatias Congenitas De La Infancia*. Fresneda: Havana, M.V; 1948.
49. Christidès C, Cabrol C. *Anatomie Des Arteres Coronaires Du Coeur*. Paris: Les Editions J. B. Baillière; 1976.
50. Clark EB, Markwald RR, Takao A. *Developmental Mechanisms of Heart Disease*. Armonk, NY: Futura Publishing Co, Inc; 1995.
51. Clark EB, Takao A. *Developmental Cardiology, Morphogenesis and Function*. Mount Kisco, NY: Futura Publishing Company, Inc; 1990.
52. Cooley DA, Hallman GL. *Surgical Treatment of Congenital Heart Disease*. Philadelphia: Lea & Febiger; 1966:1–213.
53. Corone P. *Cardiopathies Congenitales*. Paris: Maloine SA Editeur; 1972.
54. Cotran RS, Kumar V, Robbins SL, eds. *Robbins Pathologic Basis of Disease*. Philadelphia: W.B. Saunders Co; 1994.
55. Crupi G, Parenzan L, Anderson RH, eds. *Perspectives in Pediatric Cardiology.* Vol. 2. Pediatric Cardiac Surgery; Mt Kisco, NY: Futura Publishing Company, Inc.; 1989, 1990. Parts 1–3.
56. Davies MJ, Anderson RH, Becker AE. *The Conduction System of the Heart*. London: Butterworths; 1983.
57. Davis JA, Dobbing J. *Scientific Foundations of Paediatrics*. Philadelphia: W.B. Saunders Co; 1974.
58. Davila JC. *Second Henry Ford Hospital International Symposium on Cardiac Surgery*. New York: Appleton-Century-Crofts; 1977.
59. DeHaan RL, Ursprung H, eds. *Organogenesis*. New York: Holt, Rinehart, and Winston; 1965.
60. De la Cruz y Toyos MV, Munoz Castellanos L, Espino Vela J, Attie Cury F. *Inversiones Ventriculares*. Madrid: Editorial Cientifico - Medica; 1971.
61. De Medeiros Sobrinho JH. *Embriologia e Taxonomia das Malformacoes Cardiovasculares*. Sarvier: Sao Paulo; 1977.
62. De Vivie ER, Hellberg K, Ruschewski W, eds. *Herzchirurgie*. 3rd. Oeynhausen: TM - Verlag; 1982.
63. Donzelot E, D'Allaines F, eds. *Traité Des Cardiopathies Congénitales*. Paris: Masson & Co; 1954.
64. Dordevic BS, Kanjuh VI, Saradnici I. *Urodjene Srcane Mane*. Belgrade: Redakcijski Odbor; 1974.
65. Doyle EF, Engle MA, Gersony WM, Rashkind WJ, Talner NS. *Pediatric Cardiology, Proceedings of the Second World Congress*. New York: Springer-Verlag; 1986.
66. Dupuis C, Kachaner J, Freedom RM, Payot M, Davignon A, eds. *Cardiologie Pédiatrique*. Paris: Médecine-Sciences Flammarion; 1991.
67. Edwards JE, Carey LS, Neufeld HN, Lester RG. *Congenital Heart Disease, Correlation of Pathologic Anatomy and Angiocardiography*. Philadelphia: W.B. Saunders Co; 1965.
68. Edwards JE, Lev M, Abell MR, eds. *The Heart*. Baltimore: Williams & Wilkins Co; 1974.
69. Eldredge WJ, Goldberg H, Lemole GM. *Current Problems in Congenital Heart Disease*. New York: SP Medical & Scientific Books; 1979.
70. Elliott LP, Schiebler GL. *X-Ray Diagnosis of Congenital Heart Disease*. Springfield: Charles C. Thomas; 1968.
71. Emmanouilides GC, Riemenschneider TA, Allen HD, Gutgesell HP. *Moss and Adams Heart Disease in Infants, Children, and Adolescents, Including the Fetus and Young Adult*. 5th ed. Baltimore: Williams & Wilkins; 1995.
72. Engle MA, ed. *Pediatric Cardiovascular Disease*. Philadelphia: FA Davis Co; 1981.
73. Fawcett DW. *The Cell, its Organelles and Inclusions - an Atlas of Fine Structure*. Philadelphia: W.B. Saunders Co; 1966.
74. Feigenbaum H. *Echocardiography*. Philadelphia: Lea & Febiger; 1976.
75. Feldt RH, ed. *Atrioventricular Canal Defects*. Philadelphia: W.B. Saunders Co; 1976.
76. Fengolio JJ, ed. *Endomyocardial Biopsy: Techniques and Applications, Boca Raton*. Florida: CRC Press, Inc; 1982.
77. Ferencz C, Rubin JD, Loffredo CA, Magee CA, eds. *Epidemiology of Congenital Heart Disease, the Baltimore-Washington Infant Study*. Perspectives in Pediatric Cardiology; Vol. 4. Mount Kisco, NY: Futura Publishing Co, Inc; 1993:1981–1989.
78. Fitzgerald MJT. *Human Embryology: A Regional Approach, New York*. Hagerstown, Maryland: Harper & Row; 1978.
79. Fontana RS, Edwards JE. *Congenital Cardiac Disease: A Review of 357 Cases Studied Pathologically*. Philadelphia: W.B. Saunders Co; 1962.
80. Fraser FC, Nora JJ. *Genetics of Man*. Philadelphia: Lea & Febiger; 1975.
81. Freedom RM, Benson LN, Smallhorn JF. *Neonatal Heart Disease*. London: Springer-Verlag; 1992.
82. Freedom RM, Culham JAG, Moes CAF. *Angiocardiography of Congenital Heart Disease*. New York: Macmillan Publishing Company; 1984.

83. Friedman WF, Lesch M, Sonnenblick EH, eds. *Neonatal Heart Disease*. New York: Grune & Stratton; 1973.
84. Fyler DC, ed. *Nadas' Pediatric Cardiology*. Philadelphia: Hanley and Belfus, Inc; 1992.
85. Garson A, Bricker JT, McNamara DG, eds. *The Science and Practice of Pediatric Cardiology*. Philadelphia: Lea & Febiger; 1990.
86. Gasser RF. *Atlas of Human Embryos, Hagerstown*. Maryland: Harper & Row; 1975.
87. Gasul BM, Arcilla RA, Lev M, eds. *Heart Disease in Children, Diagnosis and Treatment*. Philadelphia: JB Lippincott Co; 1966.
88. Giuliani ER, Gersh BJ, McGoon MD, Hayes DL, Schaff HV. *Mayo Clinic Practice of Cardiology*. St Louis: Mosby; 1996.
89. Godman MJ, ed. *Paediatric Cardiology*. Vol. 4. Edinburgh: World Congress London; 1980:1981.
90. Goodwin JF, ed. *Heart Muscle Disease*. Lancaster: MTP Press Ltd; 1985.
91. Goor DA, Lillehei CW. *Congenital Malformations of the Heart -- Embryology, Anatomy, and Operative Considerations*. New York: Grune & Stratton; 1975.
92. Gould SE, ed. *Pathology of the Heart and Blood Vessels*. Springfield: Charles C Thomas; 1968.
93. Grant JCB. *A Method of Anatomy, Descriptive and Deductive*. Baltimore: Williams & Wilkins Co; 1948.
94. Grant JCB. *An Atlas of Anatomy*. Baltimore: Williams & Wilkins Co; 1947.
95. Gray H. In: Pick TP, Howden R, eds. *Anatomy, Descriptive and Surgical, A Revised American from the Fifteenth English Edition*. New York: Bounty Books; 1977.
96. Gross RE. *The Surgery of Infancy and Childhood, its Principles and Techniques*. Philadelphia: WB Saunders Co; 1953.
97. Gross RE. *An Atlas of Children's Surgery*. Philadelphia: WB Saunders Co; 1970.
98. Hallman GL, Cooley DA. *Surgical Treatment of Congenital Heart Disease*. Philadelphia: Lea & Febiger; 1975.
99. Ham AW, Leeson TS. *Histology*. Philadelphia: JB Lippincott Co; 1961.
100. Hamilton HL. *Lillie's Development of the Chick, an Introduction to Embryology*. New York, Holt: Rinehart and Winston; 1965.
101. Hamilton WJ, Mossman HW, Hamilton B, Mossman's Human Embryology. *Prenatal Development of Form and Function*. Baltimore: Williams & Wilkins Co; 1972.
102. Harris P, Heath D. The human pulmonary circulation, its form and function. *Health and Disease*. Edinburgh: E & S Livingstone Ltd; 1962.
103. Hernández Rodríguez M, ed. *Pediatría*. Madrid: Ediciones Díaz de Santos, SA; 1994.
104. Hamburger V. *A Manual of Experimental Embryology*. Chicago: The University of Chicago Press; 1966.
105. Hudson REB. *Cardiovascular Pathology*. Baltimore: Williams & Wilkins Co; 1965.
106. Hyman LH. *Comparative Vertebrate Anatomy*. Chicago: University of Chicago Press; 1964.
107. Jones KL. *Smith's Recognizable Patterns of Human Malformation*. Philadelphia: WB Saunders Co; 1988.
108. Kahn DR, Strang RH, Wilson WS. *Clinical Aspects of Operable Heart Disease*. New York: Appleton-Century-Crofts; 1968.
109. Keck EW. *Pädiatrische Kardiologie, Herzkrankheiten im Säughlings - und Kindesalter*. Munich: Urban & Schwarzenberg; 1972.
110. Keibel F, Mall FP, eds. *Manual of Human Embryology*. Philadelphia: JB Lippincott Co; 1910.
111. Keith JD, Rowe RD, Vlad P, eds. *Heart Disease in Infancy and Childhood*. New York: Macmillan Publishing Co, Inc; 1958:1967–1978.
112. Kidd BSL, Keith JD, eds. *The Natural History and Progress in Treatment of Congenital Heart Defects*. Springfield: Charles C Thomas; 1971.
113. Kidd BSL, Rowe RD, eds. *The Child with Congenital Heart Disease after Surgery*. Mount Kisco, NY: Futura Publishing Co, Inc; 1976.
114. Kirklin JW, ed. *Advances in Cardiovascular Surgery*. New York: Grune & Stratton; 1973.
115. Kirklin JW, Barratt-Boyes BG. In: *Cardiac Surgery - Morphology, Diagnostic Criteria, Natural History, Techniques, Results, and Indications*. 2nd ed. New York: Churchill Livingstone; 1993.
116. Kirklin JW, Karp RB. *The Tetralogy of Fallot, from a Surgical Viewpoint*. Philadelphia: WB Saunders Co; 1970.
117. Kissane JM, ed. *Pathology of Infancy and Childhood*. St Louis: CV Mosby Co; 1975.
118. Kjellberg SR, Mannheimer G, Rudhe U, Jonsson B. *Diagnosis of Congenital Heart Disease, a Clinical and Technical Study by the Cardiologic Team of the Pediatric Clinic, Karolinska Sjukhuset*. Stockholm. Chicago: The Year Book Publishers, Inc; 1955.
119. Kreutzer EA, Flores JE, Viegas C. *Radiologia Cardiovascular en Pediatría, Correlación Clínica Y Fisiopatológica*. Buenos Aires: Editorial Medica Panamericana SA; 1982.
120. Kreutzer EA. *y Col: Cardiologia Y Cirugia Cardiovascular Infantil*. Buenos Aires: Doyma Argentina SA; 1993.
121. Krovetz LJ, Gessner IH, Schiebler GL. *Handbook of Pediatric Cardiology*. New York: Harper & Row; 1969.
122. Langman J, Medical Embryology. *Human Development—Normal and Abnormal*. Baltimore: Williams & Wilkins Co; 1969.
123. Lansing AI, ed. *The Arterial Wall*. Baltimore: Williams & Wilkins Co; 1959.
124. Lev M. *Autopsy Diagnosis of Congenitally Malformed Hearts*. Springfield: Charles C Thomas; 1953.
125. Lewis T. *Diseases of the Heart, Described for Practitioners and Students*. London: Macmillan & Co; 1949.
126. Lieberman M, Sano T, eds. *Perspectives in Cardiovascular Research. Volume 1: Development and Physiological Correlates of Cardiac Muscle*. New York: Raven Press; 1976.
127. Litwin SB. *Color Atlas of Congenital Heart Surgery*. St Louis: Mosby; 1996.
128. Lock JE, Keane JF, Fellows KE. *Diagnostic and Interventional Catheterization in Congenital Heart Disease*. Boston: Martinus Nijhoff Publishing; 1987.
129. Long WA, ed. *Fetal and Neonatal Cardiology*. Philadelphia: W.B. Saunders Co; 1990.
130. Lozsádi K. *A Veleszületett Szívbetegségek Klinikopatologiaja*. Budapest: Medicina Könyvkiadó; 1983.
131. Lue H-C, Takao A, eds. *Subpulmonic Ventricular Septal Defect*. Tokyo: Springer-Verlag; 1983.
132. Macartney FJ, ed. *Congenital Heart Disease*. Lancaster: MTP Press Ltd; 1986.
133. Marino B, Dallapiccola B, Mastroiacovo P. *Cardiopatie Congenite e Sindromi Genetiche*. Milan: McGraw-Hill Libri Italia srl; 1995.
134. Marino B, Thiene G. *Atlante di Anatomia Ecocardiografica Delle Cardiopatie Congenite*. Florence: USES Edizioni Scientifiche Firenze; 1990.
135. Markowitz M, Gordis L. In: *Rheumatic Fever*. 2nd ed. Philadelphia: WB Saunders Co; 1972.
136. Mavroudis C, Backer CL, eds. *Pediatric Cardiac Surgery*. St. Louis: Mosby; 1994.
137. McKusick VA. *Cardiovascular Sound in Health and Disease*. Baltimore: Williams & Wilkins Co; 1958.

138. McKusick VA. *Heritable Disorders of Connective Tissue*. 3rd ed. Saint Louis: CV Mosby Co; 1966.
139. Meszaros WT. *Cardiac Roentgenology, Plain Films and Angiocardiographic Findings*. Springfield: Charles C Thomas; 1969.
140. Miller SW. *Cardiac Angiography*. Boston: Little, Brown & Co; 1984.
141. Minot CS. *A Laboratory Text-Book of Embryology*. Philadelphia: Blakiston's Son & Co; 1910.
142. Moller JH. *Essentials of Pediatric Cardiology*. Philadelphia: F.A. Davis Co; 1973.
143. Moller JH, Neal WA, eds. *Fetal, Neonatal, and Infant Cardiac Disease*. Norwalk, CT: Appleton & Lange; 1990.
144. Moss AJ, Adams FH, eds. *Heart Disease in Infants, Children and Adolescents*. Baltimore: Williams & Wilkins Co; 1968.
145. Moss AJ, Adams FH, Emmanouilides GC, eds. *Heart Disease in Infants, Children, and Adolescents*. 2nd ed. Baltimore: Williams & Wilkins Co; 1977.
146. Moulaert AJMG. *Ventricular Septal Defects and Anomalies of the Aortic Arch*. Leiden: Drukkerij Luctor Et Emergo; 1974.
147. Nadas AS. *Pediatric Cardiology, Philadelphia*; 1957,1963.
148. Nadas AS, Fyler DC. *Pediatric Cardiology*. Philadelphia: WB Saunders Co; 1972.
149. Nebesar RA, Kornblith PL, Pollard JJ, Michels NA. *Celiac and Superior Mesenteric Arteries, A Correlation of Angiograms and Dissections*. Boston: Little, Brown & Co; 1969.
150. Neill CA, Clark EB, Clark C. *The Heart of a Child - what Families Need to Know about Heart Disorders in Children*. Baltimore: The Johns Hopkins University Press; 1992.
151. Netter FH. The Ciba Collection of Medical Illustrations. *A Compilation of Paintings on the Normal and Pathologic Anatomy and Physiology, Embryology, and Diseases of the Heart*. Vol. 5. New York: Ciba Pharmaceutical Co; 1969.
152. Netter FH. *Atlas of Human Anatomy, Summit*. New Jersey: Ciba - Geigy Corp; 1989.
153. Neufeld HN, Schneeweiss A. *Coronary Artery Disease in Infants and Children*. Philadelphia: Lea & Febiger; 1983.
154. Nichols DG, Cameron DE, Greeley WJ, Lappe DG, Ungerleider RM, Wetzel RC, eds. *Critical Heart Disease in Infants and Children*. St. Louis: Mosby; 1995.
155. Nishimura H, Okamoto N, eds. *Sequential Atlas of Human Congenital Malformations, Observations of Embryos, Fetuses and Newborns*. Tokyo: Igaku Shoin Ltd; 1976.
156. Nora JJ, Fraser FC. *Medical Genetics: Principles and Practice*. Philadelphia: Lea & Febiger; 1974.
157. Nora JJ, Takao A. *Congenital Heart Disease: Causes and Processes*. Mount Kisco, NY: Futura Publishing Co; 1984.
158. Norman JC, ed. *Cardiac Surgery*. New York: Appleton-Century-Crofts; 1967.
159. Okamoto N. *Congenital Anomalies of the Heart - Embryologic, Morphologic and Experimental Teratology*. Tokyo: Igaku-Shoin; 1980.
160. Olsen EGJ. *The Pathology of the Heart*. New York: Intercontinental Medical Book Corp; 1973.
161. Ongley PA, Sprague HB, Rappaport MB, Nadas AS. *Heart Sounds and Murmurs, a Clinical and Phonocardiographic Study*. New York: Grune & Stratton; 1960.
162. Parenzan L, Carcassonne M, eds. *Open Heart Surgery in Infancy, Proceedings of the International Symposium Held in Bergamo*. Milan: Sapil Sp A; 1974.
163. Patten BM. *Human Embryology*. New York: MGraw-Hill Book Co Inc; 1953.
164. Pearson AA, Sauter RW, eds. *The Development of the Cardiovascular System*. Portland, Oregon: University of Oregon Medical School; 1968.
165. Perloff JK. *The Clinical Recognition of Congenital Heart Disease*. Philadelphia: WB Saunders Co; 1970:1994.
166. Pexieder T. *Cell Death in the Morphogenesis and Teratogenesis of the Heart*. Berlin: Springer-Verlag; 1975.
167. Pexieder T, ed. *Mechanisms of Cardiac Morphogenesis and Teratogenesis. Perspectives in Cardiovascular Research*. Vol. 5. New York: Raven Press; 1981.
168. Pierson RN, Kriss JP, Jones RH, Macintyre WJ, eds. *Quantitative Nuclear Cardiography*. New York: John Wiley & Sons; 1975.
169. Pomerance A, Davies MJ, eds. *The Pathology of the Heart*. Oxford: Blackwell Scientific Publications; 1975.
170. Pongpanich B, Sueblinvong V, Vongprateep C, eds. *Pediatric Cardiology - Proceedings of the III World Congress of Pediatric Cardiology, Bangkok*. Amsterdam: Excerpta Medica; 1990: 26 November - 1 December 1989.
171. Potter EL. *Pathology of the Fetus and the Newborn*. Chicago: The Year Book Publishers, Inc; 1952.
172. Potter EL, Craig JM. *Pathology of the Fetus and Infant*. Chicago: Year Book Medical Publishers, Inc; 1975.
173. Pugh L. *Color Atlas of Pathology - Prepared under the Auspices of the US Naval Medical School of the National Naval Medical Center*. Bethesda, Maryland, Philadelphia: JB Lippincott Co; 1944.
174. Quero Jiménez M, Arteaga Martínez M, eds. *Paediatric Cardiology - Atrioventricular Septal Defects*. Madrid: Ediciones Norma, SA; 1988.
175. Rashkind WJ, ed. *Benchmark Papers in Human Physiology/16, Congenital Heart Disease*. Stroudsburg, PA: Hutchinson Ross Publishing Co; 1982.
176. Ravitch MM, ed. *The Papers of Alfred Blalock*. Baltimore: The Johns Hopkins Press; 1966.
177. Robb GP. *An Atlas of Angiocardiography, Prepared for the American Registry of Pathology*. Bethesda: Armed Forces Institute Of Pathology; 1951 (American Registry of Pathology).
178. Robb JS. *Comparative Basic Cardiology*. New York: Grune & Stratton; 1965.
179. Robbins SL. *Textbook of Pathology, with Clinical Applications*. Philadelphia: WB Saunders Co; 1957.
180. Romanoff AL. *The Avian Embryo, Structural and Functional Development*. New York: The Macmillan Co; 1960.
181. Rosenquist GC, Bergsma D, eds. *Morphogenesis and Malformation of the Cardiovascular System*. New York: Alan R Liss, Inc; 1978.
182. Rowe RD, Freedom RM, Mehrizi A, Bloom KR. *The Neonate with Congenital Heart Disease*. Philadelphia: WB Saunders Co; 1981.
183. Rowe RD, Mehrizi A. *The Neonate with Congenital Heart Disease*. Philadelphia: WB Saunders Co; 1968.
184. Roberts WC, ed. *Congenital Heart Disease in Adults*. Philadelphia: FA Davis Co; 1979.
185. Rudolph AM. Congenital Diseases of the Heart. In: *Clinical-Physiologic Considerations in Diagnosis and Management*. Chicago: Year Book Medical Publishers, Inc; 1974.
186. Rushmer RF. *Cardiovascular Dynamics*. Philadelphia: WB Saunders Co; 1961.
187. Sabiston DC, Spencer FC, eds. *Gibbon's Surgery of the Chest*. Philadelphia: WB Saunders Co; 1976.

188. Sade RM, Cosgrove DM, Castaneda AR. *Infant and Child Care in Heart Surgery. Clinical Manual of the Department of Cardiovascular Surgery, Children's Hospital Medical Center.* Boston, Massachusetts. Chicago: Year Book Medical Publishers, Inc; 1977.
189. Shaher RM. *Complete Transposition of the Great Arteries.* New York: Academic Press; 1973.
190. Simeunovic SD. *Plucna Hipertenzija, U Urodenim Srcanim Manama - Dijagnostika, Procena, Lecenje.* Belgrade: M Gembarovski; 1984.
191. Smith CA. *The Physiology of the Newborn Infant.* Springfield: Charles C Thomas; 1959.
192. Spitzer A. The architecture of normal and malformed hearts, A phylogenetic theory of their development. Translated, summarized, and analysed by Lev M and Vass A, based on: uber Den Bauplan Des Normalen Und Missbildeten Herzens. Versuch Einer Phylogenetischen Theorie. *Virchows Arch f Pathol Anat.* 1923;243:81–201; Springfield, 1951, Charles C Thomas.
193. Squarcia U, ed. *Progressi in Cardiologia Pediatrica.* Milan: Casa Editrice Ambrosiana; 1978.
194. Stark J, de Leval M, eds. *Surgery for Congenital Heart Defects.* London: Grune & Stratton; 1983.
195. Starling EH. *Starling on the Heart, Facsimile Reprints, Including the Linacre Lecture on the Law of the Heart, Analysis and Critical Comment by Chapman CB and Mitchell JH.* London: Dawsons of Pall Mall; 1965.
196. Stewart JR, Kincaid OW, Edwards JE. *An Atlas of Vascular Rings and Related Malformations of the Aortic Arch System.* Springfield: Charles C Thomas; 1964.
197. Smith DW. *Recognizable Patterns of Human Malformation - Genetic, Embryologic, and Clinical Aspects.* Philadelphia: WB Saunders Co; 1970.
198. Takahashi M, Wells WJ, Lindesmith GC, eds. *Challenges in the Treatment of Congenital Cardiac Anomalies.* Mount Kisco, NY: Futura Publishing Co Inc; 1986.
199. Taran M. *Collected Works on Rheumatic Fever.* Flushing, NY: International Professional Publications, Inc; 1967.
200. Taussig HB. Congenital Malformations of the Heart. New York, The Commonwealth Fund, 1947, Volume I: General Considerations. Volume II: Specific Malformations. Cambridge, Massachusetts: Harvard University Press; 1960.
201. Thiene G, Frescura C. *Codificazione Diagnostica E Atlante Delle Cardiopathie Congenite.* Trieste: Edizioni Lint; 1984.
202. Tucker BL, Lindesmith GC, eds. *First Clinical Conference on Congenital Heart Disease.* New York: Grune & Stratton; 1979.
203. Tucker BL, Lindesmith GC, Takahashi M. *Obstructive Lesions of the Right Heart. Third Clinical Conference on Congenital Heart Disease.* Baltimore: University Park Press; 1984.
204. Van Mierop LHS, Oppenheimer-Dekker A, Bruins CLDC. Boerhaave Series for Postgraduate Medical Education. *Embryology and Teratology of the Heart and the Great Arteries: Conducting System; Transposition of the Great Arteries; Ductus Arteriosus.* Vol. 13. The Hague: Leiden University Press, Martinus Nijhoff Medical Division; 1978.
205. Van Praagh R, Takao A, eds. *Etiology and Morphogenesis of Congenital Heart Disease.* Mount Kisco, NY: Futura Publishing Co; 1980.
206. Van Praagh R, Van Praagh S, eds. *Diagnostic and Surgical Pathology of Congenital Heart Disease.* Vols. 1 and 2. Washington DC: Health Video Dynamics Inc; 1991.
207. Venables AW. *Essentials of Paediatric Cardiology.* Springfield: Charles C Thomas; 1964.
208. Vince DJ. *Essentials of Pediatric Cardiology.* Philadelphia: JB Lippincott Co; 1974.
209. Vlodaver Z, Neufeld HN, Edwards JE. *Coronary Arterial Variations in the Normal Heart and in Congenital Heart Disease.* New York: Academic Press Inc; 1975.
210. Wagenvoort CA, Heath D, Edwards JE. *The Pathology of the Pulmonary Vasculature.* Springfield: Charles C Thomas; 1964.
211. Walmsley R, Watson H. *Clinical Anatomy of the Heart.* Edinburgh: Churchill Livingstone; 1978.
212. Watson H, ed. *Paediatric Cardiology.* Saint Louis: CV Mosby Co; 1968.
213. Wenink ACG, Oppenheimer-Dekker A, Moulaert AJ, eds. *Boerhaave Series for Postgraduate Medical Education.* The Ventricular Septum of the Heart; Vol. 21. The Hague: Leiden University Press; 1981.
214. White PD. *Heart Disease.* New York: Macmillan Co; 1951.
215. Williams RG, Bierman FZ, Sanders SP. *Echocardiographic Diagnosis of Cardiac Malformations.* Boston: Little, Brown & Co; 1986.
216. Williams RG, Tucker CR. *Echocardiographic Diagnosis of Congenital Heart Disease.* Boston: Little, Brown & Co; 1977.
217. Wolstenholme GEW, O'Connor M, eds. *Ciba Foundation Symposium: Cardiomyopathies.* Boston: Eyre & Spottiswoode; 1964.
218. Wood P. *Diseases of the Heart and Circulation.* London: Eyre & Spottiswoode; 1957.
219. Zimmerman HA. *Intra Vascular Catheterization.* Springfield: Charles C Thomas; 1959.
220. Majno G. *The Healing Hand, Man and Wound in the Ancient World.* Cambridge, Massachusetts: A Commonwealth Fund Book, Harvard University Press; 1975.
221. Lyons AS, Petrucelli RJ, eds. *Medicine, an Illustrated History.* New York: Harry N. Abrams, Inc; 1987.
222. East T. *The Story of Heart Disease. The FitzPatrick Lectures for 1956 and 1957 Given before the Royal College of Physicians of London.* London: William Dawson & Sons Ltd; 1958.
223. Harris CRS. *The Heart and the Vascular System. Ancient Greek Medicine - from Alcmaeon to Galen.* Oxford: Clarendon Press; 1973.

SECTION II

Cardiovascular Development

2

Embryology and Etiology

In the human, an **embryo** may be defined as the developing organism from fertilization until the end of the second month of gestation, that is, from 0 to 60 days of life.

THE FIRST WEEK OF LIFE

The salient events of the first week of life (Fig. 2.1) are (1) ovulation, (2) fertilization, (3) segmentation, (4) blastocyst formation, and (5) the beginning of implantation.

A living human ovum surrounded by its corona radiata is shown in Fig. 2.2. **The single-celled ovum stage** is Streeter's **horizon 1.**[1] This ovum is thought to be 1.25 days old or less. One cannot tell by inspection whether this ovum has been fertilized. Fertilization normally occurs in the distal fallopian tube (see Fig. 2.1).

When fertilization has occurred, the next stage is known as **cleavage**. The large single-celled ovum undergoes mitotic division forming two cells (Fig. 2.3). A rapid succession of mitotic divisions produces a progressively larger number of smaller cells known as **blastomeres** (*blastos* = offspring or germ, and *meros* = part, Greek). A **morula** is shown in Fig. 2.4. A morula consists of 16 cells with no central cavity. Morula means "little mulberry" (*morus* = mulberry, Latin). This solid mass of blastomeres, formed by the cleavage of a fertilized ovum, fills all the space occupied by the ovum before cleavage. The stage of cleavage (Figs. 2.3 and 2.4) is Streeter's **horizon 2**. Cleavage occurs during the voyage of the zygote down the fallopian tube and into the uterine cavity. It is thought to take 3 to 4 days to reach the morula stage.

Then the morula develops a cavity, forming a **blastocyst** (Fig. 2.5). Blastocyst literally means "offspring" or "germ" (*blastos*, Greek) plus "bladder" (*kystis*, Greek). The formation of a cavity (bladder) separates the thick **inner cell mass** (future individual) from the thin-walled **trophoblast** (future placenta). Trophoblast means "nourishment" (*trophe*, Greek) plus "offspring" or "germ" (*blastos*, Greek). The blastocyst stage is reached by 4½ to 6 days of age and constitutes Streeter's **horizon 3**.

Parenthetically, etymologies are included to help the reader to remember these terms. If one understands what a designation really means (its etymology), then it is much easier to remember.

The blastocyst begins to implant in the uterine mucosa at about 7 days of age, that is, 7 days after ovulation (Figs. 2.1 and 2.6). **Implantation** is Streeter's **horizon 4**.

THE SECOND WEEK OF LIFE

The principal developments during the second week of life are summarized diagrammatically in Fig. 2.7:

1. Implantation is completed.
2. A bilaminar disc of ectoderm and endoderm develops out of the inner cell mass.
3. The amniotic cavity appears.
4. The yolk sac develops.
5. Primitive villi of the developing placenta make their appearance.

At the beginning of the second week, that is, at about 7½ days of age, the zygote normally is implanted, but the trophoblast still has no villi. This stage is **horizon 5** (Fig. 2.8).

About 2 days later, that is, at 9 days of age, primitive villi are seen (Fig. 2.9). The embryonic disc is now bilaminar, consisting of columnar ectodermal cells and cuboidal endodermal cells. The amniotic cavity and the yolk sac can now be seen. This is Streeter's **horizon 6**. The embryo shown in Fig. 2.9 closely resembles the diagram of Fig. 2.7.

Although the cardiovascular system is the first organ system to reach functional maturity, during the first two weeks of life, humans have no heart and no vascular system; that is, the cardiovascular system does not yet exist.

What germ layer does the cardiovascular system come from? From the mesoderm. But where does the mesoderm come from? As will soon be seen, from the ectoderm.

Ectoderm means "outside skin" (*ektos* = outside + *derma* = skin, Greek). *Endoderm* means "inside skin" (*endon* = within or inside + *derma* = skin, Greek). *Mesoderm* means "middle skin" (*mesos* = middle + *derma* = skin, Greek).

THE THIRD WEEK OF LIFE

The main events during the third week of embryonic life from the cardiovascular standpoint normally are:

1. the development of the mesoderm from the ectoderm on the 15th day of life,
2. the appearance of the cardiogenic crescent of precardiac mesoderm on the 18th day of life,

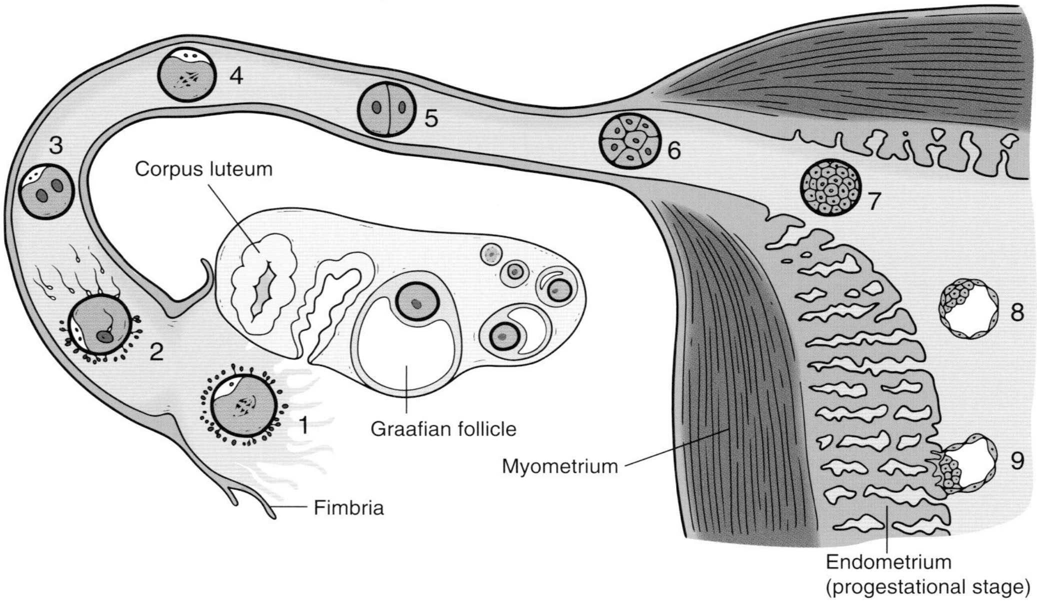

Fig. 2.1 Schematic representation of the events taking place during the first week of human development. (1) Oocyte immediately after ovulation. (2) Fertilization approximately 12–24 hours after ovulation. (3) Stage of the male and female pronuclei. (4) Spindle of the first mitotic division. (5) Two-cell stage, approximately 30 hours of age. (6) Morula containing 12–16 blastomeres, approximately 3 days of age. (7) Advanced morula stage reaching the uterine lumen, approximately 4 days of age. (8) Early blastocyst stage, approximately 4½ days of age. The zona pellucida surrounding the zygote has now disappeared. (9) Early phase of implantation, blastocyst approximately 6 days of age. The ovary shows the stages of transformation from a primary follicle to a graafian follicle to a corpus luteum. The uterine endometrium is depicted in the progestational stage. (From Langman J. *Medical Embryology*. Baltimore: Williams & Wilkins; 1963, with permission.)

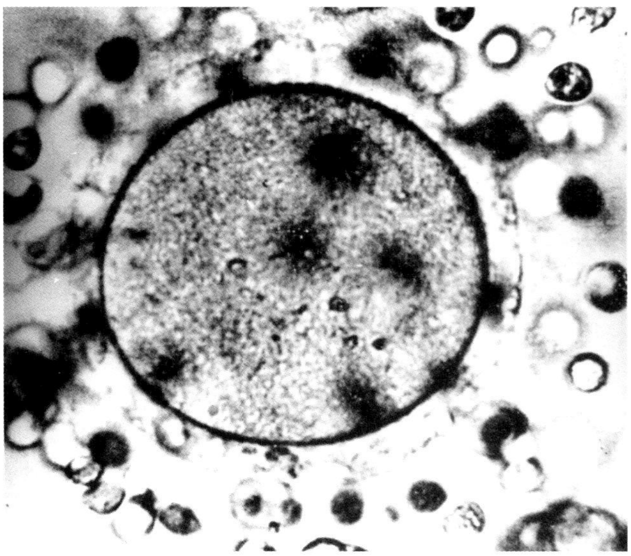

Fig. 2.2 Photomicrograph of a living human ovum, surrounded by the corona radiata, recovered from the uterine tube. This is the single-cell stage, horizon 1, 24 hours of age or less. (From Hamilton WJ, Mossman HW. *Human Embryology*. 4th ed. Baltimore: Williams & Wilkins: 1972, with permission.)

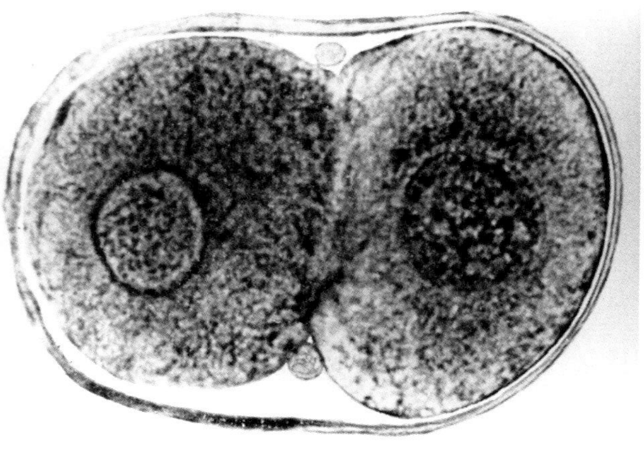

Fig. 2.3 The two-cell stage of the human zygote, estimated age approximately 30 hours. The two spherical blastomeres are of approximately equal size. Two polar bodies are also seen. In this photomicrograph, the human zygote has been fixed, this being the work of Drs. Hertig and Rock. (From Hamilton WJ, Mossman HW. *Human Embryology*. 4th ed. Baltimore: Williams & Wilkins: 1972, with permission.)

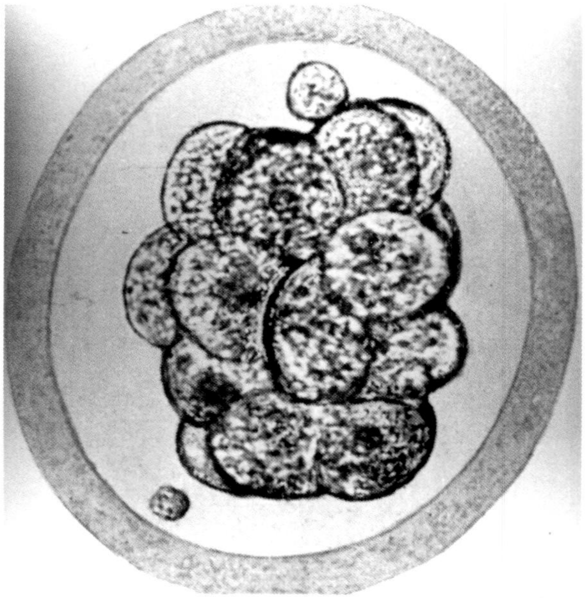

Fig. 2.4 Living morula, containing 16 cells, of a macaque monkey. Note the two polar bodies. This was the work of Drs. Lewis and Hartman. (From Hamilton WJ, Mossman HW. *Human Embryology.* 4th ed. Baltimore: Williams & Wilkins: 1972, with permission.)

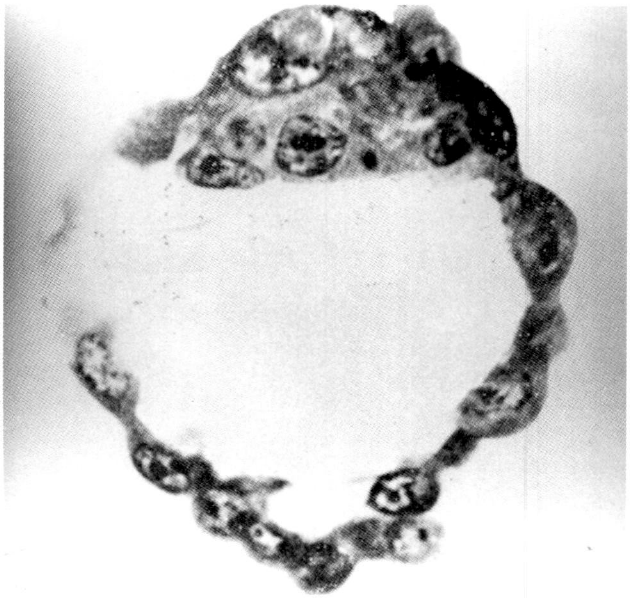

Fig. 2.5 Human blastocyst, photomicrograph of a section prepared by Drs. Hertig and Rock, estimated age approximately 5 days. This is horizon 3, in which the blastocyst is 5 to 6 days of age. (From Hamilton WJ, Mossman HW. *Human Embryology.* 4th ed. Baltimore: Williams & Wilkins: 1972, with permission.)

3. the development of the intra-embryonic celom on the 18th day of life,
4. the development of the straight heart tube at 20 days of age,
5. the beginning of D-loop formation in normal development, or the beginning of L-loop formation in abnormal development, at 21 days of age, and
6. the initiation of the heartbeat at the straight tube stage or at the early D-loop stage.

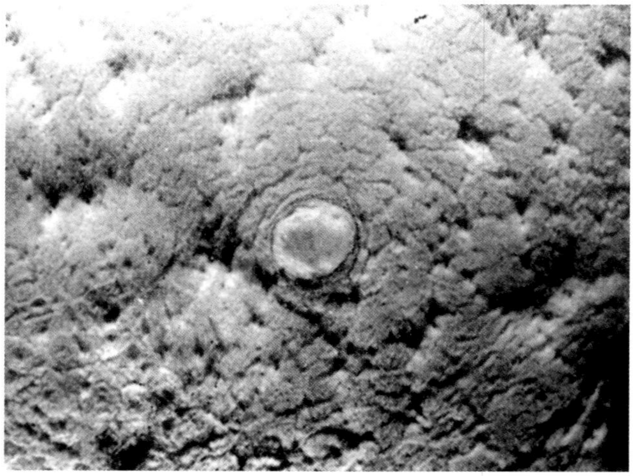

Fig. 2.6 Implantation of a 12½-day human embryo. The mouths of the uterine glands are prominent. The zygote is the slightly raised circular area. Implantation is Streeter's horizon 4. (From Hertig AT, Rock J. Two human ova in the pre-villous stage, having an ovulation age of about 11 and 12 days, respectively. Washington: *Contrib Embryol Carnegie Inst.* 1941;29:127, with permission.)

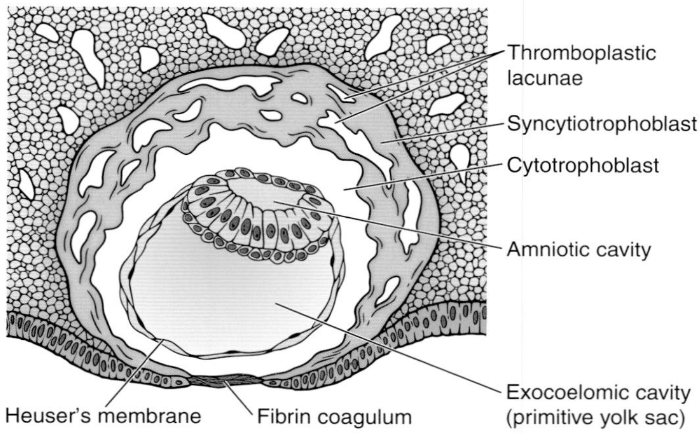

Fig. 2.7 The second week of life. The implanted bilaminar disc consists of columnar ectoderm and cuboidal endoderm. The mesoderm has not as yet appeared. Note also the amniotic cavity and the primitive yoke sac. (From Langman J. *Medical Embryology.* Baltimore: Williams & Wilkins; 1963, with permission.)

In somewhat greater detail, the main events in the development of the cardiovascular system during the third week of embryonic life are as follows:

1. The **mesoderm** develops from the ectoderm, appearing in the normal human embryo on the 15th day of life (Fig. 2.10). Note that the villi are branching and that the primitive streak has appeared, these being the features that typify **horizon 7.**

The primitive streak is a depression that marks the long axis of the embryo when viewed from the dorsal aspect (Fig. 2.11). As the mesoderm buds off from the ectoderm, the right-sided mesoderm migrates rightward and then cephalically, while the left-sided mesoderm migrates leftward and then cephalically. Since the mesoderm remains ipsilateral (right remains right sided and left remains left sided), rather than crossing

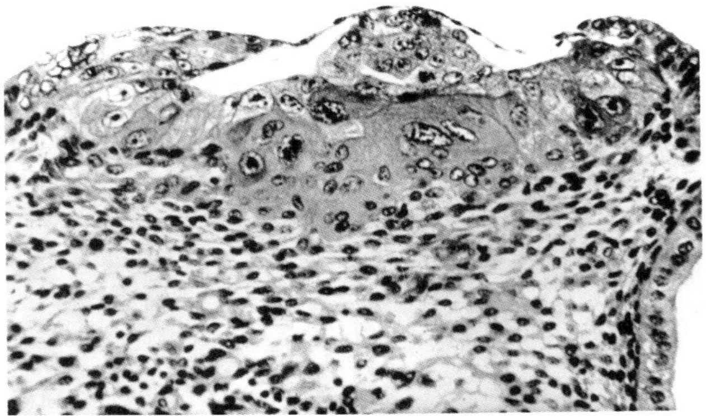

Fig. 2.8 Embryo implanted, but without villi, this being horizon 5. This section is through the middle of Carnegie embryo Mu-8020, estimated to be 7½ days old. The trophoblast (future placenta) consists of a thick proliferating disc without villi, growing into the endometrial stroma and with the embryo being covered by a thin mesothelial-like layer. The inner cell mass (the embryo) is represented by an oval mass of cells without obvious organization into cell layers. (From Hertig AT, Rock J. Two human ova in the pre-villous stage, having an ovulation age of about 11 and 12 days, respectively. Washington: *Contrib Embryol Carnegie Inst.* 1941;29:127, with permission.)

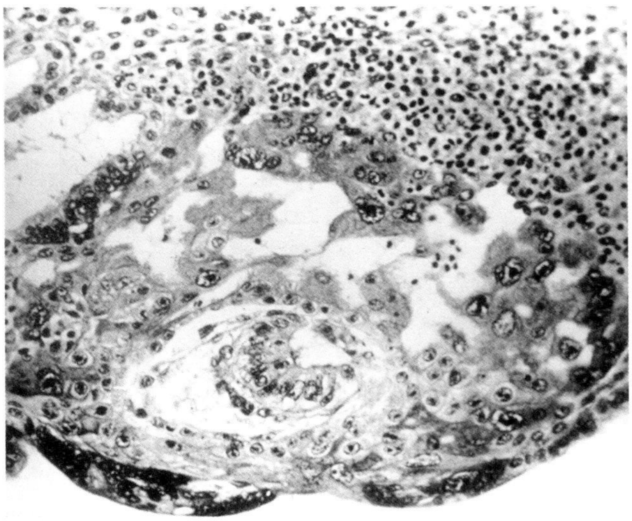

Fig. 2.9 Section through the middle of a human embryo showing primitive villi, distinct yolk sac, amniotic sac, and a bilaminar disc consisting of columnar ectoderm and cuboidal endoderm, but with no intervening mesoderm, estimated age 9 days, Streeter's horizon 6. (From Hertig AT, Rock J. Two human ova in the pre-villous stage, having an ovulation age of about 11 and 12 days, respectively. Washington: *Contrib Embryol Carnegie Inst.* 1941;29:127, with permission.)

the midline, the result is a depression between the right-sided and left-sided mesoderm—the primitive streak—that marks the long axis of the embryo when viewed from its dorsal or amniotic sac aspect (Figs. 2.11 and 2.12). This lateral and then cephalic migration of the mesoderm bilaterally can be well documented in explanted chick embryos by cinephotomicrography. I have made many movies of this process.

2. **The cardiogenic crescent of precardiac mesoderm** appears on day 18 in the normal human embryo. The

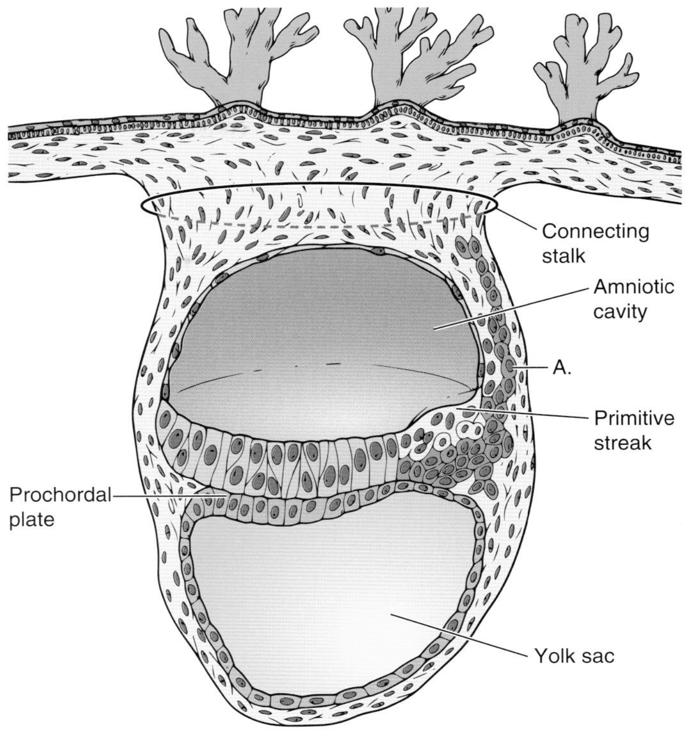

Fig. 2.10 The appearance of the mesoderm, from which the cardiovascular system will arise, at 15 days of age. The mesoderm (meaning "middle skin") buds off from the ectoderm. This is a schematic drawing of a longitudinal section, left lateral view, through the Edwards-Jones-Brewer embryo. This stage is horizon 7, characterized by a primitive streak and branching villi. The mesoderm migrates into the embryo (intra-embryonic mesoderm) and also into the connecting stalk at *A* (extra-embryonic mesoderm). (From Hamilton WJ, Mossman HW. *Human Embryology.* 4th ed. Baltimore: Williams & Wilkins: 1972, with permission.)

left-sided and right-sided precardiac mesoderm unite in front of the developing brain, forming a horseshoe-shaped crescent of precardiac mesoderm, as in Carnegie embryo 5080 of Davis[2] (Fig. 2.13). The reconstruction of this embryo is shown in Fig. 2.14. This embryo was 1.5 mm in length. The first pair of somites was just forming. This stage corresponds to Streeter's late **horizon 8** (no somites) and early **horizon 9** (one to three pairs of somites), that is, at the junction of horizons 8 and 9 (horizon 8/9). A late horizon 9 embryo with three pairs of somites is shown in Fig. 2.15.

The **notochord** gives our phylum its name: **Phylum Chordates**. This phylum includes all animals with a notochord and is essentially synonymous with the craniates and the vertebrates.

The **prochordal plate**, as its name indicates, lies anterior to (in front of) the notochord. The prochordal plate consists of ectoderm and endoderm, is never normally invaded by mesoderm, and subsequently breaks down, contributing to the formation of the mouth.

The **cloacal membrane** caudally also is normally not invaded by mesoderm. This membrane subsequently breaks down to help create the cloacal opening.

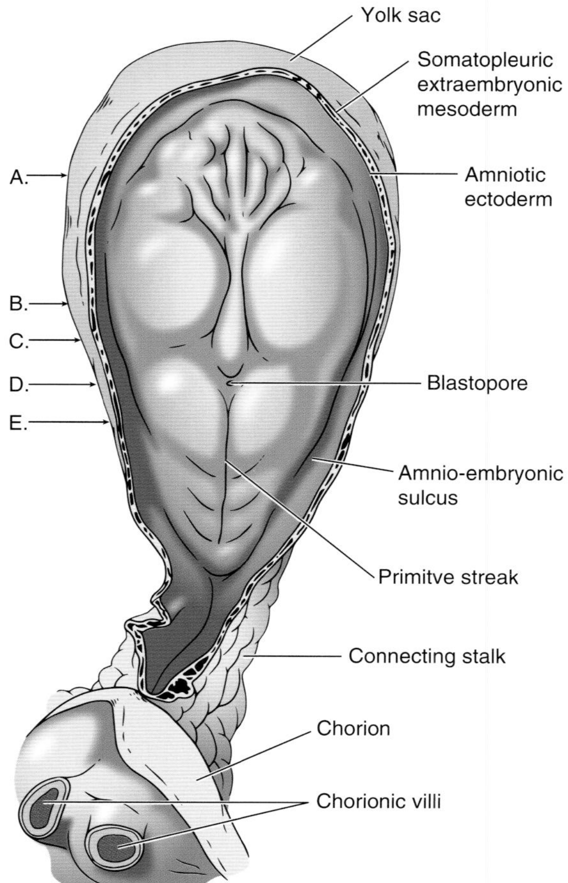

Fig. 2.11 Dorsal aspect of the model of an 18-day presomite human embryo showing the primitive streak. (From Hamilton WJ, Mossman HW. *Human Embryology*. 4th ed. Baltimore: Williams & Wilkins: 1972, with permission.)

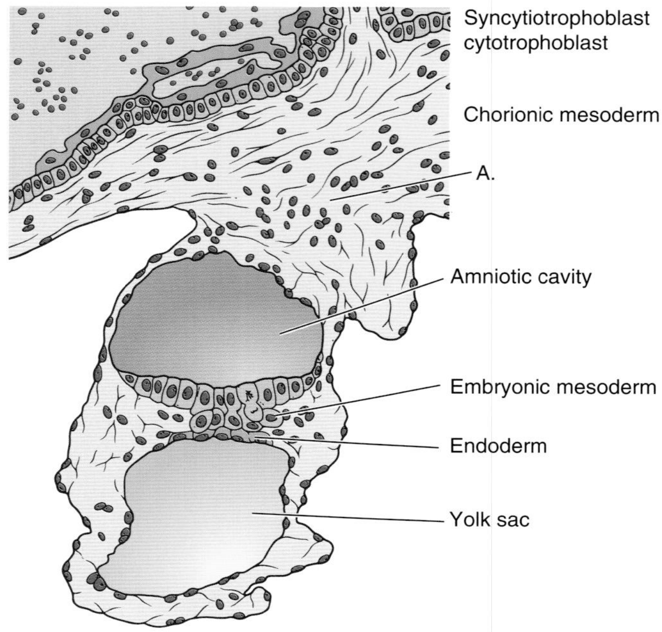

Fig. 2.12 Diagram of transverse section through the caudal part of the Edwards-Jones-Brewer embryo showing the mesoderm budding off from the ectoderm, based on Brewer JI: A human embryo in the bilaminar blastodisc stage (the Edwards-Jones-Brewer ovum). Contrib Embryol Carnegie Inst 1938;27:85.

3. The **intraembryonic celom** appears on the 18th day of life, in horizon 9, because the mesoderm cavitates (see Fig. 2.15). The mesoderm splits into dorsal and ventral layers, which are separated by the intraembryonic celom (or space). The dorsal layer of the mesoderm is called the **somatopleure** because this layer is adjacent to the body wall and forms, for example, the pericardial sac. (*Soma* = body + *pleura* = side, Greek.) The ventral layer of the mesoderm is known as the **splanchnopleure** because this layer is on the inside, that is, on the visceral side. (*Splanchnos* = viscus + *pleura* = side, Greek.) The splanchnopleure forms, for example, the myocardium.

The intraembryonic celom communicates with the extraembryonic celom (Fig. 2.15, arrows). The intraembryonic celom forms all of the body cavities, which at this stage are not divided from each other. The intraembryonic celom includes the future pericardial, pleural, and peritoneal cavities. Note that even the somites, which form the future skeletal muscles, contain small central cavities (see Fig. 2.15). The ability to form cavities is one of the more important characteristics of mesoderm.

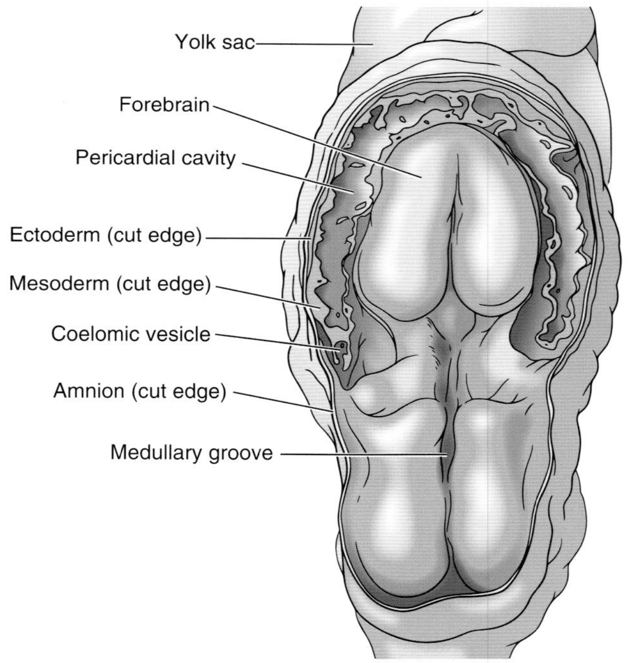

Fig. 2.13 Human cardiogenic crescent, dorsal view. The dorsal somatopleuric mesoderm has been dissected away, exposing the underlying splanchnopleuric mesoderm. This is a drawing of Carnegie embryo 5080, in which the first pair of somites is appearing; the length is 1.5 mm, and this embryo is at the junction of horizons 8 and 9. (From Davis CL. Development of the human heart from its first appearance to the stage found in embryos of 20 paired somites. *Contrib Embryol Carnegie Inst.* 1927;19:245.)

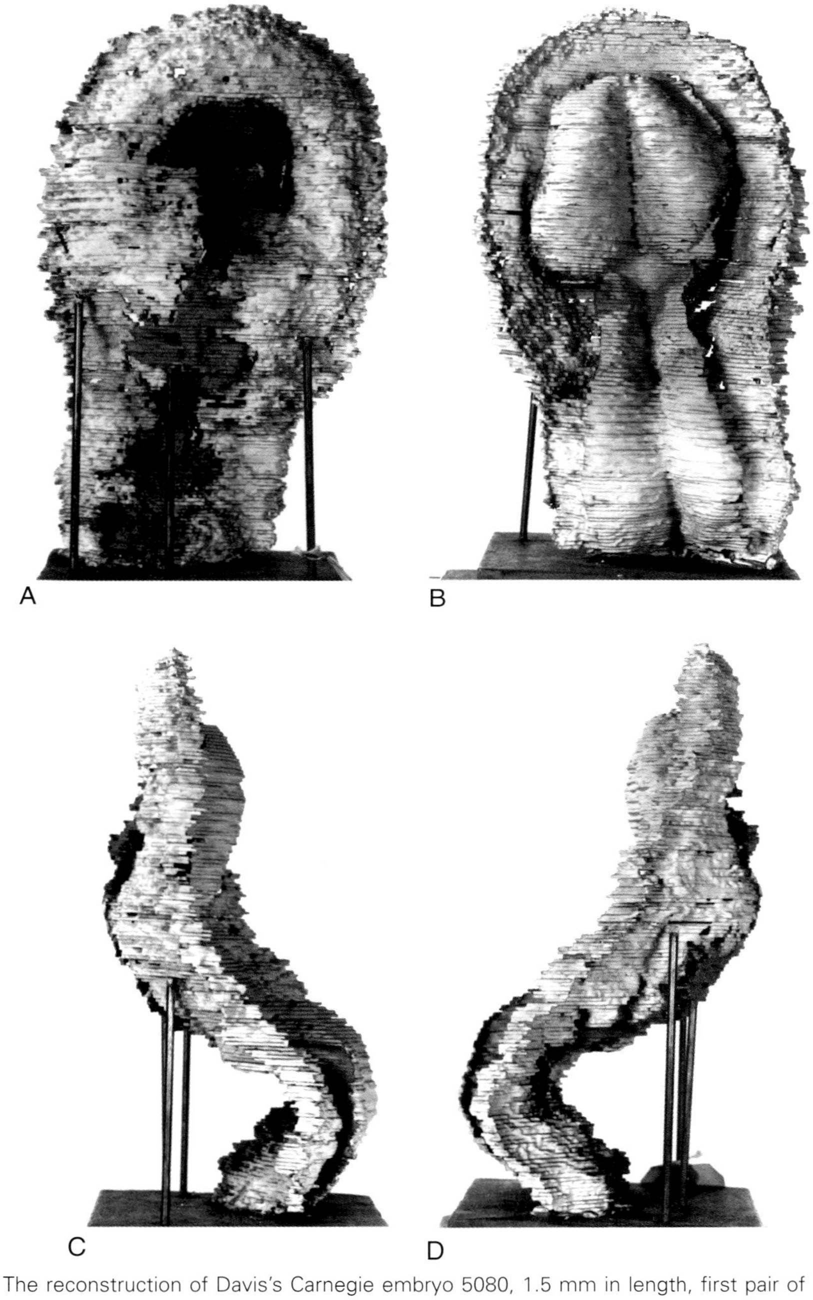

Fig. 2.14 The reconstruction of Davis's Carnegie embryo 5080, 1.5 mm in length, first pair of somites just forming, horizon 8/9. (A) Ventral view with foregut, mid-gut, and hind-gut endoderm darker than more lateral and rostral cardiogenic crescent. (B) Dorsal view, shown diagrammatically in Fig. 2.13. (C) Left lateral view of reconstruction. (D) Right lateral view of reconstruction.

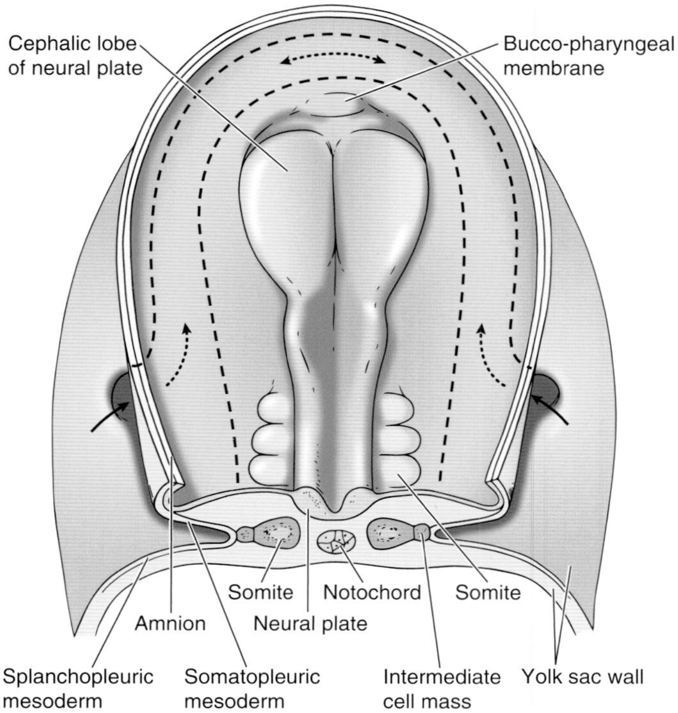

Fig. 2.15 Schematic presentation of the cranial part of an embryo with three pairs of somites, dorsal view, to show the intra-embryonic celom *(broken arrows)* and the communication of the intra-embryonic celom with the extra-embryonic celom *(black solid arrows)*. The cardiogenic crescent of precardiac mesoderm is shaped like a horseshoe *(broken lines)*. The longitudinal axis of the embryo is indicated by the notochord. Just lateral to the notochord lies the paraxial mesoderm from which the somites form (future skeletal muscles). Lateral to the paraxial mesoderm is the lateral plate mesoderm of the cardiogenic crescent.

In Fig. 2.15, *buccopharyngeal membrane* is another name for the prochordal plate. The intermediate cell mass is early kidney (see Fig. 2.15). The brain is still a *neural plate*, not having formed a tubular structure as yet. The notochord indicates the long axis of the embryo. The *somites* (*soma* = body, Greek) form from the *paraxial mesoderm*, the mesoderm that is beside (*para* = beside, Greek) the long axis of the body, indicated by the notochord. By contrast, the heart forms from the *lateral plate mesoderm*, so called because it is lateral to the paraxial mesoderm (see Fig. 2.15). The precardiac mesoderm of the cardiogenic crescent then continues to migrate cephalically on the foregut endoderm to form a straight heart tube (Fig. 2.16).

4. The **straight heart tube** or preloop stage normally occurs in the human embryo at 20 days of age (Fig. 2.17). The straight heart tube stage can be achieved in the human embryo by **horizon 9**, in Carnegie embryo 1878 of Davis and Ingalls that had two pairs of somites and was 1.38 mm in length (Fig. 2.18). However, the straight tube stage often is not reached until **horizon 10**, as in Carnegie embryo 3709 (Fig. 2.19), with four pairs of somites, 2.5 mm in length, estimated age 20 to 22 days, and as in Carnegie embryo Klb (Fig. 2.20), with six pairs of somites and a length of 1.8 mm.

   At the straight tube stage, note that the endocardial lumina of the left and right "half hearts" may be largely unfused (Fig. 2.20) or incompletely fused (see Fig. 2.19). The space between the myocardium and the endocardium is filled with cardiac jelly. As the precardiac mesoderm migrates cephalically and medially onto the foregut endoderm to form a straight heart tube, the foregut endoderm is growing caudally or posteriorly, as is well shown by my time-lapse movies in the chick embryo.

5. **D-loop formation** normally begins at the end of the third week of embryonic life in humans (see Figs. 2.16 and 2.17). By analogy with other vertebrates, it seems very likely that this is when the heart in human embryos starts to beat: Carnegie embryo 4216 (Fig. 2.21), seven pairs of somites, 2.2 mm in length, horizon 10 (20–22 days of age); Carnegie embryo 391 (Fig. 2.22), eight pairs of somites, 2 mm in length, horizon 10 (day 20–22); and Carnegie embryo 3707 (Fig. 2.23), 12 pairs of somites, 2.08 mm in length, horizon 10 (20–22 days of age). When D-loop formation begins—the heart bending convexly to the right—the endocardial tubes have fused forming a single endocardial lumen. (*Dexter, dextra, dextrum* are the masculine, feminine, and neuter adjectives, respectively, meaning "right sided," Latin.)

   At the horizon 10 stage (see Figs. 2.21–2.23), the future morphologically right ventricle (RV), which develops from the proximal bulbus cordis, is superior to the future morphologically left ventricle (LV), which develops from the ventricle of the bulboventricular loop. The future interventricular septum—between the bulbus cordis and the ventricle of the straight bulboventricular tube—lies in an approximately horizontal position. If an arrest in development were to occur at the horizon 10 stage (20–22 days of age), **superoinferior ventricles** would result, with the RV superior to the LV and the ventricular septum approximately horizontal. The atrioventricular canal, which is in common (not divided into mitral and tricuspid valves) at this stage, opens superiorly only into the ventricle—future LV. Hence, **common-inlet LV** is potentially present during horizon 10 (see Figs. 2.21–2.23). Both future great arteries originate only from the bulbus cordis (future RV). Thus, **double-outlet RV** would result from an arrest of development during horizon 10 (20–22 days of age).

   To put it another way, **common-inlet LV, superoinferior ventricles, and double-outlet RV are all normal findings at the horizon 10 (20–22 day) stage.** This understanding illustrates why a knowledge of normal cardiovascular embryology appears to be so relevant to the understanding of the pathologic anatomy of complex congenital heart disease.

   However, it must also be borne in mind that much remains to be learned concerning the etiology and morphogenesis of congenital heart disease.[2] For example, if developmental arrest really is a pathogenetic mechanism leading to congenital heart disease, as is widely assumed, it remains to be proved when and why such developmental arrests occur in the human embryo. We think we know *when*—but this is only an extrapolation based on normal cardiovascular development—and we often have no idea *why*. Hence, in this chapter, I am not

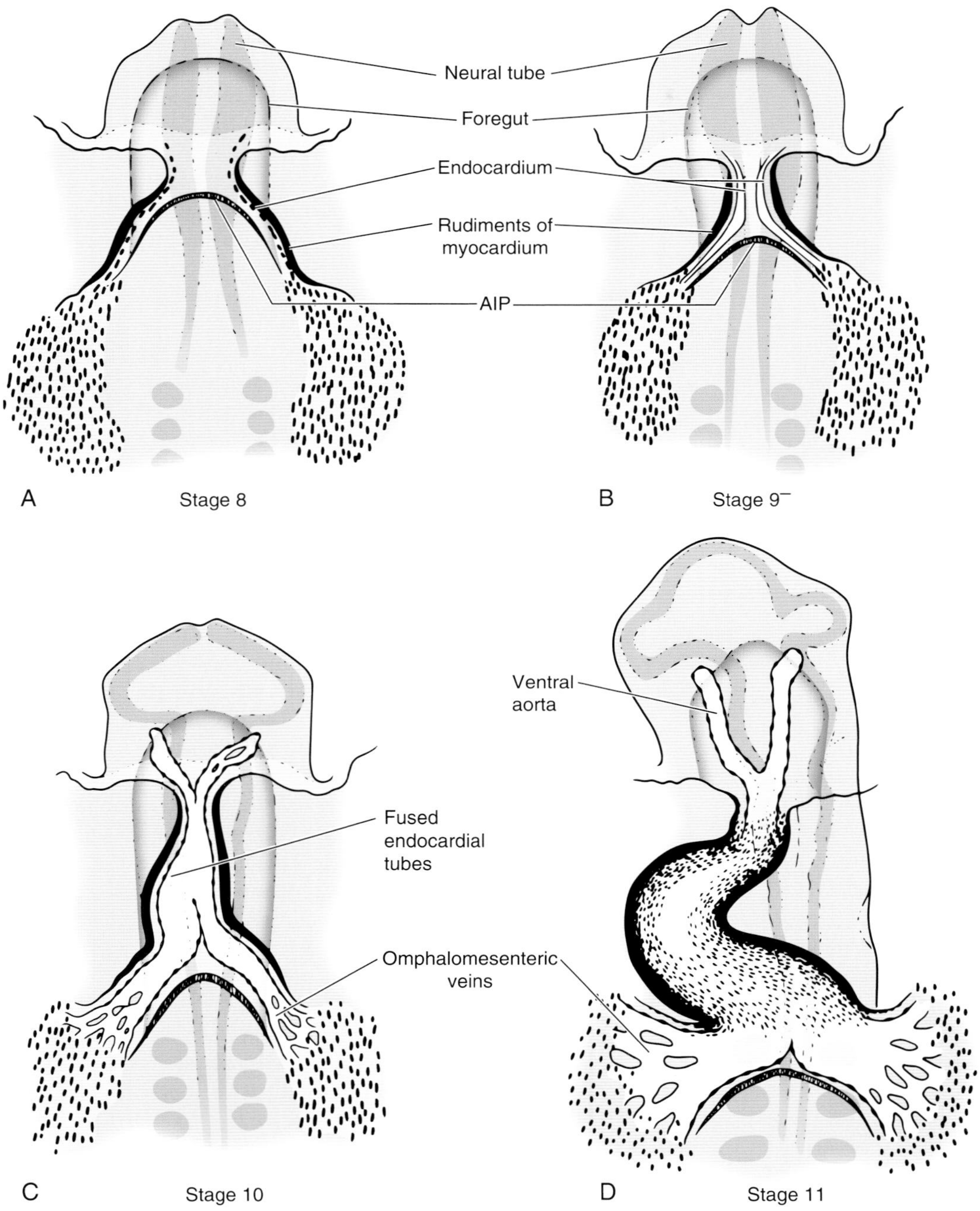

Fig. 2.16 (A) Cardiogenic crescent, at Hamilton-Hamburger stage 8 in the chick embryo. (B) Developing straight heart tube at Hamilton-Hamburger stage 9^{-}. (C) Straight heart tube becoming early D-loop, at Hamilton-Hamburger stage 10. (D) D-loop. In these ventral views of the developing chick heart, undifferentiated precardiac mesoderm is indicated with vertical hatching. *AIP,* Anterior intestinal portal. (From DeHaan RL, Ursprung H, eds. *Organogenesis.* New York: Holt, Rinehart, and Winston; 1965.)

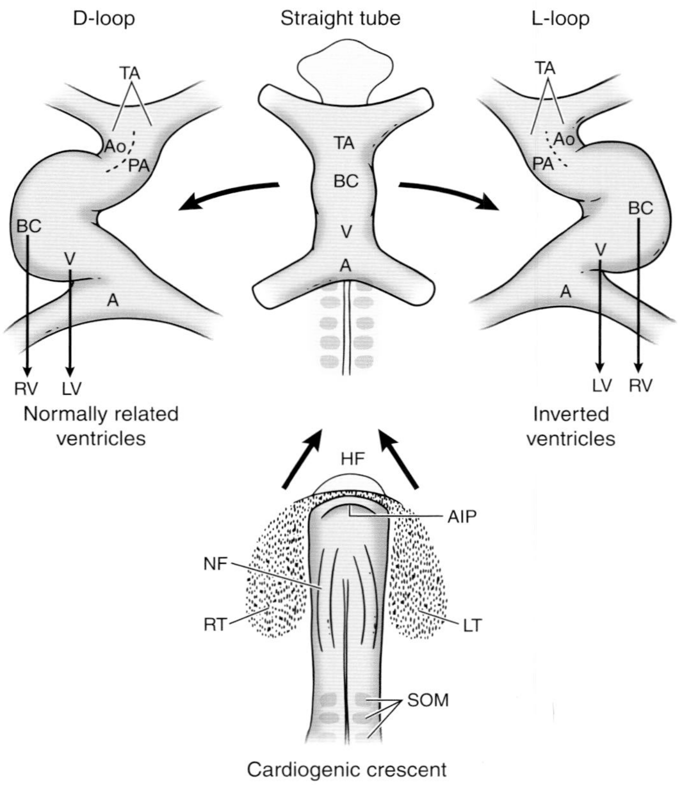

Fig. 2.17 Cardiac loop formation. Cardiogenic crescent of precardiac mesoderm. Straight heart tube or preloop stage. D-loop, with solitus (noninverted) ventricles. L-loop with inverted (mirror-image) ventricles. *A,* Atrium; *AIP,* anterior intestinal portal; *Ao,* aorta; *BC,* bulbus cordis; *HF,* head fold; *LT,* left; *LV,* morphologically left ventricle; *NF,* neural fold; *PA,* (main) pulmonary artery; *RT,* right; *RV,* morphologically right ventricle; *SOM,* somites; *TA,* truncus arteriosus. (From Van Praagh R, Weinberg PM, Matsuoka R, et al. Malposition of the heart. In Adams FH, Emmanouilides GC, eds. *Heart Disease in Infants, Children, and Adolescents.* 3rd ed. Baltimore: Williams & Wilkins; 1983, with permission.)

endeavoring to make implications concerning the causation of congenital heart disease. Instead, I am presenting factual data concerning normal cardiovascular development. The precise relevance of this understanding to the etiology and morphogenesis of human congenital heart disease remains to be proved. Nonetheless, when obvious correlations appear to exist, I will point them out, with the aforementioned mental reservations being understood.

THE FOURTH WEEK OF LIFE

The main features of normal cardiovascular development during the fourth week of embryonic life are:

1. the completion of D-loop formation,
2. the beginning of the development of the morphologically LV and of the morphologically RV,
3. the beginning of the circulation, and
4. the initiation of cardiovascular septation.

In somewhat greater detail, the salient features of normal human cardiovascular development during the fourth week of embryonic life, that is, from day 22 to day 28 inclusive, include the changes that occur during Streeter's horizons 11 to 13, inclusive (Fig. 2.24). It is noteworthy that each of **Streeter's horizons** covers an approximately 2-day time interval. One doubles the horizon number to find the embryonic age in days at the beginning of the horizon. For example, horizon 11 indicates the stage beginning at an age of 22 days (11 × 2), which lasts for 2 days—from day 22 to day 24 inclusive (22 + 2) (see Fig. 2.24).

The diagram (see Fig. 2.24) also makes it possible to estimate the approximate age of an embryo (on the horizontal axis) from its length in millimeters (on the vertical axis). For example, an embryo with a crown–rump length of 5 mm falls into the middle of horizon 13, which corresponds to an embryonic age of 26 to 28 days (see Fig. 2.24).

Streeter's horizons are an aging and staging system not just for the heart but for all organ systems (see Fig. 2.24).

D-loop formation normally is completed in horizon 11 (22–24 days), as is seen in Carnegie embryo 470, which is 3.3 mm long and has 16 pairs of somites (Figs. 2.25 and 2.26).

Fig. 2.26 shows a reconstruction of the lumen of this embryo, like a perfect angiocardiogram. Note that the future ventricular apex points rightward following the completion of D-loop formation; that is, **dextrocardia** is present. The blood flows from the right atrium (RA) to the left atrium, as in **tricuspid atresia**. The blood then flows from the left atrium only into the future LV, similar to **common-inlet or double-inlet LV**. The development of the LV sinus is somewhat more advanced than is that of the RV sinus. The developing LV is anterior (ventral) relative to the RV, as the right lateral and left lateral views demonstrate. Hence, the anterior (ventral) ventricle is not necessarily the RV, contrary to what works on angiocardiography often say. Following D-looping, the ventral ventricle is the LV, and the dorsal ventricle is the RV, because dextrocardia with a rightward pointing apex is present.

Note also that the right atrial appendage lies to the left of the vascular pedicle; that is, **left-sided juxtaposition of the atrial appendages** is present.

A reconstruction of the atria of the same embryo (Carnegie embryo 470 of Davis) is shown in Fig. 2.27. When the dorsal walls of the atria are removed, revealing the interior, the floor of the morphologically RA strongly resembles that seen in typical **tricuspid atresia** (see Fig. 2.27, right panel). The atrioventricular canal opens from the left atrium into the LV.

In Fig. 2.25, it will be seen that the vitelline veins are adjacent to the yolk sac (*vitellus* = yolk, Latin). The right and left umbilical veins are lateral to the right and left vitelline veins, respectively. The umbilical veins plus the vitelline veins are together known as the omphalomesenteric veins. The septum transversum is the embryonic diaphragm. The anterior intestinal portal leads into the foregut behind the heart. Note the pericardial sac, the first pair of aortic arches, and the pharyngeal membrane.

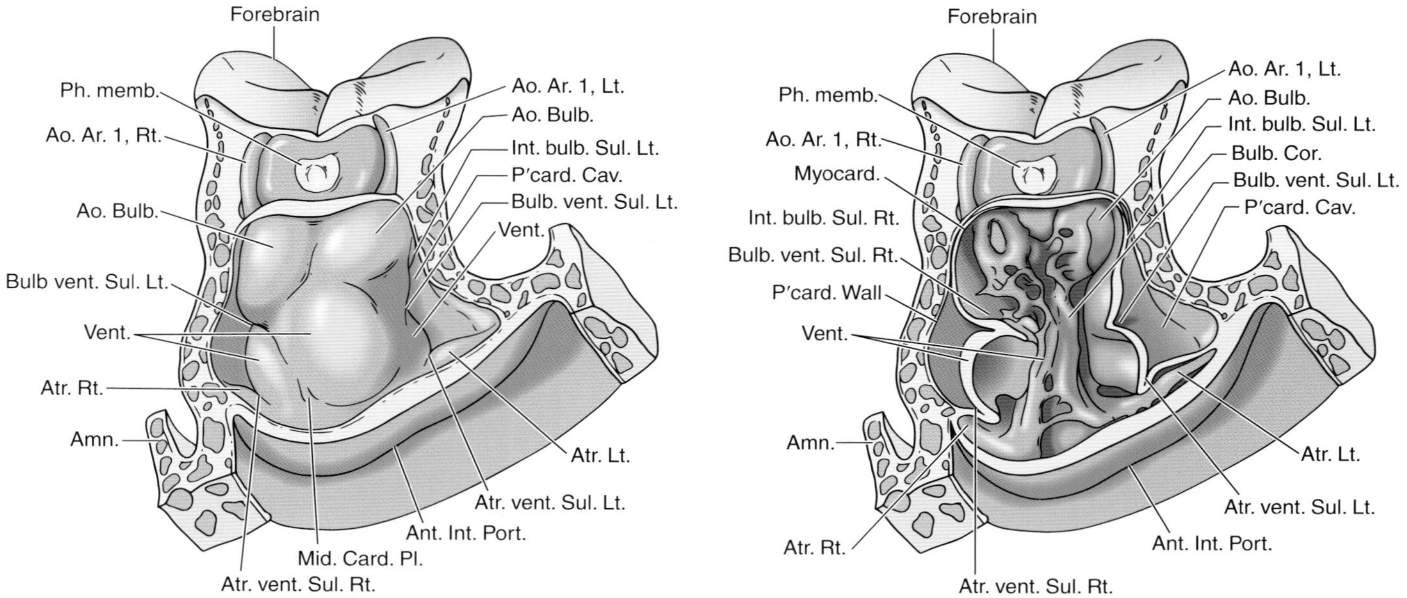

Fig. 2.18 Straight tube stage, Carnegie embryo 1878, two pairs of somites, 1.38 mm in length, horizon 9. The left panel shows the outside ventral view of the myocardium, with the pericardial sac removed. The right-sided panel shows the interior of the heart with the ventral myocardial wall removed. The space between the myocardium and the endocardial tubes is filled with cardiac jelly. *Amn,* Amnion; *AoAr 1, Lt,* aortic arch 1, left; *AoAr 1, Rt,* aortic arch 1, right; *Ao Bulb,* aortic bulbus; *Ant Int Port,* anterior intestinal portal; *Atr L,* atrium, left; *Atr R,* atrium, right; *Atr vent Sul Lt,* atrioventricular sulcus, left; *Atr vent Sul, Rt,* atrioventricular sulcus, right; *Bulb vent Sul, Lt,* bulboventricular sulcus, left; *Bulb vent Sul, Rt,* bulboventricular sulcus, right; *Int bulb Sul, Lt,* interbulbar sulcus, left; *Mid Card Pl,* midcardiac plate; *Myocard,* myocardium; *P'card Cav,* pericardial cavity; *Ph memb,* pharyngeal membrane; *Vent,* ventricle. (From Davis CL. Development of the human heart from its first appearance to the stage found in embryos of 20 paired somites. *Contrib Embryol Carnegie Inst.* 1927;19:245.)

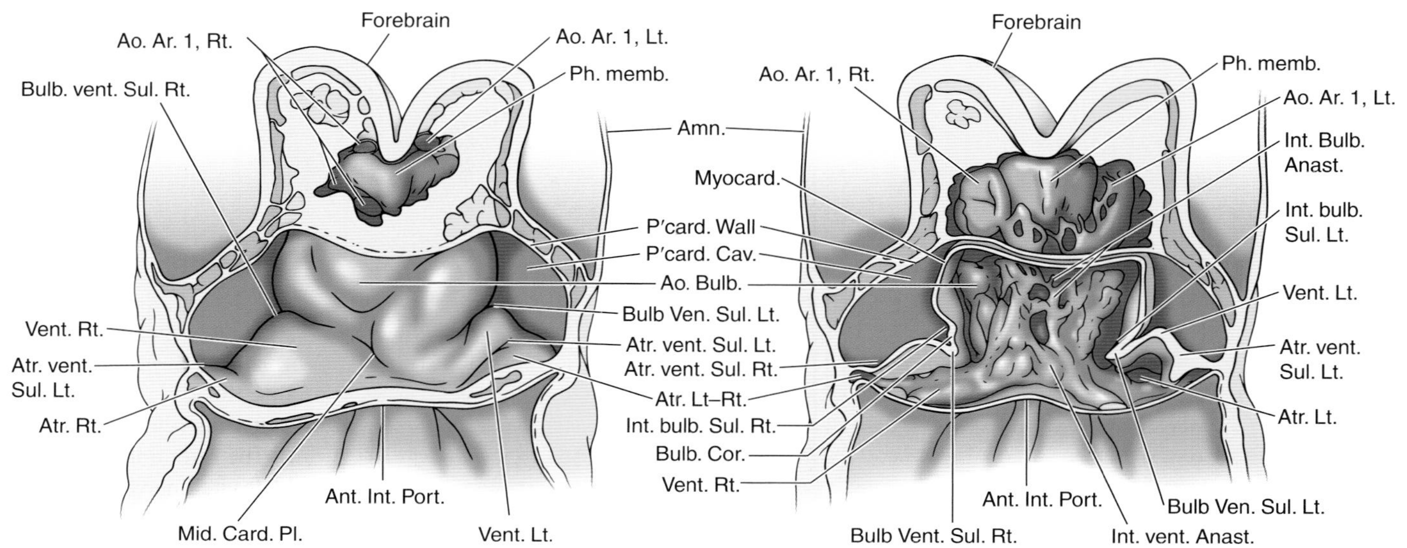

Fig. 2.19 Early straight tube stage, the left-sided and right-sided cardiac primordia are incompletely fused into a straight tube, Carnegie embryo 3709, four pairs of somites, 2.5 mm in length, horizon 10, estimated age 20 to 22 days. Ventral view, left-sided panel with pericardial sac removed, right-sided panel with ventral myocardium removed. *Int Bulb Anast,* Interbulbar anastomosis; *Int vent Anast,* interventricular anastomosis; other abbreviations as previously. (From Davis CL. Development of the human heart from its first appearance to the stage found in embryos of 20 paired somites. *Contrib Embryol Carnegie Inst.* 1927;19:245.)

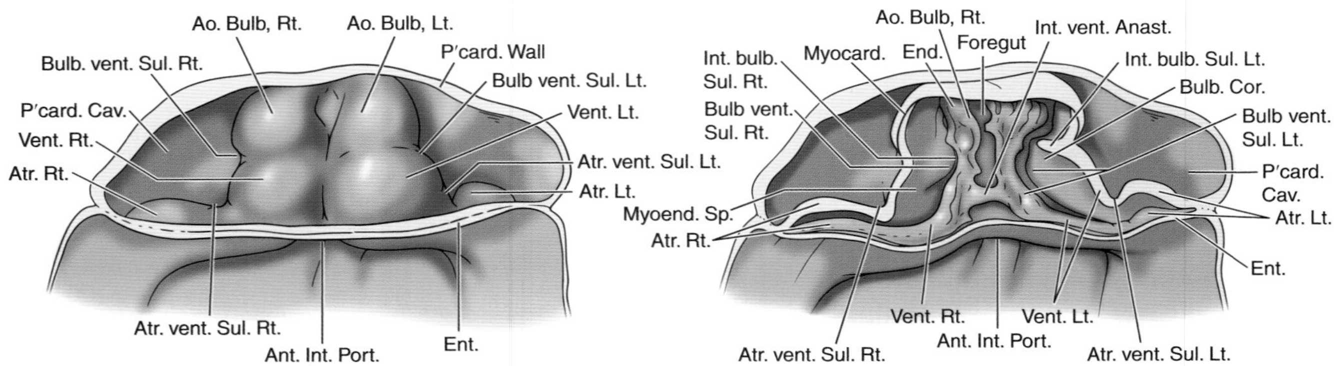

Fig. 2.20 Early straight tube stage, left-sided and right-sided cardiogenic primordia incompletely fused. Left-sided panel shows prominent vertical fusion furrow between left-sided and right-sided primordia. Right-sided panel with ventral myocardium removed shows marked lack of fusion of left-sided and right-sided endocardial tubes. This is Carnegie embryo Klb of Davis, six pairs of somites, 1.8 mm in length, horizon 10. *End,* Endocardium; *Ent,* enteron; other abbreviations as previously. (From Davis CL. Development of the human heart from its first appearance to the stage found in embryos of 20 paired somites. *Contrib Embryol Carnegie Inst.* 1927;19:245.)

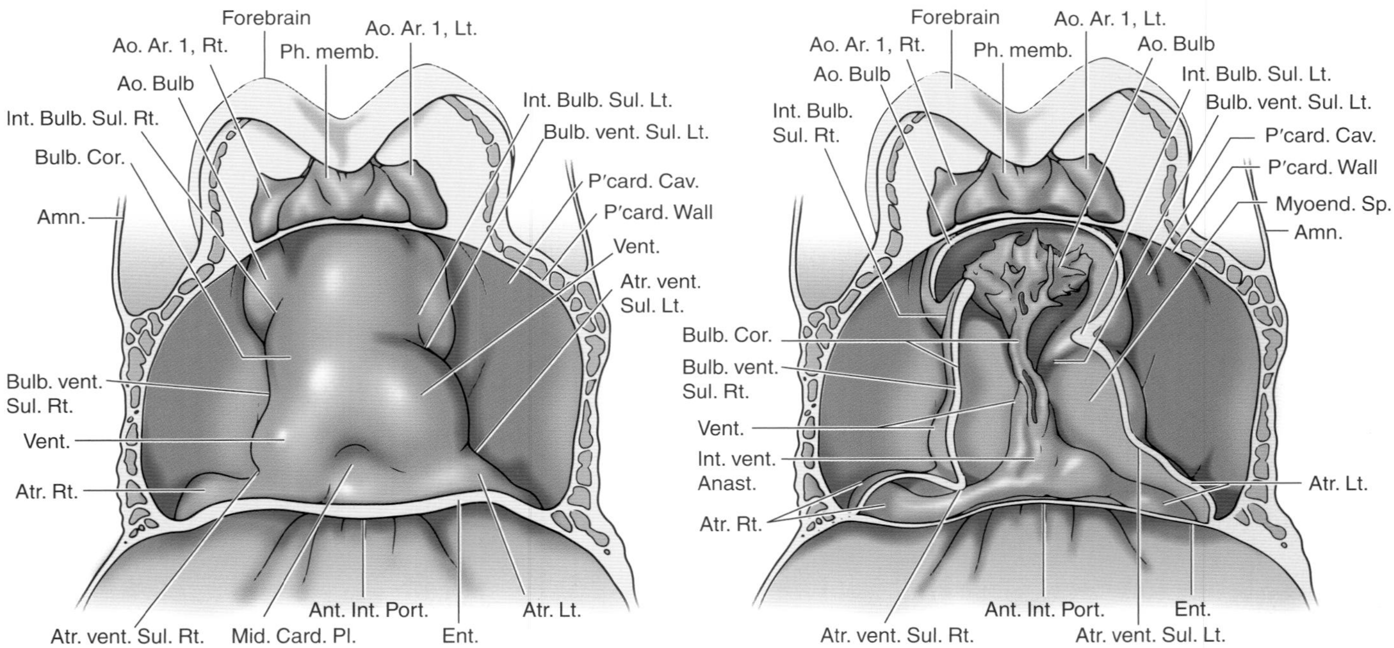

Fig. 2.21 Straight tube stage showing fusion of left-sided myocardial and endocardial primordia. Carnegie embryo 4216 of Davis, this being the Davis-Payne embryo, seven pairs of somites, 2.2 mm in length, horizon 10. *Bulb Cor,* Bulbus cordis; *Myoend sp,* myoendocardial space (filled with cardiac jelly); other abbreviations as previously. (From Davis CL. Development of the human heart from its first appearance to the stage found in embryos of 20 paired somites. *Contrib Embryol Carnegie Inst.* 1927;19:245.)

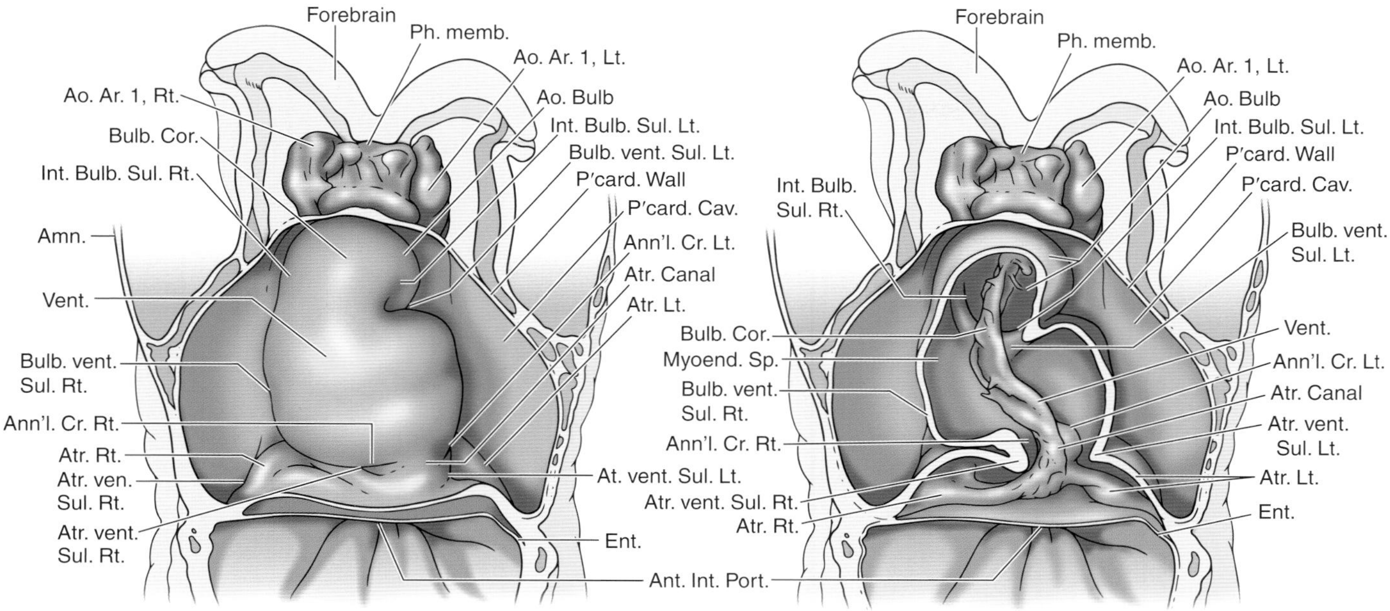

Fig. 2.22 Early D-loop, Carnegie human embryo 391, eight pairs of somites, 2 mm in length, horizon 10, estimated age 20 to 22 days. The atria open superiorly into the ventricle (future morphologically left ventricle), which in turn opens superiorly into the bulbus cordis (future morphologically right ventricle) which in turn gives rise to the future great arteries. *Atr canal,* Atrial canal; *Ann'l Cr, Lt,* annular crease, left; *Ann'l Cr, Rt,* annular crease, right; other abbreviations as previously. (From Davis CL. Development of the human heart from its first appearance to the stage found in embryos of 20 paired somites. *Contrib Embryol Carnegie Inst.* 1927;19:245.)

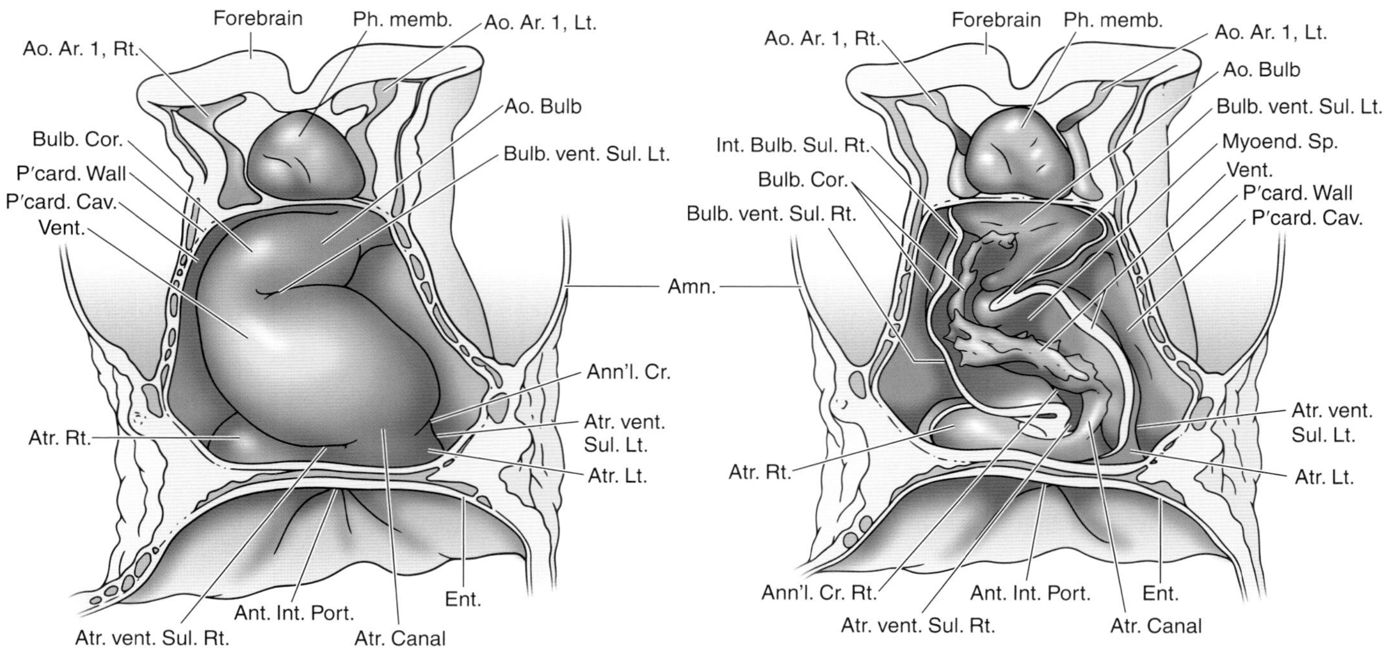

Fig. 2.23 D-loop formation more than half completed. Carnegie human embryo 3707 of Davis, 12 pairs of somites, 2.08 mm in length, horizon 10, estimated age 20 to 22 days. Note that the left bulboventricular sulcus has become a deep inwardly protruding spur, the future bulboventricular flange, and that the right bulboventricular sulcus has flattened out and has almost disappeared. Abbreviations as previously. (From Davis CL. Development of the human heart from its first appearance to the stage found in embryos of 20 paired somites. *Contrib Embryol Carnegie Inst.* 1927;19:245.)

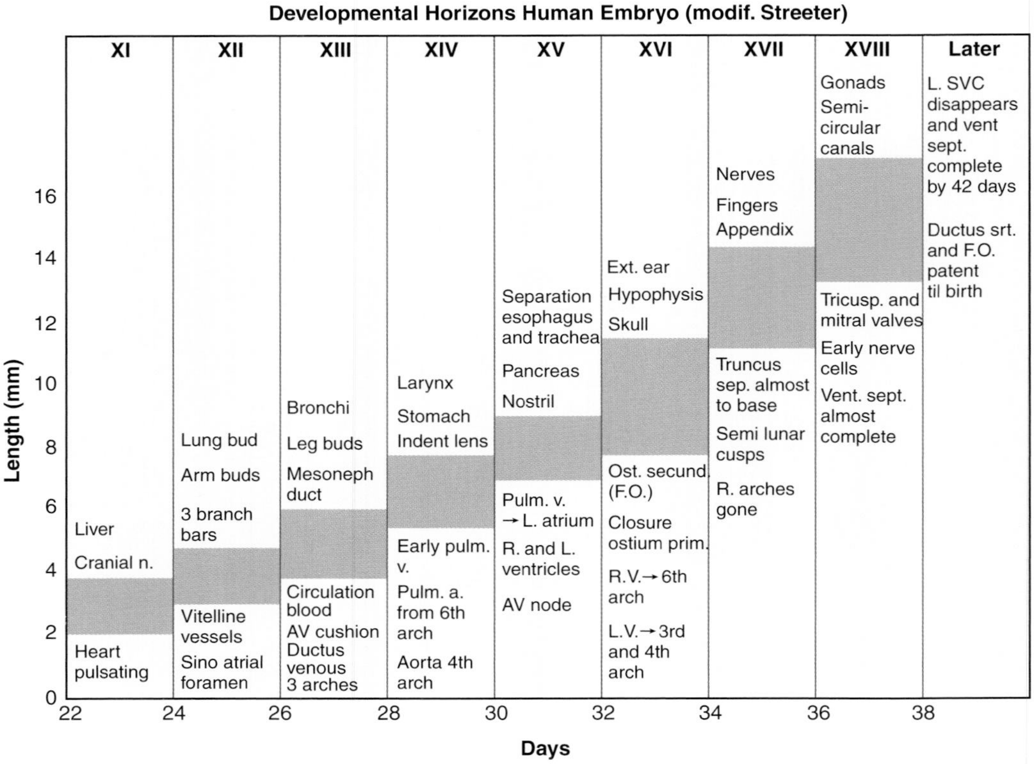

Fig. 2.24 Developmental horizons (stages) in the human embryo, modified from Streeter. Horizons are indicated at the top in Roman numerals. Embryonic ages are shown at the bottom in days. Embryonic lengths are given at the left in millimeters (mm). The salient features of each horizon are indicated. *AV,* Atrioventricular; *ductus art,* ductus arteriosus; *FO,* foramen ovale; *L,* left; *LSVC,* left superior vena cava; *n,* nerves; *R,* right; *pulm v,* pulmonary vein; *ost,* ostinum secundum; *tricusp,* tricuspid; *v,* vein; *vent sept,* ventricular septum. (From Neill CA. Development of the pulmonary veins with reference to the embryology of anomalies of pulmonary venous return. *Pediatrics.* 1956;18:880, with permission.)

By 26 to 28 days of age (horizon 13), as illustrated by Carnegie embryo 836 (Figs. 2.28 and 2.29), the ventricular D-loop has descended relative to the atria. Development of the LV is more advanced than that of the RV. The ventricular apex is still pointing to the right. The LV remains ventral to the RV. The RA opens only into the left atrium, as in tricuspid atresia. The left atrium opens only into the LV. The LV ejects into the RV. And both future great arteries—still undivided—originate only from the RV.

A true circulation, as opposed to ebb and flow, is thought to begin at this stage. This is the ancient **in-series circulation**, as in aquatic vertebrates such as sharks. It is a single, as opposed to a double, circulation. It is called an in-series, as opposed to an in-parallel, circulation because the blood passes in series from RA to LA to LV to RV to the undivided great artery. Note that aortic arches 2 and 3 have appeared, whereas the first pair of aortic arches have undergone involution (see Fig. 2.29).

In Figs. 2.26, 2.28, and 2.29, note that there is a smooth or nontrabeculated area between the LV and the RV that will become the smooth crest of the muscular interventricular septum. The trabeculated portions of the greater curvature of the D-loop evaginate (pouch outward), forming the ventricular sinuses. The smooth or nontrabeculated portion of the bulboventricular D-loop do not evaginate.

The development of the aortic arches during the fourth week of embryonic life is presented in Figs. 2.30 to 2.32, inclusive.[3] At the beginning of the fourth week (horizon 11), the first pair of aortic arches appears, as in Carnegie embryo 2053, 3 mm long, 20 pairs of somites. Each first aortic arch passes above (cephalad to) the first pharyngeal pouch on either side (see Fig. 2.30). The second pair of aortic arches is beginning to form.

At this stage, the heart is a cervical organ. The aortic arches are related to the gill arches of our aquatic vertebrate ancestors. Arrest of development at the fourth week stage appears to result in **cervical ectopia cordis**. Subsequently, the heart descends into the thorax.

Later in the fourth week of life, the second, third, and an early fourth pair of aortic arches appear, as in Carnegie embryo 836 (early horizon 13, 26 days of age, 4 mm in length, 30 pairs of somites present) (see Fig. 2.31). Each aortic arch passes cephalad to its pharyngeal pouch. Note the thoracic location of the stomach and the large tracheo-esophageal communication ("fistula") that are normal at this stage.

By late in the fourth week, as in Carnegie embryo 1380 (see Fig. 2.32), the third and fourth pairs of aortic arches have developed, aortic arches 1 and 2 have involuted, and the sixth aortic arches are developing. In this embryo 1380 (5 mm in length, horizon 13), the right ductus arteriosus (sixth arch) is

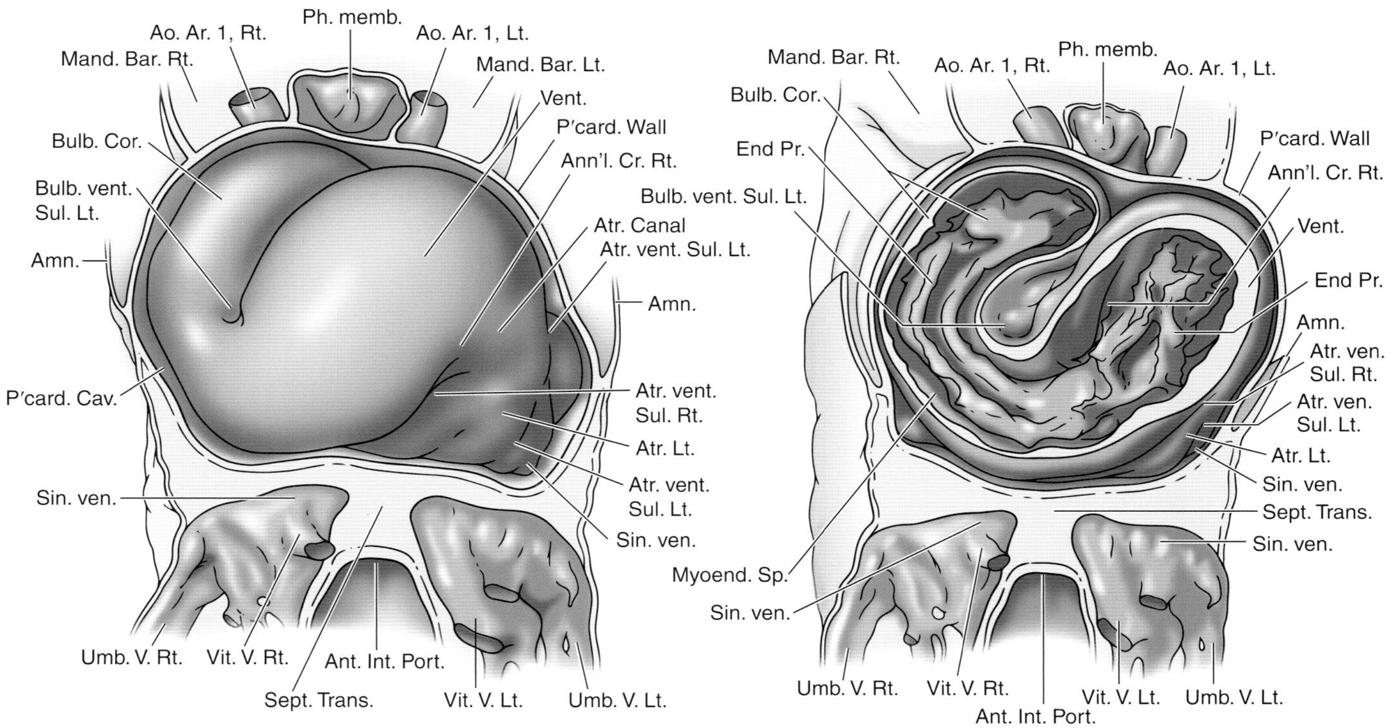

Fig. 2.25 D-loop formation has been completed, the bulboventricular loop now being convex to the right. Carnegie human embryo 470 of Davis, 16 pairs of somites, 3.3 mm in length, horizon 11, estimated age 22 to 24 days following ovulation. *End Pr,* Endocardial protrusion; *Mand bar Lt,* mandibular bar, left; *Mand bar, Rt,* mandibular bar, right; *Sept Trans,* septum transversum; *Sin Ven,* sinus venosus; *Umb V, Lt,* umbilical vein, left; *Umb V, Rt,* umbilical vein, right; *Vit V Lt,* vitelline vein, left; *Vit V Rt,* vitelline vein, right. Other abbreviations as previously. (From Davis CL. Development of the human heart from its first appearance to the stage found in embryos of 20 paired somites. *Contrib Embryol Carnegie Inst.* 1927;19:245.)

completely formed, but the left ductus arteriosus still has not formed.

Note that both the left and the right pulmonary artery branches have formed, despite the fact that a complete left sixth aortic arch is not present (see Fig. 2.32, left panel). This appears to explain why it is possible to have pulmonary artery branches present in association with congenital absence of the ductus arteriosus. The pulmonary artery branches initially arise as outpouching from the aortic sac (i.e., from the aorta), not from the sixth arches (as has often been said). Later, as will be seen, the pulmonary artery branches appear to originate from the sixth aortic arches. But the point I seek to make is that this is not where the pulmonary artery branches start from (see Fig. 2.32). Note also that the pulmonary vein has appeared. Hence, in the fourth week of life, all of the foregoing are normal findings: dextrocardia, tricuspid atresia, an undivided atrioventricular canal from the left atrium to the LV, an in-series circulation, and an undivided great artery that arises only above a poorly developed RV sinus.

THE FIFTH WEEK OF LIFE

The salient cardiovascular developments during the fifth week of embryonic life (from day 29 to day 35 inclusive, i.e., from horizon 14 to horizon 17 inclusive, see Fig. 2.24) are:

1. continuation of the development of the LV, RV, and ventricular septum;
2. approximation of the aorta to the interventricular foramen, the mitral valve, and the LV;
3. separation of the aorta and pulmonary artery;
4. separation of the mitral and tricuspid valves;
5. enlargement of the RV sinus;
6. movement of the muscular ventricular septum to the left, beneath the atrioventricular canal;
7. opening of the tricuspid valve into the RV; and
8. closure of the ostium primum by the endocardial cushions of the atrioventricular canal, thereby separating the atria; and leftward movement of the ventricles and ventricular apex, thus "curing" dextrocardia and resulting in mesocardia (a ventrally or anteriorly pointing ventricular apex).

Fig. 2.33 is a diagram of the heart of Carnegie embryo 3385 in horizon 15 (day 30–32), 8.3 mm in length. Fig. 2.15 presents the reconstruction of this embryo photographically. Note that the development of the RV sinus is starting to catch up with that of the LV sinus. The ventricles and the ventricular apex are swinging leftward. The atrioventricular canal is still opening into the larger LV. Left-sided juxtaposition of the atrial appendages is no longer present, the large RA now lying to the right of the great arteries that are undergoing septation longitudinally. Aortic arches 3, 4, and 6 are now

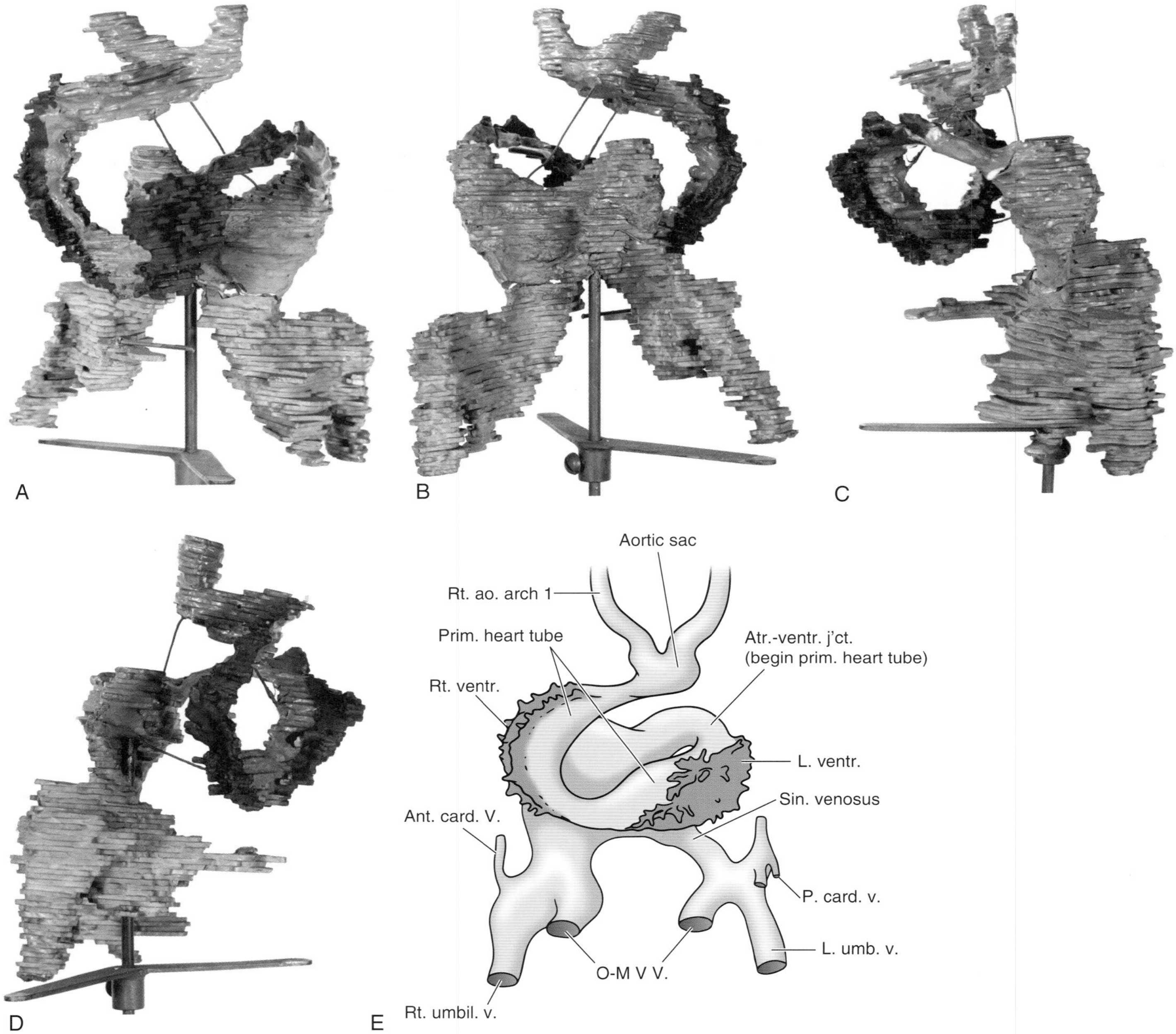

Fig. 2.26 Reconstruction of the lumen of Carnegie embryo 470 (shown in Fig. 2.25). This is like a perfect frozen angiocardiogram. The trabecular zones of the ventricle and of the bulbus cordis are darker than the rest of the reconstruction. (A) is a ventral view; (B) is a dorsal view; (C) is a left lateral view; and (D) is a right lateral view. (E) The diagram of Carnegie embryo 2053, also horizon 11, serves to illustrate and label the reconstruction of Carnegie embryo 470. *Ant Card V,* Anterior cardinal vein; *Atr-Ventr j'ct,* atrioventricular junction; *L Umb V,* left umbilical vein; *L Ventr,* left ventricle; *O-M VV,* omphalomesenteric veins; *P Card V,* posterior cardinal vein; *Prim heart tube,* primary heart tube; *Rt Umbil V,* right umbilical vein; *Rt Ventr,* right ventricle; *Sin Venosus,* sinus venosus. Other abbreviations as previously. Heart reconstruction photographs by the author; diagram of the reconstruction of the lumen of Carnegie embryo 2053. (From Streeter GL. Developmental horizons in human embryos, age groups XI–XXIII, embryology reprint. Washington, DC: *Carnegie Inst.* II;1951, with permission.)

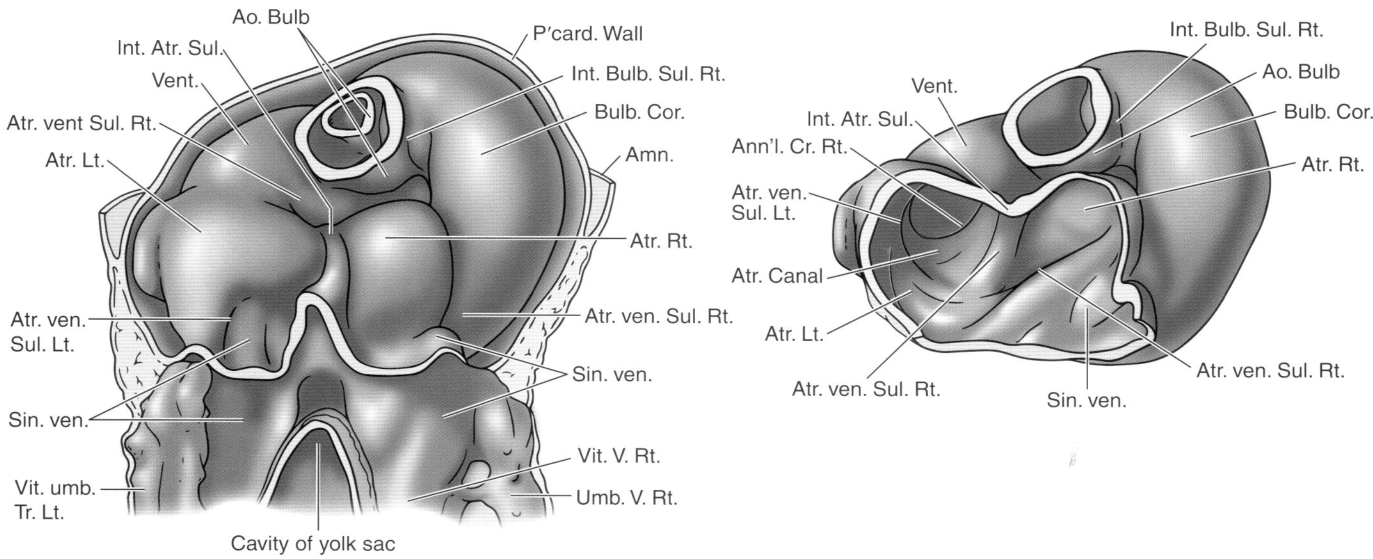

Fig. 2.27 Dorsal view of the atria of Carnegie human embryo 470, 3.3 mm in length, 16 pairs of somites, horizon 11, estimated age 22 to 24 days, left panel with posterior atrial free walls intact, and right panel with posterior atrial free walls removed to permit view of the interior of the developing atria. Note the resemblance to typical tricuspid atresia. *Int Atr Sul,* Interatrial sulcus. (From Davis CL. Development of the human heart from its first appearance to the stage found in embryos of 20 paired somites. *Contrib Embryol Carnegie Inst.* 1927;19:245.)

present, as are small, downward dangling pulmonary artery branches (Fig. 2.34).

Fig. 2.35 shows the heart of Carnegie embryo 6510 diagrammatically, this embryo being in horizon 16 (32–34 days of age), with a length of 10.1 mm. The reconstruction of this embryo (Fig. 2.36) shows that RV growth is catching up with that of the LV. The ventricular septum now lies in an approximately anteroposterior plane; that is, mesocardia is now present. In the right and left lateral views of this reconstruction, one can see that the ostium primum is now very small and is being closed by the endocardial cushions of the atrioventricular canal. Fig. 2.37 is a reconstruction of the ventricular lumina of this embryo, which confirms the presence of mesocardia and shows that the right and left ventricular sinuses are now approximately the same size.

In Fig. 2.35 it is noteworthy that the atrioventricular canal is starting to undergo septation, dividing it into the mitral and tricuspid valves. Note also that the tricuspid valve is starting to open into the RV, instead of into the LV. Thus, as the RV sinus enlarges, double-inlet LV is being "cured."

In the human embryo, the superior and inferior endocardial cushions of the atrioventricular canal normally fuse in horizon 17 (days 34–36 of age), thereby dividing the common atrioventricular valve into the mitral and tricuspid valves, as is shown by the elegant microdissections of human embryos by Asami[4] (Fig. 2.38).

Note the changes in the relationship between the developing semilunar valves that are occurring during the fifth week of life. By days 30 to 32 (horizon 15), the semilunar interrelationships between the great arteries are like those of **D-transposition of the great arteries:** the developing aortic valve is anterior and to the right, whereas the developing pulmonary valve is posterior and to the left (see Fig. 2.38, top left panel).

By day 33 (horizon 16a), the pulmonary valve has been carried from posterior and to the left of the developing aortic valve to a side-by-side and left position, similar to that seen in the **Taussig–Bing malformation**. Thus, the pulmonary valve has been carried atop the developing subpulmonary part of the conus to a leftward and side-by-side position, whereas the developing aortic valve moves almost not at all (see Fig. 2.38, left middle panel). The aortic valve swivels and keeps facing the anteriorly (ventrally) migrating pulmonary valve, but otherwise the aortic valve does not move. We think this is because the subaortic part of the conus normally does not grow and actually resorbs, whereas the subpulmonary part of the conus normally does grow, elevating the pulmonary valve superiorly (cephalad) and protruding it anteriorly (ventrally).

By day 33 (horizon 16b), the pulmonary valve is now somewhat anterior to the aortic valve, as in typical **tetralogy of Fallot** (see Fig. 2.38, left lower panel). Note that the atrioventricular canal is still in common (not divided) and that the common atrioventricular valve is opening mainly into the LV but also a little bit into the RV.

By days 34 to 36 (horizon 17), the pulmonary valve is now normally anterior and to the left of the aortic valve, and the common atrioventricular canal has now divided into mitral and tricuspid valves (see Fig. 2.38, top right). It should be understood that the mitral and tricuspid valves of the embryo are very different from the mitral and tricuspid valves of the postnatal individual. For example, the leaflets of

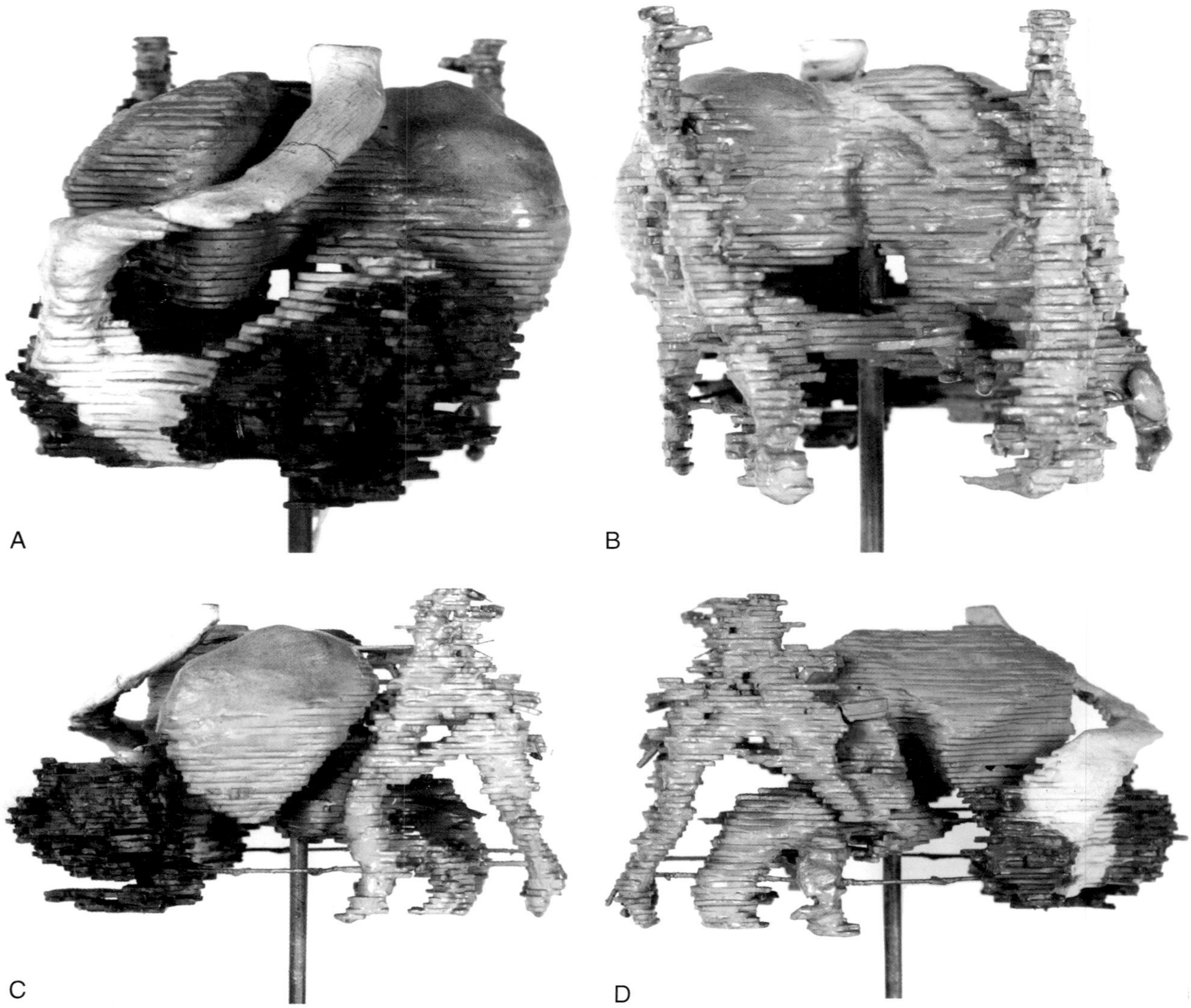

Fig. 2.28 This is a reconstruction of the exterior of the atria and veins, but of the lumen of the bulboventricular loop of Carnegie human embryo 836, 30 pairs of somites, 4 mm in length, horizon 13, estimated age 26 to 28 days. Note that the tip of the right atrial appendage is still somewhat to the left of the vascular pedicle, that is, left-sided juxtaposition of the atrial appendages is still present (as in Fig. 2.26). However, the ventricular portion of the heart has descended somewhat relative to the atria (compare with Fig. 2.26). The dark-colored trabecular zones of the left and right ventricles are developing. The apex of the heart is still oriented rightward. Note that the site of the future interventricular septum is a light colored band between the adjacent dark colored trabeculations of the left and right ventricles. Right ventricular development lags behind that of the left ventricle. The right ventricle is dorsal (posterior) to the left ventricle at this stage, as the right lateral view of this reconstruction shows (right upper panel). Note also that the blood flow is still in-series (as in Fig. 2.26): from right atrium to left atrium to left ventricle to right ventricle to the developing great arteries.

the atrioventricular valves of the embryo are relatively thick, like little flippers, which is why these embryonic leaflets are called endocardial "cushions." The designation "cushions" is intended to convey the fact that these early leaflets are relatively thick (like cushions), not thin and delicate like small leaves ("leaflets").

In Fig. 2.38, lower right panel, the normally related great arteries are seen from behind and above. Normally related great arteries are usually described as twisting about each other. But in fact, they are *untwisting* about each other. Why *un*twisting? The fixed frame of reference between the aorta and the pulmonary artery is distally, at the aortic arch and pulmonary bifurcation. Here, because aortic arches 4 are cephalad to pulmonary arches 6, the aorta always arches over (cephalad to) the pulmonary bifurcation. This is the only fixed, unvarying aorto–pulmonary relationship, as long as both the aortic arch and the pulmonary bifurcation are present. By contrast, the aorto–pulmonary spatial relationship at the level of the semilunar valves is highly variable, as their fifth embryonic week spatial relationships show (see Fig. 2.38). No matter what the semilunar interrelationship of the great arteries is proximally, at the fixed aortic arch/pulmonary bifurcation site distally—the pulmonary artery must be posteroinferior to the aortic arch.

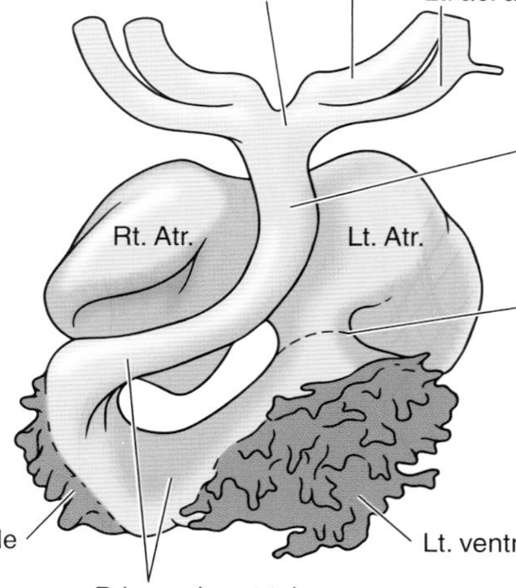

Fig. 2.29 Diagram of human Carnegie embryo 836 (presented photographically in Fig. 2.28), which shows that aortic arches 2 and 3 have appeared and that aortic arch 1 has involuted. This diagram looks at the reconstruction somewhat from above and in front. (From Streeter GL. Developmental horizons in human embryos, age groups XI–XXIII, embryology reprint. Washington, DC: *Carnegie Inst.* II;1951, with permission.)

What happens during normal fifth-week development is that the pulmonary valve rotates clockwise from posterior and left to anterior and left relative to the aortic valve, as viewed from behind and above (see Fig. 2.38). This twisting in a clockwise direction at the semilunar valve level (as seen from above) must be undone by an equal and opposite counterclockwise untwisting of the fibroelastic great arteries as they pass from the semilunar valves proximally to the aortic arch/pulmonary bifurcation level distally, because the great arteries are fixed at this distal level by the aortic arch 4/6 relationship. This is why the great arteries normally must passively untwist as they pass from the semilunar valves proximally to the aortic arch/pulmonary bifurcation distally. This untwisting equals, in degrees, the difference between the variable aorto–pulmonary semilunar interrelationship proximally and the fixed aorto–pulmonary interrelationship distally at the level of the aortic arch/pulmonary bifurcation.

Viewed from the front and below, as in a subxiphoid two-dimensional echocardiogram, the semilunar interrelationship in horizon 15 (see Fig. 2.38) is similar to that of D-transposition of the great arteries shown diagrammatically in Fig. 2.39; the semilunar valves have rotated only 40 degrees to the right relative superoinferior plane (+40 degrees). If the semilunar interrelationship remains as in D-transposition, then the proximal aorto–pulmonary relationship at the semilunar valves and the

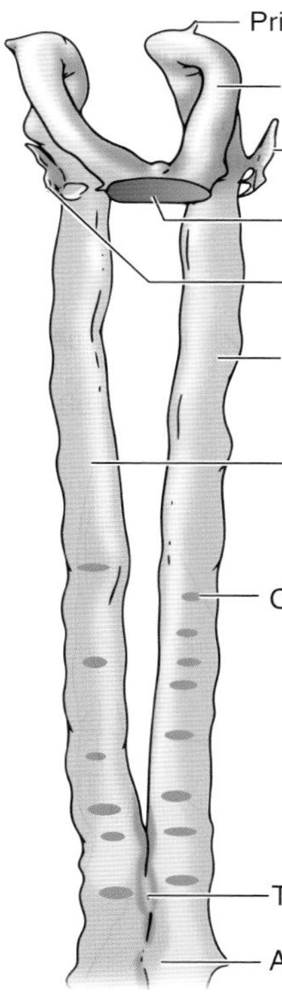

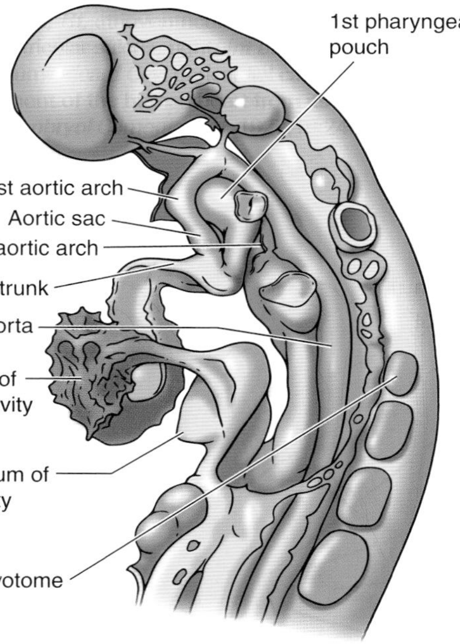

Fig. 2.30 The aortic arches of Carnegie human embryo 2053 (shown diagrammatically in Fig. 2.26), 20 pairs of somites, 3 mm in length, horizon 11, estimated age since ovulation 22 to 24 days. A double aortic arch with left and right dorsal aortae is present. Note that the left first aortic arch arches over the first pharyngeal pouch and that the second aortic arch above the second pharyngeal pouch is just forming. Note the left optic vesicle and the left otic vesicle, which is at the level of the left first aortic arch. Myotome is a synonym for somite. (From Congdon ED. Transformation of the aortic-arch system during the development of the human embryo. *Contrib Embryol. Carnegie Inst.* 1922;14:47, with permission.)

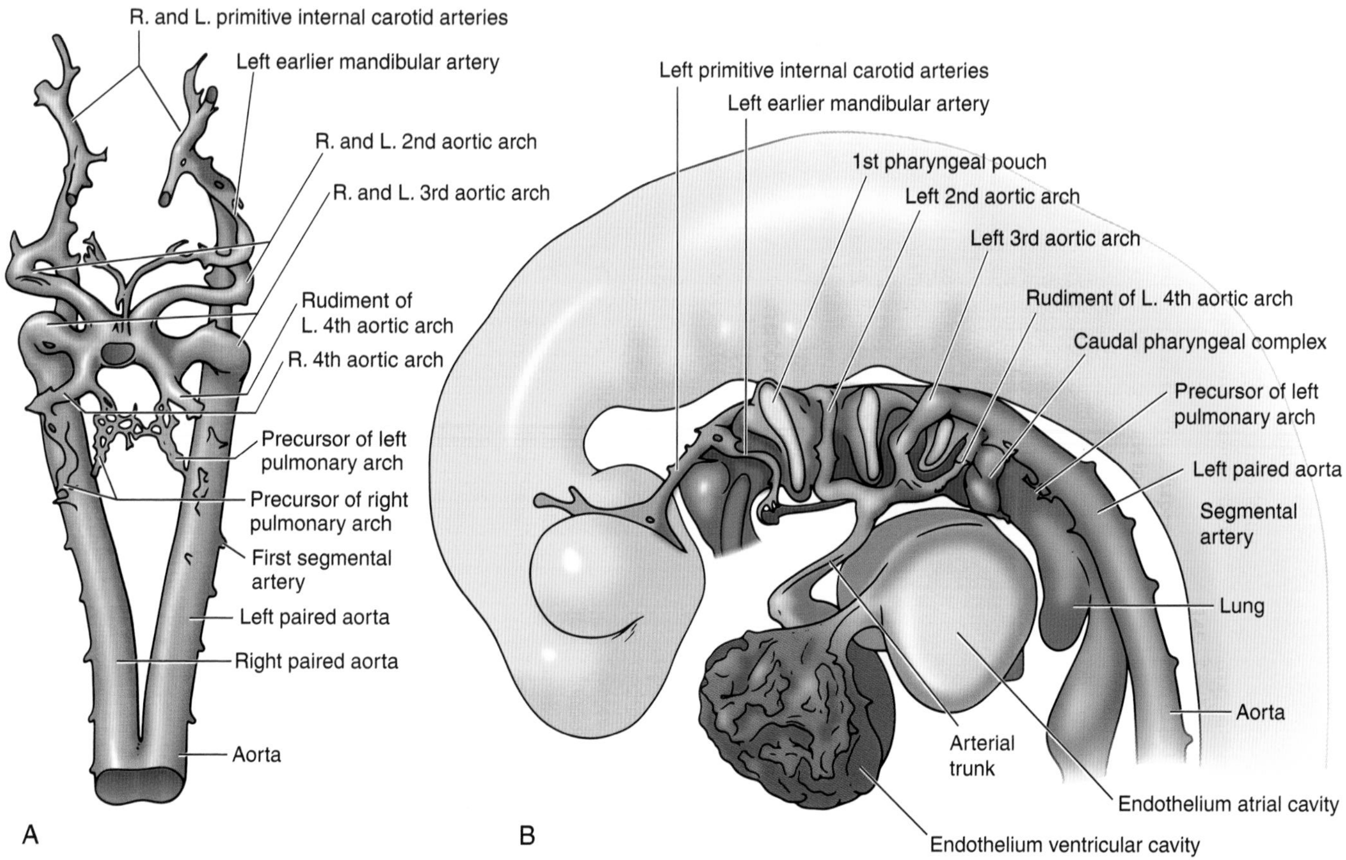

Fig. 2.31 The aortic arches of Carnegie human embryo 836 of Congdon, 30 pairs of somites, 4 mm in length, horizon 13, estimated age 26 to 28 days (same embryo as shown in Fig. 2.28). Note that the left first aortic arch (left earlier mandibular artery) is still present arching over the first pharyngeal pouch and that the left second and third aortic arches also arch over the second and third pharyngeal pouches, respectively. The left fourth arch has not quite formed. There is no evidence of a left fifth arch. The left sixth arch also has not formed as yet beneath the caudal pharyngeal complex, which is also known as the ultimobranchial body—the telescoped and partially fused fourth and fifth pharyngeal pouches. The right fourth arch has formed completely. Note that the left and right pulmonary arterial branches are both present and are heading down to the lung buds, before the right and left dorsal sixth arches (the ductus arteriosi) have formed. Note also the large communication between the lung and the esophagus (a large tracheoesophageal communication being normal at this stage), as is the intrathoracic stomach. (From Congdon ED. Transformation of the aortic-arch system during the development of the human embryo. *Contrib Embryol. Carnegie Inst.* 1922;14:47, with permission.)

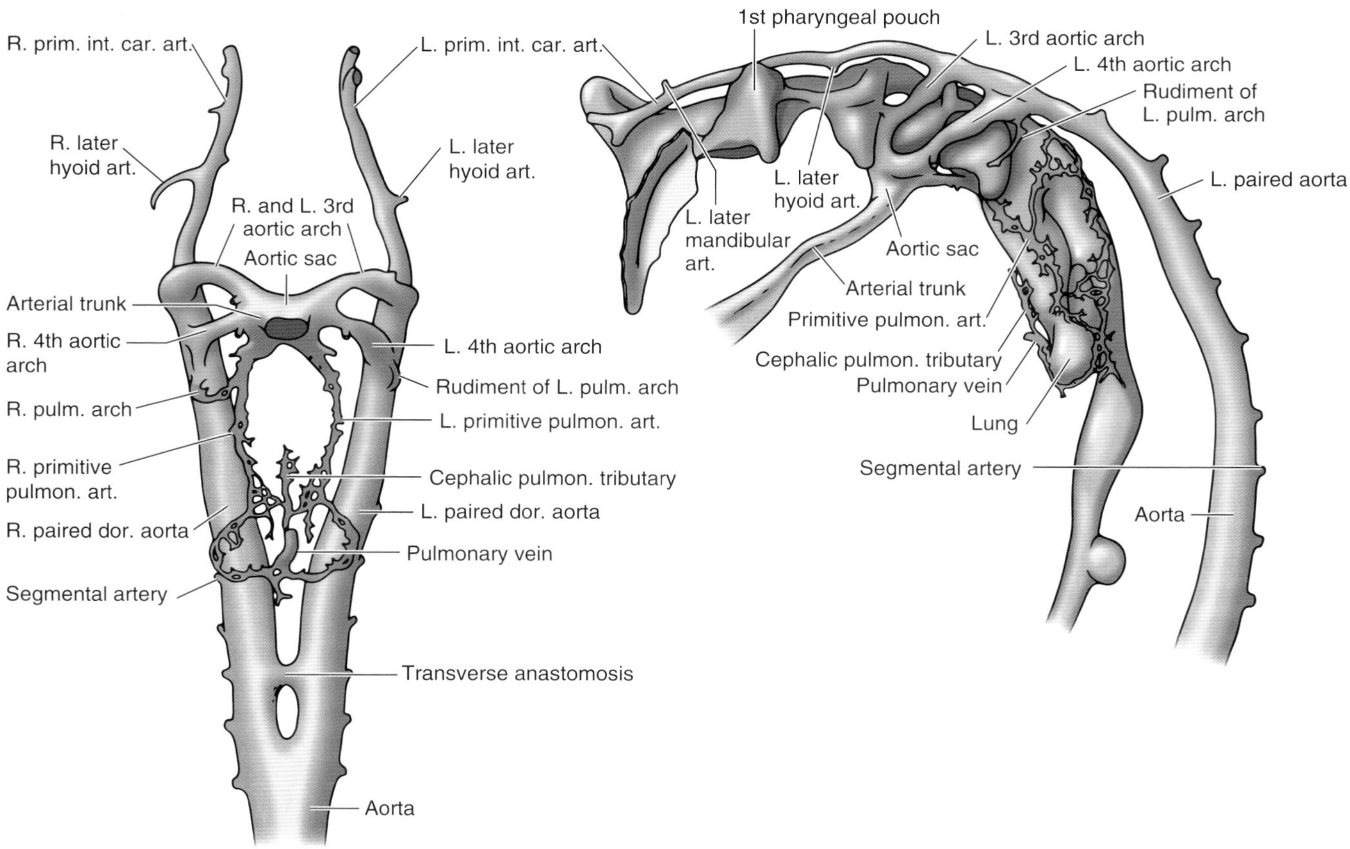

Fig. 2.32 The aortic arches of Carnegie human embryo 1380 of Congdon, 5 mm in length, horizon 13, estimated age since ovulation 26 to 28 days. The left panel is a ventral view, and the right panel is a left lateral view. Note that the mandibular arteries (first arches) have involuted. So too have the hyoid arteries (second arterial arches). Left aortic arches 3 and 4 are present, arching above the third and fourth pharyngeal pouches, respectively. The left sixth aortic arch (the pulmonary arch or ductus arteriosus) is incomplete. However, the right sixth arch has completely formed. Even in the absence of complete sixth arches, the pulmonary arteries have grown down to the lung buds and the common pulmonary vein has appeared. A double aortic arch is still present. (From Congdon ED. Transformation of the aortic-arch system during the development of the human embryo. *Contrib Embryol. Carnegie Inst.* 1922;14:47, with permission.)

distal aorto–pulmonary relationship at the aortic arch/pulmonary bifurcation level remain quite similar (only 40 degrees different). Consequently, as the great arteries pass from proximally at the semilunar valves to distally at the aortic arch/pulmonary bifurcation level, the great arteries have little untwisting to do: only 40 degrees of levorotation (see Fig. 2.39). Hence, with D-transposition, the great arteries and the aortopulmonary septum appear relative parallel, or straight (not twisted about each other).

But as the pulmonary valve continues to move anteriorly on the left (as in horizon 16a, Fig. 2.38, and +90 degrees rotation, Fig. 2.39), then the difference between the semilunar interrelationship proximally and the fixed aorto–pulmonary relationship distally is greater: 90 degrees when the semilunar valves are side by side (see Fig. 2.39). Consequently, the fibroelastic great arteries have twice as much passive untwisting to do as in typical D-transposition (90 degrees of levorotation, as opposed to 40 degrees of levorotation, Fig. 2.39). So, when the semilunar valves are side by side, the great arteries do seem to be twisted around each other but to a subnormal degree.

As the pulmonary valve continues its normal ventral morphogenetic movement in horizons 16b and 17 (see Fig. 2.38), the pulmonary valve gets more and more anterior, while the aortic valve gets relatively more posterior, as a normal semilunar interrelationship is achieved: horizon 17 (see Fig. 2.38) and +150 degrees (see Fig. 2.39). When the great arteries are normally related, they have to untwist through about 150 degrees to return to the fixed aorto–pulmonary relationship distally at the level of the aortic arch/pulmonary bifurcation (see Fig. 2.39).

Asami[4] showed that the same progression of the pulmonary valve from posteriorly on the left to anteriorly on the left relative to the almost stationary aortic valve also occurs in the normal development of the heart of the rat embryo (Fig. 2.40).

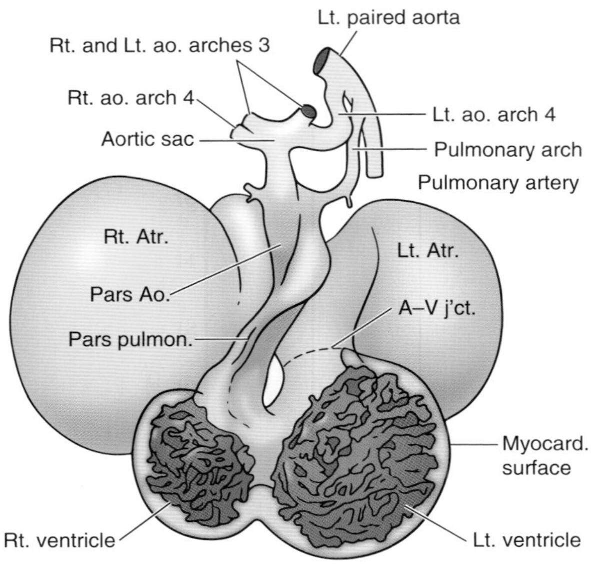

Fig. 2.33 Diagram of reconstruction of Carnegie human embryo 3385, ventral view, showing the exterior of the right and left atria, and with the reconstruction of the interior of the left and right ventricles, the great arteries and the aortic arches. Note that the development of the right ventricle is starting to catch up with that of the left ventricle. The ventricular portion of the heart is swinging leftward. The ventricular septum is oriented approximately ventrodorsally, as in mesocardia. The atrioventricular junction still opens only into the left ventricle, but the main pulmonary artery (pars Pulmon) and the ascending aorta (pars Ao) are becoming distinct. Other abbreviations as previously. (From Streeter GL. Developmental horizons in human embryos, age groups XI–XXIII, embryology reprint. Washington, DC: *Carnegie Inst.* II;1951, with permission.)

Sometimes people have trouble understanding what we mean by saying that normally, the great arteries are *passively untwisting* about each other because of the difference between the proximal aortopulmonary relationship at the semilunar valves compared with the distal aortopulmonary relationship at the aortic arch and pulmonary bifurcation. "What are we trying to get at? What's the point?" they ask.

The point is as follows: It has often been said that normally related great arteries, which appear to spiral around each other, result from spiral growth and development of the truncoconal ridges, whereas transposition of the great arteries results from straight growth and development of the truncoconal ridges. In this classical concept, spiral or straight development of the aortopulmonary and infundibular (truncoconal) ridges is thought to be the morphogenetic cause of normally related or transposed great arteries, respectively. This classical view may be called the *malseptation concept* of the morphogenesis of transposition of the great arteries, in which the growth and development of the aortopulmonary septum is regarded as the primary developmental mechanism causing transposition of the great arteries.

Our view is very different. My colleagues and I do not think that aortopulmonary malseptation is the primary morphogenetic mechanism causing transposition of the great arteries and the other conotruncal anomalies. Instead, we think that aortopulmonary septation in transposition of the great arteries is normal per se. We think that the malseptation or straight aortopulmonary septum hypothesis concerning the morphogenesis of transposition of the great arteries is wrong. We think that whether the aortopulmonary septum is spiral or straight depends on the proximal aortopulmonary relationship at the semilunar valves compared with the distal fixed aortopulmonary relationship at the aortic arch and pulmonary bifurcation.

1. When the proximal and distal relationships are very similar, as in transposition of the great arteries, then the great arteries appear parallel, straight, not twisted.
2. But when the proximal and distal relationships are very different, as with normally related great arteries, then the great arteries appear twisted around each other. In fact, the fibroelastic great arteries are untwisting about each other, as they must, because the distal aortopulmonary relationship at the aortic arch/pulmonary bifurcation is fixed by the aortic arches 4/6 relationship. The normal untwisting of the great arteries is a passive, not an active, process.

The great arteries are where the torque or twist normally is taken out of the ventriculoinfundibular system, which is fixed both proximally, at the atrioventricular valves, and distally at the aortic arch/pulmonary bifurcation. The combination of ventricular D-loop formation plus asymmetrical development of the distal or subsemilunar part of the conus (growth of the subpulmonary part, with lack of growth and absorption of the subaortic conal free wall) together produces about 150 degrees of dextrorotation (rotation in a rightward direction) at the semilunar valves.

Normally, the aortic valve is posterior, inferior, and to the right relative to the pulmonary valve. But the aortic arch is anterior and superior relative to the pulmonary bifurcation. So, what has to happen? The ascending aorta and main pulmonary artery have to untwist around each other, going through approximately 150 degrees of levorotation (rotation in a leftward direction) as they proceed from the semilunar valve level to the aortic arch/pulmonary bifurcation level, in order to undo the torque or twist that was put into the ventriculoinfundibular system by the musculature involved in D-loop formation of the ventricles and development of the subpulmonary part only of the conus. Thus, ventriculoinfundibular musculature appears to be the source of the 150 degrees of dextrorotation at the semilunar valves, whereas the fibroelastic tissue of the great arteries permits passive untwisting of about 150 degrees of levorotation to occur between the semilunar valves and the aortic arch/pulmonary bifurcation.

In the evolution from ancient fish (such as sharks) to mammals (such as humans), the musculature of the conus arteriosus has receded from the branchial (gill or aortic) arches to the infundibulum. This demuscularization of the ascending (ventral) aorta was necessary in order for the appearance of fibroelastic (demuscularized) great arteries in reptiles, birds, and mammals. If our great arteries had remained coated in muscle

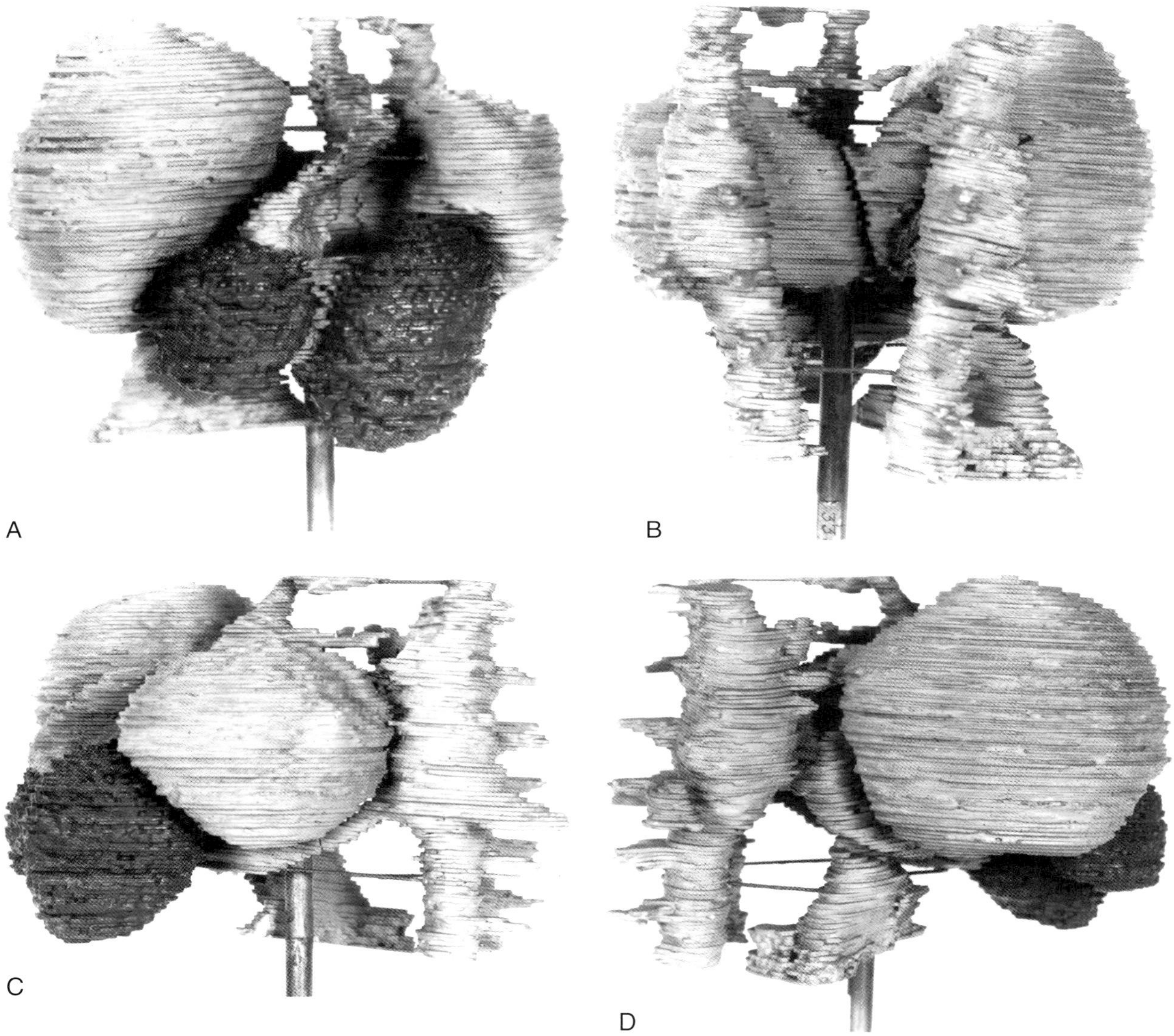

Fig. 2.34 This is the reconstruction of Carnegie human embryo 3385 (shown diagrammatically in Fig. 2.33). The actual reconstruction of the ventricular lumina confirms the progressing development of the right ventricular cavity. The space between the left and right ventricular cavities is occupied by the developing interventricular septum. Image A is a ventral view that shows this best. Image B is the dorsal view, image C is the left view of this reconstruction, and image D is the right lateral view.

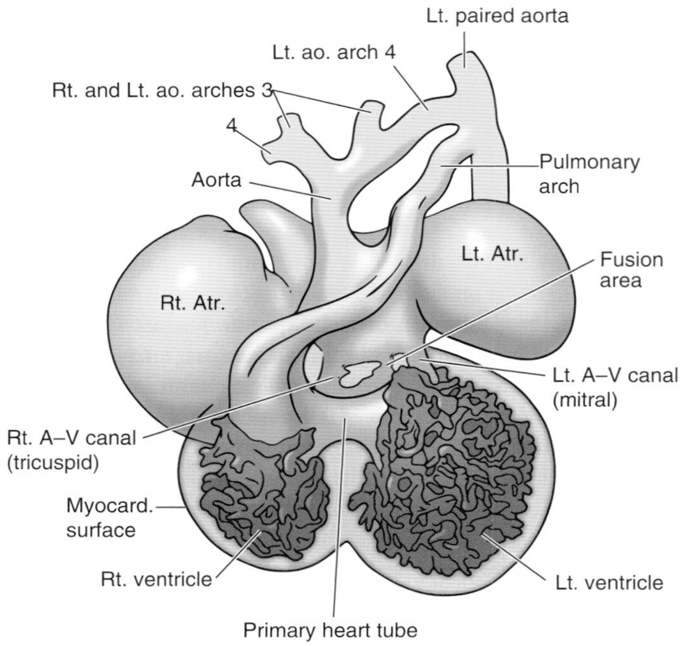

Fig. 2.35 This is a diagram of the ventral view of Carnegie human embryo 6510, horizon 16. Note that the atrioventricular canal is beginning to undergo division (fusion area) into tricuspid and mitral canals or valves. The tricuspid valve is starting to open into the developing right ventricle. (From Streeter GL. Developmental horizons in human embryos, age groups XI–XXIII, embryology reprint. Washington, DC: *Carnegie Inst.* II;1951, with permission.)

("muscle bound"), then the necessary untwisting of fibroelastic great arteries described heretofore might well have been impossible.

It is helpful to understand that the *conus arteriosus* (arterial cone) is well named. This musculature comes from the great arteries, literally. The conus arteriosus muscle attaches the great arteries to the ventricles. The conus arteriosus is really part of the great arteries (the conotruncus, in embryologic parlance) not part of the ventricles. This is why the conus can form a crista supraventricularis (supraventricular crest) that normally is above the morphologically RV sinus but that abnormally can be above the morphologically LV sinus—as in anatomically corrected malposition of the great arteries and double-outlet LV. The conus arteriosus is not an intrinsic and inseparable part of the morphologically RV. Instead, the conus arteriosus forms the outflow tract of *both* ventricles. The conus arteriosus can straddle the ventricular septum to any degree. The conal connector attaches both ventricles below to both great arteries above. Normally, the conus arteriosus appears to be located almost exclusively above the morphologically RV, because the part of the conus above the morphologically LV—the subaortic conal free wall—has failed to grow and has undergone resorption, resulting in aortic-to-mitral direct fibrous continuity. This negative conal development (lack of growth and resorption) is necessary to connect the aortic valve with the mitral valve and the LV sinus. Conversely, positive conal development (normal growth of the subpulmonary conus) is also necessary to connect the pulmonary valve with the morphologically RV sinus.

To summarize this important point, phylogenetically the conus arteriosus comes from the great arteries and is part of the great arterial segment, the conotruncus (not part of the ventricles, meaning the ventricular sinuses or inflow tracts that are the main pumping portions). The conal connector between the ventricular sinuses and the great arteries normally undergoes both positive development (growth of the subpulmonary conus) and negative development (lack of growth and resorption of the subaortic conal free wall).

What is a ventricle? The essence of a ventricle is its sinus or inflow tract—its main pumping portion: no ventricular sinus means no ventricle. The proximal connector of the ventricular sinus (the atrioventricular canal or junction) and the distal connector of the ventricular sinus (the conus arteriosus—developed or resorbed) do not constitute a ventricle anatomically or physiologically. When the ventricular pumping portion (the sinus) is absent, the ventricle is absent anatomically and functionally.

This **conal connector** is of crucial importance to the understanding of normally and abnormally related (i.e., connected) great arteries. Whether the aortopulmonary semilunar relationship is very different from or similar to the aortic arch/pulmonary bifurcation relationship is largely determined by the development of the subsemilunar conal connector.

Thus, the formation of the truncoconal ridges is not the primary morphogenetic mechanism in transposition of the great arteries (and the other conotruncal malformations). Instead, the primary morphogenetic mechanism in transposition involves abnormal development (growth, lack of growth, and absorption) of the subsemilunar conal free walls (not the septum). The famously eye-catching aortopulmonary septum, which may be spiral or straight, is one of the passive secondary effects of subsemilunar conal development, not the primary morphogenetic mechanism of the conotruncal malformations such as transposition of the great arteries.

The development of the atrioventricular canal and of the conotruncus (infundibulum and great arteries) is presented diagrammatically in Figs. 2.41 to 2.45, inclusive:

At the end of the fourth week (27 days), 4 to 5 mm, horizon 13, the atrioventricular canal is in common (undivided) and opens only into the developing LV; that is, common-inlet LV normally is present (see Fig. 2.41, left panel). Aortic arches 1 to 6 are seen. Note the aortic arches 1 and 2 have involuted. Arches 3 and 4 are completely present. Arch 5 is not present, and arch 6 is just beginning—very incomplete at this stage. The conus and truncus arteriosus are present but are entirely undivided (see Fig. 2.41, right panel).

At the beginning of the fifth week (29 days, 6–7 mm), horizon 14, the endocardial cushions of the atrioventricular canal are somewhat better developed, but the common atrioventricular

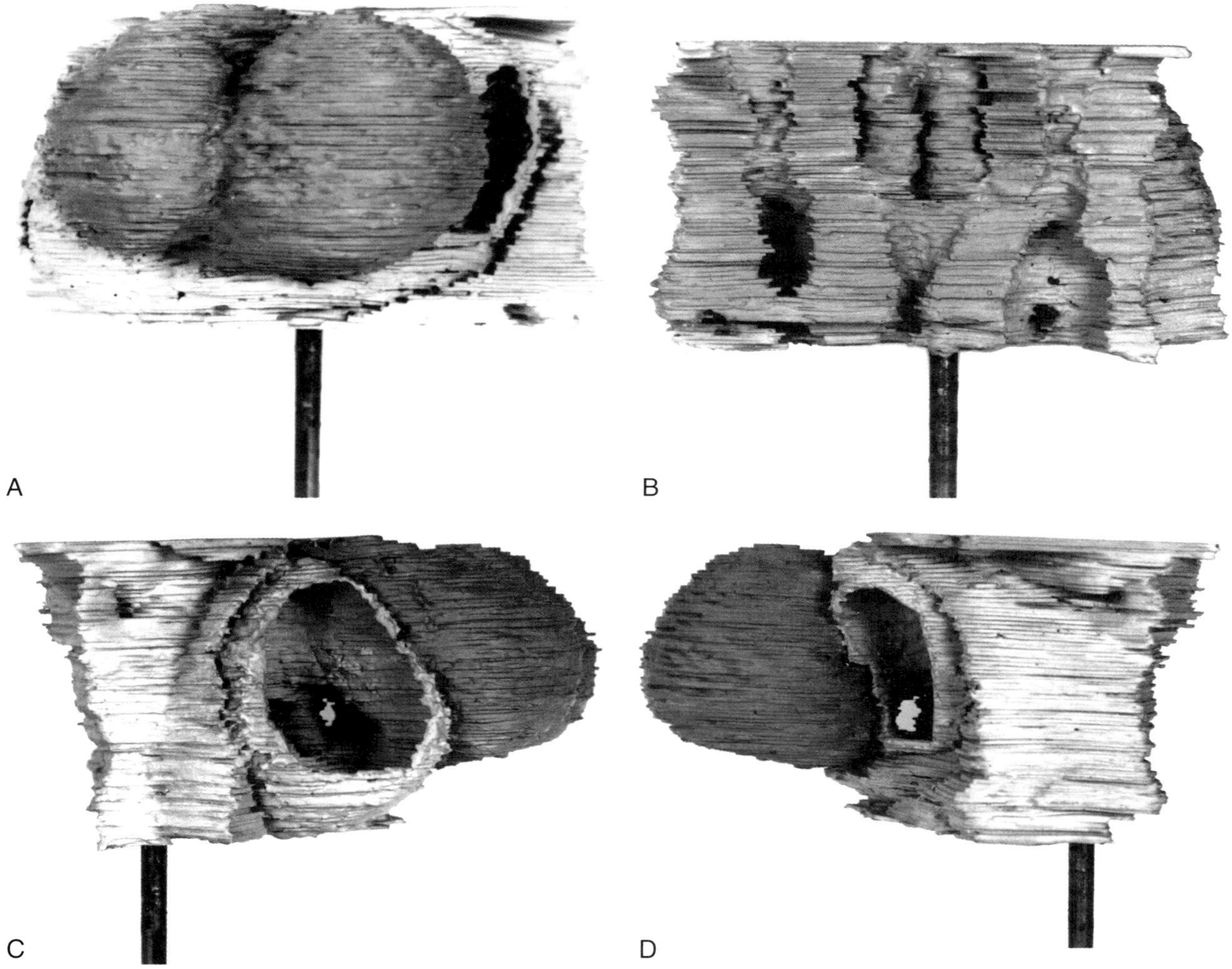

Fig. 2.36 Reconstruction of Carnegie human embryo 6510, 10.1 mm in length, horizon 16, estimated age 32 to 34 days. This is the same embryo that is presented diagrammatically in Fig. 2.35. Note that the lumen of the right ventricle is almost equal in size to that of the left ventricle (A, ventral view). In the right lateral view through the opened right atrium (D) and in the left lateral view through the opened left atrium (C), note that the ostium primum is now very small and is about to close as part of the subdivision of the atrioventricular canal by the endocardial cushions. Thus, mesocardia is present, and the septum of the atrioventricular canal has almost formed completely. B is a dorsal view of the reconstruction. The ventricles seen in the other three panels show the exterior or ventricular myocardial aspect as seen from outside the heart.

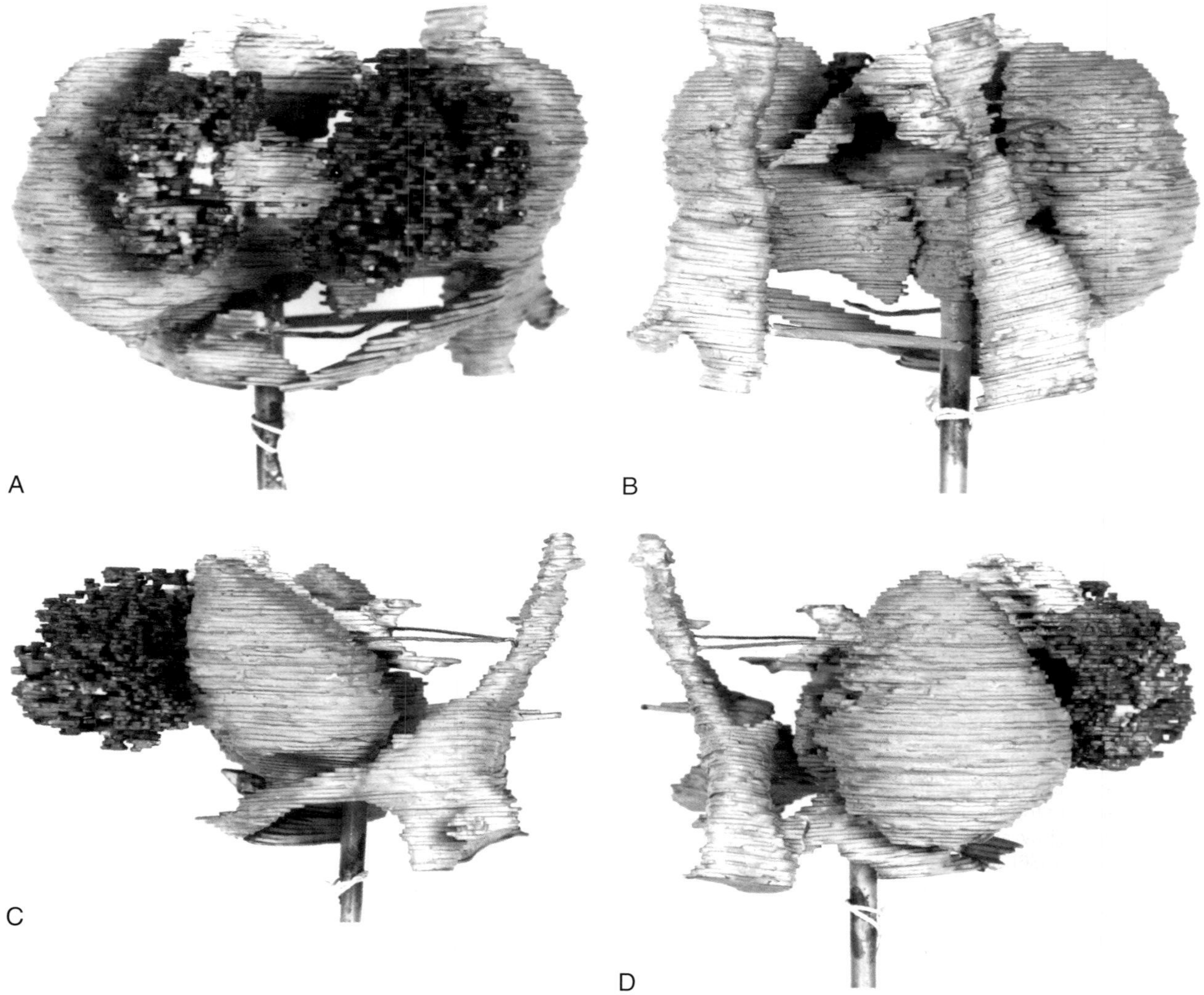

Fig. 2.37 Reconstruction of the outside of the atria and veins and of the lumina of the right and left ventricles of Carnegie human embryo 6510, horizon 16 (also shown in Figs. 2.35 and 2.36). This ventricular luminal reconstruction confirms the accuracy of the diagram (Fig. 2.35) and of the external reconstruction of the ventricles (Fig. 2.36). A, ventral view; B, dorsal view; C, left lateral view; and D, right lateral view.

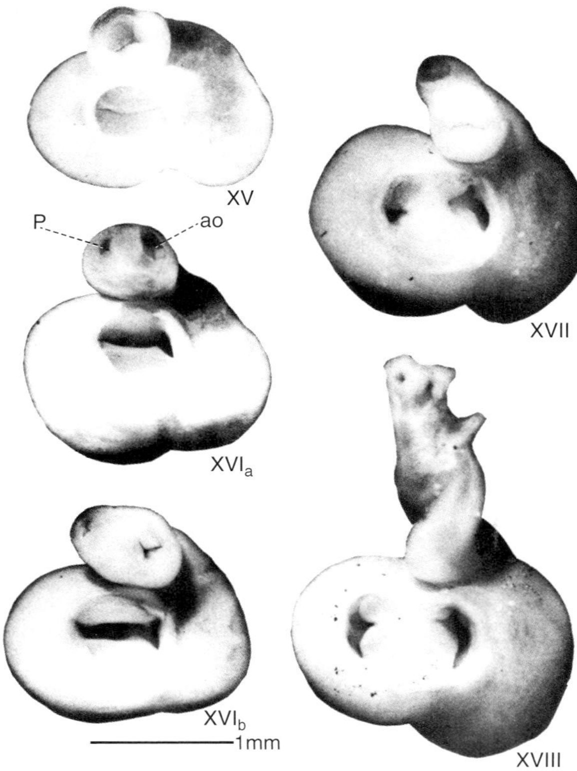

Fig. 2.38 Morphogenetic movement of the developing pulmonary valve in normal human embryos from horizon 15 (day 30–32) to horizon 17 (day 34–36). The normal septation of the atrioventricular canal is also seen. The free walls and the septum of the great arteries have been removed above the level of the semilunar valves, and the atrial free walls and septum have been removed above the developing atrioventricular valves. Ventral is toward the top, dorsal toward the bottom, right toward the viewer's right hand, and left toward the viewer's left hand. In horizon 15, the developing pulmonary valve is posterior and to the left of the developing aortic valve. Early in horizon 16 (16A, day 32–33), the pulmonary valve has moved from posteriorly on the left to side by side on the left of the developing aortic valve *(ao)*. Late in horizon 16 (day 33–34), the pulmonary valve has been carried atop the developing subpulmonary infundibulum to a position slightly anterior to the developing aortic valve. By horizon 17 (days 34–36), the pulmonary valve has been carried by the developing subpulmonary infundibulum to a position normally anterior and to the left of the developing aortic valve. During this posterior to anterior progression of the pulmonary valve, the aortic valve moves almost not at all, only swiveling to keep on facing the anteriorly moving pulmonary valve. Note that the aorticopulmonary septum at the semilunar valve level is absent in horizon 15 but has appeared early in horizon 16. Note also that the superior and inferior endocardial cushions are unfused normally in horizon 16 but fused in horizon 17 (days 34–36). The human embryo in horizon 18 (days 36–38) shows the normal untwisting of the fibroelastic great arteries as they progress from the semilunar valves proximally to the aortic arch and pulmonary bifurcation distally, where the aorta is always cephalad relative to the pulmonary artery bifurcation because of the aortic arches 4/6 relationship. (From Asami I. Partitioning of the arterial end of the embryonic heart. In Van Praagh R, Takao A, eds. *Etiology and Morphogenesis of Congenital Heart Disease*. Mt Kisco, NY: Futura Publishing Co.; 1980:51, with permission.)

canal is still opening only into the developing LV (see Fig. 2.42, left panel). Aortic arches 3, 4, and 6 are all completely present.

The conal and truncal swellings have appeared (see Fig. 2.42). The two conal swellings are dextrodorsal and sinistroventral. The two truncal swellings are dextrosuperior and sinistroinferior. Note that dextrodorsal conal swelling is confluent with the dextrosuperior truncal swelling. Similarly, the sinistroventral conal swelling is confluent with the sinistroinferior truncal swelling. (This is the terminology of Dr. Lodewyk H.S. ["Bob"] Van Mierop, who collaborated with Dr. Frank H. Netter to produce these elegant diagrams.)

At the 31st day (8–9 mm, horizon 15), the superior and inferior endocardial cushions of the atrioventricular canal are beginning to approach each other (see Fig. 2.43, left panel). The still common atrioventricular valve now opens somewhat into the RV, even though it still opens mainly into the LV.

The dextrodorsal conal swelling plus the dextrosuperior truncal swelling and the sinistroventral conal swelling plus the sinistroinferior truncal swelling both are becoming much more prominent (see Fig. 2.43, right panel). Nonetheless, the ascending aorta and the main pulmonary artery are still in common (not divided).

At 33 days of age (10 mm, horizon 16), the superior and inferior endocardial cushions are close together but have not fused; common atrioventricular canal is still present (see Fig. 2.44). Although the common atrioventricular valve opens somewhat into the RV, it still opens mostly into the LV.

At 35 days of age (12 mm in length, horizon 17), the superior and inferior endocardial cushions have fused, dividing the common atrioventricular valve into mitral and tricuspid valves (see Fig. 2.45). Note that the right and left conal cushions have fused distally, at the semilunar valve level. However, more proximally, the right conal cushion (also known as the right bulbar ridge) and the left conal cushion (also known as the left bulbar ridge) remain unfused. Both the interventricular foramen (the ventricular septal defect) and the interconal foramen (the conal septal defect) are normally still patent.

At 34 to 36 days of age (horizon 17), aortic arches 3, 4, and 6 are present, as are the left and right pulmonary artery branches (Fig. 2.46, Carnegie embryo 1121, 11 mm). Note that the ascending aorta and main pulmonary artery are divided (no longer in common).

Hence, the fifth week of life in utero is when the phylogenetically primitive, single, in-series circulation typical of aquatic vertebrates is largely converted to the phylogenetically more recent, double, in-parallel, systemic, and pulmonary circulations of air-breathing vertebrates. It is in the fifth embryonic week that **common atrioventricular canal, transposition of the great arteries, double-outlet RV, tetralogy of Fallot, and other conotruncal anomalies** either are avoided by normal

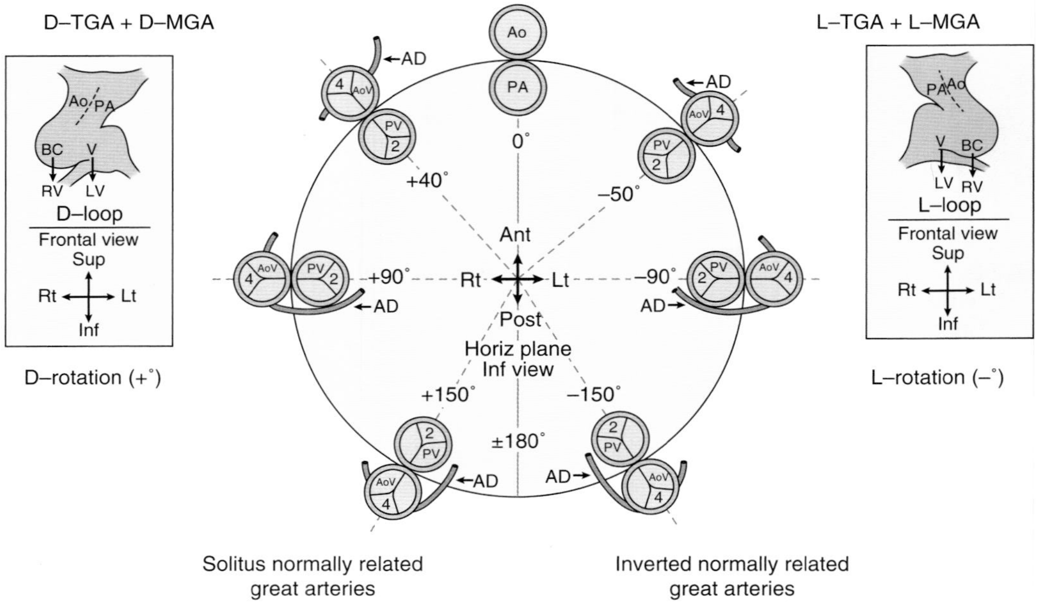

Fig. 2.39 Untwisting of the great arteries as they proceed from the variable semilunar interrelationships proximally between the pulmonary valve *(PV)* and the aortic valve *(AoV)* to the fixed relationship between the aortic arch *(Ao)* and the pulmonary artery bifurcation *(PA)* distally. The untwisting of the great arteries equals, in degrees, the difference between the variable semilunar interrelationship proximally and the fixed aortic arch/pulmonary artery bifurcation relationship distally. Solitus normally related great arteries normally undergo approximately 150 degrees of rotation to the right relative to the aortic arch/pulmonary artery bifurcation, dextrorotation of the semilunar valves being expressed in positive degrees, that is, +150 degrees. Consequently, the fibroelastic great arteries must untwist through 150 degrees in the opposite direction (levorotation) as they proceed from the valves proximally to the aortic arch/pulmonary bifurcation distally. Inverted normally related great arteries undergo approximately 150 degrees of levorotation relative to the aortic arch/pulmonary artery bifurcation, levorotation being expressed in negative degrees, that is, −150 degrees. Consequently, inverted normally related great arteries must untwist through approximately 150 degrees in the opposite direction (dextrorotation) as they proceed from the variable valve level relationship proximally to the fixed aortic arch/pulmonary artery bifurcation relationship distally. Abnormally related great arteries undergo less dextrorotation or less levorotation at the semilunar valve level. Consequently, such great arteries have less untwisting to do as they proceed from the variable relationship at the semilunar valves proximally to the fixed relationship at the aortic arch/pulmonary artery bifurcation distally. When the semilunar valves are side by side, they have undergone only 90 degrees rotation—to the right or to the left—relative to the aortic arch/pulmonary artery bifurcation. Thus, such great arteries have to untwist through only 90 degrees (in the direction opposite to the rotation of the semilunar valves) as they proceed from the valves proximally to the aortic arch/pulmonary artery bifurcation distally. Typical D-transposition of the great arteries *(D-TGA)* or L-transposition of the great arteries *(L-TGA)* has undergone even less rotation—to the right or to the left—relative to the aortic arch/pulmonary artery bifurcation distally. Hence, in transposition, the great arteries have even less untwisting to do as they proceed from the valves proximally to the aortic arch/pulmonary artery bifurcation distally, and consequently the great arteries in transposition appear essentially parallel, straight, or uncrossed—not untwisting about each other. In this diagram, the semilunar valves and the aortic arch/pulmonary artery bifurcation are depicted as in a short-axis view. The diagrams of the D-loop and the L-loop ventricles are shown in a ventral or frontal view. *AD,* Anterior descending coronary artery; *D-MGA,* D-malposition of the great arteries, as for example in double-outlet right ventricle; *L-MGA,* L-malposition of the great arteries. Other abbreviations as previously. (From Van Praagh R. Approccio segmentario alla diagnosi delle cardiopatie congenite. In Squarcia U, ed. *Progressi in Cardiologia Pediatrica.* Milan: Casa Editrice Ambrosiana; 1978:7.)

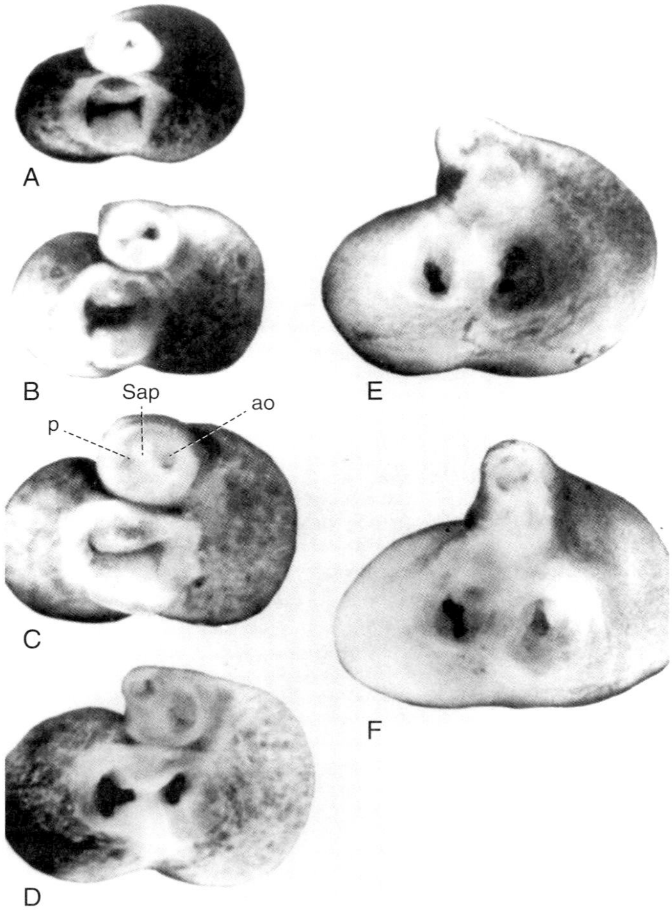

Fig. 2.40 Dorsal views of the embryonic rat heart after removal of the atria and great arteries above the semilunar valves. (A) 12½ days. (B) 12¾ days. (C) 13 days. (D) 13¾ days. (E) 14½ days. (F) 15½ days. The major part of the rotation of the semilunar valves takes place on the side of the developing pulmonary valve *(p)*, whereas the developing aortic valve *(ao)* moves only slightly. *Sap,* Septum aortopulmonale (aortopulmonary septum). Note that the progression of the developing pulmonary valve from posteriorly on the left relative to the developing aortic valve to side by side on the left and then to anteriorly on the left is essentially identical to what also happens in the human embryo (Fig. 2.38). Note also that the common atrioventricular canal divides into mitral and tricuspid orifices at 13¾ days in the rat and by 14½ days has been completed, the cleft in the anterior leaflet of the mitral valve having disappeared. (From Asami I. Partitioning of the arterial end of the embryonic heart. In Van Praagh R, Takao A, eds. *Etiology and Morphogenesis of Congenital Heart Disease.* Mt Kisco, NY: Futura Publishing Co.; 1980:51, with permission.)

development (see Figs. 2.38 and 2.40) or occur with abnormal development.

Other important developmental considerations include:
1. the presence or absence of infundibular apoptosis; and
2. **congenital heart equations.**

THE SIXTH AND SEVENTH WEEKS OF LIFE

The main cardiovascular developments during the sixth and seventh weeks of intrauterine life are) closure of the conotruncal (infundibuloarterial) septum and closure of the membranous part of the interventricular septum.

The formation of the aortopulmonary septum begins distally at the junction of the aortic arches 4 and the pulmonary arches 6 (see Fig. 2.46, left). Fusion of the truncoconal ridges proceeds from distally to proximally.

By six weeks of age (12 mm in length), the fusion of the left and right truncoconal ridges has reached approximately the stage.

During the seventh week (14.5 to 20 mm in length), the left and right truncoconal ridges normally complete their fusion proximally, thereby completing the formation of the conal or infundibular septum.

The space between the infundibular septum above and the ventricular septum below normally is filled by fibrous tissue that is closely related to the anterior leaflet of the tricuspid valve, thus forming the membranous portion of the ventricular septum. The *pars membranacea septi* (membranous part of the septum, Latin) has two parts:
1. below the annular attachment of the tricuspid valve, this being the **interventricular portion of the membranous septum**; and
2. above the annular attachment of the tricuspid valve, this being the **atrioventricular portion of the membranous septum.**

Although closure of the rightmost end of the interventricular foramen usually is achieved between 38 and 45 days of age, this event can be delayed until shortly following birth, resulting in so-called **spontaneous closure** of a ventricular septal defect, "spontaneous" meaning medically or surgically unassisted.

In a 37-day-old embryo (16 mm) diagrammed by Netter (Fig. 2.47), both the conal and the ventricular septa appear to be closed. However, in a reconstruction of Carnegie embryo 6520 (14.2 mm, horizon 18), the interventricular foramen is still open (Fig. 2.48). Note that RV growth has caught up with LV growth (see Fig. 2.48). The ventricular apex is now pointing to the left; that is, levocardia has been achieved.

Thus, the sixth and seventh weeks of embryonic life are when cardiac septation is usually completed, the systemic and pulmonary circulations being completely separated—except for the patent foramen ovale and the patent ductus arteriosus. Normally, the latter two communications do not close until following birth. Normally, development during the sixth and seventh weeks of intrauterine life avoids **aortopulmonary window, conal septal defect,** and **ventricular septal defect**; whereas abnormal development at this time can result in the aforementioned anomalies. The importance of developmental events during the sixth and seventh embryonic weeks is emphasized by the realization that ventricular septal defect appears to be by far the most common form of congenital heart disease.

Embryology of the Aortic Arch System

The normal development of the aortic arch system in human embryos is summarized in Fig. 2.49.[3]

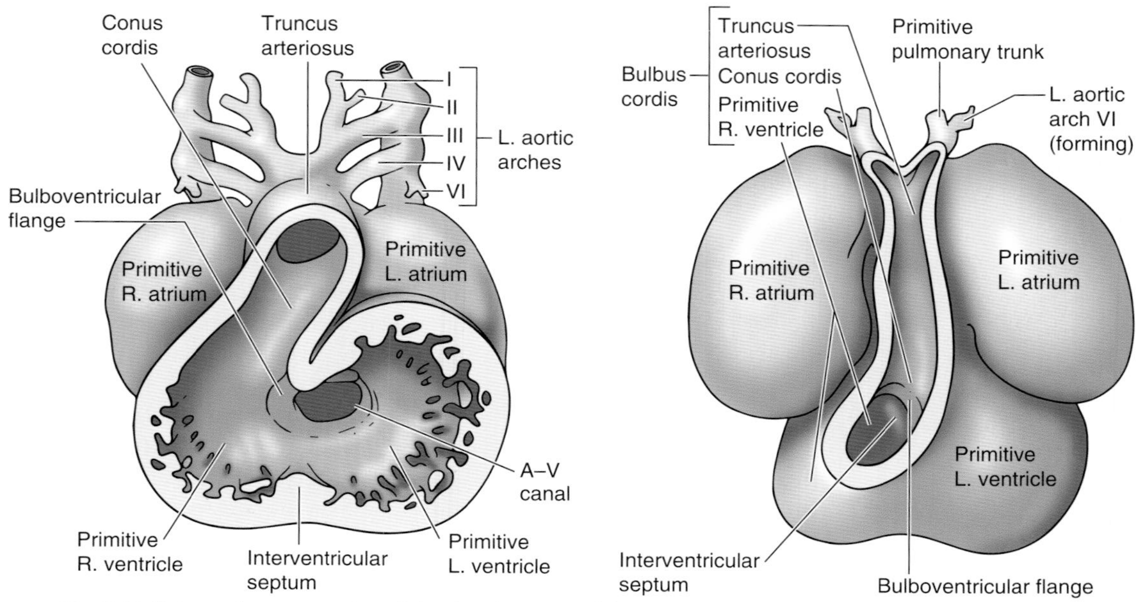

Fig. 2.41 Schematic presentation of the development of the atrioventricular canal, conus, and truncus arteriosus, 4–5 mm in length, approximately 27 days of age, horizon 13, view from the front in the left panel showing the AV canal and the conus, and view from above in the right panel showing the truncus arteriosus. (From Frank Netter: The Netter Collection of Medical Illustrations, Volume 5, HEART, 1969, with permission.)

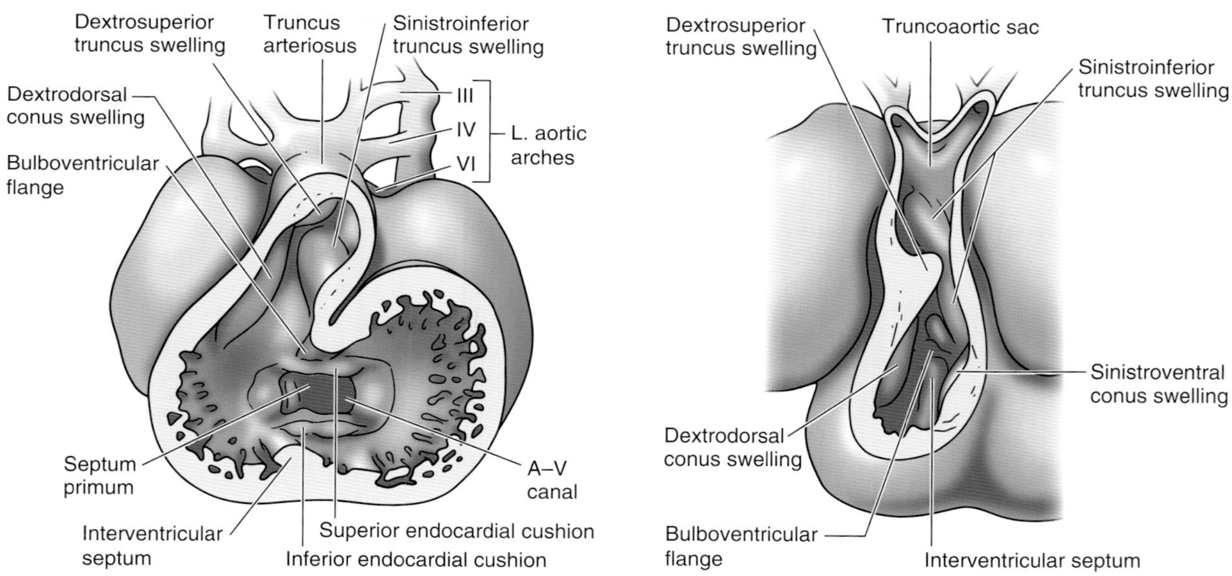

Fig. 2.42 6–7 mm in length, approximately 29 days of age, horizon 14, left panel viewed from the front, right panel from above. The atrioventricular canal (A–V canal) is still in common and opens only into the left ventricle. The dextrodorsal and sinistroventral conal swellings have appeared. The dextrosuperior and sinistroinferior truncal swellings are also now present. (From Frank Netter: The Netter Collection of Medical Illustrations, Volume 5, HEART, 1969, with permission.)

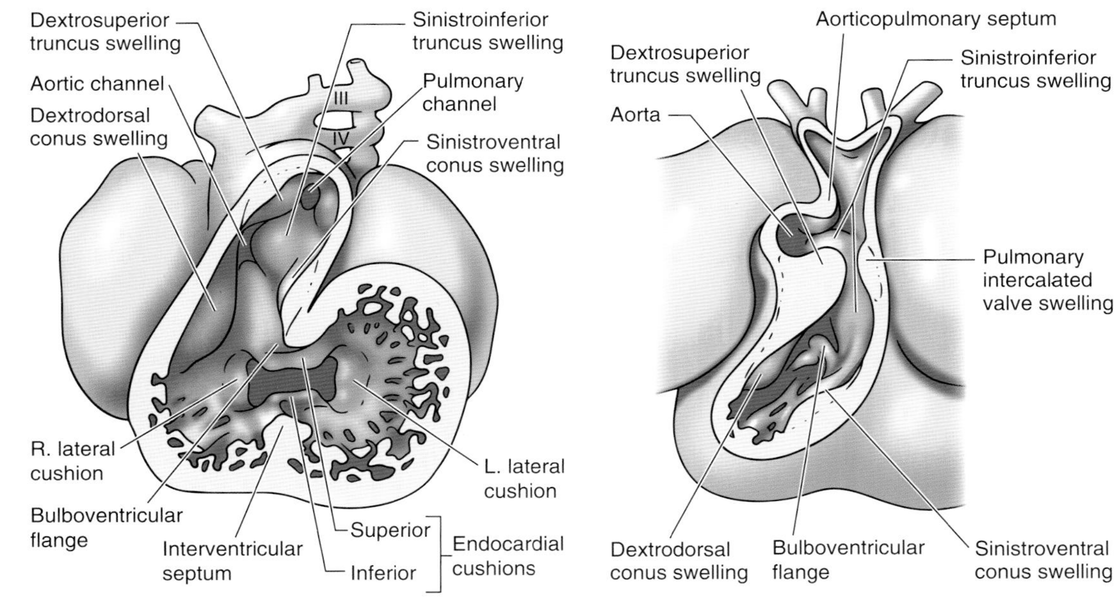

Fig. 2.43 Diagram of human embryo 8 to 9 mm in length, approximately 31 days of age, horizon 15, left panel as seen from the front, right panel as viewed from above. Note that the atrioventricular canal is still in common but is now beginning to open into the right ventricle. The truncal and conal swellings are becoming more pronounced. (From Frank Netter: The Netter Collection of Medical Illustrations, Volume 5, HEART, 1969, with permission.)

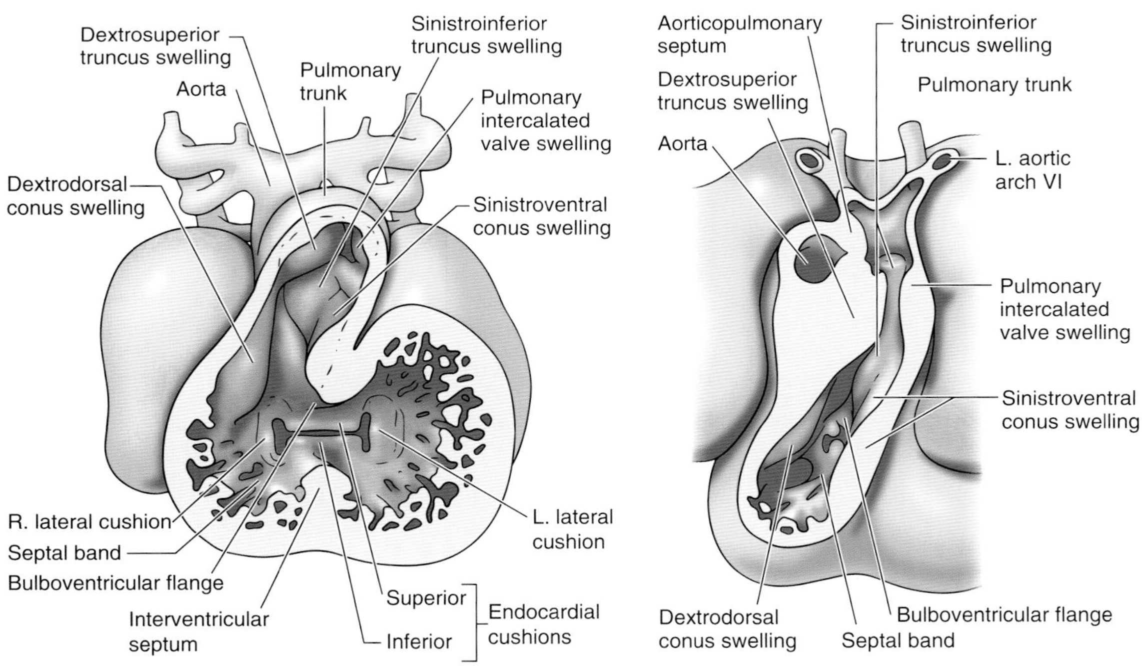

Fig. 2.44 10 mm human embryo, estimated age 33 days, horizon 16. (A) ventral view. (B) coronal section showing view of the interior as seen from the front. Note that the superior and inferior endocardial cushions have approximated but not fused and that the atrioventricular canal now opens somewhat into the right ventricle. (From Frank Netter: The Netter Collection of Medical Illustrations, Volume 5, HEART, 1969, with permission.)

There are four normal aortic arch interruptions (Figs. 2.49–2.51):

1. and 2. involution of the dorsal aortae on the right and left sides between aortic arches 3 and 4, this segment of the dorsal aorta being known as the ductus caroticus (*carotid ductus,* Latin); compare diagram 12 (see Fig. 2.51), in which these normal interruptions have not occurred, with diagram 13, in which these normal interruptions have occurred;

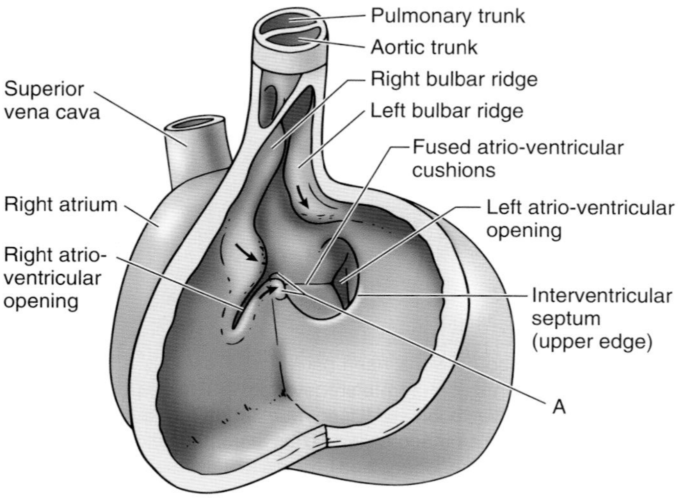

Fig. 2.45 Diagram of a 12 mm human embryo as seen from the front (ventral view), estimated age 35 days, horizon 17. Note that the superior and inferior endocardial cushions have fused, dividing the common atrioventricular canal into mitral and tricuspid valves. The right and left conal (bulbar) ridges have fused distally (cephalically), and this process of fusion is progressing inferiorly or caudally. (From Hamilton WJ, Mossman HW. *Human Embryology*. 4th ed. Baltimore: Williams & Wilkins: 1972, with permission.)

3. involution of the right ductus arteriosus (right dorsal sixth arch) (diagram 13, see Fig. 2.51); and
4. involution of the right dorsal aorta, *distal* to the seventh intersegmental artery that is part of the right subclavian artery (diagram 14, see Fig. 2.49).

Which type of aortic arch one has (left or right) depends on which dorsal aorta persists. Normally in humans, the left dorsal aorta persists, whereas in birds (which are feathered reptiles), the right aortic arch normally persists.

If the right dorsal aorta undergoes involution *proximal* to the seventh intersegmental artery (diagram 13, see Fig. 2.51), this results in an **aberrant right subclavian artery** arising as the last brachiocephalic artery with a left aortic arch.

Both fourth aortic arches normally persist: the left fourth arch as part of the left aortic arch and the right fourth arch as part of the right subclavian artery. Which aortic arch is present does *not* depend on which fourth aortic arch persists—this being a common error in the literature but on which dorsal aorta persists.

A left aortic arch passes over the left main stem bronchus. **A right aortic arch** passes over the right main stem bronchus. These are the definitions of a left aortic arch and a right aortic arch, respectively.

At the aortic arch 3, 4, 6 stage, a **fifth aortic arch** is present in about one-third of human embryos (asterisk, diagram 8, see Fig. 2.51).

This summary diagram of Congdon (see Fig. 2.51)—in my judgment the best that has ever been done of the development of the normal human aortic arch system, and certainly the most realistic—is the key to understanding **vascular rings.** **A double aortic arch** is seen in Fig. 2.49, right (Carnegie embryo 940 of Congdon, 14 mm, horizon 18, 36–38 days of

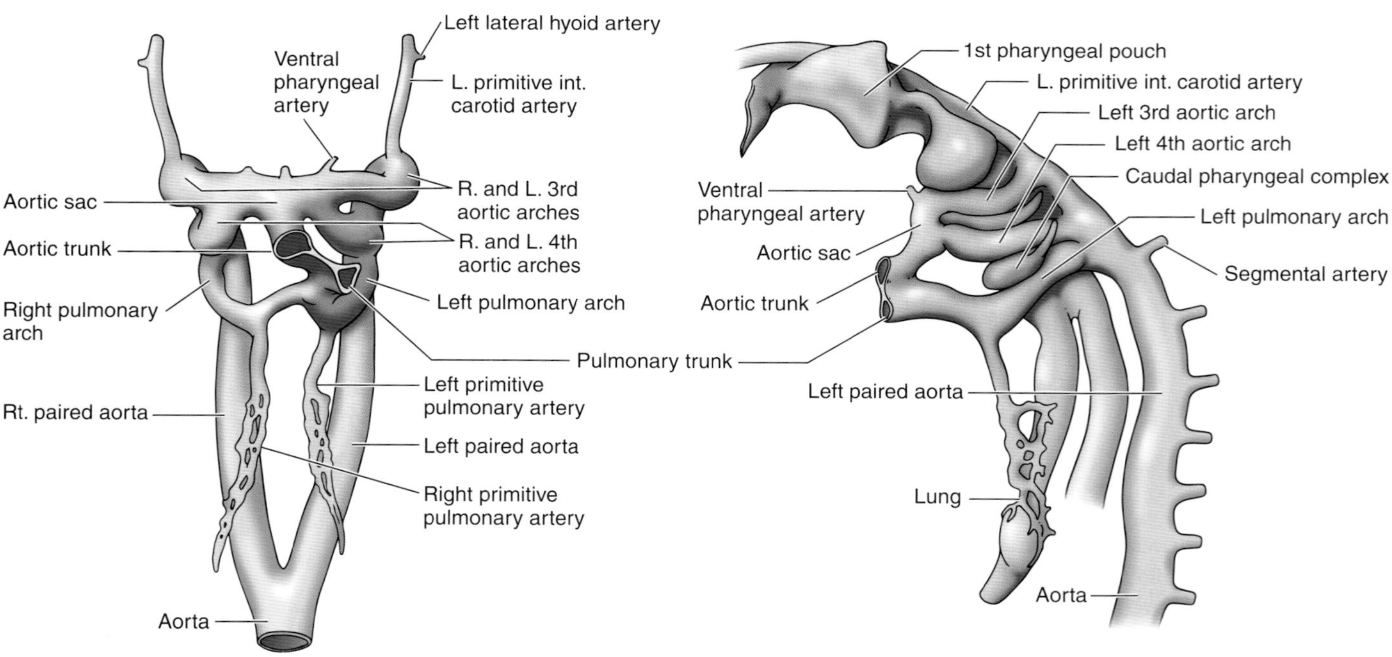

Fig. 2.46 Arterial arches of Carnegie human embryo 1121, 11 mm in length, horizon 17, estimated age 34 to 36 days. This is the aortic arch 3, 4, and 6 stage. Aortic arches 1 and 2 have involuted. Aortic arch 5 is not present. Left panel ventral view, right panel left lateral view. Distal aortopulmonary septation is well seen (left). Both ductus arteriosi (sixth arches) and both dorsal aortae are still intact. (From Congdon ED. Transformation of the aortic-arch system during the development of the human embryo. *Contrib Embryol. Carnegie Inst.* 1922;14:47, with permission.)

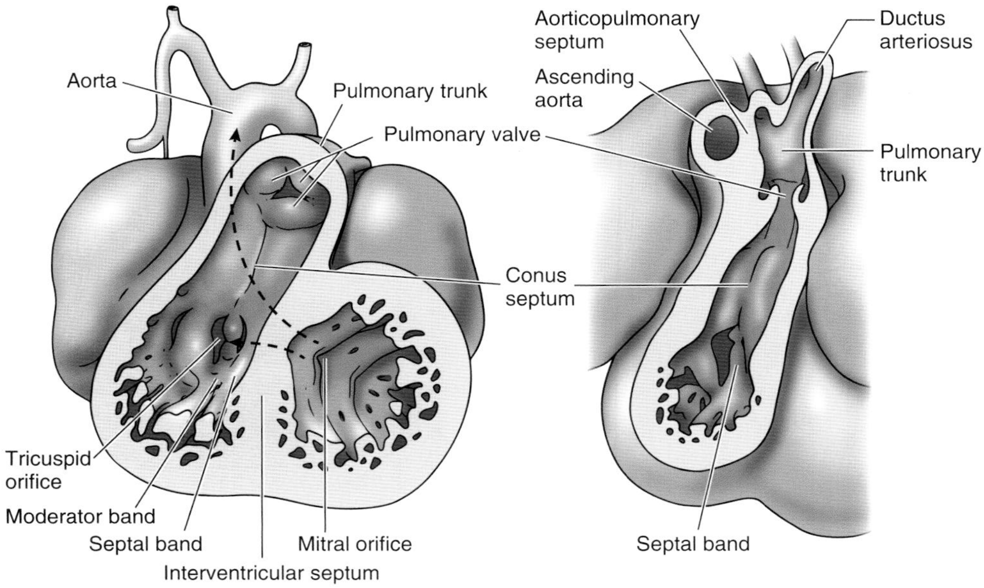

Fig. 2.47 16 mm in length, approximate age 37 days, horizon 18. Note that the aorticopulmonary septum has formed, separating the great arteries. The pulmonary and aortic valves are now also separate. The conal septum is well formed by fusion of the right and left conal ridges. The atrioventricular canal is now separated into mitral and tricuspid orifices. However, the interventricular foramen (potential ventricular septal defect) is still open *(inferior horizontal arrow, left-sided panel)*. (From Frank Netter: The Netter Collection of Medical Illustrations, Volume 5, HEART, 1969, with permission.)

age). Normally, by horizon 20 (40–42 days), the right dorsal aorta has involuted, resulting in a left aortic arch (see Fig. 2.50, right, Carnegie embryo 1390, 18 mm in length).

ABNORMAL MAMMALIAN CARDIOVASCULAR EMBRYOLOGY: THE *IV/IV* MOUSE

Because almost all of the foregoing account is concerned with *normal* human cardiovascular embryology, whereas this book is concerned mainly with *abnormal* human hearts, a brief introduction to the salient features of the *iv/iv* mouse model of congenital heart disease[5-8] is included here (Figs. 2.52–2.62). *iv/iv* means that this mouse model is thought to be homozygous for the situs inversus gene, *iv* being the gene symbol for *inversus*. All of the following scanning electron micrographs (Fig. 2.52–2.62, inclusive) are courtesy of Dr. William M. Layton and his colleagues,[5-8] with whom I had the pleasure and privilege to work.

In Fig. 2.52, note the median fusion furrow that still demarcates the contributions coming from the left and right sides of the cardiogenic crescent.

In Fig. 2.53, a straight tube or preloop heart is seen, without a median fusion furrow.

In Fig. 2.54, an early D-loop is seen. In Fig. 2.55, another early D-loop is seen. The bulbus cordis (future RV) is superior and to the right of the ventricle (future LV). The indentation between the bulbus cordis and the ventricle indicates the site of the future ventricular septum, which is still almost horizontal—as is typical of superoinferior ventricles. Note also the right and left dorsal aortae beneath the neural plate and the septum transversum (embryonic diaphragm) that separates the thorax from the abdomen.

In Fig. 2.56, a normal-looking bulboventricular D-loop is seen, which is convex to the right. The bulbus cordis lies to the right of the ventricle. Hence, it is anticipated that the future morphologically RV (from the bulbus cordis) and the future morphologically LV (from the ventricle) of this D-loop would be solitus or noninverted.

In Fig. 2.58, an abnormal-looking D-loop (convex to the right) is seen. Fig. 2.58 presents another abnormal looking D-loop.

In Fig. 2.59, an L-loop is seen. Note that the greater curvature of the bulboventricular loop is convex to the left.

In Fig. 2.60, another L-loop—convex to the left—is seen. The bulbus cordis (future morphologically RV) lies to the left of the ventricle (future morphologically LV). Hence, bulboventricular L-loop formation is considered to be the developmental basis for **ventricular inversion** or **mirror-image ventricles**. The undivided great artery bifurcates beneath the pharynx. Each arterial arch opens upward into a dorsal aorta on either side of the pharynx.

Another abnormal-appearing D-loop is seen in Fig. 2.61. In Fig. 2.62, there are sketches of normal-appearing (n) D-loops at 9½ days of age and at 10½ days of age in utero (left-sided drawings), compared with abnormal-appearing D-loops (middle and right-sided drawings).

In conclusion, why is an understanding of cardiovascular embryology important? Because it makes possible the understanding of the pathologic anatomy of congenital heart disease, which in turn is the basis of accurate diagnosis and successful management. An understanding of cardiovascular embryology may also provide clues to the etiologies of congenital heart

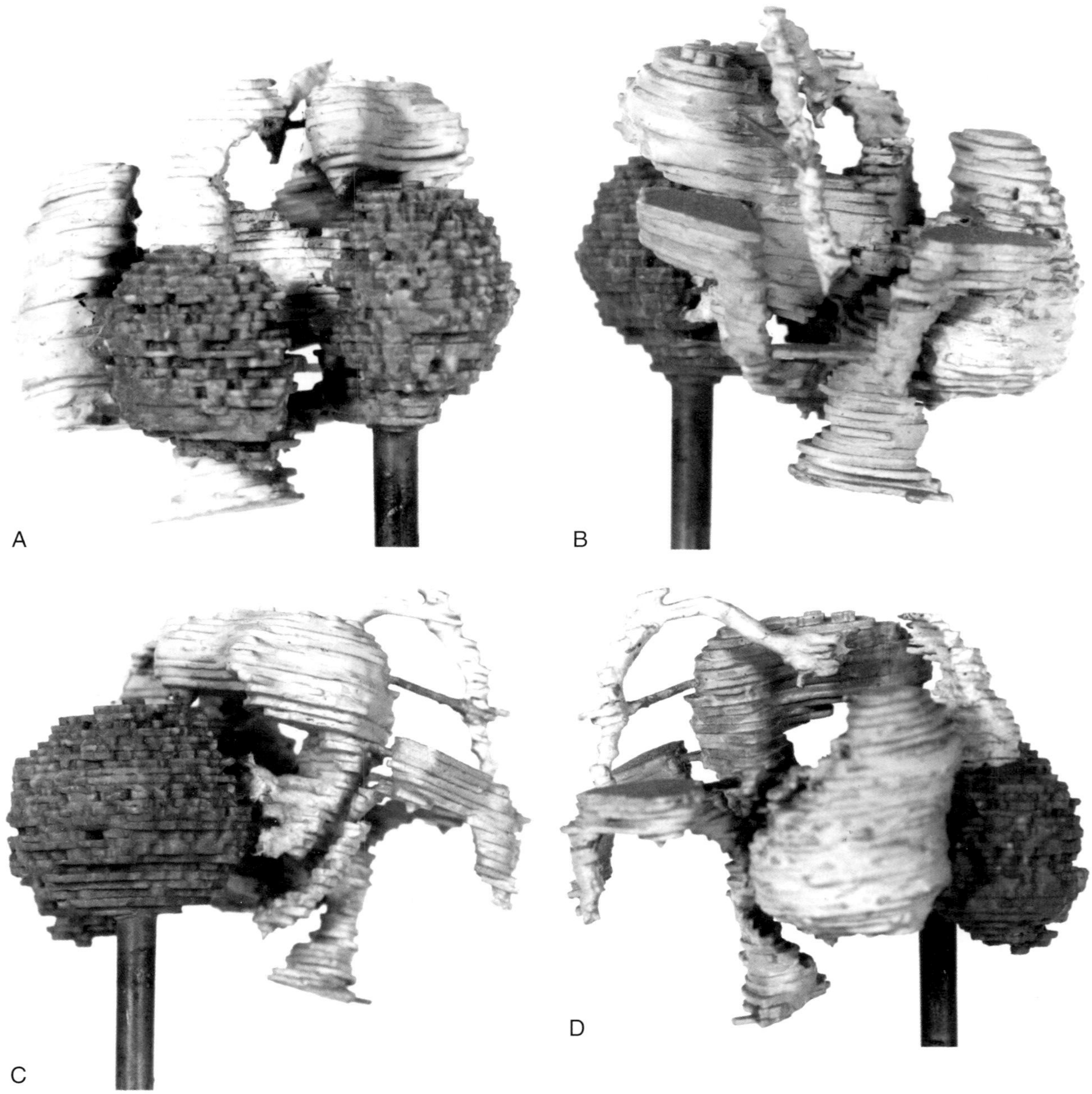

Fig. 2.48 Luminal reconstruction of Carnegie human embryo 6520, 14.2 mm in length, horizon 18, 36 to 38 days of age. A, ventral view; B, dorsal view; C, left lateral view; D, right lateral view. Note that right ventricular growth has now caught up with left ventricular growth. The ventricular septum is the space between the left and right ventricular cavities. The ventricular apex now points leftward, normal levocardia having been achieved by this stage. However, the interventricular foramen (potential ventricular septal defect) is still patent.

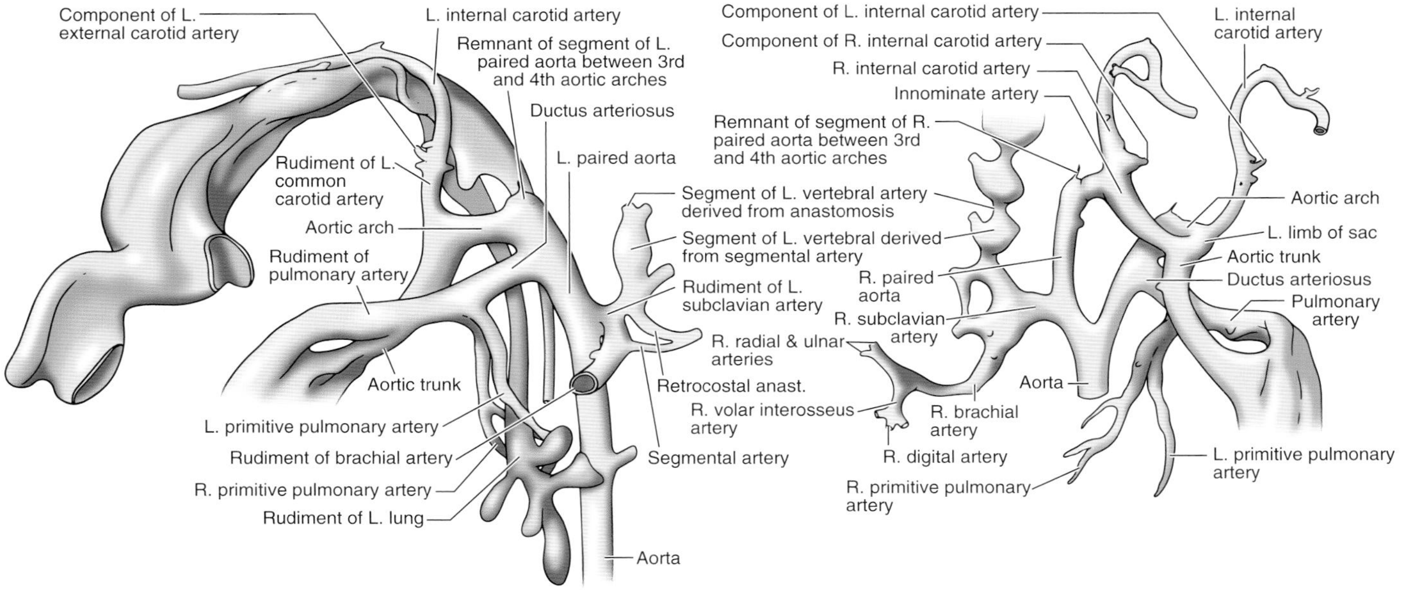

Fig. 2.49 Aortic arch system of Carnegie human embryo 940, 14 mm in length, horizon 18, 36 to 38 days of age. Left lateral view, left panel; right anterior oblique view, right panel. Double aortic arch is still present. Right ductus arteriosus has involuted. Definitive right subclavian artery normally consists of right fourth arch, right dorsal aorta, and seventh intersegmental artery (right panel). Note how the vertebral artery is formed from vertical intersegmental arterial anastomoses (right panel). (From Congdon ED. Transformation of the aortic-arch system during the development of the human embryo. *Contrib Embryol. Carnegie Inst.* 1922;14:47, with permission.)

diseases, which in turn may facilitate prediction and prevention. At the present time, much more remains to be learned.

Literature

In addition to the textbooks on embryology referred to in Chapter 1, there are many fascinating papers that will greatly augment the reader's understanding. These references are cited approximately chronologically in order to make possible a comprehension of the growth of understanding over time.[9-223] These references are by no means all that have appeared but are rather a sampling of papers that I have found helpful.

Embryology of Specific Anomalies

For our best present understanding of the embryology of specific forms of congenital heart disease, please see the anomaly in question.

Recent Etiologic Insights

We are witnessing an explosion in the understanding of the *etiology* (mostly genetic) of normal and abnormal development. For example, a gene called *"nodal"* decides which will be the tail end of a developing individual.[222] If mutated in a certain way, then there is no head. Nodal sets up the spine and determines which will be the left side and which the right side. The role of nodal has been conserved throughout our phylum (Chordata) and has been passed from fish to amphibia to reptiles, birds, and mammals. Nodal decides whether organs will be left sided or right sided.

The heart is considered to be a good example of this, according to Tabin[222]: "In birds and mammals, it initially forms a tube in the middle of the embryo. Then a signal from the protein made by the nodal gene determines which way the tube bends or loops as it develops into a chick's or human's heart.

"If the loop is to the right, the heart will form on the left, as it does in the vast majority of cases. If the tube loops to the left, the heart becomes located on the right side."

Although the foregoing statements are good generalizations, exceptions are not rare. D-loop ventricles may remain right sided, resulting in isolated dextrocardia. L-loop ventricles may remain left sided, as in the classical form of congenitally physiologically corrected transposition of the great arteries. Nonetheless, just as Tabin says, the rule is that D-loop ventricles end up in the left chest pointing leftward (normal levocardia), whereas L-loop ventricles end up in the right chest pointing rightward (dextrocardia, as *in situs inversus totalis*).

Nodal and other genes determine the "handedness" of the stomach and the direction of coiling of the intestine. Tabin[222] says, "Every organ makes an independent decision about its left- or right-handedness. The heart doesn't determine what the stomach or the liver will do; the latter organs respond separately to 'go left' or 'go right' signals." Nodal does not act alone. Many genes switch on and off during development. We are just beginning to understand the genetics of normal and abnormal cardiac morphogenesis; hence the frantic and fascinating revolution through which we are living.

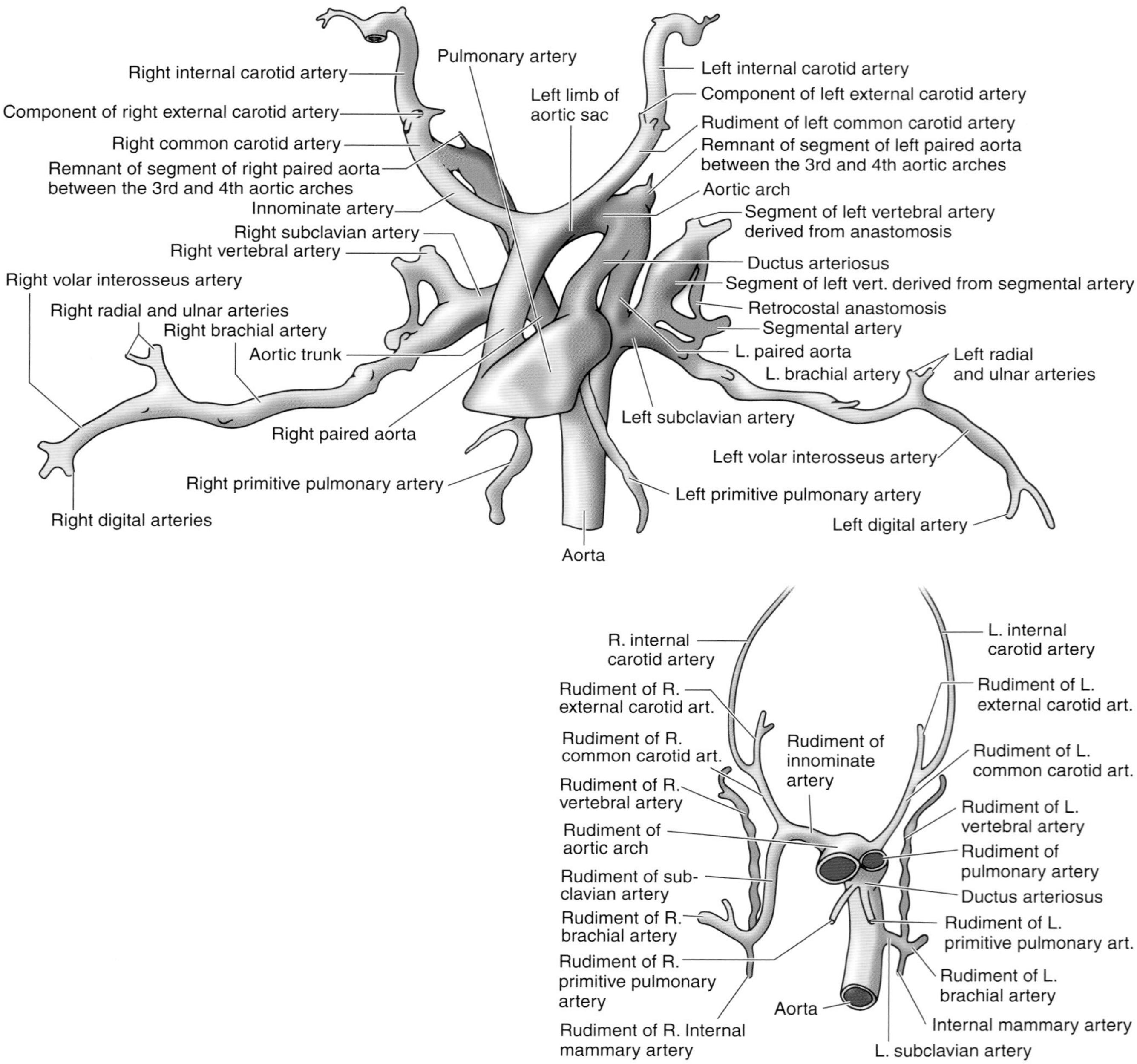

Fig. 2.50 Congdon's Fig. 2.39 (left panel) is Carnegie human embryo 940, 14 mm in length, horizon 18, 36 to 38 days of age. Congdon's Fig. 2.40 (right panel) is Carnegie human embryo 1390, 18 mm in length, horizon 20, estimated age 40 to 42 days. Although a double aortic arch is present in the left panel, it is not seen in the right panel because the right dorsal aorta has undergone normal involution distal to the origin of the right seventh intersegmental artery. Note that the left seventh intersegmental artery (subclavian artery) is also still quite low and has to ascend up to the level of the distal aortic arch. (From Congdon ED. Transformation of the aortic-arch system during the development of the human embryo. *Contrib Embryol. Carnegie Inst.* 1922;14:47, with permission.)

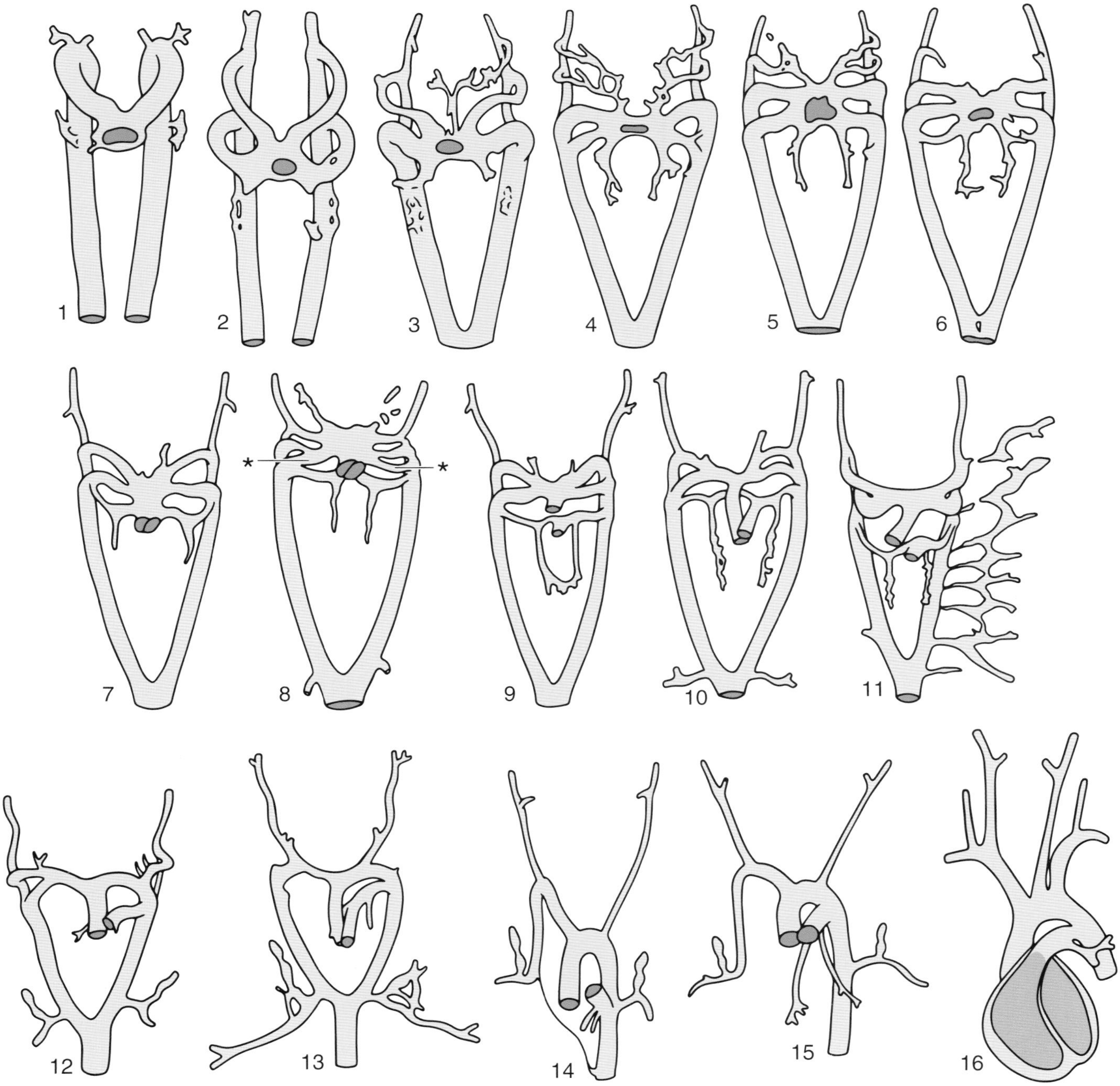

Fig. 2.51 Diagrammatic summary of the evolution of the aortic arches, ventral view. In diagram 8, the asterisks indicate a fifth aortic arch bilaterally. The first of the four normal aortic arch interruptions is involution of the right ductus arteriosus (diagram 12, horizon 17, 34–36 days of age). The second and third normal aortic arch interruptions are noted in diagram 13, horizon 18, 36 to 38 days of age, namely, the involution of the ductus caroticus bilaterally, that is, the dorsal aorta between aortic arches 3 that head cephalically and aortic arches 4 that head caudally. The last of the normal interruptions of the aortic arch system is shown in diagram 14, horizon 18 (late) or 19 (early), 38 to 39 days of age, namely, the involution of the right dorsal aorta distal to the right seventh intersegmental artery, which determines the normal presence of a left aortic arch. (From Congdon ED. Transformation of the aortic-arch system during the development of the human embryo. *Contrib Embryol. Carnegie Inst.* 1922;14:47, with permission.)

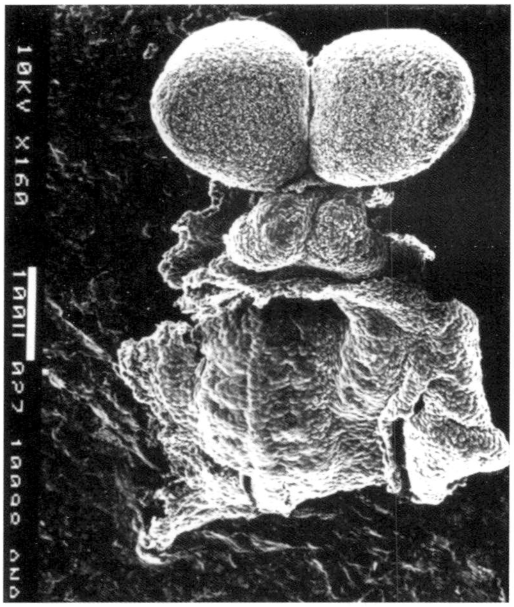

Fig. 2.52 8½-day-old *iv/iv* mouse embryo, low power scanning electron microscopy, ventral view, with the pericardium removed. The heart lies between the developing fore-brain above and the septum transversum (embryonic diaphragm) and the anterior intestinal portal below. The left-sided and right-sided heart rudiments have fused, but one can still see the line of fusion between the left-sided and right-sided primordia. (From Layton, WM, Manasek FJ. Cardiac looping in early *iv/iv* mouse embryos. In Van Praagh R, Takao A, eds. *Etiology and Morphogenesis of Congenital Heart Disease.* Mt Kisco, NY: Futura Publishing Co.; 1980:109, with permission.)

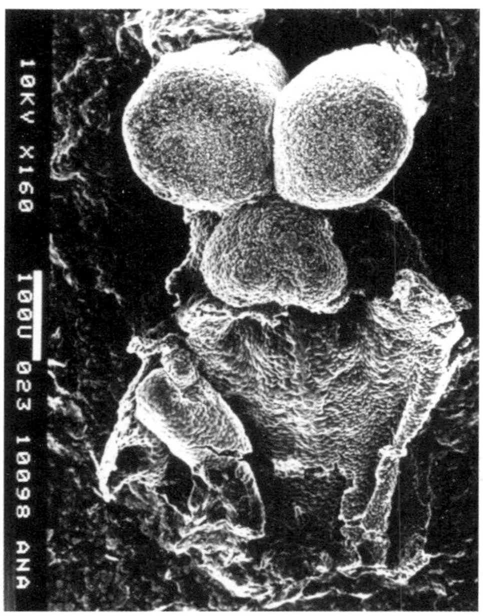

Fig. 2.53 As the heart enlarges, the fusion line disappears. This is the straight tube or preloop phase. (From Layton, WM, Manasek FJ. Cardiac looping in early *iv/iv* mouse embryos. In Van Praagh R, Takao A, eds. *Etiology and Morphogenesis of Congenital Heart Disease.* Mt Kisco, NY: Futura Publishing Co.; 1980:109, with permission.)

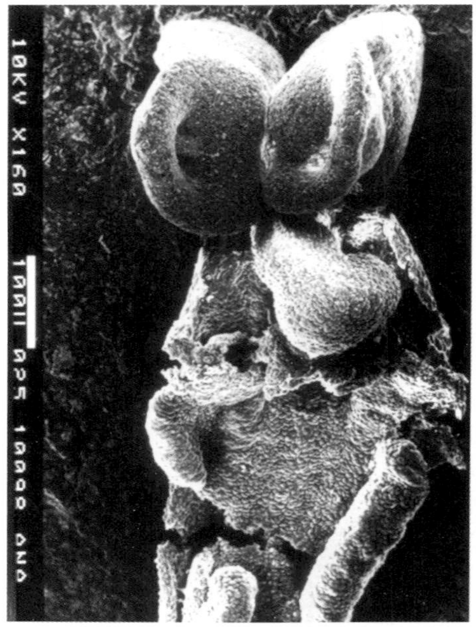

Fig. 2.54 The early D-loop phase. The heart has elongated, and the left ventricular bulge has appeared. (From Layton, WM, Manasek FJ. Cardiac looping in early *iv/iv* mouse embryos. In Van Praagh R, Takao A, eds. *Etiology and Morphogenesis of Congenital Heart Disease.* Mt Kisco, NY: Futura Publishing Co.; 1980:109, with permission.)

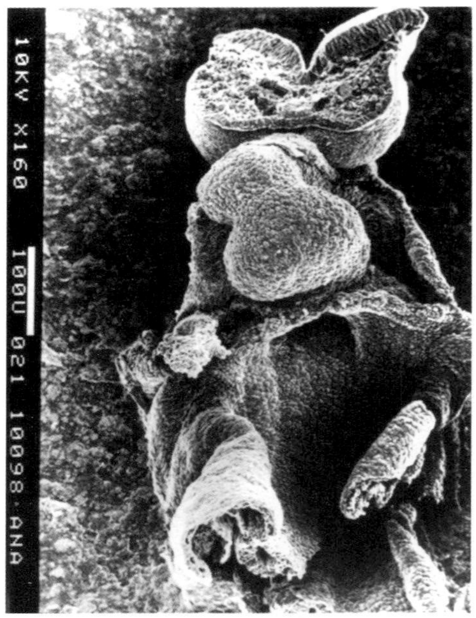

Fig. 2.55 The heart of this *iv/iv* mouse embryo displays a slight but definite dextral convex curvature, that is, very early D-loop formation. The bulbus cordis (future right ventricle) is superior to the ventricle (future left ventricle), and the future interventricular septal region is almost horizontal. This stage is very similar to superoinferior ventricles in which the right ventricle is superior, the left ventricle inferior, and the ventricular septum approximately horizontal. (From Layton, WM, Manasek FJ. Cardiac looping in early *iv/iv* mouse embryos. In Van Praagh R, Takao A, eds. *Etiology and Morphogenesis of Congenital Heart Disease.* Mt Kisco, NY: Futura Publishing Co.; 1980:109, with permission.)

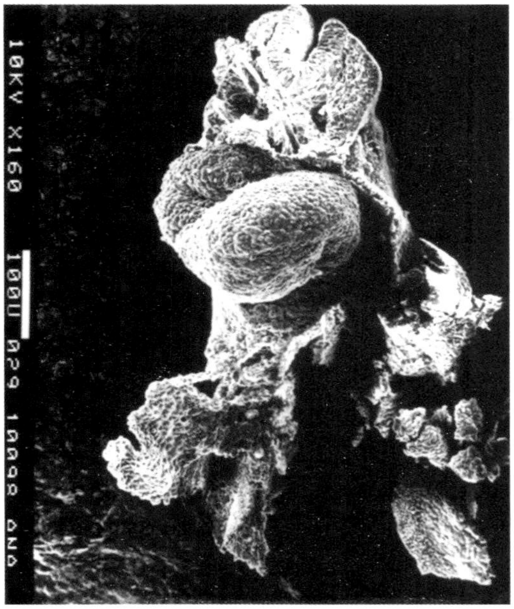

Fig. 2.56 D-loop formation has been achieved, the bulboventricular loop being convex to the right. The left and right dorsal aortae can be seen above the heart loop and the brain is in the process of becoming a tubular structure. (From Layton, WM, Manasek FJ. Cardiac looping in early *iv/iv* mouse embryos. In Van Praagh R, Takao A, eds. *Etiology and Morphogenesis of Congenital Heart Disease*. Mt Kisco, NY: Futura Publishing Co.; 1980:109, with permission.)

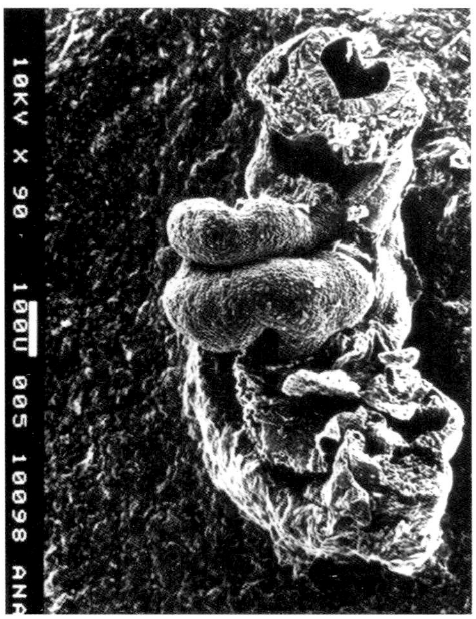

Fig. 2.57 Distorted D-loop of *iv/iv* mouse embryo at 9½ days of age. The bulbus cordis (future right ventricle) is superior and the ventricle (future left ventricle) is inferior. (From Layton, WM, Manasek FJ. Cardiac looping in early *iv/iv* mouse embryos. In Van Praagh R, Takao A, eds. *Etiology and Morphogenesis of Congenital Heart Disease*. Mt Kisco, NY: Futura Publishing Co.; 1980:109, with permission.)

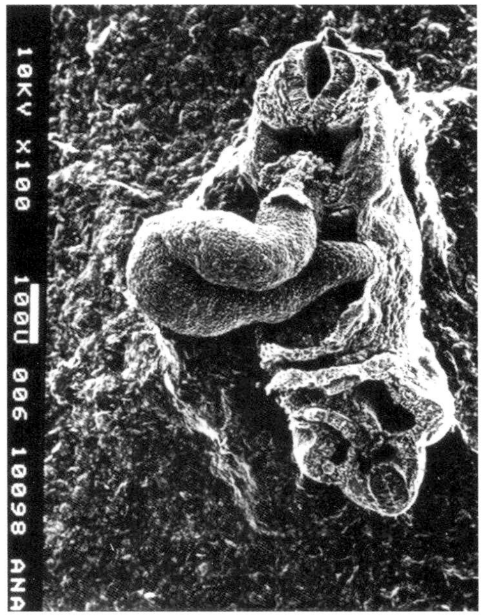

Fig. 2.58 Another distorted ventricular D-loop in an *iv/iv* mouse embryo. (From Layton, WM, Manasek FJ. Cardiac looping in early *iv/iv* mouse embryos. In Van Praagh R, Takao A, eds. *Etiology and Morphogenesis of Congenital Heart Disease*. Mt Kisco, NY: Futura Publishing Co.; 1980:109, with permission.)

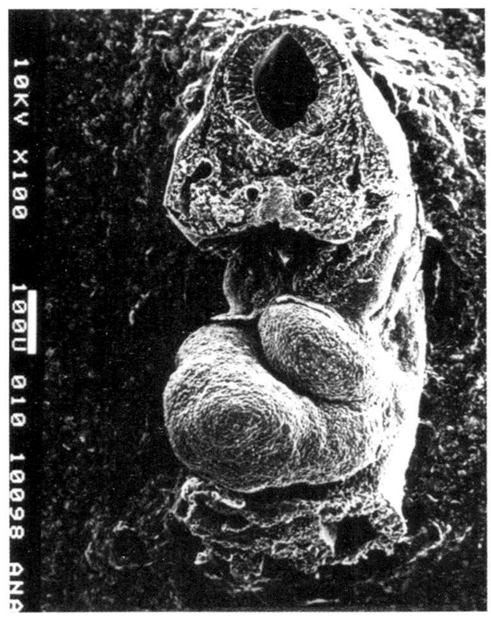

Fig. 2.59 Ventral view of a ventricular L-loop in an *iv/iv* mouse embryo. Note that the bulboventricular loop is convex to the left but otherwise appears unremarkable, that is, an ordinary-appearing L-loop (Theiler stage 14). (From Layton, WM, Manasek FJ. Cardiac looping in early *iv/iv* mouse embryos. In Van Praagh R, Takao A, eds. *Etiology and Morphogenesis of Congenital Heart Disease*. Mt Kisco, NY: Futura Publishing Co.; 1980:109, with permission.)

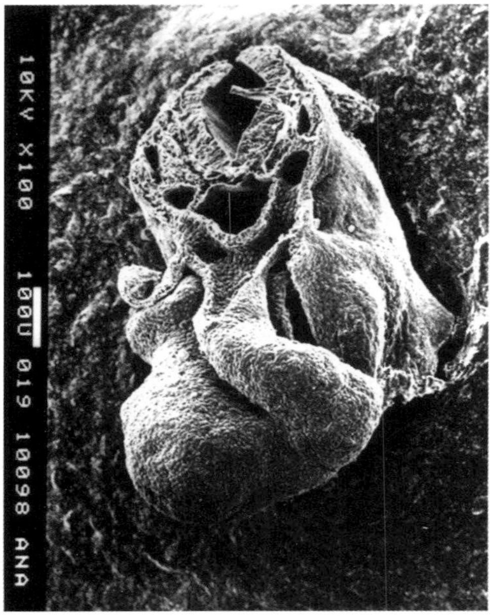

Fig. 2.60 Ventral view of an L-loop in an *iv/iv* mouse embryo, Stage 15. Again, this is an ordinary appearing L-loop. Note the left and right aortic arches that are ascending on either side of the pharynx to join the right and left dorsal aortae. (From Layton, WM, Manasek FJ. Cardiac looping in early *iv/iv* mouse embryos. In Van Praagh R, Takao A, eds. *Etiology and Morphogenesis of Congenital Heart Disease.* Mt Kisco, NY: Futura Publishing Co.; 1980:109, with permission.)

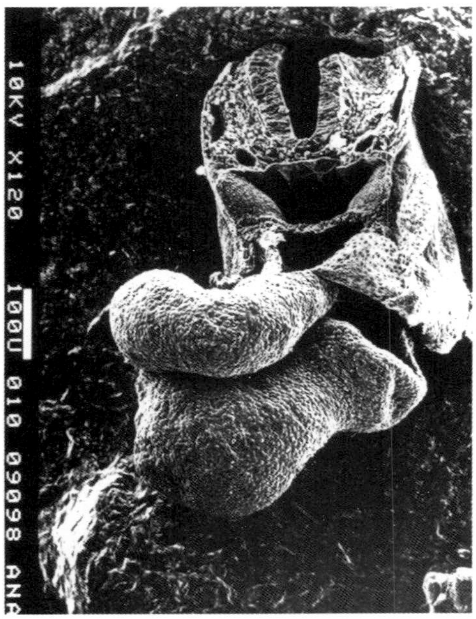

Fig. 2.61 Ventral view of a ventricular D-loop in an *iv/iv* mouse in stage 15. This D-loop is somewhat atypical in appearance. (From Layton, WM, Manasek FJ. Cardiac looping in early *iv/iv* mouse embryos. In Van Praagh R, Takao A, eds. *Etiology and Morphogenesis of Congenital Heart Disease.* Mt Kisco, NY: Futura Publishing Co.; 1980:109, with permission.)

The molecular genetic revolution involves all organ systems. For example, a protein made by the *sonic hedgehog gene* (named after a computer game) forms the bones that make up the trunk.[222] Sonic also shapes the brain and the spinal cord.

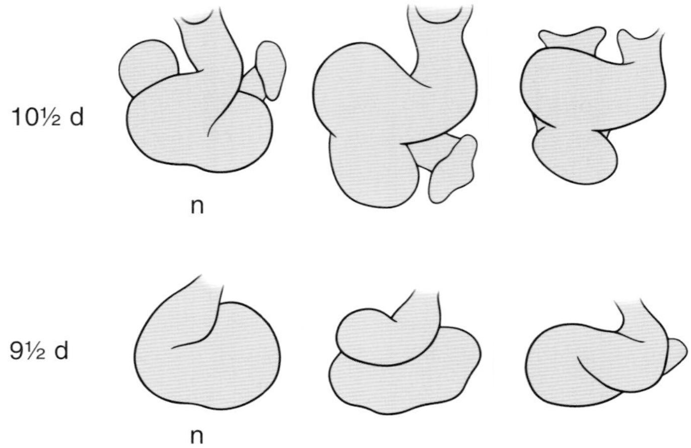

Fig. 2.62 Outline drawings of cardiac loops of 9½ day (bottom row) and 10½ day (top row) *iv/iv* mouse embryos. The loops at the left, labeled *n*, are normal in appearance. The others show the typical loop distortion found in some of the *iv/iv* embryos. (From Layton, WM, Manasek FJ. Cardiac looping in early *iv/iv* mouse embryos. In Van Praagh R, Takao A, eds. *Etiology and Morphogenesis of Congenital Heart Disease.* Mt Kisco, NY: Futura Publishing Co.; 1980:109, with permission.)

The sonic hedgehog gene is known to turn on the nodal gene in birds.

Amid the enthusiasm of discovery, a word of caution is in order: These are early days. Much more work needs to be done before the etiology of the many forms of congenital heart disease will be established with certainty.

Nonetheless, the current enthusiasm appears entirely justified. For example, concerning Layton's *iv/iv mouse model*[5-7] that my colleagues and I helped to describe and interpret,[3-8] it is now known that the *iv/iv* mouse (thought to be homozygous for the *i*nversus *v*iscerum gene, hence *iv*) has a mutation of an axonemal dynein gene.[223] Allelic mouse mutations *iv* and legless (*lgl*) both have left–right inversion (*situs inversus*) in half of liveborn homozygotes. The inference is that the *iv* gene product determines correct left–right anatomic organization (*situs solitus*), and that in the absence of the *iv* gene product, the pattern of visceral anatomic organization develops at random: phenotypically, the pattern of anatomic organization may be normal (*situs solitus*), a mirror image of normal (*situs inversus*), or ambiguous (*situs ambiguus*).

At the molecular level, the normally asymmetrical patterns of expression of *nodal* and *lefty* are randomized in *iv* mutant embryos, suggesting that the *iv* gene functions early in the genetic program of left–right organization.[224] *Left/right-dynein (lrd)*, an axonemal dynein heavy chain gene, is defective in both the *iv* and *lgl* mutations. *lrd* encodes a 14 to 16 kilobase (kb) message.

Analysis of a 7 kb coding sequence revealed 67% identity and 81% similarity to sea urchin axonemal dynein b heavy chain gene, compared with only 31% identity and 54% similarity to rat cytoplasmic dynein heavy chain gene.[223] Does this surprising finding suggest genetic phylogenetic regression in the *iv* mouse mutant, with greater similarity to sea urchins than to rats?

The *lrd* gene is known to be tightly linked to *iv* and is deleted in *lgl*. Supp and her colleagues[223] identified a missense mutation in *lrd* resulting in glutamic acid to lysine substitution. This glutamic acid residue is conserved in every known dynein heavy chain sequence. *lrd* mRNA is found in oocytes, one-cell embryos, two-cell embryos, and in blastocysts, prior to the expression of *nodal* and *lefty*. Hence, an axonemal dynein is believed to play a role in determining left–right asymmetry.[223]

Another example of the importance of molecular genetics to the understanding of the etiology of congenital heart disease is provided by the following recent discovery. Axial patterning and lateral asymmetry both are controlled by a signaling pathway mediated by type IIB activin receptors.[224] For this to be understood, one needs to appreciate that vertebrate animals exhibit both asymmetrical segmented axial skeletons (the vertebral column), and asymmetrical lateral (right–left) visceral patterning. The segmental identity of individual vertebrae is believed to be determined by the *Hox genes* that have defined expression boundaries along the cephalocaudal axis, known as the axial Hox code. Disturbance of the Hox code by ectopic expression or mutation of Hox genes often leads to transformation of the vertebrae. It has recently been shown by Oh and Li[224] that disruption of the type IIB activin receptor by gene targeting ("knockout") leads to altered expression of multiple Hox genes, resulting in abnormal vertebral patterns. Although these knockout mice without activin receptor IIB (Act R $IIB^{-/-}$) live up to and through birth, they die shortly thereafter because of the coexistence of complex congenital heart disease characterized by randomized heart position, malposition of the great arteries (similar to human transposition of the great arteries and double-outlet RV), and visceral heterotaxy with asplenia.

It should be recalled that the *iv/iv* mouse model[5-8] is really a model of visceral heterotaxy, with many homozygotes having the heterotaxy syndrome with polysplenia, some having visceral heterotaxy with asplenia (about 5%), and others phenotypically having situs inversus viscerum (hence the gene symbol *iv*).

Although the *iv* mouse model displays disturbance of lateral asymmetry only, the disrupted type IIB activin receptor model[224] displays disruption of both asymmetries: axial (cephalocaudal) and lateral (right–left).

Activins are members of the transforming growth factor-β (TGF-β) superfamily that exert a diverse range of biological effects on cell growth and differentiation.[225]

Recent investigations using both transgenic and knockout mice have identified more than 20 genes that are essential for normal cardiogenesis.[226,227]

As these words are being written, we are about to begin what might be called "the human *iv/iv* gene project." We hope to be able to isolate DNA from formalin-fixed heart specimens, amplify the DNA by polymerase chain reaction, and sequence various promising candidate genes in an effort to discover the etiology of various types of human congenital heart disease. Congenital heart collections, such as that in the Cardiac Registry of Children's Hospital in Boston, appear to be largely unrecognized and entirely untapped "gold mines" of genetic information.

REFERENCES

1. Streeter GL. Development horizons in human embryos. Description of Age Group XI, 13-20 Somites, and Age Group XII, 21-29 Somites. *Contrib Embryol Carnegie Inst Washington.* 1942;30:211.
2. Van Praagh R, Takao A, eds. *Etiology and Morphogenesis of Congenital Heart Disease.* Mt Kisco, NY: Futura Publishing Co; 1980.
3. Congdon ED. Transformation of the aortic-arch system during the development of the human embryo. *Contrib Embryol Carnegie Inst Washington.* 1922;14:47.
4. Asami I. Partitioning of the arterial end of the embryonic heart. In: Van Praagh R, Takao A, eds. *Etiology and Morphogenesis of Congenital Heart Disease.* Mt Kisco, NY: Futura Publishing Co; 1980:51.
5. Layton WM. Random determination of a developmental process. Reversal of normal visceral asymmetry in the mouse. *J Hered.* 1976;67:336.
6. Layton WM. Heart malformations in mice homozygous for a gene causing situs inversus. In: Bergsma D, ed. *Abnormal Cardiac Morphogenesis: Birth Defects, Original Article Series.* Vol 14. New York: Alan R Liss, Inc; 1978:277.
7. Layton WM, Manasek FJ. Cardiac looping in early *iv/iv* mouse embryos. In: Van Praagh R, Takao A, eds. *Etiology and Morphogenesis of Congenital Heart Disease.* Mt Kisco, NY: Futura Publishing Co; 1980:109.
8. Van Praagh R, Layton WM, Van Praagh S. The morphogenesis of normal and abnormal relationships between the great arteries and the ventricles: pathologic and experimental data. In: Van Praagh R, Takao A, eds. *Etiology and Morphogenesis of Congenital Heart Disease.* Mt Kisco, NY: Futura Publishing Co; 1980:271.
9. Rose C. Beiträge zur vergleichenden Anatomie des Herzens der Wirbelthiere. *Morphol Jahrb.* 1890;16:27.
10. Buxton BH. Photographs of the series of sections of an early human embryo. *J Anat Physiol.* 1899;33:381.
11. Cunningham DJ. The significance of anatomical variations. *J Anat Physiol.* 1899;33:1.
12. Flint JM. Development of the lungs. *Am J Anat.* 1906;6:1–1907.
13. Tandler J. The development of the heart. In: Keibel F, Mall FP, eds. *Manual of Human Embryology.* Vol 2. Philadelphia and London: JB Lippincott Co; 1912:534.
14. Mall FP. On the development of the human heart. *Am J Anat.* 1912;13:249.
15. Robertson JI. Development of the heart and vascular system of lepidosiren paradoxa. *Quart J Microsc Sci.* 1913;59:53.
16. Brown AJ. The development of the pulmonary vein in the domestic cat. *Anat Rec.* 1913;7:299.
17. Parker KM. The early development of the heart and anterior vessels in marsupials, with special reference to Permales. *Proc Zool Soc.* 1915:459. London.
18. Squier TL. On the development of the pulmonary circulation in the chick. *Anat Rec.* 1915-16;10:425.
19. Schulte VW. The fusion of the cardiac anlages and the formation of the cardiac loop in the cat (*felis domestica*). *Am J Anat.* 1916;20:45.
20. Frazer JE. The formation of the pars membranacea septi. *J Anat.* 1916;51:19.
21. Wang CC. The earliest stages the of development of the blood vessels and of the heart in ferret embryos. *J Anat.* 1917–1918;52:107.
22. Waterston D. The development of the heart in man. *Trans R Soc Edinburgh.* 1917–1921;52, part 2:42.

23. Murray HA. Development of the cardiac loop in the rabbit, with special reference to the bulboventricular groove and origin of the interventricular septum. *Am J Anat.* 1919;26:29.
24. Morrill CV. Symmetry reversal and mirror-imaging in monstrous trout and a comparison with similar conditions in human double monsters. *Anat Rec.* 1919;16:265.
25. Huntington GS. The morphology of the pulmonary artery in the mammalia. *Anat Rec.* 1919–1920;17:165.
26. O'Donoghue CH. The blood vascular system of the Tuatara, Sphenodon punctatus. *Phil Trans Roy Soc London.* 1920–1921;210 (B):175.
27. Yoshinaga T. A contribution to the early development of the heart in mammalia, with special reference to the Guinea pig. *Anat Rec.* 1921;21:239.
28. Swett FH. Situs inversus viscerum in double trout. *Anat Rec.* 1921;22:183.
29. Buell CE. Origin of the pulmonary vessels in the chick. *Contrib Embryol Carnegie Inst Washington.* 1922;14:13.
30. Congdon ED. Transformation of the aortic-arch system during the development of the human embryo. *Contrib Embryol Carnegie Inst Washington.* 1922;14:47.
31. Patten BM. The formation of the cardiac loop in the chick. *Am J Anat.* 1922;30:373.
32. Takahashi S. Notes on the formation of the cardiac septa in the chick. *J Anat (London).* 1923;57:168.
33. Watson KM. The origin of the heart and blood vessels in *felis domestica. J Anat (London).* 1924;58:105.
34. Johnstone PN. Studies on the physiologic anatomy of the embryonic heart. II. An inquiry into the development of the heartbeat in chick embryos, including development of irritability to electrical stimulation. *Johns Hopkins Hosp Bull.* 1925;36:299.
35. Copenhaver WM. Experiments on the development of the heart of *amblystoma punctatum. J Exp Zool.* 1926;43:321.
36. Davis CL. Development of the human heart from its first appearance to the stage found in embryos of 20 paired somites. *Contrib Embryol Carnegie Inst Washington.* 1927;19:245.
37. Streeter GL. Development of the mesoblast and notochord in pig embryos. *Contrib Embryol Carnegie Inst Washington.* 1927;19:73.
38. Bremer JL. Part II. The left aorta of reptiles. *Am J Anat.* 1928;42:338.
39. M'Intyre D. The development of the vascular system in the human embryo prior to the establishment of the heart. *Trans Roy Soc Edinburgh.* 1926-1928;55:77.
40. O'Donoghue CH, Abbott EB. The blood vascular system of the spiny dogfish, squalus acanthias linné, and squalus sucklii gill. *Trans Roy Soc Edinburgh.* 1928;55:823.
41. Girgis A. The development of the heart in the rabbit. *Proc Zool Soc.* 1930; part 2:755.
42. Patten BM, Kramer TC. The initiation of contraction in the embryonic chick heart. *Am J Anat.* 1933;53:349.
43. Llorca FO. Quelques remarques à propros du développement des artères pulmonaires chez l'embryon humain. *Ann d'anat path.* 1933;10:935.
44. Girgis A: A further contribution on the development of the heart in the rabbit. *Proc Zool Soc London.*1933;421.
45. Goss CM. Double hearts produced experimentally in rat embryos. *J Exp Zool.* 1935;72:33.
46. Davies F, MacConaill MA. Cor biloculare, with a note on the development of the pulmonary veins. *J Anat.* 1937;71:437.
47. Goss CM. The first contractions of the heart in rat embryos. *Anat Rec.* 1937-1938;70:505.
48. Odgers PNB. The development of the pars membranacea septi in the human heart. *J Anat (London).* 1938;72:247.
49. Copenhaver WM. Initiation of beat and intrinsic contraction rates in the different parts of the Amblystoma heart. *J Exp Zool.* 1939;80:193.
50. Odgers PNB. The development of the atrio-ventricular valves in man. *J Anat (London).* 1939;73:643.
51. Dwinnell LA. Physiological contraction of double hearts in rabbit embryos. *Proc Soc Exp Biol & Med.* 1939;42:264.
52. Kramer TC. The partitioning of the truncus and conus and the formation of the membranous portion of the interventricular septum in the human heart. *Am J Anat.* 1942;71:343.
53. Barry A. The intrinsic pulsation rates of fragments of the embryonic chick heart. *J Exp Zool.* 1942;91:119.
54. Bacon RL. Self-differentiation and induction in the heart of Amblystoma. *J Exp Zool.* 1945;98:87.
55. Field EJ. Early development of the sheep heart. *J Anat.* 1946;80:75.
56. Arey LB. *Developmental Anatomy, a Textbook and Laboratory Manual of Embryology.* 5th ed. Philadelphia and London: WB Saunders Co; 1946:55.
57. Auër J. The development of the human pulmonary vein and its major variations. *Anat Rec.* 1948;101:581.
58. Streeter GL. Developmental Horizons in Human Embryos. Description of Age Groups XV, XVI, XVII, and XVIII. Vol. 32. Washington: Contrib Embryol Carnegie Inst; 1948:133.
59. Keith A. *Human Embryology and Morphology.* 6th ed. Baltimore: Williams & Wilkins Co; 1948:427.
60. Butler H. Some derivatives of the foregut venous plexus of the albino rat, with reference to man. *J Anat.* 1952;86:95.
61. Butler JK. *An Experimental Analysis of Cardiac Loop Formation in the Chick. Thesis Presented to the Faculty of the Graduate School of the University of Texas in Partial Fulfillment of the Requirements for the Degree of Master of Arts.* Vol. 31. University of Texas; 1952. August.
62. Hamilton WJ, Boyd JD, Mossman HW. *Human Embryology.* Baltimore: Williams & Wilkins Co; 1952:71.
63. Goss CM. Development of the median coordinated ventricle from the lateral hearts in rat embryos with 3 to 6 somites. *Anat Rec.* 1952;112:761.
64. Sangvichien S. Experimental reversal of the heartbeat in chick embryos. *Anat Rec.* 1952;112:529.
65. Licata RH. The human embryonic heart in the ninth week. *Am J Anat.* 1954;94:73.
66. Wilens S. The migration of heart mesoderm and associated areas in *Amblystoma Punctatum. J Exp Zool.* 1955;129:579.
67. Foxon GEH. Problems of the double circulation in vertebrates. *Biol Rev.* 1955;30:196.
68. Neill CA. Development of the pulmonary veins with reference to the embryology of anomalies of pulmonary venous return. *Pediatrics.* 1956;18:880.
69. Los JA. *De embryonale ontwikkeling van de venae pulmonales en de sinus coronarius bij de mens (the development of the pulmonary veins and the coronary sinus in the human embryo).* Leiden: Luctor et Emergo; 1958 (thesis).
70. Willis RA. The growth of young embryos transplanted whole into the brain in rats. *J Pathol Bacteriol.* 1958;76:337.
71. DeHaan RL. Cardia bifida and the development of pacemaker function in the early chick heart. *Devel Biol.* 1959;1:586.
72. Mulherkar L. The effects of trypan blue on chick embryos cultured in vitro. *J Embryol Exp Morph.* 1960;8:1.

73. Silver PHS. Special problems of experimenting *in* ovo on the early chick embryo, and a solution. *J Embryol Exp Morph.* 1960;8:369.
74. McKenzie J, Ebert JD. The inhibitory action of antimycin A in the early chick embryo. *J Embryol Exp Morph.* 1960;8:314.
75. Rychter Z, Lemez L. The vascular system of the chick embryo. VIII. On the relation of the experimentally produced left archus aortae to the right ventricle. *Csl Morfol.* 1961;1:55.
76. Rychter Z. The vascular system of the chick embryo. IX. Experimental occlusion of 4 and 5 aortic arches on the fourth embryonic day. *Csl Morfol.* 1961;9:69.
77. Rychter Z. The vascular system of the chick embryo. X. Experimental occlusion of 2 and 3 aortic arches on the fourth embryonic day. *Csl Morfol.* 1961;9:294.
78. Rychter Z, Lemez L. The vascular system of the chick embryo. XI. Experimental aortic coarctation as influenced by occlusion of some aortic arches. *Csl Morfol.* 1961;9:311.
79. Yamada T. A chemical approach to the problem of the organizer. *Advances in Morphogenesis.* Vol. 1. New York and London: Academic Press; 1961:1.
80. DeHaan RL. Differentiation of the atrioventricular conducting system of the heart. *Circulation.* 1961;24(2):458.
81. Snellen HA, Dankmeijer J, Dekker A, van Ingen HC, Loss JA, Wielanga J. *Embryonic development and congenital cardiovascular anomalies. Memorias del IV Congresso Mundial de Cardiologia.* Vols. 1-A. Mexico: *Impresora Galve SA*; 1962:132.
82. DeHaan RL. Organization of the cardiogenic plate in the early chick embryo. *Acta Embryol Morphol Exper.* 1963;6:26.
83. Baron MG, Wolf BS, Steinfeld L, Van Mierop LHS. Endocardial cushion defects. Specific diagnosis by angiocardiography. *Am J Cardiol.* 1964;13:162.
84. Pankey GA, Mogabgab WJ. Contracting chick embryo heart cells in tissue culture. Effect of viruses and other agents. *Am Heart J.* 1965;70:94.
85. DeHaan RL. Morphogenesis of the vertebrate heart. In: DeHaan HL, Ursprung H, eds. *Organogenesis.* New York: Holt, Rinehart, and Winston; 1965:377.
86. Rosenquist GC. A radioautographic study of labeled grafts in the chick blastoderm. Development from primitive-streak stages to stage 12. *Contrib Embryol Carnegie Inst, Washington.* 1966,38:71.
87. De la Cruz MV, Campillo-Sainz C, Munoz-Armas S. Congenital heart defects in chick embryos subjected to temperature variations. *Circ Res.* 1966;18:257.
88. Kleinfeld M, Schade O, Gruen F. Effects of digitoxin and isoproterenol on the rhythmicity and contractility of cultured chick heart cells. *Circulation.* 1966;34(suppl III):146.
89. Van Mierop LHS, Bertuch CJ. Development of arterial blood pressure in the chick embryo. *Am J Physiol.* 1967;212:43.
90. DeHaan RL. Regulation of spontaneous activity in growth of embryonic chick heart cells in tissue culture. *Develop Biol.* 1967;16:216.
91. Jaffee OC. The development of the arterial outflow tract in the chick embryo heart. *Anat Rec.* 1967;158:35.
92. Marcarian HQ, Smith RD, Barton J, Jenkins TW. A rapid method for studying vascular patterns three-dimensionally and histologically. *Am Heart J.* 1967;74:219.
93. Jensh RP, Brent RL. An analysis of the growth retarding effects of trypan blue in the albino rats. *Anat Rec.* 1967;159:453.
94. Okamoto N, Ikeda T, Satow Y, Sawasaki M, Inoue A. Effects of fast neutron irradiation on the developing rat embryo. *Hiroshima J Med Sci.* 1968;17:169.
95. Okamoto N. Morphology and classification of the cardiovascular anomalies induced by 14.1 MeV neutron irradiation. *Proc Research Inst Nuclear Med Biol.* 1968;9:25.
96. Nora JJ, Sommerville RJ, Fraser FC. Homologies for congenital heart disease: murine models, influenced by dextroamphetamine. *Teratology.* 1968;1:413.
97. Nishimura H, Takano K, Tanimura T, Yasuda M. Normal and abnormal development of human embryos: first report of the analysis of 1,213 intact embryos. *Teratology.* 1968;1:281.
98. DeHaan RL, Gottlieb SH. The electrical activity of embryonic chick heart cells isolated in tissue culture singly or in interconnected cell sheets. *J Gen Physiol.* 1968;52:643.
99. Shepard TH, Tanimura T, Robkin M. In vitro study of rat embryos. I. Effects of decreased oxygen on embryonic heart rate. *Teratology.* 1969;2:107.
100. Berns MW. Reconstruction using photographed serial sections. *Anat Rec.* 1967;159:405.
101. Priest JH. Human cell culture: an important tool for the diagnosis and understanding of disease. *J Pediat.* 1968;72:415.
102. Manasek FJ. Embryonic development of the heart. I. A light and electron microscopic study of myocardial development in the early chick embryo. *J Morph.* 1968;125:329.
103. Manasek FJ. Embryonic development of the heart. II. Formation of the epicardium. *J Embryol Exp Morph.* 1969;22:333.
104. Stalsberg H. The origin of heart asymmetry: right and left contributions to the early chick embryo heart. *Develop Biol.* 1969;19:109.
105. Donald I. Sonar as a method of studying prenatal development. *J Pediat.* 1969;75:326.
106. Van Mierop LHS, Gessner IH. The morphologic development of the sinoatrial node in the mouse. *Am J Cardiol.* 1970;25:204.
107. Sissman NJ. Developmental landmarks in cardiac morphogenesis: comparative chronology. *Am J Cardiol.* 1970;25:141.
108. DeHaan RL. Cardiac development: a problem in need of synthesis. *Am J Cardiol.* 1970;25:139.
109. Smith RB. Development of innovation of coronary arteries in human foetus up until 230 mm stage (midterm). *Br Heart J.* 1970;32:108.
110. Lieberman M. Physiologic development of impulse conduction in embryonic cardiac tissue. *Am J Cardiol.* 1970;25:279.
111. Halle W, Wollenberger A. Differentiation and behavior of isolated embryonic and neonatal heart cells in a chemically defined medium. *Am J Cardiol.* 1970;25:292.
112. Klein RL, Horton CR, Thureson-Klein A. Studies on nuclear amino acid transport and cation content in embryonic myocardium of the chick. *Am J Cardiol.* 1970;25:301.
113. Gessner IH, Van Mierop LHS. Experimental production of cardiac defects: the spectrum of dextroposition of the aorta. *Am J Cardiol.* 1970;25:272.
114. Stalsberg H. Mechanism of dextral looping of the embryonic heart. *Am J Cardiol.* 1970;25:265.
115. Manasek FJ. Sulfated extracellular matrix production in the embryonic heart and adjacent tissues. *J Exp Zool.* 1970;174:415.
116. Rosenquist GC, DeHaan RL. Migration of precardiac cells in the chick embryo: a radioautographic study. *Contrib Embryol Carnegie Inst Washington.* 1966;38:111.
117. Manasek FJ. Myocardial cell death in the embryonic chick ventricle. *J Embryol Exp Morph.* 1969;21:271.
118. Rosenquist GC. Cardia bifida in chick embryos: anterior and posterior defects produced by transplanting tritiated thymidine-labeled grafts medial to the heart-forming regions. *Teratology.* 1970;3:135.

119. Barrow MV, Taylor WJ. The production of congenital heart defects with the use of antisera to rat kidney, placenta, heart, and lung homogenates. *Am Heart J.* 1971;82:199.
120. Barrow MV, Willis LS. Ectopia cordis (ectocardia) and gastroschisis induced in rats by the lathyrogen, beta-amino propionitrile (BAPN). *Am Heart J.* 1972;83:518.
121. Birch GE. An elegant transplant. *Am Heart J.* 1971;81:573.
122. Goor DA, Dische R, Lillehei CW. The conotruncus. I. Its normal inversion and conus absorption. *Circulation.* 1972;46:375.
123. Los JA. Analysis of persistent interventricular communication in a human embryo of 19.8 mm CR length. A helpful record in the study of the components participating in heart septation. *Acta Morph Neerl-Scand.* 1972;9:179.
124. Harh JY, Paul MH, Gallen WJ, Friedberg DZ, Kaplan S. Experimental production of hypoplastic left heart syndrome in the chick embryo. *Am J Cardiol.* 1973;31:51.
125. Corone P. Bases embryologique utiles à la compréhension des cardiopathies congenitales. *Coeur.* 1973; Numero Special:1.
126. Manasek FJ, Burnside MB, Waterman RE. Myocardial cell shape change as a mechanism of embryonic heart looping. *Develop Biol.* 1972;29:349.
127. Lieberman M, Manasek FJ, Sawanobori T, Johnson EA, Cytochalasin B. Its morphological and electrophysiological actions on synthetic strands of cardiac muscle. *Develop Biol.* 1973;31:380.
128. Castro-Quezada A, Nadal-Ginard B, de la Cruz MV. Experimental study of the formation of the bulboventricular loop in the chick. *J Embryol Exp Morph.* 1972;27:623.
129. Los JA. The heart of the five days' chick embryo during dilatation and contraction. A functional hypothesis based on morphological observations. *Acta Morph Neerl-Scand.* 1971 and 1972;9:309.
130. Dor X, Corone P. Le role du conus dans la morphogenèse cardiaque. Essai d'etude sur l'embryon de poulet. *Coeur.* 1973;4:207.
131. Marx JL. Embryology: out of the womb—into the test tube. *Science.* 1973;182:811.
132. Manasek FJ. *Some Comparative Aspects of Cardiac and Skeletal Myogenesis, Developmental Regulation, Aspect of Cell Differentiation.* New York: Academic Press, Inc; 1973:193.
133. Manasek FJ, Reid M, Vinson W, Seyer J, Johnson R. Glycosaminoglycan synthesis by the early embryonic chick heart. *Develop Biol.* 1973;35:332.
134. Anderson RH, Wilkinson JL, Arnold R, Lubkiewicz K. Morphogenesis of bulboventricular malformations. I. Consideration of embryogenesis in the normal heart. *Br Heart J.* 1974;36:242.
135. Johnson RC, Manasek FJ, Vinson WC, Seyer JM. The biochemical and ultrastructural demonstration of collagen during early heart development. *Develop Biol.* 1974;36:252.
136. De Terra N. Cortical control of cell division. *Science.* 1974;184:530.
137. McMahon D. Chemical messengers in development: a hypothesis. *Science.* 1974;185:1012.
138. Weiss J, Morad M. Single cell layered heart: electromechanical properties of the heart of Boltenia overifera. *Science.* 1975;186:750.
139. Dor X, Corone P. Embryologie normale et genese des cardiopathies congenitales. *Encycl Méd Chir Paris.* 1981;3:11001, C10, 11001 C20, 11001 C30.
140. Wahn HL, Lightbody LE, Tchen TT, Taylor JD. Induction of neural differentiation in cultures of amphibian undetermined presumptive epidermis by cyclic AMP derivatives. *Science.* 1975;188:366.
141. Ishikawa S, Takao A, Ando M, Mori K. The teratogenic effect of centrifugal force on the cardiovascular system of chick embryo. *Congenital Anom.* 1975;15:11.
142. Manasek FJ. The extracellular matrix of the early embryonic heart. In: Lieberman M, Sano T, eds. *Developmental and Physiological Correlates of Cardiac Muscle.* New York: Raven Press; 1975:1.
143. Pexieder T. Cell death in the morphogenesis and teratogenesis of the heart. *Adv Anat, Embryol Cell Biol.* 1975;51:6.
144. Los JA, van Eijndthoven E. The fusion of endocardial cushions in the heart of the chick embryo. A light-microscopical and electron-microscopical study. *Z Anat Entwickl-Gesch.* 1973;141:55.
145. Los JA. A case of heart septum defect in a human embryo of 27 mm C.R. Length, as a helpful record in studying the components participating in heart septation. *Acta Morphol Neerl-Scand.* 1970/71;8:161.
146. Manasek FJ. Macromolecules of the extracellular compartment of embryonic and mature hearts. *Circ Res.* 1976;38:331.
147. Argüello C, de la Cruz MV, Sánchez Gómez C. Experimental study of the formation of the heart tube in the chick embryo. *J Embryol Exp Morph.* 1975;33:1.
148. Hendrix MJC, Morse DE. Atrial septation. 1. Scanning electron microscopy in the chick. *Develop Biol.* 1977;57:345.
149. Manasek FJ. Glycoprotein synthesis and tissue interactions during establishment of the functional embryonic chick heart. *J Mol Cell Biol.* 1976;8:389.
150. Dor X. *Études des torsions distales de l'ébauche cardiaque, développement normal et malformations expérimentales réalisées chez l'embryon de poulet. Thesis, Université Pierre et Marie Curie.* Paris, France: Faculté de Médecine Pitié-Salpètrière; 1976.
151. Dor X, Corone P. Le rôle du conus dans la morphogenèse cardiaque. Essai d`étude sur l`embryon de poulet. *Coeur.* 1973;4:207.
152. Dickmann Z, Spilman CH. Prostaglandins in rabbit blastocysts. *Science.* 1975;190:997.
153. Okamoto N, Ikeda T, Miyabara S. *Morphology of Abnormal Cardial Looping Induced by Fast Neuron in the Rat Embryo. Acta Universitatis Carolimae Monographis.* Europ Teratology Soc; 1973:56–57.
154. Okamoto N, Ikeda T, Satow Y. Effects of 14.1-MEV fast-neutron irradiation on the cardiovascular system of the rat fetus. In: Sikov MR, Mahlum DD, eds. *Radiation Biology of Fetal and Juvenile Mammals.* Oakridge:, U.S. Atomic Energy Commission;1969: 325.
155. Okamoto N, Satow Y. Cell death in bulbar cushion of normal and abnormal developing heart. In: Lieberman M, Sano T, eds. *Developmental and Physiological Correlates of Cardiac Muscle.* New York: Raven Press; 1975:51.
156. Okamoto N, Ikeda T, Satow Y, Shimada K. Early effects of 14.1 MeV fast neutron irradiation on rat embryo, with reference to teratogenesis. *Hiroshima J Med Sci.* 1972;21:101.
157. Laane HM. The arterial pole of the embryonic heart. I. Nomenclature of the arterial pole of the embryonic heart. II. *Septation of the Arterial Pole of the Embryonic Chick Heart.* Amsterdam & Lisse: Swets & Zeitlinger BV; 1978.
158. Chuaqui JB, Bersch W. The periods of determination of cardiac malformations. *Virchows Arch A Pathol Anat.* 1972;356:95.
159. Wenink ACG. Development of the human cardiac conducting system. *J Anat.* 1976;121:617.
160. Allwork SP. *The Embryological Basis of Congenital Malformations of the Outflow Tracts of the Human Heart, Thesis.* London: Royal Postgraduate Medical School; 1975.

161. Ishikawa S, Takao A, Ando M, Mori K. The teratogenic effect of centrifugal force on the cardiovascular system of chick embryo. *Cong Anom.* 1975;15:11.
162. Halbert SA, Tam PY, Blandau RJ. Egg transport in the rabbit oviduct: the roles of cilic and muscle. *Science.* 1976;191:1052.
163. Van Mierop LHS, Patterson DF, Schnarr WR. Hereditary conotruncal septal defects in keeshound dogs: embryologic studies. *Am J Cardiol.* 1977;40:936.
164. Lemanski LF, Marx BS, Hill CS. Evidence for abnormal heart induction in cardiac-mutant salamanders (Amblystoma mexicanum). *Science.* 1977;196:894.
165. Kulikowski RR, Manasek FJ. Cardiac mutant salamanders: evidence for heart induction. *J Exper Zool.* 1977;201:485.
166. Manasek FJ. Structural glycoproteins of the embryonic cardiac extracellular matrix. *J Mol Cell Cardiol.* 1977;9:425.
167. De la Cruz MV, Sánchez Gómez C, Arteaga MM, Argüello C. Experimental study of the development of the truncus and the conus in the chick embryo. *J Anat.* 1977;123:661.
168. Goor DA, Dische R, Lillehei CW. The conotruncus. I. Its normal inversion and conus absorption. *Circulation.* 1972;46:375.
169. Nakamura A, Manasek FJ. Experimental studies of the shape and structure of isolated cardiac jelly. *J Embryol Exp Morph.* 1978;43:167.
170. Thompson RP, Fitzharris TP. Morphogenesis of the truncus arteriosus of the chick embryo heart. The formation and migration of mesenchymal tissue. *Am J Anat.* 1979;154:545.
171. Thompson RP, Fitzharris TP. Morphogenesis of the truncus arteriosus of the chick embryo heart. Tissue reorganization during septation. *Am J Anat.* 1979;156:251.
172. Pexieder T, Paschoud N. La stabilité phylogénétique des zones de la mort cellulaire physiologique dans l'organogenèse du coeur. *Acta Anat.* 1973;86:321.
173. Pexieder T. Prenatal development of the endocardium: a review. *Scanning Electron Microsc.* 1981;2:223.
174. Seidl W, Steding G. Contribution to the development of the heart. Part III: the aortic arch complex. Normal development and morphogenesis of congenital malformation. *Thorac Cardiovasc Surg.* 1981;29:359.
175. Wenink ACG. Development of the ventricular septum. In: Wenink ACG, et al., ed. *The Ventricular Septum of the Heart.* The Hague: Martinus Nighoff; 1981:23.
176. Dor X, Corone P. *Embryologie normale et genèse des cardiopathies congenitales.* Paris: Encyclopédie Medico-Chiru-rgicale; 1981.
177. Corone P. Introduction à l`embryologie cardiaque: "le fer à cheval". Vers une classification embryologique des cardiopathies congenitales. *Coeur.* 1982;13:285.
178. Wenink ACG, Gittenberger-de Groot AC. Left and right ventricular trabecular patterns. Consequence of ventricular septation and valve development. *Br Heart J.* 1982;48:462.
179. Dor X, Corone P. Migration et cloisonnement du cono-truncus. Etude expérimentale sur le coeur d`embryon de poulet. *Coeur.* 1982;13:453.
180. De la Cruz MV, Quero-Jiménez M, Martinez MA, Cayré R. Morphogénèse du septum interventriculair. *Coeur.* 1982;13:443.
181. Pexieder T. The tissue dynamics of heart morphogenesis. II. Quantitative investigations. B. Cell death foci. *Ann Embryol Morph.* 1973;6:335.
182. Thompson RF, Wong YMM. A computer graphic study of cardiactruncal septation. *Anat Rec.* 1983;206:207.
183. De la Cruz MV, Giménez-Ribotta M, Saravalli O, Cayré R. The contribution of the inferior endocardial cushion of the atrioventricular canal to cardiac septation and to the development of the atrioventricular valves: study in the chick embryo. *Am J Anat.* 1983;166:63.
184. Yokoyama H, Matsuoka R, Bruyère HJ, Gilbert EF, Uno H. Light and electron-microscopic observations of theophylline-induced aortic aneurysms in embryonic chicks. *Am J Pathol.* 1983;112:258.
185. Bruyère HJ, Matsuoka R, Carlsson E, Cheung MO, Dean R, Gilbert EF. Cardiovascular malformations associated with administration of prenalterol to young chick embryos. *Teratology.* 1983;28:75.
186. Wenink ACG. Embryology of the ventricular septum: separate origin of its components. *Virchows Arch A Path Anat Histol.* 1981;390:71.
187. Hawkins JA, Hu N, Clark EB. Effect of caffeine on hemodynamic function in the stage 24 chick embryo. *Circulation.* 1983;68(III):394.
188. Freinkel N, Lewis NJ, Akazawa S, Roth SI, Gorman L. The honeybee syndrome—implications of the teratogenicity of mannose in rat-embryo culture. *N Eng J Med.* 1984;310:223.
189. Villée CA. Birth defects and glycolysis. *N Eng J Med.* 1984;310:254.
190. Wenink ACG, Oppenheimer-Dekker A, Moulaert AJ, eds. *The Ventricular Septum of the Heart.* The Hague: Leiden University Press; 1981.
191. De la Cruz MV, Gómez CS, Arteaga MM, Arguello C. Experimental study of the development of the truncus and the conus in the chick embryo. *J Anat.* 1977;123:661.
192. Thompson RP, Wong YMM, Fitzharris TP. Patterns of tensile stress in the developing cardiac truncus. In: Nora JJ, Takao A, eds. *Congenital Heart Disease, Causes and Processes.* Mount Kisco, NY: Futura Publishing Company; 1984:387.
193. Asami I, Koizumi K. The development of the aortic channel when it arises from the right ventricle: an analytical experimental approach to the morphogenesis of transposition of the great arteries. In: Nora JJ, Takao A, eds. *Congenital Heart Disease, Causes and Processes.* Mount Kisco, NY: Futura Publishing Co; 1984:531.
194. Clark EB, Takao A, eds. *Developmental Cardiology, Morphogenesis and Function.* Mount Kisco, NY: Futura Publishing Co; 1990.
195. Van Mierop LHS, Kutsche LM. Development of the ventricular septum of the heart. *Heart Ves.* 1985;1:114.
196. O'Rahilly R, Müller F. Embryonic length and cerebral landmarks in staged human embryos. *Anat Rec.* 1984;209:265.
197. Binder M. The teratogenetic effects of a bis (dichloroacetyl) diamine on hamster embryos, aortic arch anomalies and the pathogenesis of the DiGeorge syndrome. *Am J Pathol.* 1985;118:179.
198. Thompson RP, Fitzharris TP. Division of cardiac outflow. In: Ferrans V, Rosenquist G, Weinstein C, eds. *Cardiac Morphogenesis.* Elsevier Science Publishing Co, Inc; 1985:169.
199. Thompson RP, Sumida H, Abercombie V, Satow Y, Fitzharris TP, Okamoto N. Morphogenesis of human cardiac outflow. *Anat Rec.* 1985;213:578.
200. Van Praagh R. Cardiac embryology: the conotruncus. *Heart Ves.* 1985;1:193.
201. Dor X, Corone P. Migration and torsions of the conotruncus in the chick embryo heart: observational evidence and conclusions drawn from experimental intervention. *Heart Ves.* 1985;1:195.
202. O'Rahilly R. The embryonic period. *Teratology.* 1986;34:119.
203. Besson WT, Kirby ML, Van Mierop LHS, Teabeaut JR. Effects of the size of lesions of the cardiac neural crest at various embryonic ages on incidence and types of cardiac defects. *Circulation.* 1986;73:360.

204. Vuillemin M, Pexieder T. Normal stages of cardiac organogenesis in the mouse: I. Development of the external shape of the heart. *Am J Anat.* 1986;184:101.
205. Vuillemin M, Pexieder T. Normal stages of cardiac organogenesis in the mouse: II. Development of the internal relief of the heart. *Am J Anat.* 1989;184:114.
206. Saunders S, Jalkanen M, O'Farrell S, Bernfield M. Molecular cloning of syndecan, an integral membrane proteoglycan. *J Cell Biol.* 1989;108:1547.
207. Pexieder T, Wenink ACG, Anderson RH. A suggested nomenclature for the developing heart. *Int J Cardiol.* 1989;25:255.
208. De la Cruz MV, Sánchez-Gómez, Palomino MA. The primitive cardiac regions in the straight tube heart (stage 9-) and their anatomical expression in the mature heart: an experimental study in the chick embryo. *J Anat.* 1989;165:121.
209. Ben-Shachar G, Arcilla RA, Lucas RV, Manasek FT. Ventricular trabeculations in the chick embryo heart and their contribution to ventricular muscular septal development. *Circ Res.* 1985;57:759.
210. Pexieder T. Pathogenese der angeborenen Herzfehler: Dichtung und Wahrheit. *Z Kardiol.* 1990;79:315.
211. Kirby ML, Waldo KL. Role of neural crest in congenital heart disease. *Circulation.* 1990;82:332.
212. Moscoso G, Pexieder T. Variations in microscopic anatomy and ultra structure of human embryonic hearts subjected to three different modes of fixation. *Pathol Res Pract.* 1990;186:768.
213. Martin-Rodriguez JC, Perez-Miguelsanz J, Maestro C, Murillo J, Puerta J. Study of the first cells seen in the cardiac jelly using monoclonal antibody 13F4. *Cardiol Young.* 1993;3:I-125.
214. Keller B, Tinney J, Hu N, Clark E. Embryonic ventricular pressure-volume relations in the stage 16 to 21 chick embryo. *Cardiol Young.* 1993;3:I-2.
215. Lamers WH, Wessels A, Verbeek FJ, et al. New findings concerning ventricular septation in the human heart, implications for maldevelopment. *Circulation.* 1992;86:1194.
216. De la Cruz MV, Sánchez Gómez C, Cayré R. The developmental components of the ventricles: their significance in congenital cardiac malformations. *Cardiol Young.* 1991;1:123.
217. Angelini P. Embryology and congenital heart disease. *Tex Heart Inst J.* 1995;22:1.
218. Schatteman GC, Li T, Loushin C. Platelet derived growth factor-A is required for normal murine cardiovascular development: *in vivo* assessment of putative regulators of development. *Circulation.* 1995;92:(Suppl I-118).
219. Hixon RL, Leatherbury L, Scamber P, Wolfe RR, Stadt HA, Kirby ML. Morphologic and hemodynamic assessment of tuple 1 gene attenuated chick embryos. *Pediatrics.* 1996;98:(suppl 534).
220. Van Splunder P, Stijnen T, Wladimiroff JW. Fetal atrioventricular flow-velocity wave forms and their relation to arterial and venous flow-velocity wave forms at 8 to 20 weeks of gestation. *Circulation.* 1996;94:1372.
221. Clark EB, Markwald RR, Takao A, eds. *Developmental Mechanisms of Heart Disease.* Armonk, NY: Futura Publishing Co, Inc; 1995.
222. Cromie WJ. Genes put your heart in the right place. *Harvard University Gazette*; 1997;42:8.
223. Supp DM, Witte DP, Potter SS, Brueckner M. Mutation of an axonemal dynein affects left-right asymmetry in inversus viscerum mice. *Nature.* 1997;389:963.
224. Oh SP, Li E. The signaling pathway mediated by the type II B activin receptor controls axial patterning and lateral asymmetry in the mouse. *Genes Dev.* 1997;11:1.
225. Mathews LS. Activin receptors and cellular signaling by the receptor serine kinase family. *Endocr Rev.* 1994;15:310.
226. Olson EN, Srivastava D. Molecular pathways controlling heart development. *Science.* 1996;272:671.
227. Rossant J. Mouse mutants and cardiac development: new molecular insights into cardiogenesis. *Circ Res.* 1996;78:349.

SECTION III

Anatomic and Developmental Approach to Diagnosis

3

Morphologic Anatomy

An understanding of normal morphologic anatomy is basic to the accurate diagnosis of congenital heart disease. One of the diagnostic problems posed by complex congenital heart disease is that any cardiac chamber, valve, or vessel can be virtually "anywhere." Consequently, the diagnostic identification of the cardiac chambers cannot be based on relative position (such as right sided or left sided) nor on function (such as venous or arterial), because position and function are variables in congenital heart disease. For example, a ventricle may be described as left-sided and arterial. But the question then arises, which ventricle is it? Is it a morphologically left ventricle or a morphologically right ventricle? A **positionally** left ventricle may be a **morphologically** left ventricle or a **morphologically** right ventricle. Morphologic anatomic identification of cardiovascular structures is essential to accurate diagnosis.

The **morphologic method** of diagnosis in congenital heart disease was pioneered by Lev[1] in 1954, who emphasized the septal surface morphologies. The morphologic method of chamber identification was expanded by Van Praagh and his colleagues between 1964 and 1972.[2-4] The latter investigators emphasized both the septal surface and the free-wall morphologies, which made it possible to diagnose the anatomic types of single ventricle,[2] and also made it possible to diagnose any heart—no matter where it may be located in space.[3,4]

THE ATRIA

The anatomic features of the morphologically right atrium and of the morphologically left atrium are presented in Figs. 3.1 to 3.8. Their morphologic anatomic features are summarized in Table 3.1.

Whenever we say right atrium or left atrium without further qualification, **morphologically right atrium** or **morphologically left atrium** should be understood. When referring to the cardiac chambers (atria or ventricles), **right** and **left** refer to morphologic characteristics, not to relative position. When advantageous for clarity, the relative position in space may also be indicated specifically, as in: right atrium (left sided).

The Morphologically Right Atrium

Angiocardiographically, the broad triangular shape of the right atrial appendage, both in the posteroanterior view (Fig. 3.1) and in the left lateral view (Fig. 3.2), is highly characteristic.

Anatomically, the **external appearance** of the right atrium is characterized by a broad triangular right atrial appendage (Fig. 3.3). The right atrial appendage resembles Snoopy* looking to his left. The bridge of Snoopy's nose is formed by the tinea sagittalis (which is seen on the interior of the right atrium). Normally, the inferior vena cava and the superior vena cava are also visible externally, returning to the right atrium. The inferior vena cava is a highly reliable diagnostic marker of the right atrium, whereas the superior vena cava is not. The atrium with which the inferior vena cava connects is always the morphologically right atrium, to the best of our present knowledge. By contrast, the superior vena cava connects, not rarely, with the left atrium because of unroofing of the coronary sinus.

Note that the inferior vena cava can *drain* into the left atrium, for example, when a prominent right venous valve (Eustachian valve) is associated with a deficient or absent septum primum. But in this situation, the inferior vena cava *connects* normally with the right atrium. It is important to distinguish between *connections* and *drainage*.

Externally, the **sulcus terminalis** indicates the termination of the medial, venous, sinus venosus component of the right atrium and the beginning of the more lateral, muscular, contractile portion of the right atrium. The sulcus terminalis, or **sinoatrial sulcus**, lies just lateral to the ostia of the superior vena cava and the inferior vena cava. This shallow furrow runs superoinferiorly on the posterior external aspect of the right atrium, between the venous component of the right atrium medially that joins the superior and inferior vena caval ostia and the musculi pectinati (pectinate muscle) portion of the right atrial appendage that lies more laterally. The sulcus terminalis (terminal sulcus), also known as the sinoatrial sulcus, corresponds to the crista terminalis (terminal crest) that is seen on inspection of the interior of the right atrium.

The importance of the sulcus terminalis is that this is where the **sinoatrial node**, the pacemaker of the heart, resides. Although not visible upon external inspection, the head of the sinoatrial node is located to the right of, or lateral to the superior vena cava (in visceroatrial situs solitus), just beneath the epicardium, in the sulcus terminalis. The tail of the sinoatrial node extends like the tail of a comet—almost down to the level of the inferior vena cava. Hence, the sinoatrial node is so called because it lies at the junction of the sinus venosus medially and the atrium (appendage) laterally; thus, the pacemaker really is sinoatrial in location.

Because the sinoatrial node is invisible upon careful external inspection, one must know where it is—particularly if one is a surgeon about to do a right atriotomy.

*Dog, one of the characters in *Peanuts*, created by American cartoonist Charles M. Schulz (born 1922).

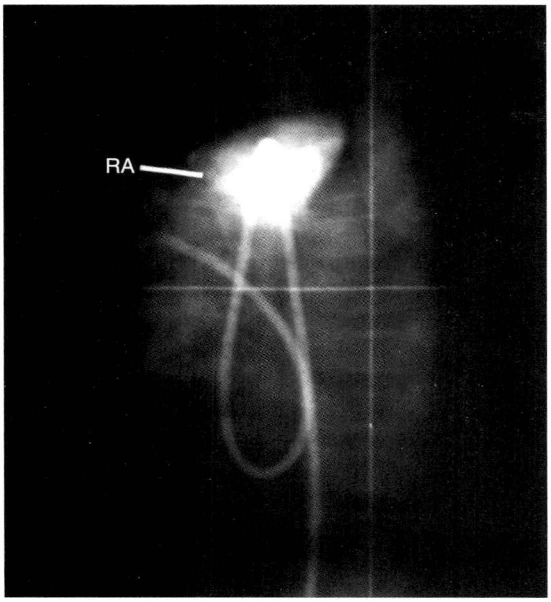

Fig. 3.1 Angiocardiogram of morphologically right atrium *(RA)*, posteroanterior projection. Note the broad triangular shape of the RA appendage. (From Van Praagh R. The segmental approach to diagnosis in congenital heart disease. In Bergsma D, ed. *Birth Defects: Original Article Series*. 1972;8:4; with permission.)

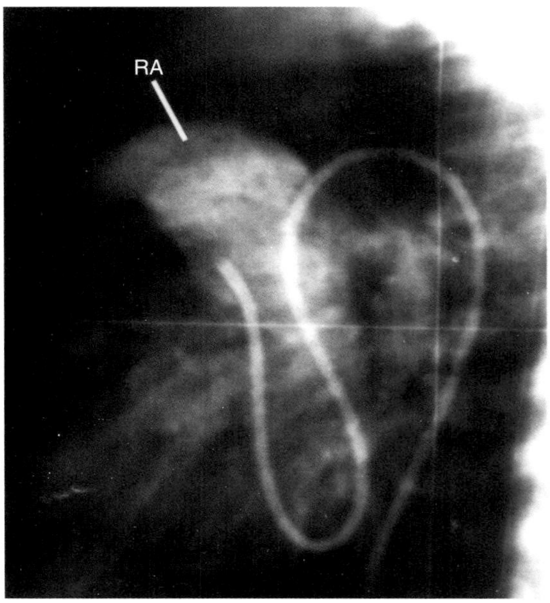

Fig. 3.2 Angiocardiogram of morphologically right atrium *(RA)*, left lateral projection, showing the pyramidal shape of the RA appendage. Interruption of the inferior vena cava from the renal veins to the hepatic veins accounts for the "candy cane" or "shepherd's crook" course of the catheter in the large azygos vein that returns the venous blood from the lower body to the superior vena cava and thence to the RA. (From Van Praagh R. The segmental approach to diagnosis in congenital heart disease. In Bergsma D, ed. *Birth Defects: Original Article Series*. 1972;8:4; with permission.)

What is the blood supply of the sinoatrial node? The answer is: about 55% from the right coronary artery and about 45% from the left coronary artery, typically from the left circumflex branch.

The sinoatrial nodal artery runs through the sinoatrial node like a shish kabob skewer. The sinoatrial nodal tissue is located around the sinoatrial nodal artery. Surgically, if at all possible, one should avoid producing thrombosis of the sinoatrial nodal artery in order to avoid sick sinus syndrome. Dr. "Billy" Kreutzer, the famous congenital heart surgeon from Buenos Aires and coinventor of the Fontan–Kreutzer procedure, told me how he avoids the sinoatrial node. Just after he has put cardioplegia solution into the aortic root, he watches very carefully to see if the sinoatrial nodal artery is coming from the right coronary artery and into the "front door" of the head of the sinoatrial node or if the sinoatrial nodal artery is coming from the left circumflex coronary artery, in which case it can come around behind the superior vena cava to enter the sinoatrial node via "the back door." Cardioplegia solution usually is water clear; so a surgeon who watches carefully at this point in the procedure often can identify exactly where the sinoatrial nodal artery is. It is not enough just to avoid surgical transection of the sulcus terminalis. The surgeon must also, if possible, avoid transection of the sinoatrial nodal artery **before** it reaches the sinoatrial node in the sulcus terminalis.

The external appearance of the right atrium (see Fig. 3.3) is so characteristic that an experienced eye usually needs only a quick glance to make this morphologic anatomic identification.

The **internal appearance** of the morphologically right atrium is equally distinctive (Fig. 3.4). The most highly reliable diagnostic features of the right atrium are: (1) the ostium of the inferior vena cava, (2) the ostium of the coronary sinus, (3) the superior limbic band of septum secundum, and (4) the large broad triangular right atrial appendage and its musculi pectinati (pectinate muscles).

Normally, the superior vena cava enters the right atrium (see Fig. 3.4). However, if a persistent left superior vena cava is present in visceroatrial situs solitus and if the coronary sinus is unroofed due to the presence of a coronary sinus septal defect, then the persistent left superior vena cava will drain into the morphologically left atrium. Hence, the superior vena cava is not as highly reliable a diagnostic marker of the right atrium as is the inferior vena cava.

Lateral to the entry of the superior vena cava—to the right in visceroatrial situs solitus (see Fig. 3.4) and to the left in visceroatrial situs inversus—lies the **crista terminalis (terminal crest)**. The crista terminalis internally (see Fig. 3.4) corresponds to the sulcus terminalis externally (see Fig. 3.3), which is where the sinoatrial node is located. If deep sutures are put into the crista terminalis, for example, while doing the Mustard procedure or the Fontan–Kreutzer procedure, then the sinoatrial nodal artery may be traumatized. Thrombosis of the sinoatrial nodal artery results in ischemic necrosis of the sinoatrial node, which in turn leads to the **sick sinus syndrome**.

The **tinea sagittalis** intersects with the crista terminalis just anterior to the entry of the superior vena cava (see Fig. 3.4). Externally, the tinea sagittalis corresponds to the bridge of Snoopy's nose. From the practical standpoint, right behind the tinea sagittalis is a favorite place for the tips of cardiac catheters to get caught. A little injudicious push of the cardiac catheter at this point can lead to perforation of the right atrial appendage.

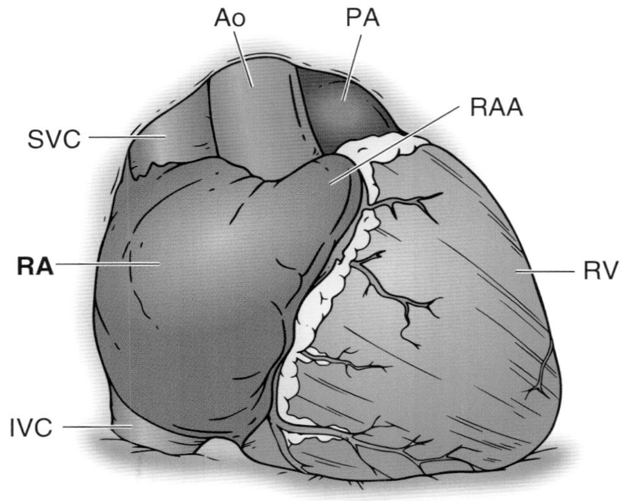

Fig. 3.3 Exterior of the morphologically right atrium *(RA)*. Because the right atrial appendage *(RAA)* is well incorporated into the RA, the RA is triangular or pyramidal in shape—very different from the left atrial appendage. *Ao,* Ascending aorta; *IVC,* inferior vena cava; *PA,* main pulmonary artery; *RV,* morphologically right ventricle; *SVC,* superior vena cava. (From Van Praagh R, Vlad P. Dextrocardia, mesocardia, and levocardia: the segmental approach to diagnosis in congenital heart disease. In Keith JD, Rowe RD, Vlad P, eds. *Heart Disease in Infancy and Childhood.* 3rd ed. New York: Macmillan Publishing; 1978:638.)

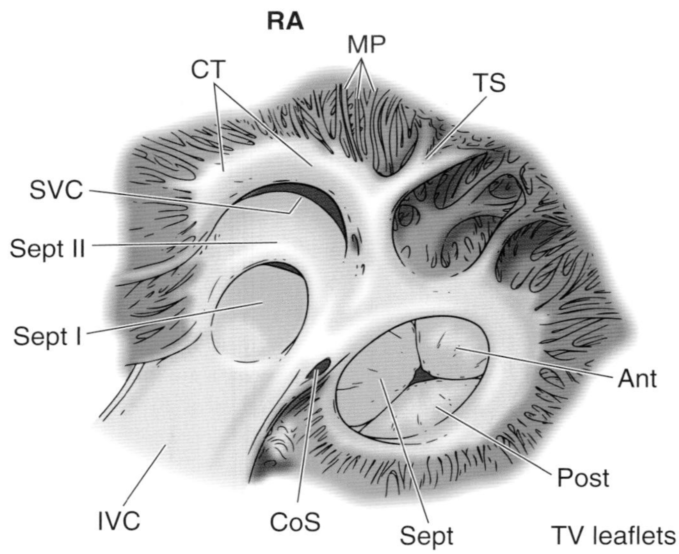

Fig. 3.4 Interior of morphologically right atrium *(RA)*. The RA is the atrium that has the following morphologic features: (1) Its septal surface displays the superior limbic band of septum secundum *(Sept II)*. (2) Its appendage is broad, triangular, and well incorporated into the RA, displaying numerous musculi pectinati *(MP)* or pectinate muscles, a tinea sagittalis *(TS)*, and a crista terminalis *(CT)* lateral to the entry of the superior vena cava *(SVC)*. (3) The inferior vena cava *(IVC)* connects directly with the RA. (4) The ostium of the coronary sinus *(CoS)* opens into the RA. (5) Septum primum *(Sept I)* opens away from the RA and into the morphologically left atrium. Normally, the anterior *(Ant)*, posterior *(Post)*, and septal *(Sept)* leaflets of the tricuspid valve *(TV)* can be seen from the right atrial aspect. (From Van Praagh R, Vlad P. Dextrocardia, mesocardia, and levocardia: the segmental approach to diagnosis in congenital heart disease. In Keith JD, Rowe RD, Vlad P, eds. *Heart Disease in Infancy and Childhood.* 3rd ed. New York: Macmillan Publishing; 1978:638.)

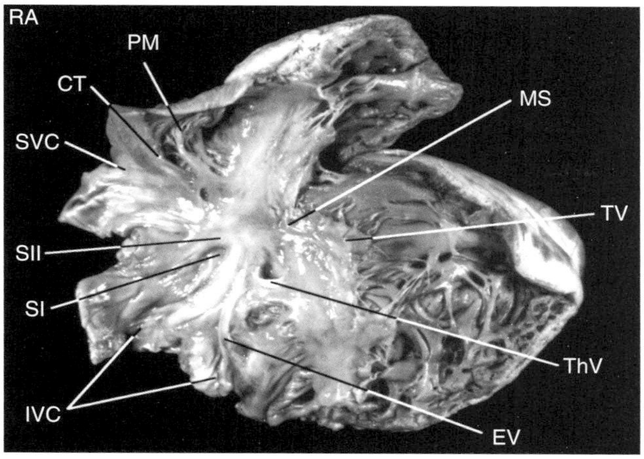

Fig. 3.5 Photograph of the interior of the morphologically right atrium *(RA)* showing the inferior vena cava *(IVC)*, the superior vena cava *(SVC)*, the crista terminalis *(CT)* lateral to the entry of the SVC, the superior limbic band of septum secundum *(SII)*, septum primum *(SI)*, the eustachian valve *(EV)* of the IVC, the thebesian valve *(ThV)* of the coronary sinus, the pectinate muscles *(PM)*, the septal leaflet of the tricuspid valve *(TV)*, and the membranous septum *(MS)* between the anterior and septal leaflets of the TV. The atrioventricular node and the unbranched portion of the His bundle lie on a straight line between the ostium of the coronary sinus (which is covered by the ThV) and the MS. The triangle of Koch is formed by the tendon of Todaro (anterior extension of the EV, toward the viewer's right-hand side), the ThV, and the origin of the septal leaflet of the TV.

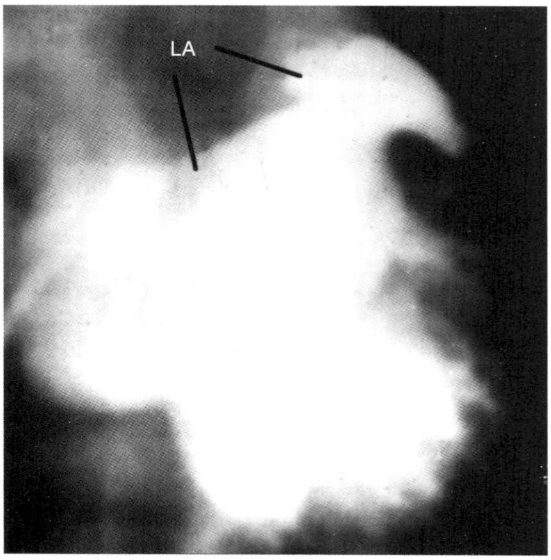

Fig. 3.6 Angiocardiogram of morphologically left atrium *(LA)*, posteroanterior projection. (From Van Praagh R. The segmental approach to diagnosis in congenital heart disease. In Bergsma D, ed. *Birth Defects: Original Article Series*. 1972;8:4; with permission.)

In the posteroanterior image intensifier, the catheter tip may seem to be quite far to the left. But looking in the lateral image intensifier reveals that the catheter tip is very anterior—rather than more posterior, as the left atrium is. If in doubt concerning the position of the catheter tip, the catheteer should also look at the color of the blood—dark red meaning right atrium, bright red indicating left atrium. Hence, checking the location of the catheter tip in both the posteroanterior and lateral projections and checking the oxygen saturation of the blood will help to avoid a perforation of the right atrial appendage.

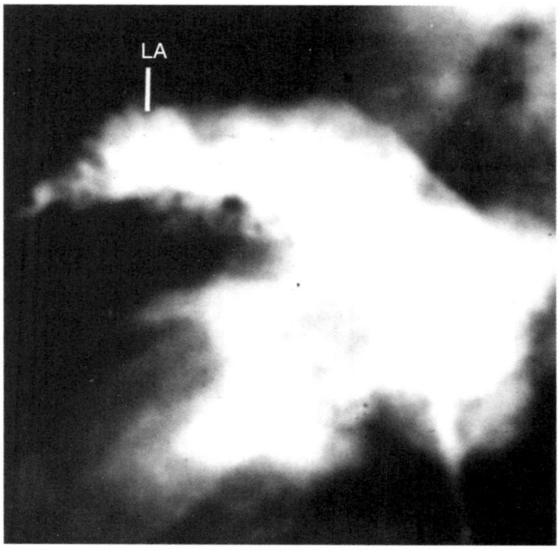

Fig. 3.7 Angiocardiogram of left atrium *(LA)*, left lateral projection. Note the characteristically long, thin, poorly incorporated left atrial appendage—like a pointing finger, which is better seen in the lateral than in the posteroanterior projection. (From Van Praagh R. The segmental approach to diagnosis in congenital heart disease. In Bergsma D, ed. *Birth Defects: Original Article Series*. 1972;8:4; with permission.)

But let us say you have just perforated the right atrial appendage with a cardiac catheter. What do you do now? The answer is: nothing. Don't quickly retract the catheter, pulling it out of the hole in the right atrial appendage. The wall of the right atrial appendage, particularly between the pectinate muscles, is very thin—less than 1 mm in thickness. Instead, leave the catheter where it is. Call your surgical colleagues. Prepare to do a pericardiocentesis. The anatomic point I seek to make is that the right atrial appendage free wall is very thin and may bleed into the pericardial sac following removal of the perforating cardiac catheter. Unfortunately, the right atrial free wall is not a self-sealing "tire," as the much thicker ventricular walls often are. So, the risk of cardiac tamponade following removal of a perforating cardiac catheter is greater following atrial free-wall perforation than following ventricular free-wall perforation. This, then, is the practical importance of the tinea sagittalis. Perhaps it should be added that right atrial perforations can also occur at many other sites; they do not occur only behind the tinea sagittalis.

The **atrioventricular node** and the proximal unbranched portion of the **atrioventricular (or His) bundle** unfortunately are invisible. So you have to know where they are, particularly if you are a catheteer, an electrophysiologist, or a cardiac surgeon. **The atrioventricular node and the atrioventricular bundle lie between the ostium of the coronary sinus posteriorly and the membranous septum anteriorly** (Figs. 3.4 and 3.5).

Where is the membranous septum? From the right atrial standpoint, the membranous septum lies between the anterior and septal leaflets of the tricuspid valve (see Figs. 3.4 and 5). The **atrioventricular portion** of the membranous septum extends

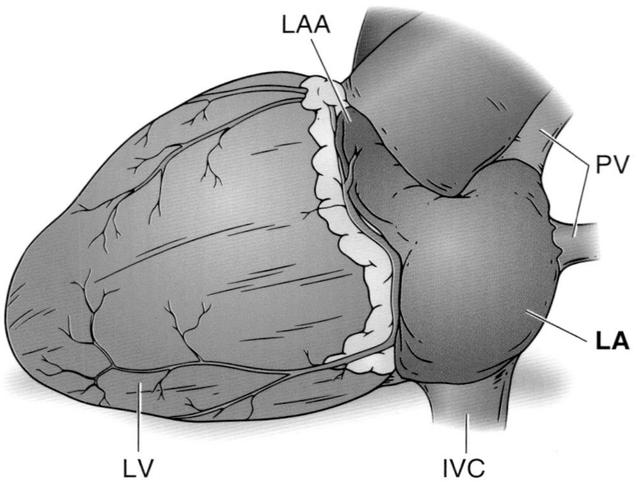

Fig. 3.8 External appearance of morphologically left atrium *(LA)*. The left atrial appendage *(LAA)* is relatively long, thin, and tubular because it is poorly incorporated into the cavity of the LA. The pulmonary veins *(PV)* normally connect with the LA but can be partially or totally anomalous. (From Van Praagh R, Vlad P. Dextrocardia, mesocardia, and levocardia: the segmental approach to diagnosis in congenital heart disease. In Keith JD, Rowe RD, Vlad P, eds. *Heart Disease in Infancy and Childhood.* 3rd ed. New York: Macmillan Publishing; 1978:638, with permission.)

TABLE 3.1 Morphologic Anatomic Features of Right Atrium and Left Atrium

Anatomic Features	Right Atrium	Left Atrium
Veins	Inferior vena cava, constant Superior vena cava, variable Coronary sinus, variable	Pulmonary veins, variable
Appendage	Broad, triangular	Narrow, finger-like
Musculi pectinati	Many	Few
Crista terminalis	Present	Absent
Tinea sagittalis	Present	Absent
Septal surface	Septum secundum	Septum primum
Conduction system	Sinoatrial node Atrioventricular node and bundle	

above the commissure between the anterior and septal leaflets of the tricuspid valve and separates the left ventricle below from the right atrium above. A defect in the atrioventricular portion of the membranous septum results in a **left ventricular-to-right atrial shunt**, often referred to as a Gerbode defect. The **interventricular portion** of the membranous septum lies just below the anterior leaflet/septal leaflet commissure of the tricuspid valve. A defect of the interventricular portion of the membranous septum results in a **membranous ventricular septal defect**.

So, the **atrioventricular node and the proximal unbranched portion of the His bundle** extend in a straight line from the ostium of the coronary septum posteroinferiorly to the membranous septum anterosuperiorly. The tail of the atrioventricular node may extend a short way into the ostium of the coronary sinus. Hence, a coronary sinus rhythm may represent a high nodal rhythm. If you are a cardiac surgeon and if you are showing a younger colleague where the atrioventricular conduction system is, don't point with a sucker. As the late Dr. Bill Mustard (of Mustard procedure fame) once told me, the tip of a sucker can easily become stuck and adherent to the right atrial endocardium. Then, when you have to pull the sucker away from the right atrial endocardium, complete and permanent heart block can result, because the atrioventricular node and His bundle are immediately subendocardial. So, point out the location of the atrioventricular node and His bundle with a probe or some other instrument that will not inadvertently injure the conduction system.

When the His bundle reaches the region of the membranous septum, the His bundle dives or penetrates just proximal to the membranous septum. The **penetrating portion** of the atrioventricular bundle normally passes behind and below the membranous septum.

When the atrioventricular bundle reaches the ventricular level, it branches. The **branching portion** of the His bundle first gives off the left posterior radiation, then the left middle radiation, then the left anterior radiation, and lastly the right bundle branch.

Another approach to localizing the grossly invisible atrioventricular node and the proximal unbranched portion of the atrioventricular bundle is the **triangle of Koch** (see Fig. 3.5). The sides of this triangle are as follows: (1) the tendon of Todaro, which is the anterior extension of the eustachian valve of the inferior vena cava; (2) the thebesian valve of the coronary sinus; and (3) the attachment of the septal leaflet of the tricuspid valve.

The difficulties associated with the triangle of Koch are as follows: (1) The tendon of Todaro is invisible grossly, although it is well seen histologically. However, if one grasps the eustachian valve of the inferior vena cava and pulls down gently in the direction of the inferior vena cava, then the tendon of Todaro (pronounced tod′-a-ro) stands out clearly in the floor of the right atrium. (2) The eustachian valve of the inferior vena cava can be small or absent. But even in such cases, one can usually see where the eustachian valve "should" have been. (3) The thebesian valve of the coronary sinus can be small or absent. Nonetheless, knowing where the ostium of the coronary sinus is, one can usually see where the thebesian valve of the coronary sinus "should" have been. (4) The origin of the septal leaflet of the tricuspid valve can be downwardly displaced, distinctly below the right atrioventricular junction.

Consequently, the triangle of Koch can have poorly demarcated sides, and it is quite large. The largeness of the triangle of Koch can be reduced by the understanding that the atrioventricular node and the proximal unbranched portion of the His bundle are located toward the apex of the triangle of Koch—remote from the thebesian valve that forms the base of this triangle.

Because the tendon of Todaro is invisible, and because the eustachian, thebesian, and septal tricuspid leaflets are quite variable, we have found that the **coronary sinus–membranous septum line** is the easiest and most accurate method of localizing the atrioventricular node and the proximal unbranched portion of the His bundle.

The conduction system is considered in greater detail in Chapter 28.

If my friend and mentor, the late Dr. Maurice Lev, were writing this chapter, he would say that the morphologically right atrium is the atrium that on its septal surface displays the **superior limbic band of septum secundum** (see Figs. 3.4 and 3.5). By contrast, as will be seen, the morphologically left atrium is the atrium that on its septal surface displays septum primum.

When we speak of **septum secundum**, we mean the **superior limbic band** of septum secundum (see Figs. 3.4 and 3.5). **Limbus** means border (Latin). The superior limbic band forms the superior border of the foramen ovale or fossa ovalis. The superior limbic band is a muscular structure. It is the anterior interatrial plica (fold) of muscle, between the right and left atrial appendages. Normally, the ascending aorta lies just in front of the superior limbic band of septum secundum. If one excises septum secundum completely, one ends up outside the heart, in the pericardial cavity, or one can cut into the ascending aorta. Thus, in doing a surgical atrial septectomy, one should excise the membranous septum primum, but one should avoid generous excision of septum secundum's superior limbic band in the anterosuperior direction. Usually septum secundum can be left untouched.

Septum secundum is said also to have an **inferior limbic band** that forms the inferior border of the foramen ovale or fossa ovalis (see Figs. 3.4 and 3.5). The inferior limbic band begins as a venous structure. The inferior limbic band is part of the origin of septum primum—also a venous structure. Later in development, the inferior limbic band undergoes muscularization. Hence, the septum secundum, as ordinarily defined, is a composite structure: The superior limbic band is muscular, whereas the inferior limbic band is primarily venous.

In utero, the atrial septum is a valve, normally, a unidirectional flap valve that permits only right-to-left blood flow. The atrial septum may be likened to a door that normally opens only from the right atrium into the left atrium. Septum primum is the door. Septum secundum is the door jamb.

There are seven valves in the heart. In addition to the four obvious ones, the other three valves are: (1) the eustachian valve of the inferior vena cava, (2) the thebesian valve of the coronary sinus, and (3) the atrial septum in utero.

The septum spurium (spurious septum) is the superior commissure of the sinoatrial valve. The right venous valve (i.e., the right leaflet of the sinoatrial valve) runs along the inferior rim of the crista terminalis. The left venous valve runs over the superior limbic band of septum secundum to the left of the entry of the superior vena cava. The right and left venous valves come together, forming the superior commissure of the sinoatrial valve, where the crista terminalis and the superior limbic band of septum secundum unite. When unusually prominent, this superior commissure of the sinoatrial valve has been called the septum spurium.

The tendon of Todaro is part of the inferior commissure of the sinoatrial valve.

The superior limbic band of septum secundum is also called the **crista dividens** (the dividing crest) of the perinatal physiologists. When the oxygenated blood from the placenta comes up the inferior vena cava and enters the right atrium, the placental blood stream divides on the superior limbic band of septum secundum, which functions as a dividing crest. This crest divides the oxygenated placental blood stream into the **via sinistra** (the left road) and the **via dextra** (the right road). The via sinistra goes to the left atrium, left ventricle, ascending aorta, and the brain, whereas the via dextra sends blood to the right ventricle, pulmonary artery, and via the patent ductus arteriosus to the abdominal viscera.

The inferior rim of the superior limbic band of septum secundum is the **limbic ledge** in the catheterization laboratory. If one wishes to cross the atrial septum with a catheter, one can advance the catheter from the inferior vena cava up into the superior vena cava, then turn the catheter tip toward the left atrium and slowly withdraw the catheter. As the tip passes under the superior limbic band, the tip then moves leftward, against septum primum. Immediately beneath this limbic ledge is where one may wish to do a Brockenbrough procedure to cross an intact atrial septum into the left atrium.

If there is a crista dividens (dividing crest), there should be a crista reuniens (reuniting crest). But where is it? Where do the via sinistra and the via dextra reunite? The answer is: at the aortic isthmus/patent ductus arteriosus junction. This is the aortic arch 4–aortic arch 6 junction. The crista reuniens is the spur between the aortic isthmus and the patent ductus arteriosus.

Developmentally, what is the morphologically right atrium? The right atrium consists of three main embryonic components: (1) **the sinus venosus**, that is, the ostium of the inferior vena cava; the ostium of the superior vena cava, the smooth or venous-like tissue between these two ostia medially (the right sinus horn); and the ostium of the coronary sinus (the left sinus horn); (2) **the primitive atrium**, which forms the right atrial appendage; and (3) **the common atrioventricular canal**, which contributes to the septum of the atrioventricular canal (the atrioventricular septum) and the tricuspid valve leaflets.

So, what is the morphologically right atrium? It consists of the dominant horn of the sinus venosus (normally the right sinus horn), a large triangular well-incorporated atrial appendage, and an atrioventricular canal component. This is why the ostium of the inferior vena cava, the ostium of the coronary sinus, and a well incorporated (large, triangular) atrial appendage are its cardinal diagnostic features.

Etymologies and History. Some of the terms that have been used in Figs. 3.3, 3.4, and 3.5 are likely to be strange and unfamiliar to you. But as soon as you know the root meanings of these terms, they become much easier to understand and to remember. Each of the words we use has a story. (Parenthetically, this section is intended for those readers who are interested in the deep understanding provided by a knowledge of the relevant history and root meanings of our terminology. However, those readers not enthralled by history and language should feel free to skip this section.)

Atrium is derived from ancient Roman architecture. The earliest Roman house was a circular one-roomed hut with wattled walls and a conical thatched roof. Later, the ancient Roman house became rectangular, built of cubical bricks faced with stucco. The roof was tiled, usually sloped inward, and beneath a central opening in the roof was a tank for collecting rainwater. This house contained only one chamber—the living-room or **atrium**,[5] in which all the activities of daily life went on. It got its name from **ater** (black, Latin), the color that was imparted to the interior by the circling smoke of the hearth fire. Chimneys were unknown until very late, and windows were few and small. Hence, *atrium* literally means black room.

In later Republican times, enormous mansions were built, but they followed the earlier plan. The entrance door opened into a hall that led to the atrium, along the side of which tiny windowless bedrooms were partitioned off. At the rear of the atrium was a private office where the father of the family kept his papers and money. Beside the private office there were passages leading to an open courtyard—with lawn, flower bed, and central fountain. The dining room opened off the courtyard. At the back of the house were the kitchens, bathrooms, and service quarters. Often there was a second and even a third story, where the household slaves lived. These mansions were solidly built of concrete faced with slabs of colored marble. The walls were carefully smoothed and covered with mural paintings, and the floors were made of concrete finished with mosaics.[5]

Consequently, **atrium** acquired the connotation of the room that one entered first, which then led elsewhere.

In even earlier ancient Greek, *atrion* meant entrance hall. Much medical Latin was derived directly from Greek, often via Claudius Galen (130–201, CE), a Greek from Pergamos in Asia Minor who spent much of his professional life in Rome.

Thus, both in Greek and Roman usage, *atrion* or *atrium* was the place one entered first in a house, which then led elsewhere.

Vena cava means hollow vein [Latin].

Pectinate muscles means comblike muscles (*pecten* = comb, in Latin). In the right atrial appendage, the pectinate muscles tend to be parallel and straight, like the teeth of a comb or like a cock's comb. The crista terminalis is like the spine of a comb, whereas the pectinate muscles resemble its teeth (see Fig. 3.4).

Tinea sagittalis means sagittal worm. *Sagitta* means arrow (Latin). The sagittal plane is thus the anteroposterior plane, as though an arrow were shot straight through the body from front to back from ventral surface to dorsal surface). Hence, the tinea sagittalis is a wormlike muscle that lies in the sagittal plane (see Fig. 3.4).

Tricuspid means three points (*cuspis* = a point, especially of a spear, in Latin). *Tricuspid* in Greek is *triglochin*. The meaning of *glochin* was any projecting point, such as the end of a yoke strap or the barb of an arrow. **Erasistratos** (Erasistratus in Latin), the brilliant young Alexandrian contemporary of Herophilos (c 300 BCE), discovered, described, and named the tricuspid valve and the mitral (or bicuspid) valve. It was also Erasistratos who discovered that the heart is a pump.

Coronary means encircling like a crown (*corona*, Latin). The Greek precursor of *corona* was *stephanos*, meaning wreath—as in the laurel or wild olive wreath of ancient Greek Olympic champions. The coronary sinus and the coronary arteries encircle the head of the heart (its base) like an Olympic wreath. **Sinus** means a bending, curve, or fold (in Latin). Thus, the **coronary sinus** literally means a fold that encircles the head of the heart like a garland.

The triangle of Koch honors the German surgeon Walter Koch, born in 1880. The atrioventricular node has been referred to as **Koch's node**. The atrioventricular node has also been called **Aschoff's node** and the **node of Aschoff and Tawara**.

The tendon of Todaro immortalizes **Francesco Todaro**, an Italian anatomist who lived from 1839 to 1918.

The sinoatrial node is also known as **Keith's node**, or as **the node of Keith and Flack**.

Although **Aristotle** (384–322 BCE) discovered the cardiovascular system (please see Chapter 1), he thought that the human heart normally has three ventricles, by which he meant three chambers.[6] Aristotle did not include what we call the right atrium as part of the heart. He thought that the right atrium is a dilatation of the great vein, that is, the inferior vena cava plus the superior vena cava. Aristotle thought that the heart begins at what we call the right ventricle and the left atrium.

Herophilos (c 300 BCE) (Herophilus in Latin), the Greek physician who founded the medical school at Alexandria in

Egypt, was one of the earliest proponents of the idea that the atria really are part of the heart, not just a dilatation of the great veins.

Some 300 years later, during the time of Jesus Christ, **Rufus of Ephesus** called what we term the base of the heart the *head* of the heart. Rufus, who was also a Greek, observed that of the two ventricles, the left is thicker and artery-like, while the right is thinner and vein-like but has the larger volume. It is noteworthy that Rufus recognized only *two* ventricles (not three, as Aristotle had).

Rufus of Ephesus stated: "On each side of the head of the heart are things like wings. They are hollow and soft and pulsate with the rest of the heart and are called its ears." This was because these structures were on either side of the head of the heart. "Ears" are "auricles" (auricula in Latin). So it was that the ears or auricles were definitely identified as parts of the heart and distinguished from the ventricles. *Venter* means "belly" (Latin). *Ventriclus* means "little belly" or "womb" (Latin).

However, Galen opposed this new understanding of Rufus of Ephesus. Galen continued to regard the tricuspid valve as "the insertion of the vena cava into the heart."

Consequently, the discovery of Rufus of Ephesus that the atria are indeed parts of the heart, but significantly different from the ventricles, had to wait for 1500 years for confirmation and acceptance by **Leonardo da Vinci** (1452–1519). In his investigation of the heart, Leonardo described "lower ventricles," "upper ventricles," and "ears." His upper ventricles are our atria. His "ears" are our auricular appendages.

Finally, the concept of Rufus of Ephesus was fully accepted by **Andreas Vesalius** (1514–1564) in the first edition of his *De Humani Corporis Fabrica* in 1543. For Vesalius, there were two atria and two ventricles, period.

Thus, it took about 1500 years for the right atrium to be accepted as a part of the heart.

The Morphologically Left Atrium

Angiocardiographically, the morphologically left atrium has an appendage that is long and thin—poorly incorporated into the main cavity of the left atrium (Figs. 3.6 and 3.7). The left atrial appendage looks like a pointing finger or a map of Central America or a windsock at an airport. The characteristic shape of the left atrial appendage is often better seen in the lateral projection (see Fig. 3.7) than in the posteroanterior projection (see Fig. 3.6).

Anatomically, the left atrial appendage is long and thin (Fig. 3.8), very different from the external appearance of the right atrial appendage (see Fig. 3.3). Normally, the pulmonary veins also connect with the left atrium (see Fig. 3.8). However, because of totally and partially anomalous pulmonary venous connections, the pulmonary veins are not a highly reliable diagnostic marker of the morphologically left atrium. For example, totally anomalous pulmonary venous connection makes it clear that it is possible for a morphologically left atrium to exist with no pulmonary venous connection being present.

The internal anatomy of the left atrium is distinctive (Figs. 3.9 and 3.10)—very different from that of the right atrium (see Figs. 3.4 and 3.5). The left atrial septal surface displays septum primum (see Figs. 3.9 and 3.10), the flap valve of the foramen ovale. This is the "door" of the interatrial communication, which is on the left atrial septal surface because septum primum (the first septum) opens into the left atrium out of the right atrium.

The left atrial appendage normally is so poorly incorporated into the main cavity of the left atrium that one can barely see the

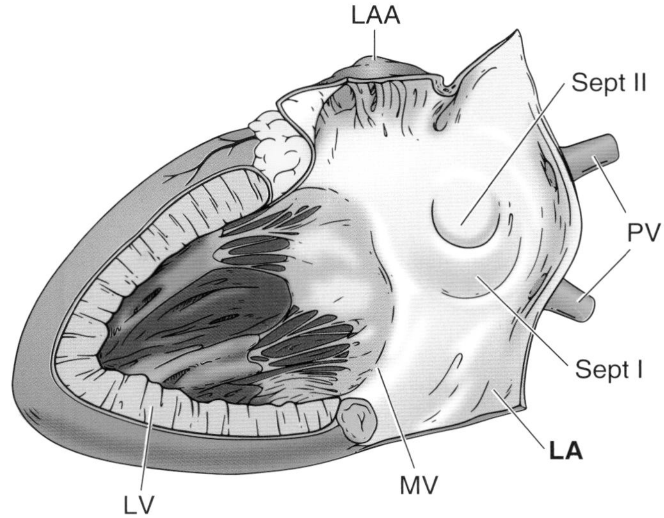

Fig. 3.9 The interior of the morphologically left atrium *(LA)*. The LA is characterized by septum primum *(Sept I)*—the flap valve of the foramen ovale—on its septal surface, because septum primum opens into the LA, away from the right atrium *(RA)*. Septum primum and septum secundum *(Sept II)* together form a unidirection flap valve that opens out of the RA and into the LA. The pulmonary veins *(PV)* normally connect with the dorsal wall of the LA. The left atrial appendage *(LAA)* is so poorly incorporated into the LA that few pectinate muscles are visible from within the cavity of the LA, unless the LAA is cut open. Note that the opened mitral valve *(MV)* and the opened left ventricle *(LV)* can also be seen. (From Van Praagh R, Vlad P. Dextrocardia, mesocardia, and levocardia: the segmental approach to diagnosis in congenital heart disease. In Keith JD, Rowe RD, Vlad P, eds. *Heart Disease in Infancy and Childhood.* 3rd ed. New York: Macmillan Publishing; 1978:638, with permission.)

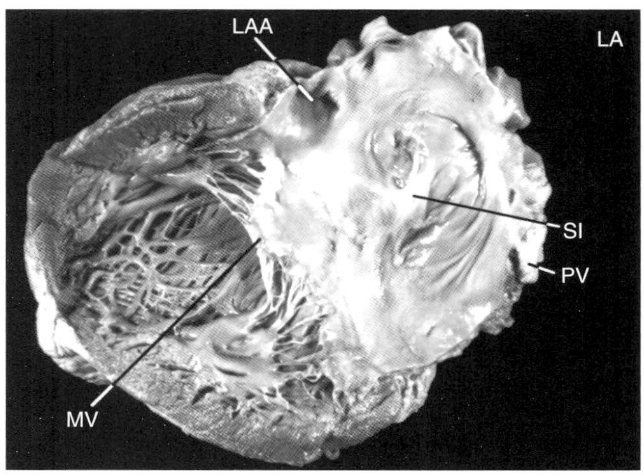

Fig. 3.10 Photograph of the interior of the morphologically left atrium *(LA)* showing the flap of the foramen ovale—septum primum *(SI)*—on the septal surface, the normal connection of the pulmonary veins *(PV)*, the left atrial appendage *(LAA)* that is not incorporated into the cavity of the LA, the pectinate muscles barely visible within the LAA, and the deep anterior leaflet of the mitral valve *(MV)*.

pectinate muscles of the left atrial appendage from the center of the left atrial cavity (see Fig. 3.9).

Because this interatrial "door" opens from the right atrium into the left atrium, the right atrial septal surface is characterized by septum secundum—the door jamb (see Fig. 3.4), whereas the left atrial septal surface is characterized by septum primum—the door (see Fig. 3.8).

What is septum primum really? We think that the answer to this question is: Septum primum is the main component of the left venous valve mechanism, that is bifid (it consists of two parts).[7] In other words, septum primum is a big venous valve—normally the largest venous valve leaflet in the body. This is why septum primum normally is directly continuous with the left wall of the inferior vena cava.[7] The other, normally much smaller component of the left venous valve mechanism is known as the **left venous valve**. It is applied to the right atrial surface of septum primum inferiorly and is often difficult to see grossly. When visible, there may be an **interseptovalvular space**, a space between septum primum to the left and the left venous valve to the right.[7]

Because septum primum is really a large venous valve, this appears also to explain why septum primum often contains numerous very small **fenestrations**. Venous valves, like septum primum, often also contain small fenestrations.

Have you ever thought how very strange it is that the largest venous valve in the body, the sinoatrial valve, is normally grossly incompetent (regurgitant)? We are aware of no other vascular valve in the body that *normally* is severely regurgitant. We think that this interpretation is not really true as far as the sinoatrial valve is concerned. Septum primum, which is the main component of the left leaflet of the sinoatrial valve,[7] normally prevents regurgitation from the *left* atrium into the right atrium and the venae cavae. Consequently, **the body's largest venous valve, the sinoatrial valve, normally is not incompetent**. The sinoatrial valve only becomes incompetent if septum primum is deficient, thereby creating an ostium secundum type of atrial septal defect. Aristotle and Galen thought that what we call the right atrium is part of the great vein (superior vena cava plus inferior vena cava), because the right atrium is not separated by valves from the venae cavae but instead is confluent with these great veins.

Septum primum is the flap valve of the foramen ovale that is torn during balloon atrial septostomy, which was developed by Dr. Bill Rashkind to increase mixing at the atrial level in physiologically uncorrected transposition of the great arteries.

Septum primum grows upward (cephalically)[7] not downward, as many textbooks of embryology say.

Septum primum does not grow downward to close ostium primum, as has been stated erroneously. The septum of the atrioventricular canal is closed initially by the endocardial cushions of the atrioventricular canal. Common atrioventricular canal is an endocardial cushion defect (not a septum primum defect). It is possible to have a complete form of common atrioventricular canal with a normally formed septum primum. The atrial septum may be intact, even though a large atrioventricular septal defect coexists.

Deficiency of septum primum is the most common cause of an ostium secundum type of atrial septal defect. Other causes of a secundum type of atrial septal defect include a deficient superior limbic band of septum secundum, as with left-sided juxtaposition of the atrial appendages; deficiency of both septum primum and the superior limbic band of septum secundum; and distention of the right atrium, as with a vein of Galen shunt in the head but without deficiency of either septum primum or septum secundum. In the latter situation, the secundum atrial septal defect undergoes spontaneous closure following successful clipping of the vein of Galen shunt, with volume unloading of the right atrium and disappearance of right atrial distention.

Thus, a secundum atrial septal defect may be associated with deficiency of septum primum, deficiency of septum secundum (superior limbic band), or both—or neither (with right atrial distention).

What is a patent foramen ovale? An open (patent) oval foramen (foramen ovale) is a communication between the right and left atria through which a probe can be passed. The probe passes beneath the downwardly facing concavity of the superior limbic band of septum secundum (see Figs. 3.4 and 3.5) and above the upwardly facing concavity of septum primum (see Figs. 3.9 and 3.10). The patent foramen ovale has some right-left length, as it passes beneath septum secundum and above septum primum. A patent foramen ovale typically does not permit left-to-right shunting; otherwise the communication would be regarded as an ostium secundum type of atrial septal defect. Hence, patent foramen ovale has the connotation that it is a probe-patent interatrial communication that does not permit shunting.

An intact atrial septum is known as a **fossa ovalis** (oval ditch or depression). A fossa ovalis has the connotation that it cannot possibly permit any kind of shunting (left-to-right or right-to-left) no matter how distended the atria may become, because the atrial septum is anatomically sealed. Some people speak of a fossa ovalis type of atrial septal defect. We regard this designation as an oxymoron.

What is the difference between a patent foramen ovale and an ostium secundum? A patent foramen ovale is an interatrial communication with some right-left length. It passes under the superior limbic band of septum secundum (see Figs. 3.4 and 3.5), and it passes over the superior margin of septum primum (see Figs. 3.9 and 3.10). In contrast, ostium secundum is the space above the superior margin of septum primum (see Figs. 3.9 and 3.10). Ostium secundum does not extend beneath the superior limbic band of septum secundum. Ostium secundum has almost no right-to-left length, being only as wide as septum primum. Fenestrations or defects in septum primum are called that. (We do not call them ostia secunda. As will be explained in Chapter 9 on interatrial communications, we think that the conventional account of the formation of ostium secundum is incorrect.)

Embryologically, the left atrium consists of three main components:

1. The venous component is the common pulmonary vein, which normally is incorporated into the left atrium up to just beyond the primary division of each branch. There is really only one pulmonary vein, not four (two left and two right) or five (two left and three right). The appearance of four or five pulmonary veins is produced by the incorporation of the left and right branches of the common pulmonary vein up to just beyond the first division of each branch.[7] The common

pulmonary vein normally appears at 27 days in the human embryo.[7]

2. The primitive atrial component is the atrial appendage.
3. The atrioventricular canal component consists of the mitral valve and the lower portion of the atrial septum, that is, that portion of the atrioventricular septum that lies between the mitral annulus below and the atrial septum (inferior limbic band component) above.

Why do the right and left atrial appendages have such different shapes? (See Fig. 3.3 versus Fig. 3.8.) We think that the answer, at least in part, is hemodynamics. The blood flows from the placenta, up the inferior vena cava and into the right atrium, distending the right atrial appendage and thereby incorporating the appendage into the main cavity of the right atrium.

Some of the inferior vena caval return arches over the top of septum primum like a waterfall. On the left atrial side, the blood passes down through the mitral valve and into the left ventricle. In other words, the blood of the via sinistra passes downward *behind* the left atrial appendage as it passes through the mitral valve and into the left ventricle. The blood that arches over septum primum does not flow into the left atrial appendage, distending it. The right-to-left cascade of the via sinistra occurs behind the left atrial appendage. Consequently, the left atrial appendage remains an appendix to the left atrial cavity rather than being distended and incorporated into it.

In the heterotaxy syndrome with asplenia, why may both atrial appendages look quite rightish?

Conversely, in the heterotaxy syndrome with polysplenia, why may both atrial appendages look quite leftish? Again, we think the answer is hemodynamics. **In the asplenia syndrome**, the inferior vena cava almost always is intact (not interrupted). Consequently, the blood from the placenta flows up the inferior vena cava and into the right atrium. Because the atrial septum is often very defective and common atrioventricular canal frequently coexists, the blood returning to the heart by way of the inferior vena cava flows into both atrial appendages, distending both and making both look rightish.

By contrast, **in the polysplenia syndrome**, the inferior vena cava is often interrupted from the renal veins below to the hepatic veins above. Consequently, the blood from the lower body must return to the heart by way of the azygos vein(s). The azygos vein can be right sided, left sided, or even bilateral. Hence, the blood from the placenta and lower body returns to the heart via a markedly enlarged azygos vein that joins a superior vena cava. The blood then passes down the superior vena cava, into the atrium, and passes *behind* both atrial appendages as it goes through an atrioventricular valve to reach the ventricular level. Since the augmented superior vena caval blood flow does not flow into either atrial appendage—but instead passes behind the appendages—consequently both atrial appendages remain undistended and hence both appear leftish.

We think that the concept of atrial isomerism, or atrial appendage isomerism, is wrong.[8] The right atrium, or the right atrial appendage, is not really bilateral. Similarly, the left atrium, or the left atrial appendage, also is not really bilateral. In some, but by no means all cases of viscera heterotaxy with asplenia or polysplenia, bilaterally similar appearing appendages can be found—we think for the aforementioned hemodynamic reasons. In many cases of visceral heterotaxy with asplenia or polysplenia, however, the atria and the atrial appendages are morphologically very different (not "isomeric").[9]

Hence, we think that just as each human being has only one morphologically left ventricle and one morphologically right ventricle, so too each human being has only one morphologically right atrium or right atrial appendage and only one morphologically left atrium or left atrial appendage.

Once one understands that the concept of atrial or atrial appendage isomerism is erroneous, then it is readily possible to diagnose the morphologic identities of the atria in virtually all cases of the polysplenia syndrome and in the majority of cases of the asplenia syndrome.[9] Diagnoses such as "atrial situs ambiguus," "right atrial isomerism," "right atrial appendage isomerism," "left atrial isomerism," or "left atrial appendage isomerism" mean that the morphologic anatomic identities of the atria are *un*diagnosed. All such cases await accurate morphologic anatomic diagnosis (see Figs. 3.3, 3.4, 3.7, and 3.8). For detailed consideration of the heterotaxy syndromes with asplenia, polysplenia, and occasionally with a normally formed spleen, please see Chapter 29.

The morphologic anatomic features of the right atrium and left atrium are summarized in Table 3.1.

The Morphologically Right Ventricle

Angiocardiographically, the morphologically right ventricle is the coarsely trabeculated one (Fig. 3.11). The infundibulum (or

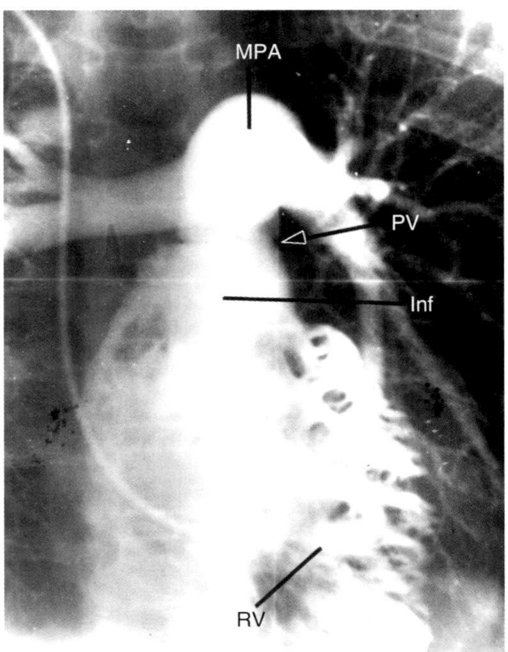

Fig. 3.11 Morphologically right ventricle *(RV)* as seen by selective right ventricular angiocardiography, posteroanterior projection. Noteworthy are the coarse trabeculations, the well expanded infundibulum *(Inf)*, and the good-sized pulmonary valve *(PV)* and main pulmonary artery *(MPA)*. (From Van Praagh R, Van Praagh S, Nebesar RA, et al. Tetralogy of Fallot: underdevelopment of the pulmonary infundibulum and its sequelae. *Am J Cardiol*. 1970;26:25, with permission.)

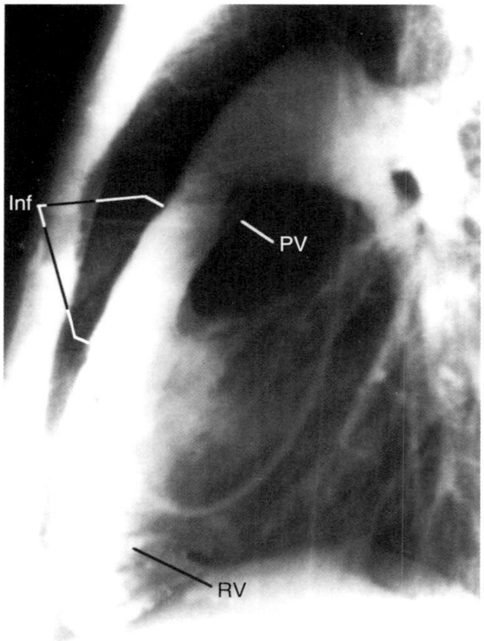

Fig. 3.12 Morphologically right ventricle *(RV)* as seen by selective right ventricular angiocardiography, left lateral projection. The subpulmonary infundibulum *(Inf)* is better seen in the lateral projection than in the posteroanterior projection. The normal pulmonary valve *(PV)* sits high and anteriorly atop the well-expanded subpulmonary conus. (From Van Praagh R, Van Praagh S, Nebesar RA, et al. Tetralogy of Fallot: underdevelopment of the pulmonary infundibulum and its sequelae. *Am J Cardiol.* 1970;26:25, with permission.)

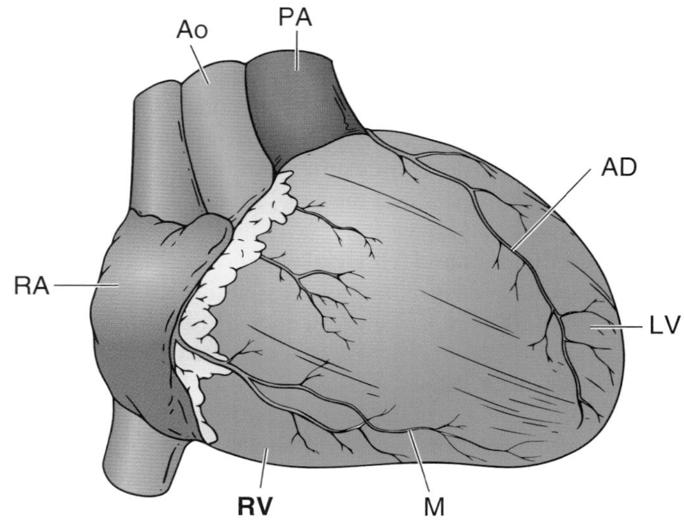

Fig. 3.13 Morphologically right ventricle *(RV)*, exterior view. Like the right atrium *(RA)*, the RV also has a triangular or pyramidal external shape. The anterior and diaphragmatic surfaces of the RV meet, forming an angle of less than 90 degrees—an acute angle. Hence the anteroinferior margin of the RV is known as the acute margin. The distribution of the coronary arteries is highly characteristic of the RV. Note in particular the acute marginal branch *(M)* of the right coronary artery, plus the preventricular branch and the conal branch (most superiorly). *Ao,* Aorta; *AD,* anterior descending coronary artery; *LV,* morphologically left ventricle; *PA* pulmonary artery. (From Van Praagh R, Vlad P. Dextrocardia, mesocardia, and levocardia: the segmental approach to diagnosis in congenital heart disease. In Keith JD, Rowe RD, Vlad P, eds. *Heart Disease in Infancy and Childhood.* 3rd ed. New York: Macmillan Publishing; 1978:638, with permission.)

conus) normally appears relatively smooth and well expanded in the posteroanterior projection.

Infundibulum means funnel (Latin), this being the inside appearance of the right ventricular outflow tract. **Conus** means cone (Latin), this being the outside appearance of the right ventricular outflow tract, as in an embryonic reconstruction. This is why *infundibulum* has more of an anatomic connotation, whereas *conus* has more of an embryologic connotation, but both terms are used as synonyms.

The right ventricular sinus (body, or inflow tract) is usually better seen in the posteroanterior projection (see Fig. 3.11), whereas the infundibulum often is better seen in the lateral projection (Fig. 3.12).

Anatomically, the external appearance of the morphologically right ventricle appears triangular, as viewed externally from the front (Fig. 3.13). In this respect it resembles the right atrium, which also has a triangular external appearance (see Fig. 3.13). The right ventricle, viewed from the front, resembles a pyramid. The base of the pyramid rests on the diaphragm, whereas the apex of the pyramid blends with the main pulmonary artery.

Along the base of this pyramid, the anterior surface of the right ventricle merges with the diaphragmatic surface. This margin of the right ventricle, between the anterior and diaphragmatic surfaces, is known as the **acute margin** (*margo acutis*, Latin), because these two surfaces meet at an angle of less than 90 degrees. (As in geometry, an angle less than 90 degrees is regarded as an acute angle, whereas an angle greater than 90 degrees is considered to be an obtuse angle.)

The epicardial branches of the right coronary artery are also distinctive and hence diagnostically helpful. Note the conal or preventricular branches and the acute marginal branch of the right coronary artery (see Fig. 3.13). The acute marginal branch is so called because it runs along the acute margin of the right ventricle.

Particularly when somewhat hypertrophied, the right ventricle often has a somewhat bulbous external appearance, reminiscent of its origin from the bulbus cordis. (Amusingly enough, *bulbus* in Latin means onion.)

The superficial myocardial fibers of the right ventricular free wall tend to run horizontally parallel to the diaphragm.

Consequently, all of the foregoing features often make it possible to make the diagnosis of morphologically right ventricle based on external inspection only. This is a very useful game for surgeons to learn how to play as soon as the pericardium is open: What is the ventricular shape? What does the pattern of the epicardial coronary arteries suggest? Is the ventricular margin acute (or obtuse)? Does the ventricle look bulbous? What is the orientation of the superficial myocardial fibers (horizontal or oblique)?

Anatomically, the internal appearance of the morphologically right ventricle (Figs. 3.14 through 3.16) displays **trabeculae carneae** (fleshy ridges, Latin) that are relatively coarse, few, and straight (compared with those of the morphologically

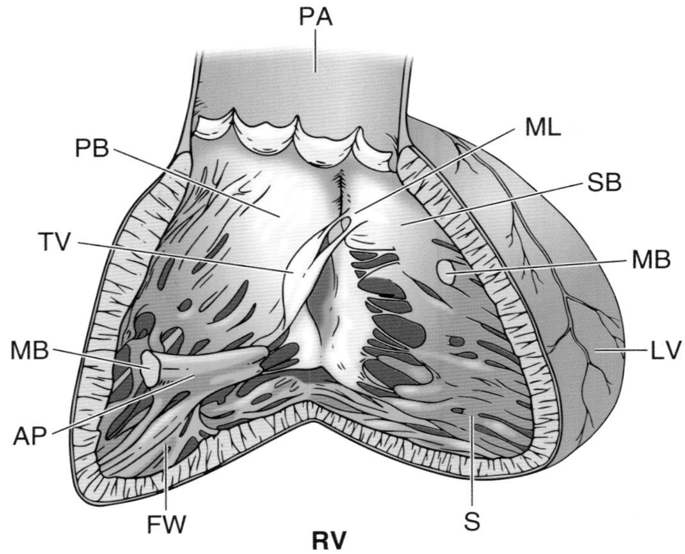

Fig. 3.14 Morphologically right ventricle *(RV)*, diagrammatic interior view. The trabeculae carneae (fleshy ridges) of the RV are few, coarse, and straight compared with those of the left ventricle *(LV)*. The papillary muscles of the RV are numerous, small, and arise from the septal surface *(S)* and from the free-wall surface *(FW)*. The anterior papillary muscle *(AP)* is the only relatively large papillary muscle of the RV. The tricuspid valve *(TV)* attaches to both the septal and the free-wall surfaces, its leaflets being of approximately the same depth. The septal band *(SB)* runs on the anterosuperior portion of the right ventricular septal surface. The moderator band *(MB)* runs from the septal band medially to the superior portion of the anterior papillary muscle group laterally. The right bundle branch (RBB) of the atrioventricular conduction system emerges on the septal band just beneath the papillary muscle of the conus—also known as the muscle of Lancisi or the muscle of Luschka *(ML)*. The RBB runs down the septal band, close to its inferior margin, to the moderator band, on which it crosses from the septal surface to the anterior papillary muscle group and thence as the Purkinje network onto the right ventricular free wall. The RV normally ejects into the pulmonary artery *(PA)*. The pulmonary valve above and the tricuspid valve below are separated by the subpulmonary conus or infundibulum. The conal septum, which lies beneath the septal commissure of the pulmonary valve (at the aortopulmonary septum), extends out onto the parietal or free wall of the RV as the parietal band *(PB)*. Note the line of fusion or "suture" between the parietal band (conal septum) laterally and the septal band medially. The parietal band is also known as the crista supraventricularis (supraventricular crest) and as the ventriculoinfundibular fold. The septal band plus the moderator band are also known collectively as the trabecula septomarginalis or the septomarginal trabeculation. (From Van Praagh R, Vlad P. Dextrocardia, mesocardia, and levocardia: the segmental approach to diagnosis in congenital heart disease. In Keith JD, Rowe RD, Vlad P, eds. *Heart Disease in Infancy and Childhood.* 3rd ed. New York: Macmillan Publishing; 1978:638, with permission.)

left ventricle). The **papillary muscles** of the right ventricle are numerous and small, attaching to both the right ventricular septal surface and to the right ventricular free-wall surface. The smallness of the right ventricular papillary muscles makes right ventriculotomy readily possible.

The **tricuspid valve** leaflets are all of approximately the same depth. The anterior leaflet is a bit deeper than the others, but the difference is not great.

The tricuspid valve is **"septophilic"**; it "likes" the ventricular septum and attaches to it as well as to the free wall.

The number of tricuspid valve leaflets varies from two to four. In infants, the tricuspid valve often has only two leaflets—a parietal or free-wall leaflet and a septal leaflet. Throughout most of life, however, the tricuspid valve has three leaflets, because the parietal (free-wall) leaflet becomes subdivided into anterior and posterior portions by the insertion of the chordae tendineae (tendinous strings, Latin) from the anterior papillary muscle group. Late in life, after episodes of heart failure, an infundibular leaflet may appear between the anterior and septal leaflets of the tricuspid valve. An infundibular leaflet (beneath the infundibular septum) may also be associated with a ventricular septal defect.

The tricuspid valve reminds one of the riddle of the Sphinx, who asked all passersby: "What walks on four feet in the morning, on two feet at noon, and on three feet in the evening?" The Sphinx killed all who failed to answer her question, until Oedipus solved the riddle by saying, "Man crawls on all fours as a baby, walks upright in the prime of life, and uses a cane in old age." Similarly, the tricuspid valve has two leaflets in infancy, three leaflets in the prime of life, and four leaflets in old age.

Consequently, one cannot reliably identify the tricuspid valve simply by counting leaflets, contrary to what has often been said.

The right ventricular sinus (body, or inflow tract) normally is the lung pump. The tricuspid valve opens into it (see Fig. 3.15).

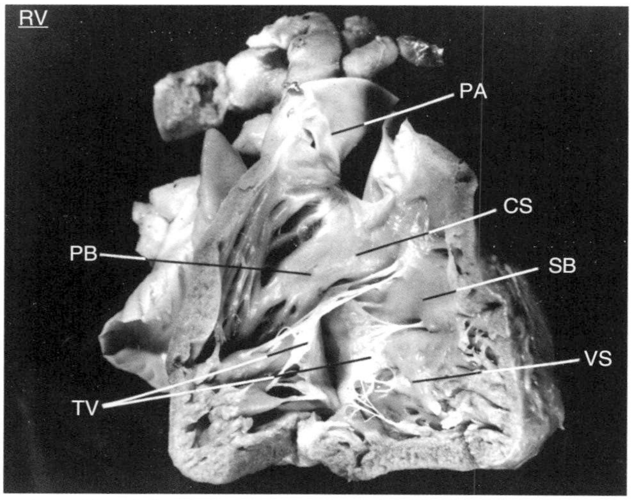

Fig. 3.15 Morphologically right ventricle *(RV)*, photographic interior view. The tricuspid valve *(TV)* attaches to the ventricular septum *(VS)* (the TV is "septophilic") as well as to the free wall. The papillary muscles are numerous but small. The trabeculations are few, coarse, and straight. There is pulmonary-tricuspid fibrous discontinuity because of the interposition of the normal subpulmonary conus. The conal septum *(CS)* extends onto the right ventricular parietal or free wall as the parietal band *(PB)*. The septal band *(SB)* is also well seen. The fusion line between the distal conal septum and the septal band is distinctly visible. The RV is the lung pump that normally ejects into the main pulmonary artery *(PA)*. (From Van Praagh R, Van Praagh S, Vlad P, et al. Anatomic types of congenital dextrocardia, diagnostic and embryologic implications. *Am J Cardiol*. 1964;13:510, with permission.)

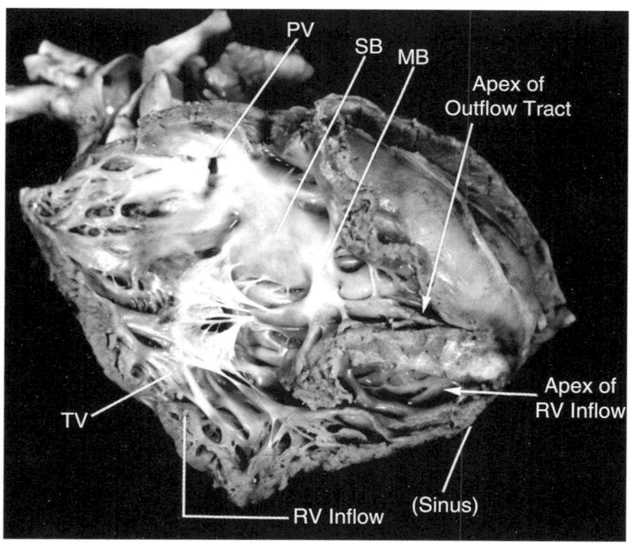

Fig. 3.16 The two apices of the morphologically right ventricle *(RV)*. The right ventricular sinus or inflow tract has an apex that is proximal (or upstream) relative to the septal and moderator bands. The infundibulum or outflow tract also has an apex, which is distal (or downstream) relative to the septal and moderator bands. The RV sinus and its apex and the infundibulum and its apex are most clearly exemplified by double-chambered right ventricle. *MB*, Moderator band; *PB*, parietal band; *PV*, pulmonary valve; *SB*, septal band; *TV*, tricuspid valve. (From Van Praagh R, Plett JA, Van Praagh S. Single ventricle - pathology, embryology, terminology and classification. *Herz*. 1979;4:113, with permission.)

The right ventricular sinus or pumping portion is smaller than is usually understood.

The right ventricular sinus below is demarcated from the infundibulum above by a ring of conal (infundibular) muscle. This **conal or infundibular ring** (see Fig. 3.15) consists of the conal septum that extends laterally on the free (or parietal) wall as the parietal band, the septal band, and the moderator band. This conal ring marks the beginning of the infundibulum, conus, or outflow tract that extends up to the semilunar valve level (normally, the pulmonary valve).

The **conal septum** lies beneath the septal commissure of the pulmonary and aortic valves, the **septal commissure** being located at the aortopulmonary septum. The septal commissure of the aortic valve is the intercoronary commissure. The **conal septum** normally separates the pulmonary valve above from the tricuspid valve below (see Figs. 3.14 through 3.16). The conal septum divides the pulmonary and aortic outflow tracts. From the right ventricular standpoint, the conal septum extends out onto the right ventricular parietal (free) wall. Hence, this structure is also known as the **parietal band**. The conal septum and parietal band plus the adjacent subsemilunar conal free wall together constitute the **distal or subsemilunar part of the conus.**

The septal band and the moderator band together constitute the **proximal or apical part of the conus.**

The distal or subsemilunar conus is the part that is abnormal in the conotruncal anomalies, such as transposition of the great arteries and double-outlet right ventricle.

The proximal or apical part of the conus is the portion that is abnormal in double-chambered right ventricle (also known as anomalous muscle bundles of the right ventricle).

The **septal band** is so called because it runs on the anterosuperior portion of the right ventricular septal surface.

The **moderator band** was so named by King[10] in 1837 because he thought that this extension from the septal band to the anterior papillary muscle group and the right ventricular free wall would moderate the degree of possible distention of the right ventricle in diastole. We now know that one of the functions of the moderator band is to carry the **right bundle** of the atrioventricular conduction system from the right ventricular septal surface to the anterior papillary muscle group and thence via the Purkinje network to the right ventricular free wall.

It is noteworthy that the right ventricle really has **two apices** (see Fig. 3.16). The apex of the right ventricular sinus (inflow tract) lies proximal and inferior to the moderator band. The apex of the infundibulum (conus, or outflow tract) lies distal and superior to the moderator band. This distinction between the right ventricular sinus and its apex and the infundibulum and its apex is seen most clearly in **double-chambered right ventricle.** This condition represents a failure of incorporation of the conus arteriosus into the right ventricle. Consequently, there is an obstructive separation between the right ventricular sinus proximally and the malincorporated conus distally, resulting in stenosis at mid-right ventricular level, that is, at the level of the septal and moderator bands.

The normal definitive right ventricle is very much a **composite structure**. The essence of the right ventricle is the right ventricular sinus or pump. The right ventricular sinus is its sine qua non. Without the right ventricular sinus—without the pumping portion—from the functional standpoint, one really does not have a right ventricle.

The right ventricular sinus can be absent, resulting in single (unpaired) left ventricle. The proximal or atrioventricular valve connector is present; hence, the tricuspid valve opens into the left ventricle, resulting in double-inlet left ventricle. The distal or conal connector is also present. Consequently, an infundibular outlet chamber is typically present, despite absence of the right ventricular sinus, emphasizing the composite nature of the normal definitive right ventricle. The right ventricular sinus is different from the atrioventricular canal (tricuspid valve) and is also different from the conus. The atrioventricular canal, the right ventricular sinus, and the conus arteriosus are really three different structures that normally blend in the definitive right ventricle.

The tricuspid valve and right ventricular sinus can both be atretic but with a normal subpulmonary infundibulum, as in typical tricuspid atresia. This again emphasizes that the right ventricular sinus and the infundibulum are really two different structures. Tricuspid atresia again illustrates the composite nature of the normal definitive right ventricle.

The tricuspid valve and the right ventricular sinus can both be dysplastic but with a normal infundibulum and great arteries, as in typical Ebstein anomaly of the tricuspid valve (and right ventricular sinus). Again, the composite nature of the definitive right ventricle is illustrated clearly.

The parietal band has also been called the ventriculoinfundibular fold. We think that the parietal band is an infundibular fold, not really a *ventriculo*infundibular fold. However, the parietal band is an infundibular fold that borders on the underlying ventricle—normally the right ventricle (that is, the right ventricular sinus). Hence, the parietal band is an infundibular fold at the ventriculoinfundibular junction.

The septal band and the moderator band have collectively been called the **trabecula septomarginalis**, or the **septomarginal trabeculation**. Trabecula septomarginalis was the term that Julius Tandler applied in 1913 to what in English is known as the moderator band. Literally, *trabecula septomarginalis* (Latin) means septomarginal trabeculation, that is, the *trabeculation* that runs from the *septum* to the acute *margin* of the right ventricle. Accurately speaking, as Tandler[11] used it in 1913, this is the structure that in English is known as the moderator band. Recently, however, septomarginal trabeculation has been used to mean **the septal band plus the moderator band.** The "trabecular zone" of the right ventricle has been used to refer to the septal band, which is a broad smooth *non*trabeculated structure (see Figs. 3.14 through 3.16). The trabeculations of the right ventricular septal surface lie below the septal band.

There are four components that together make up the normal definitive right ventricle (Fig. 3.17):

1. the common atrioventricular canal,
2. the right ventricular sinus,

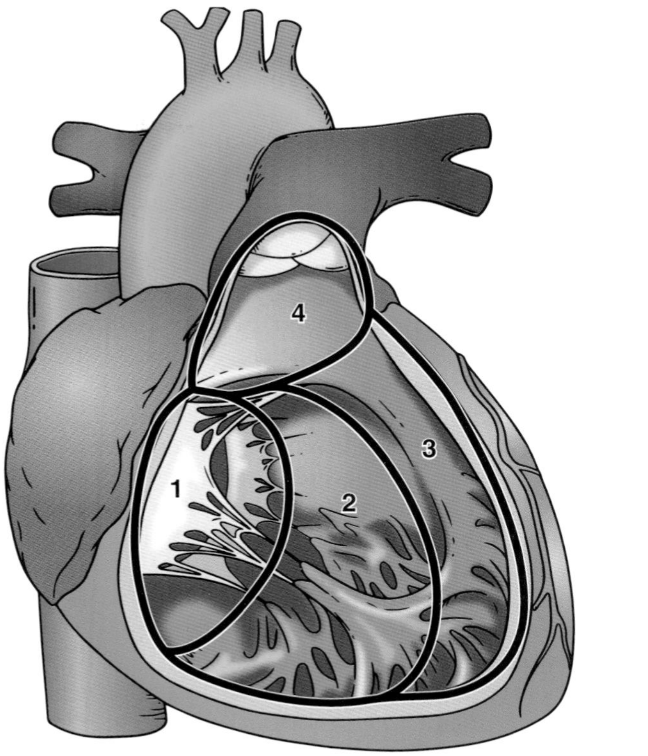

Fig. 3.17 The four component parts of the morphologically right ventricle: Component 1 is the atrioventricular canal. Component 2 is the right ventricular sinus or body. Component 3 is the septal band and moderator band. Component 4 is the conal septum and the parietal band. Components 1 and 2 together constitute the right ventricular inflow tract or inlet. Components 3 and 4 together constitute the conus, infundibulum, outflow tract, or outlet. (From Van Praagh R, Geva T, Kreutzer J. Ventricular septal defects: how shall we describe, name and classify them? *J Am Coll Cardiol.* 1989;14:1298, with permission.)

3. the septal band and moderator band, and
4. the conal septum and parietal band.

Components 1 and 2 together make up the **right ventricular inflow tract**. Components 3 and 4 make up the **right ventricular outflow tract.**

In different words, component 2, the right ventricular sinus or pump, is the sine qua non of the right ventricle. The proximal connector of the right ventricular sinus is the atrioventricular canal, component 1. The distal connector of the right ventricular sinus (component 2) is the conus—components 3 and 4. The proximal or septal band part of the conus, component 3, is important for incorporating the conus arteriosus into the right ventricular sinus. This septal band and moderator band component is malformed when the conus arteriosus is malincorporated into the right ventricular sinus, as in double-chambered right ventricle. The distal or parietal band part of the conus, component 4, is important for performing Mother Nature's arterial switch operation. The distal or subsemilunar part of the conus is malformed in the so-called conotruncal malformations, which are really just conal malformations (the great arteries per se being normal), such as typical transposition of the great arteries and the Taussig–Bing type of double-outlet right ventricle.

The understanding of the four main components of the right ventricle (see Fig. 3.17) is important for the understanding of **ventricular septal defects**. This understanding (see Fig. 3.17) explains why ventricular septal defects are located where they are. Ventricular septal defects occur at the junctions of these four components. Ventricular septal defects also occur when one or more of these four components are deficient or absent.

The conduction system of the right ventricle is the right bundle branch. This is the superior radiation. In the right ventricle, there is no inferior radiation. The conduction system corresponds to the papillary musculature. In the right ventricle, there is often only one well-formed papillary muscle group—the anterior, to which the right bundle branch runs. The other right ventricular papillary muscles are often little more than enlarged trabeculae carneae. The right bundle appears just beneath the papillary muscle of the conus (also known as the muscle of Lancisi, the muscle of Luschka, or the medial papillary muscle). The right bundle branch then courses down the septal band to the moderator band and thence to the anterior papillary muscle group and the right ventricular free wall.

The right bundle is often visible macroscopically, particularly where it emerges just beneath the papillary muscle of the conus and courses down the septal band, parallel with and closer to the inferior margin than to the superior margin of the septal band. The right bundle branch looks like a linear streak, 1 mm or less in diameter, brownish white in fixed heart specimens and creamy white in fresh heart specimens and in the operating room. Because the right bundle can be visualized with practice, it is possible to avoid transfixing the right bundle with needles and sutures in the operating room during, for example, patch closure of ventricular septal defects, thereby avoiding right bundle branch block.

It is often said that the right ventricle is a one-coronary ventricle—the right coronary artery. This is almost true, except for the small conal branch, which is really the artery of the conus arteriosus. So, the right ventricle often has **two coronary arteries** in the right coronary sinus of Valsalva of the aortic valve: a large right coronary artery to the right and a smaller conal artery to the left.

The stratum spongiosum/stratum compactum ratio is large. There is often more trabeculated (spongiosum) than compact (compactum) myocardium in the right ventricular free wall.

The Morphologically Left Ventricle

Angiocardiographically, the morphologically left ventricle appears minimally or finely trabeculated both in the posteroanterior and in the lateral projections (Fig. 3.18). The aortic valve

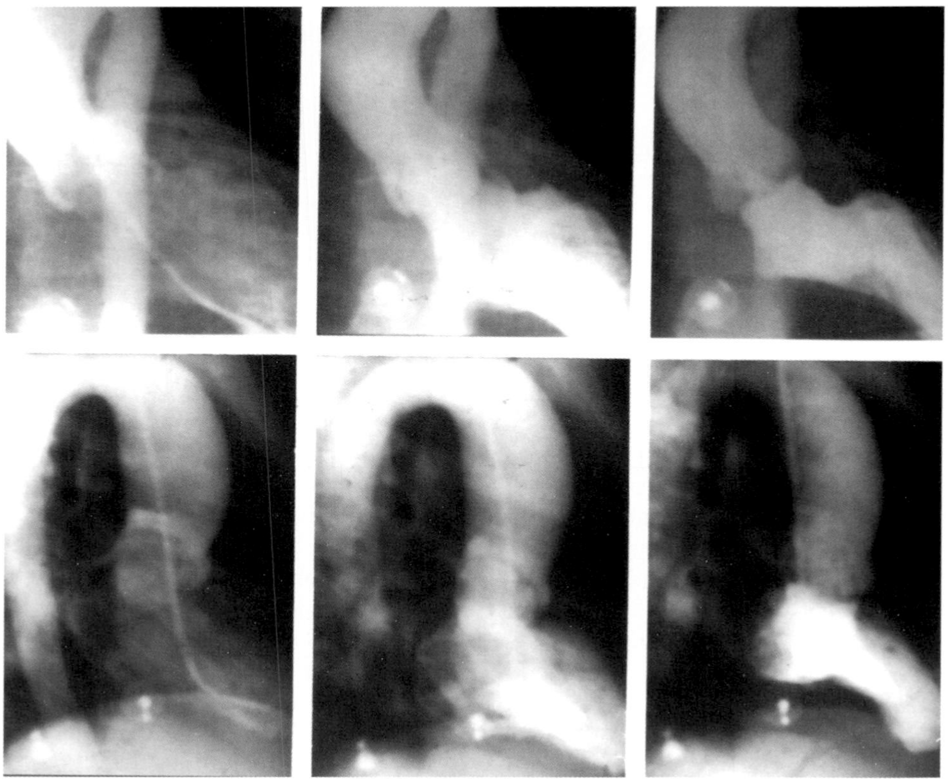

Fig. 3.18 Morphologically left ventricle, viewed angiocardiographically: top row, posteroanterior projection; bottom row, simultaneous right lateral projection. Note the ellipsoidal shape and minimal trabeculation of the left ventricle. The normally related aortic valve is low and posterior, close to the mitral valve, reflecting the normal absence of subaortic conal free-wall musculature, which permits the normal aortic-mitral approximation and fibrous continuity. (From Van Praagh R. Conotruncal malformations. In Barratt-Boyes BG, Neutze JM, Harris EA, eds. *Heart Disease in Infancy, Diagnosis and Surgical Treatment.* Edinburgh and London: Churchill Livingstone; 1973:141, with permission.)

normally is low and posterior, on top of the mitral valve, reflecting the normal absence of subaortic conal musculature.

Anatomically, the external appearance of the morphologically left ventricle is specific (Fig. 3.19). The shape of the left ventricle is like a bullet or a torpedo. Consequently, the left ventricular free wall has what is described as an obtuse margin, that is, it forms an angle of greater than 90 degrees.

The coronary arteries also are characteristic. The anterior and posterior descending coronary arteries indicate where the ventricular septum is. The free-wall branches tell you where the anterolateral and posteromedial papillary muscle groups are located. The superior free-wall branch is known as the diagonal artery. It usually arises from the left anterior descending coronary artery and supplies the region of the anterolateral papillary muscle group. The inferior free-wall artery is known as the obtuse marginal branch. It arises from the left circumflex coronary artery and helps to supply—along with the posterior descending—the posteromedial papillary muscle group.

Hence, the shape and distribution of the coronary arteries of the left ventricle are specific (see Fig. 3.19) and very different from those of the right ventricle (see Fig. 3.13).

The internal appearance of the morphologically left ventricle is distinctive (Figs. 3.20 and 3.21). The left ventricular septal surface superiorly is smooth (nontrabeculated). The apical third to half of the left ventricular septal surface displays numerous fine oblique trabeculae carneae that form a lattice-like mesh. The smallness of these trabeculations explains why the left ventricle appears minimally trabeculated by angiocardiography (see Fig. 3.18).

The papillary muscles of the left ventricle are few, but large (see Figs. 3.20 and 3.21). Both papillary muscle groups—the anterolateral and the posteromedial—arise from the left ventricular free wall. **The anterolateral group** is superior and remote from the septum, whereas **the posteromedial** group is inferior and adjacent to the septum.

The anterolateral papillary muscle group receives the superior (or anterior) radiation of the left bundle branch of the atrioventricular conduction system. The posteromedial papillary muscle group receives the inferior (or posterior) radiation of the left bundle branch of the atrioventricular conduction system.

Hence, the radiations of the conduction system and the papillary muscles correspond to each other. The left ventricle has superior and inferior radiations of the left bundle branch, corresponding to the superior and inferior papillary muscle groups of the left ventricle; whereas the right ventricle has a superior radiation only (the right bundle branch), corresponding to the superior (anterior) papillary muscle group of the right ventricle. There is no inferior radiation of the right bundle branch; perhaps this is because the inferior (posterior) papillary muscles of the right ventricle are little more than enlarged trabeculations, there usually being no well-formed posterior papillary muscle group.

Because the papillary muscles of the left ventricle are large, they fill the interior of the left ventricular free wall to a major degree, making left ventriculotomy difficult or impossible, except at the apex, or high paraseptally (coronary artery branches permitting).

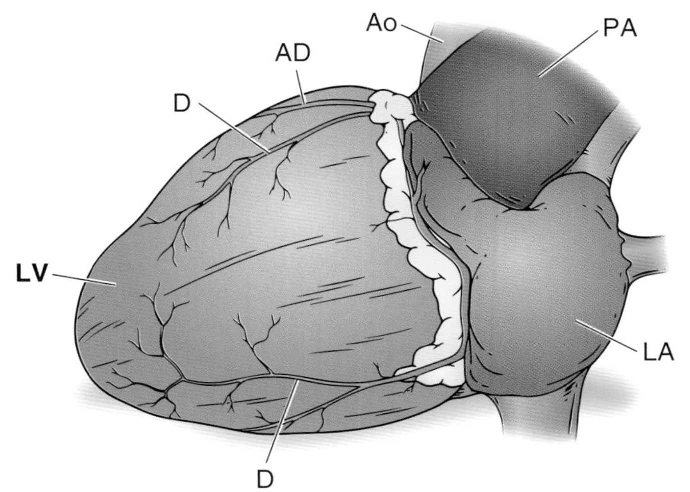

Fig. 3.19 Morphologically left ventricle *(LV)*, exterior view. Note that the LV is shaped like a bullet or a torpedo. The anterior descending *(AD)* coronary artery indicates the location of the interventricular septum. Running diagonally across the left ventricular wall are two coronary artery branches. The superior is known as the diagonal artery *(D)*, usually a branch of the AD that supplies the territory of the superior (anterolateral) papillary muscle group. The inferior free-wall artery, known as the obtuse marginal coronary, is a branch of the left circumflex that helps to supply the territory of the inferior (posteromedial) papillary muscle group. *Ao,* Ascending aorta; *LA,* morphologically left atrium; *PA,* pulmonary artery. (From Van Praagh R, Vlad P. Dextrocardia, mesocardia, and levocardia: the segmental approach to diagnosis in congenital heart disease. In Keith JD, Rowe RD, Vlad P, eds. *Heart Disease in Infancy and Childhood.* 3rd ed. New York: Macmillan Publishing; 1978:638, with permission.)

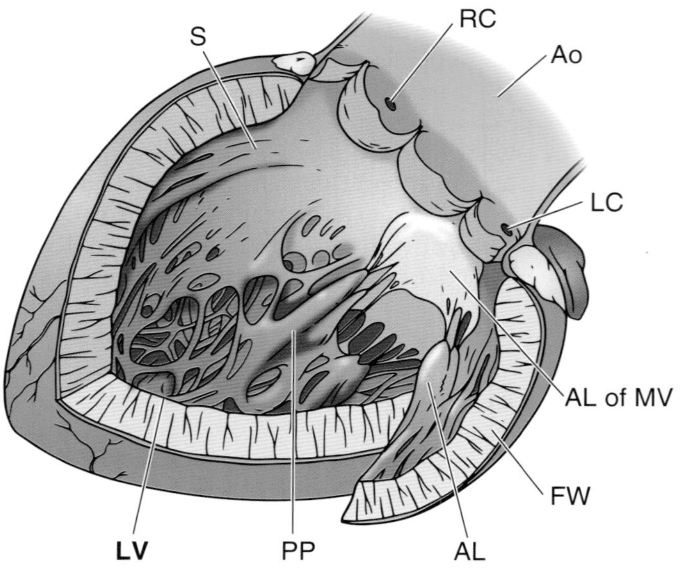

Fig. 3.20 Morphologically left ventricle *(LV)*, diagrammatic view of the interior. The superior septal surface *(S)* is smooth, whereas the inferior septal surface is characterized by numerous small, oblique trabeculations that form a lattice-like mesh. The superior or anterolateral *(AL)* and the inferior or posteromedial *(PP)* papillary muscle groups are large and originate only from the left ventricular free wall *(FW)*. The noncoronary-left coronary *(LC)* commissure of the aortic valve normally sits above the middle of the anterior leaflet of the mitral valve *(AL of MV)*. The noncoronary-right coronary *(RC)* commissure normally sits above the membranous portion of the interventricular septum. Immediately beneath the membranous septum is the left bundle of the atrioventricular conduction system. The superior and inferior radiations of the left bundle can often be seen as whitish streaks arching across the smooth superior portion of the left ventricular septal surface, heading toward the superior *(AL)* and the inferior *(PP)* papillary muscle groups, respectively. (From Van Praagh R, Vlad P. Dextrocardia, mesocardia, and levocardia: the segmental approach to diagnosis in congenital heart disease. In Keith JD, Rowe RD, Vlad P, eds. *Heart Disease in Infancy and Childhood*. 3rd ed. New York: Macmillan Publishing; 1978:638, with permission.)

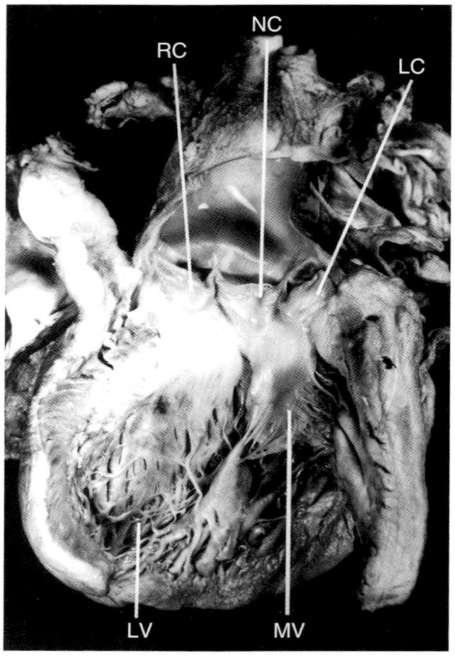

Fig. 3.21 Morphologically left ventricle *(LV)*, interior photographic view. Note the smooth left ventricular septal surface superiorly, the finely trabeculated septal surface inferiorly, the two large papillary muscle groups arising from the free wall only, the normal aortic-mitral fibrous continuity, the noncoronary-left coronary *(NC-LC)*, commissure that sits above the middle of the deep anterior leaflet of the mitral valve *(MV)*, and the noncoronary-right coronary *(NC-RC)*, commissure that sits above the membranous septum, which in turn is just above the left bundle branch of the atrioventricular conduction system. (From Van Praagh R, Van Praagh S, Nebesar RA, et al. Tetralogy of Fallot: underdevelopment of the pulmonary infundibulum and its sequelae. *Am J Cardiol*. 1970;26:25, with permission.)

Although it is usually said that there are only two papillary muscle groups in the left ventricle (the anterolateral and the posteromedial), in fact there is often a third group between the anterolateral and the posteromedial groups. This **middle group** also arises from the left ventricular free wall only. Normally, the chordae tendineae from the middle papillary muscle group run to the posterior leaflet of the mitral valve, typically to the central portion of the posterior mitral leaflet.

The mitral valve and its tensor apparatus (papillary muscles and chordae tendineae) may be described as **"septophobic."** Normally, the mitral valve does not attach to the ventricular septum. However, the posteromedial papillary muscle is often paraseptal—very close to the left ventricular septal surface.

The morphology of the atrioventricular valves corresponds to the ventricles of entry, not to the atria of exit, when there is single inlet each ventricle. For example, when an atrioventricular valve opens into a morphologically left ventricle, it is a **mitral valve**, even if the atrioventricular valve is opening out of a morphologically right atrium that is left sided in visceroatrial situs inversus. Similarly, when an atrioventricular valve opens into a morphologically right ventricle, it is a **tricuspid valve**, even if the atrioventricular valve is opening out of a morphologically left atrium that is right sided in visceroatrial situs inversus. Corrected transposition of the great arteries in situs solitus and in situs inversus illustrates the foregoing clearly.

Consequently, the atrioventricular valves are helpful in prenatal echocardiographic identification of the morphologically right and left ventricles. Is the atrioventricular valve "septophilic"—attaching to the ventricular septum, indicating that this valve is the tricuspid valve and hence that this ventricle is the right ventricle? Or is the atrioventricular valve "septophobic"—not attaching to the ventricular septum, indicating that this valve is the mitral valve and consequently that this ventricle is the left ventricle?

Just as one can often see with the naked eye the right bundle branch as it courses down the septal band, close to its inferior margin and heading toward the moderator band, so too one can often grossly see the superior and inferior radiations of the left bundle branch of the atrioventricular conduction system as they arch across the smooth superior portion of the left ventricular septal surface, heading toward the anterolateral and the posteromedial papillary muscle groups, respectively (see Fig. 3.20).

The left ventricle is almost all sinus, body, or inflow tract, that is, pumping portion. Normally, there is no subaortic conal free-wall musculature, thereby permitting direct aortic-mitral fibrous continuity (see Figs. 3.20 and 3.21). The noncoronary and left coronary leaflets of the aortic valve are in direct fibrous continuity with the anterior leaflet of the mitral valve. From the developmental standpoint, these aortic valve leaflets are in fibrous continuity with the superior endocardial cushion component of the anterior mitral leaflet, as the anomaly of common atrioventricular canal makes clear.

If one is resecting a subaortic fibrous membrane through the aortic valve, the following normal relationships are important (see Figs. 3.20 and 3.21):

The noncoronary/left coronary commissure of the aortic valve normally sits above the middle of the anterior leaflet of the mitral valve.

The noncoronary/right coronary commissure sits directly above the membranous septum (sometimes called the undefended space because it consists of fibrous tissue, without muscle), and the membranous septum in turn sits right above the left bundle branch of the atrioventricular conduction system. The subcoronary arc that extends anteriorly from beneath the right coronary ostium to beneath the left coronary ostium is the safest subaortic area in terms of surgical resection. Nonetheless, the superior radiation of the left bundle passes close beneath the subcoronary arc. The foregoing relations are all of importance to the surgeon to avoid trauma to the anterior leaflet of the mitral valve, to the membranous septum, to the muscular portion of the interventricular septum, and to the left bundle branch of the atrioventricular conduction system.

The mitral valve is both an inflow valve and an outflow valve. The deep anterior leaflet of the mitral valve is part of the left ventricular inflow tract and part of the left ventricular outflow tract. In contrast, the tricuspid valve is an inflow valve only.

The fact that the anterior mitral leaflet is an important part of the left ventricular outflow tract is relevant to the understanding of **hypertrophic obstructive cardiomyopathy** (also known as **idiopathic hypertrophic subaortic stenosis**). Asymmetric hypertrophy of the interventricular septum, an important feature of hypertrophic obstructive cardiomyopathy, reduces the space that normally exists between the left ventricular septal surface and the anterior leaflet of the mitral valve. Normally, the reason that the anterolateral papillary muscle of the left ventricle is anterior and *lateral*—that is, remote from the ventricular septum—is to create this interseptovalvular space that is necessary to have an unobstructed left ventricular outflow tract.

Asymmetric septal hypertrophy bulges into this space, reducing or even obliterating it. The anterolateral papillary muscle group and this portion of anterior leaflet of the mitral valve become antero*medial* relative to the left ventricular septal surface—not antero*lateral* as they normally should be. The anterior portion of the anterior mitral leaflet and the anterolateral papillary muscle group become much too close to the ventricular septum because of its asymmetric hypertrophy. Hence, the anterior leaflet of the mitral valve now becomes part of the left ventricular outflow tract obstruction during ventricular systole, resulting in systolic anterior movement of the mitral valve's anterior leaflet, often also with mitral regurgitation.

The foregoing is merely one example of why it is important to understand that the anterior leaflet of the mitral valve is a significant part of the left ventricular outflow tract.

The anterior leaflet of the mitral valve is a deep semicircular structure—much deeper than the posterior leaflet (see Fig. 3.9). In contrast, all of the tricuspid leaflets are of approximately the same depth (see Figs. 3.4, 3.5, 3.14, and 3.15). This leads to the question: Why is there this striking difference?

Our best present understanding is as follows: The anterior leaflet of the mitral valve is a dual or composite structure formed by the fusion of the superior and inferior endocardial cushions of the atrioventricular canal (as complete and partial forms of common atrioventricular canal demonstrate). The anterior mitral leaflet is a "doublet," formed from two components, whereas all other atrioventricular valve leaflets are "singletons," formed by only one component, that is, by adjacent atrioventricular endocardial cushion tissue (without fusion with other valve-forming tissue).

The anterior leaflet of the mitral valve normally is formed by the fusion of two components to form a semicircular door-like occluder that can close an approximately circular systemic atrioventricular orifice (see Fig. 3.9). The anterior mitral leaflet is the "door," whereas the much shallower posterior mitral leaflet is the "door jamb."

The tricuspid valve does not have a deep, semicircular, composite, doorlike anterior leaflet. Each of the tricuspid valve's leaflets are "singletons" (one-component structures) that are adequate for closing an approximately semicircular tricuspid orifice prenatally—when the ventricular septum is straight up and down (because right and left ventricular pressures are equal). The "singleton" tricuspid leaflets are also adequate to close the crescentic tricuspid orifice postnatally—when the ventricular septum bulges convexly into the right ventricular cavity (because left ventricular pressure is greater than right ventricular pressure).

So, the mitral and tricuspid valves are well designed for what each is normally required to do. But the tricuspid valve is not well designed to serve as a systemic atrioventricular valve, occluding an approximately circular atrioventricular orifice—as the tricuspid valve is required to do in atrial switch repairs for transposition of the great arteries (Mustard or Senning procedures). Not surprisingly, the tricuspid valve may permit central leak, and this tricuspid regurgitation may later present as right ventricular pump failure (dilated congestive cardiomyopathy).

Hence, the differences in the structure of the mitral and tricuspid valves are an important part of the reasons **an arterial switch procedure for transposition of the great arteries is preferable to an atrial switch procedure.** It is not only that the left ventricle appears to be better designed as a long-term systemic pump than is the right ventricle, but it is also that the mitral valve is better designed to serve as a systemic atrioventricular valve and to occlude an approximately circular orifice than is the tricuspid valve.

The papillary muscles of the left ventricle are a well-balanced pair—the anterolateral and the posteromedial, both of which arise from the free-wall surface of the left ventricle (see Figs. 3.20 and 3.21). By contrast, the papillary muscles of the right ventricle are not a well-balanced pair. They arise both from the septal and the free-wall surfaces. Many of the papillary muscles of the right ventricle are little more than enlarged trabeculae carneae.

If the right ventricle becomes distended for any reason, the tensor apparatus of the tricuspid valve may be pulled too far apart, because the tricuspid valve attaches to both the septum and the free wall, resulting in tricuspid regurgitation. Distention of the left ventricle, in contrast, is less likely to cause mitral regurgitation because all of the papillary muscles arise from the left ventricular free wall. Consequently, distention is less likely to pull the tensor apparatus too far apart, resulting in mitral regurgitation.

The left ventricle is a two-coronary ventricle: the anterior descending coronary artery and the left circumflex coronary artery. In contrast, the right ventricle has only one good-sized coronary artery, the right coronary.

Thus, virtually all features of the morphologically left ventricle are distinctive and different from those of the morphologically right ventricle. The salient morphologic anatomic differences are summarized in Table 3.2.

Although the morphologic anatomic details are very different between the anatomically left and right ventricles, nonetheless the left ventricle also consists of four main anatomic and developmental components (Fig. 3.22), as does the right ventricle (see Fig. 3.17).

The four main components of the morphologically left ventricle are (see Fig. 3.22):

1. the common atrioventricular canal, labeled component 1;
2. the finely trabeculated left ventricular sinus, labeled component 2;
3. the smooth left ventricular septal surface component, labeled part 3 and regarded as proximal conus (in direct continuity with the septal band of the right ventricle); and
4. the subsemilunar conal septum that lies beneath the right coronary leaflet of the normally related aortic valve, labeled component 4.

The left ventricular inflow tract is composed of components 1 and 2, and the left ventricular outflow tract consists of components 3 and 4 medially and component 1 (the anterior leaflet of the mitral valve) laterally (see Fig. 3.22).

Hence, both the right and left ventricles appear to consist of four main components (see Figs. 3.17 and 3.22), not three components as some have suggested. In order to avoid misunderstanding due to terminologic differences, we have simply

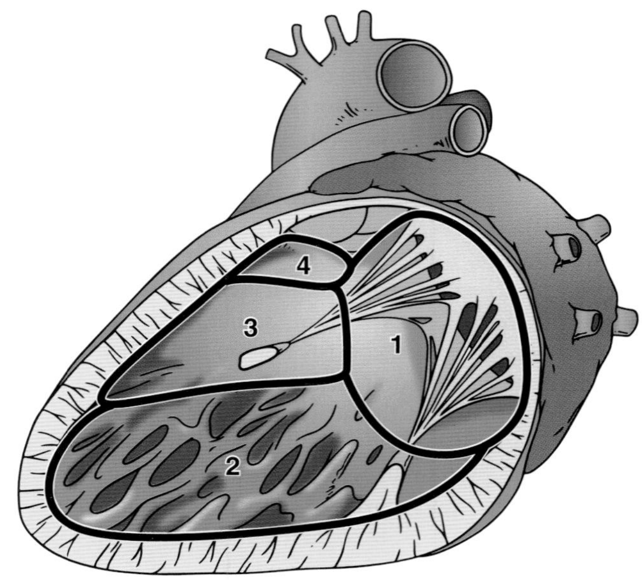

Fig. 3.22 The four component parts of the morphologically left ventricle (compare with Fig. 3.17). Component 1 is the atrioventricular canal. Component 2 is the finely trabeculated left ventricular sinus. Component 3 is the smooth superior component of the interventricular septum, continuous with the septal band of the right ventricle, and regarded as the proximal portion of the conus. Component 4 is the distal, subsemilunar conal septum. Components 1 and 2 together constitute the left ventricular inflow tract or inlet. Components 3 and 4, plus the anterior leaflet of the mitral valve make up the left ventricular outflow tract, or outlet. (From Van Praagh R, Geva T, Kreutzer J. Ventricular septal defects: how shall we describe, name and classify them? *J Am Coll Cardiol*. 1989;14:1298, with permission.)

TABLE 3.2 Morphologic Anatomic Features of the Right Ventricle and Left Ventricle

Anatomic Features	Right Ventricle	Left Ventricle
Trabeculae carneae	Coarse Few Straight	Fine Numerous Oblique
Papillary muscles	Numerous Small Septal and free wall	Two Large Free-wall origins only
Atrioventricular valve leaflets	Three Approximately equal depth	Two Very unequal depths
Infundibulum	Well developed	Absent
Semilunar-atrioventricular fibrous continuity	Absent	Present
Coronaries	One (right coronary artery)	Two (left anterior descending and circumflex branch of left coronary)
Conduction system radiations	One	Two

numbered the components from 1 to 4.[12] This is how the right ventricle (see Fig. 3.17) and left ventricle (see Fig. 3.22) really "come apart" with various malformations, revealing their component parts.

The malformations or "natural experiments" that are particularly revealing concerning the four components that make up both ventricles are:

1. common atrioventricular canal, complete and partial forms, that almost always have an atrioventricular septal defect involving the septum of the atrioventricular canal (component 1, see Figs. 3.17 and 3.22);
2. midmuscular ventricular septal defects between components 2 and 3 (see Figs. 3.17 and 3.22);
3. conoventricular type of ventricular septal defect, which may or may not be paramembranous, between component 4 above and component 3 below (see Figs. 3.17 and 3.22); and
4. conal septal defects, which are subpulmonary or subsemilunar, and are defects of component 4 (see Figs. 3.17 and 3.22).

Thus, Figs. 3.17 and 3.22 illustrate the four component parts of the right and left ventricles. This understanding in turn facilitates comprehension of the various anatomic types of ventricular septal defect.

Variations of the Conus Arteriosus

The anatomy of the conus arteriosus or infundibulum is exceedingly variable.

The four main anatomic types of conus are (Fig. 3.23):

1. **subpulmonary**, with normally related great arteries;
2. **subaortic**, with typical transposition of the great arteries;
3. **bilateral**—subpulmonary and subaortic, with typical double-outlet right ventricle; and
4. **bilaterally absent or very deficient**, neither subpulmonary nor subaortic, with some forms of double-outlet left ventricle.

The presence or absence of subsemilunar conal musculature prevents or permits semilunar-atrioventricular fibrous continuity, respectively (see Fig. 3.23).

1. **The normal subpulmonary conus** prevents pulmonary-atrioventricular fibrous continuity, whereas absence of subaortic conal free-wall musculature (remote from the conal septum) permits the normal aortic-mitral fibrous continuity. Normally, there is also a tenuous aortic-tricuspid fibrous continuity via the pars membranacea septi, because the membranous septum is intimately related to the tricuspid valve. The membranous septum essentially is tricuspid valve tissue. This will come as no surprise once it is recalled that the interventricular foramen normally closes only at its rightmost end, that is, at its tricuspid valve end.
2. **The subaortic conus** prevents aortic-atrioventricular valvar fibrous continuity, whereas absence of the subpulmonary conal free-wall musculature (remote from the conal septum) permits pulmonary-mitral fibrous continuity, as in typical transposition of the great arteries.

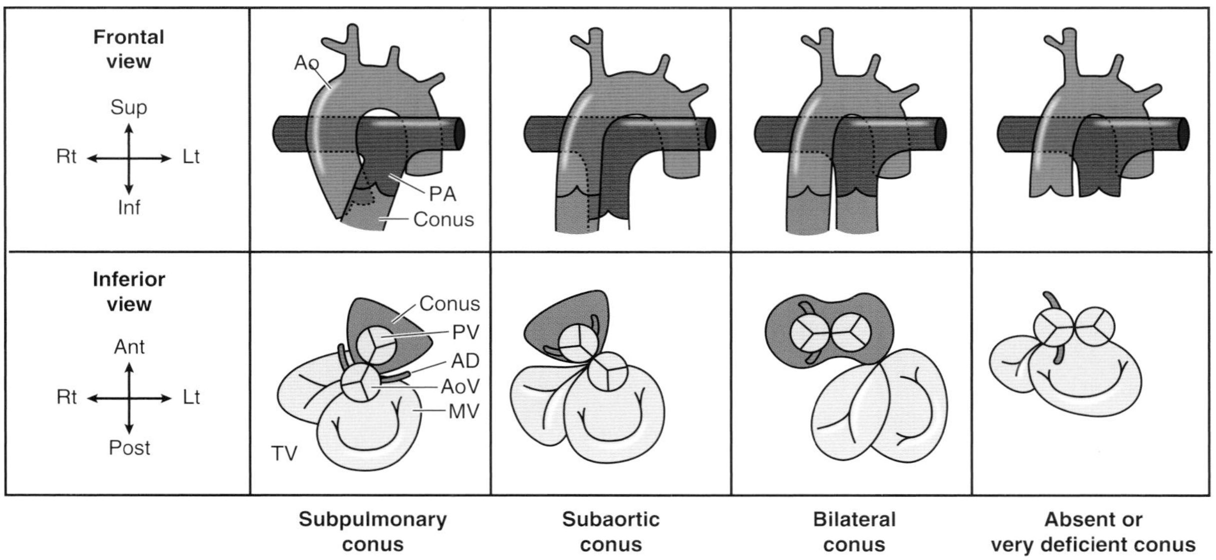

Fig. 3.23 Anatomic types of conus or infundibulum, upper row as seen from the front, lower row as viewed from below—as in short-axis subxiphoid two-dimensional echocardiogram, conal musculature indicated by hatching. The four main anatomic types of conus are: (1) **subpulmonary conus**, with fibrous continuity between aortic valve *(AoV)* and mitral valve *(MV)*, typically with normally related great arteries; (2) **subaortic conus**, with pulmonary-mitral fibrous continuity, with typical transposition of the great arteries; (3) **bilateral conus**—subaortic and subpulmonary, with no semilunar-atrioventricular fibrous continuity, often with double-outlet right ventricle; and (4) **bilaterally absent or very deficient conus**—with no or little subaortic and subpulmonary conus, permitting aortic-mitral and pulmonary-mitral fibrous continuity in double-outlet left ventricle, or aortic-tricuspid and pulmonary-mitral fibrous continuity in a rare form of transposition of the great arteries. *Ao,* Aorta; *AD,* anterior descending coronary artery; *PV,* pulmonary valve. (From Van Praagh R. Congenital heart disease: embryology, anatomy, and approach to diagnosis. In Van Praagh R, Van Praagh S, eds. *Diagnostic and Surgical Pathology of Congenital Heart Disease,* video series with syllabus. Boston: Children's Hospital and Harvard Medical School, 1991;1:48, with permission.)

3. **The bilateral conus**, characterized by the conal septum plus subaortic and subpulmonary conal free-wall musculature, prevents any semilunar-atrioventricular fibrous continuity, as in typical double-outlet right ventricle.
4. **The bilaterally absent conus**, in which the subaortic and the subpulmonary conal free-wall musculature is absent or very deficient, permits semilunar-to-atrioventricular fibrous continuity. There may be aortic-mitral and pulmonary-mitral direct fibrous continuity, as in a rare form of double-outlet left ventricle.[13] Or there may be aortic-tricuspid and pulmonary-mitral fibrous continuity, as in a rare form of transposition of the great arteries.[14]

Just as the anatomic types of atria and ventricles can readily be diagnosed because of their distinctive and different morphologic characteristics (see Figs. 3.1 through 3.22), so too the anatomic types of infundibulum (see Fig. 3.23) can also be readily diagnosed by angiocardiography or echocardiography or by magnetic resonance imaging, etc. Fig. 3.23 should also be understood to be a realistic diagram of the variation in the anatomy of the conus arteriosus (infundibulum). This is not a diagram of embryology, nor is it a developmental hypothesis.

The anatomic variations in conal anatomy do, however, have considerable developmental relevance. Briefly, the development of the conal connector between the ventricles (ventricular sinuses) and the great arteries appears to largely determine the ventriculoarterial alignments (which ventricle ejects into which great artery).[15] The so-called conotruncal anomalies (transposition, double-outlet right ventricle, double-outlet left ventricle, etc.) appear to be conal (infundibular) anomalies only. The great arteries per se seem to be normal. The malpositions of the great arteries appear to be secondary to the malformations of the conus, from which the great arteries arise.[15] This is thought to explain why aortopulmonary septal defect—a definite malformation of the great arteries involving the aortopulmonary septum—is so very rare in association with transposition or double-outlet right ventricle, etc. Aortopulmonary "window" is, we think, almost unknown in these "conotruncal" anomalies because the aortopulmonary septum is really normally formed in transposition and double-outlet right ventricle, contrary to what most books still say.

Examples of anatomic variations in the conus are:

Tetralogy of Fallot is characterized by a small-volume subpulmonary conus, well seen both angiocardiographically (Figs. 3.24, 3.25, and 3.26) and anatomically (Figs. 3.27 and 3.28). The hypoplastic subpulmonary conus of tetralogy is very different from the normal subpulmonary conus (see Figs. 3.11, 3.12, 3.14, and 3.15). Indeed, this is what we think tetralogy of Fallot really is: a hypoplastic small-volume subpulmonary conus and the sequelae thereof[16] (please see Chapter 20).

Transposition of the great arteries typically has a well-developed subaortic conus, preventing aortic-atrioventricular fibrous continuity, and absence of the subpulmonary conal free-wall muscle, permitting pulmonary-mitral fibrous continuity. Both the subaortic conus and the absence of a subpulmonary conal free wall are well seen angiocardiographically (Figs. 3.28

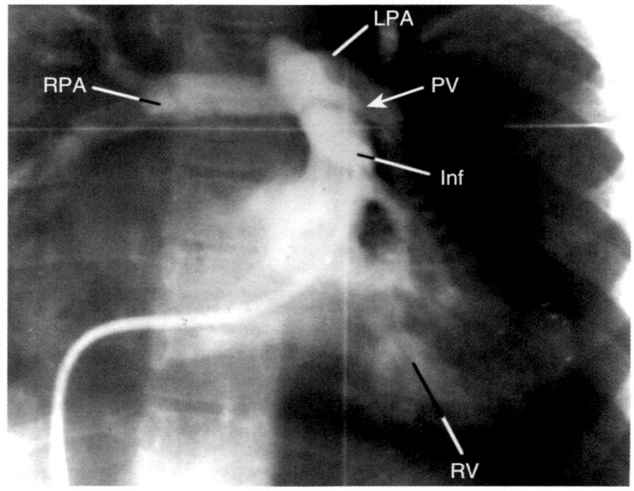

Fig. 3.24 The small-volume subpulmonary conus or infundibulum *(Inf)* in typical tetralogy of Fallot, shown by selective right ventricular angiocardiography, posteroanterior projection. Compare with Fig. 3.11. *LPA,* Left pulmonary artery; *PV,* pulmonary valve; *RPA,* right pulmonary artery. (From Van Praagh R. The segmental approach to diagnosis in congenital heart disease. In Bergsma D, ed. *Birth Defects: Original Article Series.* 1972;8:4; with permission.)

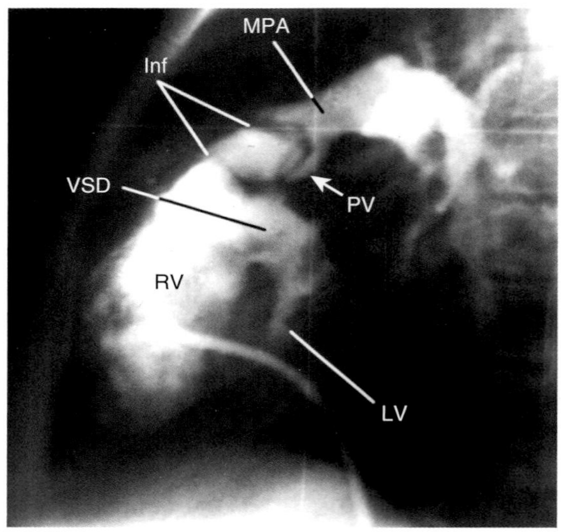

Fig. 3.25 The small-volume subpulmonary infundibulum *(Inf)* in typical tetralogy of Fallot, shown by selective right ventricular angiocardiography, left lateral projection (simultaneous with Fig. 3.24). Compare with Fig. 3.12. Note that the subpulmonary infundibulum in tetralogy of Fallot is distinctly smaller in both the posteroanterior and the lateral projections than normal. The somewhat thickened pulmonary valve *(PV)* in tetralogy is lower and more posterior than the normal, sitting atop the hypoplastic subpulmonary conus that has not elevated the pulmonary valve superiorly nor protruded it anteriorly to a normal degree. The anterosuperior malalignment of the hypoplastic conal septum is seen. The main pulmonary artery *(MPA)* and its branches are somewhat hypoplastic compared with normal (see Figs. 3.11 and 3.12). The right-to-left shunting of contrast from the right ventricle *(RV)* into the left ventricle *(LV)* through the ventricular septal defect *(VSD)* is also well seen. (From Van Praagh R. The segmental approach to diagnosis in congenital heart disease. In Bergsma D, ed. *Birth Defects: Original Article Series.* 1972;8:4; with permission.)

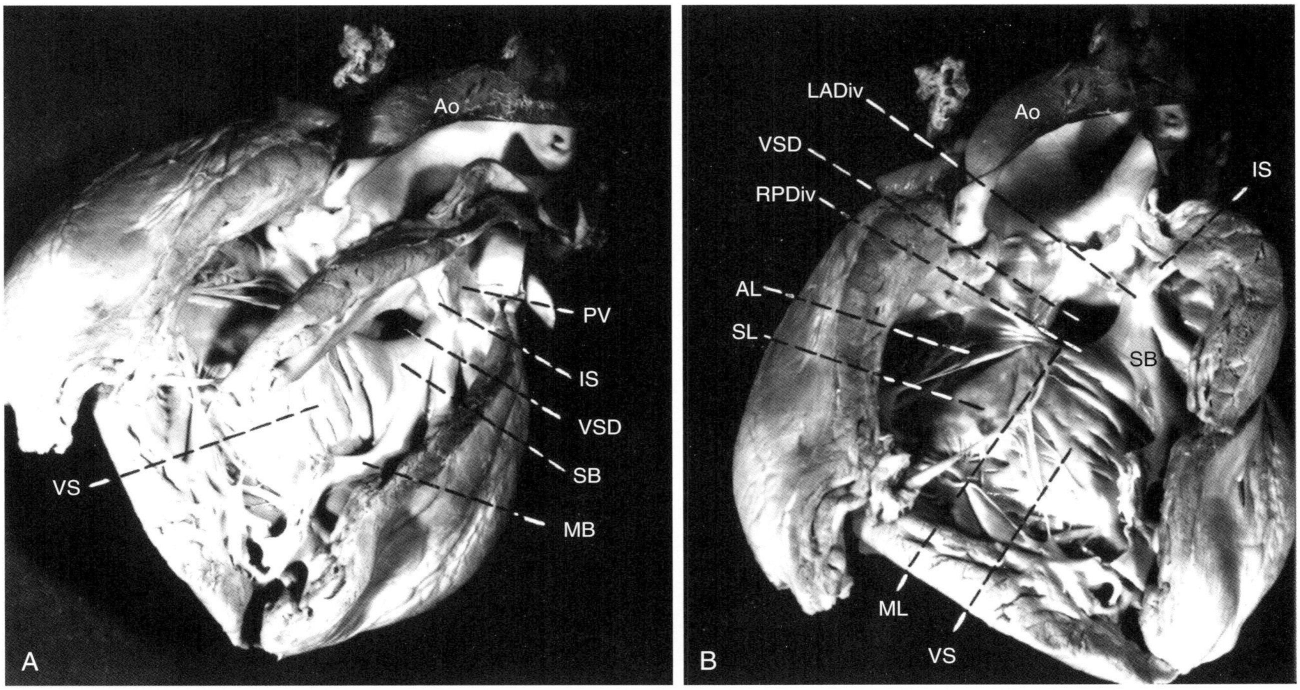

Fig. 3.26 Tetralogy of Fallot with moderate pulmonary outflow tract stenosis. The opened right ventricle in (A) shows the pulmonary outflow tract and in (B) shows the outflow tract into the overriding aorta. In (A), note the hypoplastic infundibular septum *(IS)*, the bicuspid pulmonary valve *(PV)*, and the right ventricular hypertrophy. In (B), the hypoplasia and anterosuperior malalignment of the IS are well seen. The IS is so anterosuperiorly displaced that it intersects with the left anterior division *(LADiv)* of the septal band *(SB)*, instead of filling the space above the SB, resulting in a ventricular septal defect *(VSD)*. *Ao*, Aorta; *AL*, anterior leaflet of the tricuspid valve; *MB*, moderator band; *ML*, muscle of Lancisi, also known as the papillary muscle of the conus; *RPDiv*, right posterior division of the septal band; *SL*, septal leaflet of the tricuspid valve; *VS*, ventricular septum. (From Van Praagh R, Van Praagh S, Nebesar RA, et al. Tetralogy of Fallot: underdevelopment of the pulmonary infundibulum and its sequelae. *Am J Cardiol*. 1970;26:25, with permission.)

and 3.29) and anatomically (Figs. 3.30 and 3.31). This is what we think typical transposition of the great arteries really is: a well-developed subaortic conus with absence of the subpulmonary conal free wall and the sequelae thereof[15,17,18] (please see Chapter 20).

Double-outlet right ventricle of the Taussig-Bing type[19,20] has a bilateral conus—subaortic and subpulmonary—that is well seen both angiocardiographically (Figs. 3.32 and 3.33) and anatomically (Figs. 3.34 and 3.35). We think that the development of a bilateral conus is important in the embryonic morphogenesis of the Taussig-Bing malformation (please see Chapter 23).

Double-outlet left ventricle with an intact ventricular septum[13] has a blind right ventricular outflow tract and a bilaterally absent conus with aortic-mitral and pulmonary-mitral fibrous continuity. The semilunar-mitral approximation, reflecting bilateral absence of subsemilunar conal musculature, is evident both angiocardiographically (Figs. 3.36 and 3.37) and anatomically (Fig. 3.38). We think that lack of development of conal musculature beneath both semilunar valves is an important part of the embryonic morphogenesis of this rare form of double-outlet left ventricle[13] (please see Chapter 24).

What is the basis of the morphologic anatomic differences between the left ventricle and the right ventricle? For example, why is the morphologically right ventricle the ventricle with the infundibulum or conus, whereas the morphologically left ventricle almost always has very little conus associated with it?

We think that the answer to this question is: Developmentally, the right ventricle is the superior ventricle, derived from the bulbus cordis (see Chapters 2 and 27). The conus arteriosus is cephalic and adjacent to the developing right ventricle. Consequently, from a **spatial standpoint**, the conus arteriosus can readily connect with the superior right ventricle. However, the left ventricle is the inferior ventricle, derived from the ventricle of the bulboventricular loop. Spatially, therefore, the conus arteriosus is close only to the superior right ventricle but not to the inferior left ventricle. Hence, the conus usually is incorporated mostly into the right ventricle and only minimally into the left ventricle.

From an **evolutionary standpoint**, it seems likely that the right ventricular sinus evolved from the proximal portion of the bulbus cordis; that is, the right ventricular sinus (the lung pump) may well have evolved beneath the septal and moderator bands. In this sense, the septal and moderator band regions of the proximal conus arteriosus may be regarded as the evolutionary "mother" of the right ventricular sinus. Consequently, there is a very close linkage between the septal and moderator bands above and the right ventricular sinus that normally pouches out

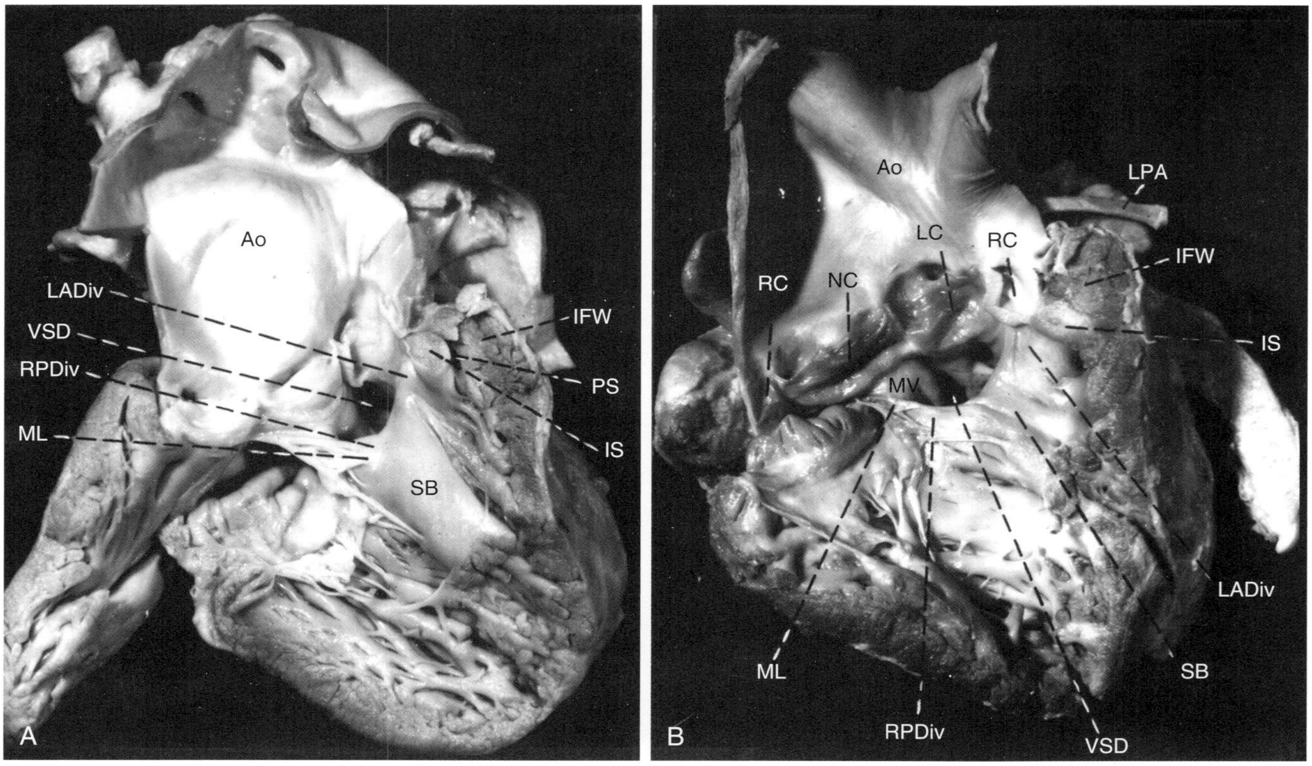

Fig. 3.27 Tetralogy of Fallot with severe pulmonary outflow tract obstruction in (A) and tetralogy of Fallot with pulmonary outflow tract atresia in (B). View of opened right ventricles and aortas. In (A), the infundibular septum *(IS)* is very close to the infundibular free wall *(IFW)*, resulting in severe infundibular and valvar pulmonary stenosis *(PS)*. The infundibular septum intersects with the ventricular septum somewhat anterior to the left anterior division *(LADiv)* of the septal band *(SB)*, leaving the space above the SB wide open, resulting in a large subaortic ventricular septal defect *(VSD)*. In (B), the IS and the infundibular free wall *(IFW)* are fused, resulting in pulmonary infundibular atresia. Note how small the left pulmonary artery *(LPA)* is and how large the ascending aorta *(Ao)* is. *LC*, Left coronary leaflet of the aortic valve; *ML*, muscle of Lancisi; *MV*, mitral valve; *NC*, noncoronary leaflet of the aortic valve; *RC*, right coronary leaflet of the aortic valve; *RPDiv*, right posterior division of the septal band. (From Van Praagh R, Van Praagh S, Nebesar RA, et al. Tetralogy of Fallot: underdevelopment of the pulmonary infundibulum and its sequelae. *Am J Cardiol.* 1970;26:25, with permission.)

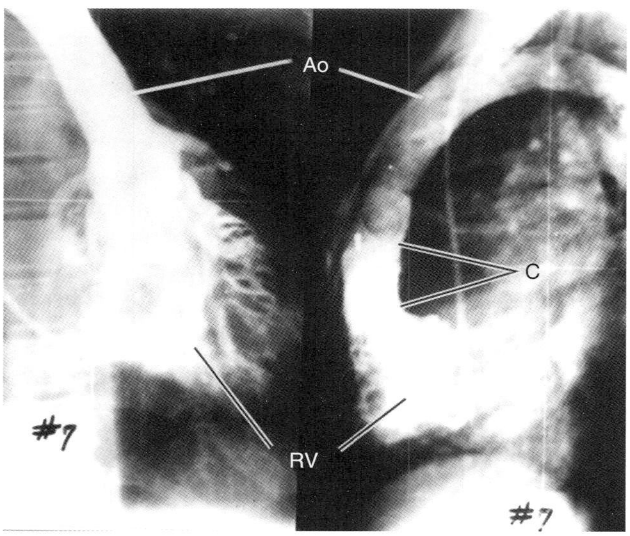

Fig. 3.28 The well-developed subaortic conus *(C)* of typical transposition of the great arteries, *left panel,* posteroanterior projection; *right panel* simultaneous left lateral projection, selective right ventricular angiocardiogram. The valve of the transposed aorta *(Ao)* sits high and anteriorly atop the subaortic conus above the coarsely trabeculated right ventricle *(RV)*. (From Van Praagh R. The segmental approach to diagnosis in congenital heart disease. In Bergsma D, ed. *Birth Defects: Original Article Series.* 1972;8:4; with permission.)

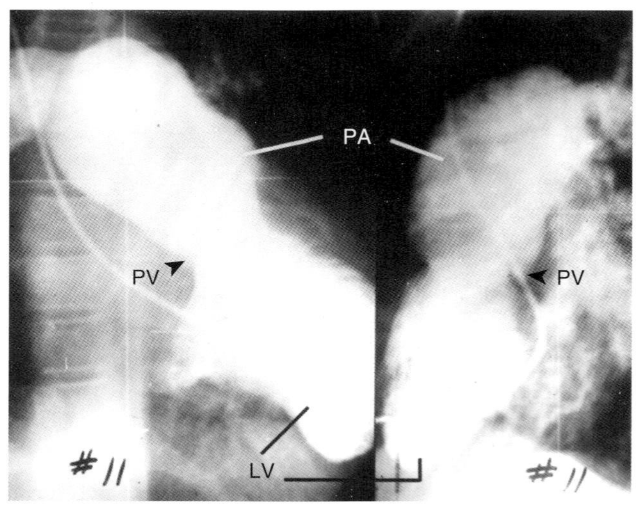

Fig. 3.29 Absence of the subpulmonary conal free wall in typical transposition of the great arteries permits the pulmonary valve *(PV)* to be in direct fibrous continuity with the mitral valve, which explains why the transposed pulmonary artery *(PA)* sits low and posteriorly above the morphologically left ventricle *(LV)*. *Left panel,* anteroposterior projection; *right panel* simultaneous left lateral projection, selective left ventricular angiocardiogram. (From Van Praagh R. The segmental approach to diagnosis in congenital heart disease. In Bergsma D, ed. *Birth Defects: Original Article Series.* 1972;8:4; with permission.)

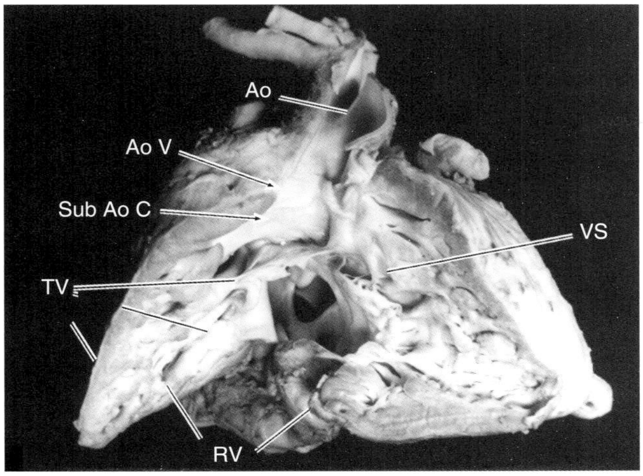

Fig. 3.30 The well-developed muscular subaortic conus *(Sub Ao C)* of typical D-transposition of the great arteries (D-TGA). The transposed aortic valve is widely separated from the tricuspid valve *(TV)* by the subaortic conal musculature. *Ao,* Aorta; *RV,* right ventricle; *VS,* ventricular septum. (From Van Praagh R. Transposition of the great arteries: history, pathologic anatomy, embryology, etiology, and surgical considerations. In Mavroudis C, Backer CL, eds. *Cardiac Surgery: State of the Art Reviews.* 1991;5:7, with permission.)

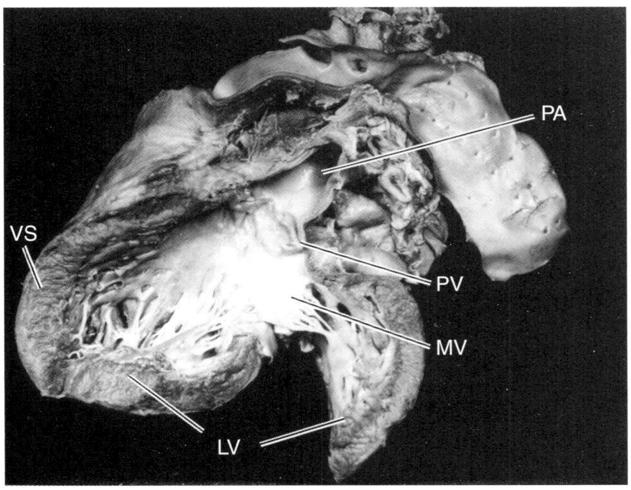

Fig. 3.31 The absence of subpulmonary conal free-wall musculature (remote from the conal septum) in typical transposition of the great arteries that permits direct fibrous continuity between the transposed pulmonary valve *(PV)* and the normally located mitral valve *(MV)*. *LV,* Left ventricle; *VS,* ventricular septum. (From Van Praagh R. Transposition of the great arteries: history, pathologic anatomy, embryology, etiology, and surgical considerations. In Mavroudis C, Backer CL, eds. *Cardiac Surgery: State of the Art Reviews.* 1991;5:7, with permission.)

immediately below these bands. Anatomically, we have never seen a case in which there was dissociation between the septal and moderator bands on the one hand and the right ventricular sinus on the other. By contrast, the distal portion of the conus—the parietal band or subsemilunar part—can and does dissociate from the right ventricle. The distal or subsemilunar part of the conus can straddle the ventricular septum to any degree (straddling conus), and the distal or subsemilunar part of the conus can be located predominantly above the left ventricular sinus—as in anatomically corrected malposition of the

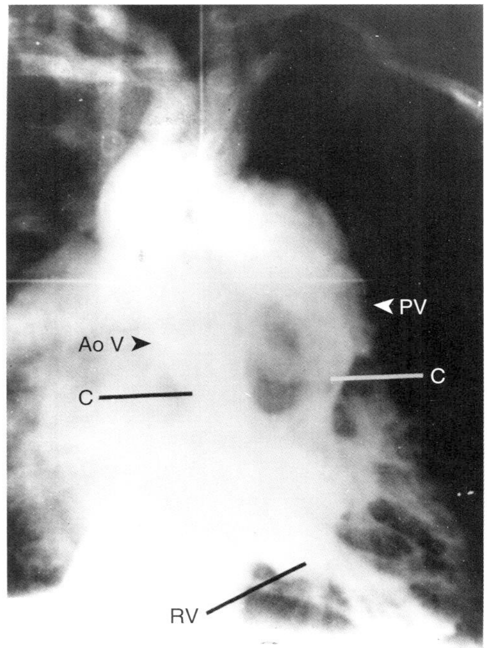

Fig. 3.32 Angiocardiogram, Taussig-Bing malformation, showing the well-developed conus *(C)* beneath the aortic valve *(Ao V)* and the pulmonary valve *(PV)*. Both great arteries arise above the morphologically right ventricle *(RV)*. Note the prominent conal septum between the subaortic and the subpulmonary outflow tracts. Selective RV injection, posteroanterior projection. (From Van Praagh R. The segmental approach to diagnosis in congenital heart disease. In Bergsma D, ed. *Birth Defects: Original Article Series.* 1972;8:4; with permission.)

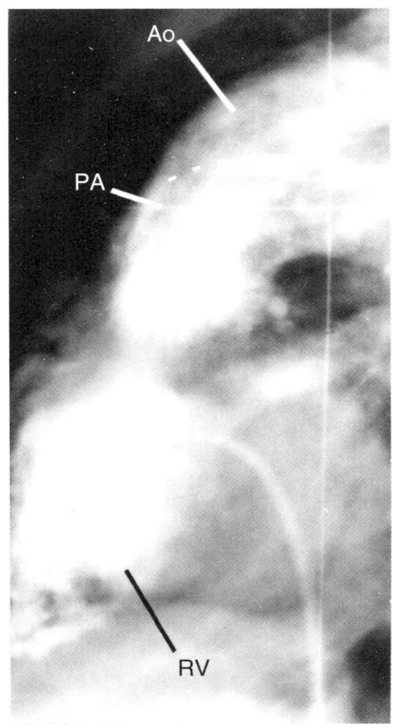

Fig. 3.33 Angiocardiogram, Taussig-Bing malformation, selective right ventricular injection, left lateral projection, simultaneous with frame shown in Fig. 3.32. Note that the aorta *(Ao)* and the pulmonary artery *(PA)* originate side by side above the right ventricle *(RV)*. (From Van Praagh R. The segmental approach to diagnosis in congenital heart disease. In Bergsma D, ed. *Birth Defects: Original Article Series.* 1972;8:4; with permission.)

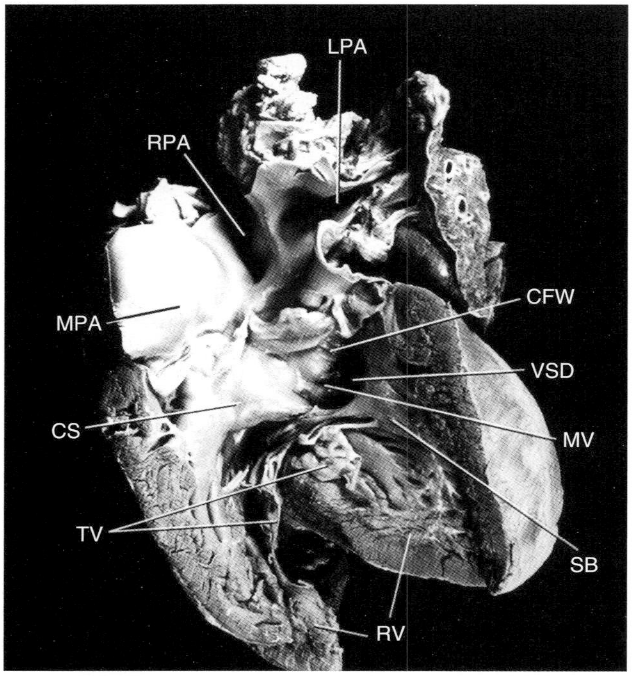

Fig. 3.34 The original Taussig-Bing heart showing opened right ventricle *(RV)* and outflow tract to the main pulmonary artery *(MPA)*. The conal septum *(CS)* and subpulmonary conal free-wall myocardium *(CFW)* prevent fibrous continuity between the pulmonary valve and the tricuspid valve *(TV)* or the mitral valve (not seen, opens normally into the left ventricle). The ventricular septal defect *(VSD)* is subpulmonary. The CS intersects with the right posterior division of the septal band *(SB)*. There is marked hypertrophy of the RV and dilatation of the MPA and its branches. *LPA,* Left pulmonary artery; *MV,* mitral valve; *RPA,* right pulmonary artery. (From Van Praagh R. What is the Taussig-Bing malformation? *Circulation*. 1968;38:445, with permission.)

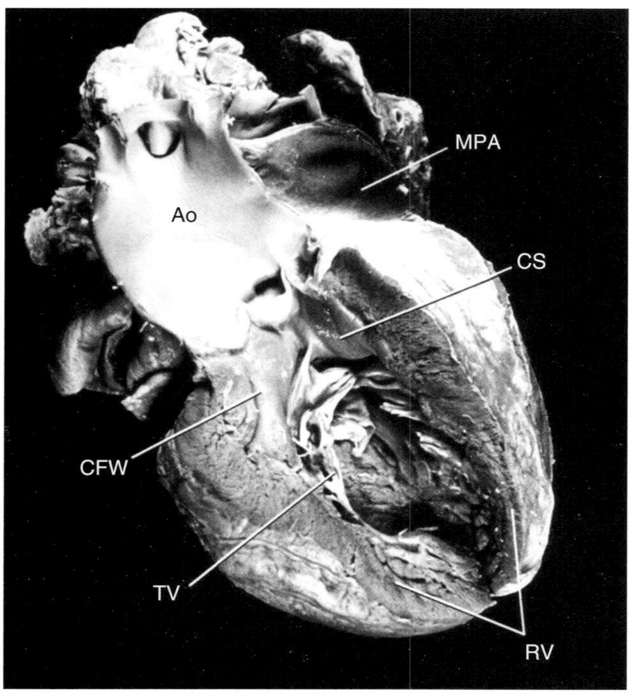

Fig. 3.35 The original Taussig-Bing heart showing opened right ventricle *(RV)* and outflow tract to the ascending aorta *(Ao)*, which lies to the right of the outflow tract to the main pulmonary artery *(MPA)* (see Fig. 3.34). Note the right side of the conal septum *(CS)* and the subaortic conal free-wall myocardium *(CFW)* that separate the malposed aortic valve from the tricuspid valve *(TV)*, preventing aortic-tricuspid fibrous continuity. (From Van Praagh R. What is the Taussig-Bing malformation? *Circulation*. 1968;38:445, with permission.)

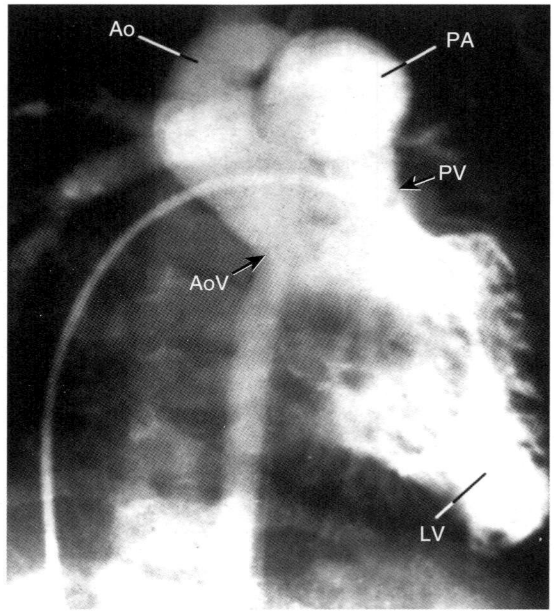

Fig. 3.36 Double-outlet left ventricle (DOLV) with intact ventricular septum and absence of conal musculature beneath the pulmonary valve *(PV)*, permitting aortic-mitral and pulmonary-mitral direct fibrous continuity. This is the rare Paul type of DOLV. Selective left ventricular angiocardiogram, posteroanterior projection. *Ao,* Aorta; *PA,* pulmonary artery. (From Paul MH, Muster AJ, Sinha SN, et al. Double-outlet left ventricle with an intact ventricular septum, clinical and autopsy diagnosis and developmental implications. *Circulation*. 1970;41:129, with permission.)

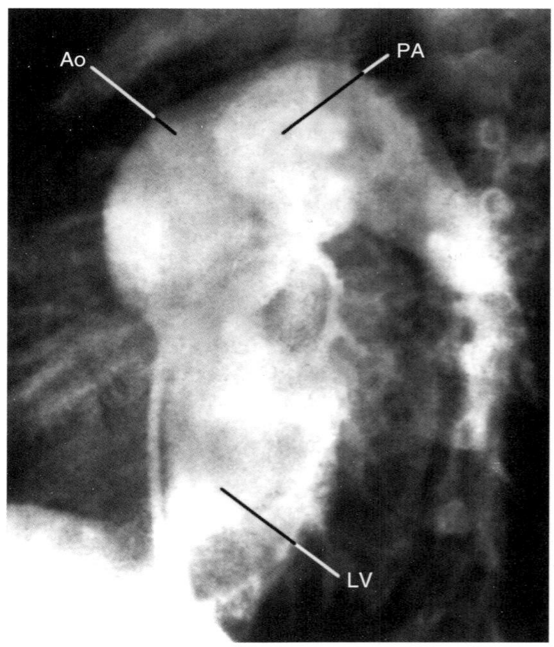

Fig. 3.37 The Paul type of double-outlet left ventricle, same case as in Fig. 3.36, simultaneous left lateral projection showing that the ventricular septum is intact. Both the aorta *(Ao)* and the pulmonary artery *(PA)* originate entirely above the left ventricle *(LV)*. (From Paul MH, Muster AJ, Sinha SN, et al. Double-outlet left ventricle with an intact ventricular septum, clinical and autopsy diagnosis and developmental implications. *Circulation*. 1970;41:129, with permission.)

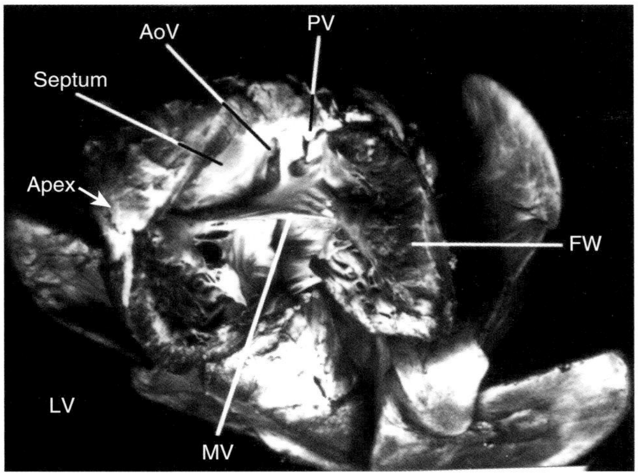

Fig. 3.38 The Paul type of double-outlet left ventricle with intact ventricular septum *(Septum)* and absence of subsemilunar conal musculature, permitting direct fibrous continuity between both the aortic valve *(AoV)* and the pulmonary valve *(PV)* and the anterior leaflet of the mitral valve *(MV)*. View of the opened free wall *(FW)* of the left ventricle *(LV)*, as seen from the ventricular apex (short-axis view). (From Paul MH, Muster AJ, Sinha SN, et al. Double-outlet left ventricle with an intact ventricular septum, clinical and autopsy diagnosis and developmental implications. *Circulation*. 1970;41:129, with permission.)

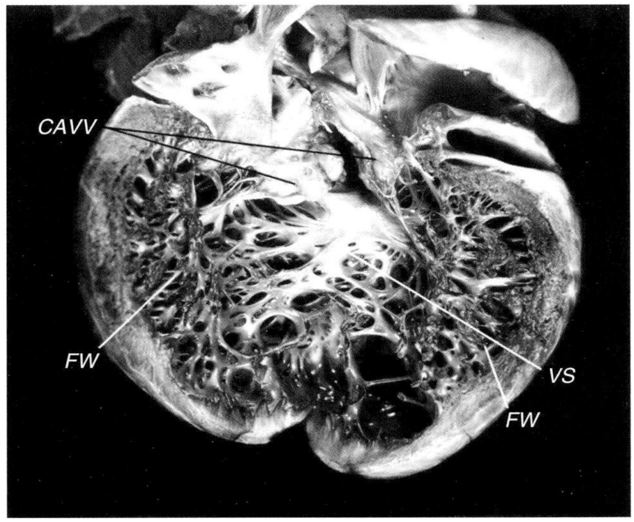

Fig. 3.39 Spongiosum heart in situs inversus totalis, showing the opened right-sided morphologically left ventricle (LV). The trabeculae carneae of the stratum spongiosum of each ventricle underwent differentiation but failed to resorb, thereby showing in a postnatal heart the situation normally seen only in the early embryonic heart. The left ventricular septal surface *(VS)* is smooth superiorly—this being a normal feature of the morphologically LV. The cavity of the LV is full of numerous fine oblique trabeculations of the spongy layer of the LV myocardium. The compact layer of the LV free wall *(FW)* is relatively thick (compared with that of the morphologically right ventricle). The left ventricular papillary muscles are not well differentiated, and the patient has a common atrioventricular canal with a common atrioventricular valve *(CAVV)*. (From Van Praagh R, Ongley PA, Swan HJC. Anatomic types of single or common ventricle in man, morphologic and geometric aspects of 60 necropsied cases. *Am J Cardiol*. 1964;13:367, with permission.)

great arteries (Chapter 25) and as in double-outlet left ventricle (Chapter 24). But the proximal part of the conus (the septal and moderator bands) and the right ventricular sinus never dissociate, in our experience.

Thus, phylogenetically and ontogenetically, there is a very close relationship between the conus and the right ventricular sinus. Embryologically (ontogenetically), the conus arteriosus and the right ventricular sinus are both derived from different parts of the same structure, the bulbus cordis: the conus from the distal bulbus cordis and the right ventricular sinus from the proximal bulbus cordis.

But why is the myocardial morphology of the left ventricle so different from that of the right ventricle? Why are the trabeculae carneae of the morphologically left ventricle numerous, fine, and oblique, whereas those of the right ventricle are much fewer, coarser, and straighter? Why is the compact myocardium of the left ventricle so much thicker than that of the right ventricle?

It is interesting to note that these morphologic differences are evident even in the human embryo at the 9 mm stage (horizon 16, estimated age 32 to 34 days). Hence, the morphologic differences between the left and right ventricles are present from their earliest appearance.

The "spongiosum heart" is also highly relevant. Rarely is it possible to have persistence of the stratum spongiosum in a postnatal heart (Figs. 3.39 and 3.40). Normally, most of the stratum spongiosum is resorbed—leaving only the trabeculations, but rarely, the stratum spongiosum can persist, filling the ventricular cavities. The left ventricular trabeculations are indeed numerous, fine, and oblique, forming a lattice-like mesh (see Fig. 3.39); whereas the right ventricular trabeculations are much fewer and far coarser (see Fig. 3.40). The left ventricular stratum compactum—the compact or cortical layer—is much thicker in the left ventricle (see Fig. 3.39) than in the right ventricle (see Fig. 3.40).

We do not know the *basic* reason for these differences. However, for reasons still unknown, these morphologic differences are really the differences between the architecture of the ventricle (left ventricle) as opposed to that of the proximal bulbus cordis (right ventricle). Since the left and right ventricles are derived from different parts of the bulboventricular loop, we think that these morphologic differences are not surprising. Indeed, it would be surprising if there were no morphologic differences between the left and right ventricles, in view of their different embryologic origins.

Hence, we think that these distinctive and characteristic morphologic differences between the left and right ventricles are not due to hemodynamics, as some have suggested. Hemodynamic factors result in hypertrophy or hypoplasia, but neither changes the anatomic pattern of the morphologically left and right ventricles. For example, whether hypertrophied or hypoplastic, the anatomic patterns of the morphologically left and right ventricles remain basically unaltered.

Our hypothesis is that the characteristic anatomic features of the morphologically left and right ventricles are related to their different sites of origin in the bulboventricular loop. In turn, we think that these differences between the left ventricle (derived

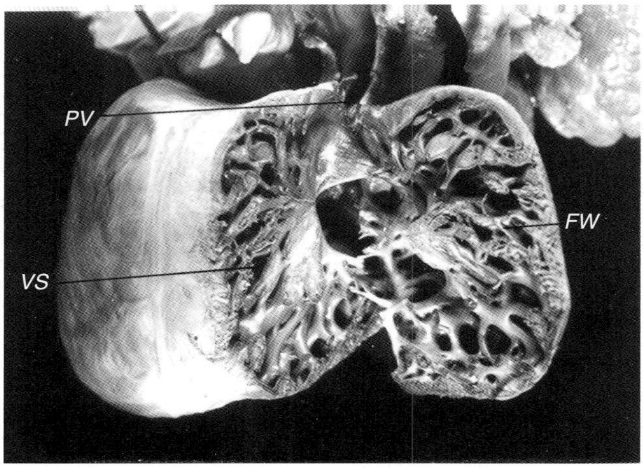

Fig. 3.40 Spongiosum heart in situs inversus totalis, showing the opened left-sided morphologically right ventricle (RV) and pulmonary artery. The trabeculations of the RV myocardium are much thicker and fewer than are those of the left ventricle (Fig. 3.39), as in the early human embryo. The compact layer of the RV myocardium is much thinner than that of the left ventricular myocardium (Fig. 3.39)—as in the early human embryo. Note the hypoplastic pulmonary valve *(PV)* and the anterosuperior displacement of the smooth conal septum. This patient had mirror-image tetralogy of Fallot with common atrioventricular canal in situs inversus totalis, in addition to the persistence of early morphologic characteristics of the left and right ventricular myocardium. *FW,* Free wall; *VS,* ventricular septum. (From Van Praagh R, Ongley PA, Swan HJC. Anatomic types of single or common ventricle in man, morphologic and geometric aspects of 60 necropsied cases. *Am J Cardiol.* 1964;13:367, with permission.)

from the ventricle of the bulboventricular loop) and the right ventricle (derived from the bulbus cordis of the bulboventricular loop) are largely determined by genetic factors.

Phylogenesis or Evolution of the Left and Right Ventricles

(This section is included for those readers who are interested in in-depth understanding but may be skipped by those who prefer to focus only on the morphologic anatomy of the heart.)

From the phylogenetic or evolutionary standpoint, are there any important differences between the morphologically left and right ventricles? *Homo sapiens sapiens* (man wise wise, Latin)—our modest scientific name for our species—belongs to the **phylum Chordata**, which includes all animals with a notochord (*noton* = back and *chorde* = cord, Greek) (please see Chapter 2). The notochord marks the long axis of the embryo, indicating where the brain and vertebrae will develop. Hence, the chordates are synonymous with the vertebrates.

But first, **who really discovered evolution**? Was it Charles Robert Darwin (1809–1882) and/or Alfred Russel Wallace (1823–1913), as is usually said?[21] Fascinating to relate, the answer is no. To the best of our present knowledge, evolution was discovered by **Empedocles**, the brilliant pre-Socratic physicist who lived from 495 to 435 BCE in Acragas (now Agrigento) in Sicily, which at that time was part of Magna Graecia (Great Greece). Empedocles realized not only the existence of the evolution or mutability of species, but he also grasped how it works: the occurrence of favorable changes by **chance**.[22,23]

It is now also clear that the mutability of species was understood even prior to Empedocles. **Anaximander** (c. 611 to c. 547 BCE), who was born in Miletus and was a student of Thales, thought that humans had evolved from other animals. This idea is even older than Anaximander: the Syrians, to whom he refers, worshipped fish as their ancestor. Thus, the theory of evolution antedates Darwin and Wallace by at least 2500 years.

The significant aspect of Empedocles' theory was not the concept of evolution per se. By his time, that idea was several hundred years old. The significant thing is that Empedocles understood that what superficially looked like the workings of purpose (teleology) was in fact achieved by chance—what in modern terminology is known as the natural selection of variations occurring by chance. This was the brilliant and original part of Empedocles' theory of evolution.

If it seems unlikely that an ancient Greek such as Empedocles could have stated the theory of evolution as early as the 5th century BCE, perhaps it should be recalled that the atomic theory of matter was conceived by Leucippus, another 5th century BCE physicist. The atomic theory was then advocated by his student Democritus (c. 460 to c. 370) of Abdera, who made this theory famous.

Remarkably enough, it turns out that the Syrians referred to by Anaximander were right: We *are* descended from fish! Phylogenetically, our remote ancestors are now thought to have been the **ancient fish** of the Ordovician period and the upper Devonian period—some 500 million to 345 million years ago.[24,25] In craniate vertebrates, the heart began as a specialized part of the primary longitudinal ventral blood vessel. This pulsatile part of the primary longitudinal ventral blood vessel pumped venous blood from the ducts of Cuvier (the common cardinal veins) forward and upward through the gills, where oxygenation took place. As long as our vertebrate ancestors "breathed" water, there was a single circulation with a single ventricle and no need for a second ventricle (future right ventricle).

Amphibians evolved in the early Carboniferous period, about 325 million years ago. These animals developed lungs and so could breathe air, but they still had only one ventricle for the systemic and pulmonary circulations. Also, they had to breed in the water, like modern frogs.

Some of these primitive amphibians evolved not only modern amphibians but also fully terrestrial animals that did not need to breed in the water. These were the **Amniota**—all animals with an amniotic sac (please see Chapter 2). The amniotic sac surrounded a "mare internum" (internal sea) of amniotic fluid in which the embryo and later the fetus floated, like our aquatic vertebrate ancestors.

The terrestrial Amniota then evolved into **reptiles**, **birds**, and **mammals**. Birds are essentially feathered reptiles, whereas mammals are furry or hairy reptiles. Mammals evolved during the Jurassic period, about 180 million years ago, when reptiles—including the giant dinosaurs—were the lords of the earth. Although fish and amphibia do not have a right ventricle, higher reptiles (such as alligators and crocodiles), birds, and mammals normally all do have a right ventricle.

The evolution of the right ventricle from the proximal portion of the conus arteriosus (bulbus cordis) was one of the most important cardiovascular adaptations of the Amniotic vertebrates to air-breathing. The right ventricular sinus became the lung pump. The ancient ventricle of our phylum (the Chordates) remained the body pump.

Why did the newly evolved pulmonary pump become the **right** ventricle? And why did the ancient "professional" pump of our phylum, the systemic pump, become the **left** ventricle? The answer to these questions is: D-loop formation. In all Amniotic vertebrates, D-loop formation places the conus arteriosus—beneath which the pulmonary ventricular sinus develops—to the **right** of the ventricle of the bulboventricular loop, from which the systemic ventricular sinus develops (please see Chapter 2). Consequently, D-loop formation normally makes the pulmonary ventricle the right ventricle and the systemic ventricle the left ventricle.

Since amphibia have two atria, right and left, the evolution of the right ventricular sinus was an important part of the development of a **double circulation** (systemic and pulmonary) in fully terrestrial vertebrates. By contrast, in aquatic and amphibious vertebrates, there is only a **single circulation**, the systemic, which also supplies the organs of respiration (gills, lungs, and skin).

In addition to the evolution of the right ventricular sinus, another critically important cardiovascular adaptation to land-living and air-breathing was the evolution of **asymmetrical development of the conus arteriosus: subpulmonary only—not subaortic** (see Fig. 3.23). Asymmetrical development of the conus was the original arterial switch operation, which prevented transposition of the circulations (please see Chapters 2 and 27). Elevation of the pulmonary valve superiorly and anteriorly atop the developing subpulmonary conus switches the pulmonary valve away from the interventricular foramen and the left ventricular blood stream. Failure of the development and resorption of the subaortic conal free wall keeps the aortic valve low and posterior, permitting aortic-mitral fibrous continuity. Hence, development of the subpulmonary conus, plus failure of development of the subaortic conal free wall, switches the aortic valve close to the left ventricle. Then closure of the interventricular foramen at its rightmost end by tricuspid valve tissue forms the membranous septum, thereby completing the separation of the left and right ventricles.

To summarize, the evolution of the right ventricle included three of the most important cardiovascular adaptations to air-breathing and land-living: (1) the development of the right ventricular sinus—**the lung pump**; (2) the development of the asymmetrical conus beneath the pulmonary artery only—**the natural arterial switch process**; and (3) an important contribution to **septation**—the conal septum, part of the muscular interventricular septum, and the membranous septum.

Is the evolution of the right ventricle important to human congenital heart disease? The answer is a definite yes, in the following sense. In our phylum Chordata, the morphologically left ventricle is the ancient professional pump. It is at least 500 million years old, and it is seldom involved in primary malformation.

By contrast, in evolutionary terms, the morphologically right ventricle is a "Johnny Come Lately"—a relative newcomer that is only about 180 million years old. The right ventricle is only slightly more than one-third as old as the left ventricle (36%); moreover, the right ventricle is much more prone to malformation than is the left ventricle, perhaps because it is phylogenetically so much more recent.

Indeed, many of the anomalies that collectively are known as congenital heart disease really are malformations involving one or more components of the right ventricle (see Fig. 3.17) or anomalies involving septation. These are malformations involving our adaptations to air-breathing and land-living. Some of these anomalies are: absence of the right ventricular sinus, resulting in single left ventricle with double-inlet left ventricle; tricuspid atresia; Ebstein anomaly of the tricuspid valve and right ventricular sinus; Uhl disease; congenitally unguarded tricuspid orifice; hypoplasia of the right ventricular sinus, with or without straddling tricuspid valve, with or without superoinferior ventricles, with or without crisscross atrioventricular relations; double-chambered right ventricle; membranous ventricular septal defect; conoventricular type of ventricular septal defect; conal septal defect; tetralogy of Fallot; transposition of the great arteries; double-outlet right ventricle; double-outlet left ventricle; and anatomically corrected malposition of the great arteries.

Thus, an in-depth understanding of the right ventricle is the key to the understanding of much of congenital heart disease.

On the Importance of Examining Heart Specimens

You must, if possible, examine heart specimens for yourself—many heart specimens. There is no substitute. Only then will you be able to make the **accurate diagnosis** of, for example, single left ventricle (absent right ventricular sinus) or single right ventricle (absent left ventricular sinus). It is not always easy. Accurate anatomic diagnosis is a skill that takes time and experience to learn. The heart specimens are the best teachers.

REFERENCES

1. Lev M. Pathologic diagnosis of positional variations in cardiac chambers in congenital heart disease. *Lab Invest.* 1954;3:71.
2. Van Praagh R, Ongley PA, Swan HJC. Anatomic types of single or common ventricle in man. Morphologic and geometric aspects of 60 necropsied cases. *Am J Cardiol.* 1964;13:367.
3. Van Praagh R, Van Praagh S, Vlad P, Keith JD. Anatomic types of congenital dextrocardia, diagnostic and embryologic implications. *Am J Cardiol.* 1964;13:510.
4. Van Praagh R. The segmental approach to diagnosis in congenital heart disease. In: Bergsma D, ed. *Birth Defects: Original Article Series.* 1972:4:8.
5. Hamilton DE, Carlisle JO. *Latin For Secondary Schools.* Toronto: WJ Gage & Co., Ltd; 1946:191.
6. Van Praagh R, Van Praagh S. Aristotle's "triventricular" heart and the relevant early history of the cardiovascular system. *Chest.* 1983;84:462.

7. Van Praagh R, Corsini I. Cor triatriatum: pathologic anatomy and a consideration of morphogenesis based on 13 postmortem cases and a study of normal development of the pulmonary vein and atrial septum in 83 human embryos. *Am Heart J.* 1969;78:379.
8. Van Praagh R, Van Praagh S. Atrial isomerism in the heterotaxy syndromes with asplenia, or polysplenia, or normally formed spleen: an erroneous concept. *Am J Cardiol.* 1990;60:1504.
9. Van Praagh S, Santini F, Sanders SP. Cardiac malpositions with special emphasis on visceral heterotaxy (asplenia and polysplenia syndromes). In: Fyler DC, ed. *Nadas' Pediatric Cardiology*. Philadelphia: Hanley & Belfus, Inc; 1992:589.
10. King TW. An essay on the safety-valve function in the right ventricle of the human heart; and on the gradations of this function in the circulation of warm-blooded animals. *Guy's Hosp Rep.* 1837;2:104.
11. Tandler J. Anatomie Des Herzens. Jena. *Verlag von Gustav Fischer.* 1913;62.
12. Van Praagh R, Geva T, Kreutzer J. Ventricular septal defects: how shall we describe, name, and classify them? *J Am Coll Cardiol.* 1989;14:1298.
13. Paul MH, Muster AJ, Sinha SN, Cole RB, Van Praagh R. Double-outlet left ventricle with an intact ventricular septum: clinical and autopsy diagnosis and developmental implications. *Circulation.* 1970;41:129.
14. Pasquini L, Sanders SP, Parness IA, et al. Conal anatomy in 119 patients with D-loop transposition of the great arteries with ventricular septal defect: an echocardiographic and pathologic study. *J Am Coll Cardiol.* 1993;21:1712.
15. Van Praagh R, Layton WM, Van Praagh S. The morphogenesis of normal and abnormal relationships between the great arteries and the ventricles: pathologic and experimental data. In: Van Praagh R, Takao A, eds. *Etiology and Morphogenesis of Congenital Heart Disease*. New York: Mt Kisco: Futura; 1980:317.
16. Van Praagh R, Van Praagh S, Nebesar RA, Muster AJ, Sinha SN, Paul MH. Tetralogy of fallot: underdevelopment of the pulmonary infundibulum and its sequelae, report of a case with cor triatriatum and pulmonary sequestration. *Am J Cardiol.* 1970;26(25).
17. Van Praagh R, Van Praagh S. Isolated ventricular inversion, a consideration of the morphogenesis, definition, and diagnosis of nontransposed and transposed great arteries. *Am J Cardiol.* 1966;17:395.
18. Van Praagh R, Vlad P, Keith JD. Complete transposition of the great arteries. In: Keith JD, Rowe RD, Vlad P, eds. *Heart Disease in Infancy and Childhood*. 2nd ed. New York: Macmillan; 1967:682.
19. Taussig HB, Bing RJ. Complete transposition of the aorta and a levoposition of the pulmonary artery. *Am Heart J.* 1949;37:551.
20. Van Praagh R. What is the Taussig-Bing malformation? *Circulation.* 1968;38:445.
21. Darwin C. *The Origin of Species*. New York: Mentor Books, the New American Library; 1958: originally published in 1859.
22. Van Praagh R. *Survival, A New Approach From The Life Sciences To The Major Problem Of Our Time*. Phoenix: Falcon Press; 1985:96.
23. Aristotle. *The Physics. Vol IV, Books I-IV, with English translation by PW Wicksteed and FM Cornford*. London and Cambridge: W. Heinemann Ltd, Harvard University Press, The Loeb Classical Library;1970:168.
24. Robb JS. *Comparative Basic Cardiology*. New York and London: Grune & Stratton; 1965.
25. Norman D. *Prehistoric Life, The Rise Of The Vertebrates*. New York: Macmillan; 1994.

4

Segmental Anatomy

The segmental approach to the diagnosis of congenital heart disease is based on an understanding of the morphologic and segmental anatomy of the heart. The **morphologic anatomy** of the heart is summarized in Chapter 3. The **segmental anatomy** of the heart is presented here. The segment-by-segment or step-by-step approach to diagnosis greatly simplifies the diagnostic problem posed even by the most complex forms of congenital heart disease.

THE CARDIAC SEGMENTS

The cardiac segments are the anatomic and developmental "building blocks" out of which all hearts—normal and abnormal—are made.

The three main cardiac segments are the atria, the ventricles, and the great arteries.

The two connecting cardiac segments are the atrioventricular canal or junction and the infundibulum or conus.

Hence, there are five diagnostically and surgically important cardiac segments: (1) the atria, (2) the atrioventricular canal, (3) the ventricular sinuses, (4) the infundibulum or conus, and (5) the great arteries.

ATRIAL SITUS

Where is the morphologically right atrium (RA)? Where is the morphologically left atrium (LA)? To answer these diagnostic questions, an understanding of the two main types of visceroatrial situs is helpful (Fig. 4.1):

1. **In visceroatrial situs solitus**, the liver is predominantly right sided, the stomach and spleen are left sided, the right lung is trilobed, the left lung is bilobed, the right bronchus is eparterial, the left bronchus is hyparterial, the RA is right sided, and the LA is left sided.
2. **In visceroatrial situs inversus**, the liver is predominantly left sided, the stomach and spleen are right sided, the left-sided lung is trilobed, the right-sided lung is bilobed, the left-sided bronchus is eparterial, the right-sided bronchus is hyparterial, the RA is left sided, and the LA is right sided.
3. **In "situs ambiguus" or visceral heterotaxy**—often but not always associated with the asplenia or the polysplenia syndrome—the liver can be bilaterally symmetrical; the stomach may be left sided, right sided, or midline because of a common gastrointestinal mesentery (in which the stomach is not "tacked down"); the lungs may be bilaterally trilobed with bilaterally eparterial bronchi—often with the asplenia syndrome; or the lungs may be bilaterally bilobed with bilaterally hyparterial bronchi—often with the polysplenia syndrome; and the superior venae cavae may be bilateral.

In Fig. 4.1, note **the visceroatrial situs concordances**, the situs (pattern of anatomic organization) of the viscera (abdominal and thoracic) and of the atria usually being the same: both solitus (usual, ordinary, customary—therefore normal), both inversus (a mirror image of situs solitus), or both ambiguus—as can occur with the heterotaxy syndromes (with asplenia, polysplenia, or occasionally with a normally formed spleen).

"Situs ambiguus" or visceral heterotaxy is not a third type of visceroatrial situs.

There are only two basic types of visceroatrial situs (see Fig. 4.1): situs solitus and situs inversus. "Situs ambiguus" (visceral heterotaxy) is the poorly lateralized or abnormally symmetrical pattern of visceral organization that can occur with the asplenia and polysplenia syndromes. However, on careful study, the heterotaxy syndromes appear to have either basically situs solitus of the viscera and atria or basically situs inversus of the viscera and atria.[1] "Situs ambiguus" is now much less ambiguous than it used to be.

Visceral heterotaxy and "situs ambiguus," when not otherwise qualified, indicate that the basic types of visceral situs and atrial situs have not been diagnosed. These are cases awaiting diagnosis of their anatomic types of visceroatrial situs.

The concepts of **atrial isomerism** and of **atrial appendage isomerism**, as mentioned in Chapter 3, are wrong. To summarize, bilaterally right atria or bilaterally left atria have never been documented. In the heterotaxy syndromes of asplenia and polysplenia, in terms of size, shape, and position, the atrial appendages often are not mirror image; that is, atrial appendage isomerism (mirror imagery) often is not present. Also, it should be understood that *partial* isomerism (e.g., of the atrial appendages only) is not isomerism. For example, D-glucose and L-glucose would not be isomers if only some of their atoms were mirror images but others were not. Isomerism is like pregnancy; it is either present or absent—but not partial. Partial isomerism (e.g., of the atrial appendages only) is a contradiction in terms—an error in logic. The realization that the old concept of atrial-level isomerism is erroneous is important, because this

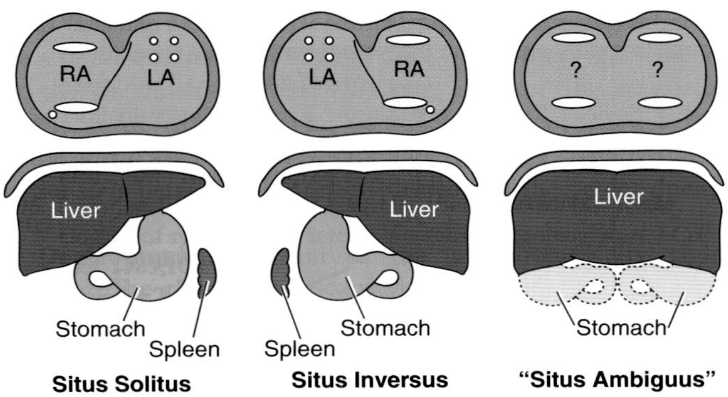

Fig. 4.1 The two types of visceroatrial situs, situs solitus (the usual, hence, the normal pattern of visceral and atrial organization) and situs inversus (the mirror-image pattern of visceroatrial organization). Diagnostically, the type of visceroatrial situs is important for atrial localization. In so-called situs ambiguus, the type of atrial situs is undiagnosed. *LA*, Morphologically left atrium; *RA*, morphologically right atrium. (From Van Praagh R. The segmental approach to diagnosis in congenital heart disease. In: Bergsma D, ed. *March of Dimes. Birth Defects: Original Article Series.* 1972;8:4, with permission.)

understanding then "opens the door" to diagnosing the atrial situs. Atrial-level "isomerism" masks the fact that the atrial situs is undiagnosed.

However, it should also be emphasized that whenever one encounters two atrial appendages that both look "rightish" (broad, triangular, pyramidal), one should immediately think of the asplenia syndrome as a strong diagnostic possibility. Similarly, whenever one sees two atrial appendages that both look "leftish" (long, thin, finger-like), one should immediately think of the polysplenia syndrome as a diagnosis to consider. This bilateral right sidedness or bilateral left sidedness appearance of the atrial appendages is thus diagnostically very helpful.

But one should also understand that the patient really does not have two right atrial appendages (one on each side) nor two left atrial appendages (one on each side). Instead, the foregoing are diagnostically helpful anatomic *appearances*, not real anatomic *facts*. For example, the polysplenia syndrome can occur in visceroatrial situs inversus. The morphologically RA is left sided, but it may well have a finger-like tip to its appendage. Nonetheless, this is a left-sided RA, not a left-sided atrium that is mostly RA but with an LA tip of its appendage. If the latter situation were in fact the case, then this left-sided atrium would be a chimera: mostly RA, but with an LA tip of its appendage. Instead, the LA (including its appendage) is right sided, and the RA is left-sided, just as one would expect in visceroatrial situs inversus, despite the "leftish" appearance of both atrial appendages.

Thus, Dr. Jesse Edwards' "bilateral right sidedness" and "bilateral left sidedness" concepts are very helpful when correctly understood as teaching mnemonics to help one to remember the various features of the asplenia and polysplenia syndromes, respectively. However, these ideas should not be "oversold" at the atrial level as anatomic facts, because they are not. Each human being has only one RA and one RA appendage, just as each human being has only one LA and one LA appendage.

In the asplenia syndrome, for example, when we are unable to diagnose the morphologic anatomic identity of the atria and hence are unable to diagnose the anatomic type of atrial situs, we make the diagnosis of *situs ambiguus of the atria*, which means that we do not know what the atrial situs is. The latter is an honest statement, which we think is vastly preferable to the diagnosis of "right atrial isomerism" or "right atrial appendage isomerism," because the latter diagnoses are erroneous in terms of literal anatomic accuracy.

Anatomic accuracy is the "gold standard" that we have endeavored to employ throughout this study. Accuracy we regard as the basic principle of science. Congenital heart disease is so complex that the only way to avoid confusion is by anatomic accuracy. Accurate pathologic anatomy is the basis of diagnosis in congenital heart disease.

An accurate physiologic diagnosis is also of great importance. But in congenital heart disease, the pathologic anatomy usually determines the *pathophysiology*. Consequently, accurate pathologic anatomy remains the basis of diagnosis in congenital heart disease. For example, cyanosis with decreased pulmonary blood flow and venoarterial shunting can have many different anatomic causes, which must be diagnosed accurately and treated effectively. Hence, the anatomic details are of paramount practical importance.

Occasionally in the heterotaxy syndromes, the situs of the abdominal viscera and the situs of the atria can be different, that is, **visceroatrial situs discordance** can occur.[1,2]

Although **visceroatrial situs concordance** is the rule in situs solitus and in situs inversus (see Fig. 4.1), **visceroatrial situs discordance** can occur in the heterotaxy syndromes.

Inversion is defined in anatomy as mirror imagery. In **situs inversus**, there is right–left reversal but without anteroposterior or superoinferior change (see Fig. 4.1), as in a mirror image. The mirror is the sagittal plane between the diagrams of situs solitus and situs inversus in Fig. 4.1.

The first of the main cardiac segments is thus the viscera and the atria—not just the atria. This is why the diagnosis of the anatomic type of visceroatrial situs (see Fig. 4.1) usually is helpful for atrial localization. If the plain posteroanterior chest x-ray shows situs solitus (the usual arrangement) of the viscera—with liver shadow to the right and stomach bubble to the left (Fig. 4.2), then very probably the atria are also in situs solitus—with RA to the right and LA to the left.

Conversely, if the liver shadow is to the left and the stomach bubble is to the right (Fig. 4.3), situs inversus of the viscera strongly suggests that the atria also will be in situs inversus.

But if the liver shadow is bilaterally symmetrical (Fig. 4.4), this strongly suggests "situs ambiguus," or the heterotaxy syndrome of the viscera and of the atria.

Although the diagnosis of the anatomic type of visceroatrial situs (solitus, inversus, or "ambiguus," see Fig. 4.1) is a useful first approximation concerning atrial identification, in complex cases one must go much further:

1. **Where is the inferior vena cava (IVC)?** Is it right sided or left sided? Does it switch sides at the level of the liver? The atrium to which the IVC connects directly, in our experience, always has been the RA.

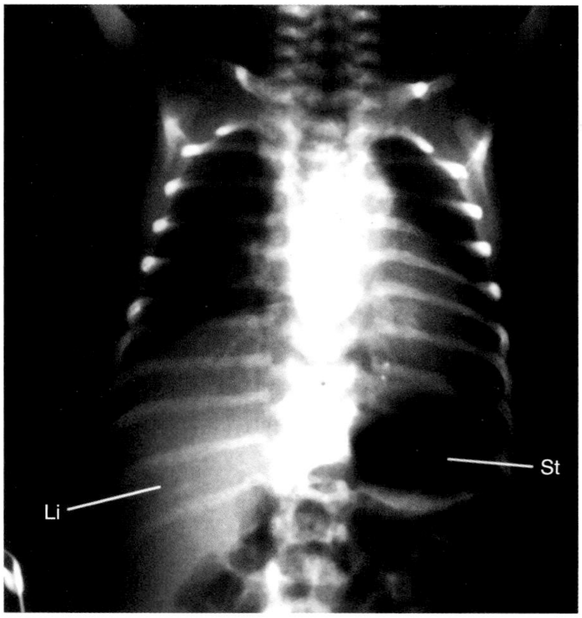

Fig. 4.2 Frontal chest x-ray in visceroatrial situs solitus, with right-sided liver shadow *(Li)* and left-sided stomach bubble *(St)*. Since the viscera are in situs solitus, very probably the atria also are in situs solitus, because of the visceroatrial concordances (see Fig. 4.1). (From Van Praagh R. The segmental approach to diagnosis in congenital heart disease. In: Bergsma D, ed. *March of Dimes. Birth Defects: Original Article Series.* 1972;8:4, with permission.)

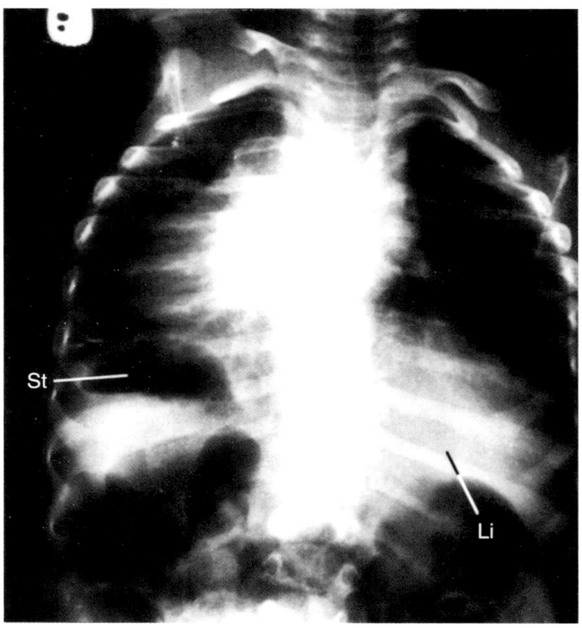

Fig. 4.3 Frontal chest x-ray in visceroatrial situs inversus with left-sided liver shadow *(Li)*, right-sided stomach bubble *(St)*, and dextrocardia. Because the abdominal viscera are in situs inversus, the atria also very probably are in situs inversus, in view of the visceroatrial concordances (see Fig. 4.1). (From Van Praagh R. The segmental approach to diagnosis in congenital heart disease. In: Bergsma D, ed. *March of Dimes. Birth Defects: Original Article Series.* 1972;8:4, with permission.)

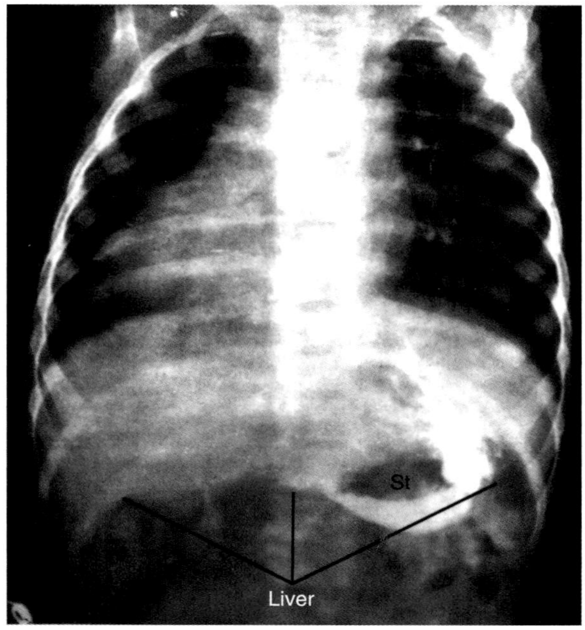

Fig. 4.4 Frontal chest x-ray in a patient with the heterotaxy syndrome and congenital asplenia, with visceroatrial "situs ambiguus" (meaning that the basic type of visceral and atrial situs is not diagnosed). Note the symmetrical liver shadow, with the right lobe and left lobe being approximately of the same size. The stomach *(St)*, localized with barium swallow, changed in position from x-ray to x-ray because of a common gastrointestinal mesentery, the gastrointestinal tract therefore not being normally "tacked down." This abnormally symmetrical liver is highly characteristic of "situs ambiguus" and should suggest the asplenia syndrome. (From Van Praagh R. The segmental approach to diagnosis in congenital heart disease. In: Bergsma D, ed. *March of Dimes. Birth Defects: Original Article Series.* 1972;8:4, with permission.)

2. **Where is the ostium of the coronary sinus?** The atrium into which the ostium of the coronary sinus opens always has proved to be the RA. (A coronary sinus septal defect—or an unroofed coronary sinus—must not be mistaken for the right atrial ostium of the coronary sinus.)
3. **What is the shape and size of the atrial appendage?** Is the appendage large, triangular, and anterior? If so, this is typical of the RA. Is the appendage small, finger-like, and posterior? If so, this is typical of the LA.
4. **What is the morphology of the atrial septal surface?** Is it characterized by septum secundum's superior and inferior limbic bands? If so, this is typical of the RA. Is septum primum well seen on the atrial septal surface? If so, this is typical of the LA.

(Please see Chapter 3 for more details concerning the morphologic anatomy of the RA and the LA.)

For convenience and brevity, situs solitus of the viscera and atria may be abbreviated as **S**. Situs inversus of the viscera and atria may be symbolized as **I**. "Situs ambiguus" of the viscera and atria may be abbreviated as **A**.

The three main cardiac segments—the atria, the ventricles, and the great arteries—may be regarded as the elements of a set. The standard mathematical symbol meaning "the set of" is braces: {}.

The segmental situs set is written in sequential, blood-flow order: {atria, ventricles, great arteries}. The three elements of the set are separated by commas, this being conventional set notation.

The segmental situs set thus may begin as {S,-,-} or as {I,-,-} or as {A,-,- —meaning situs solitus of the viscera and atria (S), or situs inversus of the viscera and atria (I), or "situs ambiguus" of the viscera and atria (A), respectively.

The diagnostic questions concerning atrial localization (where is the morphologically RA, and where is the morphologically LA?) are answered by determining the anatomic type(s) of visceral situs and atrial situs that is (are) present (see Fig. 4.1). In situs solitus and in situs inversus, there virtually always is visceroatrial situs concordance: the situs of the viscera and the situs of the atria are both the same, both solitus, or both inversus. But, as noted heretofore, in the heterotaxy syndromes (asplenia, polysplenia, and heterotaxy with a normally formed spleen), there can be visceroatrial situs discordance. The situs of the viscera and the situs of the atria can be different[1-3]—a fact that is relevant to diagnostic atrial localization. To the best of our present knowledge, the atrium with which the IVC connects always is the morphologically RA. (Please see Chapter 3 for the other anatomic features of the morphologically right and left atria.)

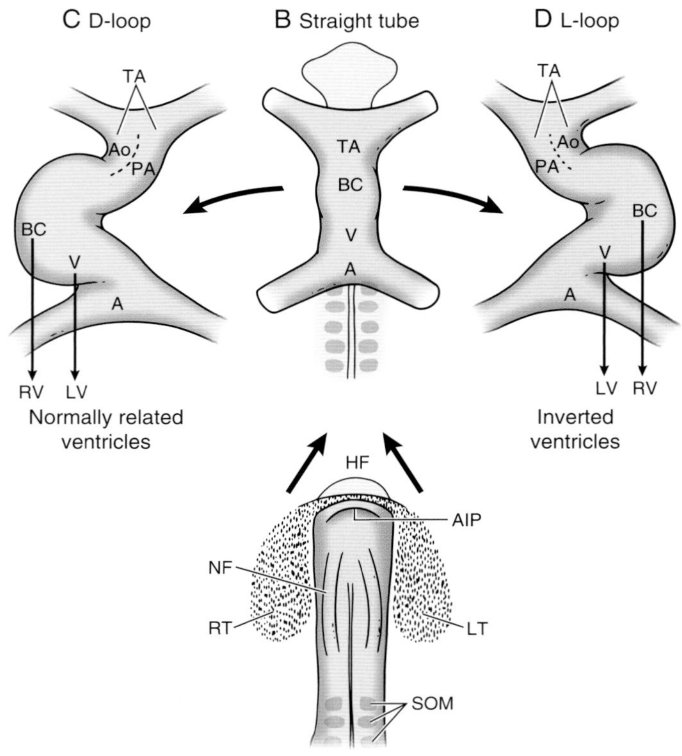

Fig. 4.5 Cardiac loop formation. (A) Cardiogenic crescent of precardiac mesoderm. (B) Straight heart tube or pre-loop stage. (C) D-loop, with solitus (noninverted) ventricles. (D) L-loop with inverted (mirror-image) ventricles. *A*, Atrium; *AIP*, anterior intestinal portal; *Ao*, aorta; *BC*, bulbus cordis; *HF*, head fold; *LT*, left; *LV*, morphologically left ventricle; *NF*, neural fold; *PA*, main pulmonary artery; *RT*, right; *RV*, morphologically right ventricle; *SOM*, somites; *TA*, truncus arteriosus. (From Van Praagh R, Weinberg PM, Matsuoka R, et al. Malpositions of the heart. In: Adams FH, Emmanouilides GC, eds. *Heart Disease in Infants, Children, and Adolescents.* 4th ed. Baltimore: Williams & Wilkins; 1983, with permission.)

VENTRICULAR SITUS

Where is the morphologically right ventricle (RV) and where is the morphologically left ventricle (LV)? The answers to these diagnostically important questions are largely determined by establishing the type of ventricular loop that is present (Fig. 4.5).

With D-loop ventricles, the RV typically is right-sided and somewhat anterior relative to the LV (see Fig. 4.5).

With L-loop ventricles, the RV usually is left sided relative to the LV (see Fig. 4.5). Whether the RV is anterior, side by side, posterior, or superior to the LV is variable.

For example, with superoinferior ventricles[4] and crisscross atrioventricular relations,[5] the spatial relationship between the RV and the LV cannot be described in right–left terms. For example, with superoinferior ventricles[4] in which the ventricular septum is approximately horizontal, the RV is superior to the LV; the right-versus-left approach does not work.

This is why we proposed **chirality or handedness** in 1980.[6] **The D-loop RV is right handed** in the following sense (Fig. 4.6): The thumb of the right hand passes through the tricuspid valve, the fingers of the right hand pass through the RV outflow tract, the palm of only the right hand faces the right ventricular septal surface, and the dorsum of only the right hand faces the right ventricular free wall.

Conversely, the L-loop RV is left handed in the following sense (Fig. 4.7): The thumb of your left hand passes through the left-sided tricuspid valve, the fingers of your left hand pass through the RV outflow tract, the palm of only the left hand faces the right ventricular septal surface, and the dorsum of only the left hand faces the right ventricular free wall.

Hence, the D-loop RV and the L-loop RV are stereoisomers, as are the right and left hands.

Chirality works just as well for the LV as it does for the RV.

The D-loop LV is left-handed: With the thumb through the mitral valve and the fingers in the left ventricular outflow tract, the palm of only the left hand faces the left ventricular septal surface, and the dorsum of only the left hand faces the left ventricular free wall.

The L-loop LV is right handed: With one's thumb (literally or figuratively) through the right-sided mitral valve and one's fingers in the left ventricular outflow tract, the palm of only the right hand faces the left ventricular septal surface, and the dorsum of only the right hand faces the left ventricular free wall.

When not otherwise specified, chirality or handedness should be assumed to be referring to the RV (see Figs. 4.6 and 4.7), even though chirality works just as well for the LV.

Parenthetically, chirality also applies to the atria: **In situs solitus of the viscera and atria, the RA is right handed.** The thumb of the right hand passes (literally or figuratively) into the superior vena cava and the fingers of the right hand pass out into the right atrial appendage. The palm of only the right hand faces the right atrial septal surface, and the dorsum of only the right hand faces the right atrial free wall.

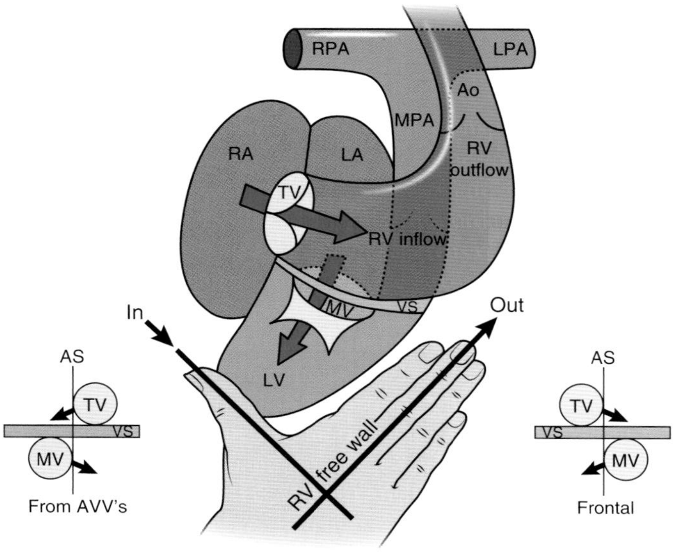

Fig. 4.6 The D-loop or solitus right ventricle is right handed. Figuratively or literally, the thumb of the right hand goes through the tricuspid valve *(TV)*, indicating the right ventricular *(RV)* inflow tract *(IN)*. The fingers of the right hand go into the right ventricular outflow tract *(OUT)*. The palm of only the right hand faces the right ventricular septal surface. The dorsum of the right hand is adjacent to the right ventricular free wall. *Ao,* Aorta; *AS,* atrial septum; *AVV's,* atrioventricular valves; *LA,* morphologically left atrium; *LPA,* left pulmonary artery; *LV,* morphologically left ventricle; *MPA,* main pulmonary artery; *MV,* mitral valve; *RA,* morphologically right atrium; *RPA,* right pulmonary artery; *TV,* tricuspid valve; *VS,* ventricular septum. (From Van Praagh S, LaCorte M, Fellows KE, et al. Supero-inferior ventricles, anatomic and angiocardiographic findings in ten postmortem cases. In: Van Praagh R, Takao A, eds. *Etiology and Morphogenesis of Congenital Heart Disease.* Mt Kisco, NY: Futura Publishing Co.; 1980:317, with permission.)

Conversely, **in situs inversus of the viscera and atria, the RA is left handed.** The thumb of the left hand passes into the superior vena cava, the fingers of the left hand pass out into the right atrial appendage, the palm of only the left hand faces the right atrial septal surface, and the dorsum of only the left hand faces the right atrial free wall.

Similarly, **in visceroatrial situs solitus, the LA is left handed.** The thumb of the left hand passes into the pulmonary veins, the fingers of the left hand pass out into the left atrial appendage, the palm of only the left hand faces the left atrial septal surface, and the dorsum of only the left hand faces the left atrial free wall.

In visceroatrial situs inversus, the LA is right handed. The thumb of the right hand passes into the pulmonary veins; the fingers of the right hand pass out into the left atrial appendage; the palm of only the right hand faces the left atrial septal surface; and the dorsum of only the right hand faces the left atrial free wall.

To return to the ventricles, the important point is that **D-loop ventricles** and **L-loop ventricles** refer to the *situs* of the ventricles—that is, to the pattern of anatomic organization of the ventricles—not to their *spatial relations.* For example, with **superoinferior ventricles,**[4] the RV is above, the LV is below, and the ventricular septum is approximately horizontal. Since the RV extends both to the right and to the left, and the LV also extends both to the right and to the left, what type of ventricular loop is present: D-loop ventricles or L-loop ventricles?

One must not confuse spatial relations (such as right–left relations) with situs (handedness). What you really want to know is the situs of the ventricles (see Figs. 4.6 and 4.7), no matter what their spatial relations may be.

So how do you diagnose the ventricular situs (D-loop/L-loop) with superoinferior ventricles? Just look at the RV. Is it right handed (see Fig. 4.7)? That is the answer.

With crisscross atrioventricular relations,[5,7] the RV may start on the right side but may extend far to the left, and the LV may begin on the left but may proceed far to the right. What kind of ventricular loop is that? Again, remember that you are not concerned with spatial relations such as right–left. What you want to know is the intrinsic pattern of anatomic organization of the ventricle—the ventricular situs, no matter how bizarre their spatial relations may be. So, look at the RV. Is it right handed and therefore a D-loop (see Fig. 4.6)?[6] Or is it left handed and therefore an L-loop (see Fig. 4.7)?[6]

Consider **single RV**, with no identifiable vestige of LV anywhere. How can you prove where the absent LV should have been in order to establish what type of ventricular loop is present? Again, just look at the big RV. Is it a right-handed RV (see Fig. 4.6)? If so, the ventricular situs is solitus, that is, D-loop ventricles. Is it a left-handed RV (see Fig. 4.7)? If so, one is dealing with L-loop ventricles that are assumed to be inverted.

Although it is quick, easy, and convenient to describe D-loop ventricles and L-loop ventricles in terms of their spatial relations, as we did at the outset (D-loop ventricles = right-sided RV, L-loop ventricles = left-sided RV), one must understand that this is just a handy short cut. It usually works (in uncomplicated cases). But this convenient shortcut breaks down in complex cases, such as those aforementioned (superoinferior ventricles, crisscross AV relations, and single RV). It is the complex cases that teach one the difference between ventricular **spatial relations** and **ventricular situs** (D-loop/L-loop ventricles). It is the complex cases that teach one that ventricular spatial relations and ventricular situs are really **two different variables.** It is the complex cases that teach one to use **ventricular chirality** (see Figs. 4.6 and 4.7) to make the diagnosis of D-loop ventricles or L-loop ventricles—and not to be confused by ventricular spatial relations.

Why do we not just talk about *situs solitus* of the ventricles (instead of *D-loop* ventricles) and *situs inversus* of the ventricles (instead of *L-loop* ventricles)?

D-loop ventricles are, to the best of our knowledge, always *solitus* ventricles, that is, as in situs solitus totalis.

L-loop ventricles appear to be *truly inverted* ventricles when they occur as part of situs inversus totalis. For the ventricles to be truly inverted, one must postulate right–left reversal of the ventricular primordia.

Consider a straight heart tube. Label the right side x and the left side y (see Fig. 4.5).[8] D-loop formation places x on the greater curvature of the loop that bulges convexly to the right, whereas y is located on the lesser curvature to the left.

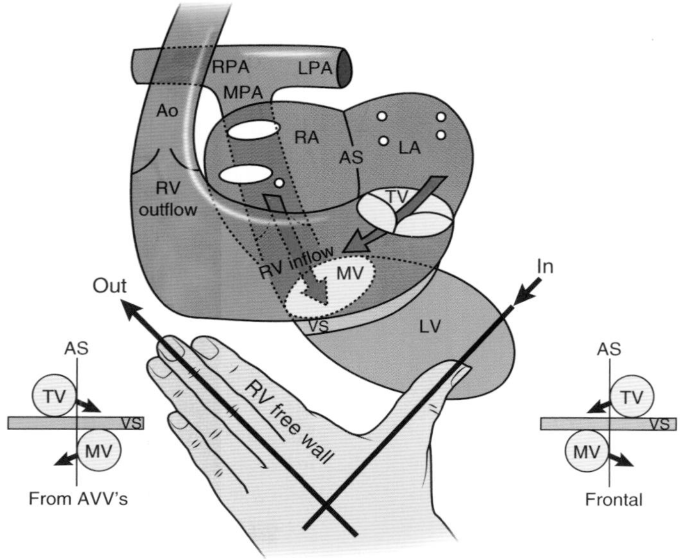

Fig. 4.7 The L-loop or inverted right ventricle is left handed. Figuratively or literally, the thumb of one's left hand goes through the tricuspid valve, indicating the right ventricular inflow tract *(IN)*. The fingers of the left hand go into the right ventricular outflow tract *(OUT)*. The palm of only one's left hand faces the right ventricular septal surface, and the dorsum of the left hand is adjacent to the right ventricular free wall. Abbreviations as previously. (From Van Praagh S, LaCorte M, Fellows KE et al. Supero-inferior ventricles, anatomic and angiocardiographic findings in ten postmortem cases. In: Van Praagh R, Takao A, eds. *Etiology and Morphogenesis of Congenital Heart Disease.* Mt Kisco, NY: Futura Publishing Co.; 1980:317, with permission.)

If the same straight heart tube folds convexly to the left, y occupies the greater curvature bulging convexly to the left, while x occupies the lesser curvature to the right (see Fig. 4.5).[8]

Now compare this D-loop and this L-loop (see Fig. 4.5). Labeling the sides x and y makes it clear that the L-loop is not really a mirror image of the D-loop. For this L-loop to be a true mirror image of this D-loop, one would have to postulate right–left reversal of the anlagen at (or before) the straight tube stage, prior to L-loop formation. If x and y were right–left reversed at (or before) the straight tube stage, only then would the L-loop be a true mirror image of the D-loop. Only then would this L-loop be truly inverted compared with this D-loop (see Fig. 4.5).[8]

If x and y were *not* right–left reversed at or before the straight tube stage, then this L-loop is not a true mirror image of this D-loop, as comparison of the x and y labels makes clear.

So then it became obvious, at least in theory, that there could be two very different kinds of L-loop ventricles (see Fig. 4.5)[8]:

- those that are truly inverted and
- those that are only apparently inverted, that is, solitus heart tubes that have undergone malrotation with looping to the left instead of to the right.

What do the anatomic data suggest? Mirror-image dextrocardia, as part of situs inversus totalis, appears to have truly inverted ventricles. If one photographs these ventricles, reverses the negatives, and prints them reversed, then these "uninverted" images do look like normal noninverted ventricles. Or more simply, take your slides of the ventricles in mirror-image dextrocardia, front-back reverse them, and project them reversed. Again, these "uninverted" images look like ordinary solitus D-loop ventricles. If there is a ventricular septal defect (VSD), the atrioventricular conduction system runs *below* the VSD—in the normal and in the inverted normal way.

If one does the same thing to photos of the ventricles in classical corrected transposition of the great arteries, the "uninverted" images of the ventricles often do not look like normal solitus D-loop ventricles. This might be because the ventricles in corrected transposition often are abnormal; so their "uninverted" images cannot look normal.

But there may well be more to it than that. For example, in classical corrected transposition, the atrioventricular bundle of His typically runs *above* and *in front of* a VSD—instead of behind and below the VSD, which is normal both in situs solitus and in situs inversus totalis. In this respect, the ventricles in corrected transposition clearly are not a mirror image of D-loop ventricles.

In the right-sided LV of classical corrected transposition, the superior papillary muscle often is antero*medial* (instead of antero*lateral*, which is normal). The inferior papillary muscle is often postero*lateral* (instead of postero*medial*, which is normal).

These observations can be explained by postulating that the ventricular sinuses are not inverted (right–left reversed) but upside down, because a solitus heart tube underwent L-loop formation (instead of D-loop formation, which is normal in the development of a solitus straight heart tube). In classical corrected transposition, if the right-sided LV were upside down, this would explain why the AV conduction system is above the VSD, why the upper papillary muscle is paraseptal (antero*medial*), and why the lower papillary muscle is remote from the septum (postero*lateral*).

If the ventricles in classical corrected transposition are malrotated with L-loop formation (but not really inverted), then the RV sinus is also upside down (as is the LV sinus). Perhaps this is why the left-sided RV sinus is so often malformed in classical corrected transposition. If one remembers that the development of the tricuspid valve is intimately related to the development of the RV sinus, this may help to explain the very high prevalence of left-sided tricuspid valve anomalies in classical corrected transposition.

The upside-down orientation of the RV sinus in classical corrected transposition may be masked by the downgrowth of the subaortic conal musculature from above, making it look as though the left-sided RV is right side up.

If this hypothesis is true, then the subaortic conus would be connecting with the bottom of the RV sinus rather than with the top of the RV sinus, as occurs normally.

How could this happen? Perhaps this connection of the conus with the caudal aspect of the RV sinus (instead of with the cephalic end of the RV sinus, which is normal) might be explained by remodeling in utero. The conotruncus may twist upward and migrate from a caudal to a cephalic position (similar to the caudocranial migration of the embryonic subclavian arteries) in order for the conotruncus to originate above the upside-down ventricular sinuses.

We are not sure that this hypothesis is true. Instead, the point is that **the ventricles in classical corrected transposition may not be truly inverted**. This may apply to all discordant L-loop ventricles, that is, to all cases with situs solitus of the viscera and atria, with discordant L-loop ventricles. The point is that in classical corrected transposition, for example, the ventricular part of the heart clearly has looped in a leftward direction: an L-loop definitely is present. But whether these L-loop ventricles are truly inverted—or only apparently inverted—remains unknown at the present time.

Consequently, in our diagnosis and designation of the ventricular part of the heart in congenital heart disease, we have deliberately chosen to use the designations *D-loop* ventricles and *L-loop* ventricles, defined anatomically in terms of chirality (see Figs. 4.6 and 4.7), because these terms are thought to be anatomically and embryologically accurate. We have deliberately chosen not to use the designations *noninverted* ventricles and *inverted* ventricles, because the anatomic and developmental accuracy of the latter term appears to be very uncertain. Discordant L-loop, in particular, may or may not prove to be inverted. Hence, in the interests of anatomic accuracy, we thought it wise to avoid the ventricular *noninversion/inversion* hypothesis because of its highly uncertain validity.

Other problems associated with ventricular *noninversion/inversion* were that these terms were usually employed in an atrial-situs-dependent sense. This meant that ventricular *inversion* meant one thing in visceroatrial situs solitus (L-loop ventricles), the opposite thing in visceroatrial situs inversus (D-loop ventricles), and nothing in visceroatrial situs ambiguus—because the atrial situs, which was the frame of reference, was itself uncertain or unknown.

Others used ventricular *inversion* not in a visceroatrial-situs-dependent sense. For them, ventricular *inversion* meant that the pattern of ventricular anatomic organization was as in situs inversus totalis.

Consequently, we realized in 1964[8] that the designation ventricular *inversion* suffered from confusion in usage: Some used this diagnosis in an atrial-situs-dependent sense, whereas others did not. We thought it would be absurd for us to tell other investigators what they should mean by ventricular *inversion*.

This is why we introduced the diagnostic terms atrioventricular *concordance* and atrioventricular *discordance* in 1964.[9] For example, in physiologically corrected transposition in situs inversus, whether one wished to regard these (D-loop) ventricles as *inverted for situs inversus* or as *noninverted in situs inversus*, everyone would agree that these ventricles are *discordant* relative to the atria, because the RA opened into the LV (both left sided) and the LA opened into the RV (both right sided).

In order to facilitate **diagnostic data analysis** in large series of complex cases of congenital heart disease, one needs to have simple anatomic terms that do not change in meaning or become meaningless, depending on the type of visceroatrial situs that coexists. This is why we introduced *D-loop* and *L-loop* ventricles in 1964.[10] The meanings of D-loop ventricles (see Fig. 4.6) and of L-loop ventricles (see Fig. 4.7) never change or become meaningless; this immutability of meaning greatly facilitates diagnostic data analysis.

The really new feature of the **segmental approach to diagnosis**[8,9,11] was that the ventricles and the great arteries are diagnosed and designated per se rather than being expressed in terms of the atrial situs. Consequently, the ventricular and great arterial diagnoses do not change or become meaningless, depending on the atrial situs.

Why not express the ventricular situs (D-loop ventricles/L-loop ventricles) in terms of atrioventricular concordance/discordance?

First, like ventricular *noninversion/inversion*, atrioventricular *concordance/discordance* is an atrial-situs-dependent approach. Consequently, the meaning of (for example) *atrioventricular discordance* changes or becomes meaningless, depending on the type of visceroatrial situs that coexists. For example, in visceroatrial situs solitus, *AV discordance* means *L-loop ventricles*. In visceroatrial situs inversus, *AV discordance* means *D-loop ventricles*. In visceroatrial situs ambiguus, *AV discordance* is *meaningless* (Fig. 4.8).

Second, there are many anomalies in which the concept of AV concordance *or* discordance does not apply accurately:

1. In *straddling tricuspid valve*, RA to RV is concordant, while RA to LV is discordant. Hence, the AV alignments are both concordant *and* discordant (not either/or).
2. In *double-inlet LV*, the AV alignments are both concordant (LA to LV) *and* discordant (RA to LV)—not either/or.
3. In *straddling mitral valve*, the AV alignments are both concordant (LA to LV) *and* discordant (LA to RV)—again, not either concordant *or* discordant.
4. In *double-inlet RV*, the AV alignments are both concordant (RA to RV) and discordant (LA to RV)—not either/or.

Third, there are even rare anomalies in which the concept of AV concordance *or* discordance does apply accurately but in which the AV alignments predict the type of ventricular situs *wrongly*:

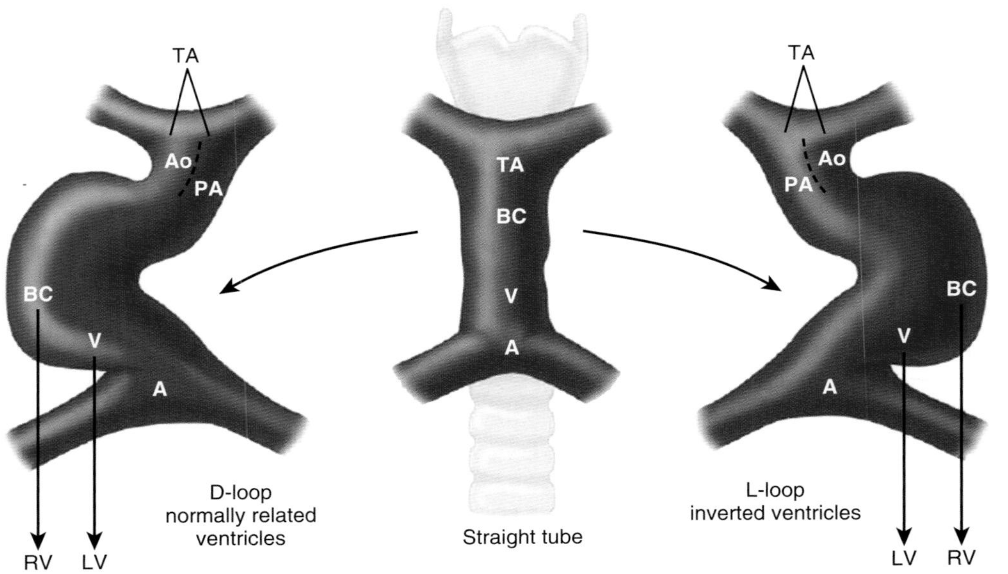

Fig. 4.8 The two general types of bulboventricular loop. Following the straight tube stage, the loop normally protrudes initially to the right forming a dextro or D-loop. Abnormally, the straight tube may protrude or fold convexly to the left, forming an L-loop. Since the morphologically right ventricle *(RV)* develops from the proximal portion of the bulbus cordis *(BC)*, and the morphologically left ventricle *(LV)* develops from the ventricle *(V)* of the bulboventricular loop, consequently D-loop formation is associated with solitus or noninverted ventricles, whereas L-loop formation is associated with inverted or mirror-image ventricles. If one labels the right side of the heart at the straight tube stage "X" and the left side of the heart "Y," note the locations of X and Y following D-loop formation and L-loop formation. Note that an L-loop is not necessarily a mirror image of a D-loop. Indeed, an L-loop is a mirror image of a D-loop only if the primordia of the L-loop are right–left reversed (inverted) at and probably prior to the straight tube stage. The L-loop that is diagrammed is not a mirror image of the D-loop that is diagrammed, as comparison of the X and Y labels indicates. True mirror imagery does not result from L-loop formation. Rather, L-loop formation is characteristic of an inverted straight heart tube, as in situs inversus totalis. However, the L-loop ventricles in classical corrected transposition of the great arteries {S,L,L} may well not have true inversion of the ventricles. However, these ventricles are definitely L-loop ventricles, whether they are truly or only apparently inverted. *A*, Atrium; *Ao*, future aorta; *PA*, future main pulmonary artery; *TA*, truncus arteriosus. (From Van Praagh R, Ongley PA, Swan HJC. Anatomic types of single or common ventricle in man, morphologic and geometric aspects of sixty necropsied cases. *Am J Cardiol.* 1964;13:367, with permission.)

- It is possible to have AV concordance between solitus atria and L-loop ventricles.[6]
- It is also possible to have AV discordance between solitus atria and D-loop ventricles.[6]

The fact that AV alignments rarely can predict the ventricular situs (D-loop/L-loop ventricles) wrongly[6,12] has been confirmed by Anderson.[13]

These, then, are the main reasons that we think the ventricular situs should be diagnosed specifically as D-loop or L-loop ventricles—not as ventricular noninversion or inversion and not by means of AV concordance or discordance. D-loop/L-loop ventricles always applies accurately, and its usage is not confused.

For convenient brevity, the ventricular situs is listed as the second element in the segmental situs set of {atria, ventricles, great arteries}. **D-loop ventricles** are symbolized as **D**: {-,D,-}. **L-loop ventricles** are symbolized as **L**: {-,L,-}.

GREAT ARTERIAL SITUS

This section has to do with the pattern of anatomic organization (the situs) of the great arteries.

Parenthetically, it is noteworthy that *situs* is a fourth declension masculine Latin noun that literally means site or location. Being a fourth declension (not a second declension) noun, *situs* is both singular and plural. Similarly, *ductus* is also a fourth declension masculine Latin noun. The plural of *ductus arteriosus* is *ductus arteriosi*. Hence, it is correct to speak of the atrial, ventricular, and great arterial *situs*.

The main anatomic types of great arterial situs are:

1. **solitus normally related great arteries,** symbolized as **S**;
2. **inversus normally related great arteries,** abbreviated as **I**;
3. **D-transposition or D-malposition of the great arteries,** symbolized as **D**;
4. **L-transposition or L-malposition of the great arteries,** abbreviated as **L**; and
5. **A-transposition or A-malposition of the great arteries,** symbolized as **A**.

The great arterial situs is the third element of the segmental situs set: {atria, ventricles, great arteries}. Thus, solitus normally related great arteries is symbolized as {-,-,S}; inverted normally related great arteries as {-,-,I}; D-transposition or D-malposition of the great arteries as {-,-,D}; L-transposition or L-malposition of the great arteries as {-,-,L}; and A-transposition or A-malposition of the great arteries as {-,-,A}.

A diagram of various types of human heart is presented in Fig. 4.9.

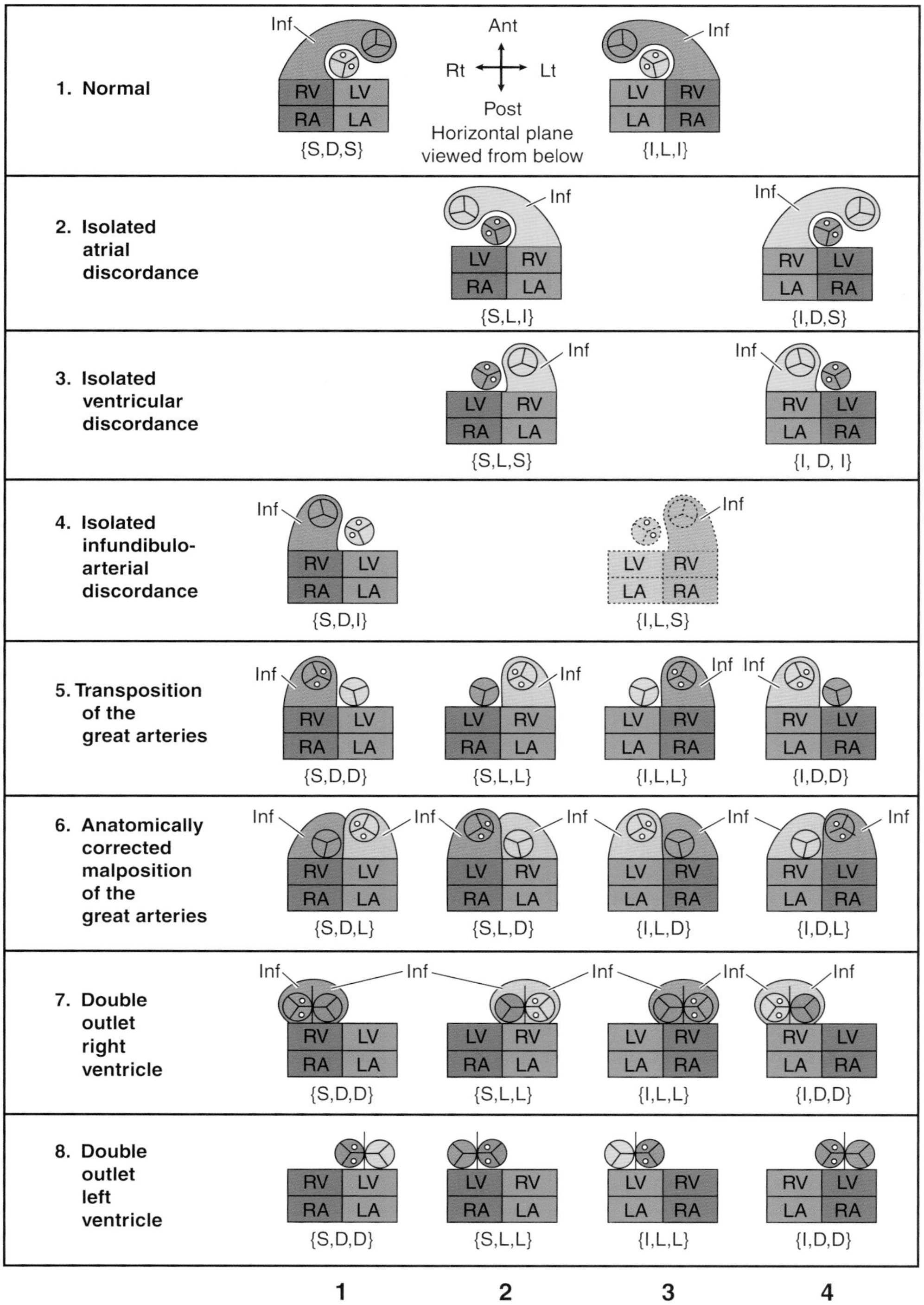

Fig. 4.9 Types of human heart: segmental sets and alignments. Heart diagrams are viewed from the front and below, similar to a subxiphoid two-dimensional echocardiogram. *Ant,* Anterior; *Inf,* infundibulum; *L,* left; *LA,* morphologically left atrium; *LV,* morphologically left ventricle; *Post,* posterior; *R,* right; *RA,* morphologically right atrium; *RV,* morphologically right ventricle. The aortic valve is indicated by the coronary ostia; the pulmonary valve is indicated by absence of coronary ostia. Braces {} mean "the set of." The segmental sets are explained in the text. Rows 1–4 and 6 have ventriculoarterial *(VA)* concordance. Row 5, transposition of the great arteries, has VA discordance. Rows 7 and 8 have double-outlet RV and LV, respectively. Columns 1 and 3 have atrioventricular (AV) concordance, {S,D,-} and {I,L,-}, respectively. Columns 2 and 4 have AV discordance, {S,L,-} and {I,D,-}, respectively. (From Foran RB, Belcourt C, Nanton MA, et al. Isolated infundibuloarterial inversion {S,D,I}: a newly recognized form of congenital heart disease. *Am Heart J.* 1988;116:1337, with permission.)

Solitus normally related great arteries, {-,-,S}, typically have a pulmonary valve that is anterior, superior, and to the left of the aortic valve (Fig. 4.10).[14] There is a subpulmonary muscular conus, absence of the subaortic conal free wall musculature, pulmonary-atrioventricular fibrous discontinuity, and aortic-mitral fibrous continuity. The fibroelastic great arteries untwist through approximately 150 degrees in a clockwise direction (as viewed from the front) as the great arteries pass from the semilunar relationship proximally to the aortic arch/pulmonary bifurcation relationship distally (Fig. 4.11).[14]

The solitus normal heart is {S,D,S}, which means the set of solitus atria, D-loop ventricles, and solitus normally related great arteries (see Fig. 4.9). As one would expect with this segmental anatomy, there is **atrioventricular concordance** and **ventriculoarterial concordance**. Typically, there are no associated malformations.

Inverted normally related great arteries, {-,-,I}, typically have a pulmonary valve that is anterior, superior, and to the right of the aortic valve (see Fig. 4.10).[14] There is a muscular subpulmonary conus, absence of the subaortic conal free wall musculature, pulmonary-atrioventricular fibrous discontinuity, and aortic-mitral fibrous continuity. The fibroelastic great arteries untwist through approximately 150 degrees in a counterclockwise direction (as viewed from the front) as the great arteries pass from the semilunar relationship proximally to the aortic arch/pulmonary bifurcation relationship distally (see Fig. 4.11).[14]

The inverted "normal" heart is **{I,L,I}**, which means the set of inverted atria, L-loop ventricles, and inverted normally related great arteries (see Fig. 4.9). As one would expect with this segmental anatomy, there is **atrioventricular concordance** and **ventriculoarterial concordance**. Typically, dextrocardia is present as part of situs inversus totalis, and associated malformations may or may not be present.[9]

D-transposition of the great arteries usually is **TGA {S,D,D}**, which means transposition of the great arteries with the set of solitus atria, D-loop ventricles, and D-transposition in which the transposed aortic valve is to the right (dextro, or D

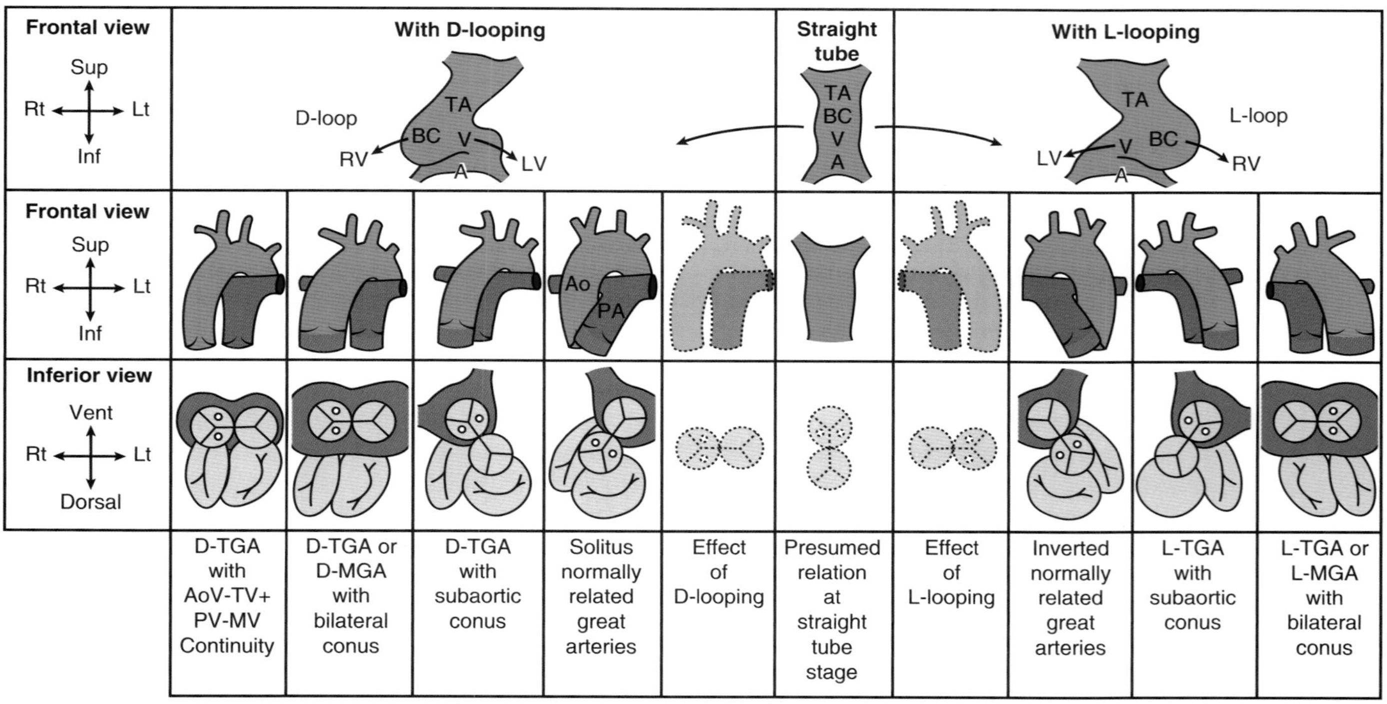

Fig. 4.10 Morphogenesis of normally and abnormally related great arteries. **Top row**: The straight heart tube normally folds in a rightward (dextral) direction forming a D-loop, but abnormally can fold in a leftward (levo) direction, forming an L-loop. *A,* Atrium; *BC,* bulbus cordis; *LV,* morphologically left ventricle; *RV,* morphologically right ventricle; *TA,* truncus arteriosus; *V,* ventricle. D-loop formation is associated with solitus (noninverted) ventricles, whereas L-loop formation is associated with inverted (mirror-image) ventricles. Hearts are viewed from the ventral aspect. **Second row from the top**: Great arteries seen from the front. *Ao,* Aorta; *Inf,* inferior; *Lt,* left; *PA,* pulmonary artery; *Rt,* right. Conal musculature is indicated by subsemilunar hatching. Dotted lines indicate postulated effect of D- or L-looping only, that is, without the effect of conal development. **Third row from the top**: View from below (inferior view) of semilunar valves (aortic valve indicated by coronary ostia), atrioventricular valves, and conal musculature (hatching), with D-loop ventricles and with L-loop ventricles. **Bottom row: Note that solitus normally related great arteries** are associated with a subpulmonary conus and with absence of subaortic conal free-wall musculature. The presence of a subpulmonary conus results in pulmonary valve-atrioventricular valve fibrous discontinuity, aortic valve-mitral valve direct fibrous continuity, and aortic-tricuspid fibrous continuity via the membranous septum. **Typical transpositions of the great arteries** (**D- and L-**) have a muscular subaortic conus and no subpulmonary conal free-wall musculature. The subaortic conus results in aortic-atrioventricular fibrous discontinuity and in pulmonary-mitral fibrous continuity. D-TGA and L-TGA can have a bilateral conus (subaortic and subpulmonary conal musculature) resulting in no semilunar-atrioventricular fibrous continuity. **D- or L-malposition of the great arteries** can be associated with **double-outlet right ventricle** or **double-outlet left ventricle** or **anatomically corrected malposition of the great arteries.** (From Van Praagh R. Approccio segmentario alla diagnosi delle cardiopatie congenite. In: Squarcia U, ed. *Progressi in Cardiologia Pediatrica*. Milan: Casa Editrice Ambrosiana; 1978:7, with permission.)

= right, Latin) relative to the transposed pulmonary valve (see Fig. 4.9). As one would expect, there is **atrioventricular concordance** and **ventriculoarterial discordance**. *Transposition* of the great arteries means ventriculoarterial discordance.[15]

TGA {S,D,D} is classical **complete transposition** of the great arteries. *Partial* transposition was coined by Vierordt[16] in 1898. In *partial* transposition, only one of the great arteries is transposed, that is, placed across the ventricular septum. Partial transposition is now called more specifically either *double-outlet right ventricle* (DORV) or *double-outlet left ventricle* (DOLV) (see Fig. 4.9). Abbott[17] introduced *complete* transposition, as opposed to *partial* transposition, into the English medical literature in 1915. *Complete* transposition means that both great arteries are placed across the ventricular septum and so arise above the anatomically inappropriate ventricles: aorta (Ao) above the morphologically RV and pulmonary artery (PA) above the morphologically LV.

Transposition is derived from the Latin verb *transponere*: *trans* = across, and *ponere* = to place. *Positio* is the Latin noun meaning *position* or *placement*, which is related to the Latin verb

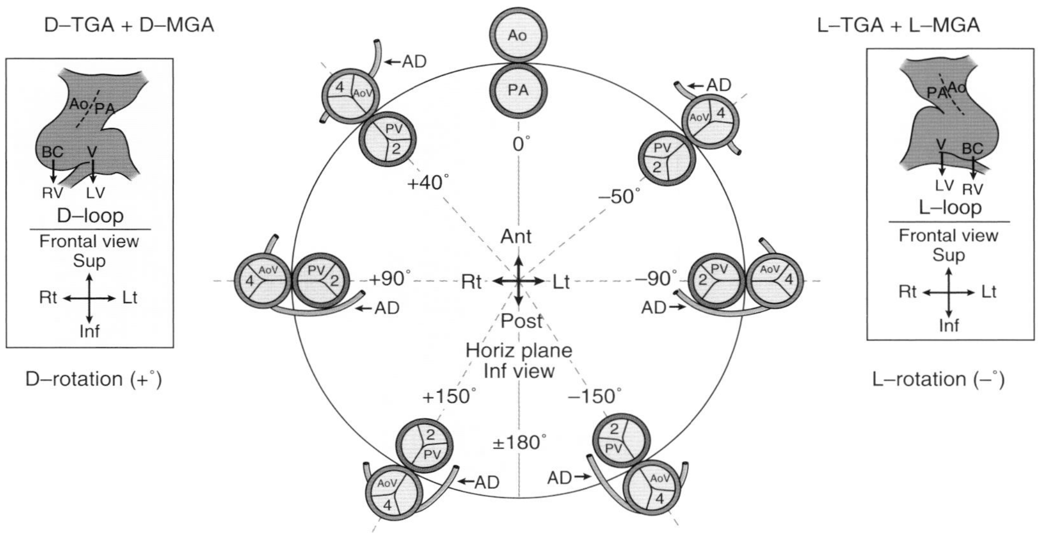

Fig. 4.11 The untwisting of the great arteries as they pass from the highly variable semilunar interrelationship proximally to the fixed aortic arch/pulmonary bifurcation relationship distally. **Solitus normally related great arteries** untwist through approximately 150 degrees of clockwise rotation as seen from below (+150 degrees). **Inverted normally related great arteries** also untwist through approximately 150 degrees, but in the opposite direction—counterclockwise rotation as seen from below (-150 degrees). **Abnormally related great arteries** have to untwist much less than normal as the great arteries proceed from the valves proximally to the aortic arch/pulmonary bifurcation distally, because the aorto-pulmonary relationship proximally at the semilunar valves is closer to the fixed distal relationship at the aortic arch/pulmonary artery bifurcation. **D- and L-transposition of the great arteries** both have to untwist much less than normal, and consequently transposed great arteries appear relatively parallel, straight, uncrossed or untwisted. **When the semilunar valves are side by side, as in double-outlet right ventricle**, then the great arteries have to untwist more than in typical transpositions but less than with normally related great arteries. *AD*, Anterior descending coronary artery; *Ant*, anterior; *Ao*, aorta; *AoV*, aortic valve; *D-MGA*, D-malposition of the great arteries, including double-outlet right ventricle, double-outlet left ventricle, and anatomically corrected malposition of the great arteries in which the aortic valve lies to the right of the pulmonary valve; *D-TGA*, D-transposition of the great arteries; *Inf*, inferior; *L-MGA*, L-malposition of the great arteries, including double-outlet right ventricle, double-outlet left ventricle, and anatomically corrected malposition in which the malposed aortic valve lies to the left of the malposed pulmonary valve; *L-TGA*, L-transposition of the great arteries; *Lt*, left; *LV*, morphologically left ventricle; *PA*, pulmonary artery; *Post*, posterior; *PV*, pulmonary valve; *Rt*, right; *RV*, morphologically right ventricle; *Sup*, superior. The nonseptal pulmonary leaflet is conventionally numbered as leaflet 2. The nonseptal and normally noncoronary aortic leaflet is conventionally numbered leaflet 4. **The two-four semilunar diameter** is helpful in measuring the semilunar interrelationship relative to the sagittal plane. D-TGA may display 40 degrees dextrorotation at the semilunar valves relative to the sagittal plane (+40 degrees). L-TGA may display a semilunar interrelationship 50 degrees to the left of the sagittal plane (−50 degrees). Taussig-Bing malformation with a side-by-side relationship may have a 2/4 semilunar diameter that makes a right angle to the right of the sagittal plane (+90 degrees). Double-outlet right ventricle with L-loop ventricles may display a rotation at the semilunar valves of 90 degrees to the left of the sagittal plane (−90 degrees). Solitus and inversus normally related great arteries display +150 degrees and −150 degrees rotation at the semilunar valves relative to the sagittal plane, respectively. (From Van Praagh R. Approccio segmentario alla diagnosi delle cardiopatie congenite. In: Squarcia U, ed. *Progressi in Cardiologia Pediatrica.* Milan: Casa Editrice Ambrosiana; 1978:7, with permission.)

ponere. *Transposition* of the great arteries thus literally means *across placement* of the great arteries, the ventricular septum being the implicit frame of reference.

As the term *transposition* of the great arteries is now used,[15] all transpositions are *complete* (as opposed to partial) because the *partial* transpositions of the late 19th and the 20th centuries are now known as *DORV* and as *DOLV* (see Fig. 4.9). *Physiologically uncorrected* and *physiologically corrected* transpositions are both *complete* transpositions.

However, in Abbott's[17] classification of TGA, there were three types: (1) *complete* TGA, meaning the classical physiologically uncorrected TGA; (2) *partial* TGA, which we would now call DORV; and (3) *corrected* TGA. Abbott's[17] usage has stuck; this is why *complete TGA*, when not otherwise specified, means classical complete physiologically uncorrected TGA {S,D,D} (see Fig. 4.9).

Following the work of Spitzer[18] in 1923, it was understood that TGA {S,D,D} is complete *noninverted* TGA. Why "noninverted"? Because in D-TGA, the aortic valve lies to the right (*dextro* or *D*) relative to the pulmonary valve. This is normal in visceroatrial situs solitus: In solitus normally related great arteries, the aortic valve lies to the *right* of the pulmonary valve (see Fig. 4.9). Hence, typical D-TGA, that is, TGA {S,D,D} is a *noninverted* transposition because there is no right–left reversal of the semilunar valves compared with what is normal in visceroatrial situs solitus. In typical D-TGA, the great arteries are transposed (ventriculoarterial discordance is present), but the great arteries are not inverted (right–left reversal is not present on comparison with what is normal in situs solitus).

Hence, **TGA {S,D,D}** (see Fig. 4.9) is typical complete, physiologically uncorrected, noninverted D-TGA. Associated malformations may or may not coexist.[19] When associated malformations are present, one can have **TGA {S,D,D} with VSD**; or **TGA {S,D,D} with VSD and pulmonary outflow tract stenosis (PS)**; or **TGA {S,D,D} with VSD of the AV canal type, straddling tricuspid valve, hypoplastic RV**, etc.[19]

DORV was regarded as a *partial* transposition because only one of the great arteries (not both) is transposed (see Fig. 4.9). In DORV, only the aorta is transposed relative to the ventricular septum; it is normal for the pulmonary artery to arise above the RV.

DOLV may also be regarded as a *partial* transposition, again because only one great artery (rather than both) is transposed (see Fig. 4.9). In DOLV, only the pulmonary artery is transposed relative to the ventricular septum; it is normal for the aorta to originate above the LV.

D-malposition of the great arteries is a broad term meaning only that the malposed aortic valve lies to the right (*dextro* or D) relative to the malposed pulmonary valve. D-transposition may be regarded as one specific type of D-malposition of the great arteries. Ordinarily, however, D-TGA is specifically so designated.

Where the concept of D-malposition of the great arteries is particularly helpful is in those situations in which the great arteries are malposed but *not* transposed, accurately speaking: DORV, DOLV, and anatomically corrected malposition of the great arteries (ACM) (see Fig. 4.9). For example:

DORV {S,D,D}, which is the most common anatomic type of DORV (see Fig. 4.9), means double-outlet right ventricle with the set of solitus atria, D-loop ventricles, and D-malposition of the great arteries. A bilateral conus (subaortic and subpulmonary) often is present, which precludes semilunar-atrioventricular fibrous continuity. The atrioventricular alignments are typically those of **atrioventricular concordance**, which is what one would expect from the segmental anatomy: {S,D,-}. The ventriculoarterial alignments are those of **DORV**, as is indicated in the brief diagnosis in front of the segmental situs set: DORV {S,D,D}. Associated malformations typically include a VSD that may be subaortic, or subpulmonary, or beneath both great arteries, or remote from both great arteries, or absent—the only outlet from the LV being an LV-to-RA shunt.[20,21] Hence, the diagnosis of a case, briefly expressed, was: **DORV {S,D,D} with subpulmonary VSD, bilateral conus, and systemic pulmonary hypertension. This is the Taussig-Bing type of DORV.**[22,23]

DOLV {S,D,D}, another example of D-malposition of the great arteries, means double-outlet left ventricle with the set of solitus atria, D-loop ventricles, and D-malposition of the great arteries (see Fig. 4.9). Again, there is **atrioventricular concordance**, as one would expect from the segmental anatomy: {S,D,-}. The ventriculoarterial alignments are those of **DOLV**, as the brief diagnosis indicates: DOLV {S,D,D}. As far as associated malformations are concerned, a VSD is common, as is great arterial outflow tract obstruction.[23] Hence, the diagnosis of a case, briefly expressed, was: **DOLV {S,D,D} with subaortic VSD, and PS (infundibular and valvar). This is the most common form of DOLV—the so-called tetralogy of Fallot type of DOLV** (because it has frequently been mistaken for tetralogy of Fallot).

Anatomically corrected malposition of the great arteries affords another example of D-malposition of the great arteries. **ACM {S,L,D}** (see Fig. 4.9) means anatomically corrected malposition of the great arteries with the set of solitus atria, L-loop ventricles, and D-malposition of the great arteries. There is **atrioventricular discordance**, as the segmental anatomy indicates {S,L,-}. There is **ventriculoarterial concordance**, as the brief diagnosis indicates: ACM {S,L,D}. *Anatomically corrected malposition of the great arteries* means two things: (1) The great arteries are malposed. (2) But despite their malposition, each great artery nonetheless arises above the anatomically correct ventricle: RV to PA and LV to Ao. Consequently, ACM means ventriculoarterial concordance. The conus is either bilateral (subaortic and subpulmonary) or subaortic only.[24,30] As far as associated malformations are concerned, ACM usually has a VSD.

Hence, the diagnosis of such a case may be expressed briefly as follows: **ACM {S,L,D} with bilateral conus, VSD, aortic outflow tract stenosis, preductal coarctation of the aorta, and large PDA (patent ductus arteriosus).**

ACM {S,L,D} is physiologically uncorrected. There is only one alignment discordance, at the atrioventricular level. There is ventriculoarterial concordance, by definition. Hence, an atrial switch procedure (Senning or Mustard procedure) achieves both a physiologic correction and an anatomic correction.

L-transposition of the great arteries means two things: (1) TGA is present. (2) The transposed aortic valve is to the left (*levo* or *L* = left, Latin) relative to the transposed pulmonary valve.

Examples of L-TGA are as follows (see Fig. 4.9):

1. **Classical physiologically corrected transposition is TGA {S,L,L}**, which means transposition of the great arteries with the set of solitus atria, L-loop ventricles, and L-transposition. Typically, there is atrioventricular discordance, as the segmental anatomy suggests: {S,L,-}. There is **ventriculoarterial discordance**, by definition (TGA). Two right–left switching errors (alignment discordances) cancel each other physiologically, associated malformations permitting. Consequently, the destinations of the venous blood streams should be physiologically correct: venae cavae to the pulmonary artery and pulmonary veins to the aorta. Associated malformations are frequent. The diagnosis of such a case may be expressed briefly as follows: **TGA {S,L,L} with subpulmonary VSD and severe left-sided tricuspid regurgitation (Ebstein-like anomaly of the left-sided tricuspid valve).**

TGA {S,L,L} is a *complete* transposition (not a partial transposition); it is a *congenitally physiologically corrected* transposition (because there are two alignment discordances that cancel each other); and it is an *inverted* TGA, because the aortic valve is to the *left* of the pulmonary valve, which is right–left switched on comparison with what is normal in situs solitus (in which the aortic valve is to the *right* of, posterior to, the pulmonary valve, see Fig. 4.9).

Although all three of the foregoing attributes of TGA {S,L,L} should be understood, by far the most important is that TGA {S,L,L} is *congenitally physiologically corrected* (at least in theory, if associated malformations do not uncorrect the potential physiologic correction). The fact that TGA {S,L,L} is a *complete* TGA is now of little or no importance because *all* transpositions are complete (not partial). The fact that TGA {S,L,L} is an *inverted* TGA in situs solitus is interesting but not very useful from a practical standpoint, because the concept of *inverted TGA* (like *ventricular inversion*) does not apply clearly and unambiguously to congenital heart disease as a whole:

Inverted TGA, for example, does not apply at all in visceroatrial situs ambiguus, because the basic type of visceroatrial situs is uncertain or unknown. Similarly, the concepts of *physiologically uncorrected* TGA and *physiologically corrected* TGA also do not apply in visceroatrial situs ambiguus, because both are atrial-situs-dependent concepts. By contrast, *D*-TGA and *L*-TGA do apply in visceroatrial situs ambiguus because *D*-TGA and *L*-TGA are not atrial-situs-dependent concepts.

The usage of *inverted* TGA in visceroatrial situs inversus is confused. Some feel that *D*-TGA is an inverted TGA for visceroatrial situs inversus; this is an atrial-situs-dependent interpretation. *D*-TGA is right–left reversed compared with what is "normal" in situs inversus, in which the aortic valve normally is to the *left* of and posterior to the pulmonary valve (Fig. 4.9). Others feel that *D*-TGA is a *noninverted* TGA in situs inversus; this is an atrial-situs-independent interpretation. This confusion in usage and meaning associated with *noninverted/inverted* TGA is entirely avoided by *D-/L*-TGA. Hence, *noninverted/inverted* TGA[18] will not be considered further.

2. **Physiologically uncorrected ("complete") transposition of the great arteries in situs inversus is TGA {I,L,L}**, which means transposition of the great arteries with the set of inverted atria, L-loop ventricles, and L-transposition. Typically, the **atrioventricular alignments are concordant**: {I,L,-}. The **ventriculoarterial alignments are discordant**, by definition (TGA). Since there is only one segmental alignment discordance (at the AV level), the circulations are physiologically uncorrected. Associated malformations may or may not be present.
3. **TGA {S,D,L}** means transposition of the great arteries with the set of solitus atria, D-loop ventricles, and L-position of the aorta. The atrioventricular alignments are concordant, as the segmental anatomy suggests: {S,D,-}. The **ventriculoarterial alignments** are discordant, by definition (TGA). Since there is only one alignment discordance (at the ventriculoarterial level), the circulations are physiologically uncorrected. Associated malformations are frequent. This is a specific type of physiologically uncorrected TGA with characteristic surgical challenges.[25] The diagnosis, briefly put, in one such case was: **TGA {S,D,L} with subaortic VSD, PS (subvalvar and valvar), underdevelopment of the RV sinus, and superoinferior ventricles.**

L-malposition of the great arteries, like D-malposition of the great arteries, occurs in three different conotruncal anomalies: (1) DORV, (2) DOLV, and (3) ACM.

Examples of each are as follows:

1. **DORV {S,L,L}** means double-outlet right ventricle with the set of solitus atria, L-loop ventricles, and L-malposition of the great arteries. Typically, there is **atrioventricular discordance**, as the segmental anatomy suggests: {S,L,-}. The ventriculoarterial alignments are those of **DORV**, by definition. Associated malformations are frequent.[26]
2. **DOLV {S,L,L}** briefly indicates double-outlet left ventricle with the set of solitus atria, L-loop ventricles, and L-malposition of the great arteries. There is **atrioventricular discordance** as the segmental anatomy suggests: {S,L,-}. The ventriculoarterial alignments are those of **DOLV**, as the brief diagnosis indicates: DOLV {S,L,L}. Associated malformations may include VSD and pulmonary outflow tract stenosis or atresia.
3. **ACM {S,D,L}** briefly indicates anatomically corrected malposition with the set of solitus atria, D-loop ventricles, and L-malposition of the great arteries. There is **AV concordance**: {S,D,-}. There is VA concordance, by definition (ACM). Associated malformations include a VSD (virtually always), subaortic stenosis, etc. ACM {S,D,L} is the most common anatomic type of ACM.

A-Transposition and A-Malposition

Occasionally, the transposed or malposed aortic valve may lie directly anterior (*antero* or *A*) to the transposed or malposed pulmonary valve. Hence, you will occasionally see cases of **TGA {S,D,A}, DORV {S,D,A}, and DOLV {S,D,A}**, etc.

To summarize, the semilunar interrelationships can be (see Figs. 4.9 through 4.11):

1. solitus normal (S),
2. inversus normal (I),
3. D-transposition or D-malposition (D),
4. L-transposition or L-malposition (L), and
5. A-transposition or A-malposition (A).

It is noteworthy that **S** and **I** are reserved for normally related great arteries only (solitus normal and inversus normal, respectively), and **D**, **L**, and **A** are used for abnormally related great arteries. **A** also is used to indicated abnormally formed atria: non-S and non-I. So the third symbol in the segmental situs set immediately indicates whether the great arteries are normally or abnormally related: for example, {S,D,**S**} and TGA {S,D,**D**}.

If the ventriculoarterial alignments are abnormal, then the type of abnormal ventriculoarterial alignment is indicated immediately in front of the segmental situs set: for example **TGA** {S,D,D} or **DORV** {S,D,D}, etc.

If the ventriculoarterial alignments are normal, no indication of this is placed before the segmental situs set. For example, we do not write NRGA {S,D,S}, meaning normally related great arteries with the set of.... "NRGA" is redundant, because this is what the S in the third element of {S,D,**S**} means.

By contrast, when the segmental situs set is {S,D,D}, it is essential to indicate the type of ventriculoarterial alignment because D as the third element in the set, {S,D,**D**}, indicates only the semilunar relationship, that is, that the aortic valve is to the right (*dextro* or *D*) of the pulmonary valve. The third symbol in an abnormal segmental situs set does not indicate the type of ventriculoarterial alignment. This is why **TGA** {S,D,D}, **DORV** {S,D,D}, and **DOLV** {S,D,D} are essential (not redundant).

Segmental Alignments

We often speak loosely about "normally related" great arteries and about "abnormally related" great arteries. But what we really mean is **normally aligned great arteries** and **abnormally aligned great arteries**. What matters both hemodynamically and surgically is the type of ventriculoarterial alignment, not the spatial relations between the great arteries.

Similarly, we sometimes speak loosely about atrioventricular "connections" and ventriculoarterial "connections." What we really mean is **atrioventricular alignments** and **ventriculoarterial alignments**. The atria and the ventricles do not connect muscle to muscle (except at the AV bundle of His) because of the interposition of the fibrous atrioventricular canal or junction. Similarly, the ventricles (ventricular sinuses or pumping portions) and the great arteries do not connect tissue to tissue because of the interposition of the conus arteriosus or infundibulum.

The three main cardiac segments—the atria, the ventricular sinuses, and the great arteries—are connected and separated by the two connecting cardiac segments: the atrioventricular canal or junction and the conus or infundibulum.

The distinction between segmental alignments and connections is important in the interests of anatomic and embryologic accuracy.

Have you ever considered what would happen if the atria and the ventricles really did connect muscle to muscle (instead of being separated by the fibrous atrioventricular junction)? If during cardiogenesis in utero the RA connected with the RV and the LA connected with the LV, then discordant L-loop ventricles would be developmentally impossible. It is because the atria and the ventricles are *not* connected directly that discordant L-loop ventricles and discordant D-loop ventricles can occur. Also, direct atrioventricular muscular connections would facilitate ventricular pre-excitation, resulting in the Wolff-Parkinson-White syndrome. Electrophysiologically, it is very important that the atria and the ventricles do not connect directly, muscle to muscle, except at the atrioventricular bundle of His. One of the functions of the fibrous atrioventricular junctional segment is to separate and to electrically insulate the ventricles from the atria, except at the His bundle.

Hence, the concept of AV *alignments* is anatomically and developmentally accurate, whereas the concept of AV *connections* is not.

Have you ever thought how important it is developmentally that the ventricles (i.e., the ventricular sinuses or pumping portions) do not connect directly, tissue to tissue, with the great arteries? During cardiogenesis in utero, if the RV connected directly with the PA, and if the LV connected directly with the Ao, then the VA alignments would always be concordant; that is, ventriculoarterial malalignments of all types (see Fig. 4.9) would be developmentally impossible.

Thus, for the understanding of the conotruncal anomalies, it is very important to appreciate that the ventricular sinuses and the great arteries really do not connect directly. This is why the growth and development of the **conal connector** is so important to the understanding of the developmental biology of normal and abnormal ventriculoarterial alignments.[14] If the growth and development of the conal connector is abnormal, then the ventriculoarterial alignments are abnormal.[14]

But isn't the conus arteriosus or infundibulum an intrinsic part of the RV? Not really. The conus arteriosus forms the outflow tract of *both* ventricles (not just of the RV). In a variety of anomalies, the distal or subsemilunar part of the conus can be partly or even entirely above the LV, proving that the conus and the RV sinus can and do dissociate. Anomalies in which the distal (subsemilunar) part of the conus often is above the LV include DOLV[23] and ACM.[24]

Note that the great arteries arise **above** the ventricles, not **from** the ventricles.

The main cardiac segments—the atria, the ventricles, and the great arteries—are like "bricks." The connecting cardiac segments—the atrioventricular canal or junction, and the conus arteriosus or infundibulum—are like "mortar." This is why the main cardiac segments may be aligned in so many different ways—because they do not connect directly. Instead, the main cardiac segments are connected and are separated by the interposed connecting segments.

The Segmental Approach to Diagnosis

The segmental approach to the diagnosis of congenital heart disease[8,9,11] is based on an understanding of the morphologic cardiac anatomy (Chapter 3) and the segmental cardiac anatomy (the present chapter).

This segment-by-segment or step-by-step approach is a **sequential approach**[27] to diagnosis in the sense that one proceeds in a venoarterial sequence from atria to ventricles to great arteries. The segment-by-segment approach is also a **systematic approach** to diagnosis.[28]

The new feature of the segmental approach to diagnosis is that the patterns of anatomic organization (the situs) of the atria, of the ventricles, and of the great arteries are diagnosed independently. The ventricular anatomy and the great arterial anatomy are not diagnosed relative to the atrial situs. Because the segmental approach is *not* an atrial-situs-dependent method, the meanings of the terms used to describe the ventricular situs (D-loop/L-loop ventricles) and the meanings of the terms used to describe the great arterial situs (S, I, D, L, A) never change or become meaningless. Consequently, the segmental approach facilitates accurate diagnostic **data analysis** in large series of complex cases. For example, the segmental approach now makes it possible to answer questions such as: How many anatomic types of transposition of the great arteries are there, and what are they?[19]

Segmental set analysis is also facilitated by the segmental approach. For example, is TGA **{S,D,L}** statistically significantly different from TGA **{S,D,D}**, and if so, in what respects?[25] Different segmental situs sets (combinations) often have specific and very different associated malformations on comparison with other segmental situs sets. TGA {S,D,L} proved to have six statistically significant differences on comparison with the usual type of TGA, that is, TGA {S,D,D}.[25] Why is TGA **{S,L,L}** so much more prone to single LV (absence of the RV sinus) than is TGA **{S,D,D}**?[19] At present, to our knowledge, no one knows the answer. But the point is that **segmental set analysis** is a promising new research method that is facilitated by the segmental approach to diagnosis.

In concluding this chapter, we would like to acknowledge that the diagnostic approach to the diagnosis of congenital heart disease that is currently used worldwide has been built by many hands. It is a **segment-by-segment, alignment-by-alignment, and connection-by-connection method. Associated malformations** are regarded as very important. **Functional aspects** are emphasized: How does this combination of cardiac segments, alignments, and connections—with or without associated malformations—function? Although the anatomic diagnosis is emphasized in this book, the physiologic diagnosis is considered to be equally as important.

Lev[29] introduced the morphologic method of chamber diagnosis and designation, emphasizing septal surface morphologies. **Van Praagh et al.**[8-12] extended the morphologic method, including not only the *septal surface morphologies* but also the *free wall* morphologies, and they applied the morphologic method in a systematic, segment-by-segment way to facilitate accurate diagnosis. **Kirklin et al.**[30] and **Shinebourne et al.**[27] emphasized the hemodynamic, clinical, and surgical importance of atrioventricular and ventriculoarterial concordance or discordance. **De la Cruz** and **Da Rocha**[31] focused attention on ventricular D-loops and L-loops. **Otero Coto** and **Quero Jiménez**[32] pointed out that there are really *five* diagnostically important cardiac segments—atria, atrioventricular canal, ventricles (ventricular sinuses), infundibulum or conus, and great arteries, not just *three*—atria, ventricles, and great arteries. Anderson and his colleagues[7,13] made important contributions, both terminologic and anatomic.

This diagnostic approach is eminently applicable to all imaging techniques, such as cardiac catheterization and angiocardiography, echocardiography (one-, two-, and three-dimensional), and magnetic resonance imaging. It also works very well under direct vision, as in the operating room.

REFERENCES

1. Van Praagh S, Santini F, Sanders SP. Cardiac malpositions with special emphasis on visceral heterotaxy (asplenia and polysplenia syndromes). In: Fyler DC, ed. *Nadas' Pediatric Cardiology*. St. Louis: Hanley & Belfus, Inc, Philadelphia, and Mosby-Yearbook, Inc; 1992:589.
2. Hastreiter AR, Rodriguez-Coronel A. Discordant situs of thoracic and abdominal viscera. *Am J Cardiol.* 1968;22:111.
3. Clarkson PM, Brandt PWT, Barratt-Boyes BG, Neutze JM. Isolated atrial inversion: visceral situs solitus, visceroatrial discordance, discordant ventricular d-loop without transposition, dextrocardia: diagnosis and surgical correction. *Am J Cardiol.* 1972;29:877.
4. Van Praagh S, LaCorte M, Fellows KE, et al. Supero-inferior ventricles, anatomic and angiocardiographic findings in 10 postmortem cases. In: Van Praagh R, Takao A, eds. *Etiology and Morphogenesis of Congenital Heart Disease*. Mt Kisco: Futura Publishing Co; 1980:317.
5. Foran RB, Belcourt C, Nanton MA, et al. Isolated infundibuloarterial inversion {S,D,I}: a newly recognized form of congenital heart disease. *Am Heart J.* 1988;116:1337.
6. Van Praagh R, David I, Gordon D, Wright GB, Van Praagh S. Ventricular diagnosis and designation. In: Godman M, ed. *Paediatric Cardiology 1980*. Edinburgh: Churchill Livingstone; 1981:153.
7. Anderson RH, Shinebourne ER, Gerlis LM. Criss-cross atrioventricular relationships producing paradoxical atrioventricular concordance or discordance: their significance to nomenclature of congenital heart disease. *Circulation.* 1974;50:176.
8. Van Praagh R, Ongley PA, Swan HJC. Anatomic types of single or common ventricle in man, morphologic and geometric aspects in 60 autopsied cases. *Am J Cardiol.* 1964;13:367.
9. Van Praagh R, Van Praagh S, Vlad P, Keith JD. Anatomic types of congenital dextrocardia, diagnostic and embryologic implications. *Am J Cardiol.* 1964;13:510.
10. Van Praagh R, Plett JA, Van Praagh S. Single ventricle: pathology, embryology, terminology, and classification. *Herz.* 1979;4:113.
11. Van Praagh R. The segmental approach to diagnosis in congenital heart disease. In: Bergsma D, ed. *Birth Defects: Original Article Series*. 1972;8:4.
12. Van Praagh R. When concordant or discordant atrioventricular alignments predict the ventricular situs wrongly. I. Solitus atria, concordant alignments, and L-loop ventricles. II. Solitus atria, discordant alignments, and D-loop ventricles. *J Am Coll Cardiol.* 1987;10:1278.
13. Anderson RH, Smith A, Wilkinson JL. Disharmony between atrioventricular connections and segmental combination, unusual variants of "crisscross" hearts. *J Am Coll Cardiol.* 1987;10:1273.
14. Van Praagh R, Layton WM, Van Praagh S. The morphogenesis of normal and abnormal relationships between the great arteries and the ventricles: pathologic and experimental data. In: Van Praagh R,

Takao A, eds. *Etiology and Morphogenesis of Congenital Heart Disease.* Mt Kisco: Futura Publishing Company; 1980:271.
15. Van Praagh R, Pérez-Treviño C, López-Cuellar M, et al. Transposition of the great arteries with posterior aorta, anterior pulmonary artery, subpulmonary conus and fibrous continuity between aortic and atrioventricular valves. *Am J Cardiol.* 1971;28:621.
16. Vierordt H. Die angeborenen herzkrankheiten. In: *Nothnagel's Spec Path Therapie.* 1898:1.
17. Abbott ME. Congenital cardiac diseases. In: Osler W, McCrae T, eds. *Modern Medicine.* Philadelphia: Lea & Febiger; 1915:323.
18. Spitzer A. Über den Bauplan des normalen und missbildeten Herzens. Versuch einer phylogenetischen Theorie. *Virchows Arch Pathol Anat.* 1923;243:81. [Spitzer A: The Architecture of Normal and Malformed Hearts: a Phylogenetic Theory of Their Development, with a Summary and Analysis of the Theory by M. Lev and A. Vass, Springfield, Charles C. Thomas, 1951.]
19. Van Praagh R. Transposition of the great arteries: history, pathologic anatomy, embryology, etiology, and surgical considerations. In: Mavroudis C, Backer CL, eds. *Cardiac Surgery, the Arterial Switch Operation, State of the Art Reviews.* Philadelphia: Hanley & Belfus, Inc; 1991:5–7.
20. Megarity A, Chambers R, Calder AL, Van Praagh S, Van Praagh R. Double-outlet right ventricle with left ventricular-right atrial communication: fibrous obstruction of left ventricular outlet by membranous septum and tricuspid leaflet tissue. *Am Heart J.* 1972;84:242.
21. Taussig HB, Bing RJ. Complete transposition of the aorta and a levoposition of the pulmonary artery. Clinical, physiological, and pathological findings. *Am Heart J.* 1949;37:551.
22. Van Praagh R. What is the Taussig-Bing malformation? *Circulation.* 1968;38:445.
23. Van Praagh R, Weinberg PM, Srebro J. Double outlet left ventricle. In: Adams FH, Emmanouilides GC, Riemenschneider TA, eds. *Moss' Heart Disease in Infants, Children and Adolescents.* 4th ed. Baltimore: Williams & Wilkins; 1989:461.
24. Van Praagh R, Van Praagh S. Anatomically corrected transposition of the great arteries. *Br Heart J.* 1967;29:112.
25. Houyel L, Van Praagh R, Lacour-Gayet F, et al. Transposition of the great arteries {S,D,L}: pathologic anatomy, diagnosis, and surgical management of a newly recognized complex. *J Thorac Cardiovasc Surg.* 1995;110:613.
26. Van Praagh S, Davidoff A, Chin A, Shiel FS, Reynolds J, Van Praagh R. Double outlet right ventricle: anatomic types and developmental implications based on a study of 101 autopsied cases. *Coeur.* 1982;13:389.
27. Shinebourne EA, Macartney FJ, Anderson RH. Sequential chamber localization—logical approach to diagnosis in congenital heart disease. *Br Heart J.* 1976;38:327.
28. Rao PS. Systematic approach to differential diagnosis. *Am Heart J.* 1981;102:389.
29. Lev M. Pathological diagnosis of positional variations in cardiac chambers in congenital heart disease. *Lab Invest.* 1964;3:71.
30. Kirklin JW, Pacifico AD, Bargeron LM, Soto B. Cardiac repair in anatomically corrected malposition of the great arteries. *Circulation.* 1973;48:154.
31. De la Cruz M, DaRocha JP. An ontogenetic theory for the explanation of congenital malformations involving the truncus and conus. *Am Heart J.* 1956;51:782.
32. Otero Coto E, Quero Jiménez M. Approximación segmentaria al diagnóstico y clasificación de las cardiopatías congénitas, *Fundamentos y utilidad. Rev Esp Cardiol.* 1977;30:557.

SECTION IV

Congenital Heart Disease

5

The Congenital Cardiac Pathology Database

An accurate, statistically analyzed database is considered to be of fundamental importance in the effort to make our field more quantitative. At present, almost no book on pediatric cardiology, pediatric cardiac surgery, or pediatric cardiac pathology has a database. We initially thought that Abbott's[1] epochal *Atlas of Congenital Cardiac Disease,* based on 1000 postmortem cases, was an exception.

However, on further investigation we found that this classic was, to a major degree, a literature review,[2] not a consecutive series of personally studied cases.

Fortunately, however, there are at least four excellent exceptions:

- *The Report of the New England Regional Infant Cardiac Program* (RICP) by Fyler and his associates[3]
- *The Baltimore-Washington Infant Study* (BWIS) of Ferencz and her colleagues[4,5]
- *The Pathology of Congenital Heart Disease* by Bharati and Lev[6]
- *Necropsied Cases of Japanese Patients with Congenital Heart Disease* by Ando and his coworkers[7]

The publications of Fyler[3] and Ferencz[4,5] are epidemiologic studies, whereas the books by Bharati and Lev[6] and Ando[7] are pathology studies. To the best of our present knowledge, these are the only published data with which our own findings can be compared statistically.

Although terminology, the understanding of etiology and morphogenesis, and the methods of diagnosis and treatment of congenital heart disease all will change to some extent over time, nonetheless the pathologic anatomy appears to be a virtual constant. Hence, the primary emphasis of the present study is on pathologic anatomic *data*.

Table 5.1 is a summary of the congenital cardiac pathology database, based on personal study of 3216 consecutive cases. These cases were studied at the Children's Hospital in Boston, from 1951 to 1997 inclusive, a consecutive 47-year period. We have seven cases between 1944 and 1950, but the consecutive series did not begin until 1951. Cases from 1965 and earlier were studied retrospectively, whereas patients from 1966 on were examined prospectively.

How many anatomic types of congenital heart disease are there?

Table 5.1 attempts to answer this "impossible" question. In Table 5.1, 203 different anatomic types of congenital cardiovascular disease are summarized.

In the present series (see Table 5.1), 68 ranks were found, ranging from the most common—**ventricular septal defect** (VSD), 36.23% (34.56%–37.90% being the 95% confidence interval)—to the rarest (0.03%). Table 5.1 represents a *summary* of the material basis of most of this book. The chapters that follow serve as illustration, explanation, and commentary.

Table 5.1 will repay careful study. Even the *cognoscenti* of congenital heart disease will find "gems" here—entities that they may never have heard of or seen.

The numbers are intriguing. For example, there has been considerable discussion about what the most common form of congenital heart disease really is. Some have favored bicuspid (bicommissural) aortic valve. Although they may perhaps be right in the population of all living people (p), in our sample of this population (p), VSD was by far the most common anatomic type of congenital heart disease (36.23%, 34.56%–37.90%, see Table 5.1), whereas **bicuspid aortic valve** ranked 13th in prevalence (8.02%, 7.08%–8.96%, see Table 5.1).

It has often been said that **tetralogy of Fallot** (TOF) is the most common form of cyanotic congenital heart disease, ranking sixth in our database (13.31%, 12.14%–14.48%, see Table 5.1). We were therefore surprised to find that **transposition of the great arteries** (TGA) appears to be slightly more common (15.17%, 13.94%–16.40%, see Table 5.1).

The three most common forms of congenital heart disease (see Table 5.1)—VSD (36.23%), **secundum atrial septal defect** (24.66%), and **patent ductus arteriosus** (17.57%)—all may be regarded as the abnormal postnatal persistence of normal prenatal states.

However, as will be seen, the reasons for the postnatal persistence of these prenatal flow pathways are congenital malformations.

Hence, Table 5.1 merits careful consideration, because it represents a summary of "the big picture," in numerical perspective.

The limitations of Table 5.1 also merit mention. Because this table is a summary, it is lacking in analysis and context. For example, although VSD was the most common anomaly found in this series, one also wants to know the answers to several other questions: In how many of these patients was the diagnosis *isolated* VSD? And in how many of these cases was the VSD merely part of *complex congenital heart disease*, such as TGA or double-outlet right ventricle (DORV)? In the latter cases, the main diagnosis was TGA or DORV—not VSD.

It should be stated explicitly that we have not seen a case of *isolated* VSD at autopsy in many years. This is what I mean by saying that *analysis* and *context* are also essential to clinical

TABLE 5.1 **The Congenital Cardiac Pathology Database (n = 3216)**

Entity Number	Rank Order	Type of Congenital Heart Disease	Number of Patients	% of Series	95% Confidence Interval
1	1st	Ventricular septal defect, all types	1165	36.23	34.56–37.90
2	2nd	Atrial septal defect, ostium secundum type	793	24.66	23.17–26.15
3	3rd	Patent ductus arteriosus (>2 weeks of age)	565	17.57	16.26–18.88
4	4th	Transposition of the great arteries, all types	488	15.17	13.94–16.40
5	5th	Common atrioventricular canal, all types	481	14.96	13.73–16 .19
6	6th	Tetralogy of Fallot	428	13.31	12.14–14.48
7	7th	Aortic stenosis, all types	398	12.38	11.24–13.52
8	8th	Persistent left/right superior vena cava	415	12.90	11.74–14.06
9	9th	Coarctation of aorta, all types	379	11.78	10.67–12.89
10	10th	Pulmonary stenosis, all types	338	10.51	9.45–11.57
11	11th	Double-outlet right ventricle, all types	265	8.24	7.29–9.19
12	12th	Coronary artery anomaly, all types	261	8.12	7.18–9.06
13	13th	Bicuspid (bicommissural) aortic valve	258	8.02	7.08–8.96
14	14th	Bicuspid (bicommissural) pulmonary valve	248	7.71	6.79–8.63
15	15th	Aortic atresia, valvar	235	7.31	6.41–8.21
16	16th	Right aortic arch in situs solitus or left aortic arch in situs inversus	225	7.00	6.12–7.8
17	17th	Mitral stenosis, congenital	224	6.97	6.09–7.5
18	18th	Mitral regurgitation	216	6.72	5.85–7.59
19	18th	Endocardial fibroelastosis of the left ventricle	216	6.72	5.85–7.59
20	19th	Totally anomalous pulmonary venous connection	203	6.31	5.47–7.15
21	20th	Pulmonary atresia with ventricular septal defect, all types (tetralogy of Fallot excluded)	198	6.16	5.33–6.99
22	21st	Mitral atresia	183	5.59	4.89–6.49
23	22nd	Aberrant right or left subclavian artery	170	5.29	4 .52–6.06
24	23rd	Dextrocardia	120	3.73	3.08–4.38
25	24th	Hypoplasia or absence of the left ventricle	113	3.51	2.87–4.15
26	24th	Tricuspid regurgitation, congenital	113	3.51	2.8 7–4.15
27	25th	Tricuspid atresia	111	3.45	2.82–4.08
28	25th	Truncus arteriosus	111	3.45	2.82–4.08
29	26th	Common atrium	108	3.36	2.74–3.98
30	27th	Asplenia syndrome	94	2.92	2.34–3.50
31	28th	Pulmonary atresia with intact ventricular septum	88	2.74	2.18–3.30
32	29th	Ebstein anomaly	83	2.58	2.03–3.13
33	29th	Tricuspid stenosis, congenital	83	2.58	2.03–3.13
34	30th	Single left ventricle with infundibular outlet chamber	81	2.52	1.98–3.06
35	30th	Right ventricular hypoplasia, primary	81	2.52	1.98–3.06
36	31st	Interrupted aortic arch	67	2.08	1.59–2.57
37	31st	Major aortopulmonary collateral arteries	67	2.08	1.59–2.57
38	32nd	Aortic regurgitation, congenital	64	1.99	1.51–2.47
39	33rd	Unicuspid (unicommissural) aortic valve	63	1.96	1.48–2.44
40	34th	Polyvalvular disease	62	1.93	1.45–2.41
41	35th	Absent ductus arteriosus	59	1.83	1.37–2.29
42	36th	Polysplenia syndrome	57	1.77	1.31–2.23
43	37th	Cleft mitral valve	43	1.34	0.94–1.74
44	38th	Interrupted inferior vena cava	42	1.31	0.92–1.70

Continued

TABLE 5.1 **The Congenital Cardiac Pathology Database (n = 3216)—cont'd**

Entity Number	Rank Order	Type of Congenital Heart Disease	Number of Patients	% of Series	95% Confidence Interval
45	38th	Partially anomalous pulmonary venous connection	41	1.27	0.88–1.66
46	39th	Straddling tricuspid valve	41	1.27	0.88–1.66
47	40th	Juxtaposition of the atrial appendages, left-sided	38	1.18	0.81–1.55
48	41st	Coronary sinus septal defect	36	1.12	0.76–1.48
49	41st	Premature closure of the foramen ovale	36	1.12	0.76–1.48
50	42nd	Anomalous muscle bundles of the right ventricle	33	1.03	0.68–1.38
51	42nd	Sinusoids	33	1.03	0.68–1.38
52	43rd	Absent pulmonary valve leaflets	31	0.96	0.62–1.30
53	44th	Double-orifice mitral valve	28	0.87	0.55–1.19
54	45th	Hypertrophic cardiomyopathy	26	0.81	0.50–1.12
55	45th	Single right ventricle (left ventricle absent)	26	0.81	0.50–1.12
56	45th	Hypoplastic mitral valve	26	0.81	0.50–1.12
57	46th	Brachiocephalic arteries, anomalies of	25	0.78	0.48–1.08
58	46th	Left ventricular outflow tract obstruction	25	0.78	0.48–1.08
59	47th	Heart block, complete, congenital	24	0.75	0.45–1.05
60	48th	Potentially parachute mitral valve with common atrioventricular canal	23	0.72	0.43–1.01
61	48th	Straddling mitral valve	23	0.72	0.43–1.01
62	48th	Left ventricular inlet and outlet obstruction	23	0.72	0.43–1.01
63	49th	Superoinferior ventricles	22	0.68	0.40–0.96
64	50th	Vascular ring	21	0.65	0.37–0.93
77	55th	Anterolateral muscle of the left ventricle (muscle of Moulaert), prominent	13	0.40	0.18–0.62
78	55th	Marfan syndrome	13	0.40	0.18–0.62
79	55th	Absence of a pulmonary artery branch	13	0.40	0.18–0.62
80	55th	Scimitar syndrome	13	0.40	0.18–0.62
81	56th	Cor triatriatum (sinistrum)	12	0.37	0.16–0.58
82	57th	Double aortic arch	11	0.34	0.14–0.54
83	58th	Sinus venosus defect	10	0.31	0.12–0.50
84	58th	Quadricuspid aortic valve	10	0.31	0.12–0.50
85	58th	Supramitral stenosing ring	10	0.31	0.12–0.50
86	58th	William syndrome	10	0.31	0.12–0.50
87	58th	Crisscross hearts	10	0.31	0.12–0.50
88	58th	Aneurysms of sinus venosus	10	0.31	0.12–0.50
89	59th	Aneurysm of the left ventricle, congenital	9	0.28	0.10–0.46
90	60th	Bicuspid truncal valve	9	0.28	0.10–0.46
91	60th	Ectopia cordis	9	0.28	0.10–0.46
92	60th	Isolated levocardia	9	0.28	0.10–0.46
93	60th	Lung, absence of	9	0.28	0.10–0.46
94	60th	Uhl disease of the right ventricle	9	0.28	0.10–0.46
95	61st	Left ventricular dysplasia	8	0.25	0.08–0.42
96	61st	Pulmonary artery sling	8	0.25	0.08–0.42
97	62nd	Blood cyst, prominent	7	0.22	0.06–0.38
98	62nd	Typical congenital mitral stenosis with left ventricular outflow tract obstruction	7	0.22	0.06–0.38
99	62nd	Quadricuspid pulmonary valve	7	0.22	0.06–0.38
100	62nd	Absence or atresia of the right superior vena cava	7	0.22	0.06 to .38

TABLE 5.1 The Congenital Cardiac Pathology Database (n = 3216)—cont'd

Entity Number	Rank Order	Type of Congenital Heart Disease	Number of Patients	% of Series	95% Confidence Interval
101	63rd	Common-inlet right ventricle	6	0.19	0.04–0.34
102	63rd	Cantrell syndrome	6	0.19	0.04–0.34
103	63rd	Left ventricular to right atrial shunt	6	0.19	0.04–0.34
104	63rd	Myxomatous mitral valve	6	0.19	0.04–0.34
105	63rd	Absence or hypoplasia of left ventricular papillary muscle, without parachute mitral valve	6	0.19	0.04–0.34
106	63rd	{S,L,S}, i.e., isolated ventricular inversion	6	0.19	0.04–0.34
107	64th	Anatomically corrected malposition {S,D,L}	5	0.16	*
108	64th	Anomalous muscle bundles of the left ventricle	5	0.16	
109	64th	Double-outlet infundibular outlet chamber	5	0.16	
110	64th	Discontinuous pulmonary artery branches	5	0.16	
111	64th	{I,D,S}, i.e., situs inversus of atria, D-loop ventricles, solitus normally related great arteries	5	0.16	
112	64th	Rhabdomyoma	5	0.16	
113	65th	Absence of main pulmonary artery	4	0.12	
114	65th	Obstructive bulboventricular foramen	4	0.12	
115	65th	Chiari network, prominent	4	0.12	
116	65th	Displaced septum primum	4	0.12	
117	65th	Isolation of the left atrial appendages	4	0.12	
118	65th	Retroaortic innominate vein	4	0.12	
119	65th	Left ventricular diverticulum, apical	4	0.12	
120	65th	Absence or defect of pericardium	4	0.12	
121	65th	Pulmonary artery branch from ascending aorta ("hemitruncus")	4	0.12	
122	65th	Functionally single right ventricle, i.e., diminutive left ventricle present	4	0.12	
123	66th	Congenitally unguarded tricuspid orifice, i.e., absent tricuspid leaflets	3	0.09	
124	66th	Diverticulum of Kommerell	3	0.09	
125	66th	Double-outlet right atrium, i.e., one atrioventricular valve opening into each ventricle	3	0.09	
126	66th	Intussusception of the left atrial appendage (inside-out appendage)	3	0.09	
127	66th	Isolated left subclavian artery	3	0.09	
128	66th	Right atrial outlet atresia, i.e., right-sided "mitral" atresia with large left ventricle	3	0.09	
129	66th	Raghib syndrome	3	0.09	
130	66th	{S,L,I}, i.e., solitus atria, L-loop ventricles, with inverted normally related great arteries	3	0.09	
131	67th	Aneurysm of sinus of Valsalva	2	0.06	
132	67th	Annuloaortic ectasia	2	0.06	
133	67th	Adherent mitral valve (plastered against left ventricular septal surface)	2	0.06	
134	67th	Isolated ostium primum type of atrial septal defect (without cleft mitral valve or ventricular septal defect of atrioventricular canal type)	2	0.06	

Continued

TABLE 5.1 **The Congenital Cardiac Pathology Database (n = 3216)—cont'd**

Entity Number	Rank Order	Type of Congenital Heart Disease	Number of Patients	% of Series	95% Confidence Interval
135	67th	{A(S),L,I} i.e., situs ambiguus of the viscera, solitus atria, L-loop ventricles, and inverted normally related great arteries	2	0.06	
136	67th	Ostial stenosis of pulmonary arterial branch	2	0.06	
137	67th	Atrioventricular situs discordance with atrioventricular alignment concordance	2	0.06	
138	67th	Common-inlet left ventricle	2	0.06	
139	67th	Crossed pulmonary arteries	2	0.06	
140	67th	Common ventricle (ventricular septum absent)	2	0.06	
141	67th	Endocardial fibroelastosis of the left ventricle, familial	2	0.06	
142	67th	{I,L,I}, i.e., situs inversus of viscera and atria, L-loop ventricles, and inverted normally related great arteries	2	0.06	
143	67th	Inferior vena cava, narrowing of at level of liver	2	0.06	
144	67th	Moderator band of left ventricle	2	0.06	
145	67th	Innominate vein anterior to thymus	2	0.06	
146	67th	Malincorporation of common pulmonary vein	2	0.06	
147	67th	Right atrium, idiopathic dilatation of	2	0.06	
148	67th	Right ventricular dysplasia syndrome	2	0.06	
149	67th	Right ventricle, small chambered and thick walled (without pulmonary atresia and intact ventricular septum)	2	0.06	
150	67th	Straddling of both tricuspid valve and mitral valve	2	0.06	
151	67th	{S,D,I}, i.e., isolated infundibuloarterial inversion	2	0.06	
152	67th	Subclavian artery as first branch of aortic arch	2	0.06	
153	67th	Right superior vena cava draining into left atrium	2	0.06	
154	67th	Triple-orifice mitral valve	2	0.06	
155	67th	Triple-orifice tricuspid valve	2	0.06	
156	67th	Muscular tricuspid valve	2	0.06	
157	68th	Acardia (in twin)	1	0.03	
158	68th	Aneurysm, coronary sinus	1	0.03	
159	68th	Acommissural aortic valve	1	0.03	
160	68th	Absence of aortic valve leaflets	1	0.03	
161	68th	{A(I),L,I}, i.e., situs ambiguus of the viscera, inverted atria, L- loop ventricles and inverted normally related great arteries	1	0.03	
162	68th	{A(I),L,S}, i.e., isolated infundibuloarterial noninversion	1	0.03	
163	68th	Absence of left atrial appendage	1	0.03	
164	68th	{A,L,I}, i.e., situs ambiguus of viscera and atria, L-loop ventricles, and inverted normally related great arteries	1	0.03	
165	68th	Alagille syndrome, i.e., peripheral pulmonary stenosis, cholestasis, and odd facies	1	0.03	
166	68th	Cervical aortic arch	1	0.03	
167	68th	Cor triatriatum dextrum	1	0.03	
168	68th	Double-inlet and double-outlet right ventricle	1	0.03	

TABLE 5.1 **The Congenital Cardiac Pathology Database (n = 3216)—cont'd**

Entity Number	Rank Order	Type of Congenital Heart Disease	Number of Patients	% of Series	95% Confidence Interval
169	68th	Double-outlet left atrium, i.e., one atrioventricular valve to each ventricle	1	0.03	
170	68th	Fifth aortic arch, persistent	1	0.03	
171	68th	Glycogen storage disease (Pompe disease)	1	0.03	
172	68th	Infundibular atresia, isolated	1	0.03	
173	68th	Carotid artery, isolated	1	0.03	
174	68th	{I,D,I}, i.e., isolated ventricular noninversion	1	0.03	
175	68th	Left innominate artery, isolated	1	0.03	
176	68th	{IS,D,S} with polysplenia, i.e., situs inversus of the viscera, situs solitus of the atria, D-loop ventricles, and solitus normally related great arteries	1	0.03	
177	68th	Interseptovalvular space, prominent	1	0.03	
178	68th	Inferior vena cava, right-to-left switching of (at liver)	1	0.03	
179	68th	Inferior vena cava draining into left atrium via coronary sinus septal defect	1	0.03	
180	68th	Levoatrial cardinal vein	1	0.03	
181	68th	Left atrium, absence of	1	0.03	
182	68th	Left subclavian artery, ostial stenosis of	1	0.03	
183	68th	Microcardia	1	0.03	
184	68th	Multiple orifice common atrioventricular valve	1	0.03	
185	68th	Multiple orifice tricuspid valve	1	0.03	
186	68th	Congenitally unguarded mitral orifice, i.e., absence of mitral leaflets	1	0.03	
187	68th	Mitral valve causing left ventricular outflow tract obstruction	1	0.03	
188	68th	Mitral valve, partly muscular	1	0.03	
189	68th	Normally related great arteries with bilateral conus	1	0.03	
190	68th	Origin of the right and left pulmonary artery branches from ascending aorta	1	0.03	
191	68th	Overriding tricuspid valve	1	0.03	
192	68th	Pseudocoarctation of the aorta	1	0.03	
193	68th	Premature closure of the ductus arteriosus	1	0.33	
194	68th	Patent ductus venosus	1	0.33	
195	68th	Premature narrowing of the foramen ovale	1	0.03	
196	68th	Rendu-Osler-Weber disease, i.e., pulmonary arteriovenous fistulae and familial hemorrhagic telangiectasia	1	0.03	
197	68th	Solitary aorta arising above the right ventricle with absence of the main pulmonary artery	1	0.03	
198	68th	Supramitral band, congenital	1	0.03	
199	68th	Submitral network	1	0.03	
200	68th	Senger syndrome, i.e., nonobstructive hypertrophic cardiomyopathy with cataracts	1	0.03	
201	68th	Teratoma, intrapericardial	1	0.03	
202	68th	Umbilical vein running anteriorly and superiorly to the liver	1	0.03	
203	68th	Vascular vice with totally anomalous pulmonary venous connection	1	0.03	

*95% confidence intervals not given when the number of the proportion, np 5, to avoid inaccuracy.[8]

relevance. Such analysis and context are provided in the chapters that follow.

Also, one may say that TGA is somewhat more common in our experience than is TOF. However, this is a comparison of *all* cases of TGA (physiologically uncorrected and congenitally physiologically corrected) versus all cases of TOF. In considering cyanotic congenital heart disease, one may well wish to exclude corrected transposition (even though it too can be cyanotic). Again, this type of analytic data is provided in the chapters that follow.

Another possible criticism of Table 5.1 is: This is an institutional database, not a regional database. Moreover, this is a pathology database, not a live-patient database. Hence, our pathology-based data may be skewed in the direction of "badness," that is, unusually severe disease. In view of these limitations, why should one suppose that our institutional pathology database bear any relationship to what happens in the real world?

Our answer: It is because of these concerns that our data are statistically compared, whenever possible, with the aforementioned epidemiologic and pathologic studies.[3 7] As will be seen concerning VSD, for example, our data typically are not statistically significantly different from those of epidemiologic studies, such as the RICP.[3] When they differ, our epidemiologic colleagues think that our pathologic data are probably more accurate, because there is nothing "harder" than good pathology data. The fact that our pathology data have been gathered over such a long period (47 years), through so many different medical and surgical eras at a hospital that is de facto a regional and a world center, may explain why the findings in our pathology database typically are not statistically significantly different from the epidemiologic data of Fyler et al.[3] that were gathered from the same region during part of the same time. Nonetheless, statistical comparison of our data with those of the other investigators is an integral part of the present study. However, such statistical comparisons are not always possible. It should be understood that the data of the present study are much more detailed than have been published in most previous epidemiologic, clinical, and laboratory studies.

If one is wondering, "Why do the percentages in Table 5.1 not add up to 100%?," the answer is because this table is a list of congenital cardiovascular anomalies, not a list of the main diagnoses in these 3216 patients. Most patients had more than one anomaly.

REFERENCES

1. Abbott ME. Atlas of congenital cardiac disease. *Am Heart Assoc.* 1936:1–62.
2. Bauer D de F, Astbury EC. Congenital cardiac disease bibliography of the 1,000 cases analyzed in Maude Abbott's atlas, with an index. *Am Heart J.* 1944;27:688–732.
3. Fyler DC, Buckley LP, Hellenbrand WE, Cohn HE. Report of the New England regional infant cardiac program. *Pediatrics.* 1980;65(suppl):377–461.
4. Ferencz C, Rubin JD, Loffredo CA, Magee CA, eds. *Epidemiology of Congenital Heart Disease. The Baltimore-Washington Infant Study 1981-1989. Perspectives in Pediatric Cardiology.* Vol. 4. Mount Kisco, NY: Futura Publishing Company, Inc; 1993:1–353.
5. Ferencz C, Loffredo CA, Correa -Villasenor A, Wilson PD, eds. *Genetic and Environmental Risk Factors of Major Cardiovascular Malformations: The Baltimore-Washington Infant Study: 1981-1989. Perspectives in Pediatric Cardiology.* Vol. 5. Armonk, NY: Futura Publishing Company, Inc; 1997:1–463.
6. Bharati S, Lev M. *The Pathology of Congenital Heart Disease, a Personal Experience with More than 6,300 Congenitally Malformed Hearts.* Armonk, NY: Futura Publishing Company, Inc; 1996:1–1554.
7. Ando M. *Necropsied Cases of Japanese Patients with Congenital Heart Disease. Tokyo Women's Medical College.* Tokyo: Heart Institute of Japan; 1984:1–626.
8. Glantz SA. In: *Primer of Biostatistics.* 2nd ed. New York: McGraw -Hill, Inc; 1987:183.

6

Systemic Venous Anomalies

We shall begin the specific anomalies section with systemic venous malformations because this book is organized in a venoarterial or blood-flow sequence—segment by segment, alignment by alignment, and connection by connection. The first question we must endeavor to answer is, **What are the systemic venous anomalies?** The answer to this question turns out to be stranger and more fascinating than anything one is likely to be able to imagine. Because most standard textbooks do not have a chapter that deals adequately with this topic, the present chapter is something of an exploration of *terra incognita*. Fortunately, the Cardiac Pathology Database (Table 6.1) and the medical journal literature will make it possible to answer this question.

PERSISTENT LEFT OR RIGHT SUPERIOR VENA CAVA

Persistent left superior vena cava (LSVC) in visceroatrial situs solitus and persistent right SVC (RSVC) in visceroatrial situs inversus are remarkably frequent anomalies (Fig. 6.1). Indeed, persistence of the contralateral superior vena cava (SVA) was the eighth most common form of congenital heart disease in the cardiac pathology database (Chapter 5, Table 5.1), being found in 415 of the 3216 patients with congenital heart disease (12.90% of this series, 95% confidence interval [CI] 11.74% to 14.06%).

The sex ratio was male-to-female = 221:184 (1.2:1), with the sex being unknown in 10 cases.

The median age at death in 397 patients was 2 months, ranging from 0 months (fetuses and stillbirths) to 413 months (34.41 years). The age at death was not known to us in 18 cases.

What kinds of congenital heart disease are persistent LSVC or RSVC associated with? The answer to this question is summarized in Table 6.2. You will note that persistent LSVC or RSVC is associated with 45 different forms of congenital heart disease. When ranked in order of prevalence from most common to most rare, 18 different ranks were found.

The asplenia syndrome with visceral heterotaxy ranked second in prevalence, 45 cases (10.84%, see Table 6.2).

Ventricular septal defect (VSD) was the third most common form of congenital heart disease associated with persistent left or RSVC (43 cases, 10.36%), with many of these patients having multiple congenital anomalies (MCAs).

The remainder of Table 6.2 speaks for itself and will not be reiterated here. But the questions remain: Why are common atrioventricular (AV) canal (6.99%), transposition of the great arteries (TGA) (6.27%), polysplenia syndrome with visceral heterotaxy (4.82%), and hypoplastic left heart syndrome (17.83%)—including preductal coarctation of the aorta (6.27%), mitral atresia (3.61%), mitral and aortic atresia (3.37%), aortic valvar atresia with mitral hypoplasia (1.93%), aortic stenosis (1.45%), and interrupted aortic arch (1.2%)—so relatively commonly associated with persistent left or RSVC?

As with so many "Why?" questions, we really do not know the answer. But our speculative thoughts are as follows. In visceroatrial situs solitus, persistence of the LSVC is normal both anatomically and hemodynamically in many vertebrates (e.g., mice and rats). All humans normally have bilateral SCVs in utero. In this sense, bilateral SVCs are "normal"—but not postnatally, one must add.

We suspect that persistent left or RSVC may indicate a developmental arrest at the time in utero when bilateral SVCs normally are present (i.e., fairly early in cardiogenesis). For example, the spleen normally appears in humans in horizons 15 to 17 (i.e., between 30 and 36 days of gestational age), as Ivemark[1] showed. Bilateral superior venae cavae (SVCs) normally are present at this age. Assuming that the asplenia syndrome reflects a developmental arrest that becomes manifest in utero, probably for genetic reasons, at or before the beginning of horizon 15 (30 days of age), and assuming that the polysplenia syndrome similarly becomes manifest in utero somewhat later, during horizons 16 (32 to 34 days of age) or 17 (34 to 36 days of age), this hypothesis could explain why bilateral SCVs are so common in both the asplenia syndrome (that ranked second) and the polysplenia syndrome (that ranked sixth) (see Table 6.2).

Similarly, common AV canal was a common form of congenital heart disease associated with bilateral SVA (ranking fourth, see Table 6.2). Developmentally, it is known that the superior and inferior endocardial cushions of the common AV canal normally fuse in horizon 17 (days 34 to 36), dividing the common AV canal into mitral and tricuspid canals (see Chapter 2, Figure 2-39). The inference therefore is that common AV canal may well become manifest in utero, probably for genetic reasons, at or before horizon 17 (i.e., at or before 34 to 36 days of age).

However, it is also noteworthy that persistent left or RSVC did not occur in any cases of pulmonary atresia with intact ventricular septum (see Table 6.2). This observation strongly suggests that persistence of the left or RSVC is a nonrandom event. In the Congenital Heart Database (Chapter 5), pulmonary atresia with intact ventricular septum ranked 28th in prevalence, very close to the asplenia syndrome, which ranked 27th in prevalence (see

TABLE 6.1 Systemic Venous Anomalies

No.	Prevalence	Anomaly	No. of Cases	% of Series	95% CI
1	1	Persistent L or R SVC	415	12.90	11.74–14.06
2	2	Interruption of IVC[a]	42	1.31	0.92–1.70
3	3	Atresia or stenosis of CoS ostium	20	0.62	0.35–0.89
4	4	Aneurysm of sinus venosus	9	0.28	0.10–0.46
5	5	Absence or atresia of RSVC	7	0.22	0.06–0.38
6	6	Absence of left innominate vein	5	0.16	0.15–0.17
7	7	Left innominate vein anterior to thymus	3	0.09	0.08–0.10
8	8	Raghib syndrome	2	0.06	0.05–0.07
9	8	Right SVC to LA	2	0.06	0.05–0.07
10	9	Retroaortic innominate vein	1	0.03	0.02–0.04
11	9	Left-to-right switching of IVC	1	0.03	0.02–0.04
12	9	Umbilical vein to coronary sinus	1	0.03	0.02–0.04
13	9	"Portal vein" to azygos vein	1	0.03	0.02–0.04

[a]Heterotaxy syndrome with polysplenia was excluded.
CI, Confidence interval; *CoS,* coronary sinus; *IVC,* inferior vena cava; *L,* left; *LA,* morphologically left atrium; *No.,* number; *R,* right; *RSVC,* right superior vena cava; *SVC,* superior vena cava.

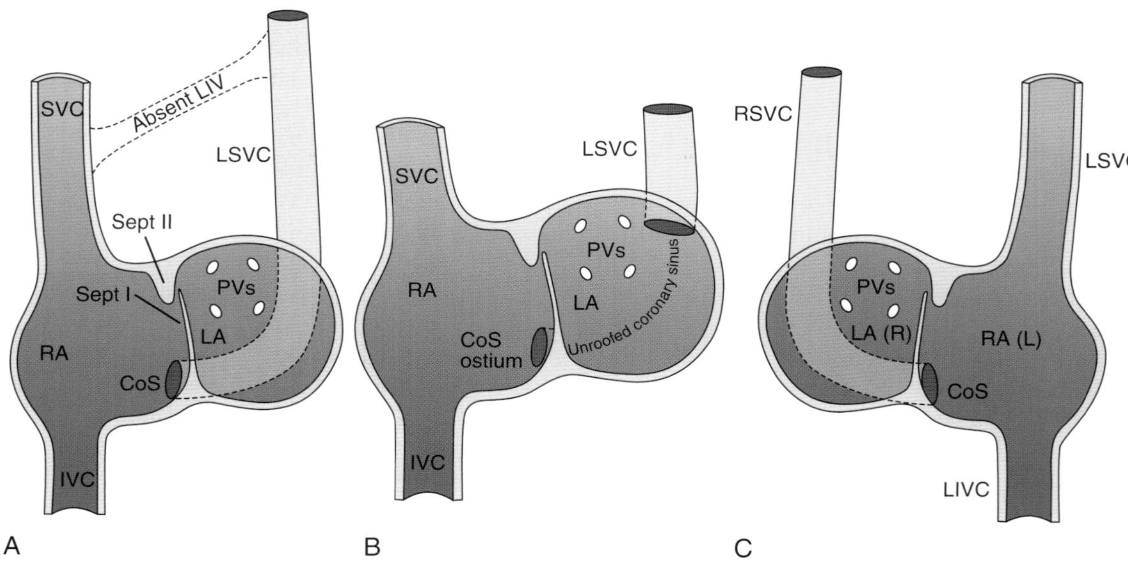

Fig. 6.1 (A) Diagram, as seen from the front, of persistent left superior vena cava *(LSVC)* connecting with the coronary sinus *(CoS)* and draining into the morphologically right atrium *(RA)* in visceroatrial situs solitus. The inferior vena cava *(IVC)* is right-sided, as is the normal single right superior vena cava *(SVC)*. Hence, bilateral SVCs are present, and the left innominate vein *(LIV)*, also known as the left brachiocephalic vein, is absent (indicated by *dashed lines*). The morphologically left atrium *(LA)* lies to the left of the RA. Septum primum *(Sept I)*, the flap valve of the patent foramen ovale, lies to the left of septum secundum *(Sept II)*, and the pulmonary veins *(PVs)* connect normally with the LA. (B) Persistent LSVC with unroofed coronary sinus, that is, large coronary sinus septal defect; hence the persistent LSVC drains into the LA. Note the large low posterior ostium of the CoS; this interatrial communication typically permits left-to-right shunting because the coronary sinus is unroofed. With a persistent LSVC, a large CoS ostium is usual; hence this interatrial communication is a normal opening, not an atrial septal defect, that is, not an abnormal opening in the atrial septum. This trilogy of developmentally interrelated anomalies—persistent LSVC, unroofed CoS, and large lower posterior interatrial communication—is often referred to as the Raghib syndrome.[4] Note that the left innominate vein is absent—a frequent finding with bilateral SVCs. Other abbreviations as previously. (C) Diagram of persistent right SVC *(RSVC)* in visceroatrial situs inversus. The persistent RSVC connects with the CoS and drains into morphologically right atrium which is left-sided *[RA (L)]*. Note that the morphologically left atrium is right-sided *[LA (R)]*. There is a left-sided inferior vena cava *(LIVC)*, a LSVC, PVs connecting with the LA (R), septum primum (the flap valve of the foramen ovale) lying to the right of septum secundum, and absence of the innominate (brachiocephalic) vein, typical of bilateral SVCs. (From Van Praagh S, Carrera ME, Sanders SP, et al. Sinus venosus defects: Unroofing of the right pulmonary veins—anatomic and echocardiographic findings and surgical treatment. *Am Heart J.* 1994;128:365-379; with permission.)

TABLE 6.2 **What Is Persistent Left or Right Superior Vena Cava Associated With? n = 415**

Rank	Entity	No. of Cases	% of Series	Rank	Entity	No. of Cases	% of Series
1	Tetralogy of Fallot	66	15.90	16	DORV {S,L,L}	3	0.72
2	Asplenia syndrome	45	10.84	16	Totally anomalous pul venous connection	3	0.72
3	Ventricular septal defect	43	10.36	16	Trisomy 18	3	0.72
4	Common AV canal (complete and incomplete)	29	6.99	17	Aortic isthmic atresia	2	0.48
5	TGA {S,D,D/A/L}	26	6.27	17	Agenesis of right lung	2	0.48
5	Preductal coarctation of aorta	26	6.27	17	Aberrant right subclavian artery	2	0.48
6	Polysplenia syndrome	20	4.82	17	Vascular ring	2	0.48
7	DORV {S,D,D}	18	4.34	17	{I,D,S}	2	0.48
8	Mitral atresia	15	3.61	17	Pulmonary valvar stenosis with IVS	2	0.48
9	Mitral and aortic atresia	14	3.37	17	Ebstein anomaly	2	0.48
10	Truncus arteriosus	12	2.89	17	Conjoined twins	2	0.48
10	Tricuspid atresia	12	2.89	17	Holmes heart	2	0.48
10	Left-sided juxtaposition of atrial appendages	12	2.89	17	Ellis-van Creveld syndrome	2	0.48
				17	{I,L,I}	2	0.48
11	ASD II	11	2.65	18	Dextrocardia	1	0.24
12	Aortic valvar atresia (with patent MV)	8	1.93	18	Right-sided JAA syndrome	1	0.24
				18	Primary EFE of LV	1	0.24
13	Aortic stenosis	6	1.45	18	DOLV {S,D,D}	1	0.24
13	TGA {S,L,L/D}	6	1.45	18	Sinus venosus defect	1	0.24
14	Interrupted aortic arch	5	1.20	18	PAPVC	1	0.24
14	Scimitar syndrome	5	1.20	18	PDA	1	0.24
14	DORV {I,L,L}	5	1.20	18	Hypertrophic cardiomyopathy	1	0.24
15	Normal heart with L/RSVC	4	0.96	18	{S,L,I}	1	0.24
16	HLH without other discrete anomaly	3	0.72	18	Pulmonary artery sling	1	0.24

ASD II, Atrial septal defect, ostium secundum type; *AV*, atrioventricular; *CI*, confidence interval; *CoS*, coronary sinus; *DOLV {S,D,D}*, double-outlet left ventricle with the segmental anatomic set of situs solitus of the viscera and atria, D-loop ventricles, and D-malposition of the great arteries; *DORV {I,L,L}*, double-outlet right ventricle with the segmental anatomic set of situs inversus of the viscera and atria, concordant L-loop ventricles, and L-malposition of the great arteries; *DORV {S,D,D}*, double-outlet right with the set of solitus viscera and atria, concordant D-loop ventricles, and D-malposition of the great arteries; *DORV {S,L,L}*, double-outlet right ventricle with solitus viscera and atria, discordant L-loop ventricles, and L-malposition of the great arteries; *EFE*, endocardial fibroelastosis; *HLHS*, hypoplastic left heart syndrome; *{I,D,S}*, the segmental anatomic set of situs inversus of the viscera and atria, discordant D-loop ventricles, and solitus normally related great arteries; *{I,L,I}*, the segmental anatomic set of inverted viscera and atria, concordant L-loop ventricles, and inverted normally related great arteries; *IVC*, inferior vena cava; *IVS*, intact ventricular septum; *JAA*, juxtaposition of the atrial appendages; *L*, left; *LA*, morphologically left atrium; *LV*, morphologically left ventricle; *MV*, mitral valve; *PAPVC*, partially anomalous pulmonary venous connection; *PDA*, patent ductus arteriosus; *Pul*, pulmonary; *No.*, number; *R*, right; *RSVC*, right superior vena cava; *{S,L,I}*, the segmental anatomic set of solitus viscera and atria, discordant L-loop ventricles, and inverted normally related great arteries; *SVC*, superior vena cava; *TGA {S,D,D/A/L}*, transposition of the great arteries with the segmental anatomic set of situs solitus of the viscera and atria, concordant D-loop ventricles, and D-transposition or A-transposition or L-transposition of the great arteries; and *TGA {S,L,L}*, TGA with the segmental anatomic set of solitus viscera and atria, discordant L-loop ventricles, and L-transposition of the great arteries.
Note: Tetralogy of Fallot was by far the most common form of congenital heart disease associated with persistent left or right superior vena cava, 66 of 415 postmortem cases (15.90%).

Table 5-1). Nonetheless, in these two anomalies with very similar prevalence, asplenia was the second most common form of congenital heart disease associated with persistent left or RSVC (see Table 6.2), whereas pulmonary atresia with intact ventricular septum was never associated with persistent left or RSVC (see Table 6.2) ($p < .0001$).

Why this very marked difference? We think that the answer may well be that whereas the asplenia syndrome occurs early in cardiac morphogenesis (at or before horizon 15, i.e., 30 days of age), when bilateral SVC normally are present, pulmonary atresia with intact ventricular septum occurs significantly later in utero, after closure of the interventricular foramen, which usually occurs between 38 and 45 days in normal cardiac morphogenesis, when the contralateral SVA (left or right) normally has undergone involution. Hence, we think that bilateral SVC indicate a relatively early developmental arrest, at or before horizon 17 (34 to 36 days of age), when bilateral SVC are normally present in utero.

What is the prevalence of persistent LSVC in normal people with visceroatrial situs solitus? Examination of 112 normal control heart specimens revealed persistence of the LSVC in none. However, cases with a persistent LSVC may have been

TABLE 6.3 Prevalence of Persistent Left or Right Superior Vena Cava With Various Types of Congenital Heart Disease

Rank	Entity	No.	Percentage	Rank	Entity	No.	Percentage
1	{I,L,I}	2/2	100.00	20	Vascular ring	2/21	9.52
2	Ellis-van Creveld	2/3	66.67	21	Mitral atresia	15/183	8.20
3	Asplenia	45/94	47.87	22	Preductal coarctation	26/328	7.93
4	DORV {I,L,L}	5/12	41.67	23	TGA {S,D,D/A/L}	28/361	7.76
5	{I,D,S}	2/5	40.00	24	CAVC (C & I)	29/385	7.53
6	Scimitar syndrome	5/13	38.46	25	Interrupted aortic arch	5/67	7.46
7	Polysplenia	20/57	35.09	26	DOLV {S,D,D}	1/14	7.14
8	{S,L,I}	1/3	33.33	27	TGA {S,L,L}	5/84	5.95
9	Conjoined twins	2/9	22.22	28	Trisomy 18	3/51	5.88
9	Agenesis of Rt lung	2/9	22.22	29	Rt JAA	1/18	5.55
10	DORV {S,L,L}	3/16	18.75	30	Hypertrophic CM	1/26	3.85
11	DORV {S,D,L}	2/11	18.18	31	VSD	43/1165	3.69
12	TGA {S,L,D}	1/6	16.67	32	AoAt with MV hypopl	8/235	3.40
13	Tetralogy of Fallot	66/428	15.42	33	MAt & Ao At	14/418	3.35
14	Atretic isthmus of aorta	2/14	14.29	34	PAPVC	1/41	2.44
15	PA sling	1/8	12.50	35	Ebstein	2/83	2.41
16	DORV {S,D,D}	16/143	11.19	36	Aortic stenosis (Valv, Supravalv, Sub Valv)	6/398	1.51
17	DORV {I,D,D}	1/9	11.11	37	TAPVC	3/203	1.48
18	Truncus arteriosus	12/111	10.81	38	ASD II	11/793	1.39
18	Tricuspid atresia	12/111	10.81	39	Aberrant RS art	2/170	1.18
19	Sinus venosus defect	1/10	10.00	40	Dextrocardia	1/119	.84
19	EFE of LV, primary	1/10	10.00	41	PDA	1/565	.18

AoAt, Aortic atresia; *ASD II,* atrial septal defect, ostium secundum type; *AV,* atrioventricular; *CAVC (C&I),* common atrioventricular canal (complete and incomplete); *CI,* confidence interval; CM, cardiomyopathy; *CoS,* coronary sinus; *DOLV {S,D,D},* double-outlet left ventricle with the segmental anatomic set of situs solitus of the viscera and atria, D-loop ventricles, and D-malposition of the great arteries; *DORV {I,L,L},* double-outlet right ventricle with the segmental anatomic set of situs inversus of the viscera and atria, concordant L-loop ventricles, and L-malposition of the great arteries; *DORV {I,D,D},* double-outlet right ventricle with the segmental anatomic set of situs inversus of the viscera and atria (I), discordant D-loop ventricles (D), and D-malposition of the great arteries (D); *DORV {S,D,D},* double-outlet right with the set of solitus viscera and atria, concordant D-loop ventricles, and D-malposition of the great arteries; DORV {S,L,D}, double-outlet right ventricle with the segmental anatomic set of situs solitus of the viscera and atria (S), discordant L-loop ventricles (L), and D-malposition of the great arteries (D); *DORV {S,D,L},* double-outlet right ventricle with the segmental anatomic set of situs solitus of the viscera and atria (S), concordant D-loop ventricles (D), and L-malposition of the great arteries (L); *DORV {S,L,L},* double-outlet right ventricle with solitus viscera and atria, discordant L-loop ventricles, and L-malposition of the great arteries; *EFE,* endocardial fibroelastosis; *HLHS,* hypoplastic left heart syndrome; hypopl, hypoplasia; *{I,D,S},* the segmental anatomic set of situs inversus of the viscera and atria, discordant D-loop ventricles, and solitus normally related great arteries; *{I,L,I},* the segmental anatomic set of inverted viscera and atria, concordant L-loop ventricles, and inverted normally related great arteries; *IVC,* inferior vena cava; *IVS,* intact ventricular septum; *JAA,* juxtaposition of the atrial appendages; *L,* left; *LA,* morphologically left atrium; *LV,* morphologically left ventricle; *MAt,* mitral atresia; *MV,* mitral valve; *PAPVC,* partially anomalous pulmonary venous connection; *PDA,* patent ductus arteriosus; *Pul,* pulmonary; *No.,* number; *R,* right; *Rt JAA,* right-sided juxtaposition of the atrial appendages; *RS Art,* right subclavian artery; *RSVC,* right superior vena cava; *{S,L,I},* the segmental anatomic set of solitus viscera and atria, discordant L-loop ventricles, and inverted normally related great arteries; *SVC,* superior vena cava; *TAPVC,* totally anomalous pulmonary venous connection; *TGA {S,D,D/A/L},* TGA with the segmental anatomic set of situs solitus of the viscera and atria, concordant D-loop ventricles, and D-transposition or A-transposition or L-transposition of the great arteries; and *TGA {S,L,L},* TGA with the segmental anatomic set of solitus viscera and atria, discordant L-loop ventricles, and L-transposition of the great arteries; *VSD,* ventricular septal defect.
Note: Horizontal line between ranks 33 and 34: conditions above the line (ranks 1 to 33, inclusive) are statistically significantly different from the normal prevalence of 0.3%, whereas conditions below the horizontal line (ranks 34–41, inclusive) are not statistically significantly different from normal (see text).

excluded from our normal collection because such hearts are not entirely normal. Hence, our impression is that the prevalence of persistent left LSVC or RSVC in the "normal" postnatal population is less than 1%. This impression is supported by the literature, in which the prevalence of persistent LSVC in unselected autopsies was found to be 0.3%: 1 in 348 patients (0.29%),[2] and 0.3% in more than 4000 unselected autopsies.[3]

Using the criterion that the normal prevalence of persistent LSVC or RSVC equals 0.3%, it becomes possible to establish which of the aforementioned main diagnoses listed in Table 6.2 have an elevated prevalence of persistent contralateral SVC (Table 6.3). This table requires comment:

1. In view of the very small number of cases, we do not feel confident that situs inversus {I,L,I} always has a persistent RSVC, even though both of our cases did (2/2 cases, 100%; see Table 6.3).
2. Similarly, in view of our very limited experience with the Ellis-van Creveld syndrome, we do not feel confident that a persistent

LSVC typically is present in this syndrome, even though this was found in 2 of our 3 cases (66.67%, see Table 6.3).

3. In contrast, we are sure that bilateral SVC are often present in the asplenia syndrome: 45 of 94 cases, 47.87% (see Table 6.3). Asplenia may be the most common form of congenital heart disease with bilateral SVC. As in Table 6.2, asplenia was more commonly associated with bilateral SVC than was polysplenia (35.09%; see Table 6.3). Tetralogy of Fallot (TOF) (15.42%) was more commonly associated than was physiologically uncorrected TGA {S,D,D/A/L} (7.76%, see Table 6.3). Almost equal in prevalence was common AV canal (7.53%; see Table 6.3). Congenitally physiologically corrected TGA {S,L,L} was only slightly less prevalent (5.95%; see Table 6.3).

When the various types of double-outlet right ventricle (RV) were added together, DORV (see Chapter 4) (14.14%, see Table 6.3) was almost as common as tetralogy and twice as common as transposition. VSD (3.69%) ranked only 31st in Table 6.3, compared with 3rd in Table 6.2. Nonetheless, this prevalence of persistent left or RSVC with VSD (3.69%) is 10 times the normal prevalence (0.3%).

Of the 41 entities listed in Table 6.3, which are statistically significantly different from normal? Remembering that a persistent LSVC occurred in only 1 of 348 unselected autopsies (0.287%), statistical analysis using the chi-square (χ^2) test, which is nonparametric, showed that the condition of mitral atresia plus aortic atresia (14/415, 3.37%; see Table 6.3) is statistically significantly different from normal: $\chi^2 = 9.478$, $p = 0.002$. All conditions above the horizontal line in Table 6.3 (i.e., ranks 1 to 33) are statistically significantly different from normal, whereas those entities below the horizontal line (i.e., ranks 34 to 41) are not statistically significantly different from normal.

Nonsyndromic Multiple Congenital Anomalies

Malformations involving the cardiovascular system and one or more other organ systems (but excluding Down syndrome, scimitar syndrome, agenesis of the right lung, and trisomy 18—well-known syndromes in their own right) were found in 108 of these 415 patients (26.02%).

Down syndrome coexisted in 21 of these 415 patients (5.06%) with persistent LSVC or RSVC. The occurrence of Down syndrome was nonrandom: Persistent LSVC + Down syndrome + complete common AV canal occurred together in 11 of 17 patients with completely common AV canal (64.71%). However, Down syndrome did not coexist in any of the 12 patients with incompletely common AV canal.

The asplenia syndrome and the polysplenia syndrome with visceral heterotaxy are considered subsequently (Chapter 29) and hence will not be considered further here.

TOF with persistent LSVC occurred in 66 patients, many of whom had MCAs. To state these relationships as simply as possible:

$$\text{TOF} + \text{LSVC} = 66$$

$$\text{TOF} + \frac{\text{LSVC}}{\text{Total TOF} = \frac{66}{428(15.42\%)}} \quad \text{(see Table 6.3)}$$

$$\text{TOF} + \text{LSVC} + \text{MCA} = 32$$

$$\text{TOF} + \text{LSVC} + \frac{\text{MCA}}{\text{TOF}} + \text{LSVC} = \frac{32}{66\,(48.48\%)}$$

In other words, almost half (48%) of our patients with TOF and persistent LSVC also had MCAs.

But what proportion are these cases relative to all of our patients with TOF? The answer is:

$$\text{TOF} + \text{LSVC} + \frac{\text{MCA}}{\text{Total TOF} = \frac{32}{428}} \quad (7.48\%)$$

Was Down syndrome common in our patients with TOF and persistent LSVC? Briefly, no:

$$\text{TOF} + \text{LSVC} + \text{Down} = 4\text{TOF} + \text{LSVC} + \text{Down} = 4$$

$$\text{TOF} + \text{LSVC} + \frac{\text{Down}}{\text{TOF}} + \text{LSVC} = \frac{4}{66} \quad (6.06\%)$$

$$\text{TOF} + \text{LSVC} + \frac{\text{Down}}{\text{Total TOF} = \frac{4}{428}} \quad (0.93\%)$$

Thus, TOF with persistent LSVC frequently had MCA (48%), but seldom had Down syndrome (6%).

What does **MCA** in association with TOF and persistent LSVC really mean? To answer this question specifically, we reviewed 50 cases of TOF with persistent LSVC or RSVC in detail.

First, what kinds of patients with tetralogy were these? There were 28 males and 22 females, males-to-females = 1.27:1. The segmental anatomic set was the usual **TOF** {S,D,S} in 47 patients (94%). {S,D,S} means the segmental anatomic set of solitus atria (S), D-loop ventricles (D), and solitus normally related great arteries (S), resulting in AV and ventriculoarterial (VA) concordance.

The segmental anatomic set of **TOF** {I,D,S} was found in 2 of these patients (4%). {I,D,S} means the segmental anatomic set of situs inversus of viscera and atria (I), discordant D-loop ventricles (D), and solitus normally related great arteries (S), resulting in AV discordance and VA concordance. Hence, these were like usual patients with TOF, except that the viscera and atria were inverted, resulting in AV discordance plus a tetralogy type of conotruncus. From a physiologic standpoint, because there is one segmental discordance (AV discordance), the systemic and pulmonary arterial circulations are physiologically uncorrected, as in physiologically uncorrected (complete) TGA. Hence, from the functional standpoint, TOF {I,D,S} resembles complete TGA with VSD and pulmonary outflow tract obstruction (stenosis or atresia). However, in TOF {I,D,S}, because there is VA concordance, the physiologically uncorrected systemic and pulmonary arterial circulations should be corrected with an atrial switch procedure (Senning or Mustard), not with an arterial switch type of operation, because VA concordance is present in TOF {I,D,S}. This rare form of tetralogy, TOF {I,D,S}, illustrates the important point that physiologic uncorrection of the circulations can occur without TGA. One segmental discordance that physiologically uncorrects the circulations can occur at the AV junction, as in TOF {I,D,S}, rather than at the much more frequent VA junction, as in TGA {S,D,D} or in TGA {I,L,L}.

Finally, the segmental anatomic set of **TOF** {I,L,I} was encountered in 1 patient (2%). {I,L,I} means the segmental anatomic set of situs inversus of the viscera and atria {I}, concordant L-loop ventricles (L), and inverted normally related great arteries (I), resulting in both AV and VA concordance. Hence, this was a patient with situs inversus totalis with inverted TOF. Such a patient should be treated surgically as with a mirror-image TOF.

Patients with situs inversus of the viscera and atria, in which the morphologically right atrium (RA), the SVC, and the inferior vena cava (IVC) are all *left-sided* (i.e., in mirror-image positions), had persistent RSVC, as in TOF {I,D,S} and as in TOF {I,L,I}. Thus, a persistent RSVC was present in 3 patients with TOF (6%).

Pulmonary outflow tract atresia was present in 13 patients (26%). A bicuspid pulmonary valve was noted in 13 patients (26%). A secundum type of atrial septal defect (ASD) (pentalogy of Fallot) was found in 12 cases (24%). A right aortic arch (in visceroatrial situs solitus) was present in 11 patients (23%). Major aortopulmonary collateral arteries were found in 7 patients (14%). A patent ductus arteriosus (PDA), often small, was present in 7 cases (14%). Additional muscular VSDs coexisted in 5 patients (10%). An unroofed coronary sinus, also known as a coronary sinus septal defect, was present in 5 patients (10%); consequently, the systemic venous blood carried by the LSVC was able to flow into the left atrium (LA), and the left atrial blood was able to flow into the RA through the enlarged coronary sinus ostium. Unroofing of the coronary sinus plus a large low posterior defect in the atrial septum, which is the enlarged right atrial ostium of the unroofed coronary sinus, is known as the *Raghib syndrome*.[4] Completely common AV canal was found in 4 cases (8%), 1 of whom had a common atrium (2%). An aberrant right subclavian artery originating as the last branch from the aortic arch occurred in 4 patients (8%).

The following anomalies were found in two patients each (4%): anomalous left innominate vein, retroaortic in one, and anterior to the ductus arteriosus and beneath the aortic arch in the other; absent left innominate vein; congenital mitral stenosis; absent ductus arteriosus; absent left coronary ostium, resulting in a "single" right coronary artery; bicuspid aortic valve, due to absence of the right coronary-noncoronary commissure in 1 patient and absence of the left coronary-noncoronary commissure in the other; a unicommissural and hence unicuspid pulmonary valve; and absent pulmonary valve leaflets with aneurysmal dilatation of the pulmonary artery and branches.

The following malformations were found in one patient each (2%) of these 50 patients with TOF and persistent LSVC or RSVC: high left coronary artery ostium; hypoplasia of both coronary ostia; dextrocardia; potentially parachute mitral valve in the setting of common AV canal, with all chordae tendineae inserting into the anterolateral papillary muscle of the left ventricle (LV); preductal coarctation of the aorta; anomalous muscle bundles of the RV; left aortic arch in visceroatrial situs inversus; commissural cleft of the anterior leaflet of the mitral valve, the cleft pointing superiorly toward the anterolateral commissure (not oriented approximately horizontally, as in a common AV canal type of cleft); myxomatous aortic valve leaflets; aortic regurgitation due to the presence of a small leaflet at the right coronary-noncoronary commissure, separating the right coronary and noncoronary leaflets, preventing their coaptation (quadricuspid aortic valve); Ebstein anomaly of the tricuspid valve; aneurysm of the coronary sinus (the left horn of the sinus venosus), underlying the LV and communicating with the left ventricular cavity via slit-like openings behind and beside the posteromedial papillary muscle group, this being a previously unknown and unreported malformation, to our knowledge (Figs. 6.2 and 6.3); totally anomalous pulmonary venous connection to the RA; polyvalvular disease; RSVC draining into the LA in visceroatrial situs solitus (via a sinus venosus defect); suprasystemic RV with small, slit-like VSD surrounded by muscle, due to the presence of a prominent, muscular right posterior division of the septal band, the VSD being conoventricular but not paramembranous (not confluent with the tricuspid valve's leaflet tissue); brachiocephalic trunk giving origin to all brachiocephalic arteries except the left subclavian artery; interruption of the IVC, associated with the polysplenia syndrome, the segmental anatomic set being {A,S,D,S}, meaning that there was visceral heterotaxy with situs ambiguus (A), the atria being in situs solitus (S), with concordant D-loop ventricles (D), and solitus normally related great arteries (S); left subclavian artery as the first branch from a right aortic arch; and absence of the iliac arteries.

MCAs result from the presence of additional malformations involving systems other than the cardiovascular system, that is, *multisystem malformations.*

Some well-known syndromes are characterized by multisystem malformation, such as (see Table 6.3): Ellis-van Creveld syndrome, the asplenia syndrome, the polysplenia syndrome, the scimitar syndrome, conjoined twins, and agenesis of the lung. Speaking of well-known syndromes, it should be stated that 4 of these 50 patients had Down syndrome (8%) and 1 patient (2%) had familial Down syndrome. One neonate with TOF and persistent LSVC also had a history of familial congenital heart disease, with his mother having had valvar pulmonary stenosis.

However, what we are really after here are the MCAs that do not constitute a presently well-known syndrome. These may be called **"nonsyndromic" MCAs**. (We strongly suspect that many of the anomalies to be summarized hereafter do in fact constitute unrecognized syndromes. Part of the fascination of MCAs is the desire to find recognizable patterns—the hope of introducing order into chaos.)

- Four patients (8% of this series) had tracheo-esophageal fistula with esophageal atresia.
- Three patients (6%) displayed each of the following anomalies: absent left kidney and ureter, central nervous system dysplasia and dysfunction, and imperforate anus.
- Two patients (4%) had each of the following: Cantrell syndrome, congenital deafness, cranial synostosis, clinodactyly, bilaterally undescended testes, and cleft palate.
- One patient (2%) exhibited each of the following: the amnion rupture syndrome; complete thoracic ectopia cordis; pelvic kidney; multicystic kidney with ureteral atresia; horseshoe kidney; fusion of the kidneys, left-sided, with hydronephrosis

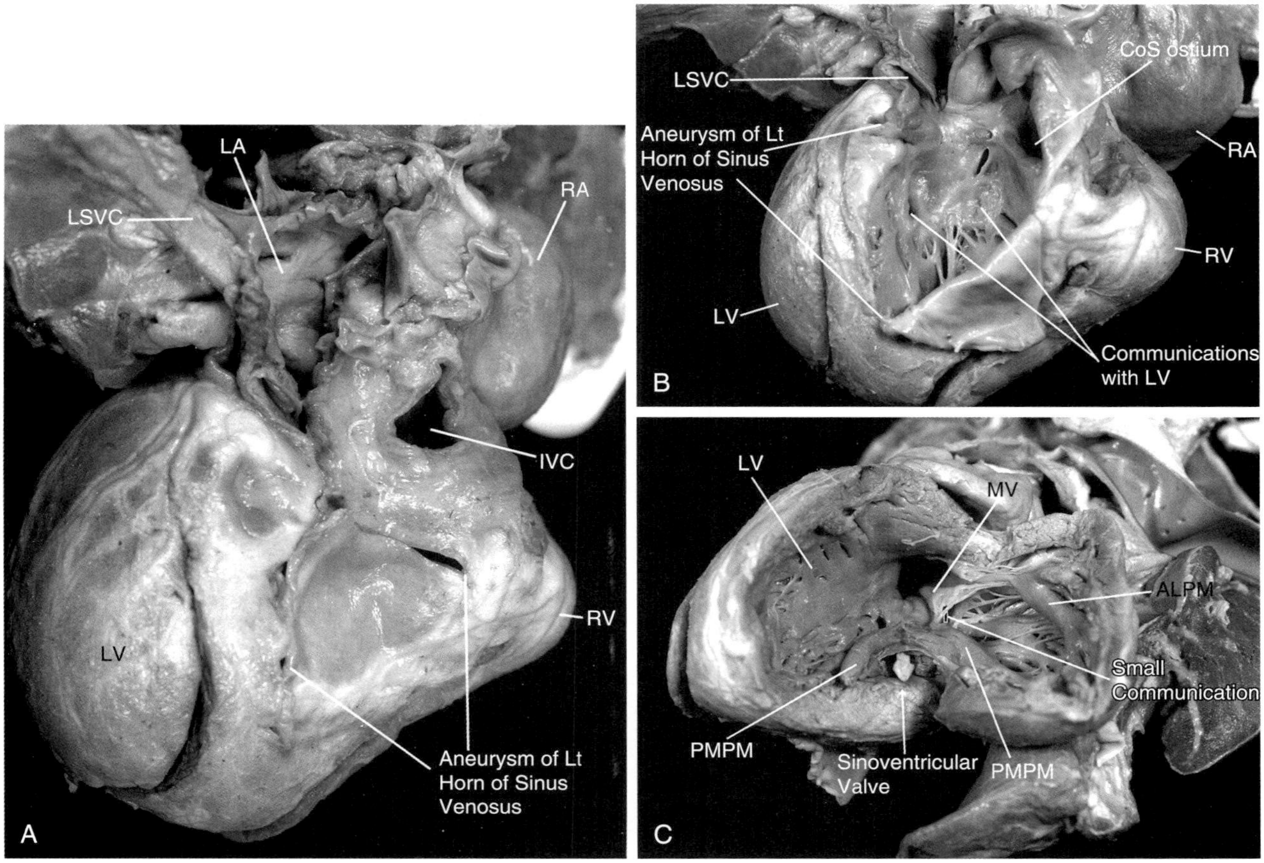

Fig. 6.2 Aneurysm of left horn of sinus venosus, that is, of coronary sinus, in 23-month-old girl with tetralogy of Fallot (TOF), moderate infundibular pulmonary stenosis, persistent left superior vena cava *(LSVC)* to coronary sinus *(CoS)* to right atrium *(RA)* (see Case 5, Table 6.4), case of Dr. Victor A. Saldivar. (A) Posterior view of the heart showing the opened left atrium *(LA)*, the RA, the large persistent LSVC, the transected inferior vena cava *(IVC)*, the left ventricle *(LV)*, the right ventricle *(RV)*, and the large (3 cm in dorsoventral length × 2 cm in right-left width), thin-walled aneurysm of the left sinus horn or CoS that underlies the LV. (B) Opened aneurysm of the left horn of the sinus venosus. Note that the free wall of the aneurysm is very thin (1 to 2 mm in thickness) and smooth-walled. The opened LSVC above the aneurysm is seen, as is the very enlarged ostium (18 mm in diameter) of the CoS that opens into the RA. Although the "floor" (inferior wall) of the CoS aneurysm is smooth and thin-walled, the "roof" (superior wall) is thick and coarsely trabeculated. In this trabeculated roof, two small communications with the overlying LV are present. The more leftward communication is the larger, having an oval orifice that measures 5 mm in length. This orifice is 2 to 3 mm in depth. The more rightward orifice is tiny, almost closed, and measures only 1.0 to 1.5 mm in diameter. (C) The opened LV shows unremarkable septal and free wall architecture, with a well-developed anterolateral papillary muscle *(ALPM)* and mitral valve *(MV)*. However, the posteromedial papillary muscle *(PMPM)* is bifid. Between the two "legs" of the PMPM group the larger of the two communications between the CoS and the LV emerges *(white arrow head)*. This communication is guarded by two fibrous leaflets with short chordae tendineae that insert into the overlying PMPM and into the adjacent LV musculature. Hence a small sinoventricular valve is present between the underlying sinus venosus aneurysm and the overlying LV. A second tiny communication was found adjacent to the MV (small communication). These CoS aneurysm-to-LV communications were misdiagnosed angiocardiographically as apical muscular ventral septal defects.

and hydroureter due to ureterovesical stenosis; common urinary and intestinal outflow tract (cloaca); lissencephaly, familial; megacolon; double right bronchus; absent gallbladder; bronchus suis (pig bronchus, i.e., right upper lobe bronchus arising directly from the trachea); chromosome 17 translocation; balanced translocation from chromosome 8 to chromosome 13; supernumerary digits; scoliosis; cystic lung disease; rectourethral fistula; rectovaginal fistula; VACTERL syndrome (vertebral defects, anal atresia, cardiac defects, tracheo-esophageal fistula, renal anomalies, and limb abnormalities); hydrocephalus; hypospadias; left diaphragmatic hernia, foramen of Bochdalek type; double left renal artery; short terminal phalanges, hand; cleft palate, forme fruste; micrognathia; glossoptosis; claw foot; Klippel-Feil syndrome; hypoplasia of the lower extremities; and agenesis of the uterus.

To summarize, the foregoing is the picture of **TOF with persistent left or RSVC—as it really is,** including not only the cardiovascular anomalies, but also the very important extracardiac anomalies.

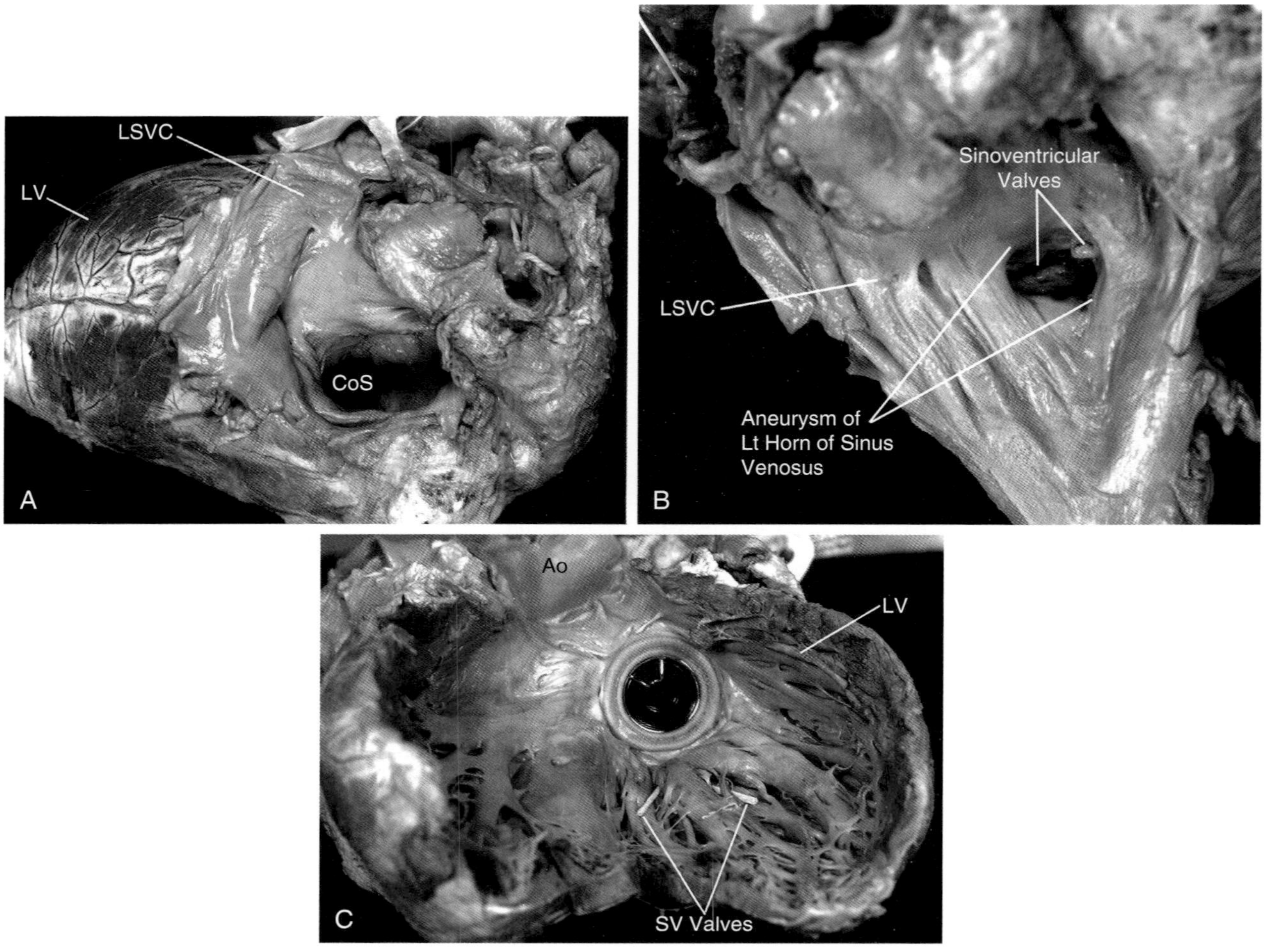

Fig. 6.3 Aneurysm of the left horn of the sinus venosus or coronary sinus *(CoS)*, with persistent left superior vena cava *(LSVC)* draining into the CoS to the right atrium, and with two sinoventricular *(SV)* valves communicating between CoS aneurysm and left ventricle *(LV)*, the SV valves opening through and between the posteromedial papillary muscle group of the LV, in a 15 9/12–year-old young woman with complete common atrioventricular (AV) canal type A of Rastelli, patient of Dr. Peter Vlad and Dr. Subramanian at the Buffalo Children's Hospital. The patient underwent three cardiac operations: (1) at 6 9/12 years of age (10/28/1968), exploratory cardiotomy with mitral and tricuspid valvuloplasties; (2) at 7 years of age (2/21/1969), patch closure of atrial septal defects (ASDs) and ventricular septal defects (VSDs) with mitral valve replacement using a Starr-Edwards valve; and (3) at 14 11/12 years of age (1/5/1977), mitral valve replacement with Bjork-Shiley prosthesis. Continuing low cardiac output led to death on 10/11/1977. The aneurysm of the CoS and the SV valves opening from the CoS into the LV were surprise postmortem findings. (A) Left posterolateral view showing the large opened LSVC connecting with the very large CoS. (B) Interior of persistent LSVC and CoS showing the aneurysm of the left sinus horn that measures 17 × 8 mm. Two SV valves can be seen within the aneurysm, a large one to the left (closer to the LSVC), and a very much smaller one to the right. The great cardiac vein can be seen opening into the enlarged CoS—between the LSVC to the left and the aneurysm with SV valves to the right (mentally extend the LSVC leader). (C) The opened LV showing the Bjork-Shiley mitral valve prosthesis, the LV free wall to the viewer's right, the LV septal surface toward the viewer's left, and the ascending aorta *(Ao)*. The two SV valves, containing probes, open into the LV cavity behind and between the musculature of the posteromedial papillary muscle group. The LV orifice of the larger SV valve measures 8 × 6 mm. These two SV valves were separated from the mitral valve by a cuff of LV myocardium. The aneurysm of the left horn of the sinus venosus and these two SV valves were thought not to have been of any clinical, or hemodynamic, or surgical importance. Because these two SV valves were located very close to the right atrium (RA), this heart could be considered to have *triple-outlet RA* (the tricuspid component of the common AV valve plus the two SV valves) and *triple-inlet LV* (the mitral component of the common AV valve and the two SV valves). However, our preferred diagnosis is simply aneurysm of the CoS with two SV valves between the CoS and the LV.

As the foregoing detailed study of persistent LSVC or RSVC with TOF indicates, persistent SVC often does not occur alone; it frequently has plenty of company.

Literature Review and Discussion

Although standard textbooks have little information on systemic venous anomalies in general, and on bilateral SVC in particular, much can be learned from a review of the medical journal literature.[4-86] Highlights are as follows.

In 1965, Raghib, Ruttenberg, Anderson, Amplatz, Adams, and Edwards[4] published a paper entitled, "Termination of the LSVC in Left Atrium, ASD, and Absence of Coronary Sinus—A Developmental Complex." This is the group of anomalies that is now often referred to as the **Raghib syndrome.** We think that the large low posterior defect in the atrial septum is the enlarged right atrial ostium of the unroofed coronary sinus. The coronary sinus is "absent," that is, unrecognizable, because of the large coronary sinus septal defect—the "unroofing" of the coronary sinus that reflects failure of formation of the partition between the coronary sinus posteriorly and the LA anteriorly. The opening in the atrial septum is not really an ASD, that is, an abnormal opening or defect in the atrial septum. Instead, this is a normal opening in the atrial septum (i.e., the ostium of the coronary sinus [not a septal "defect"]). Nonetheless, this normal but enlarged coronary sinus ostium functions like an ASD because of the coexistence of a large coronary sinus septal defect that unroofs the coronary sinus that is not truly absent.

Hence, the coronary sinus septal defect that unroofs the coronary sinus is responsible both for the right-to-left shunting of the persistent LSVC blood and the coronary sinus blood into the LA, and for the left-to-right shunting of the left atrial blood into the RA. The Raghib syndrome is thus a persistent LSVC to the coronary sinus with a large coronary sinus septal defect, and the hemodynamic sequelae thereof.

In 1965, Rastelli, Ongley, and Kirklin[7] published a paper entitled, "Surgical Correction of Common Atrium with Anomalously Connected Persistent Left Superior Vena Cava: Report of a Case." Rastelli et al[7] concluded that persistent LSVC is an unusual anomaly, occurring in 9 of 3452 cases (0.26%), confirming the previously mentioned prevalence of approximately 0.3%. These authors reported the first surgical correction of the Raghib syndrome.

Totally anomalous systemic venous connection does not exist. Although such a case was reported in 1965,[8] we think that totally anomalous systemic venous connection does not occur. In the patient in question,[8] the left-sided atrium received a LSVC, a left IVC, and the coronary sinus, plus all of the pulmonary veins. Not described were the visceral situs, the atrial septum, and the type of bulboventricular loop. We thought that the patient[8] probably had situs inversus of the atria, with totally anomalous pulmonary venous drainage. In our experience, any chamber to which both the IVC and the ostium of the coronary sinus are connected has always proved to be the morphologically RA, which in this case was left-sided; hence our conclusion that atrial inversion and totally anomalous pulmonary venous connection were present.

In 1969, another case was published[11] that was thought to have totally anomalous systemic venous drainage into the LA. We thought that this 15-year-old boy really had cor triatriatum dexter and a secundum ASD, resulting hemodynamically in totally anomalous systemic venous drainage into the LA. We think this patient anatomically did not have totally anomalous systemic venous connection. Hence, cor triatriatum dexter (a prominent and obstructive right venous valve) plus a secundum ASD is yet another way of getting a large amount of systemic venous blood into the LA via a very large right-to-left shunt at the atrial level, but without totally anomalous systemic venous connection.

Idiopathic dilatation of the superior vena cava was reported in 1972 by Franken[15] and by Ream and Giardina.[16]

Absence of the RSVC associated with a large persistent LSVC connecting with the coronary sinus was reported in 1972 by Harris, Gialafos, and Jefferson.[17] This report illustrated that a persistent LSVC does not necessarily mean that bilateral SVCs are present. This paper also considered the difficulties associated with transvenous pacing in this situation.

Congenital communications between the coronary sinus and the LA were considered in 1974 by Rose, Beckman, and Edwards.[21] In discussing coronary sinus septal defect, these authors focused on three physiologically different situations:

1. A coronary sinus septal defect (unroofing of the coronary sinus) decompressing the LA in association with mitral atresia and a sealed foramen ovale;
2. A coronary sinus septal defect associated with stenosis of the right atrial ostium of the coronary sinus; and
3. A coronary sinus septal defect in association with tricuspid atresia and a sealed foramen ovale.

Does persistent LSVC have any electrophysiologic significance? In 1976, James, Marshall, and Edwards[24] published a paper entitled, "De Subitaneis Mortibus [On Sudden Death]. XX. Cardiac Electrical Instability in the Presence of a Left Superior Vena Cava." This was a study of two patients. Patient 1 had a small sinoatrial node. The AV node contained numerous venous lacunae and was stretched out beneath the enlarged coronary sinus ostium. The AV node and the His bundle were found to be dispersed within the central fibrous body, this being the fetal pattern. Fragments of the AV node were also found on the crest of the muscular ventricular septum.

The second patient with a persistent LSVC who experienced sudden unexpected death had a VSD and palpitation. After closure of the VSD, there were multiple postoperative arrhythmias leading to death. Autopsy revealed that the sinoatrial node was normal, but that the sinoatrial nodal artery contained a polypoid fibromuscular mass that virtually occluded the arterial lumen. The AV node and the His bundle in the central fibrous body again displayed a dispersed fetal pattern.

Is it possible for the RSVC to drain into the LA, with no other associated congenital heart disease? The answer is yes. Vázquez-Pérez and Frontera-Izquierdo[28] in 1979 published a report entitled, "Anomalous Drainage of the Right Superior Vena Cava Into the Left Atrium as an Isolated Anomaly: Rare Case Report." The patient, a 7-month-old boy, was thought at that time to be the fifth known case of this anomaly.

Developmentally, how is this possible? Our hypothesis is that this patient had a sinus venosus defect, which made it possible for the RSVC to drain into the LA. We speculate that a prominent right venous valve—the valve of the SVC—was also present, closing the sinus venosus defect on its right atrial side. Consequently, the right upper and middle lobe pulmonary veins were not unroofed and hence did not drain into the RA, and there was no interatrial communication. (See Chapter 9 for a detailed consideration of sinus venosus defect.) It should be emphasized that the foregoing developmental interpretation is a *hypothesis*.

Can a persistent LSVC drain into the LA because of unroofing of the coronary sinus but without an interatrial communication? The answer is rarely yes. In 1978, Lozsádi[29] published a report based on two heart specimens, both of which had a persistent LSVC that opened into the LA because of a coronary sinus septal defect that unroofed the coronary sinus. But the remarkable finding in both cases was atresia of the right atrial ostium of the coronary sinus (i.e., there was no interatrial communication). Previously, it had been thought that an ASD was a necessary part of this anomaly. Hence, Lozsádi[29] reported two cases of the Raghib syndrome *without* an interatrial communication.

Developmentally, how is this possible? Lozsádi[29] hypothesized that this opening—the right atrial ostium of the coronary sinus—was closed by septum primum (the flap valve of the foramen ovale).

Our suggestion would be that this opening was closed by an adherent Thebesian valve of the coronary sinus, which is part of the right venous valve. Septum primum typically is superior and somewhat anterior to the coronary sinus ostium, whereas the right and left venous valves are ideally located to seal closed the right atrial ostium of the coronary sinus, if these valve leaflets develop abnormally.

Anomalous drainage of a LSVC into the LA as an isolated anomaly—without an interatrial communication—was confirmed in 1978 by Dupuis, Frontera, Pernot, Vasquez-Perez, and Verney.[32] These authors stated that as of 1978, there were 3 previously reported cases of LSVC draining into the LA as an isolated anomaly, to which they added 6 new cases. They also noted that as of that time, there were 4 previously reported cases of RSVC draining into the LA. They reported that LSVC to LA usually was a well-tolerated right-to-left shunt. Mild cyanosis was characteristic. Clubbing and shortness of breath could occur, but congestive heart failure was infrequent. The cardiac silhouette was normal. Left ventricular hypertrophy was noted electrocardiographically. Diagnosis at that time was made by cardiac catheterization and angiocardiography (but now would be made by two-dimensional echocardiography), and treatment was surgical by ligation of the persistent LSVC just above the LA.

What is cor triatriatum dexter? In 1979, Ott, Cooley, Angelini, and Leachman[33] published a paper entitled, "Successful Surgical Correction of Symptomatic Cor Triatriatum Dexter." The patient was a 67-year-old woman. Surgical removal of the obstructive right venous valve between the medial caval compartment (the sinus venosus) and the more right lateral tricuspid valve and right atrial appendage compartment not only removed the supratricuspid stenosis but also cured the patient's supraventricular tachycardia.

Cor triatriatum dexter (i.e., right-sided cor triatriatum) is a systemic venous anomaly. Why? Because the sinus venosus is the systemic venous confluence, and the right leaflet of the sinoatrial valve (briefly known as the right venous valve) demarcates the junction of the systemic venous confluence (where the ostia of the superior vena cava, the IVC, and the coronary sinus converge) and the right atrial appendage (which represents the primitive atrium). Hence, the right venous valve, which is obstructive in cor triatriatum dexter, is a systemic venous valve. In this sense, therefore, cor triatriatum dexter really is a systemic venous anomaly and hence is mentioned in this chapter on anomalies of the systemic veins.

Normally, the right venous valve is largely incompetent. The valve of the SVC (that fortunately has no eponym attached to it) and the valve of the IVC (the Eustachian valve) both are normally incompetent. The valve of the coronary sinus (the Thebesian valve), which also is derived from the right venous valve, may or may not be competent.

But *why* is the right venous valve mostly incompetent, at least insofar as the venae cavae are concerned? We think that the answer is: If the right venous valve is competent and prevents regurgitation into the venae cavae, then the right venous valve is also obstructive, resulting in what is known as cor triatriatum dexter. In order not to be obstructive, the right venous valve must be relatively poorly formed and hence incompetent.

In 1979, Battle-Diaz, Stanley, Kratz, Fouron, Guérin, and Davignon[35] published a paper entitled, "Echocardiographic Manifestations of Persistence of the Right Sinus Venosus Valve." The patient was a female infant whose cor triatriatum dexter was repaired surgically by removal of the obstructive right leaflet of the sinus venosus valve.

For clarity, it should be mentioned that the *sinus venosus valve* is the same thing as the *sinoatrial valve;* the latter designation indicates that this valve is located at the junction of the sinus venosus and the primitive atrium, which forms the right atrial appendage.

For the uninitiated, "right sinus venosus valve" or "right venous valve" may be confusing because these terms suggest that there is also a left sinus venosus valve or a left venous valve. One may then wonder, "Are there *two* venous valves—a right and left?" At this point, it becomes essential to understand what *valve* really means, that is, its etymology. The English word *valve* is derived from the Latin *valva,* which means leaf of a folding door. In this original sense, a valve (valva) meant either of the halves of a double door, or any of the leaves of a folding door (*Webster's New World Dictionary,* College Edition, 1958, page 1609). Hence *valve* has come to mean either an orifice guarded by one or more leaflets or the leaflets themselves.

The sinus venosus valve or the venous valve is thus being analogized to double door with two halves or leaves. The right and left venous valves refer to the leaflets, not to the orifice. There is only one orifice, with right and left leaflets or valves, in the original Latin sense *(valva).*

Congenital aneurysms of the superior vena cava were considered by Modry, Hidvegi, and LaFleche[38] in 1980. These authors concluded that there are two types: fusiform and saccular. (Fusiform means spindle-shaped, derived from Latin *fusus,* a spindle + *forma,* a shape.) Congenital superior vena caval aneurysms do not enlarge, rupture, or thrombose, and hence should be treated conservatively. Diagnosis by radiologic evaluation is based on size variation with respiration. It is important to recognize congenital SVC aneurysms so as to avoid needless thoracotomy.

Surgical correction of anomalous RSVC to the LA was described by Alpert, Rao, Moore, and Covitz[40] in 1981. The technique involved excision of the upper portion of the atrial septum that separated the SVC from the RA. A pericardial patch was attached along the caudal margin of the created ASD, and the cephalad margin of the patch was sutured to the junction of the SVC and the LA. Thus, the RSVC blood flow was diverted to the right of the patch into the RA.

Biatrial drainage of the RSVC with stenosis of the pulmonary veins was reported in 1984 by Bharati and Lev.[46] The authors stated that this was the first autopsy-proved case in the English literature in which all of the following features coexisted:

RSVC entering both atria; obstruction of the entry of the RSVC into the RA; aneurysmal dilatation of the RSVC; entry of the stenosed right upper pulmonary vein into the superior vena caval aneurysm; and drainage of all other pulmonary veins into the LA, these pulmonary veins being markedly stenosed.

Abnormal position of the left innominate vein was reported in 1985 by Smallhorn, Zielinsky, Freedom, and Rowe.[48] The left innominate (brachiocephalic) vein passed beneath the left aortic arch. In 1990, Choi et al[67] reported a subaortic position of the left innominate vein in almost 1% (0.98%) of individuals—a much higher prevalence than previously reported. A subaortic innominate vein was more common in patients with TOF, with or without pulmonary atresia, and such patients were more likely to have a right aortic arch.

Intrapericardial blood cyst is a rare form of systemic venous anomaly. In 1984, Cabrera, Martinez, and Del Campo[50] reported the case of a 21-month-old girl who had an intrapericardial venous cyst that was an egg-shaped mass measuring 4.5 × 3.5 cm. This venous cyst was connected by a patent pedicle with the left innominate vein. In addition, 100 mL of fluid was present within the pericardial sac. The venous cyst was ligated and resected.

Surgical repair of LSVC draining into the LA was described by Sand et al[52] in 1986. These authors constructed a simple tunnel to the RA, which has become the definitive surgical repair of this anomaly.

Coronary sinus septal defect with tricuspid atresia was reported in 1986 by Rumisek et al[55] as a rare cause of right-to-left shunting following the modified Fontan procedure.

Aneurysm of the left horn of the sinus venosus (coronary sinus) was reported by DiSegni, Siegal, and Katzenstein[57] in 1986. The patient had mitral atresia and hypoplastic left heart syndrome. The coronary sinus diverticulum penetrated the posterior wall of the RV and communicated with the right ventricular cavity. Communicating aneurysm of the coronary sinus results in a rare form of **double-outlet RA.** Congenital diverticulum of the coronary sinus was also reported in 1988 by Petit, Eicher, and Louis.[58] Coronary venous aneurysms and accessory AV connections were described in 1988 by Ho, Russell, and Rowland.[64]

Can a persistent LSVC draining into the coronary sinus cause a subdivided LA? Ascuitto et al[59] answered this question affirmatively in 1987.

When a persistent LSVC drains into the LA, must the coronary sinus be unroofed? We think that the correct answer is yes. However, as Looyenga et al[62] reported in 1986, occasionally a vein interpreted as persistent LSVC can connect with the left pulmonary veins, draining in this way into the LA, without unroofing of the coronary sinus. We think that this vessel was a levoatrial cardinal vein, not a persistent LSVC.

A closed technique for the repair of RSVC draining into the LA was reported in 1993 by Nazem and Sell.[71] The patient, a 26-year-old woman, also had the right upper lobe pulmonary veins connecting with the RSVC and the atrial septum was intact. Without cardiopulmonary bypass, the authors divided the azygos vein, transected the superior vena cava above the anomalous right pulmonary veins, and anastomosed the superior part of the RSVC end-to-side to the right atrial appendage.

In 1994, Raissi et al[72] repaired drainage of the RSVC into the LA without cardiopulmonary bypass, using excluding clamps.

Diverticulum of the superior vena cava was reported by Sai et al[74] in 1994. The patient, a 14-year-old girl, was thought to have a tumor. Instead, at surgery a venous diverticulum was found arising from the junction of the left innominate vein and the RSVC. The diverticulum was closed with sutures and then resected.

What is the best way of diagnosing coronary sinus septal defect (unroofed coronary sinus)? Chin and Murphy[77] in 1992 answered: color-flow Doppler echocardiography, a method that has subsequently proved to be of considerable assistance in making this diagnosis.

Can a dilated coronary sinus produce left ventricular inflow obstruction, and is this an unrecognized entity? Answering both questions affirmatively, Cochrane, Marath, and Mee[78] in 1994 introduced surgical reduction of the enlarged coronary sinus as treatment for this condition. We think that this entity is the same as subdivided LA, mentioned previously.[59]

Extracardiac techniques for the surgical correction of LSVC draining into the LA were described in 1997 by Reddy, McElhinney, and Hanley[85]: (1) anastomosis of the LSVC to the right atrial appendage; (2) passing the transected LSVC under the aortic arch and over the pulmonary artery, with anastomosis of the end of the LSVC to the side of the RSVC; and (3) a bidirectional left cavopulmonary anastomosis.

Absence of the RSVC in visceroatrial situs solitus was considered in 1997 by Bartram, Van Praagh, Levine, Hines, Bensky, and Van Praagh.[86] Based on 9 new cases and a literature review of 121 previously published cases, these authors found that absence of the RSVC in situs solitus is rare (0.07% to 0.13% of congenital cardiovascular anomalies). When the RSVC was absent, typically there was a persistent LSVC to the coronary sinus draining into the RA and a left-sided azygos vein draining into the LSVC. Less constant features were additional cardiovascular malformations (46%) and rhythm abnormalities (36%) that usually appeared related to complications of old age.

Prior to invasive medical or surgical procedures, echocardiographic diagnosis of absence of the RSVC is of considerable practical importance in many procedures, such as implantation of a transvenous pacemaker, placement of a monitoring pulmonary artery catheter, systemic venous cannulation for extracorporeal membrane oxygenation, systemic venous cannulation for cardiopulmonary bypass, performance of partial or total cavopulmonary anastomoses, obtaining endomyocardial biopsy samples, and the performance of orthotopic cardiac transplantation.

INTERRUPTION OF THE INFERIOR VENA CAVA

In this series of 3216 postmortem cases of congenital heart disease, interruption of the IVC occurred in 42 cases (1.31%; 95% CI 0.92% to 1.70%). Interrupted IVC was the 38th most frequent form of congenital cardiovascular disease in our Congenital Cardiac Pathology Database (Chapter 5, Table 5.1).

What is interruption of the IVC? From the pathologic anatomic standpoint, it is absence of the IVC between the renal

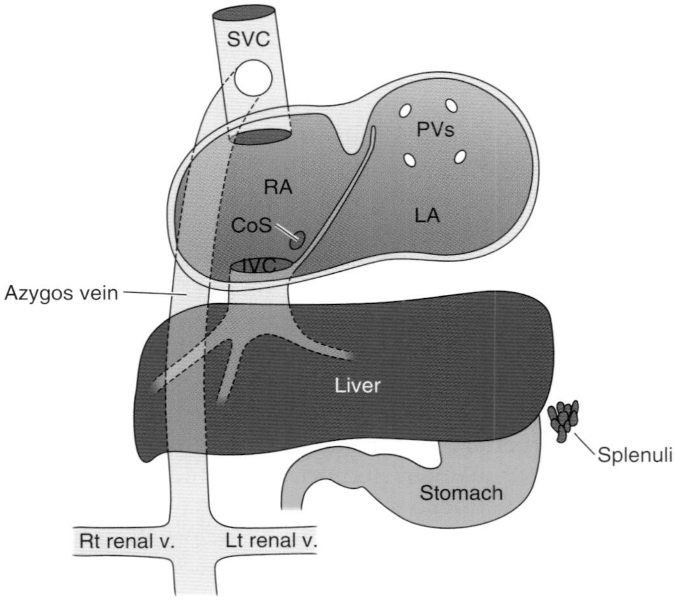

Fig. 6.4 Diagram of Interruption of the Inferior Vena Cava *(IVC)* in the Heterotaxy Syndrome With Polysplenia. Although the liver shows abnormal bilateral symmetry, the basic type of visceroatrial situs is situs solitus. The suprahepatic segment of the IVC and the coronary sinus *(CoS)* both connect with the right-sided right atrium *(RA)*, as does the superior vena cava *(SVC)*. Note that the IVC is interrupted from the renal veins below to the suprahepatic segment of the IVC above, the IVC blood stream returning to the SVC via a markedly enlarged azygos vein. The stomach is left-sided, as are multiple splenuli adjacent to its greater curvature. The septum primum lies to the left of the septum secundum, and the left atrium *(LA)* and pulmonary veins *(PVs)* are to the left of the RA and the venae cavae. *Lt Renal V,* Left renal vein; *Rt Renal V,* right renal vein. (From Van Praagh S, Kakou-Guikahue M, Kim H-S, et al. Atrial situs in patients with visceral heterotaxy and congenital heart disease: Conclusions based on findings in 104 postmortem cases. *Coeur.* 1988;19:483-502; with permission.)

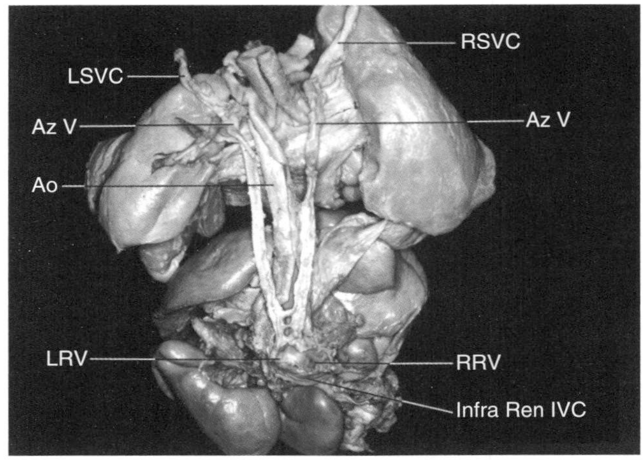

Fig. 6.5 The Right-Sided Inferior Vena Cava (IVC) Is Interrupted. Bilateral azygos veins *(Az V)* connect with bilateral superior venae cavae (SVCs). The right SVC *(RSVC)* entered the right atrium (RA) directly. The left SVC *(LSVC)* continued into the coronary sinus, which drained normally into the morphologically RA. All pulmonary veins also drained into the right-sided morphologically RA. Multiple fenestrations in septum primum and a moderate-sized membranous ventral septal defect permitted blood to enter the left heart. *Ao,* Aorta; *IVC,* inferior vena cava; *LRV,* left renal vein; *RRV,* right renal vein. (Reproduced with permission from Van Praagh S, Santini F, Sanders SP. Cardiac malpositions with special emphasis on visceral heterotaxy [asplenia and polysplenia syndromes]. In: Fyler DC ed. *Nadas' Pediatric Cardiology.* Philadelphia, PA: Hanley & Belfus; 1992:589.)

veins below and the hepatic veins above. The systemic venous blood is returned from the lower body to the heart by a greatly enlarged azygos vein that drains into the LSVC or RSVC (Fig. 6.4). Occasionally, the azygos vein can be bilateral—both left-sided and right-sided, draining into the LSVC and RSVC (Fig. 6.5).

This greatly enlarged azygos vein, which substitutes for the absent IVC, is often called "an azygos extension to the superior vena cava." In fact, the azygos vein always drains into the superior vena cava, but it is not nearly as prominent (large) as is an azygos extension of the lower IVC to the superior vena cava, this being the difference between an ordinary azygos vein and an azygos extension.

Azygos is a Greek word meaning unpaired or unmatched: *a,* not + *zygon,* a yoke. The basic idea is that a pair of oxen are joined by a yoke. *Zygote* means yoked, or paired, or matched—a cell formed by the union of two gametes. The azygos vein is unpaired in the sense that normally, only one such vein (the right) goes all the way up on the dorsal body wall to drain into the SVC. The other such vein (the left) goes only part way up and then crosses over from the left side to the right side to drain into the azygos vein. The left-sided dorsal body wall vein that goes only part way up toward the SVC and then crosses from left to right is known as the *hemiazygos vein,* meaning that it is like half an azygos vein—the lower (caudal) half.

Thus, any dorsal body wall vein, right-sided or left-sided, that drains into a superior vena cava (right or left) is an azygos vein (right or left). In other words, just because such a vein is left-sided does not mean that it is the hemiazygos vein; if such a vein drains into a superior vena cava, it is an azygos vein, be it right-sided or left-sided.

Funnily enough, when both azygos veins persist and both drain into bilateral SVC, these veins are still called the right and left azygos veins, even though they are not, literally speaking, *a + zygos,* that is, unpaired or unmatched. Bilateral SVCs seldom are associated with bilateral azygos veins.

Etymologically, what does *vena cava* mean? *Vena* = vein and *cava* = hollow (the feminine of *cavus,* Latin). So, vena cava literally means "hollow vein." This is perhaps a little amusing because all veins are hollow. However, in an adult, the venae cavae are so large that when one peers into them, they do indeed appear cavernous or hollow.

Azygos is the correct Greek spelling that ordinarily is used in anatomic nomenclature. *Azygous* is the English spelling. In medical literature, azygos vein and hemiazygos vein are preferred.

From the embryologic standpoint, the definitive IVC normally is composed of five different developmental and anatomic components, which form caudally to cephalically and are as follows[5]:

1. the anastomosis between the right and left posterior cardinal veins,
2. the right supracardinal vein,

3. the intersubcardinal anastomosis,
4. the mesenteric part of the IVC, and
5. the hepatic and suprahepatic segment of the IVC, derived from the hepatic and the vitelline veins.

The mesenteric part, that is, the renal vein to hepatic vein part (component 4 above), is the essence of the IVC. The cephalic pole of the right mesonephros lies close to the liver. As Patten states,[5] a fold of dorsal body-wall tissue early makes a bridge between the right mesonephros and the liver. This is the caval plica (fold) of the mesentery through which the mesenteric part of the IVC, indicated by small crosses in Fig. 6.5, develops between the right side of the intersubcardinal anastomosis and the liver. In interruption of the IVCs, it is this all-important mesenteric part of the IVC that is missing. Without this mesenteric component, one has an interrupted IVC.

This mesenteric component is the part of the vena cava that leaves the plane of the body wall dorsally and ventures out into the peritoneal cavity ventrally as it grows cephalically and ventrally to unite with the hepatic venous confluence that forms the hepatic and suprahepatic segment of the IVC. This is the shortcut of the systemic venous blood from the lower body to the RA. Without this shortcut to the RA, the lower systemic venous blood has to take the "longer way home" via the azygos vein to the SVC and thence to the RA.

The IVC is one of the most highly reliable diagnostic markers of the morphologically RA, as noted heretofore. "But does this apply," one may wonder, "with interruption of the IVC?" The answer is yes, it does, because the hepatic and suprahepatic segment of the IVC connects with the RA, just as it does with an uninterrupted (intact) IVC. Thus, selective right atrial angiocardiography in interrupted IVC will show you the suprahepatic segment of the IVC receiving hepatic veins from the liver. The same findings can be observed with two- or three-dimensional echocardiography and with magnetic resonance imaging. Hence, even with interruption, the IVC remains a very highly reliable diagnostic marker of the morphologically RA because the hepatic and suprahepatic segment of the IVC is always present. It is the segment below that—the renal vein–to–hepatic vein anastomosis—that is absent in interruption of the IVC.

Of the 42 patients with interruption of the IVC, visceral heterotaxy with the polysplenia syndrome was present in 31 cases (73.8%), and visceral heterotaxy with the asplenia syndrome was found in 1 rare case (2.4%). Thus, visceral heterotaxy, almost always with polysplenia, was present in 76% of cases with interruption of the IVC.

What proportion of patients with the polysplenia syndrome did *not* have interruption of the IVC? The answer is 26 of 57 (45.6%). Conversely, 54.4% of patients with polysplenia did have interruption of the IVC.

Visceral heterotaxy with polysplenia and asplenia are presented in detail in Chapter 29, they will not be described further here.

Interruption of the IVC Without Visceral Heterotaxy and Polysplenia. Of the 42 patients with interruption of the IVC, 10 did not have visceral heterotaxy with polysplenia or asplenia (23.81%). However, interruption of the IVC with situs solitus of the viscera and atria never occurred in isolation. Also, there was no case of interruption of the IVC without visceral heterotaxy that occurred in visceroatrial situs inversus.

The sex ratio was males-to-females = 2:7 (0.29:1). The age at death ranged from 3 hours to 17 months, with the median being 19 days.

The associated anomalies found with interruption of the IVC in situs solitus were as follows:

1. MCAs in 5 patients (50%);
2. accessory spleen or spleens in 4 cases (40%) (in addition to a normally formed spleen and without visceral heterotaxy);
3. VSD in 4 patients (40%), of the conoventricular type in 3 and muscular in 1; and
4. PDA in 3 (30%), causing death in 1 patient from congestive heart failure.
5. Two patients each (20%) had the following: TGA {S,D,D}, double-outlet RV {S,D,D}, totally anomalous pulmonary venous connection to the RA, ASD of the ostium secundum type, preductal coarctation of the aorta, omphalocele, bilateral conus (subaortic and subpulmonary), and aberrant right subclavian artery.
6. One patient (10%) had each of the following: hypoplastic and abnormally serpentine right and left pulmonary arteries; partially anomalous pulmonary venous connection from the left lung to a subdiaphragmatic suprahepatic venous plexus and thence via the liver and hepatic veins to the RA, associated with major aortopulmonary collateral arteries arising from the abdominal aorta above the celiac axis and supplying the right lower lobe region and the left lower lobe region of the lungs; abnormal lobulation of the spleen; hypoplasia of the lungs; multiple hemangiomata of the skin and lips; absence of the ligamentum teres; hypoplasia of the RSVC; absence of the RSVC; absence of the portal vein; the Raghib syndrome[4] (persistent LSVC to the coronary sinus, with unroofing of the coronary sinus, and with a large low posterior opening in the atrial septum representing the right atrial ostium of the enlarged and unroofed coronary sinus); completely common AV canal, type A of Rastelli; common-inlet LV; truncus arteriosus type A2; congenital absence of the ductus arteriosus; right aortic arch; intrahepatic gallbladder; malrotation of the colon with persistence of the mesocolon of the ascending and descending colon; pulmonary outflow tract atresia (with D-TGA); hydrocephalus; short neck; spina bifida; micrognathia; talipes equino varus; scoliosis; absent left innominate vein; mitral atresia; right hemifacial microsomia; pectus excavatum; 13 ribs bilaterally; bifid upper thoracic vertebrae; and clinodactyly.

The enlarged azygos vein was right-sided, connecting with the RSVC in 7 patients (70%), left-sided connecting with the LSVC in 2 patients (20%), and not recorded in 1 case.

Thus, what does the finding of interruption of the IVC suggest from the diagnostic standpoint?

1. If situs ambiguus with visceroatrial heterotaxy is present, one should consider the polysplenia syndrome, or rarely the asplenia syndrome (see Chapter 29).
2. If situs solitus of the viscera and atria is present, one should search carefully for additional cardiovascular and noncardiovascular anomalies (as mentioned earlier).

Literature Review and Discussion

The medical journal literature dealing with anomalies of the IVC[87-97] contains information of interest, some of which may be summarized as follows.

Is there electrocardiographic evidence of interruption of the IVC? In 1972, Van der Horst and Gotsman[87] pointed out that in a patient with congenital heart disease, coronary sinus or left atrial rhythm should suggest interruption of the IVC with azygos continuation to the superior vena cava. Coronary sinus rhythm was present in 4 of 8 cases (50%), left atrial rhythm in 2 (25%), an inverted P vector in 1 (12.5%), and a normal P vector in 1 (12.5%).

These findings were confirmed in 1973 by Merrill, Pieroni, Freedom, and Ho.[89] In a series of 18 cases, they found a coronary sinus rhythm in 56%. They also noted a prominent azygos-SVC confluence radiologically. Either or both electrocardiographic and radiologic clues were present in 89% of these cases.

Can interruption of the IVC manifest as a thoracic tumor? The answer is yes. In 1974, Bernal-Ramirez, Hatch, and Bower[90] reported the case of a 46-year-old man whose chest x-ray films showed a right hilar mass produced by the abnormally prominent azygos-SVC junction.

Can anomalous development of the IVC be associated with pulmonary thromboembolism? Again, the answer is yes. In 1975, Miller et al[91] reported the case of a 23-year-old man with duplication of the IVC. The left IVC joined the left renal vein and crossed anterior to the aorta to join the right IVC. Several clots formed in the left IVC, resulting in recurrent pulmonary thromboembolism. The patient was treated by interruption of both IVCs just below the renal veins. The presence of bilateral IVC was attributed to the persistence of the supracardinal veins bilaterally. (The supracardinal vein is also known as the thoracolumbar line vein, the important part that persists being the paraureteric segment of this vein.) An alternative therapeutic approach to ligation or clipping of the duplicated IVC is the placement of a Mobin-Uddin umbrella filter beneath the renal veins bilaterally.

Is the lateral chest film a reliable indicator of an azygos continuation of the IVC? In 1976, O'Reilly and Grollman[93] stated that the answer to this question is no. In 7 patients with an angiocardiographically proved azygos continuation, 5 cases (71%) had a clearly recognized IVC shadow on lateral chest film x-ray studies. In a sixth patient, the IVC shadow was faintly visualized. In a control series of 100 normal patients, no IVC shadow was identified in two lateral chest films; and in 7 other controls, the IVC shadow was poorly seen or absent because of adjacent diaphragmatic, pleural, or pulmonary parenchymal abnormality.

We agree with these authors[93] because in patients with interruption of the IVC, between the renal veins below and the hepatic veins above, the suprahepatic segment of the IVC is *always* present. Otherwise, the hepatic venous blood would have no way of returning to the heart.

Consequently, the suprahepatic segment of the IVC remains a highly reliable diagnostic marker of the morphologically RA, even in patients with interruption of the IVC.

What is the prevalence of interruption of the IVC? In our postmortem series, it will be recalled that the prevalence of interruption of the IVC was 42 of 3216 cases of congenital heart disease (1.31%; 95% CI 0.92% to 1.70%). Nedeljkovic et al[96] found that in 586 cases of congenital heart disease studied at autopsy, there were 4 patients with interruption of the IVC (0.6%). Among 368 patients with congenital heart disease studied by cardiac catheterization and angiocardiography, 2 had interruption of the IVC (0.5%).

What is the best noninvasive method of diagnosing interruption of the IVC with azygos continuation? The answer to this question may well continue to change with progressive technological improvements. However, in 1983, Ritter and Bierman[97] advocated the combination of two-dimensional echocardiography for anatomic detail, combined with gated pulsed color Doppler interrogation for blood flow characteristics.

ATRESIA OR STENOSIS OF CORONARY SINUS OSTIUM

Absence of a discrete right atrial ostium of the coronary sinus is frequent in association with common AV canal. For example, inability to find a right atrial ostium of the coronary sinus was specifically noted in the following six cases: A61-214, A63-236, A73-188, A77-90, A89-83, and C73-386. (A = autopsy; C = consult. For example, A89-83 means autopsy performed in 1989, number 83; in other words, the 83rd autopsy performed in 1989.) Incomplete common AV canal was present in 1 patient (A63-236), with the other 5 having complete common AV canal.

Although absence of a right atrial ostium of the coronary sinus was specifically noted in the aforementioned 6 patients with complete or incomplete common AV canal, we suspect that it is much more usual for the examiner in such a case not to note that he or she is unable to find the right atrial ostium of the coronary sinus. The presence of common AV canal is so eye-catching that one is very likely not to realize that the right atrial ostium of the coronary sinus cannot be identified. Consequently, we (alas) do not have reliable statistics concerning the frequency of absence of the right atrial ostium of the coronary sinus in association with the common AV canal. However, our impression is that inability to find (interpreted as absence of) the right atrial ostium of the coronary sinus in association with common AV canal is quite frequent—the rule, rather than the exception. We suspect that cardiac venous blood may open into the LA via single or multiple ostia. We are aware of no rigorous study of this anomaly. Nonetheless, it is also our impression that absence of a discrete right atrial ostium of the coronary sinus in the common AV canal seems not to matter; such absence has no hemodynamic or surgical consequences of which we are aware.

Indeed, absence of the right atrial ostium of the coronary sinus in association with common AV canal is a largely unknown diagnosis at the present time. We are deliberately drawing attention to this diagnosis because it may prove to have significant hemodynamic or surgical consequences that are now unrecognized.

Among the 3216 patients in this series with congenital heart disease, 20 had congenital atresia (Fig. 6.6) or stenosis of the right atrial ostium of the coronary sinus (0.62%; 95% CI 0.35% to 0.89%).

It is necessary to specify *congenital* atresia or stenosis of the coronary sinus because two patients had *iatrogenic* coronary sinus atresia after cardiac surgery: C74-40 and A87-25. The first was a 4½-year-old girl with TGA {S,D,D} and a VSD of the conoventricular type. At 2 months of age, the patient underwent a Blalock-Hanlon atrial septectomy, followed at 2 7/12 years of age by a Mustard procedure and patch closure of the VSD. The Mustard baffle totally occluded the lumen of the coronary sinus approximately 3 mm to the left of its ostium.

The other patient with iatrogenic coronary sinus atresia was a 19 4/12–year-old man with double-outlet RV {S,D,D} with a persistent LSVC to the coronary sinus, left-sided juxtaposition of the atrial appendages, small ASD of the ostium secundum type, large VSD of the confluent conoventricular plus AV canal type, and pulmonary stenosis (valvar and subvalvar). At 18 10/12 years of age, a modified Rastelli procedure was performed. The VSD was closed using an intraventricular conduit to the aorta, an aortic homograft conduit was placed from the right ventricular free wall to the main pulmonary artery, and direct suture closure of the ASD was performed. Two subsequent operations were required to close residual VSDs and to replace the aortic valve. The noncoronary leaflet of the aortic valve had been torn, and aortic valvuloplasty was followed by severe aortic regurgitation. Despite two reoperations, continuing low cardiac output persisted due to severe biventricular dysfunction, leading to death.

Autopsy revealed total occlusion of the coronary sinus 8 to 10 mm to the left of its dilated right atrial orifice, with complete thrombotic occlusion of the persistent LSVC.

In both of these cases, iatrogenic occlusion of the coronary sinus was thought to be an important cause of postoperative death because of its deleterious effect on myocardial function.

But what we are focusing on here is *congenital* (not acquired) obstruction of the coronary sinus: coronary sinus atresia and coronary sinus stenosis. Among these 20 patients, congenital coronary sinus atresia was present in 14 (70%) (see Fig. 6.6), and congenital coronary sinus stenosis was found in 6 (30%).

Sex Ratio: The ratio in congenital coronary sinus atresia was males-to-females = 8:5 (1.6:1), with the sex being unknown in 1. The sex ratio in patients with congenital coronary sinus stenosis was males-to-females = 4:2 (2:1). The sex ratio in congenital coronary sinus obstruction as a whole, including both atresia and stenosis, was males-to-females = 12:7 = 1.7:1, with the sex being unknown in 1. Hence, in this small series (sex known in 19 cases), there was a strong male preponderance.

Age at Death: In the 20 patients with congenital coronary sinus atresia, the age at death was known in 19: median = 43 days (1.4 months), ranging from 0 (30 weeks gestation in 1 fetus) to 3680 days, that is, 10 1/12 years. In the 6 patients with congenital coronary sinus stenosis, the age at death was known in all: median = 135 days (4.5 months), ranging from 10 days to 12 years. In the series as a whole (coronary sinus atresia and stenosis), the median age at death was 75 days (2.5 months), ranging from 0 to 12 years.

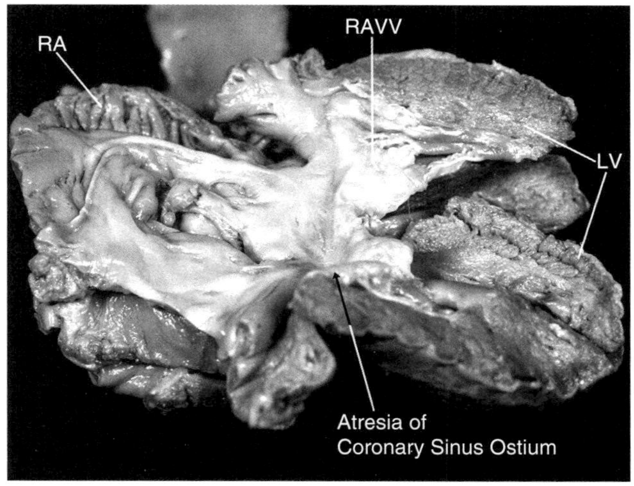

Fig. 6.6 Atresia of Right Atrial Ostium of Coronary Sinus. A small persistent left superior vena cava (SVC) connected with the obstructed coronary sinus. The presence or absence of a left innominate vein between the left and right SVCs was not recorded. At autopsy, the presence of coronary sinus ostial atresia was not identified as a clinical or hemodynamic problem. This 2½-month-old girl also had transposition of the great arteries (TGAs) {S,D,D}, left atrial outlet ("mitral") atresia, a large surgically created atrial septal defect, a hypertrophied and enlarged morphologically right atrium *(RA)* opening through a right atrioventricular valve *(RAVV)* into a single morphologically left ventricle *(LV)*, absence of the morphologically right ventricular sinus, subaortic infundibular outlet chamber, bilateral conus with widely patent outflow tract from the single LV into the large and banded main pulmonary artery, moderate obstruction of the bulboventricular foramen between the single LV and the infundibular outlet chamber produced by insertion of the RAVV into the conal septum, small subaortic muscular infundibulum, hypoplasia of the ascending aorta and aortic arch with preductal coarctation of the aorta (2 to 3 mm in internal diameter), large but functionally closing patent ductus arteriosus (PDA) (2 mm in internal diameter), large and high ostium of left coronary artery. Thus, apparently asymptomatic coronary sinus ostial atresia was associated with complex congenital heart disease, the cardiac venous blood returning to the right heart via a small persistent left SVC and other (unidentified) systemic venous tributaries. Death resulted from preductal coarctation of the aorta and a functionally closing ductus arteriosus, depriving the lower body of circulation.

Discussion: Coronary sinus ostial atresia never occurred in isolation. These 14 postmortem-proved cases constituted only 0.44% of the 3216 cases of congenital heart disease in this series as a whole. Congenital coronary sinus atresia (see Fig. 6.6) was associated with the following forms of congenital heart disease: persistent RSVC or RSVC in 8 (57%), persistent LSVC in visceroatrial situs solitus in 7, and persistent RSVC in visceroatrial situs inversus in 1; VSD in 8 (57%), being of the conoventricular type in 4, of the muscular type in 3, and of the AV canal type in 1; mitral atresia in 6 (43%); aortic atresia in 5 (36%); with mitral atresia and aortic atresia coexisting in 5 cases (36%); ASD of the ostium secundum type in 4 (29%); PDA in 4 (29%); and TGA {S,L,L} in 2 (14%); 1 patient (7%) had each of the following: TGA {S,D,D}, double-outlet RV {S,D,D}, double-outlet RV {I,L,L}, double-outlet LV {S,D,D}, dextrocardia, absence of the main pulmonary artery, discontinuity of the right and left pulmonary artery branches, common AV canal opening mostly into the morphologically RV, aortic stenosis (valvar), pulmonary stenosis (valvar), coronary sinus septal defect (unroofing of the coronary sinus), a small third coronary artery, absence of the left anterior descending coronary artery after the origin of the left circumflex coronary artery, endocardial fibroelastosis of the left and RV, complete heart block, monozygotic twin, hydrops fetalis (severe intrauterine congestive heart failure), fetal demise, straddling tricuspid valve (right-sided), straddling tricuspid valve (left-sided), tricuspid regurgitation (right-sided), tricuspid regurgitation (left-sided), preductal coarctation of the aorta, bilateral PDA, prematurity, aberrant right subclavian artery, coronary sinus luminal atresia with patent right atrial ostium, muscularized Eustachian valve of the IVC, and pulmonary atresia with intact ventricular septum.

The foregoing documents the complexity of the congenital heart disease that was associated with coronary sinus atresia.

Comment: Can we make any sense of this? What can we learn from the foregoing? Well, first of all, we should confess that before doing this study, we knew little about coronary sinus ostial atresia except that it occurs; hence this investigation was a voyage of discovery.

The high prevalence of **persistence of a superior vena cava connecting with the coronary sinus** certainly makes sense hemodynamically. In several cases, it was appreciated that the blood flowed in a retrograde direction because of atresia of the right atrial ostium of the coronary sinus. The cardiac venous blood flowed retrogradely in the coronary sinus, up the (typically left) SVA, rightward via the (left) innominate vein into the (right) SVC and thence downward into the RA. In other words, the cardiac venous return followed a "snowman" pathway, reminiscent of supracardiac totally anomalous pulmonary venous connection. In coronary sinus atresia, the pulmonary veins were always normally connected. It was the *cardiac* venous return (not the pulmonary venous return) that flowed in this supracardiac "snowman" pathway.

But not always. For example, in one patient there was a coronary sinus septal defect that unroofed the coronary sinus, permitting the coronary sinus blood and that of the persistent LSVC to flow into the LA, rather than flowing retrogradely into the RA via the supracardiac "snowman" venous pathway. The coronary sinus septal defect permits right-to-left shunting into the LA, whereas coronary sinus atresia without unroofing of the coronary sinus has no shunt, even though the cardiac venous blood "takes the long way home" via the supracardiac venous pathway.

We think the high prevalence of **VSD** (57%) reflects the complexity of the congenital heart disease with which coronary sinus atresia typically is associated.

But the real surprise of this study was the relatively high prevalence of the **hypoplastic left heart syndrome** in association with coronary sinus atresia: mitral atresia in 43%, with mitral atresia and aortic atresia coexisting in 36%. Prior to this review, we had no idea of the existence of this association between coronary sinus atresia and mitral atresia.

From the developmental perspective, what might this association between coronary sinus atresia and mitral atresia mean? First, it should be said that we really do not know; a definite answer to this question awaits future study. Our speculative thoughts are as follows. Mitral atresia typically involves failure of normal formation of the mitral portion of the common AV canal. The coronary sinus wraps around the outside of the mitral canal. Our speculative hypothesis is that failure of normal formation of the mitral canal may be associated with failure of normal formation of the immediately adjacent coronary sinus, resulting anatomically in mitral and coronary sinus atresia. This essentially unknown association between mitral atresia and coronary sinus atresia invites further study.

Coronary sinus stenosis was identified in only 6 of the 3216 cases of congenital heart disease making up this series as a whole (0.19%). Congenital stenosis of the right atrial ostium of the coronary sinus was associated with the following forms of congenital heart disease: VSD in 3 cases (50%), of the conoventricular type in 2 and of the AV canal type (but without common AV canal) in 1; persistent LSVC to the coronary sinus in 2 (33%); mitral atresia in 2 (33%); aortic stenosis in 2 (33%), valvar in 1 and subvalvar in the other; secundum type of ASD in 2 (33%); single LV with infundibular outlet chamber in 2 (33%); TGA {S,D,D} in 2 (33%); and 1 patient (17%) having each of the following: TGA {S,D,L}, transportation of the great arteries {S,L,L}, stenosis of the origin of the left coronary artery (arising from the right coronary sinus of Valsalva), double-orifice mitral valve (50/50 division of the mitral orifice by a tongue of fibrous tissue), aortic atresia (valvar), PDA, coronary sinus septal defect (unroofed coronary sinus), preductal coarctation of the aorta, and aberrant location of the stenotic coronary sinus ostium (abnormally rightward and anterior).

Embryologically, congenital atresia and stenosis of the right atrial ostium of the coronary sinus appear to reflect an abnormality of the right venous valve. If the Thebesian valve, which is derived from the right venous valve, becomes partially or totally adherent to the right atrial ostium of the coronary sinus, the result is stenosis or atresia, respectively, of the ostium of the coronary sinus. Anatomically, one can often see the head of a small probe shining through the narrowed or atretic coronary sinus ostium that is veiled by the abnormally adherent and hence obstructive Thebesian valve or Eustachian valve (when separate Thebesian and Eustachian valves are not present). Why the right venous valve becomes obstructive remains unknown at present.

Comment: Congenital stenosis of the right atrial ostium of the coronary sinus appears to be the forme fruste of congenital atresia of the coronary sinus. In this small series (n = 6), we again found relatively high prevalences of many of the same associated forms of congenital heart disease: VSD (50%), persistent LSVC to the coronary sinus (33%), mitral atresia (33%), and aortic stenosis (33%) and atresia (17%).

The natural history of patients with congenital coronary sinus stenosis (median age at death 4.5 months, ranging from 10 days to 12 years) was somewhat better than that of patients with congenital coronary sinus atresia (median age at death 1.4 months, ranging from 0 [a fetus of 30 weeks gestational age] to 10 1/12 years).

Nonetheless, it is our impression that congenital coronary sinus atresia and stenosis probably are usually of little or no clinical importance, because the cardiac venous return seems to find alternative routes of returning to the cardiac lumen. Difficult-to-find Thebesian veins often are invoked. Injection or other studies to clarify this question remain to be done. In only 1 of our 6 cases (17%) of congenital coronary sinus stenosis was the coronary sinus described in the fresh state (at the time of autopsy, prior to fixation) as dilated.

In none of our 20 cases of *congenital* atresia or stenosis of the coronary sinus was obstruction of the coronary sinus blood flow thought to be a significant cause of the patient's death. This is in sharp contrast to *acquired* atresia or severe stenosis of the coronary sinus postoperatively, in which iatrogenic obstruction of the coronary sinus always appeared to be a major cause of the patient's death, apparently because of the lack of other communications between the coronary sinus and the cardiac lumen after the normal involution of the persistent LSVC into the ligament of Marshall.

Finally, it must be added that congenital coronary sinus atresia or severe stenosis may in fact be clinically important in certain circumstances. Because these are diagnoses that are seldom made in life, it should be understood that we may well have much to learn concerning these two largely unrecognized anomalies.

Literature Review and Discussion

Reports in the medical journal literature concerning atresia of the right atrial ostium of the coronary sinus[98-103] were of considerable interest, as the following briefly indicates.

Can atresia of the right atrial ostium of the coronary sinus occur without a persistent LSVC, and if so, how? In 1972, Falcone and Roberts[98] reported 4 cases, all autopsy-proved, with atresia of the right atrial ostium of the coronary sinus and without a persistent LSVC. Of these 4 patients, 3 had a *left* atrial ostium of the coronary sinus, permitting a right-to-left shunt at the atrial level and explaining how long-term survival was possible without a persistent LSVC. One of these patients had two small openings in a small cardiac vein that drained into the right atrial appendage. The coronary sinus and associated veins were markedly distended. Clinically, this patient was thought to have an idiopathic myocardial disease with cardiomegaly. Except for the latter patient, the other 3 had additional forms of congenital heart disease. All 4 were adults, ranging from 27 to 63 years of age.

Atresia of the right atrial ostium of the coronary sinus was thought to be of no clinical significance in the 3 patients with unobstructed openings of the coronary sinus into the LA. However, the patient with no left atrial opening of the coronary sinus and with only an apparently obstructive opening into the right atrial appendage was thought to have a primary myocardial disease with idiopathic cardiomegaly, probably secondary to the stenotic (and ectopic) egress from the cardiac venous system. Hence, atresia or stenosis of the right atrial ostium of the coronary sinus is of no clinical importance, as long as there is an unobstructed exit for the cardiac venous blood somewhere else.

Is cardiac venous hypertension associated with increased risk for coronary arterial thrombosis? The report of Gerlis et al[99] in 1984 suggested that the answer is perhaps. These authors reviewed 14 previously reported cases of coronary sinus atresia associated with a persistent LSVC, adding 2 new cases of their own. In their Case 1, a 43-year-old woman, the persistent LSVC was small—only 4 mm in diameter (compared with a RSVC that was 12 mm in diameter). The coronary sinus was dilated (8 mm in diameter). A larger medial branch of the left anterior descending coronary artery was occluded by an old, firmly adherent thrombus that was associated with a massive myocardial infarction. Histologically, this thrombosed coronary artery showed no significant disease of the vessel wall.

In discussing this mysterious finding of coronary thrombosis in a histologically unremarkable left anterior descending coronary artery, Gerlis et al[99] noted that Falcone and Roberts[98] had stated the hemodynamic consequences of coronary venous hypertension (due to the obstructively small persistent LSVC in this patient) would be predominantly reflected into the left coronary artery because 75% of its blood flow enters the coronary sinus.

Thus, Gerlis et al[99] raise the important possibility that coronary sinus atresia may be associated with thrombosis in a normal left coronary arterial system if the draining LSVC is small and hence obstructive. This was the first such case reported in the literature; further experience is needed in order to assess this hypothesis. Thus, the inference appears to be that coronary sinus atresia associated with a persistent LSVC may not be an entirely benign condition in adult life if the left superior vena is obstructively small. Again, more experience is needed to test this hypothesis.

Can atresia of the coronary sinus orifice be diagnosed in life? Yes. In 1985, Watson[100] reported what he thought was the second case diagnosed by angiocardiography into the coronary sinus via a persistent LSVC. The first case diagnosed in life was that of Fudemoto et al[103] in 1976. In reviewing 37 known cases of coronary sinus atresia, Watson[100] found that approximately half were not associated with any other form of congenital heart disease. Exit of the coronary sinus blood in these 37 patients was as follows:

1. a persistent LSVC in 16 (43%);
2. an unroofed coronary sinus opening into the LA in 9 (24%);
3. venous channels draining into the right or LA in 9 (24%); and
4. combinations of the above in 3 (8%).

Also in 1985, Yeager et al[101] reported angiographic diagnosis of coronary sinus atresia in a term infant with pulmonary atresia, intact ventricular septum, and sinusoidal communications between the right ventricular cavity and the coronary arteries, with retrograde coronary arterial filling.

In terms of echocardiographic diagnosis, Yeager et al[101] noted in retrospect that the persistent LSVC was visualized, but not the coronary sinus or the coronary sinus ostium. They concluded that the only echocardiographic clue to the diagnosis of coronary sinus ostial atresia was absence of the dilated coronary sinus that usually is associated with a persistent LSVC. They added that although not performed in their patient, Doppler interrogation of the LSVC should reveal reversal of the usual direction of blood flow.[101]

Although coronary sinus atresia with a persistent LSVC typically is of no clinical importance, is it of any surgical significance?

Unfortunately, the answer is yes. As was reported in 1989 by Yokota et al,[102] inadvertent division of a small persistent LSVC (4 mm in diameter) in a 4 11/12-year-old boy in the process of performing an arterial switch procedure for TGA resulted in death on the fifth postoperative day. Autopsy revealed no kinking or distortion of the implanted coronary arteries. Congestion and hemorrhage of the myocardium were described as massive, with infarction of the right ventricular free wall. The surprise finding of the autopsy was atresia of the coronary sinus orifice.

These authors[102] concluded that the only way to prevent this unusual but fatal complication during surgery is to bear in mind the possibility that the LSVC may be the only outlet for the cardiac venous blood and to determine the patency of the coronary sinus orifice whenever a persistent LSVC is ligated or divided.

ANEURYSMS OF THE SINUS VENOSUS

Aneurysms of the left horn of the sinus venosus (i.e., of the coronary sinus) and of the right horn of the sinus venosus (i.e., of the systemic venous component of the morphologically RA) are rare and consequently largely unknown at the present time. In this study of 3216 cases of congenital heart disease, aneurysms of the left and right horns of the sinus venosus were found in 10 patients (0.31%). Of these, 6 cases (66.7%) had congenital aneurysms of the left sinus horn, that is, of the coronary sinus (see Figs. 6.2 and 6.3). All 6 patients were female. The mean age at death was 1104 days (3.02 years), ranging from 1 day to 15 9/12 years. The median age at death was 90 days.

All 6 patients had complex congenital heart disease (Table 6.4). Major anomalies of the AV valves were present in 4 of these 6 cases (66.7%): mitral atresia in 2, tricuspid atresia in 1, and common AV valve in 1.

Communications between the coronary sinus aneurysm and the ventricular cavities were present in 3 of these 6 patients (50%): between the coronary sinus aneurysm and the left ventricular cavity in 2 (see Cases 5 and 6; Table 6.4) (see Figs. 6.2 and 6.3) and between the coronary sinus aneurysm and the right ventricular cavity in 1 (see Case 4; Table 6.4).

The oldest patient in this series, a 15 9/12–year-old young woman, had a **valved** communication between the coronary

TABLE 6.4 Aneurysms of the Left Horn of the Sinus Venosus (Coronary Sinus Aneurysms)

Case No.	Sex and Age	Diagnosis
1	F 2.5 mo	Tricuspid atresia type Ib; ventricular septal defect, conoventricular, small (3 × 2 mm); **enlarged coronary sinus with small coronary sinus aneurysm;** prominent right venous valve forming rete Chiari; aberrant right subclavian artery; anterior descending coronary artery from right coronary artery via conus coronary artery
2	F 3½ mo	Mitral atresia; double-outlet right ventricle {S,D,D}; ventricular septal defect, conoventricular, subaortic, small (2 × 2 mm); ventricular septal defect, muscular (2 × 8 mm); secundum type of atrial septal defect, small; **coronary sinus aneurysm (6 × 12 mm) communicating with middle cardiac vein (posterior interventricular vein)**
3	F 8 days	Double-outlet right ventricle {S,D,D} with subpulmonary infundibulum, aortic-tricuspid fibrous continuity, mitral atresia, tiny left atrium with no left atrial appendage, diminutive left ventricle (DORV with hypoplastic left heart and unilateral conus—in this case subpulmonary only = infantile type of DORV); bilateral superior venae cavae, with absent left innominate vein, and persistent left superior vena cava to coronary sinus to right atrium; bilateral azygos veins; partially anomalous pulmonary venous connection: all pulmonary veins to coronary sinus, and right upper lobe pulmonary vein also to left atrium via a small side branch; rete Chiari; tricuspid regurgitation; subaortic narrowing with tubular hypoplasia of aortic arch and discrete coarctation of aorta; **small venous aneurysm arising from inferior surface of coronary sinus adjacent to right atrium, aneurysm underlying diaphragmatic surface of left ventricle; Wolff-Parkinson-White syndrome with orthodromic reentrant tachycardia**
4	F 1 day	Conjoined twin B, left-sided, joined from level of diaphragm caudad, with single liver, duplicated small bowel, common colon, and remnant of leg fused posteriorly: omphaloischiopagus tripus; hydrocephalus with Dandy-Walker malformation (atresia of the foramen of Magendie); oligohydramnios; severe congestive heart failure with biventricular dysfunction, pleural and pericardial effusions; bilateral superior venae cavae with absence of left innominate vein; right atrial hypertrophy and enlargement, extreme; tricuspid regurgitation, mild; **small aneurysm of coronary sinus arising from inferior surface of coronary sinus adjacent to the right atrium and communicating with right ventricular cavity just inferior to the posterior leaflet of the tricuspid valve;** ventricular septal defect, conoventricular and paramembranous, without pulmonary stenosis (Eisenmenger complex); patent ductus arteriosus, large, 1 day old; intraoperative death of twin B while separating conjoined twins
5	F 23 mo	Tetralogy of Fallot with moderate infundibular pulmonary stenosis; persistent left superior vena cava to coronary sinus to right atrium; **large coronary sinus aneurysm (30 × 20 mm, free wall 1–2 mm thick); 2 valvelike communications between aneurysm and left ventricular cavity close to posteromedial papillary muscle group (misdiagnosed as muscular ventricular septal defects) (see Fig. 6.2)**
6	F 159/12 y	Complete common atrioventricular canal, type A; **large coronary sinus aneurysm with valved communication between aneurysm and left ventricular cavity behind the posteromedial papillary muscle group;** sinoventricular valve measures 17 × 8 mm from right atrial aspect, and 8 × 6 mm from left ventricular aspect; persistent left superior vena cava to coronary sinus to right atrium and to left ventricle; sinoventricular valve is separated by left ventricular muscle from mitral component of common atrioventricular valve (see Fig. 6.3)

F, Female; *M*, male; *mo*, months; *y*, year.

sinus aneurysm and the left ventricular cavity (see Case 6; Table 6.4). This accessory sinoventricular valve measured 17 × 8 mm from the right atrial aspect and 8 × 6 mm from the left ventricular aspect.

In a 23-month-old girl, two valve-like communications between the coronary sinus and the left ventricular cavity, which were located behind the posteromedial papillary muscle group, were mistaken angiocardiographically for muscular VSDs (see Case 5; Table 6.4).

In one of these patients (16.7%), Wolff-Parkinson-White syndrome[104] with orthodromic reentrant tachycardia was present (see Case 3; Table 6.4).

In none of these cases was there any vestige of valvar leaflet tissue between the aneurysm and the more cephalic portion of the coronary sinus or the RA, that is, the neck leading into the coronary sinus aneurysm was always entirely unguarded by valvar leaflet tissue.

Right atrial aneurysms involving the right horn of the sinus venosus (Fig. 6.7) were found in 4 of these 10 patients (40%) (Table 6.5). All but one were males, with the ages at death being 2 days, 5 weeks, 6 months, and 4 years.

Again, these right atrial aneurysms involving the right sinus horn never occurred in isolation; they were always associated with complex congenital heart disease (see Table 6.5). Of these

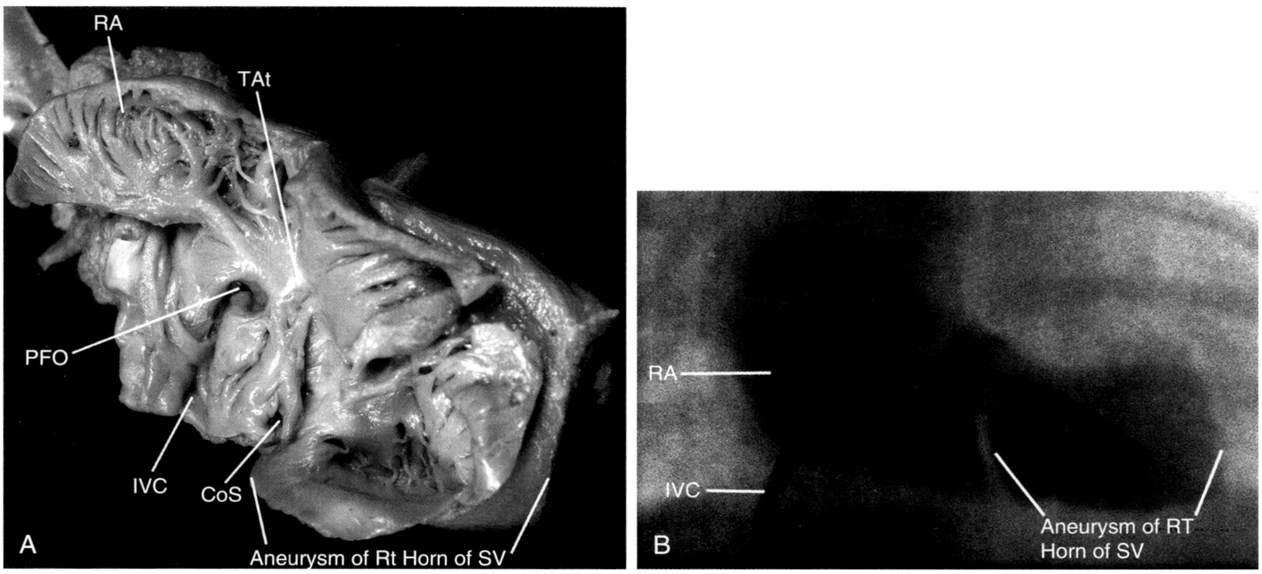

Fig. 6.7 (A) Aneurysm of the right (Rt) horn of the sinus venosus *(SV)* in a 5-week-old girl with tricuspid atresia *(TAt)*. Note how thin-walled and smooth the aneurysmal free wall is. (B) Selective angiocardiographic injection into the aneurysm of the right horn of the sinus venosus. The contrast refluxes freely into the right atrium, there being no valve-like tissue between the aneurysm and the RA. There is no anterograde flow of contrast, and no communication with a ventricle. *CoS,* Coronary sinus; *IVC,* inferior vena cava; *PFO,* patent foramen ovale; *RA,* right atrium; *Rt,* right; *SV,* sinus venosus. (Patient of Dr. James Reynolds, Southern Baptist Hospital, New Orleans, LA.)

TABLE 6.5 Aneurysms of Right Horn of Sinus Venosus

Case No.	Sex and Age	Diagnosis
1	M 6 mo	Infantile Ebstein anomaly with marked tricuspid stenosis; ventricular septal defect, muscular, apical, huge (12 × 10 mm); **large aneurysm of the right horn of the sinus venosus** 39 mm long, 25 mm wide, and free wall 2 mm thick; orifice between the aneurysm and right atrium 22 × 13 mm; ventricular septum dysmorphic and thickened (20–23 mm)
2	M 2 days	Transposition of the great arteries {S,D,D} with polysplenia syndrome, bilaterally bilobed lungs, and bilateral hyparterial bronchi; ventricular septal defect, conoventricular type, with posterior overriding pulmonary artery; muscular ventricular septal defect; bicuspid aortic valve; isthmic hypoplasia; and patent ductus arteriosus (at 2 days of age); **thin-walled aneurysm communicated with the right atrium**.
3	M 4 y	Ebstein anomaly with anomalous muscle bundles of the right ventricle; ventricular septal defect, conoventricular type; double-orifice mitral valve with accessory anterolateral and main posteromedial orifices; left ventricular dysplasia with thickened endocardium; prominent right venous valve of superior and inferior venae cavae, without cor triatriatum; polyvalvular disease (tricuspid and mitral valves); biventricular myocardial dysplasia; familial cardiomyopathy; **sinus venosus aneurysm,** located beneath right ventricular sinus (inflow tract), communicating with right atrium via two slit-like orifices, aneurysm containing bizarre trabeculations ("stalactites" and "stalagmites"); aneurysm of no hemodynamic significance
4	F 5 wk	Tricuspid atresia {S,D,S}, with smooth thin-walled aneurysm of right sinus horn (see Fig. 6.8).

3 patients, 2 had Ebstein anomaly (see Cases 1 and 3; Table 6.5). None of these right atrial aneurysms was associated with a significant arrhythmia, and none communicated with a ventricular cavity.

Literature Review and Discussion

Ho et al[105] reported 2 patients with aneurysm of the coronary sinus in 1983, this being the first known report of this entity. Two years later, Gerlis et al[104] linked coronary sinus aneurysms with ventricular preexcitation, demonstrating histologically the presence of accessory AV connections, a finding that was subsequently confirmed by Ho et al[106] in 1988.

To the best of our present knowledge, valvelike communications between coronary sinus aneurysms and both ventricular cavities are reported here for the first time.

The Anatomy and Terminology of the Cardiac Veins. In order to understand and describe the aneurysms of the left and right horns of the sinus venosus, a brief review of the anatomy and terminology of the cardiac veins is helpful. Because many pediatric cardiologists and cardiac surgeons do not know even the names of the major cardiac veins, let us start at the beginning.

They are called the **cardiac veins,**[107] not the *coronary* veins. However, some investigators[108] have applied the term *coronary* to the arteries and the veins of the heart. The English word *coronary* is derived from the Latin term *corona,* meaning *garland* or *crown,* which in turn is derived from the Greek word *korone* or *stephanos,* meaning wreath. Hence, the literal meaning of coronary is encircling in the manner of a crown. Claudius Galenus (130–200 CE), known in English as Galen, was a Greek from Pergamos in Asia Minor whose medical and scientific career climaxed in Rome. Here, he introduced many Greek medical terms into Latin, one of which was *corona.* The root meaning of corona is *wreath,* as worn about the head of an Olympic champion, and, thus, similar to a crown. In Greek, the coronary arteries were called *stephaniaia angia,* meaning wreath-like vessels. It was this term that Galen then translated into Latin as *corona.*

It will also be recalled (Chapter 1) that Rufus of Ephesus, at about the beginning of the current era (approximately 1 to 25 CE), had named what we call the "base" of the heart, the "head" of the heart. From this it followed that the atrial appendages became known as the "ears" (auricles, from *auricula,* Latin) because they are located on either side of the "head" of the heart. The coronary arteries do indeed wrap around the "head" of the heart like a wreath or a crown. However, the cardiac veins do not (Fig. 6.8). From the anterior interventricular sulcus to the acute margin of the heart, the right AV sulcus contains the right coronary artery, but normally no major cardiac vein. Thus, the arteries of the heart are crownlike, whereas the veins are not, hence coronary arteries, but not coronary veins. Instead, they are cardiac veins.[107]

Following J.C. Boileau Grant[107] (see Fig. 6.7), who was my Professor of Anatomy, the anterior interventricular cardiac vein is known as the *great vein,* or the *left vein,* because it normally flows leftward in the left AV groove and then proceeds posteriorly, where it flows into the coronary sinus. The coronary sinus normally has four tributaries (see Fig. 6.8): (1) the *great or left cardiac vein,* mentioned previously; (2) the *oblique vein*

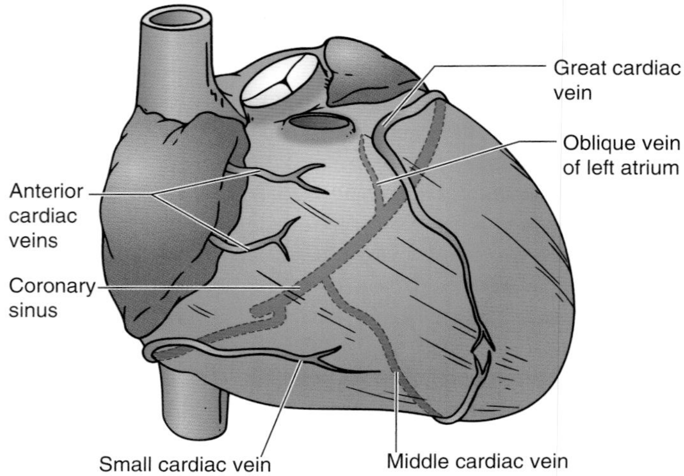

Fig. 6.8 **Diagram of the Cardiac Veins.** How can the names and the distributions of these five cardiac veins be remembered? There are two naming systems here. One system is in terms of size: small, middle, great. The other approach is positional—to group them into right and left cardiac veins. The right cardiac veins include the small, the middle, and the anterior and mostly drain the right ventricle. The left cardiac veins include the great and the oblique veins and mostly drain the left heart, the great (or left) cardiac vein draining the left ventricle and the oblique vein draining the left atrium. (From Grant JCB. *An Atlas of Anatomy.* 6th ed. Baltimore, MD: Williams & Wilkins; 1972:diagram 438 with permission.)

coming in from above and leftward, the oblique vein being a remnant of the LSVC, which normally involutes and becomes the ligament of Marshall; (3) the *middle cardiac vein,* which is the posterior interventricular vein that flows into the coronary sinus from below; and (4) the *small cardiac vein,* which comes from the acute margin of the RV and flows rightward and then posteriorly to reach the undersurface of the coronary sinus just to the left of its right atrial ostium.

One or two *anterior cardiac veins* from the conus arteriosus and the anterior right ventricular free wall "jump" across the right AV sulcus anteriorly and drain directly into the RA (see Fig. 6.8).

Not shown in Fig. 6.8 are the *inferior ventricular veins* that help to drain the diaphragmatic surfaces of the ventricles into the coronary sinus; and the *Thebesian veins,* which are minute vessels that begin in the heart wall and open directly into the chambers of the heart.

The previously mentioned ligament of Marshall commemorates **John Marshall,** an English anatomist (1818–1891), whose work on the development of the SVC accounts for the eponym.[109] The Thebesian veins honor the memory of **Adam Christian Thebesius,** a German physician (1686–1732).

Embryology of the Cardiac Veins. To understand aneurysms of the sinus venosus, particularly those that communicate with the left or right ventricular cavity, an acquaintance with the relevant embryology and phylogeny is very helpful. Much of our present understanding of the development and evolution of the cardiac veins stems from the work of R.T. Grant[108,110] and of R.T. Grant and M. Regnier.[111]

The first cardiac vessels to appear in rabbit embryos are the cardiac veins,[108] the earliest remnant being seen in embryos of 7 mm total length as an endothelial outgrowth from the left horn of the sinus venosus. The endothelial proliferation pierces the thin muscular wall of the sinus venosus and so comes to lie in the developing connective tissue between the sinus venosus, the atria, and the ventricles. The first outgrowth is quickly followed by others, so that in the 8-mm embryo there are three or four such openings from the sinus venosus that unite in the loose connective tissue and form a *wide and irregular sinus*.

Normally, this wide and irregular venous sinus then branches to the right and medially, where it forms the beginning of the small and middle cardiac veins (see Fig. 6.7). In the adult rabbit, the small and middle cardiac veins open together into the coronary sinus, whereas in humans these two cardiac veins open separately into the coronary sinus (see Fig. 6.2).

In the 8.5-mm rabbit embryo, the left or great cardiac vein has also appeared. The small and left cardiac veins then extend toward the right and left AV grooves, respectively, and the middle cardiac vein passes down the dorsal interventricular furrow toward the ventricular apex. The cardiac veins spread as capillary plexuses, from which the main cardiac venous trunks later emerge. The cardiac veins are confined to the sulci and lie in the developing connective tissue on the surface of the myocardium, which, as yet, they do not enter.

By the 10-mm stage in the rabbit embryo, the main cardiac veins are distinct. The middle cardiac vein has reached the ventricular apex, and the small and left cardiac veins have passed around the right and left AV grooves, respectively, and now lie on the right and left sides of the bulbus cordis (conus arteriosus). Branches then proceed outward from the main cardiac veins, passing over the developing ventricular myocardium and inward toward the AV orifices. A few branches also pass to the atria. The terminal portions of all of these main branches then enter the myocardium.

By the 8.5-mm stage in the rabbit embryo, outgrowths from the atrial endocardium have grown outward, piercing the myocardium. A little later, similar outgrowths occur from the ventricular endocardium, forming extensions of the intertrabecular spaces that Minot[112] called "sinusoids," which in turn give rise to epicardial capillaries. At the 10-mm stage, the cardiac veins are not continuous with the epicardial capillaries, which, however, do connect with the cavities of the heart. These atrial and ventricular vessels then develop further and branch beneath the epicardium.

Later, the subepicardial atrial vessels connect with the atrial branches of the cardiac veins, thereby forming the **Thebesian veins** of the adult atria. The subepicardial ventricular vessels join with each other and with the ventricular branches of the cardiac veins. At the same time, the ventricular branches of the cardiac veins that have entered the myocardium communicate with the intertrabecular spaces and thence with the ventricular cavities, as Grant[108] was able to show histologically in an 11-mm rabbit embryo.

Our hypothesis concerning the embryology of sinus venosus aneurysms, therefore, is as follows:

1. An aneurysm of the sinus venosus appears to represent persistence of the wide and irregular sinus, which is the earliest stage in the development of the cardiac veins after the proliferation and outgrowth of the endothelium from the left horn of the sinus venosus.[108] This hypothesis appears able to explain aneurysms of the coronary sinus (the left horn of the sinus venosus). We postulate that similar endothelial outgrowths may also occur from the right horn of the sinus venosus, thereby accounting for aneurysms that are confluent with the venous portion—the right sinus horn component—of the RA.
2. Communications between coronary sinus aneurysms and the ventricular cavities appear to represent persistence of the early sinusoidal communications between the cardiac veins and the intertrabecular spaces of the ventricular cavities.

The cause of these developmental arrests is unknown at present.

Parenthetically, it is of interest to note that the **coronary arteries** develop a little later than do the cardiac veins, first appearing at the 10- to 11-mm stage in rabbit embryos. After making contact with the aortic lumen within the sinuses of Valsalva, the coronary arteries pass first to the bulbus cordis (conus arteriosus), and then spread over the rest of the heart, uniting with the capillary network already formed by the intertrabecular spaces and the cardiac veins.

Condensation or compaction of the myocardium, that is, the development of the stratum compactum, reduces most of the intertrabecular spaces to capillaries.

Grant and Regnier[111] pointed out that in lamprey eels *(Cyclostomata)*, coronary arteries are entirely absent; that is, the heart is *avascular*. The heart is nourished by blood passing through the intertrabecular spaces between the myocardial fibers. The muscle of the ventricle consists only of stratum spongiosum (spongy muscle), there being no superficial cortex of stratum compactum (compact muscle), that requires a coronary circulation.

In the *Amphibia*, the ventricle is entirely spongy and is largely free of coronary arteries. Those capillaries that do reach the base of the ventricle remain in the epicardium and do not penetrate the myocardial wall. The bulbus cordis, however, has a well-developed coat of compact muscle and hence is well supplied with coronary arteries.

In other vertebrates, such as the *Torpedo*, a genus of several cartilaginous fish related to the skates and rays that give electric shocks (*torpedo*, Latin meaning torpor, lethargy, inertness, numbness), and the rabbit, a completely spongy myocardium is found only during development. Coronary vessels do not appear until the cortical condensation of the ventricular muscle has begun. Coronary vessels are absent in Torpedo embryos of less than 16 mm and in rabbit embryos less than 7 mm.[111]

Regarding coronary sinus aneurysms with ventricular communication(s), a focal lack of formation of compact myocardium (stratum compactum) may well permit persistence of a primitive type of communication between the cardiac veins and the ventricular cavities.[108]

ABSENCE OR ATRESIA OF THE RIGHT SUPERIOR VENA CAVA

Absence or atresia of the RSVC occurred in 7 of 3216 patients with congenital heart disease, accounting for 0.22% of these cases of cardiac anomalies, the 95% CI varying from 0.06% to 0.38% (see Table 6.1). Absence or atresia of the RSVC was the fifth most common systemic venous anomaly in our cardiac pathology database (see Table 6.1). Of these 7 cases, the heart specimens were available for reexamination in 6.

Sex: In this small series, the male-to-female ratio was 4:2 (2:1).

Age at Death: Mean 7.7 ± 10.1 months; range 5.5 hours to 20.75 months; and median 2.5 months.

Segmental Situs Sets: {S,D,S} in 2 of 6 (33%); TGA {S,D,D} in 1 of 6 (17%); TGA {S,L,L} in 1 of 6 (17%); DORV {A(S),L,L} with asplenia in 1 of 6 (17%); and DORV {A(I),L,L} with asplenia in 1 of 6 (17%).

It is noteworthy that absence of the right-sided superior vena cava is "normal" with atrial situs inversus, as in DORV {A(I),L,L} with asplenia. Consequently, one may say that the denominator should be reduced from 6 cases to 5 cases with absent RSVC, in which absence of the RSVC is abnormal. Hence, the segmental anatomy in this small series may be modified as follows: {S,D,S} in 2 of 5 (40%); TGA {S,D,D} in 1 of 5 (20%); and DORV {A(S),L,L} with asplenia in 1 of 5 (20%).

Cardiac Position: Levocardia in 4 of 6 (67%) and dextrocardia in 2 of 6 (33%).

Left SVC: LSVC to coronary sinus to RA (right-sided) in 4 of 6 patients (67%), 2 of whom had unroofing of the coronary sinus (i.e., a coronary sinus septal defect); LSVC to LA (left-sided) because of unroofing of the coronary sinus, with heterotaxy syndrome and asplenia, in 1 of 6 patients (17%); and LSVC to RA (left-sided), with heterotaxy syndrome and asplenia, in 1 of 6 patients (17%). (In the latter case, absence of the right-sided SVC draining into the right-sided atrium may be regarded as "normal," because the atrial situs in this patient with asplenia was thought to be inversus. Similarly, drainage of an LSVC into a left-sided RA is also "normal" for visceroatrial situs inversus. Hence, the latter patient could be deleted from the present study because these atria with situs ambiguus and asplenia probably basically had atrial situs inversus.)

Main Diagnosis: Absence or atresia of the RSVC below the level of the left innominate vein and below the entry of the azygos vein was never the main cardiovascular diagnosis. Indeed, absence or atresia of the RSVC always occurred in the setting of complex congenital heart disease. The main cardiovascular diagnoses were as follows:

Case 1: Congenital aortic valvar stenosis with bicommissural aortic valve (absence of the intercoronary commissure) and atresia of the aortic arch distal to the left subclavian artery.

Case 2: Heterotaxy syndrome with asplenia, DORV {A(I),L,L}, single RV (LV absent), pulmonary atresia, common AV valve, common-inlet RV, right aortic arch, bilateral patent ductus arteriosi.

Case 3: Left atrial outlet atresia (functionally identical to mitral atresia), intact atrial septum, coronary sinus septal defect (unroofing of the coronary sinus being the only outlet from this "blind" LA), common AV valve opening into both ventricles, common AV valve inserting only into the anterolateral papillary muscle group of the LV (also known as potentially parachute mitral valve—following possible surgical repair of common AV canal), and VSD of AV canal type.

Case 4: Dextrocardia with TGA {S,L,L}; pulmonary atresia; unroofing of the coronary sinus; common AV canal; common-inlet RV; LV hypoplasia; totally anomalous pulmonary venous connection to the left innominate vein with obstruction (connecting vein to left innominate vein 1 mm in diameter); small ASD II; PDA, right-sided, closing (cause of death); and right aortic arch.

Case 5: TGA {S,D,D}; left-sided juxtaposition of the atrial appendages (i.e., levomalposition of the right atrial appendage); pulmonary stenosis, infundibular; bilateral conus; and aneurysm of membranous septum contributing to subpulmonary stenosis.

Case 6: Heterotaxy syndrome with asplenia; DORV {A(S),L,L} with pulmonary atresia; totally anomalous pulmonary venous connection with obstruction; dextrocardia; common-inlet RV; and PDA, closing (cause of death).

Multiple Congenital Anomalies: Present in 2 of these 6 patients (33%): Cases 1 and 2.

Case 1 also had hydrocephalus, the Arnold-Chiari malformation, thoracoabdominal meningomyelocele with spina bifida, paraplegia without control of bladder or bowel sphincters.

Case 2, in addition to asplenia, also had occipital meningocele, bilateral microphthalmia, bilateral cleft lip and cleft palate, low-set ears, micrognathia, polydactyly of hands and feet, bilateral talipes equino varus, hypoplasia of the pelvis, omphalocele, bilateral multicystic kidneys, penile hypoplasia with hypospadias, cryptorchidism, and a normal male karyotype.

Literature Review

In 1997, Bartram et al,[86] based on 121 known cases of absent RSVC in visceroatrial situs solitus (including 9 new cases and 95 references), found that this anomaly typically is characterized by persistence of the LSVC connecting with the coronary sinus and draining to the RA, and by a left-sided azygos vein draining into the LSVC.

Less constant features were additional cardiovascular malformations (46%) and rhythm abnormalities (36%) that usually appeared to be related to old age.

These authors[86] concluded that **the majority of cases have otherwise structurally normal hearts.** This is one of the most important findings of this study.[86]

When one excludes cases with the heterotaxy syndrome and asplenia (Cases 2 and 6, previously), even when the atria appear to be in situs solitus (as in Case 6), and when one excludes cases with other multisystem anomalies in visceroatrial situs solitus (e.g., Case 1), then the prevalence of additional congenital heart disease declines to less than half (46%), just as Bartram et al[86] found.

When additional congenital heart disease is present, no specific pattern relating to absence of the RSVC was found.[86]

Because absence of the RSVC is clinically silent, the status of this great vein should be assessed echocardiographically prior to invasive medical or surgical procedures, such as implantation of a transvenous pacemaker, placement of a pulmonary artery catheter without fluoroscopy for intraoperative or intensive care unit monitoring, systemic venous cannulation for extracorporeal membrane oxygenation (ECMO), systemic venous cannulation for cardiopulmonary bypass, partial or total cavopulmonary anastomoses, endomyocardial biopsies, and orthotopic cardiac transplantation.[86]

ABSENCE OF LEFT INNOMINATE VEIN

Absence of the left innominate vein often (see Fig. 6.1A) is associated with bilateral SVC, apparently because of disuse atrophy. For example, when a persistent LSVC drains into the coronary sinus and thence into the RA, no left innominate vein is needed to convey the left jugular and left subclavian blood to the RSVC and thence to the RA. Because the venous blood is conveyed from left to right by the persistent LSVC and the coronary sinus, there is no hemodynamic need for the left innominate vein to remain large and patent. Instead, it typically is small or absent when there is persistence of the LSVC draining into a large coronary sinus. However, when the LSVC becomes atretic and involutes beneath the level of the left innominate vein, the left innominate vein normally persists as a large brachiocephalic vein, and the coronary sinus becomes a normally small common cardiac vein.

The size of cardiovascular structures (arteries, veins, and cardiac chambers) appears to vary directly in size with flow per unit time (e.g., mL/min/M^2). Absence of the left innominate (brachiocephalic) vein appears to be another example of the previously mentioned principle: low flow, facilitated by persistence of the LSVC, leads to involution of the left innominate vein.

Bilateral SVC, each draining into a common atrium, also are often associated with absence of (i.e., apparent involution or failure of development of) the left innominate vein, as in the heterotaxy syndromes with asplenia or polysplenia. In such a common atrium, often associated with a common AV valve and common AV canal, the coronary sinus is absent (i.e., not identifiable because of being unroofed). Hence, an identifiable coronary sinus is not necessary for absence of the left innominate vein.

Unfortunately, absence of the left innominate vein was recorded in only 5 of 3216 cases of congenital heart disease (see Table 6.1), constituting 0.19% of congenital heart disease cases, with a 95% CI of 0.18% to 0.20%. We think that absence of the left innominate vein is very underrepresented in our records; that is, we often failed to record this anomaly. Absence of something can easily be overlooked, whereas the presence of an anomaly is much more eye catching. With apologies for the small size of this sample, let us look at these patients with absence of the left innominate vein:

Sex: Males-to-females = 4:1.

Age at Death: The mean age at death was 3.73 ± 2.23 months, ranging from 5 days to 5.75 months, and the median age at death was 3.75 months.

Types of Cases: What kinds of cases had absence of the left innominate (or brachiocephalic) vein? All 5 cases had bilateral SVC, this being the only finding that all cases had in common.

A persistent LSVC connected with the coronary sinus and drained into the RA (right-sided) in 2 of these 5 patients. A third patient also had a persistent LSVC to coronary sinus to RA; but in addition, this patient also had totally anomalous pulmonary venous connection to the persistent LSVC. This totally anomalous pulmonary venous connection was obstructed by the vascular vice mechanism. Prior to connecting with the LSVC, this anomalous pulmonary venous connection ran behind the left pulmonary artery and in front of the left mainstem bronchus, where the anomalous pulmonary venous structure was squeezed or compressed between the left pulmonary artery and the bronchus. Hence, 3 of these 5 patients with absence of the left innominate vein had bilateral SVCs with persistent LSVC to coronary sinus to a right-sided RA (60%).

One patient with visceral heterotaxy and the polysplenia syndrome had a persistent LSVC that drained into the LA (left-sided) because of the coexistence of a large coronary sinus septal defect that unroofed the coronary sinus and permitted drainage of the LSVC into the LA (20%).

The fifth patient had the heterotaxy syndrome with asplenia, bilateral SVCs, and absence of the left innominate vein. There was a persistent RSVC that drained into the right-sided LA because of a coexisting large coronary sinus septal defect (typical of the asplenia syndrome) (20%). Hence, there were bilateral SVCs, each draining into the ipsilateral atrium.

Apart from bilateral SVCs, these 5 patients had nothing else in common.

Case 1 (A86-184) had heterotaxy syndrome with polysplenia, {S,D,S}, LSVC unroofed into the LA, interrupted IVC, right azygos vein to RSVC, incompletely common AV canal (common atrium, cleft mitral valve, mild mitral regurgitation), mild valvar pulmonary stenosis, necrotizing enterocolitis, and PDA (that was ligated).

Case 2 (A90-134) was a twin, probably identical. Familial congenital heart disease was present, in the sense that the co-twin had a large VSD. Case 2, a 3.5-month-old boy, had MCAs: anal stenosis (treated with dilation), bilateral hydronephrosis, bilateral ureteropelvic obstruction, bilateral ureteral reflux, and congenital heart disease. This patient had DORV {S,D,L}; persistent LSVC to coronary sinus to RA; left juxtaposition of the atrial appendages; a large secundum ASD, overriding without straddling of the tricuspid valve; hypoplasia of the RV sinus; a large VSD (confluent conoventricular and AV canal types); pulmonary outflow tract atresia; PDA, small; and hypoplasia of the mitral valve.

Case 3 (A92-15) had the heterotaxy syndrome with asplenia; DORV {A(I),D,D}; persistent RSVC to LA (R); incompletely common AV canal (ASD I and cleft mitral valve); imperforate Ebstein anomaly of the tricuspid valve; double-orifice mitral valve with smaller accessory orifice in the superior leaflet of the mitral valve (above the cleft); all primary mitral chordae tendineae inserting into the anterolateral papillary muscle of the LV (i.e., potentially parachute mitral valve); subpulmonary fibrous stenosis; VSD of the conoventricular type (not of the AV canal type); and hydrocephalus due to acquired stenosis of the aqueduct of Silvius, probably secondary to cerebral intraventricular hemorrhage.

Case 4 (A88-81) had totally anomalous pulmonary venous connection with obstruction produced by a vascular vice. The anomalous vein passed between the left pulmonary artery anteriorly and the left mainstem bronchus posteriorly. Then the anomalous pulmonary vein curled antero-inferiorly and connected with the LSVC, which in turn continued into a large coronary sinus and thence into the RA. Hence, this was a rare form of totally anomalous pulmonary venous connection: to a persistent LSVC, but with obstruction of the anomalous pulmonary venous pathway by a vascular vice. The left innominate vein was absent. In addition, the following were noteworthy: {S,D,S}; large ASD II; moderate valvar PS with bicuspid pulmonary valve; two VSDs, membranous and mid-muscular; aberrant right subclavian artery; and Alagille syndrome (arteriohepatic dysplasia) with hyperbilirubinemia and jaundice related to severe hypoplasia of the common bile duct and the hepatic bile duct with hepatomegaly, marked cholestasis, and hepatic fibrosis.

Case 5 (A71-100) had pulmonary atresia with intact ventricular septum; {S,D,S}; small PDA; congenital tricuspid stenosis; right atrial hypertrophy and enlargement, marked; bicuspid aortic valve due to absence of the right coronary-noncoronary commissure; and prematurity (birth weight 3 lb and 13 oz, i.e., 1.73 kg).

Conclusions

Apart from the presence of bilateral SVCs, we were not able to discern any other common denominators in these 5 patients with absence of the left innominate vein. Absence of the left innominate vein occurs with many different forms of congenital heart disease. Whenever one encounters bilateral SVCs, one should expect the left innominate vein to be absent or small, apparently because with bilateral SVCs, the left jugular and left subclavian venous blood streams do not need a left innominate vein to reach the atrial level of the heart.

INNOMINATE VEIN ANTERIOR TO THE THYMUS

In our records there are 3 rare and surprising cases in which the left innominate vein ran in an anomalous course anterior to the thymus, constituting 3 of 3216 cases of congenital heart disease (0.09%, 95% CI 0.08 to 0.10; see Table 6.1). We believe these numbers (1) because this is a positive finding and hence likely to be noted and recorded, as opposed to a negative finding (e.g., absence of the left innominate vein) that may not be noted and recorded; and (2) because initially we could not remember ever having seen that before (although we obviously had, having made the diagnosis). So, we think that a left innominate vein running anterior to the thymus is, in fact, as rare as our statistics suggest.

Sex: All 3 patients were female; hence the male-to-female ratio in this very small series was 0:3.

Age at Death: Mean 38 ± 51 hours, ranging from 0 (a 38-week stillborn fetus) to 96 hours (a 4-day-old newborn).

What kind of patients had the left innominate vein running anterior to the thymus? (Normally, the left innominate vein is inferior and posterior to the thymus. Hence normally, the thymus "sits" on the left innominate vein.) Not only were all 3 patients female, but all had *MCAs.*

Case 1 (A81-169) was a newborn girl who died at 18 hours of age. She was the product of a 37-week gestation; had a birth weight of 2450 g (5.4 lb); and had multiple dysmorphic features, including webbed neck, shield chest, widely spaced nipples, nonpitting edema of the lower extremities, microcephaly, microphthalmia, epicanthal folds, low-set ears, micrognathia, bilateral simian creases, and third toe overlapping the fourth toe bilaterally. Her karyotype was normal, 46XX. The heart showed polyvalvular disease, all valve leaflets being thickened and myxomatous. The tricuspid valve had an Ebstein-like anomaly with a deep curtain-like anterior leaflet and a marked paucity of interchordal spaces, but with only mild downward displacement of the septal leaflet. Thickening and rolling of the anterior margins of the anterior and septal leaflets suggested tricuspid regurgitation. There was massive hepatomegaly and leftward bowing of the atrial septum. Thickening of the closing margins of the pulmonary leaflets suggested probable pulmonary valvar stenosis. Myxomatous changes of the anterior and posterior mitral leaflets with reduction of interchordal spaces resulted in some degree of mitral stenosis (no hemodynamic data available in this patient who died at 18 hours of age). Thickening of the aortic leaflets, particularly along their closing margins, suggested aortic valvar stenosis. A secundum type of ASD was due to multiple fenestrations of septum primum and enlargement of ostium secundum. The ductus arteriosus appeared normal for this age, probe patent but functionally closing.

The anomalous left innominate vein running anterior to the thymus, although a rare and eye-catching anomaly, was of no functional significance.

In view of the phenotypic anomalies mentioned earlier, this patient was clinically thought to have either Turner syndrome or Noonan syndrome. When the karyotype with chromosomal banding proved to be normal, and when the ovaries at autopsy were found to be unremarkable, the diagnosis of Turner syndrome (45 XO) was abandoned. Some thought that, by default, the diagnosis of Noonan syndrome should be made. However, because of atypical features such as the presence of polyvalvular disease (with a normal karyotype), in the final anatomic diagnosis of our Pathology Department, the diagnosis of Noonan syndrome was not made. It was generally agreed, however, that this was a case of MCAs, not entirely typical of any identified syndrome.

Our conclusion is that Case 1 had a Noonan-like syndrome with MCAs.

Case 2 (A83-21) was a 4-day-old female infant with **MCAs and persistent fetal circulation.** The patient experienced multiple episodes of cyanosis and hypoxemia, had suprasystemic pulmonary arterial hypertension, and showed a marked increase in the smooth muscle of the acinar pulmonary arteries with peripheral extension. The patient had bilateral pulmonary congestion and edema, right ventricular hypertrophy, bilateral pleural effusions, and anasarca. Additional findings included a small persistent LSVC to the coronary sinus to the RA, left innominate vein running anterior to the thymus, aberrant right subclavian artery, medial deviation of the 4th and 5th toes of the right foot, and imperforate anus.

Case 3 (C82-459) was a 38-week stillborn female with **MCAs.** Clinically she was thought possibly to have trisomy 13-15; however, skin fibroblasts failed to grow, and thus the karyotype could not be established. The patient was thought to have had an intrauterine infection, with multiple pustules of the skin. The patient had a left cleft lip, a bilaterally cleft palate, low-set ears, left innominate vein anterior to the thymus, TOF with moderate pulmonary valvar stenosis, completely common AV canal (type C of Rastelli), a tissue-deficient mitral valve component of the common AV valve with regurgitation, a secundum type of ASD due to deficiency and fenestrations of septum primum (pentalogy of Fallot), right aortic arch, congenital isolation of the left subclavian artery originating from the left pulmonary artery via a probe-patent left PDA, and congenital absence of the right ductus arteriosus (with a right aortic arch).

Conclusion

The only common denominator that we were able to perceive among these 3 female infants with left innominate vein anterior to the thymus was that all had major (but very different) MCAs.

THE RAGHIB SYNDROME

The Raghib syndrome was found in 2 patients, that is, 0.06% of 3216 patients with congenital heart disease, with 95% CI 0.05% to 0.07% (see Table 6.1).

The Raghib syndrome[4] may be defined as a persistent SVC (a persistent LSVC in visceroatrial situs solitus, or a persistent RSVC in visceroatrial situs inversus), and a coronary sinus septal defect that unroofs the persistent SVC into the morphologically LA, which are associated with a large low posterior interatrial communication that is thought to be the enlarged right atrial ostium of the unroofed coronary sinus (see Fig. 6.1B).

Case 1 (A88-44) was a 7-day-old female infant with MCA and a normal karyotype (46,XX); dysmorphic facies with a broad flat nasal bridge; right microtia; right hemifacial microsomia; anteverted nares; retrognathia; pectus excavatum; short sternum; webbed neck; two-vessel umbilical cord; 13 ribs bilaterally; upper thoracic bifid vertebrae; clinodactyly; umbilical hernia; hypoplasia of the left lobe of the thymus; interrupted IVC, with left-sided azygos vein to left SVC; absence of the RSVC; large coronary sinus septal defect unroofing the coronary sinus into the LA, with large posteroinferior ostium of coronary sinus within the atrial septum (the Raghib syndrome); complete form of common AV canal (type A of Rastelli); common-inlet LV with relatively small RV; normal segmental situs set {S,D,S}; truncus arteriosus type A2; thick myxomatous bicuspid and bicommissural truncal valve; left aortic arch with aberrant right subclavian artery; congenital absence of the ductus arteriosus; and abnormal brachiocephalic arteries. The first brachiocephalic artery arose above the ostium of the left pulmonary artery and supplied a relatively small right common carotid artery. The second brachiocephalic branch was a left innominate artery that supplied the left common carotid artery and the left subclavian artery. The third and last brachiocephalic artery was the aberrant right subclavian (previously mentioned).

Thus, this was a rare form of truncus arteriosus type A2 because of the coexistence of completely common AV canal, a relatively small RV with common-inlet LV, interruption of the IVC, a left-sided azygos venous extension, the Raghib syndrome, absence of the RSVC, abnormal brachiocephalic arteries, absence of the ductus arteriosus, MCAs, familial congenital heart disease (father with repaired VSD), and familial noncardiovascular anomalies (mother with posterior dislocation of the right temperomandibular joint, and maternal uncle with tracheo-esophageal fistula who died at 3 weeks of age). Our patient developed necrotizing enterocolitis that led to death at 7 days of age. Autopsy was limited to heart and lungs. Abdominal ultrasound in life showed a normally located spleen. We were not sure whether polysplenia with multiple attached splenuli could be identified by ultrasound; hence, we were not certain that the heterotaxy syndrome with polysplenia was excluded.

Case 2 (A89-12) was a 28 11/12–year-old man with dextrocardia and inverted TOF {I,L,I}. The findings included severe pulmonary stenosis with a bicuspid and bicommissural pulmonary valve and a persistent RSVC draining into the LA (right-sided) because of a large coronary sinus septal defect, and a large low posterior opening in the atrial septum (the coronary sinus ostium). Hence, a mirror-image (inverted) Raghib syndrome was present. A LSVC and an innominate vein were both also present. The patient had multiple VSDs: the high subaortic TOF type of conoventricular defect and an apical muscular VSD. A right aortic arch was present, usual for situs inversus totalis.

The patient died on the second postoperative day after repair of TOF at almost 29 years of age. Prior to this time, he had a left Blalock-Taussig shunt at 11 years of age, a right Blalock-Taussig anastomosis at 20 years of age, intermittent seizures, an auto accident at 24 years of age because of seizures, and a right occipital brain abscess at 26 years of age.

The history of this patient illustrates very clearly why we are now endeavoring to correct TOF upon diagnosis in infancy, as advocated by Dr. Aldo Castañeda and colleagues, rather than performing multiple palliative procedures.

Conclusion

In both of our patients, the Raghib syndrome occurred in the setting of complex congenital heart disease. Case 1 had visceroatrial situs solitus with MCAs. Case 2 had visceroatrial situs inversus, which also may be viewed as a coordinated form of MCAs.

RIGHT SUPERIOR VENA CAVA DRAINING PARTLY INTO THE LEFT ATRIUM

In a patient with visceroatrial situs solitus, the RSVC drained partly into the morphologically LA. This anomaly is also known as biatrial drainage of the RSVC.

Sex: Male.

Age at Death: 3 days.

Diagnoses: The patient was a 3-day-old male identical twin with a vein of Galen aneurysm, an overriding RSVC that drained predominantly into the LA, a sinus venosus defect, right pulmonary veins confluent with the RSVC, hence partially anomalous pulmonary venous drainage, and an intact interatrial septum with septum primum and septum secundum fused. The RSVC was unroofed into the right pulmonary veins, which connected normally with the LA. Hence, the RSVC and the right pulmonary veins were not separated; that is, they were confluent. Because the right pulmonary veins connected normally with the LA, the lack of separation of the RSVC anteriorly and the right pulmonary veins posteriorly had two different effects: (1) partially anomalous pulmonary venous *drainage* of some of the right pulmonary venous blood stream into the RSVC and thence into the RA, despite normal *connection* of the right pulmonary veins with the LA; and (2) partially anomalous systemic venous *drainage* of some of the RSVC blood stream into the LA, despite normal *connection* of the RSVC with the RA.

Thus, we have partially anomalous pulmonary venous drainage and partially anomalous systemic venous drainage, despite normal pulmonary venous and SVC connections. Why these anomalous venous drainages? There are two reasons: (1) because the right pulmonary veins posteriorly and the SVC anteriorly are confluent (not separated, i.e., unroofed into each other); and (2) because of the normal venous connections. Some of the right pulmonary venous blood drains into the RA because the RSVC connects normally with the RA. Some of the RSVC blood drains into the LA because the right pulmonary veins connect normally with the LA.

This new understanding explains why we used to think (and many still do) that when the RSVC drains partly into the LA, this is due to leftward malalignment of the right horn of the sinus venosus relative to the atrial septum. In other words, we used to think that the RSVC really is too far leftward and hence drains partially into the LA. Now, thanks to the new understanding of Stella Van Praagh, M.D., and her colleagues,[113] we now realize that our old hypothesis (real leftward displacement of the RSVC) was due to misleading appearances, not to anatomic and embryologic reality. Our present understanding is that the RSVC is normally located and normally connected with the RA. However, because the partition between the posteriorly running right pulmonary veins and the more anteriorly situated RSVC is absent, consequently the RSVC appears to run directly into the dilated right pulmonary veins that open widely into the LA. This confluence of the RSVC with the right pulmonary veins makes it look as though the inferior portion of the RSVC is more leftward than normal. In fact, this posterior and leftward wall is the normal posterior wall of the right pulmonary veins as they connect with the LA. Hence, the inferior portion of the RSVC is not really more leftward than normal; instead, it is the right pulmonary veins' posterior wall that is leftward, and this, of course, is normal.

The real problem is that the sinus venosus defect is invisible: When the partition between the RSVC and the right pulmonary veins is absent, these two venous structures simply become confluent. One is not left with discrete margins of this defect, hence invisibility.

The high and posterior opening into the LA is not the sinus venosus defect, contrary to what is conventionally taught. Instead, this high posterior interatrial communication—through which the RSVC may drain into the LA—is the ostium of the right pulmonary veins. The real sinus venosus defect is what the surgeon patches. He or she creates the missing partition between the superior vena cava anteriorly and the right pulmonary veins posteriorly (Fig. 6.9).

To summarize this new understanding[113]:

1. The high posterior interatrial communication above the atrial septum is the ostium of the right pulmonary veins.
2. The sinus venosus defect is the missing partition between the RSVC and the right pulmonary veins.
3. Hence, the sinus venosus defect is a right-sided unroofing defect (in visceroatrial situs solitus), analogous to the Raghib syndrome, which is a left-sided unroofing defect (a coronary sinus septal defect).
4. In both unroofing defects (right-sided and left-sided), the interatrial communications are normal venous ostia (not abnormal defects in the atrial septum). In sinus venosus defect, the interatrial communication is the ostium of the right pulmonary veins. In the Raghib syndrome, the interatrial communication is the ostium of the coronary sinus.

From the foregoing it should be apparent that the distinction between venous *drainage* and *connection(s)* is very important. The concepts are different, and both are important. In right SVC to LA, right pulmonary venous and RSVC drainages are anomalous, whereas the venous connections with the atria are normal.

However, the essential anomaly in right SVC to LA is the sinus venosus unroofing defect. When the unroofing defect is high, the right pulmonary veins are unroofed into the RSVC (and vice versa), and hence the RSVC can drain anomalously into the LA. But when the unroofing defect is lower, the right pulmonary veins are unroofed into the RA, and consequently the RSVC does not appear to drain into the LA.

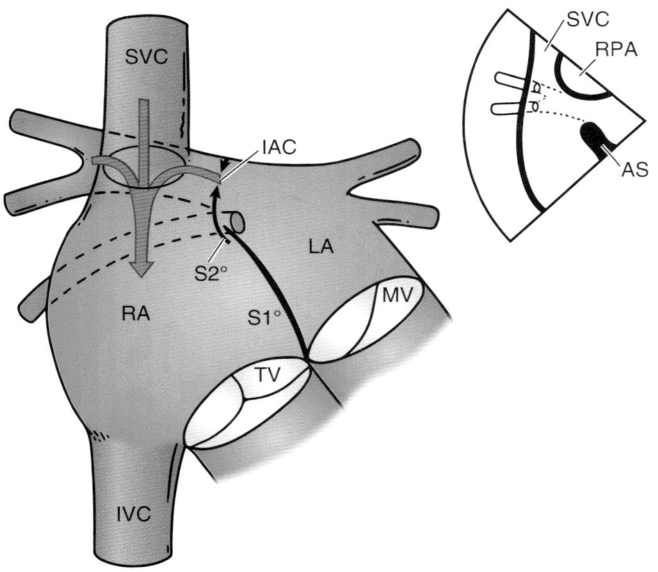

Fig. 6.9 Typical sinus venosus defect, which is really a cavopulmonary venous defect: the oval orifice between the superior vena cava *(SVC)* anteriorly and the right upper and middle pulmonary veins posteriorly, through which cavopulmonary venous shunting occurs *(arrows)*. The normal orifice of the right upper and middle pulmonary vein entering the left atrium *(LA)* is an interatrial communication *(IAC)* because of the coexistence of cavopulmonary venous defect. The right lower pulmonary vein enters the LA normally and typically is not involved in the cavopulmonary venous defect; consequently, the right lower pulmonary vein does not function as an IAC. The IAC is a normal orifice, not an atrial septal defect. The IAC is not a sinus venosus defect. The real defect is the cavopulmonary venous defect that the surgeon patches. *AS,* Atrial septum; *IVC,* inferior vena cava; *MV,* mitral valve; *RPA,* right pulmonary artery; *S1°,* septum primum; *S2°,* septum secundum; *TV,* tricuspid valve. (Reproduced with permission from Geva T, Van Praagh S. Anomalies of the pulmonary veins. In: Allen HD, Clark EB, Gutgesell HP, Driscoll DJ, eds. *Moss and Adams' Heart Disease in Infants, Children, and Adolescents, Including the Fetus and Young Adult.* 6th ed. Philadelphia, PA: Lippincott Williams & Wilkins; 2001:736.)

There are two different anatomic types of sinus venosus unroofing defect:

1. the higher or low right SVC type; and
2. the lower or high RA type.

RSVC to LA occurs only with the higher or low RSVC type of sinus venosus unroofing defect.

Parenthetically, we think that **the so-called IVC type of sinus venosus defect** is a mistake, that is, an entirely different kind of anomaly, without an unroofing defect and without partially anomalous right pulmonary venous drainage. When septum primum (the flap valve of the foramen ovale) is more or less totally absent, then the interatrial communication is confluent with the IVC. (An interatrial communication that is confluent with either the SVC or the IVC is the old, simplistic definition of sinus venosus defect. This unsatisfactory definition indicates little or no deep understanding of the anomaly.) The so-called IVC type of sinus venosus defect is a very large secundum type of ASD, often also called a common atrium. The interatrial communication is an ASD due to virtual absence of the septum primum with or without a prominent Eustachian valve (not a normal venous ostium as is associated with a sinus venosus defect). Septum primum grows *upward* from the IVC.[114] Consequently, when septum primum is absent, a huge secundum type of ASD extends down to the IVC and is confluent with it.

In Case 1, the segmental situs set was unremarkable: {S,D,S}. A PDA was probe patent and appeared to be functionally closing.

Secondary to the cerebral arteriovenous malformation with a vein of Galen aneurysm, there was marked cardiomegaly with hypertrophy and enlargement of all cardiac chambers, particularly involving the LA and LV, due to the presence of high-output congestive heart failure.

The patient suffered from recurrent seizures that did not respond to anticonvulsive medication. Delivery had been by breech extraction. Autopsy revealed a large subarachnoid hematoma in the posterior fossa, and microcephaly with necrotic cerebral hemispheres, extensive gliosis, and old and recent hemorrhagic infarctions.

To summarize from the cardiovascular standpoint, the huge cerebral arteriovenous malformation resulting in a vein of Galen aneurysm was by far the clinically most important anomaly. The patient had bounding pulses, bilateral rales and rhonchi, marked cardiomegaly, and hepatosplenomegaly, and was described as much less vigorous than his normal twin, our patient having "marked acrocyanosis" and "poor color." Although cardiac catheterization and neurosurgery were not performed after carotid arteriography, we speculated at autopsy that the rapid cerebral transit time would have permitted little unsaturation to occur, hence the absence of frank central cyanosis.

Thus, the RSVC drained predominantly into the LA, with an intact but dysplastic-looking atrial septum, in a patient with a huge cerebral arteriovenous malformation and a vein of Galen aneurysm, who died from high-output congestive heart failure at 3 days of age. Hence, in this patient, the biatrial connection of the RSVC was part of multiple cardiovascular anomalies.

Discussion

Unroofing of the right pulmonary veins, that is, absence of the common party wall between the right upper and middle pulmonary veins posteriorly and the superior vena cava and the right sinus horn part of the RA anteriorly, results in several interrelated phenotypes:

1. **Typical so-called sinus venosus defect.** The right upper and middle pulmonary veins connect with the RSVC or with the superior part of the RA (systemic venous component). The interatrial communication is the ostium of the unroofed right pulmonary veins. This interatrial communication is not an ASD (an abnormal opening in the atrial septum). This interatrial communication also is not a "sinus venosus defect." This conventional concept of a sinus venosus defect is simply wrong and is based on lack of anatomic and developmental understanding. The real defect in this anomaly is the unroofing of the right pulmonary veins (absence of the common party wall), not the ostium of the right pulmonary

veins (which is a normal structure). The real defect is what the surgeon fixes. The surgeon partitions ("reroofs") the right pulmonary veins posteriorly, separating the right pulmonary veins from the RSVC and the RA anteriorly. After this surgical reroofing procedure, the right pulmonary venous blood then flows through the former interatrial communication (the right pulmonary venous ostium) into the LA. If the right pulmonary venous ostium into the LA is too small (hypoplastic because of shunting into the SVC and RA), this ostium may need to be enlarged to provide an unobstructed right pulmonary venous pathway (the Warden procedure).

2. **Biatrial drainage of the RSVC.** The RSVC can drain into both the RA and the LA. Because the right pulmonary veins are unroofed, the RSVC flows into the top of the right pulmonary veins, which then connect normally with the LA. This creates the phenotype of biatrial drainage of the RSVC. The opening of the RSVC into the LA can be large, and the opening of the RA can be relatively small. The atrial septum is intact.
3. **Left atrial drainage of the RSVC.** The RSVC can communicate via the unroofed right pulmonary veins only with the LA. The RSVC does not open at all into the RA, and the atrial septum is intact (Fig. 6.10).

Much of this new understanding concerning nonseptation of the right pulmonary veins posteriorly from the RSVC and the sinus venosus component of the RA anteriorly has recently been summarized by Geva and Van Praagh.[115,116]

In view of the fact that the conventional understanding of sinus venosus defect—often called sinus venosus ASD—is anatomically erroneous (as earlier), it is proposed that the high type of sinus venosus defect involving the RSVC, but not the RA, may accurately be called **cavopulmonary venous defect.** The low type of sinus venosus defect involving the sinus venosus portion of the RA and the right pulmonary veins may accurately be called **sinopulmonary venous defect.** The term *sinus venosus defect,* at best, is only half right because it omits the right pulmonary venous component of the defect, which is not regarded as sinus venosus tissue. Consequently, the designations *cavopulmonary venous defect* and *sinopulmonary venous defect* are preferred because of their anatomic accuracy and clarity.

A change in terminology is indicated because the conventional meaning of "sinus venosus ASD" is wrong: The interatrial communication is the unroofed, but otherwise normal, right pulmonary vein ostium (not a sinus venosus type of ASD). The real defect, which is not referred to in the conventional meaning, is what the surgeon patches.

It is also noteworthy that the low type of defect and the high type of defect may be hemodynamic opposites. From the hemodynamic standpoint, the low defect (the sinopulmonary venous defect) is predominantly a left-to-right shunt, that is, a partially anomalous drainage of the right pulmonary veins into the low RSVC and RA. By contrast, the high defect (the cavopulmonary venous defect) may be predominantly a right-to-left shunt, with flow of the RSVC blood into the LA, particularly when the junction of the RSVC and the RA is stenotic or atretic. In other words, when cavopulmonary venous defect occurs *without* stenosis of the RSVC-RA junction (see Fig. 6.9),[115] the atrial-level shunt may be predominantly left to right or bidirectional. But when cavopulmonary venous defect occurs *with* stenosis or atresia of the RSVC-RA junction (see Fig. 6.10),[116] the atrial-level shunt is either predominantly or entirely right to left, respectively.

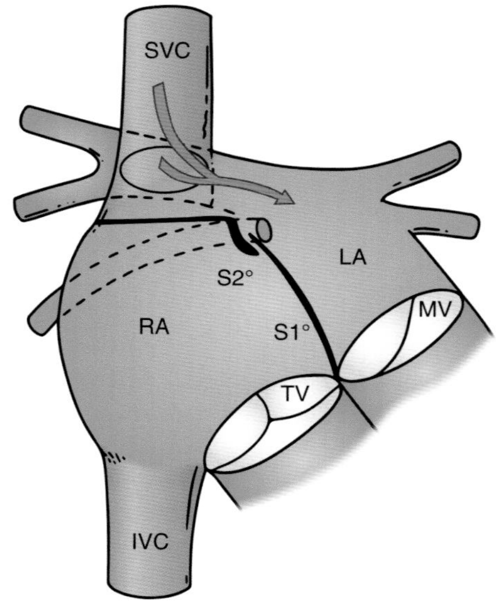

Fig. 6.10 Right superior vena cava *(SVC)* draining into the left atrium *(LA)* via a cavopulmonary venous defect: the oval orifice through which cavopulmonary venous shunting occurs *(arrows).* Because atresia of the SVC at the right atrial *(RA)* junction coexists, the shunting is only right-to-left from the right SVC into the LA. There is no interatrial defect. *IVC,* Inferior vena cava; *MV,* mitral valve; *S1°,* septum primum; *S2°,* septum secundum; *TV,* tricuspid valve. (Reproduced with permission from Geva T, Van Praagh S. Abnormal systemic venous connections. In: Allen HD, Clark EB, Gutgesell HP, Driscoll DJ, eds. *Moss and Adams' Heart Disease in Infants, Children, and Adolescents, Including the Fetus and Young Adult.* 6th ed. Philadelphia, PA: Lippincott Williams & Wilkins; 2001:773.)

RETROAORTIC INNOMINATE VEIN

The left innominate (or left brachiocephalic) vein ran behind the upper ascending aorta and beneath the beginning of the transverse aortic arch in one patient, constituting 0.03% of this series of congenital heart disease (1/3216 cases; 95% CI 0.02% to 0.04%) (see Table 6.1).

From the embryologic standpoint, how can the left innominate (brachiocephalic) vein run behind and beneath the junction of the ascending and arch portions of the aorta? The left innominate vein normally appears in the human embryo during the seventh week of gestation. This vein normally runs above the developing pericardial sac, slightly above the aortic arch, and crosses just in front of the base of the innominate (brachiocephalic) artery and connects with the left side of the right jugular vein. Hence, the left innominate vein normally passes in front of the trachea and esophagus. However, as is pointed out by Marshall[109] and well illustrated in his Plate V, the persistent LSVC runs just to the left of the aortic arch and the ductus arteriosus. Normally, the left end of the innominate vein originates high enough to pass above the aorta and in front of the innominate artery. But if the left innominate vein arises sufficiently low from the LSVC, just above the pericardial sac, the left innominate vein, which begins as a diminutive venous connection, would have to pass behind and beneath the aorta to connect with the RSVC. Hence, our hypothesis is that a retroaortic innominate vein results from abnormally caudal or inferior formation of the bridging left innominate vein.

How could a retroesophageal innominate vein—referred to by Marshall[109]—be understood developmentally? The anatomy suggests that a left innominate vein running behind both the trachea and the esophagus may be explained by an abnormally high and posterior formation of this vein. Cephalically, the left internal jugular vein extends somewhat posteriorly to the esophagus.

Hence, we hypothesize that the cephalocaudal height at which the left innominate vein forms may explain both a retroaortic innominate vein (abnormally low formation) and a retroesophageal innominate vein (abnormally high formation).

Definitions

The **left innominate vein** is the bridging vein between the left jugular vein, at the level of the left subclavian vein, that extends to the right jugular vein, somewhat below the level of the right subclavian vein. But what is the **right innominate vein**? Briefly, it is the inferior prolongation of the right jugular vein that extends from the level of the right subclavian vein superiorly to the level of the left innominate vein inferiorly.

Where does the **SVC** begin? The superior extent of the RSVC is normally indicated by the insertion of the left innominate vein. Hence, the **RSVC** lies between the level of the left innominate vein superiorly and the RA inferiorly.

The **LSVC** is less precisely defined because, in visceroatrial situs solitus with bilateral SVC, the left innominate vein is often absent; hence, the upper limit of the LSVC cannot be defined in terms of the innominate vein. In this situation, we use the left subclavian vein as an arbitrary marker of the LSVC (below) and the left jugular vein (above). The LSVC is delimited inferiorly by the **coronary sinus,** which runs in the left posterior AV groove or sulcus.

What really is the coronary sinus? Is it the cardiac venous confluence? Or is it the left horn of the sinus venosus? Or is it the left common cardinal vein, also known as the left duct of Cuvier? The short answer is all or some of the above. The coronary sinus always is the cardiac venous confluence (see Fig. 6.2). When there is no persistent LSVC, the left horn of the sinus venosus (alias the left common cardinal vein or the left duct of Cuvier) has involuted and makes no contribution to the coronary sinus. However, when a persistent LSVC connects with the coronary sinus, the left sinus horn persists (does not involute) and is responsible for the characteristic enlargement of the coronary sinus that is associated with a persistent LSVC.

An enlarged coronary sinus should suggest at least four diagnostic possibilities:

1. a persistent (typically left) superior vena cava,
2. a coronary sinus septal defect,
3. totally or partially anomalous pulmonary venous connection to the coronary sinus, or
4. some combination of the foregoing.

Now, let us return to our rare case of retroaortic innominate vein.

Sex: Male

Age at Death: 4 weeks

Diagnoses: This patient had a normal segmental situs set, that is {S,D,S}, with MCAs. Pregnancy was complicated by chronic abruptio placentae, and birth was by cesarean section at 36 weeks gestation, with a birth weight of 2.8 kg. The MCAs consisted of abnormal facies with hypertelorism, low-set ears, small mouth with down-turned corners, and small chin; cleft palate; hypospadias; retroaortic innominate vein; interrupted aortic arch type B (of Celoria and Patton[117]); aberrant right subclavian artery from the top of the descending thoracic aorta; mild subaortic narrowing due to leftward and posterior malalignment of the conal septum, which in turn was related to malalignment of the whole conotruncus with the pulmonary valve abnormally anterior and rightward, whereas the aortic valve was abnormally posterior and leftward; small aortic annulus, with tricommissural aortic valve; two VSDs consisting of a small, slit-like conoventricular VSD, 3 mm in length, between the conal septum (parietal band) above and the right posterior division of the septal band below, and a large muscular VSD (6 to 7 mm in diameter) behind the septal leaflet of the tricuspid valve (but not confluent with the tricuspid annulus); and a large PDA (not closing).

At 3 days of age, via a left thoracotomy and a median sternotomy, a 7 mm in diameter Gore-Tex conduit was placed between the ascending and descending aorta to repair the interrupted aortic arch, with ligation of the PDA and banding of the main pulmonary artery. The surgeons observed that the thymus appeared moderately hypoplastic, raising the question of DiGeorge syndrome.

The postoperative period was characterized by chronic poor perfusion with cool and edematous extremities. The gradient across the pulmonary artery band site was 30 to 40 mm Hg. There was also mild stenosis of the aortic outflow tract and across the conduit (25 mm Hg), with mild kinking at the proximal conduit anastomosis (cardiac catheterization). The postoperative course was characterized by oliguria, hypotension, pleural effusions, and azotemia, treated by peritoneal dialysis. The patient experienced intermittent episodes of bradycardia, and death occurred 30 days postoperatively, despite all therapeutic endeavors.

Autopsy revealed that the proximal ostium leading from the ascending aorta into the conduit measured only 3 mm in internal diameter in the fresh state, whereas the distal anastomosis with the descending thoracic aorta measured 7 mm in internal diameter. Extensive antemortem thrombosis was found involving the SVC, the retroaortic left innominate vein, the IVC, and the descending thoracic aorta. No thrombosis was present in the aortic-arch conduit.

In the final autopsy report, it was agreed that the DiGeorge syndrome was present.

Summary

A retroaortic left innominate vein occurred in the setting of MCAs, including the DiGeorge syndrome with interrupted aortic arch type B, aberrant right subclavian artery, multiple VSDs (two), cleft palate, and hypospadias. The retroaortic left innominate vein was clinically and hemodynamically silent.

LEFT-TO-RIGHT SWITCHING OF THE INFERIOR VENA CAVA

Left-to-right switching of the IVC, at the level of the renal veins (left-sided below the renal veins, right-sided above the renal veins) was observed in 1 of 3216 cases of congenital heart disease (0.03%; 95% CI 0.02% to 0.04%; see Table 6.1).

Embryologically, how is it possible for the IVC to shift sides—from left to right (as in our case), or from right to left—at the level of the renal veins? Normally the posterior cardinal veins drain preferentially into the *right* supracardinal vein, which then flows into the *right* portion of the intersubcardinal anastomosis and thence into the new anastomotic vein or the mesenteric part of the IVC that arises from the cephalic end of the *right* side of the intersubcardinal anastomosis, between 6 and 8 weeks of gestational age. In our case, the posterior cardinals via the iliac anastomosis flowed predominantly into the *left* supracardinal vein, which then flowed into the left part of the intersubcardinal anastomosis, but exited from the *right* cephalic end of the intersubcardinal anastomosis via a normally *right-sided* new anastomotic vein or the mesenteric part of the IVC. Hence, the definitive IVC appears to shift from left to right at the level of the renal veins. Thus, the intersubcardinal anastomosis is the site of switching (left to right, or right to left) between contralateral supracardiac component and new anastomotic venous component of the definitive IVC.

Sex: Female

Age at Death: 1 day

Diagnoses: This patient had major MCAs, that is, Cantrell syndrome[118] with thoracoabdominal ectopia cordis and TOF. In somewhat greater detail, the patient had facial dysmorphism with low-set ears, large tongue, webbed neck, puffy eyelids, and wide-set nipples. The patient had Cantrell syndrome,[118] characterized by thoracoabdominal ectopia cordis with a large unruptured omphalocele containing liver, small bowel, and the cardiac apex. There was a half-moon–shaped anterior diaphragmatic defect associated with absence of the diaphragmatic pericardium. The lungs were markedly hypoplastic bilaterally, with atelectasis, congestion, edema, hemorrhage, and occasional foci of hyaline membrane formation. The heart had TOF with moderate pulmonary outflow tract stenosis (hypoplasia), bicuspid pulmonary valve because of rudimentary right septal-nonseptal commissure, almost total absence of septum primum resulting in a very large secundum type of ASD or common atrium (pentalogy of Fallot), and absence of the ductus arteriosus or ligamentum arteriosum. The gallbladder was absent, although the extrahepatic bile ducts were present and patent.

Summary

Left-to-right switching of the IVC at the level of the renal veins occurred in the setting of MCAs, but was not per se clinically or hemodynamically important.

UMBILICAL VEIN TO CORONARY SINUS

The umbilical vein connected with the coronary sinus and drained into the RA in 1 patient (A81-76) (0.03%; 95% CI 0.02% to 0.04%; see Table 6.1). This anomalous umbilical vein ran adjacent to the right lobe of the liver, where it received several small hepatic veins.

Embryologically, how is it possible for the umbilical vein to connect directly with the coronary sinus? At 4 weeks of gestational age, the left and right umbilical veins connect directly with the left and right common cardinal veins, respectively. Normally, however, by 5½ weeks gestational age, these direct connections of the umbilical veins with the common cardinal veins have undergone involution. Hence, by 5½ weeks of age, the umbilical veins normally flow into the liver, where they join the portal venous system that flows into the ductus venosus and thence into the suprahepatic segment of the IVC and finally into the RA. Thus, by 5½ weeks of age the normal definitive connections of the umbilical veins that do not bypass the liver have been achieved. Rarely, however, as in the present case, the initial direct connection of the umbilical vein with the coronary sinus can persist, bypassing the liver, as in the normal 4-week human embryo. How and why this normal 4-week gestational-age situation can persist to the neonatal period is, to the best of our present knowledge, unknown. Thus, although the *morphogenesis* of the umbilical vein connecting with the coronary sinus is clear, the *cause* of this anomaly is unknown.

Sex: Male.

Age at Death: 10 days.

Other Diagnoses: This patient was born postmature at 42 weeks gestational age and had the persistent fetal circulation syndrome. The segmental anatomy was unremarkable: {S,D,S}. The SVC and IVC returned normally to the RA. Other findings included a secundum ASD due to deficiency of septum primum, PDA, right atrial hypertrophy and enlargement, right ventricular hypertrophy and enlargement, and the previously mentioned anomalous systemic venous return—extrahepatic course of the umbilical vein to the right atrial ostium of the coronary sinus.

ANOMALOUS “PORTAL” VEIN TO AZYGOS VEIN

Absence of the hepatic portal venous system was observed in 1 patient (A53-114) (0.03%, 95% CI 0.02% to 0.04%; see Table 6.1). Instead, there was an anomalous “hepatic portal” venous connection between the splenic vein and the superior mesenteric vein and the azygos vein (Fig. 6.11).

Sex: Female.

Age at Death: 6½ years.

Discussion: In greater detail, before opening the abdomen, a plexus of prominent veins was seen in the right lower quadrant,

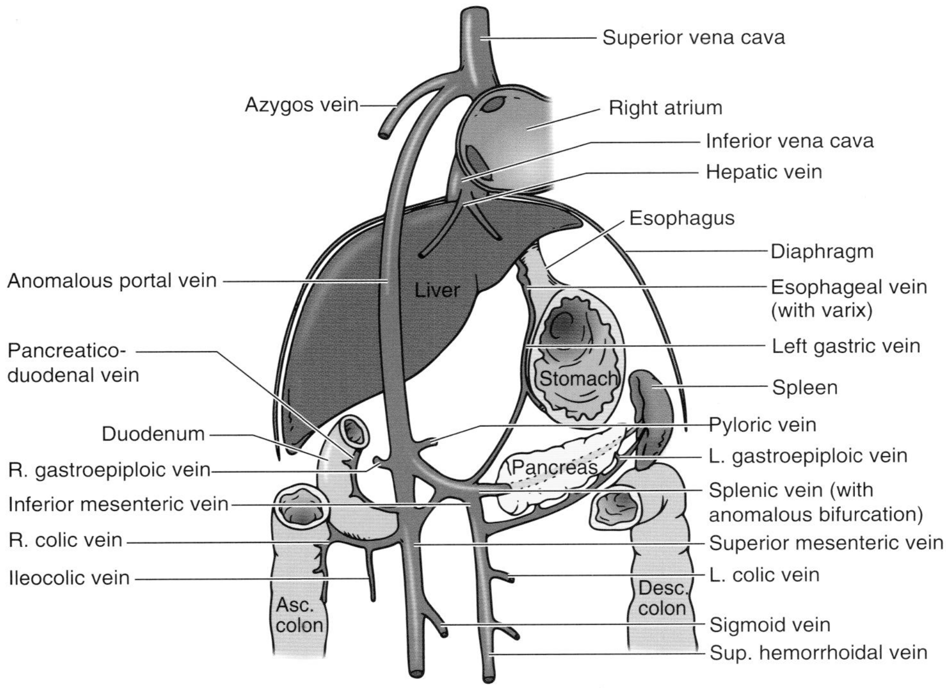

Fig. 6.11 Absence of the portal vein to the liver, with anomalous "portal" vein connecting with the azygos vein, resulting in portal venous hypertension with marked splenomegaly (140/58 g) and esophageal varices. The cause of death of this 6½-year-old girl was a ruptured esophageal varix. (Diagram reproduced from an autopsy protocol of Boston Children's Hospital, Boston, Massachusetts. *ASC,* ascending; *DESC,* descending; *ESOPH,* esophagus; *l,* left; *r,* right; *RT,* right; *v,* vein. Courtesy of the Department of Pathology, Boston Children's Hospital, Boston, MA)

visible through the skin. On opening the abdomen and having inspected the viscera, the esophagus was transected, revealing large esophageal varices that coursed the length of the esophagus and joined with the left superior intercostal vein and the left hemiazygos vein. Injection of the splenic vein with saline resulted in the distention of the inferior varices, also revealing two tiny defects in these varices, from which bleeding had occurred in life. Opening of the esophagus revealed large blood clots in this area, and the stomach was also filled with fresh blood.

The autopsy protocol by Drs. N.I. Donell and B.H. Landing continues as follows:

In an attempt to find the source of the esophageal varices, the portal system is dissected out and traced, and the following remarkable anomaly is found. The portal vein is identified with the splenic vein entering it from the spleen, and the superior mesenteric vein entering it from the mesentery and the usual smaller vessels. However, the splenic vein instead of entering by one channel, appears to fork shortly before it reaches the portal vein, and enters the portal vein through two channels, which are equal in diameter. A very small valve-like ridge is present in one of the forks; however, no obstruction appears to be present. The wall of the vein is uniformly thin and smooth. The portal vein is then followed towards the liver, and instead of entering the liver in the normal fashion, it passes up through the diaphragm joining the right azygos [vein] and entering the RSVC before that vessel enters the heart.... The portal vein, itself, appears to be uniformly thin-walled, smooth, with no valves present, and no obstruction found. The venous system is traced through the splenic vein into the splenic hilum and shows many anastomosing channels, none of which appears to be obstructed or shows any thickening of the walls.

The hepatic artery entered the liver normally. The course of this anomalous portal vein that flowed into the azygos vein is shown diagrammatically in Fig. 6.11, which is taken from the original autopsy protocol.

There was marked splenomegaly (140/58 g), with splenic fibrosis. Anomalous portal venous hypertension was thought to constitute the pathogenesis of the patient's splenomegaly and esophageal varices that ruptured, leading to death.

Although this rare patient may be regarded as having an anomalous portal vein (see Fig. 6.11), an alternative interpretation is that the hepatic portal vein was in fact absent and hence did not flow into the porta hepatis. We think that the portal hypertension leading to esophageal varices with fatal rupture in this 6½-year-old girl was related to the small caliber of the azygos vein to which the anomalous portal vein connected.

INFERIOR VENA CAVA NEVER CONNECTS DIRECTLY WITH LEFT ATRIUM

Thus far, all of this chapter has been devoted to 13 different anatomic types of systemic venous anomalies, that is, malformations of the systemic veins that we are sure do indeed happen (see Table 6.1). (Perhaps it should be stated explicitly that we have been exceedingly careful not to include any anomaly unless we are certain that what we are saying is anatomically accurate. We also know that to err is human, and that inevitably we will make mistakes. But we have been as careful and as critical as we know how to be.) However, the present section focuses on an anomaly that, although reported in the literature, we think does not in fact exist, namely, the IVC connecting directly with the morphologically LA.

In 1955, a very influential autopsied case was published concerning a 32-year-old married woman in whom the IVC was described as connecting directly with the LA, with this finding being documented only with a diagram (authors' Fig. 3), not with a photograph.[118] Even in this diagram, the wall of the "IVC" looked remarkably thick and muscular, several times thicker than the transected walls of the aorta and of the main pulmonary artery in the authors' adjacent Figure 4. The wall of the transected "IVC" measures 1 to 4 mm in thickness (authors' Fig. 3), whereas the transected walls of the aorta and pulmonary artery (authors' Fig. 4) measure 1 mm and less than 1 mm in thickness, respectively. These observations suggested to us that the structure identified as the IVC by the authors was in fact not the IVC, because its wall was far too thick and it appeared muscular; the wall of the IVC was shown as four times as thick as the wall of the ascending aorta. We realized that it was highly improbable that the wall of the true IVC would be up to four times as thick as that of the ascending aorta.

Consequently, we wrote to the senior author, requested the heart specimen for reexamination, and in due time the heart specimen was kindly sent to us. In our consultation (C91-41) concerning this scientifically important case, we found that both the RA and the LA had been cut in a frontal (coronal) plane, but at a level too anteriorly (ventrally). Large segments of the posterior walls of the right and left atria were missing posteroinferiorly (Figs. 6.12 and 6.13). Consequently, no remnant of the IVC connecting with the RA could be found.

Nevertheless, a small eustachian valve of the IVC (a right venous valve remnant) and a left venous valve remnant with multiple fenestrations were readily identified within the RA, and were photographed (see Fig. 6.12). The presence of the eustachian valve and the left venous valve indicate that the IVC connected normally with the RA between the eustachian valve to the right and the left venous valve to the left (see Fig. 6.12).

The orifices of the right and left pulmonary veins could be recognized in the posterosuperior wall of the LA (see Fig. 6.13), indicating that the pulmonary veins connected normally with the LA.

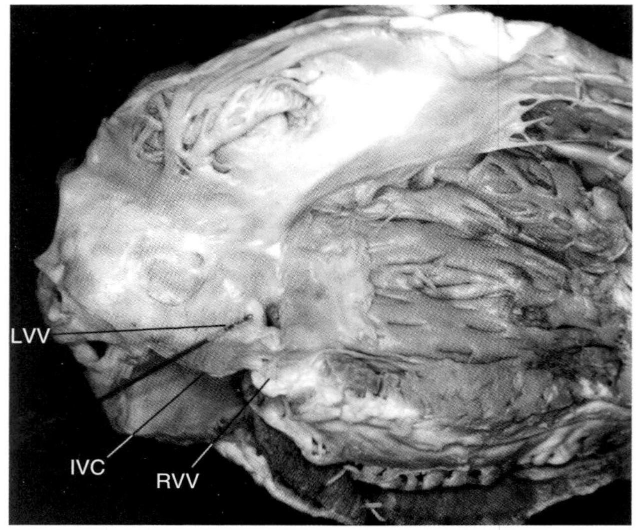

Fig. 6.12 The case of Gardner and Cole,[119] published in 1955 as a case in which the inferior vena cava *(IVC)* was thought to connect directly with the left atrium. This photograph shows the opened right atrium, tricuspid valve, and right ventricular inflow tract. We think that the thin-walled IVC connected directly with this right atrium, between the remnant of the right venous valve *(RVV),* known as the eustachian valve to the right, and the left venous valve *(LVV)* to the left. The ostium of the coronary sinus (unlabeled) lies anterior and superior to the RVV and the LVV. The atrial and ventricular septa are intact. (Reproduced with permission from Geva T, Van Praagh S, Gardner DL, Cole L. Long survival with inferior vena cava draining into left atrium. *Br Heart J.* 1955;17:93.)

The posteroinferior wall of the LA was missing, due to a postmortem artifact that may well have been produced when the heart was removed from the chest by the prosector. As indicated previously, it appears as though the incision was made too far anterosuperiorly, above the level of the IVC, with removal of a portion of the posteroinferior walls of both atria. The defect in the left atrial wall was approximated by a stitch posteroinferiorly, which inadvertently changed this defect into an apparently oval orifice (see Fig. 6.13) that was subsequently thought to represent the orifice of the IVC.

Reexamination also revealed that the margins of this putative IVC were not composed of thin venous tissue consistent with the wall of the IVC. Instead, this wall consisted of an inner 1-mm-thick layer of whitish fibrous tissue representing the left atrial endocardium, and an outer 3-mm-thick layer of left atrial myocardium; hence, the wall of this "IVC" had a total thickness of 4 mm (see Fig. 6.13). Also, right or left venous valve remnants were not found within the LA, only within the RA (see Fig. 6.12).

But why, then, was this famous patient cyanotic and clubbed? If her IVC had not connected with her LA and the atrial septum was intact, grasping at straws we speculated whether this was a case of pulmonary arteriovenous malformations. Subsequently, the paraffin blocks were found (approximately 40 years later!), recuts were made, and the histologic slides were kindly sent to us and examined by Professor Lynne M. Reid, an internationally known authority on the pulmonary vasculature.

Her report read, in part, "The preacinar arteries give the impression of being dilated. In the alveolar region, in addition

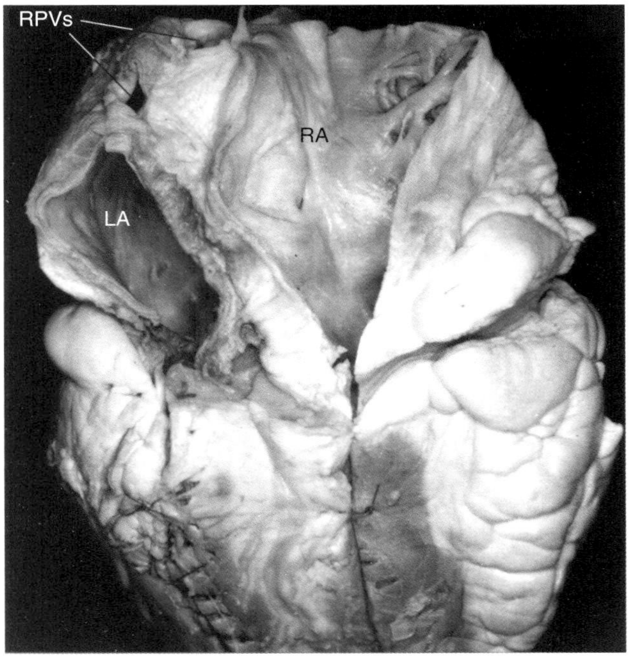

Fig. 6.13 Posteroinferior view of the case of Gardner and Cole[119] showing the opened right atrium *(RA)* and left atrium *(LA)*. The right pulmonary veins *(RPVs)* can be seen connecting normally with the LA. This large opening in the posteroinferior wall of the LA was interpreted as the site of connection of the IVC with the LA.[118] However, the wall of this "IVC" was 4 mm thick: a whitish internal layer 1 mm thick (the endocardium of the LA); and an outer muscular layer 3 mm thick (the myocardium of the LA wall). This wall is not thin and venous, as the wall of the IVC would be. Also, no right or left venous valve remnants were found within the LA, only within the RA (see Fig. 6.7). *Conclusion:* The opening into the LA is the transected LA free wall, not the IVC. Instead, the IVC connected with the RA normally, as the eustachian valve of the IVC (RVV) and the left venous valve (LVV) indicate (see Fig. 6.9). For other important details, please see text. (Reproduced with permission from Geva T, Van Praagh S, Gardner DL, Cole L. Long survival with inferior vena cava draining into left atrium. *Br Heart J.* 1955;17:93.)

to diffuse congestion, the sections show numerous small, dilated vessels, and near the pleura these are sometimes in several layers. The appearance is suggestive of numerous small AV fistulae and consistent with the clinical features. We cannot of course be certain from such an examination, but one can at least say 'suggestive.'"

Professor Donald Heath agreed entirely that there were no signs of pulmonary vascular obstructive disease with pulmonary hypertension. As was pointed out by Professor Dugald L. Gardner, the senior author of this famous case report, "Dr. Reid's observations of the numerous dilated pre-acinar arteries and veins agree very closely with the findings that Dr. Frank Carey and I made originally."

Professor Gardner also helped reconstruct this case in a letter to Dr. Stella Van Praagh on June 16, 1993, that said, in part,

The answers to your questions are as follows:

1. *The case was brought to my attention as a Coroner's autopsy. I can only surmise that the case was brought to Dr. Cole's attention by a General Practitioner, since Dr. Cole was the senior cardiologist to the Addenbrooks Hospital, Cambridge in the years 1953/54.*
2. *Forty years is a long time over which to cast one's memory, but I am reasonably certain that, recognizing that there was a cardiac anomaly, the heart was fixed in formalin by packing the chambers with cotton wool immersed in this fluid. By that time, of course, the heart had been excised and the autopsy report submitted to the Coroner. There was no opportunity of going back to repeat the anatomical investigation and no anomaly of the great vessels was recognized during the autopsy.*

So, with the very kind and generous assistance of Professor Dugald Gardner, we think that this half-century old mystery is solved. Everyone assumed that the patient must have had some form of cyanotic congenital heart disease; hence, the heart specimen was sent to Professor Gardner. But the prosector in this Coroner's case (of sudden and unexpected death) artifacted the posteroinferior atrial walls during removal of the heart, well before Gardner and Cole saw the heart specimen.

We would like to thank Professor Gardner and his colleagues for their kindness and generosity. Without their help, the foregoing reappraisal would not have been possible. Professor Gardner favored publication of this reassessment, to set the scientific record straight. Consequently, photographs of the heart specimen of Gardner and Cole,[119] that I took in 1991, were included in a subsequent publication by T. Geva and S. Van Praagh.[116]

Other astute observers such as Drs. Russell V. Lucas, Jr. and Kimberly A. Krabill[120] have recently stated: "In the absence of situs abnormalities, entrance of a right-sided IVC into the LA is not possible from an embryologic point of view."

We agree, and might add the following: *direct connection* of the IVC with the LA does not occur, to the best of our present knowledge. However, *drainage* of the IVC blood stream into the LA can occur in two different situations (which Lucas and Krabill[120] understand):

1. A prominent eustachian valve of the IVC can baffle IVC blood into the LA via a patent foramen ovale, or via a secundum ASD with deficiency of septum primum.
2. Rarely, the IVC can connect with the left horn of the sinus venosus (the coronary sinus); if the coronary sinus is unroofed, the IVC blood stream drains into the LA, even though the IVC connects with the sinus venosus. If the coronary sinus is not unroofed (no coronary sinus septal defect), the IVC blood drains normally into the RA, as is well shown angiocardiographically in a patient of Dr. Luis E. Alday, pediatric cardiologist of Cordoba, Argentina.

Does the foregoing account include all the systemic venous anomalies that exist? The answer is no. There are other rare and fascinating malformations that we have not seen pathologically but merit mention.

Is it possible to have two, complete, uninterrupted IVCs? Accurately speaking, we think that the answer is no, in the sense that the *true* IVC seems always to be unilateral, apparently because the essence of the IVC (that is absent in interrupted IVC); that is, the new anastomotic pathway from the intersubcardinal anastomosis to the vitelline veins that become the hepatic sinusoids and the hepatic segment of the IVC seems always to be unilateral, to the best of our present knowledge. It will be recalled that the IVC is normally derived, from below upward, from the following five components: (1) the posterior cardinal veins; (2) the supracardinal veins; (3) the subcardinal veins; (4) the anastomotic pathway or mesenteric component of the IVC; and (5) the vitelline veins (hepatic sinusoids). So, when we speak of the *true* IVC, we mean a vein derived from the previously mentioned five venous systems.

However, Dr. Stephen Sanders and Dr. John Murphy, when they were working at the Aldo Castañeda Institute of the Clinique de Genolier in Switzerland, encountered a patient who did indeed have what appeared to be two complete uninterrupted IVCs, based on documentation by cardiac catheterization, angiocardiography, and two-dimensional echocardiography (personal communication, circa 1996). Drs. Russell Lucas and Kimberly Krabill[120] have documented pathologically a case of **double IVC** entering the RA (their Figure 60.17).

The question then becomes, How can one understand double IVC developmentally? We think that Lucas and Kraybill's diagrams (Figs. 6.14 and 6.15) help make this very rare anomaly comprehensible embryologically. Fig. 6.14 reviews key features of normal venoatrial development, and Fig. 6.15 shows what is thought to happen with **anomalous termination of the left or right umbilical vein and absence of the ductus venosus.**

Initially, the left and right umbilical veins connect with the left and right common cardinal veins, outside the liver, at 4 weeks of age. However, by 5½ weeks, the extrahepatic portions of both umbilical veins have involuted, the umbilical veins now being incorporated into the enlarging liver along with the vitelline (yolk sac) veins. The combined umbilical and vitelline veins are then known as the omphalomesenteric veins, because the umbilical veins travel via the umbilicus (*omphalos* = umbilicus, Greek) and the vitelline (yolk sac) veins become the mesenteric veins. This stage of the normal atrophy of the cephalic extrahepatic portions of the left and right umbilical veins is well shown in Fig. 6.14D. Note also that the ductus venosus is rapidly enlarging beneath the liver, that the ductus venosus is essentially a direct extension of the large caudal portion of the left umbilical vein, and that the left umbilical vein and ductus venosus are flowing rightward and posteriorly toward the right vitelline vein and the right horn of the sinus venosus and thence to the RA.

But what happens if the ductus venosus fails to form? Fig. 6.15 answers this question. The cephalic portion of the left umbilical vein enlarges, instead of undergoing atrophy, and may connect with the left horn of the sinus venosus (the coronary sinus) either via the original extrahepatic route (see Fig. 6.15A) or the somewhat later intrahepatic route (see Fig. 6.15B). Alternatively, the right umbilical vein may persist and enlarge, connecting with the right horn of the sinus venosus (the venous component of the RA) (see Fig. 6.15C) or with the IVC (see Fig. 6.15D).

You may be thinking, "Fine. But that still does not explain double IVC." We would agree. The last step in the puzzle involves an anomalous connection of right or left umbilical vein with the right or left iliac vein, respectively (Fig. 6.16B). We hypothesize that the left umbilical vein connects anomalously with the left common iliac vein, which is part of the posterior cardinal venous system. This anomalous connection of the left umbilical vein results in enlargement of the left posterior cardinal vein (instead of the normal involution). Consequently, this anomalous left umbilical vein plus left posterior cardinal extension courses cephalically, passing either outside or inside the left lobe of the liver (see Fig. 6.15A or B, respectively), then connecting with the coronary sinus and flowing into the RA if the coronary sinus septum is intact or draining into the LA if there is a coronary sinus septal defect (unroofed coronary sinus), as in the patient of Drs. Stephen Sanders and John Murphy. The latter patient also has the heterotaxy syndrome, with uncertain splenic status.

Thus, we approve of the diagnosis of double IVCs, with the understanding that this anomaly consists of a normal true IVC plus an abnormal vena cava consisting of an anomalous left umbilical vein, with left posterior cardinal venous extension, plus absence of the ductus venosus, with or without unroofing of the coronary sinus. There may ultimately prove to be other anatomic types of double IVC.

Hence, we conclude that double IVC consists of one normal (true) IVC and one anomalous IVC-like vessel. **Absence of the ductus venosus may well be the fundamental anomaly in double IVC** (see **Fig. 6.15**).[120]

Persistence of the ductus venosus is another rare anomaly that we have not identified but that has been seen by others.[120] Postnatally patent ductus venosus allows portal venous blood to bypass the liver and shunt directly into the IVC. Patent ductus venosus can be associated with dysplasia of the portal vein branches.[120]

Congenital caput medusae—a venous plexus surrounding the umbilicus—has been observed in association with an anomalous right umbilical vein connecting with the RSVC (see Fig. 6.16A).

Caput Medusae means the head of Medusa (Latin). In Greek mythology, Medusa was the most famous of the three monstrous Gorgon sisters. Once a beautiful woman, Medusa offended Athena, who changed her hair into snakes and made her face so hideous that all who looked at her were turned to stone.

In medicine, caput medusae means dilatation and stasis of the periumbilical veins, seen mainly in newborns and in patients with cirrhosis of the liver. In the patient diagrammed in Fig. 6.16A, again the ductus venosus was absent. Whether this anomalous right umbilical vein was stenotic at its connection with the RSVC was not addressed.[120]

Right umbilical vein connecting with the right portal vein is diagrammed in Fig. 6.16C.[120] The marked dilatation of the anomalous right umbilical vein and of both the right and left

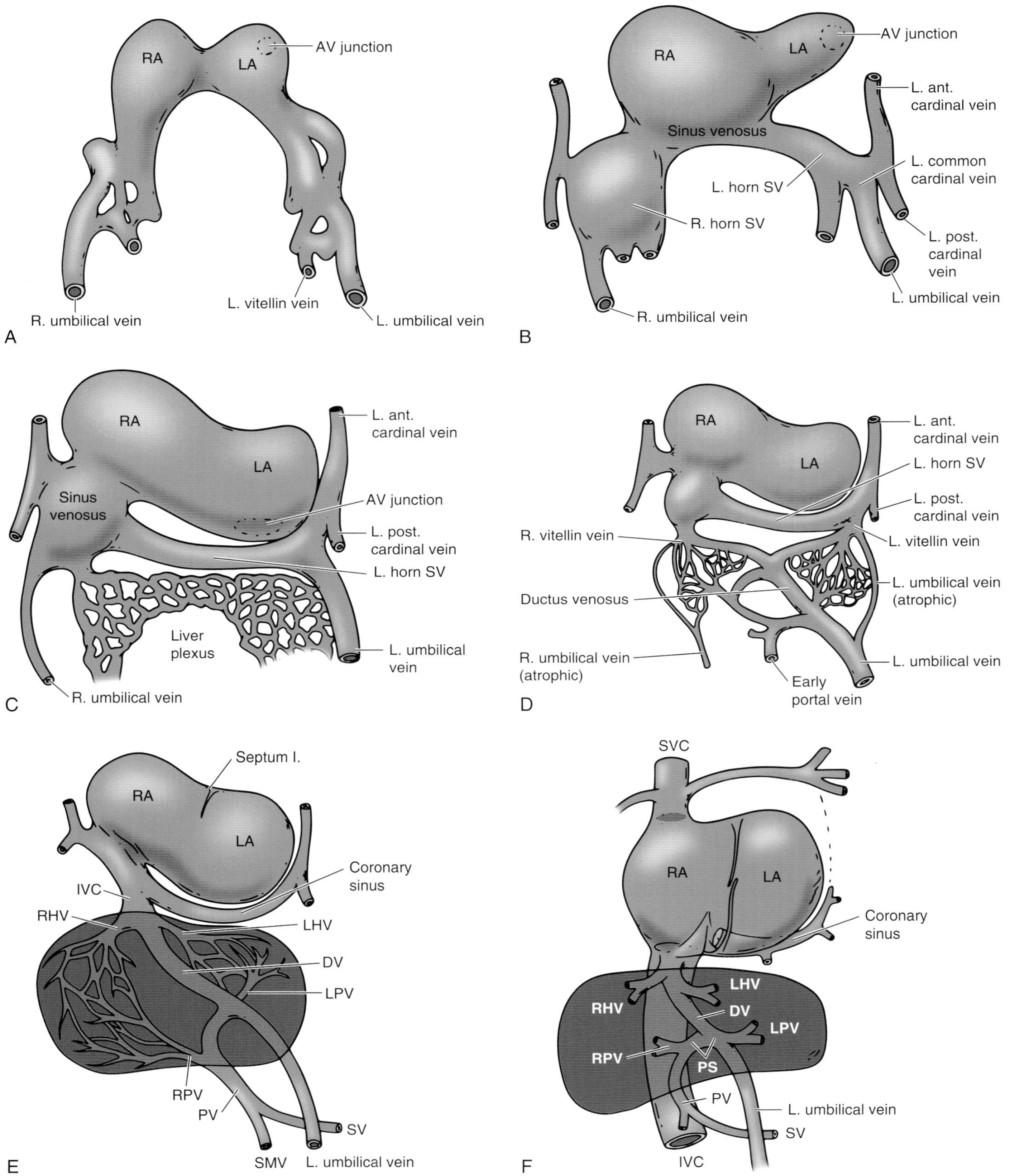
RA
LA
AV junction
R. umbilical vein
L. vitellin vein
L. umbilical vein
A
RA
LA
AV junction
L. ant. cardinal vein
Sinus venosus
L. common cardinal vein
L. horn SV
R. horn SV
L. post. cardinal vein
L. umbilical vein
R. umbilical vein
B
RA
LA
L. ant. cardinal vein
Sinus venosus
AV junction
L. post. cardinal vein
L. horn SV
Liver plexus
L. umbilical vein
R. umbilical vein
C
RA
LA
L. ant. cardinal vein
L. horn SV
L. post. cardinal vein
R. vitellin vein
L. vitellin vein
Ductus venosus
L. umbilical vein (atrophic)
R. umbilical vein (atrophic)
L. umbilical vein
Early portal vein
D
Septum I.
RA
LA
Coronary sinus
IVC
RHV
LHV
DV
LPV
RPV
PV
SV
SMV
L. umbilical vein
E
SVC
RA
LA
Coronary sinus
LHV
RHV
DV
LPV
RPV
PS
PV
L. umbilical vein
SV
IVC
F

Continued

Fig. 6.14 Embryology of the Systemic Veins. (A) In the 4 mm (3.6 week) human embryo, the right umbilical vein *(R. Umbilical V.)* and the left umbilical vein *(L. Umbilical V.)* are lateral to the right vitelline vein (unlabeled) and the left vitelline vein *(L. Vitelline V.)*, respectively. The umbilical veins are the first to appear in the human embryo. They flow from the placenta via the umbilical cord and pass through the umbilicus (*omphalikos* = umbilicus, Greek). The right and left umbilical veins then flow symmetrically, outside the liver, into the right and left common cardinal veins (see Fig. 6.5A). The vitelline veins originate more medially, in the wall of the yolk sac (*vitellus* = yolk, Latin) (see Fig. 6.5G). Slightly later in development, the lateral umbilical veins and the medial vitelline veins become confluent. They are then known as the omphalomesenteric veins, *omphalo* indicating that these veins are formed partly from the umbilical veins, and *mesenteric* denoting that these veins are formed partly from the vitelline veins that are midgut veins traveling via the mesentery. The umbilical and vitelline veins flow into the ipsilateral common cardinal veins (unlabeled), which in turn join the developing morphologically right atrium *(RA)* on the right side and developing morphologically left atrium *(LA)* on the left side. The atrioventricular *(AV)* junction exits from the LA in a superior (cephalad) direction, where it opens into the ventricle (future morphologically left ventricle) of the bulboventricular D-loop (not shown). (B) By the 4.5-mm stage (3.8 weeks) in the human embryo, asymmetry is appearing. The right horn of the sinus venosus *(R. Horn SV)* is becoming bigger than the left horn of the sinus venosus *(L. Horn SV)*. The right and left common cardinal veins, also known as the ducts of Cuvier, are important components of each sinus horn. The left anterior cardinal vein *(L. Ant. Cardinal V.)* and the left posterior cardinal vein *(L. Post. Cardinal V.)* flow into each other, forming the left common cardinal vein *(L. Common Cardinal V.)*. The same process is also occurring on the right side (unlabeled). Also flowing into each sinus horn is the umbilical vein laterally and the vitelline vein medially. Blood flow in the left umbilical vein is becoming greater than in the right umbilical vein; hence, the left umbilical vein is enlarging, while the right umbilical vein is beginning to atrophy. An indentation is appearing between the LA and the left sinus horn that will soon separate these two structures. The right and left vitelline veins have begun their evolution into hepatic sinusoids (not shown). (C) In the 5-mm (4 week) human embryo, the left umbilical vein is distinctly larger than the right umbilical vein, the left horn of the sinus venosus is now completely separated from the LA, and the sinus venosus now opens into the RA only. (D) In the 6-mm (4.5 week) human embryo, the left umbilical vein is large, whereas the right umbilical vein is atrophic. Both umbilical veins have now established communications with the vitelline veins forming the hepatic sinusoids, and the extrahepatic communications of the left and right umbilical veins with the left and right horns of the sinus venosus have normally become atrophic. The large left umbilical vein (postnatally the ligamentum teres or round ligament) travels in the inferior rim of the falciform ligament, passes to the left of the quadrate lobe of the liver and flows into the left portal vein *(LPV)*, that has just appeared. This large venous channel from the placenta then continues posteriorly to the left of the caudate lobe of the liver. Posteriorly or dorsal to the LPV, this venous extension of the left umbilical vein is known as the ductus venosus (*DV*, venous duct); postnatally, this vein normally becomes the ligamentum venosum (venous ligament). The DV flows posteriorly to the left of the caudate lobe of the liver, and then it wraps itself around the posterior surface of the caudate lobe and passes rightward to connect with the inferior vena cava, and thence to the RA. Hence, the large left umbilical vein flows posteriorly and rightward, through the LPV and via the DV to the right vitelline veins, the suprahepatic segment of the inferior vena cava *(IVC)*, the sinus venosus, and the RA. En route, the left umbilical vein and its DV extension communicate not only with the LPV but also with the left and right vitelline veins. (E) In the 9-mm (5.2 week) human embryo, the extrahepatic right umbilical vein normally has completely involuted, as has the extrahepatic portion of the left umbilical vein. The portal venous system has now formed. The splenic vein *(SV)*, the superior mesenteric vein *(SMV)*, and the inferior mesenteric vein (not shown) become confluent to form the PV, which then branches into the right portal vein *(RPV)* and the LPV. The left umbilical vein and its posterior (dorsal) extension, the DV flow through (or anastomose with) the LPV. The distal portion of the hepatic sinusoids form the right hepatic veins *(RHV)* and the left hepatic veins *(LHV)*, which then flow into the suprahepatic segment of the IVC, adjacent to the connection of the DV. Note that the retrohepatic and infrahepatic segments of the IVC have not formed as yet. (F) Just before birth, the RPV and LPV are supplied both by the left umbilical vein and the PV. Shortly after birth, the left umbilical vein is interrupted and its extension, the DV, closes adjacent to the IVC. Normally, the LPV and the hepatic veins remain widely patent. The retrohepatic and infrahepatic segments of the IVC have formed, and the left anterior (superior) cardinal vein normally undergoes involution, forming the ligament of Marshall. The left horn of the sinus venosus is normally represented only by the coronary sinus (Cor. Sin.). *PS*, Portal sinus. (Reproduced with permission from Lucas RV, Krabill KA. Abnormal systemic venous connections. In: Emmanouilides GC, Riemenschneider TA, Allen HD, Gutgesell HP, eds. *Moss and Adams Heart Disease in Infants, Children, and Adolescents, Including the Fetus and Young Adult*. 5th ed. Baltimore, MD: Williams & Wilkins; 1995:899.)

portal venous branches to about three times their normal size was associated with obstruction due to absence of the ductus venosus and hence no direct pathway of the right umbilical venous blood to the RA.

The status of the ductus venosus should be diagnosed carefully and specifically. Absence of the ductus venosus may be associated with anomalous left and right umbilical veins and with double IVCs.

The references of this chapter merit mention in several respects:

1. They are organized chronologically, so that the interested reader can follow the growth and development of the understanding of any of these topics.
2. References 7 to 86 are concerned mainly with anomalies of the SVC.
3. References 87 to 97, and 118 to 137 focus mainly on malformations of the IVC.
4. References 98 to 105 are concerned primarily with anomalies of the coronary sinus.
5. The reader is urged to consider the references with care because the literature is an inexhaustible gold mine of information, containing data that we ourselves have not seen or literature that in the interests of brevity we have not commented on previously[121-139]; for example:
   a. umbilical vein entering the RA,[122]
   b. membranous obstruction of the suprahepatic segment of the IVC and its treatment,[124-126,129,134-137]
   c. hepatic veno-occlusive disease in a newborn infant of a woman drinking herbal tea,[131]
   d. cor triatriatum dexter, that is, an obstructive right leaflet of the sinoatrial valve,[66,132] and
   e. Chiari network (remnants of right leaflet of sinoatrial valve) entrapping thromboemboli and acting like a congenital filter of the IVC.[134]

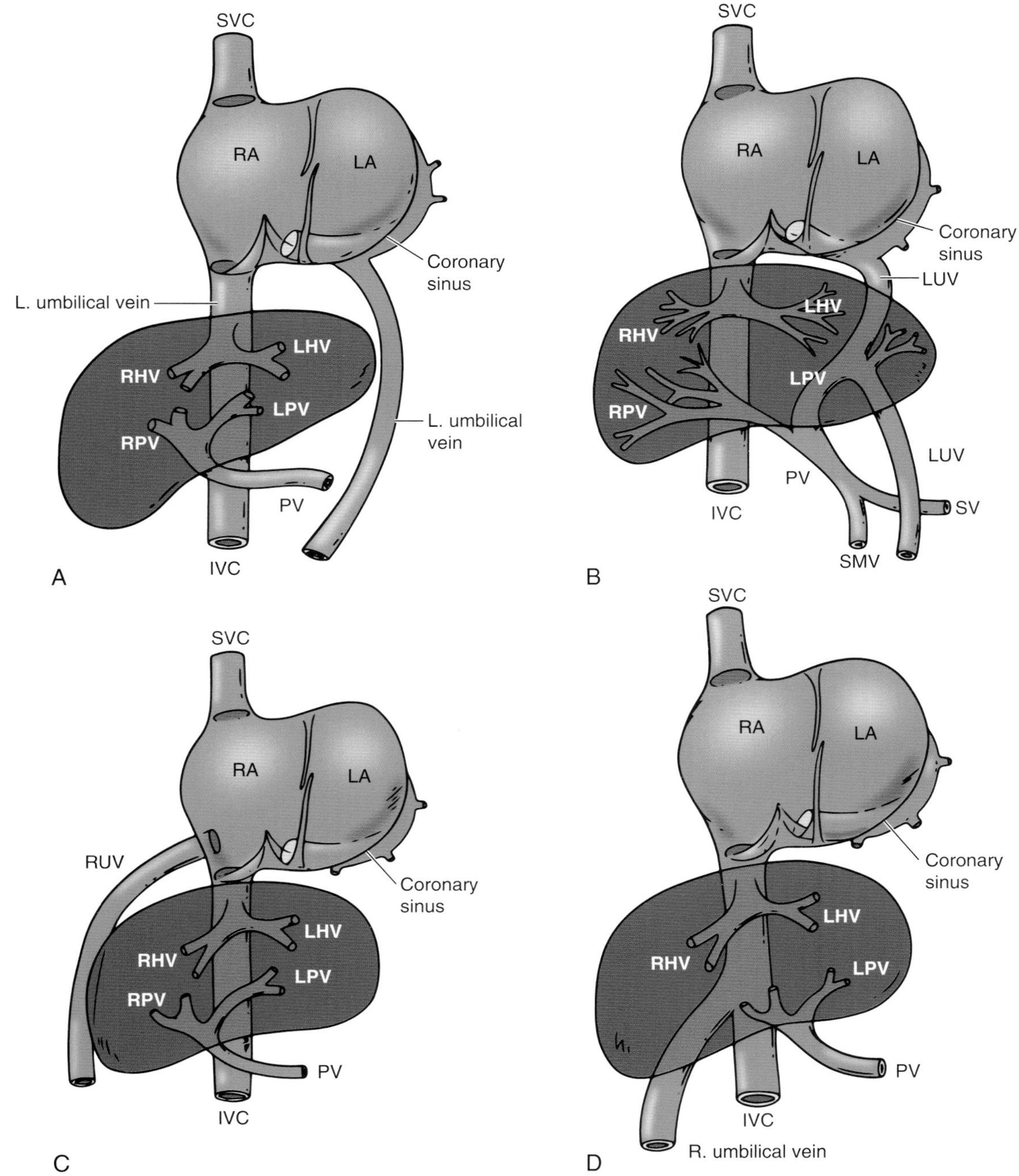

Fig. 6.15 Absence of the Ductus Venosus With Anomalous Termination of an Umbilical Vein. When the ductus venosus is absent, this may force the left umbilical vein *(LUV)* to terminate in the coronary sinus (A). This anomaly represents persistence of the normal stages shown in Fig. 6.11B–C (embryonic age of 4 weeks or slightly earlier). Or the LUV can terminate in the left portal vein *(LPV),* which is normal (B). However, when the ductus venosus is absent, this forces the LPV to remain a large vein, to pursue an intrahepatic course within the left lobe of the liver, and to anastomose with a large left-sided extrahepatic segment of the LUV, and thence to drain into the coronary sinus (B). Thus, when the ductus venosus is absent, the LUV can drain into the coronary sinus either by pursuing an entirely extrahepatic course (A), or a partially intrahepatic course (B). Similarly, when the ductus venosus is absent, the right umbilical vein *(RUV)* can pursue an entirely extrahepatic course, terminating in the sinus venosus component of the morphologically right atrium *(RA)* (C). This anomaly represents persistence of the normal stages shown in Figs. 6.11B–C (embryonic age of 4 weeks or slightly earlier). Or the right umbilical vein (R. Umb. V.) can pursue a partially intrahepatic, within or just below the right lobe of the liver, terminating in the inferior vena cava *(IVC)* (D). The anomalous left and right umbilical vein seem always to terminate in the left and right sides of the sinus venosus *(SV),* respectively; that is, their anomalous terminations appear always to be ipsilateral (never contralateral), apparently for embryologic reasons (see Fig. 6.11). *LA,* Left atrium; *LHV,* left hepatic vein; *PV,* pulmonary vein, *RHV,* right hepatic vein; *RPV,* right portal vein; *SVC,* superior vena cava. (Reproduced with permission from Lucas RV, Krabill KA. Abnormal systemic venous connections. In: Emmanouilides GC, Riemenschneider TA, Allen HD, Gutgesell HP, eds. *Moss and Adams Heart Disease in Infants, Children, and Adolescents, Including the Fetus and Young Adult.* 5th ed. Baltimore, MD: Williams & Wilkins; 1995:899.)

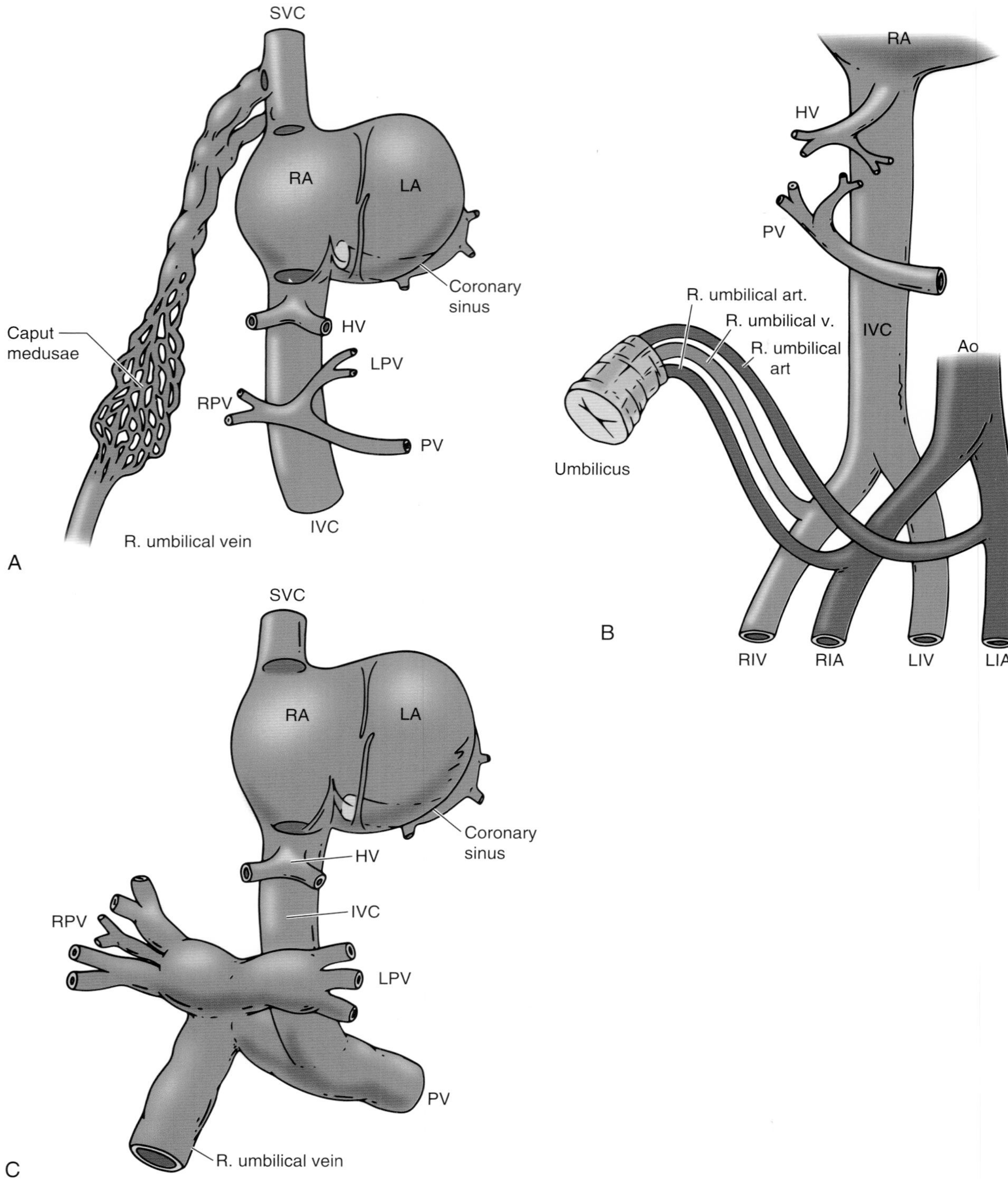

Fig. 6.16 When the ductus venosus is absent, other anomalous terminations of the right umbilical vein include the right superior vena cava *(SVC)* (A), the right iliac vein *(RIV)* (B), and the right portal vein (C). The anomaly shown in A represents termination of the right umbilical vein into the right anterior (superior) cardinal vein. Whether or not the periumbilical caput medusae was related to stenosis of the junction between the anomalous right umbilical vein and the SVC remains unknown. The malformation shown in B represents an anomalous termination of the right umbilical vein into the right posterior cardinal vein. The anomaly depicted in C is a mirror-image of normal development. Normally, the left umbilical vein becomes dominant and anastomoses with the left portal vein *(LPV),* as in Fig. 6.12E. Here, however, the right umbilical vein has become dominant and has anastomosed with the right portal vein *(RPV).* Absence of the ductus venosus is associated with dilatation of the RPV and LPV, respectively. Note that in all three of these diagrams, the portal vein *(PV)* has no dorsal extension, that is, no ductus venosus. The PV and its right and left branches resemble a diminutive main pulmonary artery with its right and left branches, but with no "patent ductus arteriosus" running dorsally (A–C). Absence of the ductus venosus is an important diagnosis that merits recognition. *Ao,* Aorta; *HV,* hepatic vein; *IVC,* inferior vena cava; *LA,* left atrium; *LIA,* left innominate artery; *LIV,* left innominate vein; *RA,* right atrium; *RIA,* right innominate artery. (Reproduced with permission from Lucas RV, Krabill KA. Abnormal systemic venous connections. In: Emmanouilides GC, Riemenschneider TA, Allen HD, Gutgesell HP, eds. *Moss and Adams Heart Disease in Infants, Children, and Adolescents, Including the Fetus and Young Adult.* 5th ed. Baltimore, MD: Williams & Wilkins; 1995:899.)

SUMMARY

In our cardiac pathology database, 13 different anomalies of the systemic veins were found (see Table 6.1):

1. persistent LSVC or RSVC, 415 of 3216 patients (12.9%);
2. interruption of the IVC (excluding the heterotaxy syndrome with polysplenia in 42 patients [1.31%]);
3. atresia or stenosis of the coronary sinus ostium in 20 patients (0.62%);
4. aneurysm of the sinus venosus in 10 cases (0.31%);
5. absence or atresia of the RSVC in 7 patients (0.22%);
6. absence of the left innominate vein in 5 patients (0.16%);
7. left innominate vein running anterior to the thymus in 3 cases (0.09%);
8. the Raghib syndrome in 2 patients (0.06%);
9. right SVC draining in part into the left atrium in 1 patient (0.03%);
10. retroaortic innominate vein in 1 patient (0.03%);
11. left-to-right switching of the IVC in 1 patient (0.03%);
12. umbilical vein connecting anomalously with the coronary sinus in 1 patient (0.03%); and
13. anomalous "portal vein" bypassing the liver and connecting anomalously with the azygos vein in 1 patient (0.03%).

The pathologic anatomic findings were correlated with diagnostic and surgical considerations. Some of the literature was reviewed and discussed. A relatively new understanding of sinus venosus defect was presented. Evidence was provided that supports the view that the IVC does not connect directly with the LA, but can drain anomalously into the LA in at least two different situations.

REFERENCES

1. Ivemark BI. Implications of agenesis of the spleen on the pathogenesis of conotruncus anomalies in childhood. *Acta Pediatr Scand*. 1955;44(suppl):1.
2. Sanders JM. Bilateral superior vena cava. *Anat Rec*. 1946;94:657.
3. Geissler W, Albert M. Persistierende linke obere hohlvene und mitralstenose. *Z Gesamte Inn Med*. 1956;11:865.
4. Raghib G, Ruttenberg HD, Anderson RC, Amplatz K, Adams Jr P, Edwards JE. Termination of left superior vena cava in left atrium, atrial septal defect, and absence of coronary sinus—a developmental complex. *Circulation*. 1965;31:906.
5. Patten BM. *Human Embryology*. 2nd ed. New York: McGraw-Hill Book Company, Inc; 1953:639.
6. Ruscazio M, Van Praagh S, Marrass AR, Catani G, Iliceto S, Van Praagh R. Interrupted inferior vena cava in asplenia syndrome and a review of the hereditary patterns of visceral situs abnormalities. *Am J Cardiol*. 1998;81:111.
7. Rastelli GC, Ongley PA, Kirklin JW. Surgical correction of common atrium with anomalously connected persistent left superior vena cava: report of a case. *Mayo Clin Proc*. 1965;40:528.
8. Miller GA, Ongley PA, Rastelli GC, Kirklin JW. Surgical correction of total anomalous systemic venous connection: report of a case. *Mayo Clin Proc*. 1965;40:532.
9. Meadows WR, Sharp JT. Persistent left superior vena cava draining into the left atrium without arterial oxygen unsaturation. *Am J Cardiol*. 1965;16:273.
10. Overy HR, Steinbicker PG, Blount SG. Anomalous systemic venous drainage with hypoplasia of the right ventricular myocardium. *Circulation*. 1966;33:613.
11. Gueron M, Hirsh M, Borman J. Total anomalous systemic venous drainage into the left atrium. Report of a case of successful surgical correction. *J Thorac Cardiovasc Surg*. 1969;58:570.
12. Kilman JW, Williams TE, Kakos GS, Molnar W, Ryan JM. Budd-Chiari syndrome due to congenital obstruction of the Eustachian valve of the inferior vena cava. *J Thorac Cardiovasc Surg*. 1971;62:226.
13. Jones RN, Niles NR. Spinnaker formation of sinus venosus valve. Case report of a fatal anomaly in a ten-year-old boy. *Circulation*. 1968;38:468.
14. van der Horst RL, Winship WS, Gotsman MS. Drainage of left hepatic vein into coronary sinus associated with other systemic venous anomalies. *Br Heart J*. 1971;33:164.
15. Franken EA. Idiopathic dilatation of the superior vena cava (superior vena cava dilatation). *Pediatrics*. 1972;49:297.
16. Ream CR, Giardina A. Congenital superior vena cava aneurysm caused by infectious mononucleosis. *Chest*. 1972;62:755.
17. Harris A, Gialafos J, Jefferson K. Transvenous pacing in presence of anomalous venous return to heart. *Br Heart J*. 1972;34:1189.
18. Freed MD, Rosenthal A, Bernhard WF. Balloon occlusion of a persistent left superior vena cava in the preoperative evaluation of systemic venous return. *J Thorac Cardiovasc Surg*. 1973;65:835.
19. Horowitz S, Esquivel J, Attie F, Lupi E, Espino-Vela J. Clinical diagnosis of persistent left superior vena cava by observation of jugular pulses. *Am Heart J*. 1973;86:759.
20. Farr JE, Anderson WT, Brundage BH. Congenital aneurysm of the superior vena cava. *Chest*. 1974;65:566.
21. Rose AG, Beckman CB, Edwards JE. Communication between coronary sinus and left atrium. *Br Heart J*. 1974;36:182.
22. DeLeval MR, Ritter DG, McGoon DC, Danielson GK. Anomalous systemic venous connection, surgical considerations. *Mayo Clin Proc*. 1975;50:599.
23. Crenshaw R, Okies JE, Phillips SJ, Bonchek LI, Starr A. Partial anomalous systemic venous return, report of surgical treatment in two cases. *J Thorac Cardiovasc Surg*. 1975;69:433.
24. James TN, Marshall TK, Edwards JE. De subitaneis mortibus. XX. Cardiac electrical instability in the presence of a left superior vena cava. *Circulation*. 1976;54:689.
25. Ezekowitz MD, Alderson PO, Bulkley BH, et al. Isolated drainage of the superior vena cava into the left atrium in a 52-year-old man, a rare congenital malformation in the adult presenting with cyanosis, polycythemia, and an unsuccessful lung scan. *Circulation*. 1978;58:751.
26. Snider AR, Ports TA, Silverman NH. Venous anomalies of the coronary sinus: detection by M-mode, two-dimensional and contrast echocardiography. *Circulation*. 1979;60:721.
27. Foster ED, Baeza OR, Farina MF, Shaher RM. Atrial septal defect associated with drainage of left superior vena cava to left atrium and absence of the coronary sinus. *J Thorac Cardiovasc Surg*. 1978;76:718.

28. Vázquez-Pérez J, Frontera-Izquierdo P. Anomalous drainage of the right superior vena cava into the left atrium as an isolated anomaly. Rare case report. *Am Heart J.* 1979;97:89.
29. Lozsádi LK. A morphogenetic consideration of congenital malformation of the coronary sinus. *Magyar Pediat.* 1978;12(suppl 4):30.
30. Blieden LC, Deutsch V, Neufeld HN. Unusual forms of interatrial communication and of systemic venous communication with the atria. *Magyar Pediat.* 1978;12(suppl 4):16.
31. Zuberbuhler JR, Shinebourne EA. Diagnosis and treatment of left atrial to left superior vena caval shunt. *Magyar Pediat.* 1978;12(suppl 4):12.
32. Dupuis C, Frontera P, Pernot C, Vasquez-Perez J, Verney R. Anomalous drainage of the superior vena cava into the left atrium as an isolated anomaly. French-Spanish cooperative study of six cases. *Magyar Pediat.* 1978;12(suppl 4):11.
33. Ott DA, Cooley DA, Angelini P, Leachman RD. Successful surgical correction of symptomatic cor triatriatum dexter. *J Thorac Cardiovasc Surg.* 1979;78:573.
34. Konstam MA, Levine BW, Strauss HW, McKusick KA. Left superior vena cava to left atrial communication diagnosed with radionuclide angiocardiography and with differential right to left shunting. *Am J Cardiol.* 1979;43:149.
35. Battle-Diaz J, Stanley P, Kratz C, Fouron JC, Guérin R, Davignon A. Echocardiographic manifestations of persistence of the right sinus venosus valve. *Am J Cardiol.* 1979;43:850.
36. Foale RA, Baron DW, Richards AF. Isolated congenital absence of coronary sinus. *Br Heart J.* 1979;42:355.
37. Lenox CC, Zuberbuhler JR, Park SC, et al. Absent right superior vena cava with persistent left superior vena cava: implications and management. *Am J Cardiol.* 1980;45:117.
38. Modry DL, Hidvegi RS, LaFleche LR. Congenital saccular aneurysm of the superior vena cava. *Ann Thorac Surg.* 1980;29:258.
39. Shapiro EP, Al-Sadir J, Campbell NPS, Thilenius OG, Anagnostopoulos CE, Hays P. Drainage of right superior vena cava into both atria. Review of the literature and description of a case presenting with polycythemia and paradoxical embolization. *Circulation.* 1981;63:712.
40. Alpert BS, Rao PS, Moore HV, Covitz W. Surgical correction of anomalous right superior vena cava to the left atrium. *J Thorac Cardiovasc Surg.* 1981;82:301.
41. Laslett LJ, Ikeda RM, Mason DT. Female adolescent Buerger's disease: objective documentation and therapeutic remission. *Am Heart J.* 1981;102:452.
42. Huhta JC, Smallhorn JF, Macartney FJ, Anderson RH, de Leval M. Cross-sectional echocardiographic diagnosis of systemic venous return. *Br Heart J.* 1982;48:388.
43. Freedom RM, Schaffer MS, Rowe RD. Anomalous low insertion of right superior vena cava. *Br Heart J.* 1982;48:601.
44. Park HM, Summerer MH, Preuss K, Armstrong WF, Mahomed Y, Hamilton DJ. Anomalous drainage of the right superior vena cava into the left atrium. *J Am Coll Cardiol.* 1983;2:358.
45. Yeager SB, Chin AJ, Sanders SP. Subxiphoid two-dimensional echocardiographic diagnosis of coronary sinus septal defects. *Am J Cardiol.* 1984;54:686.
46. Bharati S, Lev M. Direct entry of the right superior vena cava into the left atrium with aneurysmal dilatation and stenosis at its entry into the right atrium with stenosis of the pulmonary veins: a rare case. *Pediatr Cardiol.* 1984;5:123.
47. Russel GA, Stovin PGI. Coronary sinus type atrial septal defect in a child with pulmonary atresia and Ebstein's anomaly. *Br Heart J.* 1985;53:465.
48. Smallhorn JF, Zielinsky P, Freedom RM, Rowe RD. Abnormal position of the brachiocephalic vein. *Am J Cardiol.* 1985;55:234.
49. Schick EC, Lekakis J, Rothendler JA, Ryan TJ. Persistent left superior vena cava and right superior vena cava drainage into the left atrium without arterial hypoxemia. *J Am Coll Cardiol.* 1985;5:374.
50. Cabrera A, Martinez P, Del Campo A. Intrapericardial haematic cyst, a rare form of left superior vena cava atresia. *Br Heart J.* 1984;52:352.
51. Stanford W, Doty DB. The role of venography in the management of patients with superior vena cava obstruction. *Ann Thorac Surg.* 1986;41:158.
52. Sand ME, McGrath LB, Pacifico AD, Mandke NV. Repair of left superior vena cava entering the left atrium. *Ann Thorac Surg.* 1986;42:560.
53. O'Callaghan WG, Colavita PG, Ellenbogen KA, Gilbert MR, German LD. Persistent left superior vena cava: localization of site of ectopic atrial pacemaker and associated atrioventricular accessory pathway. *Am Heart J.* 1986;111:1200.
54. Choi JY, Anderson RH, Macartney FJ. Absent right superior caval vein (vena cava) with normal atrial arrangement. *Br Heart J.* 1987;57:474.
55. Rumisek JD, Pigott JD, Weinberg PM, Norwood WI. Coronary sinus septal defect associated with tricuspid atresia. *J Thorac Cardiovasc Surg.* 1986;92:142.
56. Reinus WR, Gutierrez FR. Duplication of the inferior vena cava in thromboembolic disease. *Chest.* 1986;90:916.
57. DiSegni E, Siegal A, Katzenstein M. Congenital diverticulum of the heart arising from the coronary sinus. *Br Heart J.* 1986;56:380.
58. Petit A, Eicher JC, Louis P. Congenital diverticulum of the right atrium situated on the floor of the coronary sinus. *Br Heart J.* 1988;59:721.
59. Ascuitto RJ, Ross-Ascuitto NT, Kopf GS, et al. Persistent left superior vena cava causing subdivided left atrium: diagnosis, embryological implications, and surgical management. *Ann Thorac Surg.* 1987;44:546.
60. Llorente A, Martinez P, del Campo A, Chouza M, Agosti J. Differential diagnosis of intrapericardial mass identified as venous ectasia. *Texas Heart Inst J.* 1986;13:209.
61. Oguni H, Hantano T, Yamada T, et al. A case of absent right superior vena cava with persistent left superior vena cava: cross-sectional echocardiographic diagnosis. *Heart Ves.* 1985;1:239.
62. Looyenga DS, Lacina SJ, Gebuhr CJ, Stockinger FS. Persistent left superior vena cava communicating with the left atrium through a systemic-pulmonary venous malformation. *J Am Coll Cardiol.* 1986;8:621.
63. Akalin H, Uysalel A, Özyurda Ü, et al. The triad of persistent left superior vena cava connected to the coronary sinus, right superior vena cava draining into the left atrium, and atrial septal defect: report of a successful operation for a rare anomaly. *J Thorac Cardiovasc Surg.* 1987;94:151.
64. Ho SY, Russell G, Rowland E. Coronary venous aneurysms and accessory atrioventricular connections. *Br Heart J.* 1988;60:348.
65. Arsenian MA, Anderson RA. Anomalous venous connection of the superior vena cava to the left atrium. *Am J Cardiol.* 1988;62:989.
66. Imachi T, Arimitsu K, Minami M, Hayakawa M, Kawagucyi A. Cor triatriatum dexter with anomalous pulmonary venous drainage and sinus venosus atrial septal defect. *J Thorac Cardiovasc Surg.* 1988;95:734.

67. Choi JY, Jung MJ, Kim YH, Noh CI, Yun YS. Anomalous subaortic position of the brachiocephalic vein (innominate vein): an echocardiographic study. *Br Heart J.* 1990;64:385.
68. Wiles HB. Two cases of left superior vena cava draining directly to a left atrium with a normal coronary sinus. *Br Heart J.* 1991;65:158.
69. King RE, Plotnick GD. Isolated right superior vena cava into the left atrium detected by contrast echocardiography. *Am Heart J.* 1991;122:583.
70. Molina JE. Surgery for effort thrombosis of the subclavian vein. *J Thorac Cardiovasc Surg.* 1992;103:341.
71. Nazem A, Sell JE. Closed technique for repair of right superior vena cava draining to left atrium. *Ann Thorac Surg.* 1993;55:1568.
72. Raissi K, Meraji M, Sadeghi HM, Firoozabady SH. Case report of isolated and abnormal drainage of right superior vena cava into left atrium. *J Thorac Cardiovasc Surg.* 1994;108:387.
73. Chin AJ. Subcostal two-dimensional echocardiographic identification of right superior vena cava connecting to left atrium. *Am Heart J.* 1994;127:939.
74. Sai S, Yoshida I, Itoh Y, et al. Diverticulum of the superior vena cava. *Ann Thorac Surg.* 1994;58:889.
75. Mill MR, Wilcox BR, Detterbeck FC, Anderson RH. Anomalous course of the left brachiocephalic vein. *Ann Thorac Surg.* 1993;55:600.
76. Sunaga Y, Hayashi K, Okubo N, et al. Transesophageal echocardiographic diagnosis of coronary sinus type atrial septal defect. *Am Heart J.* 1992;124:1657.
77. Chin AJ, Murphy JD. Identification of coronary sinus septal defect (unroofed coronary sinus) by color Doppler echocardiography. *Am Heart J.* 1992;124:1655.
78. Cochrane AD, Marath A, Mee RBB. Can a dilated coronary sinus produce left ventricular inflow obstruction? An unrecognized entity? *Ann Thorac Surg.* 1994;58:1114.
79. Pathi V, Guererro R, MacArthur KJD, Jamieson MPG, Pollack JCS. Sinus venosus defect: single patch repair with caval enlargement. *Ann Thorac Surg.* 1995;59:1588.
80. Berstein HS, Moore P, Stanger P, Silverman NH. The levoatriocardinal vein: morphology and echocardiographic identification of the pulmonary-systemic connection. *J Am Coll Cardiol.* 1995;26:995.
81. Adatia I, Gittenberger-de Groot AC. Unroofed coronary sinus and coronary sinus orifice atresia. Implications for management of complex congenital heart disease. *J Am Coll Cardiol.* 1995;25:948.
82. Rusk RA, Bexton RS, McComb JM. Persistent left sided and absent right sided superior vena cava complicating permanent pacemaker insertion. *Heart.* 1996;75:413.
83. Komai H, Naito Y, Fujiwara K. Operative technique for persistent left superior vena cava draining into the left atrium. *Ann Thorac Surg.* 1996;62:1188.
84. Nü M, Matsuoka S, Mori K, Hayabuchi Y, Tatara K, Kuroda Y. Digital subtraction angiography, magnetic resonance imaging and echocardiographic findings in patients with an anomalous subaortic left brachiocephalic vein. *Cardiol Young.* 1997;7:172.
85. Reddy VM, McElhinney DB, Hanley FL. Correction of left superior vena cava draining to the left atrium using extracardiac techniques. *Ann Thorac Surg.* 1997;63:1800.
86. Bartram U, Van Praagh S, Levine JC, Hines M, Bensky AS, Van Praagh R. Absent right superior vena cava in visceroatrial situs solitus. *Am J Cardiol.* 1997;80:175.
87. Van der Horst RL, Gotsman MS. Abnormalities of atrial depolarization in infradiaphragmatic interruption of inferior vena cava. *Br Heart J.* 1972;34:295.
88. Roberts KD, Edwards JM, Astley R. Surgical correction of total anomalous systemic venous drainage. *J Thorac Cardiovasc Surg.* 1972;64:803.
89. Merrill WH, Pieroni DR, Freedom RM, Ho CS. Diagnosis of infrahepatic interruption of the inferior vena cava. *Hopkins Med J.* 1973;133:329.
90. Bernal-Ramirez M, Hatch HB, Bower PJ. Interruption of the inferior vena cava with azygos continuation. *Chest.* 1974;65:469.
91. Miller SW, Baker AR, Raffin TA, van Houten FX. Recurrent pulmonary emboli with duplication of the inferior vena cava. *New Engl J Med.* 1975;292:408.
92. Benrey J, Williams RL, Reul GJ. Hemiazygos continuation to coronary sinus with normal left innominate vein. Cardiovasc Diseases. *Bull Texas Heart Inst.* 1975;2:325.
93. O'Reilly RJ, Grollman JH. The lateral chest film as an unreliable indicator of azygos continuation of the inferior vena cava. *Circulation.* 1976;53:891.
94. Krayenbuhl CU, Lincoln JCR. Total anomalous systemic venous connection, common atrium, and partial atrioventricular canal, a case report of successful surgical correction. *J Thorac Cardiovasc Surg.* 1977;73:686.
95. Encarnacao AF, Leiria G, Lima M, Sampayo F. Angiography in interruption of inferior vena cava with azygos system continuation. *Magyar Pediat.* 1978;12(suppl 4):16.
96. Nedeljkovic V, Papic R, Tucakovic G, Kanjuh V, Mogic M. Infrahepatic interruption of inferior vena cava with azygos continuation. *Magyar Pediat.* 1978;12(suppl 4):17.
97. Ritter SB, Bierman FZ. Noninvasive diagnosis of interrupted inferior vena cava: gated pulsed Doppler application. *Am J Cardiol.* 1983;51:1796.
98. Falcone MW, Roberts WC. Atresia of the right atrial ostium of the coronary sinus unassociated with persistence of the left superior vena cava: a clinicopathologic study of four adult patients. *Am Heart J.* 1972;83:604.
99. Gerlis LM, Gibbs JL, Williams GL, Thomas GDH. Coronary sinus orifice atresia and persistent left superior vena cava. A report of two cases, one associated with atypical coronary artery thrombosis. *Br Heart J.* 1984;52:648.
100. Watson GH. Atresia of the coronary sinus orifice. *Pediatr Cardiol.* 1985;6:99.
101. Yeager SB, Balian AA, Gustafson RA, Neal WA. Angiographic diagnosis of coronary sinus ostium atresia. *Am J Cardiol.* 1985;56:996.
102. Yokota M, Kyoku I, Kitano M, et al. Atresia of the coronary sinus orifice. Fatal outcome after intraoperative division of the drainage left superior vena cava. *J Thorac Cardiovasc Surg.* 1989;98:30.
103. Fudemoto Y, Kobayashi T, Wakasugi S, Joh T, Fujimoto K, Toyama S. Atresia of the right coronary sinus orifice with persistent left superior vena cava diagnosed by coronary angiography. *Respir Circ.* 1976;24:625.
104. Gerlis LM, Davies MJ, Boyle R, Williams G, Scott H. Pre-excitation due to accessory sinoventricular connexions associated with coronary sinus aneurysms, a report of two cases. *Br Heart J.* 1985;53:314.
105. Ho SY, Gupta I, Anderson RH, Lendon M, Kerr I. Aneurysm of the coronary sinus. *Thorax.* 1983;38:686.
106. Ho SY, Russell G, Rowland E. Coronary venous aneurysms and accessory atrioventricular connections. *Br Heart J.* 1988;60:348.

107. Grant JCB. *An Atlas of Anatomy*. 6th ed. Baltimore: Williams & Wilkins Co, diagram; 1972:438.
108. Grant RT. Development of the coronary vessels in the rabbit. *Heart*. 1926;13:261.
109. Marshall J. On the development of the great anterior veins in man and remnants of foetal structures found in the adult, a comparative view of these great veins in the different mammalia, and an analysis of their occasional peculiarities in the human subject. *Phil Trans Roy Soc London*. 1850;140(133).
110. Grant RT. An unusual anomaly of the coronary vessels in the malformed heart of a child. *Heart*. 1926;13:273.
111. Grant RT, Regnier M. The comparative anatomy of the cardiac coronary vessels. *Heart*. 1926;13:285.
112. Minot CS. On a hitherto unrecognized form of blood circulation without capillaries in the organs of vertebrata. *Proc Boston Soc Nat History*. 1901;29:185.
113. Van Praagh S, Carrera ME, Sanders SP, Mayer JE, Van Praagh R. Sinus venosus defects: unroofing of the right pulmonary veins—anatomic and echocardiographic findings and surgical treatment. *Am Heart J*. 1994;128:365.
114. Van Praagh R, Corsini I. Cor triatriatum: pathologic anatomy and a consideration of morphogenesis based on 13 postmortem cases and a study of normal development of the pulmonary vein and atrial septum in 83 human embryos. *Am Heart J*. 1969;78:379.
115. Geva T, Van Praagh S. Anomalies of the pulmonary veins. In: Allen HD, Clark EB, Gutgesell HP, Driscoll DJ, eds. *Moss and Adams' Heart Disease in Infants, Children, and Adolescents, Including the Fetus and Young Adult*. 6th ed. Philadelphia: Lippincott Williams & Wilkins; 2001:736 (Chapter 35).
116. Geva T, Van Praagh S. Abnormal systemic venous connections. In: Allen HD, Clark EB, Gutgesell HP, Driscoll DJ, eds. *Moss and Adams' Heart Disease in Infants, Children, and Adolescents, Including the Fetus and Young Adult*. 6th ed. Philadelphia: Lippincott Williams & Wilkins; 2001:773 (Chapter 36).
117. Celoria GC, Patton RB. Congenital absence of the aortic arch. *Am Heart J*. 1959;58:407.
118. Cantrell JR, Haller JA, Ravitch MM. A syndrome of congenital defects involving the abdominal wall, sternum, diaphragm, pericardium, and heart. *Surg Gynecol Obstet*. 1958;107:602.
119. Gardner DL, Cole L. Long survival with inferior vena cava draining into left atrium. *Br Heart J*. 1955;17:93.
120. Lucas RV, Krabill KA. Abnormal systemic venous connections. In: Emmanouilides GC, Riemenschneider TA, Allen HD, Gutgesell HP, eds. *Moss and Adams Heart Disease in Infants, Children, and Adolescents, Including the Fetus and Young Adult*. 5th ed. Baltimore: Williams & Wilkins; 1995:899.
121. Gantam HP. Left atrial inferior vena cava with atrial septal defect. *J Thorac Cardiovasc Surg*. 1968;55:827.
122. Monie IW. Umbilical vein entering the right atrium: comments on a previously reported human case. *Teratology*. 1971;4:461.
123. Singh A, Doyle EF, Danilowicz D, Spencer FC. Masked abnormal drainage of the inferior vena cava into the left atrium. *Am J Cardiol*. 1976;38:261.
124. Riggs T, Hirschfeld S, Borkat G, Liebman J. Inferior vena cava obstruction secondary to indwelling venous catheters: two cases. *Pediatrics*. 1976;58:446.
125. Taneja A, Mitra SK, Moghe PD, Rao PN, Samanta N, Kumar L. Budd-Chiari syndrome in childhood secondary to inferior vena caval obstruction. *Pediatrics*. 1979;63:808.
126. Frinpong-Boateng K, Luhmer I, Walterbusch G, Oelert H. Congenital obliteration of the suprahepatic inferior vena cava. *J Thorac Cardiovasc Surg*. 1982;84:110.
127. Amodeo A, DiDonato R, Dessanti A, et al. Relief of membranous obstruction of the inferior vena cava in a 5-year-old child. *J Thorac Cardiovasc Surg*. 1986;92:1101.
128. Sanchez HE, Human DG. Drainage of the inferior vena cava to the left atrium. *Pediatr Cardio*. 1986;16:207.
129. Van Praagh R, Van Praagh S. Does connection of the IVC with the LA exist? *Pediatr Cardiol*. 1987;8:151.
130. Murphy JP, Gregoric I, Cooley DA. Budd-Chiari syndrome resulting from a membranous web of the inferior vena cava: operative repair using profound hypothermia and circulatory arrest. *Ann Thorac Surg*. 1987;43:212.
131. Roulet M, Laurini R, Rivier L, Calame A. Hepatic veno-occlusive disease in a newborn infant of a woman drinking herbal tea. *J Pediatr*. 1988;112:433.
132. Alboliras ET, Edwards WD, Driscoll DJ, Seward JB. Cor triatriatum dexter: two-dimensional echocardiographic diagnosis. *J Am Coll Cardiol*. 1987;9:334.
133. Chang C-H, Lee M-C, Shieh MJ, Chang J-P, Lin PJ. Transatrial membranotomy for Budd-Chiari syndrome. *Ann Thorac Surg*. 1989;48:409.
134. Goedde TA, Conetta D, Rumisek JD. Chiari network entrapment of thromboemboli: congenital inferior vena cava filter. *Ann Thorac Surg*. 1990;49:317.
135. Chan P, Lee C-P, Lee YH. Complete membranous obstruction of the inferior vena cava treated successfully by King's biotome and balloon angioplasty. *Am J Cardiol*. 1993;72:241.
136. Odell JA, Rode H, Millar AJW, Hoffman HP. Surgical repair in children with the Budd-Chiari syndrome. *J Thorac Cardiovasc Surg*. 1995;110:916.
137. De DH, Pezzella AT, Nguyenduy T. Membranous obstruction of hepatic venous flow. *Texas Heart Inst J*. 1995;22:320.
138. Mori K, Matsuoka S, Hayabuchi Y, Kuroda Y, Kitagawa T. Absence of the inferior vena cava in a patient with omphalocele: two-dimensional echocardiographic and cineangiographic findings. *Heart Ves*. 1996;11:104.
139. Van Praagh S, Santini F, Sanders SP. Cardiac malpositions with special emphasis on visceral heterotaxy (asplenia and polysplenia syndromes). In: Fyler DC, ed. *Nadas' Pediatric Cardiology*. Philadelphia: Hanley & Belfus, Inc; 1992:589.

7

Pulmonary Venous Anomalies

TOTALLY ANOMALOUS PULMONARY VENOUS CONNECTION/DRAINAGE

Definition

Totally anomalous pulmonary venous connection (TAPVC) is an anomaly in which none of the pulmonary veins connect normally with the morphologically left atrium (LA).[1]

TAPVC used to be known as total anomalous pulmonary venous *drainage*. Then, Dr. Jesse Edwards and colleagues proposed that total anomalous pulmonary venous *connection* would be a more anatomically accurate diagnosis. This proposal seemed correct and was generally adopted. Hence, TAPV*C* and TAPV*D* were initially regarded as synonymous.

As will be seen, later we would realize that it is possible for the pulmonary veins to be normally *connected,* but to have totally anomalous pulmonary venous *drainage* (TAPVD). Examples include marked levomalposition of the atrial septum to the left of the left pulmonary veins (LPVs), and mitral atresia with an intact atrial septum and decompression of the LA via a levoatrial cardinal vein into a left vertical vein (LVV) and then into the left innominate vein (LIV) and the right superior vena cava (RSVC) and thence to the right atrium (RA). Such cases are presented subsequently (Figs. 7.1 and 7.2).

Classification

In 1957, Darling, Rothney, and Craig[2] classified TAPVC into four anatomic types: (1) **supracardiac,** (2) **cardiac,** (3) **infracardiac,** and (4) **mixed.**

Historical Note. Dr. John Craig, the senior author of this landmark paper,[2] was my principal teacher of pediatric pathology at the Children's Hospital Medical Center (as it was then called) in Boston, from 1956 to 1957. Dr. Bill Rothney was a Senior Resident in Pathology. I did not know Dr. Darling.

In 1962, when I was taking the oral part of the examination for the American Sub-board of Pediatric Cardiology, Dr. Abraham Rudolph asked me, "What is the embryologic basis of anomalous pulmonary venous drainage?" I replied by telling Dr. Rudolph the Darling, Rothney, and Craig classification of TAPVC,[2] which seemed to satisfy him. Years later, I realized that my answer had been not wrong but certainly superficial, as will soon be seen.

Embryologically, TAPVC represents failure of development of the common pulmonary vein, as was appreciated by Lucas et al[3] in 1962. As a consequence of failure of development of the common pulmonary vein, an anastomosis almost always persists and enlarges between the pulmonary venous plexus of the lung buds and the systemic veins.

As the classification of TAPVC[2] indicates, such pulmonary venous–to–systemic venous anastomoses can occur at the *supracardiac* level between the lungs and the anterior cardinal veins (Fig. 7.3),[1] at the *cardiac* level between the lungs and the sinus venosus, at the *infracardiac* level between the lungs and the ductus venosus (see Fig. 7.3), or at several of the previously mentioned levels in the *mixed* form of TAPVC.

These normal anastomoses between the pulmonary venous plexus and the systemic venous plexus usually undergo involution after the development of the common pulmonary vein. But if the common pulmonary vein fails to develop, these pulmonary-systemic venous anastomoses can persist, resulting in TAPVC.

It will be seen that the previously mentioned classification of TAPVC is a very general classification. There are multiple different anatomic subtypes of supracardiac, cardiac, infracardiac, and mixed TAPVC (see Fig. 7.3).[1]

Embryology

The normal development of the common pulmonary vein and of the sinus venosus in humans is depicted diagrammatically in Fig. 7.4.[4] We were able to identify the common pulmonary vein with certainty in human embryos at the 4.6-mm stage (crown-rump length), when the estimated age since ovulation was 27 days (Fig. 7.5).[5] Normally, the common pulmonary vein appears to grow outward from the dorsal atrial wall into the lung buds. Note that the common pulmonary vein is located within a "horseshoe" formed by the right and left horns of the sinus venosus (see Fig. 7.4).[4]

When the TAPVC pathway is supracardiac or infracardiac, the anomalous venous pathway is much longer than normal. The common pulmonary vein (see Figs. 7.4 and 7.5) provides a much shorter route for the pulmonary venous return from the lungs to the LA. This normal shortcut provided by the common pulmonary vein appears to lead to the involution through disuse atrophy of the various anastomoses between the pulmonary and the systemic veins.

From a developmental standpoint, these so-called anomalous pulmonary venous connections are neither anomalous nor pulmonary. They are normal embryonic pathways. But in

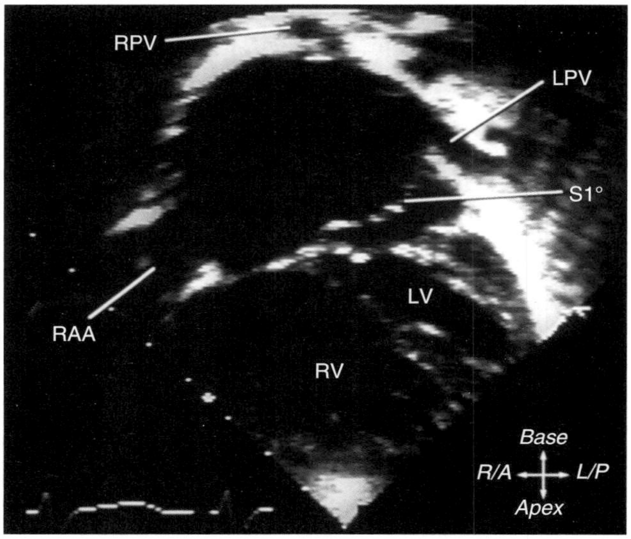

Fig. 7.1 Marked Leftward Malposition of the Septum Primun *(SI°)*. Both a left pulmonary vein *(LPV)* and a right pulmonary vein *(RPV)* can be seen entering the right atrium to the right of the SI° in this apical four-chamber view of the heart of a 2-year-old infant with tetralogy of Fallot {S,D,S}. Also seen are the openings into the right atrial appendage *(RAA)*, the right ventricle *(RV)*, and the left ventricle *(LV)*. Note that there is a large angle between the plane of the ventricular septum and the plane of SI° (130 degrees). It is because of this marked leftward malposition of SI° that all pulmonary veins drain to the right of SI° into the "right" atrium, which is really the right atrium plus much of the left atrium (extending from just to the right of the RPV to SI°). The "left" atrium (to left of SI°) is very small. In addition to the septum primum malposition atrial septal defect (between SI° and the posterior atrial wall), there are also multiple fenestrations within SI°. The marked malposition of SI° may suggest the erroneous diagnosis of common atrium with a supramitral membrane, or cor triatriatum sinister. The surgical treatment of leftward malposition of SI° involves excision of the displaced SI° and replacement with a prosthetic atrial septum—probably using a pericardial patch—in the normal location. (From Van Praagh S, Carrera ME, Sanders S, Mayer Jr JE, Van Praagh R. Partial or total direct pulmonary venous drainage to right atrium due to malposition of septum primum: Anatomic and echocardiographic findings and surgical treatment—A study based on 36 cases. *Chest.* 1995;107:1488, with permission.)

the postnatal individual, they are abnormal, that is, not usual. These totally anomalous pulmonary venous pathways are not pulmonary veins. In TAPVC, the basic problem is usually that the common pulmonary vein is absent or atretic.

It is also noteworthy that one can have normal pulmonary venous connections to the LA coexisting with anomalous pulmonary venous connection in the same patient: to the RSVC in one of our patients and to the left superior vena cava (LSVC) and thence to the coronary sinus in another patient. Thus, *normal and anomalous pulmonary venous connections rarely can coexist in the same patient,* if the normal early embryonic anastomoses between the lungs and the systemic veins fail to involute. Although such rare patients have anomalous pulmonary venous connections that resemble TAPVC, they cannot be said to have TAPVC because the pulmonary veins are also normally connected. Can such rare patients be said to have partially anomalous pulmonary venous connection (PAPVC)? We think that the answer is no—because all parts of both lungs appear to have both normal and anomalous pulmonary venous connection and drainage. There is no part of either lung that drains only anomalously.

Consequently, we think that such rare patients have a newly recognized anomaly: the coexistence of normally connected and anomalously connected pulmonary veins.[1]

What really is TAPVC? The short (and incomplete) answer to this question is absence of the common pulmonary vein and the sequelae thereof (i.e., the persistence of various anastomoses between the pulmonary veins and the systemic veins). This is not the whole story.

But what do we really mean when we say that the common pulmonary vein is "absent"? Failure of the common pulmonary vein to develop in TAPVC may be due to several different processes: (1) agenesis—failure to appear; (2) involution—disappearance; or (3) atresia—appearance, but remaining an uncanalized cordlike strand (Fig. 7.6).[1] In the great majority of cases (97%), no remnant of the common pulmonary vein was found, supporting the hypotheses that most patients with TAPVC have agenesis, or involution of the common pulmonary vein.[1]

In dealing with postnatal anatomy, most of us are used to the notion that normally there are four or five pulmonary veins—one from each lobe of the lungs: two pulmonary veins from the left lung and two or three pulmonary veins from the right lung.

Developmentally, however, there is really only *one* pulmonary vein, which normally is incorporated into the LA up to just beyond the primary division of each branch. The incorporation of the common pulmonary vein into the LA in normal human embryos is shown in Fig. 7.7.[5]

The *horizontal vein* (see Fig. 7.3) that runs from pulmonary hilum to hilum in TAPVC—except in some mixed types—is not the common pulmonary vein, which is absent in TAPVC.[1,3]

Thus, this is why we talk about the *horizontal pulmonary vein* (see Fig. 7.3), not the common pulmonary vein, because the common pulmonary vein typically is absent in TAPVC.

OBSTRUCTION

In a detailed study published in 1976 of 93 autopsied cases of TAPVC, Delisle et al[1] found that TAPVC is often a rapidly lethal disease and that obstruction of the anomalous venous pathway adversely effects longevity. This was perhaps best indicated by the median ages at death: whole series, 7 weeks; isolated TAPVC with obstruction of the anomalous venous pathway, 3 weeks; and isolated TAPVC without obstruction of the anomalous venous pathway, 3 months.[1]

In the supracardiac type of isolated TAPVC, we were surprised to find that the incidence of obstruction was remarkably high, at 50%.[1]

In the "snowman" type of supracardiac isolated TAPVC, obstruction occurred at two sites: (1) behind the left pulmonary artery (LPA) and in front of the left mainstem bronchus, which Dr. Jesse Edwards and colleagues graphically called the vascular vise, as in Fig. 7.3A; and (2) at the junction of the LIV with the RSVC, as in Fig. 7.3B.

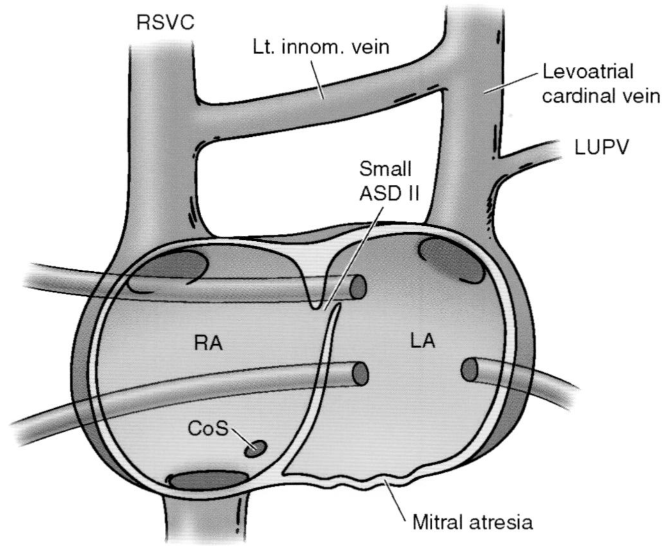

Fig. 7.2 Levoatrial cardinal vein apparently decompressing a hypertensive left atrium *(LA)* in a patient with mitral atresia and a small ostium secundum type of atrial septal defect *(ASD II)*. The levoatrial cardinal vein is confluent with the left upper pulmonary vein *(LUPV)*. The LUPV is unusually large and connects normally with the LA. The LUPV flows superiorly into the large levoatrial cardinal vein, which connects with a large left innominate vein *(Lt innom vein)*, which is also known as the left brachiocephalic vein. The Lt innom vein then connects with the right superior vena cava *(RSVC)* and thence to the right atrium *(RA)*. Thus, a "snowman"—like anomalous pulmonary venous drainage pathway is present. It is noteworthy that a large Lt innom vein is present. All of the pulmonary veins are normally *connected* with the LA, but they all *drain* anomalously via the levoatrial cardinal vein, the Lt innom vein, and the RSVC to the RA. The ostium of the coronary sinus *(CoS)* is normally small, and there is no communication between the CoS and the LA (no CoS septal defect, also known as unroofing of the CoS), and no communication between the LUPV–levoatrial cardinal vein and the CoS. The LUPV–levoatrial cardinal vein pathway is so large that we initially mistook this venous pathway for a persistent left superior vena cava (LSVC). *Why is this pathway not a persistent LSVC?* For several reasons: It communicates too posteriorly and superiorly with the LA, because it is in fact the normally connected, if enlarged, LUPV. A true persistent LSVC always originates more anteriorly, immediately behind the left atrial appendage. A persistent LSVC also communicates with the CoS. *What really is the levoatrial cardinal vein?* It is a persistent pulmonary-to-systemic venous anastomosis between the LUPV (the pulmonary venous plexus) and the Lt innnom vein (the systemic venous plexus). The Lt innom vein always persists when a levoatrial cardinal vein is present; whereas the Lt innom vein typically is absent with bilateral superior venae cavae. In the left-sided venous pathway, the blood flows in opposite directions in these two different anomalies: *cephalad* with a levoatrial cardinal vein and *caudal* with a persistent LSVC. This patient was a 20-day-old boy with multiple congenital anomalies: prominent helix of the right ear; dysplastic toenails; sacral dimple; membranous mitral atresia with single papillary muscle group of the left ventricle (parachute mitral valve with mitral atresia); aortic atresia, valvar, with intact ventricular septum; juxtaductal coarctation of the aorta; patent ductus arteriosus, large; postoperative status, Norwood procedure; familial congenital anomalies, patient's father being the fourth generation with Waardenburg syndrome; mother also deaf, the cause of the maternal deafness was not known to us; and the patient's brother was also congenitally deaf. This was also a case of familial congenital heart disease: a cousin had congenital heart disease (no other details known to us). Thus, this case of partially anomalous pulmonary venous drainage (LUPV via levoatrial cardinal vein to Lt innom vein and RSVC to RA) could also be viewed as a case of totally anomalous pulmonary venous connection (with normal pulmonary venous connections), explaining why the left-sided anomalous venous pathway was so large (and hence resembling a persistent LSVC). This anomalous pulmonary venous pathway and drainage was only one part of multiple congenital anomalies (cardiac and extracardiac) in this patient, and in the family. (From Van Praagh S, Carrera ME, Sanders SP, Mayer JE, Van Praagh R. Sinus venosus defects: Unroofing of the right pulmonary veins—anatomic and echocardiographic findings and surgical treatment. *Am Heart J.* 1994;128:365-379; with permission.)

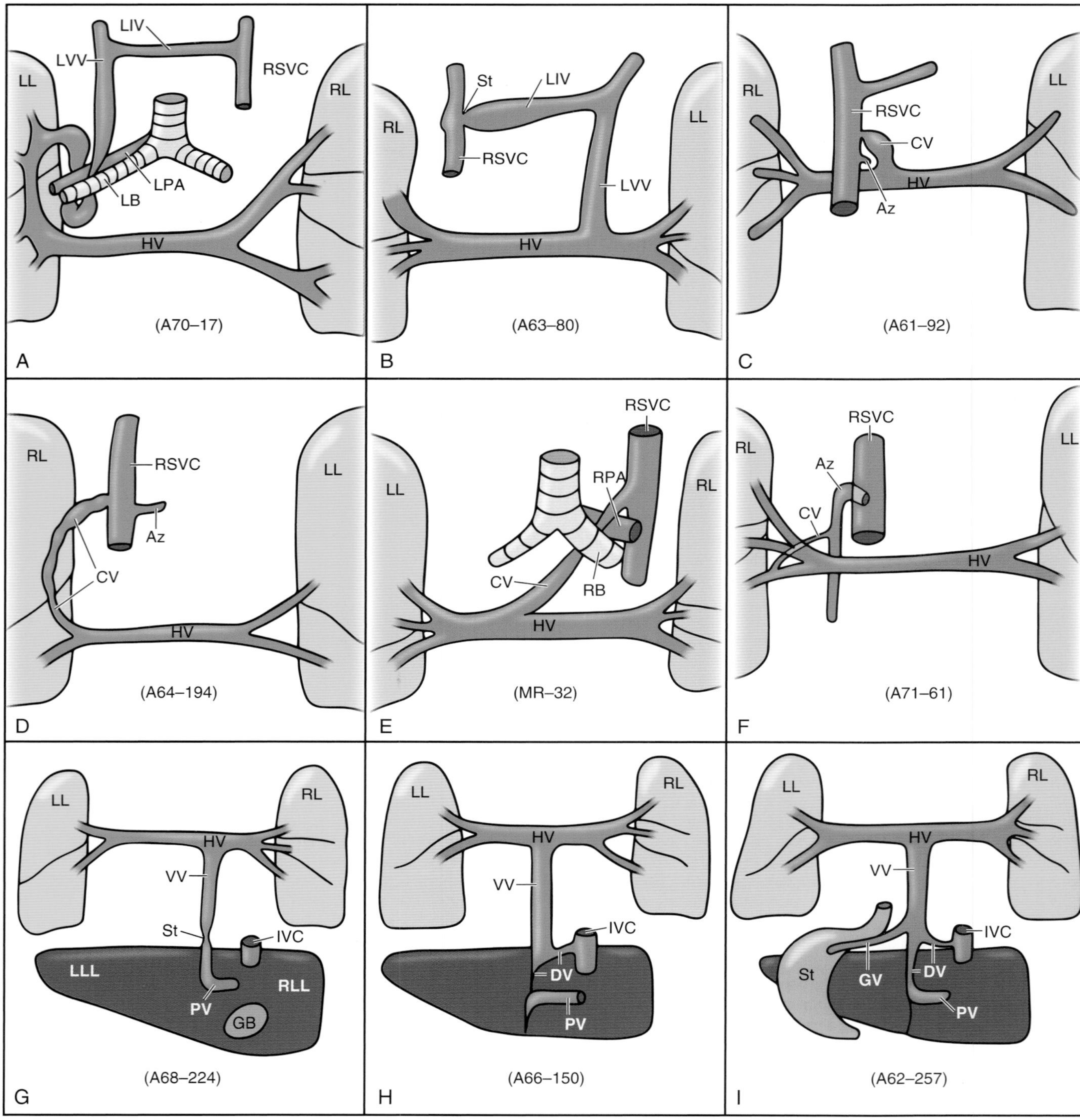

Fig. 7.3 Diagrams of various types of obstruction of anomalous venous pathway in totally anomalous pulmonary venous connection (TAPVC). (A–F) Supracardiac TAPVC with obstruction. (G–I) Infracardiac TAPVC with obstruction. Rare cases of cardiac TAPVC are not shown. Diagrams are views from either the back (posterior view), with the left lung *(LL)* to the left and the right lung *(RL)* to the right, as in A, E, G to I or the front (frontal views) with the RL to the right and LL to the left, as in B to D and F. (A) In the "snowman" type of supracardiac TAPVC with obstruction, the pulmonary venous blood from the RL passes via the horizontal vein *(HV)* to the LL. The anomalous pathway then turns superiorly and receives pulmonary veins from the LL. Then the anomalous pathway turns inferiorly and then curls again superiorly, passing between the left pulmonary artery *(LPA)* anteriorly and the left bronchus *(LB)* posteriorly, where it is compressed and obstructed. This form of obstruction is known as a vascular vise because the obstruction is produced in part by a vascular structure, the LPA. In the unobstructed form of snowman supracardiac TAPVC, the left vertical vein *(LVV)* passes anteriorly to the LPA (not posteriorly). Then the LVV flows into the left innominate vein *(LIV)* and thence into the

Fig. 7.3, cont'd right superior vena cava *(RSVC)* and right atrium (not shown). *(A70-17)* means autopsy performed in 1970, number 17. (B) Snowman type of supracardiac TAPVC showing stenosis *(St)* at the junction of the LIV and the RSVC, with poststenotic dilatation of the right lateral wall of the RSVC opposite the jet from the junctional stenosis. (C) RSVC type of supracardiac TAPVC with stenosis. The communicating vein *(CV)* between the HV and the RSVC is hypoplastic and hence stenotic. The hypoplastic ostium of the CV into the RSVC was just above the ostium of the azygos vein *(Az)*. (D) In the RSVC type of supracardiac TAPVC, note the hypoplasia, resulting in stenosis of the intrapulmonary and extrapulmonary parts of the CV. (E) Rarely, a vascular vise type of stenosis can occur with the RSVC type of supracardiac TAPVC: when the CV from the HV to the RSVC runs between the *right* pulmonary artery *(RPA)* anteriorly and the *right* bronchus *(RB)* posteriorly. (F) Another rare form of supracardiac TAPVC with obstruction: a diminutive and hence highly obstructive CV runs between a right lower lobe pulmonary venous branch and the Az vein. (G) In the infracardiac type of TAPVC, the vertical vein *(VV)* runs inferiorly from the HV, adjacent to the esophagus (not shown). At the diaphragm, the VV is compressed, resulting in stenosis. Below the diaphragm, the anomalous pulmonary venous pathway flows into the portal vein *(PV)*, because the extrahepatic part of the ductus venosus connecting with the inferior vena cava *(IVC)* has closed. Consequently, the pulmonary venous blood stream must percolate through the hepatic sinusoids—a second site of increased resistance (hence obstruction) before reaching the IVC via the hepatic veins and then returning to the right atrium. A simplified view of the undersurface of the liver shows the right lobe of the liver *(RLL)*, the left lobe of the liver *(LLL)*, and the gallbladder *(GB)*. (H) In another case of TAPVC below the diaphragm, the VV flows into the ductus venosus *(DV)*. Because the portion of the DV that connects with the portal vein is atretic, all of the pulmonary venous return must pass through a small and acutely angulated portion of the DV that connects with the IVC and thence to the right atrium. The small size and acute angulation of the patent portion of the DV results in stenosis of the anomalous pulmonary venous pathway. (I) In this patient with infracardiac TAPVC with obstruction of the anomalous pulmonary venous pathways, the HV opened into the inferiorly running VV that then opened into the DV. The DV opened through small communications with the IVC, the portal vein, and a large gastric vein *(GV)*. (From Delisle G, Ando M, Calder AL, Zuberbuhler JR, Rockenmacher S, Alday LE, Mangini O, Van Praagh S, Van Praagh R. Total anomalous pulmonary venous connection: Report of 93 autopsied cases with emphasis on diagnostic and surgical considerations. *Am Heart J*. 1976; 91:99, with permission.)

Why is the type of TAPVC shown in Fig. 7.3A–B known as the snowman type? Because, after about 4 months of age, one can often see a shadow above the cardiac silhouette on the plain posteroanterior chest x-ray film that is formed by the prominent LVV, LIV, and RSVC. The heart shadow forms the "body," and the venous shadow forms the "head" of the snowman.

In the snowman type of TAPVC, the vascular vise (between the LPA anteriorly and the left bronchus posteriorly, see Fig. 7.3A) was the more common form (75%).[1] When the LVV passed from the horizontal vein upward and *in front of* the LPA, as it usually does, the snowman type of TAPVC was not associated with obstruction at this site.

In Fig. 7.3A, the anomalous pulmonary venous pathway is viewed from behind. From the left end of the horizontal vein, the anomalous pathway heads superiorly, just beneath the pleura of the left lung. Then the venous pathway emerges into the mediastinum, turns inferiorly, and then curls superiorly and passes between the LPA anteriorly and the left bronchus posteriorly. In contrast with Fig. 7.3A, Fig. 7.3B is viewed from the front. Noting the labels of the lungs (*LL* = left lung, *RL* = right lung; see Fig. 7.3) makes it immediately obvious whether the TAPVC is being viewed from the front (see Fig. 7.3B–D, F) or from behind (Fig. 7.3A, E, G–I).

In one-third of these obstructed snowmen, there was marked poststenotic dilatation of the LVV above the level of the LPA and the left mainstem bronchus (Figs. 7.8 and 7.9), as was also observed by Kauffman et al.[6]

Why are we talking about the *LVV* (see Fig. 7.3)? Isn't this vein derived embryologically from the left anterior cardinal vein? We think that the answer is yes. Why then do we not call this vein the LSVC? The answer is because it does not return to the heart as a persistent LSVC does, either to the coronary sinus in visceroatrial situs solitus or to the left-sided morphologically RA in visceroatrial situs inversus. We think there must be developmental differences between the LVV (see Fig. 7.3) and LSVC. Inferiorly, at the level of the left bronchus and the LPA, the LVV may not be derived from the left anterior cardinal vein, accounting for the anatomic differences between the LVV in TAPVC (see Fig. 7.3) and a typical persistent LSVC.

In the less common site of obstruction of the snowman type of supracardiac TAPVC, the opening of the LIV into the RSVC can be remarkably small: only 2 mm in diameter, with marked poststenotic dilatation of the RSVC opposite the stenotic orifice of the LIV.[1] The cause of this stenosis remained unclear.

In the RSVC type of supracardiac isolated TAPVC, the majority were obstructed (67%). Two patients had severe stenosis at the point of entry of the oblique connecting vein into the RSVC (see Fig. 7.3C). Another had stenosis (hypoplasia) of the anomalous venous pathway, both within the right lung and within the mediastinum—between the right lung and the RSVC (see Fig. 7.3D).[1]

An additional patient had a *right-sided* vascular vise because the oblique connecting vein ran from the horizontal vein inferiorly and passed superiorly and rightward between the *right* pulmonary artery (RPA) anteriorly and the *right* bronchus posteriorly to reach the RSVC (see Fig. 7.3E).[1]

In the azygos vein type of supracardiac isolated TAPVC, both patients had severe obstruction. In one, there was severe

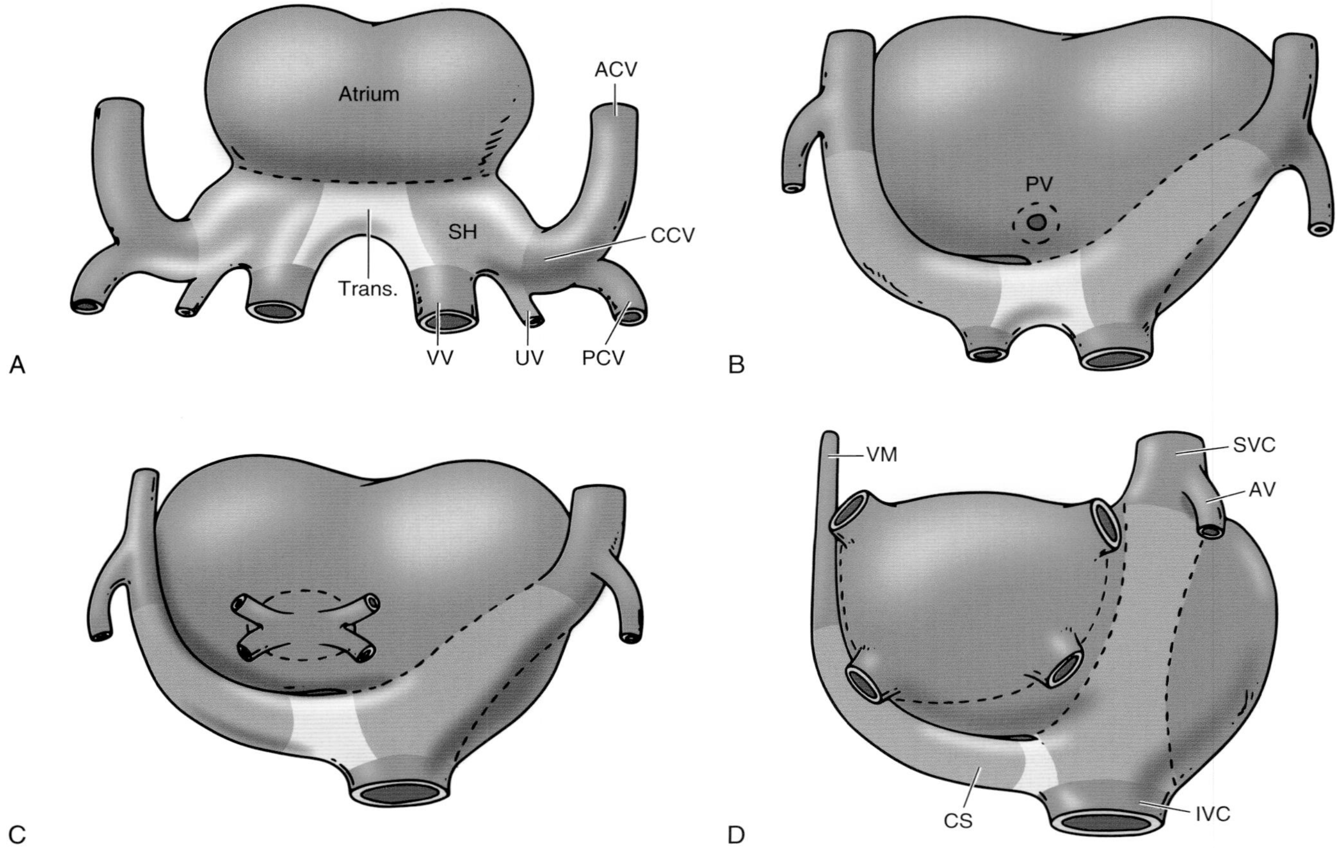

Fig. 7.4 Development of the Pulmonary Veins and Sinus Venosus, Posterior View (Diagrammatic). (A) Human embryo 3-mm crown-rump length, estimated gestational age 23 days shows a symmetrical sinus venosus, an undivided common atrium, and no pulmonary vein. (B) At 5-mm, 27 days gestational age, the pulmonary vein *(PV)* has appeared, just above the transverse portion of the sinus venosus, between the right and left sinus horns. The right sinus horn is now slightly larger than the left sinus horn. The umbilical and vitelline veins have merged bilaterally, forming the omphalomesenteric veins (unlabeled), right larger than left. (C) At 12 mm, 35 days gestation age, the pulmonary vein and its branches are becoming incorporated into the left atrium. The right sinus horn is larger than the left. The common pulmonary vein and its branches are now slightly to the left of and slightly above the transverse portion of the sinus venosus. (D) In the newborn infant, the common PV and its branches are now fully incorporated into the left atrium, forming its dorsal wall. The pulmonary vein and its branches lie in the arms of a sinus venosus "horseshoe," the large right sinus horn to the right and the normally much smaller left sinus horn to the left. Flowing into the large right sinus horn and the morphologically right atrium (RA) are the inferior vena cava *(IVC)*, the right superior vena cava *(SVC)*, and the azygos vein *(AV)*. Connecting with the much smaller left sinus horn is the vein of Marshall *(VM)*, which is the left SVC. Normally, this structure is ligamentous postnatally, that is, the ligament of Marshall. The coronary sinus *(CS)* is the normally greatly reduced left sinus horn. The remnant of the transverse portion of the sinus venosus surrounds the right atrial ostium of the coronary sinus. *ACV,* Anterior cardinal vein; *CCV,* common cardinal vein (duct of Cuvier); *PCV,* posterior cardinal vein; *SH,* sinus horn (stippled); *Trans,* transverse portion of sinus venosus (cross hatched) between right sinus horn and left sinus horn; *UV,* umbilical vein; *VV,* vitelline vein. (From Van Mierop LHS, Wiglesworth FW. Isomerism of the cardiac atria in the asplenia syndrome. *Lab Invest.* 1962;11:1303, © U.S.–Canadian Academy of Pathology, with permission.)

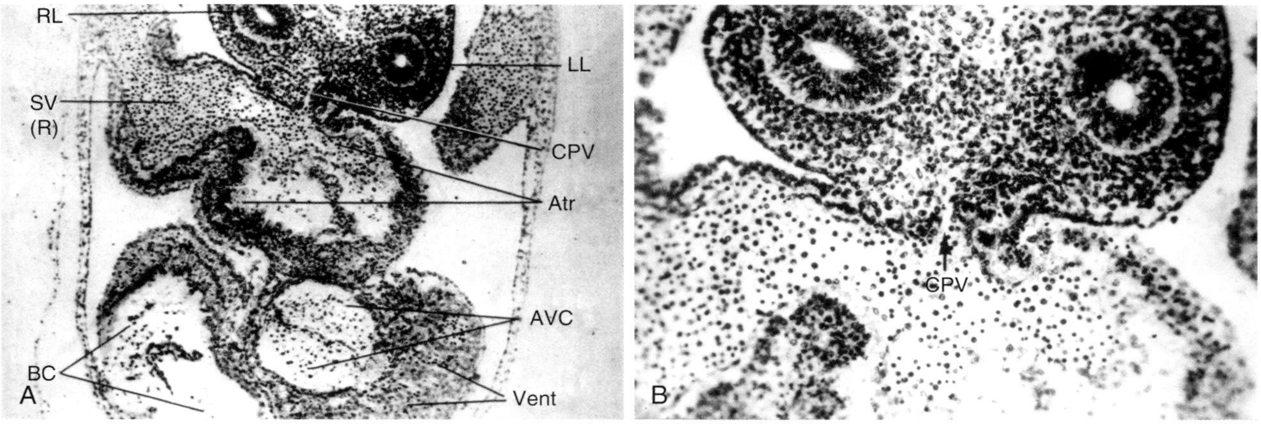

Fig. 7.5 Development of the Pulmonary Vein in the Human Embryo, Horizontal (Transverse) Section. (A) Youngest embryo in whom the common pulmonary vein *(CPV)* was definitely identified (Harvard Embryo, Minot Collection, No. 2321, 4.6 mm, estimated age since ovulation 27 days, section 257). *Atr,* Primitive undivided atrium; *AVC,* atrioventricular canal showing ventral (anterior) and dorsal (posterior) endocardial cushions; *BC,* bulbus cordis or future right ventricle, showing conal cushions and endocardially lined lumen; *LL,* left lung bud; *(R),* right horn of the sinus venosus; *RL,* right lung bud; *SV,* sinus venosus; *Vent,* ventricle of bulboventricular D-loop, which is the future morphologically left ventricle. (Alum cochineal and orange G stain, original magnification ×150.) (B) Same embryo, close-up of CPV (original magnification ×250). (From Van Praagh R, Corsini I. Cor triatriatum: Pathologic anatomy and a consideration of morphogenesis based on 13 postmortem cases and a study of normal development of the pulmonary vein and atrial septum in 83 human embryos. *Am Heart J.* 1969;78:379-405, with permission.)

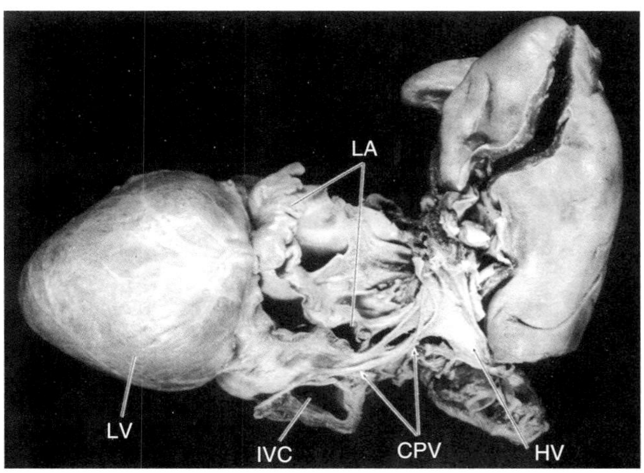

Fig. 7.6 Atretic cordlike common pulmonary vein *(CPV)* running from horizontal vein *(HV)* dorsally to inferior surface of morphologically left atrium *(LA)* ventrally, passing immediately to the left of the inferior vena cava *(IVC)*, left lateral view. This is the normal location of the CPV early in its development. It is very uncommon to find evidence of an atretic CPV. This rare case supports the view that the supracardiac and infracardiac forms of totally anomalous pulmonary venous connection (TAPVC) result from agenesis, involution, or atresia of the CPV, with persistence of an early anastomotic pathway between the pulmonary venous plexus and the systemic venous plexus. *LV,* Morphologically left ventricle. (From Delisle G, Ando M, Calder AL, Zuberbuhler JR, Rockenmacher S, Alday LE, Mangini O, Van Praagh S, Van Praagh R: Total anomalous pulmonary venous connection: Report of 93 autopsied cases with emphasis on diagnostic and surgical considerations. *Am Heart J.* 1976;91:99, with permission.)

hypoplasia of the oblique connecting vein, the diameter being less than 1 mm (see Fig. 7.3).[1] The other patient had marked stenosis of the entry of the azygos vein into the RSVC.

In the coronary sinus type of cardiac isolated TAPVC (Fig. 7.10), none had obstruction.[1] An example of *familial TAPVC* was found in this type: a 1½-month-old white male infant had a sibling who had died 2 years previously from subdiaphragmatic TAPVC.[1]

In the ductus venosus type of infracardiac isolated TAPVC (see Fig. 7.3G–I), obstruction was thought to be 100% (n = 14).[1] The anomalous pulmonary venous pathway always led to the ductus venosus and then continued as follows: (1) to the left portal vein in 8 patients (see Fig. 7.3G); (2) to the inferior vena cava (IVC) in 3 cases (see Fig. 7.3H); (3) to the left portal vein and the IVC in 1 patient, because both portions of the ductus venosus (leading to the left portal vein and to the IVC) were patent; (4) to the left portal vein, to the IVC, and to the left gastric vein in 1 patient (see Fig. 7.3I); and (5) with no continuation whatever in 1 case because of closure[3,7] of the ductus venosus leading both to the left portal vein and to the IVC (Fig. 7.11).[1] This patient was a male identical twin; the other twin was normal.

How was it possible for this patient with atresia of both parts of the ductus venosus (see Fig. 7.11) to survive for 6 days postnatally? (*Atresia* literally means *a* "absence of" *tresis* "a hole," Greek.) We really do not know the answer to this question. We speculated that perhaps pulmonary-to-bronchial venous anastomoses with retrograde blood flow may have facilitated this

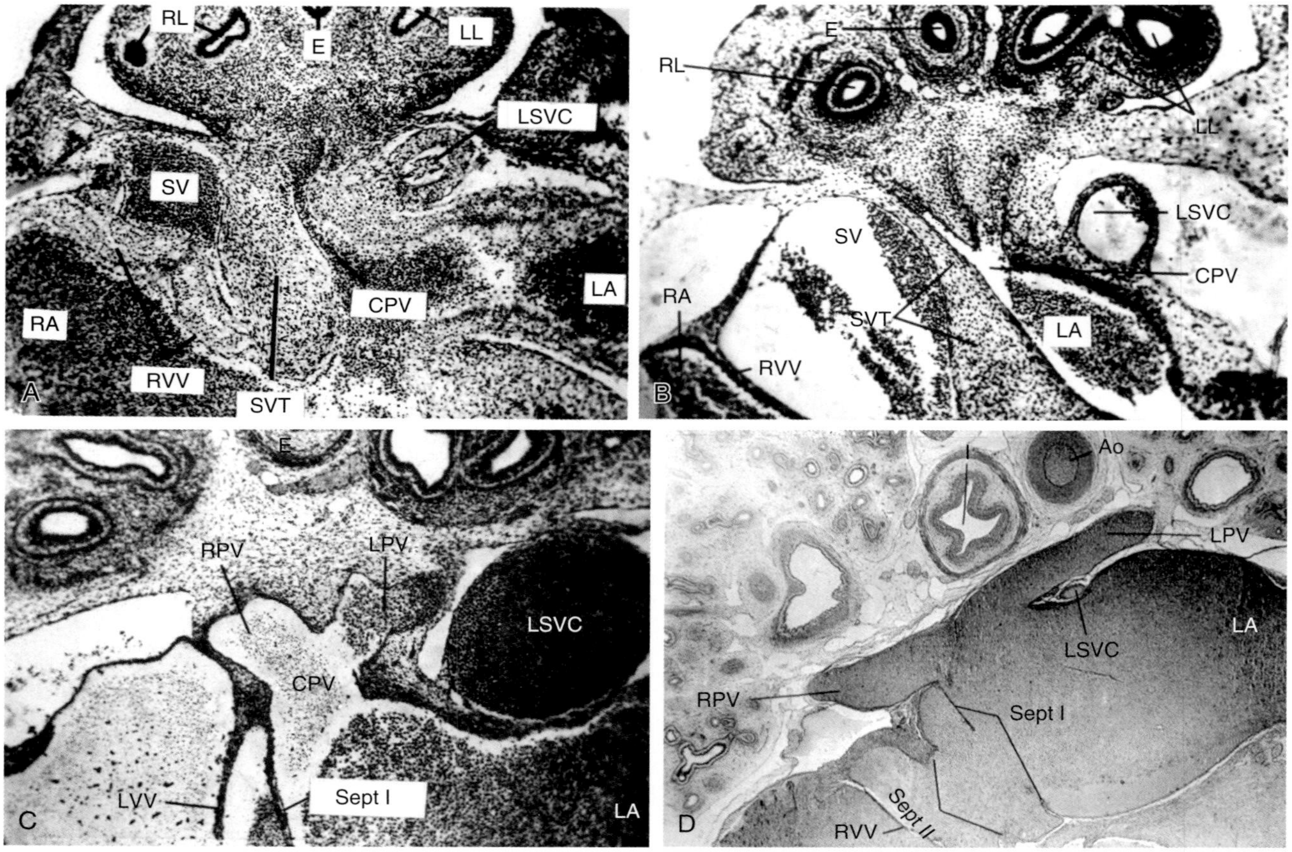

Fig. 7.7 Incorporation of the Common Pulmonary Vein *(CPV)* Into the Left Atrium *(LA)*. (A) Horizontal plane (transverse) section shows the CPV leaving the LA immediately to the left of a prominent mass of sinus venosus tissue *(SVT)* of the right sinus horn. Incorporation of the CPV into the LA has not begun as yet. The CPV communicates directly with the lung buds (*RL*, right lung; *LL*, left lung), anterior (ventral) to the esophagus. The left superior vena cava *(LSVC)* is moderately small. The lumen of the right horn of the sinus venosus (SV) is relatively prominent and is seen to the left of the right venous valve *(RVV)*. Morphologically right atrium *(RA)* lies to the right of the RVV. (Harvard Minot Collection human embryo no. 1005, 9.4 mm, 33 days, section 331, borax carmine and Lyons blue stain, original magnification, ×130.) (B) The CPV is beginning to be incorporated into the LA. Note that the CPV is trifurcating in the broad dorsal mesocardium, the right branch apparently draining the RL, the left branch draining the LL, and the middle branch raining the central region. The CPV lies immediately to the left of the broad mass of SVT from the right sinus horn. The septum primum and the left venous valve both growth upward from this mass of SVT. Both the septum primum and the left venous valve *(LVV)* are cephalad to this plane of section and hence are not seen. In other words, the CPV lies below and immediately to the left of the septum primum. (Harvard Minot Collection human embryo no. 2313, 11.9 mm, 35 days, section 510, cochineal and orange G stain, original magnification ×130.) (C) Incorporation of the CPV and its branches—the right pulmonary vein *(RPV)* and the left pulmonary vein *(LPV)*—into the LA is progressing. In this somewhat more cephalad section (compared with Fig. 7.7B), one can see that the CPV lies to the left of the septum primum *(Sept I)*. Note the intimate relation between the LVV and Sept I. The space between Sept I and the LVV is known as the interseptovalvular space. The LSVC in this embryo is large. (Harvard Minot Collection human embryo no. 2155, 17.6 mm, 38 days, section 789, cochineal and orange G stain, original magnification ×130.) (D) The pulmonary vein is midline, as always; note its relation to the trachea *(T)*. The pulmonary vein branches—the RPV and the LPV—are still not fully incorporated into the LA. The LSVC is very small, but not quite atretic. A left aortic arch *(Ao)* is present. Sept I lies to the left of the superior limbic band of septum secundum *(Sept II)*. The RVV lies to the right of the Sept II. (Harvard Minot Collection human embryo no 2128, 45 mm, 63 days, section 2035, cochineal and orange G stain, original magnification ×40.) *E*, enlargement; *LV*, left ventricle. (From Van Praagh R, Corsini I. Cor triatriatum: Pathologic anatomy and a consideration of morphogenesis based on 13 postmortem cases and a study of normal development of the pulmonary vein and atrial septum in 83 human embryos. *Am Heart J*. 1969;78:379, with permission.)

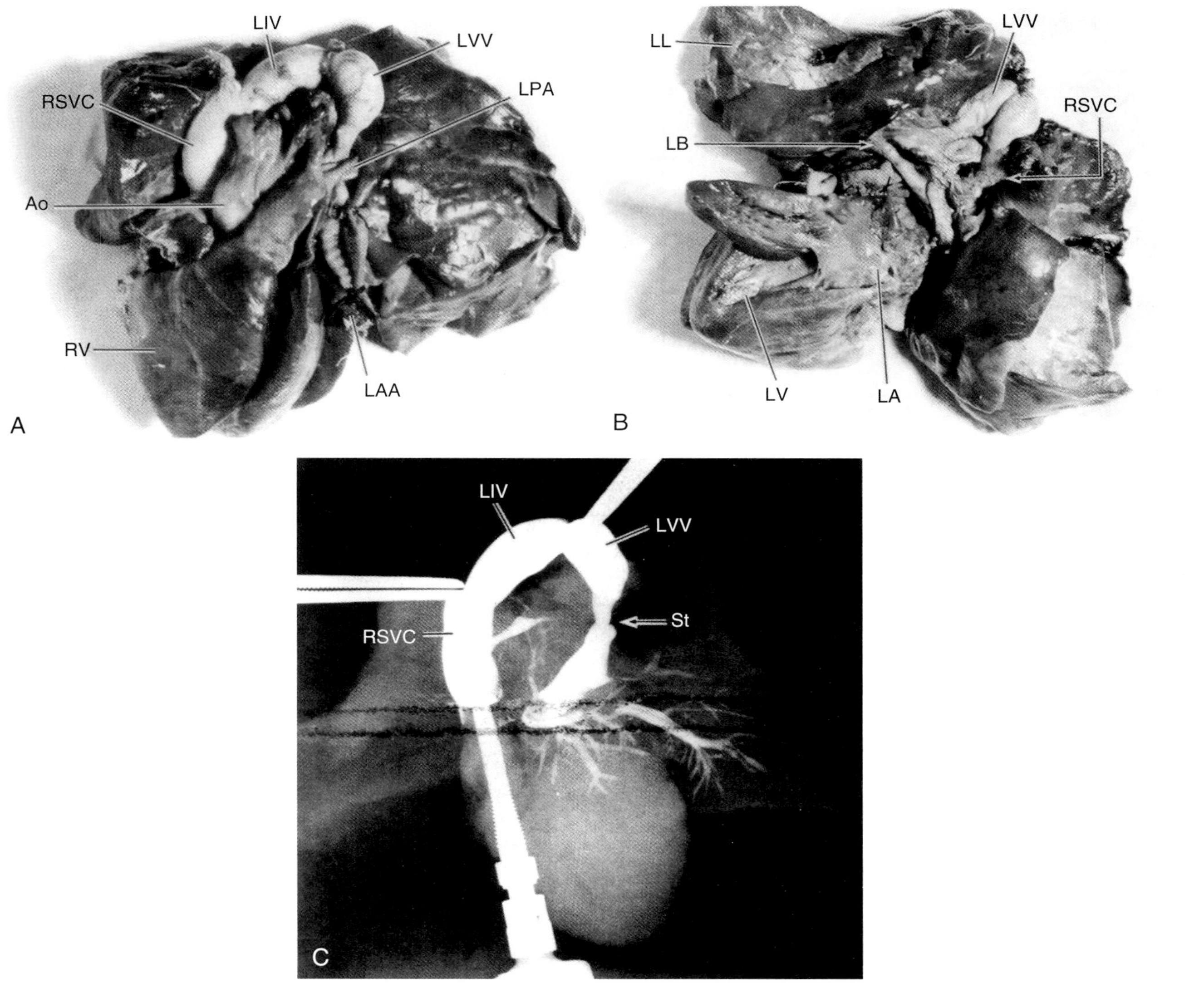

Fig. 7.8 "Snowman" type of supracardiac totally anomalous pulmonary venous connection (TAPVC) with the vascular vise type of obstruction of the left vertical vein *(LVV)* between the left pulmonary artery *(LPA)* anteriorly and the left bronchus *(LB)* posteriorly. (A) Anterior view. (B) Posterior view of autopsied specimen of heart and lungs. Usually the LVV passes anteriorly to the LPA; hence, no obstruction. The snowman pathway is formed by the LVV, the left innominate vein *(LIV)*, and the right superior vena cava *(RSVC)*. (C) Postmortem angiogram of the snowman pathway, anterior view, confirming the presence of stenosis *(St)* where the LVV passes between the left pulmonary artery anteriorly and the left bronchus posteriorly. *Ao,* Ascending aorta; *LA,* left atrium; *LAA,* left atrial appendage; *LL,* left lung; *LV,* left ventricle; *RV,* right ventricle. (From Delisle G, Ando M, Calder AL, Zuberbuhler JR, Rockenmacher S, Alday LE, Mangini O, Van Praagh S, Van Praagh R. Total anomalous pulmonary venous connection: Report of 93 autopsied cases with emphasis on diagnostic and surgical considerations. *Am Heart J.* 1976;91:99, with permission.)

infant's survival. It is also true that we do not know when the ductus venosus became atretic; the ductus venosus may have been patent for some portion of this patient's postnatal life. Alternatively, the ductus venosus may have closed prenatally, the circulation depending on a patent ductus arteriosus (PDA). If the ductus venosus closed prenatally, the patient had a ductus arteriosus–dependent circulation. Hence, postnatal patency of the ductus arteriosus may well have contributed to this patient's postnatal survival.

This patient (see Fig. 7.11) makes it clear that TAPVC below the diaphragm is **a ductus venosus–dependent anomaly.** The natural history is if the ductus venosus closes completely (Fig. 7.12), and the ductus arteriosus also closes, the patient dies.

The infracardiac type of TAPVC can be obstructed not only by the narrowing or closure of the ductus venosus, but also by extrinsic compression of the paraesophageal vertical vein at the diaphragm. *Stenosis at the diaphragm* (see Fig. 7.3G) was found in 3 of these 14 patients (21%).[1]

When the obstruction of the anomalous pulmonary venous connection is very severe or complete (i.e., when atresia is present), diagnostic studies such as cardiac catheterization and angiocardiography can be diagnostically misleading, as

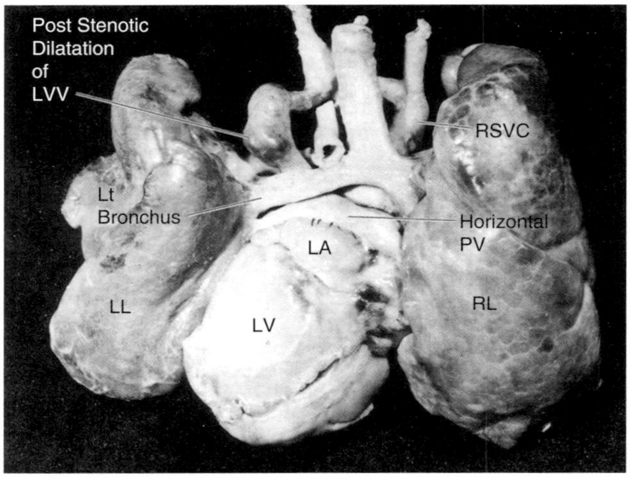

Fig. 7.9 Posterior View of an Obstructed "Snowman" Type of Supracardiac Totally Anomalous Pulmonary Venous Connection. The left vertical vein *(LVV)* arises from the left end of the horizontal pulmonary vein. The LVV passes anteriorly to the left *(Lt)* bronchus. Note the poststenotic dilatation of the LVV just above the level of the Lt bronchus, confirming the presence of a stenotic vascular vise. The horizontal pulmonary vein *(PV)* (the "surgeon's friend") has been anastomosed to the dorsal wall of the left atrium *(LA)*. Note that the perilobular venules and lymphatics of the right lung *(RL)* are visibly more prominent than normal, confirming the preoperative presence of obstruction of the totally anomalous pulmonary venous pathway. *LL,* Left lung; *LV,* left ventricle; *RSVC,* right superior vena cava. (From Delisle G, Ando M, Calder AL, Zuberbuhler JR, Rockenmacher S, Alday LE, Magini O, Van Praagh S, Van Praagh R. Total anomalous pulmonary venous connection: Report of 93 autopsied cases with emphasis on diagnostic and surgical considerations. *Am Heart J.* 1976;91:99, with permission.)

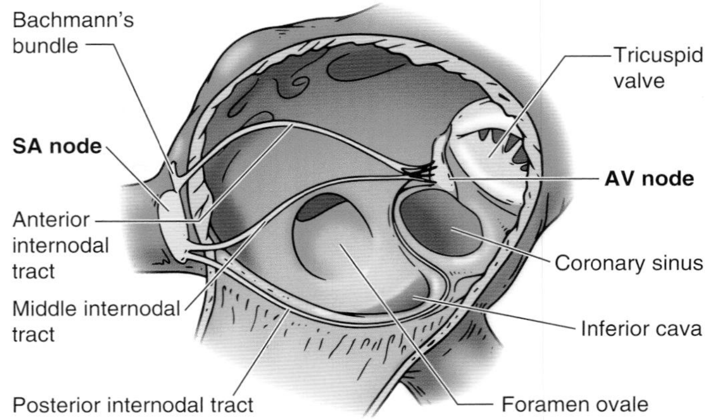

Fig. 7.10 Opened right atrium in a patient with totally anomalous pulmonary venous connection to the coronary sinus, positioned as seen at the surgery with the superior vena cava (SVC) to the left and the inferior vena cava to the right. Note how enlarged the ostium of the coronary sinus is, reflecting the markedly increased blood flow into the coronary sinus. The foramen ovale is patent. Note the positions of the sinoatrial *(SA)* node, lateral to the SVC in the SA sulcus; the atrioventricular *(AV)* node and the proximal unbranched portion of the atrioventricular (His) bundle, running from the ostium of the coronary sinus to the commissure between the anterior and septal leaflets of the tricuspid valve, where the membranous septum is located and beneath which the penetrating portion of the His bundle passes; and the anterior internodal tract or preferential conduction pathway that runs from the anterosuperior end of the SA node to the AV node. Also coming from the anterior end of the SA node is the Bachmann bundle or preferential conduction pathway to the left atrium; the middle internodal tract or preferential conduction pathway passes from the posteroinferior end of the SA node and courses along the superior limbic band of septum secundum above the patent foramen ovale (or fossa ovalis, if closed) to reach the AV node; and the posterior internodal tract or preferential conduction pathway, which also passes from the posteroinferior end of the SA node and courses along the SA sulcus (crista terminalis) to reach the AV node. Whether the internodal pathways are anatomically defined tracts or merely preferential conduction pathways remains controversial; hence, both terminologies are used here to acknowledge this difference of opinion. Unfortunately, none of these conduction system–related structures is visible to the naked eye (the SA node, the AV node, and the preferential internodal pathways/tracts). Hence, they are drawn in here—as though they were visible—to help the surgeon and the electrophysiologist locate these important structures. *LL,* Left lung. (From Van Praagh R, Harken AH, Delisle G, Ando M, Gross RE. Total anomalous pulmonary venous drainage to the coronary sinus: A revised procedure for its correction. *J Thorac Cardiovasc Surg.* 1972;64:132, with permission.)

occurred in the patient shown in Figs. 7.11 and 7.12. The posteroanterior chest x-ray film (Fig. 7.13) showed a normal-sized heart with "ground-glass" lung fields, accurately suggesting the correct diagnosis of TAPVC with atresia of the anomalous connection. However, cardiac catheterization revealed no localized oxygen step-up and angiocardiography showed no anomalous pulmonary venous pathway—both because this connection was atretic (see Figs. 7.11 and 7.12). Information from the cardiac catheters led to the erroneous conclusion that this patient probably had lung disease, not congenital heart disease.

Dr. Ed Neuhauser, our Chief of Radiology at that time, took one look at the chest x-ray film (see Fig. 7.13) and said, "Totally anomalous pulmonary venous connection below the diaphragm with obstruction, right?" It took an autopsy to prove that this diagnosis was indeed right (see Fig. 7.11 and 7.12). In retrospect, we understood that one should *expect* negative cardiac catheterization and angiocardiography findings in TAPVC with severe obstruction.

Twins occurred twice in these 14 patients with TAPVC to the ductus venosus. Both were identical twins, and in both pairs the co-twin was normal.[1]

The mixed type of TAPVC was always isolated and was occasionally obstructed (20%). In the study of Delisle et al,[1] 5 of 93 cases (5%) had anomalous pulmonary venous connections at more than one level:

1. a snowman pathway from both lungs to the RSVC that also had a stenotic connection from both lungs to the coronary sinus;
2. a snowman connection that also had anomalous connections from the right upper lobe to the RSVC;
3. the left lung draining via a snowman pathway and the right lung draining into the coronary sinus;
4. an infracardiac connection to the portal vein and a small snowman connection; and
5. a subdiaphragmatic connection to the portal vein, with connections from the right upper lobe to the RSVC.

The latter 2 patients with anomalous connections to the ductus venosus were both thought to have an obstruction. **Isolated TAPVC** means that no other congenital heart disease is present. **Nonisolated TAPVC** means that another congenital heart disease coexists.

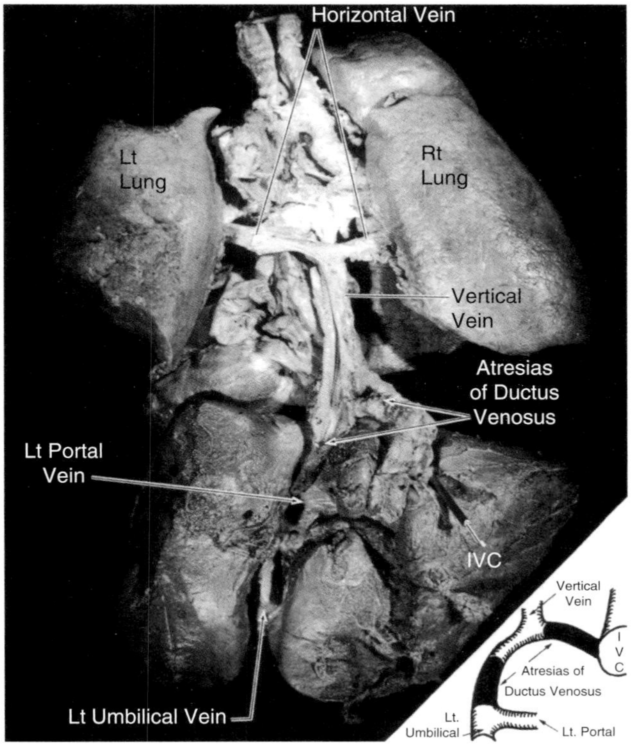

Fig. 7.11 Atresia or occlusion of both parts of the ductus venosus leading to the inferior vena cava *(IVC)* and to the left *(Lt)* portal vein resulting in total obstruction of the paraesophageal vertical vein in a patient with totally anomalous pulmonary venous connection below the diaphragm. *Rt,* Right. (From Delisle G, Ando M, Calder AL, Zuberbuhler JR, Rockenmacher S, Alday LE, Mangini O, Van Praagh S, Van Praagh R. Total anomalous pulmonary venous connection: Report of 93 autopsied cases with emphasis on diagnostic and surgical considerations. *Am Heart J.* 1976;91:99, with permission.)

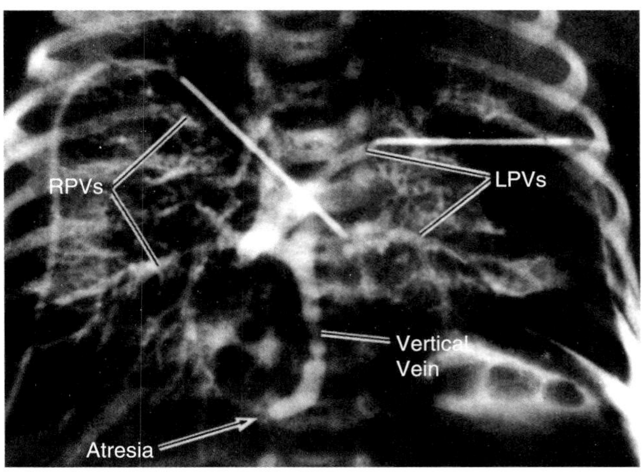

Fig. 7.12 Postmortem angiogram in a patient with totally anomalous pulmonary venous connection below the diaphragm showing total obstruction due to atresia of the paraesophageal vertical vein at the ductus venosus. This is the same patient as in Fig. 7.11. *LPVs,* Left pulmonary veins; and *RPVs,* right pulmonary veins. (From Delisle G, Ando M, Calder AL, Zuberbuhler JR, Rockenmacher S, Alday LE, Mangini O, Van Praagh S, Van Praagh R. Total anomalous pulmonary venous connection: Report of 93 autopsied cases with emphasis on diagnostic and surgical considerations. *Am Heart J.* 1976;91:99, with permission.)

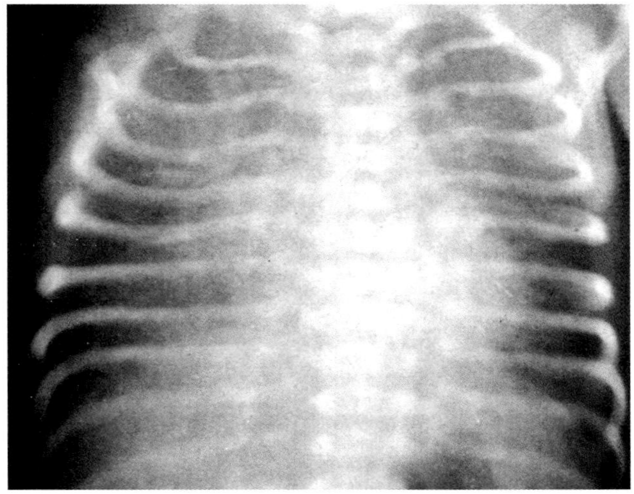

Fig. 7.13 Posteroanterior chest x-ray film showing normal heart size with severe bilateral "ground-glass" lung fields. These two findings strongly suggest totally anomalous pulmonary venous connection below the diaphragm with severe obstruction. (Same case as in Figs. 7.11 and 12.) (From Delisle G, Ando M, Calder AL, Zuberbuhler JR, Rockenmacher S, Alday LE, Mangini O, Van Praagh S, Van Praagh R. Total anomalous pulmonary venous connection: Report of 93 autopsied cases with emphasis on diagnostic and surgical considerations. *Am Heart J.* 1976;91:99, with permission.)

Delisle et al[1] appreciated this distinction between isolated and nonisolated TAPVC. They also understood that there are two different groups within nonisolated TAPVC: without heterotaxy and with heterotaxy.

Nonisolated Totally Anomalous Pulmonary Venous Connection Without Heterotaxy

In this series of 93 autopsied cases, there were 12 (13%) that had nonisolated TAPVC with congenital heart disease but without heterotaxy: double-outlet right ventricle (DORV) with pulmonary stenosis in 3; D-transposition of the great arteries (TGA) in 3; mitral atresia in 2; and tricuspid atresia, double-inlet left ventricle (LV), and pulmonary artery sling in 1 case each.[1]

Extracardiac anomalies included cat eye syndrome, conjoined twins, and agenesis of the right lung with anomalous pulmonary venous drainage. The latter situation may be called *total partially anomalous pulmonary venous connection.*

TAPVC with intact atrial septum is very rare. Such a case was found in this group. A persistent LSVC drained into the coronary sinus, as did all of the pulmonary veins. The cephalic end of the LSVC was markedly dilated (Fig. 7.14). Although the atrial septum was intact, there were multiple ventricular septal defects (VSDs), making it possible for oxygenated blood to reach the left heart and the systemic circulation. Hastreiter et al[8] published a similar case: TAPVC with an intact atrial septum and a PDA.

Nonisolated Totally Anomalous Pulmonary Venous Connection With Heterotaxy

There were 23 such cases (25% of the series)[1]: asplenia, 14 cases; polysplenia and rudimentary spleen, 8 cases; and heterotaxy with a normally formed spleen, 1 patient.

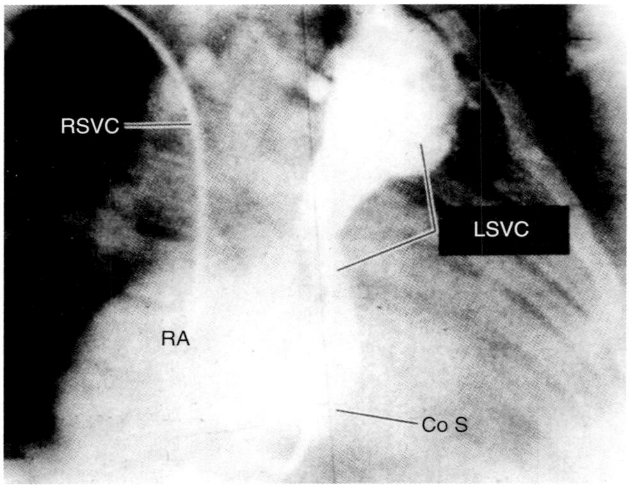

Fig. 7.14 Angiogram in a patient with totally anomalous pulmonary venous connection to the coronary sinus *(CoS)* and with a persistent left superior vena cava *(LSVC)* to the CoS to the right atrium *(RA)*. This patient had the rare findings of an intact atrial septum, multiple ventricular septal defects (VSDs) (one conoventricular type of VSD and one conal septal defect type of VSD), with marked hypertrophy and enlargement of the right atrium and right ventricle. Note the unusual and marked enlargement of the cephalic end of the LSVC, which may reflect elevated right-sided pressures and resistances associated with connections of all pulmonary veins and the LSVC to the CoS, plus absence of a patent foramen ovale or secundum atrial septal defect (with consequent inability to decompress the right atrium by right-to-left shunting), plus elevated right ventricular pressures (related to right ventricular volume overload and multiple VSDs). Thus, marked dilatation of the LSVC connecting with the CoS should suggest that persistence of the LSVC may not be isolated and that right-sided pressures may be unusually elevated. *RSVC,* Right superior vena cava. (From Delisle G, Ando M, Calder AL, Zuberbuhler JR, Rockenmacher S, Alday LE, Mangini O, Van Praagh S, Van Praagh R. Total anomalous pulmonary venous connection: Report of 93 autopsied cases with emphasis on diagnostic and surgical considerations. *Am Heart J.* 1976;91:99, with permission.)

CLASSIFICATION OF TOTALLY ANOMALOUS PULMONARY VENOUS CONNECTION

The salient anatomic findings in these 93 postmortem cases of TAPVC are summarized in Tables 7.1 to 7.4.

Surgical Considerations

From the surgical standpoint, how true is the generalization that it does not really matter what anatomic type of TAPVC is present or whether it is obstructed, because there always is a horizontal vein running from pulmonary hilum to hilum (see Fig. 7.3) that the surgeon can anastomose to the dorsal wall of the LA, as is seen in Fig. 7.9? Specifically, is the "surgeon's friend"—the horizontal vein (see Fig. 7.3)—always present, just "waiting" to be anastomosed to the LA? The answer is that typically there is a horizontal vein, but with the following exceptions:

1. TAPVC to the RA,
2. TAPVC to the coronary sinus, and
3. occasionally in the mixed type of TAPVC.

TAPVC to RA. In TAPVC to the RA, there is no discrete horizontal vein that can be anastomosed to the LA in the usual way. The pulmonary veins connect directly with what has been interpreted in the past as the dorsal wall of the RA, without forming a horizontal vein. From the anatomic standpoint, one approach to surgical repair is atrial septectomy, followed by surgical construction of a new atrial septum that will direct the pulmonary venous return into the

TABLE 7.1 Classification of 93 Cases of TAPVC by Frequency

Frequency	Site of Anomalous Connection	No. of Cases	% of Series
1	To left innominate vein ("snowman")	24	26
2	To ductus venosus (infracardiac)	22	24
3	To coronary sinus	17	18
4	To right superior vena cava	14	15
5	To right atrium[a]	7	8
6	To more than one level (mixed)	5	5
7	To azygos vein	2	2
8	To left superior vena cava	2	2

[a]Totally anomalous pulmonary venous drainage (TAPVD), not connection, to the right atrium.[9]

TABLE 7.2 Classification of 93 Cases of TAPVC by Presence or Absence of Other Congenital Heart Disease

	% of Series	No. of Cases
Isolated TAPVC	58	62
Nonisolated TAPVC	35	38
Without heterotaxy	12	13
With heterotaxy[a]	23	25

TAPVC, Totally anomalous pulmonary venous connection.
[a]Asplenia, 14 cases; polysplenia and rudimentary spleen, 8 cases; asplenia-like heterotaxy with normally formed spleen, 1 case.

TABLE 7.3 Classification of 93 Cases of TAPVC by Site of Connection and by Presence or Absence of Other Congenital Heart Disease

Site of Connection	Isolated	Nonisolated	No. of Cases	%
Supracardiac				
To left innominate vein (snowman)	20	4	24	26
To right superior vena cava	6	8	14	15
To azygos vein	2	0	2	2
To left superior vena cava	0	2	2	2
Cardiac				
To coronary sinus	11	6	17	18
To right atrium[a]	0	7	7	8
Infracardiac				
To ductus venosus	14	8	22	24
Mixed				
To more than one level	5	0	5	5

[a]Totally anomalous pulmonary venous drainage (not connection) to the right atrium.[9]

TABLE 7.4 Obstruction of Anomalous Venous Pathway in Isolated TAPVC[a]

	OBSTRUCTED		NOT OBSTRUCTED		MEDIAN AGE AT DEATH	
Site of Connection	**No. of Cases**	**% of Group**	**No. of Cases**	**% of Group**	**Obstructed**	**Not Obstructed**
Left innominate vein (snowman)	8	40	12	60	4 wk	14 wk
Right superior vena cava	4	67	2	33	2 wk	2 1/2 y[a]
						9 1/3 y[a]
Azygos vein	2	100	0	0	36 h	
						23 d
Coronary sinus	0	0	11	100	0	7 wk
Ductus venosus	14	100	0	0	3 wk	0
Mixed	2	40	3	60	17 d	5 mo
					8 wk	

[a]Surgical deaths. When there are only 2 cases in a group, both ages at death are given, rather than the median.
TAPVC, Totally anomalous pulmonary venous connection.

LA and/or to the physiologically appropriate atrioventricular (AV) valve.

In 1995, S. Van Praagh et al[24] published a study of 36 patients, 21 with postmortem confirmation and 15 living patients, in which there was partially anomalous (44%) or totally anomalous (56%) pulmonary venous drainage into the RA because of displacement of the septum primum into the LA. Displacement of the septum primum—leftward in atrial situs solitus or rightward in atrial situs inversus—was present in all patients and appeared to be responsible for the anomalous pulmonary venous drainage.

For example, in visceroatrial situs solitus, when the septum primum was displaced to the left so that the atrial septum lay between the right and LPVs, this created the appearance known as *ipsilateral pulmonary veins*,[24] which is characteristic of the polysplenia syndrome and has led to the (we think erroneous) interpretation of bilaterally left atria or left atrial isomerism (Fig. 7.15) in visceral heterotaxy with polysplenia.

When the atrial septum is displaced even further to the left so that the septum primum lies to the left of all of the pulmonary veins, this creates the appearance generally known as TAPVC to the RA (see Fig. 7.1)[24] (see Tables 7.1 to 7.3). The atrial septum can be displaced so far to the left that it resembles a *supramitral membrane* and can result physiologically in significant supramitral stenosis and LV hypoplasia. Surgically, such a markedly malpositioned atrial septum should be excised and replaced with a normally located atrial septum—currently fashioned from glutaraldehyde-fixed pericardium.

Does this mean that the conventional diagnosis of "TAPVC to the RA" is wrong? We now think that the answer is yes.[24] This diagnosis should be modified to TAPVD[24] to the RA. Accurately speaking, ipsilateral pulmonary veins have partially anomalous pulmonary venous *drainage* (not connection).[24]

Whenever the pulmonary veins connect with the atria, within the "horseshoe" formed by the right and left horns of the sinus venosus (see Fig. 7.4), we think that the pulmonary veins are *connected normally*. However, the pulmonary venous drainage can be partially anomalous (see Fig. 7.15) or totally anomalous (Fig. 7.16), depending on how malpositioned the septum primum is. In Figs. 7.1 and 7.15, note how malpositioned the atrial septum is relative to the ventricular septum (which is normally located). Normally, the atrial septum is approximately parallel with the ventricular septum, not markedly angulated as it is in Figs. 7.1 and 7.15. Displacement of septum primum into the LA often can be more obvious echocardiographically than it is anatomically.

From the right atrial view, the septum primum is much too easy to see, that is, much better seen from the right atrial perspective than normally is the case (see Fig. 7.16). (This intriguing fact was first pointed out to us by Dr. Luis Alday of Cordoba, Argentina.) Why is this so? We think that the answer is because the superior limbic band of the septum secundum, which normally covers the upper part of the septum primum, is poorly developed or absent. This is particularly true in patients with polysplenia and visceral heterotaxy.[24] Rarely, this can also occur in patients with asplenia or with a normally formed spleen and visceral hetertoaxy.[24]

Why can septum primum be displaced into the morphologically LA, resulting in partially or TAPVD? Our hypothesis is as follows: When the superior limbic band of the septum secundum is absent or very poorly formed, the upwardly growing septum primum[5] has no septum secundum to attach to superiorly, and consequently systemic venous blood flow from the IVC and SVC can displace the unattached septum primum into the LA.

This new understanding of the role of malposition of the septum primum[24] has several significant sequelae:

1. TAPVC and TAPVD are two different things. What was formerly thought to be TAPV*C* to the RA is now thought to be TAPV*D* to the RA, with normally pulmonary venous connections and malposition of the septum primum.[24]
2. *Septum primum malposition of the atrial septal defect* (ASD) (see Fig. 7.1)[24] is a newly recognized anatomic type of ASD that lies between the posterior margin of the malpositioned septum primum and the posterior wall of the LA.

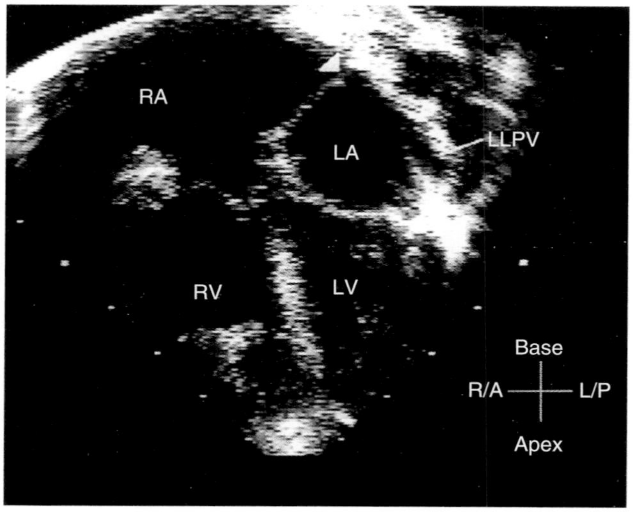

Fig. 7.15 Leftward malposition of the septum primum, resulting in the right pulmonary veins draining into the right atrium *(RA)*, as was shown with color-flow Doppler mapping. The left atrium *(LA)* appears to be smaller than normal and receives all of the left pulmonary veins, the left lower lobe pulmonary vein *(LLPV)* being seen to enter the LA in this view. In this apical four-chamber view of the heart of a living 3 9/12-year-old child with normal segmental anatomy, that is, {S,D,S}, normally the plane of the atrial septum should be essentially parallel to that of the ventricular septum between the right ventricle *(RV)* and the left ventricle *(LV)*. Instead, the atrial septum of this patient is angulated 55 degrees to the left of the plane of the ventricular septum, resulting in ipsilateral pulmonary venous drainage (right pulmonary veins to RA and left pulmonary veins to LA). Although there is partially anomalous pulmonary venous *drainage* involving the right pulmonary veins, all of the pulmonary veins appear to be normally *connected* at the atrial level within the "horseshoe" formed by the right and left horns of the sinus venosus. Septum primum malposition is the cause of this partially anomalous pulmonary venous drainage, not partially anomalous pulmonary venous connection. Septum primum malposition is a newly recognized cause of anomalous pulmonary venous drainage at the cardiac level. An interatrial communication, a *septum primum malposition defect (arrowhead)*, lies between the posterior margin of the malpositioned septum primum and the posterior atrial wall. A septum primum malposition defect is a newly recognized form of interatrial communication. The structure labeled *RA* consists of the RA plus the medial portion of the LA, which extends from just to the right of the right pulmonary veins dorsally (unlabeled) to the leftwardly malpositioned septum primum. Hence, the LA is not really small; it just looks small because of the leftwardly displaced septum primum. *L/P*, Left and posterior; *R/A*, right and anterior. (From Van Praagh S, Carrera ME, Sanders S, Mayer Jr JE, Van Praagh R. Partial or total direct pulmonary venous drainage to right atrium due to malposition of septum primum: Anatomic and echocardiographic findings and surgical treatment—A study based on 36 cases. *Chest*. 1995;107:1488, with permission.)

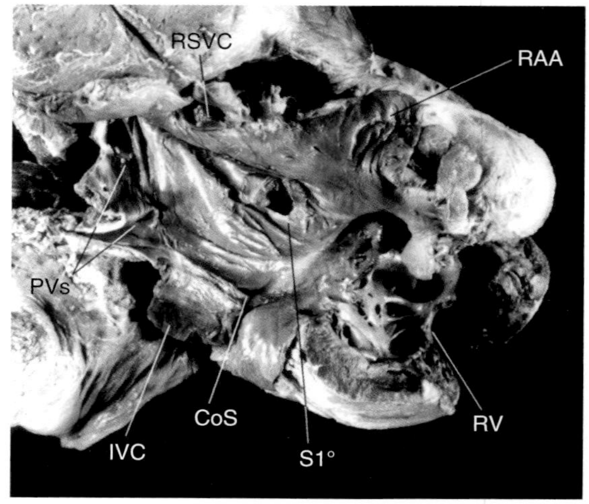

Fig. 7.16 Marked Leftward Malposition of Septum Primum *(SI°)*, With All of the Systemic Veins and All of the Pulmonary Veins Draining Into the Right Atrium. This is a right lateral view of the opened right atrium, tricuspid valve, and right ventricle *(RV)* of the heart of a 7 2/12 year-old-girl with visceral heterotaxy, right-sided polysplenia, and normal cardiac segmental anatomy, that is, {S,D,S}. There was a small membranous ventricular septal defect, not seen in this view. Note that septum primum *(SI°)* is unusually well seen from the right atrial view, we think because the superior limbic band of septum secundum is poorly formed. Usually, SI° is seen this well only from the left atrial perspective. In this heart, S1° was not seen from the left atrial view[24] (not shown). These unusual findings, that is, S1° well seen from the right atrial perspective, but not from the left atrial perspective (the opposite of normal), we have found to be characteristic of heterotaxy with polysplenia, often with malposition of the septum primum, as in this patient. The interatrial communication lies between the upper border of S1° and the posterior atrial wall. The RV is very hypertrophied. *CoS*, Coronary sinus; *IVC*, inferior vena cava; *PVs*, pulmonary veins; *RAA*, right atrial appendage; *RSVC*, right superior vena cava. (From Van Praagh S, Carrera ME, Sanders S, Mayer JR JE, Van Praagh R. Partial or total direct pulmonary venous drainage to right atrium due to malposition of septum primum: Anatomic and echocardiographic findings and surgical treatment—A study based on 36 cases. *Chest*. 1995;107:1488, with permission.)

3. *This is a new understanding of TAPVC/D.*[24] The supracardiac and infracardiac forms of TAPVC do indeed appear to result from failure of development of the common pulmonary vein, almost always leading to the persistence of early embryonic anastomoses between the pulmonary and the systemic veins, as described earlier.

But what is TAPVC to the coronary sinus? The common pulmonary veins may have developed and connected abnormally with the left sinus horn, because of anomalous development of the common pulmonary vein, abnormal development of the left sinus horn (coronary sinus), or both. Does the common pulmonary vein grow out dorsally from the atrial wall to tap into the pulmonary venous plexus, as Fig. 7.4 suggests? Or does the common pulmonary vein grow in both directions (dorsally from the heart and ventrally from the developing lungs)? Are there species differences? All of these questions have been answered positively. Consequently, we think that definitive resolution of these questions embryologically may well help clarify the morphogenesis of TAPVC to the coronary sinus.

The pulmonary veins in TAPVC to the coronary sinus look like *pulmonary veins*, suggesting that the common pulmonary vein did not fail to develop. By contrast, the common pulmonary vein does appear to be absent in the supracardiac and infracardiac forms of TAPVC.

Hypothesis. If the foregoing hypothesis is correct, this means that the supracardiac and infracardiac forms of TAPVC are indeed characterized by failure of development of the common pulmonary vein, whereas the cardiac forms of TAPVC and TAPVD are not. TAPVD to the RA appears to have normally connected pulmonary veins, with malposition of the septum primum into the LA. In TAPVC to the coronary sinus, the common pulmonary vein appears to have developed and connected abnormally to the immediately subjacent left sinus horn (see Fig. 7.4).

For us, the foregoing is a new developmental insight, namely, that TAPVC and TAPVD appear to result from three different morphogenetic processes:

1. failure of development of the common pulmonary vein, resulting in the supracardiac and infracardiac forms of TAPVC;
2. atrial septal malposition, resulting in partially or TAPVD to the RA; and
3. abnormal connection of the common pulmonary vein, resulting in TAPVC to the coronary sinus.

It is understood that there may ultimately prove to be more than three developmental mechanisms that can result in TAPVC and TAPVD. However, the foregoing is our best present understanding.

We would like to pay tribute to Dr. Jesse Edwards, who in 1953 proposed the concept that TAPVD may be due to malposition of the atrial septum:

> *Anomalous connection [of the pulmonary veins] with the superior portion of the RA may be explained on the basis of abnormality of the atrial septum. If the septum develops farther to the left than is normal, that outpouching of the sinoatrial region which joins the pulmonary vessels may lie to the right of the atrial septum and the entire venous system of the lungs will then connect with the right atrium. Lesser degrees of abnormal positioning of the atrial septum may account for cases in which the left pulmonary veins enter the LA while those of the right lung enter the right atrium.*

This concept was reaffirmed by Moller et al[11] in 1967. After our study[24] had been completed in 1994, we were delighted to rediscover Edwards' forgotten hypothesis[10,11] and to be able to demonstrate that the pathologic anatomic findings do indeed show septum primum malposition,[24] just as Edwards had foreseen. Now we must continue with those anomalies in which there is no horizontal vein for surgical anastomosis with the LA.

TAPVC to the Coronary Sinus. In TAPVC to the coronary sinus, there is no discrete horizontal vein. However, the coronary sinus can function as a horizontal vein from the surgical standpoint, and a large "window" can readily be made between the coronary sinus and the LA (see Figs. 7.10 and 7.17).[12] **The operative steps are as follows (see** Fig. 7.17**).**[12]

The RA is opened horizontally, from the right atrial appendage anteriorly and extending the incision posteriorly, stopping anterior to the sulcus terminalis to avoid injury to the tail of the sinoatrial (SA) node and to the posterior internodal tract or preferential internodal pathway. From the surgeon's perspective in the operating room, the SVC is to the left, the IVC is to the right, and the right atriotomy incision appears to be in a longitudinal or vertical direction, as opposed to a latitudinal or horizontal direction. This opening incision avoids both the SA node lateral to the entry of the SVC and the sulcus terminalis and crista terminalis where the posterior internodal tract or preferential pathway runs (see Figs. 7.10 and 7.17A). The aim of this careful placement of the right atriotomy is to avoid sick sinus syndrome or other atrial arrhythmias postoperatively.

The coronary sinus is relatively huge and has a cornucopia-like shape. A right-angle clamp is inserted into the markedly enlarged coronary sinus (see Figs. 7.17A and 7.17B). The apposed (conjoined) anterior wall of the coronary sinus and the posterior wall of the LA are then pushed up with the tip of the clamp so that the conjoined wall is displaced and can be seen through the patent foramen ovale (see Fig. 7.17B).

This tented-up wall is then grasped with toothed forceps and a piece is cut out, leaving an opening of at least 15 mm in diameter (see Fig. 7.17C). In this manner, a wide and sutureless opening is created between the coronary sinus posteriorly and the LA anteriorly (see Fig. 7.17D). This opening is made well within the coronary sinus, to the left of the orifice of the coronary sinus, so as not to injure the posterior internodal pathway or preferential tract that courses near the ostium of the coronary sinus (see Fig. 7.10).

The ostium of the coronary sinus is then closed with a running horizontal mattress stitch, placing the sutures at least 4 to 5 mm inside the ostium (see Fig. 7.17E), to avoid injury to the AV node and the internodal preferential conduction pathways (see Fig. 7.10). Alternatively, the coronary sinus ostium may be closed using a patch, placed well inside the large coronary sinus, to avoid any distortion of the surgically created coronary sinus septal defect—the "window" between the coronary sinus posteriorly and the LA anteriorly.

The patent foramen ovale is then sutured closed (see Fig 7.17F), placing the sutures through the *left* side of the superior limbic band of septum secundum to spare the middle internodal preferential conduction pathway that runs along the right side of the superior limbic band of septum secundum.

Parenthetically, it should be added that whether the internodal tracts shown in Fig. 7.10 actually exist as anatomically discrete internodal tracts or alternatively are preferential internodal conduction pathways (but not anatomically discrete tracts) remains controversial. This is why we have referred to them both as internodal *tracts* and as internodal *preferential conduction pathways*. Within either interpretation, these internodal regions are thought to be electrophysiologically important and hence should not be inadvertently damaged surgically.

The foregoing operation for the correction of TAPVC to the coronary sinus (Fig. 7.17)[12] is now known as the **Van Praagh procedure.** This operation was "born" in the Cardiac Registry of Children's Hospital Boston. The surgeon had attempted to redirect the coronary sinus blood flow through a surgically enlarged patent foramen ovale using a

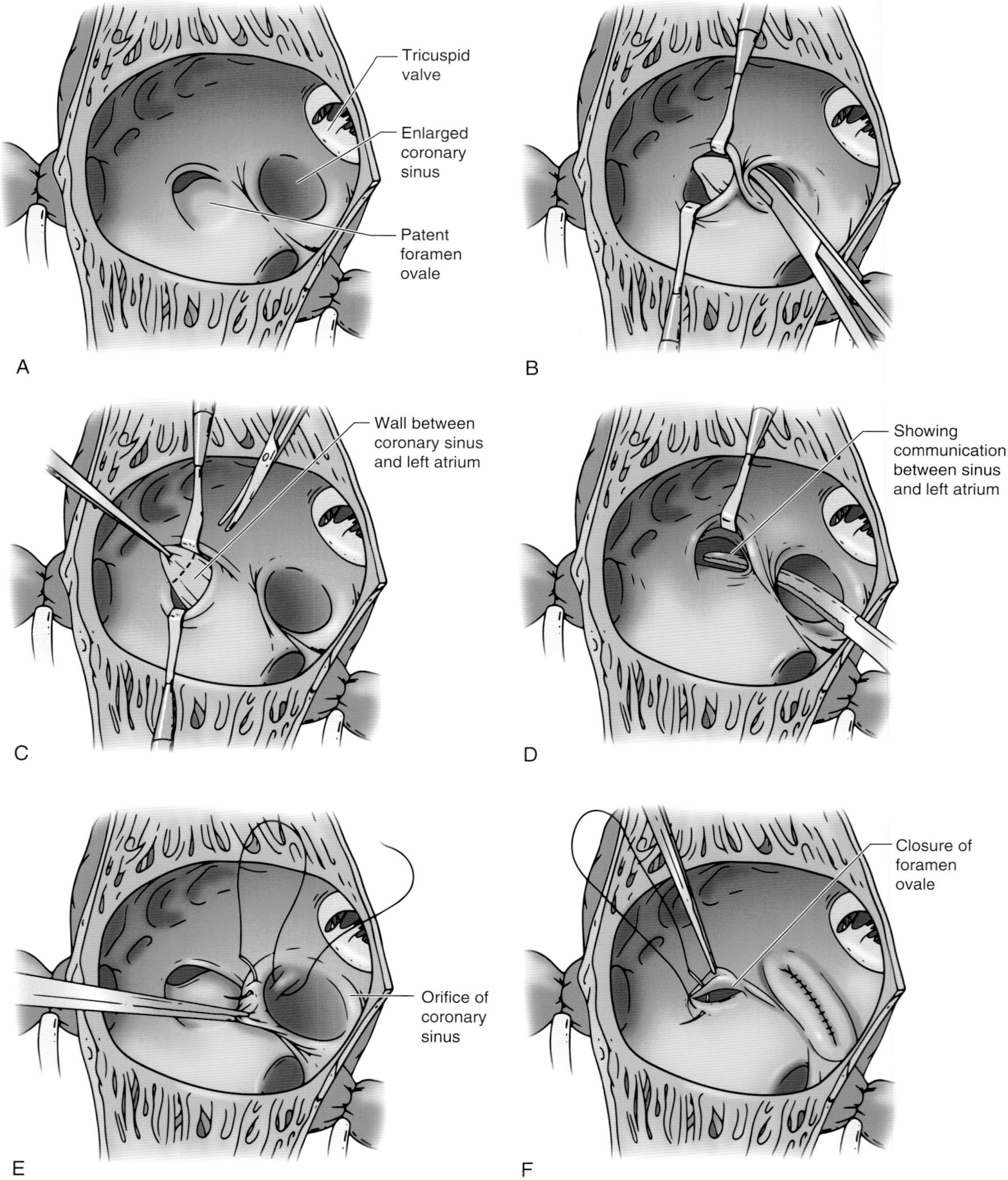
Tricuspid valve
Enlarged coronary sinus
Patent foramen ovale
A
B
Wall between coronary sinus and left atrium
C
Showing communication between sinus and left atrium
D
Orifice of coronary sinus
E
Closure of foramen ovale
F

Fig. 7.17 Surgical Repair of Totally Anomalous Pulmonary Venous Connection to the Coronary Sinus, Operative Technique.[12] (A) Right atriotomy. The lateral wall of the right atrium is opened quite anteriorly, to avoid the posterior internodal pathway that runs in the region of the sulcus terminalis and the crista terminalis (see Fig. 7.10). (B) Careful placement of a right-angle clamp into the enlarged coronary sinus and protrusion of the wall between the coronary sinus and the left atrium so this wall can be seen through the patent foramen ovale. (C) Grasping the tented-up wall between the coronary sinus and the left atrium, a large piece of this common wall is excised *(dotted line)*. (D) Demonstration of the large communication that has been created between the coronary sinus and the left atrium, that is, a large surgically created coronary sinus septal defect. (E) Running-suture closure of the enlarged ostium of the coronary sinus. The stitches are placed well to the left, within the orifice of the coronary sinus, to avoid injury to the atrioventricular node and the internodal conduction pathways. Alternatively, the enlarged coronary sinus ostium may be closed with a pericardial patch, placed well to the left, inside the coronary sinus. Patching may produce less alteration of adjacent anatomic structures than a running-suture closure. (F) Suture closure of the patent foramen ovale. The stitches are placed through the leftward portion of the superior limbic band of the septum secundum to avoid damaging the middle internodal pathway (see Fig. 7.10). This method of repair of totally anomalous pulmonary venous connection to the coronary sinus is known as the Van Praagh procedure. (From Van Praagh R, Harken AH, Delisle G, Ando M, Gross RE. Total anomalous pulmonary venous drainage to the coronary sinus: A revised procedure for its correction. *J Thorac Cardiovasc Surg*. 1972;64:132, with permission.)

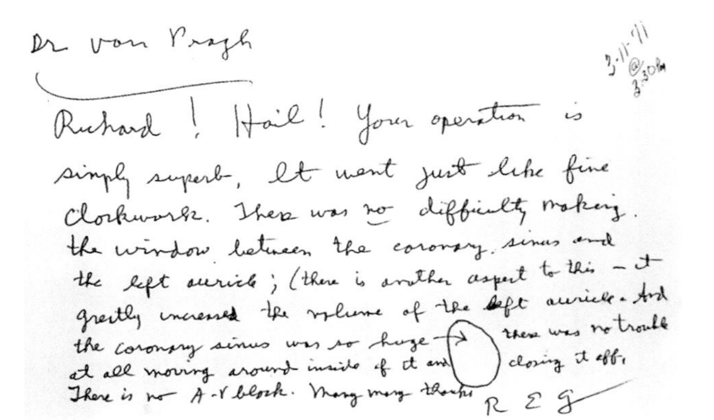
Dr van Praagh
3-17-71 @ 3:30pm
Richard! Hail! Your operation is simply superb, It went just like fine clockwork. There was no difficulty making the window between the coronary sinus and the left auricle; (there is another aspect to this — it greatly increased the volume of the left auricle. And the coronary sinus was so huge — there was no trouble at all moving around inside of it and closing it off. There is no A-V block. Many many thanks
R E G

Fig. 7.18 Dr. Robert E Gross's note to Dr. R. Van Praagh, just after Dr. Gross had operated on the first patient with totally anomalous pulmonary venous connection to the coronary sinus using the new technique illustrated in Figure 7.17.[12] (From Van Praagh R, Harken AH, Delisle G, Ando M, Gross RE. Total anomalous pulmonary venous drainage to the coronary sinus: A revised procedure for its correction. *J Thorac Cardiovasc Surg*. 1972;64:132.)

large U-shaped conduit between the coronary sinus ostium below and enlarged patent foramen ovale above. Autopsy revealed that the large U-shaped conduit had obstructed the IVC blood stream almost totally, leading to the death of the patient. The operation described previously was designed (1) to avoid vena caval obstruction, (2) to avoid pulmonary venous obstruction, and (3) to avoid interruption of the preferential internodal electrophysiologyic pathways between the SA and AV nodes.

On March 17, 1971, Dr. Robert E. Gross, the legendary pioneer of congenital heart surgery who first ligated a PDA in Lorraine Sweeney on August 26, 1938, sent me the following note (Fig. 7.18):

> *Dr. Van Praagh. Richard! Hail! Your operation is simply superb. It went just like fine clockwork. There was no difficulty making the window between the coronary sinus and the left auricle. There is another aspect to this—it greatly increases the volume of the left auricle. And the coronary sinus was so huge there was no trouble at all moving around inside of it and closing it off. There is no A-V block. Many thanks. REG*

Mixed Type of TAPVC. **In the mixed type of TAPVC,** occasionally there is no horizontal vein for the surgeon to suture to the LA. In the study by Delisle et al,[1] this situation was found in only 1 of 5 cases of mixed TAPVC (20%): the left lung drained via a snowman connection, and the right lung drained into the coronary sinus.

Agenesis of the right lung with anomalous pulmonary venous connection of the left lung merits mention. There were two such patients in the study by Delisle et al[1]: a snowman connection in one, and a coronary sinus connection in the other. However, the reason that this situation is noteworthy is that it can *mimic a vascular ring*. Agenesis of the right lung resulted in extrinsic dextrocardia. Because the heart was abnormally right sided, the normal left aortic arch compressed the tracheobronchial tree anteriorly and superiorly. To make matters worse, the large LPA was *posterior* to the left bronchus. (Normally, the LPA is anterior to the left bronchus.) Hence, the large LPA compressed the left bronchus posteriorly and inferiorly. The ligamentum arteriosum, and in one case an aberrant right subclavian artery, facilitated the external tracheobronchial compression.

From the surgical standpoint, in addition to correction of the anomalous pulmonary venous connection, steps to relieve the vascular tracheobronchial compression also may well be necessary, such as:

1. division of the ligamentum arteriosum, and
2. division of an aberrant right subclavian artery, if present, and aortopexy—attaching the aorta anteriorly in a subcostal or substernal location to reduce or eliminate the anteroposterior tracheobronchial compression.

Thus, with agenesis of the right lung, tracheobronchial compression appeared to be as important as the TAPVC, suggesting that both problems should be managed surgically.

With the exception of the aforementioned new morphogenetic understanding (three different mechanisms), the foregoing is essentially what we knew before undertaking the present study for this book. That which follows is what we have learned very recently by reviewing all of our data.

FINDINGS

This is a study of 204 postmortem cases of TAPVC and TAPVD that includes the 93 cases of Delisle et al[1] referred to previously.

Prevalence: TAPVC/D constitutes 6.34% of the cases of congenital heart disease in this study (204 of 3216).

Sex: The sex was known in 199 cases. Males = 121/199 (60.8%). Females = 78/199 (39.2%). Males-to-females = 121/78 = 1.55:1.0. Thus, there was a male predominance (61% versus 39%).

Age at Death: The age at death was known in 196 patients: mean = 448 · 959 ±
1239 · 519 days, that is, 1.23 years ± [1 standard deviation] 3 · 40 years, ranging from 0 (fetal demise) to 22.63 years. The median age at death was 39 days (1.3 months).

Heart position: The heart position was known in 202 patients: levocardia, 161 cases (79.70%); dextrocardia, 38 cases (18.81%); and mesocardia, 3 cases (1.49%).

Types of Patient: What types of patient had TAPVC/D? In other words, how many had *isolated TAPVC/D,* that is, with no other congenital heart disease and with no other associated malformations? How many had *nonisolated TAPVC/D,* that is, with other congenital heart disease and/or with associated malformations? And in the nonisolated TAPVC/D group, what were the other forms of congenital heart disease and/or associated malformations? These questions are answered briefly in Table 7.5.

Isolated TAPVC/D accounted for only slightly more than half of this series (51%; see Table 7.5). Nonisolated TAPVC/D was prominent (49%; see Table 7.5). It is interesting how different these numbers are from our earlier study of 93 postmortem cases of TAPVC/D[1] (see Table 7.2), in which isolated TAPVC accounted for 62% and nonisolated TAPVC for 38% (p = .07, i.e., not significant, but close).

In the present study, done in 2003, no case was omitted for any reason. The size of the nonisolated group was somewhat increased by the number of patients with visceral heterotaxy (n = 68; see Table 7.5). Heterotaxy accounted for 69% of the nonisolated group of TAPVC (see Table 7.5), similar to the earlier study (66%)[1] (see Table 7.2).

Table 7.6 conveys the anatomic complexity of these cases of TAPVC:

1. 7 different kinds of heart with normally related great arteries (solitus normally related, or inversus normally related);
2. 6 different kinds of heart with TGA;
3. 12 different kinds of heart with DORV;
4. 2 different types of double-outlet infundibular outlet chamber (with absence or marked hypoplasia of the right ventricular sinus, body, or inflow tract); and
5. 2 different types of anatomically corrected malposition of the great arteries.

TABLE 7.5 Types of Patients With TAPVC/D (n = 11)

Type of Patient	No. of Cases	% of Series
Isolated	102	51
Nonisolated	98	49
Heterotaxy with asplenia	58	29
Multiple congenital anomalies	23	11.5
Heterotaxy with polysplenia	8	4
Conjoined twin	5	2.5
Heterotaxy with normal spleen	2	1
Congenital heart block	1	0.5
Ellis-van Creveld syndrome	1	0.5

TAPVC/D, Totally anomalous pulmonary venous connection/drainage.

Anatomic Types of TAPVC/D

Perhaps the most important realization of the present study is that the anatomic types of TAPVC/D are linked to the type of visceroatrial situs that is present. The anatomic types of some forms of TAPVC/D are significantly different, depending on the anatomic type of visceroatrial situs that coexists (Tables 7.7 to 7.11).

For example, in visceroatrial situs solitus, the most common form of TAPVC/D was the snowman type to the LIV (38 cases, 30.16% of 126 cases; Table 7.7). By contrast, the snowman type of TAPVC was the rarest form in heterotaxy with asplenia (1 case, 1.72% of 58 cases; Table 7.8). TAPVC to the LIV (the snowman type) did not occur at all in the other nonsolitus types of visceroatrial situs: heterotaxy with polysplenia (n = 8; Table 7.9); heterotaxy with a normally formed spleen (n = 2; Table 7.10); and situs inversus of the viscera and atrial (n = 4; Table 7.11). This difference in the prevalence of the snowman type of TAPVC in visceroatrial situs solitus compared with nonsolitus types of visceroatrial situs is statistically highly significant ($p < .0001$, $x^2 = 23.97$).

Conclusions. TAPVC to the LIV (snowman type) was common in visceroatrial situs solitus (38; see Table 7.7), but rare in heterotaxy with asplenia (1.7%; see Table 7.8), and was not observed in small series of heterotaxy with polysplenia (see Table 7.9), heterotaxy with normally formed spleen (see Table 7.10) or in visceroatrial situs inversus (see Table 7.11).

By contrast, the prevalence of TAPVC to the ductus venosus was approximately the same in visceroatrial situs solitus (25.4%; see Table 7.7) and visceral heterotaxy with asplenia (27.6%; see Table 7.8). TAPVC to the ductus venosus was not observed in heterotaxy with polysplenia (see Table 7.9) or in heterotaxy with a normally formed spleen (see Table 7.10), but did occur in visceroatrial situs inversus (25%; see Table 7.11).

The data suggest that **TAPVC to the ductus venosus** is approximately equally as frequent in solitus and nonsolitus visceroatrial situs.

TAPVC to the coronary sinus occurred only in visceroatrial situs solitus (19%; see Table 7.7) but not in visceral heterotaxy (see Tables 7.8 to 7.10) and not in situs inversus (see Table 7.11) ($p < .0001$).

TABLE 7.6 Segmental Anatomy and Associated Malformations (n = 202)
1. **Normally Related Great Arteries (Solitus/Inversus) = 121 (59.90%)**
a. **{S,D,S},** n = 112 (55.45%)
Multiple congenital anomalies = 17 (8.42%)
Polysplenia = 3
Polysplenia without visceral heterotaxy = 1
Accessory spleen = 2
Ellis-van Creveld syndrome = 1
Holt-Oram syndrome = 1
Conjoined twin = 1
b. **{A(I),L,I},** n = 1 (0.5%)
Asplenia = 1
c. **{A,L,I},** n = 1 (0.5%)
Asplenia = 1
Sister with asplenia (i.e., familial asplenia)
d. Truncus arteriosus {S,D,S}, n = 2 (0.99%)
Multiple congenital anomalies = 1
e. **{S,L,S},** n = 2 (0.99%)
Asplenia = 1
Multiple congenital anomalies = 1
f. **{I,D,I},** n = 1 (0.5%)
Heterotaxy with normally formed spleen
g. **{I,D,S},** n = 2 (0.99%)
Polysplenia = 1
Congenital complete heart block = 1
2. **Transposition of the Great Arteries** = 16 (7.92%)
a. **TGA {S,D,D},** n = 6 (2.97%)
Asplenia = 2
Conjoined twins = 1
b. **TGA {S,L,L},** n = 1 (0.5%)
c. **TGA {A(S),L,L},** n = 2 (0.99%)
Asplenia = 2
d. **TGA {A (I), L,L},** n = 1 (0.5%)
Asplenia = 1
e. **TGA {I,D,D},** n = 1 (0.5%)
f. **TGA {A(I),D,D},** n = 5 (2.48%)
Asplenia = 4/5
Familial asplenia = 1 (brother with asplenia)
3. **Double-Outlet Right Ventricle** = 62 (30.69%)
a. **DORV {S,D,D},** n = 13 (6.44%)
Asplenia = 5
Conjoined twin = 3
Conjoined & asplenia = 1
Polysplenia = 1
Multiple congenital anomalies and DiGeorge syndrome = 1
b. **DORV {A(S),D,D},** n = 12 (5.94%)
Asplenia = 10
Familial asplenia = 1
Polysplenia = 2
c. **DORV {A,D,D},** n = 7 (3.47%)
Asplenia = 7
Twin = 1
d. **DORV {A,D,L},** n = 1 (0.5%)
Asplenia = 1
e. **DORV {I,L,L},** n = 3 (1.49%)
f. **DORV {A(I),L,L},** n = 7 (3.47%)
Asplenia = 5
Asplenia & trisomy 13 = 1
Polysplenia = 2
g. **DORV {A(I),L,A},** n = 1 (0.5%)
? Asplenia = 1 (autopsy limited to heart and lungs)
h. **DORV {A(I),L,D},** n = 1 (0.5%)
Asplenia = 1
i. **DORV {A,L,L},** n = 3 (1.49%)
Asplenia = 3
j. **DORV {A(S),L,L},** n = 6 (2.97%)
Asplenia = 6
k. **DORV {A(I),D,D},** n = 7 (3.47%)
Asplenia = 6
Heterotaxy with normally formed spleen = 1
l. **DORV {I(S),D,D},** n = 1 (0.5%)
Common gastrointestinal mesentery
4. **Double-Outlet Infundibular Outlet Chamber** = 3 (1.49%)
a. **DOIOC {S,D,D},** n = 2 (0.99%)
Multiple congenital anomalies = 1
Asplenia and conjoined twin = 1
b. **DOIOC {I,D,D},** n = 1 (0.5%)
Asplenia = 1
5. **Anatomically Corrected Malposition of the Great Arteries** = 2 (0.99%)
a. **ACM {A(I),D,L},** n = 1 (0.5%)
Asplenia = 1
b. **ACM {A,D,L},** n = 1 (0.5%)
Asplenia = 1

TAPVC to the coronary sinus occurred only in visceroatrial situs solitus.

The **mixed type of TAPVC** occurred both in visceroatrial situs solitus (10.3%; see Table 7.7) and in heterotaxy with asplenia (5.2%; see Table 7.8) and polysplenia (12.5%; see Table 7.9), but not in visceroatrial situs inversus (see Table 7.11) (p = NS, i.e., 0.25).

The prevalence of the **mixed type of TAPVC** in visceroatrial situs solitus and in visceroatrial situs nonsolitus (heterotaxy and situs inversus) was not significantly different.

TAPVC to SVC occurred in visceroatrial situs solitus (9.5%; see Table 7.7) but was much more common in heterotaxy with asplenia (53.5%; see Table 7.8), heterotaxy with polysplenia (25%; see Table 7.9), heterotaxy with a normally

TABLE 7.7 TAPVC/D in Visceroatrial Situs Solitus (n = 126/198, 63.64%)

Anatomic Type of TAPVC/D	No. of Cases	% of 126 Cases
1. Snowman to left innominate vein	38	30.16
2. To ductus venosus	32	25.40
3. To coronary sinus	24	19.05
4. Mixed	13	10.32
5. To right superior vena cava	11	8.73
6. To right atrium	5	3.97
7. To azygos vein	2	1.59
8. To left superior vena cava	1	0.79

TAPVC/D, Totally anomalous pulmonary venous connection/drainage.

TABLE 7.8 TAPVC/D With Heterotaxy and Asplenia (n = 58/198, 29.29%)

Anatomic Type of TAPVC/D	No. of Cases	% of 58 Cases
1. To superior vena cava, right or left	31	53.45
2. To ductus venosus	16	27.59
3. To right atrium, right- or left-sided	6	10.34
4. Mixed	3	5.17
5. Snowman, to left innominate vein	1.72	
6. To right side of common atrium	1	1.72

TAPVC/D, Totally anomalous pulmonary venous connection/drainage.

TABLE 7.9 TAPVC/D With Heterotaxy and Polysplenia (n = 8/198, 4.04%)

Anatomic Type of TAPVC/D	No. of Cases	% of 8 Cases
1. To right atrium	5	62.5
2. To right superior vena cava	2	25.0
3. Mixed	1	12.5

TAPVC/D, Totally anomalous pulmonary venous connection/drainage.

TABLE 7.10 TAPVC/D With Heterotaxy and Normally Formed Spleen (n = 2/198, 1.01%)

Anatomic Type of TAPVC/D	No. of Cases	% of 2 Cases
1. To superior vena cava—right atrial junction, left-sided	1	50
2. To right atrium, left-sided	1	50

TAPVC/D, Totally anomalous pulmonary venous connection/drainage.

TABLE 7.11 TAPVC/D With Visceroatrial Situs Inversus (n = 4/198, 2.02%)

Anatomic Type of TAPVC/D	No. of Cases	% of 4 Cases
1. To superior vena cava, left or right	2	50
2. To right atrium, left-sided	1	25
3. To ductus venosus	1	25

TAPVC/D, Totally anomalous pulmonary venous connection/drainage.

formed spleen (50%; see Table 7.10), and visceroatrial situs inversus (50%; see Table 7.11). Indeed, TAPVC to SVC (right or left) was by far the most common type of TAPVC in visceral heterotaxy (34/68, i.e., 50%; see Tables 7.8 through 7.10). These differences in the prevalence of TAPVC to SVC in visceroatrial situs solitus and in visceroatrial situs nonsolitus are very highly statistically significant ($p < .0001$, $x^2 = 38.62$).

TAPVC to the SVC is common in visceral heterotaxy and in situs inversus (see Tables 7.8 to 7.11) but is much less frequent in visceroatrial situs solitus (see Table 7.7).

TAPVC/D to the RA is infrequent in visceroatrial situs solitus (4%; see Table 7.7), but is more common in visceral heterotaxy with asplenia (10%; see Table 7.8), in heterotaxy with polysplenia (62.5%; see Table 7.9), in heterotaxy with a normally formed spleen (50%; see Table 7.10), and in visceroatrial situs inversus (25%; see Table 7.11). In our earlier study of 93 postmortem cases with Dr. Georges Delisle et al[1] in 1976, we never found TAPVC/D to the RA in the isolated form with visceroatrial situs solitus (see Table 7.3). Consequently, we concluded that TAPVC/D to the RA is characteristic of the nonisolated form, typically with visceral heterotaxy and asplenia or polysplenia.[1]

The present larger study of 198 (of a total of 204) autopsied cases of TAPVC/D shows that it is indeed possible to have TAPVC to the RA in visceroatrial situs solitus, that is, without visceral heterotaxy or situs inversus (3.97%; see Table 7.7). Nonetheless, the prevalence of TAPVC/D to the RA in visceroatrial situs nonsolitus (13/72, i.e., 18.05%) (see Tables 7.8 to 7.11) remains a statistically highly significant difference ($p < .001$, $x^2 = 10.98$) compared with the findings in visceroatrial situs solitus (see Table 7.7).

TAPVC/D to the RA is significantly more frequent in visceral heterotaxy (with asplenia, or polysplenia, or with a normal spleen) and in visceroatrial situs inversus than in visceroatrial situs solitus.

To summarize, TAPVC/D more frequently found in visceroatrial situs solitus includes:

1. TAPVC to the LIV (snowman type) ($p < .0001$) and
2. TAPVC to the coronary sinus ($p < .0001$).

TAPVC/D more frequently found in visceral heterotaxy and in situs inversus includes:

1. TAPVC to a SVC ($p < .0001$) and
2. TAPVC/D to the RA ($p < .001$).

TAPVC/D with prevalences that were not significantly different in visceroatrial situs solitus and nonsolitus (heterotaxy with asplenia, heterotaxy with polysplenia, heterotaxy with normal spleen, and visceroatrial situs inversus) include:

1. mixed TAPVC/D ($p = .25$, i.e., NS) and
2. TAPVC to the ductus venosus ($p = .78$, i.e., NS).

Associated Malformations

In Visceroatrial Situs Solitus (n = 126)

1. **TAPVC to the LIV (snowman type).** Obstruction was present in 9 of 38 cases (23.7%). Agenesis of the right lung was observed in 1 patient, and agenesis of the left lung in another case.

2. **TAPVC to the ductus venosus.** Atresia of the anomalous pulmonary venous pathway was present in 3 of 32 patients (9.4%). A conjoined twin was present in 3 other cases (9.4%), and multiple congenital anomalies (MCAs) were found in 2 patients (6.25%).
3. **TAPVC to the coronary sinus.** Obstruction of the anomalous pulmonary venous pathway was observed in 1 patient (A76-008), who had agenesis of the LPVs. Where the right pulmonary veins (RPVs) joined the coronary sinus, the junction was obstructive. This patient also had DORV {S,D,D}, with the DiGeorge syndrome and MCAs. This case proves that it is indeed possible to have TAPVC to the coronary sinus with congenital obstruction (stenosis or atresia), unrelated to prior surgery. Prior to this patient, we had thought (erroneously) that congenital obstruction did not occur with TAPVC to the coronary sinus.[1]
4. **Mixed TAPVC.** MCAs were present in 2 of these 13 patients (15.4%).
5. **TAPVC to the RSVC.** Obstruction was present in 3 of these 11 patients (27.3%). MCAs were found in 2 other patients (18.2%).
6. **TAPVD to the RA.** Of these 5 patients, 2 (40%) had MCAs, 1 of which had the Ellis-van Creveld syndrome.
7. **TAPVC to the azygos vein.** Both of these patients had severe stenosis of the anomalous pulmonary venous pathway (100%).

In Visceral Heterotaxy With Asplenia (n = 58)

1. **TAPVC to the RSVC.** Obstruction was present in 6 of these 20 patients (30%).
2. **TAPVC to the LSVC.** Obstruction was present in 4 of these 11 patients (36.4%).

In these 31 cases with TAPVC to a right or left SVC, obstruction was present in a total of 10 patients (32.3%).

3. **TAPVC to the ductus venosus.** Although some degree of obstruction may well have been present in all 16 cases (100%), it was particularly marked in 2 (12.5%).

Systemic Veins

Just as the types of pulmonary venous anomalies were linked to the types of visceroatrial situs that were present (as earlier), so too the types of systemic venous malformations were also linked to the types of visceroatrial situs that coexisted, as follows.

Situs Solitus of the Viscera and Atria (Present in 122 of 198 Cases of TAPVC/D [61.6%])

1. **Normal systemic veins** were present in 97 of 122 patients (79.5%). Abnormalities of the systemic veins were found in 25 cases (20.5%).
2. **Persistent LSVC to the coronary sinus to the RA** was present in 18 of 122 patients (14.75%). Although an abnormality, this anomaly led to no physiologic derangement because all of the systemic venous blood did indeed return to the morphologically RA.
3. **Interruption of the IVC** was found in 2 of these 122 patients with visceroatrial situs solitus (1.6%). The interrupted IVC was right-sided in 1 patient and left-sided in the other.
4. **Bilateral SVC with unroofing of the coronary sinus** was present in 1 patient (0.8%). Because of the large coronary sinus septal defect (unroofing of the coronary sinus), the blood of the left SVC drained into the LA.
5. **Bilateral SVC with hypoplasia of the right SVC** was found in 1 patient (0.8%). Bilateral SVC was observed in 2 of 122 patients with situs solitus of the viscera and atria (1.6%).
6. **Left SVC to LA, absence of an identifiable coronary sinus, and atresia of the right SVC** were present in 1 patient (0.8%). Unroofing of the coronary sinus explains why the left SVC drained into the LA and why a discrete coronary sinus was not found.
7. **Absence of the coronary sinus** was observed in 1 patient (0.8%) with visceroatrial situs solitus and TAPVC/D.
8. **Absence of the ductus venosus** was noted in 1 patient (0.8%).
9. **A small arteriovenous fistula between the descending aorta and the IVC** was present in 1 patient (0.8%).

Systemic Veins in Visceroatrial Heterotaxy With Asplenia.

Of the 198 patients with TAPVC in which the data were suitable for analysis, visceral heterotaxy with asplenia was present in 59 cases (29.8%). The complexity of the systemic venous anatomy is so great that it almost defies brief summary. Of these 59 cases with heterotaxy and asplenia, 1 patient was excluded because the systemic veins were not well described. Hence, the following is an analysis of 58 patients with TAPVC, heterotaxy, and asplenia.

In how many of these 58 cases of the asplenia syndrome did we think we could identify the anatomic type of atrial situs? The answer is in 46 of 58 patients (79.3%). We were not able to diagnose the atrial situs with confidence in 12 of 58 cases (20.7%).

The key to the understanding of the systemic veins in these patients is to diagnose, when possible, the basic anatomic type of visceroatrial situs that is present, despite the coexistence of visceral heterotaxy (anomalies of lateralization or asymmetry). The anatomic pattern of the systemic veins is linked to the visceroatrial situs and indeed is an expression of the visceroatrial situs.

What is (are) the basic type (s) of visceroatrial situs in the heterotaxy syndrome with asplenia? This is one of the mysteries of contemporary pediatric cardiology. Let us see what these cases suggest:

The atrial situs was diagnosed in 46 patients:

1. basically situs solitus of the atria, that is, {A(S,-,-}, in 26 of 46 cases (56.52%); and
2. basically situs inversus of the atria, that is, {A(I),-,-}, in 20 of 46 patients (43.48%).

This ratio of the proportions of atrial situs solitus to atrial situs inversus suggests an almost random distribution:

$$\frac{\text{Solitus}}{\text{inversus}} = \frac{56.52\%}{43.48\% \left(\frac{1.30}{1.0}\right)}$$

Now let us look at the 12 cases in which the atrial situs was not diagnosed but was recorded as situs ambiguus, not otherwise qualified, that is, {A,-,-}. The sidedness of the IVC was recorded in 9 patients:

TABLE 7.12 Systemic Venous Anomalies With TAPVC, Visceral Heterotaxy, and Asplenia

With Solitus Atria: {A(S),-,-}, n = 26/58 (44.8%)

Anomaly	No. of Cases	% of Series
Bilateral SVC	13	22.4
Left-sided IVC	4	6.9
IVC switches L→R at liver	1	1.7
Absent coronary sinus[a]	4	6.9
Unroofed coronary sinus [a]	3	5.2
Left-sided hepatic vein(s)	4	6.9
LSVC to CoS to RA	2	3.4
Atretic RSVC and LSVC to LA	1	1.7
Interrupted IVC	1	1.7

{A(S),-,-}, Situs ambiguus of the viscera with solitus atria; *CoS,* coronary sinus; *IVC,* inferior vena cava; *LA,* morphologically left atrium; *L→R,* left to right; *LSVC,* left superior vena cava; *RA,* morphologically right atrium; *RSVC,* right superior vena cava; *SVC,* superior vena cava; *TAPVC,* totally anomalous pulmonary venous connection.
[a]"Absent" and "unroofed" coronary sinus are essentially the same anomaly. The status of coronary sinus was not specified in the other 19 cases.

1. left-sided IVC6
2. right-sided IVC3

If one accepts that the sidedness of the IVC strongly suggests the basic type of visceroatrial situs that is present (right-sided IVC = probable situs solitus, and left-sided IVC = probable situs inversus), the findings become:

$$\text{Situs inversus} = \frac{26}{55\,(47.27\%)}, \text{ and}$$

$$\text{Situs inversus} = \frac{26}{55}\,(47.27\%)$$

Hence, the ratio of the proportions of situs solitus/situs inversus in this sample of the asplenia syndrome becomes 1 · 115, that is., quite close to 1:1, a randomized distribution of atrial situs. Thus, these findings suggest that **in visceroatrial heterotaxy with asplenia, the basic types of situs are approximately 1 to 1, or 50/50 (in percentages), that is, essentially randomized.**

If the aforementioned data are representative and the inferences are valid, this means that visceroatrial situs ambiguus with asplenia is much less ambiguous than it used to be just a few years ago. However, it is also noteworthy that there are some cases of the asplenia syndrome in which we were not able to diagnose the basic type of atrial situs with confidence, that is, {A,-,-} = 12/58 (20.7%).

The systemic venous anomalies found within each group, that is, {A(S),-,-}, {A(I),-,-}, and {A,-,-} are summarized in Tables 7.12, 7.13, and 7.14, respectively.

TABLE 7.13 Systemic Venous Anomalies With TAPVC, Visceral Heterotaxy, and Asplenia

With Inversus Atria: {A(I),-,-}, n = 20/58 (34.5%)

Anomaly	No. of Cases	% of Series
Bilateral SVC	7	12.1
Atresia of RSVC	5	8.6
Absent CoS	4	6.9
Unroofed CoS	4	6.9
Right-sided hepatic veins	5	8.6
RSVC to LA (R)	2	3.4
R→L switch of IVC to RA (L)	1	1.7
Interrupted IVC	1	1.7

{A(I),-,-}, Situs ambiguus of viscera with inversus atria; *CoS,* coronary sinus; *IVC,* inferior vena cava; *LA (R),* morphologically left atrium, right-sided; *RA (L),* morphologically right atrium, left-sided; *RSVC,* right superior vena cava; *SVC,* superior vena cava; *TAPVC,* totally anomalous pulmonary venous connection.

TABLE 7.14 Systemic Venous Anomalies With TAPVC, Visceral Heterotaxy, and Asplenia

With Undiagnosed Atrial Situs: {A,-,-}, n = 12/58 (20.7%)

Anomaly	No. of Cases	% of Series
Bilateral SVC	8	13.8
Left-sided IVC	6	10.3
Right-sided IVC	3	5.2
Absent CoS	3	5.2
Unroofed CoS	1	1.7
Right-sided hepatic vein(s)	2	3.4
Left-sided hepatic vein(s)	1	1.7
Left-sided hepatic vein to LIVC	1	1.7

{A,-,-}, Visceroatrial situs ambiguus, atrial situs not diagnosed; *CoS,* coronary sinus; *IVC,* inferior vena cava; *LIVC,* left-sided inferior vena cava; *TAPVC,* totally anomalous pulmonary venous connection.

Systemic Veins in Visceroatrial Heterotaxy With Polysplenia. In 198 well-documented cases of TAPVC, 9 had visceral heterotaxy with polysplenia (4.5%). The atrial situs was solitus, that is, {A(S),-,-}, in 6 patients (66.7%) and was inversus, or {A(I),-,-}, in 3 cases (33.3%). Although atrial situs solitus was more predominant in polysplenia (66.7%) than in asplenia (56.5%), this difference was not statistically significant (p = .25, NS, Fisher's exact test).

Thus, in this sample of visceral heterotaxy, patients with asplenia and patients with polysplenia both had atrial situs solitus and atrial situs inversus. The status of the spleen (asplenia versus polysplenia) cannot be used to infer the type of atrial situs present.

It is noteworthy that in this small series of patients with polysplenia, the atrial situs was *always* diagnosed with confidence. This is a characteristic difference between polysplenia (atrial situs can be diagnosed with confidence always, or almost always) and asplenia (atrial situs may not be diagnosed with confidence in ≈ 20% of cases). It also should be understood that because the concept of atrial isomerism is erroneous, it is therefore possible to diagnose the atrial situs of polysplenia patients almost always and to diagnose the atrial situs of asplenic patients usually (≈ 80%).

The salient associated systemic venous anomalies in the 6 patients with TAPVC, heterotaxy with polysplenia, and atrial situs solitus were as follows:

1. LSVC to coronary sinus, to RA, 4 of 6 (66.7%);
2. interruption of the IVC, 2 of 6 (33.3%); and
3. bilateral superior venae cava, 1 of 6 (16.7%).

One of these patients with polysplenia and visceroatrial situs solitus did not have heterotaxy. **Polysplenia without visceroatrial heterotaxy** is noteworthy and rare.

The salient associated systemic venous anomalies in the 3 patients with TAPVC, heterotaxy with polysplenia, and atrial situs inversus were as follows:

1. interruption of the IVC in all 3 (100%),
2. RSVC to coronary sinus to left-sided RA in 2 (66.7%),
3. bilateral SVC in 1 (33.3%), and
4. hepatic veins draining into the morphologically LA in 1 patient (33.3%).

Interruption of the IVC with an enlarged azygos vein to a SVC was observed in 5 of these 9 polysplenic patients (56%).

Systemic Veins in Visceral Situs Inversus. In 198 well-documented cases of TAPVC, situs inversus of the viscera was present in 6 patients (3.03%). The salient visceroatrial findings were the following:

1. The atrial situs was inversus in 5 of 6 patients (83%), just as one would expect.
2. In 1 patient, a 3-day-old boy, the IVC was left-sided, as expected, but it switched from left to right at the level of the liver to connect with a right-sided morphologically RA. In other words, there was **visceroatrial situs discordance of the {I(S),-,-} type.** The segmental anatomy was DORV {I(S),D,D}. The patient had a RSVC, with nonobstructive TAPVC to the RSVC, bilaterally trilobed lungs, a normally formed right-sided spleen, common gastrointestinal mesentery, common atrium, common AV valve opening into a single morphologically RV, absent morphologically LV, bilateral conus, pulmonary outflow tract atresia, absent left anterior descending coronary artery, left aortic arch (abnormal for visceral situs inversus), and a PDA (3 mm). This case is recorded in detail because of its rarity.
3. A persistent RSVC, resulting in bilateral SVCs, was found in 2 patients (33.3%).
4. Congenital complete heart block was observed in 1 patient (16.7%).

Systemic Veins in Visceral Heterotaxy With a Normally Formed Spleen. Of 198 well-documented cases of TAPVC, 2 (1.01%) had visceral heterotaxy with a normally formed spleen. The salient features of these 2 rare cases were as follows.

One was a 6-month-old girl with dextrocardia. The segmental anatomy was {A(I),D,I}, i.e., isolated ventricular noninversion. The IVC was right-sided, but it switched from right to left at the level of the liver and connected with the left-sided morphologically RA. The stomach and normally formed spleen were left sided. The SVC was left-sided and the coronary sinus was absent. There was TAPVC to the left-sided morphologically RA. The lobation of the lungs was solitus. A common atrium was present in association with completely common AV canal, type A of Rastelli. A single LV was present due to absence of the right ventricular sinus. Common-inlet LV was present. From the infundibular outlet chamber an atretic pulmonary artery originated. The aortic arch was right-sided, but the descending thoracic aorta was left-sided. A left-sided PDA connected the LPA and the left innominate artery (left PDA being inappropriate for situs inversus).

The other patient was a 7 4/12–year-old boy with dextrocardia and DORV {A(I),D,D}. The right-sided IVC switched from right to left at the liver and connected with the left-sided morphologically RA. The stomach and normally formed spleen were left-sided (echocardiographic observations, the autopsy being limited to heart and lungs). The coronary sinus was absent and there were bilateral SVCs. There was TAPVC to the junction of the LSVC with the left-sided morphologically RA, without obstruction. The right lung had 4 lobes and the left lung had 3. There was a partially common AV canal with an ostium primum type of ASD. The tricuspid component of the common AV valve was large and regurgitant. The mitral component of the common AV valve was adherent to the crest of the ventricular septum and was atretic. There was no VSD. The patient had a functionally single morphologically RV. The morphologically LV was minute, with neither inlet nor outlet. There was a subaortic conus, pulmonary atresia, and a left aortic arch.

Thus, visceral heterotaxy rarely does occur with a normally formed spleen, as these two cases of complex congenital heart disease illustrate.

PARTIALLY ANOMALOUS PULMONARY VENOUS CONNECTION/DRAINAGE

The main questions for consideration are:

1. What really is PAPVC/D?
2. How many anatomic types of PAPVC/D are there?
3. What are their relative prevalences?
4. Is PAPVC/D usually isolated? Or is it usually accompanied by other associated malformations (nonisolated PAPVC/D)?
5. Among the patients with nonisolated TAPVC/D, are there any patterns among the associated cardiac or noncardiac malformations?
6. Are some types of PAPVC/D clinically and therefore surgically important, whereas other types are far less important? This is a study of 45 postmortem cases of PAPVC/D.

Prevalence: PAPVC/D constituted 1.40% of the cases of congenital heart disease in this study (45 of 3216). PAPVC/D was much less frequent than TAPVC/D: 1.4% versus 6.34%.

Sex: The sex was known in all 45 cases: males, 21 (47%) and females 24 (53%). The male-to-female ratio was 21:24 (0.875). Thus, PAPVC/D was characterized by a female preponderance.

These findings are the opposite of those encountered with TAPVC/D, which had a male predominance: males, 121/199, 60.8%; females, 78/199, 39.2%; and male-to-female ratio = 1.55:1.0. However, these sex differences between PAPVC/D and TAPVC/D did not quite reach statistical significance (p = .08).

Age at Death: mean = 966 · 15 days, that is, 2.65 years ± [1 standard deviation] 2332 · 59 days, that is, ± 6.39 years, ranging from 0 (fetal death) to 25 years. The median age at death of patients with PAPVC/D was 75 days (2.5 months).

For comparison, the median age at death of patients with TAPVC/D was 39 days (1.3 months).

Scimitar Syndrome: Because the scimitar syndrome seems to be a real entity, whereas many of the other anatomic types of PAPVC/D may be random events, that is, failures of separation of the pulmonary venous and systemic venous plexuses (see later), we thought it might be useful to look at the data for patients with the scimitar syndrome in isolation, not admixed with data from the other anatomic types of PAPVC/D:

Sex: males, 3; females, 10; and male-to-female ratio = 3/10 (0.3:1.0).

Age at Death: mean = 151 days, that is, 5 months ± [1 standard deviation] 294 days, that is, ± 9.8 months, ranging from 0 postnatal days (fetal abortion) to 820 days, that is, 2.25 years. The median age at death of these 13 patients with scimitar syndrome was 10 days.

Comment:

1. The median age at death in patients with the scimitar syndrome (10 days) was much less than the median age at death in patients with PAPVC/D who did not have the scimitar syndrome (116 days, or 3.87 months).
2. The male-to-female ratio in patients with the scimitar syndrome (0.3) was very different from the ratio found in patients with PAPVC/D who did not have scimitar syndrome (18/14 = 1.3) ($p < .05$).

The anatomic types of partially anomalous pulmonary venous connection or drainage (PAPVC/D) that were found in 46 postmortem cases are summarized, in order of decreasing frequency, in Table 7.15. As Table 7.15 shows, we found 14 anatomically different types of PAPC/D, with the scimitar syndrome being the most common type in this series:

1. typical right-sided scimitar syndrome in 12 patients (26%), and
2. 1 rare case of left-sided scimitar syndrome (2%).

Hence, the total prevalence of the scimitar syndrome in this series was 28%.

TABLE 7.15 Anatomic Types of PAPVC/D (n = 45)

Anatomic Type	No. of Cases	% of Series[a]
1. Scimitar syndrome, right-sided	12	27
2. Right upper pulmonary vein to RSVC	12	27
3. Left upper pulmonary vein to left vertical vein to left innominate vein to RSVC	6	13
4. Sinus venosus defect, right atrial type	4	9
5. Sinus venosus defect, superior vena caval type	1	2
6. Ipsilateral pulmonary veins	2	4
7. Right pulmonary veins to RA with leftward malposition of septum primum and deficient septum secundum	1	2
8. All right pulmonary veins to RSVC immediately above SVC/RA junction	1	2
9. Right pulmonary veins to coronary sinus and right upper lobe vein also to left atrium	1	2
10. Right pulmonary veins and left lower lobe pulmonary vein via vertical vein to RSVC	1	2
11. Right pulmonary vein to azygos vein	1	2
12. Left upper pulmonary vein to coronary sinus	1	2
13. Left upper pulmonary veins to levoatrial cardinal vein to left innominate vein to RSVC	1	2
14. Left pulmonary veins through diaphragm to hepatic venous confluence on the upper surface of the liver to the right-sided inferior vena cava via stenotic orifice (left-sided scimitar syndrome)	1	2

PAPVC/D, Partially anomalous pulmonary venous connection/drainage; *RSVC,* right-sided superior vena cava; *SVC,* superior vena cava.
[a]Percentages are rounded off to the nearest whole number.

Scimitar Syndrome

The scimitar syndrome was christened in 1960 by Drs. Catherine Neill, Charlotte Ferencz, David Sabiston, and H. Sheldon[14] because of the curvilinear density that may be seen in the lower right lung field in the plain chest x-ray film of such patients. This curvilinear shadow—that is somewhat reminiscent of a curved oriental sword (scimitar)—is cast by the anomalous RPV that drains most or all of the right lung into the IVC just above or just below the diaphragm (Fig. 7.19).

Other cardinal features of the scimitar syndrome are an anomalous systemic arterial blood supply arising from the region of the celiac axis of the abdominal aorta and passing through the diaphragm to supply the lower right lung, a reciprocally small right pulmonary artery (RPA), hypoplasia of the right lung, and dextrocardia secondary to the smallness of the right lung. The detailed findings in these 12 cases of right-sided scimitar syndrome are summarized in Table 7.16.

Left-Sided Scimitar Syndrome. Our findings in what may be called the left-sided scimitar syndrome involved a 3-day-old female infant[15] and may be summarized as follows. A scimitar vein draining all of the left pulmonary venous blood passed through the diaphragm and into a hepatic venous confluence on the superior surface of the liver. From there, the anomalous left pulmonary venous pathway traveled rightward and joined the suprahepatic segment of the IVC via a stenotic orifice that was 3 mm in diameter. A single RPV connected with the LA. Numerous small pulmonary venous collaterals bilaterally connected with the intercostals veins.

Two relatively large systemic arteries from the abdominal aorta above the celiac axis penetrated the diaphragm and supplied the lower portions of the left lung and the right lung. Other smaller systemic collateral arteries from the descending thoracic aorta supplied the lungs bilaterally; that is, major aortopulmonary collateral arteries (MAPCAs) were present both from above and below the diaphragm.

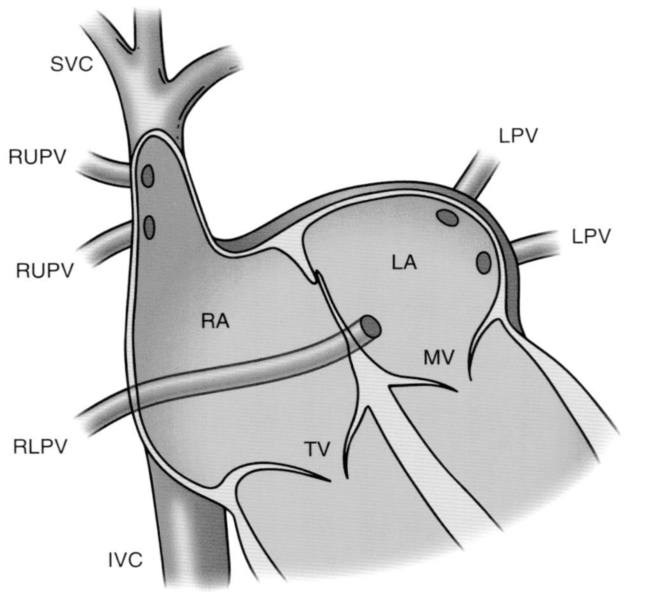

Fig. 7.19 Diagram of Right Upper Pulmonary Veins *(RUPV)* Connecting Anomalous With the Right Superior Vena Cava *(SVC)*. The right lower pulmonary veins *(RLPV)* and the left pulmonary veins *(LPV)* connect normally with the morphologically left atrium *(LA)*. *IVC*, Inferior vena cava; *MV*, mitral valve; *RA*, right atrium; *TV*, tricuspid valve. (From Van Praagh S, Carrera ME, Sanders SP, Mayer JE, Van Praagh R. Sinus venosus defects: Unroofing of the right pulmonary veins—Anatomic and echocardiographic findings and surgical treatment. *Am Heart J*. 1994;128:365-379; with permission.)

The RPA and LPA branches were strikingly hypoplastic and serpentine, we thought because of the major systemic arterial collateral blood supply to both lungs.

The IVC was interrupted, with absence of its renal-to-hepatic venous segment. An enlarged right-sided azygos vein connected with the RSVC. The spleen was normally located and normally formed.

We reported this rare case in 1979[15] because it represented a most unusual basis for persistence of the fetal pattern of the circulation. At autopsy, the PDA was small and appeared to be closing.

What Really Is the Scimitar Syndrome? As Table 7.16 shows, the scimitar syndrome typically is an anomaly of the right lung that almost always has a scimitar vein draining into the IVC (in 11 of 12 patients, 92%; see Table 7.16). The one exception had an anomalous RPV draining into the RA. In this case, the hypoplastic right lung received four moderately large systemic arteries from the celiac axis below the diaphragm that supplied 60% to 70% of the arterial blood supply of the hypoplastic right lung. Dextrocardia was present, secondary to the right pulmonary hypoplasia. The normally related great arteries produced severe tracheal compression anteriorly (treated with aortopexy), again secondary to the right pulmonary hypoplasia and the secondary dextrocardia. In view of all of the previously mentioned findings, we thought that this case should be regarded as a closely related variant of the scimitar syndrome, even though the signature finding—the scimitar vein—was not present in this rare case.

Thus, the main point is that the scimitar syndrome really is an anomaly typically of the right lung, with characteristic malformations of the systemic veins, and often with anomalous systemic arterial blood supply (in 58% of these cases; see Table 7.16).

The next point is that **both lungs can be abnormal,** as in 33% of our cases of right-sided scimitar syndrome (see Table 7.16) and as in our patient with left-sided scimitar syndrome.

Rarely is it possible to have a **scimitar vein with a normal ipsilateral lung.** Our case had a left-sided scimitar vein that ran behind the LA and then passed through the diaphragm and connected with the suprahepatic segment of the right-sided IVC. This patient (whom we are currently in the process of reporting) had elective surgical closure of a secundum ASD at 10 years of age. At 22 years of age, she had side-to-side anastomosis of the left pulmonary venous confluence with the LA, with ligation and division of the left-sided scimitar vein to the right of the anastomosis. Six years postoperatively, cardiac magnetic resonance imaging (MRI) showed that the anastomosis was widely patent. Ten years postoperatively, the patient remains asymptomatic. (This is a living and currently unpublished patient.)

Pulmonary pathologists regard typical scimitar syndrome as a special form of *intralobar sequestration*. We made the diagnosis of sequestration of the right lung—meaning that the right lung did not communicate normally with the right bronchus (hence the right lung was sequestered or separated from its bronchus)—in only 1 case (8%).

Familial congenital anomalies were noted in 1 of these patients (8%) and consanguinity (first cousin marriage) was recorded in 1 case (8%).

Although one usually thinks of the scimitar syndrome as occurring in isolation, it is noteworthy that **other forms of congenital heart disease frequently coexisted (see Table 7.16):** secundum type of ASD in 5 patients (42%); persistent LSVC to the coronary sinus in 4 (33%); preductal coarctation of the aorta in 3 (25%); muscular VSD in 3 (25%); conoventricular type of VSD in 2 (17%); mitral atresia in 2 (17%); polysplenia in 2 (17%), without visceral heterotaxy in 1 (8%); and truncus arteriosus, aberrant left coronary artery, right aortic arch Wolff-Parkiknson-White syndrome, and absent RPA in 1 case each (8%).

Perhaps even more impressive, **MCAs,** that is, malformations involving not only the cardiovascular system but also one or more additional systems, were present in more than half of these patients with the scimitar syndrome (58%; see Table 7.16).

Diagnostic and Surgical Implications

The scimitar syndrome is clearly a very serious clinical form of PAPVC because it is so much more than "just" a PAPVC.

TABLE 7.16 Findings In Right-Sided Scimitar Syndrome (n = 12)

Finding	No. of Cases	% of Series
Hypoplastic right lung	11	92
Bilaterally unilobed lungs	4	33
All right pulmonary veins to IVC	7	58
All right pulmonary veins to ductus venosus, to hepatic sinusoids, to RA	1	8
Inferior scimitar vein to IVC and superior vein to RSVC	1	8
Inferior scimitar vein to IVC and right upper pulmonary veins to LA	2	17
Right lower pulmonary vein to RA, all other pulmonary veins to LA	1	8
Anomalous arteries from abdominal aorta	7	58
Dextrocardia	6	50
Mesocardia	1	8
Ostium secundum type of ASD	5	42
LSVC to coronary sinus to RA	4	33
Preductal coarctation of the aorta	3	25
Mitral atresia	2	17
Conoventricular type of VSD	2	17
Muscular type of ventricular septal defect	3	25
Polysplenia {S,D,S}	2	17
Polysplenia without heterotaxy	1	8
Bicuspid aortic valve	2	17
Truncus arteriosus type A1	1	8
Truncal valvar regurgitation	1	8
Eccentric coronary ostia within sinuses of Valsalva	2	17
Aberrant left coronary from pulmonary artery bifurcation	1	8
Stenosis of left upper pulmonary vein	1	8
Right aortic arch	1	8
Wolff-Parkinson-White syndrome	1	8
Absent right pulmonary artery	1	8
Severe pulmonary hypertension, bilateral	1	8
Familial scimitar syndrome	1	8
Multiple congenital anomalies (i.e., more than the cardiovascular system involved)	7	58
Horseshoe kidneys, forme fruste (i.e., fibrous union at lower poles)	1	8
Microcephaly with lissencephaly	1	8
Bilateral cataracts	1	8
Septated vagina with uterus bilocularis	2	17
Multicystic right kidney	1	8
Left diaphragmatic hernia, foramen of Bochdalek type	2	17
Eventration of right leaf of diaphragm	2	17
Left umbilical vein passing through hepatic substance (not fissure) to reach porta hepatis	1	8
Right adrenal separated from right kidney	1	8
Left ovary extending up to left-sided spleen	1	8
Coloboma, left iris	1	8
Absent gallbladder, biliary tree otherwise normal	1	8

ASD, Atrial septal defect; *IVC,* inferior vena cava; *LA,* morphologically left atrium; *RA,* morphologically right atrium; *RSVC,* right superior vena cava; *{S,D,S},* the set of situs solitus *(S)* of the viscera and atria, D-loop ventricles *(D),* and solitus normally related great arteries *(S)*; *truncus arteriosus type A1, A,* ventricular septal defect *(VSD)* present, 1 = remnant of aortopulmonary septum present.

Diagnostically, one should not only document the scimitar vein but also search for additional anomalous right pulmonary venous connections. Also high on one's mental must-exclude list should be anomalous systemic arteries from below the diaphragm, or from above it, or from both sites of origin; additional types of congenital heart disease; and a wide variety of possible multisystem anomalies (see Table 7.16).

Surgically, although one would like to treat such patients as conservatively as possible—by baffling the scimitar venous return into the LA and by interrupting the anomalous systemic arterial blood supply typically from the region of the celiac axis (by surgical ligation or interventional coils)—one may be forced to do a right pneumonectomy, because typical scimitar syndrome is really a sick right lung, not just PAPVC, with or without anomalous systemic arterial blood supply from below the diaphragm.

Thus, in our experience, the scimitar syndrome is not only the most frequent form of PAPVC (13/45 patients, 29%), but also diagnostically and surgically the most serious form (see Table 7.16).

RUPV to RSVC. The right upper pulmonary vein (RUPV) draining anomalously into the RSVC was the second most common form of PAPVC that was encountered in the present series: 12 of 45 patients (27%; see Table 7.15).

In RUPV to RSVC (see Fig. 7.19), only one pulmonary vein drains anomalously. Consequently, RUPV to RSVC is a less severe form of PAPVC than is the scimitar syndrome, in which typically all RPVs drain anomalously.

Other differences from the scimitar syndrome are as follows: RUPV to RSVC typically is *not* associated with an abnormal right lung, right pulmonary hypoplasia, secondary dextrocardia, or anomalous systemic arterial blood supply.

What, then, is typical of RUPV to RSVC? It often is not the main diagnosis and consequently may be overlooked diagnostically and surgically. Prominent "main" diagnoses associated with RUPV to RSVC are presented in Table 7.17.

Thus, RULPV to RSVC was overshadowed by other more important diagnoses in 7 of these 11 cases (64%; see Table 7.17).

In addition to these seven major forms of congenital heart disease (see Table 7.17), other cardiovascular anomalies also coexisted with RULPV to RSVC (Table 7.18).

These 11 patients with RUPV to RSVC were associated with additional interesting data:

1. Abnormal lobation of the lungs was present in 3 cases (27%). In 1 case, both lungs had abnormal lobation. These findings indicate that RULPV to RSVC can be associated with abnormal lungs.
2. One of these patients was an identical twin; the co-twin was normal.
3. Familial congenital heart disease was present in 2 patients (18%). One had a brother with VSD and mild pulmonary stenosis. The other had a brother with tetralogy of Fallot (TOF) and pulmonary atresia.

What is the anatomic difference between RULPV to the RSVC, and sinus venosus defect of the SVC type? In RULPV to RSVC, the RULPV is anomalously connected to the RSVC typically at approximately the level of the azygos vein, and there is usually no interatrial communication. Indeed, an interatrial communication typically must be created by the surgeon to permit the RUPV blood to reach the LA.

TABLE 7.17 Prominent "Main" Diagnoses Associated With Right Upper Pulmonary Vein to Right Superior Vena Cava (n = 11)

Main Diagnosis	No. of Cases	% of Series
Truncus arteriosus	2	18
Type A1	1	
Type A3	1	
Tetralogy of Fallot	1	9
Pulmonary stenosis (very severe) with intact ventricular septum	1	9
Heterotaxy with asplenia and DORV {A(S),D,D}	1	9
Aortic atresia and mitral atresia with intact ventricular septum	1	9
Transposition of the great arteries {S,D,D} with VSD of AVC type, LVOTO (mitral tissue), PS (valvar and subvalvar) and cleft MV	1	9

AVC, Atrioventricular canal; *DORV {A(S),D,D},* double-outlet right ventricle with the segmental set of visceroatrial situs ambiguus, with the atria in situs solitus {A(S),-,-}, D-loop ventricles {-,D,-}, and D-malposition of the great arteries {-,-,D}; *LVOTO,* left ventricular outflow tract obstruction; *MV,* mitral valve; *PS,* pulmonary stenosis; *{S,D,D},* with the segmental set of situs solitus of the viscera and atria S,-,-], D-loop ventricles {-,D,-}, and D-transposition of the great arteries {-,-,D}; truncus arteriosus type A1,[17] ventricular septal defect (VSD) present (type A), with aortopulmonary septal remnant (type1); truncus arteriosus type A3,[17] ventricular septal defect (VSD) present (type A), with absence of a pulmonary artery branch (type 3).

By contrast, in sinus venosus defect of the SVC type, the right upper and often the right middle lobe pulmonary veins open somewhat lower into the RSVC, and there is a characteristic interatrial communication. This interatrial communication is the orifice of the RPVs into the LA. From the right atrial aspect, this interatrial communication is located above and behind the foramen ovale (or fossa ovalis, when the foramen ovale is sealed). From the left atrial aspect, this interatrial communication is just behind and somewhat above the septum primum. In sinus venosus defect, the pulmonary veins are thought to be normally connected with the LA. But the right upper and right middle pulmonary veins drain anomalously into the RSVC because of absence of the partition that normally separates the RPVs posteriorly from the RSVC anteriorly. In other words, the RPVs are "unroofed" into the RSVC because of absence of the partition that normally separates them.[9]

Thus, RUPV to RSVC is characterized by anomalous pulmonary venous *connection* and *drainage,* whereas a sinus venosus defect has anomalous pulmonary venous *drainage* with normal pulmonary venous *connection.*

Diagnostically and surgically, these differences are of critical importance. Generations of pediatric and adult cardiologists and cardiac surgeons have been erroneously taught that

TABLE 7.18 Other Forms of Congenital Heart Disease Coexisting With Right Upper Lobe Pulmonary Vein to Right Superior Vena Cava (n = 11)

Type of Congenital Heart Disease	No. of Cases	% of Series
Right pulmonary vein from right hilum to RSVC	1	9
Left superior vena cava to coronary sinus to right atrium	2	18
Common atrium	1	9
Ostium secundum type of ASD	1	9
Common AV canal	3	27
Mitral atresia with intact atrial septum	1	9
Ventricular septal defect	3	27
Membranous	1	
Conoventricular	1	
AV canal type	1	
Single right ventricle	1	9
Sinusoid from infundibular apical recess to left anterior descending coronary artery	1	9
Hypoplastic and bicuspid aortic valve (rudimentary right coronary/noncoronary commissure)	1	9
Preductal coarctation of aorta	1	9
Congenital absence of the ductus arteriosus	1	9
Aberrant right subclavian artery	1	9
Right aortic arch	1	9
Major aortopulmonary collateral arteries	1	9
Prominent right venous valve	1	9

ASD, Atrial septal defect; *AV*, atrioventricular; *RSVC*, right superior vena cava.

the interatrial communication is the sinus venosus ASD. In fact, this interatrial communication is the normal opening of the RPVs into the LA.[9] The partition that the surgeon creates to baffle the right pulmonary venous blood through the interatrial communication, which may or may not need enlarging, into the LA repairs the real sinus venosus defect.[9] The surgeon "re-roofs" the unroofed RPVs, thereby repairing the real sinus venosus defect between the RPVs posteriorly and the RSVC (or RA) anteriorly.

To summarize this point concerning differential diagnosis, if there is an interatrial communication posterosuperior to the foramen ovale (or fossa ovalis or septum primum), one is dealing with a sinus venosus unroofing defect of the RPV(s). However, if there is no characteristically located interatrial communication, one is dealing with RUPV to RSVC, which is the persistence of a normal embryonic connection of the right pulmonary venous plexus with the systemic venous system. Why such normal embryonic venous connections persist abnormally into the postnatal period remains unknown.

LUPV to the LVV to the LIV to the RSVC to the RA. This was the third most common anatomic type of PAPVC/drainage, occurring in 6 of these 45 patients (13%; see Table 7.15).

An LUPV connected anomalously with a LVV (Fig. 7.20). What is the LVV? Developmentally, it is the left anterior cardinal vein. Then why do we not call the LVV the LSVC? Dr. Jesse Edwards and colleagues thought that this vein should not be called the LSVC because it does not return to the heart the way the LSVC does. In other words, below the connection of the LUPV, this left anterior cardinal vein typically has undergone involution and is consequently either absent or atretic. So this is the understanding that lies behind the designation *LVV.*

The *left innominate vein* is a strange name, if one thinks about it. *Innominate* of course mean "nameless," or "no name." (If we can have a No-Name Restaurant, why not a no-name vein or artery?) The other name for the LIV is the left brachiocephalic vein.

The LULPV blood returns to the heart via the *snowman pathway.* Why is the LIV to the LIV to the RSVC to the RA called the *snowman pathway*? This term was coined for the typical form of supracardiac TAPVC. As mentioned previously, by about 4 months of age, this supracardiac anomalous pulmonary venous pathway becomes visible on the plain posteroanterior chest x-ray film. Then, with a little imagination, the cardiovascular shadow resembles a snowman, the heart shadow forming the body and the supracardiac venous shadow forming the head of the snowman.

The salient anatomic findings associated with LUPV to LVV to LIV to RSVC to RA are summarized in Table 7.19. Table 7.19 should be self-explanatory, with perhaps several exceptions.

What is TGA {S,D,L}? Just as the segmental anatomy suggests, there is AV concordance {S,D,-} and VA discordance—this being the definition of TGA. But the interesting and unusual feature is that the aortic valve is anterior and to the *left* relative to the pulmonary valve, that is, TGA {S,D,*L*} (Fig. 7.21)

The question is why is the transposed aortic valve to the left of the transposed pulmonary valve? The answer appears to be because the bulboventricular loop is malpositioned—not just the conus, but also the ventricles.

TGA {S,D,L} is a recently recognized distinctive form of complete or physiologically uncorrected TGA that is characterized by six additional interrelated anomalies[18]: (1) VSD, usually conoventricular, in 96%; (2) malalignment of the conal septum, typically leftward and posteriorly, in 80%; (3) right ventricular hypoplasia, in 50%; (4) pulmonary outflow tract stenosis, in 27%; (5) ventricular malposition, such as superoinferior ventricles, in 23%; and (6) absent left coronary ostium resulting in "single" right coronary artery, in 23%. Each of these six interrelated anomalies was associated significantly more frequently with TGA {S,D,L} than with the classic form of TGA {S,D,D} ($p < .01$ to $< .02$).[18] These characteristics associated malformations largely determined the surgical management of patients with TGA {S,D,L}.[18]

Mixed PAPVC was encountered in 2 of these patients (see Table 7.19). In addition to the LULPV to LVV to LIV to RSVC to RA pathway (the "snowman" pathway), 1 patient also had an anomalous RPV to the RSVC. Another patient also had a diminutive vein from the LVV to the coronary sinus.

Before reviewing these cases (see Table 7.19), we thought that the *mixed* type of anomalous pulmonary venous connection

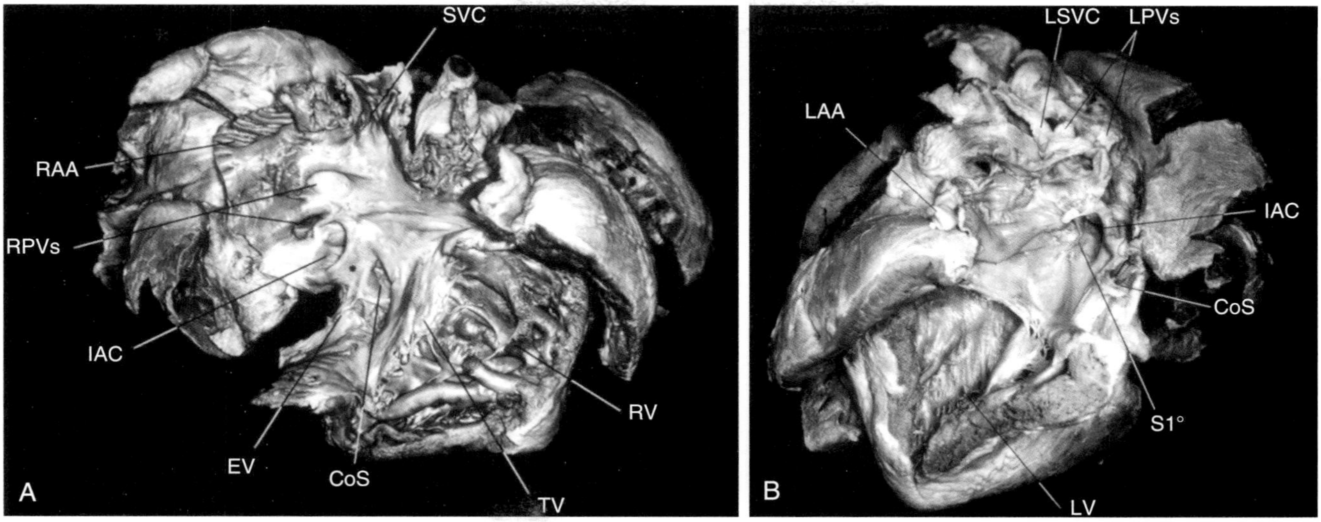

Fig. 7.20 Sinus Venosus Defect of the Inferior or Right Atrial Type. (A) Opened right atrium (RA), tricuspid valve *(TV)*, and right ventricle *(RV)*. The right pulmonary veins *(RPVs)* are unroofed into the RA because of absence of the partition that normally separates the RPVs posteriorly from the RA anteriorly. The coronary sinus *(CoS)* is enlarged because it receives a persistent left superior vena cava *(LSVC)*. The superior vena cava *(SVC)* connects normally with the RA. The Eustachian valve *(EV)* indicates the normal location of the inferior vena cava. The interatrial communication *(IAC)* is separated from the EV by the tissue of the septum primum *(SI°)*. *RAA,* Right atrial appendage. (B) Opened left atrium, mitral valve, and left ventricle *(LV)*. Note that the IAC lies directly posterior to the SI°, the IAC being in the location normally occupied by the ostia of the RPVs. Indeed, the IAC is the ostia of the RPVs. These right pulmonary venous ostia function as an IAC because the anterior wall of the RPVs and the adjacent posterior wall of the RA are both absent, this being the unroofing defect that creates a congenital window between the normally connected RPVs posteriorly and the RA anteriorly. The persistent LSVC is located anteriorly to the normally connected left pulmonary veins (LPVs). Thus, the IAC is the normal right pulmonary venous ostia (not a sinus venosus type of atrial septal defect, as has conventionally been taught). The real defect is not the IAC, but the unroofing defect or window between the RPVs posteriorly and the RA anteriorly. This is the real defect, that the surgeon repairs, by "re-roofing" the right pulmonary veins. This defect is misnamed: much more than sinus venosus (right atrial) tissue is involved because the anterior walls of the RPVs are also missing. Hence, the conventional understanding of so-called sinus venosus defect is significantly erroneous.[9] (From Van Praagh S, Carrera ME, Sanders SP, Mayer JE, Van Praagh R. Sinus venosus defects: Unroofing of the right pulmonary veins—Anatomic and echocardiographic findings and surgical treatment. *Am Heart J.* 1994;128:365, with permission.)

applied only to TAPVC. But these cases indicate that it is indeed possible for PAPVCs to be multiple and to occur at different sites.

The second case, mentioned previously, also very strongly suggests that the LVV in this anatomic type of PAPVC is indeed the LSVC, because the LVV connects with the coronary sinus (via a diminutive vein), just as a persistent LSVC does.

You will note that there were 2 cases of mitral atresia (33%; see Table 7.19). But 1 of these patients had left atrial outlet atresia, not really mitral atresia (see Table 7.19).

What is left atrial outlet atresia with a large morphologically LV and a small morphologically right ventricular sinus? We think that this rare entity is different from typical mitral atresia that has a diminutive LV. In this case of left atrial outlet atresia (that resembles mitral atresia), the LA is located above the LV free wall; consequently the left atrial outlet is blind. Pulmonary venous blood passed from LA to the RA (atrial septum was found to be surgically excised at autopsy). The RA opened into the large LV via an AV valve that was mitral in morphology. (This is why we think that mitral atresia really is not present.) The right ventricular sinus was small (not absent) and received no entering AV valve or tensor apparatus. This patient, a 4-month-old boy, also had TGA {S,D,L}, stenosis of the left atrial ostium of the common pulmonary vein, and diffuse hypoplasia of all pulmonary veins, without evidence of acquired pathological conditions. This patient also had mixed PAPVC: LUPV to LVV, and a diminutive vein from the LVV to the coronary sinus with an obstructive right atrial ostium of the coronary sinus.

So, what is left atrial outlet atresia with a large LV? Based on the previously mentioned anatomic description, we think that from the developmental standpoint, this entity represents *rightward malalignment* of a very abnormal bulboventricular loop relative to the atria. The result of rightward ventricular malalignment relative to the atria is that the outlet of the LA is blind because it is located above the left ventricular free wall. The AV valve opening from the RA into the LV is of mitral morphology; hence, our disinclination to make the conventional diagnosis of mitral atresia in this situation (with a large LV and an AV valve of mitral morphology). Why the bulboventricular loop is malaligned to the right relative to the atria remains unknown.

This entity was first reported, to our knowledge, by Quero.[19] In his case, the right ventricular sinus was absent, resulting in the arresting combination of "mitral atresia" with single LV,

TABLE 7.19 Salient Anatomic Findings Associated With Left Upper Pulmonary Vein to Left Vertical Vein to Left Innominate Vein to Right Superior Vena Cava to Right Atrium (n = 6)

Anatomic Finding	No. of Cases	% of Series
Conoventricular VSD	3	50
Muscular VSD	1	17
Transposition of the great arteries {S,D,L} (Figure 7.21)	2	33
Mitral atresia	2	33
Left atrial outlet atresia with large LV and small RV	1	
Poor incorporation of common pulmonary vein into left atrium	2	33
Nonstenotic junction with LA	1	
Tricuspid atresia	1	17
Ostium secundum type of ASD	1	17
Obstructive ostium of coronary sinus	1	17
Anomalous right pulmonary vein to RSVC, i.e., *mixed PAPVC*	117	
Mixed PAPVC	1	17
Diffuse hypoplasia of pulmonary veins	1	17
Patent ductus arteriosus, left-sided	1	17
Right aortic arch	1	17
Polysplenia	1	17
Aortic atresia with mitral atresia and intact ventricular septum	1	17
Truncus arteriosus type A2	1	17
Regurgitant quadricuspid truncal valve	1	17
Preductal coarctation of aorta	1	17
Multiple congenital anomalies: pectus excavatum, widely spaced nipples, increased carrying angle, shield-shaped chest	1	17

ASD, Atrial septal defect; *LA,* morphologically left atrium; *LV,* morphologically left ventricle; *LVV,* left vertical vein; *PAPVC,* partially anomalous pulmonary venous connection; *RSVC,* right superior vena cava; *RV,* morphologically right ventricle; *truncus arteriosus type A2,*[17] with ventricular septal defect (type A), and without aortopumonary septal remnant (type 2); *TGA {S,D,L},* transposition of the great arteries with the segmental anatomic set of visceroatrial situs solitus {S,-,-}, with D-loop ventricles {S,D,-}, and with L-transposition of the great arteries {S,D,L}; *VSD,* ventricular septal defect.

infundibular outlet chamber, and TGA, that is, TGA {S,D,D}. Quero[19] wanted to convince the medical world (and he certainly did) that single ventricle could indeed coexist with AV valve atresia. Single or common ventricle used to be defined as follows[20]: both AV valves or a common AV valve opens entirely or predominantly into one ventricle (Fig. 7.22) This old premorphologic definition of single ventricle tacitly excludes AV valve atresia. Quero's point was that this old definition of single ventricle[20] is unsatisfactory in this respect (see Figure 7.22)

We agree with Quero[19] about this. Even if mitral atresia is not really present in this entity (as earlier), we now know that single ventricle should be diagnosed in terms of its ventricular myocardial morphology, not in terms of the AV valves. For example, Quero's patient[19] had single RV (because the RV sinus was absent), whereas our patient did not (because the RV sinus was merely hypoplastic). Both Quero's case[19] and the present patient had "mitral atresia" or left atrial outlet atresia. The latter diagnosis we think is more accurate, as suggested earlier. This entity is merely one example of the importance of **ventriculoatrial malalignment.**

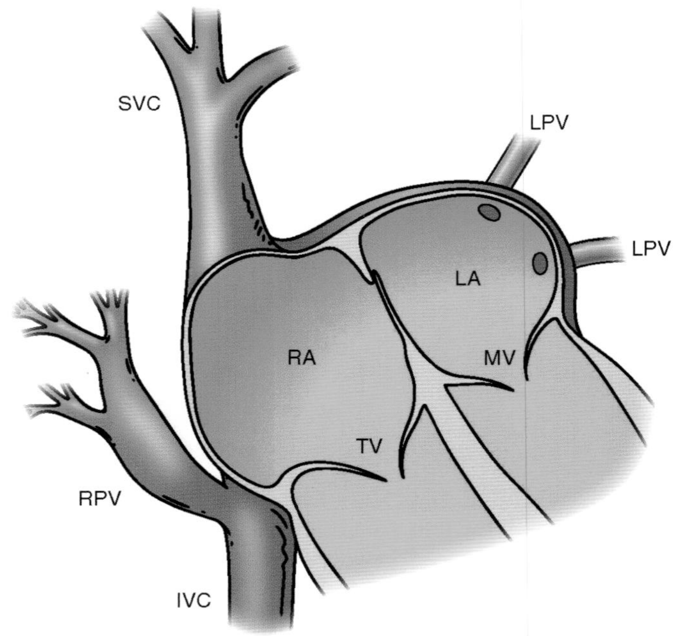

Fig. 7.21 Diagram of the Scimitar Syndrome. All of the right pulmonary veins *(RPVs)* typically connect anomalously with the inferior vena cava *(IVC),* just below the morphologically right atrium *(RA).* Only the left pulmonary veins *(LPVs)* connect normally with the morphologically left atrium *(LA).* The superior vena cava *(SVC)* typically connects normally with the RA. There may or may not be anomalous systemic arterial blood supply, typically from the celiac axis of the abdominal aorta to the lower right lung. The right pulmonary artery and the right lung may be hypoplastic. The heart may be abnormally right-sided, because of right pulmonary hypoplasia. The anomalously connected RPVs often create a curvilinear density in the posteroanterior chest x-ray film that is reminiscent of a scimitar—a curved oriental sword; hence the name of the syndrome.[14] The dextroposition of the heart may obscure the scimitar sign. *MV,* Mitral valve; TV, tricuspid valve. (From Van Praagh S, Carrera ME, Sanders SP, Mayer JE, Van Praagh R. Sinus venosus defects: Unroofing of the right pulmonary veins—Anatomic and echocardiographic findings and surgical treatment. *Am Heart J.* 1994;128:365-379; with permission.)

Sinus Venosus Defect, Right Atrial Type. This was the fourth most frequent type of PAPVD, occurring in 4 of these 45 cases (9%) (see Table 7.15). As was indicated in Chapter 6 concerning systemic venous anomalies, **sinus venosus defect** is absence of the partition that normally separates the RPV posteriorly from the RA anteriorly[9] (see Fig. 7.20). Consequently, the RUPV and right lower pulmonary vein (RLPV) drain anomalously into the RA.[9] However, the RPVs are connected normally with the LA, the posterior wall of the RPVs connecting normally with

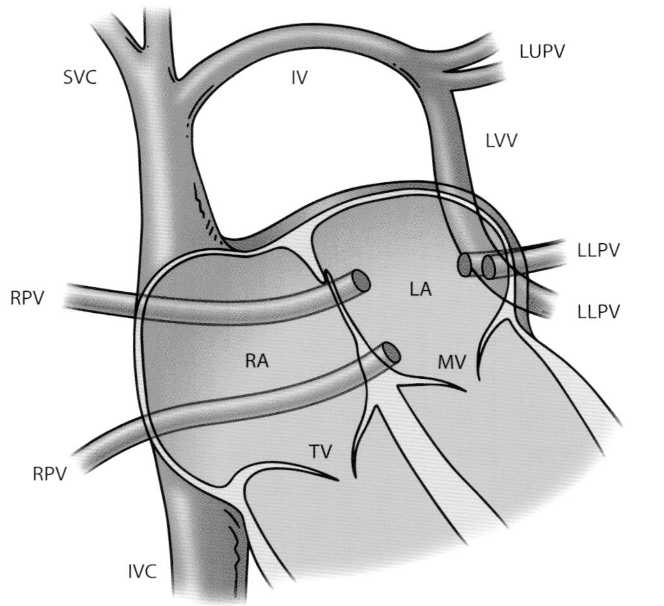

Fig. 7.22 Diagram of anomalous connection of the left upper pulmonary veins *(LUPV)* to the left vertical vein *(LVV)* and thence by the left innominate vein *(IV)* to the right superior vena cava *(SVC)* and right atrium *(RA)*. *IVC,* Inferior vena cava; *LA,* left atrium; *LLPV,* left lower pulmonary vein; *MV,* mitral valve; *RPV,* right pulmonary vein; *TV,* tricuspid valve. (From Van Praagh S, Carrera ME, Sanders SP, Mayer JE, Van Praagh R. Sinus venosus defects: Unroofing of the right pulmonary veins—Anatomic and echocardiographic findings and surgical treatment. *Am Heart J.* 1994;128:365-379; with permission.)

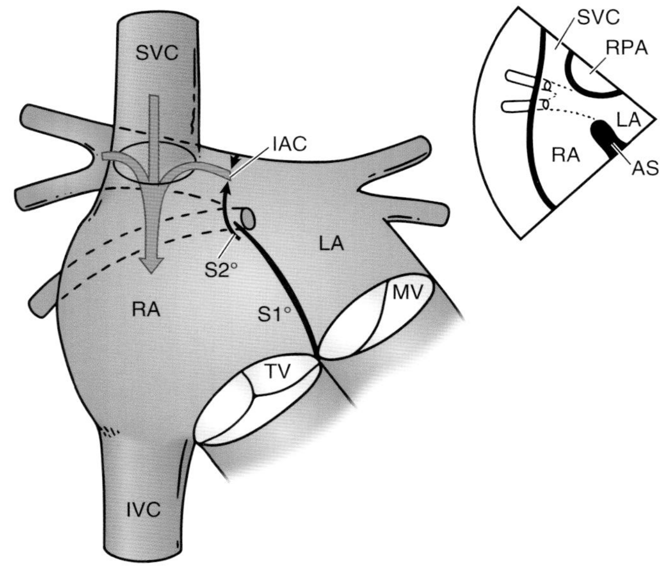

Fig. 7.23 Diagrammatic Representation of Sinus Venosus Defect of the Superior, or Superior Vena Caval, Type. Absence of the common wall between the superior vena cava *(SVC)* anteriorly and the right upper pulmonary vein posteriorly permits left-to-right shunting of blood from the right upper pulmonary vein into the SVC and right atrium *(RA)*. The interatrial communication *(IAC)* is not an atrial septal defect. Instead, it is the orifice of the right upper pulmonary vein *(arrowheads)*. *Inset* shows the normal course of the right upper pulmonary vein behind the inferior portion of the SVC, explaining why absence of the common wall between these two contiguous structures results in a sinus venosus defect of the SVC type. *AS,* Atrial septum; *IVC,* inferior vena cava; *MV,* mitral valve; *RPA;* right pulmonary artery; *S1°,* septum primum; *S2°,* septum secundum; *TV, tricuspid* valve. (From Geva T, Van Praagh S. Anomalies of the pulmonary veins. In: Allen HD, Clark EB, Gutgesell HP, Driscoll DJ, eds. *Moss and Adams' Heart Disease in Infants, Children and Adolescents, Including the Fetus and Young Adult.* 6th ed. Philadelphia, PA: Lippincott Williams & Wilkins; 2001:736, with permission.)

the posterior wall of the morphologically LA,[9] as is also true in the SVC type of sinus venosus defect (Fig. 7.23). The interatrial communication is the ostium of the RPVs, which is located posteriorly and superiorly relative to the foramen ovale and septum primum.[9]

This interatrial communication plus the absence of the intervenous partition between the RPVs posteriorly and the SVC and/or RA anteriorly combine to function like an ASD, typically permitting left-to-right shunting at the atrial level.[9]

Surgical repair of sinus venosus defect involves the prosthetic creation of the missing intervenous partition, thereby closing the sinus venosus defect, with or without enlargement of the right pulmonary venous ostium where it enters the LA (the interatrial communication). The right pulmonary venous ostium into the LA may be smaller than normal apparently because of extensive left-to-right shunting from the RPVs into the RSVC and/or RA.

The foregoing is a relatively new understanding of sinus venosus defect.[9] Previously it was thought that the interatrial communication was the sinus venosus "ASD." We now understand that this interatrial communication is not an atrial septal *defect*. Instead, it is a normal opening posterosuperior to the septum primum (see Fig. 7.20B); that is, it is the normal opening of the RPVs where they connect with, and open into, the LA.

It is the unroofing of the RPVs (the absence of the intervenous partition) that makes this normal right pulmonary venous ostium function like an ASD.

A sinus venosus defect is the *right-sided* venous unroofing defect. Unroofing of the coronary sinus, including the Raghib syndrome, is the *left-sided* unroofing defect, that is, absence of the partition between the coronary sinus posteriorly and the LA anteriorly. The characteristic large, low, posterior interatrial communication of the Raghib syndrome again is not an ASD. Instead, it is an interatrial communication, that is, the ostium of the unroofed coronary sinus.

Thus, there are two venous unroofing defects: right-sided (sinus venosus defect) and left-sided (unroofing of the coronary sinus).

Finally, it should be understood that the so-called *inferior vena caval type of sinus venosus defect* is an error. The real problem here is absence of septum primum. Hence, the interatrial communication is very large and extends very caudally—right

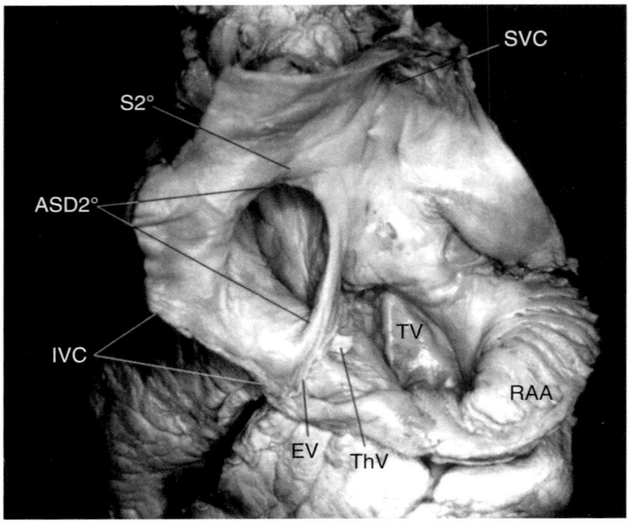

Fig. 7.24 **Huge Ostium Secundum Type of Atrial Septal Defect *(ASD2°)* in a 35-Year-Old Woman, Opened Right Atrial View.** The septum primum, the flap valve of the foramen ovale, is totally absent. Consequently, the lower border of the ASD2° is confluent with the inferior vena cava *(IVC)* and the Eustachian valve *(EV)* of the IVC. We think that the concept of a sinus venosus defect of the IVC type (meaning confluent with the IVC) is erroneous. Instead, such defects are secundum ASDs that are confluent with the IVC when the septum primum is absent, as in this patient. There is no "unroofing" defect in huge secundum-type ASDs that are confluent with the IVC. *RAA,* Right atrial appendage, *S2°,* septum secundum; *SVC,* superior vena cava; *ThV,* Thebesian valve of the coronary sinus; *TV,* tricuspid valve. (From Van Praagh S, Carrera ME, Sanders SP, Mayer JE, Van Praagh R. Sinus venosus defects: Unroofing of the right pulmonary veins—Anatomic and echocardiographic findings and surgical treatment. *Am Heart J.* 1994;128:365, with permission.)

down to the IVC—because the septum primum is absent[9] (Fig. 7.24). Thus, the so-called IVC type of sinus venosus defect is really a large ostium secundum type of ASD, due to absence of the septum primum. None of the RPVs are unroofed. The RPVs may well *drain* anomalously into the RA because of the absence of the septum primum.

Sinus venosus defects of the SVC and/or right atrial type have partially anomalous pulmonary venous drainage of the RPVs into the RA, but with normal pulmonary venous connections of the RPVs with the LA—and hence the characteristic posterosuperior interatrial communication (i.e., the right pulmonary venous ostium into the LA).

Sinus venosus defects are also considered in detail in Chapter 6 concerning systemic venous anomalies, because sinus venosus defects are both systemic venous anomalies (Chapter 6) and pulmonary venous anomalies (this chapter).

The salient anomalies associated with sinus venosus defect of the right atrial type (n = 4) are summarized in Table 7.20. Sinus venosus defects may be regarded as *nonisolated* (associated with other clinically significant congenital heart disease) or as *isolated* (not associated with other clinically significant congenital heart disease).

Thus, sinus venosus defect of the right atrial type usually was nonisolated (75%; see Table 7.20).

TABLE 7.20 Anatomic Findings Associated With Sinus Venosus Defect of the Right Atrial Type (n = 4)

Finding	No. of Cases	% of Series
Nonisolated	3	75
Incomplete form of common AV canal with ASD I, cleft MV, congenital MS, small LV, and TR	1	
Dextrocardia, DORV {S,L,L}, CA, CCAVC type C, unroofed CoS, PS (subvalvar and valvar, with bicuspid PV), IIVC with azygos vein to RSVC, large spleen (multilobed and horse-shoe shaped), right aortic arch	1	
Multiple congenital anomalies: tracheal origin of RUL bronchus, and AV malformation of scalp	1	
Isolated		25
Persistent LSVC to CoS to RA	1	

ASD I, Atrial septal defect of ostium primum type (one type of partial AV septal defect); *AV,* atrioventricular; *CA,* common atrium; *CCAVC,* completely common AV canal; *CoS,* coronary sinus; *DORV {S,L,L},* double-outlet right ventricle with the set of situs solitus of the viscera and atria, L-loop ventricles, and L-malposition of the great arteries; *IIVC,* interrupted inferior vena cava; *LSVC,* left superior vena cava; *LV,* morphologically left ventricle; *MV,* mitral valve; *PS,* pulmonary stenosis; *PV,* pulmonary valve; *RA,* morphologically right atrium; *RSVC,* right superior vena cava; *RUL,* right upper lobe (of lung); *TR,* tricuspid regurgitation.

Sinus Venosus Defect, Superior Vena Caval Type. Of these 45 patients with PAPVC/D, 1 had a sinus venosus defect of the SVC type (2%; see Table 7.15). The RUPV was unroofed into the RSVC–right atrial junction (Fig. 7.25A). The posterior wall of this RUPV connected normally with the LA and limited the interatrial communication posteriorly (see Fig. 7.25B). The foramen ovale was probe patent but functionally closed (see Fig. 7.25B). All of the other pulmonary veins connected normally with the LA (see Fig. 7.25B). This 10 10/12-year-old girl had a sinus venosus defect of the SVC type that was otherwise isolated (no other clinically significant cardiac or noncardiac anomalies). Note that in the normal LA, the normally located RUPV—the largest of the three ostia adjacent to the septum primum (S1°; see Fig 7.25C)—is in the exact location of the interatrial communication in sinus venous defects (see Figs. 7.20B and 7.25B).

The total incidence of sinus venosus defect, that is, of the SVC type and of the right atrial type, was 5 of 46 patients (11%; see Table 7.15).

Ipsilateral Pulmonary Veins. In this series of 45 patients with PAPVC/D, 2 had ipsilateral pulmonary veins (4%; see Table 7.15). *Ipsilateral* is derived from *ipse* meaning "self" (Latin), plus *lateralis* from *latus* meaning "side" (Latin). Thus, the designation *ipsilateral pulmonary veins* means that the pulmonary veins drain into the atrium of the same side: right-sided pulmonary veins drain into the right-sided atrium, and left-sided pulmonary veins drain into the left-sided atrium (Fig. 7.26).

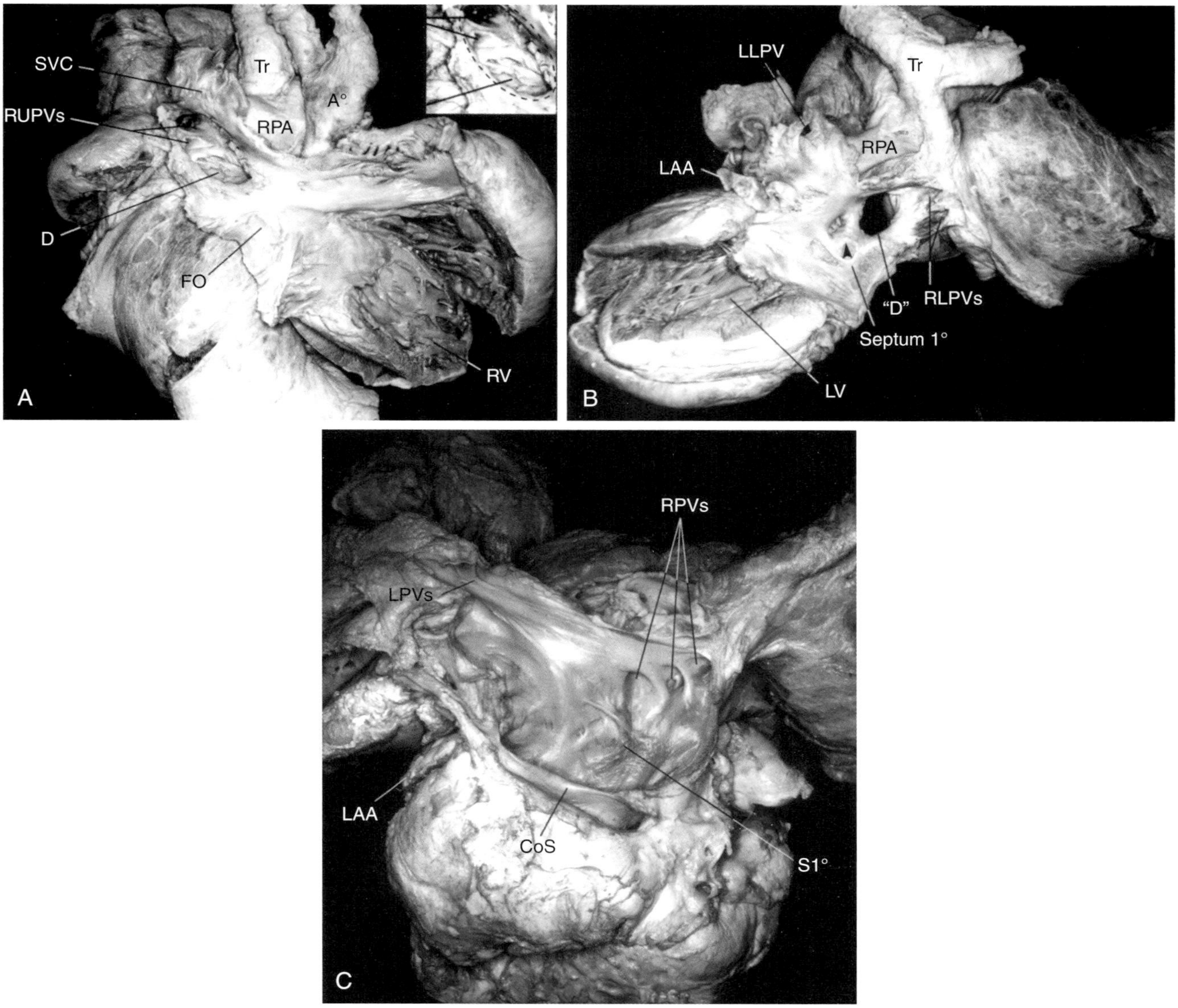

Fig. 7.25 Sinus Venosus Defect, Superior Vena Caval Type, in the Heart of a 10 10/12-Year-Old Girl. (A) The opened right atrium, tricuspid valve, and right ventricle *(RV)*. The ostia of the right upper pulmonary veins *(RUPVs)* are seen through a large defect *(D)* in the common wall between the RUPVs posteriorly and the right superior vena cava *(SVC)* anteriorly. This "unroofing" or "window" defect (D) lies beneath the right pulmonary artery *(RPA)*, where the right pulmonary veins are located. This defect (D), magnified in the *inset*, is located well above the fossa ovalis *(FO)*—the location of typical ostium secundum type of atrial septal defects. The left end of this D leads to the left atrium (LA) and constitutes the interatrial communication (IAC). (B) The opened LA, mitral valve, and left ventricle *(LV)*. Note that the interatrial communication (IAC) is located immediately posterosuperior to the septum primum *(septum 1°)*. (C) The opened normal left atrium of a 6 4/12-year-old girl with tetralogy of Fallot. It is noteworthy that this is exactly where the ostium of the RUPVs is located normally. The ostium of the RUPV is the largest of the three ostia of the right pulmonary veins (RPVs) seen in C. Consequently, we have concluded that the IAC is the ostium of the RUPV. Because of the "unroofing" defect, the ostia of the RPVs function as an IAC. This is why the conventional teaching has been that the sinus venosus type of ASD is located well above the FO, because the ostium of the RUPV heading into the LA is located above the FO. The IAC is not the sinus venosus defect; the IAC is the normal ostium of the RUPV. Instead, the real sinus venosus defect is the "unroofing" or "window" defect between the RUPV and the right SVC that lies to the right of the IAC and that the surgeon closes with a patch, thereby separating the RUPV and its branches from the right SVC. The surgical repair leads the RUPV return through the IAC into the LA. Thus, the surgeon does not close the IAC. Instead, he uses it as the ostium of the RUPVs—which it is. By separating the RUPV and the right SVC with a patch, the surgeon closes the sinus venosus defect, which lies to the right of the IAC. *CoS,* Coronary sinus; *LAA,* left atrial appendage; *LLPV,* left lower pulmonary vein; *RLPV,* right lower pulmonary vein. (From Van Praagh S, Carrera ME, Sanders SP, Mayer JE, Van Praagh R. Sinus venosus defects: Unroofing of the right pulmonary veins—Anatomic and echocardiographic findings and surgical treatment. *Am Heart J.* 1994;128:365, with permission.)

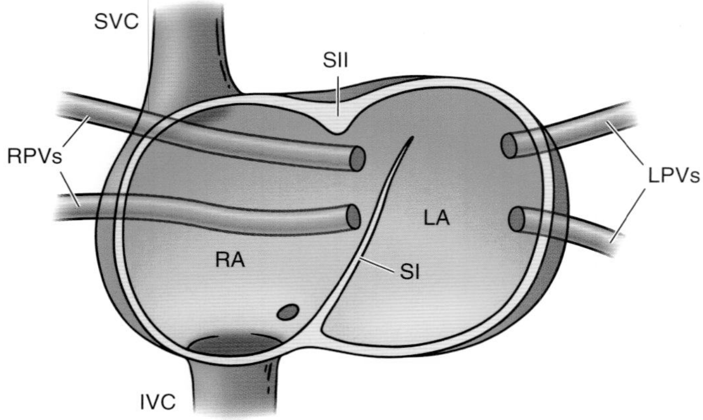

Fig. 7.26 Diagram of the Concept of Ipsilateral Pulmonary Veins. The right-sided pulmonary veins *(RPVs)* drain into the right-sided atrium, and the left-sided pulmonary veins *(LPVs)* drain into the left-sided atrium. Thus, the pulmonary veins of the side (right or left) drain into the atrium of the same side (right or left, respectively). The septum primum *(SI)* often is displaced or malpostioned into the morphologically left atrium *(LA)*. The septum secundum *(SII)* frequently appears underdeveloped, and SI does not attach normally on the left side of SII. Ipsilateral pulmonary veins often are associated with visceral heterotaxy with polysplenia. Pulmonary veins draining into both the left-sided and right-sided atrium are suggestive of bilaterally left-sided atria or left atrial "isomerism." Bilateral "left-sidedness" is regarded as a helpful teaching mnemonic (memory aid), but not as accurate anatomy. This form of partially anomalous pulmonary venous drainage, that is, ipsilateral pulmonary venous drainage, should certainly suggest the possibility of the polysplenia syndrome with visceral heterotaxy. With ipsilateral pulmonary venous *drainage,* we think the pulmonary venous *connections* are normal. We think that ipsilateral pulmonary venous drainage is due to leftward malposition of SI. Although the suprahepatic segment of the inferior vena cava *(IVC)* is present, the IVC frequently is interrupted between the renal and hepatic veins, with an enlarged azygos vein—often called an azygos extension—bringing the systemic venous return from the lower body to the superior vena cava *(SVC)* and thence to the morphologically right atrium *(RA)*. We think that the concept of ipsilateral pulmonary veins is prone to misinterpretation and misunderstanding in two main respects. (1) The pulmonary veins do not *connect* with opposite atria. Instead, they *drain* into opposite atria because of malposition of the septum primum. Ipsilateral pulmonary veins are *normally connected* with the dorsal wall of the LA. (2) The presence of ipsilateral pulmonary veins does not mean that the atria really have bilateral left-sidedness, that is, that there is an LA on both the right and left sides (left atrial isomerism). Anatomically accurate left atrial isomerism has never been documented in a single individual (conjoined twins excluded). But ipsilateral pulmonary veins should remind one of the mnemonic of bilaterally left atria and hence should suggest the possibility of visceral heterotaxy with polysplenia, which was present in both of our cases.

Both of these patients had visceral heterotaxy with the polysplenia syndrome. One was a 3-month-old girl with the segmental anatomic set of {A,D,S}, bilateral SVC, interrupted IVC, left-sided azygos vein to the LSVC, and suprahepatic IVC to the right-sided atrium. The morphology of the atrial septum was bizarre: neither septum primum nor septum secundum was clearly recognizable. It looked as though the septum primum and septum secundum were abnormally fused to each other, with both the right-sided and left-sided atrial septal surfaces being curiously featureless or "faceless." Neither side displayed either a right atrial or a left atrial septal surface morphology. The completely common AV canal type A was present. The coronary sinus was absent. The cardiac veins had multiple openings into the left-sided atrium. Biventricular hypertrophy, widely patent pulmonary and aortic outflow tracts, left aortic arch, and a large PDA (5 mm, internal diameter) were present. Other findings included a symmetrical liver (right lobe slightly larger than the left), right-sided stomach, three right-sided splenuli (4/14 g; i.e., hyposplenia), common gastrointestinal mesentery, appendix in the right lower quadrant, and bilaterally bilobed lungs.

The other patient with ipsilateral pulmonary veins was a 3-day-old boy, also with visceral heterotaxy and the polysplenia syndrome. The segmental anatomy was {A(I,S),L,I}. This segmental situs set is fascinating. There was visceral heterotaxy with situs ambiguus: {*A*-,-,-}. The abdominal visceral situs was thought to be basically situs inversus: {A (*I*,-,-}. The liver was symmetrical with a left-sided gallbladder. The stomach and the polysplenia were right-sided.

The atrial situs was thought to be solitus: {A (I,*S*),-,-}. The right-sided atrium had RA morphology, receiving the suprahepatic segment of the interrupted IVC, the RSVC (that received an enlarged azygos vein), the coronary sinus, and the RPVs. The left-sided atrium was small, had the morphologic appearance of a LA, and received only the LPVs. There was right-sided juxtaposition of the atrial appendages. The atrial septum was intact and malformed, with the septum primum and septum secundum being indistinct. Premature closure of the foramen ovale was present.

L-loop ventricles were present: {A(I,S),*L*,-}. The great arteries were inverted and normally related: {A(I,S),L,*I*}. Hence, there was **visceroatrial situs discordance,** with abdominal situs inversus and atrial situs solitus. **Isolated atrial noninversion** was also present; only the atria were not inverted.

Superoinferior ventricles were also noted. The small RV was superior, left-sided and left-handed, whereas the large LV was inferior, right-sided, and right-handed. The lungs were bilaterally trilobed (not bilobed, which is more usual with the polysplenia syndrome).

Comment: Ipsilateral pulmonary veins are where the concept of *bilateral left-sidedness* or *left atrial isomerism* comes from. This was part of Dr. Jesse Edwards' helpful teaching mnemonic that the polysplenia syndrome is characterized by "bilateral left-sidedness." The ipsilateral pulmonary veins were supposed to suggest that a LA is present bilaterally—because pulmonary veins are reminiscent of the morphologically LA on both the right and the left sides.

Other features of "bilateral left-sidedness" typically found with the polysplenia syndrome include bilaterally bilobed lungs (not present in this case), absence of the gallbladder (not present in this case), and interruption or "absence" of the IVC (present in this case).

As mentioned elsewhere, we think that the concepts of "bilateral right-sidedness" in the asplenia syndrome and "bilateral left-sidedness" in the polysplenia syndrome are helpful memory aids that should not be regarded as accurate anatomy. In the heterotaxy syndromes with asplenia and polysplenia, there is a good deal of crossover or overlap of morphologic features, as the case just presented illustrates.

It is also noteworthy that **right-sided juxtaposition of the atrial appendages** (i.e., dextromalposition of the left atrial appendage in atrial situs solitus) often is associated with left-sided hypoplasia,[21] as in the latter patient who had hypoplastic left-sided tricuspid valve and RV.

Conversely, **left-sided juxtaposition of the atrial appendages** (i.e., levomalposition of the right atrial appendage in atrial situs solitus) often is associated with hypoplasia of right-sided structures (AV valves and ventricles).[22,23]

Ipsilateral pulmonary veins are characteristic of visceral heterotaxy with polysplenia (see Chapter 29) and are underrepresented here.

From the developmental standpoint, S. Van Praagh et al[24] presented the hypothesis that whenever pulmonary veins connect at the atrial level, above the coronary sinus and between the SVCs, they are connected normally. We think that **malposition of the septum primum** accounts for ipsilateral pulmonary veins.[24] In the 2 patients presented earlier, the suprahepatic IVC was right-sided, leading to our diagnostic impression that the atria probably were basically in situs solitus.

In typical cases of the polysplenia syndrome (Chapter 29), the superior limbic band of septum secundum is poorly developed or absent, which is important because the septum primum normally attaches to the left side of the superior limbic band. When the septum secundum is poorly developed or absent, the septum primum has nothing to attach to superiorly. Consequently, the septum primum can get blown into the LA by the IVC blood stream, displacing the septum primum to the left of the RPVs and resulting in ipsilateral pulmonary veins (Figs. 7.15 and 7.26).

If our understanding of ipsilateral pulmonary veins is correct, this is a form of PAPVD (into the morphologically RA) with normal pulmonary venous *connections* because of malposition of the septum primum into the LA, to the left of the RPVs (in atrial situs solitus). Thus, PAPVC and PAPVD are two different concepts (not synonyms), as ipsilateral pulmonary venous drainage illustrates.

RPVs to RA With Leftward Malposition of Septum Primum and Deficient Septum Secundum. A 5-month-old boy had all RPVs draining into the RA, with leftward malposition of the septum primum and deficient development of the superior limbic hand of the septum secundum (1/45 patients, 2%; see Table 7.15). The segmental anatomy was {S,D,S}, and the spleen was normally formed. A persistent LSVC connected with the coronary sinus. The LA received the LPVs. Additional cardiovascular anomalies included mild to moderate congenital aortic stenosis, a bicuspid but nonstenotic pulmonary valve, and stenosis of the orifice of the right upper lobe pulmonary vein (RULPV) (<1 mm in internal diameter). This patient also had MCAs: hypospadias, polydactyly with six fingers on the left hand, and bilateral inguinal hernias. This patient could also be regarded as having *ipsilateral pulmonary veins* as in the previous discussion (see Table 7.15). However, we thought this patient merited separate presentation because heterotaxy with polysplenia was not present and because this patient had multiple noncardiovascular anomalies. Alternatively, this patient supports the view that ipsilateral pulmonary veins occur both with and without the polysplenia syndrome. But if polysplenia is not present, another multisystem malformation coexists. In other words, the anomaly of ipsilateral pulmonary veins was always nonisolated; that is, associated malformations were always present.

All RPVs to the RSVC Immediately Above the RSVC-RA Junction. Of these 45 patients with PAPVC/D, 1 (2%) had all RPVs connecting with the RSVC immediately above its junction with the RA (see Table 7.15; Fig. 7.27). This 2-day-old boy had MCAs: valvar pulmonary atresia with intact ventricular septum; Ebstein anomaly of the tricuspid valve with absence of the septal and posterior leaflets; and a deep, curtain-like anterior leaflet with greatly reduced interchordal spaces; Uhl disease of the RV with extreme thinning of the right ventricular free wall; secundum ASD with multiple fenestrations of the septum primum; partially common AV canal with primum ASD; cleft anterior mitral leaflet with thickening and rolling of the cleft free margins consistent with mitral regurgitation; parachute mitral valve with all primary chordae tendineae inserting into the anterolateral papillary muscle group; three left ventricular papillary muscle groups, that is, anterolateral and posteromedial (the two normal left ventricular papillary muscle groups), plus an anterosuperior papillary muscle group (unusual finding); double-orifice mitral valve with an accessory posteromedial orifice; PDA; origin of both carotid arteries from a single orifice and aberrant right subclavian artery; and hypospadias.

RPVs to Coronary Sinus and RULPV Also to LA. In 1 of 45 patients (2%; Table 7.15), an 8-day-old girl, almost all RPVs connected with the coronary sinus and thence to the RA, with one RULPV also connecting normally with the LA (Fig. 7.28). Again, this anatomic type of PAPVC was only one of many different kinds of congenital cardiovascular disease in this 8-day-old girl: DORV {S,D,D}; mitral atresia; diminutive LA with no left atrial appendage; patent foramen ovale; bilateral SVCs with LSVC to coronary sinus and RA, with absence of the LIV; small sinus venosus aneurysm from inferior surface of coronary sinus close to the RA and underlying diaphragmatic surface of the LV; bilateral azygos veins; rete Chiari; diminutive LV; right ventricular hypertrophy and enlargement, marked; tricuspid regurgitation; subpulmonary infundibulum with aortic-tricuspid fibrous continuity; subaortic conoventricular type of VSD; subaortic stenosis between conal septum anteriorly and tricuspid valve posteriorly; tubular hypoplasia of transverse aortic arch with discrete coarctation of the aorta (1.5 to 2 mm, internal diameter); large PDA, functionally closed or closing; and Wolff-Parkinson-White syndrome with episodes of reentrant orthodromic tachycardia. Low cardiac output and metabolic acidosis led to death. Bilaterally trilobed lungs were present. The state of the spleen was not observed (autopsy limited to heart and lungs).

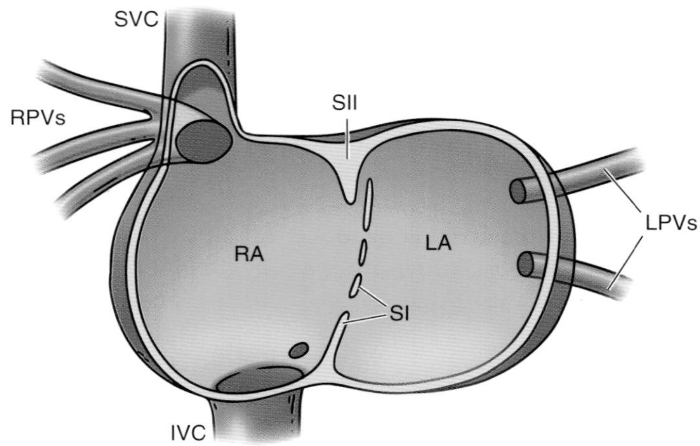

Fig. 7.27 All right pulmonary veins *(RPVs)* connect with the right superior vena cava *(SVC)* immediately above the SVC–right atrial *(RA)* junction. The left pulmonary veins *(LPVs)* connect normally with the left atrium *(LA)*. There is a secundum type of atrial septal defect (ASD II) due to multiple fenestrations in septum primum *(SI)*. This patient had multiple congenital anomalies, including hypospadias; pulmonary atresia (valvar) with an intact ventricular septum; partially common atrioventricular canal with an ostium primum type of ASD (ASD I) and cleft anterior leaflet of the mitral valve; parachute mitral valve with all primary chordae tendineae inserting into the anterolateral papillary muscle of the left ventricle; double-orifice of the mitral valve with severe mitral regurgitation; Ebstein anomaly of the tricuspid valve with a deep curtain-like anterior leaflet and absence of the septal and posterior leaflets of the tricuspid valve; Uhl disease of the right ventricular free wall; aberrant right subclavian artery; and origin of both carotid arteries from one orifice. *IVC,* inferior vena cava; *SII,* septum secundum.

Hence, this was a typical case of **DORV with hypoplastic left heart and a unilateral (subpulmonary) conus** with subaortic outflow tract stenosis and preductal coarctation of the aorta. This is Dr. Richard Rowe's *infantile type of DORV,* that is, with hypoplastic left heart (mitral atresia and marked LV hypoplasia). Why typical? Because the conus is unilateral, not bilateral as is usual with DORV and two well-developed ventricles.

Does the unilateral conus (in this case, subpulmonary) matter clinically? Very much so, because the unilaterality of the conus results in great arterial outflow tract obstruction. In this patient, there was aortic-tricuspid fibrous continuity because of the absence of subaortic conal free-wall musculature. This in turn led to subaortic stenosis because the aortic outflow tract was squeezed between the conal septum anteriorly and the tricuspid valve posteriorly. Subaortic stenosis led to reduced anterograde aortic blood flow, resulting in tubular hypoplasia of the aortic arch and predisposing to discrete coarctation of the aorta. The presence of a well-developed subpulmonary conus was associated with a widely patent pulmonary outflow tract and a large PDA.

Why did this patient die at 8 days of age? In addition to the presence of aortic outflow tract obstruction described previously, the ductus arteriosus was functionally closed. This meant that the lower body was deprived of adequate arterial blood flow, resulting in low cardiac output and metabolic acidosis, leading to death.

The presence of significant aortic outflow tract obstruction meant that the circulation was ductus arteriosus dependent. From a therapeutic standpoint, in this situation prostaglandin E1 and a Norwood procedure are urgently needed.

It is the presence of DORV with a unilateral (subpulmonary only) conus that leads to aortic outflow tract stenosis, which in turn makes the patient duct dependent. So, in DORV with hypoplastic left heart, the unilaterality of the conus can be very important if it sets up aortic outflow tract stenosis, as in this patient. This is as typical a type of DORV as is the Taussig-Bing malformation, but the infantile type of DORV remains largely unknown. This patient illustrates the very poor natural history of this type of DORV (hence nicknamed the "infantile" type) and why the natural history is so poor (duct dependency).

In this patient, the coexistence of PAPVC (almost all RPVs to the coronary sinus) would have been a physiologic advantage in view of the mitral atresia and the normally formed atrial septum (probably obstructive). This patient's PAPVC is physiologically reminiscent of the **Sterling Edwards procedure,** in which the atrial septum was repositioned between the RPV and LPV to force the RPVs to drain into the RA, thereby increasing atrial-level mixing, as was done in the early days of the surgical management of TGA. The Sterling Edwards procedure created ipsilateral pulmonary veins; so too did this patient's PAPVC.

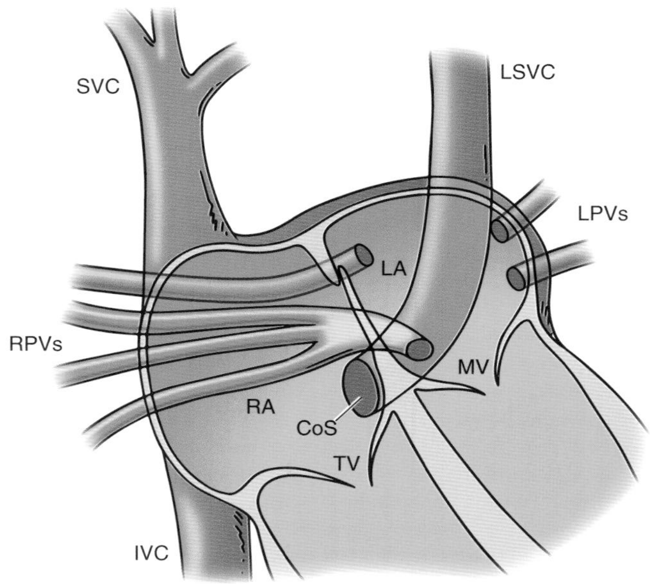

Fig. 7.28 Right pulmonary veins *(RPVs)* connecting with coronary sinus *(CoS)* and right upper lobe pulmonary vein also connecting normally with the left atrium *(LA)*. CoS is markedly enlarged because it also receives a persistent left superior vena cava *(LSVC)*. The left pulmonary veins *(LPVs)* connect normally with the LA. This rare form of partially anomalous pulmonary venous connection was just one part of complex congenital heart disease that included double-outlet right ventricle (DORV). The segmental anatomy was DORV {S,D,D}. Mitral atresia coexisted, this being the infantile type of DORV (so called because of its very unfavorable natural history). As is typical of the infantile type of DORV, the conus was unilateral (not bilateral): subpulmonary. There was aortic valve–tricuspid valve direct fibrous continuity (reflecting absence of subaortic conal musculature). The posteroinferior subaortic outflow tract was squeezed between the conal septum anteriorly and the tricuspid valve posteriorly, resulting in subaortic stenosis and reflected by the coexistence of coarctation of the aorta. Stenosis of the posterior great arterial outflow tracts is typical of the infantile type of DORV with a unilateral conus (subpulmonary or subaortic). There was a conoventricular type of ventricular septal defect (VSD) that opened into a hypoplastic left ventricle. The bilateral superior vena cavae *(SVC)* had bilateral azygos veins and absence of the left innominate vein. A small sinus venosus aneurysm extended downward from the CoS and underlay the left ventricle. The patient had Wolff-Parkinson-White syndrome. The lungs were bilaterally trilobed, but the status of the spleen was unknown because the autopsy permission was limited. *IVC,* Inferior vena cava; *MV,* mitral valve; *RA,* right atrium; *TV,* tricuspid valve.

RPVs and Left Lower Lobe Pulmonary Vein via Vertical Vein to RSVC. Of these 45 patients with PAPVC/D, 1 (2%; see Table 7.15) had all RPVs and the left lower lobe pulmonary vein (LLLPV) connecting via a vertical vein with the RSVC (Fig. 7.29). In this 20-week fetus, this type of PAPVC was but one part of complex congenital heart disease and MCAs: visceral heterotaxy with asplenia; TGA {A(S),D,D}; partially common AV canal with an ostium primum defect and common atrium (the presence or absence of a cleft anterior mitral leaflet remained uncertain because of artifact); absence of the coronary sinus; marked hypoplasia of the mitral valve and LV; pulmonary outflow tract atresia; hypoplasia of the PDA; bilaterally trilobed lungs; symmetrical liver with the right lobe slightly larger than the left; absence of the gallbladder (rare in asplenia); and cleft lip.

RPV to Azygos Vein and to the LA via the Stenotic Orifice. Of these 45 patients with PAPVC/D (2%; see Table 7.15), a 6¾-month-old boy had the RPVs connecting with the azygos vein and with the LA via a stenotic orifice (Fig. 7.30). The LPVs connected with the LA via a stenotic single orifice.

Again, this type of PAPVC was but one part of complex congenital heart disease and MCAs: DORV {S,D,D}; subpulmonary conus with aortic-tricuspid fibrous continuity and subaortic stenosis; mitral atresia; LV hypoplasia; conoventricular type of VSD and slit-like muscular VSD; and incomplete lobation of both lungs. It is noteworthy that this patient also had the infantile type of DORV with a hypoplastic left heart, a unilateral subpulmonary conus, and subaortic stenosis.

Therapeutically, this patient received a Damus-Kaye-Stansel procedure (for subaortic stenosis) and a central shunt to supply

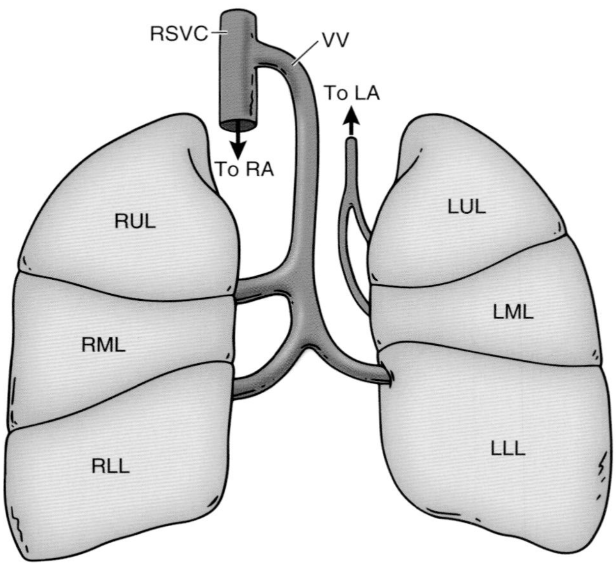

Fig. 7.29 All of right pulmonary veins from the right upper lobe *(RUL)*, right middle lobe *(RML)*, and right lower lobe *(RLL)*, and the left lower lobe *(LLL)* pulmonary vein connected with a vertical vein *(VV)* that in turn connected with the right superior vena cava *(RSVC)*. Small veins from the left upper lobe *(LUL)* and the left middle lobe *(LML)* connected with the left atrium *(LA)*. The patient was a 20-week-old male fetus with visceral heterotaxy and asplenia with transposition of the great arteries {A(S),D,D}. The salient findings were a common atrium with a partially common atrioventricular canal with marked hypoplasia (functional stenosis) of the mitral valve; marked hypoplasia of the left ventricle; enlargement of the right ventricle; absence of the coronary sinus; bilaterally trilobed lungs with eparterial bronchi; abnormally symmetrical liver with the right lobe somewhat larger than the left; absent gallbladder (rare with asplenia); presence or absence of mitral cleft uncertain because of artifact; cleft lip; pulmonary arterial outflow tract atresia; bilateral conus (subaortic and subpulmonary) with widely patent aortic outflow tract; left aortic arch; small left-sided patent ductus arteriosus (1 mm in diameter); right-sided atrial appendage larger and more anterior than left atrial appendage; inferior vena cava right-sided; no left SVC, and no ventricular septal defect. *RA*, Right atrium.

the pulmonary artery branches; a surgical attempt was made to relieve the ostial stenoses of the RPV and LPV that connected with the LA.

LUPV to Coronary Sinus. Of the 45 patients (2%), a 14-hour-old boy had the left upper lobe pulmonary vein connecting with the coronary sinus and thence to the RA. All other pulmonary veins connected normally with the LA (Fig. 7.31).

Again, this patient had MCAs (i.e., multisystem anomalies), including multiple cardiovascular malformations; choanal atresia; micrognathia; caudal displacement of external ears; absent gallbladder; normal segmental anatomy, that is, {S,D,S}; LSVC to the IVC above the diaphragm; normal spleen; truncus arteriosus with quadricuspid truncal valve and single coronary orifice; large secundum ASD; conoventricular type of VSD (associated with truncus arteriosus); and congenital absence of the ductus arteriosus.

LUPVs to Levoatrial Cardinal Vein to LIV to RSVC to RA. Of these 45 patients with PAPVC/D, 1 had the previously mentioned anatomic pattern (2%; see Table 7.15).

You may well be wondering, "What is a *levoatrial cardinal vein*? Just as the name suggests, this is an anomalous vein that runs from the LA (hence *levoatrial*) to the left anterior cardinal vein (hence *cardinal*). A levoatrial cardinal vein typically is present, apparently to decompress the LA, such as when mitral atresia coexists (as in this patient), with a functionally intact ASD (as in this patient) (see Fig. 7.2).

A levoatrial cardinal vein is different from a persistent LSVC inferiorly or caudally. A levoatrial cardinal vein (see Fig. 7.2) connects with the LA, not with the coronary sinus, which remains normally small; whereas a persistent LSVC connects with an enlarged coronary sinus, not with the LA. Superiorly or cranially, both a levoatrial cardinal vein and a persistent LSVC connect with the LIV (if the latter is present).

As is usual with PAPVC, this patient had **MCAs (multisystem malformations) and multiple other types of cardiovascular anomalies:** prominent helix of the right ear; dysplastic toenails; sacral dimple; familial congenital anomalies, that is, congenital deafness, patient's father being the fourth generation with Waardenburg syndrome, the cause of the patient's mother's deafness being unknown, and the patient's brother being congenitally deaf; familial congenital heart disease, a cousin having congenital heart disease; and this patient having hypoplastic left heart syndrome with mitral atresia, small secundum ASD (previously mentioned), aortic stenosis, intact ventricular septum, large PDA, juxtaductal coarctation of the aorta, and LULPVs to levoatrial cardinal vein to LIV to RSVC to RA (previously mentioned). The patient was treated with a modified Norwood procedure.

DISCUSSION OF PARTIALLY ANOMALOUS PULMONARY VENOUS CONNECTION AND PARTIALLY ANOMALOUS PULMONARY VENOUS DRAINAGE

In this series of 45 postmortem cases of PAPVC/D, 14 different anatomic types emerged (see Table 7.15). If one combines right-sided and left-sided scimitar syndrome cases (see Table 7.15), this reduces the anatomic types of TAPVC/D to 13.

Do we really think that there are only 13 different anatomic types of PAPVC/D? No. We strongly suspect that other anatomic types probably exist that are not represented in our series.

Nonetheless, the present study (see Table 7.15) represents the first attempt, to our knowledge, to answer the questions: How many anatomic types of PAPVC and/or PAPVD are there? What are they? And what are their relative prevalences?

Where did the PAPVCs arise from? The answer to this question is summarized in Table 7.21.

These 45 patients had 49 sites of origin of PAPVC. Origins of partially anomalous pulmonary veins from the right lung (38/49, 78%; see Table 7.21) were much more common than from the left lung (11/49, 22%). The ratio of right lung origins to left lung origins was 38/11 (3.45:1).

Why do PAPVCs arise so much more often from the right lung than from the left lung (see Table 7.21)? The answer to

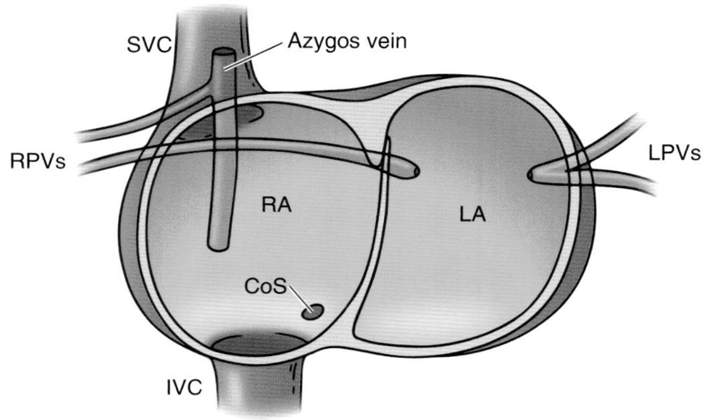

Fig. 7.30 Partially anomalous pulmonary venous connection (PAPVC): right pulmonary veins *(RPVs)* connect with azygos vein, this being a stenotic and anomalous connection. RPVs also connecting normally with the left atrium *(LA)* via a single stenotic orifice. All left pulmonary veins *(LPVs)* connect with the LA via a single stenotic orifice. Thus, there was congenital stenosis of all pulmonary venous ostia, one of which was connected anomalously from the right lung to the azygos vein. This patient was a 6¾-month-old boy with double-outlet right ventricle (DORV) {S,D,D} with mitral atresia, an unremarkable tricuspid valve, right atrial *(RA)* hypertrophy and enlargement, hypoplastic LA, surgically resected atrial septum, left ventricular (LV) hypoplasia, right ventricular hypertrophy and enlargement, two ventricular septal defects (1 VSD conoventricular in type, 4 to 5 mm in diameter, subaortic and 1 VSD mid-muscular, 1 × 6 mm), subpulmonary conus with aortic valve–tricuspid valve fibrous continuity. Hence, this patient had DORV with a hypoplastic left heart (mitral atresia and hypoplastic LV), that is, the infantile type of DORV (of Richard D. Rowe, MD) with a unilateral (not a bilateral) conus, that is, a subpulmonary (only) conus, permitting aortic-tricuspid fibrous continuity, which did not result in subaortic stenosis. The pulmonary outflow tract was also widely patent. The patient was status post Damuss-Kaye-Stansel procedure, that is, main pulmonary artery anastomosed end-to-side to the ascending aorta to circumvent the hypoplastic left heart, unnecessary in this case because of the coexistence of DORV without aortic outflow tract obstruction. The lungs were supplied by a patent central shunt. The azygos vein was surgically ligated at its entry into the superior vena cava *(SVC)*. The stenotic pulmonary venous ostia connecting with the LA were surgically cut back to enlarge them. The diagram reflects the preoperative anatomy. Thus, this case of obstructed PAPVC was associated with complex congenital heart disease, as earlier. *CoS,* Coronary sinus; *IVC,* inferior vena cava.

this question is thought to be as follows. Sinus venous defects in visceroatrial situs solitus always are right-sided. Malposition of the septum primum always occurs in a leftward direction in visceroatrial situs solitus, often resulting in ipsilateral pulmonary veins. Both of these malformations result in anomalous drainage of only the RPVs.

Spatial geometry also may be important:

1. The right lung is farther from the LA than is the left lung. This greater right lung–to-LA distance may predispose to a greater prevalence of right lung than left lung to PAPVCs.
2. The great systemic veins (IVC and SVC) are right-sided, perhaps making PAPVCs more likely from the right lung than from the left lung.
3. The systemic venous confluence, that is, the right horn of the sinus venosus, is right-sided and is an integral part of the morphologically RA. The right-sidedness of the normal systemic venous confluence may well predispose to a greater prevalence of PAPVCs from the right lung than from the left lung. The right-sidedness of the normal systemic venous confluence in visceroatrial situs solitus may well also explain why sinus venosus defects always involve the right lung and the RPVs and never involve the left lung and the LPVs (to the best of our present knowledge).

Where do the PAPVC/Ds go to? The answer to this question is summarized in Table 7.22. These 45 patients with PAPVC/drainage had 48 terminations or destinations of the anomalous veins that are presented in order of decreasing prevalence (see Table 7.22).

Of these 45 patients with PAPVC or drainage, only 3 were **isolated** (7%), whereas the vast majority were **nonisolated** (42 patients, 93%).

Isolated PAPVC/D means that no other significant cardiac or noncardiac anomaly was present; whereas *nonisolated* PAPVC/D means that other significant cardiac or noncardiac malformation coexisted. As the detailed analysis of these 45 patients with PAPVC/D indicated, PAPVC/D typically was associated with other congenital anomalies, cardiac and extracardiac.

Typically, PAPVC/D was but part of multiple cardiovascular anomalies, often also associated with noncardiovascular

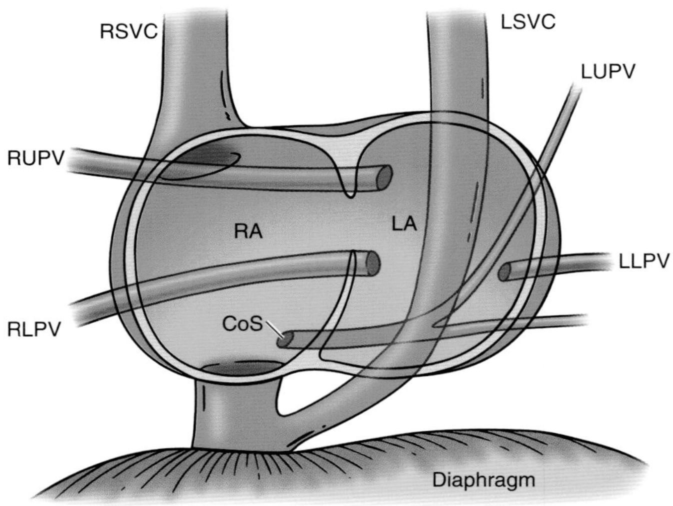

Fig. 7.31 Partially Anomalous Pulmonary Venous Connection (PAPVC). The left upper pulmonary vein *(LUPV)* connects with the coronary sinus *(CoS)*, the other pulmonary veins connecting normally with the left atrium *(LA)*: left lower pulmonary vein *(LLPV)*, right upper pulmonary vein *(RUPV)*, and right lower pulmonary vein *(RLPV)*. The systemic veins were also partially anomalous anatomically, but not physiologically. There were bilateral superior venae cavae: right superior vena cava *(RSVC)* and left superior vena cava *(LSVC)*. The left innominate vein was absent, there being no connecting vein between the LSVC and the RSVC. The LSVC communicated, via an anomalous systemic venous pathway, with the suprahepatic segment of the inferior vena cava (IVC) above the diaphragm. The LSVC did not communicate with the CoS. The LSVC connecting directly with the IVC above the diaphragm is an exceedingly rare anomaly. This patient was a 14-hour-old boy with normal segmental anatomy, {S,D,S}, a normally formed spleen, and multiple congenital anomalies: choanal atresia, absent gallbladder, absent ductus arteriosus, micrognathia, caudal displacement of the external ears, truncus arteriosus, quadricuspid truncal valve, single coronary arterial ostium, and large secundum type of atrial septal defect. Thus, the presence of PAPVC (LUPV to CoS) was only one of many congenital malformations, both cardiac and extracardiac, in this patient. *RA*, Right atrium.

TABLE 7.21 Origins of Partially Anomalous Pulmonary Venous Connections (n = 49)

Site of Origin	No.	Percentage
Right lung	38	78
Left lung	11	22

malformations (93%). So, PAPVC/D should be seen not in isolation, but as an integral part of more extensive cardiovascular and noncardiovascular anomalies.

These findings in PAPVC/D are in sharp contrast with those in TAPVC/D. It will be recalled (see Table 7.5) that TAPVC/D was isolated in 102 of 200 patients (51%) and nonisolated in 98 of 200 cases (49%). These differences concerning the isolation or nonisolation of the anomalous pulmonary venous drainage on comparison of TAPVC/D with PAPVC/D are statistically very highly significant ($p < .0001$, $x^2 = 29.4959$) (Table 7.23).

TABLE 7.22 Terminations of Partially Anomalous Pulmonary Venous Connections or Drainages (n = 48)

Termination	Percentage	No.
1. Right superior vena cava	16	33
2. Inferior vena cava	11	23
3. Morphologically right atrium	8	17
4. Left vertical vein to left innominate vein	6	12.5
5. Coronary sinus	3	6
6. Ductus venosus	1	2
7. Vertical vein to right superior vena cava	1	2
8. Azygos vein	1	2
9. Levoatrial cardinal vein to left innominate vein	1	2

TABLE 7.23 Isolated or Nonisolated?

Comparison of PAPVC/D and TAPVC/D

	PAPVC/D No.	%	TAPVC/D No.	%	*p* Value
Isolated	3	7	102	51	<0.0001
Nonisolated	42	93	98	49	49

DISCUSSION AND LITERATURE REVIEW ON PARTIALLY ANOMALOUS PULMONARY VENOUS CONNECTION AND DRAINAGE

In addition to the references already cited,[1-24] many more concerning pulmonary venous anomalies merit inclusion.[25-374] As usual, the references have been arranged approximately chronologically, from the earliest to the most recent, making it possible for the interested reader to trace the growth of the understanding of TAPVC/D, PAPVC/D, and other pulmonary venous anomalies.

Who first described TAPVC? To the best of our knowledge, it was Mr. James Wilson,[25] an English surgeon, in 1798. Mr. Wilson's fascinating case was communicated to the Royal Society of London on May 3 by Dr. Matthew Baillie, who only 5 years previously had discovered what we now call TGA and had presented this newly recognized anomaly to the Royal Society.

Mr. Wilson's case was complex indeed. The patient died at 7 days of age, and autopsy confirmed the presence of an omphalocele with the heart in the epigastrium. There was absence of the central fibrous tendon portion of the diaphragm and absence of the diaphragmatic portion of the pericardium. (This is a good description of thoracoabdominal ectopia cordis with an omphalocele and a large symmetrical diaphragmatic hernia, which is now known as the **Cantrell syndrome.**[26])

Wilson's patient[25] had a common atrium, right-sided juxtaposition of the atrial appendages, single ventricle, and truncus arteriosus. The RVP and LPV both connected with the LSVC, which also received a left azygos vein. The state of the spleen was not described. Our interpretation is based both on Wilson's description and on his diagram.

This case appears to be the earliest known description of not only TAPVC but also thoracoabdominal ectopia cordis, right-sided juxtaposition of the atrial appendages, common atrium, single ventricle, and truncus arteriosus.

How accurate is our interpretation of the pathologic anatomy of Wilson's case[25] likely to be? Here is the evidence. The heart was described as being in the epigastrium and associated with an omphalocele. The defects of the diaphragm and of the diaphragmatic pericardium were convincingly described. The TAPVC to the LSVC is depicted diagrammatically (Wilson's Fig. 7.3).[25] So too is the right-sided juxtaposition of the atrial appendages. The common atrium is called "single atrium" by Wilson.[25] The single ventricle is described as "single ventricle." But what about our diagnosis of truncus arteriosus, a diagnosis that Wilson did not make? Here is Wilson's[25] description:

> *A large arterial trunk arose from the ventricle, and ascended into the thorax, between the pleurae, immediately behind the thymus gland: it soon divided into two large branches, one of which continued to ascend, forming the aorta; the other passed backwards, and proved, upon examination to be the pulmonary artery.*

Note that the pulmonary artery arose from the *ascending* aorta, not from the aortic arch, nor from the descending thoracic aorta. Hence, Wilson's[25] "pulmonary artery" is likely to be just that, not a PDA, and not MAPCAs. Also, his description does not sound like an aortopulmonary window (i.e., an aortopulmonary septal defect). These, then, are our reasons for concluding that Wilson's patient had truncus arteriosus.

Several papers, among them that of Smith[29] in 1951, attribute the first description of anomalous pulmonary venous connection to **Winslow in 1739** (Mém. Acad. roy. d.sc. 1739, p 113). But when we chased this reference down, with the help of the Rare Books Department of the Countway Library of Medicine of Harvard Medical School, we discovered that the article referred to was really by M. Lémery entitled, *Sur Le Trou Ovale, Second Mémoire [On the Foramen Ovale, Second Memoire].* On page 113 (referred to in the reference), paragraph two may be translated from French as follows. M. (the abbreviation for Monsieur or Mister) Lémery writes:

> *Consequently, when one finds no foramen ovale in a fetus, otherwise well formed, which is very rare, it is necessary that there is some supplement to (or replacement for) the foramen ovale, and this supplement must not be searched for in the size of the patent ductus arteriosus; Mr. Winslow points out one for us, consisting of small holes of communication through which blood is able to pass from the superior vena cava into the pulmonary vein, and these little openings he has sometimes observed in the adult.*

And that's all that Lémery wrote about this topic. As one can see, Lémery was not reporting a case of TAPVC/D, nor of PAPVC/D. Nor did the famous Danish anatomist Jacob Benignus Winslow (1669–1760), who worked in Paris and has been immortalized by the eponymic foramen of Winslow. (His friends in Paris called him Jacques-Benigne.) We also perused Winslow's textbook, *Exposition Anatomique de la Structure du Corps Humain* (1732), but were unable to find any description of TAPVC or PAPVC or drainage therein. This, then, is why we tentatively regard the publication of Mr. James Wilson[25] of London in 1798 as the earliest known *definite* reference to TAPVC.

Who first described sinus venosus defect? It was first described by Dr. Thomas B. Peacock[31] of London, England in 1858. His patient was an acyanotic 6-year-old girl who died of scarlet fever, bronchitis, and pulmonary edema. "An opening nearly circular in form and six lines [12.7 mm] in diameter exists at the upper part of the septum atriorum, above the fossa ovalis, and the latter passage is closed, except that a small valvular communication still exists."

Almost 100 years later, in 1956, this anomaly was named *the sinus venosus type of ASD* by Mr. Donald N. Ross,[32] the eminent English surgeon. This name has stuck, probably because one needs a designation to specify this type of interatrial communication as opposed to the other three types (ostium secundum, ostium primum, and common atrium).

It took almost another 40 years, in 1994, before Dr. Stella Van Praagh and her colleagues[9] understood this anomaly well enough to appreciate that it is not really an ASD (although it acts like one), and that the real malformation is absence of the normal partition between the RPVs posteriorly, and the SVC and RA anteriorly. As explained previously, surgical repair involves replacement of the missing intervenous partition so that the right pulmonary venous blood flows through the right pulmonary venous ostium (the high interatrial communication), rather than shunting left-to-right into the RA.

We realized[9] that the term **sinus venosus defect** is at least half right**.** Sinus venosus tissue is involved anatomically; that is, the posterior missing wall of the RSVC and of the sinus venosus (or systemic venous) component of the RA. However, this term is also half wrong. Not mentioned is the missing anterior wall of the unroofed pulmonary veins.

In an effort to change terminology minimally, we have supported the designation **sinus venosus defect** (instead of sinus venosus ASD), in the interests of anatomic accuracy, as ealier.[9]

Accurately speaking, the SVC type of sinus venosus defect has a **cavopulmonary venous defect.** The right atrial type of sinus venosus defect has a **right atriopulmonary venous defect.** Again, these designations are included here in the interests of clear and accurate anatomic understanding.

Who first described sinus venosus defect of the right atrial type? This was first described by Dr. Arthur Keith,[33] in 1909, before he became Sir Arthur Keith (Fig. 7.32)

Swan, Kirklin, Becu, and Wood[30] described a sinus venosus defect of the SVC type in 1957, with excellent photographic documentation of the right and left atrial appearances. These authors captured the essence of the malformation: anomalous drainage of the RPVs into the low RSVC, plus a high interatrial communication above and behind the foramen ovale or fossa ovalis.

Who first understood what the sinus venosus defect really is? No, it was not us in 1994, although we did not learn this

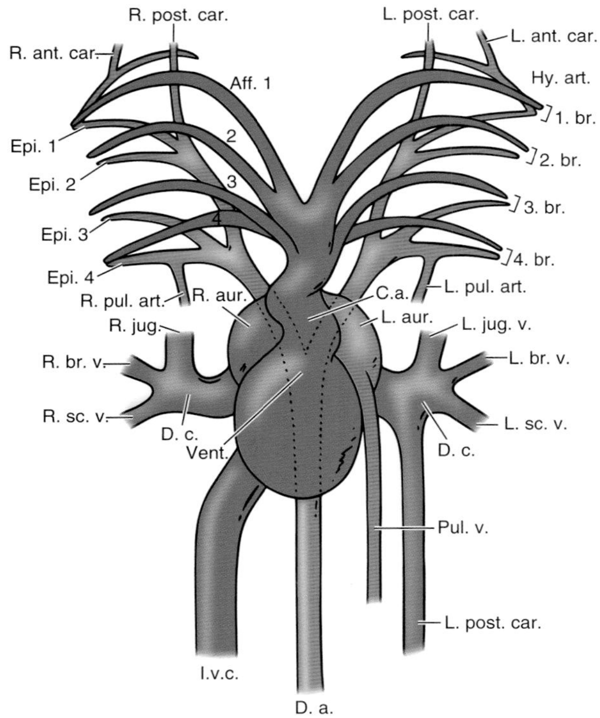

Fig. 7.32 **Diagram of the Heart and Blood Vessels of the Lungfish, *Ceratodus fosteri*.** Venous blood is shown as light in color; arterial blood is black. *Aff 1–4,* Afferent vessels of branchial bars 1 to 4; *1br–4br,* branchial bars 1 to 4; *c.a.,* conus arteriosus; *D.a.,* dorsal aorta; *D.c.,* ductus of Cuvier; *Epi. 1–4,* epibranchial vessels 1 to 4; *Hy. Art.,* hyoid artery; *I.v.c.,* inferior vena cava; *L. ant. car.,* left anterior cardinal artery; *L. aur.,* left auricle; *L. br. v.,* left brachial vein; *L. jug. v.,* left jugular vein; *L. post. car.,* left posterior cardinal artery; *L. pul. art.,* left pulmonary artery; *L. sc. v.,* left subclavian vein; *R. ant. car.,* right anterior cardinal artery; *R. aur.,* right auricle; *R. br. v.,* right brachial vein; *R. jug. v.,* right jugular vein; *R. post. car.,* right posterior cardinal artery; *R. pul. art.,* right pulmonary artery; *R. sc. v.,* right subclavian vein; *Vent,* ventricle. Lungs appear for the first time in lungfish, evolving from the swim bladder. Lungfish represent an early stage in vertebrate evolution, just after cartilaginous and bony fish, and just before amphibia, which were followed by reptiles, birds, and mammals. Even at this very early vertebrate evolutionary stage represented by the lungfish, many of the features of the normal human cardiovascular system had developed. The unsaturated venous blood of the inferior vena cava (IVC) and both ducts of Cuvier open into the right atrium (RA). The oxygenated blood of the pulmonary vein opens into the left atrium (LA). Both atria are partially divided. They open through a partially divided common atrioventricular valve into a single ventricle. The single ventricle ejects into a spiral conus arteriosus, that is partly divided into the two pathways by a spiral valve. The more oxygenated blood from the LA is directed into branchial arches 1 and 2, the less oxygenated blood stream from the RA flowing preferentially to branchial arches 3 and 4. The left and right pulmonary arteries originate from the most distal branchial arches 4. Thus, the lungs and two atria evolved before two ventricles did. The right ventricular sinus (inflow tract)—the lung pump—is an evolutionary "Johnny come lately." The right ventricular sinus did not evolve until the vertebrate stage of Reptilia had been reached. From an evolutionary standpoint, the conus arteriosus is much older than the right ventricular sinus. The lungfish has a "double aortic arch." The lungfish may be regarded as the earliest amphibian. Thus, from the very onset of air breathing, the pulmonary vein has been a left-sided or left atrial structure.

until after our paper[9] was published. Dr. Stella Van Praagh was rereading Maude Abbott's *Congenital Cardiac Disease*[34] (1915), and there it was, an understanding identical to our own. Abbott wrote, "Paltauf thought that the hole in the septum was not a defect at all, but represented the orifice of the RPV, which entered here directly above the septum, with the superior vena cava."

Exactly right, we thought. But Abbott gave no reference to Paltauf. Finally, with the help of Mr. Jack Eckert, MA, MLS, Rare Book Librarian, Countway Library of Medicine, Harvard Medical School, we found Paltauf's paper that was published in 1913.[35] **Richard Paltauf** (1858–1924) was an eminent Austrian pathologist and bacteriologist who founded a well-known school of pathologic anatomy in Vienna.

Nützel[36] (1914) and von Hackensellner[37] (1955) both also published papers presenting essentially the same understanding of this anomaly as that of Paltauf[35] (1913) and Van Praagh et al[9] (1994). The drawing of Kiss et al[38] of sinus venosus defect of the SVC type shows the pathologic anatomy of this anomaly with great clarity (Fig. 7.33). It is our intention to honor our Austrian and German predecessors Paltauf,[35] Nützel,[36] and von Hackensellner[37] and to give them credit for figuring out what so-called sinus venosus defect really is from the anatomic and developmental standpoints.

Cavopulmonary venous defect[39] occurs at three different levels and is associated with four different phenotypes:

1. When the cavopulmonary venous defect occurs at the right atrial level, between the venous or sinus venosus component of the RA and the RPVs, the phenotype that results is known as **sinus venosus defect of the right atrial type** (see Fig. 7.20).
2. When the cavopulmonary venous defect occurs at the SVC–right atrial junction, the phenotype that results is that of **sinus venosus defect of the SVC type** (see Figs. 7.23, 7.25, 7.33).
3. When the cavopulmonary venous defect occurs at the SVC level,[39] above the SVC–right atrial junction, the resulting phenotype is either:
   a. biatrial drainage of the SVC, or
   b. left atrial drainage of the (right) SVC.

We think that the latter phenotype occurs when RSVC-to-left atrial flow predominates (when left atrial pressure and/or resistance is [are] less than right atrial pressure and/or resistance). We hypothesize that when RSVC-to–left atrial flow predominates, the normal RSVC-to–right atrial orifice may become stenotic or atretic. When atretic, the RSVC drains exclusively into the LA.[39]

All four of the previously mentioned phenotypes result from failure of development or involution of the normal cavopulmonary venous partition, resulting in a cavopulmonary venous defect. The variable is the height at which the cavopulmonary venous defect occurs (as earlier).

We suggest the term **cavopulmonary venous defect** as an alternative to sinus venosus defect because cavopulmonary venous defect is anatomically more accurate. It is also all-inclusive. Sinus venosus defect does not include two of the four phenotypes: (1) biatrial drainage of the RSVC (without interatrial communication) and (2) left atrial drainage of the RSVC

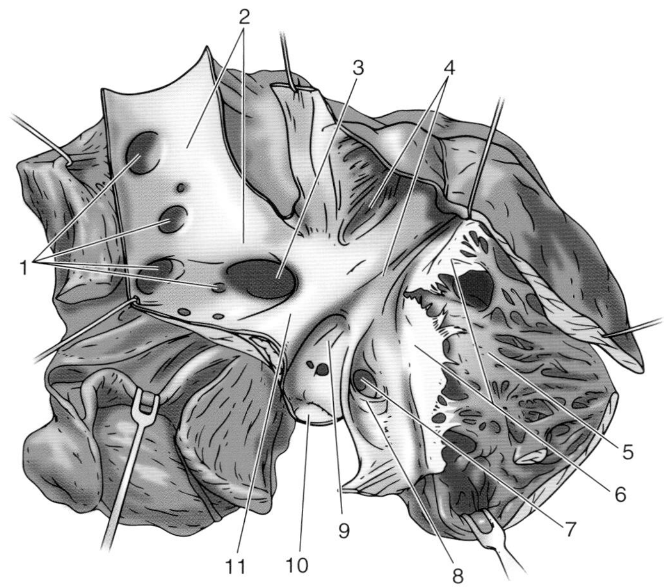

Fig. 7.33 Sinus Venosus Defect of the Superior Vena Caval Type, Drawing of Opened Right Heart. *1,* Right pulmonary veins; *2,* superior vena cava; *3,* communication with left atrium; *4,* right atrium; *5,* right ventricle; *6,* septal leaflet of tricuspid valve; *7,* ostium of coronary sinus; *8,* Thebesian valve of coronary sinus; *9,* fossa ovalis formed by closed septum primum; *10,* confluence of inferior vena cava (excised, below) with septum primum that forms the floor of the fossa ovalis; and *11,* superior limbic band of septum secundum, also known as the tubercle of Lower. The right pulmonary veins *(1)* have been unroofed into the superior vena cava *(2);* that is, the partition that normally separates the right pulmonary veins posteriorly *(1)* from the more anterior superior vena cava *(3)* has failed to form. What looks like a superior atrial septal defect confluent with the superior vena cava, traditionally called a sinus venosus atrial septal defect *(3),* is the normal ostium of the right pulmonary veins opening into the left atrium. This normal right pulmonary venous ostium into the left atrium acts as an interatrial communication or atrial septal defect because of congenital absence of the right pulmonary venous–right superior vena caval partition. The surgical repair of this pulmonary–caval venous partition defect is to replace the absent partition, typically at the present time with glutaraldehyde-treated pericardium. The left-to-right shunt at the atrial level is due not only to left-to-right shunting through the unroofed right pulmonary venous ostium *(3),* but also to right pulmonary venous blood *(1)* pouring into the superior vena cava *(2)* and thence directly into the right atrium *(4).* Because of this superior vena caval component of the "left-to-right" shunt, the right pulmonary venous ostium leading into the left atrium *(3)* may be restrictively small, and may need to be enlarged as part of the surgical reconstruction (the Warden procedure). Thus, *the right horn of the sinus venosus* may be defective (its posterior wall), resulting in nonpartition from the right pulmonary veins, known as a sinus venosus defect; and *the left horn of the sinus venosus* may be defective (its anterior wall), resulting in nonpartition of the coronary sinus from the left atrium and a large low posterior interatrial communication (the ostium of the unroofed coronary sinus), known as the Raghib syndrome, or as a coronary sinus septal defect, or as unroofing of the coronary sinus. Hence, both right and left sinus venosus horns have clinically and surgically important unroofing or partitioning defects, with interatrial communications that are really normally structures, not septal defects (abnormalities). It is the partitioning defects that make these normal structures (right pulmonary vein ostium and coronary sinus ostium) behave hemodynamically like septal defects. Hence, the "chapter heading" should be *Interatrial Communications,* not Atrial Septal Defects, because they are not all atrial septal *defects.* (From Kiss A, Partilla H, Pernkopf E. Die transposition der venenmündungen [eine entwicklungsgeschichtliche analyse, vorgenommen an hand eines falles von pulmonalinsuffizienz mit vorhofsseptumdefekt und partieller transposition der lungenvenenmündungen]. *Virchows Arch.* 1954;324:707, with permission.)

(without interatrial communication). With the high (SVC) type of cavopulmonary venous defect, the RPVs are unroofed into the RSVC above the atria. Consequently, the RPVs pass above and behind RA and connect only with the LA[39]; hence, there is no interatrial communication.

Perhaps the main advantage of the term and concept *cavopulmonary venous defect* is that it focuses on the real anatomic defect, not on the interatrial communication, which is the RPV orifice, not an ASD due to failure of normal lateralization of the right horn of the sinus venosus, causing the sinus venosus to override the atrial septum and resulting in a so-called sinus venosus type of ASD. Once one understands what the interatrial communication really is, that is, the orifice of the RPV(s), then it becomes possible to understand so-called sinus venosus defect, which really is a cavopulmonary venous "window" or partition defect. The real problem with the designation *sinus venosus defect* is that this whole interpretation or understanding is wrong. The interatrial communication is not a septal defect, and it is not the real anomaly.

However, we are well aware that old errors die hard. Our minimalist hope is that even if people continue to use the terms *sinus venosus defect* or *sinus venosus atrial septal defect,* they will understand that the interatrial communication is *not* the defect, and that what the surgeon patches *is* the defect. Our more optimistic hope, in the interests of anatomic accuracy, is that *cavopulmonary venous defect* will be understood and found to be useful.

Does the literature contain any large and carefully done study of partial anomalous pulmonary venous drainage and TAPVD? Yes. The paper of Blake, Hall, and Manion[43] is noteworthy. It is based on 113 postmortem cases that display 27 different anatomic variations.

Severe Pulmonary Vascular Obstructive Disease

Levy et al[44] published the case of a 5-month-old girl with severe pulmonary arteriolar intimal proliferation secondary to TAPVC that resulted in marked pulmonary arterial hypertension. We have not seen pulmonary vascular obstruction (PVO) secondary to TAPVC/D at this young age.

Incomplete Scimitar Syndrome

In the scimitar syndrome, all of the RPVs do not necessarily drain into the IVC. In 1969, Gazzaniga et al[59] reported the case of a 53-year-old woman in whom the RPVs connected with the IVC and also with the LA. The patient's atrial septum was intact. At that time, these authors[59] thought that theirs was the third known such case. We encountered several incomplete, partial, or variant forms of the scimitar syndrome (see Table 7.16):

1. all RPVs to the ductus venosus, in 1 of 12 cases (8%);
2. inferior scimitar vein to the IVC and a superior RPV to the RSVC, in 1 of 12 patients (8%);
3. inferior scimitar vein to the IVC and RUPVs to the LA, in 2 of 12 patients (17%); and
4. RLPV to the low RA, all other pulmonary veins connecting with the LA, in 1 of 12 patients (8%).

All of the RPVs connected with the IVC, resulting in **typical scimitar syndrome,** in only 7 of these 12 patients (58%) (see Table 7.16). Anomalous systemic arteries from the abdominal aorta supplied the lower right lung in 7 of these 12 patients (58%) (see Table 7.16). Thus, **partial or variant forms of scimitar syndrome** were quite common, being found in 5 of these 12 patients (42%).

In 1970, Gathman and Nadas[63] published a clinical and physiologic study of 75 pediatric patients with TAPVC/D. They concluded that pulmonary venous obstruction is an important feature of this defect, a point with which we strongly concur (see Fig. 7.3). They also stated that pulmonary venous obstruction "can occur with anomalous return to any site." Although this is true, it also should be understood that pulmonary venous connection to the coronary sinus is very seldom obstructed in an unoperated patient. (But it can happen, as reported earlier.)

In 1971, Gomes, Feldt, McGoon, and Danielson[64] from the Mayo Clinic reported long-term results after correction of TAPVC/D. In a series of 59 cases ranging from 2 months to 37 years of age with a median of 5 years of age, the mortality rate under 1 year of age was 47% and over 1 year of age was 7%. Among survivors, the long-term results were excellent. These were good results for that time, but clearly there was much room for improvement.

In 1970, Roe[65] reported further experience with a left posterolateral thoracotomy approach to the repair of TAPVC/D, his patients ranging from 3 months to 46 years of age. The patient was lying on his/her right side with the left side up. Arterial cannulation was done via the descending thoracic aorta, and the venous cannula was placed into the dilated right ventricular outflow tract. Then an anastomosis was made between the horizontal vein (running from pulmonary hilum to hilum; see Fig. 7.3) and the dorsal wall of the LA. Roe[65] stated that "exposure is excellent, suturing can be done comfortably, cardiac displacement is unnecessary, and retraction is limited to the lung."

In using a left posterolateral thoracotomy approach, the surgeon is taking advantage of what is known as the **Taussig maneuver.** Because the LA is not connected with the pulmonary veins (preoperatively), but only by the venae cavae, the heart can be rotated from left to right—like turning the page of a book. Just a little of this rotational movement, but not enough to kink the venae cavae, gives excellent exposure to the back of the heart, that is, to the dorsal wall of the LA and the horizontal pulmonary vein.

(Please note that it is not our intention to try to tell present and future cardiac surgeons how they should repair TAPVC/D. Instead, an understanding of the Taussig maneuver and its anatomic basis may well be of use surgically, no matter what approach the surgeon may prefer.)

From an anatomic standpoint, perhaps the easiest approach would be to use the usual median sternotomy, with the patient supine, to facilitate venous and arterial cannulation and then for the surgeon to stand on the patient's *left side,* where the surgeon would have excellent exposure to the back of the heart—because of the Taussig maneuver.

Roe[65] made another point of considerable importance: "When the connection between the common venous trunk [the horizontal vein] and the LA is made larger than the mitral valve area, pulmonary congestion does not occur and the communicating vein can be ligated." From a morphometric standpoint, the cross-sectional area of the anastomosis must be larger than the cross-sectional area of the mitral orifice, to avoid iatrogenic supramitral stenosis and pulmonary venous hypertension.

TABLE 7.24 **Age in TAPVC/D at Death, Operation, or Last Follow-up[69]**

Age at Death (y)	%
<1	70
1–2	5
2–10	20
11–20	3
>21	1

Natural History of Totally Anomalous Pulmonary Venous Connection and Drainage

In 1971, Jensen and Blount[69] reviewed 27 cases of TAPVC/D, reporting 3 in detail. One of these patients was a 46-year-old man with the supracardiac snowman type, the oldest case of TAPVC/D known up to that time. At the time of this report,[69] the patient was alive and was improved by the administration for the first time of digitalis and diuretics. These authors pointed out that absence of pulmonary venous obstruction, absence of pulmonary arterial hypertension, and adequate intracardiac communication (such as a patent foramen ovale or secundum type of ASD) favored longevity. Jensen and Blount's meta-analysis of longevity in TAPVC/D[69] is summarized in Table 7.24.

TAPVC/D and Age. The chances of an untreated patient with TAPVC/D living to see an internist are less than 5%. But such cases do occur.[64,65,69]

In 1977, Pastore et al[121] published the case of a 52-year-old man with the snowman type of TAPVC and severe calcific pulmonary stenosis. In addition to being the oldest known patient with unoperated TAPVC reported up to that time, this patient also clarified the factors promoting **longevity in TAPVC.** A large ASD permits adequate systemic arterial blood flow. The ASD in this patient measured 6 × 3 cm.

Normal or nearly normal pulmonary arterial blood pressure is also very advantageous. Distal to the stenotic pulmonic valve, the pressure in the main pulmonary artery was 20/5 mm Hg. To have normal pulmonary arterial blood pressure, it is important not to have stenosis of the anomalous pulmonary venous pathway. It is also important not to have markedly increased pulmonary arterial blood flow, which predisposes to pulmonary arteriolar intimal proliferation that in turn becomes pulmonary vascular obstructive disease with pulmonary hypertension.

If one has TAPVC with a large ASD and with normal pulmonary artery pressure, does this mean that the natural history is benign and that surgery can be avoided? Unfortunately not. As the 52-year-old man reported by Pastore et al[121] illustrated, one is then highly vulnerable to paradoxical embolization through the large ASD. It was a cerebrovascular accident and other prior systemic embolic events that led to the surgical repair of the supracardiac TAPVC, the associated large ASD, and the calcified pulmonary valvar stenosis.

In 1982, McManus et al[169] topped the foregoing by reporting a 62-year-old man with the snowman type of supracardiac TAPVC who had survived without surgical intervention. This patient also had a common atrium—promoting venoarterial mixing at the atrial level—and a bicuspid aortic valve but with normal function.

Mystery Cases

Mystery cases exist in the literature, despite all of our knowledge and understanding of TAPVC/D. For example, what did the patient reported by Shadravan et al[72] in 1971 really have? This 22-month-old black boy was found at successful surgery to have the following. The pulmonary veins from the right lower lobe, left upper lobe, and left lower lobe drained into a thin-walled chamber behind the RA. This thin-walled chamber had only a minute opening into the RA; hence, this communication with the RA was highly stenotic. The junction of the RSVC with the RA was also very stenotic. The RULPV connected with the RSVC above the stenotic RSVC–right atrial junction. The RSVC blood and the blood from the anomalous right upper lobe vein returned to the IVC via enlarged azygos and hemiazygos veins. The thin-walled chamber was opened and anastomosed to the LA.

But the question remains, What was the thin-walled chamber that received all of the left lung pulmonary veins and the right lower lobe pulmonary vein? We speculate that this structure may perhaps have been a distended horizontal pulmonary vein—distended because of severe stenosis of its communication with the RA. Coexisting pulmonary venous and systemic venous (at the RSVC–right atrial junction) stenoses are fortunately very rare. Is our interpretation of this rare case[72] correct? We are not certain that it is, and that is the point. Could the thin-walled chamber that received most of the pulmonary veins have been a persistent right horn of the sinus venosus, with which most of the pulmonary veins connected anomalously? We really do not know. The point is that there still may be anatomic types of TAPVC/D that remain unknown because they may not have been adequately described. We think that we have never seen a case like that described by Shadravan et al.[72]

Tajik et al[85] reported a similar case in a 22-year-old woman who had TAPVC to the RA via an unidentified small posterior chamber. The authors stated that all pulmonary veins connected with "a small posterior chamber which in turn drained into the RA." We thought that this chamber probably represented **persistence of the right horn of the sinus venosus.** It also could be called a sinus venosus aneurysm involving the right sinus horn. (However, we are speculating. We do not know for sure.)

Left Atrial and Left Ventricular Volumes in Totally Anomalous Pulmonary Venous Connection and Drainage

In 1972, Graham et al[74] found in TAPVC that LV end-diastolic volume was less than 67% of normal in 5 of 15 patients preoperatively (33%). However, the average for the entire group was not significantly different from normal. Left atrial volume was only 55% of normal, presumably because the normal common pulmonary vein component of the LA is absent in TAPVC. By contrast, in large ASDs, Graham et al[74] found that the left ventricular end-diastolic volume averaged only 87% of normal (significantly decreased). However, left atrial volume was normal.

Thus, these results showed that in TAPVC, left atrial volume is significantly reduced preoperatively and that left ventricular volume and output can be diminished preoperatively. However, bad surgical results could no longer be "explained" by claiming that TAPVC/D has significant left ventricular hypoplasia, that is, that it is a type of hypoplastic left heart syndrome. The findings of Dr. Tom Graham et al[74] did not support this widespread but erroneous impression.

Scimitar Syndrome Expanded?

Hayward et al[75] in 1972 published 2 cases of the scimitar syndrome and attempted to further clarify it. They called this syndrome the **vena cava–bronchovascular complex** and noted that it can consist of (1) the scimitar vein to the IVC, with or without the RPV to the LA; (2) anomalous systemic arterial blood supply from the abdominal aorta; (3) right pulmonary hypoplasia; (4) right bronchial anomalies; and (5) an accessory right-sided fibrous diaphragm (interpreted as an anomaly of the embryonic septum transversum). We think that this paper[75] is noteworthy because we had not previously been aware that an accessory fibrous diaphragm could be associated with and perhaps a part of the scimitar syndrome. It has been stated that the scimitar syndrome in humans resembles the normal situation in teleosts (ordinary bony fish) and in lungfish.[77] If true, this insight might provide a phylogentic understanding of the scimitar syndrome. Unfortunately, our investigation does not provide support for this intriguing hypothesis. Ordinary fish (teleosts) do not have lungs and hence do not have anything closely analogous to the pulmonary veins. In lungfish, such as dipnoi, the pulmonary vein returns from the swim bladder (lung) and empties directly into the left side of the atrium (Fig. 7.34).[80] Robb[80] quotes Goodrich as follows:

> *The sinus venosus receives the venous blood from two ductus Cuvieri and a median vein formed by the union of a vena cava inferior with hepatic veins; but an important new departure is the separation of the return stream from the lung-like air bladder. For the two pulmonary veins join, as in amphibia, to a single vessel which, passing along the dorsal wall of the sinus, empties aerated blood directly into the left side of the atrium. Into the right side of the atrium the sinus empties the venous blood, and there extends from behind and above a muscular septum which subdivides the atrial cavity almost completely into larger right and smaller left auricular spaces.*

So, as you can see, in lungfish the pulmonary vein returns to the LA (see Fig. 7.34),[80] not to the IVC. In the ascending evolution of vertebrate phylogeny, the lungfish is the lowest stage at which a pulmonary vein and atrial septum appear.

However, in an effort to understand what Behdad and Folger[77] meant by analogizing the scimitar syndrome in humans and the normal pulmonary venous anatomy in lungfish, note this (once again from Dr. Jane Sand Robb's[80] superb *Comparative Basic Cardiology*) concerning lungfish: "The pulmonary artery

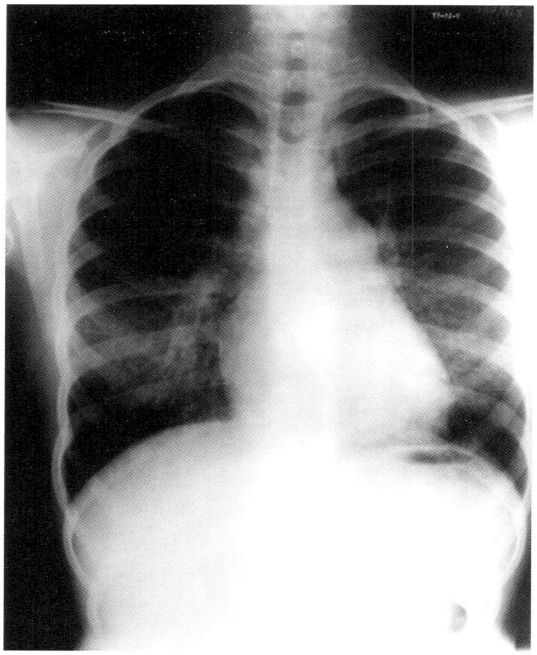

Fig. 7.34 Pulmonary veno-occlusive disease, posteroanterior chest radiograph, in a girl who died at 13 3/12 years of age. Note the bilateral pulmonary parenchymal densities observed shortly before death.

springs from the dorsal aorta. Blood returns in a special pulmonary vein to the left side of the *sinus venosus*." The italics are ours. Note that some authors still regard the partially septated atrium of the lungfish as the sinus venosus, whereas others regard this structure as the partly divided atrium. But no one, to our knowledge, has equated the LA (or the left side of the sinus venosus) with the IVC. However, the IVC is a major tributary flowing into the right horn of the sinus venosus.[81]

In summary, the pulmonary vein in lungfish normally connects with the LA and the atrial part of the heart is septated into LA and RA, thereby separating the oxygenated pulmonary venous return from the unoxygenated systemic venous return. These two features (left atrial connection of the pulmonary vein and atrial septation) have been highly conserved throughout vertebrate evolution.

Anomalous Pulmonary Venous Drainage With Pulmonary Atrioventricular Fistula(s)

In 1973, Mertens, Clapp, and Ferris[96] published the case of a 74-year-old white woman with anomalous pulmonary venous drainage of the snowman type (into the LIV and RSVC, well demonstrated angiographically) and with a minute pulmonary arteriovenous fistula of the left upper lobe.

Our initial impression was that Mertens et al[96] were reporting the oldest known patient with TAPVC/D (of the snowman type) who also had a minute pulmonary arteriovenous fistula of the left upper lobe. But on rereading their paper, we realized that our first impression was wrong. These authors[96] stated that their patient had anomalous pulmonary venous drainage in association with a minute left upper lobe pulmonary arteriovenous fistula. They did not say that their patient had TAPVC of the snowman type (even though the angiocardiogram showing the LIV and RSVC full of contrast certainly looks like this type of TAPVC). These authors did not say that no pulmonary veins connect with the LA.

Mertens et al[96] refer to the description and classification of pulmonary arteriovenous aneurysms and fistulas of Anabtawi, Ellison, and Ellison[97]:

1. multiple small AV fistulas without aneurysm;
2. large AV aneurysm, peripheral;

3A. large AV aneurysm, central;
3B. large AV aneurysm with anomalous venous drainage;
3C. multiple small AV fistulas with anomalous venous drainage;
4A. large venous aneurysm with systemic artery communication;
4B. large venous aneurysm without fistula; and
5. anomalous venous drainage without fistula.

Mertens et al[96] thought that their patient had a type 3C arteriovenous fistula, despite the fact that their patient had a single (not a multiple) arteriovenous fistula. They point out that the normal (adult) lung has pulmonary arteriovenous shunts of between 35 and 200 microns in diameter. Minute abnormal arteriovenous fistulas range between 500 microns and 2 mm in diameter.

Thus, it is important to bear in mind that pulmonary arteriovenous fistulas may or may not be associated with anomalous venous drainage, as mentioned earlier.[96,97]

Mertens et al[96] point out that the anomalous pulmonary venous connections (which may be associated with pulmonary arteriovenous fistulas) usually are *congenital* but can be acquired. The patient of Mertens et al[96] probably had a snowman type of congenital anomalous pulmonary venous connection and drainage but also with normal pulmonary venous connections with the LA. Consequently, this 74-year-old woman may be regarded as having PAPVC/D, because she presumably also had normally connected pulmonary veins.

This type of PAPVC/D[96] (associated with pulmonary arteriovenous fistula[s][97] and with normally connected pulmonary veins) is unfamiliar to pediatric cardiologists and cardiac surgeons. The existence of this entity is also noteworthy for cardiologists and cardiac surgeons dealing with congenital heart disease in the adult.

Familial Totally Anomalous Pulmonary Venous Connection

Familial TAPVC/D was reported by Nakazawa et al.[100] A 1-month-old boy was found to have the supracardiac (snowman) type of TAPVC. One year later, his sister was diagnosed as having TAPVC to the coronary sinus. TAPVC in siblings is rare, this being the fourth known case in the English literature up to that time (1972–1973).[100] The topic of familial TAPVC/D was addressed by Paz and Castilla in 1971.[101]

Displacement of the "Atrial Septum" With Partially Anomalous Pulmonary Venous Connection and Drainage

Utley, Noonan, Walters, and Frist[112] published the case of a 2½-year-old boy in which the "atrial septum" was so displaced to the left and posteriorly that both the tricuspid and the mitral valves opened from the RA into the appropriate ventricles. There was a small low defect in the atrial septum that resembled a small ostium primum type of ASD. No coronary sinus opened into the RA. When the small and posteriorly located "atrial septum" was excised surgically, the ostia of three pulmonary veins were seen. There was an additional channel opening into the "LA" that consisted of a persistent LSVC. The LULPV connected with the persistent LSVC.

In this complex case, the authors[112] were not entirely sure of the correct diagnosis. They mentioned the possibility that the patient may in fact have had a common atrium, explaining absence of the atrial septum between the AV valves, with cor triatriatum that received an unroofed persistent LSVC, that in turn received an aberrant LULPV. Excision of the "atrial septum" cured the cor triatriatum and decompressed all of the pulmonary veins and the persistent LSVC. The surgeon ligated the LSVC above the connection of the LULPV and then patched all of the pulmonary veins to flow through the mitral valve, thereby curing the patient. This case is mentioned to indicate how difficult it can be occasionally to identify the atrial septum with certainty. For a structure to be the atrial septum—or some remnant thereof—must lie between the AV valves. This was true in all of the cases presented earlier in which the upper portion of the atrial septum was displaced to the left, resulting in PAPVD or TAPVD. In other words, the base of the atrial septum lies between the tricuspid and mitral valves, no matter how leftwardly displaced the superior or upper portion of the atrial septum may be.

Also, an ostium primum type of ASD (to the best of our present knowledge and understanding) cannot lie well to the left and posteriorly relative to the mitral valve. Consequently, we think that the patient of Utley et al[112] had a common atrium (hence, no remnant of atrial septal tissue between the AV valves), unroofing of the coronary sinus (thus, no coronary sinus ostium opening into the RA), persistent LSVC opening into the unroofed coronary sinus, anomalous LULPV connecting with the LSVC, and cor triatriatum (the small and unrestrictive "ostium primum type of ASD" being the restrictive exit from the common pulmonary vein chamber of the cor triatriatum that also received the persistent LSVC).

To summarize, we think that the lesson of this publication[112] is that PAPVC to a persistent LSVC and cor triatriatum can coexist. When common atrium is present, that is, absence of the atrial septum, the cor triatriatum can resemble a posteriorly and leftwardly displaced atrial septum, and the stenotic low opening of the common pulmonary vein chamber of cor triatriatum can resemble an ostium primum type of defect.

Unilateral Emphysema With Totally Anomalous Pulmonary Venous Connection

Sulayman, Thilenius, Replogle, and Arcilla[113] reported the case of a 3½-month-old girl with TAPVC to the LIV (snowman type). The LVV usually runs anteriorly to the LPA, and when it does, the LVV is not obstructed. Occasionally, the LVV runs behind the LPA and in front on the left main bronchus. In this situation, the LVV is in the middle, sandwiched between the LPA anteriorly and the left bronchus posteriorly, resulting in stenosis of the LVV (see Fig. 7.3A); hence, Dr. Jesse Edwards' graphic description: *vascular vise*.

Rarely, however, as in this patient,[113] the LVV can run posteriorly to the left mainstem bronchus. This means that the bronchus is in the middle, compressed between the LPA anteriorly and the vertical vein posteriorly. In this patient, there was a *bronchial vise,* and compression of the left main bronchus led to unilateral emphysema involving the left lung. Dr. Robert Repogle repaired this patient successfully by anastomosing the horizontal vein to the LA and by enlarging the LA with a Dacron patch.

Is Totally Anomalous Pulmonary Venous Connection Below the Diaphragm Always Obstructed?

No, as in the 10-year-old girl reported by Duff, Nihill, Vargo, and Cooley,[115] it is rarely possible to have TAPVC to the ductus venosus and thence to the IVC without obstruction. This patient also had a large secundum ASD, a VSD, and a PDA. This was also the first patient with Goldenhar syndrome known to have TAPVC.

Gastrointestinal Hemorrhage: Unusual Complication of Totally Anomalous Pulmonary Venous Connection

King and Marchildon[124] reported a 3-day-old boy with esophageal atresia and tracheo-esophageal fistula who also had mixed TAPVC. The right upper lobe connected via a small anomalous pulmonary vein with the RSVC. All of the other pulmonary veins, from the right middle lobe, right lower lobe, and all of the left lung, connected via a large anomalous pulmonary vein to the distal esophagus and terminated in the proximal stomach. Exsanguinating fatal hemorrhage occurred from massive esophageal and gastric varices. Postmortem angiography showed that these varices ultimately terminated in the portal venous system and did not communicate with the IVC. At postmortem angiography, contrast poured into the stomach from these ruptured varices.

Surgical Correction of Totally Anomalous Pulmonary Venous Connection in Premature Neonates

Can surgical correction be performed successfully in premature neonates? This question was answered affirmatively in 1976 by Sparrow, Mohan, and Gonzalez-Lavin,[125] who reported the successful surgical correction of a 2.5-kg 16-day-old girl with TAPVC to the coronary sinus. She was the smallest patient to undergo successful correction up to that time.

Surgical Correction of Totally Anomalous Pulmonary Venous Connection Below the Diaphragm

In 1978, Porter, Vargo, McNamara, and Cooley[133] reported one of the first patients with infradiaphragmatic TAPVC who had been successfully corrected surgically. At that time, the patient had a 14-year follow-up. The patient had undergone surgery at 7 weeks of age in 1961. Why report such a success in 1978?[133] Because the surgical results had been so bad. Now, we tend to forget what a very tough fight this was from the surgical perspective. For example, in 1977, the same distinguished group[131] from Houston, Texas reported a surgical mortality rate for infradiaphragmatic TAPVC of 66%. Porter et al[133] made another important point concerning TAPVC below the diaphragm, namely, the distinction between *prehepatic* drainage and *posthepatic* drainage. Prehepatic drainage goes to the portal vein and then to the liver and is much more likely to be obstructed than is posthepatic drainage via the ductus venosus to the IVC. Their patient with TAPVC below the diaphragm had posthepatic drainage to the IVC and hence had a benign clinical course. So, too, did the patient of Duff et al[115] referred to earlier.

The clinical picture that one tends to think of in association with TAPVC below the diaphragm—a chest radiograph with a relatively small heart, ground-glass lung fields (pulmonary congestion and edema), severe pulmonary arterial hypertension, and systemic or suprasystemic right ventricular pressure—is the clinical picture of TAPVC below the diaphragm *with prehepatic drainage* into the portal vein and through the hepatic sinusoids. This is the clinical picture of severe pulmonary venous obstruction. This is not the clinical picture of TAPVC below the diaphragm with posthepatic drainage into the IVC without significant pulmonary venous obstruction. It must be added that TAPVC below the diaphragm with posthepatic drainage into the IVC can be obstructed if the ductus venosus or its junction with the IVC is restrictively small. Nonetheless, the distinction between prehepatic and posthepatic drainage of infradiaphragmatic TAPVC is important.[133]

To comprehend how and why TAPVC below the diaphragm can be either prehepatic or posthepatic, an understanding of the ductus venosus is essential, as is explained previously (see Fig. 7.11).

Totally Anomalous Pulmonary Venous Connection: A Form of Cyanotic Congenital Heart Disease

One does not ordinarily think of TAPVC as a form of cyanotic congenital heart disease because it is characterized by a large left-to-right shunt at the supracardiac, cardiac, or infracardiac levels or at a mixture of these levels.[2] However, as was pointed out by Batisse, Landau, Piechaud, and Kachaner[139] in 1978, when TAPVC in the newborn is obstructed, the patient has severe and intractable cyanosis and pulmonary edema, pulmonary hypertension, and systemic or suprasystemic right ventricular hypertension. The severe cyanosis typically is due to right-to-left shunting at the atrial level through either a patent foramen ovale or a secundum ASD, secondary to the obstruction of the pulmonary venous pathway and the resulting severe right-sided hypertension. In a series of 17 patients with obstructed TAPVC, the pressure in the main pulmonary artery was equal to or greater than systemic in 15 (88%), the mean pulmonary artery–to–systemic artery pressure ratio being 1.25:1.

Should Totally Anomalous Pulmonary Venous Connection Be Treated With Initial Balloon Atrial Septostomy?

In 1978, McNamara, Duff, Mullins, and Cooley[140] argued that patients with TAPVC should be treated with balloon atrial septostomy (BAS). Their impression was that BAS can be life-saving in patients with TAPVC and that BAS often advantageously permits delay of definitive surgery. Of 13 patients with TAPVC who received initial BAS, 11 survived surgical repair (85%). Of 80 patients with TAPVC who did not receive initial BAS, only 56 survived surgical correction (70%). However, this difference was not statistically significant ($p = .16$, Fisher's exact test). Nonetheless, it will be recalled that a good-sized interatrial communication was one of the two factors favoring longevity in unoperated TAPVC,[121] as mentioned previously.

The Essence of the Scimitar Syndrome

In 1978, Drs. Catherine Neill and Lulu Haroutunian[147] made a presentation that crystallized the essence of the scimitar syndrome. This was an unusually authoritative communication, not only because of Neill's expertise concerning the development of the pulmonary veins[148] but also because she and her colleagues had named and described this syndrome in 1960.[14] The view of Neill and Haroutunian was that the scimitar syndrome is not only an anomaly of the RPVs. Instead it is an anomaly of right lung development, involving both its arterial blood supply and its venous drainage.

The Statistics of Pulmonary Venous Anomalies

The statistics of pulmonary venous anomalie were published by Kanjuh et al[149] from Belgrade in 1978. Kanjuh et al looked at a total of 12,160 autopsies.[149] Of these, 586 or 4.8% were congenital heart disease autopsies. Of the 586 congenital heart disease autopsies, 32 or 5.5% were anomalies of pulmonary veins. The anomalies of the pulmonary veins can be divided by isolated anomalies of pulmonary veins (12 or 37.5%) and nonisolated anomalies of pulmonary veins (20 or 62.5%). Eighteen (56.25%) anomalies were totally anomalous pulmonary venous connection while eight (25%) were partially anomalous pulmonary venous connection. Other anomalies noted were cor triatriatum, unincorporated common pulmonary vein, hypoplastic and stenotic pulmonary veins with anomalous course, asplenia, polysplenia, and hyperplastic and anomalously lobated spleen.[149]

It is noteworthy that TAPVC/D and PAPVC/D constituted 81% of all the pulmonary venous anomalies reported in this series.[149]

Pulmonary Vascular Disease With Totally Anomalous Pulmonary Venous Connection

Newfeld, Wilson, Paul, and Reisch[155] reported a remarkable amount of PVO disease involving the pulmonary resistance vessels (arterioles) associated with TAPVC. Even in infants 4 weeks of age or younger, 12 of 13 (92%) had intimal changes of the pulmonary resistance vessels. By 6 months of age, plexiform lesions and extensive pulmonary arteriolar occlusion were found, especially when pulmonary venous obstruction was also present. Hence, Newfeld et al[155] emphasized that extensive and rapidly developing PVO involving the pulmonary arterioles is frequently associated with TAPVC.

Rare Site of Obstruction in Totally Anomalous Pulmonary Venous Connection

Arciniegas, Henry, and Green[158] reported a rare site of obstruction in TAPVC to the coronary sinus, namely, the right atrial ostium of the coronary sinus. This we have not seen. It will be recalled that in our experience, TAPVC to the coronary sinus occurred only in visceroarterial situs solitus (never in visceroarterial situs inversus, nor in situs ambiguus with visceral heterotaxy), was never obstructed (0/11 cases; see Table 7.4), and typically has a huge right atrial ostium of the coronary sinus (see Fig. 7.10). Consequently, the patient of Arciniegas et al[158] is rare and noteworthy.

Partially Anomalous Pulmonary Venous Connection and Drainage With Intact Atrial Septum: A Dangerous Duo

The combination of PAPVC/D and an intact atrial septum is dangerous, particularly in the adult, because of the risk for severe PVO disease involving the pulmonary arterioles. Babb et al[161] reported 3 patients with this combination, and the 2 adults had severe PVO.

Prenatal Damage to Pulmonary Vascular Bed and to Extrapulmonary Veins in Obstructed Totally Anomalous Pulmonary Venous Connection

In a pathologic morphometric study of 6 cases of obstructed TAPVC (5 infradiaphragmatic and 1 to the RA), Haworth[166] found the following:

1. The mean percentage of the pulmonary arterial medial thickness was greater than normal in all.
2. Within the lung, the mean percentage of pulmonary vein wall thickness was significantly increased in all 6 cases.
3. Intimal proliferation occurred in preacinar veins in 2 of the 6 cases (33%).
4. The extrapulmonary veins were smaller than normal in all 5 cases of infradiaphragmatic TAPVC.
5. Microscopically, these extrapulmonary veins were abnormally thick-walled in 4 of 5 (80%), with intimal proliferation in 3 of 5 (60%).
6. The descending vertical vein was severely narrowed or occluded in 2 of 5 cases (40%).
7. The prenatal increase of intrapulmonary arterial and venous muscularity may facilitate episodic pulmonary hypertensive crises postoperatively.
8. In infradiaphragmatic TAPVC, prenatal structural changes in the extrapulmonary veins may predispose to the later development of pulmonary vein stenosis, despite a successful surgical repair.

Thus, Haworth's conclusion[166] was that in newborns with obstructed TAPVC, prenatal pulmonary vascular disease is present and should be anticipated.

Does Left Ventricular Size Help Determine Survival in Totally Anomalous Pulmonary Venous Connection?

Lima et al[171] concluded that it probably does.

Surgical Experience With Totally Anomalous Pulmonary Venous Connection in Infancy

In 1983, Mazzucco et al[172] from Padua reported their results, based on 20 patients. Major intracardiac anomalies were present in 4 infants (20%) with complex TAPVC, and isolated TAPVC was found in 16 (80%). The 4 with complex TAPVC all had pulmonary venous obstruction, and additional associated malformations were as follows: critical pulmonary valvar stenosis, 1 case; multiple VSDs, 1 case; mitral atresia, 1 case; and the asplenia syndrome, 1 case. Mortality with complex TAPVC was 4 of 4 (100%), whereas mortality with isolated TAPVC was 2 of 16 (12.5%). The classification of Mazzucco et al[172] of TAPVC into **isolated** and **complex** subgroups remains clinically highly relevant.

TAPVC with drainage of one lung by the other. In 1983, Brenner, Bharati, Berman, and Lev[173] reported a rare form of TAPVC in a patient with visceral heterotaxy and asplenia, dextrocardia, and TGA {A,L,L} with pulmonary outflow tract atresia. The left-sided lung drained by a horizontal pulmonary vein into the right-sided lung and thence to the RSVC via a small orifice. Their patient closely resembles that of Delisle et al[1] that is diagrammed in Fig. 7.3D.

Left pulmonary artery branch stenoses in the scimitar syndrome. Hypoplasia or stenosis of the RPA is typical of the scimitar syndrome, particularly when an anomalous systemic arterial blood supply from below the diaphragm supplies the right lower lung. In contrast to this familiar association, Platia and Brinker[175] in 1984 reported the rare situation of peripheral *left* pulmonary arterial branch stenoses in a 19-year-old woman with scimitar syndrome. This unusual case provides further evidence that in the scimitar syndrome, the anomalies are not exclusively right-sided.

Surgical repair of PAPVC to the SVA. In 1984, Williams et al.[177] from Atlanta reported a conceptually beautiful and simple way of surgically repairing PAPVC to the RSVC in children. The repair consisted of connecting the superior part of the SVC—above the anomalously connected pulmonary veins—to the RA via a conduit consisting of an atrial flap and pericardium. Then the unmoved pulmonary veins were tunneled to the LA. How well would this repair work? Only future follow-up could tell. Our concerns about using the right atrial appendage as a conduit to direct SVC blood to the RA would be that such conduits often become stenotic over time. However, this is why the right atrial appendage was amplified with pericardium—to make conduit stenosis less likely. On the positive side of our guesstimate, the conduit consists, in part, of living tissue (the right atrial appendage) and hence should grow and hopefully enlarge over time. Moreover, if stenosis developed in this SVC-to-RA conduit, perhaps the stenosis could be dealt with by stenting. Suffice it to say that at that time (1984), this ingenious repair seemed very appealing. (Our purpose is to present an accurate history of important developments in this field, not to endorse or advocate particularly therapeutic approaches.)

Does PGE_1 open the ductus venosus (as it opens the ductus arteriosus)? Bullaboy et al[180] thought so. Their patient was a

3-day-old boy with TAPVC to the portal system. In their patient, PGE_1 appears to have opened the ductus venosus. Hence they suggested[180] that PGE_1 may have a new therapeutic role in lessening the obstruction of TAPVC below the diaphragm by opening the ductus venosus.

Balloon angioplasty for obstructed TAPVC? Yes, it can help. In 1985, Rey et al[190] reported the case of a 3-month-old boy with supracardiac TAPVC. There was stenosis where the vertical vein entered the LIV. Balloon dilation helped.

Obstructed TAPVC to the coronary sinus? Yes, said Jonas et al[201] in 1987. In a series of 27 patients, stenosis was present in 6 (22%). This is important both diagnostically and surgically because it means that pulmonary venous obstruction can be present in all forms of TAPVC—supracardiac, cardiac, and infracardiac.

Surgical repair of the scimitar syndrome. In 1987, Tsuchida et al[213] presented an intraatrial conduit repair of the scimitar vein. In a 26-year-old woman, these authors used a woven Dacron graft that was 14 mm wide and 6 cm long to direct the pulmonary venous return of the scimitar vein into the LA. This conduit type of repair within the RA became the standard surgical approach to the rerouting of the scimitar venous return into the LA.

Balloon dilation of narrowed pulmonary veins in TAPVC? In 1988, Lucas, Lock, Tandon, and Edwards[217] reported their findings in a series of 49 patients. Pulmonary venous obstruction was present in all cases (100%) of TAPVC below the diaphragm and in 53% of cases of TAPVC above the diaphragm. Their conclusion at that time was that balloon dilation of the narrowed pulmonary veins did not work.

Surgical Results in TAPVC. I will never forget a meeting at the Hospital for Sick Children in Toronto when I was a fellow in pediatric cardiology (1960 to 1963). Dr. William T. Mustard was presenting his surgical results in TAPVC. Seeing me in the audience and knowing how interested I was in cardiac pathology, Dr. Mustard interrupted his presentation and said to me "Richard, these results are so bad they should be presented by a pathologist!" (Laughter.) If memory serves me correctly, the surgical mortality was around 50% at that time. These results were typical of what the surgical pioneers were able to achieve in those early days. By 1989, however, Sano, Brawn, and Mee[219] from Melbourne, Australia were able to report a series of 44 patients with a surgical mortality of only 2.3%—a remarkable improvement.

How can TAPVC below the diaphragm be repaired? In 1990, Phillips et al[225] answered this question as follows: Anastomose the horizontal vein (that goes from pulmonary hilum to hilum) with the dorsal wall of the LA in the following manner. The horizontal vein and the vertical vein that passes below the diaphragm form a Y. Rotate the long inferiorly running limb of the Y anteriorly and superiorly, thereby enlarging the LA. The anastomosis should be larger than the mitral orifice. As these authors stated,[225] "Use of the descending vein as an integral part of the reconstruction and enlargement of the LA was the major technical factor leading to a successful outcome in these patients and eliminating a patch or transposition of the atrial septum." From an anatomic standpoint, making the anastomosis larger than the mitral orifice appears to be key, thereby avoiding iatrogenic pulmonary venous stenosis postoperatively.

PAPVC and Turner syndrome: Is there an association? In 1990, Moore et al[227] reported 12 patients with Turner syndrome. Of these, 3 (25%) had PAPVC with intact atrial septum. Of these 3 patients, 1 also had moderate congenital aortic stenosis. These data suggest that there may be a nonrandom association between Turner syndrome and PAPVC.

How is it possible to repair TAPVC in patients with visceral heterotaxy and the asplenia syndrome? Okita et al[237] solved this problem in a case by anastomosing the LVV to the LPA, the RSVC to the RPA, and the horizontal vein to the LA.

What is TAPVC from a developmental viewpoint? Becher, Rockenmacher, and Marin-Padilla[250] in 1992 supported the view (that we have long shared) that TAPVC results from atresia, involution, or agenesis of the common pulmonary vein and its sequelae. These investigators favored the concept of atresia of the common pulmonary vein (as opposed to involution or agenesis). We remain agnostics in this regard. No matter how and why the common pulmonary vein failed to develop, the resulting sequela appears to be that almost always, early embryonic communications between the pulmonary venous plexus and the systemic venous plexus persist and enlarge at the supracardiac, cardiac, or infracardiac level, or at a mixture of these levels. Rarely, no pulmonary venous–to–systemic venous communication persists, resulting in atresia and hence total obstruction of the anomalous pulmonary venous pathway (see Figs. 7.11 and 7.12).[1]

Stenosis of individual pulmonary veins in patients with TAPVC. Jenkins et al[256] found in 1993 that the size of individual pulmonary veins in infants with TAPVC is a strong independent predictor of survival or mortality. In a series of 32 patients, 6 (18.8%) died before hospital discharge and 8 (25.0%) died subsequently, the overall mortality being 43.8%. A study was undertaken in an effort to discover why the mortality rate was so high. Measuring the pulmonary veins carefully by two-dimensional echocardiography, these investigators found that of 8 late deaths, 6 (75.0%) had stenosis of individual pulmonary veins at sites remote from the anastomosis to the LA. They concluded that in patients with TAPVC and small individual pulmonary veins, the anomaly may not be correctable by surgical creation of an anastomosis between the pulmonary venous confluence and the LA.[256] Thus, morphometric measurements of the individual pulmonary veins at diagnosis in TAPVC may help to predict patient outcomes.

With uncorrected TAPVC, is it possible to have a successful pregnancy? Yes, said Misumi et al[257] in 1994. Their patient was a 29-year-old woman with a snowman type of supracardiac TAPVC. The authors thought that the additional volume load associated with pregnancy may have caused the pulmonary congestion that they noted and treated with digoxin and diuretics. In addition, they treated their patient with home oxygen to ameliorate her pulmonary diffusion problem associated with pulmonary edema. Labor was induced at 38 weeks with oxytoxcin because of a suspicion of mild intrauterine growth restriction. Epidural anesthesia was used to minimize pain and anxiety. Antibiotic prophylaxis was given. The mother delivered a 2500-g normal boy vaginally with vacuum extraction, and her postpartum course was unremarkable. This was the first reported case of a successful pregnancy in a mother with uncorrected TAPVC.[257]

Surgical risk factors in TAPVC. In 1995, Bando et al[270] pointed out that the presence of a small pulmonary venous confluence (horizontal pulmonary vein) with diffuse pulmonary vein stenosis remains a risk factor for adverse outcome. Their findings confirmed those of Jenkins et al.[256]

Reclassification of TAPVC. As Dudell et al[271] suggest, TAPVC should be reclassified as follows. TAPVC occurs at the following levels: supracardiac, cardiac, infracardiac, mixed, and **none.** These authors[271] presented 5 cases of TAPVC without any communication with systemic veins at any level. They diagnosed their patients has having **common pulmonary vein atresia.**[271] These cases of atresia of the common pulmonary vein, without persistence of any pulmonary venous–to–systemic venous communication, that is, without a functional anomalous pulmonary venous pathway, are the very rare exceptions. The employment of extracorporeal membrane oxygenation (ECMO) led to improvement in all 5 patients. Surgery was attempted in 3, with 2 successes.[271]

Surgical management of pulmonary vein stenosis. Until recently, the medical and surgical management of stenosis of the pulmonary veins with or without TAPVC has been a disaster, with no known long-term survivors. But in 1996, a ray of hope appeared. Lacour-Gayet, Rey, and Planché[273] from the Marie Lannelongue Cardiac Surgical Center in Paris, France published what may well prove to be a brilliant solution to this problem. Their patient was a 2½-year-old boy with obstructed TAPVC below the diaphragm. He was first operated on at 6 days of age, but by 15 months, reoperation had become necessary because of stenosis of both RPVs and of the LLPV. Conventional pulmonary venous endovenectomies were performed, but 1 year later it had become clear that recurrent pulmonary venous stenosis was present. This is what usually happened with pulmonary venous stenosis. Thus, when the patient was 2½ years of age, Lacour-Gayet et al[273] performed a new operation using deep hypothermia and circulatory arrest, the main steps of which were as follows:

1. The RA was incised along its posterior border.
2. The atrial septum was excised as posteriorly as possible to gain access to the LA.
3. The RPVs were transected about 10 mm outside the LA. Here, the RPVs appeared normal (not stenotic).
4. The RPVs were then incised back to the pericardium.
5. A large part of the posterior left atrial wall, including the RPV ostia and the atrial septum were resected.
6. The RA was then closed from the atrial septum to the right atrial free wall posteriorly using a GoreTex patch. This left a large opening leading into the LA.
7. The right part of the pericardium (to which the RPVs were attached) was then sutured to the inferior border of the IVC and to the RA. Consequently, the RPVs drained through the pericardial cavity and into the LA.

The LLPV had moderate ostial stenosis, which was resected by conventional endovenectomy, with the usual result—restenosis 6 months later. Repeat cardiac catheterization and angiocardiography 6 months postoperatively showed that the result of this new operation on the RPVs was excellent. Their diameters were normal and the mean pulmonary artery pressure was 25 mm Hg. Longer follow-up is of course necessary, plus many more cases.

Lacour-Gayet et al[273] think that the advantage of this new technique is that no sutures are placed in the stenotic veins. The authors[273] state that this new procedure was inspired by the Senning procedure in which the pulmonary venous return is led to the right heart by an extensive nonobstructive pulmonary venous pathway fashioned out of pericardium.

These authors[273] have also applied a similar technique to stenotic LPVs. The stenotic LPV was incised from its left atrial ostium all the way back to the left pulmonary hilum. The LPV was left open, draining freely into a septated pericardial cavity and thence to the LA.

This "sutureless" technique (no sutures in the pulmonary veins) applies to native or primary pulmonary venous stenosis, as well as to postoperative pulmonary venous stenosis in patients with TAPVC, as in their case.[273] Time and further experience[279,280] are of course needed to assess the efficacy of this new and promising approach to the surgical repair of stenosis of the pulmonary veins.

TAPVC to the coronary sinus with an unroofed coronary sinus. In 1996, Banitt[274] reported the case of a 24-year-old man with TAPVC to the coronary sinus who also had a coronary sinus septal defect (congenital unroofing of the coronary sinus). Surgical repair consisted only of patching the coronary sinus ostium, to close what was physiologically tantamount to an ASD with left-to-right shunting. The patient was left with a small right-to-left shunt from the coronary sinus into the LA. This case is reminiscent of the Van Praagh procedure for the repair of TAPVC to the coronary sinus (Fig. 7.18),[12] except that in this rare patient[274] there was no need to surgically create a coronary sinus septal defect.

Anomalous pulmonary venous return to the RA due to malposition of the septum primum into the LA. In 1995, Hiramatsu et al[282] understood the idea of Dr. Stella Van Praagh et al[24] and acted on it. Hiramatsu et al[282] corrected the displacement of the atrial septum into the LA by correctly positioning the septum primum, thereby redirecting all of the pulmonary venous return into the LA, without using a patch.

Normal development of the pulmonary veins in human embryos and the morphogenesis of sinus venosus defects. Blom, Gittenberger-de Groot, and colleagues[285] published a study of these subjects in 2001, based on 20 human embryos, 4 to 7 weeks of age. Their salient conclusions were as follows:

1. At 4 weeks (28 days) of age, the orifice of the nonlumenized common pulmonary vein is visible as an endothelial invagination within the sinus venosus segment. The study of Van Praagh and Corsini,[5] based on 83 human embryos, is in approximate agreement concerning the timing of the first appearance of the common pulmonary vein (see Fig. 7.5A–B): 27 days estimated ovulation age. However, in our case the common pulmonary vein was not nonlumenized; a small lumen was present (see Fig. 7.5A–B). Perhaps more important, we did not think that the common pulmonary vein was connected with the sinus venosus. Instead, we thought that the developing pulmonary vein was located *above* the sinus venous (not within the sinus venosus) and communicated with the primitive atrium (see Fig. 7.4), as has long been thought. If the common pulmonary vein begins by connecting with the sinus venosus, Blom et al[285] do not explain why the pulmonary veins normally do not connect with the coronary sinus (the left sinus horn) or with the RA (partly composed of the right sinus horn).
2. Blom et al[285] state that the development of the septum primum and a ventral proliferation of extracardiac mesenchyme from the dorsal mesocardium position the common pulmonary vein into the LA. We would agree about the importance of the development of the septum primum,[5] and we also think that Blom et al[285] are probably right that the dorsal mesocardium may well play a role (see Fig. 7.5A–B). So the effort to understand the normal development of the common pulmonary vein continues.
3. Blom et al[285] conclude that a deficiency of the wall between the sinus venosus in the RA and the adjacent pulmonary vein explains the development of sinus venosus defects. The understanding of Blom et al[285] concerning the morphogenesis of sinus venosus and our own understanding (Am Heart J 1994;128:365; see Chapter 6) seem to be very close.

Improved surgical management of the scimitar syndrome. In 2003, Brown et al[293] published an improved approach to the surgical management of the scimitar syndrome. They reported 9 patients (1 male and 8 female), operated on between 1990 and 2000, with a mean age of 11.5 years.

Using a right thoracotomy through the right fifth intercostal space, all patients had direct reimplantation of the scimitar vein into the LA, without cardiopulmonary bypass. Two patients also had resection of a right lower lobe pulmonary sequestration. Follow-up was complete. Mortality was zero, and reoperations were zero. Follow-up was a mean of 55 ± 46 months. Echocardiography at follow-up showed that all patients had a patent anastomosis, without evidence of restenosis. Thus, long intraatrial baffles that are prone to stenosis and cardiopulmonary bypass can be avoided, with excellent results to date.[293] An important technical detail of this revised operative technique is that the surgeon spatulated the scimitar vein and did an end-to-side anastomosis so that the anastomosis was twice the diameter of the scimitar vein.[293] As always, more time and further follow-up are needed to obtain a long-term assessment of this promising new approach.

PULMONARY ARTERIOVENOUS FISTULAE

We have only 3 cases of pulmonary arteriovenous fistulae (fistulas) in our cardiovascular pathology database (3/3216 = 0.09%). This is a very small sample, suggesting that pulmonary arteriovenous fistulae and congenital heart disease seldom coexist. We suspect that most of the cases of pulmonary arteriovenous fistulae that have been examined over the years by the Pathology Department of Children's Hospital Boston did not have congenital heart disease, and hence we in the Cardiac Registry did not have the privilege of examining them. However, the small number in this series also means that we have the unusual luxury of describing each case individually and trying to learn the diagnostic and management lesions of each case—just as we always do with every individual case.

Cases

Case 1. Case 1 was a 7 10/12-year-old white girl with TOF {A(S),D,S} with the heterotaxy syndrome and left-sided polysplenia. As the segmental anatomy indicates, there was some degree of ambiguity of the visceral situs (A), but it was thought to be basically situs solitus (S). The atria were also thought to be basically in situs solitus, hence TOF {A(S),D,S}.

The descending colon was freely mobile (not normally "tacked down"). The lungs were bilaterally bilobed. The liver was predominantly right-sided. The IVC was interrupted. An enlarged azygos vein connected with the LSVC. The RSVC was small and did not connect directly with the underlying RA. The LIV was well developed, carrying the RSVC blood to the LSVC. Precisely how the LSVC connected with the atria was uncertain at autopsy because of considerable postoperative change (a bidirectional Glenn procedure, described later). We think that the large LSVC probably connected with the atria via an unroofed coronary sinus, but we could not prove that because the LSVC had been transected and anastomosed end-to-side with the LPA (the bidirectional Glenn).

The suprahepatic segment of the IVC connected with the atrium inferiorly and posteriorly, approximately in the midline. A common atrium was present, no vestige of the atrial septum being found. The pulmonary veins appeared to connect normally with the LA, posteriorly and to the left.

The right-sided atrial appendage was relatively large and triangular, whereas the left-sided atrial appendage was comparatively small, long, and finger-like—supporting the interpretation of basically situs solitus of the atria. Completely common AV canal, type C was present (echocardiography).

TOF was present with a small subpulmonary infundibulum. The conal septum was displaced anteriorly, superiorly, and to the left. There was considerable aortic overriding; but the aortic valve was rightward, posterior, and inferior relative to the pulmonary valve, and there was direct fibrous continuity between the overriding aortic valve and the superior leaflet of the common AV valve.

A right aortic arch with mirror-image branching of the brachiocephalic arteries was present. Mesocardia was found, the heart being centrally located within the chest. **How was this patient with complex tetralogy of Fallot managed (in the**

1980s)? At 5 months of age, a 4-mm central shunt was constructed at another institution between the ascending aorta and the pulmonary artery. At 2 11/12 years of age, the central shunt was taken down and a left-sided bidirectional Glenn shunt was done.

At 3 2/12 years, mild regurgitation of the common AV valve was detected echocardiographically. At 5 3/12 years of age, to reduce the flow work of the heart, the main pulmonary artery was ligated. When the patient was 7½ years of age, multiple small pulmonary arteriovenous fistulae were found by cardiac catheterization and angiocardiography, this being 4½ years after the bidirectional Glenn procedure. Clinically, the patient had developed progressive, severe cyanosis and physical limitation.

At 7½ years of age, an intraatrial conduit was placed, rerouting the hepatic venous blood to the pulmonary artery. This was a Fontan completion procedure, designed to expose the lungs to hepatic venous blood, with the thought that absence of hepatic venous blood to the lungs may have played an etiologic role in the development of the numerous small pulmonary arteriovenous fistulae. At the same procedure, the regurgitant common AV valve was replaced with a 33-mm St. Jude prosthetic valve.

Postoperatively, the patient failed to regain consciousness and a bihemispheric encephalopathy developed, leading to death 21 days postoperatively. Neuropathology of the central nervous system revealed numerous neurons with shrunken nuclei and hypereosinophilic cytoplasm characteristic of recent hypoxic or ischemic necrosis. These findings were widespread in the cerebral gray matter, in the posterior fossa, and also in the spinal cord.

What happened during the Fontan completion procedure? We were never entirely certain. The cardiac arrest time had been undesirably long (1 hour and 29 minutes). We could not exclude the possibility of air embolism. Suffice it to say that the immediate cause of death was massive hypoxic central nervous system necrosis. In regard to lessons of this case, ideally, how should this patient have been managed?

1. Do not treat TOF with chronic palliation with either an aortopulmonary shunt or a bilateral Glenn procedure.
2. Instead of chronic palliation, repair the patient, if necessary in stages.
   a. For example, something similar to a reverse Mustard procedure would have been necessary at the atrial level because the large persistent LSVC probably entered the common atrium quite far to the left via an unroofed coronary sinus. Also, the hepatic segment of the IVC was posterior and centrally located (which is really normal). Thus, in septating the common atrium, the LSVC blood stream would have to be baffled rightward.
   b. The completely common AV canal type C would have to be repaired at the same time.
   c. And the pulmonary infundibular and valvar pulmonary stenosis, typical of TOF, would also have to be repaired.

The foregoing is a lot of surgery to do in one procedure, which may be why our surgeons elected not to attempt this in 1990. Even now it would not be easy. Perhaps atrial septation and completely common AV canal repair, leaving the VSDs open and the pulmonary outflow tract stenosis unrepaired, might constitute the first stage. The second stage would then consist of VSD closure and unobstruction of the pulmonary outflow tract.

However, we strongly suspect that our surgeons would now prefer to correct everything at one operation, this being made safely possible by improved cerebral protection against hypoxia.

Nonetheless, the point of this case is that TOF in the setting of the heterotaxy syndrome with polysplenia can be a complex and difficult surgical problem.

We have not done anything about the diffuse bilateral small pulmonary arteriovenous fistulae that presumably were induced by lack of the *hepatic factor*[294-296] because the patient had received a chronic bidirectional Glenn procedure. To the best of our present knowledge, the postulated "hepatic factor" has not as yet been identified biochemically.

Do pulmonary arteriovenous fistulae regress on exposure to IVC blood and, if so, how long does this take? At the present time, we do not know the answers to these important questions. Clearly, it seems to be better to *avoid* the development of pulmonary arteriovenous fistulae by repairing such patients, rather than palliating them with a chronic bidirectional Glenn operation.

Thus, this patient is yet another example of the **Castañeda principle**[297] that palliation often is more hazardous than complete repair. But the practical problem remains: How best to do the complete repair?

The pulmonary pathologic issues in this patient merit mention. As soon as barium was injected into the pulmonary arteries, almost simultaneously it appeared in the pulmonary veins. Normally, the barium solution remains confined to the pulmonary arteries and arterioles; it does not grossly and densely fill the pulmonary veins. The latter finding is typical of pulmonary arteriovenous malformations. Histologically, the number of pulmonary vessels was thought not to be significantly increased.

Case 2. This patient was a 4 2/12-year-old white girl who also had heterotaxy with polysplenia but who had no Glenn or Fontan procedure before the appearance of diffuse bilateral pulmonary arteriovenous malformations at 2½ years of age. This history suggests that even unoperated patients with the polysplenia syndrome may be at increased risk for the development of pulmonary arteriovenous malformations. The first known case of polysplenia with pulmonary arteriovenous malformations in an unoperated patient without intracardiac shunts was reported by Papagiannis et al[298] in 1993.

In somewhat greater detail, the present patient was born at 37 weeks gestation with a birth weight of 2.5 kg. On the first day of life, duodenal atresia was diagnosed and surgically corrected. During surgery, polysplenia was diagnosed, there being five small splenuli in the right upper quadrant. The stomach was also right-sided.

The patient had chronic congestion and wheezing, was treated with bronchodilators, and at 18 months of age a secundum ASD was closed surgically at another institution. On discharge from hospital, her atrial saturation was 97%.

She did well until 2½ years of age, when she was noted to be cyanotic. At 3 years of age, the patient was examined by a pediatric cardiologist, who found clubbing, cyanosis, and dyspnea on exertion. On room air, her systemic arterial oxygen saturation was 84% with a pH of 7.30, pO_2 of 53 mm Hg, and a pCO_2 of 31 mm Hg. Cardiac catheterization at an outside institution revealed an intact atrial septum, an interrupted IVC with an azygos continuation to the RSVC, and connection of the suprahepatic segment of the IVC with the right-sided RA. At 3 5/12 years of age, repeat cardiac catheterization at another outside institution revealed bilateral pulmonary arteriovenous malformations. The patient was started on home oxygen therapy that increased her oxygen saturations to 97% to 99%.

At 3 8/12 years of age, she was admitted for an episode of lower gastrointestinal bleeding, the cause of which was unclear. She had a normochronic, normocytic anemia (hematocrit 27.3%, hemoglobin 9.4 g/100 mL, mean corpuscular volume 87.5 m^3, mean corpuscular hemoglobin 30.1 μg, and mean corpuscular hemoglobin concentration 34.4%). Although chest x-ray films showed a normal cardiovascular silhouette and normal pulmonary vascularity, there was diffuse prominence of the pulmonary interstitium with possible fibrosis, atelectasis, or infiltrative disease. She was then listed for lung transplantation.

Her subsequent clinical course was characterized by progressive deterioration with falling systemic arterial oxygen saturations (78% to 80% at 4½ years of age) and increasing respiratory effort.

Bilateral lung transplantation was performed at 4 2/12 years of age. The donor was a 10-month-old infant with diabetic ketoacidosis. The operation took 11 hours, including 1 hour of cardiopulmonary bypass. The postoperative course was complicated by pulmonary hypertension, systemic hypotension, and combined metabolic and respiratory acidosis. Consequently, she was placed on ECMO immediately postoperatively. Multiorgan failure then occurred, leading to death on the eighth postoperative day.

Autopsy confirmed many of the previously mentioned findings and revealed others: visceral heterotaxy with right-sided polysplenia. Cardiac segments {A(S),D,S}, with some ambiguity (A) of visceral situs but with solitus atria (S); interruption of the IVC with enlarged azygos vein to the RSVC; ostium secundum type of ASD; surgically closed right-sided stomach; duodenal atresia, well-repaired; status postsurgical correction of malrotated intestine, with multiple intestinal and fibrous adhesions; short globular pancreas; incompletely annular pancreas (associated with duodenal atresia); massive gastrointestinal hemorrhage, diffuse, with focal thickening of small bowel and colonic wall; acute pulmonary alveolar damage with extensive hemorrhage and infarcts; and narrowing of anastomosis between native and donor LPA (5 mm in diameter).

The lessons from this case are as follows:

1. Perhaps the most important lesson is that diffuse bilateral pulmonary arteriovenous malformations can occur in patients with polysplenia who have *not* undergone a Glenn or Fontan procedure.[298] Because the suprahepatic segment of the interrupted IVC connected normally with the right-sided morphologically RA, the hepatic factor should have been delivered normally to the lungs. (The segmental anatomy was normal, i.e., {S,D,S}, with AV and VA concordance.) Consequently, it seems difficult, if not impossible, to explain the diffuse bilateral pulmonary arteriovenous malformations on the basis of absence of the hepatic factor in the lungs, at least in this case. Hence, there may be more to the cause of pulmonary arteriovenous malformations than the postulated hepatic factor. Are pulmonary arteriovenous malformations really part of the polysplenia syndrome? Before it will be possible to answer this question with certainty, we will need more carefully studied patients (with this question specifically in mind). For now, we regard nonsurgically related pulmonary arteriovenous malformations as a *rare association* of visceral heterotaxy with polysplenia.[298]
2. We think that bilateral lung transplantation was the appropriate therapy in this case. This case occurred relatively early in our lung transplant experience (1992). We thought that the donor was too small (a 10-month-old donor for a 4-year-old patient). Consequently, the surgery was difficult and took too long (11 hours). However, all of these lung transplantation problems are important technical details that can be improved. The real problem is the scarcity of appropriate donors.

Case 3. The patient was born prematurely at 31½ weeks gestation. His mother had a history of a pulmonary arteriovenous fistula that had been resected 10 years before this pregnancy, and there was a strong family history of Osler-Weber-Rendu disease (hereditary hemorrhagic telangiectasia). The patient was cyanotic at birth. Two-dimensional echocardiography showed normal cardiac anatomy with dilation of the LPA and veins. MRI revealed a pulmonary arteriovenous malformation of the left lung versus a hemangioma. At 20 days of age, his oxygen saturation values were 43% to 60% on room air. Arterial blood gas values were pH 7.25, pCO_2 36 mm Hg, and pO_2 31 mm Hg.

Cardiac catheterization and angiocardiography at 2 days of age showed a large pulmonary arteriovenous malformation of the left upper lobe. A small ASD with left-to-right shunting was also noted. Fourteen coils were used to embolize the arteriovenous malformation, but some residual right-to-left intrapulmonary shunting was observed. His saturations improved to mid-70% and low 80%.

By 2 months of age, his oxygen saturation values were 55% to 60%, a new T wave inversion was noted electrocardiographically, and his arterial blood gas values were pH 7.37, pCO_2 45 mm Hg, and pO_2 24 mm Hg. With oxygen administration (100% by face mask), there was no increase in systemic arterial oxygen saturations. Nine coils were placed to embolize the residual arteriovenous malformations in the left upper and left lower lobes. The posterolateral segment of the left lower lobe and the right lung were thought to be free of arteriovenous malformations. Systemic arterial oxygen saturations increased from 40% to 62% before embolization to 85% after embolization. At 6 months of age, increasing cyanosis and a saturation of 56% were noted. Physical examination showed moderate tachypnea, a hyperdynamic precordium, and continuous murmurs throughout the chest. Cardiac catheterization and angiocardiography showed multiple residual arteriovenous malformations of the left upper and lower lobes that were embolized with 11 coils. The patient's oxygen saturation increased to 89%, and the Qp/Qs ratio increased from 0.6:1 to 1:1.

At 7 months of age, he had a mild episode of bronchiolitis due to respiratory syncytial virus. At 8 months, he had wheezing and fever. His expiratory phase was prolonged, he had crackles over the left chest, and his cyanosis was more marked. Blood culture grew pneumococcus sensitive to penicillin. He was discharged home on oral penicillin and prednisone. At 9 months of age he was readmitted with lethargy, vomiting, fever, and decreased oral intake. Fever persisted despite antibiotics. The patient developed bradycardia and hypotension and expired despite all resuscitative efforts.

Autopsy showed marked cardiomegaly, right ventricular enlargement, and left ventricular hypertrophy and enlargement. The LPA was markedly dilated (16 mm in diameter), and the LUPV was even more dilated (19 mm).

The left upper lobe of the lung was markedly enlarged and firm, with an irregular surface and focal areas of hemorrhage. Multiple dilated arteries and veins were visible, with coils in place, and with multiple recent antemortem thrombi. The left lower lobe was hypoplastic, with no evidence of arteriovenous malformations, and the right lung was normal.

Histologically, the left upper lobe's parenchyma displayed numerous large and closely spaced blood vessels. These vessels consisted of prominent thick-walled pulmonary arteries with lamellated elastic fibers, smaller muscular arteries with well-defined internal and external elastic membranes, and large thick-walled pulmonary veins with absence of (or only scanty) elastic tissue components. Occasional thick-walled vessels with partial investment by layered elastic tissue were also observed, these structures being suggestive of abnormal pulmonary arteriovenous connections. The pulmonary arteries showed eccentric intimal fibrous plaques and areas of thrombosis in many different stages, from unorganized occlusive thrombi, to thrombi with organization and recanalization, and other thrombi with obstruction and fibrous obliteration of the vascular lumen.

Extensive perivascular fibrosis of the left upper lobe also extended into the alveolar parenchyma, with reduction of functional respiratory tissue. One prominent focus of acute parenchymal necrosis and infarction was also seen; there was no evidence of reparative response. Acute or subacute pneumonia was not identified. Bacteria were not identified with bacterial stains, and fungi were not seen.

The lessons of the case were as follows:

1. The left lower lobe was hypoplastic and was not involved by pulmonary arteriovenous fistulae, contrary to our clinical diagnostic impression.
2. We thought that a left upper lobectomy should have been done, instead of placing 34 coils on three different occasions into the left upper lobe arteriovenous fistulae. It is our impression that coils are more likely to be successful when the arteriovenous malformation is relatively small (rather than when it is large or huge, as in the present case). It also should be mentioned that this was relatively early in our experience with coil occlusion of pulmonary arteriovenous malformations (1992).
3. This 9-month-old boy almost certainly had Osler-Weber-Rendu disease, as his mother did. The pulmonary arteriovenous malformations of Osler disease are probably different from those that may occur after chronic Glenn shunts: those of Osler-Weber-Rendu disease tend to be much larger than post-Glenn arteriovenous malformations.
4. Central cyanosis, present at or shortly after birth, is not always due to congenital heart disease. One should know that pulmonary arteriovenous malformations belong on one's list of the causes of neonatal or infantile central cyanosis.
5. A large right-to-left intrapulmonary shunt existed during fetal life, explaining the left ventricular hypertrophy and enlargement that is characteristic of large pulmonary arteriovenous fistulae, as in Case 3.[299-301]
6. The large right-to-left intrapulmonary shunt results in a steal phenomenon, blood being shunted away from the pulmonary vascular system, that consequently may be hypoplastic[301] as the left lower lobe was in Case 3.

Pulmonary arteriovenous fistulae occur in approximately 15% of patients with Osler-Weber-Rendu disease.[302] Hereditary hemorrhagic telangiectasia is an autosomal dominant condition. At least three genes are capable of causing this disorder. Two have been mapped to chromosome 9q33-q34 and to chromosome 3p22. Thus, by mutation detection or linkage analysis, presymptomatic and prenatal diagnosis is now possible.[303]

STENOSIS OF THE PULMONARY VEINS

Our database reveals that 35 patients had stenosis of the pulmonary veins. We then carefully restudied these cases and excluded all those in whom pulmonary venous stenosis was thought to be iatrogenic, that is, after the Mustard procedure or Senning procedure, produced by a mitral valve prosthesis, or secondary to any other surgical operation. Our desire was to study congenital or perhaps naturally acquired pulmonary stenosis (but not postoperative pulmonary vein stenosis, in the belief that iatrogenic pulmonary venous stenosis can be avoided by better surgical technique in patients who did not have pulmonary vein stenosis preoperatively). Consequently, 14 cases were excluded. Hence, this study of pulmonary vein stenosis is based on 21 patients (21/3216 of congenital heart disease = 0.65%).

How many anatomic types of pulmonary venous stenosis did we find? The answer is seven, and they are summarized in Table 7.25.

Stenosis of Individual Pulmonary Veins

This was the most common type of pulmonary vein stenosis in this series (9/21 patients, 42.9%, see Table 7.25). In this small series of this rare disease, there was a strong male preponderance: males-to-females = 7/2 (3.5:1). The ages at death ranged from 26 hours to 12.3 years, with a mean of 23 months and a median of 8 months.

Stenosis of individual pulmonary veins involved the following veins:

1. all of the pulmonary veins in 5 of 9 patients (55.5%);
2. the LPV, both upper lobe and lower lobe branches, in 2 of 9 patients (22.2%);
3. the LULPV, the LLPV, and the RULPV, but with the RLLPV being widely patent, in 1 of 9 patients (11.1%); and

TABLE 7.25 Anatomic Types of Pulmonary Venous Stenosis (n = 21)

Anatomic Types	No. of Cases	% of Series
1. Stenosis of individual pulmonary veins	9	42.9
2. With heterotaxy and asplenia	5	23.8
3. TAPVC to left innominate vein	2	9.5
4. TAPVC below the diaphragm	2	9.5
5. Stenosis with scimitar syndrome	1	4.8
6. Functional stenosis of pulmonary veins	1	4.8
7. Poor incorporation of common pulmonary vein into LA with hypoplasia of all pulmonary veins	1	4.8

LA, left atrium; *TAPVC*, totally anomalous pulmonary venous connection.

4. the LULPV only in 1 of 9 patients (11.1%).

Stenosis of individual pulmonary veins was a primary cause of death in all of the previously mentioned 9 patients, except for the last, who had stenosis of the LULPV only. Thus, stenosis of individual pulmonary veins was a highly lethal abnormality: 8 of 9 patients (89%).

It may be noteworthy that we never saw stenosis of the RPVs only, whereas we had 3 patients (33%) in whom only the LPVs were involved. Hence, the LPVs may be more prone than the RPVs to stenosis of individual pulmonary veins; however, more experience with this rare and poorly understood entity is needed before any firm conclusions can be reached in this regard.

When all of the pulmonary veins were involved by stenosis, several noteworthy findings were encountered:

1. In a female infant who died at 26 hours of age, the youngest patient in this series, RLPV and LLPV opened into a common chamber that in turn emptied into the LA via a restrictive communication (4 × 5 mm). The RUPV and LUPV did not enter this common chamber; instead, each connected with the LA by a stenotic orifice that measured 2 mm in internal diameter. Thus, this patient had what may be called **"hemi-cor triatriatum"** because only half of the pulmonary veins connected with the stenotic chamber that communicated with the LA. Hemi-cor triatriatum is an exceedingly rare anomaly.
2. Stenosis of individual pulmonary veins involving all of the pulmonary veins can coexist with **PAPVC,** as in a 6.75-month-old male infant. The LPVs and RPVs were stenotic at their junction with the LA. However, the RPVs also had a wide and unobstructed communication with the azygos vein.
3. Stenosis of individual pulmonary veins, which are normally (not anomalously) connected, typically occurs at the pulmonary venous–left atrial junction, where the pulmonary veins pass through the left atrial wall to drain into the left atrial cavity. Occasionally, however, the stenosis of the individual pulmonary veins occurs **at the pericardial reflections.** This location is quite far out, very peripheral relative to the left atrial wall. This abnormality was found in a 13.5-month-old boy. This gross appearance suggested extrinsic constriction of the pulmonary veins by, or close to, the pericardial reflection. Grossly, the pulmonary veins appeared to be stenotic, not where they passed through the left atrial wall, but peripherally, at the level of the pericardial reflection, that is, at the level of the primary division of the LPV and the RPV into two branches on each side. Hence, the gross appearance suggested *pericardial constriction of the LVPs and RPVs.*

Histologic examination, done by the author and Dr. Ruthellen Fried (our pulmonary pathologist in the early 1980s) revealed a broader picture. There was very marked fibrosis about the pulmonary veins, both within the lungs, at the pericardial reflections, and also where the pulmonary veins pass through the left atrial wall. The pulmonary venous intima per se appeared normal, that is, thin and unremarkable. But the subintimal layer was enormously thickened with fibrous tissue. No abnormal myocytes were recognized. There was no suggestion of inflammation—no mononuclear or polymorphonuclear leukocytes. No thrombosis was seen. Pulmonary veno-occlusive disease was not present.

So the question became: What is the cause of this marked and extensive *subintimal pulmonary venous fibrosis*? We could not tell. Consequently, we tentatively concluded that stenosis of individual pulmonary veins is idiopathic subintimal pulmonary venous fibrosis (more about histology later). Other cases amplified this understanding.

In a 12 3/12-year-old boy, the oldest patient in this series, three veins were involved (left upper, left lower, and right upper), but the fourth (RLPV) was widely patent. In somewhat greater detail, the LLPV was highly stenotic, the lumen being only 1 mm in internal diameter. The LUPVs and RUPVs were totally occluded by old thrombus at their junction with the left atrial wall. Peripheral to the left atrial wall (i.e., closer to the lungs), the internal diameters of pulmonary veins were not stenotic: LLPV, 3.0 mm; LUPV, 4.5 mm; RUPV, 5.0 mm; and RLPV, 14.0 mm (dilated). Each pulmonary vein wall measured less than 1 mm in thickness.

Histologic examination of the LLPV, LUPV, and RUPV in this patient revealed an increase in fibrous tissue and a decrease in elastic tissue that appeared coarser and more widely spaced than normal.

The lessons of this patient were thought to be as follows:

1. Stenosis of individual pulmonary veins, if chronic, can progress to **pulmonary venous atresia** at the pulmonary venous–left atrial junction.
2. The mechanism of atresia appeared to be **thrombosis** at the pulmonary venous–left atrial junction.

Other histologic interpretations were as follows:

1. In a 9-month-old boy with severe stenosis of the LPVs only (1 mm in internal diameter), the histologic findings showed considerable noncellular intimal proliferation of both large and small veins of the left lung.
2. In a 3-month-old boy with severe stenosis of all pulmonary veins as they entered the LA (RPV < 1 mm in internal diameter, LPV 1 to 2 mm in internal diameter associated with circumferential nodularities), the histologic finding at the pulmonary venous–left atrial junction was described as showing moderate to severe cellular intimal thickening composed of loose myoxid connective tissue with elastic tissue.

TABLE 7.26 **Stenosis of Individual Pulmonary Veins (n = 9)**

Case No.	Case Description
1	Multiple congenital anomalies: polyvalvar disease (karyotype unknown) with redundant MV without MR, redundant TV with mild TR, redundant AoV with mild AR; ASD II; VSD (conoventricular, paramembranous) with mild anterior deviation of conal septum; PDA; microcephaly with developmental delay; premature closure of cranial sutures with increasing hydrocephalus; bronchiolitis due to RSV, 4 mo, treated with ribovirin; severe progressive stenosis of all PVs, L > R, 11-mo-old girl
2	TGA {S,D,D} with IVS + PS (valvar, bicuspid, rudimentary septal commissure, myxomatous PV), abnormal TV with absent interchordal spaces + mild TR; bronchiolitis at 2 months; stenotic LUPV (1 mm), 8-mo-old boy. Died after Mustard procedure because of coexisting pulmonary valvar stenosis with IVS. Stenosis of LUPV not important as cause of death.
3	Multiple congenital anomalies: anal atresia with rectourethral fistula; right undescended testicle overlying right kidney; bilaterally symmetrical liver with normally formed spleen; absent gallbladder and cystic duct with normal bile ducts; malrotation of bowel with cecum and appendix in LUQ with Ladd bands; VSD (conoventricular, high, large, subaortic, with anterior malalignment of conal septum, i.e., Eisenmenger's complex); LSVC to CoS to RA; ASD II; Meckel's diverticulum of ileum; no visceral heterotaxy, (i.e., {S,D,S}). 9-mo-old boy, severe stenosis of LPVs only; left lung markedly consolidated
4	Congenital aortic valvar stenosis (unicuspid, unicommisural—only LC/NC commissure well formed); small-chambered, thick-walled LV with severe EFE of LV; moderate congenital MS; premature closure of foramen ovale; sinusoid between left ventricular cavity and posterior descending coronary artery; ropelike anterior descending coronary artery; tubular hypoplasia of transverse aortic arch; preductal coarctation of aorta; large PDA; pulmonary lymphangiectasia. 26-hr-old female infant with stenosis of all PVs, RLPV and LLPV opening to a common chamber (hemi-cor triatriatum) that drained through a restrictive orifice (4 × 5 mm) into LA, RUPV = 2 mm, LUPV = 2 mm (both drained through stenotic orifices into the LA)
5	Mitral atresia ({S,D,S}; restrictive atrial septum; VSD (conoventricular, Eisenmenger complex); linear midmuscular VSD; subaortic stenosis (produced by MAt and TV leaflet tissue). 6.75-mo-old boy, stenosis of all pulmonary veins, RPVs also having wide unobstructed connection with azygos vein (i.e., partially anomalous pulmonary venous connection)
6	Twin; full term but small for gestational age (1660 g); TGA {S,D,D} with VSD (conoventricular, paramembranous, 4 mm, partly obstructed by tricuspid valve tissue), aortic arch hypoplasia with preductal coarctation, PDA; reactive pulmonary hypertension (R_{PA} = 10 WU, room air and 2 WU, 90% O_2); PA bronchiolitis due to RSV. 7-mo-old boy, stenosis of left pulmonary veins only (diagnosed at 7 mo of age). SIPVs: congenital? vs. acquired?
7	Isolated stenosis of all PVs, 3-mo-old boy
8	Isolated stenosis of all PVs, 13.5-mo-old boy
9	Isolated stenosis of left lower pulmonary vein, with thrombotic occlusion of left upper and right upper pulmonary veins, right lower pulmonary vein widely patent + dilated. Right carotid aneurysm, intracranial, with recanalized thrombus (presumed thromboembolism from thrombosed pulmonary veins)

AR, Aortic regurgitation; *ASDII*, ostium secundum type of atrial septal defect; *AoV*, aortic valve; *CoS*, coronary sinus; *EFE*, endocardial fibroelastosis; *IVS*, intact ventricular septum; *L>R*, left greater than right; *LA*, morphologically left atrium; *LC/NC*, left coronary-noncoronary; *LPV*, left pulmonary vein; *LLPV*, left lower pulmonary vein; *LSVC*, left superior vena cava; *LUPV*, left upper pulmonary vein, *LUQ*, left upper quadrant; *LV*, morphologically left ventricle; *MAt*, mitral atresia; *MR*, mitral regurgitation; *MS*, mitral stenosis; *MV*, mitral valve; *PA*, pulmonary artery; *PDA*, patent ductus arteriosus; *PS*, pulmonary stenosis; *PVs*, pulmonary veins; R_{PA}, resistance in the pulmonary artery; *RA*, morphologically right atrium; *RLPV*, right lower pulmonary vein; *RPVs*, right pulmonary veins; *RSV*, respiratory syncytial virus; *RUPV*, right upper pulmonary vein; *{S,D,S}*, the segmental anatomic set of situs solitus of the viscera and atria, D-loop ventricles, and solitus normally related great arteries, with atrioventricular and ventriculoarterial concordance being assumed, unless stated to the contrary; *SIPVs*, stenosis of individual pulmonary veins; *TGA {S,D,D,}*, transposition of the great arteries with the segmental anatomic set of situs solitus of the viscera and atria, D-loop ventricles, and D-transposition of the great arteries, with atrioventricular concordance assumed unless stated to the contrary and with ventriculoarterial discordance understood (the meaning of TGA); *TR*, tricuspid regurgitation; *TV*, tricuspid valve; *VSD*, ventricular septal defect; *WU*, Wood units.

The foregoing descriptions of the histologic findings in stenosis of individual pulmonary veins make it clear that this disease process is not completely understood:

1. Is the stenosing fibroelastic tissue intimal or subintimal or does it originate from somewhere else and migrate to an intimal or subintimal site (see later)?
2. What is the cause of this excessive fibroelastic pulmonary venous tissue?

We hope that future investigation will clarify these unresolved questions.

Associated Malformations. What kind of patients were these cases with stenosis of individual pulmonary veins? In other words, did stenosis of individual pulmonary veins (SIPVs) typically occur in isolation (isolated SIPVs), or did SIPVs characteristically occur with other significant associated malformations (nonisolated SIPVs)? The answer to these important questions are given in Table 7.26.

As Table 7.26 indicates, stenosis of individual pulmonary veins often occurred with significant associated malformations:

1. nonisolated SIPVs occurred in 6 of these 9 patients (66.7%) (Cases 1 to 6, inclusive; see Table 7.26), and
2. isolated SIPVs was found in 3 of these 9 patients (33.3%) (Cases 7 to 9, inclusive; see Table 7.26).

Stenosis of the Pulmonary Veins With Visceral Heterotaxy and Asplenia

This was the second most common anatomic type of pulmonary venous stenosis in this series (5/21 patients, 23.8%; see Table 7.25). In all 5 patients, a hypoplastic and hence stenotic communicating vein connected with the SVC:

1. to the RSVC in 3 of 5 patients (60%), and
2. to the LSVC in 2 of 5 patients (40%).

One of these patients with a hypoplastic communicating vein to the LSVC was very rare—perhaps unique—and hence merits more detailed description. The patient was a 4-month-old girl with visceral heterotaxy and asplenia who also had the **Goldenhar syndrome** (oculoauriculovertebral dysplasia). This is the only patient of whom we are aware who has had both the asplenia and the Goldenhar syndromes. The heterotaxy syndrome in this patient was quite typical with DORV {A(I),D,D}, left-sided IVC and SVC, larger triangular left-sided atrial appendage (consistent with a morphologically RA, left-sided and anterior), and a smaller right-sided finger-like atrial appendage (consistent with a morphologically LA, right-sided and posterior). There was a common atrium, and a common AV valve canal opened into a large, right-sided morphologically RV, that is, common-inlet RV. The morphologically LV was diminutive, left-sided and posterior. There was a bilateral conus with no pulmonary or aortic outflow tract obstruction (rare not to have pulmonary outflow tract stenosis or atresia). All 5 of these patients with visceral heterotaxy and asplenia had DORV. The segmental anatomy was as follows:

1. DORV {A(S),D,D} in 2,
2. DORV {A(I),D,D} in 1, and
3. DORV {A,L,L} in 2. One of the latter patients had "D"ORV {A,L,L} because the main pulmonary artery (MPA) was absent, the RPA and LPA branches were discontinuous, and small bilateral PDAs were present. Purists might prefer to regard this patient has having **solitary aortic outlet RV** because the MPA was in fact absent. We prefer the more familiar diagnosis of **"D"ORV with absence of the MPA.** However, the diagnoses are equivalent in anatomic meaning and hence either is satisfactory.

For those desiring more information concerning visceral heterotaxy with asplenia, see Chapter 36.

Congenital Pulmonary Venous Stenosis With Totally Anomalous Pulmonary Venous Connection to the Left Innominate Vein

This was the third anatomic type of pulmonary venous stenosis that was found in this series: 2 of 21 patients (9.5%; see Table 7.25).

The first of these patients, a 32-day-old girl, had a **typical vascular vise.** The LVV was compressed between the LPA anteriorly and the left mainstem bronchus posteriorly (see Fig. 7.3A).[1]

The second patient, a 12-day-old boy, was unique in our experience. Two very hypoplastic, thread-like veins originated from within the left pulmonary parenchyma, behind the left mainstem bronchus, and ran superiorly and medially to connect with the LIV. These two oblique communicating veins were less than 1 mm in diameter and were therefore highly stenotic. There was no typical LVV. In addition, this patient had complex congenital heart disease: a large ostium secundum type of ASD, a closing PDA (after the ill-advised administration of indomethacin to close the ductus), a bicuspid aortic valve (because of a rudimentary right coronary-noncoronary commissure), and preductal coarctation of the aorta. Thus, after functional closure of the ductus arteriosus, the right heart circulation was markedly obstructed by the extremely hypoplastic oblique communicating pulmonary veins, explaining the marked right atrial and right ventricular hypertrophy and enlargement. The oblique communicating pulmonary veins were so hypoplastic that they were not visualized echocardiographically. Consequently, the presence of marked congenital pulmonary venous stenosis was not understood diagnostically, which in turn led to the administration of indomethacin, functionally closing the ductus, thereby making obstruction of the right heart circulation worse. Because the patient also had preductal coarctation of the aorta, both right heart and left heart circulations were significantly obstructed.

Severe biventricular obstruction is not a viable situation. The differences between the prenatal circulation, that the patient survived, and the postnatal circulation, that the patient could not survive, are thought to be as follows:

1. Functional closure of the PDA deprived the right heart of its "escape hatch"—right-to-left shunting through the PDA.
2. Reduction of the pulmonary arteriolar resistance postnatally suddenly made the extremely hypoplastic communicating pulmonary veins a factor of major importance, that is, unmasking high-grade pulmonary venous stenosis that had not been of hemodynamic importance prenatally.

Congenital Pulmonary Venous Stenosis With Totally Anomalous Pulmonary Venous Connection Below the Diaphragm

This is the fourth anatomic type of congenital pulmonary venous stenosis encountered in this series: 2 of 21 patients (9.5%; see Table 7.25). This form of congenital pulmonary venous stenosis has been discussed previously in connection with TAPVC; hence, the following is brief.

The first patient was a 3-week-old girl who had obstruction of the vertical paraesophageal vein at the diaphragmatic crus (see Fig. 7.3G).[1]

The second patient, a 9-day-old girl, had TAPVC to the portal vein. The ductus venosus connecting with the IVC underwent closure, forcing all of the pulmonary venous blood to return to the RA via the hepatic sinusoids, resulting in pulmonary venous stenosis. Spontaneous closure of the ductus arteriosus meant that the pulmonary circulation was denied this potential "escape hatch" (no right to left ductal shunting). Consequently, all of the pulmonary arterial blood had to percolate through the restrictive hepatic sinusoids.

This patient also had complex congenital heart disease in addition to the obstructed subdiaphragmatic TAPVC: a secundum type of ASD, an aberrant right subclavian artery (without dysphagia), a forme fruste of right juxtaposition of the atrial appendages, and right atrial and right ventricular hypertrophy and enlargement, reflecting TAPVC with obstruction.

In these patient descriptions, if additional associated anomalies are not mentioned, one may assume that no other associated malformations were present (as in the first patient described earlier).

Functional Pulmonary Venous Stenosis With the Scimitar Syndrome

This, to our knowledge, is a unique case of a 6-month-old girl with MCAs. She had the scimitar syndrome with all RPVs connecting with the IVC immediately below the diaphragm. There was anomalous systemic arterial blood supply to both lobes of the right lung from the abdominal aorta. The right lung was bilobed, the large upper lobe and middle lobe components forming the right upper lobe, and with marked hypoplasia of the right lower lobe. Sequestration was not present because the tracheobronchial tree connected with all lobes of both lungs. Mesocardia was present, secondary to mild hypoplasia of the right lung. The RPA was larger than is often seen in this condition.

The right scimitar pulmonary vein was obstructed functionally (but not anatomically) because of marked stenosis of the IVC at its junction with the RA. The hepatic segment of the IVC was encircled by liver tissue, the internal diameter of the IVC-RA junction measuring less than 1 mm. Small "vegetations" (nonbacterial) were noted at this highly stenotic IVC-RA junction. Angiocardiography revealed retrograde (caudad) blood flow in the superior portion of the IVC. Multiple collateral anastomoses were present with right and left paravertebral veins. There was generalized hypoplasia of the entire IVC; and the azygos vein was enlarged and returned normally to the RSVC.

There was also stenosis of the Lupus at their junction with the LA, associated with one small "vegetation" (small, raised, nonbacterial nodule). There was possible stenosis of the LLPVs, with one small "vegetation" at the pulmonary venous ostium. Cardiac catheterization revealed pulmonary hypertension at systemic or suprasystemic levels that was thought to be due not only to the anomalous systemic arterial blood supply to the right lung but also to the obstruction of both the RPV and LPV returns.

Again, it should be emphasized that the right pulmonary scimitar vein per se was not stenotic; instead, the stenosis involved the IVC-RA junction. Nonetheless, the hemodynamic effect was stenosis of the RPV blood stream. This is why we referred earlier to this as *functional* pulmonary venous stenosis (as opposed to *anatomic* pulmonary venous stenosis). Purists may prefer to delete this as a case of pulmonary venous stenosis because the RPVs themselves were not stenotic. In a similar anatomically accurate sense, this is a very rare case of **stenosis of the IVC-RA junction.**

This patient, who was the product of a first-cousin marriage (consanguinity), also had a forme fruste of horseshoe kidneys with fibrous attachment of the lower renal poles. The hypoplastic IVC indented the lower pole of the right kidney. Bilateral hydropelvis and hydroureter were present. This patient had clinical evidence of psychomotor retardation with probable microcephaly (head circumference and body weight were both well below the third percentile), micropolygyria, bilateral cataracts, simian crease of the left palm, and arachnodactyly (?Marfan syndrome).

To summarize, we thought that the truly interesting features of this case were as follows:

1. the marked hypoplasia of the entire IVC;
2. obstruction of the markedly hypoplastic IVC at two places:
   a. at the IVC-RA junction; and
   b. somewhat below this junction in association with encircling hepatic tissue; and
3. bilateral pulmonary venous obstruction in a patient with scimitar syndrome.

At the time we did this autopsy (in 1970), we had never before seen any of these three previously mentioned features. I remain just as impressed by this case today (in 2003) as I was 51 years ago. As is so often the case, we told ourselves that this case *has* to be reported, but we did not do it until now, hence, this book (there are so many unreported "reportable" cases like this).

Functional Stenosis of the Pulmonary Veins

Functional stenosis (as opposed to anatomic stenosis) of normally connected pulmonary veins occurred in a 14-day-old boy (1/21 patients, 4.8%; see Table 7.25) with mitral atresia and a highly obstructive atrial septum. There was a probe-patent foramen ovale with a muscularized septum primum that bulged aneurysmally into the cavity of the RA. Hence, there was significant obstruction of the pulmonary venous blood stream because of the coexistence of mitral atresia and a highly restrictive atrial septum. There was no stenosis of the pulmonary veins per se. Hence, this patient suffered from functional (but not anatomic) pulmonary venous stenosis.

Again, purists might prefer to delete this patient from any discussion of pulmonary venous stenosis (which was not present in an anatomically precise sense, but which was very important clinically and hemodynamically).

In somewhat greater detail, there were multiple fenestrations of the septum primum. A persistent LSVC connected with the coronary sinus and returned to the RA.

DORV {S,D,D} was present with a subpulmonary conus. There was aortic valve–to–tricuspid valve fibrous continuity. As expected with mitral atresia, there was marked hypoplasia of the morphologically LV and a small subaortic VSD.

There was subvalvar and valvar aortic stenosis. The subaortic stenosis was produced by narrowing of the aortic outflow tract between the clonal septum anteriorly, superiorly, and to the left and the underlying tricuspid valve. There was also marked aortic annular stenosis (hypoplasia) with tubular hypoplasia of the transverse aortic arch and preductal coarctation of the aorta (internal diameter 1.5 mm). The PDA was large.

So what is this? This is the **infantile type of DORV,** so-named by the late Dr. Richard Rowe; that is, this is DORV with hypoplastic left heart. Mitral atresia is typical. One of the more important aspects of this understanding is that DORV with hypoplastic left heart (e.g., mitral atresia) typically has a unilateral (not a bilateral) conus:

1. When there is a subpulmonary conus, with no subaortic conal free wall and hence with aortic-tricuspid fibrous continuity (as in this patient), there usually is aortic outflow tract obstruction with preductal coarctation.
2. When the unilateral conus is subaortic, with no subpulmonary coal free wall, there is pulmonary-tricuspid fibrous continuity and pulmonary outflow tract obstruction between the conal septum anterosuperiorly and the tricuspid valve posteroinferiorly.

To summarize, when mitral atresia is associated with a restrictive atrial septum, functional (as opposed to anatomic) pulmonary venous obstruction is clinically and hemodynamically very important. Balloon or surgical atrial septostomy/septectomy is urgently needed and can be lifesaving.

Poor Incorporation of the Common Pulmonary Vein Into the Left Atrium

A 4-month-old boy had poor incorporation with stenosis of the common pulmonary vein at its junction with the LA. This patient also had PAPVC (mixed) with an LVV running from the LUPV to the LIV, and a diminutive vein from the LVV to the coronary sinus with stenosis of the right atrial ostium of the coronary sinus. Hence, this patient had a stenotic ostium of a poorly incorporated common pulmonary vein that coexisted with a stenotic mixed PAPVC.

This patient also had TGA {S,D,L} with left atrial outlet atresia ("mitral" atresia). There was a large morphologically LV. The LA was located above the left ventricular free wall. Consequently, the LA was "blind" and had no AV valve opening into the LV. The right-sided AV valve had mitral morphology and opened only into the large LV. A small right ventricular sinus was present, which received no AV valve leaflets or chordae tendineae. This small RV sinus had no papillary muscles. The only inlet into this small RV was via a restrictive slit-like conoventricular type of VSD that measured 5 mm in horizontal length, but only 1 to 2 mm in vertical height. There was a subaortic conus, with pulmonary–AV valvar direct fibrous continuity. The restrictive slit-like VSD constituted subaortic stenosis and was associated with tubular hypoplasia of the transverse aortic arch, severe preductal coarctation of the aorta, and a large PDA. There appeared to be rightward malalignment of the ventricular part of the heart relative to the atria, resulting in left atrial outlet atresia because the bottom of the LA "opened" into the LV free wall (instead of into the LV cavity), creating the appearance of "mitral" atresia. We think that mitral atresia really is not present because the right-sided AV valve was of mitral morphology and opened only into the large LV.

Consequently, our interpretation of the findings is that the LA has no outlet because of ventriculoatrial malalignment with rightward displacement of the bulboventricular loop relative to the atria. We think that the lack of a left atrial AV outflow is not because of mitral atresia. This is also why the LV is large. With true mitral atresia, the LV is diminutive.

Briefly, this patient had left atrial outlet atresia with a large LV, that is, the **Quero anomaly**.[19] Consequently, at 3 weeks of age (in 1992) the patient underwent surgical division of the PDA, repair of the coarctation of the aorta using an extended end-to-side anastomosis (between the transected end of the descending thoracic aorta and the opened underside of the hypoplastic transverse aortic arch), atrial septectomy, pulmonary venoplasty to remove the obstructive membrane between the unincorporated common pulmonary vein and the LA, and banding of the MPA.

Postoperative cardiac catheterization revealed residual pulmonary venous stenosis (20 mm Hg) and stenosis between the pulmonary venous confluence and the LIV (30 mm Hg).

At 3 months of age, stent placement was attempted at the connection of the pulmonary veins with the LA. One stent migrated into the LA and then into the left ventricle. A second stent occluded the RPV and led to arterial desaturation with cardiac arrest of short duration. Emergent cardiac surgery led to the removal of both stents, one at the junction of the RPV with the LA causing obstruction, and the other from the tensor apparatus of the right AV valve in the LV. Venoplasty was then performed of the anastomosis between the RPVs and the LA.

Repeat cardiac catheterization at 4 months of age showed what was interpreted as severe discrete stenosis between all pulmonary veins and the LA. The gradient between the LPVs and the LA was 22 mm Hg. Because of the restrictive VSD, the gradient between the LV and the aortic root was 60 mm Hg, and left ventricular end-diastolic pressure was elevated to 17 mm Hg. In view of the previously mentioned findings, it was decided in consultation with the family to abandon further "heroic" therapeutic efforts and the patient expired shortly thereafter.

At autopsy we were surprised to find that the previously mentioned diagnostic impression was significantly erroneous, as follows: Discrete stenosis of all of the pulmonary veins at their junction with the LA was not found. Indeed, these anastomoses could not have been better, we thought. The anastomosis of the common pulmonary vein with the LA was widely patent, 7 mm in internal diameter.

The surprise finding at autopsy was diffuse hypoplasia of all pulmonary veins. The pulmonary veins were thin and delicate, but very small. The internal diameters of the pulmonary veins at autopsy in the fresh state (not formalin fixed) were as follows: RUPV, 2.5 mm; RLPV, 2.5 mm; LUPV, 3.0 mm; left middle pulmonary vein, 1.5 mm; and LLPV, 2.0 mm.

The diagnostic and surgical lessons of this case are as follows:

1. Our initial diagnostic impression, that is, poorly incorporated common pulmonary vein with stenosis at the pulmonary venous–left atrial junction, was not wrong. But it was significantly incomplete.
2. The finding of severe, generalized pulmonary venous hypoplasia and hence stenosis at autopsy was a total surprise to all of us.
3. This surprising, unexpected, and very important finding reminded us of what Dr. Stephen Sanders,[256] our superb echocardiographer at that time, had been saying, namely, when patients with TAPVC do not do well postoperatively, it often is not because the anastomosis between the horizontal vein (the pulmonary venous confluence) is too small, but rather because significant hypoplasia of the pulmonary veins coexists.
4. From the diagnostic standpoint, when one makes the diagnosis of discrete stenosis of pulmonary veins at the left atrial junction, one should also look very carefully for coexisting hypoplasia/stenosis of the pulmonary veins remote from their left atrial junction.[256]
5. From the therapeutic standpoint, we thought that the only strategy that might succeed in this type of patient might be a heart and lung transplant.

The Literature

In addition to the literature already referred to, other papers concerning stenosis of the pulmonary veins merit mention.[304-333]

Isolated Versus Nonisolated. In 1966, Dr. James H. Moller et al[304] presented a postmortem case of stenosis of individual pulmonary veins without other congenital heart disease. In our series of 21 cases of pulmonary venous stenosis, only 3 (14%) had *isolated* pulmonary vein stenosis. The great majority had *nonisolated* pulmonary vein stenosis (18/21; 86%). Thus, isolated pulmonary vein stenosis is rare in our experience: 3 of 3216 (0.09%).

Congenital or Acquired? In 1967, Dr. George Contis et al[305] presented a postmortem patient who had pertussis, followed by two episodes of pneumonia, leading these authors to suggest that the stenosis of the individual pulmonary veins may have been acquired (not congenital). In our 3 patients, two appeared to be definitely congenital. In the third patient, who had pertussis followed by pneumonias,[305] the pathologist who signed this case out—Dr. Gordon Vawter—thought that the stenosis of the individual pulmonary veins probably was congenital but that there was some possibility that it could have been acquired. Thus, our impression—based on these 3 rare cases of isolated stenosis of individual pulmonary veins—is that this condition is congenital, rather than postnatally acquired.

Sclerosing Mediastinitis. Nasser et al[306] in 1967 reported sclerosing mediastinitis as an acquired cause of pulmonary venous obstruction. This we did not see in our series, but one should be aware of this possibility.

Is Surgical Cure Possible? In 1972, Binet et al[307] from Paris reported what they thought was the first recorded case of successful diagnosis and surgical management of congenital unilateral pulmonary venous stenosis. First seen at 3½ months of age, this little girl had a history of repeated episodes of hemoptysis. Angiocardiography revealed a to-and-fro motion of contrast in the right pulmonary artery. At surgery, bypass was not used. One large pulmonary vein was found. A pericardial patch was used to widen the lumen at the bifurcation of the RPVs. This report was published when the patient was 8 years of age and doing well. Later on, stenosis of individual pulmonary veins would be discovered to have a very dismal therapeutic prognosis; however, this patient of Dr. Jean Paul Binet[307] appears to have done well, at least until 8 years of age.

However by 1982, Driscoll et al[315]—based on a series of 8 patients that they had tried to treat by transvenous balloon dilatation—concluded that the prognosis of congenital stenosis of individual pulmonary veins is poor and that "treatment is an enigma."

With Transposition of the Great Arteries. In 1984, Vogel et al[317] noted that when unilateral congenital pulmonary vein stenosis complicates TGA, the stenosis in their experience was always left-sided. The question, of course, is why. These authors[317] hypothesized that the preferential blood flow to the right lung postnatally in patients with TGA may predispose to hypoplasia and hence to stenosis of the lower flow LPVs. (I remain unpersuaded because there are so many patients with D-TGA who do *not* have stenosis of the LPVs.)

Therapeutic Hope. In 1984, Bini et al[318]—including Drs. John W. Kirklin and Al Pacifico—concluded, based on a series of 10 patients, that rapid restenosis of the pulmonary veins occurred in all cases and that no surgical repair was successful.

However in 1986, Reid et al[322] reported the case of a young woman who was not correctly diagnosed as having unilateral pulmonary vein stenosis until she was 16 years of age. Successful surgical therapy consisted of pneumonectomy. Admittedly, pneumonectomy is a pretty drastic form of "successful surgical therapy," but considering the alternative, pneumonectomy certainly merits mention.

In 1993, Luhimo et al[327] reported good long-term results in 6 patients using encircling endocardectomy. All were well 5 to 15 years postoperatively.

In 1996, Lacour-Gayet et al[273] introduced a new sutureless surgical technique that was used in situ pericardium (described in detail earlier).

In 1998, Najm et al[279] from the Hospital for Sick Children in Toronto reported a favorable experience with this new sutureless technique.

In 1999, Lacour-Gayet et al[289] in Paris applied this new technique to the repair of progressive pulmonary venous obstruction after the surgical reconstruction of TAPVC, which occurred in 16 of 178 such patients (9%). The new approach worked well, and these authors called their operation **in situ pericardial pouch plasty.**

At the present time (2003), in situ pericardial pouch plasty appears very promising as a potential therapeutic solution to the difficult problem posed by stenosis of the pulmonary veins. However, longer follow-up and more experience are needed before we will be able to assess this approach definitively.

Secondary Pulmonary Vascular Changes. Congenital pulmonary venous stenosis may induce pulmonary vascular changes, as Endo et al[330] reported in 2000. These investigators found progressive medial thickening and intimal fibrosis of pulmonary arteries and veins, plus pulmonary lymphangectasia. However, they found no plexiform lesions or more advanced stages of pulmonary arterial and arteriolar obstructive disease, which may explain the reversibility of pulmonary hypertension caused by congenital pulmonary venous obstruction.

Chemotherapy. In 2001, Jenkins et al[290] concluded that isolated progressive pulmonary venous stenosis may be caused by myofibroelastic proliferation.[326] These investigators treated such patients with vinblastine and methotrexate. They reported a mortality rate of 72%.[290] Thus, at the present time, chemotherapy does not appear to be a promising approach to the treatment of pulmonary venous stenosis.

Small Intrapulmonary Arteries. When totally anomalous pulmonary connection has an obstructed pulmonary venous pathway, the small pulmonary arteries within the pulmonary parenchyma may be significantly hypoplastic. Maeda et al[332] found that in 10 patients with TAPVC and pulmonary venous obstruction, the radius of the small pulmonary arteries within the lung measured on average 47.0 ± 21.8 μm, whereas the radius of small pulmonary arteries within the lung in normal controls averaged 75.9 ± 9.8 μm ($p < .001$). These findings suggest that even when pulmonary venous obstruction is successfully repaired in such patients, some obstruction of the pulmonary circulation with pulmonary arterial hypertension may persist because of hypoplasia of the small pulmonary arteries within the lungs. Further data are needed concerning this surprising and (to us) new possibility.

PULMONARY VENO-OCCLUSIVE DISEASE

What is pulmonary veno-occlusive disease? In the following text, we are going to do our utmost to answer this question. But, as you will see, much mystery remains.

First we must mention what pulmonary veno-occlusive disease is not. Pulmonary veno-occlusive disease is not *congenital* atresia or marked hypoplasia of the connecting vein in TAPVC. (We blush to confess that we had 2 cases like that, misfiled as pulmonary veno-occlusive disease. One died at 13 hours of age [A91-29] and the other died at 30 hours of age [A71-61].) Congenital atresia or severe hypoplasia (marked stenosis) of the anomalous pulmonary venous pathway in TAPVC is not what is meant by pulmonary veno-occlusive disease.

Instead, pulmonary veno-occlusive disease is an *acquired* disorder (not a congenital one) involving a structurally normal cardiovascular system with normally formed pulmonary veins.

We have only 1 case of pulmonary veno-occlusive disease in our entire database: 1/3400 = 0.029%. Or, because we have 3216 cases of congenital heart disease and 184 cases of acquired cardiovascular disease in our database, because pulmonary veno-occlusive disease is an acquired disorder, it may well be more accurate to report its incidence as 1/184 (0.54%). However, suffice it to say that this disease is very rare in our experience. Because we have studied only one such case, we have the unusual opportunity to provide a detailed account of this one patient—in the hope that such an account will make this case as unforgettable for you as it has been for us.

The patient was a 13 3/12-year-old young woman (A70-249). Clinically, she was thought to have familial primary pulmonary hypertension. When our patient was 2 years of age, her older brother died at the age of 12 years with what was thought probably to be pulmonary vascular obstructive disease. Unfortunately, no autopsy was performed of her older brother and consequently the true nature of her older brother's illness remains unknown.

Because of her brother's death, our patient underwent cardiac catheterization when she was 2 years of age. The results of the cardiac catheterization were completely normal, with normal right ventricular and pulmonary artery pressures. Her present illness seemed to begin in the spring of 1969, when she was 11 8/12 years of age. Complaining of a mild decrease in exercise tolerance, she was seen by an experienced pediatric cardiologist in another city who concluded that the patient was normal based on her physical examination, chest x-ray films, and electrocardiogram. However, 1 year later in the spring of 1970, at 12 8/12 years of age, she became markedly symptomatic and tired on climbing a flight of stairs.

At 13 1/12 years of age, physical examination revealed a loud single second heart sound and mild peripheral desaturation. Arterial oxygen saturation by ear oximetry was 93% at rest and 86% on exercise. In the opinion of one of our radiologists, Dr. Thorne Griscom, the pulmonary parenchyma showed a reticular, nodular appearance—not characteristic of primary pulmonary hypertension, which was the patient's diagnosis at this time. Other radiologists disagreed. Subsequent chest x-rays films, however, bore out the diagnostic impression that the patient had a diffuse, nodular, bilateral pulmonary parenchymal disease. The electrocardiogram showed right ventricular hypertrophy with ST and T wave changes.

Cardiac catheterization revealed a near systemic level of pulmonary hypertension. Although there was no evidence of intracardiac right-to-left or left-to-right shunts, there was mild desaturation (88%) of the pulmonary veins and systemic arteries that was thought to be due to intrapulmonary shunts. The patient was discharged on priscoline 25 mgm orally three times a day.

One month later, she was readmitted because of a marked increase in shortness of breath and continuous nausea. Chest x-ray films now showed diffuse reticular nodular infiltrates in both lung fields (see Fig. 7.34). The differential diagnosis included possible tuberculosis, fungal disease, vasculitis, or hemosiderosis. Because of the development of hepatomegaly, the patient was digitalized. Intravenous steroids were begun. Evidence of low cardiac output and respiratory distress further increased, leading to bradycardia and death on December 14, 1970 at 13 3/12 years of age.

In our discussion of this case immediately after the autopsy, I said:

> **Type of Case:** *I don't know what type of case this is. . . . The pulmonary parenchymal findings do not fit the diagnosis of primary pulmonary hypertension. None of us has ever seen lungs that grossly look like this: small red to bluish to occasionally blackish nodules, varying from less than 1 mm in diameter to as much as 4 mm, and averaging approximately 2 mm in diameter. These hemorrhagic raised palpable nodules are scattered diffusely over the pleural surfaces of both lungs. Cutting into the left lower lobe, the same sort of nodules are found scattered throughout relatively normal looking, well aerated pulmonary parenchyma.*

We were seeing something that none of us had ever seen before, something that was very striking and unforgettable. Each of us tried to describe what we were looking at. Richard Van Praagh said, "It looks as though the lungs have the measles" (referring to the cutaneous rash of measles). Roberta Williams, MD, the Cardiology fellow rotating through the Cardiac Registry, said, "They look like leopard lungs" (referring to the dark, blue-black spots). Louise Calder, MD, who was then one of our Cardiac Registry fellows, added, "Lumpy leopard lungs" (referring to the fact that the lesions are not just spots, but are really nodules). Richard Van Praagh, MD, director of the Cardiac Registry, agreed, but remarked that these lumpy spots are mainly reddish to bluish, not black. We noted that these red-blue-black nodules are located in the lungs only and nowhere else. Today, more than 30 years later, we still clearly remember these startling "**leopard lungs.**"

We hoped, of course, that histologic examination would give us a nice, clear-cut, straight-forward answer to our central question, that is, what is this disease? Here is how Dr. Gordon Vawter (Associate Pathologist-in-Chief) and Dr. Abraham (fellow in Pathology) signed this case out: Primary pulmonary hypertension (?familial), pulmonary artery sclerosis and pulmonary arteriolar sclerosis (grade IV), pulmonary veno-occlusive disease with pseudo-angiomatoid collateral circulation in the lung, and right ventricular and right atrial hypertrophy and enlargement.

The RPA was perfused with radiopaque material (barium solution) at postmortem, maintaining a pressure of 65 mm Hg by Dr. Luisa Stigol, our pulmonary pathologist. The radiograph obtained after postmortem examination showed a marked decrease in background haze, as is typical in cases with pulmonary hypertension. Even more interesting, injection of the RPVs with contrast at postmortem showed blockage of many small pulmonary venules (Fig. 7.35).

Because this was a very unusual and perplexing case, at the urging of Amnon Rosenthal, MD (the patient's cardiologist), Hubert Jockin, MD (one of our general pathologists) hand-carried this patient's histologic slides to Prof Case A. Wagenvoort, an expert in pulmonary pathology at the University of Amsterdam in the Netherlands, for a consultation. As it happened, Prof and Mrs. Wagenvoort had just published a paper in *Circulation* in late 1970 concerning primary pulmonary hypertension, including pulmonary veno-occlusive disease.[335]

Prof Wagenvoort's conclusion was that this is a case of pulmonary veno-occlusive disease, because of the following histologic features: focal interstitial fibrosis, increase of bronchial mucus cells, occlusion of pulmonary veins and venules, and thrombotic lesions in the pulmonary arteries.

In somewhat greater detail, Prof Wagenvoort thought that the relevant findings were as follows:

In the lungs, there are multiple circumscribed foci of interstitial fibrosis; mild infiltration of polymorphonuclear leukocytes and a few lymphocytes in these foci; congestion of lung tissue and mild hemosiderosis, particularly in these foci; bronchi somewhat dilated with an increased number of mucus (goblet) cells; marked lymphocyte peribronchial infiltration; and thickening of the pleura and interlobular septa, containing numerous dilated lymphatics.

The pulmonary arteries showed marked intimal fibrosis of the patchy eccentric type; sometimes the formation of intraluminal septa indicative of organized thrombi or emboli, sometimes subtotal obliteration of smaller arterioles, and mild atherosclerosis of elastic pulmonary arteries with one small fairly recent thrombus. *The pulmonary veins* revealed intimal fibrosis, particularly in many pulmonary venules, some of which are occluded by loose fibrous tissue.

The previously mentioned vascular lesions—arterial and venous—are particularly severe in the foci of interstitial fibrosis (our "lumpy leopard nodules"), but are not confined to these lesions.

Prof Wagenvoort stated, "This is not a case of 'primary pulmonary hypertension.'" However, in their 1970 paper, Wagenvoort and Wagenvoort[333] included 5 postmortem cases of pulmonary veno-occlusive disease in their study of 156 autopsied cases of primary pulmonary hypertension. Certainly, the cause of our apparently familial case of pulmonary hypertension is

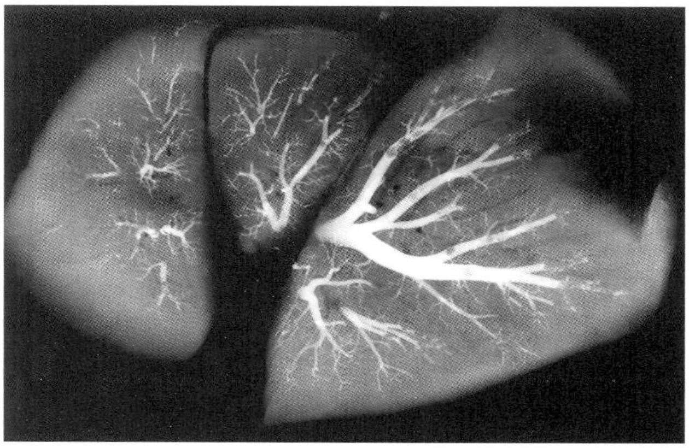

Fig. 7.35 Injection of pulmonary veins at autopsy with contrast medium in 13 3/12-year-old girl with pulmonary veno-occlusive disease, showing numerous blocked small pulmonary veins.

"primary" (unknown). The fact that this disease killed two siblings at approximately the same age suggests that this idiopathic familial pulmonary hypertension may well have a genetic or metabolic basis that targets males and females in early adolescence: our patient was 13, and her brother was 12 years of age at death.

Wagenvoort and Wagenvoort[333] summarized their 5 autopsied cases of pulmonary veno-occlusive disease as follows: males-to-females = 2/3; average age = 16.2 years; and thrombotic lesions: recent = 1/5, and with septa (old recanalized thrombi) = 2.5.

The Wagenvoorts[333] suggested that pulmonary veno-occlusive disease might have a viral cause, but they added that this possibility is purely speculative.

Since the time of our case (1970), several informative studies have been published concerning primary pulmonary hypertension in general and about pulmonary veno-occlusive disease specifically.[334-338] In 1977, Edwards and Edwards[335] pointed out that there are three pathologic types of primary pulmonary hypertension:

1. plexogenic pulmonary arteriopathy,
2. recurrent pulmonary thromboembolism, and
3. pulmonary veno-occlusive disease.

1. **Plexogenic pulmonary arteriopathy**[335] appears to result from pulmonary arteriolar vasoconstriction, as was pointed out by Wagenvoort, Heath, and Edwards in their splendid book in 1964.[339] Pulmonary arteriolar vasoconstriction leads to medial hypertrophy, intimal fibrosis, luminal narrowing and/or occlusion, and ultimately plexiform lesions that bypass the occluded arterioles. This is the most common form of primary pulmonary hypertension. Prof Wagenvoort was sure that our patient did not have this disease, which is what he meant by saying that our patient did not have (the common form of) primary pulmonary hypertension.
2. **Recurrent pulmonary thromboembolism,**[335] the second pathologic type of primary pulmonary hypertension, our patient also did not have. This is the kind of primary pulmonary hypertension that can result from unrecognized multiple small pulmonary thromboemboli from pelvic and/or leg veins.

3. **Pulmonary veno-occlusive disease**[335] is a rare form of primary pulmonary hypertension. Even though we did not recognize it at the time, in retrospect, our patient was a classic example of pulmonary veno-occlusive disease. Why?

As Edwards and Edwards[335] point out, this disease may well be of thrombotic origin. Organized thrombi of the pulmonary veins often lead to large recanalized channels, to partially obstructive intimal pads, or to luminal fibrous plugs that may be loose and edematous or densely fibrotic.

Proximal to the thrombotic or later fibrotic obstruction, a pulmonary vein or venule may respond to increased luminal pressure by developing medial hypertrophy. This is known as arterialization of the pulmonary veins. Such secondary changes may resemble those seen with mitral stenosis.

Because the pulmonary capillaries and lymphatics are obstructed by the pulmonary venous thrombotic and fibrotic disease, the histologic picture in pulmonary veno-occlusive disease is very different from that seen either with plexogenic or thromboembolic pulmonary hypertension. Pulmonary capillaries are engorged, dilated, and tortuous. Alveolar hemorrhages are occasionally seen and, as a result, pulmonary hemosiderosis may be extensive.

Pulmonary lymphatics and pleural lymphatics are dilated, and the interlobular septa are edematous. Fibrovascular pleural adhesions are common and may afford collateral routes of egress of the pulmonary venous blood from the lungs.

In response to the elevated pressure, muscular pulmonary arteries develop medial hypertrophy. Thrombi, recent or organized, are occasionally found in small pulmonary arteries. Typically, plexiform lesions are absent. Patchy interstitial fibrosis and interstitial pneumonia may be seen.[335]

In 1988, Rich[336] made it clear that in pulmonary veno-occlusive disease, chest x-rays characteristically show *increased bronchovascular markings and Kerley B lines* that reflect the chronically increased pulmonary capillary pressures. This insight explains our patient's chest x-ray findings (see Fig. 7.35). Increased pulmonary bronchovascular markings and Kerley B lines are typical only of pulmonary veno-occlusive disease, but of neither other type of primary pulmonary hypertension.

Rich[336] also clarified that at cardiac catheterization, the pulmonary wedge pressure may be normal or elevated, depending on the severity or the pulmonary venous occlusion that is present. He also noted that one can obtain different pulmonary wedge pressures at different sites, again depending on variable degrees of pulmonary venous occlusion.

Rich[336] stated that pulmonary veno-occlusive disease has been reported in siblings, which we think is the case concerning the patient we are reporting.

Swensen et al[337] in 1996 reported the computerized tomography (CT) findings in 8 patients with pulmonary veno-occlusive disease, finally helping to clarify what we were looking at in 1970. These authors found that the most common CT findings were smooth interlobular septal thickening, diffuse multifocal regions of ground-glass opacity, pleural effusions, enlarged central pulmonary arteries, and pulmonary veins of normal caliber.

Swensen et al[337] confirmed that chest x-ray films show a prominent interstitial infiltrative process with Kerley B lines. They noted that the Kerley B lines correspond to the smoothly thickened interlobular septa. The thickened interlobular septa form ill-defined nodules that tend to be distributed around bronchioles.

So at long last we really understood the lumpy leopard lungs of our patient with pulmonary veno-occlusive disease. The obstructed pulmonary veins and venules (see Fig. 7.35) resulted in engorged lymphatics, edematous interlobular septa, with engorged, tortuous, and occasionally hemorrhagic pulmonary capillaries. Our nodules were pulmonary lobules, separated from relatively normal lung tissue by thickened, edematous interlobular septa. The various colors of the nodules—pink, red, blue, and black—depended on the age of the capillary engorgement and/or hemorrhage, be it recent (red), old (black), or intermediate (blue). The bilateral reticular pattern on the pulmonary chest x-ray films with prominent Kerley B lines (see Fig. 7.34) indicates severe pulmonary congestion and edema, in the absence of left heart failure or cardiac obstruction.

Thus, Kerley B lines, without left heart obstruction (such as cor triatriatum, mitral stenosis, or aortic stenosis) or left heart failure, should strongly suggest the diagnosis of pulmonary venous stenosis or occlusion—that is, pulmonary veno-occlusive disease.

At the present time (2004), untreated pulmonary veno-occlusive disease is uniformly fatal. The current treatment of choice is lung transplantation.[337,338]

The case of our patient was published in 1973 by Rosenthal, Vawter, and Wagenvoort.[340] Their summary is so good that we would like to include it here,

> *The outstanding features of this condition are symptoms and signs of postcapillary pulmonary hypertension, roentgenographic findings of diffuse bilateral pulmonary edema with or without discrete peripheral densities, absence of structural heart disease, pulmonary venous unsaturation, and, usually, normally pulmonary arterial wedge pressure.*[340]

Rosenthal, Vawter, and Wagenvoort[340] also stated that they had documented,

> *For the first time that intra-pulmonary veno-occlusive disease may be an acquired condition because cardiac catheterization, performed 10 years before the onset of symptoms, had normal pulmonary artery pressure. However, they added that a genetic role in the pathogenesis of the disease is suggested by the death of a sibling of our patient from a similar illness.*[340]

This raises the important question, **What is the cause of intrapulmonary veno-occlusive disease?** Unfortunately, the answer to this question remains unclear. Here are some of the possibilities:

1. Pulmonary veno-occlusive disease may result from pulmonary interstitial fibrosis involving fibrosis of the pulmonary venous bed. Changes in the pulmonary venous intima may predispose to thrombosis in situ, resulting in pulmonary venous narrowings or occlusions.[341] Note that pulmonary interstitial fibrosis was present in our patient. However, it is also possible that pulmonary venous occlusion may cause pulmonary interstitial fibrosis[342] rather than vice versa.[341]

2. Mediastinal fibrosis can involve virtually every level of the pulmonary venous bed, from the small pulmonary venules to the large pulmonary veins where they enter the LA.[342] Our patient, however, did not have mediastinal fibrosis, and the pulmonary veno-occlusive disease was intrapulmonary, not intrapulmonary and extrapulmonary.
3. Viral illness can be followed by pulmonary veno-occlusive disease with morphologic changes suggesting a causal relationship.[344]
4. Chemotherapy also can be followed by pulmonary veno-occlusive disease, again suggesting a causal relationship.[345]
5. Toxin exposure can be followed by pulmonary veno-occlusive disease.[346]
6. A still unidentified genetic cause is suggested by the occurrence of familial pulmonary veno-occlusive disease, with the deaths of siblings at widely different times, without known prior exposures of either sibling to viral illness, chemotherapy, or other toxins, as in our family.

Other cases of familial pulmonary veno-occlusive disease have been reported.[347,348] Thus, from the etiologic standpoint, there appear to be multiple different types of pulmonary veno-occlusive disease,[341-348] just as there are several different types of primary pulmonary hypertension.[333-336]

Although much more has been written and could be said about pulmonary veno-occlusive disease,[349-356] as Wagenvoort[351] suggested in 1976, pulmonary veno-occlusive disease appears to be a syndrome, rather than a single entity. This disorder can, for example, follow therapy for malignant neoplasms,[354] and it can occur after the use of oral contraceptives.[356] However, the form of pulmonary veno-occlusive disease seen in infants and children typically is idiopathic and can be familial (as earlier).

Atresia or Absence of the Pulmonary Veins

Pulmonary vein atresia was diagnosed in 2 of these 3216 autopsied patients with congenital heart disease (0.06%), and **pulmonary vein absence** was found in 3 patients (0.09%).

Pulmonary Vein Atresia

Patient 1. Atresia of the RPVs was found in a 7-day-old boy, who also had premature closure of the foramen ovale. The right and left atrial septal surfaces displayed no delineation between the septum primum (normally the flap valve of the foramen ovale) and septum secundum (the superior limbic band). Thus, the atrial septal surfaces were *featureless,* which is typical of so-called premature closure of the foramen ovale (which appears really to be a malformation of the atrial septum, not just premature closure of the foramen ovale).

The LPVs connected normally with a hypoplastic LA. A hypoplastic mitral valve led to a hypoplastic LV that ejected into a mildly hypoplastic ascending aorta. The ductus arteriosus was probe patent and was thought to be functionally closing. Right ventricular hypertrophy was present.

Thus, atresia of only the RPVs is rare and did not occur in isolation. Instead, atresia of the RPVs was associated with an unusual form of the hypoplastic left heart syndrome, that is, premature closure of the foramen ovale.

Patient 2. A 5-week-old boy with TAPVC below the diaphragm to the ductus venosus and thence to the IVC had a small fibrous cord running from the superior bifurcation of the anomalous pulmonary venous pathway to the LA (Fig. 7.36). This small fibrous cord was interpreted as the *atretic common pulmonary vein.*

We regard this as a very important case because here one can actually see that the common pulmonary vein was atretic, leading in turn to the persistence of an anomalous pulmonary venous pathway, that is, TAPVC below the diaphragm. This case is part of the proof (not just hypothesis) that TAPVC results from atresia or agenesis or the common pulmonary vein. The pathology resident who did the case was Dr. David Murphy, who went on to become an outstanding congenital heart surgeon in Halifax, Canada, and this figure is based on his diagram (see Fig. 7.36).

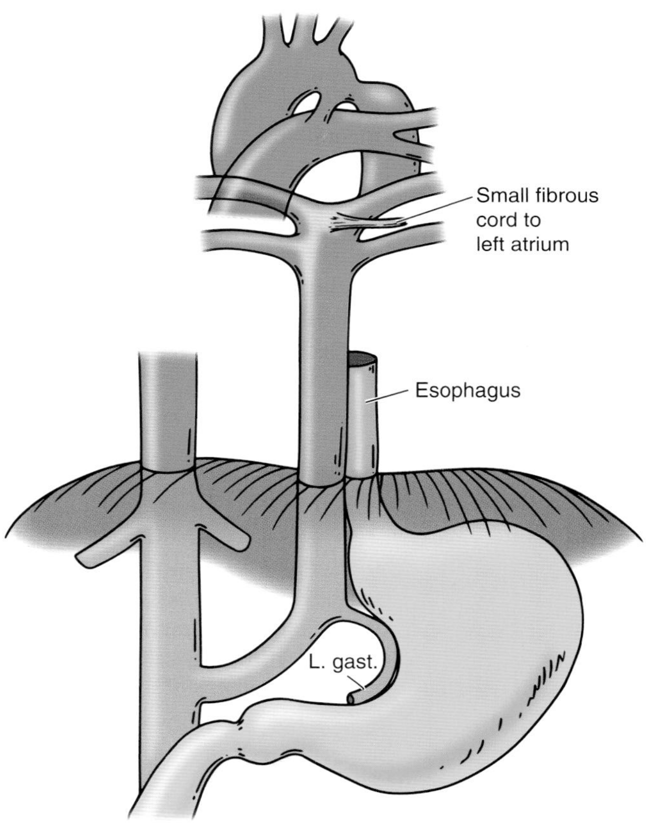

Fig. 7.36 Atresia of the Common Pulmonary Vein. Based on a diagram made at autopsy showing small fibrous cord (the atretic common pulmonary vein) running from the dorsal wall of the left atrium to the top of the vertical paraesophageal vein running below the diaphragm in a case of infracardiac totally anomalous pulmonary venous connection in a 5-week-old boy. A small patent ductus arteriosus (unlabeled) is also shown. *L. gast.,* left gastric vein.

This patient also had a small PDA (see Fig. 7.36), right ventricular hypertrophy, with pulmonary congestion, and hemorrhages.

This case is noteworthy because almost never can one find and demonstrate atresia of the common pulmonary vein in patients with TAPVC (see Fig. 7.36). We think that all cases of supracardiac and infracardiac TAPVC have atresia or agenesis of the common pulmonary vein—resulting in TAPVC, but we can almost never prove it, except in rare cases such as this.

Note also that atresia of pulmonary vein *branches only* can be associated with normally connected pulmonary veins. In patient 1, only the RPVs were atretic and the pulmonary veins were connected normally with the LA. In patient 2, however, *atresia of the common pulmonary vein (all of it)* typically results in TAPVC. This is what TAPVC typically is.

Pulmonary Vein Absence. The pulmonary veins can be partially or totally absent in several very different scenarios.

Patient 1. A 47-day-old boy with MCAs had absence of the LPVs in association with agenesis of the left lung. This patient also had the Arnold-Chiari malformation, a large leaking lumbosacral meningomyelocle, hydrocephalus, talipes equinovarus (club foot deformity), and congenital heart disease.

There was levoposition of the heart associated with absence of the left lung, the cardiac apex pointing leftward and somewhat posteriorly. The segmental anatomy was normal {S,D,S}. Despite the fact that the great arteries were normally related to the underlying ventricles and AV valves, the ascending aorta was anterior and to the right relative to the MPA that was posterior and to the left, superficially resembling D-TGA. Thus, the spatial relationship between the great arteries was very abnormal because of the secondary cardiac levoposition. The patient also had a large conoventricular type of VSD, with mild hypoplasia and mild anterior displacement of the conal septum, but without pulmonary outflow tract stenosis.

The right lung was greatly enlarged. Autopsy revealed aspiration of gastric contents into the deformed tracheobronchial tree with generalized pneumonitis. The left mainstem bronchus was short and blind. Both the LPA and the LPVs were absent. There were multiple hemivertebrae and 13 ribs bilaterally.

To summarize, absence of the LPVs was associated with agenesis of the left lung and other major associated malformations.

Patient 2. A 10-day-old boy with MCAs had agenesis of the LPVs, absence of the morphologically LA, anomalous connection of the RPVs to the coronary sinus with stenosis of this right pulmonary venous connection, mitral atresia with no evidence of the mitral valve, a subaortic VSD, and DORV {S,D,D} with a subpulmonary conus, aortic-tricuspid fibrous continuity, with mild subaortic stenosis, and mild to moderate hypoplasia of the ascending aorta and aortic arch, without coarctation of the aorta.

In addition, this patient had crossed origins of the pulmonary artery branches. The ostium of the LPA was superior and to the right, relative to the ostium of the right pulmonary artery that was inferior and to the left. The patient had the DiGeorge syndrome with thymus hypoplasia, apparent absence of the parathyroid glands (none found), and hypocalcemia. The infant was dysmorphic, with low-set ears, microphthalmia, microcornea, and hypoplastic optic nerves.

The patient's mother had toxemia of pregnancy, cervical incompetence treated with a Shirodkar wire that was removed before induction of labor, and quiescent ocular toxoplasmosis (of uncertain significance).

From the cardiovascular standpoint, this patient had **a previously unknown form of TAPVC:** absence of the LPVs, with absence of the LA, and an anomalous connection of the RPVs to the coronary sinus with obstruction of the RPVs. Thus, the left pulmonary venous obstruction was total, and the right pulmonary venous stenosis was severe. Up until this time (1976) we did not know that it is possible for **the LA to be congenitally absent.**

It is also noteworthy that this patient had the *infantile type of* DORV {S,D,D} with a unilateral (not a bilateral) conus, subpulmonary only, with aortic-tricuspid fibrous continuity. As is typical of DORV with a unilateral conus (subpulmonary or subaortic, but not both), hypoplastic left heart coexisted (mitral atresia).

Patient 3. This newborn girl died at 20 minutes of postnatal age. Autopsy revealed normal segmental anatomy {S,D,S} and a horizontal vein running from the right pulmonary hilum to the left pulmonary hilum, but with no communicating vein at any level (surpacardiac, cardiac, or infracardiac). The horizontal pulmonary vein was thick-walled, with a small lumen. The LA was abnormally small, lacking the normal pulmonary venous component. The foramen ovale was probe patent and unremarkable. There were right ventricular hypertrophy and enlargement, a PDA and coarctation of the aorta (the internal diameter of the aortic isthmus was less than 2 mm).

There were very prominent pulmonary perilobular venules and lymphatics, producing the appearance of "*strawberry lung.*" The external surface of both lungs displayed numerous, fine, elevated protuberances reminiscent of the external appearance of a strawberry. As far as we could tell, pulmonary venous obstruction was total.

It is worth recalling that the horizontal pulmonary vein ("the surgeon's friend") is not the common pulmonary vein. Instead, the common pulmonary vein is absent, creating the hemodynamic problem. But so too are all of the usually present communicating veins, at all levels.

What should we call this anomaly? Accurately speaking, it is not TAPVC because there is no anomalous pulmonary venous connection. Our suggestion, consistent with anatomic accuracy, would be (1) absence of the common pulmonary vein, with (2) absence of communicating veins at all levels. Because this situation is so rare and hence so unfamiliar, one might add that this is like TAPVC with a horizontal hilum-to-hilum vein but with no communicating pulmonary-to-systemic veins, and thus with total pulmonary venous obstruction.

A designation that has been used in the literature for the foregoing anomaly is *atresia of the common pulmonary vein.* This means that the RPVs and LPVs are present and confluent, but that the common pulmonary vein—that normally connects with the LA—is atretic. In the interests of anatomic accuracy, we would prefer to call this malformation *absence of the common pulmonary vein* because typically there is no cord-like atresia of the common pulmonary vein. Instead, there is no vestige of the common pulmonary vein. However, as often used in the literature (see following section), common pulmonary vein atresia means (1) absence of the common pulmonary vein, with the RPVs and LPVs present and confluent; and (2) absence of any communicating vein from the pulmonary venous branches to any other structure (atrium or systemic vein).

The Literature

Papers concerning atresia or absence of the pulmonary veins merit mention.[357-366]

In 1972, Hawker et al[357] described 2 patients very similar to our patient 3 (immediately earlier). Both of their patients had a horizontal pulmonary vein with no communicating vein at any level. Accurate diagnosis was achieved angiocardiographically and attempted surgical repair in their case 2 was unsuccessful.

These authors[357] diagnosed their patients as having "common pulmonary vein atresia." They called the horizontal pulmonary vein, that is, the confluent RPV and LPV branches the "common pulmonary vein," apparently not realizing that this horizontal pulmonary vein is not really the common pulmonary vein, as explained earlier. By saying that their "common pulmonary vein" was atretic, they meant that it did not communicate with the LA or with any systemic vein at any level. The horizontal vein had a small lumen and a thick wall just like our patient 3 did; that is, the horizontal vein per se was not atretic. These points are mentioned in the interests of clarity of understanding.

In 1972, it was not widely understood that TAPVC typically results (1) from atresia, absence, or involution of the common pulmonary vein; plus (2) persistence of a communicating vein or veins from a pulmonary vein branch to one or more systemic veins, the coronary sinus, or the RA.

In 1974, Mody and Folger[108] presented a very similar patient with a horizontal vein and only a tiny communicating vein to the RSVC. Most understandably, they also diagnosed their patient as having "atresia of the common pulmonary vein," just as Hawker et al[357] had done 2 years earlier. A 5-mm anastomosis was constructed between the horizontal vein and the dorsal left atrial wall, but this patient too died soon postoperatively.

Hence, as mentioned heretofore, *"atresia of the common pulmonary vein"* in the literature[108,357] can mean a horizontal pulmonary vein, with absence of the common pulmonary vein that normally connects with the LA (hence TAPVC—meaning no pulmonary vein connecting with the LA), and with essentially no communicating vein connecting the horizontal pulmonary vein with any systemic vein (hence, essentially total pulmonary venous obstruction).

In 1975, Nasrallah et al[358] reported the case of a 16-month-old boy with atresia of the RPVs who was successfully treated with right pneumonectomy. Selective wedge cineangiography of the pulmonary artery to the right lower lobe showed atresia of the pulmonary veins. There was delayed emptying of the contrast via a fine tortuous network of bronchial veins that drained into the azygos vein. Histologic examination revealed marked intimal proliferation and medial hypertrophy of the totally obstructed RPVs.

In 1977, Dye et al[359] reported occlusion of the right lower and middle pulmonary veins due to sclerosing mediastinitis in a 32-year-old black woman. The patient had severe hemoptysis. Diagnosis was established at thoracotomy. Right lower and middle lobectomy was performed. The pulmonary veins from these two lobes were found to be totally occluded by invading hard, fibrous tissue. The most impressive microscopic findings were dense fibrous tissue with many foci of acute and chronic inflammatory cells. This process also surrounded and invaded the adjacent bronchus. The patient's postoperative course was uncomplicated.

There is no similar case of mediastinal fibrosis with pulmonary venous occlusion in our series of mostly pediatric patients. In 1978, Ledbetter et al[360] reported 3 more patients with absence ("atresia") of the common pulmonary veins, 1 of whom had asplenia. In 1983, Beerman et al[361] reported 3 patients with unilateral pulmonary vein atresia. Case 1, a 10-year-old white girl, had angiocardiographically proved RPV atresia. However, no surgical intervention was undertaken because the patient had normal pulmonary artery pressure and no cardiovascular or respiratory symptoms. This case was very illuminating: *It is possible to have unilateral pulmonary vein atresia and to be asymptomatic.*

Case 2[361] was a 4-year-old white boy with a VSD, a PDA, and LPV atresia. In addition to surgical repair of the VSD and PDA, the confluence of the left superior and inferior pulmonary veins was opened just outside the LA. A diaphragm obstructing both veins was removed, and patch enlargement of the area was performed. Postoperatively, the patient was greatly improved with a considerable increase in his exercise tolerance and reduction of his pulmonary hypertension. However, his LPVs were found to remain completely occluded.

Case 3,[361] a 6½-year-old white boy, had LPV atresia. The patient had persistent hemoptysis from the left lung, but no perfusion of this lung, and hence left pneumonectomy was performed with a good postoperative course. Histologic examination revealed marked intimal hyperplasia of the pulmonary veins, with mounds of fibroblasts and collagen filling the lumina of the large LPVs.

In 1983, Kingston et al[362] also reported 3 children with unilateral atresia or absence of the pulmonary veins, and they reviewed 7 previously reported cases. These authors emphasized that this diagnosis should be considered in patients with recurrent unilateral pulmonary infection or edema. They advocated pulmonary arteriography as being necessary for diagnosis, and they noted that artery wedge angiography is the most informative diagnostic procedure. Their Case 1 had isolated left pulmonary venous atresia. Their Case 2 had TGA {S,D,D} with atresia of the LPVs. Their Case 3 had pulmonary valve atresia with an intact ventricular septum and atresia or absence of the LPVs.

In their review of 10 cases,[362] unilateral pulmonary venous absence/atresia was right-sided in 5 and left-sided in 5. Other forms of congenital heart disease were absent in 4 patients but coexisted in 6.

In 1986, Shrivastava, Moller, and Edwards[363] presented the case of a 7-year-old boy with atresia of the LPVs, for which left pneumonectomy was done at age 3½ years. Four years later, the patient developed intrapulmonary veno-occlusive disease of the right lung, leading to death. This is an exceedingly rare combination: pulmonary vein atresia of one lung, followed by intrapulmonary veno-occlusive disease of the other lung.

In 1987, Kelley et al[364] reported the case of a white male infant with surgically corrected TAPVC to the coronary sinus who developed postnatal atresia of the extraparenchymal LPVs. The patient also developed ipsilateral intraparenchymal pulmonary arteritis that was thought to be secondary to the left-sided pulmonary venous atresia. Both immunoglobulin G (IgG; 250 μg/mL; normal <30) and IgM (326 μg/mL; normal <30) were markedly elevated. This was the first report of a patient with unilateral pulmonary vein atresia with ipsilateral necrotizing pulmonary arteritis.

Cullen et al[365] reported 2 patients with isolated pulmonary vein atresia. In their Case 2, right pneumonectomy was considered but deferred in a 7-year-old boy until after his adolescent growth spurt, to avoid scoliosis.

In 1992, Mehta and Chidambaram[366] published the case of a male newborn with LPV atresia who was treated with left pneumonectomy and PDA ligation. This patient had thoracolumbar hemivertebrae. Scoliosis developed postoperatively, which may have been related to the left pneumonectomy, or the hemivertebrae, or both. From the cardiovascular standpoint, at 22 months of age this patient remained asymptomatic, with no evidence of pulmonary hypertension.

The foregoing completes our literature sample concerning atresia or absence of the common pulmonary vein, RPVs, or LPVs. Note that we are aware of no references concerning atresia or absence of all pulmonary veins (common, and right, and left).

MISALIGNMENT OF PULMONARY VEINS WITH ALVEOLAR CAPILLARY DYSPLASIA

Although we have no cases of misalignment of the pulmonary veins with alveolar capillary dysplasia in our congenital and acquired heart disease database, we think nonetheless that we should briefly consider this rare cause of primary pulmonary hypertension in neonates because pediatric cardiologists may well be consulted concerning these rare and fatally affiliated newborns.[367,368] What is misalignment of the pulmonary veins (MPVs) with alveolar capillary dysplasia? Briefly, it is a rare and fatal form of neonatal pulmonary hypertension. The pulmonary lobules are maldeveloped. The air spaces are abnormally large and simple. The epithelial cells are prominent. The air space walls are abnormally wide and very deficient in capillaries. The pulmonary veins are malpositioned, running next to pulmonary artery branches, instead of in the interlobular septa, which is normal.

Failure of formation and ingrowth of alveolar capillaries that do not make contact with the alveolar epithelium results in pulmonary hypertension and poor alveolar gas exchange. The pulmonary hypertension related to the paucity of pulmonary alveolar capillaries and the misaligned pulmonary veins is associated with hypertrophy of the media of the small pulmonary arteries, muscularization of the intra-acinar arteries, and right ventricular hypertrophy. These pulmonary histologic changes can be diffuse or patchy. Although diagnosis can be made only by histologic examination of lung tissue, the diagnosis can be missed on lung biopsy with only partial MPV.

Thus, in newborns with persistent pulmonary hypertension in whom no predisposing factor can be found (such as obvious intrinsic lung disease, sepsis, or prolonged hypoxemia), one should consider the diagnostic possibility of MPV. Unfortunately, this entity is uniformly fatal. Patients with partial misalignment can survive for 1 to 3 months. Lung transplantation may offer the hope of palliation.

Thus, MPVs with alveolar capillary dysplasia and a marked paucity of alveolar capillaries is a rare but very serious cause of clinically idiopathic primary pulmonary hypertension in the neonate. First reported in 1981 by Janney et al,[369] almost all of these infants have been full-term with uncomplicated deliveries. More than 50% have had associated anomalies involving the genitourinary, gastrointestinal, and/or the cardiovascular systems. Respiratory distress appears within the first 2 days of life, but the severity of illness and the age at death have varied considerably.[367,368]

PULMONARY VARIX

Aneurysmal dilatation of a pulmonary vein (pulmonary varix) is another abnormality that we have found in the literature[370,371] but not in our database. A pulmonary varix has been reported in a 25-year-old woman[370] and in a 33-year-old woman with rheumatic mitral regurgitation.[371] The importance of being aware of this abnormality is that a pulmonary varix can be mistaken on chest x-ray films for a pulmonary neoplasm. This diagnostic suspicion could, in turn, lead to an unnecessary and potentially dangerous percutaneous needle biopsy attempt or to an unnecessary thoracotomy. A pulmonary varix can also simulate a granuloma, lymphadenopathy, or pulmonary arteriovenous fistula.

Pulmonary angiography has been regarded as diagnostically definitive because it demonstrates its pulmonary venous nature, and it excluded early filling typical of an arteriovenous fistula. We would anticipate that more modern and less invasive diagnostic modalities such as cine MRI may be used to diagnose and follow such patients.

Pulmonary varices are thought probably to be congenital anomalies that typically have a benign course. However, 4 such patients have died as a result of their pulmonary varices, either from rupture and exsanguination or from thromboembolism—clots being found in the varix at autopsy.[371]

NORMAL ANATOMIC VARIATIONS OF THE PULMONARY VEINS

A careful study of the architecture of the pulmonary veins was done by Ho et al[372] in 2001, with special reference to radiofrequency ablation and the maze procedure in the treatment of atrial fibrillation. These workers demonstrated the highly variable architecture of the normal pulmonary veins.

Using magnetic resonance angiography, in 2003 Wittkampf et al[373] found that the left pulmonary venous ostia normally are oval, whereas the right pulmonary venous ostia normally are more circular. These workers found that pulmonary venous ostia can be very narrow anteroposteriorly, despite a normal venogram appearance during catheter ablation procedures. They concluded that to know what the true pulmonary ostia are, three-dimensional imaging, such as MRI or computer tomography, is necessary.

RECENT INVESTIGATIONS CONCERNING THE DEVELOPMENT OF THE PULMONARY VEINS

Terwolbeck et al[374] and Blom et al[285] have published contributions concerning the embryology of the pulmonary veins. Blom et al[285] found that at 28 days the orifice of the nonlumenized common pulmonary vein normally is visible as an endothelial invagination within the sinus venous. Our reaction was that this is an important statement. With which part of the sinus venosus does the common pulmonary vein normally connect—with the right horn or with the left horn? The authors[285] do not say. If with the right horn, one would expect the result to be TAPVC with the RA. If with the left horn, one would expect the result to be TAPVC with the coronary sinus. Perhaps the authors were using the term *sinus venosus* loosely, meaning that until the septum primum appears, one cannot tell exactly where the dorsal wall of the LA is or will be. So let's call it all "sinus venosus." This point is important because we currently think that if the common pulmonary vein connects with either the right or left horn of the sinus venosus, TAPVC is present, by definition. Perhaps the authors[285] mean that before the appearance of the common pulmonary vein and septum primum, the dorsal well of the primitive common atrium all may be regarded as sinus venosus tissue—because the systemic venous sinus long antedates the appearance of the common pulmonary vein at about 27 days of age (see Fig. 7.5).

These workers observed that development of the septum primum and ventral proliferation of extracardiac mesenchyme from the dorsal mesocardium normally position the common pulmonary vein into the LA.

Our reaction was that this statement is true for the normal heart. Abnormally, however, the septum primum can be malpositioned into the LA, resulting in partially or totally anomalous pulmonary vein drainage.[24] Hence, the LA can lie on *both* sides of the septum primum—not just to its left (in visceroatrial situs solitus), as was presented in Chapter 6.

The right wall of the common pulmonary vein contributes to the posterior part of the atrial septum and is continuous with the dorsal sinuatrial fold (the future left venous valve).

By 7 weeks of age, the proximal part of the RUPV normally becomes part of the common wall between the right-sided sinus venosus and the common pulmonary vein.

A deficiency of the wall between the sinus venosus in the RA and the right branch(es) of the common pulmonary vein explains the development of sinus venosus defects.

Thus, Blom, Gittenberger-de Groot, and colleagues[285] in 2001 agreed with the findings and interpretation of Van Praagh et al[9] in 1994 that sinus venosus defects represent a failure of formation of the wall between the sinus venosus part of the RA and the RPVs. This understanding of sinus venosus defects is presented in detail in Chapter 6. We mention sinus venous defects again here because they represent an anomaly not only of the right atrial part of the sinus venosus but also of the RPVs.[9,285]

REFERENCES

1. Delisle G, Ando M, Calder AL, et al. Total anomalous pulmonary venous connection: report of 93 autopsied cases with emphasis on diagnostic and surgical considerations. *Am Heart J.* 1976;91:99.
2. Darling RC, Rothney WB, Craig JM. Total pulmonary venous drainage into the right side of the heart: report of 17 autopsied cases not associated with other major cardiovascular anomalies. *Lab Invest.* 1957;6:44.
3. Lucas RV, Woolfrey BF, Anderson RC, Lester RG, Edwards JE. Atresia of the common pulmonary vein. *Pediatrics.* 1962;29:729.
4. Van Mierop LHS, Wigglesworth FW. Isomerism of the cardiac atria in the asplenia syndrome. *Lab Invest.* 1962;11:1303.
5. Van Praagh R, Corsini I. Cor triatriatum: pathologic anatomy and a consideration of morphogenesis based on 13 postmortem cases and a study of normal development of the pulmonary vein and atrial septum in 83 human embryos. *Am Heart J.* 1969;78:379.
6. Kauffman SL, Ores CN, Anderson DH. Two cases of total anomalous pulmonary venous return of the supracardiac type with stenosis simulating infradiaphragmatic drainage. *Circulation.* 1962;25:376.
7. Nakib A, Moller JH, Kanjuh VI, Edwards JE. Anomalies of the pulmonary veins. *Am J Cardiol.* 1967;20:77.
8. Hastreiter AR, Paul MH, Molthan ME, Miller RA. Total anomalous pulmonary venous connection with severe pulmonary venous obstruction, a clinical entity. *Circulation.* 1962;25:916.
9. Van Praagh S, Carrera ME, Sanders SP, Mayer JE, Van Praagh R. Sinus venosus defects: unroofing of the right pulmonary veins—anatomic and echocardiographic findings and surgical treatment. *Am Heart J.* 1994;128:365.
10. Edwards JE. Symposium on anomalous pulmonary venous connection (drainage): pathologic and developmental considerations in anomalous pulmonary venous connection. *Proc Staff Meetings Mayo Clin.* 1953;28:441.
11. Moller JH, Nakib A, Anderson RC, Edwards JE. Congenital cardiac disease associated with polysplenia: a developmental complex of bilateral "left-sidedness." *Circulation.* 1967;36:789.
12. Van Praagh R, Harken AH, Delisle G, Ando M, Gross RE. Total anomalous pulmonary venous drainage to the coronary sinus: a revised procedure for its correction. *J Thorac Cardiovasc Surg.* 1972;64:132.
13. Rutledge JM, Hiatt PW, Vick GW, Grifka RG. A sword for the left hand: an unusual case of left-sided scimitar syndrome. *Pediatr Cardiol.* 2001;22:350.
14. Neill CA, Ferencz C, Sabiston DC, Sheldon H. The familial occurrence of hypoplastic right lung with systemic arterial supply and venous drainage: "scimitar syndrome." *Johns Hopkins Med J.* 1960;107:1.
15. Goldstein JD, Rabinovitch M, Van Praagh R, Reid L. Unusual vascular anomalies causing persistent pulmonary hypertension in a newborn. *Am J Cardiol.* 1979;43:962.

16. Wagenvoort CA, Heath D, Edwards JE. Sequestration of lung, intralobar sequestration: "scimitar syndrome." In: *In the Pathology of the Pulmonary Vasculature*. Springfield, Illinois: Charles C Thomas; 1964:392.
17. Van Praagh R, Van Praagh S. The anatomy of common aorticopulmonary trunk (truncus arteriosus communis) and its embryologic implications, a study of 57 necropsied cases. *Am J Cardiol*. 1965;16:406.
18. Houyel L, Van Praagh R, Lacour-Gayet F, et al. Transposition of the great arteries {S,D,L}: pathologic anatomy, diagnosis, and surgical management of a newly recognized complex. *J Thorac Cardiovasc Surg*. 1995;110:641.
19. Quero M. Coexistence of single ventricle with atresia of one atrioventricular orifice. *Circulation*. 1972;46:794.
20. Van Praagh R, Ongley PA, Swan HJC. Anatomic types of single or common ventricle in man, morphologic and geometric aspects in sixty autopsied cases. *Am J Cardiol*. 1964;13:367.
21. Van Praagh S, O'Sullivan J, Brili S, Van Praagh R. Juxtaposition of the morphologically right atrial appendage in solitus and inversus atria: a study of 35 postmortem cases. *Am Heart J*. 1996;132:382.
22. Van Praagh S, O'Sullivan J, Brili S, Van Praagh R. Juxtaposition of the morphologically left atrial appendage in solitus and inversus atria: a study of 18 postmortem cases. *Am Heart J*. 1996;132:391.
23. Melhuish BPP, Van Praagh R. Juxtaposition of the atrial appendages, a sign of severe cyanotic congenital heart disease. *Br Heart J*. 1968;30:269.
24. Van Praagh S, Carrera ME, Sanders SP, Mayer JE, Van Praagh R. Partial or total direct pulmonary venous drainage to right atrium due to malposition of septum primum: anatomic and echocardiographic findings and surgical treatment—a study based on 36 cases. *Chest*. 1995;107:1488.
25. Wilson J. *A Description of A Very Unusual Formation of the Human Heart, Phil Trans Royal Soc London, Part II*; 1798:346.
26. Cantrell JR, Haller JA, Ravitch MM. A syndrome of congenital defects involving the abdominal wall, sternum, diaphragm, pericardium, and heart. *Surg Gynecol Obstet*. 1958;107:602.
27. Brody H. Drainage of the pulmonary veins into the right side of the heart. *Arch Path*. 1942;33:221.
28. Brantigan OC. Anomalies of the pulmonary veins, their surgical significance. *Surg Gynecol Obstet*. 1947;84:653.
29. Smith JC. Anomalous pulmonary veins. *Am Heart J*. 1951;41:561.
30. Swan HJC, Kirklin JW, Becu LM, Wood EH. Anomalous connection of right pulmonary vein to superior vena cava with interatrial communications: hemodynamic data in eight cases. *Circulation*. 1957;16:54.
31. Peacock TB. Malformations dependent on arrest of development at an early period of fetal life. In: Peacock TB, ed. *Malformations of the Human Heart*. London: John Churchill; 1858:24–25.
32. Ross DN. The sinus venosus type of atrial septal defect. *Guy's Hosp Rep*. 1956;105:376.
33. Keith A. The Hunterian lectures on the malformation of the heart. Lecture III. *Lancet*. 1909;2:519.
34. Abbott ME. Congenital cardiac disease. In *Osler & McCrae's Modern Medicine*. Vol 4. Philadelphia: Lea & Febiger; 1915:323.
35. Paltauf R. *Über einen seltenen Defekt in der Vorhofscheidewand*. Verhandlungen der Deutschen Pathologischen Gesellschaft; 1913:249.
36. Nützel H. Beitrag zurkenntnis der missbildungen im bereiche der oberen hohlvene. *Frankfurt Z Pathol*. 1914;15(1).
37. von Hackensellner HA. Abnorme einmündung von lungenvenen in die vena cava cranialis. *Virchows Arch*. 1955;327:603.
38. Kiss A, Partilla H, Pernkopf E. Die transposition der venenmündungen (eine entwicklungsgeschichtliche analyse, vorgenommen an hand eines falles von pulmonalinsuffizienz mit vorhofsseptumdefekt und partieller transposition der lungenvenenmündungen). *Virchows Arch*. 1954;324:707.
39. Van Praagh S, Geva T, Lock JE, del Nido PJ, Vance MS, Van Praagh R. Biatrial or left atrial drainage of the right superior vena cava: anatomic, morphogenetic, and surgical considerations. Report of three new cases and literature review. *Pediatr Cardiol*. 2003;24:350.
40. Anderson HN, Guntheroth WG, Winterscheid LC, Merendino KA. Congenital communications of the right pulmonary veins with the azygos vein. Report of a case with surgical correction. *Circulation*. 1964;30:439.
41. Whitaker W, Watson DA, Keates PG. Total anomalous pulmonary venous drainage into the left innominate vein associated with transposition of the great vessels. *Circulation*. 1964;30:918.
42. Mehrizi A, Dekker A, Ottesen OE. Angiocardiographic feature of total anomalous venous return into coronary sinus simulating tricuspid atresia or stenosis. *J Pediat*. 1964;65:615.
43. Blake HA, Hall RJ, Manion WC. Anomalous pulmonary venous return. *Circulation*. 1965;32:406.
44. Levy AM, Naeye RL, Tabakin BS, Hanson JS. Far-advanced intimal proliferation and severe pulmonary hypertension secondary to total anomalous pulmonary venous drainage. *Am J Cardiol*. 1965;16:280.
45. Scott LP, Welch CC. Factors influencing survival in total anomalous pulmonary venous drainage in infants. *Am J Cardiol*. 1965;16:286.
46. Mohiuddin SM, Levin HS, Runco V, Booth RW. Anomalous pulmonary venous drainage. A common trunk emptying into the left atrium and inferior vena cava. *Circulation*. 1966;34:46.
47. Nathan H, Eliakin M. The junction between the left atrium and the pulmonary veins. An anatomic study of human hearts. *Circulation*. 1966;34:412.
48. Kalke BR, Carlson RG, Ferlic RM, Sellers RD, Lillehei CW. Partial anomalous pulmonary venous connections. *Am J Cardiol*. 1967;20:91.
49. Kiely B, Filler J, Stone S, Doyle EF. Syndrome of anomalous venous drainage of the right lung to the inferior vena cava. A review of 67 reported cases and three new cases in children. *Am J Cardiol*. 1967;20:102.
50. Jegier W, Charrette E, Dobell ARC. Infradiaphragmatic anomalous pulmonary venous drainage. Normal hemodynamics following operation in infancy. *Circulation*. 1967;35:396.
51. Llewellyn MA, Cullum PA, Thomas JB, Anderson IM. Infracardiac total anomalous pulmonary venous drainage. *Brit Med J*. 1968;3:35.
52. Frye RL, Krebs M, Rahimtoola SH, Ongley PA, Hallermann FJ, Wallace RB. Partial anomalous pulmonary venous connection without atrial septal defect. *Am J Cardiol*. 1968;22:242.
53. Snellen HA, van Ingen HC, Hoefsmit CCM. Patterns of anomalous pulmonary venous drainage. *Circulation*. 1968;38:45.
54. Bonham-Carter RE, Capriles M, Noe Y. Total anomalous pulmonary venous drainage. A clinical and anatomical study of 75 children. *Brit Heart J*. 1969;31:45.
55. Bruschke AVG, Bloch A. Anomalous pulmonary venous drainage associated with mitral valve disease. *Am Heart J*. 1969;78:437.

56. Mody MR, Gallen WJ, Lepley D. Total anomalous pulmonary venous drainage below the diaphragm. Successful surgical correction in an infant. *Am J Cardiol.* 1969;24:575.
57. Glancy DL, Braunwald NS, O'Brien KP, Roberts WC. Scimitar syndrome associated with patent ductus arteriosus, aortic coarctation, and irreversible pulmonary hypertension. *Johns Hopkins Med J.* 1968;123:297.
58. Serratto M, Bucheleres HG, Bicoff P, Miller RA, Hastreiter RA. Palliative balloon atrial septostomy for total anomalous pulmonary venous connection in infancy. *J Pediat.* 1968;73:734.
59. Gazzaniga AB, Matloff JM, Harken DE. Anomalous right pulmonary venous drainage into the inferior vena cava and left atrium. *J Thorac Cardiovasc Surg.* 1969;57:251.
60. Takayasu S, Sato T, Nishida H, Obunai Y, Ishihara A, Takao A. Partial anomalous pulmonary venous return with intact atrial septum. *Bull Heart Inst Japan.* 1970:78.
61. Gomes MMR, Feldt RH, McGoon DC, Danielson GK. Total anomalous pulmonary venous connection. Surgical considerations and results of operation. *J Thorac Cardiovasc Surg.* 1970;60:116.
62. Halpern BL, Murray GC, Conti CR, Humphries JO, Gott VL. Continuous murmur due to the combination of rheumatic mitral stenosis and a rare type of anomalous pulmonary venous drainage. *Circulation.* 1970;42:165.
63. Gathman GE, Nadas AS. Total anomalous pulmonary venous connection. Clinical and physiologic observations of 75 pediatric patients. *Circulation.* 1970;42:143.
64. Gomes MMR, Feldt RH, McGoon DC, Danielson GK. Long-term results following correction of total anomalous pulmonary venous connection. *J Thorac Cardiovasc Surg.* 1971;61:253.
65. Roe BB. Posterior approach to correction of total anomalous pulmonary venous return. Further experience. *J Thorac Cardiovasc Surg.* 1970;59:748.
66. Joffe HS, O'Donovan TG, Glaun BP, Chesler E, Shrire V. Subdiaphragmatic total anomalous pulmonary venous drainage: report of a successful surgical correction. *Am Heart J.* 1971;81:250.
67. Friedli B, Davugnon A, Stanley P. Infradiaphragmatic anomalous pulmonary venous return. Surgical correction in a newborn infant. *J Thorac Cardiovasc Surg.* 1971;62:301.
68. Joffe HS, Chesler E, O'Donovan TG, Schrire V. Successful correction of supradiaphragmatic total anomalous pulmonary venous drainage with obstruction in a 3-month-old infant. *J Thorac Cardiovasc Surg.* 1971;62:238.
69. Jensen JB, Blount SG. Total anomalous pulmonary venous return. A review and report of the oldest surviving patient. *Am Heart J.* 1971;82:387.
70. Gersony WM, Bowman FO, Steeg CN, Hayes CJ, Jesse MJ, Malm JR. Management of total anomalous pulmonary venous drainage in early infancy. *Circulation.* 1971;43:I–19.
71. Klint R, Weldon C, Hartmann A, Schad N, Hernandez A, Goldring D. Mixed-type total anomalous pulmonary venous drainage. Report of a successful surgical correction and review of the literature. *J Thorac Cardiovasc Surg.* 1972;63:164.
72. Shadravan I, Baucum R, Fowler RL, Villadiego R, Puyau FA. Obstructed anomalous pulmonary venous return. *Am Heart J.* 1971;82:232.
73. Freidli B, Guerin R, Davignon A, Fouron JC, Stanley P. Surgical treatment of partial anomalous pulmonary venous drainage, a long-term follow-up study. *Circulation.* 1972;45:159.
74. Graham TP, Jarmakani JM, Canent RV. Left ventricular volume characteristics with a right ventricular volume overload. Total anomalous pulmonary venous connection and large atrial septal defect. *Circulation.* 1972;45:389.
75. Hayward RH, Martt JM, Brewer LM, Inmon TM, Best EB. Surgical correction of the vena cava—bronchovascular complex. Developmental pulmonary, arterial, and venous anomalies with accessory diaphragm. *J Thorac Cardiovasc Surg.* 1972;64:203.
76. El-Said G, Mullins CE, McNamara DG. Management of total anomalous pulmonary venous return. *Circulation.* 1972;45:1240.
77. Behdad M, Folger GM. Scimitar syndrome with anatomic variations. *Am J Cardiol.* 1972;29:252.
78. Woody JN, Graham TP, Bredford WD, Sabiston DC, Carnent RV. Hypoplastic right lung with systemic blood supply and anomalous pulmonary venous drainage: reversal of pulmonary hypertension with surgical management in infancy. *Am Heart J.* 1972;83:82.
79. Buckley MJ, Behrendt DM, Goldblatt A, Laver MB, Austen WG. Correction of total anomalous pulmonary venous drainage in the first month of life. *J Thorac Cardiovasc Surg.* 1972;63:269.
80. Robb JS. The heart in chordates. In: Robb JS, ed. *Comparative Basic Cardiology.* New York and London: Grune & Stratton; 1965:41.
81. Los JA. *The Development of The Pulmonary Veins and The Coronary Sinus in the Human Embryo. Luctor et Emergo, Publisher.* Leiden: [M.D. Thesis, University of Leiden, in Dutch with English summary.]; 1958.
82. Behrendt DM, Aberdeen E, Waterston DJ, Bonham-Carter RE. Total anomalous pulmonary venous drainage in infants. I. Clinical and hemodynamic findings, methods, and results of operation in 37 cases. *Circulation.* 1972;46:347.
83. Silove ED, Behrendt DM, Aberdeen E, Bonham-Carter RE. Total anomalous pulmonary venous drainage. II. Spontaneous functional closure of interatrial communication after surgical correction in infancy. *Circulation.* 1972;46:357.
84. Engle MA. Total anomalous pulmonary venous drainage. Success story at last. *Circulation.* 1972;46:209.
85. Tajik AJ, Gau GT, Schattenberg TT. Echocardiogram in total anomalous pulmonary venous drainage. Report of case. *Mayo Clin Proc.* 1972;47:247.
86. Guller B, Ritter DG, Kincaid OW. Tricuspid atresia with pulmonary atresia and total anomalous pulmonary venous connection to the right superior vena cava. *Mayo Clin Proc.* 1972;47:105.
87. Puig-Massona M, Murtra M, Revuelta JM. A new technique in the correction of partial anomalous pulmonary venous drainage. *J Thorac Cardiovasc Surg.* 1972;64:108.
88. Ikeda T, Ishihara T, Yoshimatsu H, et al. Accessory diaphragm associated with congenital posterolateral diaphragmatic hernia, aberrant systemic artery to the right lower lobe, and anomalous pulmonary vein. *J Thorac Cardiovasc Surg.* 1972;64:18.
89. Mascarenhas E, Javier RP, Samet P. Partial anomalous pulmonary venous connection and drainage. *Am J Cardiol.* 1973;31:512.
90. Lemoine G, Glaser F, Louville Y, et al. Retour veineux pulmonaire total anormal chez le nourisson: traitement chirurgical. *Coeur (NS).* 1973;467.
91. Stanley P, Davignon A, Kratz C, Fouron JC, Guerin R, Chartrand C. Traitment chirurgical du retour veineux pulmonaire anormal total du nourisson. *Coeur NS.* 1973;477.
92. Bharati S, Lev M. Congenital anomalies of the pulmonary veins. *Cardiovasc Clin.* 1973;5:23.
93. Neirotti R, Gonzalez-Lavin L, Ross DN. Anomalous pulmonary venous connexions of left lung associated with valvular heart disease. Report of two cases. *Br Heart J.* 1972;34:969.
94. Mullins CE, El-Said GM, Neches WH, et al. Balloon atrial septostomy for total anomalous pulmonary venous return. *Br Heart J.* 1973;35:752.

95. Steeg CN, Ellis K, Gersony WM. Total anomalous pulmonary venous drainage with ventricular septal defect. *Am Heart J.* 1973;86:341.
96. Mertens MA, Clapp PR, Ferris EJ. Abnormal pulmonary vessels in a patient with chest pain. *Chest.* 1973;64:758.
97. Anabtawi IN, Ellison RG, Ellison LT. Pulmonary arteriovenous aneurysms and fistulas. *Ann Thorac Surg.* 1965;1:277.
98. de Leval MR, Stark J, Bonham-Carter RE. Total anomalous pulmonary venous drainage to superior vena cava associated with preductal coarctation of aorta. Successful correction in a 12-day-old infant. *Br Heart J.* 1973;35:1098.
99. Radley-Smith R, Yacoub M. Primary surgical correction of total anomalous pulmonary venous drainage in infants. *Br Heart J.* 1973;35:866.
100. Nakazawa M, Mori K, Mimori S, Takao A. A familial case of total anomalous pulmonary venous return. *Bull Heart Inst Japan.* 1972;14(125):1973.
101. Paz JE, Castilla EE. Familial total anomalous pulmonary venous return. *J Med Genet.* 1971;8:312.
102. Breckenridge IM, de Leval M, Stark J, Waterston DJ. Correction of total anomalous pulmonary venous drainage in infancy. *J Thorac Cardiovasc Surg.* 1973;66:447.
103. Kawashima Y, Nakano S, Matsuda H, Miyamoto T, Manabe H. Successful correction of total anomalous pulmonary venous drainage with a new surgical technique. *J Thorac Cardiovasc Surg.* 1973;66:959.
104. Hordof AJ, Hayes CJ, Bowman FO, Malm JR, Gersony WM. Hemodynamic assessment of total anomalous pulmonary venous connection (TAPVC) following correction during infancy. *Am J Cardiol.* 1974;33:144.
105. Rao PS, Silbert DR. Superior vena caval obstruction in total anomalous pulmonary venous connexion. *Br Heart J.* 1974;36:228.
106. Barratt-Boyes BG. Primary definitive intracardiac operations in infants: total anomalous pulmonary venous connection. In: Kirklin JW, ed. *Advances in Cardiovascular Surgery*. New York: Grune & Stratton; 1973:127.
107. Dische MR, Teixeira ML, Winchester PH, Engle MA. Horseshoe lung associated with a variant of the "scimitar" syndrome. *Br Heart J.* 1974;36:617.
108. Mody GT, Folger GM. Atresia of the common pulmonary vein: report of one case. *Pediatrics.* 1974;54:62.
109. Higashino SM, Shaw GG, May JA, Ecker RR. Total anomalous pulmonary venous drainage below the diaphragm. Clinical presentation, hemodynamic findings, and surgical results. *J Thorac Cardiovasc Surg.* 1974;68:711.
110. Tynan M, Behrendt D, Urquhart W, Graham GR. Portal vein catheterization and selective angiography in diagnosis of total anomalous pulmonary venous connexion. *Br Heart J.* 1974;36:1155.
111. Chia B-L, Tau N-C, Tan LKA. Total anomalous pulmonary venous drainage. Case presenting with prominent right supraclavicular thrill and loud continuous murmur. *Am J Cardiol.* 1974;34:851.
112. Utley JR, Noonan JA, Walters LR, Frist RA. Anomalous position of atrial septum with anomalous pulmonary and systemic venous drainage. Correction including ligation of persistent left superior vena cava. *J Thorac Cardiovasc Surg.* 1974;67:730.
113. Sulayman R, Thilenius O, Replogle R, Arcilla RA. Unilateral emphysema in total anomalous pulmonary venous return. *J Pediat.* 1975;87:433.
114. Paquet M, Gutgesell H. Echocardiographic features of total anomalous pulmonary venous connection. *Circulation.* 1975;51:599.
115. Duff DF, Nihill MR, Vargo TA, Cooley DA. Infradiaphragmatic total anomalous pulmonary venous return. Diagnosis and surgical repair in a 10-year-old child. *Br Heart J.* 1975;37:1093.
116. Alpert JS, Dexter L, Vieweg WVR, Haynes FW, Dalen JE. Anomalous pulmonary venous return with intact atrial septum. Diagnosis and pathophysiology. *Circulation.* 1977;56:870.
117. Mathew R, Thilenius OG, Replogle RL, Arcilla RA. Cardiac function in total anomalous pulmonary venous return before and after surgery. *Circulation.* 1977;55:361.
118. Chartrand C, Payot M, Davignon A, Guerin R, Stanley P. A new surgical approach for correction of partial anomalous venous drainage into the superior vena cava. *J Thorac Cardiovasc Surg.* 1976;71:29.
119. Noonan JA, Srivastava TN, Trinkle K, Castellos JM. Total anomalous pulmonary venous return with associated patent ductus arteriosus, two cases with successful correction. *Chest.* 1976;70:683.
120. Pritchard DA, Tajik AJ, Rutherford BD, Harrison CE, Pluth JR, Danielson GK. Partial anomalous pulmonary venous connection (intact atrial septum) associated with mitral regurgitation. *Am Heart J.* 1977;94:209.
121. Pastore JO, Akins CW, Zir LM, Buckley MJ, Dinsmore RE. Total anomalous pulmonary venous connection and severe pulmonic stenosis in a 52-year-old man. *Circulation.* 1977;55:206.
122. Haworth SG, Reid L. Structural study of pulmonary circulation and of heart in total anomalous pulmonary venous return in early infancy. *Br Heart J.* 1977;39:80.
123. Nakazawa M, Jarmakani JM, Gyepes MT, Prochazka JV, Yabek SM, Marks RA. Pre and postoperative ventricular function in infants and children with right ventricular volume overload. *Circulation.* 1977;55:479.
124. King DR, Marchildon MB. Gastrointestinal hemorrhage, an unusual complication of total anomalous pulmonary venous drainage. *J Thorac Cardiovasc Surg.* 1977;73:316.
125. Sparrow AW, Mohan K, Gonzalez-Lavin L. Successful correction of total anomalous pulmonary venous connection in a 2.5 kilogram premature neonate. *Am J Cardiol.* 1976;37:108.
126. Billig DM, Peguero FA. Total anomalous pulmonary venous return. Successful total correction in a 44 year old man with subtotal absence of interatrial septum, tricuspid insufficiency, and cardiac dextroversion. *Chest.* 1976;69:687.
127. Munier C. *Intervention De Van Praagh Sur Un Cas De Retour Veineux Pulmonaire Anormal Total: Étude Hemodynamique Des Suites Immediates, Thèse Pour Le Doctorat En Medecine, Université Paris.* Faculté de Medecine Broussais-Hotel-Dieu; 1975.
128. Anderson PD, Glasser SP, Czarnecki S, Hopeman AR. Three unusual complications resulting from attempted repair of partial anomalous pulmonary venous drainage. *Chest.* 1976;69:384.
129. Clarke DR, Stark J, de Leval M, Pincott JR, Taylor JFN. Total anomalous pulmonary venous drainage in infancy. *Br Heart J.* 1977;39:436.
130. Mortera C, Tynan M, Goodwin AW, Hunter S. Infradiaphragmatic total anomalous pulmonary venous connection to portal vein. Diagnostic implications of echocardiography. *Br Heart J.* 1977;39:685.
131. Duff DF, Nihill MR, McNamara DG. Infradiaphragmatic total anomalous pulmonary venous return. Review of clinical and pathological findings and results of operation in 28 cases. *Br Heart J.* 1977;39:619.

132. Whight CM, Barratt-Boyes BG, Calder AL, Neutze JM, Brandt PWT. Total anomalous pulmonary venous connection. Long-term results following repair in infancy. *J Thorac Cardiovasc Surg.* 1978;75:52.
133. Porter CJ, Vargo TA, McNamara DG, Cooley DA. Successful surgical correction of infradiaphragmatic total anomalous pulmonary venous return into the inferior vena cava, a fourteen year follow-up. *J Thorac Cardiovasc Surg.* 1978;75:68.
134. Haworth SG, Macartney FJ. The structural and functional effect on the lung of obstruction to pulmonary venous return. *Magyar Pediat.* 1978;12(suppl 4):20.
135. Oppenheimer-Dekker A, Moulaert AJ. Anatomic patterns of abnormal pulmonary venous drainage. Infradiaphragmatic drainage of the pulmonary veins, their relation to the dorsal atrial wall and the embryological implications hereof. *Magyar Pediat.* 1978;12(suppl 4):19.
136. Orellano L, Schlemminger B, Dahn D, Kirchoff PG, Koncz J. Surgery of scimitar syndrome—report of 6 cases. *Magyar Pediat.* 1978;12(suppl 4):31.
137. Damman JF, Carpenter MA, Updike OL. Mechanisms of obstruction in anomalous pulmonary venous return above the diaphragm. *Magyar Pediat.* 1978;12(suppl 4):20.
138. Aziz KU, Paul MH, Bharati S, Lev M. Echocardiographic features of total anomalous pulmonary venous drainage into the coronary sinus. *Magyar Pediat.* 1978;12(suppl 4):21.
139. Batisse A, Landau JF, Piechaud JF, Kachaner J. Obstructed total anomalous pulmonary venous drainage in the newborn. *Magyar Pediat.* 1978;12(suppl 4):21.
140. McNamara DG, Duff DF, Mullins CE, Cooley DA. Management of total anomalous pulmonary venous return. *Magyar Pediat.* 1978;12(suppl 4):22.
141. Radley-Smith R, Yacoub M. A new anatomical type of total anomalous pulmonary venous drainage associated with other major cardiac abnormalities. *Magyar Pediat.* 1978;12(suppl 4):23.
142. Dymnicka S, Bielinska B, Erecinski J, Aleszewicz J. Clinical approach to the diagnosis of total anomalous pulmonary venous drainage in children. *Magyar Pediat.* 1978;12(suppl 4):24.
143. Sorland SJ, Rostad H, Tjonneland S, Stake G, Rosland GA. Total anomalous pulmonary venous drainage. Results of corrective surgery. *Magyar Pediat.* 1978;12(suppl 4):24.
144. Thibert M, Leca-Chetochine F, Lemoine G. Bilan de dix ans de chirurgie du retour veineux pulmonaire anormal total du nourisson. *Magyar Pediat.* 1978;12(suppl 4):25.
145. Kallfelz HC, Oelert H. Anomalous pulmonary venous drainage associated with cor triatriatum sinistrum. *Magyar Pediat.* 1978;12(suppl 4):28.
146. Vernant P, Zoumis P, Kabaker M, Nitemberg A, Casasoprana A. Le retour veineux pulmonaire anormale du poumon gauche à propos de 6 observations. *Magyar Pediat.* 1978;12(suppl 4):28.
147. Neill CA, Haroutunian LM. The scimitar syndrome; its history, current status and implications. *Magyar Pediat.* 1978;12(suppl 4):29.
148. Neill CA. Development of the pulmonary veins with reference to the embryology of anomalies of pulmonary venous return. *Pediatrics.* 1956;18:880.
149. Kanjuh V, Tucakovic G, Nedeljkovic V, Lastes-Maletic S, Papic R. An autopsy study of the anomalies of the pulmonary veins associated with other cardiac and splenic anomalies. *Magyar Pediat.* 1978;12(suppl 4):13.
150. Stevenson JG, Kawabori I, Guntheroth WG. Pulsed Doppler echocardiographic detection of total anomalous pulmonary venous return: resolution of left atrial line. *Am J Cardiol.* 1979;44:1155.
151. Yabek SM, Akl BF, Berman W. Partial anomalous pulmonary venous connection to the azygous vein with intact atrial septum. *Chest.* 1979;76:486.
152. Danilowicz D, Kronzon I. Use of contrast echocardiography in the diagnosis of partial anomalous pulmonary venous connection. *Am J Cardiol.* 1979;43:248.
153. Métras D, Ouezzin-Coulibaly A, Outtara K, Renambot J, Chauvet J. Retour veineux pulmonaire anormal total dans le sinus coronaire. Àpropos d'un cas de diagnostic difficile avec succès chirurgical. *Arch Mal Coeur.* 1979;72:908.
154. Sahn DJ, Allen HD, Lange LW, Goldberg SJ. Cross-sectional echocardiographic diagnosis of the sites of total anomalous pulmonary venous drainage. *Circulation.* 1979;60:1317.
155. Newfeld EA, Wilson A, Paul MH, Reisch JS. Pulmonary vascular disease in total anomalous pulmonary venous drainage. *Circulation.* 1980;61:103.
156. Turley K, Tucker WY, Ullyot DJ, Ebert PA. Total anomalous pulmonary venous connection in infancy: influence of age and type of lesion. *Am J Cardiol.* 1980;45:92.
157. Hammon JW, Bender HW, Graham TP, Boucek RJ, Smith CW, Erath HG. Total anomalous pulmonary venous connection in infancy. Ten years' experience including studies of postoperative ventricular function. *J Thorac Cardiovasc Surg.* 1980;80:544.
158. Arciniegas E, Henry JG, Green EW. Stenosis of the coronary sinus ostium, an unusual site of obstruction in total anomalous pulmonary venous drainage. *J Thorac Cardiovasc Surg.* 1980;79:303.
159. Škovránek J, Tůma S, Urbancová D, Šamánek M. Range-gated pulsed Doppler echocardiographic diagnosis of supracardiac total anomalous pulmonary venous drainage. *Circulation.* 1980;61:841.
160. Mardini MK, Sakati NA, Nyhan WL. Anomalous left pulmonary venous drainage to the inferior vena cava and through the pericardiophrenic vein to the innominate vein: left-sided scimitar syndrome. *Am Heart J.* 1981;101:860.
161. Babb JD, McGlynn TJ, Pierce WS, Kirkman PM. Isolated partial anomalous venous connection: a congenital defect with late and serious complications. *Ann Thorac Surg.* 1981;31:540.
162. Bove EL, de Leval MR, Taylor JFN, Macartney FJ, Szarnicki RJ, Stark J. Infradiaphragmatic total anomalous pulmonary venous drainage: surgical treatment and long-term results. *Ann Thorac Surg.* 1981;31:544.
163. Snider AR, Silverman NH, Turley K, Ebert PA. Evaluation of infradiaphragmatic total anomalous pulmonary venous connection with two-dimensional echocardiography. *Circulation.* 1982;66:1129.
164. Bauer A, Körfer R, Bircks W. Left-to-right shunt at atrial level due to anomalous venous connection of left lung. Report of seven cases. *J Thorac Cardiovasc Surg.* 1982;84:626.
165. Byrum CJ, Dick M, Behrendt DM, Rosenthal A. Repair of total anomalous pulmonary venous connection in patients younger than 6 months old. Late postoperative hemodynamic and electrophysiologic status. *Circulation.* 1982;66:I–208.
166. Haworth SG. Total anomalous pulmonary venous return. Prenatal damage to pulmonary vascular bed and extrapulmonary veins. *Br Heart J.* 1982;48:513.
167. Brosius FC, Schwartz DE, Gleason WL, Maron B, Jones M, Roberts WC. Left atrial-to-right atrial shunt without atrial septal defect or precordial murmur. Pulmonary varix and hypertrophic cardiomyopathy. *Chest.* 1982;81:91.
168. Dickinson DF, Parimelazhagen K, Tweedie MCK, et al. Total anomalous pulmonary venous connection. Repair using deep hypothermia and circulatory arrest in 44 consecutive infants. *Br Heart J.* 1982;48:249.

169. McManus BM, Luetzeler J, Roberts WC. Total anomalous pulmonary venous connection: survival for 62 years without surgical intervention. *Am Heart J*. 1982;103:298.
170. Baron P, Gutgesell H, Hawkins E, McNamara D. Infradiaphragmatic total anomalous pulmonary venous connection in siblings. *Am Heart J*. 1982;104:1107.
171. Lima CO, Valdes-Cruz LM, Allen HD, et al. Prognostic value of left ventricular size measured by echocardiography in infants with total anomalous pulmonary venous drainage. *Am J Cardiol*. 1983;51:1155.
172. Mazzucco A, Rizzoli G, Fracasso A, et al. Experience with operation for total anomalous pulmonary venous connection in infancy. *J Thorac Cardiovasc Surg*. 1983;85:686.
173. Brenner JI, Bharati S, Berman MA, Lev M. Rare type of intrapulmonary drainage of one lung by the other with total anomalous pulmonary venous return. *J Am Coll Cardiol*. 1983;2:1174.
174. Hawkins JA, Clark EB, Doty DB. Total anomalous pulmonary venous connection. *Ann Thorac Surg*. 1983;36:548.
175. Platia EV, Brinker JA. Scimitar syndrome with peripheral left pulmonary artery branch stenosis. *Am Heart J*. 1984;107:594.
176. Oakley D, Naik D, Verel D, Rajan S. Scimitar vein syndrome: report of nine new cases. *Am Heart J*. 1984;107:596.
177. Williams WH, Zorn-Chelton S, Raviele AA, et al. Extracardiac atrial pedicle conduit repair of partial anomalous pulmonary venous connection to the superior vena cava in children. *Ann Thorac Surg*. 1984;38:345.
178. Cobanoglu A, Hanlon JJ, Coombs DT, Starr A. Combined intracardiac and extracardiac repair of scimitar syndrome with anomalous pulmonary veins to both cavae. *J Thorac Cardiovasc Surg*. 1984;88:141.
179. Bexton RS, Banim SO, Rees GM, Rees RSO. Unusual form of bilateral partial anomalous pulmonary venous drainage. *Clin Cardiol*. 1984;7:175.
180. Bullaboy CA, Johnson DH, Azar H, Jennings RB. Total anomalous pulmonary venous connection to portal system: a new therapeutic role for prostaglandin E1? *Pediatr Cardiol*. 1984;5:115.
181. Cooper MJ, Teitel DF, Silverman NH, Enderlein MA. Study of infradiaphragmatic total anomalous pulmonary venous connection with cross-sectional and pulsed Doppler echocardiography. *Circulation*. 1984;70:412.
182. Rosenquist GC, Kelly JL, Chandra R, et al. Small left atrium and change in contour of the ventricular septum in total anomalous pulmonary venous connection: a morphometric analysis of 22 infant hearts. *Am J Cardiol*. 1985;55:777.
183. Galloway AC, Campbell DN, Clarke DR. The value of early repair for total anomalous pulmonary venous drainage. *Pediatr. Cardiol*. 1985;6:77.
184. Vargas FJ, Kreutzer GO. A surgical technique for correction of total anomalous pulmonary venous drainage. *J Thorac Cardiovasc Surg*. 1985;90:410.
185. Downing TP, Danielson GK, Ritter DG, Julsrud PR, Seward JB. Pulmonary artery thrombosis associated with anomalous pulmonary venous connection: an unusual complication following the modified Fontan procedure. *J Thorac Cardiovasc Surg*. 1985;90:441.
186. Vouhé PR, Baillot-Vernant F, Fermont L, Bical O, Leca F, Neveux J-Y. Cor triatriatum and total anomalous pulmonary venous connection: a rare surgically correctable anomaly. *J Thorac Cardiovasc Surg*. 1985;90:443.
187. Warden HE, Gustafson RA, Tarnay TJ, Neal WA. An alternative method for repair of partial anomalous pulmonary venous connection to the superior vena cava. *Ann Thorac Surg*. 1984;38:601.
188. Weiman DS, Lee K, Levett JM, Replogle RL. Partial anomalous pulmonary venous return: a ten-year experience. *Tex Heart Inst J*. 1985;12:239.
189. Liao PK, Su W-J, Hung J-S. Two-dimensional echocardiographic diagnosis of total anomalous pulmonary venous connection below the diaphragm. *Am J Cardiol*. 1985;56:821.
190. Rey C, Marache P, Francort C, Dupuis C. Percutaneous balloon angioplasty in an infant with obstructed total anomalous pulmonary vein return. *J Am Coll Cardiol*. 1985;6:894.
191. Schamroth CL, Sareli P, Klein HO, Davidoff R, Barlow JB. Total anomalous pulmonary venous connection with pulmonary venous obstruction: survival into adulthood. *Am Heart J*. 1985;109:1112.
192. Reardon MJ, Cooley DA, Kubrusly L, et al. Total anomalous pulmonary venous return: report of 201 patients treated surgically. *Tex Heart Inst J*. 1985;12:131.
193. Lamberti JJ, Waldman JD, Mathewson JW, Kirkpatrick SE. Repair of subdiaphragmatic total anomalous pulmonary venous connection without cardiopulmonary bypass. *J Thorac Cardiovasc Surg*. 1984;88:627.
194. Julsrud PR, Ehman RL. The "broken ring" sign in magnetic resonance imaging of partial anomalous pulmonary venous connection to the superior vena cava. *Mayo Clin Proc*. 1985;60:874.
195. Del Torso S, Goh TH, Venables AW. Echocardiographic findings in the liver in total anomalous pulmonary venous connection. *Am J Cardiol*. 1986;57:374.
196. Kissner DG, Sorkin RP. Anomalous pulmonary venous connection, medical therapy. *Chest*. 1986;89:753.
197. Canter CE, Martin TC, Spray TL, Weldson CS, Strauss AW. Scimitar syndrome in childhood. *Am J Cardiol*. 1986;58:652.
198. Schäfers H-J, Luhmer I, Oelert H. Pulmonary venous obstruction following repair of total anomalous pulmonary venous drainage. *Ann Thorac Surg*. 1987;43:432.
199. Ward KE, Mullins CE, Huhta JC, Nihil MR, McNamara DG, Cooley DA. Restrictive interatrial communication in total anomalous pulmonary venous connection. *Am J Cardiol*. 1986;57:1131.
200. Lincoln CR, Rigby ML, Mercanti C, et al. Surgical risk factors in total anomalous pulmonary venous connection. *Am J Cardiol*. 1988;61:608.
201. Jonas RA, Smolinsky A, Mayer JE, Castaneda AR. Obstructed pulmonary venous drainage with total anomalous pulmonary venous connection to the coronary sinus. *Am J Cardiol*. 1987;59:431.
202. Gikonyo DK, Tandon R, Lucas RV, Edwards JE. Scimitar syndrome in neonates: report of four cases and review of the literature. *Pediatr Cardiol*. 1986;6:193.
203. Bender HW. Diagnosis and correction of anomalous pulmonary venous return. *Ann Thorac Surg*. 1988;45:346.
204. Arciprete P, McKay R, Watson GH, Hamilton DI, Wilkinson JL, Arnold RM. Double connections in total anomalous pulmonary venous connection. *J Thorac Cardiovasc Surg*. 1986;92:146.
205. Oelert H, Schäfers H-J, Stegmann T, Kallfelz H-C, Borst HG. Complete correction of total anomalous pulmonary venous drainage: experience with 53 patients. *Ann Thorac Surg*. 1986;41:392.
206. Kirk AJB, Pollack JCS. Concomitant cor triatriatum and coronary sinus total anomalous pulmonary venous connection. *Ann Thorac Surg*. 1987;44:203.
207. Pearl W. Scimitar variant. *Pediatr Cardiol*. 1987;8:139.
208. Jennings JG, Serwer GA. Partial anomalous pulmonary venous connection to the azygos vein with intact atrial septum. *Pediatr Cardiol*. 1986;7:115.

209. Yee ES, Turley K, Hseih W-R, Ebert PA. Infant total anomalous pulmonary venous connection: factors influencing timing of presentation and operative outcome. *Circulation*. 1987;76:III-83.
210. Chin AJ, Sanders SP, Sherman F, Lang P, Norwood WI, Castaneda AR. Accuracy of subcostal two-dimensional echocardiography in prospective diagnosis of total anomalous pulmonary venous connection. *Am Heart J*. 1987;113:1153.
211. DeLeon SY, Gidding SS, Ilbawi MN, et al. Surgical management of infants with complex cardiac anomalies associated with reduced pulmonary blood flow and total anomalous pulmonary venous drainage. *Ann Thorac Surg*. 1987;43:207.
212. Lamb RK, Qureshi SA, Wilkinson JL, Arnold R, West CR, Hamilton DI. Total anomalous pulmonary venous drainage, seventeen-year surgical experience. *J Thorac Cardiovasc Surg*. 1988;96:368.
213. Tsuchida K, Anzai N, Hashimoto A, Fukushima Y, Yamada M. Intraatrial conduit repair in scimitar syndrome. *Chest*. 1987;92:1120.
214. Casta A, Wolf WJ. Echo Doppler detection of external compression of the vertical vein causing obstruction in total anomalous pulmonary venous connection. *Am Heart J*. 1988;116:1045.
215. Voegele LD, Parker EF. Pulmonary venous obstruction following atrioplasty for partial anomalous pulmonary venous drainage. *Chest*. 1987;91:791.
216. Kveselis DA, Chameides L, Diana DJ, Ellison L, Rowland T. Late pulmonary venous obstruction after surgical repair of infradiaphragmatic total anomalous pulmonary venous repair. *Pediatr Cardiol*. 1988;9:175.
217. Lucas RV, Lock JE, Tandon R, Edwards JE. Gross and histologic anatomy of total anomalous pulmonary venous connections. *Am J Cardiol*. 1988;62:292.
218. Kanjuh VI, Katkov H, Singh A, Franciosi RA, Helseth HK, Edwards JE. Atypical total anomalous pulmonary venous connection: two channels leading to infracardiac terminations. *Pediatr Cardiol*. 1989;10:115.
219. Sano S, Brawn WJ, Mee RBB. Total anomalous pulmonary venous drainage. *J Thorac Cardiovasc Surg*. 1989;97:886.
220. Gustafson RA, Warden HE, Murray GF, Hill RC, Rozar GE. Partial anomalous pulmonary venous connection to the right side of the heart. *J Thorac Cardiovasc Surg*. 1989;98:861.
221. Iga K, Hori K. Abnormal venous connection between the left upper pulmonary vein and the left brachiocephalic vein, associated with rheumatic combined valvular disease. *Heart Ves*. 1990;5:113.
222. Gleason MM. Concordant total anomalous pulmonary venous connection in dizygotic twins. *Am Heart J*. 1989;118:1338.
223. Corno A, Giamberti A, Carotti A, Giannico S, Marino B, Marcelletti C. Total anomalous pulmonary venous connection: surgical repair with a double-patch technique. *Ann Thorac Surg*. 1990;49:492.
224. Okabe H, Matsunaga H, Kawauchi M, et al. Rotation-advancement flap method for correction of partial anomalous pulmonary venous drainage into the superior vena cava. *J Thorac Cardiovasc Surg*. 1990;99:308.
225. Phillips SJ, Kongtahworn C, Zeff RH, Skinner JR, Chandramouli B, Gay JH. Correction of total anomalous pulmonary venous connection below the diaphragm. *Ann Thorac Surg*. 1990;49:734.
226. Baxter R, McFadden PM, Gradman M, Wright A. Scimitar syndrome: cine magnetic resonance imaging demonstration of anomalous pulmonary venous drainage. *Ann Thorac Surg*. 1990;50:121.
227. Moore JW, Kirby WC, Rogers WM, Poth MA. Partial anomalous pulmonary venous drainage associated with 45,X Turner's syndrome. *Pediatrics*. 1990;86:273.
228. Van Meter C, LeBlanc JG, Culpepper WS, Ochsner JL. Partial anomalous pulmonary venous return. *Circulation*. 1990;82. IV-195.
229. Saxena A, Fong LV, Lamb RK, Monro JL, Shore DF, Keeton BR. Cardiac arrhythmias after surgical correction of total anomalous pulmonary venous connection: late follow-up. *Pediatr Cardiol*. 1991;12:89.
230. Tumbarello R, Abbruzzese PA, Meloni G, Porcu M, Martelli V, Sanna A. A variant of the scimitar syndrome with stenosed drainage of the inferior vena cava. *Am Heart J*. 1991;121:616.
231. Hsu Y-H, Chien C-T, Hwang M, Chiu IS. Magnetic resonance imaging of total anomalous pulmonary venous drainage. *Am Heart J*. 1991;121:1560.
232. Fish FA, Davies J, Graham TP. Unique variant of partial anomalous pulmonary venous connection with intact atrial septum. *Pediatr Cardiol*. 1991;12:177.
233. Serraf A, Bruniaux J, Lacour-Gayet F, et al. Obstructed total anomalous pulmonary venous return, toward neutralization of a major risk factor. *J Thorac Cardiovasc Surg*. 1991;101:601.
234. Matsui M, Arai T, Horikoshi S, et al. Successful repair of a rare type of total anomalous pulmonary venous drainage. *Ann Thorac Surg*. 1991;52:131.
235. Romero-Cárdenas A, Vargas-Barrón J, Rylaarsdam M, et al. Total anomalous pulmonary venous return: diagnosis by transesophageal echocardiography. *Am Heart J*. 1991;121:1831.
236. Mehta RH, Jain SP, Nanda NC, Helmcke F, Sanyal R. Isolated partial anomalous pulmonary venous connection: echocardiographic diagnosis and a new color Doppler method to assess shunt volume. *Am Heart J*. 1991;122:870.
237. Okita Y, Miki S, Tamura T, et al. Bidirectional cavopulmonary anastomosis using vertical vein for right isomerism, pulmonary atresia, and TAPVR. *Ann Thorac Surg*. 1991;52:544.
238. Yoo SY, Nykanen DG, Freedom RM, Benson LN, Moes FCA, Burrows PE. Retrobronchial vertical vein in total anomalous pulmonary vein and its specific occurrence in right isomerism. *Cardiol Young*. 1993;3. I–146.
239. Wang JK, Chiu JH, How SW, Lue HC. Anomalous pulmonary venous pathway traversing pulmonary parenchyma—diagnosis and clinical implication. *Cardiol Young*. 1993;3. I–145.
240. Rodriguez-López AM, Marín D, Bolio A, et al. Relationship of preoperative left ventricular dimensions to the outcome of surgical repair in patients with total anomalous venous connection. *Cardiol Young*. 1993;3. I–144.
241. Korbmacher B, Rammos S, Buttgen S, Schulte HD. Long-term follow-up in repaired total anomalous pulmonary venous connection. *Cardiol Young*. 1993;3. I–142.
242. Gaynor W, Burch M, Dollery C, Sullivan I, Deanfield J, Elliott M. Repair of anomalous pulmonary venous connection to the superior caval vein by an atrial wall baffle with reimplantation of the superior caval vein. *Cardiol Young*. 1993;3. I–141.
243. Goswami KC, Shrivastava S, Saxena A, Dev V. Echocardiographic diagnosis of total anomalous pulmonary venous connection. *Am Heart J*. 1993;126:433.
244. Raisher BD, Grant JW, Martin TC, Strauss AW, Spray TL. Complete repair of total anomalous pulmonary venous connection in infancy. *J Thorac Cardiovasc Surg*. 1992;104:443.
245. Yamaki S, Tsunemoto M, Shimada M, et al. Quantitative analysis of pulmonary vascular disease in total anomalous pulmonary venous connection in sixty infants. *J Thorac Cardiovasc Surg*. 1992;104:728.

246. Black MD, Shamji FM, Goldstein W, Sachs HJ. Pulmonary resection and contralateral anomalous venous drainage: a lethal combination. *Ann Thorac Surg*. 1992;53:689.
247. Lupinetti FM, Kulik TJ, Beekman RH, Crowley DC, Bove EL. Correction of total anomalous pulmonary venous connection in infancy. *J Thorac Cardiovasc Surg*. 1993;106:880.
248. Gao Y-A, Burrows PE, Benson LN, Rabinovitch M, Freedom RM. Scimitar syndrome in infancy. *J Am Coll Cardiol*. 1993;22:873.
249. Paridon SM, Sullivan NM, Schneider J, Pinsky WW. Cardiopulmonary performance at rest and exercise after repair of total anomalous pulmonary venous correction. *Am J Cardiol*. 1993;72:1444.
250. Becher MW, Rockenmacher S, Marin-Padilla M. Total anomalous pulmonary venous connection: persistence and atresia of the common pulmonary vein. *Pediatr Cardiol*. 1992;13:187.
251. Heinemann MK, Hanley FL, Van Praagh S, et al. Total anomalous pulmonary venous drainage in newborns with visceral heterotaxy. *Ann Thorac Surg*. 1994;57:88.
252. McMullan MH, Fyke FE. Total anomalous pulmonary venous connection: surgical correction in a 66-year-old man. *Ann Thorac Surg*. 1992;53:520.
253. Dupuis C, Charaf LAC, Brevière G-M, Abou P. "Infantile" form of the scimitar syndrome with pulmonary hypertension. *Am J Cardiol*. 1993;71:1326.
254. van de Wal HJCM. Total anomalous pulmonary venous drainage by double connection corrected by ascending vein and coronary sinus repair. *J Thorac Cardiovasc Surg*. 1993;105:367.
255. Takeda S-i, Imachi T, Arimitsu K, Minami M, Hayakawa M. Two cases of scimitar variant. *Chest*. 1994;105:292.
256. Jenkins KJ, Sanders SP, Orav J, Coleman EA, Mayer JE, Colan SD. Individual pulmonary vein size and survival in infants with totally anomalous pulmonary venous connection. *J Am Coll Cardiol*. 1993;22:201.
257. Misumi K, Berdjis F, Leung C, Padilla L, Murata YCL. Adult patient with total anomalous pulmonary venous return undergoing successful pregnancy. *Am Heart J*. 1994;128:412.
258. Seliem MA, Chin AJ, Norwood WI. Patterns of anomalous pulmonary venous connection/drainage in hypoplastic left heart syndrome: diagnostic role of Doppler color flow mapping and surgical implications. *J Am Coll Cardiol*. 1992;19:135.
259. Cho YH, Lee HJ, Kim HS, et al. MRI of total anomalous pulmonary venous connections. *JCAT*. 1994;18:243.
260. Shimazaki Y, Nakano S, Kato H, et al. Mixed type of total anomalous pulmonary venous connection with hemi-pulmonary vein atresia. *Ann Thorac Surg*. 1993;56:1399.
261. Cohen AJ, Sell JE, Zurcher RP, Edwards FH. Anomalous pulmonary venous drainage of the right lung. *Ann Thorac Surg*. 1993;56:1397.
262. Caspi J, Zalstein E, Zuker N, Appelbaum A. Adjustable suture of the vertical pulmonary vein for repair of infracardiac total anomalous pulmonary venous connection. *J Thorac Cardiovasc Surg*. 1995;109:389.
263. DeLeon SY, Freeman JE, Ilbawi MN, et al. Surgical techniques in partial anomalous pulmonary veins to the superior vena cava. *Ann Thorac Surg*. 1993;55:1222.
264. Thibault C, Perrault LP, Delisle G, et al. Lobectomy in the treatment of the scimitar syndrome. *Ann Thorac Surg*. 1995;59:220.
265. Van der Velde ME, Parness IA, Colan SD, et al. Two-dimensional echocardiography in the pre- and postoperative management of totally anomalous pulmonary venous connection. *J Am Coll Cardiol*. 1991;18:1746.
266. Beitzke A, Zobel G, Rigler B, Stein JI, Suppan C. Scimitar syndrome with absence of the right pulmonary artery: a case with volume-induced, reversible, left-sided pulmonary hypertension. *Pediatr Cardiol*. 1992;13:119.
267. Correa-Villaseñor A, Ferencz C, Boughman JA, Neill CA, and the Baltimore-Washington infant study group. Total anomalous pulmonary venous return: familial and environmental factors. *Teratology*. 1991;44:415.
268. Wang J-K, Li Y-W, Young M-L, How S-W, Lue H-C. Delineation of obstruction in total anomalous pulmonary venous connection utilizing magnetic resonance imaging. *Am Heart J*. 1992;124:807.
269. Gaynor JW, Burch M, Dollery C, Sullivan ID, Deanfield JE, Elliott MJ. Repair of anomalous pulmonary venous connection to the superior vena cava. *Ann Thorac Surg*. 1995;59:1471.
270. Bando K, Turrentine MW, Sharp TG, Ensing GJ, Girod DA. Surgical repair of total anomalous pulmonary venous connection: thirty-year trends. *Circulation*. 1995;92(suppl):I–51.
271. Dudell GG, Evans ML, Krons HF, Spicer RL, Lamberti JJ. Common pulmonary vein atresia: the role of extracorporeal membrane oxygenation. *Pediatrics*. 1993;91:403.
272. Kubota H, Furuse A, Kotsuka Y, Yagyu K, Hirata K, Murakawa Y. Midterm results of the rotation-advancement flap method for correction of partial anomalous pulmonary venous drainage into the superior vena cava. *J Thorac Cardiovasc Surg*. 1996;112:1.
273. Lacour-Gayet F, Rey C, Planché C. Sténose des veins pulmonaires. Description d'une technique chirurgicale sans suture utilisant le pericarde in situ. *Arch Mal Coeur Vaiss*. 1996;89:633.
274. Banitt PF. Total anomalous pulmonary venous connection to unroofed coronary sinus in patient with no symptoms. *Am Heart J*. 1996;132:886.
275. Najm HK, Williams WG, Coles JG, Rebeyka IM, Freedom RM. Scimitar syndrome: twenty years' experience and results of repair. *J Thorac Cardiovasc Surg*. 1996;112:1161.
276. Ammash NM, Seward JB, Warnes CA, Connolly HM, O'Leary PW, Danielson GK. Partial anomalous pulmonary venous connection: diagnosis by transesophageal echocardiography. *J Am Coll Cardiol*. 1997;29:1351.
277. Delius RE, de Leval MR, Elliott MJ, Stark J. Mixed total pulmonary venous drainage: still a surgical challenge. *J Thorac Cardiovasc Surg*. 1996;112:1581.
278. Wang JK, Chiu IS, How SW, et al. Anomalous pulmonary venous pathway traversing pulmonary parenchyma, diagnosis and implication. *Chest*. 1996;110:1363.
279. Najm HK, Caldarone CA, Smallhorn J, Coles JG. A sutureless technique for the relief of pulmonary vein stenosis with the use of in situ pericardium. *J Thorac Cardiovasc Surg*. 1998;115:468.
280. Caldarone CA, Najm HK, Kadletz M, et al. Relentless pulmonary vein stenosis after repair of total anomalous pulmonary venous drainage. *Ann Thorac Surg*. 1998;66:1514.
281. Imoto Y, Kado H, Ason T, Shiokawa Y, Tominaga R, Yasui H. Mixed type of total anomalous pulmonary venous connection. *Ann Thorac Surg*. 1998;66:1394.
282. Hiramatsu T, Takanashi Y, Imai Y, et al. Atrial septal displacement for repair of anomalous pulmonary venous return into the right atrium. *Ann Thorac Surg*. 1998;65:1110.
283. van Son JAM, Hambsch J, Kinzel P, Haas GS, Mohr FW. Urgency of operation in infracardiac total anomalous pulmonary venous connection. *Ann Thorac Surg*. 2000;70:128.
284. Shiraishi I, Kato Y, Todoroki H, Satoh H, Hamaoka K. Differential color imaging technique of helical CT angiography in the diagnosis of total anomalous pulmonary venous drainage. *Circulation*. 2000;101:2017.

285. Blom NA, Gittenberger-de Groot AC, Jongeneel TH, De Ruiter MC, Poelmann RE, Ottenkamp J. Normal development of the pulmonary veins in human embryos and formulation of a morphogenetic concept for sinus venosus defects. *Am J Cardiol.* 2001;87:305.
286. van Son JAM, Hambsch J, Mohr FW. Modified repair of mixed anomalous pulmonary venous connection. *Ann Thorac Surg.* 1998;65:1441.
287. Allan LD, Sharland GK. The echocardiographic diagnosis of totally anomalous pulmonary venous connection in the fetus. *Heart.* 2001;85:433.
288. Serraf A, Belli E, Roux D, Sousa-Uva M, Lacour-Gayet F, Planché C. Modified superior approach for repair of supracardiac and mixed total anomalous pulmonary venous drainage. *Ann Thorac Surg.* 1998;65:1391.
289. Lacour-Gayet F, Zoghbi J, Serraf EE, et al. Surgical management of progressive pulmonary venous obstruction after repair of total anomalous pulmonary venous connection. *J Thorac Cardiovasc Surg.* 1999;117:679.
290. Jenkins KJ, Tan PE, Perry SB, et al. Proliferative pulmonary vein stenosis: variable patterns of progression and preliminary results using adjunct chemotherapy. *Circulation.* 2001;104(suppl II):587.
291. Greil GF, Powell AJ, Gildein HP, Geva T. Gadolinium-enhanced three-dimensional magnetic resonance angiography of pulmonary and systemic venous anomalies. *J Am Coll Cardiol.* 2002;39:335.
292. Yamagishi M, Shuntoh K, Takahashi A, Shinkawa T, Miyazaki T, Kitamura N. Intra-atrial rerouting by transference of the posterior left atrial wall for cardiac-type total anomalous pulmonary venous return. *J Thorac Cardiovasc Surg.* 2002;123:996.
293. Brown JW, Ruzmetov M, Minnich DJ, et al. Surgical management of scimitar syndrome: an alternative approach. *J Thorac Cardiovasc Surg.* 2003;125:238.
294. McFaul RC, Tajik AJ, Mair DD, Danielson GK, Seward JB. Development of pulmonary arteriovenous shunt after superior vena cava—right pulmonary artery (Glenn) anastomosis. Report of four cases. *Circulation.* 1977;55:212.
295. Cloutier A, Ash JM, Smallhorn JF, et al. Abnormal distribution of pulmonary blood flow after the Glenn shunt or Fontan procedure: risk of development of arteriovenous fistulae. *Circulation.* 1985;72:471.
296. Moore JW, Kirby WC, Madden WA, Gaither NS. Development of pulmonary arteriovenous malformations after modified Fontan operations. *J Thorac Cardiovasc Surg.* 1989;98:1045.
297. Castaneda AR, Jonas RA, Mayer JE, Hanley FL. *Cardiac Surgery of the Neonate and Infant.* Philadelphia: WB Saunders Co; 1994:230–231.
298. Papagiannis J, Kanter RJ, Effman EL, et al. Polysplenia with pulmonary arteriovenous malformations. *Pediatr Cardiol.* 1993;14:127.
299. Hall RJ, Nelson WP, Blake HA, Geiger JP. Massive pulmonary arteriovenous fistula in the newborn, a correctable form of "cyanotic heart disease;" an additional cause of cyanosis with left axis deviation. *Circulation.* 1965;31:762.
300. Clarke CP, Goh TH, Blackwood A, Venables AW. Massive pulmonary arteriovenous fistula in the newborn. *Br Heart J.* 1976;38:1092.
301. Freid R, Amberson JB, O'Loughlin JE, et al. Congenital pulmonary arteriovenous fistula producing pulmonary arterial steal syndrome. *Ped Cardiol.* 1982;2:313.
302. Hodgson CH, Burchell HB, Good CA, Clagett OT. Hereditary hemorrhagic telangectasia and pulmonary arteriovenous fistula: survey of a large family. *N Engl J Med.* 1959;261:625.
303. Pyeritz RE. Genetics and cardiovascular disease. In: Braunwald E, Zipes DP, Libby P, eds. *Heart Disease, A Textbook of Cardiovascular Medicine.* 6th ed. Philadelphia: W.B. Saunders Co; 2001:2007.
304. Moller JH, Noren GR, David PR, Amplatz K, Kanjuh VI, Edwards JE. Clinical pathologic conference. *Am Heart J.* 1966;72:530.
305. Contis G, Fung RH, Vawter GF, Nadas AS. Stenosis and obstruction of the pulmonary veins associated with pulmonary artery hypertension. *Am J Cardiol.* 1967;20:718.
306. Nasser WK, Feigenbaum H, Fisch C. Clinical and hemodynamic diagnosis of pulmonary venous obstruction due to sclerosing mediastinitis. *Am J Cardiol.* 1967;20:725.
307. Binet JP, Bouchard F, Langlois J, Chetochine F, Conso JF, Pottermain M. Unilateral congenital stenosis of the pulmonary veins. A very rare cause of pulmonary hypertension. *J Thorac Cardiovasc Surg.* 1972;63:397.
308. Park SC, Neches WH, Lenox CC, Zuberbuhler JR, Siewers RD, Bahnson JT. Diagnosis and surgical treatment of bilateral pulmonary vein stenosis. *J Thorac Cardiovasc Surg.* 1974;67:755.
309. Mortensson W, Lundström N-R. Congenital obstruction of the pulmonary veins at their atrial junctions. Review of the literature and a case report. *Am Heart J.* 1974;87:359.
310. Sade RM, Freed MD, Matthews EC, Castaneda AR. Stenosis of individual pulmonary veins. Review of the literature and report of a surgical case. *J Thorac Cardiovasc Surg.* 1974;67:953.
311. Soto B, Ceballos R. Pulmonary vein stenosis at their entrance into left atrium. *Arch Venezuelan Cardiol.* 1976;3:27.
312. Louhimo I, Tuuteri L. Congenital stenosis of individual pulmonary veins. Two cases with successful operative treatment. *Magyar Pediat.* 1978;12(suppl 4):30.
313. Bargeron LM, Allen J. Stenosis of the pulmonary veins. *Magyar Pediat.* 1978;12(suppl 4):27.
314. Bini RM, Bargeron LM. Visualization of pulmonary veins obstruction by pulmonary artery wedge injection. *Ped Cardiol.* 1982;2:161.
315. Driscoll DJ, Hesslein PS, Mullins CE. Congenital stenosis of individual pulmonary veins: clinical spectrum by transvenous balloon dilatation. *Am J Cardiol.* 1982;49:1767.
316. Geggel RL, Fried R, Tuuri DT, Fyler DC, Reid LM. Congenital pulmonary vein stenosis: structural changes in a patient with normal pulmonary artery wedge pressure. *J Am Coll Cardiol.* 1984;3:193.
317. Vogel M, Ash J, Rowe RD, Trusler GA, Rabinovitch M. Congenital unilateral pulmonary vein stenosis complicating transposition of the great arteries. *Am J Cardiol.* 1984;54:166.
318. Bini RM, Cleveland DC, Ceballos R, Bargeron LM, Pacifico AD, Kirklin JW. Congenital pulmonary vein stenosis. *Am J Cardiol.* 1984;54:369.
319. Smallhorn JF, Panperio H, Benson L, Freedom RM, Rowe RD. Pulsed Doppler assessment of pulmonary vein obstruction. *Am Heart J.* 1985;110:483.
320. Pacifico AD, Mandke NV, McGrath LB, Colvin EV, Bini RM, Bargeron LM. Repair of congenital pulmonary venous stenosis with living autologous atrial tissue. *J Thorac Cardiovasc Surg.* 1985;89:604.
321. Rey C, Marache P, Francort C, Dupuis C. Percutaneous balloon angioplasty in an infant with obstructed total anomalous pulmonary vein return. *J Am Coll Cardiol.* 1985;6:894.

322. Reid JM, Jamieson MPG, Cowan MD. Unilateral pulmonary vein stenosis. *Br Heart J.* 1986;55:599.
323. Sairanen H, Louhimo I, Tolppanen E-M. Pulmonary vein diameter in normal children. *Pediatr Cardiol.* 1986;6:259.
324. Fong LV, Anderson RH, Park SC, Zuberbuhler JR. Morphologic features of stenosis of the pulmonary veins. *Am J Cardiol.* 1988;62:1136.
325. Samdarshi TE, Morrow WR, Helmcke FR, Nanda NC, Bargeron LM, Pacifico AD. Assessment of pulmonary vein stenosis by transesophageal echocardiography. *Am Heart J.* 1991;122:1495.
326. Schürch W, Seemayer TA, Gabbiani G. Myofibroblast. In: Sternberg SS, ed. *Histology for Pathologists.* New York: Raven Press; 1992:109.
327. Luhimo I, Lundstrom U, Tuuteri L. Encircling endocardectomy in the treatment of pulmonary or hepatic venous stenosis—long-term results in six patients. *Cardiol Young.* 1993;3:I–97. (abstract 322).
328. van Son JAM, Danielson GK, Puga FJ, Edwards WD, Driscoll DJ. Repair of congenital and acquired pulmonary vein stenosis. *Ann Thorac Surg.* 1995;60:144.
329. Breinholt JP, Hawkins JH, Minich L, et al. Pulmonary vein stenosis with normal connection: associated cardiac abnormalities and variable outcome. *Ann Thorac Surg.* 1999;68:164.
330. Endo M, Yamaki S, Ohmi M, Tabayashi K. Pulmonary vascular changes induced by congenital obstruction of pulmonary venous return. *Ann Thorac Surg.* 2000;69:193.
331. Chen S-J, Wang J-K, Li Y-W, Chiu I-S, Su C-T, Lue H-C. Validation of pulmonary venous obstruction by electron beam computed tomography in children with congenital heart disease. *Am J Cardiol.* 2001;87:589.
332. Maeda K, Yamaki S, Yokota M, Murakami A, Takamoto S. Hypoplasia of the small pulmonary arteries in total anomalous pulmonary venous connection with obstructed pulmonary venous drainage. *J Thorac Cardiovasc Surg.* 2004;127:448.
333. Wagenvoort CA, Wagenvoort N. Primary pulmonary hypertension, a pathologic study of the lung vessels in 156 clinically diagnosed cases. *Circulation.* 1970;42:1163.
334. Pietra GG, Edwards WD, Kay JM, et al. Histopathology of primary pulmonary hypertension, a qualitative and quantitative study of pulmonary blood vessels from 58 patients in the National Heart, Lung, and Blood Institute, Primary Pulmonary Hypertension Registry. *Circulation.* 1989;80:1198.
335. Edwards WD, Edwards JE. Clinical primary pulmonary hypertension, three pathologic types. *Circulation.* 1977;56:884.
336. Rich S. Primary pulmonary hypertension. *Prog Cardiovasc Dis.* 1988;31:205.
337. Swensen SJ, Tasnjian JH, Myers JL, et al. Pulmonary venoocclusive disease: CT findings in eight patients. *Am J Roentgenol.* 1996;167:937.
338. Valdes L, Gonzalez-Juanatey JR, Alvarez D, et al: Diagnosis of pulmonary veno-occlusive disease: new criteria for biopsy, *Respir Med* 979, 1998.
339. Wagenvoort CA, Heath D, Edwards JE. *The Pathology of the Pulmonary Vasculature.* Springfield, IL: Charles C Thomas; 1964.
340. Rosenthal A, Vawter G, Wagenvoort CA. Intrapulmonary veno-occlusive disease. *Am J Cardiol.* 1973;31:78.
341. Wagenvoort CA, Wagenvoort N, Takahashi T. Pulmonary veno-occlusive disease: involvement of the pulmonary arteries and review of the literature. *Hum Pathol.* 1985;16:1033.
342. Andrews EC. Five cases of an undescribed form of pulmonary interstitial fibrosis caused by obstruction of the pulmonary veins. *Bull Johns Hopkins Hosp.* 1957;100:28.
343. Berry DF, Buccigrossi D, Peabody J, Peterson L, Moser KM. Pulmonary vascular occlusion and fibrosing mediastinitis. *Chest.* 1986;89:296.
344. McDonnel PJ, Summer WR, Hutchins GM. Pulmonary veno-occlusive disease. Morphological changes suggesting a viral cause. *J Am Med Assoc.* 1981;246:667.
345. Joselson R, Warnock M. Pulmonary veno-occlusive disease after chemotherapy. *Hum Pathol.* 1983;14:88.
346. Liu L, Sackler JP. A case of pulmonary veno-occlusive disease. Etiological and therapeutic appraisal. *Angiology.* 1972;23:299.
347. Voordes CG, Kuipers JRG, Elema JD. Familial pulmonary veno-occlusive disease. A case report. *Thorax.* 1977;32:763.
348. Davies P, Reid L. Pulmonary veno-occlusive disease in siblings: case reports and morphometric study. *Hum Pathol.* 1982;13:911.
349. Dainauskas JR, Hughes RL, English JT. Clinical pathologic conference. *Am Heart J.* 1971;82:817.
350. Schachter EN, Smith GLW, Cohen GS, Lee SH, Lasser A, Gee JBL. Pulmonary granulomas in a patient with pulmonary veno-occlusive disease. *Chest.* 1975;67:487.
351. Wagenvoort CA. Pulmonary veno-occlusive disease, entity or syndrome? *Chest.* 1976;69:82.
352. Anderson JL, Durnin RE, Ledbetter MK, Angevine JM, Gilbert EF, Edwards JE. Clinical pathologic conference. *Am Heart J.* 1979;97:233.
353. Massumi A, Woods L, Mullins CE, Nasser WK, Hall RJ. Pulmonary venous dilatation in pulmonary veno-occlusive disease. *Am J Cardiol.* 1981;48:585.
354. Lombard CM, Churg A, Winokur S. Pulmonary veno-occlusive disease following therapy for malignant neoplasms. *Chest.* 1987;92:871.
355. Weed HG. Pulmonary "capillary" wedge pressure not the pressure in the pulmonary capillaries. *Chest.* 1991;100:1138.
356. Townend JN, Roberts DH, Jones EL, Davies MK. Fatal pulmonary venoocclusive disease after use of oral contraceptives. *Am Heart J.* 1992;124:1643.
357. Hawker RE, Celermajer JM, Gengos DC, Cartmill TB, Bowdler JD. Common pulmonary vein atresia. Premortem diagnosis in two infants. *Circulation.* 1972;46:368.
358. Nasrallah AT, Mullins CE, Singer D, Harrison G, McNamara DG. Unilateral pulmonary vein atresia. *Am J Cardiol.* 1975;36:969.
359. Dye TE, Saab SB, Almond CH, Watson L. Sclerosing mediastinitis with occlusion of pulmonary veins. Manifestations and management. *J Thorac Cardiovasc Surg.* 1977;74:137.
360. Ledbetter MK, Wells DH, Connors DM. Common pulmonary vein atresia. *Am Heart J.* 1978;96:580.
361. Beerman LB, Oh KS, Park SC, et al. Unilateral pulmonary vein atresia: clinical and radiographic spectrum. *Pediat Cardiol.* 1983;4:105.
362. Kingston HM, Patel RG, Watson GH. Unilateral absence or extreme hypoplasia of pulmonary veins. *Br Heart J.* 1983;49:148.
363. Shrivastava S, Moller JH, Edwards JE. Congenital unilateral pulmonary venous atresia with pulmonary veno-occlusive disease in the contralateral lung: an unusual association. *Pediatr Cardiol.* 1986;7:213.
364. Kelley KM, Cheatham JP, Kugler JD, Fleming WH, McManus BM. Postnatal atresia of extraparenchymal pulmonary veins, fulminant necrotizing pulmonary arteritis and elevated circulating immune complexes. *J Am Coll Cardiol.* 1987;9:1043.

365. Cullen S, Deasy PF, Tempany E, Duff DF. Isolated pulmonary vein atresia. *Br Heart J*. 1990;63:350.
366. Mehta AV, Chidambaram B. Absent left pulmonary vein without anomalous connection: diagnosis and management in the newborn. *Am Heart J*. 1992;124:804.
367. Butler MW, Ursell PC, Wung JT, Stolar CJH. Misalignment of the pulmonary veins with alveolar capillary dysplasia as a cause of persistent neonatal pulmonary hypertension. *Cardiol Young*. 1993;3. I–18. (abstract 54).
368. Boggs S, Harris MC, Hoffman DJ, et al. Misalignment of pulmonary veins with alveolar capillary dysplasia: affected siblings and variable phenotypic expression. *J Pediatr*. 1994;124:125.
369. Janney C, Askin F, Kuhn C. Congenital alveolar capillary dysplasia: an unusual cause of respiratory distress in the newborn. *Am J Clin Pathol*. 1981;76:722.
370. Davia JE, Golden MS, Price HL, Hastings JE, Cheitlin MD. Pulmonary varix, a diagnostic pitfall. *Circulation*. 1974;49:1011.
371. Perrott WW, Shin MS. Pulmonary varix. *J Thorac Cardiovasc Surg*. 1974;68:318.
372. Ho SY, Cabrera JA, Tran VH, Farré J, Anderson RH, Sánchez-Quintana D. Architecture of the pulmonary veins: relevance to radiofrequency ablation. *Heart*. 2001;86:265.
373. Wittkampf FHM, Vonken E-J, Derksen R, et al. Pulmonary vein ostium geometry. Analysis by magnetic resonance angiography. *Circulation*. 2003;107:21.
374. Terwolbeck K, Rammos S, Wenink ACG. Early development and location of the central pulmonary vein. *Cardiol Young*. 1993;3(I-126) (abstract 436).

8

Cor Triatriatum Sinistrum (Subdivided Left Atrium) and Cor Triatriatum Dextrum (Subdivided Right Atrium)

DEFINITION

The classic form of cor triatriatum (meaning "heart with three atria") may be defined as a rare cardiac malformation in which the left atrium (LA) is subdivided into dorsal and ventral chambers by a fibromuscular diaphragm, the dorsal (posterior) chamber receiving the pulmonary veins, the ventral (anterior) chamber giving rise to the left atrial appendage and leading to the mitral valve, and the communication between the dorsal and ventral chambers being large, small, or absent, depending on the size of the opening(s) in the subdividing diaphragm.

This typical form of cor triatriatum is also known as **cor triatriatum sinistrum,** meaning left-sided triatrial heart (Latin). There is also a right-sided form of triatrial heart, known as **cor triatriatum dextrum** (Latin). As will be seen, typical cor triatriatum sinistrum has stenosis of the common pulmonary vein, with a dorsal common pulmonary vein chamber (Fig. 8.1), whereas typical cor triatriatum dextrum has a large and obstructive right venous valve between the caval compartment medially and the component of the right atrium (RA) laterally that leads to the tricuspid valve and the right atrial appendage.

Whenever the term *cor triatriatum* is used without further qualification, cor triatriatum sinistrum is meant.

It also should be understood that a heart with three atria (cor triatriatum) really does not exist, accurately speaking. These are hearts with three chambers at the atrial level, but not with three complete and separate atria.

Instead, cor triatriatum denotes **subdivided atria:** subdivided LA (cor triatriatum sinistrum, see Fig. 8.1), and subdivided RA (cor triatriatum dextrum).

Let us first consider cor triatriatum sinistrum, usually referred to for brevity simply as cor triatriatum or subdivided LA.

COR TRIATRIATUM SINISTRUM

Much has been written about cor triatriatum sinistrum.[1-128] The first clear-cut description of this anomaly was by W.S. Church[1] in 1868. His patient (Jane D) was a 38-year-old widow, the mother of four children. The opening in the subdividing diaphragm was {4/10} inch (10 mm) by {7/10} inch (18 mm). Two woodcut drawings depict cor triatriatum persuasively (Fig. 8.2).

The references are presented chronologically[1-128] so that the interested reader can gain an appreciation of how understanding of this anomaly has grown over time.

It has long been known that cor triatriatum is one of the rarest forms of congenital heart disease. In 1967, Keith, Rowe, and Vlad[73] encountered 7 patients with cor triatriatum in a series of 6647 patients with congenital heart disease, cor triatriatum constituting only 0.105% of patients with congenital heart disease in their extensive experience. Cor triatriatum was isolated in 5 patients and associated with other congenital heart disease in 2 patients.

My intense interest in cor triatriatum began in 1963, when I had the privilege of working with Dr. Maurice Lev in the Congenital Heart Disease Research and Training Center at the Hektoen Institute for Medical Research in Chicago, Illinois. This study led to a paper with Dr. Ignacio Corsini that was published in 1969.[76]

Why did Dr. Lev assign us this project? A little background will be helpful. The basic question was: What really is cor triatriatum anatomically and developmentally? At that time (1963–1965), there were two warring hypotheses concerning what cor triatriatum is: (1) stenosis of the common pulmonary vein or (2) an anomaly of septum primum (the flap valve of the foramen ovale).

We very carefully studied a series of 13 postmortem cases of cor triatriatum,[76] but initially were unable to decide which (if either) morphogenetic hypothesis was correct. The pathologic anatomy strongly suggested that the dorsal (posterior) chamber was indeed the stenotic common pulmonary vein (Figs. 8.1 to 8.4). However, the intra-atrial subdividing diaphragm always was confluent with the septum primum (see Figs. 8.4 and 8.5C), suggesting that the septum primum also must be involved in the morphogenesis of cor triatriatum.

Looking back into the literature, we found that these two conflicting developmental hypotheses went back almost to the discovery of cor triatriatum. Church,[1] who in 1868 first described the malformation that would later come to be known as cor triatriatum, expressed no hypothesis concerning the pathologic anatomy and its developmental basis. However, in 1881, Fowler[3] suggested that this anomaly resulted from overgrowth of the valve of the foramen ovale. Indeed, septum primum is an integral part of the subdividing diaphragm within the LA both grossly and histologically (Fig. 8.6).[76]

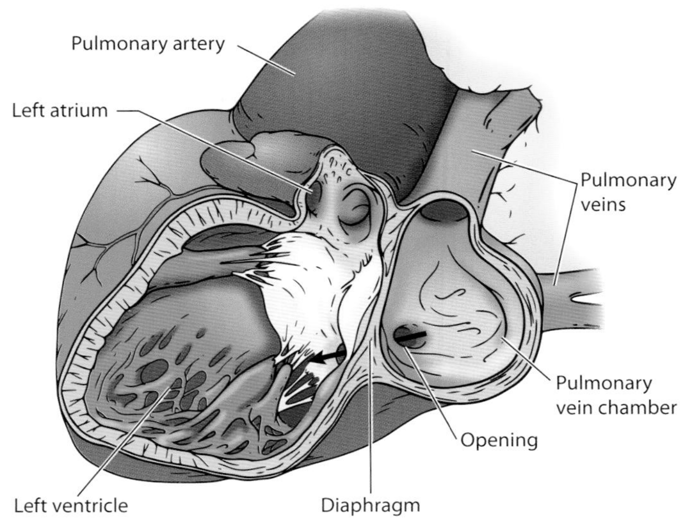

Fig. 8.1 Drawing of Cor Triatriatum Sinistrum (Subdivided Left Atrium). The dilated and hypertrophied pulmonary veins open into an hypertrophied pulmonary vein component of the left atrium (LA). This dilated, hypertrophied, and obstructed common pulmonary vein *(Pulmonary vein chamber)* is separated from the more ventral component of the LA that contains the left atrial appendage *(Left atrium)* and opens through the mitral valve (unlabeled) into the left ventricle (LV) *(Left Ventricle)* by an obliquely situated and obstructive subdividing diaphragm *(Diaphragm)*. This partition runs from superiorly and dorsally to inferiorly and ventrally. The obstructively small opening in the subdividing diaphragm lies just behind the posteromedial commissure of the mitral valve. The pulmonary artery is dilated, also reflecting that the opening in the diaphragm within the LA is obstructive, whereas the LV is not hypertrophied. (From Van Praagh R, Corsini I. Cor triatriatum: Pathologic anatomy and a consideration of morphogenesis based on 13 postmortem cases and a study of normal development of the pulmonary vein and atrial septum in 83 human embryos. *Am Heart J.* 1969;78:379-405; with permission.)

In 1903, Griffith[6] proposed that this anomaly represents failure of incorporation of the common pulmonary vein. In his own words, he wrote that this malformation appears to represent "a failure in the complete amalgamation of that part of the auricle which is said to be formed from the confluent portions of the pulmonary veins and that derived from the left-hand division of the common auricle of the embryonic heart."

Griffith[6] added, "I think it must depend on some such anomaly of development as has been suggested by Dr. Martin and myself."

What had happened is as follows. Griffith[6] presented his first case of this malformation to the Anatomical and Physiological Society of London in 1896, where he first proposed the concept of failure of incorporation of the common pulmonary vein. However, this hypothesis did not meet with the approval of the meeting so he dropped it temporarily. After the meeting, while preparing his abstract, he read Fowler's paper[3] and concluded that Fowler was right, that is, that this anomaly represents abnormal displacement of the septum primum due to abnormal streaming of the blood within the embryonic atria.

Then at the 1899 meeting of the same society, Martin[7] presented his case of the malformation, which was essentially identical to Griffith's case,[6] and Martin[7] also expressed his support for Griffith's[6] concept of malincorporation of the common pulmonary vein.

So, when Griffith[8] presented his second case of this anomaly in 1903, he returned to his original malincorporation concept because there was no evidence of acquired postnatal pathologic change. He added, "Perhaps, when the development of the pulmonary veins and their manner of junction with the left auricle is more fully understood, the explanation may become less uncertain." So, in presenting his second case, Griffith stuck to his guns (failure of incorporation), although fully understanding that much remained to be learned concerning incorporation of the pulmonary veins into the LA.

Thus, by 1903, two main morphogenetic hypotheses concerning this anomaly had emerged: (1) an *abnormality of the septum primum,* Fowler[3] in 1881; and (2) *malincorporation of the common pulmonary vein,* Griffith[6,8] in 1896 and 1903, and Martin[7] in 1899.

In 1905, Borst[10] published another definite case of this malformation and introduced the term *cor triatriatum.* Borst also proposed a third morphogenetic hypothesis: that the pulmonary vein develops to the right of the septum primum, instead of to the left of the septum primum, which he thought was normal. *Rightward malposition of the common pulmonary vein relative to the septum primum* appeared to be supported by some cases of cor triatriatum in which the common pulmonary vein chamber lies predominantly to the right of the septum primum (see Figs. 8.4 and 8.5C). However, in other cases, the common pulmonary vein chamber lies predominantly to the left of the septum primum (see Figs. 8.2C and 8.3). Both in Fowler's[3] and Borst's[10] hypotheses, the subdividing diaphragm was thought to be the septum primum.

In 1949, Loeffler[17] found that the septum primum is related normally to the septum secundum in cor triatriatum. Consequently, he decided that the subdividing diaphragm cannot

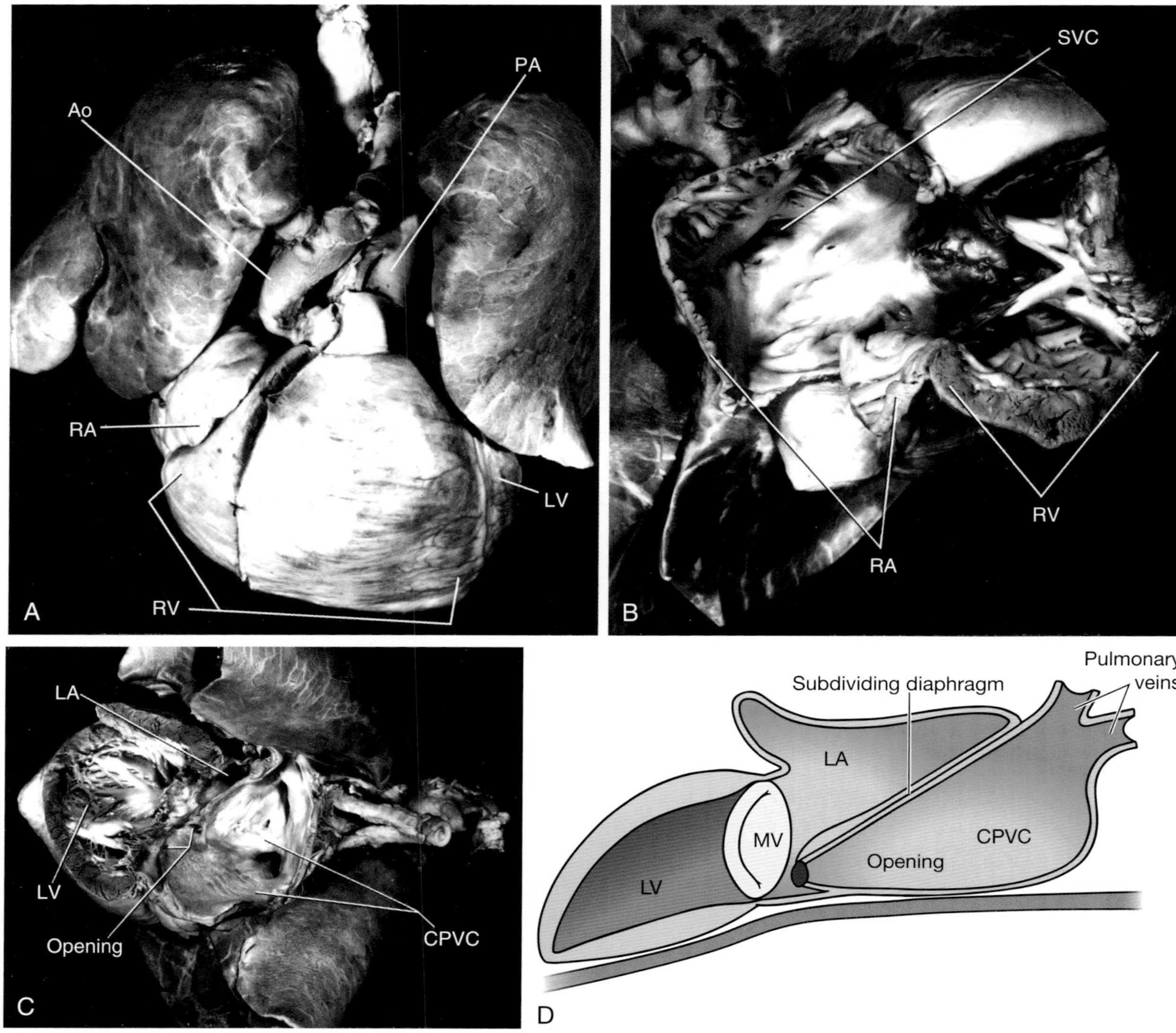

Fig. 8.2 Typical Case of Cor Triatriatum Sinistrum. (A) External frontal view of the heart and lungs. (B) Right lateral view of opened right atrium *(RA)*, tricuspid valve, and right ventricle (*RV*). (C) Left posterolateral view of the opened common pulmonary vein chamber *(CPVC)*, the stenotic opening in the subdividing diaphragm, the lower left atrium *(LA)*, the opened mitral valve *(MV)* (unlabeled), and the opened left ventricle *(LV)*. (D) diagram of the left heart chambers, obstructive subdividing diaphragm, obstructive subdividing diaphragm, and the MV. There is marked hypertrophy and enlargement of the RA and RV (A and B). The obliquity of the subdividing membrane is well seen in C and D. Because of this obliquity, the CPVC cannot be described simply as dorsal or posterior, whereas the lower LA is ventral or anterior. Although the CPVC is mostly dorsal or posterior, it also extends very ventrally or anteriorly to right behind the posteromedial commissure of the MV (D). Conversely, although the lower LA is mostly ventral or anterior, it also extends far posteriorly to just in front of the pulmonary venous branches (D). *Ao*, Aorta; *PA*, pulmonary artery; *SVC*, superior vena cava. (From Van Praagh R, Corsini I. Cor triatriatum: Pathologic anatomy and a consideration of morphogenesis based on 13 postmortem cases and a study of normal development of the pulmonary vein and atrial septum in 83 human embryos. *Am Heart J*. 1969;78:379, with permission.)

be an abnormally located septum primum. Since that time, most investigators have accepted the hypothesis of malincorporation of the common pulmonary vein that was first published in 1903 by Griffith.[8] However, Loeffler[17] was well aware that the more basic question remained unanswered, namely: Why does the common pulmonary vein fail to incorporate normally into the LA in cor triatriatum? He suggested that malincorporation of the common pulmonary vein into the LA is "caused in all probability by a disturbance of the normal growth of the posterior wall of the left atrium."[17] He concluded that the subdividing diaphragm is the abnormal posterior wall of the primitive LA.

However, not all investigators found the malincorporation hypothesis persuasive. As Sawyer et al[37] pointed out in 1957, this hypothesis fails to explain those cases in which the foramen ovale or fossa ovalis has been reported to be located in the medial wall of the dorsal (posterior) chamber. If the malincorporation hypothesis were correct, one would expect the foramen ovale (or fossa ovalis) always to open into (or to be adjacent to)

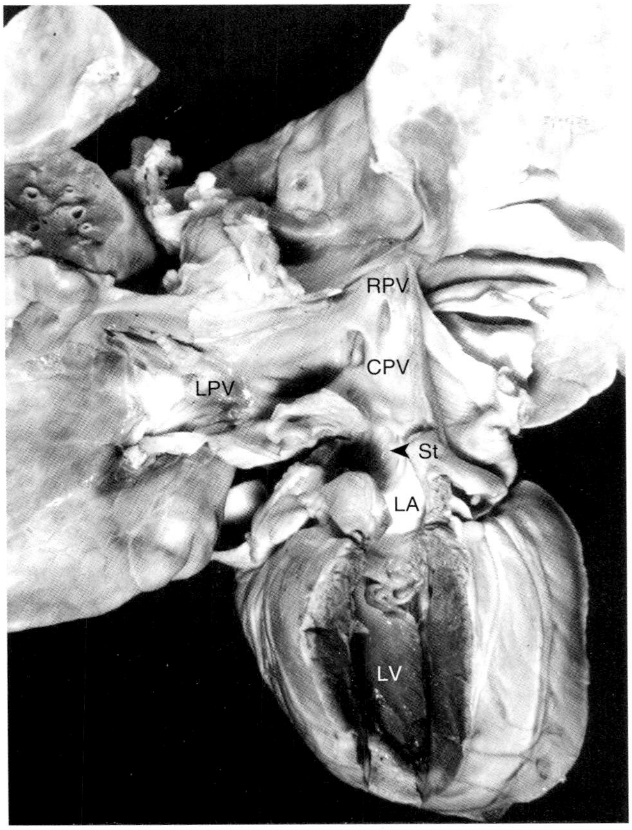

Fig. 8.3 Typical Cor Triatriatum, Opened Left Heart Chambers, Posteroinferior View. When cor triatriatum is used without other qualification, cor triatriatum sinistrum is always meant. Blood from the left pulmonary vein *(LPV)* and the right pulmonary vein *(RPV)* flowed into the common pulmonary vein and then through a stenotic orifice *(St)* into the lower left atrium *(LA)* and then across the mitral orifice (unlabeled) into the left ventricle *(LV)*. (From Van Praagh R, Corsini I. Cor triatriatum: pathologic anatomy and a consideration of morphogenesis based on 13 postmortem cases and a study of normal development of the pulmonary vein and atrial septum in 83 human embryos. *Am Heart J.* 1969;78:379, with permission.)

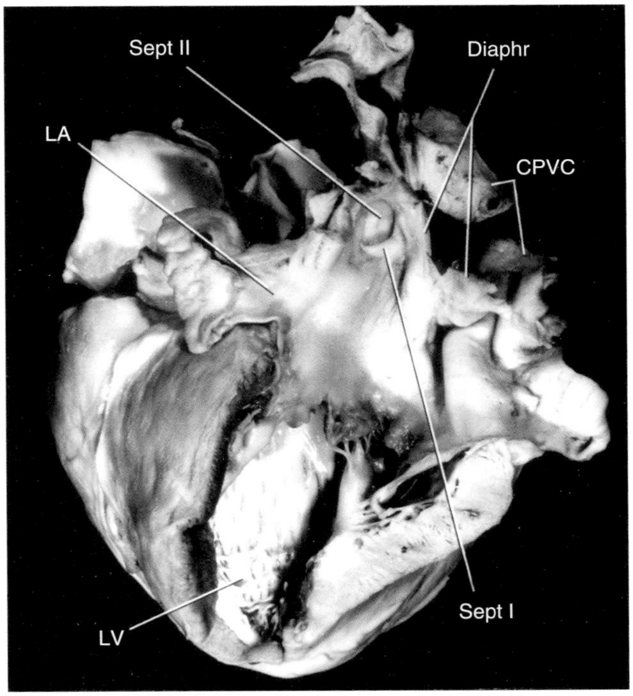

Fig. 8.4 Subdividing Diaphragm *(Diaphr)* Between Common Pulmonary Vein Chamber *(CPVC)* Dorsally and Lower Left Atrium *(LA)* Ventrally, Anterior View. The septum primum *(Sept I)* lies normally to the left of septum secundum *(Sept II)*. Sept I is in direct fibrous continuity with the subdividing diaphragm. (From Van Praagh R, Corsini I. Cor triatriatum: Pathologic anatomy and a consideration of morphogenesis based on 13 postmortem cases and a study of normal development of the pulmonary vein and atrial septum in 83 human embryos. *Am Heart J.* 1969;78:379, with permission.)

the primitive LA (the ventral chamber). This problem is exemplified by Fig. 8.7. A small opening exists between the common pulmonary vein chamber and the RA in the general region of the foramen ovale or fossa ovalis.

In view of the aforementioned confusion regarding what cor triatriatum really is anatomically and embryologically, and our inability to decide which (if any) of these three contending hypotheses is correct based on pathologic anatomic examination, we decided to undertake a study of the development of the pulmonary vein and atrial septum in 83 human embryos from the Minot Collection of Harvard Medical School. Then we attempted to correlate the pathologic anatomic findings in these 13 postmortem cases of cor triatriatum with the embryologic findings in 83 normal human embryos.[76]

EMBRYOLOGY

The youngest human embryo in which we were able to identify the common pulmonary vein with certainty had an estimated age since ovulation of **27 days** (Fig. 8.8).[76] In this horizontal plane section, note that the common pulmonary vein is an essentially midline structure and that it communicates with a still undivided common atrium. The right and left lung buds are well seen. This sinus venosus is right-sided and opens into the common atrium. The common atrium communicates with the ventricle of the bulboventricular loop via the common atrioventricular (AV) canal. The superior (ventral) and the inferior (dorsal) endocardial cushions of the common AV canal are well seen. The endocardial cushions of the bulbus cordis are seen lying to the right of the ventricle, as one would expect with a D-bulboventricular loop. In the magnification of the common pulmonary vein (see Fig. 8.8B), the erythrocytes are prominent because they are nucleated at this stage of development, resembling normoblasts of later developmental stages.

Histologically, we were unable to tell whether the common pulmonary vein grows out in a dorsal (or posterior) direction from the common atrium into the lung buds via the dorsal mesocardium, whether the common pulmonary vein grows in a ventral (or anterior) direction from the lung buds into the common atrium via the dorsal mesocardium, or whether the common pulmonary vein grows in both directions—dorsally from the common atrium and ventrally from the lung buds—to make contact in the dorsal mesocardium (the broad and short connection between the common atrium and the lung buds). Our data did not clarify the direction of growth of the common pulmonary vein. Consequently, we can make no comment on

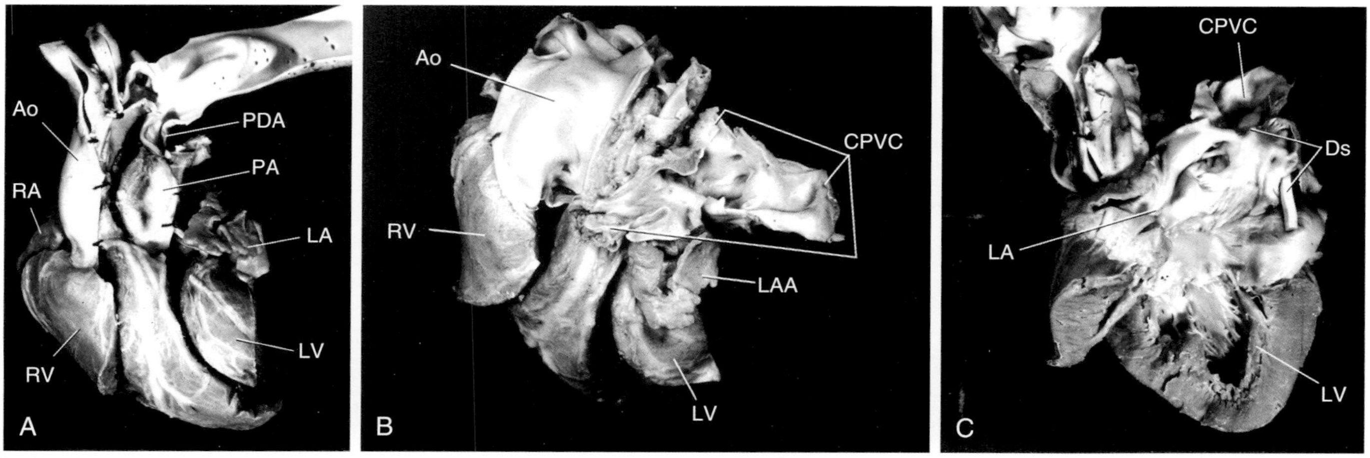

Fig. 8.5 **Cor Triatriatum With Transposition of the Great Arteries {S,D,D}.** (A) Exterior frontal view. (B) Dorsal view of the common pulmonary vein chamber *(CPVC).* (C) Ventral view of the subdividing diaphragm. (A) Note that there is situs solitus of the atria (hence {*S*,-,-}), the morphologically right atrium *(RA)* lying to the right of the morphologically left atrium *(LA).* There is a concordant ventricular D-loop (hence {S,*D*,-}), the morphologically right ventricle *(RV)* lying to the right of the morphologically left ventricle *(LV).* D-transposition of the great arteries (D-TGA) is present (hence {S,D,*D*}), the D-transposed aorta *(Ao)* lying to the right (dextro, or D) relative to the transposed pulmonary artery *(PA).* There is atrioventricular concordance with ventriculoarterial discordance. Hence, the systemic and pulmonary circulations are physiologically uncorrected, the RA and the Ao being ipsilateral (both right-sided) and the LA and PA being ipsilateral (both left-sided). This 3-month-old boy had a moderate-sized patent ductus arteriosus *(PDA),* 6 mm in circumference, that may have helped decompress the pulmonary circulation by permitting pulmonary arterial–to–descending aortic shunting. Note that the LV is more hypertrophied and enlarged than is the systemic RV, a very unusual situation in D-TGA with an intact ventricular septum and no left ventricular outflow tract obstruction. The marked left ventricular hypertrophy and enlargement is present because of the highly obstructive cor triatriatum. (B) The opening between the CPVC is not apparent, reflecting the severity of the obstruction. The left atrial appendage *(LAA)* is enlarged, going along with the severe left ventricular hypertrophy and enlargement. (C) One can see two small defects *(Ds)* in the subdividing diaphragm: the lower one, behind the posteromedial commissure of the mitral valve, measures 3 mm in diameter (opening marked with a probe), and an upper one, measuring only 0.5 mm in diameter. The septum primum (unlabeled) is continuous with the diaphragm (between the Ds). Cor triatriatum with D-TGA has predominant *left* ventricular hypertrophy and enlargement, as opposed to cor triatriatum with normally related great arteries that has prominent *right* ventricular hypertrophy and enlargement (as in Fig. 8.2A). (From Van Praagh R, Corsini I. Cor triatriatum: Pathologic anatomy and a consideration of morphogenesis based on 13 postmortem cases and a study of normal development of the pulmonary vein and atrial septum in 83 human embryos. *Am Heart J.* 1969;78:379, with permission.)

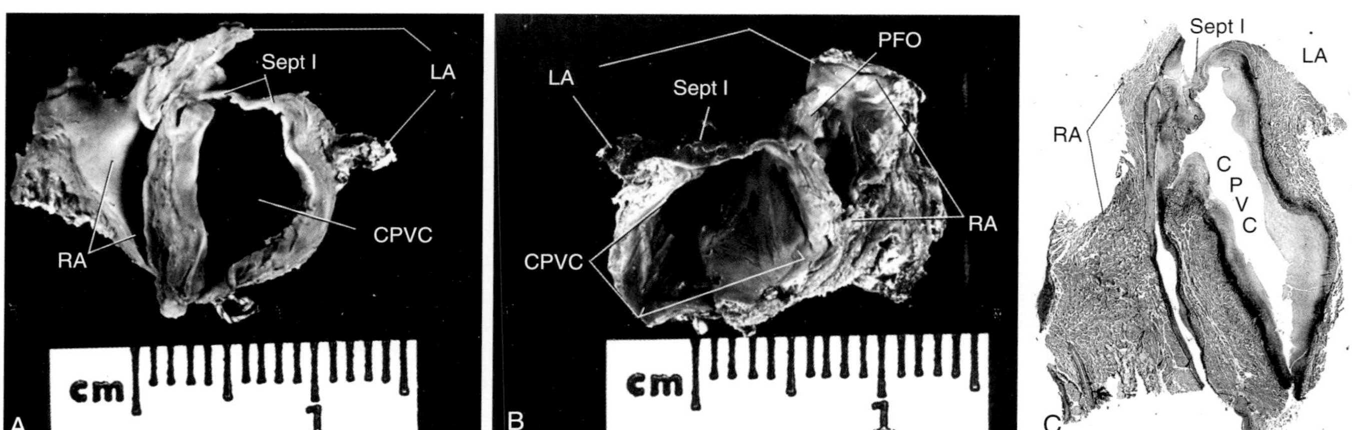

Fig. 8.6 **Frontal Section Through the Right Atrium *(RA),* Atrial Septum, Left Atrium *(LA),* Septum Primum *(Sept I),* and Common Pulmonary Vein Chamber *(CPVC)* of a Typical Case of Cor Triatriatum in a 4-Month-Old Boy.** (A) Anterior view. (B) Posterior view. (C) Histology, anterior view. The lower LA is superior, the CPVC is inferior, and the subdividing diaphragm lies between them. Sept I is confluent with the subdividing diaphragm. (B) The RA communicates with the lower LA via the patent foramen ovale *(PFO),* which lies above Sept I and the subdividing diaphragm. (A–C) One can see the markedly thickened endothelial and subendothelial layers within the hypertensive and obstructed CPVC. Sept I forms part of the roof the CPVC. (C, Verhoff-van Gieson stain, original magnification ×15.) (From Van Praagh R, Corsini I. Cor triatriatum: Pathologic anatomy and a consideration of morphogenesis based on 13 postmortem cases and a study of normal development of the pulmonary vein and atrial septum in 83 human embryos. *Am Heart J.* 1969;78:379, with permission.)

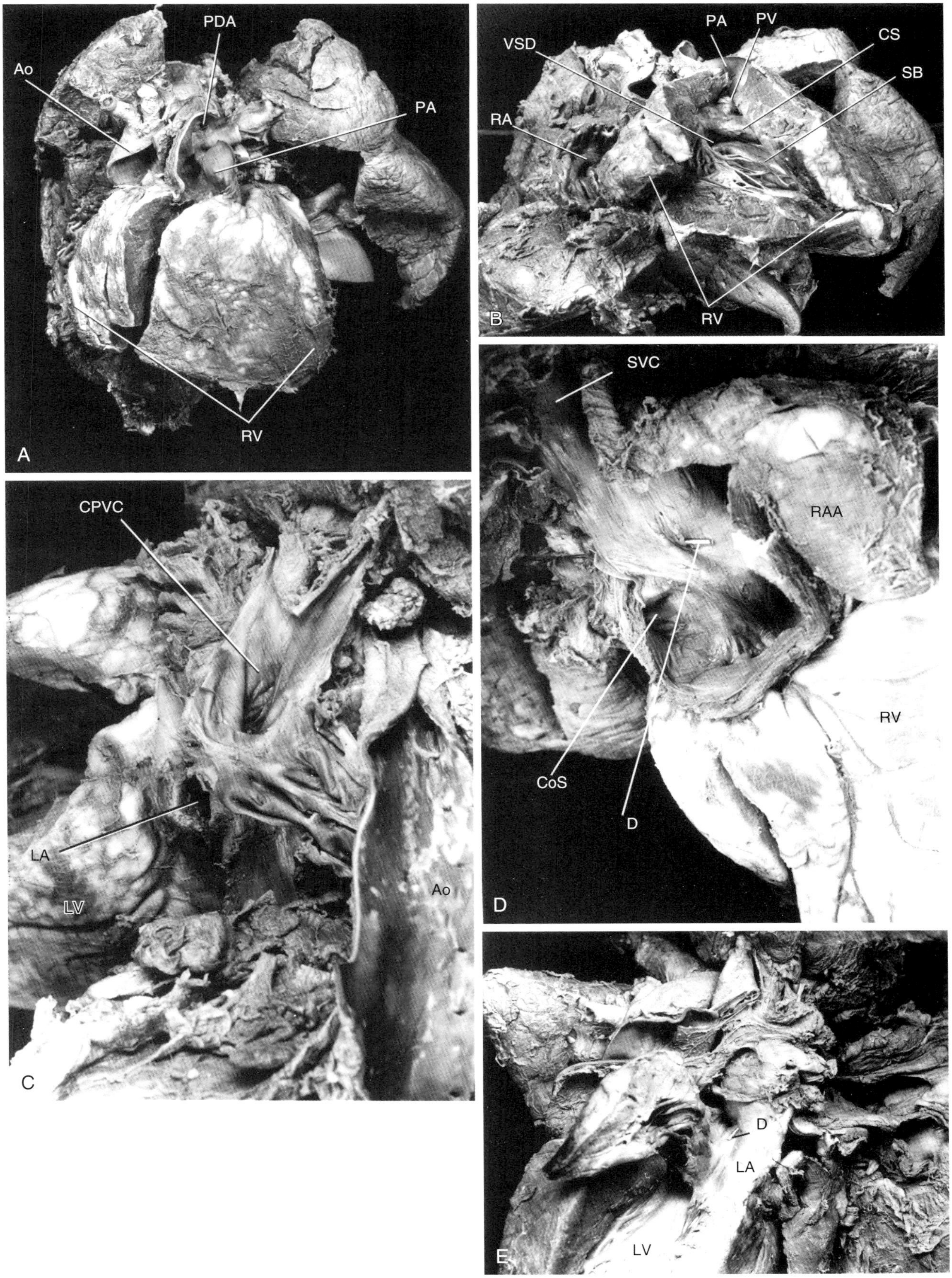
PDA
Ao
PA
RV
A
PA
PV
VSD
CS
SB
RA
RV
B
CPVC
LA
LV
Ao
C
SVC
RAA
RV
CoS
D
D
D
LA
LV
E

Fig. 8.7, cont'd

Fig. 8.7, cont'd Severe Cor Triatriatum With Tetralogy of Fallot in a 20 10/12-Year-Old Man. (A) External frontal view of heart and lungs. (B) Opened right ventricle *(RV)*. (C) Interior of common pulmonary vein chamber *(CPVC)*. (D) Interior of right atrium *(RA)*. (E) Interior of lower left atrium *(LA)*. (A) Because the main pulmonary artery *(PA)* is of approximately normal size, this heart does not look like tetralogy of Fallot (TOF) externally. A patent ductus arteriosus *(PDA)* is also seen (5 mm in diameter). (B) The opened RV reveals massive right ventricular hypertrophy. The conal septum or crista supraventricularis *(CS)* is displaced anterosuperiorly, narrowing the subpulmonary infundibulum, typical of TOF. A malalignment type of conoventricular ventricular septal defect *(VSD)* is present, because of the anterosuperior malalignment of the CS relative to the ventricular septum and septal band *(SB)*. The pulmonary valve *(PV)* is tricuspid and only mildly hypoplastic. (C) The interior of the CPVC showed no obvious communication. However, in D, inspection of the interior of the RA reveals a small defect *(D)* only 1 mm in diameter (probe), between the CPVC and the RA. This defect is interpreted as an anomalous communication, not as a patent foramen ovale. The right atrial appendage *(RAA)* is markedly hypertrophied. A persistent left superior vena cava *(SVC)* drains into the coronary sinus *(CoS)*, explaining its large ostium. (E) Careful inspection of the lower LA reveals a very small communication (D), 1 mm in diameter (probe), between the CPVC and the lower LA. Additional associated anomalies included an aberrant right subclavian artery, hypoplasia of the right middle lobe (RML) of the lung with secondary dextrocardia, partially anomalous pulmonary venous connection from the RML to the inferior vena cava, anomalous systemic artery from the descending thoracic aorta to the RML (variant of scimitar syndrome), displacement of left-sided atrial appendage posteriorly and to the right (partial form of right juxtaposition of the atrial appendages, that is, dextromalposition of the left atrial appendage), intra-aortic band beneath the ostium of the right common carotid artery (partial form of persistent 5th aortic arch), and brain abscess (large, left parietal lobe, pseudomonas). Thus, this young man had multiple cardiovascular anomalies, with nonisolated cor triatriatum. *Ao*, Aorta. (From Van Praagh R, Corsini I. Cor triatriatum: Pathologic anatomy and a consideration of morphogenesis based on 13 postmortem cases and a study of normal development of the pulmonary vein and atrial septum in 83 human embryos. *Am Heart J*. 1969;78:379, with permission.)

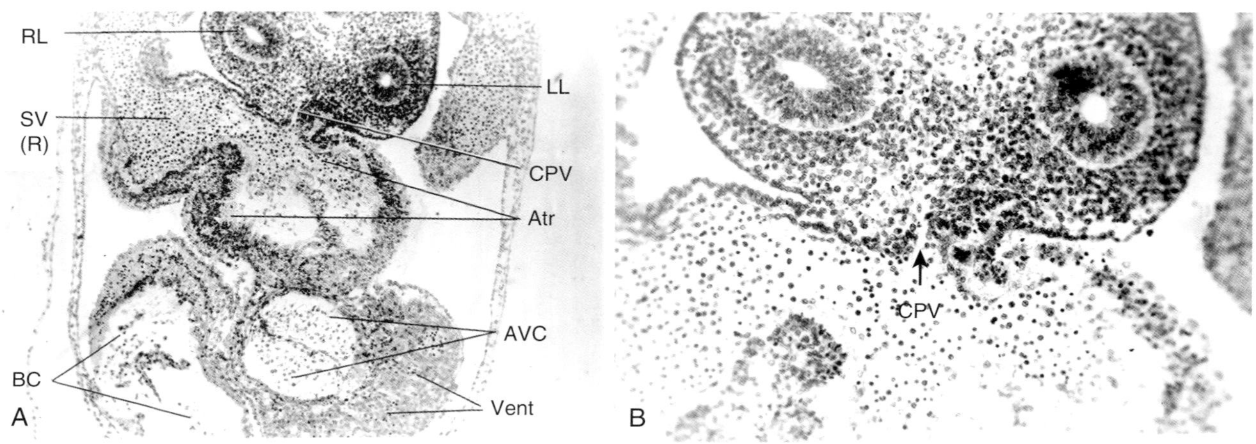

Fig. 8.8 Development of the Pulmonary Vein in Man, Horizontal Plane (Transverse) Sections. Youngest embryo in which the common pulmonary vein *(CPV)* was definitely identified (Minot Collection, Harvard Medical School, embryo no 2321, 4.6 mm crown-rump length, estimated age since ovulation 27 days, section 257). *Atr*, Primitive undivided atrium; *AVC*, atrioventricular canal consisting of undivided superior and inferior endocardial cushions; *BC*, bulbus cordis, future right ventricular outflow tract; *LL*, left lung bud; *RL*, right lung bud; *SV (R)*, sinus venosus, right horn; *Vent*, ventricle of bulboventricular loop, future left ventricle. (Alum cochineal and orange G stain, original magnification ×150; same embryo, close-up of CPV (original magnification ×250). (From Van Praagh R, Corsini I. Cor triatriatum: Pathologic anatomy and a consideration of morphogenesis based on 13 postmortem cases and a study of normal development of the pulmonary vein and atrial septum in 83 human embryos. *Am Heart J*. 1969;78:379, with permission.)

this point from our data, except to say that three possibilities exist, as mentioned earlier.

By **33 days of age,** many changes have occurred in the normal human embryo (Fig. 8.9).[76] In this horizontal plane section (see Fig. 8.9A), note that the common pulmonary vein lies immediately to the left of a prominent mass of sinus venosus fibrous tissue. The common pulmonary vein has enlarged, and it remains a midline structure ventral to the midline esophagus that lies between the developing right and left lungs. The sinus venosus (right horn) lies to the right, and a relatively small left superior vena cava (LSVC; left sinus horn) lies to the left. The right venous valve is seen, and the right and left atria are demarcated.

In a horizontal plane section from the same embryo 128 μ above that shown in Fig. 8.9A, note that the septum primum is now well formed (see Fig. 8.9B). The septum primum lies above the common pulmonary vein, both of which are essentially midline structures. The septum primum and the left venous valve both have grown upward from the mass of venous or sinus venosus fibrous tissue shown in Fig. 8.9A. The space between the septum primum and the left venous valve is known as the *interseptovalvular space* (see Fig. 8.9B).[75]

In Fig. 8.9B, note that the right horn of the sinus venosus is seen, as are the right and left venous valves—the leaflets of the body's largest venous valve. The small LSVC is again noted.

By **35 days of age** in the normal human embryo, a horizontal plane section shows that incorporation of the common pulmonary vein into the LA is beginning (Fig. 8.10).[76] Note the trifurcation of the common pulmonary vein in the dorsal mesocardium. The common pulmonary vein still lies below the septum primum and immediately to the left of the prominent mass

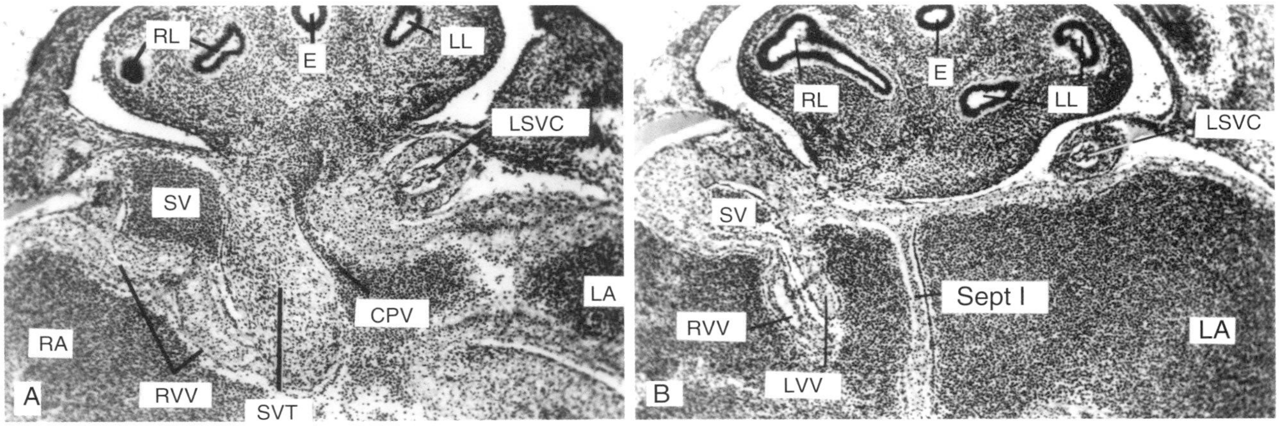

Fig. 8.9 In a 33-day-old human embryo, this horizontal plane section shows the common pulmonary vein *(CPV)* connecting with the left atrium *(LA)* immediately to the left of a prominent mass of sinus venosus tissue *(SVT)* of the right sinus horn. Incorporation of the CPV into the LA has not yet begun. (Minot Collection embryo no. 1005, Harvard Medical School, 9.4 mm, section 331, borax carmine and Lyons blue stain, original magnification ×130.) Same embryo, section 315, 128 μ above that shown in A. Septum primum *(Sept I)* is now well formed, lying above the CPV. Both Sept I and the CPV are essentially midline structures. The left venous valve *(LVV)*, that is, the left leaflet of the valve of the sinus venosus *(SV)*, and Sept I both have grown upward (cephalad) from the prominent mass of SVT seen in A. Sept I grows upward from the left side of the mass of SVT, the LVV grows upward from the right side of this mass of SVT, and the space between Sept I and the LVV is known as the interseptovalvular space, well seen in B. In the normal postnatal heart, the LVV becomes adherent to the right side of Sept I, largely obliterating the embryonic interoseptovalvular space. Persistence of the interseptovalvular space may be a rare form of nonobstruction cor triatriatum dextrum (speculation). *E*, Esophagus; *RVV*, right venous valve, that is, the right leaflet of the valve of the SV that forms the eustachian valve of the inferior vena cava and the Thebesian valve of the coronary sinus; *LL*, left lung bud; *RL*, right lung bud; *LSVC*, left superior vena cava; *RA*, right atrium. (Original magnification ×110.) (From Van Praagh R, Corsini I. Cor triatriatum: Pathologic anatomy and a consideration of morphogenesis based on 13 postmortem cases and a study of normal development of the pulmonary vein and atrial septum in 83 human embryos. *Am Heart J*. 1969;78:379, with permission.)

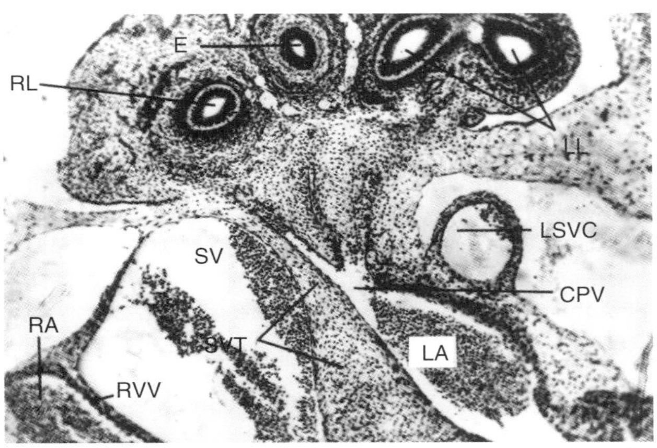

Fig. 8.10 A 35-Day-Old Human Embryo, Incorporation of the Common Pulmonary Vein *(CPV)* Into the Left Atrium *(LA)* Is Beginning. The CPV is "trifurcating" in the dorsal mesocardium. Note the developing right lung *(RL)*, left lung *(LL)*, and esophagus *(E)*. The CPV is very inferior and medial, just to the left of the mass of sinus venosus tissue *(SVT)* of the right sinus horn from which the septum primum and the left venous valve both develop and grow upward. To the right of the CPV lies the right horn of the sinus venosus *(SV)* and to the left of the CPV lies the left superior vena cava *(LSVC)*, which represent the left horn of the SV. *RA*, Right atrium; *RVV*, right venous valve. (Minot Collection embryo no. 2313, Harvard Medical School, 11.9 mm, section 510, transverse/horizontal plane, cochineal and orange G stain, original magnification ×130.) (From Van Praagh R, Corsini I. Cor triatriatum: Pathologic anatomy and a consideration of morphogenesis based on 13 postmortem cases and a study of normal development of the pulmonary vein and atrial septum in 83 human embryos. *Am Heart J*. 1969;78:379, with permission.)

of sinus venosus tissue from the right sinus horn. As frontal plane sections show *(vide infra)*, the septum primum grows upward from the left side of this mass of sinus venosus tissue and the left venous valve grows upward from the right side of this platform of sinus venosus tissue. The lungs and the midline esophagus are both developing. The right-sided sinus venosus, the right venous valve, the RA, and the LSVC are also noteworthy (see Fig. 8.10).

By **38 days of age** in the normal human embryo (Fig. 8.11), incorporation of the common pulmonary vein and its branches into the LA is progressing. Note that the common pulmonary vein now lies to the left of the septum primum instead of beneath the septum primum, as in earlier normal stages. Note that the septum primum and the left venous valve are fused at their bases. In this embryo, the left superior vena cava LSVC is still quite large (see Fig. 8.11).[76]

By **63 days of age** in the normal human embryo (Fig. 8.12),[76] this horizontal plane section shows that the common pulmonary vein is well incorporated into the LA; that is, the region of the common pulmonary vein is now so wide that it is no longer distinguishable as the common pulmonary vein because it has become incorporated as part of the dorsal wall of the LA. The right pulmonary vein enters the LA just to the left of and posterior to the septum primum. The left pulmonary vein has a separate ostium into the LA, further to the left. The fact that both pulmonary venous branches—the right and left pulmonary veins—have separate openings into the LA indicates that the common pulmonary vein has been incorporated into the LA.

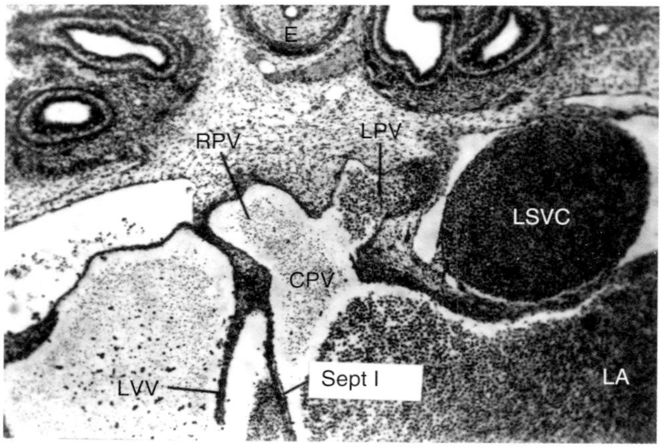

Fig. 8.11 A 38-day-old human embryo, incorporation of the common pulmonary vein *(CPV)* and its right *(RPV)* and left *(LPV)* pulmonary venous branches is progressing (compared with the stages shown in Figs. 8.8 to 8.10, inclusive). The CPV is still midline; compare with the esophagus *(E)*. The CPV now lies to the left of a thin septum primum *(Sept I)*. Note that the left venous valve *(LVV)* is the smaller rightward appendage of the LVV mechanism. Sept I and the LVV are fused dorsally. The LVV apparatus is really bifid, consisting of Sept I to the left and the LVV to the right. Sept I is the largest venous valve leaflet in the body, normally preventing left-to-right regurgitation (shunting) of blood from the left atrium *(LA)* into the right atrium (RA). The sinoatrial valve is the largest venous valve of the body, consisting (in atrial situs solitus) of the right ventricular valve to the right and the LVV and Sept I to the left. The sinoatrial valve is not normally incompetent (regurgitant), as is often said. Instead, the sinoatrial valve is normally competent between the LA to the left and the RA and venae cavae to the right. Thus, Sept I normally functions both as a valve (preventing LA-to-RA regurgitation prenatally) and as a septum (separating the LA and the RA postnatally). *LSVC,* Left superior vena cava. (Minot Collection embryo no. 2155, Harvard Medical School, 17.6 mm, section 789, horizontal plane, cochineal and orange G stain, original magnification ×130.) (From Van Praagh R, Corsini I. Cor triatriatum: Pathologic anatomy and a consideration of morphogenesis based on 13 postmortem cases and a study of normal development of the pulmonary vein and atrial septum in 83 human embryos. *Am Heart J.* 1969;78:379, with permission.)

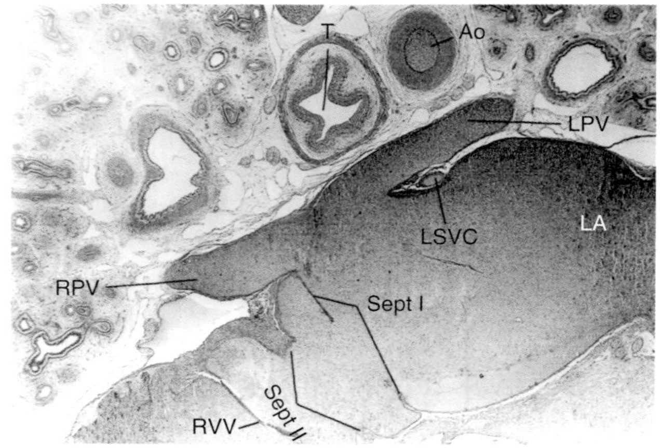

Fig. 8.12 A 63-Day-Old Human, at the End of the Embryonic Period and the Beginning of the Fetal Period (From 63 Days Until Birth). The pulmonary vein remains midline; compare with the trachea *(T)*. The right and left pulmonary vein branches (*RPV* and *LPV*) still are not fully incorporated into the left atrium *(LA)*. The septum primum *(Sept I)* to the left has become thin and membranous, whereas the superior limbic band of the septum secundum *(Sept II)* to the right is thick and muscular. Sept I and Sept II normally form a unidirectional flap valve that permits right-to-left shunting, but prevents left-to-right shunting in utero. Sept I is the interatrial valve occluder and Sept II is the valve ring. The right venous valve *(RVV)* has also become thin, like Sept I. The left superior vena cava *(LSVC)* is now much smaller than in earlier stages (see Figs. 8.8 to 8.11) but is still minimally patent. The descending thoracic aorta *(Ao)* is left-sided (relative to the trachea) and relatively thick-walled, and the pulmonary parenchyma is much more developed than previously. (Minot Collection embryo no. 2128, 45 mm, section 2035, horizontal plane of section, cochineal and orange G stain, original magnification ×40.) (From Van Praagh R, Corsini I. Cor triatriatum: Pathologic anatomy and a consideration of morphogenesis based on 13 postmortem cases and a study of normal development of the pulmonary vein and atrial septum in 83 human embryos. *Am Heart J.* 1969;78:379, with permission.)

However, at 63 days of age, incorporation of the pulmonary venous branches is incomplete. Ultimately, each pulmonary vein is incorporated into the LA up to just beyond the primary division of each branch. Postnatally, this is why there normally appear to be two left pulmonary veins (from the left upper and lower lobes of the lung), and two or three right pulmonary veins (from the right upper, middle, and lower lobes of the lung). In Fig. 8.12, both pulmonary venous ostia appear to be widely patent (nonobstructive). Note that the LSVC is now diminutive, almost a ligament of Marshall (see Fig. 8.12). The pulmonary veins remain midline structures; note the relation of the pulmonary veins to the midline trachea (see Fig. 8.12). The pulmonary parenchyma has developed considerably, as has the left aortic arch. Parts of the septum secundum and the right venous valve are also noteworthy (see Fig. 8.12).[76]

Frontal plane sections are also very helpful in understanding the normal development of the common pulmonary vein relative to that of the atrial septum (Fig. 8.13)[76] When the normal human embryo is **33 days of age** (similar in age to Fig. 8.9, which shows horizontal plane sections), one notes the prominent platform of sinus venosus tissue. From its left side, the septum primum grows upward. From its right side, the left venous valve grows upward. The right venous valve lies to the right of the inferior vena cava (IVC). Note that the common pulmonary vein is located immediately to the left of the base of the large mass of sinus venosus (fibrous) tissue. In somewhat greater detail, the common pulmonary vein runs adjacent to and partly beneath the left side of the overhanging mass of sinus venosus tissue. The tracing of this slide (see Fig. 8.13A), seen in Fig. 8.13B, makes these relationships clearer.

Thus, at **33 days of age** in the normal human embryo, the common pulmonary vein lies beneath the septum primum and the sinus venosus tissue from which the septum primum develops (see Fig. 8.13A–B). In other words, the common pulmonary vein is located as medially and as inferiorly as possible within the LA. This is the normal position of the common pulmonary vein at 33 days of age (see Fig. 8.13).[76] To indicate that this is not just one fluke section, frontal plane sections from the same 33-day-old embryo are shown 48 μ dorsal to Fig. 8.13A (see Fig. 8.13C) and 40 μ dorsal to Fig. 8.13C (see Fig. 8.13D). The small common pulmonary vein is still directly beneath septum primum and the left side of the mass of sinus venosus tissue from which the septum primum develops (see Fig. 8.13C–D).

The midline and inferior location of the common pulmonary vein in the normal 33-day-old human embryo is confirmed in

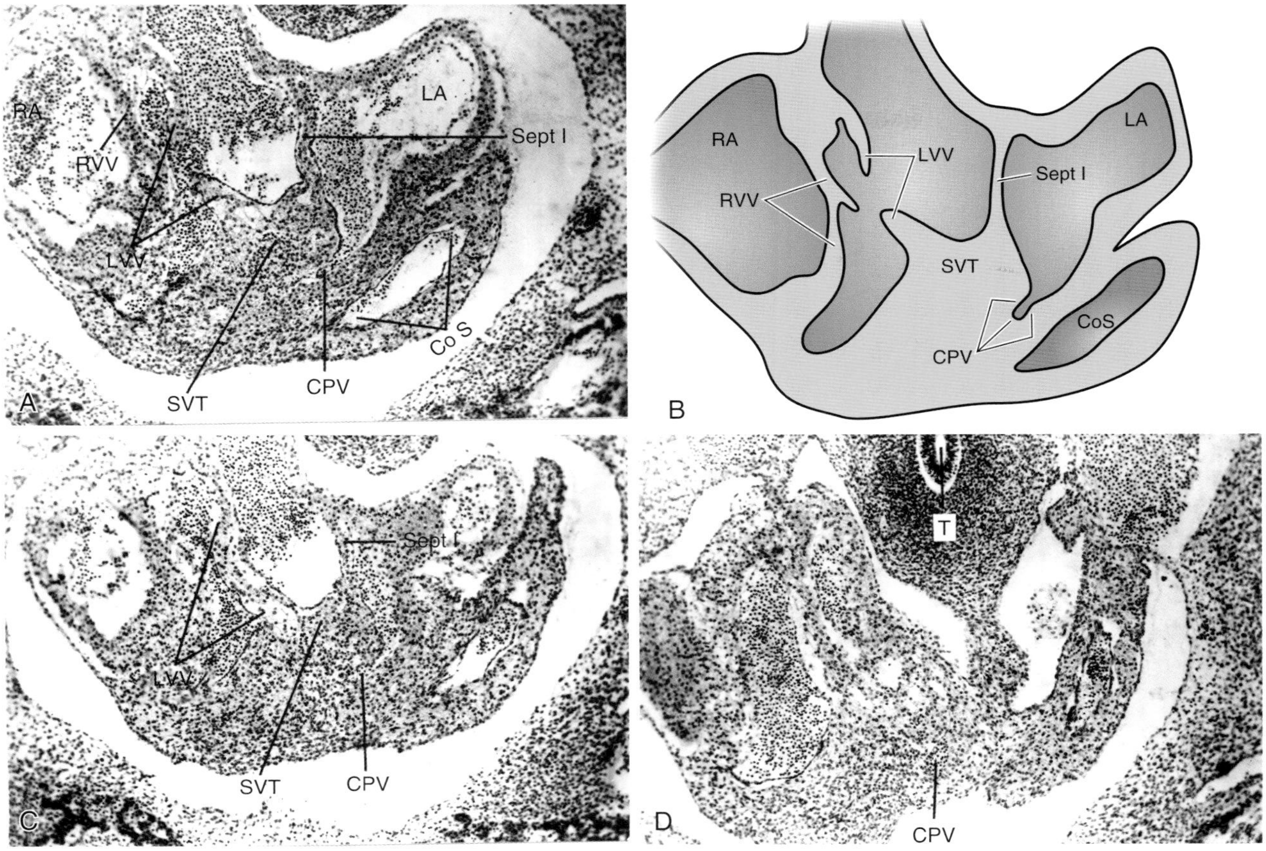

Fig. 8.13 (A) A frontal-plane section of a normal 33-day-old human embryo. The common pulmonary vein *(CPV)* is located as inferiorly and as medially within the left atrium *(LA)* as it could be. The CPV passes under an overhanging ledge of sinus venosus tissue *(SVT)*. The septum primum *(Sept I)* grows upward from the left side of this mass of SVT. The left venous valve *(LVV)* grows upward from the right side of this platform of SVT. The space between Sept I to the left and the LVV to the right is the interseptovalvar space. The CPV lies directly beneath Sept I on the left side of this SVT. The left horn of the sinus venosus, the future coronary sinus *(CoS)*, is still large. (Minot Collection, embryo no. 1919, Harvard Medical School, 10 mm, section 674, cochineal and orange S stain, original magnification ×130.) (B) Tracing of Fig. 8.13A to make clear the superior-inferior relationship between Sept I and the CPV, both midline structures at this stage (33 days of age). (C) 48 μ dorsal to the view shown in A and B; the small CPV is still directly beneath Sept I and the left side of the SVT from which both Sept I and the LVV develop. (Section 680, frontal plane, same embryo, same stain, same magnification as in A.) (D) 40 μ dorsal to C (same embryo, same stain, same plane, same magnification as A and C). The CPV is now in the dorsal mesocardium, returning from the lung buds to the LA. The midline location of the CPV is corroborated by its relation to the trachea *(T)*. *RA,* Right atrium; *RVV,* right venous valve. (From Van Praagh R, Corsini I. Cor triatriatum: Pathologic anatomy and a consideration of morphogenesis based on 13 postmortem cases and a study of normal development of the pulmonary vein and atrial septum in 83 human embryos. *Am Heart J.* 1969;78:379, with permission.)

a sagittal section of another embryo (Fig. 8.14).[76] Note that the midline location of the common pulmonary vein beneath the prominent mass of right horn sinus venosus tissue is corroborated by finding the trachea and the esophagus both cut longitudinally in the same section (see Fig. 8.14).

We are stressing the medial and inferior location of the common pulmonary vein at this early stage (27 to 33 days of age) because this is *not* how these relationships are conventionally presented. Instead, the common pulmonary vein usually is shown to appear well to the left of the septum primum and much higher (more cephalad) (Fig. 8.15). As shown previously (see Figs 8.7 to 8.14), this is *not* where we found the common pulmonary vein to appear. As will be seen, correction of this error makes it possible to understand the morphogenesis of cor triatriatum sinistrum.

But before we turn to a consideration of abnormal development, we must complete the normal development of the pulmonary vein and septum primum (Fig. 8.16).[76] When the embryo is **56 days of age,** note that the platform of sinus venosus or venous fibrous tissue has largely disappeared (compare Fig. 8.16A with Fig. 8.13). Instead, by 56 days of age, this mass of fibrous tissue has been replaced by its progeny. On the left side, the septum primum has grown upward to the left of the septum secundum, and on the right side, this less well-developed left venous valve has also grown upward (see Fig. 8.16A). The space between the septum primum to the left and the left venous valve to the right is the interseptovalvular space (see Fig. 8.16B).

Note that the septum primum and the left venous valve are both directly continuous with the left wall of the IVC (see Fig.

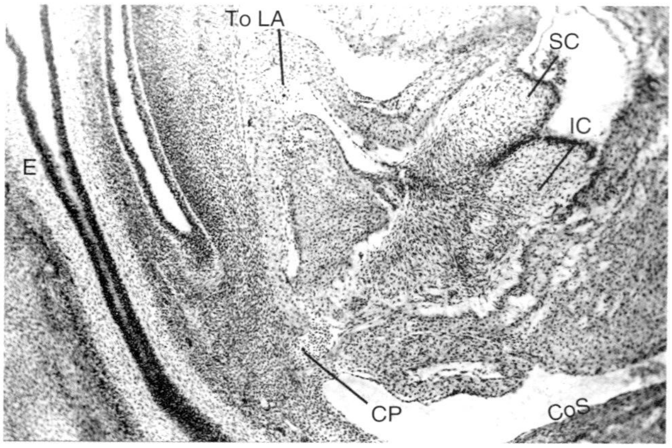

Fig. 8.14 A 33-Day-Old Human Embryo, Sagittal Section, Right Lateral View. The common pulmonary vein (CPV) leaves the left atrium *(LA)* by passing to the left of and beneath the mass of sinus venosus tissue (SVT) seen here and in Fig. 8.13. The CPV normally passes just above the left sinus horn, that is, the future coronary sinus *(CoS)*. The CPV at this age is very inferior, in the same horizontal plane as the inferior endocardial cushion *(IC)* of the common atrioventricular canal. The CPV is also very medial or midline, as is confirmed by the trachea (T) and the esophagus *(E)*, both of which are sectioned longitudinally. *CP*, common pulmonary vein; *SC*, Superior endocardial cushion of the common atrioventricular canal. (Minot Collection embryo no. 736, Harvard Medical School, 10.2 mm, section 138, borax carmine and Lyons blue stain, original magnification ×130.) (From Van Praagh R, Corsini I. Cor triatriatum: Pathologic anatomy and a consideration of morphogenesis based on 13 postmortem cases and a study of normal development of the pulmonary vein and atrial septum in 83 human embryos. *Am Heart J*. 1969;78:379, with permission.)

8.16). The right venous valve, that is, the Eustachian valve, is directly continuous with the right wall of the IVC.

The sinoatrial valve, at the junction of the sinus venosus with the RA, is the largest venous valve in the body (see Fig. 8.15). It is conventionally thought of as being incompetent; that is, it does not prevent regurgitation from the RA into the IVC or SVC.

It was during this study of human embryos that we came to understand an alternative view:

1. The left side of the sinoatrial valve is really bifid; it is composed of two leaflets—the septum primum to the left and the left venous valve to the right—that are confluent at their bases (see Figs. 8.13 and 8.16).[76] Both components of the left venous valve mechanism arise from the same platform of sinus venosus tissue (see Fig. 8.13).
2. Both components of the left venous valve mechanism grow upward (cephalad) (see Figs. 8.13 and 8.16), not downward (caudad), as is conventionally said (see Fig. 8.15). The erroneous view that the septum primum grows downward is due to misorientation of the heart in space. For example, Fig. 8.15 is easily mistaken for frontal plane views of the heart, in which the septum primum appears to grow downward. But in the embryo, the ventricles do not lie below the atria. Instead, the ventricles lie in front of (ventral to) the atria. As soon as one realizes that Fig. 8.15 is a diagrammatic *(horizontal)* plane reconstruction (not a frontal plane reconstruction), then one understands that the septum primum is really growing upward (not downward).
3. We realized that another important error in the conventional account of atrial septation is as follows. The septum primum does not grow down to close the ostium primum (see Fig. 8.15). Instead, the septum primum grows upward behind the ostium primum. The septum primum does not close the ostium primum. Instead, the ostium primum normally is closed by the endocardial cushions of the AV canal. Persistence of the ostium primum really is an endocardial cushion defect. An ostium primum defect is also correctly known as an incomplete form of common AV canal (or a partial AV septal defect).
4. The ostium secundum is the space above the upper edge of the upwardly growing septum primum (see Fig. 8.16A).[76] The ostium secundum is not formed by the timely coalescence of multiple small fenestrations within the septum primum. It should be added that there are small fenestrations within the septum primum, just as there are within other venous valves.
5. The septum primum really is a venous valve—the main component of the left venous valve apparatus. Understood in this way, the sinoatrial valve, the largest venous valve in the body, is not normally incompetent. This venous valve, because of the septum primum, is normally competent between the LA on the one hand and the RA and the venae cavae on the other.

Against the background of the previously mentioned improved understanding of the normal development of the pulmonary veins and the atrial septum, we are now ready to consider the pathologic anatomy of cor triatriatum sinistrum.

PATHOLOGIC ANATOMY

Based on our study of 13 postmortem cases of cor triatriatum sinistrum from three different medical centers that was published in 1969, the salient finds were as follows[76]:

Sex: Males = 12; females = 0; unknown, 1. The male-to-female ratio = 12:0. Thus, although this is a small series, the findings suggest that there may well be a strong male preponderance in cor triatriatum sinistrum.

Age at Death: In 12 cases (unknown in 1), mean 2.4 ± 5.8 years, ranging from 3 days to 20.8 years. The median age at death was 8.5 months.

Heart Sidedness: Left-sided in 12 of 13 cases (92%) and right-sided in 1 (8%)—a patient with secondary dextrocardia due to hypoplasia of the right lung (most marked of the right middle lobe).

Heart Size: Enlarged in all 13 cases (100%) (see Fig. 8.2A).

Right Atrium: Hypertrophied and enlarged in all (100%) (see Fig. 8.2B). The right atrial septal surface usually appeared abnormal. For example, in the case presented in Fig. 8.2, the right atrial septal surface is almost completely smooth, there being no limbic ledge formed by the septum secundum and virtually no demarcation between the septum primum and the septum secundum (see Fig. 8.2B). When obliquely probe patent, as in 8 of 13 cases (62%), the foramen ovale usually was distinctly smaller than normal, apparently because of the upward protrusion of the dor-

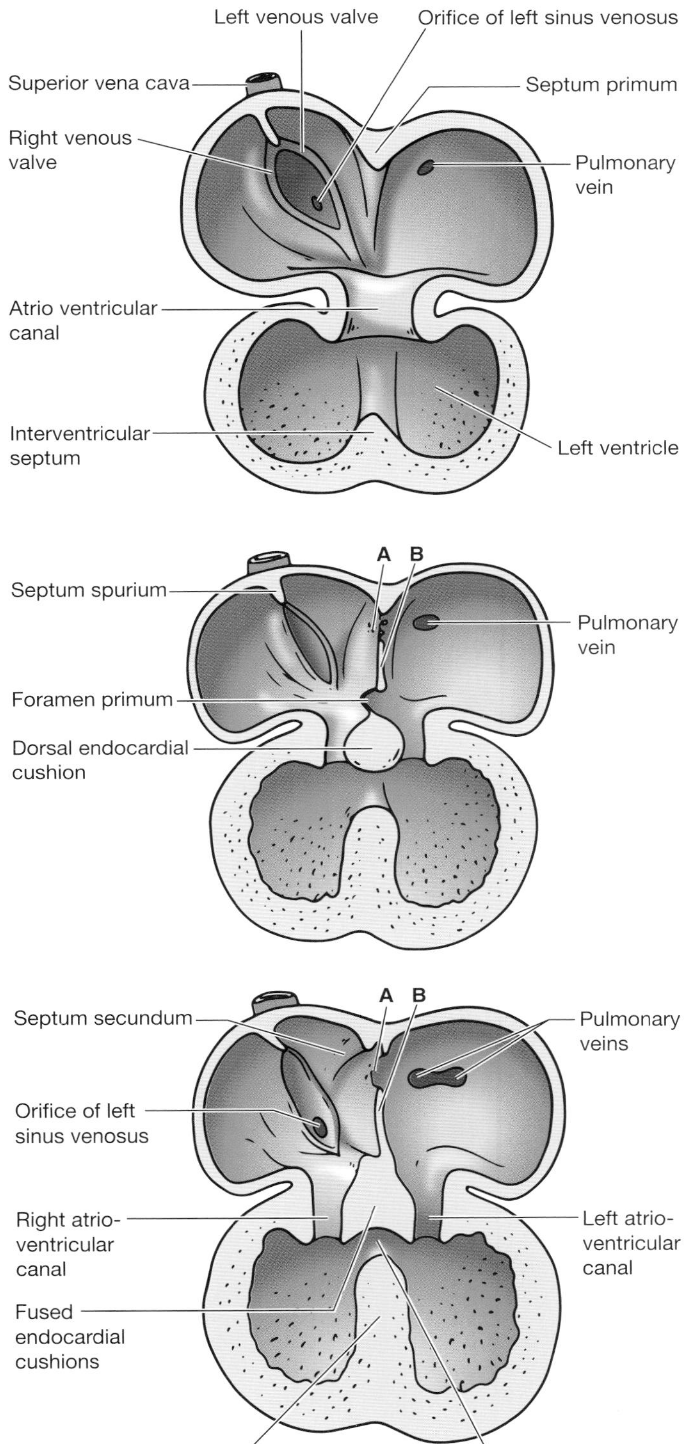

Fig. 8.15 Influential but Significantly Erroneous Conventional Diagrams of Atrial Septation and the Development of the Pulmonary Veins. Upper diagram, 5th week; middle diagram, 6th week; lower diagram, 8th week. Diagrams such as these typically are presented as coronal (frontal) sections of the embryonic heart. They show the atria to be located above the ventricles, as they are in the adult human heart. In the human embryo, however, the atria are behind (dorsal) relative to the ventricles, which are in front (ventral). The position of the normal embryonic, fetal, and neonatal heart is horizontal, not semivertical or vertical. These are schematic horizontal plane sections, not frontal plane sections. Once one understands this, then one understands that the septum primum grows upward (cephalad) not downward (caudad). This is the first important error in the conventional account of atrial septation. The *middle and lower panels* show degeneration (A) of the septum primum (B). Degeneration of the septum primum is said to lead to the formation of multiple small fenestrations that then become confluent, resulting in the formation of the ostium secundum. We think that multiple small fenestrations occur normally in the septum primum, as often also occurs in venous valves; but this is not how the ostium secundum forms. Instead, the ostium secundum is just the space above the anterosuperior margin of the upwardly growing septum primum. If the small fenestrations in the septum primum do not undergo normal obliteration, and if these fenestrations become confluent and hence significantly larger, the result is one type of ostium secundum atrial septal defect. This concept of the formation of the ostium secundum by the normal confluence of fenestrations in the septum primum is the second significant error in the conventional account of atrial septation. The third error in the usual account of atrial septation concerns the normal closure of the ostium primum (foramen primum, *middle panel*). The septum primum does not grow downward and obliterate the ostium primum by fusing with the endocardial cushions of the atrioventricular canal, as is often said. Instead, the endocardial cushions grow posterosuperiorly, thereby obliterating the ostium primum. Persistence of the ostium primum is an endocardial cushion defect, not

Fig. 8.15, cont'd a septum primum defect. The fourth error in conventional account concerning the development of the common pulmonary veins *(upper and middle panels)* is that the ostium of the common pulmonary vein is shown too far to the left, well to the left of the septum primum. Instead, as has been seen (see Figs. 8.13 and 8.14), the ostium of the common pulmonary vein is only slightly to the left of the septum primum, not well separated from it. As will be seen, we think that the almost superoinferior relationship between the septum primum and the common pulmonary vein in the 5th week of embryonic life, as in Figs. 8.13 and 8.14, is what makes cor triatriatum sinistrum possible. If the ostium of the common pulmonary vein were well to the left of the septum primum, as in the *upper and middle panels,* we think that typical cor triatriatum could not occur. These conventional diagrams also have many helpful and accurate features: the right venous valve; the left venous valve; the superior commissure of this sinoatrial valve is the septum spurium (the spurious or false septum, middle diagram); the inferior commissure of the right and left venous valves (the sinoatrial valve), which is the tendon of Todaro (unlabeled); the interseptovalvular space (unlabeled) between the septum primum to the left and the left venous valve to the right *(upper and middle panels);* the septum secundum lying to the right of the septum primum *(bottom panel);* beginning incorporation of the right and left pulmonary venous branches into the left atrium *(bottom panel);* and a ventricular septal defect of the atrioventricular canal type (*bottom panel,* labeled interventricular foramen) between the fused endocardial cushions posterosuperiorly and the crest of the muscular ventricular septum anteroinferiorly. (From Hamilton WJ, Mossman HW. *Hamilton, Boyd and Mossman's Human Embryology, Prenatal Development of Form and Function.* 4th ed. Baltimore, MD: Williams & Wilkins; 1972:246, Fig. 196, with permission.)

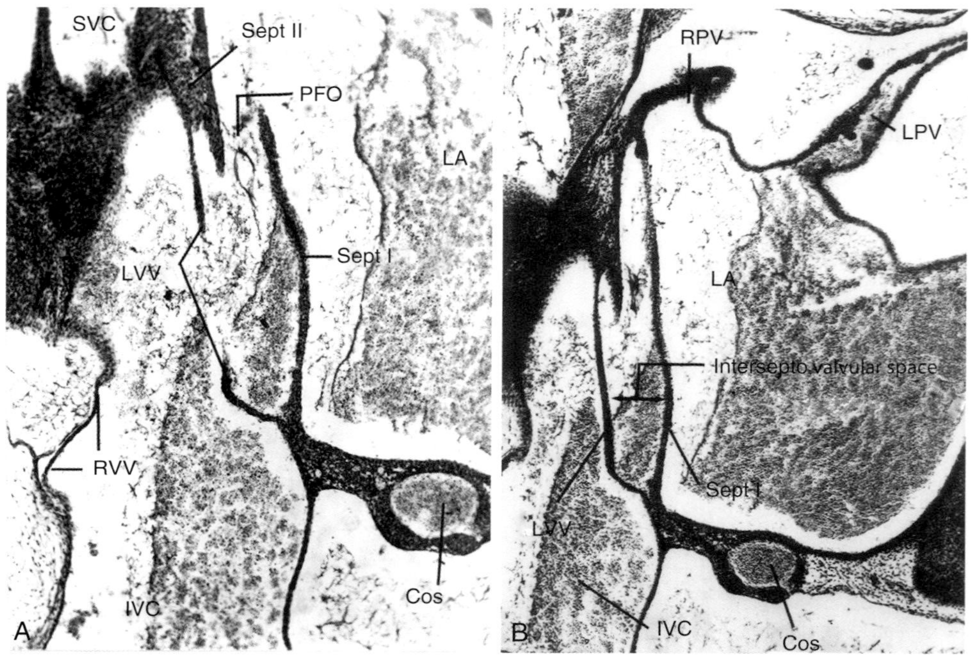

Fig. 8.16 Frontal Sections of the Venae Cavae, Atrial Septum, Coronary Sinus, and Pulmonary Veins in a 56-Day-Old Human Embryo. (A) Note the right-sided inferior vena cava *(IVC)* and superior vena cava *(SVC)*. By this age, the platform of sinus venosus tissue (see Figs. 8.13 and 14) has largely disappeared, leaving only its progeny—septum primum *(Sept I)* to the left and the left venous valve *(LVV)* to the right. Sept I and the LVV are both continuous with the left wall of the IVC. The right venous valve *(RVV)* is in direct continuity with the right wall of the IVC. Thus, Sept I, the LVV, and the RVV all appear to be derived from tissue of the right horn of the sinus venosus, whereas the coronary sinus *(CoS)* is derived from tissue of the left horn of the sinus venosus. In visceroarterial situs solitus, Sept I lies to the left of septum secundum *(Sept II)*. As is also evident in Fig. 8.12, in the prenatal circulation Sept I is the occluder of the interatrial valve and Sept II is the valve ring. The space directly above Sept I is the ostium secundum. The space between the superior rim of Sept I to the left and the inferior rim of the superior limbic band of Sept II to the right is the patent foramen ovale *(PFO)*. The section shown in B is 20 μ dorsal to that shown in A. (B) The LVV is better seen. The interoseptovalvular space lies between Sept I to the left and the LVV to the right. Postnatally, Sept I usually is much better developed than the LVV. Typically, the LVV is poorly developed and adherent to the right side of Sept I inferiorly, largely obliterating the interoseptovalvular space. Thus, the LVV mechanism of the sinoatrial valve, although embryonically bifid, usually consists postnatally of a well-developed Sept I and a rudimentary LVV. Why initially bifid? We think because both Sept I and the LVV begin by growing upward (cephalad) from the platform of sinus venosus tissue seen in Fig. 8.13, Sept I from the left side and the LVV from the right side of this platform of right horn sinus venosus tissue. By 56 days of age, both branches of the common pulmonary vein are incorporated or absorbed into the dorsal wall of the left atrium *(LA)*, creating the appearance that there are now two pulmonary veins, the right pulmonary vein *(RPV)* and the left pulmonary vein *(LPV)*. (Minot Collection, Harvard Medical School, embryo no. 914, 29 mm, section no. 490 in A and 491 in B borax carmine and Lyons blue stain, original magnification ×100.) (From Van Praagh R, Corsini I. Cor triatriatum: Pathologic anatomy and a consideration of morphogenesis based on 13 postmortem cases and a study of normal development of the pulmonary vein and atrial septum in 83 human embryos. *Am Heart J.* 1969;78:379, with permission.)

sal common pulmonary vein chamber (see Fig. 8.2D). By bulging upward, the common pulmonary vein chamber encroached on the foramen ovale from below and behind, tending to narrow or close it.

Atrial Septum: Intact, 4 (30.8%); patent foramen ovale, 8 (61.5%); and secundum atrial septal defect (ASD), 1 (7.7%).

Tricuspid Valve: Enlarged, 11 (84.6%); normal, 1 (7.7%); and tricuspid atresia, 1 (7.7%). The tricuspid valve was usually enlarged because of associated right ventricular hypertrophy and enlargement. In the 1 patient in whom the tricuspid valve was found to be normal in size (compared with normal controls), the right ventricle (RV) was thick-walled and small-chambered (and the right ventricular outflow tract and pulmonary valve were enlarged).

Ventricular Septum: Intact, 10 (76.9%); and ventricular septal defect (VSD), 3 (23.1%).

Right Ventricle: Right ventricular hypertrophy and enlargement, 11 cases (84.6%); hypoplastic, 1 (7.7%); and thick-walled and small-chambered, 1 (7.7%).

Pulmonary Valve: Enlarged, 10 (76.9%); and hypoplastic, 3 (23.1%).

Mitral Valve: Hypoplastic, 6 (46.1%); normal, 5 (38.5%); enlarged, 1 (7.7%); and absent, 1 (7.7%).

Left Ventricle: Hypoplastic, 5 (38.5%); normal, 5 (38.5%); enlarged, 2 (15.3%); and absent, 1 (7.7%).

Aortic Valve: Hypoplastic, 5 (38.5%); normal, 6 (46.1%); enlarged, 1 (7.7%); and aortic atresia, 1 (7.7%).

THE ANOMALY

The opened left heart chambers (see Figs. 8.1 and 8.2C–D) showed the following[76]:

1. **The common pulmonary vein chamber** was stenotic, dilated, and hypertrophied. It was dorsal (posterior) to, and obliquely inferior to the ventral (anterior) left atrial chamber.
2. **The fibromuscular diaphragm** was oriented obliquely from posterosuperiorly to anteroinferiorly (see Figs. 8.1 and 8.2C–D).
3. **The number of openings** in the subdividing diaphragm were: 1 in 9 cases (69.2%); 2 in 3 patients (23.1%); and none in 1 (7.7%).
4. **The size of the openings** in the diaphragm (mm in diameter): 0 mm, 1 case (1/16 = 6.25%); 0.5 mm, 2 cases (12.5%); 1 mm, 4 cases (25%); 2 mm, 3 cases (18.75%); 3 mm, 5 cases (31.25%); and 5 mm, 1 case (6.25%). The mean diameter of the opening(s) in the intra-atrial diaphragm was 1.9 ± 1.3 mm, ranging from 0 to 5 mm. The median diameter of the opening was 2.0 mm.
5. **The location of the opening** in the intra-atrial diaphragm was a short distance behind the posteromedial commissure of the mitral valve (see Figs. 8.1 and 8.2C–D). In other words, the location of the opening in the subdividing diaphragm was very inferior and very medial within the LA, that is, extremely close to the initial location of the common pulmonary vein in the early human embryo at 33 days of age (see Figs. 8.9 and 8.13), before the normal incorporation of the common pulmonary vein into the LA.

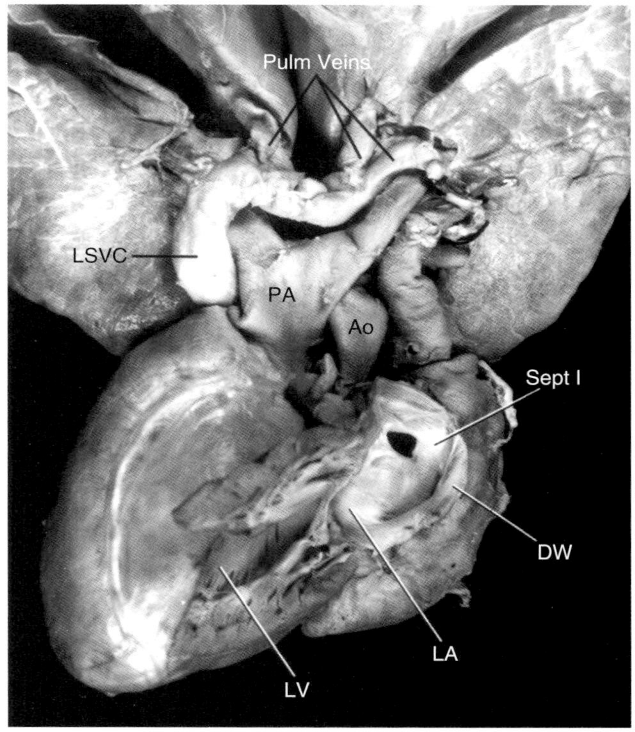

Fig. 8.17 What Does the Left Atrium *(LA)* Look Like When There Is No Common Pulmonary Vein (CPV) Component? The answer is provided by totally anomalous pulmonary venous connection (TAPVC), with this patient having a supracardiac "snowman" type of TAPVC. The septum primum *(Sept I)* is continuous with the dorsal wall *(DW)* of this small LA—small because it lacks its normal CPV component. Comparison of Sept I and the DW of this small LA with the ventral appearance of the subdividing diaphragm in typical cor triatriatum (see Fig. 8.4) reveals that both appear exceedingly similar, if not identical. These observations suggest that the subdividing diaphragm in typical cor triatriatum consists of the septum primum, DW of the LA ventrally, and the wall of the CPV dorsally. This was our hypothesis, based on gross observations, before histologic examination. *Ao,* Aorta; *LSVC,* left superior vena cava; *LV,* left ventricle. (From Van Praagh R, Corsini I. Cor triatriatum: Pathologic anatomy and a consideration of morphogenesis based on 13 postmortem cases and a study of normal development of the pulmonary vein and atrial septum in 83 human embryos. *Am Heart J.* 1969;78:379, with permission.)

6. **The septum primum was always in direct fibrous continuity with the subdividing intra-atrial diaphragm** (see Fig. 8.4). It is illuminating to note that the continuity between septum primum and the diaphragm in cor triatriatum (see Fig. 8.4) appears essentially identical to the continuity between septum primum and the dorsal wall of the LA in totally anomalous pulmonary venous connection (TAPVC) (Fig. 8.17).[76] It should be understood that the LA in TAPVC is the normal LA, minus its pulmonary venous component.

   These observations (compare Figs. 8.4 and 8.17) strongly suggest that the subdividing diaphragm in cor triatriatum is composed of the wall of the LA ventrally and the wall of the unincorporated stenotic common pulmonary vein dorsally (see Fig. 8.1 and 8.2D).
7. **Serial sections of the subdividing diaphragm** in cor triatriatum (Fig. 8.18)[76] support this interpretation. Superiorly and

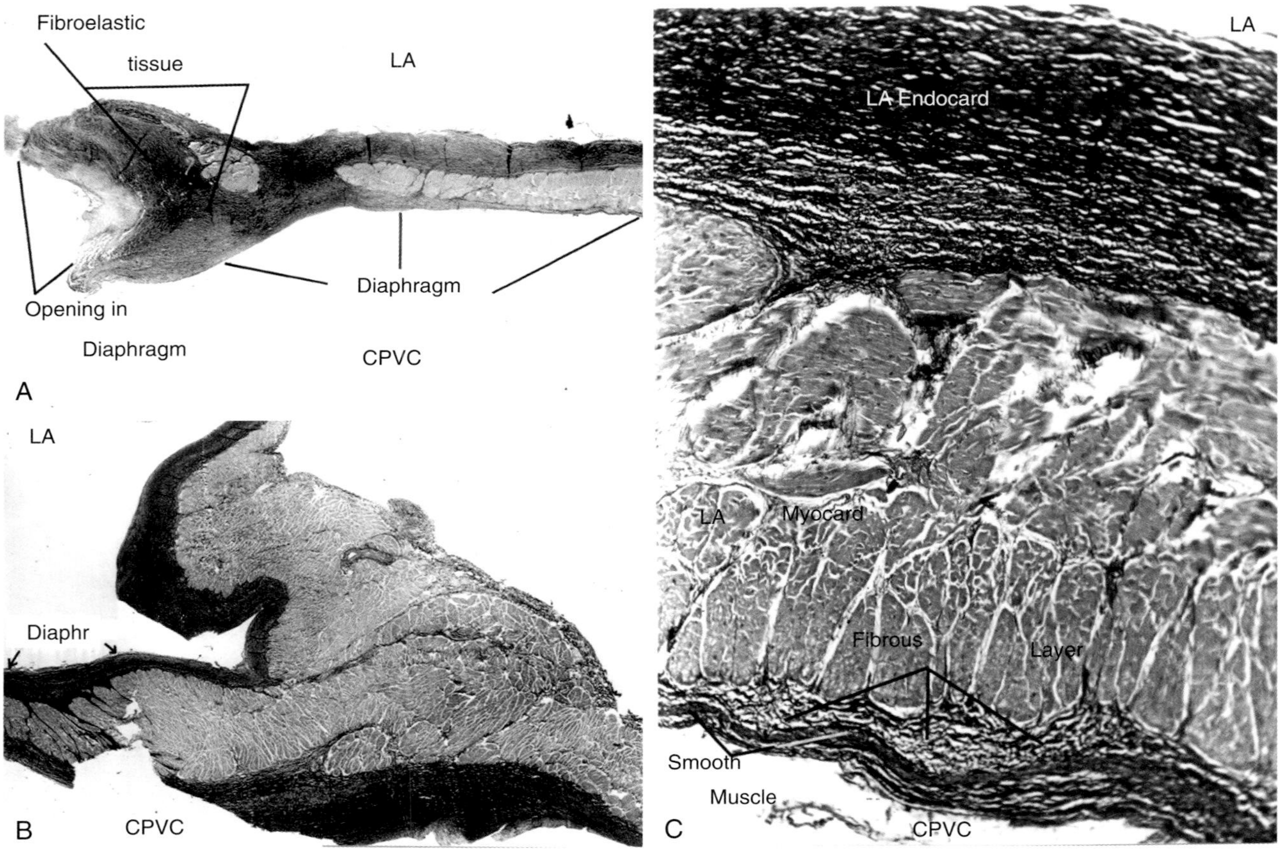

Fig. 8.18 **Histology of the Subdividing Diaphragm, Shown Grossly in Fig. 8.2C.** (A) The most anteroinferior part of the diaphragm, including the opening in the diaphragm leading into the proximal left atrium *(LA)* with the left atrial appendage, this opening being located immediately behind the posteromedial commissure of the mitral valve. Note the prominent mass of fibroelastic tissue posterosuperior to the stenotic opening in the diaphragm. For orientation, note that the obstructed common pulmonary vein chamber *(CPVC)* is inferior and posterior to the diaphragm, whereas the proximal LA is superior and anterior to the diaphragm. Histologic image of the subdividing diaphragm *(Diaphr)* at its junction with the proximal left atrial free wall (same patient as in A). (C) Higher power view of the subdividing diaphragm of the same patient, between A and B, to show greater detail. Note the thick left atrial endocardium *(LA Endocard)*, which is characteristic of the LA. The subjacent prominent layer of left atrial myocardium *(LA Myocard)* consists of striated myocardium. Beneath that is a layer of fibrous tissue *(Fibrous Layer)* that represents the left atrial epicardium and/or the adventitia of the stenotic common pulmonary vein *(CPVC)*. A prominent layer of smooth (nonstriated) muscle lies beneath the fibrous tissue layer, the smooth muscle representing the hypertrophied media of the obstructed common pulmonary vein. Most inferiorly is a layer of thickened pulmonary venous endocardium. (Verhoeff-van Gieson stain; original magnification in A and B ×12, and in C ×100.) (From Van Praagh R, Corsini I. Cor triatriatum: Pathologic anatomy and a consideration of morphogenesis based on 13 postmortem cases and a study of normal development of the pulmonary vein and atrial septum in 83 human embryos. *Am Heart J.* 1969;78:379, with permission.)

ventrally, the composition of the diaphragm is that of the left atrial free wall. Adjacent to the cavity of the ventral LA is a characteristically thick layer of left atrial endocardium. External or dorsal to this lies a prominent but discontinuous layer of striated left atrial posterior free wall myocardium. Dorsal to this there is a layer of fibrous tissue corresponding to the left atrial epicardium and the tightly apposed adventitia of the common pulmonary vein. External to this there is considerable smooth (nonstriated) muscle that occasionally forms a discrete layer (see Fig. 8.18C). This nonstriated muscle is interpreted as the hypertrophied media of the stenotic common pulmonary vein. Dorsal and inferior to that lies a layer of thickened endothelium of the common pulmonary vein chamber.

To summarize, the histologic structure of the subdividing diaphragm is bilaminar, consisting of striated and smooth muscle, supporting the concept that the diaphragm is composed of at least two structures: the dorsal left atrial free wall and the tightly opposed wall of the unincorporated common pulmonary vein.

8. **The septum primum** is a third component of the subdividing diaphragm (see Fig. 8.3A). In order to examine this aspect in greater detail, a frontal plane section was taken through the RA, atrial septum, ventral LA above, and dorsal common pulmonary vein chamber below (see Fig. 8.6A–B).[76] This biatrial (or "triatrial") frontal plane section was also examined histologically (see Fig. 8.6C). These data confirm that

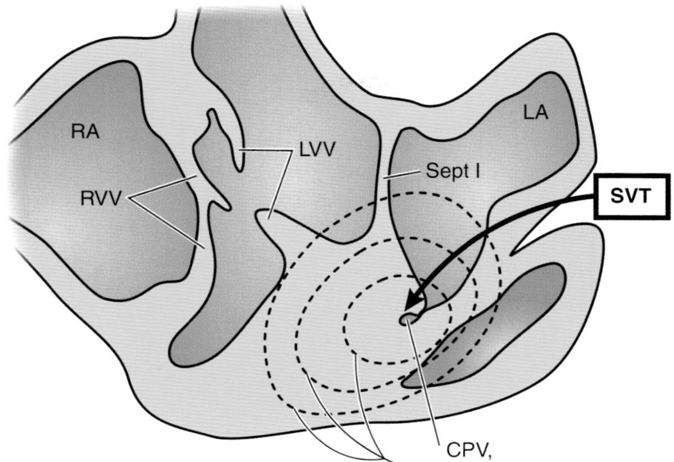

Fig. 8.19 Diagrammatic Presentation of the Pulmonary Venous Entrapment Hypothesis of the Morphogenesis of Cor Triatriatum Sinistrum. The tracing of the frontal section of the atria is very similar to that shown in Fig. 8.13B (see Fig. 8.8B in the original paper). The essential difference is that the common pulmonary vein *(CPV)* is separated from the cavity of the left atrium *(LA)* by sinus venosus tissue beneath the septum primum *(Sept I)*. It will be recalled that at this stage (33 days of age, see Fig. 8.13), before incorporation of the CPV into the dorsal part of the LA, the CPV is located as inferiorly and as medially as possible within the LA. The CPV runs just to the left of the base of an overhanging mass of sinus venosus tissue *(SVT)* (see Fig. 8.13). The hypothesis is that abnormally, the ostium of the pulmonary vein can become entrapped by this SVT, separating the CPV from the cavity of the LA. The sequelae of this entrapment are hypothesized to be as follows. The ostium of the CPV remains small or can even be obliterated by this fibrous tissue (seen histologically in Fig. 8.18A), resulting in stenosis or atresia of the ostium of the CPV. Entrapment of the ostium of the CPV prevents its incorporation into the LA, and hence the CPV remains abnormally discrete (unincorporated). Because the ostium of the CPV typically remains small, incorporation into the LA being prevented by entrapment, as the embryo and later the fetus grows, the CPV becomes progressively more obstructed, causing the CPV to dilate and become hypertrophied. Distention of the progressively more obstructed CPV causes it to impinge on the septum primum from below *(dotted circles)*. Consequently, Sept I becomes confluent with the subdividing diaphragm. In cor triatriatum, does the CPV develop abnormally far to the right, within the SVT, resulting in entrapment of the CPV? Our data do not permit us to answer this question with confidence. However, this is not our impression. The ostium of the stenotic and unincorporated CPV opens into the proximal portion of the left atrium, above the posteromedial commissure of the mitral valve, not in the plane of the atrium septum and not into the tissue of the atrial septum. Why apparent entrapment and unincorporation of the CPV occur, resulting in cor triatriatum, remains unknown. *LVV*, Left venous valve; *RA*, right atrium; and *RVV*, right venous valve. (From Van Praagh R, Corsini I. Cor triatriatum: Pathologic anatomy and a consideration of morphogenesis based on 13 postmortem cases and a study of normal development of the pulmonary vein and atrial septum in 83 human embryos. *Am Heart J.* 1969;78:379, with permission.)

the septum primum forms part of the "roof" of the common pulmonary vein chamber and part of the "floor" of the LA (Fig. 8.6A–C).[76]

9. **A prominent mass of fibroelastic tissue typically surrounds the stenotic ostium of the common pulmonary vein** (see Fig. 8.18A). We found ourselves wondering, what is all that fibroelastic tissue doing around the ostium of the common pulmonary vein? Where does the fibroelastic tissue come from? Could this mass of fibroelastic tissue around the ostium of the common pulmonary vein be causing stenosis of this vein? Could this mass of fibroelastic tissue around the pulmonary venous ostium have prevented incorporation of the common pulmonary vein into the LA?

Pulmonary Vein Entrapment Hypothesis

Correlation of the previously mentioned pathologic anatomic findings in cor triatriatum sinistrum with the data concerning the normal development of the pulmonary vein and the atrial septum in humans led to the pulmonary vein entrapment hypothesis (Fig. 8.19).[76] The frontal plane section of the embryonic heart at 33 days of age shown in this tracing is the same as that presented in Fig. 8.13B, with one exception. The overhanging mass of fibroelastic sinus venosus tissue beneath which, and just to the left of which, the common pulmonary vein normally runs (see Fig. 8.13B) is here shown as having fused with the immediately adjacent left atrial free wall (see Fig. 8.19). Consequently, the space that normally remains open above and to the left of the common pulmonary vein has been closed by fibrous tissue. Our hypothesis is that this is the fibrous tissue, from which the septum primum develops, that entraps the ostium of the common pulmonary vein, typically resulting in stenosis of the common pulmonary vein and preventing normal incorporation of the common pulmonary vein into the LA.

TABLE 8.1 **Associated Anomalies in 13 Cases of Cor Triatriatum Sinistrum**[76]

Case No.	Associated Anomalies
1	Partially anomalous pulmonary venous connection: left upper lobe pulmonary vein to left vertical vein to left innominate vein to right superior vena cava to right atrium
2	Tetralogy of Fallot with patent ductus arteriosus (5 mm in diameter), left superior vena cava to coronary sinus to right atrium, aberrant right subclavian artery, hypoplasia of right middle lobe of lung with secondary dextrocardia, partially anomalous pulmonary venous connection from right middle lobe to inferior vena cava, anomalous pulmonary arterial blood supply from descending thoracic aorta to right middle lobe, displacement of left atrial appendage to right and posteriorly, intra-aortic band beneath ostium or right common carotid artery, brain abscess (large, left parietal, pseudomonas)
3	Bicuspid aortic valve due to deficient intercoronary commissure
4	None
5	Coarctation of the aorta (moderate), atresia of right atrial ostium of coronary sinus, partially anomalous pulmonary venous connection between the left lower lobe pulmonary vein and coronary sinus, conoventricular type of ventricular septal defect (1 mm)
6	None
7	Patent ductus arteriosus (3 mm)
8	Tricuspid atresia with patent foramen ovale (8 × 5 mm), conoventricular ventricular septal defect (10 × 3 mm), moderate infundibular and valvar pulmonary stenosis with bicuspid pulmonary valve, intra-aortic band from ostium of innominate artery to ostium of left subclavian artery (persistent 5th aortic arch)[129]
9	Azygos lobe of right lung, two accessory splenuli
10	Patent ductus arteriosus (3 mm in diameter), malrotation of colon with cecum beneath gallbladder
11	No opening in intra-atrial diaphragm due to atresia of ostium of common pulmonary vein, extreme hypoplasia of left atrium, absence of mitral valve and left ventricle (single right ventricle), aortic valvar atresia, patent ductus arteriosus, aberrant right subclavian artery, persistent left superior vena cava to coronary sinus to right atrium, small accessory (third) coronary artery from proximal left pulmonary artery; intersex male with abdominal testes, short blindly ending vagina, and questionably chromatin-positive buccal smear (multiple congenital anomalies)
12	None
13	Transposition of the great arteries {S,D,D} with patent ductus arteriosus, high right coronary ostium (1 mm above sinus of Valsalva), and prominent valve of inferior vena cava

Conclusions. We ended up thinking that both of the main contending morphogenetic hypotheses contained elements of truth. The septum primum was indeed involved, as Fowler[3] had suggested in 1881. Obstruction of the common pulmonary vein appeared clearly to be present, as concluded by Griffith[6,8] in 1896 and 1903 and by Martin[7] in 1899. We thought that our study revealed a plausible mechanism that united all of the salient anatomic findings in cor triatriatum sinistrum:

1. why the common pulmonary vein typically is stenotic,
2. why the septum primum is confluent with subdividing intra-atrial diaphragm within the LA,
3. why the gross and histologic structure of the intra-atrial diaphragm is bilaminar, and
4. why the stenotic ostium of the common pulmonary vein in cor triatriatum sinistrum is located immediately behind the posteromedial commissure of the mitral valve.

Our embryologic study,[76] which was necessary to understand the morphogenesis of cor triatriatum sinistrum, also yielded surprising new information concerning the development of the atrial septum and the pulmonary vein:

1. The septum primum grows upward, not downward.
2. The septum primum and the left venous valve are both parts of a bifid left venous valve apparatus.
3. The septum primum does not grow downward and close ostium primum.
4. The starting position of the common pulmonary vein is very inferior and medial; that is, the common pulmonary vein does not begin well to the left of septum primum and relatively high up within the LA.

Associated Malformations

Associated anomalies were frequent in these 13 cases of cor triatriatum sinistrum (Table 8.1). Of these 13 cases of cor triatriatum sinistrum, 5 (38%) had clinical important associated cardiovascular anomalies (see Table 8.1: Cases 2, 5, 8, 11, and 13).

Of the 8 patients (62%) with relatively minor or no associated cardiovascular malformations, only 3 (23%) had no associated cardiovascular anomalies. In other words, 10 of these 13 patients with cor triatriatum sinistrum did have associated cardiac malformations (77%). Those patients that we regarded as having relatively minor associated cardiovascular disease were Cases 1, 2, 7, 9, and 10 (see Table 8.1).

Two of these patients with cor triatriatum and associated cardiovascular anomalies merit additional comment (see Cases 2 and 13 and Table 8.1).

Tetralogy of Fallot (TOF) with highly obstructive cor triatriatum sinistrum was found in a 20 10/12-year-old young man who died of a large left parietal lobe brain abscess caused by pseudomonas. In addition, this rare patient had the infrequent *right-sided juxtaposition of the atrial appendages,* the left atrial appendage being displaced posteriorly and to the right (see Table 8.1). In addition to a persistent LSVC to the coronary sinus and thence to the RA and an aberrant right subclavian

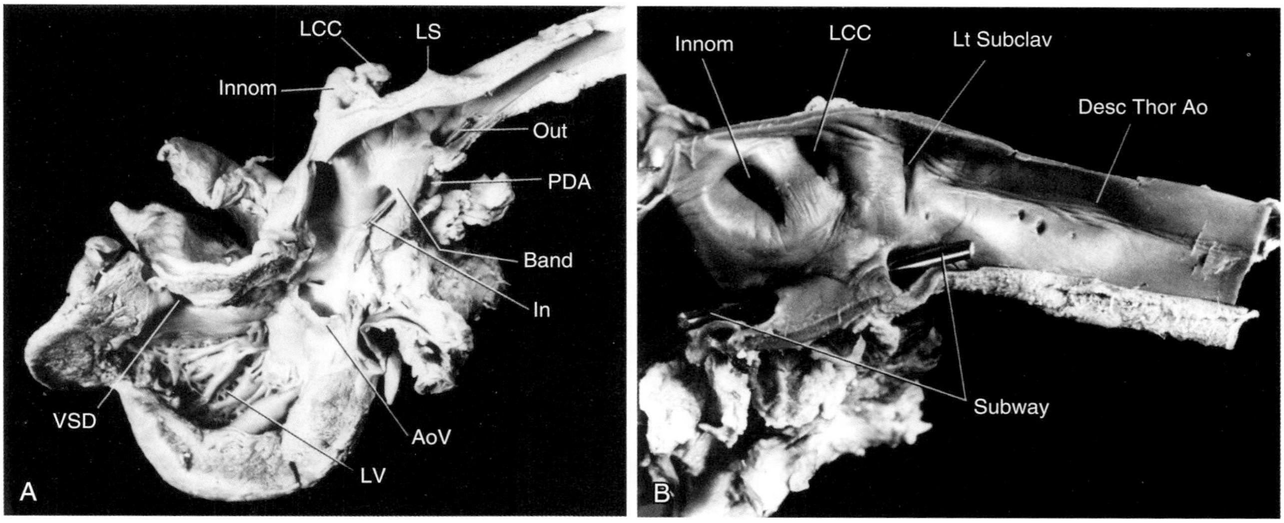

Fig. 8.20 The First Known Case of Persistent 5th Aortic Arch. (A) Opened left ventricle *(LV),* aortic valve *(AoV),* and aorta. The persistent 5th aortic arch forms a sizeable subaortic subway, containing a probe. A band, 9 mm in length, separates the normal aortic arch (4th arch) superiorly from the persistent 5th aortic arch inferiorly (probe), forming a left-sided congenital double-lumen aortic arch. The persistent 5th aortic arch begins beneath the origin of the innominate artery *(Innom),* the inlet into the 5th arch being indicated by *In.* The outlet of the 5th aortic arch is located beneath the ostium of the left subclavian artery *(LS).* The outlet of the 5th aortic arch *(Out)* is located beneath the termination of the left 4th aortic arch (the superior channel) and the outlet is just proximal to the small left patent ductus arteriosus *(PDA),* which represents the left 6th aortic arch. (B) Close-up of the interior of the aortic arch to document the relations between the beginning and end of the persistent 5th arterial arch and the brachiocephalic arteries, the beginning opposite the innominate artery *(Innom)* and the end opposite the left subclavian artery *(Lt Subclav).* The 5th arch forms a subaortic subway. *Desc Thor Ao,* Descending thoracic aorta; *LCC,* left common carotid artery; *VSD,* ventricular septal defect. (From Van Praagh R, Van Praagh S. Persistent fifth arterial arch in man, congenital double-lumen aortic arch. *Am J Cardiol.* 1969;24:279, with permission.)

artery, this patient also had a rare *partial form of the scimitar syndrome.* There was partially anomalous pulmonary venous connection (PAPVC) from the right middle lobe to the IVC; anomalous pulmonary arterial blood supply from the descending thoracic aorta to the right middle lobe of the lung; and secondary dextrocardia related to hypoplasia of the right lung, most marked of the right middle lobe.

An *intra-aortic band* beneath the ostium of the right common carotid artery is another rare and developmentally poorly understood anomaly in this patient and is of no apparent clinical significance.

This patient presented a rare constellation of anomalies: TOF with very severe pulmonary venous stenosis (cor triatriatum sinistrum), with a patent ductus arteriosus (PDA), PAPVC, and anomalous systemic arterial blood supply to the right middle lobe (see Fig. 8.7). No clinical or hemodynamic information is available to us concerning this patient who was studied in Dr. Maurice Lev's laboratory at the Congenital Heart Disease Research and Training Center, Hektoen Institute for Medical Research, Chicago, Illinois. But just consider this patient's pulmonary blood flow and the related multiple different conflicting factors.

When TOF has good congenital (or acquired) reasons for pulmonary hypertension, as in this patient, the diagnosis of TOF may well be masked. In the face of pulmonary hypertension, there may be little or no pulmonary outflow tract gradient on catheter pull back from the main pulmonary artery into the RV or as assessed by noninvasive imaging. Hence, the diagnosis of TOF may be missed and the patient may not receive appropriate surgical therapy.[76]

In this patient, the pulmonary artery was of approximately normal size (see Fig. 8.7A); consequently this heart did not look like TOF on external examination.

However, on opening this massively hypertrophied RV (see Fig. 8.7B), considerable anterosuperior deviation of the conal septum, which is typical of TOF, is seen. The pulmonary valve was tricuspid and only mildly smaller than normal.

The pulmonary veins connected with a common pulmonary vein chamber (see Fig. 8.7C) that had only two pin-hole outlets: (1) into the RA via a 1-mm opening that did not have the morphology of a patent foramen ovale (see Fig. 8.7D) and (2) into the ventral compartment of the LA via a 1-mm defect.

We think that reports of the foramen ovale opening into the dorsal common pulmonary vein chamber are misinterpretations. Instead, we think that there are abnormal communications between the common pulmonary vein chamber and the RA (not the patent foramen ovale opening into the pulmonary vein). Rather, the pulmonary veins can communicate with the systemic veins at many different sites, both extracardiac and cardiac. The medial compartment of the RA—to the left of the right venous valve (see Fig. 8.15)—is the compartment to which the right horn of the sinus venosus connects. Thus, communications between the common pulmonary vein chamber and the RA are thought to be anomalous pulmonary vein–to–sinus venosus (systemic venous component of RA) communications (see Fig. 8.7D).

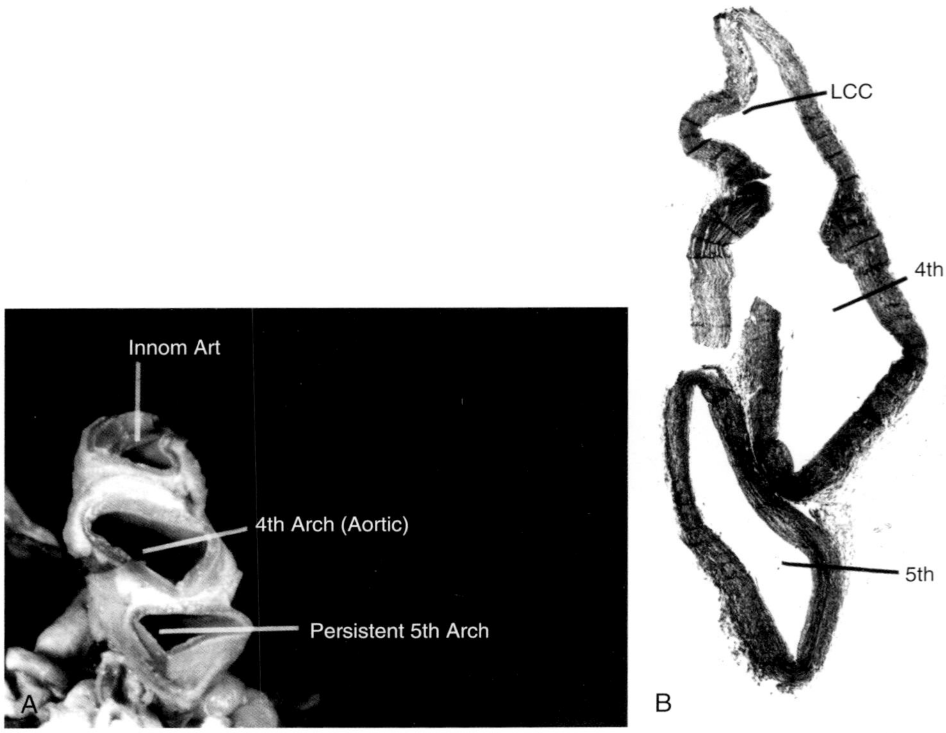

Fig. 8.21 Cross Section of Double-Lumen Aortic Arch. (A) Gross photograph, close-up, view from distal or downstream perspective, looking proximally or upstream. Note that the superior or 4th aortic arch appears completely separate from the inferior or 5th aortic arch. (B) Photomicrograph, Verhoeff-van Gieson stain, original magnification ×10. The aortic arch (4th) was opened at autopsy. The walls of both aortic arches (4th and 5th) appear structurally normal, with intervening adventitia and no evidence of aortic dissection or other acquired disease. The 5th arch is almost as big as the 4th arch, their circumferences being 12 and 16 mm, respectively. This patient, of unknown age and sex, also had tricuspid atresia; cor triatriatum sinistrum with one small opening, 3 mm in diameter, in the subdividing left atrial diaphragm; large patent foramen ovale, 8 × 5 mm, that opened into the ventral left atrial chamber; ventricular septal defect, high 10 × 3 mm; moderate pulmonary stenosis, infundibular and valvar, with bicuspid pulmonary valve; minimally patent ductus arteriosus, 1 mm in diameter. This persistent 5th aortic arch appears to have been entirely asymptomatic and of no clinical importance. Knowledge of the existence of this anomaly should prevent the potential misdiagnosis of aortic arch dissection, which could lead erroneously to unnecessary surgery. *LCC,* Left common carotid artery. (From Van Praagh R, Van Praagh S. Persistent fifth arterial arch in man, congenital double-lumen aortic arch. *Am J Cardiol.* 1969;24:279, with permission.)

In conclusion, this communication between the pulmonary vein chamber and the RA did not have the morphologic anatomic appearance of a normal patent foramen ovale; nor did this pin-hole defect look like a sinus venosus defect (of the right atrial type) (see Fig. 8.7D). Consequently, we regard this type of communication as an abnormal defect, distinct from the two previously mentioned types of communication.

Transposition of the great arteries (TGA) {S,D,D} with cor triatriatum sinistrum (see Case 13, Table 8.1) is another rare association of congenital heart diseases (see Fig. 8.5). Indeed, this 3-month-old boy was the first known case of this association.[76] When cor triatriatum sinistrum is present, typically there is marked *right* ventricular hypertrophy and enlargement (see Fig. 8.2A–B). However, when D-TGA coexists, as in this patient, marked *left* ventricular hypertrophy and enlargement are found (see Fig. 8.5A) because the obstructed pulmonary artery arises from the left ventricle (LV). A PDA is also seen. The common pulmonary vein chamber is shown from above (see Fig. 8.5B), and two openings in the intra-atrial subdividing diaphragm (3 and 0.5 mm in diameter) are seen from below (see Fig. 8.5C).

Persistent fifth aortic arch[129] was first discovered in Case 8, a patient who also had tricuspid atresia and cor triatriatum (see Figs. 8.20 and 8.21).[76] The persistent fifth aortic arch resembled a "subway" beneath the normal (fourth) aortic arch. The "subway" began beneath the ostium of the innominate artery and terminated just proximal to the ligamentum arteriosum (sixth arch)[76] (Fig. 8.22)

The foregoing is a summary of the most important lessons learned concerning cor triatriatum sinistrum in the study by Van Praagh and Corsini (1969).[76] Now let us turn to the present series, reviewed 35 years later, to see what else we have learned.

PRESENT SERIES

The present series consists of 11 postmortem cases and includes the 4 Boston Children's Hospital Medical Center (CHMC) cases that were published in 1969[76] and 1 patient that was published

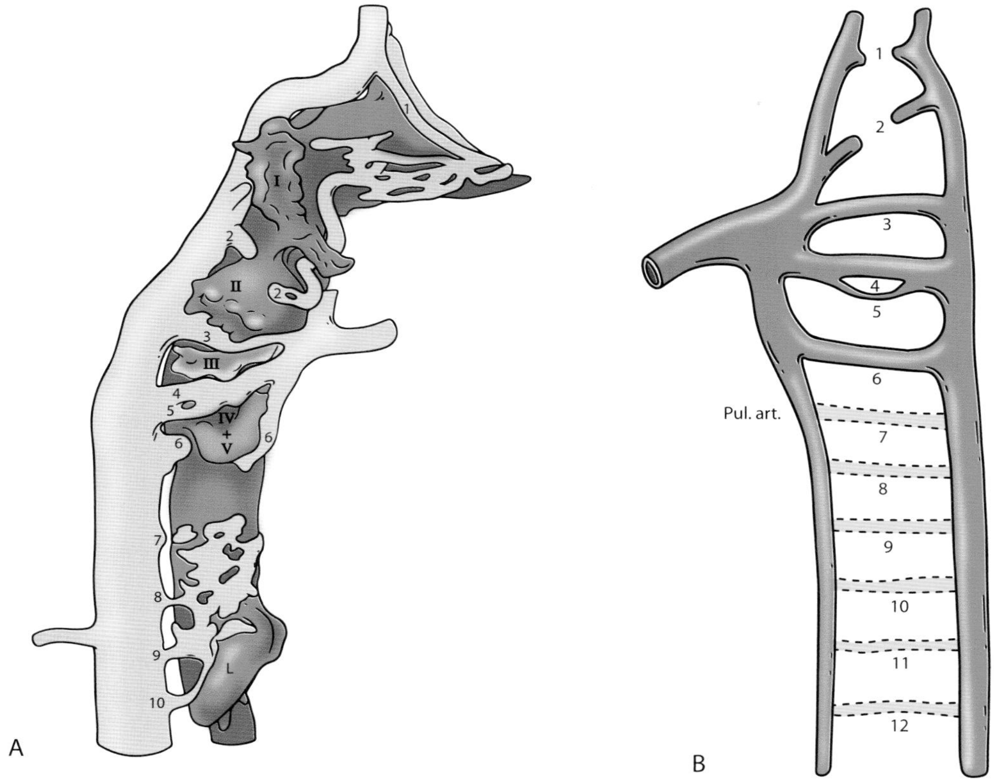

Fig. 8.22 Embryology of the 5th Aortic Arches. (A) 4-mm cat embryo, reconstruction of the right side (original magnification ×100). Aortic (arterial) arches are shown in Arabic numerals, pharyngeal pouches in Roman numerals. Most of the aortic arches pass above (cephalad to) their pharyngeal pouches: aortic arch 1 above pharyngeal pouch I, aortic arch 2 above pharyngeal pouch II, and aortic arch 3 above pharyngeal pouch III. In this embryo, aortic arches 1 and 2 are involuting and hence are no longer complete, whereas aortic arch 3 is complete. Pharyngeal pouches IV and V are fused together (IV + V), rather than separated; so too are aortic arches 4 and 5. Aortic arch 5 cannot pass above pharyngeal pouch V and below pharyngeal pouch IV because both of these pharyngeal pouches are telescoped together, with no separating groove between them. Aortic arches 3, 4, and 5 are complete. Fused pharyngeal pouches IV and V are known as the **ultimobranchial body**, that is, the last branchial body. (*Branchia* in Greek means gills. The gills of fish and other lower vertebrates are represented in mammalian embryos by the pharyngeal [or branchial] arches [or pouches], separated by clefts.) Fused pharyngeal pouches IV and V are also known as the **posterior (caudal) pharyngeal complex**, meaning that they are the last of the pharyngeal pouches. The right 6th aortic arch, that is, the right ductus arteriosus, is not completely formed, although ventral and dorsal evaginations are approaching each other, preparatory to anastomosis, thereby forming a complete right 6th arch. The 6th arches are the first postbranchial aortic arches. The right lung is labeled *L*. The intersegmental arteries 7, 8, 9, and 10 are developing. Intersegmental arteries 9 and 10 are the first blood supply to the lungs; that is, they constitute the primary pulmonary circulation, before the normal, definitive, but secondary pulmonary circulation (the pulmonary artery branches) reaches the lungs. The primary pulmonary circulation from the intersegmental arteries may persist abnormally and become important as major aortopulmonary collateral arteries (MAPCAs), particularly when there is atresia of the normal (but secondary, i.e., later developing) pulmonary arterial system. (B) Diagram of the aortic arches of the cat embryo, left side. Aortic arch 6, that is, the left ductus arteriosus, is now completely formed. The left 5th arch is becoming smaller, preparatory to its usual involution. The left pulmonary artery *(Pul. art.)* is now relatively long, extending down to the lung buds (different from A). Fig. 8.22B is almost a diagram of the persistent 5th aortic arch seen in our patient (see Figs. 8.20 and 8.21). (From Huntington GS. The morphology of the pulmonary artery in the Mammalia. *Anat Rec.* 1919-1920;17:165, with permission.)

in 1996 concerning left-sided juxtaposition of the atrial appendages due to levomalposition of the right atrial appendage (Case 1).[77] Hence, 6 new cases of cor triatriatum sinistrum are being reported in this series of 11 patients.

Incidence: 11 of 3216 autopsied cases of congenital heart disease (0.34%).

Sex: Males-to-females = 9/2 (4.5:1). One of the males was a male pseudohermaphrodite with abdominal testes, a short blind-ending vagina, and a questionably chromatin-positive buccal smear. Thus, those patients with an unequivocal sex diagnosis were males-to-females = 8/2 (4:1).

Age at Death: Mean 2.38 ± 2.61 years, ranging from 3 days to 6.5 years. The median age at death was 11 months.

Heart Position: Levocardia, 10 of 11 (90.9%); mesocardia, 1 of 11 (9.1%); and other, 0.

Segmental Anatomy: {S,D,S} = 9 of 11 (81.8%); and TGA {S,D,D} = 2 of 11 (18.2%).

Systemic Veins: Normal in 6 of 11 (55%); LSVC to coronary sinus to RA in 4 (36%); and atretic right SVC (RSVC) with LSVC to coronary sinus and coronary sinus septal defect (unroofed coronary sinus) in 1 (9%).

RA: Right atrial hypertrophy and enlargement, 11 of 11 (100%). Left-sided juxtaposition of the atrial appendages (due to levomalposition of the right atrial appendage) coexisted in 2 of 11 cases (18%).

Atrial Septum: In these 11 patients, the atrial septum was intact in 5 (45%). A large ostium secundum type of ASD was present in 2 (18%). A patent foramen ovale communicated with the LA (not the common pulmonary vein chamber) in 1 patient (9%). There was a defect between the pulmonary vein chamber and the RA in 1 (9%). An ostium primum type of AV septal defect was found in 1 patient (9%). A surgically created ASD was present in 1 (9%).

Note: For clarity and brevity, the ventral left atrial chamber that has the left atrial appendage and leads to the mitral valve will simply be called the **LA.** The dorsal left atrial chamber that receives the pulmonary veins will be called the **pulmonary vein chamber.** The advantages of these shortened terms are thought to be clarity, brevity, and anatomic accuracy.

Tricuspid Valve: Normal in 7 of 11 cases (64%); tricuspid atresia, 1, (9%); straddling into infundibular outlet chamber, 1; part of the incomplete form of common AV canal with deficient septal leaflet, 1; and part of the complete form of common AV canal (tricuspid valve not present as such), 1.

Right Ventricle: Right ventricular hypertrophy and enlargement, 9 of 11 (82%); right ventricular sinus hypoplasia with tricuspid atresia, 1 (9%); and right ventricular sinus absent with single LV, 1 (9%).

Conus Arteriosus: Subpulmonary, with normally related great arteries, in 9 of 11 (82%); and subaortic, with D-TGA, in 2 (18%).

Caliber of Right Ventricular Outflow Tract: Widely patent in 10 of 11 (91%); and stenotic, subaortic (with D-TGA and restrictive VSD) in 1 (9%).

Pulmonary Valve: Normal in 10 of 11 (91%); and pulmonary valvar atresia in 1 (9%).

Pulmonary Artery: Dilated in 8 of 11 (73%); poststenotic dilatation in 1 (9%); normal, status post main pulmonary artery banding in 1; and status post left Blalock-Taussig anastomosis and right pulmonary artery to aortic end-to-end anastomosis.

Left Atrium, Pulmonary Veins, and Cor Triatriatum Membrane: How obstructive was the cor triatriatum membrane? It had been surgically excised in 4 of 11 cases (36%); so in these patients, we could not answer this question by postmortem examination.

In the remaining 7, the findings were as follows. The cor triatriatum membrane was obstructive in 6 of 7 cases (86%). In only 1 patient was it nonobstructive, the opening measuring 15 × 10 mm. In those with obstruction, the diameter of the opening ranged from less than 1 mm (a pinhole) in 1 with functional atresia, to 10 mm in 1 with mild obstruction. The other 4 patients with severe obstruction had openings that varied from 2 to 4 mm in diameter.

Mitral Valve: Normal in 7 of 11 (64%); mitral atresia with small LV in 1 (9%); left atrial outlet atresia ("mitral" atresia) with large LV in 1; cleft mitral valve with incompletely common AV canal in 1; and incompletely common AV canal (mitral valve absent, as such) in 1.

Left Ventricle: Left ventricular hypertrophy and enlargement in 4 (36%); normal in 4; hypoplastic in 2 (18%); and single LV with infundibular outlet chamber (absent right ventricular sinus) in 1 (9%).

Ventricular Septum: Intact in 7 of 11 (64%); VSD in 4 (36%), of the conoventricular type in 2, and of the AV canal type in 2.

Caliber of the Left Ventricular Outflow Tract: Widely patent in 9 of 11 (82%); stenotic in 1 (9%), a patient with D-TGA and pulmonary stenosis because of posterior malalignment of the conal septum; and atretic in 1, a patient with pulmonary valvar atresia.

Aortic Valve: Normal in 9 of 11 (82%); bicuspid aortic valve with a rudimentary intercoronary commissure in 1 (9%); and aortic valvar atresia in 1.

Coronary Arteries: Normal in 7 of 11 (64%); usual for D-TGA in 1 (9%); eccentric right coronary ostium, but with normal course of the right coronary artery, in 1; aberrant (third) coronary artery arising from the proximal left pulmonary artery and connecting with the anterior interventricular groove, in 1; and single left coronary artery (i.e., absent right coronary arterial ostium), with intramural proximal course, in 1.

Aortic Arch and Branches: Left aortic arch in 10, and sidedness of the aortic arch not stated in 1. An aberrant right subclavian artery was present in 2 patients; and the left vertebral artery arose directly from the aortic arch in 1 patient. Mild coarctation of the aorta was found in 1.

Ductus Arteriosus/Ligamentum Arteriosum: A ligamentum arteriosum was present in 9 of 11 cases (82%), and a PDA was found in 2 patients (18%).

Isolated and Nonisolated Cor Triatriatum: In this series of 11 postmortem cases, isolated cor triatriatum was present in 5 (45%) and nonisolated cor triatriatum occurred in 6 (55%). The associated malformations (cardiovascular and noncardiovascular) are summarized in Table 8.2.

TABLE 8.2 Associated Malformations in Nonisolated Cor Triatriatum Sinistrum (n = 6)

Number	Complex Associated Malformations
1	Quero anomaly,[130] that is, left atrial outlet ("mitral") atresia with large single left ventricle. Aberrant right subclavian artery, mild coarctation of the aorta, and single left coronary artery
2	Complex D-transposition of the great arteries (D-TGA). *Case 1:* TGA {S,D,D} with pulmonary stenosis, restrictive (2 × 3 mm) subaortic ventricular septal defect (VSD) with subaortic stenosis, left-sided juxtaposition of the atrial appendages, tricuspid atresia, large secundum atrial septal defect, hypoplastic right ventricular sinus, and left superior vena cava to the coronary sinus. *Case 2:* TGA {S,D,D}, left-sided juxtaposition of the atrial appendages, intact atrial septum, left superior vena cava to coronary sinus, conoventricular VSD (12 × 6 mm), pulmonary valvar atresia, and atresia of the main pulmonary artery
3	Incompletely common atrioventricular canal, left superior vena cava to coronary sinus, unroofed coronary sinus (therefore left superior vena cava drained into left atrium)
4	Atretic right superior vena cava, left superior vena cava to coronary sinus with coronary sinus septal defect ("unroofing," 5 × 5.5 mm), completely common atrioventricular canal, type A, with mitral atresia (rightward malalignment of the ventricles relative to the atria), bicuspid aortic valve with rudimentary intercoronary commissure, multiple congenital anomalies with facial asymmetry (right larger than left) and leg asymmetry (right larger than left)
5	Maternal drugs (?progesterone) during pregnancy; infant with male pseudohermaphroditism, adrenogenital syndrome, left superior vena cava to coronary sinus, pin-hole opening in cor triatriatum membrane (almost atretic), mitral atresia, tiny left ventricle, aortic atresia (i.e., hypoplastic left heart syndrome), aberrant coronary artery from proximal left pulmonary artery, aberrant right subclavian artery and left subclavian artery from descending thoracic aorta

LITERATURE AND DISCUSSION

The early history of cor triatriatum sinistrum has been mentioned previously in connection with morphogenesis and hence will be touched on only briefly here.

Andral[2] (1829) we think does not deserve to be mentioned as perhaps the earliest describer of cor triatriatum. In a section on "Excessive Development of the Heart" he talks in very general terms about "supernumerary ventricles and atria." He writes: "In a heart with three atria, there are two lateral ones which receive the venae cavae and the pulmonary veins, and a third, in the middle, which communicates with the middle atrium." This sounds like a theoretical guesstimate, not a description of a real case of cor triatriatum sinistrum (or dextrum). Andral[2] often has been given credit, uncritically, for description of the first case of cor triatriatum sinistrum. In the kindest spirit, we think that this is simply incorrect.

In 1868, Church[1] gave the first clear description of a case of this entity, calling it an "abnormal septum in the left auricle." He did not attempt a pathogenetic explanation of this anomaly.

In 1881, Fowler[3] described what he called a "membranous band in the left auricle," ascribing it to "an overgrowth of the valve which closes the foramen ovale."

In 1986, Griffith[6] presented a heart with a "fibromuscular band" in the LA (then called the left auricle). Griffith wrote that "a small oval aperture existed in the band, which admitted the passage of a large crow-quill."

In 1899, Martin[7] showed a heart specimen "in which the left auricle was divided by a horizontal septum into a superior and inferior compartment."

In 1903, Griffith[8] reported a second example of "division of the cavity of the left auricle into the two compartments by a fibrous band," suggesting that this anomaly was due to failure of incorporation of the common pulmonary vein into the LA.

In 1904, Potter and Ranson[9] reported a heart with "a septum across the left auricle." They hotly debated the two contending morphogenetic hypotheses, favoring Fowler's[3] abnormal septum primum concept, rather than Griffith's[6,8] and Martin's[7] pulmonary venous malincorporation theory.

In 1905, Borst[10] published a well-documented case and coined the term *cor triatriatum.*

In 1911, William and Abrikossoff[13] published a well-photographed case in an 11-year-old boy calling this malformation *double LA,* that is, *linkem Doppelvorhof* in the original German.

In 1940, McLester et al[16] published the case of an 18-year-old man, calling the anomaly *congenitally double left auricle.*

In 1949, still trying to understand what this malformation really is and what it should be called, Loeffler[17] proposed the term and concept of a *heart with a pulmonary sinus.* He realized that *cor triatriatum* (triatrial heart) and *double LA* are both misnomers: the heart does not really have three atria, and the LA is not double. Instead, the LA is subdivided. Loeffler[17] accepted Griffith's[6,8] hypothesis of failure of incorporation of the pulmonary vein into the LA and suggested the following classification into three groups, based on the size of the opening in the subdividing membrane: (1) no communication, (2) one or several small openings, and (3) a large nonobstructive opening.

In 1951, Edwards et al[19] published a typical case of cor triatriatum and suggested the name *congenital stenosis of the common pulmonary vein.* We agree that this is an apt designation for the typical case. However, it does not apply well (1) when there is no opening (this is atresia of the ostium of the common pulmonary vein), or (2) when there is no stenosis of the incompletely incorporated common pulmonary vein.

In 1956, Lewis, Varco, Taufic, and Niazi[28] reported the first successful repair of cor triatriatum using inflow occlusion. The patient was a 23-year-old man who underwent surgical repair on May 24, 1955. Also in 1956, Vineberg and Gialloreto[29] reported the second successful surgical repair of stenosis of the common pulmonary vein in a 21-year-old woman who was operated upon on July 14, 1955.

In 1957, Marinozzi[33] reported 3 cases and supported the concept that cor triatriatum is really a septated LA (in the original Italian, *atrio sinistro sepimentato*). Varcasia and Patane[34] embraced the same concept and reported clinical aspects of the same 3 cases.

In 1960, Gousios and Cotton[47] reported cor triatriatum with coarctation of the aorta. Also in 1960, Therkelsen and Fabricius[43] reported a 33-year-old woman with cor triatriatum. The patient was operated on for mitral stenosis. However, the surgeon found that the mitral valve was normal, but he could not feel the pulmonary veins. This observation led to surgical opening of the subdividing membrane, resulting in a surgical cure of the patient's cor triatriatum.

As was appreciated by Manubens, Krovetz, and Adams[48] in 1960, supravalvar stenosing ring of the LA (also known as supramitral stenosing ring) is very different anatomically and developmentally from cor triatriatum. **Supramitral stenosing ring** typically is confluent with the mitral valve, lies below the level of the opening into the left atrial appendage, and is not confluent with the septum primum, whereas cor triatriatum is not confluent with the mitral valve, lies above the opening into the left atrial appendage, and is confluent with the septum primum.

Also concerning differential diagnosis, it should be pointed out that **TAPVC to the coronary sinus** is *not* a form of cor triatriatum (with no opening in the subdividing membrane and therefore no communication with the LA), contrary to the impression of some authors (e.g., Lam et al,[55] 1962). Cor triatriatum (i.e., failure of incorporation of the common pulmonary vein into the LA) and TAPVC to the coronary sinus (i.e., abnormal connection of the common pulmonary vein to the coronary sinus, and not to the LA) are two very different anatomic anomalies of abnormal connection of the common pulmonary vein. In addition, TAPVC to the coronary sinus almost always is not obstructed, whereas cor triatriatum typically is.

In 1963, Lucas et al[63] reported cor triatriatum associated with anomalous pulmonary venous connection to the left innominate vein (LIV).

In 1964, Miller, Ongley, Anderson, Kincaid, and Swan[65] clearly delineated the clinical, hemodynamic, angiocardiographic, and surgical features in 3 patients. They documented the typically severe pulmonary hypertension (78/32 to 125/75 mm Hg), the markedly elevated pulmonary arterial wedge pressures (28/20 to 65/18 mm Hg), and the normal left ventricular end-diastolic pressures.

In 1965, McGuire et al[66] emphasized that cor triatriatum can be a problem of heart disease in adults. These authors reported the case of a 19-year-old man with pulmonary edema and hemoptysis.

In 1965, Guérin and Poisson[67] urged that the following conditions be diagnosed as such and excluded from the diagnostic category of cor triatriatum: supramitral stenosing ring, supramitral aneurysm, and TAPVC to the coronary sinus. We agree with these recommendations. For those who read French, this is an excellent review, including the relevant embryology.

Concerning **the natural history of cor triatriatum**, Guérin and Poisson[67] indicated that there is a direct correlation between the size of the opening in the left atrial diaphragm and the natural history. When the diameter of the communication was less than 6 mm, there was always severe pulmonary hypertension (>100 mm Hg systolic). Survival until adulthood was possible only if the diameter of the orifice in the diaphragm was larger than 10 mm. When the size of the orifice in the diaphragm was less than 30 mm^2, the average age at death was 6 years. When less than 10 mm^2, the average age at death was approximately 1 year. When greater than 30 mm^2, the average age at death was approximately 23 years. These conclusions are not supported by detailed data or references that are evident in their paper[67]; nonetheless, these correlations seem sufficiently reasonable that they are recorded here for future consideration.

In 1966, Dr. Jane Somerville[69] introduced the concept of masked cor triatriatum, that is, that the presence of cor triatriatum can be obscured by other anomalies such as an ASD or anomalous pulmonary venous connection. In such complex situations, it is imperative to recognize the coexistence of cor triatriatum.

In 1967, Perry, Scott, and McClenathan[72] reported the successful surgical repair of the youngest patient with cor triatriatum known to that time: an 8½-month-old white boy.

In 1967, Keith, Rowe, and Vlad[73] reported that cor triatriatum "is rare, being almost the least common in our collection of 6647 patients with congenital heart disease. There are five cases in the records of the Hospital for Sick Children [in Toronto] where the malformation was relatively 'pure,' and two others in which the atrial malformation was associated with cyanotic congenital heart disease of a complex nature." Thus, their **incidence of cor triatriatum** was 7 of 6647 cases of congenital heart disease, or 0.105%.[73] In the present study, our incidence of cor triatriatum was 11 of 3216 cases of autopsy-proved congenital heart disease, that is, 0.342%. Being a pathology series, our data may be skewed in the direction of "badness." Hence, the incidence figure of Keith, Rowe, and Vlad[73] may be closer to the truth.

On the other hand, our data—being autopsy proved—may be more accurate. However, because we do not know that this is so, we report both incidence figures (0.1% and 0.3%), without favoring either. Although not identical, these incidence statistics are very close together. We hope that this range (0.1% to 0.3%) will prove to be close to the truth.

In 1968, Wolfe, Ruttenberg, Desilets, and Mulder[75] reported the youngest successfully corrected infant with cor triatriatum shown up to that time, a 3-month-old boy. The intra-atrial membrane was excised on cardiopulmonary bypass.

In 1971, Wilson, Graham, Gehweiler, and Canent[79] reported cor triatriatum with an intact subdividing diaphragm. All of the pulmonary veins connected with the dorsal common pulmonary vein chamber, except for the left inferior pulmonary vein that connected with the ventral left atrial chamber. The patient was a 9-day-old boy. This is a fascinating and puzzling case that we do not fully understand. The authors[79] regarded this patient as having PAPVC because the left lower pulmonary vein did not connect with the common pulmonary vein. However, it seems somewhat curious to regard the connection of a pulmonary vein to the LA as an *anomalous* connection.

That aside, what are we dealing with here? This case may perhaps be interpreted as **partial** or subtotal cor triatriatum. By analogy, it certainly is possible to have PAPVCs. This fact suggests that usually the development of the pulmonary veins is *unifocal,* with all of the pulmonary venous branches connecting with the common pulmonary vein. Occasionally, however, the development of the pulmonary veins can be *multifocal,* as occurs with PAPVCs. Some of the pulmonary veins are connected normally to the common pulmonary vein, but others are not connected normally. This is why Wilson et al[79] regarded the connection of the left lower pulmonary vein as anomalous, despite the fact that this vein connected with the LA. Our hypothesis is that the pulmonary veins in this patient had a *bifocal* origin. The common pulmonary vein and its branches were afflicted with malincorporation and stenosis (cor triatriatum). But the left lower pulmonary vein became detached from the common vein or may have never been attached to the common pulmonary vein. In either case, the left lower lobe developed a left lower pulmonary vein that connected with the ventral compartment of the LA. In this very rare case with bifocal development of the pulmonary veins, the main focus had cor triatriatum, but the accessory focus did not. We have not seen such a case.

In 1972, Danielson and Feldt[81] reported the first successful surgical repair of TOF with cor triatriatum in a 5-year-old white girl. At surgery, the TOF was repaired. The patient also had an ASD that led into a small left atrial chamber. Initially, the surgeons could not find the pulmonary veins. Then, they realized that they were dealing with masked cor triatriatum that had not been diagnosed preoperatively. This realization led to successful excision of the intra-atrial partition.

In 1973, Arrants et al[82] reported the youngest patient with cor triatriatum successfully corrected surgically to that date: a 10-week-old boy.

In 1974, Nimura et al[84] reported the noninvasive diagnosis of cor triatriatum in a 14-year-old boy and a 7-year-old girl using ultrasonocardiotomography and conventional echocardiography. In the same year, Gibson et al[85] reported the case of a 23-year-old man, noting that the left atrial diaphragm was shown by echocardiography but not by angiocardiography.

In 1976, Nudel et al[87] reported 2 patients in whom cor triatriatum was masked by complex congenital cardiac anomalies. Their Case 1 also had TOF, scimitar syndrome, and left ventricular outflow tract obstruction. Their Case 2 also had truncus arteriosus.

In 1976, Thilenius, Bharati, and Lev[90] published a study of 24 heart specimens with cor triatriatum. They indicated that cor triatriatum sinistrum is a subdivided LA, a view with which we and most other investigators agree.

In 1977, Jennings and Innes[89] reported a 10-week-old infant with cor triatriatum, who also had a left-sided PAPVC to the LIV. The authors stated that this was the first successful repair of this rare combination of defects.

This patient[89] had cor triatriatum *and* PAPVC. Whenever PAPVC is present, the anomalous pulmonary vein(s) does (do) not connect with the common pulmonary vein, by definition. The stenosis and failure of incorporation of the common pulmonary vein is completely present, not partially present. Thus, the cor triatriatum per se is not partial. Instead, an additional anomaly is present: PAPVC.

In any case, now you know what we think "partial" or "subtotal" cor triatriatum really is. Our view is very close to that of Wilson et al[79] (1971).

In 1978, Kachaner, Fermont, and Ribierre[92] published a study of cor triatriatum in infancy. They found that selective angiocardiography into the main pulmonary artery permitted diagnosis of cor triatriatum in 2 of their 4 patients. However, selective pulmonary angiocardiography is dangerous. One of their 2 patients died soon after this test, despite vigorous therapy. Kachaner et al[92] concluded that echocardiography is the preferable diagnostic modality, because selective pulmonary arteriography is dangerous.

In 1982, Khonsari, Saunders, Lees, and Starr[95] reported the first surgically successful repair of cor triatriatum with an imperforate left atrial membrane. They interpreted their case as having atresia of the ostium of the common pulmonary vein, and they emphasized the clinical important of immediate diagnosis and surgical intervention.

In 1983, Oglietti, Cooley, Izquierdo, Ventemiglia, Muasher, Hallman, and Ruel[96] reported their surgical results in 25 patients with cor triatriatum, who were operated on between 4 months and 38 years of age. The mortality rate was 4 of 25 (16%). Also in 1983, Schlüter et al[97] reported the advantages of transesophageal two-dimensional echocardiography for the diagnosis of cor triatriatum in the adult.

In 1984, Östman-Smith, Silverman, Oldershaw, Lincoln, and Shinebourne[102] concluded that two-dimensional echocardiography is better for the diagnosis of cor triatriatum sinistrum than cardiac catheterization and angiocardiography.

In 1985, Lang, Wagenvoort, Kupferschmid, and Kleihauer[103] reported a 17-month-old boy in whom the presence of cor triatriatum was masked by the coexistence of primary pulmonary hypertension. Interestingly, the pulmonary artery wedge pressure was not elevated, it was thought because of reduced pulmonary blood flow associated with both conditions.

In 1987, Geggel, Fulton, Chernoff, Cleveland, and Hougen[104] reported cor triatriatum associated with PAPVC to the coronary sinus. This was the first such case in the literature, amplifying the concept that cor triatriatum can indeed have various types of PAPVC.

In 1988, the findings with magnetic resonance imaging in cor triatriatum were published by Rumancik et al,[108] their patient being an 18-year-old man.

Chronic obstructive pulmonary disease in an adult can mask cor triatriatum, as in the 53-year-old Chinese woman published by Leung et al[110] in 1989.

In 1990, Yamaguchi et al[111] published a rare and surgically correctable constellation of anomalies in a 4-month-old boy consisting of cor triatriatum, VSD, and coarctation of the aorta.

In 1990, Cooley and Murphy[112] reported cor triatriatum and PAPVC (left upper lobe pulmonary vein to the LIV) in a 64-year-old man. PAPVC may be hemodynamically advantageous in association with cor triatriatum by helping to decompress the hypertensive pulmonary venous system.

In 1990, Rodefeld et al[113] reported a surgical mortality in series of 12 patients of 17%. The overall mortality was 25%. These findings focus attention on the fact that cor triatriatum is a highly lethal form of congenital heart disease, rivaling the hypoplastic left heart syndrome and much higher than most other forms of congenital heart disease.

In 1991, Tanaka et al[114] published a case on the other side of the clinical severity spectrum—a case of asymptomatic cor triatriatum that was incidentally revealed by computed tomography (CT). The patient, a 75-year-old man, was the oldest case of cor triatriatum reported up to that time and the only case to be diagnosed by CT.

In 1991, Salomone et al[115] reported a surgical mortality of 20% (3/15), again emphasizing the severe medical and surgical problem posed by cor triatriatum.

The role of intraoperative echocardiography in the diagnosis of previously unrecognized cor triatriatum was published by Hogue et al[118] in 1992 concerning a 76-year-old man, the oldest known patient with cor triatriatum published up to that time.

In 1992, Al-Fadley et al[119] reported a patient with cor triatriatum. The common pulmonary vein chamber was drained by a levoatrial cardinal vein into the LIV. Thus, the patient had a rare supracardiac form of totally anomalous venous drainage in association with cor triatriatum.

In addition, there was mitral atresia, with a restrictive interatrial communication between the LA (the ventral or "lower" chamber) and the RA.

Rarely, therefore, cor triatriatum can be associated with *totally* anomalous pulmonary venous drainage (TAPVD) (not just *partially* anomalous pulmonary venous connection/drainage [PAPVC/D]). When cor triatriatum is associated with TAPVD, this occurs via a *levoatrial-cardinal vein,* that is, an anomalous venous connection between the pulmonary venous component of the LA (hence *levoatrial*) and the cardinal venous system, that is, the LIV that flows into the RSVC, which is the right anterior cardinal vein (hence *cardinal vein*).

This patient[119] had TAPVD, not TAPVC. The levoatrial cardinal vein is not a pulmonary vein. Instead, it is a (decompressing) anastomosis between the common pulmonary vein and the systemic veins. The levoatrial-cardinal vein flows from the LA to the LSVC-LIV junction. The LSVC is the left anterior cardinal vein. Thus, *levoatrial-cardinal* vein specifies both ends of the decompressing anastomotic vein: the LA and the left anterior cardinal vein. The left innominate (or brachiocephalic) vein is the anastomosis between the left anterior cardinal vein (the LSVC) and the right anterior cardinal vein (the RSVC).

Why is the levoatrial-cardinal vein not the LSVC? The LSVC can flow into the coronary sinus and then to the RA. However, the levoatrial-cardinal vein connects inferiorly with the LA (i.e., with the common pulmonary vein component of the LA), not with the coronary sinus. Superiorly (cephalically), both the levoatrial-cardinal vein and the LSVC connect with the left end of the LIV. Inferiorly, at the level of the heart, a persistent LSVC to the coronary sinus is more anterior (ventral) than is a levoatrial-cardinal vein, the latter being more posterior (dorsal) because the levoatrial-cardinal vein connects with the pulmonary venous portion of the LA (which is very posterior). Finally, a persistent LSVC and a levoatrial-cardinal vein can coexist.

In summary, the case of Al-Fadley et al[119] had cor triatriatum with mitral atresia, a restrictive interatrial communication, a decompressing levoatrial-cardinal vein, and supracardiac TAPVD.

In 1993, van Son et al[122] reported a series of 13 cases. They concluded that echocardiography is the diagnostic method of choice and that surgical long-term results are excellent.

In 1996, Kerkar et al[124] announced **successful percutaneous balloon dilatation** of cor triatriatum sinistrum, using a double-balloon technique, in a 16-year-old woman. From an anatomic standpoint, we have long thought that cor triatriatum sinistrum could be successfully treated by percutaneous techniques. However, much more experience is needed before we will know how successful the percutaneous technique is in subdivided LA.

In 2001, Ito et al[125] reported the case of an 11-year-old boy and a 2-month-old boy with cor triatriatum and stenosis of individual pulmonary veins at their junction with the LA. For example, the 11-year-old boy, in addition to cor triatriatum, also had stenosis of the right lower lobe pulmonary vein and of the left lower lobe pulmonary vein at their junction with the LA.

The findings of Ito et al[125] appear to clarify the earlier report of Kerensky et al[123] in 1995 that we initially did not fully understand. Kerensky et al[123] had a patient with unilateral pulmonary venous obstruction. While studying this problem, they subsequently discovered that their patient also had cor triatriatum. In other words, cor triatriatum and obstruction of individual pulmonary veins can coexist. This is also the message of Ito et al.[125]

In 2002, Niccoli et al[126] reported cor triatriatum associated with an ostium primum ASD (partially common AV canal). The patient was a 44-year-old woman with a stenotic membrane partitioning the LA. The orifice in the membrane was less than 1 cm in diameter, and the patient also had severe tricuspid regurgitation. The patient died before surgery could be done.

In 2004, Keeble et al[127] appear to have discovered why patients with cor triatriatum may have mitral regurgitation. Their patient was a 27-year-old woman. Removal of the cor triatriatum membrane cured her mitral regurgitation. The jet through the opening in the cor triatriatum membrane was holding the anterior mitral leaflet open during early systole, resulting in mitral regurgitation.

In patients with cor triatriatum the mitral valve is in the poststenotic jet stream. This is thought to explain why adults with cor triatriatum are prone to mitral valve disease, as Fuster-Siebert et al[98] pointed out in 1982.

Being in the poststenotic jet stream of the entrapped and unincorporated common pulmonary vein, the anterior leaflet of the mitral valve (or wherever the jet strikes) would suffer from accentuated *hemodynamic change,* as Dr. Maurice Lev called it. *Jet lesions* are characterized by focal endocardial thickening and fibrosis. Fibrosis, in turn, leads to leaflet retraction, stiffness, and shortening. These processes would also tend to lead to mitral regurgitation. Jet lesions also may serve as foci for infective endocarditis, because the endocardium becomes thickened and roughened where the poststenotic jet strikes.

Thus, the observations of Keeble et al[127] are considered to be important, particularly in adults[98] with cor triatriatum. The poststenotic jet stream, by preventing normal mitral valve closure early in systole—with or without significant mitral valve jet lesions—is a newly discovered mechanism of mitral regurgitation in cor triatriatum sinistrum.

COR TRIATRIATUM DEXTRUM

Cor triatriatum dextrum (right-sided triatrial heart, Latin) is a RA that is subdivided by a very prominent and obstructive right leaflet of the sinoatrial valve.[131-138] The obstructing membrane is often called a right venous valve (*valva* meaning a leaf of a folding door, or either of the halves of a double door, Latin). This membrane is also often called a very prominent Eustachian and Thebesian valve (the Eustachian valve being the valve of the IVC, and the Thebesian valve being the valve of the coronary sinus).

A very prominent right venous valve can obstructively separate the caval and coronary sinus compartment medially from the more lateral compartment containing the right atrial appendage and the tricuspid valve leading into the RV. Consequently, an obstructive right venous valve can produce systemic venous stenosis and coronary sinus stenosis, if the atrial septum is intact. If the patient also has a patent foramen ovale or a secundum ASD, cor triatriatum dextrum can result in right-to-left shunting at the atrial level and central cyanosis.

Thus, cor triatriatum dextrum can be associated with two different clinical syndromes, depending on the status of the atrial septum: (1) supratricuspid stenosing membrane, with caval and coronary sinus obstruction, when the atrial septum is intact or permits minimal right-to-left shunting (classic cor triatriatum dextrum); and (2) the IVC draining to the LA, when the septum primum is deficient or absent and the right venous valve is prominent. In the latter situation, the very prominent right venous valve that ushers the IVC's blood stream into the LA is easily mistaken for the atrial septum (septum primum), when the atrial septum is in fact very deficient or absent.

Dr. Charles Baker and Dr. John Mayer, Jr. had a very rare and successfully operated patient in whom angiocardiography showed that the IVC drained into the LA. This patient, an 18-month-old boy, also had a left-sided scimitar syndrome with the scimitar vein draining into the right-sided IVC. At surgery, the IVC was divided below the entry of the scimitar vein, so that all of the pulmonary venous return went to the LA. The lower IVC was then anastomosed to the RA, to the right of the right venous valve. The cardiologist and the surgeon need to know that the IVC never connects directly with the LA. Because the right venous valve lies to the right of the IVC, and septum primum (deficient or absent) lies to the left of the IVC, it may look as though the IVC is connecting anomalously with the LA. This is the less familiar cor triatriatum dextrum syndrome.

It should be added that in this second and less familiar prominent right venous valve syndrome, there may or may not be three atrial chambers and there may or may not be IVC obstruction—depending on how deficient the septum primum (the atrial septum) is. When septum primum is essentially absent, there are only two atrial chambers (not three) and there is no IVC obstruction.

Hence, one may prefer *not* to regard such cases as having cor triatriatum dextrum, even though the RA is subdivided by a very prominent right venous valve. However, the more conventional view is that when the RA is subdivided by a prominent right venous valve, this is what is meant by "cor triatriatum dextrum."

As in the patient of Baker and colleagues mentioned earlier, the prominent right venous valve may have an opening or fenestration in it, strongly resembling an ASD.

How does one tell the septum primum (the atrial septum) from a prominent right venous valve? In visceroatrial situs solitus, the septum primum lies to the *left* of the IVC, whereas the right venous valve lies to the *right* of the IVC.

PRESENT SERIES

In this series of 3216 cases of autopsied congenital heart disease, we made the diagnosis of cor triatriatum dextrum in only 2 cases (0.06%). This suggests that cor triatriatum dextrum is one of the rarest forms of congenital heart disease.

Age at Death: 20 months in Case 1, and 5 weeks in Case 2.

Sex: Both male.

Heart Position: Levocardia in both.

Cardiac Segments: {S,D,S} in both.

Systemic Veins: Normal in both, apart from cor triatriatum dextrum.

Right Atrium: In Case 1, the RA was divided into two chambers by a prominent Eustachian valve (Fig. 8.23). In Case 2, the right venous valve was prominent and obstructed the tricuspid orifice.

Atrial Septum: Case 1 had two secundum ASDs. Case 2 had one secundum ASD.

Tricuspid Valve: Case 1 had tricuspid atresia (see Fig. 8.23). Case 2 had an Ebstein-like anomaly of the tricuspid valve.

Right Ventricle: Case 1 had an atretic right ventricular sinus (inflow tract), typical of tricuspid atresia. Case 2 had a right ventricular dysplasia, characteristic of Ebstein anomaly.

Conus: Subpulmonary in both, typical of solitus normally related great arteries.

Ventricular Septum: Case 1 had a slit-like muscular VSD. Hence, this patient had tricuspid atresia type Ib (see Fig. 8.23). Type I means that the great arteries were solitus normally related. Type b indicates that there was pulmonary outflow tract stenosis. Case 2 had an intact ventricular septum.

Caliber of the right ventricular outflow tract: Case 1 had very severe infundibular subpulmonary stenosis, with an only slightly hypoplastic pulmonary valve. Case 2 had a pulmonary valvar atresia and atresia of the main pulmonary artery.

Left Atrium and Pulmonary Veins: Unremarkable in both.

Mitral Valve: Normal in both.

Left Ventricle: Well developed in both.

Caliber of the Left Ventricular Outflow Tract: Widely patent, with unremarkable aortic valve in both.

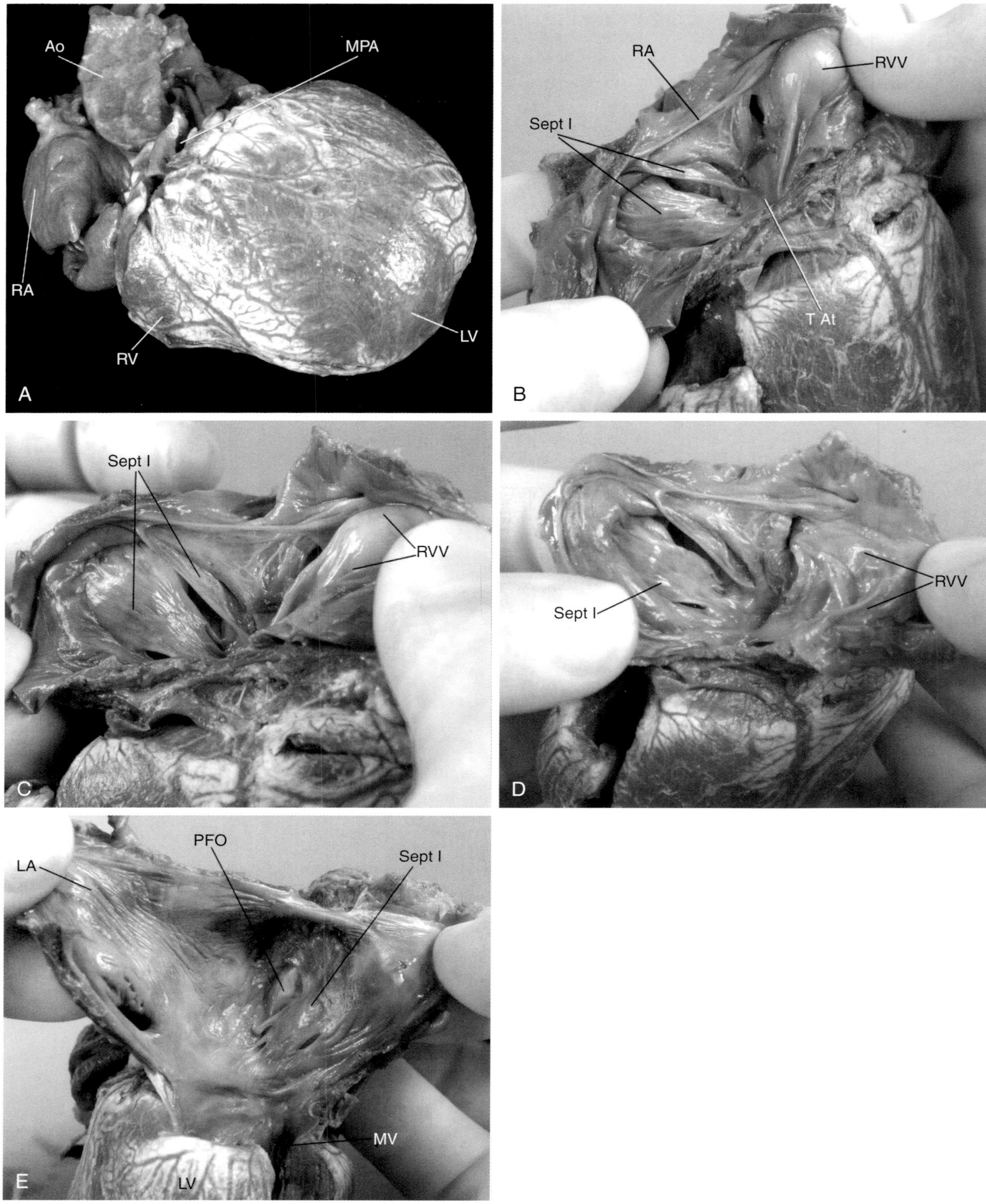

Fig. 8.23 Cor Triatriatum Dextrum (Very Large Right Venous Valve) in the Heart of a 20-Month-Old Boy With Tricuspid Atresia Type Ib (Normally Related Great Arteries, With Pulmonary Outflow Tract Stenosis). (A) The external frontal view strongly suggests tricuspid atresia. Note the markedly hypertrophied and enlarged right atrium *(RA)*, the strikingly small right ventricle *(RV)*, the very hypertrophied and enlarged left ventricle *(LV)*, the markedly rightward displacement of the left anterior descending coronary artery between the small RV and the huge LV, the small main pulmonary artery *(MPA)* suggesting pulmonary outflow tract stenosis, and the reciprocally enlarged ascending aorta *(Ao)*. The opened RA showing tricuspid atresia *(TAt)*, with the septum primum *(Sept I)* of the atrial septum to the viewer's left and a very large right venous valve *(RVV)* to the viewer's right. The RVV is distended by the examiner's index finger to show how large the RVV is. One can see that there is only a very small opening in the RVV. Sept I is artifactually torn horizontally. In this view of the RA between Sept I to the left and the RVV to the right, Sept I is better seen. In this view of the RA, the RVV is flaccid (undistended), confirming that the RVV is as large as the well-developed Sept I. The opened left atrium *(LA)*, mitral valve *(MV)*, and LV showing the well-developed Sept I and the patent foramen ovale *(PFO)* from the left atrial aspect. Multiple (three) small fenestrations are present within Sept I below the PFO. The artifactual tear in Sept 1 is not apparent because the upper and lower portions of Sept I were carefully approximated. In this patient, the presence of cor triatriatum dextrum was of no physiologic importance because of the coexistence of TAt, resulting in a total right-to-left atrial shunt.

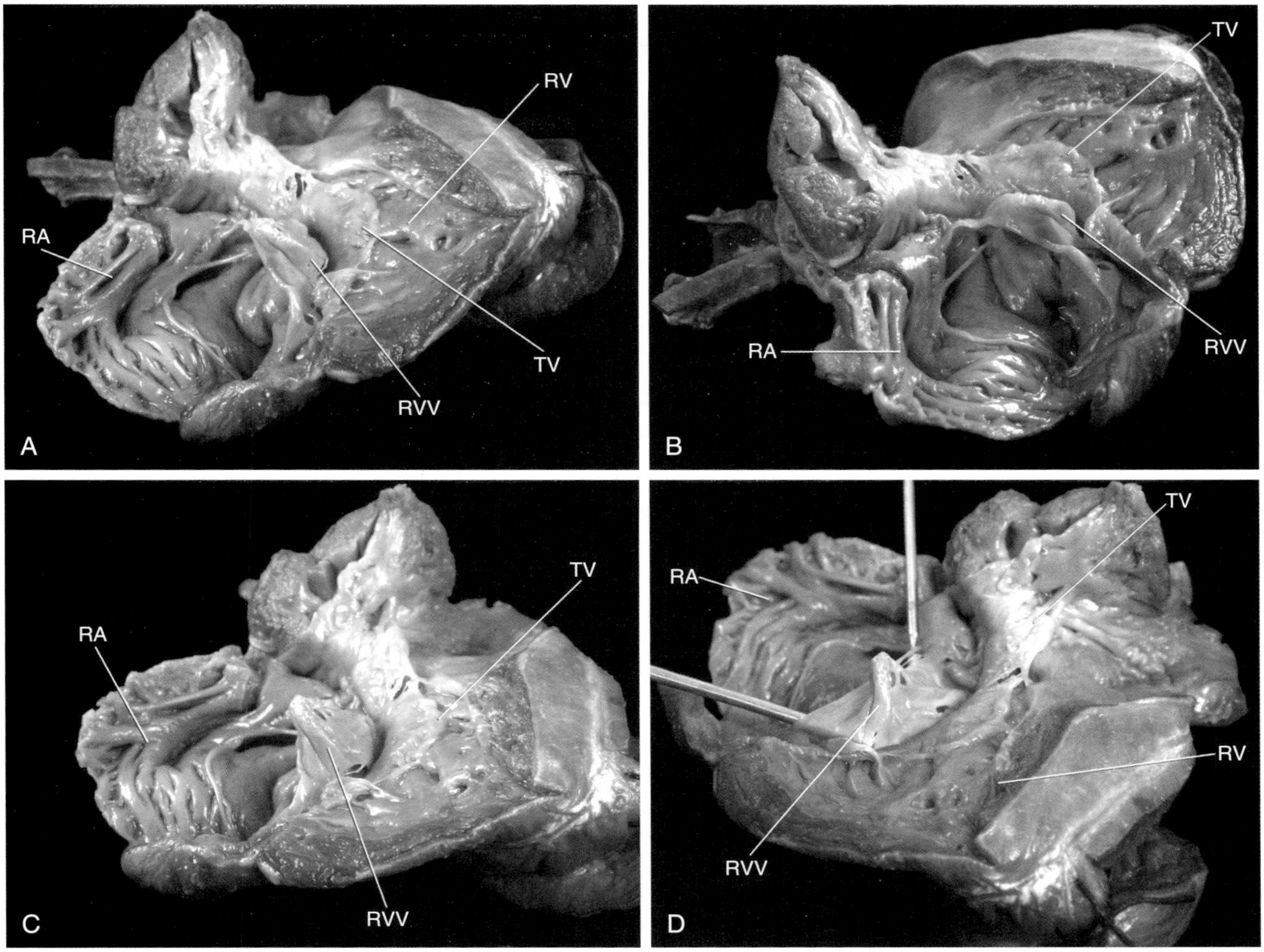

Fig. 8.24 Prominent Right Venous Valve *(RVV)* in a 15-Week-Old Girl With a Membranous Ventricular Septal Defect (5 × 7 mm). Right atrial *(RA)* view showing the unusually large RVV and the opened tricuspid valve *(TV)* and right ventricle *(RV)*. The prominent RVV can bulge down into the TV. Right ventricular view showing that the large RVV may have functioned as a supratricuspid stenosing membrane (hemodynamic data unavailable). RV view of the prominent RVV that contains two probes, the RVV looking like a spinnaker capable of bulging into the tricuspid orifice. We made the diagnosis of a prominent RVV in this case, rather than cor triatriatum dextrum, because the cavity of the RA was not subdivided. Nonetheless, the prominent RVV may have been hemodynamically significant as a supratricuspid stenosing membrane.

Coronary Arteries: In Case 1, the right coronary artery supplied both the anterior descending and the posterior descending coronary arteries. In Case 2, the right coronary ostium was absent (i.e., so-called single left coronary artery).

Aortic Arch: Left in both.

Ductus Arteriosus: Closed in both (ligamentum arteriosum).

Surgery: Case 1 had a Potts anastomosis, which was found at autopsy to be closed (cause of death). Case 2 had a Potts anastomosis and a Waterston anastomosis.

Prominent Right Venous Valve Versus Cor Triatriatum Dextrum

In Figure. 8.24, the heart specimen of a 15-week-old girl is presented in which a prominent right venous valve is well seen. However, we did not make the diagnosis of cor triatriatum dextrum in this patient because the cavity of the RA is not really subdivided into medial and lateral compartments by the unusually prominent right venous valve. Cases such as this (Fig. 8.24) are much more frequent than are cases of cor triatriatum dextrum (see Fig. 8.23).

Prominent right venous valve (see Fig. 8.24) and cor triatriatum dextrum (see Fig. 8.23) are closely related entities, the difference between them being a matter of degree and somewhat arbitrary. (How big is "big"?) Nonetheless, when the right venous valve is approximately as large as a normal septum primum and the RA is subdivided, most observers would regard this as cor triatriatum dextrum.

DISCUSSION AND LITERATURE

In our Case 1, the presence of cor triatriatum dextrum was of no hemodynamic importance because of the coexistence of tricuspid atresia type Ib with two secundum ASDs. There would have been a 100% right-to-left shunt at the atrial level, with or without cor triatriatum dextrum.

Case 2, however, was thought to exemplify **the persistent right venous valve syndrome** as described by Kauffman and Anderson[137] in 1963. This was the last paper of Dr. Dorothy Anderson, the eminent pathologist from Babies' Hospital in New York City. These authors characterized the persistent right venous valve syndrome as having pulmonary valvar atresia, a thick-walled and small-chambered RV with right ventricular myocardial dysplasia, sinusoids communicating from the right ventricular cavity with the coronary arteries, coronary arterial narrowing or occlusion at the point (s) of communication with the sinusoids, and tricuspid obstruction related to an overlying and prominent right venous valve.

Now, however, we tend to think of this as part of **the syndrome of pulmonary atresia with intact ventricular septum.** Nonetheless, Kaufmann and Anderson[137] deserve credit for having early pointed out the coexistence of this constellation of anomalies.

From a historical perspective, an obstructive right venous valve (cor triatriatum dextrum) was first reported by Leo[138] in 1886.

As will be seen from a review of the literature, cor triatriatum dextrum certainly does not always have pulmonary valvar atresia with intact ventricular septum.

From a hemodynamic standpoint, the presence of a prominent right venous valve in Case 2 also did not matter greatly because of the coexistence of pulmonary atresia with intact ventricular septum, which would have resulted in a very large right-to-left atrial shunt, with or without cor triatriatum dextrum.

Neither of our cases had relatively "pure" cor triatriatum dextrum; that is, this was not the primary diagnosis in either of our patients. But such cases rarely do exist.

In 1968, Runcie[131] published the case of a 26-year-old married woman, the mother of four children, who had a subdivided RA. The diaphragm in the RA separated the inferior and superior venae cavae medially from the tricuspid valve more laterally to the right. The opening in the right atrial membrane measured only 3 to 4 mm.

In 1982, Gussenhoven et al[133] published the case of a 13-year-old girl. Preoperatively, based on angiocardiography, she was thought to have a "benign, flexible, moving tumor" of the RA.

In 1983, Mazzucco and his colleagues[134] published the first successful surgical repair of cor triatriatum dextrum in infancy, their patient being a 5-month-old girl.

In 1990, Trakhtenbroit et al[135] showed that cor triatriatum dextrum can be accurately diagnosed by two-dimensional echocardiography. Their patient was a 56-year-old woman with cyanosis, clubbing, Ebstein malformation, and cor triatriatum dextrum.

In 1992, Raffa et al[136] published the case of a 9-year-old girl who had central cyanosis because of prominence of the Eustachian and Thebesian valves. Surgical repair consisted of ASD closure and excision of the sail-like Eustachian and Thebesian valve membrane.

To the best of our knowledge, interventional cardiologists have not as yet treated cor triatriatum dextrum with percutaneous membranotomy, with or without device closure or an associated secundum ASD. It seems likely that this interventional therapeutic step will be attempted soon.

Is there any other anatomic type of cor triatriatum dextrum, something other than a prominent and obstructive right venous valve? I wonder about the possible presence of a prominent *left* venous valve with a **persistent and recognizable interseptovalvular space** between the septum primum to the left and the left venous valve to the right. This theoretically could create three compartments at the atrial level (not really a triatrial heart, of course). No vein(s) would enter this interseptovalvular space. This hypothetical type of cor triatriatum would not be obstructive to the caval or coronary sinus blood flow. Such individuals would be asymptomatic, and this hypothetical anomaly, if it exists, would be of no clinical importance. This anatomic possibility is mentioned here because it may be possible diagnostically to visualize a prominent left venous valve and the interseptovalvular space. As has been shown, both of these structures are well developed and well seen in the human embryo (see Fig. 8.16B). We think that this rare type of cor triatriatum, which may be called **cor triatriatum intermedium** (between the left and right atria) and which is due to a persistent interseptovalvar space, may have been reported for the first time in 1976 by Thilenius, Bharati, and Lev[90]—their type C. These authors stated that this chamber received no pulmonary veins and lay between the RA and the distal portion of the LA, that is, the septum primum portion.

Thus, there appear to be *three* different anatomical types of cor triatriatum: (1) persistence of an unincorporated common pulmonary vein chamber, with stenosis, or atresia, or no obstruction of the common pulmonary vein, that is, cor triatriatum sinistrum; (2) an obstructive right venous valve, the cor triatriatum dextrum; and (3) very rarely, persistence of the interoseptovalvular space, the cor triatriatum intermedium (as earlier). We have never seen this third type of cor triatriatum with our own eyes.

How can a surgeon tell the difference between a prominent and obstructive right venous valve (cor triatriatum dextrum) and an atrial septum with a small secundum ASD? Through a right atriotomy, if one is looking at a prominent and obstructive right venous valve, one cannot see the ostia of the IVC, SVC, and coronary sinus, unless one divides the obstructing diaphragm, because the right venous valve lies to the *right* of the venae cavae, thus hiding them. Through a right atriotomy, if one is looking at the atrial septum, the ostia of the venae cavae and coronary sinus are all readily visible, because the atrial septum lies to the *left* of these venous ostia (see Fig. 8.16).

REFERENCES

1. Church WS. Congenital malformation of heart; abnormal septum in left auricle. *Trans Path Soc London*. 1868;19:188.
2. Andral G. *Précis d'Anatomie Pathologique: Excès de Developpement du Coeur, Gabon, Paris*. Vol 2; 1829:313.
3. Fowler JK. Membranous band in the left auricle. *Trans Path Soc London*. 1881;33:77.
4. Preisz H. *Beiträge zur Lehre von den angeborenen Herzenomalien Beitr path Anat*. 1890;7:245. [Cases 13 and 14].
5. Rolleston HD. Band in the left auricle of the heart. Proc Anat Soc Great Britain and Ireland. *J Anat Physiol*. 1896;30:5.

6. Griffith W. Heart with a fibromuscular band. *J Anat Physiol.* 1895-96;30:6.
7. Martin S. A heart in which the left auricle was divided by a horizontal septum into a superior and inferior compartment. Proc Anat Soc Great Britain and Ireland. *Am J Anat Physiol.* 1899;33:31.
8. Griffith TW. Note on a second example of division of the cavity of the left atrium into two compartments by a fibrous band. *J Anat Physiol.* 1902-1903;37:255.
9. Potter P, Ranson SW. A heart presenting a septum across the left auricle. *J Anat Physiol.* 1904, 1904-1905;39:69.
10. Borst M. *Ein cor triatriatum, Verhandlungen der Deutschen Pathologischen Gesellschaft.* 1905;9:178.
11. Hosch PH. Zur Lehre der Missbildungen des linker Vorhofs. I. Ein Sehnenfaden im linken Vorhof. II. Ein Herz mit linkem Doppelvorhof. *Frankfurt Z Pathol.* 1907-1908;1:563.
12. Stoeber H. Ein weiterer Fall von Cor triatriatum mit eigenartig gekreutzer Mündung der Lungenvenen. *Virchows Arch Pathol Anat Physiol Klin Med.* 1908;193:252.
13. William N, Abrikossoff A. Ein Herz mit linkem Doppelvorhof. *Virchows Arch Pathol Anat Physiol Klin Med.* 1911;203:404.
14. Palmer GA. Cardiac anomaly (so-called double left auricle). Report of a case. *Am Heart J.* 1930;6:230.
15. Helwig FC. Fenestrated hammock-like structure in the left cardiac atrium. Review of the literature and report of a case. *Arch Pathol.* 1933;15:8.
16. McLester JB, Bush JD, DuBois JS. Congenitally double left auricle. Report of a case. *Am Heart J.* 1940;19:492.
17. Loeffler E. Unusual malformation of the left atrium: pulmonary sinus. *Arch Pathol.* 1949;48:371.
18. Parsons CG. Cor triatriatum. Concerning the nature of an anomalous septum in the left auricle. *Br Heart J.* 1950;12:327.
19. Edwards JE, DuShane JW, Alcott DL, Burchell HB. Thoracic venous anomalies. III. Atresia of the common pulmonary vein, the pulmonary veins draining wholly into the superior vena cava (Case 3). IV. Stenosis of the common pulmonary vein (cor triatriatum) (Case 4). *AMA Arch Pathol.* 1951;51:446.
20. Barnes CG, Finlay HVL. Cor triatriatum. *Br Heart J.* 1952;14:283.
21. Doxiadis SA, Emery JL. A case of triatrial heart. *J Pediatr.* 1953;42:87.
22. Pedersen A, Therkelsen F. Cor triatriatum: a rare malformation of the heart, probably amenable to surgery. Report of a case, with review of literature. *Am Heart J.* 1954;47:676.
23. Haarscher A, Marcoux L. Pneumopathie gigantocellulaire traînante chez un enfant atteint d'une malformation cardiaque rare: coeur à double oreillette gauche. *Rev Méd Nancy.* 1954;79:933.
24. Déchamps G, Herbaut M. Un nouveau cas de coeur triatrial. *Acta Cardiol.* 1957;12:78.
25. Hartmann HA. Cor triatriatum (stenosis of common pulmonary vein). *AMA Arch Pathol.* 1955;59:706.
26. Becu LM, Tauxe WN, DuShane JW, Edwards JE. Anomalous connection of pulmonary veins with normal pulmonary venous drainage. Report of case associated with pulmonary venous stenosis and cor triatriatum. *AMA Arch Pathol.* 1955;59:463.
27. Nash FW, Mackinnon D. Cor triatriatum: congenital stenosis of the common pulmonary vein. *Arch Dis Child.* 1956;31:222.
28. Lewis FJ, Varco RL, Taufic M, Niazi SA. Direct vision repair of triatrial heart and total anomalous pulmonary venous drainage. *Surg Gynecol Obstet.* 1956;102:713.
29. Vineberg A, Gialloreto O. Report of a successful operation for stenosis of common pulmonary vein (cor triatriatum). *Can Med Assoc J.* 1956;74:719.
30. Vossenaar T. Cor triatriatum. *Arch Chir Neerl.* 1957;9:48.
31. Chaptal J, Latour H, Jean F, et al. Coeur triatrial. Étude anatomo-clinique. *Montpellier Méd.* 1957;52:59.
32. Barrett NR, Hickie JB. Cor triatriatum. *Thorax.* 1957;12:24.
33. Marinozzi V. Il considetto cor triatriatum (atrio sinistro sepimentato); studio anatomopatologico di tre case e contributo alla soluzione del problema patogenetico. *Arch Ital Anat E Istol Pat.* 1957;31:267.
34. Varcasia E, Patane E. Il considetto "cor triatriatum" (cuore con atrio sinistro sepimentato). Considerazioni cliniche su tre casi. *Cuore e Circol.* 1957;41:356.
35. Cottier H, Tobler W. Cor triatriatum sinister mit Stenose im anomalen Septum. *Cardiologia.* 1957;30:46.
36. Maxwell GM, Young WP, Rowe GG, Connors DM. Cor triatriatum. Report of a case with observations on surgery. *J Pediatr.* 1957;50:71.
37. Sawyer CG, Pool RS, Beck WC, Daniel LB. Cor triatriatum. *Am J Med.* 1957;23:798.
38. Latour H, Puech P, Roujon J. Coeur tri-atrial bi-auriculaire gauche. Bases du diagnostic. *Arch Mal Coeur Vaiss.* 1958;51:132.
39. Seavey PW, Dorney ER. Cor triatriatum. *Am Heart J.* 1958;55:272.
40. Keith JD, Rowe RD, Vlad P. Cor triatriatum (triatrial heart, stenosis of the common pulmonary vein). In: *Heart Disease in Infancy and Childhood.* New York: Macmillan Co; 1958:352.
41. Belcher JR, Somerville W. Cor triatriatum (stenosis of the common pulmonary vein). Successful treatment of a case. *Br Med J.* 1959;1:1280.
42. Gibbons JE, Jegier W, Murphy DR. Cor triatriatum: clinical, hemodynamic and autopsy studies and long-term observations after open surgical correction. *Circulation.* 1960;22:755 (abstract).
43. Therkelsen F. Fabricius J: Cor triatriatum. *Acta Chir Scand.* 1960;119:376.
44. Varonier HS. Le coeur triatrial. Aspect tératogénique et anatomo-clinique d'un nouveau cas avec revue de la littérature. *Pediatr Ann.* 1961;196:31.
45. Niwayama G. Cor triatriatum. *Am Heart J.* 1960;59:291.
46. Edwards JE. Stenosis of common pulmonary vein (cor triatriatum). In: Gould SE, ed. *Pathology of the Heart.* 2nd ed. Springfield: Thomas; 1960:484.
47. Gousios A, Cotton EK. Cor triatriatum associated with coarctation of the aorta. A report of a case and review of the literature. *AMA J Dis Child.* 1960;99:451.
48. Manubens R, Krovetz LJ, Adams P. Supravalvular stenosing ring of the left atrium. *Am Heart J.* 1960;60:286.
49. Redo SF, Goldberg HP. Surgical management of unusual cardiovascular anomalies. *Surg Clin N Amer.* 1961;41:417.
50. Darke CS, Emery JL, Lorber J. Triatrial heart. *Br Heart J.* 1961;23:329.
51. Abedrop E, Espino Vela J, Correa R. Estudio de un caso de corazon triauricular (cor triatriatum). *Arch Inst Cardiol Mex.* 1961;31:482.
52. Anderson RC, Varco RL. Cor triatriatum. Successful diagnosis and surgical correction in a three year old girl. *Am J Cardiol.* 1961;7:436.
53. Gialloreto OP, Vineberg A. A case of cor triatriatum studied five years after surgery. *Am J Cardiol.* 1962;9:598.

54. Magidson O. Cor triatriatum. Severe pulmonary arterial hypertension and pulmonary venous hypertension in a child. *Am J Cardiol.* 1962;9:603.
55. Lam CR, Green E, Drake E. Diagnosis and surgical correction of 2 types of triatrial heart. *Surgery.* 1962;51:127.
56. Slade PR, Tubbs OS, Wells BG. Cor triatriatum. A case successfully corrected by surgery. *Br Heart J.* 1962;24:233.
57. Grunebaum M, Yahini JH. Cor triatriatum sinistrum. *Israel Med J.* 1962;21:85.
58. James TN. Classification of triatrial hearts. *Anat Rec.* 1962;143:79.
59. Jegier W, Gibbons JE, Wiglesworth FW. Cor triatriatum: clinical, hemodynamic, and pathologic studies: surgical correction in early life. *Pediatrics.* 1963;31:255.
60. La Salle R, Ethier M, Stanley P, Davignon A. Cor triatriatum: report of a case, with emphasis on cineangiography. *Can Med Assoc J.* 1963;89:616.
61. Nadas AS. Cor triatriatum. In: *Pediatric Cardiology.* 2nd ed. Philadelphia: WB Saunders Co; 1963:592.
62. Sherman FE. Cor triatriatum. In: *An Atlas of Congenital Heart Disease.* Philadelphia: Lea and Febiger; 1963:42.
63. Lucas RV, Anderson RC, Amplatz K, Adams P, Edwards JE. Congenital causes of pulmonary venous obstruction. *Pediatr Clin N Amr.* 1963;10:781.
64. Papaioannou AC, Nihoyanopoulos J, Vlachos J. Cor triatriatum. Correlation of clinical and autopsy findings in 3 cases. *Am Heart J.* 1963;65:12.
65. Miller GHA, Ongley PA, Anderson MW, Kincaid OW, Swan HJC. Cor triatriatum. Hemodynamic and angiocardiographic diagnosis. *Am Heart J.* 1964;68:298.
66. McGuire LB, Nolan TB, Reeve R, Dammann JF. Cor triatriatum as a problem of adult heart disease. *Circulation.* 1965;31:263.
67. Guérin F, Poisson M. Le coeur triatrial. *Coeur Med Interne.* 1965;4:461.
68. Gasul BM, Arcilla RA, Lev M. Cor triatriatum. In: *Heart Disease in Children, Diagnosis and Treatment.* Philadelphia: Lippincott Co; 1966:869.
69. Somerville J. Masked cor triatriatum. *Br Heart J.* 1966;28:55.
70. Beller B, Childers R, Eckner F, Duchelle R, Ranniger K, Rabinowitz M. Cor triatriatum in the adult complicated by mitral insufficiency and aortic dissection. *Am J Cardiol.* 1967;19:749.
71. Jorgensen CR, Ferlic RM, Varco RL, Lillehei CW, Eliot RS. Cor triatriatum. Review of the surgical aspects with a follow-up report on the first patient successfully treated with surgery. *Circulation.* 1967;36:101.
72. Perry LW, Scott LP, McClenathan JE. Cor triatriatum: preoperative diagnosis and successful surgical repair in a small infant. *J Pediatr.* 1967;71:840.
73. Keith JD, Rowe RD, Vlad P. Cor triatriatum (triatrial heart, stenosis of the common pulmonary vein). In: *Heart Disease in Infancy and Childhood.* 2nd ed. New York: Macmillan Co; 1967:527.
74. Ahn C, Hosier DM, Sirak HD. Cor triatriatum. A case report and review of other operative cases. *J Thorac Cardiovasc Surg.* 1968;56:177.
75. Wolfe RR, Ruttenberg HD, Desilets DT, Mulder DE. Cor triatriatum. Total correction in an infant. *J Thorac Cardiovasc Surg.* 1968;56:114.
76. Van Praagh R, Corsini I. Cor triatriatum: pathologic anatomy and a consideration of morphogenesis based on 13 postmortem cases and a study of normal development of the pulmonary vein and atrial septum in 83 human embryos. *Am Heart J.* 1969;78:379.
77. Van Praagh S, O'Sullivan J, Brili S, Van Praagh R. Juxtaposition of the morphologically right atrial appendage in solitus and inversus atria: a study of 35 postmortem cases. *Am Heart J.* 1996;132:382.
78. Brickman RD, Wilson L, Zuberbuhler JR, Bahnson HT. Cor triatriatum. Clinical presentation and operative treatment. *J Thorac Cardiovasc Surg.* 1970;60:523.
79. Wilson JW, Graham TP, Gehweiler JA, Canent RV. Cor triatriatum with intact subdividing diaphragm and partial anomalous pulmonary venous connection to the proximal left atrial chamber (an unreported type). *Pediatrics.* 1971;47:745.
80. Maítre MJ, Otero E, Quero Jiménez M, et al. "Cor triatriatum" (studio anatomoclínico). *Rev Esp Cardiol.* 1972;25:119.
81. Danielson GK, Feldt RH. Successful repair of coexisting cor triatriatum and tetralogy of Fallot. *J Thorac Cardiovasc Surg.* 1972;63:391.
82. Arrants JE, Riopel DA, Catalano PW. Cor triatriatum: preoperative diagnosis and successful surgical correction in a ten-week-old infant. *Chest.* 1973;63:1027.
83. Marin-Garcia J, Amplatz K, Moller JH, Tandon R, Edwards JE. Clinical pathologic conference. *Am Heart J.* 1974;87:238.
84. Nimura Y, Matsumoto M, Beppu S, Matsuo H, Sakakibara H, Abe H. Noninvasive preoperative diagnosis of cor triatriatum with ultrasonocardiotomogram and conventional echocardiogram. *Am Heart J.* 1974;88:240.
85. Gibson DG, Honey M, Lennox SC. Cor triatriatum. Diagnosis by echocardiography. *Br Heart J.* 1974;36:835.
86. Marín-García J, Tandon R, Lucas RV, Edwards JE. Cor triatriatum: study of 20 cases. *Am J Cardiol.* 1975;35:59.
87. Nudel DB, Kelley MJ, Hellenbrand WE, Barash P, Stansel HC, Berman MA. Cor triatriatum masked by complex congenital cardiac anomalies. *J Thorac Cardiovasc Surg.* 1976;72:644.
88. Moodie DS, Hagler DJ, Ritter DG. Cor triatriatum, echocardiographic findings. *Mayo Clin Proc.* 1976;51:289.
89. Jennings RB, Innes BJ. Subtotal cor triatriatum with left partial anomalous pulmonary venous return. Successful surgical repair in an infant. *J Thorac Cardiovasc Surg.* 1977;74:461.
90. Thilenius OG, Bharati S, Lev M. Subdivided left atrium: an expanded concept of cor triatriatum sinistrum. *Am J Cardiol.* 1976;37:743.
91. Gharagozloo F, Bulkley BH, Hutchins GM. A proposed pathogenesis of cor triatriatum: impingement of the left superior vena cava on the developing left atrium. *Am Heart J.* 1977;94:618.
92. Kachaner J, Fermont L, Ribierre M. Cor triatriatum in infancy. *Magyar Pediat.* 1978;12(suppl 4):27.
93. Bargeron LM. Pulmonary hypertension in an infant. *Pediatr Cardiol.* 1979;1:73.
94. Arciniegas E, Farooki ZQ, Hakimi M, Perry BL, Green EW. Surgical treatment of cor triatriatum. *Ann Thorac Surg.* 1981;32:571.
95. Khonsari S, Saunders PW, Lees MH, Starr A. Common pulmonary vein atresia. Importance of immediate recognition and surgical intervention. *J Thorac Cardiovasc Surg.* 1982;83:443.
96. Oglietti J, Cooley DA, Izquierdo JP, et al. Cor triatriatum: operative results in 25 patients. *Ann Thorac Surg.* 1983;35:415.
97. Schlüter M, Langenstein BA, Thier W, et al. Transesophageal two-dimensional echocardiography in the diagnosis of cor triatriatum in the adult. *J Am Coll Cardiol.* 1983;2:1011.
98. Fuster-Siebert M, Llorens R, Arcas-Meca R, Rubio-Alvarez J, Prieto-Galán F, Garciá-Bengochea JB. Cor triatriatum with mitral valve disease in adults. *Tex Heart Inst J.* 1982;9:363.

99. Hess J, Brenken U, Eygelaar A, Martins FM. Successful management of cor triatriatum associated with anomalous pulmonary/systemic venous connection in an infant. *Pediatr Cardiol.* 1982;2:319.
100. Jacobstein MD, Hirschfeld SS. Concealed left atrial membrane: pitfalls in the diagnosis of cor triatriatum and supravalvar mitral ring. *Am J Cardiol.* 1982;49:780.
101. Richardson JV, Doty DB, Siewers RD, Zuberbuhler JR. Cor triatriatum (subdivided left atrium). *J Thorac Cardiovasc Surg.* 1981;81:232.
102. Östman-Smith I, Silverman NH, Oldershaw P, Lincoln C, Shinebourne EA. Cor triatriatum sinistrum. Diagnostic features on cross sectional echocardiography. *Br Heart J.* 1984;51:211.
103. Lang D, Wagenvoort CA, Kupferschmid C, Kleihauer E. Cor triatriatum masked by primary pulmonary hypertension. *Pediatr Cardiol.* 1985;6:161.
104. Geggel RL, Fulton DR, Chernoff HL, Cleveland R, Hougen TJ. Cor triatriatum associated with partial anomalous pulmonary venous connection to the coronary sinus: echocardiography and angiocardiographic features. *Pediatr Cardiol.* 1987;8:279.
105. Lengyel M, Árvay A, Biro V. Two-dimensional echocardiographic diagnosis of cor triatriatum. *Am J Cardiol.* 1987;59:484.
106. Wolf WJ. Diagnostic features and pitfalls in the two-dimensional echocardiographic evaluation of a child with cor triatriatum. *Pediatr Cardiol.* 1986;6:211.
107. Starc TJ, Bierman FZ, Bowman FO, Steeg CN, Wang NK, Krongrad E. Pulmonary venous obstruction and atrioventricular canal anomalies: role of cor triatriatum and double outlet right atrium. *J Am Coll Cardiol.* 1987;9:830.
108. Rumancik WM, Hernanz-Schulman M, Rutkowski MM, et al. Magnetic resonance imaging of cor triatriatum. *Pediatr Cardiol.* 1988;9:149.
109. Mori K, Dohi T. Mitral and pulmonary vein blood flow patterns in cor triatriatum. *Am Heart J.* 1989;117:1167.
110. Leung W-H, Wong C-K, Lau C-P, Cheng C-H. Cor triatriatum masked by coexisting COPD in an adult. *Chest.* 1989;96:776.
111. Yamaguchi M, Nishikawa Y, Hosokawa Y, Ohashi H, Oshima Y, Tei T. Cor triatriatum, coarctation of the aorta, and ventricular septal defect: a rare, surgically correctable anomaly. *Ann Thorac Surg.* 1990;49:473.
112. Cooley DA, Murphy MC. Cor triatriatum and anomalous pulmonary venous return—an unusual case. *Tex Heart Inst J.* 1990;17:118.
113. Rodefeld MD, Brown JW, Heimansohn DA, et al. Cor triatriatum: clinical presentation and surgical results in 12 patients. *Ann Thorac Surg.* 1990;50:562.
114. Tanaka F, Itoh M, Esaki H, Isobe J, Inoue R. Asymptomatic cor triatriatum incidentally revealed by computed tomography. *Chest.* 1991;100:272.
115. Salomone G, Tiraboschi R, Bianchi T, Ferri F, Crippa M, Parenzan L. Cor triatriatum, clinical presentation and operative results. *J Thorac Cardiovasc Surg.* 1991;101:1088.
116. Bu'Lock FA, Murphy P, Martin RP. Double partitioning of the left atrium: a previously unreported echocardiographic finding in a case in which transesophageal echocardiography aided operative resection. *Br Heart J.* 1991;66:246.
117. Papagiannis J, Harrison JK, Hermiller JB, et al. Use of balloon occlusion to improve visualization of anomalous pulmonary venous return in an adult with cor triatriatum. *Cathet Cardiovasc Diagn.* 1992;25:323.
118. Hogue CW, Barzilai B, Forstot R, Shuman TA, Cox JL. Intraoperative echocardiographic diagnosis of previously unrecognized cor triatriatum. *Ann Thorac Surg.* 1992;54:562.
119. Al-Fadley F, Galal O, Wilson N, Aloufi S. Cor triatriatum associated with total anomalous pulmonary venous drainage in the setting of mitral atresia and a restrictive interatrial communication. *Pediatr Cardiol.* 1992;13:125.
120. Gheissari A, Malm JR, Bowman FO, Bierman FZ. Cor triatriatum sinistrum: one institution's 28-year experience. *Pediatr Cardiol.* 1992;13:85.
121. Horowitz MD, Zager W, Bilsker M, Perryman RA, Lowery MH. Cor triatriatum in adults. *Am Heart J.* 1993;126:472.
122. van Son JAM, Danielson GK, Schaff HV, et al. Cor triatriatum: diagnosis, operative approach, and late results. *Mayo Clin Proc.* 1993;68:854.
123. Kerensky RA, Bertolet BD, Epstein M. Late discovery of cor triatriatum as a result of unilateral pulmonary venous obstruction. *Am Heart J.* 1995;130:624.
124. Kerkar P, Vora A, Kulkarni H, Narula D, Goyal V, Dalvi B. Percutaneous balloon dilatation of cor triatriatum sinister. *Am Heart J.* 1996;132:888.
125. Ito M, Kikuchi S, Hachiro Y, Abe T. Congenital pulmonary vein stenosis associated with cor triatriatum. *Ann Thorac Surg.* 2001;71:722.
126. Niccoli G, Heck P, Banning AP. Cyanosis, cor triatriatum, and primum atrial septal defect in an adult. *Heart.* 2002;88:136.
127. Keeble W, Lundmark E, Dargie HJ. The paradoxical finding of mitral valve incompetence and cor triatriatum: a mechanism revealed? *Heart.* 2004;90:125.
128. Reese DB. Cor triatriatum. *N Engl J Med.* 2004;350:1989.
129. Van Praagh R, Van Praagh S. Persistent fifth arterial arch in man: congenital double-lumen aortic arch. *Am J Cardiol.* 1969;24:279.
130. Quero M. Coexistence of single ventricle with atresia of one atrioventricular orifice. *Circulation.* 1972;46:794.

Cor Triatriatum Dextrum

131. Runcie J. A complicated case of cor triatriatum dexter. *Br Heart J.* 1968;30:729.
132. Verel D, Pilcher J, Hynes DM. Cor triatriatum dexter. *Br Heart J.* 1970;32:714.
133. Gussenhoven WJ, Essed CE, Bos E. Persistent right sinus venosus valve. *Br Heart J.* 1982;47:183.
134. Mazzucco A, Bortolotti U, Gallucci V, Del Torso S, Pellegrino P. Successful repair of symptomatic cor triatriatum dexter in infancy. *J Thorac Cardiovasc Surg.* 1983;85:140.
135. Trakhtenbroit A, Majid P, Rokey R. Cor triatriatum dexter: antemortem diagnosis in an adult by cross sectional echocardiography. *Br Heart J.* 1990;63:314.
136. Raffa H, Al-Ibrahim K, Taher Kayali M, Sorefan AA, Rustom M. Central cyanosis due to prominence of the Eustachian and Thebesian valves. *Ann Thorac Surg.* 1992;54:159.
137. Kauffman SL, Anderson DH. Persistent venous valves, maldevelopment of the right heart, and coronary artery-ventricular communications. *Am Heart J.* 1963;66:664.
138. Leo H. Über einen Fall von Entwicklungshemmung des Herzens. *Virchow Arch Path.* 1886;103:503.

9

Interatrial Communications

How common are interatrial communications—mostly the theostium secundum type of atrial septal defect and ostium primum type of atrial septal defect (Figs. 9.1 and 9.2)? Is atrial septal defect (ASD) a common and therefore statistically important problem, or is it a comparative rarity? As documented in Chapter 5, interatrial communications are the second most frequent anatomic type of congenital heart disease found in the present study (second only to ventricular septal defect [VSD]). The ostium secundum type of ASD occurred in 793 of 3216 autopsied cases of congenital heart disease (24.66%, 95% confidence interval 23.17% to 26.15%, Chapter 5, Table 5.1).

If one includes the incomplete form of common atrioventricular (AV) canal—the so-called ostium primum type of atrial defect, which is not really an ASD but rather an AV septal defect, but nonetheless is hemodynamically an interatrial communication—what does this do to our statistics? Several years ago, we tried to answer this question by analyzing all of our data up to that time (n = 2133, Table 9.1).

This more inclusive study (see Table 9.1) showed that interatrial communications (ASD II and ASD I) constituted 28% of our cardiac pathology database, again second only to VSD (36%), which was by far the most common form of congenital heart disease in our autopsy-proven experience.

It has been speculated by many that bicuspid aortic valve is really the most common form of congenital heart disease, a conclusion that our data do not support (11th in frequency, 8%; see Table 9.1). We suspect that this conclusion, which we think is erroneous, depends on the population that one studies and on the accuracy of one's diagnoses. Bicuspid aortic valve may well be the most common form of congenital heart disease in adults, whereas our data include some fetuses, many newborns, and many young children.

HOW MANY ANATOMIC TYPES OF INTERATRIAL COMMUNICATIONS ARE THERE?

Our answer to this question is summarized in Table 9.2. Table 9.2 contains most, if not all, of the interatrial communications that are of clinical significance.

This chapter is concerned primarily with secundum ASDs because the other forms of interatrial communication have been considered in detail elsewhere: incomplete and complete forms of the common AV canal, Chapter 11; sinus venosus defects, Chapters 6 and 7; coronary sinus septal defects, Chapters 6 and 7; atrial septum primum malposition defect, Chapter 7; and biatrial connection of the superior vena cava, Chapters 6 and 7.

OSTIUM SECUNDUM TYPE OF ATRIAL SEPTAL DEFECT

What is an ostium secundum type of ASD? The short answer is an ASD that is strongly reminiscent of the embryonic ostium secundum.

Ostium secundum is the space above septum primum (see Fig. 9.1). Septum primum is the flap valve of the foramen ovale (see Fig. 9.1). In visceroatrial situs solitus, the ostium secundum lies above the septum primum and to the left of the superior limbic band of the septum secundum (see Figs. 9.1, 9.2, and 9.3).

The superior limbic band of septum secundum is the superior muscular interatrial plica or fold between the neighboring evaginations or outpouchings of the superior walls of the right and left atria (see Figs. 9.1 to 9.3).

An ostium secundum type of ASD (ASD II) typically is a defect that is centrally located in the atrial septum. Consequently, an ASD II is not confluent with the tricuspid and mitral valves, as is an ostium primum type of ASD (ASD I) (see Fig. 9.2, lower). (An ASD I is an incomplete form of common AV valve with an incomplete AV septal defect.) An ASD II is not confluent with the superior vena cava (SVC), as is the superior type of sinus venosus defect (see Fig. 9.2, *lower*).

We used to think that an ASD II was not confluent with the inferior vena cava (IVC), as can be the lower type of sinus venosus defect. We have since learned that the foregoing statement is entirely wrong:

1. An ASD II can be confluent with the IVC if there is a low defect in the septum primum, or if the septum primum is absent, often then called the common atrium (Fig. 9.4).
2. There is no such thing as the low or IVC type of sinus venosus defect; this concept is erroneous. There is no unroofing of the right pulmonary veins (RPVs) in the so-called low type of sinus venosus defect. There is no absence of a partition or wall between the right atrium (RA) and any other structure—except for the left atrium (LA)—and absence of the partition between the RA and LA is the definition of an ASD. So there is nothing special or distinctive about such an ASD, as there is in sinus venosus defects, because in the latter the RPVs are involved (unroofed).

To put this point another way, what in the past has been called the low type of sinus venosus defect—because it is confluent with the IVC—is in fact a low defect in the septum primum or absence of the septum primum (see Fig. 9.4), which is significantly different from a sinus venosus defect in which the RPVs are directly involved that is unroofed.

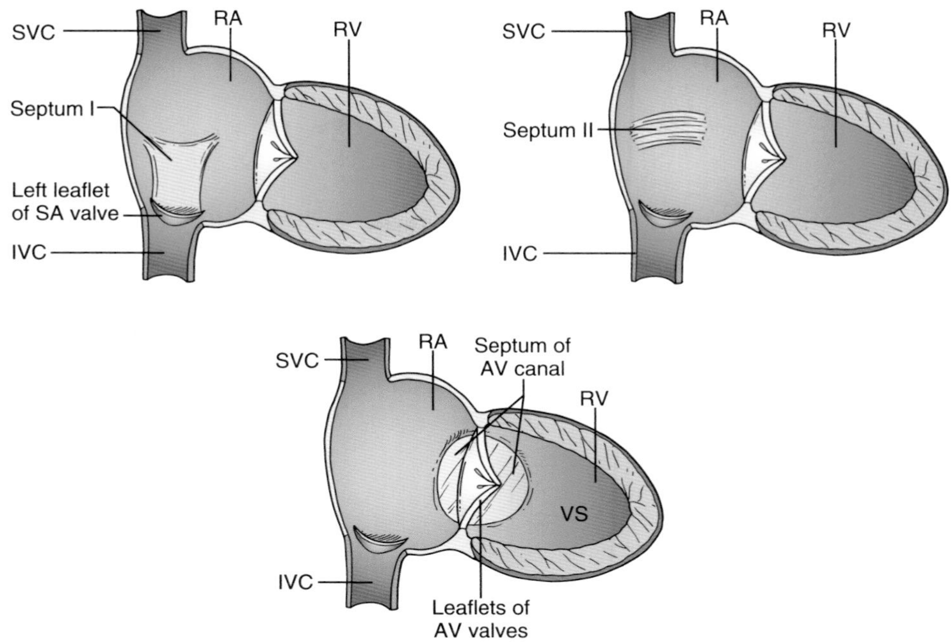

Fig. 9.1 The three main septa that make up the normal definitive interatrial septum: septum primum *(Septum I)*, the flap valve of the foramen ovale *(left upper)*; the superior limbic band of septum secundum *(Septum II)*, that forms the anterosuperior rim of the foramen ovale *(left lower)*; and the septum of the atrioventricular *(AV)* canal *(Septum of AV canal)*, that forms the anteroinferior portion of the interatrial septum and the posterior or inlet portion of the interventricular septum *(top right)*. *IVC,* Inferior vena cava; *RA,* morphologically right atrium; *RV,* morphologically right ventricle; *SA,* sinoatrial; *SVC,* superior vena cava; *VS,* ventricular septum. (From Van Praagh S, Van Praagh R. Atrial septal defects: Pathologic anatomy. In: Van Praagh R, Van Praagh S, eds. *Diagnostic and Surgical Pathology of Congenital Heart Disease.* Vol. 1. 1991;299-304. Syllabus of video series published by Health Video Dynamics. Washington, DC: Children's Hospital Boston, and Harvard Medical School, reproduced with permission.)

The foregoing distinctions are well seen echocardiographically (Fig. 9.5), as was pointed out to us by Dr. Stephen Sanders. Fig. 9.5 showed a subxiphoid long-axis view of the atria of a 4½-year-old boy. There is a large and low secundum ASD due to the absence of the septum primum. Note that this huge ASD II extends down to the Eustachian valve of the IVC, where the IVC enters the RA. Note that the RPVs are intact and connect only with the LA; that is, the RPVs are not unroofed. The partition between the RPVs and the RA is intact, as in all secundum ASDs.

The RPVs typically drain into the RA, even though the RPVs are not confluent with the RA. Such a large low ASD II that extends down to the Eustachian valve of the IVC is shown diagrammatically in Fig. 9.6.

To summarize, an ASD II can be confluent with the IVC, particularly if the ASD II is huge, resulting in a common atrium, and such an ASD that is confluent with the IVC is not a kind of sinus venosus defect. (For more information about sinus venosus defects, please see Chapters 6 and 7).

What, then, is an ASD II? It may result from the following:

1. The septum primum may be deficient, including one or more fenestrations within the septum primum (see Fig. 9.2, *lower,* and Figs. 9.7 to 9.9).[2] Deficiency of the septum primum, with or without fenestrations, is the most common cause of an ostium secundum type of ASD.
   In the normal heart (Fig. 9.10), the septum primum often is difficult to see well from the right atrial aspect (see Fig. 9.10A) but is often easier to see from the left atrial aspect (see Fig. 9.10B). However, when an ASD II is present, the deficient septum primum usually is more easily seen both from the right and left atrial perspectives (see Figs. 9.7 to 9.9), unless the septum primum is absent (see Figs. 9.4 to 9.6).
   It should be understood that ASDs are named in terms of *ostia,* not in terms of septa. Holes are named in terms of holes. Once this is appreciated, it is no longer confusing or apparently contradictory to say that the most common type of ASD II is due to deficiency of the septum primum.
2. The superior limbic band of the septum secundum can be deficient (with a well–developed septum primum), resulting in a secundum type of ASD. This is particularly common in association with the left-sided type of juxtaposition of the atrial appendages and with malposition of the septum primum[1] (Fig. 9.11).
3. Both the septum primum and septum secundum (superior limbic band) can be deficient, resulting in ASD II (see Figs. 9.2 and 9.11).
4. Rarely, neither the septum primum nor the septum secundum may be deficient, that is, the atrial septum may be normally formed. However, if there is a vein of Galen shunt in the head, resulting in a torrential left-to-right shunt, there can be a markedly increased systemic venous return down the SVC and into the heart. There can be a huge increase in the flow work of all cardiac chambers. The atria can be so

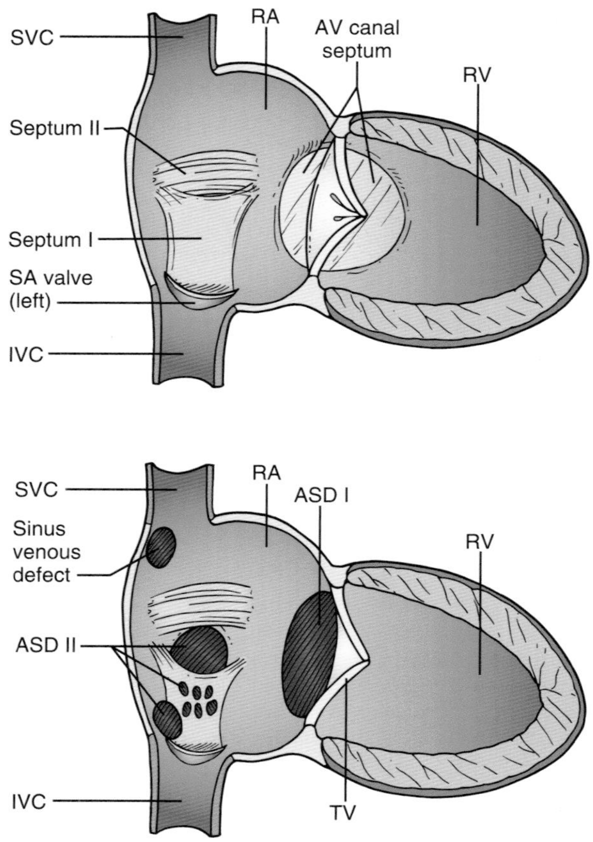

Fig. 9.2 **Anatomic Types of Interatrial Communication.** The *upper diagram* shows three fenestrations within an otherwise well-developed septum primum, resulting in one anatomic type of ostium secundum atrial septal defect (ASD). The *lower diagram* shows secundum ASDs *(ASD II),* an ostium primum type of atrial septum defect *(ASD I),* and a sinus venosus defect. The ASD II is formed by the combination of multiple defects within septum primum, plus underdevelopment of septum primum. Because septum primum is underdeveloped, there is a wide-open space above septum primum, that is, ostium secundum (the space above septum primum) is much larger than normal. Ostium secundum is the space that gives secundum ASDs their name. This underdeveloped and fenestrated septum primum results in multiple secundum ASDs: multiple fenestrations, plus an enlarged ostium secundum. This septum primum cannot occlude the central interatrial communication, thereby permitting a left-to-right atrial shunt. The superior limbic band (the upper rim) is not underdeveloped and does not contribute to the secundum ASD in this case. Only the upper sinus venosus defect (colored *black*) is a genuine sinus venosus defect, so-called. It is really the ostium of the right upper and middle pulmonary veins entering the left atrium. This right upper and middle pulmonary venous ostium entering the left atrium is visible from the right atrial side because the partition that normally separates the right superior vena cava *(SVC)* anteriorly from the right upper and middle pulmonary veins posteriorly is absent; that is, the right upper and middle pulmonary veins are "unroofed."[364] The sinus venous defect is really a sinopulmonary venous defect or window. Sinus venosus defect is not in fact an atrial septal defect; instead, this is a normal opening (not a defect) behind and above the atrial septum, which one can see from the right atrial side because the partition that normally hides the right upper and middle pulmonary veins is absent. The lower defect (in *black*) is another large, low, posterior secundum ASD, not a low or inferior vena caval *(IVC)* type of sinus venosus defect, as used to be thought. No unroofing of normally connected right pulmonary veins is involved. The ostium primum type of atrial septal defect (ASD I) is an incomplete defect in the septum of the atrioventricular canal; briefly, an incomplete atrioventricular *(AV)* septal defect. Why incomplete? Because there is no septal defect or hole below the leaflets of the tricuspid valve and mitral valve. Do these diagrams show all of the anatomic types of interatrial communication? No. Omissions include coronary sinus septal defect, that is, "unroofing" of the coronary sinus; and displacement of septum primum into the left atrium, or into the right atrium *(RA). RV,* Right ventricle; *SA,* sinoatrial. (From Van Praagh S, Van Praagh R. Atrial septal defects: Pathologic anatomy. In: Van Praagh R, Van Praagh S, eds. *Diagnostic and Surgical Pathology of Congenital Heart Disease.* Vol. 1. 1991;299-304. Syllabus of video series published by Health Video Dynamics. Washington, DC: Children's Hospital Boston, and Harvard Medical School, reproduced with permission.)

dilated and stretched that a normally formed atrial septum can have a valve-incompetent patent foramen ovale (PFO; SVC), resulting in left-to-right shunting through the central portion of the atrial septum, thus resulting in an ASD II. But when it is possible to occlude the vein of Galen arteriovenous malformation, the systemic venous return becomes normal and the heart shrinks back toward its normal size. Spontaneous closure of the ASD II may occur, because the atrial septum is intrinsically normally formed.

To summarize, an ASD II can result from deficiency of septum I, of septum II (superior limbic band), of both septum I and septum II, or rarely of neither septum I nor septum II (with marked atrial distention).

Why is deficiency of the superior limbic band of the septum secundum associated with juxtaposition of the atrial appendages?[1] When both atrial appendages lie to the left or to the right of the great arteries, the atrial appendages do not evaginate outward on either side of the vascular pedicle, as occurs

TABLE 9.1 Top 20 Types of Congenital Heart Disease (n = 2133)

Rank	Anomaly	No	%
1	Ventricular septal defect	765	36
2	**Interatrial communications***	**597**	**28**
3	Patent ductus arteriosus (>2 weeks)	409	19
4	Transposition of the great arteries	328	15
5	Tetralogy of Fallot	300	14
6	Aortic stenosis	246	12
7	Coarctation of the aorta	241	11
8	Persistent left superior vena cava	234	11
9	Pulmonary stenosis (excluding tetralogy of Fallot)	216	10
10	Completely common atrioventricular canal	179	8
11	Bicuspid aortic valve	170	8
12	Bicuspid pulmonary valve	162	8
13	Aortic atresia, valvar	153	7
14	Double-outlet right ventricle	149	7
15	Coronary arterial anomalies	146	7
16	Congenital mitral stenosis	136	6
17	Right aortic arch	133	6
17	Totally anomalous pulmonary venous connection	133	6
18	Aberrant right or left subclavian artery	117	5
18	Mitral atresia	117	5

*ASD II and ASD I (see Fig. 9.2).

TABLE 9.2 Anatomic Types of Interatrial Communications

1	Ostium secundum type of atrial septal defect
2	Ostium primum type of atrial septal defect, that is, incomplete form of common atrioventricular canal
3	Complete form of common atrioventricular canal
4	Sinus venosus defect, superior vena caval type and right atrial type
5	Coronary sinus septal defect, that is, partial or complete unroofing of the coronary sinus
6	Atrial septum primum malposition defect
7	Bilateral connection of the superior vena cava

normally. The great arteries normally act as a fixed point, on either side of which the atrial appendages expand. In the normal heart, immediately behind the aorta is the superior limbic band of septum secundum. Constrained or held in by the normally located aorta, the superior limbic band of septum secundum forms quite a tight arch with a short radius. The result is a relatively small interatrial communication that the septum primum (the flap valve of the foramen ovale) can occlude.

Not so with the left-sided juxtaposition of the atrial appendages (JAA) (see Fig. 9.11). Because both appendages typically lie to the left of the great arteries, the vascular pedicle does not constrain the superior limbic band of the septum secundum, which then forms a larger arc with a larger radius than normal. As a result, the interatrial communication is larger than normal. A normal-sized septum primum then cannot occlude the interatrial foramen. An ASD II results, which may be due predominantly or entirely to a poorly formed superior limbic band of septum secundum. However, the septum primum also can be deficient in association with JAA, that is, both factors—deficiency of the septum secundum and septum primum—can coexist (see Fig. 9.11).[1]

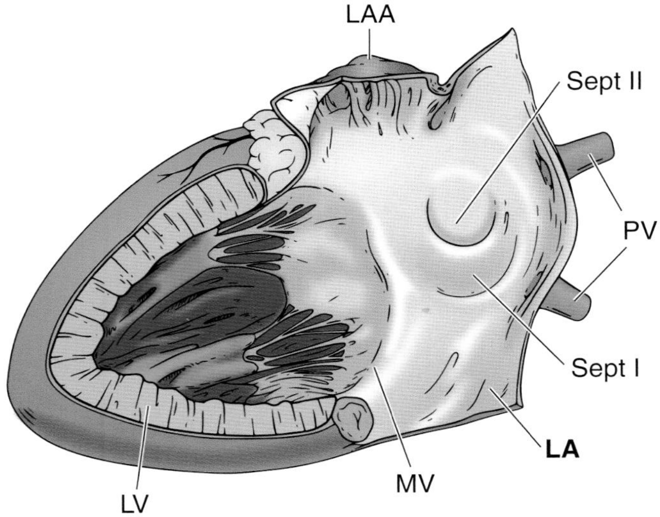

Fig. 9.3 Interior of Normal Morphologically Left Atrium. Septum primum (sept I), the flap valve of the foramen ovale (if patent) or fossa ovalis (if closed), is seen on the left atrial septal surface. The superior limbic band of septum secundum (sept II) lies to the right of the septum primum in atrial situs solitus, sept II being the anterosuperior rim of the foramen ovale or fossa ovalis. The concave upper margin of septum primum faces superiorly and slightly anteriorly when the heart specimen is oriented normally, with the left atrium *(LA)* posterior and slightly superior relative to the left ventricle *(LV)*—as in the fetus or young child (the horizontal heart position). Septum primum is oriented like a sailor's hammock. The space above septum primum is ostium secundum. Normally, the monocusp valve (sept I) and its "ring" (sept II) occlude the interatrial communication (the foramen ovale). The foramen ovale is the interatrial oval foramen with right-to-left length that extends from beneath the superior concavity of sept II on the right to above the inferior concavity of sept I on the left. *IVC,* Inferior vena cava; *LAA,* left atrial appendage; *PV,* pulmonary veins. (From Van Praagh R, Vlad P. Dextrocardia, mesocardia, and levocardia: The segmental approach to diagnosis in congenital heart disease. In: Keith JD, Rowe RD, Vlad P, eds. *Heart Disease in Infancy and Childhood.* New York, NY: MacMillan; 1978:638.)

ASD II is significantly more frequent with JAA than without JAA. In 42 autopsied patients with JAA, a secundum type of ASD was present in 30 (71%), whereas in 100 autopsied cases of transposition of the great arteries (TGA) (JAA) without JAA, a secundum type of ASD was found in "only" 23 (23%), this being a statistically highly significant difference ($p < .001$) ($\chi^2 = 29.46$).[1]

Are there other anomalies, in addition to JAA, in which abnormality of septum secundum (Sept II, i.e., the superior limbic band) may predispose to an ostium secundum type of ASD? Yes. In visceral heterotaxy with polysplenia (the polysplenia syndrome), the septum primum may be seen with unusual ease and clarity from the *right* atrial view—because the superior limbic band of septum secundum often is poorly formed or absent. Thus, in the polysplenia syndrome, the septum primum may be easily seen both from the RA and from the LA,[3] which is not normal (see Fig. 9.10). Deficiency of the superior limbic band of septum secundum may be associated with displacement of the septum primum into the LA, resulting in partially or totally anomalous pulmonary venous

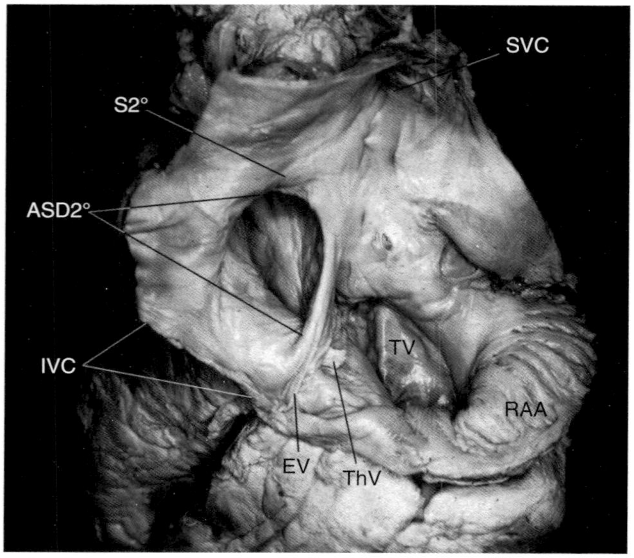

Fig. 9.4 **Huge Secundum Atrial Septal Defect *(ASD 2°)* Caused by Absence of Septum Primum, Also Known as Common Atrium (Case 395).** Right atrial view. Note that the huge secundum ASD is confluent with the inferior vena cava *(IVC)*. But this is *not* a sinus venosus defect of the IVC type, which is an erroneous concept; no right pulmonary veins are unroofed, and there is no anomalous right pulmonary venous drainage, both of which occur with typical sinus venosus defects. Thus, secundum ASDs are not always in the central portion of the atrial septum only; they can be confluent with the IVC because septum primum normally grows upward from the IVC, and if septum primum is deficient posteroinferiorly, the secundum ASD can be confluent with the IVC, as in this patient. This large secundum ASD is seen from the left atrial perspective. This 35-year-old woman died unoperated in 1982. Early misdiagnoses included functional murmur or mild valvar pulmonary stenosis. At 16 years of age, the diagnosis of secundum ASD was made and closure was advised. A second opinion was that surgery was not indicated, a course that the patient chose to follow. In her late 20s, she experienced chest tightness and shortness of breath. Slight cyanosis of the mucous membranes was noted, her systemic arterial saturation being 93%. Subsequently, angina-like chest pain occurred with decreasing exercise tolerance. Cyanosis with a slowly increasing hematocrit occurred. Severe pulmonary vascular obstruction (PVO) was diagnosed. The Eisenmenger syndrome with right-to-left atrial shunt was present. Shortly before death, severe persistent left-sided localized headache developed. Sudden death occurred, thought secondary to ventricular tachyarrhythmia. Autopsy revealed a left frontal brain abscess, right atrial and right ventricular hypertrophy and enlargement, and severe PVO (Heath-Edwards grade 5). This is a classic example of the natural history of a large secundum ASD. *EV,* Eustachian valve of the inferior vena cava; *LAA,* left atrial appendage; *LPVs,* left pulmonary veins; *RAA,* right atrial appendage; *RLPV,* right lower pulmonary vein; *S2°,* superior limbic band of septum secundum; *SVC,* superior vena cava; *ThV,* Thebesian valve of the coronary sinus; *TV,* tricuspid valve.

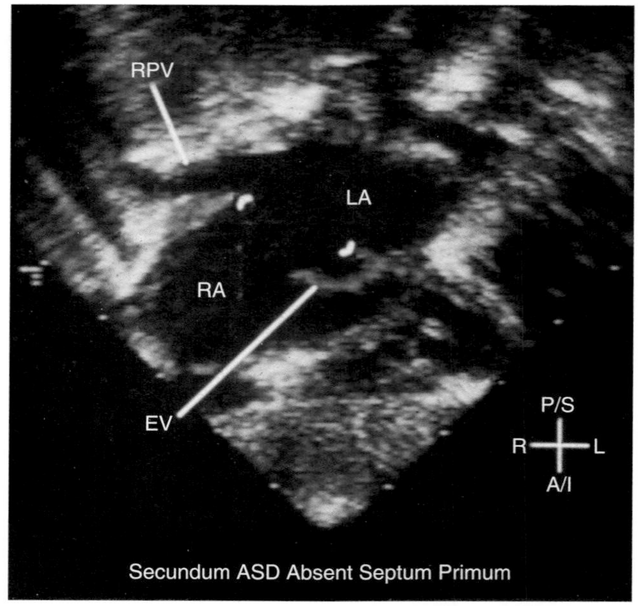

Fig. 9.5 **Two-Dimensional Echocardiogram, Subxiphoid Long-Axis View, of a Huge Low Secundum Atrial Septal Defect *(ASD)* in a 4½-Year-Old Boy.** The ASD extends down to the Eustachian valve *(EV)* of the inferior vena cava because septum primum was absent (as in Fig. 9.4). *A/I,* anteroinferior; *L,* Left; *LA,* left atrium; *P/S,* posterosuperior; *R,* right; *RA,* right atrium; *RPV,* right pulmonary vein. (Echocardiogram courtesy Stephen Sanders, MD, Boston Children's Hospital.)

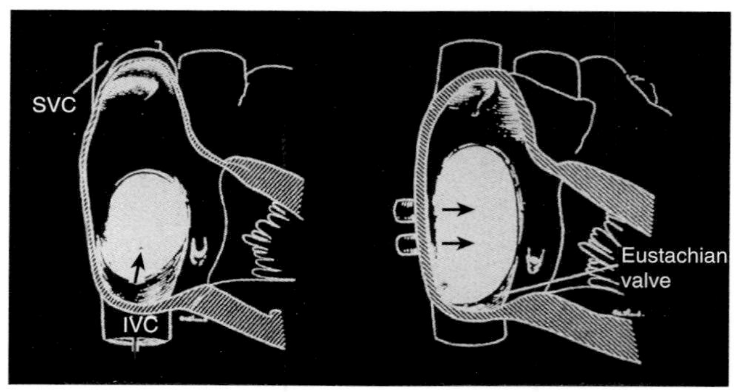

Fig. 9.6 **Diagram of Huge Secundum Atrial Septal Defect Due to Absence of Septum Primum, Right Atrial View.** The defect extends from the superior limbic band of septum secundum above to the inferior vena cava *(IVC)* and its Eustachian valve below. The *right panel* showed that the right pulmonary venous return can drain through the large defect into the right atrium. *SVC,* Superior vena cava. The Thebesian valve of the coronary sinus and the tricuspid valve are also shown (unlabeled).

drainage into the RA and an obstructive supramitral membrane (the displaced septum primum).[3] The restrictively small space between the displaced septum primum and the posterior wall of the LA we called a *septum primum malposition defect*[3] (see Chapter 7).

Pentalogy of Fallot

Pentalogy of Fallot means tetralogy of Fallot (TOF) with a secundum type of ASD. *Pentalogy* means that five anomalies are present (*pente*, five, Greek), the four anomalies of the tetralogy of Fallot (pulmonary outflow tract obstruction [stenosis or atresia], subaortic VSD, overriding aorta, and right ventricular hypertrophy) plus an ASD II. Although found in the older literature, this diagnosis is not routinely used today.

How common is an ostium secundum type of ASD found in association with TOF? In an effort to answer this question, we did a study of 100 randomly selected postmortem cases from the 1980s and 1990s. An ostium secundum type of ASD was found in 35 of these 100 cases (35%). The ASD was so large as to be regarded as resulting in common atrium in 5 of these 35 patients. Thus, a very large defect (common atrium) occurred

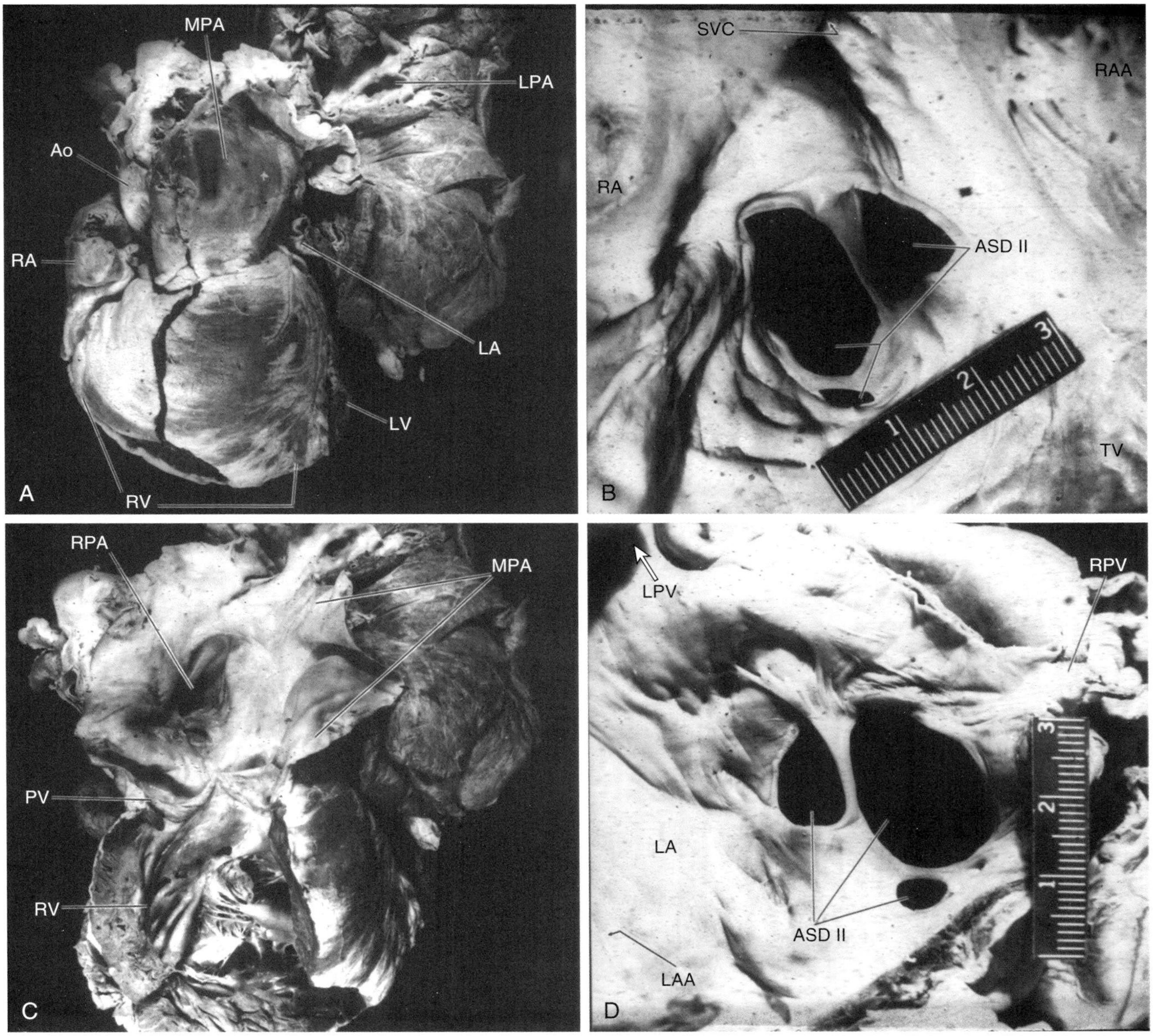

Fig. 9.7 The Heart, Lungs, and Atrial Septum of a 58-Year-Old Woman With Tetra-X Who Died of Multiple Secundum Atrial Septal Defects *(ASD II)*.[2] (A) External frontal view of heart and lungs showing right atrium *(RA)*, left atrium *(LA)*, right ventricle *(RV)*, left ventricle *(LV)*, main pulmonary artery *(MPA)*, ascending aorta *(Ao)*, and left pulmonary artery *(LPA)*. The RA and RV are markedly hypertrophied and enlarged, and the MPA and branches are dilated. (B) The three secundum ASDs from the RA perspective. (C) The opened RV and MPA confirm the marked right ventricular hypertrophy and enlargement and the dilation of the MPA and branches. The right pulmonary artery *(RPA)* is unopened. Antemortem mural thrombi were found in both atria (chronic atrial fibrillation), and organized thromboemboli were present in two small branches of the RPA. (D) The defects shown from the left atrial side. Best seen from the left atrial perspective in D, one can see that septum primum—the flap valve of the foramen ovale—is both underdeveloped (hypoplastic) and fenestrated. The enlarged ostium secundum is the most anterosuperior of the three defects; it measures 13 × 8 mm. Within the septum primum, there are two defects or fenestrations: the large one measures 22 × 17 mm, and the small one just beneath it measures 6 × 3 mm. The sum of the larger dimension of these three defects is 41 mm; thus, a large atrial septal deficiency is present. This was the 21st reported case[2] of tetra-X, the oldest known up to that time (1979), the first studied at autopsy, and the first with documented congenital heart disease. This intellectually challenged woman (IQ of 50) developed congestive heart failure at 52 years of age that progressed inexorably. Autopsy revealed marked cardiomegaly (530/270 g). The pulmonary valve *(PV)* was bicuspid, calcified, and regurgitant. Pulmonary vascular obstructive changes were found histologically (Heath-Edwards grade 2). The brain was underweight (1050/1250 g), with a generalized deficiency of hemispheric white matter. *LAA*, Left atrial appendage; *LPV*, left pulmonary vein; *RAA*, right atrial appendage; *RPV*, right pulmonary vein; *SVC*, superior vena cava. (From Keane JF, McLennan JE, Chi JG, Monedjikova V, Vawter GF, Gilles FH, Van Praagh R. Congenital heart disease in a tetra-X woman. *Chest*. 1974;66:726, reproduced with permission.)

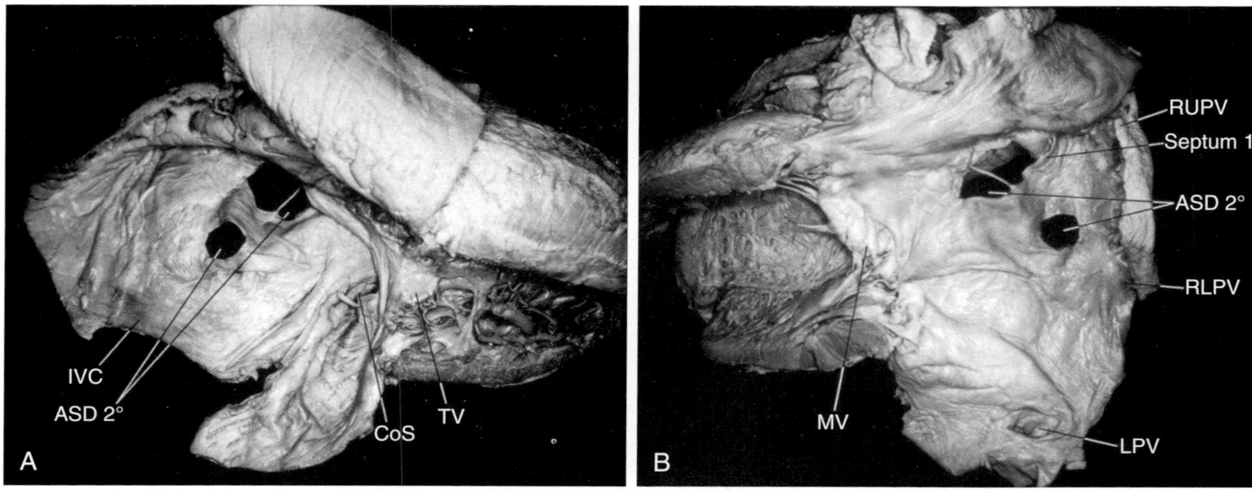

Fig. 9.8 The Heart of a 65-Year-Old Woman Who Died Because of a Large Unoperated Secundum Atrial Septal Defect *(ASD 2°)* (Case 621). (A) Interior of right atrium. (B) Interior of left atrium. The left atrial view is the best perspective for understanding secundum ASDs. Septum primum *(Septum 1°)*, the flap valve of the foramen ovale, is underdeveloped (hypoplastic). This is why the ostium secundum (the space above the upwardly pointing free margin of septum primum) is enlarged, resulting in a large ostium secundum type of atrial septal defect (32 × 15 mm). In addition, there is a large defect or fenestration within septum primum (18 × 7 mm), constituting a second secundum type of ASD. The sum of the maximal dimensions of these two defects is 50 mm, that is, a very large multiple secundum ASD. We can now examine the right atrial aspect of the atrial septum (in A) with full understanding. The larger anterosuperior defect is the enlarged ostium secundum, above the free margin of the underdeveloped septum primum. The smaller lower posteroinferior defect is the hole in the septum primum. Older patients such as this case are valuable because they illustrate the natural history[58] of a large unoccluded secundum ASD. The posterior leaflet of this patient's mitral valve *(MV)* was thickened, calcified, and prolapses into the left atrium (in B). Severe mitral regurgitation led to atrial fibrillation. She experienced hoarseness because of left atrial enlargement, with left vocal cord paralysis. Pulmonary hypertension and congestive heart failure were additional important sequelae of severe mitral regurgitation. The patient suffered a stroke two days before death because of thromboemboli that were thought probably to have arisen from the left atrium (secondary to atrial fibrillation, in turn secondary to mitral valve prolapse with severe mitral regurgitation). *Lesson:* Secundum ASD is often associated with significant acquired mitral valve pathologic findings, that in turn can have serious or fatal sequelae: mitral regurgitation, atrial fibrillation, pulmonary hypertension, congestive heart failure, systemic thromboembolism, stroke, and death. *CoS,* Coronary sinus; *IVC,* inferior vena cava; *LPV,* left pulmonary vein; *RLPV,* right lower pulmonary vein; *RUPV,* right upper pulmonary vein; *TV,* tricuspid valve.

in 14% of ASD II and in 5% of the series of tetralogy patients as a whole.

To summarize, pentalogy of Fallot occurred in approximately one-third of our autopsied cases of TOF (35%).

Common Atrium

Common atrium means, as the name indicates, that a very large ASD is present—so large that the atria are in common, that is, essentially undivided. Thus, the atrial septum is largely or totally absent.

There are **two main anatomic types of common atrium:**

1. with a divided AV canal (see Figs. 9.4 to 9.6), that is, with a separate mitral and tricuspid valve, the anterior leaflet of the mitral valve often being cleft, as in the Ellis-van Creveld syndrome (chrondoectodermal dysplasia, i.e., achondroplasia with defective development of skin, hair, and teeth; polydactyly; and defect cardiac septation in about 50%, autosomal recessive inheritance); and
2. with a common AV canal, that is, with a common AV valve and an AV septal defect (see Chapter 11). Dr. Jesse Edwards calls this type of common atrium "the forgotten type of common AV canal," in which there is an AV septal defect that typically is confluent with a large secundum type of ASD due to marked deficiency or absence of the components of the atrial septum. Thus, there are confluent secundum atrial and AV septal defects, resulting in a huge deficiency of cardiac septation.

Are there any other syndromes in which interatrial communications are characteristic? Yes. The heterotaxy syndrome with congenital asplenia, polysplenia, and right-sided but otherwise normally formed spleen spring to mind. Analysis of 95 postmortem cases of asplenia and 68 postmortem cases of polysplenia revealed the following findings (Table 9.3):

- A PFO or an intact atrial septum was much more common in the polysplenia syndrome (22%) than in the asplenia syndrome (2%) ($p < .001$) (see Table 9.3).
- An ASD II was somewhat more frequent with polysplenia (31%) than with asplenia (20%), but this difference was not statistically significant (see Table 9.3).
- An ASD I (incompletely common AV canal) was commoner with asplenia (23%) than with polysplenia (10%) ($p < .05$) (see Table 9.3).

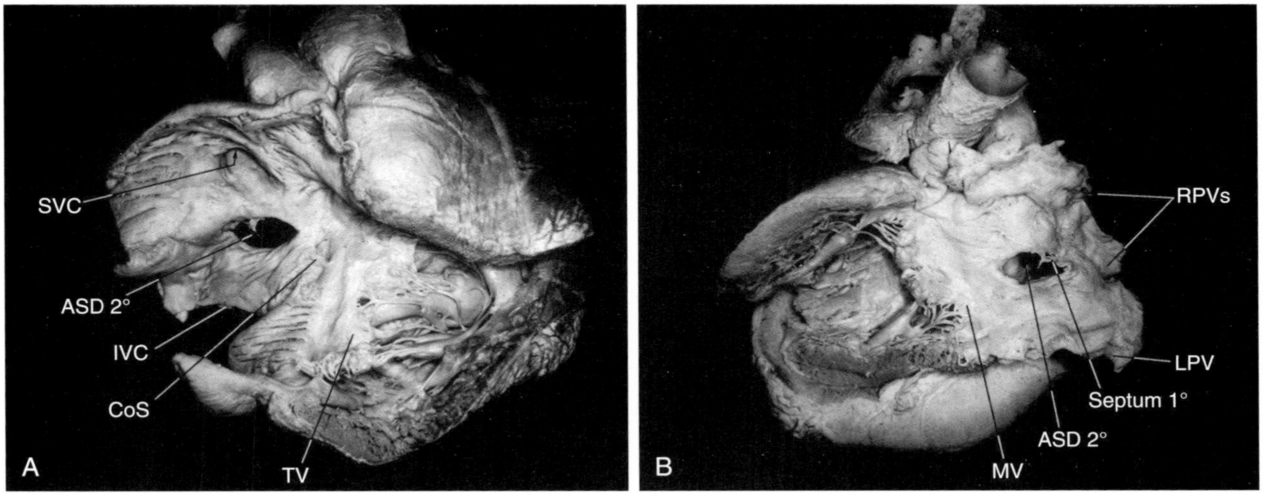

Fig. 9.9 This 1 3/12-year-old white boy with Down syndrome and a large secundum atrial septal defect (ASD) (Case 137) died in 1965 because of septicemia with meningitis (*Escherichia coli* and *Pneumococcus*) and bilateral adrenal hemorrhage (Waterhouse-Friderichsen–like syndrome, but not caused by meningococcus). (A) Right atrial view and (B) left atrial view of large secundum type of atrial septal defect *(ASD 2°)*. Septum primum *(Septum 1°)* is absent, except for a small strand of tissue seen posteriorly (in B). This trisomy 21 was a nondisjunctional mosaic. The patient also had agenesis of the gallbladder; hence this patient had mosaic trisomy 21 with multiple congenital anomalies (cardiovascular and gastrointestinal systems both involved, i.e., multisystem involvement). *Lessons:* Children with secundum ASD often have additional malformations, and they usually do not die from secundum ASD, even when it is large. *CoS,* Coronary sinus; *IVC,* inferior vena cava; *LPV,* left pulmonary vein; *MV,* mitral valve; *RPVs,* right pulmonary veins; *SVC,* superior vena cava; *TV,* tricuspid valve.

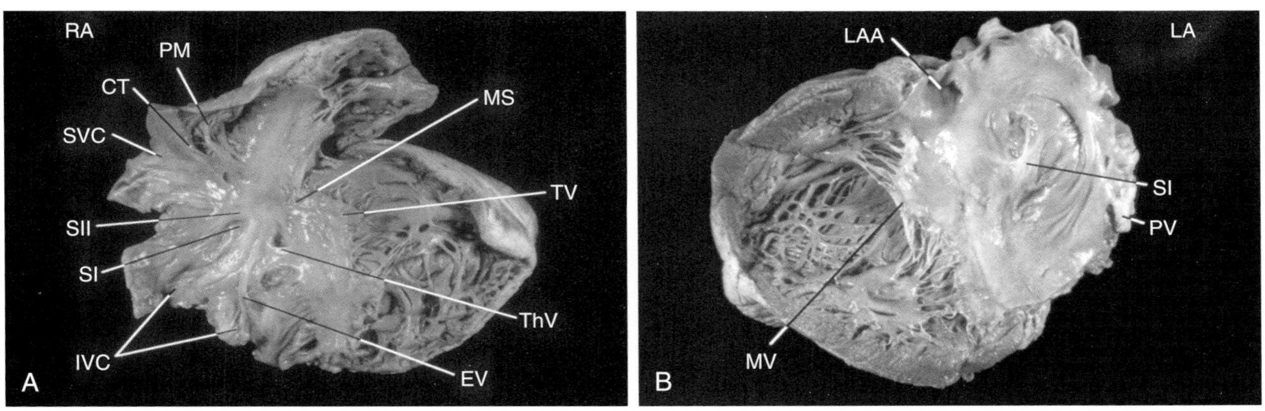

Fig. 9.10 (A) Normal morphologically right atrium *(RA)*. (B) Normal morphologically left atrium *(LA)*. (A) Note that septum primum *(SI)*—the flap valve of the foramen ovale—appears relatively small and inconspicuous. The morphology of the right atrial septal surface is dominated by septum secundum. The superior limbic band of septum secundum *(SII)* is well developed and prominent. The inferior limbic band (unlabeled) lies between septum primum posteriorly and the ostium of the coronary sinus and its Thebesian valve *(ThV)* and the Eustachian valve *(EV)* of the inferior vena cava *(IVC)* anteriorly. This is why it is often said that the RA displays septum secundum (superior and inferior limbic bands) on its septal surface, whereas the morphologically LA displays septum primum on its septal surface (in B). One can see septum primum from the RA side, and one can see septum secundum from the LA side. But the foregoing is nonetheless a useful generalization in terms of which septum—primum or secundum—is seen prominently on which septal surface. (B) Even when septum primum is fused with septum secundum, converting a foramen ovale (oval foramen) into a fossa ovals (oval fossa or depression—the right atrial appearance), nonetheless one can usually still discern septum primum and its concave, superiorly oriented upper margin. *CT,* Crista terminalis (terminal crest); *LAA,* left atrial appendage; *MS,* membranous septum; *MV,* mitral valve; *PM,* pectinate muscles; *PV,* pulmonary vein; *SVC,* superior vena cava; *TV,* tricuspid valve.

- Common atrium was much more frequent with asplenia (72%) than with polysplenia (32%) ($p < .001$) (see Table 9.3).
- Overall, visceral heterotaxy with asplenia had an interatrial communication more often (97.89%) than did visceral heterotaxy with polysplenia (77.94%) ($p < .001$) (see Table 9.3).

What about visceral heterotaxy with a normally formed but right-sided spleen? As discussed in Chapter 29, we know too little about this least frequent heterotaxy syndrome to make any statistically supported conclusions (n = 5). The data are as follows: PFO, 1 case (20%); ASD II, 1 case (20%); and common atrium, 3 cases (60%).

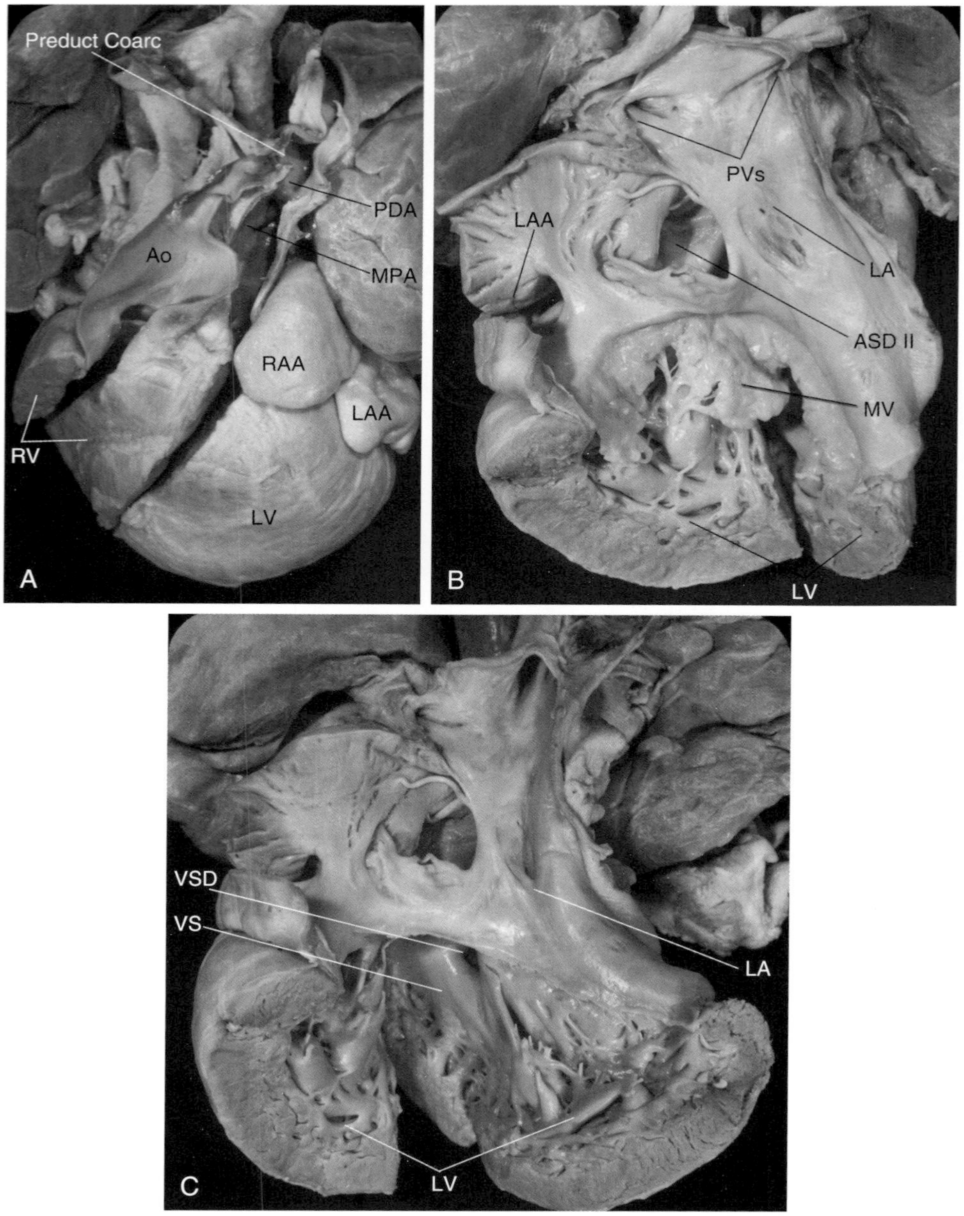

Fig. 9.11 The Heart and Lungs of a 9-Month-Old Boy With a Large Ostium Secundum Type of Atrial Septal Defect *(ASD II).* In addition, the patient had left juxtaposition of the atrial appendages, transposition of the great arteries (TGA) {S,D,D}, bilateral conus (subaortic and subpulmonary), muscular subaortic stenosis, preductal coarctation *(Preduct Coarc)* of the aorta, patent ductus arteriosus *(PDA),* thick-walled and small-chambered right ventricle *(RV)* and a conoventricular type of ventricular septal defect *(VSD)* between the conal septum above and the ventricular septum below, and a huge angle (130 degrees) between the atrial septum (60 degrees to the left of the Z axis or anteroposterior axis, projected on the horizontal plane) and the ventricular septum *(VS)* (70 degrees to the right of the Z axis, projected on the horizontal plane). (A) External frontal view. (B) Opened left atrium *(LA)* and left ventricular *(LV)* inflow tract. (C) Opened LA and LV, with mitral valve *(MV)* leaflets excised, in an effort to show the marked angulation of the VS relative to the atrial septum. The ventriculoatrial septal angle of 130 degrees is much greater than normal (median 6 degrees, mean 5 degrees ± 2 degrees, and range from 1 degree to 7 degrees).[365] (A) Note that the right atrial appendage *(RAA)* and the left atrial appendage *(LAA)* lie side by side (i.e., they are juxtaposed), both to the left of the D-transposed aorta *(Ao)* and the transposed main pulmonary artery *(MPA).* Hence, there is levomalposition of the RAA, resulting in juxtaposition of the atrial appendages. The ventricular apex (between the LV and the RV) points rightward. But dextrocardia was not apparent on the plain posteroanterior chest x-ray film, apparently because the RV was small-chambered, whereas the LV displayed marked hypertrophy and enlargement and bulged leftward. (B–C) The atrial septum is seen from the LA side. A very large ASD II is present, for two reasons: (1) septum primum (the flap valve of the foramen ovale) is almost totally absent, resulting in a very abnormally large ostium secundum (above the free margin of the vestigial septum primum). (2) Also, the superior limbic band of septum secundum is deficient, particularly superiorly. Juxtaposition of the atrial appendages (JAA) appears to predispose to underdevelopment of the superior limbic band of septum secundum (which is the "rim" of interventionist catheters, and the crista dividens of prenatal cardiovascular physiologists), apparently because the vascular pedicle (the aorta and the pulmonary artery) normally forms a fixed point or fulcrum, on either side of which the right and left atrial appendages evaginate outward, leaving a well-formed superior limbic band of septum secundum between the RAA and the LAA. But with JAA, the vascular pedicle does not lie between the RAA and the LAA. Consequently, the superior limbic band of septum secundum does not form as well; it does not form as small and tight an arc as occurs normally. Hence, the valve "ring" of the interatrial unicuspid flap valve (the foramen ovale) is larger than normal, predisposing to secundum ASD. In the study of 42 postmortem cases of JAA by Melhuish and Van Praagh,[1] the prevalence of ASD II was 71%, compared with a prevalence of 23% in a control series of 100 postmortem cases of TGA without JAA ($p < .001$). This patient has both of the main anatomic reasons for having a secundum ASD. (B–C) Deficiency of septum primum and deficiency of the superior limbic band of septum secundum. (From Melhuish BPP, Van Praagh R. Juxtaposition of the atrial appendages, a sign of severe cyanotic congenital heart disease. *Br Heart J.* 1968;30:269, reproduced with permission.)

TABLE 9.3 Atrial Septum in the Heterotaxy Syndromes

Atrial Septum	Asplenia (n = 95)	Polysplenia (n = 68)	*p* Value
1. PFO/intact	2 (2%)	15 (22%)	<.001
2. ASD II	19 (20%)	21 (31%)	NS
3. ASD I	22 (23%)	7 (10%)	<.05
4. Common atrium	68 (72%)	22 (32%)	<.001

NS, Not significant statistically; *PFO,* patent foramen ovale.

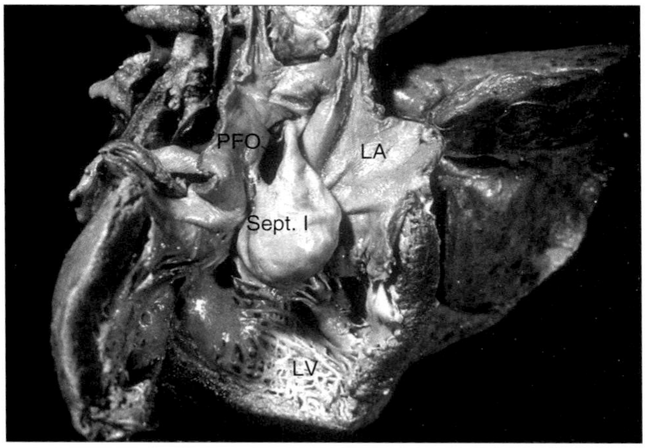

Fig. 9.12 This patient with transposition {S,D,D} and tricuspid atresia had a huge aneurysm of septum primum *(Sept I)* that bulged into the left atrium *(LA)* and then herniated downward and through the mitral valve into the left ventricular inflow tract, resulting in severe supramitral and intramitral stenosis. Why did this enormous aneurysm of septum primum occur? Our hypothesis is that septum primum was obstructive. Notice how relatively small and superior the ostium secundum is, that is, the space above the concave and superiorly oriented upper margin of the septum primum, between the anterior cornu (horn) and the posterior cornu, by which septum primum is attached to the left atrial aspect of the superior limbic band of septum secundum. Before this LA was opened, the small ostium secundum "opened" into the left atrial free wall, increasing the obstruction of the interatrial communication. Given the coexistence of tricuspid atresia, the prenatal right-to-left interatrial shunt was greater than normal. Note also that there were no fenestrations within this restrictive septum primum—which, had they been present, would have made septum primum less obstructive. This type of aneurysm of septum primum is often referred to in the literature as an atrial septal aneurysm (which it is). *PFO,* Patent foramen ovale.

Aneurysm of Septum Primum

When tricuspid atresia is associated with a PFO or a restrictive ostium secundum type of ASD, the septum primum can form a prominent aneurysm that bulges into the LA (Fig. 9.12). The aneurysm of the septum primum can form a supramitral stenosing membrane, or the aneurysm can prolapse downward into the mitral canal and into the left ventricular inlet (see Fig. 9.12), resulting in a rare form of congenital supramitral or intramitral stenosis. The septum primum appears to bulge progressively more markedly into the LA, below the ostium secundum, that is, below the superior concave rim of septum primum that delimits the so-called ostium secundum inferiorly. In advanced cases (see Fig. 9.12), the septum primum resembles a suspended bird's nest—like the nest of an oriole—that is, dangling from the anterior and posterior attachments of the septum primum to the left side of the superior limbic band of the septum. These attachments are called the anterior and posterior *horns* of the septum primum (see Fig. 9.12). The concavity of the septum primum aneurysm faces the RA and receives the thrust of right atrial systole into the concavity of the obstructive septum primum. The right atrial blood then appears to swirl upward, over the superior narrowed rim of the septum primum into the LA and then downward around the bulging convexity of the septum primum, through the obstructed mitral canal, and into the left ventricle (LV).

When there is congenital mitral atresia or severe stenosis, the septum primum can bulge in the opposite direction, into the RA. I cannot recall having seen an aneurysm of the septum primum that produced supratricuspid or intratricuspid obstruction. For reasons unknown, very impressive aneurysms of the septum primum have been associated with tricuspid atresia, as in Fig. 9.12, rather than with mitral atresia or the hypoplastic left heart syndrome (HLHS). Time may be the critical variable. Systemic venous obstruction may be better tolerated than pulmonary venous obstruction, allowing more time for the development of a leftward bulging aneurysm with tricuspid atresia than for a rightward bulging aneurysm with mitral atresia (speculation).

However, the ostium secundum type of ASD typically is associated with underdevelopment of the septum primum, with or without fenestrations of or within the septum primum. The septum primum typically is *regurgitant,* not obstructive. Prenatally, the flap valve function of the septum primum may permit significant regurgitation of blood from the left heart into the right heart, resulting in underdevelopment of the left heart, that is, **HLHS without mitral or aortic obstruction,** with overdevelopment of the right heart. We have seen patients treated surgically for the hypoplastic left heart syndrome, when the basic diagnosis was really ASD II with significant LA-to-RA regurgitation in utero and postnatally.

This is an important clinical lesson: An ASD II can manifest as HLHS. And the left heart *is* relatively hypoplastic compared with the right heart. How does one diagnostically recognize this type of HLHS? There is no stenosis or atresia at any left heart level, only hypoplasia (without dysplasia). In this type of HLHS, the basic diagnosis is ASD II with significant left-to-right regurgitation (shunting).

It is the blood of the *via sinistra* coming from the placenta up the IVC, past the right venous valve (Eustachian and Thebesian valves) to the right, past the left venous valve and septum primum to the left, and then about 60% of the IVC's blood stream goes over the concave top of the septum primum into the LA (Fig. 9.13).

This is the *via sinistra*—the left road (Latin)—of the oxygenated placental venous return that normally goes from the IVC into the left heart, and normally stays in the left heart, if the septum primum (the flap valve of the foramen ovale) is normal in form and function (essentially nonregurgitant). If the blood of the *via sinistra* then regurgitates out of the left heart, the result can be HLHS without mitral or aortic or other dysplasia ("pure" hypoplasia).

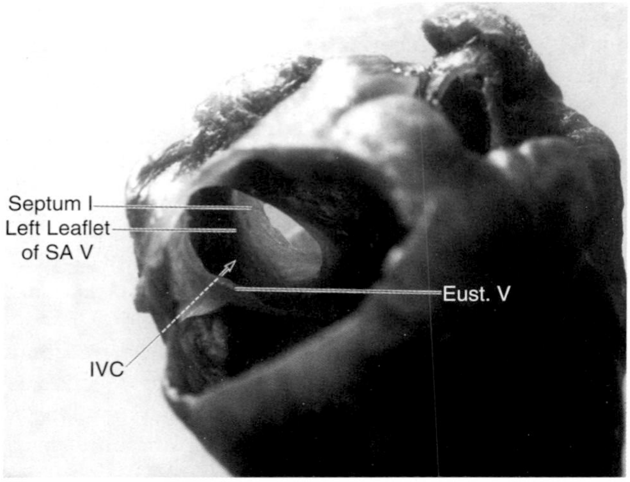

Fig. 9.13 View Through the Opened Right Atrium of a Newborn's Septum Primum (Septum I) Which Is Furthest to the Left. Slightly to the right, at the base of septum primum, is the left leaflet of the sinoatrial valve *(SA V)*, often called the left venous valve. Further to the right is the lumen of the inferior vena cava *(IVC)*. To the right of the IVC is the Eustachian valve *(Eust. V)*, which is the right leaflet of the SA V, often called the right venous valve. Thus, the left leaflet of the SA V is really bifid, consisting of two parts: septum primum and the left venous valve, which is normally vestigial. Septum primum is the largest venous valve in the body and is the main component of the bifid left venous valve mechanism. The largest venous valve in the body, the SA V, is not normally incompetent (regurgitant), as is commonly thought. Instead, because of the septum primum, the SA V is normally competent in the sense that it prevents regurgitation from left atrium to right atrium. But the SA V normally is incompetence between the right atrium and the venae cavae. Abnormally, the right venous valve can be very well developed, dividing the medial caval compartment from the more lateral appendage and tricuspid valve compartment, resulting in cor triatriatum dextrum. This is why the right venous valve is normally incompetent—so that it will not be obstructive.

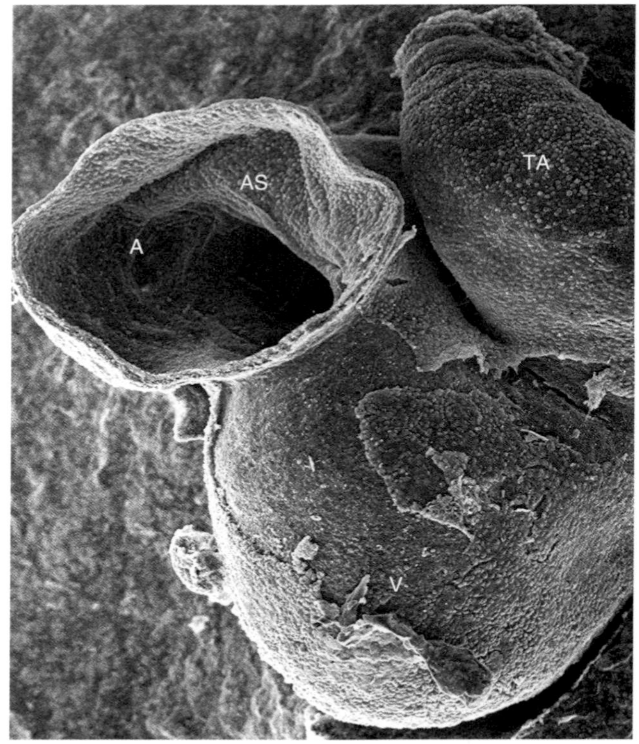

Fig. 9.14 Right Lateral View of a 3-Day-Old Embryonic Chick Heart (Hamilton-Hamburger Stage 18). The right lateral atrial wall has been removed, revealing a common (undivided) atrium *(A)*. The septum primum, the atrial septum *(AS)*, is seen cephalically and dorsally. Note that this early septum primum displays no fenestrations. The ventricle *(V)* and the truncus arteriosus *(TA)* are also seen. For correct spatial orientation, rotate this figure approximately 45 counterclockwise. The common atrium lies *behind* the ventricle, not above it. (Scanning electron micrograph ×190 by Mary Jessica Charles Hendrix in 1977, reproduced with permission from her PhD thesis, entitled *An Investigation of Atrial Septation in the Chick and Human Heart: An Electron and Light Microscopic Study*. Graduate School of Arts and Sciences, The George Washington University, Washington, DC.)

Hence, an important question for consideration is: Why can the septum primum be underdeveloped, and/or fenestrated, or absent? What is known about the development of the septum primum?

Embryology of Septum Primum

Where do all those fenestrations, holes, and deficiency in the growth of the septum primum come from that result in the great majority of ostium secundum ASDs (see Figs. 9.2, 9.4 to 9.9, and 9.11)? Is there anything known about the development of the septum primum that may make fenestrations and deficiency of the septum primum more readily understandable?

Yes indeed, there is. We were very well impressed by the Ph.D. thesis of Mary Jessica Charles Hendrix in 1977[4] that appears highly relevant to this question. In an electron and light microscopic study of the development of the atrial septum in the chick and in the human embryo, Hendrix found the following:

- In the chick embryo ("full term" or hatching in 21 days), at 3 days of age a common atrium is present. The beginnings of the septum primum (called the atrial septum) are present dorsally and cephalically, but without fenestrations in the septum primum (Fig. 9.14).[4]
- By the 4th day of incubation, fenestrations start to appear in the septum primum of the chick embryo (Fig. 9.15).[4]
- By the 5th day of gestation (incubation), multiple fenestrations have appeared in the septum primum of the chick embryo (Fig. 9.16).[4] If this were the heart of a postnatal human, we would certainly make the diagnosis of an ASD II due to multiple large fenestrations in septum primum.
- By 7 days of incubation, multiple large fenestrations are still present in the septum primum (Fig. 9.17).[4] The right venous valve is also fenestrated, forming a rete Chiari (to the right of the septum primum, unlabeled, see Fig. 9.17).[4]
- By 9 days of incubation, the septum primum is still so fenestrated in its mid-dorsal and dorsal portions that it resembles a coarse mesh of cords that are covered with endothelium (Fig. 9.18).[4] At this stage, the chick is 43% through its gestation.
- By 11 days of age, 52% of the way through gestation, the cords separating the fenestrations (foramina secunda of Hendrix) are becoming noticeably thicker, and the fenestrations are getting somewhat smaller (Fig. 9.19).[4]

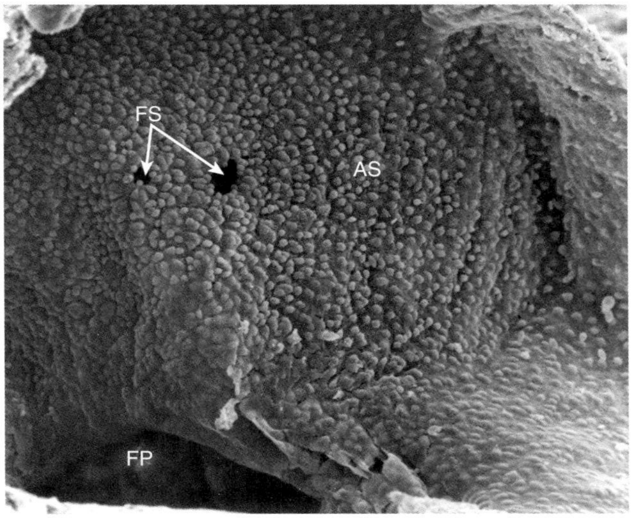

Fig. 9.15 Atrial Septum *(AS)*, That Is, Septum Primum, of a 4-Day-Old Chick Embryo (Stage 23), Left Atrial View. Fenestrations that Hendrix called foramina secundua *(FS)*, have appeared within the mid-dorsal portion of septum primum and averaged 9 microns (μ) in diameter. The interatrial communication at the anteroinferior free margin of septum primum *(FP)*, also known as ostium primum. For correct spatial orientation, rotate this figure 90 degrees clockwise. In the embryo, the ostium primum (FP) is in front of septum primum (AS), not below it. (Scanning electron micrograph ×625 by Mary Jessica Charles Hendrix in 1977, reproduced with permission from her PhD thesis, entitled *An Investigation of Atrial Septation in the Chick and Human Heart: An Electron and Light Microscopic Study*. Graduate School of Arts and Sciences, The George Washington University, Washington, DC.)

- The septum primum at 14½ days in the chick embryo is seen in Fig. 9.20. By 18½ days of gestation (88% of the way to "full term") the cords have become much thicker and the fenestrations are fewer and smaller (Fig. 9.21).
- By the time of hatching at 21 days gestation, the septum primum is normally essentially intact, with few or no remaining fenestrations (Fig. 9.22).

Comment. We thought that this careful study of the development of the septum primum (mostly in the chick embryo) was of considerable interest for several reasons. (Parenthetically, it should be understood that most chick embryologists think that there is no septum secundum in the chick; that is, the septum secundum does not grow down to help divide the atria. I agree with this viewpoint. One could also say the same of humans. The superior limbic band of the septum secundum does not grow down to help septate the atria in humans. Instead, the atria evaginate outward and upward on either side of the superior limbic band of septum secundum. So, when Hendrix[4] talks about the "atrial septum," she definitely is talking about the septum primum, not the septum secundum.)

1. The findings of Hendrix[4] strongly suggest that the presence of multiple fenestrations in the septum primum in humans may well represent the persistence of a normal earlier embryonic stage during which multiple fenestrations of the septum primum are normal.
2. Why this arrested development of the septum primum at the multiple fenestrations stage may occur in humans remains unknown, to the best of my knowledge.
3. Note that these multiple fenestrations do not normally persist and coalesce, thereby forming the ostium secundum, as in the conventional embryologic account. Instead, normally the cords that surround and separate the fenestrations become increasingly thicker until the fenestrations are obliterated. The ostium secundum is merely the space above the upper concave margin of the septum primum.
4. The septum primum grows not only in a superior direction from the IVC, but also in a ventral or anterior direction in its mid-dorsal portion, and also in an inferior direction in its cephalic portion (see Fig. 9.14). As viewed from the RA, the septum primum is shaped like a waning moon, convex dorsally and concave ventrally (see Fig. 9.14).
5. If, under pathologic circumstances, the multiple fenestrations within the septum primum do in fact coalescence and become confluent, the result would be large holes within the septum primum, resulting in a secundum type of ASD (see Figs. 9.2, 9.7-9.9, and 9.11).
6. If under pathologic circumstances, the septum primum becomes "hyperfenestrated" and if there is also very widespread coalescence of these fenestrations with dissolution of their delimiting cords, this could be the morphogenetic basis of absence of the septum primum, resulting in one anatomic type of common atrium (see Figs. 9.4 to 9.6). Another possibility is that, for reasons still unknown, the septum primum may never form in the first place. We cannot judge which of these logical possibilities is the more probable.
7. For the usual type of ASD II with multiple fenestrations or large holes in the septum primum, we think that the findings of Hendrix[4] support the hypothesis of **arrested development of the septum primum at the fenestration stage** as the probably morphogenetic basis of the most common form of secundum ASD in humans.

The Pathologic Anatomic Findings in 640 Human Cases of Secundum Atrial Septal Defect

In an effort to amplify our understanding of ASD II, a large study was undertaken of the records of 640 autopsied human patients from the Cardiac Registry of Children's Hospital Boston. All of these cardiac pathology examinations, description, and diagnoses were done by the author or by Stella Van Praagh, M.D., ably assisted over the years (1966 to 1996) by numerous excellent fellows. The heart specimens date from 1950 to 1996, inclusive. This study has not been published or presented previously.

Sex: Of these 640 patients, the sex was known in 631 (98.59%). In consultations, the patient's sex was sometimes not stated (in 9 of 640 cases, 1.4%). In these 631 patients with ASD II, there were 335 males (53%) and 296 females (47%), and the male-to-female ratio was 1.13:1.0. Thus, in this series of secundum ASD patients as a whole, there was a mild male preponderance.

Age at Death: In this series of 640 patients with ASD II, 1 case was excluded because happily this patient did not die.

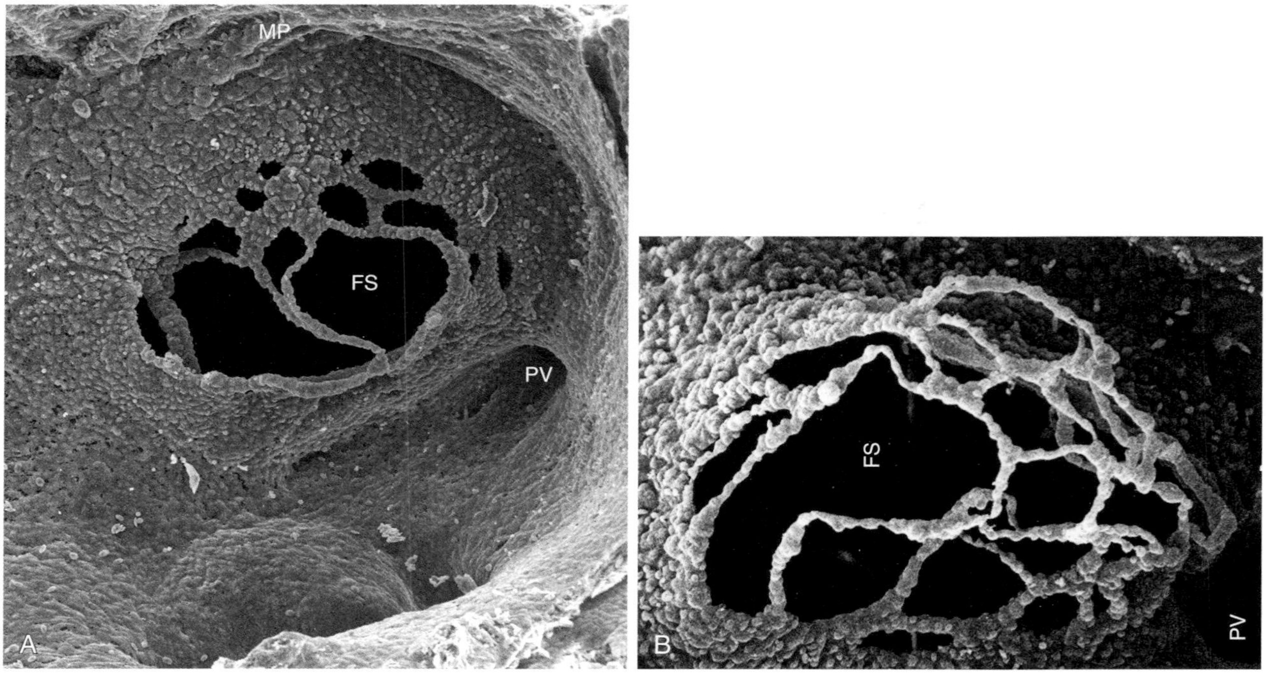

Fig. 9.16 Septum Primum of a 5-Day-Old Embryonic Chick Heart (Stage 28), Left Atrial View. (A) Fenestrations of septum primum *(FS)* are now much larger, but remain restricted to the mid-dorsal and dorsal portions of septum primum. Many minute fenestrations are also observed throughout the atrial septum. Musculi pectinati *(MP)* and the entrance of the pulmonary vein *(PV)* are also seen (×160). (B) Fenestrations of septum primum *(FS)* are even more striking in this 5½-day-old chick embryo. Fine strands of endocardium-covered septum primum separate these prominent fenestrations (×290). This figure has been rotated 90 degrees counterclockwise so that the pulmonary vein *(PV)* lies behind the fenestrated septum primum. (Scanning electron micrograph by Mary Jessica Charles Hendrix in 1977, reproduced with permission from her PhD thesis, entitled *An Investigation of Atrial Septation in the Chick and Human Heart: An Electron and Light Microscopic Study*. Graduate School of Arts and Sciences, The George Washington University, Washington, DC.)

Case number 637 (S94-2327) was a 10-year-old girl who had a Clamshell Septal Occluder Device that was explanted because of disarticulation and fracture of one right atrial arm of the device and a large right atrial thrombus associated with the right atrial umbrella. A 4-mm piece of metal was found to be sticking out of the right atrial umbrella. Also the left atrial umbrella had one unextended arm opposite the broken right atrial arm. The Clamshell device and the right atrial thrombus were removed uneventfully surgically and the secundum ASD was closed with a pericardial patch.

Of the 639 patients with secundum ASD who died, the age at death was known in 619 (97%). The mean age at death was 3.17 years. The standard deviation was ± 8.04 years. The age at death ranged from 65 years to 0 (stillbirths or fetal demises). The median age at death was 4 weeks and 5½ days, that is, 4.78 weeks, which may be rounded off to 5 weeks of age.

The median age at death (5 weeks of age) reflects much more accurately than does the mean age at death (3 years and 2.4 months of age) what really happened to these 619 patients with ASD II. The very young median age at death accurately indicates that these patients almost always had additional, more severe forms of congenital heart disease, as will be seen.

HOW IMPORTANT CLINICALLY WAS SECUNDUM ATRIAL SEPTAL DEFECT II?

Before this study, we were aware that from a statistical point of view, ASD II was the second most frequent form of congenital heart disease in our cardiac pathology database (see Table 9.1 and Chapter 5). In this sense, one might think that secundum ASD was the second most important form of congenital heart disease.

However, when one asks, **How often was secundum ASD the patient's most important clinical problem?**—the answer was very different. In our predominantly pediatric age group, we were surprised to find that ASD II was clinically the patient's most important form of disease in only 13 of these 640 patients (2.03%). A secundum ASD was an important *part* of the patient's clinical problem in an additional 8 patients (1.25%). Thus, a secundum ASD was the patient's main clinical problem or an important part of it in only 21 of these 640 patients with ASD II (3.28%). This means that some other form of disease was clinically more important than the secundum ASD in almost 97% of these patients. This finding emphasizes the importance of the distinction between statistical importance (frequency) on the one hand and clinical importance (main cause of morbidity and mortality) on the other.

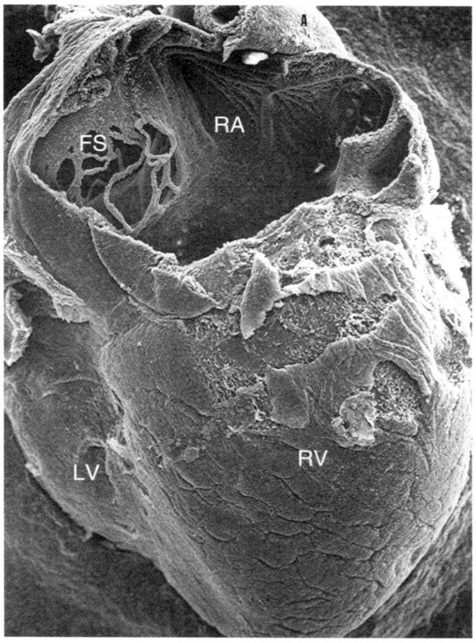

Fig. 9.17 The Atrial Septum of a 7-Day-Old Chick Embryo Heart (Stage 31), Right Posterolateral View (×125). The fenestrations in septum primum *(FS)* remain prominent in this right atrial *(RA)* view. The very fenestrated structure to the right of the fenestrated septum primum is either the left or the right venous valve (I am not sure which). Fenestration of the right or left venous valve (usually of the right venous valve) is the developmental basis of the **rete Chiari** or **Chiari's network,** when these fibrous strands persist into postnatal life and remain within the right atrium. In their development, venous valves fenestrate. Septum primum is the major leftward component of the left venous valve. The structure known as the left venous valve is the minor rightward component of the left venous valve mechanism which is bifid, having leftward (septum primum) and rightward (left venous valve) components. Here we see fenestration of both components, septum primum to the left (labeled FS) and venous valve to the right (unlabeled). For correct spatial orientation, rotate this figure about 45 degrees counterclockwise. *LV,* Left ventricle; *RV,* right ventricle. (Scanning electron micrograph by Mary Jessica Charles Hendrix in 1977, reproduced with permission from her PhD thesis, entitled *An Investigation of Atrial Septation in the Chick and Human Heart: An Electron and Light Microscopic Study.* Graduate School of Arts and Sciences, The George Washington University, Washington, DC.)

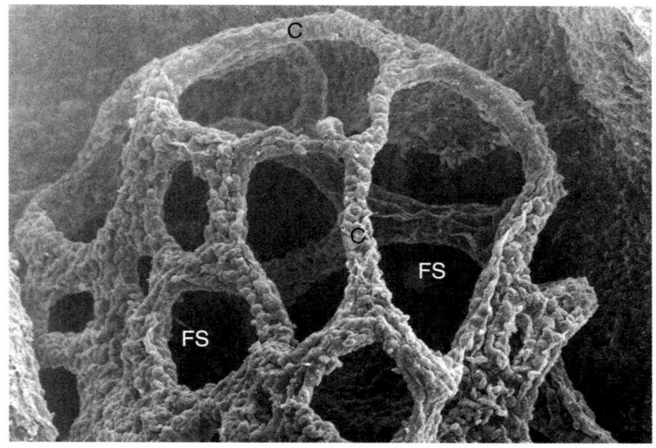

Fig. 9.18 Left Atrial View of Septum Primum During the Ninth Day of Cardiac Morphogenesis (×390). Note that the endocardium-covered cords *(C)* surrounding the fenestrations *(FS)* in septum primum are becoming coarser or thicker in appearance. (Scanning electron micrograph by Mary Jessica Charles Hendrix in 1977, reproduced with permission from her PhD thesis, entitled *An Investigation of Atrial Septation in the Chick and Human Heart: An Electron and Light Microscopic Study.* Graduate School of Arts and Sciences, The George Washington University, Washington, DC.)

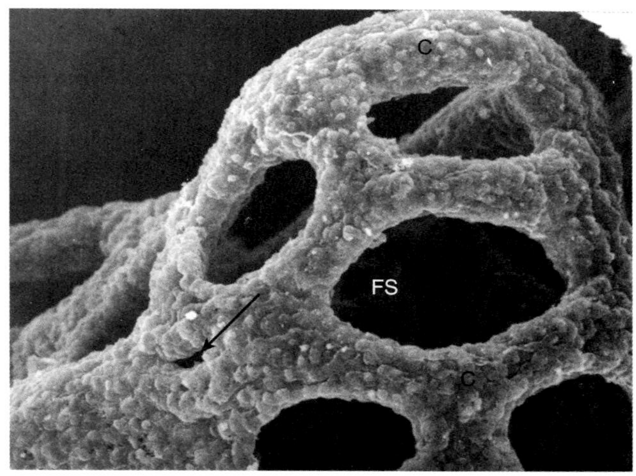

Fig. 9.19 Left Atrial View of an 11-Day-Old (Stage 37) Chick Embryo's Septum Primum (×410). The endothelium-covered cords *(C)* of septum primum are becoming thicker, averaging 38 μ in width. The fenestrations in septum primum *(FS)* average 175 μ in length and 100 μ in width. The *arrow* points at what appears to be nearly a perforation. (Scanning electron micrograph by Mary Jessica Charles Hendrix in 1977, reproduced with permission from her PhD thesis, entitled *An Investigation of Atrial Septation in the Chick and Human Heart: An Electron and Light Microscopic Study.* Graduate School of Arts and Sciences, The George Washington University, Washington, DC.)

Let us examine those patients in whom ASD II was the most important clinical problem.

When Secundum Atrial Septal Defect II Was the Most Important Clinical Problem

Sex: Male, 3 of 13 (23%); female, 10 (77%). The sex ratio was male-to-female = 3:10 (.3), or female-to-male = 10:3 (3.3/1.0). Hence, when ASD II was the main clinical problem, the expected female preponderance was found.

Age at Death: Of the 12 deceased patients (the Clamshell case, patient 637, did not die), the mean age at death was 25.39 years. The standard deviation was ± 18.14 years. The range was from 0.625 years (7½ months) to 65 years. The median age at death was 24.75 years.

These statistics concerning the age at death are very much older than those found for the series as a whole (see earlier), indicating that when a secundum ASD is the patient's main clinical problem, fatalities almost always occur in the young adult age group, not in the pediatric age range. This observation appears to explain why there are so few patients in our postmortem series in whom ASD II was the patient's primary clinical problem. Thus, secundum ASD is a "sleeper." It must be diagnosed accurately and treated effectively early in life, in order to avoid death in young adulthood.

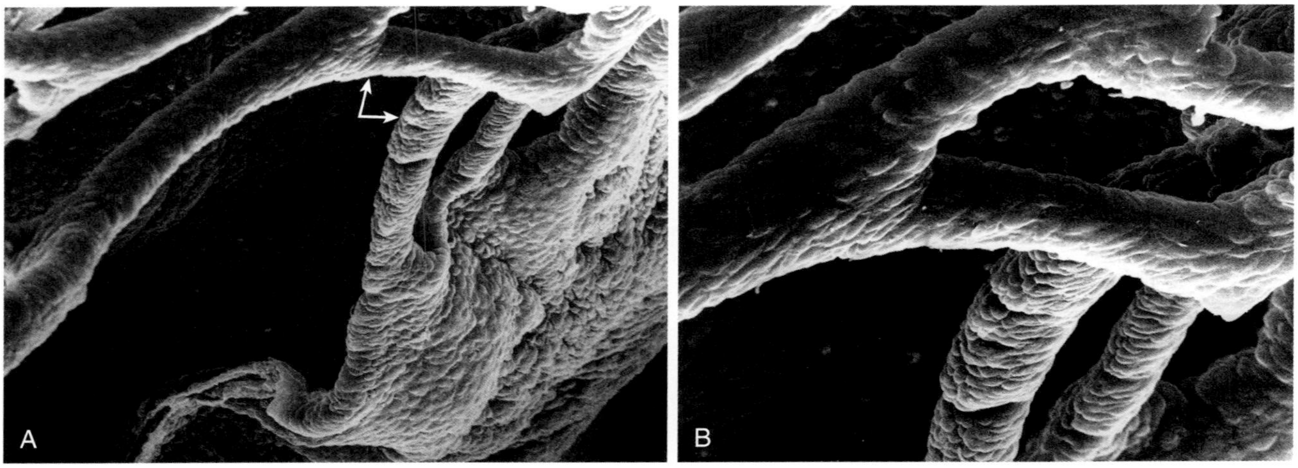

Fig. 9.20 **Left Atrial View of a Portion Of Septum Primum of a 14½-Day-Old Chick in Ovo (Stage 40+).** The endothelium-covered cords *(arrows)* surrounding the fenestrations in septum primum normally continue to thicken. (A, ×420, B, ×720.) (Electron micrograph by Mary Jessica Charles Hendrix in 1977, reproduced with permission from her PhD thesis, entitled *An Investigation of Atrial Septation in the Chick and Human Heart: An Electron and Light Microscopic Study.* Graduate School of Arts and Sciences, The George Washington University, Washington, DC.)

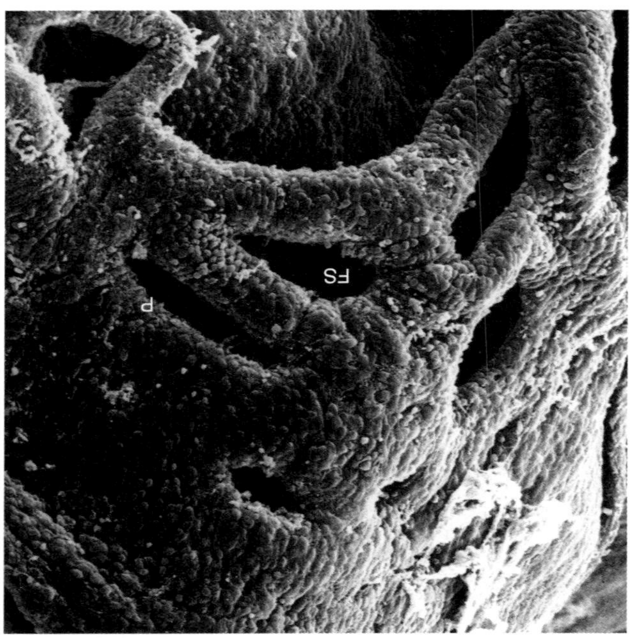

Fig. 9.21 By 18½ days of age in ovo (stage 44+), as this left atrial view of septum primum shows, the now very thick endothelium-covered cords surrounding the perforations *(FS)* are greatly reducing the size of these fenestrations (×290). This figure has been rotated through 180 degrees so that the superior free margin of septum primum will face cephalad. This is why the labels FS and *P* are upside-down. (Scanning electron micrograph by Mary Jessica Charles Hendrix in 1977, reproduced with permission from her PhD thesis, entitled *An Investigation of Atrial Septation in the Chick and Human Heart: An Electron and Light Microscopic Study.* Graduate School of Arts and Sciences, The George Washington University, Washington, DC.)

Salient Features: All 13 of these patients had *isolated* ASD II; that is, no other form of clinically significant congenital heart disease was present.

The ASD was *large* in 12 of 13 patients (92%) (Fig. 9.23). In one case, this assessment could not be made because the ASD had been surgically closed with direct sutures. Typically, the ASD was described as large, very large, or huge, with marked deficiency of the septum primum, resulting in a common atrium or almost a common atrium.

Death occurred *postoperatively* in 7 of these 13 patients (54%), early in our experience. We have not seen at autopsy a patient from our institution in whom ASD II was the primary clinical problem for the past 22 years, not since 1983.

However, we had one consultation in 1992 concerning a patient from another hospital (Case 579, C92-165). This patient was a 15 3/12-year-old young woman who had a very large ASD II. At 2 3/12 years, she underwent pericardial patch closure of her atrial defect. Postoperatively, she had sick sinus syndrome. At 10 9/12 years of age she received a pacemaker. Subsequently, she developed atrial fibrillation that spontaneously converted to normal sinus rhythm. Sudden unexpected death occurred 13 years postoperatively, in what appeared to be an arrhythmic demise. This case emphasizes the great importance of avoiding injury to the sinoatrial (SA) node and the SA nodal artery during atriotomy and atrial repair. Knowing exactly where these structures are located and taking care to avoid them (see Chapter 2) should make it possible to avoid sick sinus syndrome and its sequelae.

Pulmonary vascular obstructive disease (PVO) was very prominent in 4 of these patients. Right-to-left atrial shunting, polycythemia, cyanosis, clubbing, systemic embolization, stroke, and brain abscess all occurred.

Right-to-left shunting at any cardiac level (atrial, ventricular, or great arterial) is the *Eisenmenger reaction* of Dr. Paul Wood, who developed the Wood units in which pulmonary resistance is measured. The Eisenmenger reaction (right-to-left shunting because of elevated pulmonary vascular resistance) is not to be confused with the *Eisenmenger complex* (large subaortic VSD, aortic overriding, and right ventricular hypertrophy, but without pulmonary outflow tract obstruction

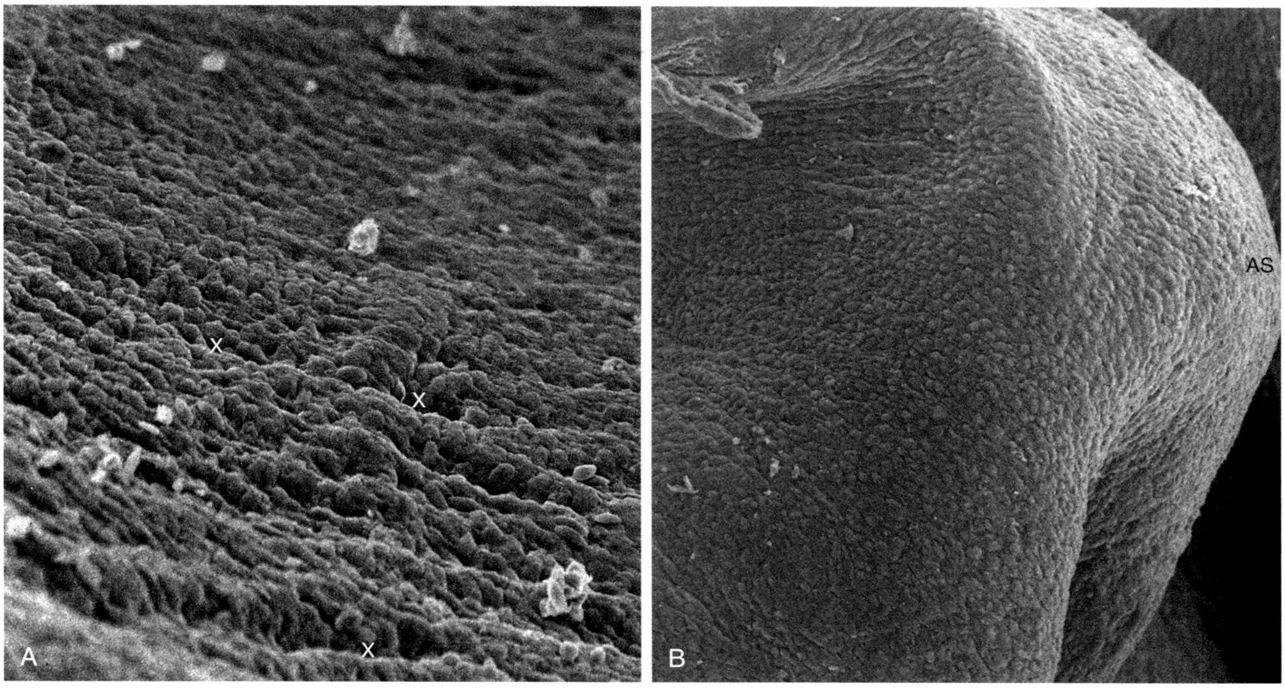

Fig. 9.22 The Chick Atrial Septum at Hatching, 21 Days Gestational Age (Stage 46), Left Atrial View of Septum Primum (×1200). (A) The depressions *(X)* in the septum were interpreted as being due to the unevenness of the fusing endocardium–covered cords that occluded the fenestrations or perforations in septum primum that are normal earlier morphologic features (see Figs. 9.15 to 9.21, inclusive). (B) By 2 days after hatching, the atrial septum *(AS)*, that is, septum primum, normally has a relatively smooth surface contour, as seen from the left atrium (×360). Thus, the appearance of multiple fenestrations in septum primum, that is part of the standard textbook account of atrial septation, turns out to be very important, not as the origin of ostium secundum, as the textbooks say. (Ostium secundum is merely the space above the concave superior free margin of septum primum). Abnormally, if they persist postnatally, these fenestrations or perforations of septum primum are by far the commonest anatomic type of secundum ASD. The standard textbook account of the embryology of atrial septation does not say anything about the gradual *disappearance* of these fenestrations in septum primum, so well documented by Hendrix. (Scanning electron micrograph by Mary Jessica Charles Hendrix in 1977, reproduced with permission from her PhD thesis, entitled *An Investigation of Atrial Septation in the Chick and Human Heart: An Electron and Light Microscopic Study*. Graduate School of Arts and Sciences, The George Washington University, Washington, DC.)

and hence distinct from TOF). Thus, late-stage ASD II typically displays the Eisenmenger reaction (but not the Eisenmenger complex).

When Atrial Septal Defect II Was an Important Part of the Patient's Main Clinical Problem

In 8 patients, the secundum ASD was an important part of the patient's main clinical problem (8/640 = 1.25%), but not the whole clinical problem.

Sex: Male, 1; females, 7; male-to-female ratio 1:7 (.14) or female-to-male ratio, 7:1 (7).

Age at Death: Mean, 15.99 years; standard deviation, ± 17.07 years; range, 5 weeks to 53 years; and median, 13 years.

Salient Features: All had large secundum ASD. *Rheumatic heart disease* had occurred in 2 of these 8 patients. One had chronic mitral regurgitation that distended the LA and enlarged the ASD II. The other had severe rheumatic mitral stenosis that had been treated (in the 1950s and 1960s) with old and recent mitral valvuloplasties. This 53-year-old woman had a large ASD II (20 mm in diameter) with a very deficient septum primum. This combination of findings—secundum ASD and mitral stenosis—is known as the **Lutembacher syndrome** (pronounced lootem-baker, i.e., in the German way), despite the fact that Rene Lutembacher (1884–1968) was a French physician from Paris who described this association in 1916, which was a very busy time in Paris.

A second patient had *mitral regurgitation*, but its cause (congenital or acquired) was not definitely established.

Down syndrome was present in 2 of these 8 patients with large secundum ASDs.

Multiple congenital anomalies (intellectual disability, hypospadias, hypoplastic penis, and cryptorchidism), *sepsis* (perirectal pelvic abscess related to *Escherichia coli* and *Aerobacter*, esophagitis, gastroenteritis, duodenal ulcers from which Monilia were cultured, tracheobronchitis, pulmonary edema, and bronchopneumonia), and *pulmonary hemorrhage* occurred in 1 patient each. Congestive heart failure and PVO were prominent in 3 patients each.

So, let us assume that most experienced observers know that ASD II can be the patient's primary clinical problem or that ASD II can be associated with other disease processes that together may constitute the patient's main clinical problem (as earlier).

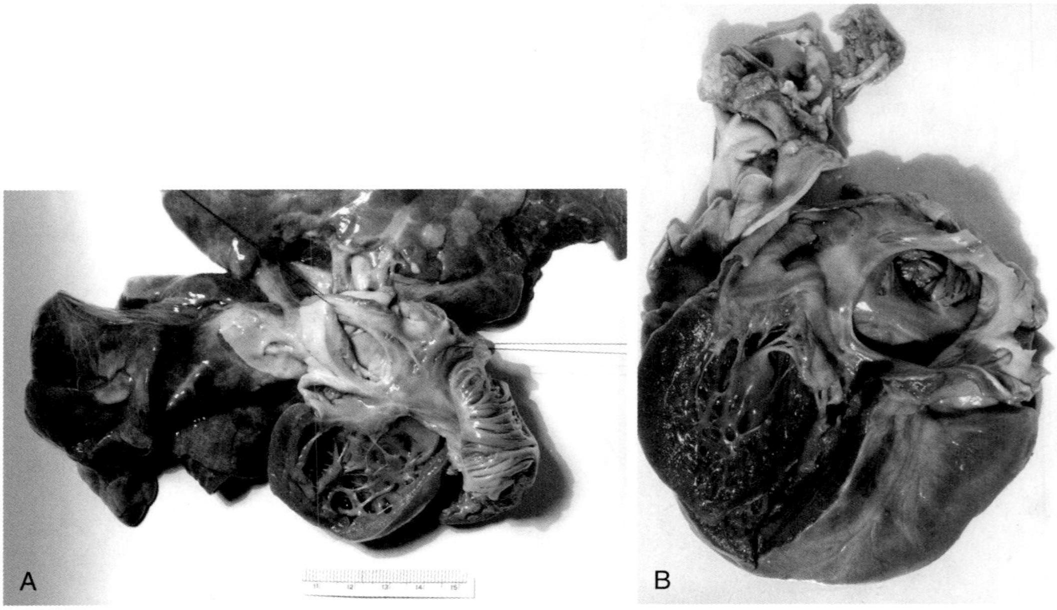

Fig. 9.23 Absence of Septum Primum Resulting in a Huge Ostium Secundum Type of Atrial Septal Defect. (A) Opened right atrium, tricuspid valve, and right ventricle of the heart of a 7½-month-old white boy with a very large secundum type of atrial septal defect (20 × 10 mm). Septum primum was absent. The patient had rapid respirations since birth (140/min). Dying in 1952 without cardiac surgery, he had severe pulmonary congestion and marked bilateral chronic pneumonitis. Thus, a large secundum atrial septal defect can cause death in infancy. (Photograph taken at the time of autopsy). (B) Opened left atrium, mitral valve, and left ventricle of a 13-year-old white girl who died in 1964 because of a huge, unoperated secundum atrial septal defect. Because of absence of septum primum, she had a common atrium with intractable congestive heart failure and ascites (500 cc). (Photograph taken at autopsy.)

But now we must consider a great unknown: What about the more than 95% of pediatric patients that have a secundum ASD, but in whom the ASD II is clinically overshadowed by other "more serious" forms of congenital heart disease? What do these patients have? What is ASD II associated with and masked by? This is what most books and papers on secundum ASD do not mention. We shall now attempt to answer these questions.

When Secundum Atrial Septal Defect II Is Present, but Not the Patient's Primary Clinical Problem

A secundum type of ASD was present in 627 of 640 patients in this study, but the ASD II was not the patient's main clinical problem (97.97%). What was? An attempt is made to answer this question in Table 9.4.

Multiple congenital anomalies were the most common main clinical problem, being present in 183 patients (29.19% of this series, see Table 9.4). "Multiple congenital anomalies" means that malformations were present in two or more systems, not in the cardiovascular system only. Other well-recognized syndromes are presented as such and are not classified as multiple congenital anomalies (see Table 9.4); for example: Down syndrome, 48 patients (7.66%); DiGeorge syndrome, 8 patients (1.28%); scimitar syndrome, 8 patients (1.28%); Noonan syndrome, 5 patients (0.8%); trisomy 18, 4 patients (0.64%); Marfan syndrome, 3 patients (0.48%); Potter syndrome, 2 patients (0.32%); Turner syndrome, 2 patients (0.32%); VACTERL (vertebral defects, anal atresia, cardiac defects, tracheo-esophageal fistula, renal anomalies, and limb abnormalities) association; CHARGE (coloboma, heart defects, atresia choanae [also known as choanal atresia], growth retardation, genital abnormalities, and ear abnormalities) association, 1 patient (0.16%), and so on.

Representative examples of "multiple congenital anomalies" are as follows: TOF with secundum ASD (pentalogy of Fallot), anomalous right subclavian artery, omphalocele, and malrotation of the intestines (Case 7); large secundum ASD (20 × 15 mm), totally anomalous pulmonary venous connection to the portal vein with patent ductus venosus, and craniosynostosis of the sagittal suture posterior to the anterior fontanelle (Case 25); secundum ASD, septum primum covering only half of the interatrial communication, pulmonary valvar stenosis with intact interventricular septum, pectus excavatum, malformation of the brain with glial nodules of the temporal lobes, diffuse ependymal gliosis, decreased cells of the dentate nucleus, and intellectual disability. This 12-year-old boy fell and sustained a skull fracture with subdural hematoma and cerebral hemorrhage (Case 26).

Thus, what is meant by *multiple congenital anomalies* is multisystem pathologic processes (not the cardiovascular systemic only), that does not constitute a well-recognized syndrome at the present time.

Table 9.4 contains a great deal of information and is essentially self-explanatory. But what this table does not do is present the many varying combinations of anomalies—cardiovascular and noncardiovascular—that occurred together.

TABLE 9.4 When Atrial Septum Defect II Was *Not* the Patient's Main Clinical Problem, What Was?

Rank Order	Condition	No. of Cases	% of Series
1	Multiple congenital anomalies	183	29.19
2	Ventricular septal defect	170	27.11
3	Transposition of the great arteries (TGA)	85	13.56
	TGA {S,D,D} = 56		
	TGA {S,D,A} = 2		
	TGA {S,D,L} = 3		
	TGA {S,L,L} = 11		
	TGA {IS,L,L} = 1		
	TGA {S,L,A} = 1		
	TGA {S,L,D} = 1		
	TGA {A(S),D,D}, asplenia = 3		
	TGA {A,D,D}, asplenia = 5		
	TGA {A(I),D,D}, asplenia = 1		
	TGA {A,L,L}, asplenia = 1		
4	Completely common AV canal	73	11.64
5	Tetralogy (pentalogy) of Fallot	68	10.85
6	Coarctation of the aorta	65	10.37
7	Totally anomalous pulmonary venous connection	56	8.93
8	Double-outlet right ventricle (DORV)	52	8.29
	DORV {S,D,D} = 23		
	DORV {S,D,A} = 1		
	DORV {S,D,L} = 4		
	DORV {S,L,L} = 1		
	DORV {S,L,D} = 1		
	DORV {I,L,L} = 2		
	DORV {I,D,D} = 3		
	DORV {A(S),D,D}, polysplenia = 2		
	DORV {A(I),L,L}, polysplenia = 2		
	DORV{A(S),D,D}, asplenia = 3		
	DORV {A,D,D} = asplenia = 3		
	DORV {A(S),D,L}, asplenia = 2		
	DORV {A(I),D,D}, asplenia = 4		
	DORV {A,L,L}, asplenia = 1		
9	Down syndrome	48	7.66
10	Tricuspid atresia	45	7.18
11	Aortic atresia, valvar	35	5.58
11	Hypoplastic left heart syndrome	35	5.58
12	Pneumonia	31	4.94
12	Incompletely common AV canal	31	4.94
13	Ebstein anomaly	29	4.63
13	Mitral atresia	29	4.63
14	Congenital mitral stenosis	28	4.47
15	Asplenia syndrome	27	4.31
16	Truncus arteriosus	26	4.15
17	Pulmonary atresia with intact VS	24	3.83
18	Left-sided juxtaposition of atrial appendages	22	3.51
18	Dextrocardia	22	3.51
19	Congenital aortic stenosis, valvar	21	3.35
20	Hypoplastic left ventricle	20	3.19
21	Interrupted aortic arch	17	2.71
	Type A = 5		
	Type B = 12		
21	Pulmonary vascular obstructive disease	17	2.71
22	Single left ventricle with DILV	16	2.55
22	Hypoplastic right ventricle	16	2.55
23	Polysplenia syndrome	15	2.39
23	Congenital mitral regurgitation	15	2.39
24	Congenital tricuspid regurgitation	14	2.23
24	Congenital tricuspid stenosis	14	2.23
25	Trisomy 13	12	1.91
26	Pulmonary valvar stenosis, isolated	11	1.75
27	Coronary sinus septal defect (unroofing)	10	1.59
28	Partially anomalous pulmonary venous connection	9	1.44
28	Patent ductus arteriosus, large	9	1.44
28	Interrupted inferior vena cava	9	1.44
28	Sepsis	9	1.44
29	DiGeorge syndrome	8	1.28
29	Cantrell syndrome	8	1.28
29	Diaphragmatic hernia	8	1.28
29	Pulmonary hemorrhage	8	1.28
29	Scimitar syndrome	8	1.28
30	Single right ventricle	7	1.12
31	Stenosis of individual pulmonary veins	6	0.96
32	Noonan syndrome	5	0.80
32	Conjoined twin	5	0.80
32	Double-outlet left ventricle	5	0.80
	DOLV {S,D,D} = 4		
	DOLV {S,D,L} = 1		
32	Double-outlet infundibular outlet chamber	5	0.80
32	Mesocardia	5	0.80
33	Persistent fetal circulation	4	0.64
33	Aortopulmonary window	4	0.64
33	Meningitis	4	0.64
33	Trisomy 18	4	0.64
33	Brain abscess	4	0.64
33	Brain hemorrhage	4	0.64
34	Pulmonary sling	3	0.48
34	Hypoplasia of left lung	3	0.48
34	Hypoplasia of both lungs	3	0.48
34	Subdural and subarachnoid hemorrhage	3	0.48
34	Marfan syndrome	3	0.48
34	Seizure disorder	3	0.48
35	Potter syndrome	2	0.32
35	Skull fracture and cerebral hemorrhage	2	0.32
35	Right-sided juxtaposition of the atrial appendages	2	0.32
35	Turner syndrome	2	0.32
35	Cerebral AV fistula (vein of Galen)	2	0.32
35	Anatomically corrected malposition of the great arteries {S,D,L}	2	0.32
35	Agenesis of right lung	2	0.32
35	Ectopia cordis, complete, thoracic	2	0.32
35	Meconium aspiration, massive	2	0.32
35	Pulmonary lymphangectasis	2	0.32
35	{S,L,I}	2	0.32
35	VACTERL association	2	0.32
35	Hypertrophic cardiomyopathy	2	0.32
35	Vascular ring	2	0.32
35	Subacute bacterial endocarditis	2	0.32
36	Bronchiolitis	1	0.16

Continued

TABLE 9.4 **When Atrial Septum Defect II Was *Not* the Patient's Main Clinical Problem, What Was?—cont'd**

Rank Order	Condition	No. of Cases	% of Series	Rank Order	Condition	No. of Cases	% of Series
36	Coronary sinus ostial stenosis	1	0.16	36	Aneurysm of ascending aorta, ruptured	1	0.16
36	Triple outlet right ventricle, conjoined twins	1	0.16	36	Dissection of aorta	1	0.16
36	Trisomy 8, mosaic	1	0.16	36	Cardiac tamponade	1	0.16
36	Primary pulmonary hypertension	1	0.16	36	Acute hemorrhagic pancreatitis	1	0.16
36	Pulmonary stenosis (valvar) and aortic stenosis (valvar)	1	0.16	36	Progeria (Cockayne syndrome)	1	0.16
36	Aneurysm of left ventricle, saccular	1	0.16	36	CHARGE association	1	0.16
36	Klippel-Feil syndrome	1	0.16	36	Cerebro-oculo-facio-skeletal (COFS) syndrome	1	0.16
36	Hypoplasia of right lung	1	0.16	36	Absence of coronary ostia and of proximal coronary arteries	1	0.16
36	Straddling mitral valve	1	0.16	36	Caudal regression syndrome	1	0.16
36	Mitral regurgitation and stenosis, congenital	1	0.16	36	Hydrops fetalis, massive	1	0.16
36	Pulmonary atresia, valvar {S,D,S} with membranous ventricular septal defect	1	0.16	36	Bronchopulmonary dysplasia	1	0.16
36	Rheumatic heart disease with mitral regurgitation and aortic regurgitation	1	0.16	36	Mitral valve prolapse	1	0.16
36	Teratoma, mediastinal	1	0.16	36	Cardiofacial syndrome	1	0.16
36	Trauma (auto accident, aortic tears)	1	0.16	36	Alagille syndrome	1	0.16
36	Stenosis of inferior vena cava, at right atrial junction	1	0.16	36	Pierre-Robin syndrome	1	0.16
36	Congenital disruption of thoracic spinal cord, complete	1	0.16	36	Cystic hydroma, neck	1	0.16
36	Leftward malposition of septum primum resulting in totally anomalous pulmonary venous drainage into RA, with polysplenia	1	0.16	36	Prune belly syndrome	1	0.16
36	{IS,D,S}, polysplenia	1	0.16	36	Anophthalmia	1	0.16
36	{AI,L,I}, polysplenia	1	0.16	36	Left ventricular apical diverticulum	1	0.16
				36	Primary endocardial fibroelastosis of right ventricle	1	0.16
				36	Straddling tricuspid valve	1	0.16
				36	Lupus erythematosus	1	0.16
				36	Sequestration, pulmonary, extralobar	1	0.16

AV, Atrioventricular; CHARGE (coloboma, heart defects, atresia choanae [also known as choanal atresia], growth retardation, genital abnormalities, and ear abnormalities); *DILV*, double-inlet left ventricle; *RA*, right atrium; *VA*, VACTERL association.

Segmental anatomy {IS,D,S} polysplenia means the segmental set of visceral situs inversus with atrial situs solitus, D-loop ventricles, and solitus normally related great arteries, with visceral heterotaxy and polysplenia, that is, visceroatrial situs discordance; **{AI,L,I} polysplenia** indicates the segmental set of visceral situs ambiguus with situs inversus of the atria, L-loop ventricles, and inverted normally related great arteries, with visceral heterotaxy and polysplenia; and **{S,L,I}** means the set of situs solitus of the viscera and atria, L-loop ventricles, and inverted normally related great arteries. In {S,L,I}, the segmental alignments are AV discordance with ventriculoarterial concordance. In words, {S,L,I} may also be called ventricular inversion with inverted normally related great arteries in visceroatrial situs solitus. {S,L,I} is a brief convenient abbreviation.

In the process of doing the study to identify the main clinical problems of these patients with ASD II, a number of rare and fascinating forms of congenital heart disease were found that merit recording here:

Ostium primum type of ASD, without a cleft in the anterior leaflet of the mitral valve (Case 113, A63-60). This case answers the question of whether it possible to have an incomplete form of common AV canal with a partial form of AV septal defect (i.e., an ostium primum ASD), but without the typical cleft in the anterior leaflet of the mitral valve. As the case of this 3-day-old girl with Down syndrome proves, the answer is, yes, rarely. The reverse, that is, a canal type of cleft in the anterior mitral leaflet but without an ostium primum type of ASD, is more frequent, but still uncommon. Thus, partial forms of common AV canal are numerous and highly variable.

Totally anomalous pulmonary venous connection (TAPVC) with physiologically normal pulmonary venous drainage. This surprising situation was found in a 1-month-old boy (Case 173, A67-216) with an ASD II (fenestrated septum primum), dextrocardia, TGA {S,L,L}, pulmonary atresia (infundibular and valvar), incompletely common AV canal, hypoplastic LV (right-sided), common-inlet right ventricle (RV) (left-sided), TAPVC to the left innominate vein, to the left SVC (LSVC), to the LA (because of a large coronary sinus septal "unroofing" defect). The aortic arch was right-sided, and the right-sided patent ductus arteriosus (PDA) was closing, leading to death. As this rare case indicates, there is a valid distinction between totally anomalous pulmonary venous *connection* (TAPVC) and totally anomalous pulmonary venous *drainage* (TAPVD).

Umbilical vein running anteriorly and superiorly to the liver to connect with the IVC. Normally the umbilical vein runs inferiorly to the liver, into the porta hepatis, where it connects with the portal vein and then continues as the ductus venosus, running to the right of and then posteriorly to the caudate lobe of the liver where the ductus venosus connects with the IVC. This anterosuperior umbilical vein was found in a 15-day-old white boy (Case 294, A76-53) with a large secundum ASD, TGA {S,D,D}, a small subpulmonary conoventricular type of VSD, and a PDA. During cardiac catheterization, the subaortic infundibulum was perforated, leading to cardiac tamponade and death.

An anterosuperior left umbilical vein running in front of and above the liver to drain into the IVC was also found in a 12-day-old girl (Case 597). She had a secundum ASD, because of multiple fenestrations in the septum primum, and a paramembranous conoventricular type of VSD. She also had multiple congenital anomalies, that is, right hydronephrosis with right ureteropelvic stenosis. In addition, this 12-day-old girl from another institution had a widely patent ductus arteriosus. Autopsy revealed that the left pulmonary artery had been ligated inadvertently and that the ductus arteriosus remained widely patent.

An anterosuperior umbilical vein is anatomically anomalous, but physiologically normal in the sense that it drains appropriately into the IVC, but without any "liver factors" (which may be important for the prevention of arteriovenous malformations).

Tracheal atresia with bronchoesophageal fistulae. Tracheal atresia is an exceedingly rare anomaly in our experience. This malformation was found in a 2½-year-old boy (Case 298, A76-121) with a small ASD II (fenestrations in the septum primum), visceral heterotaxy with polysplenia and TOF {S,D,S}, that is, pentalogy of Fallot. This patient also had hypoplasia of the stomach (microgastria), malrotation of the intestines, Meckel's diverticulum, prematurity, and severe pulmonary edema and hemorrhage. We think that tracheal atresia is very rare and uniformly lethal, at least at the present time.

Parachute mitral valve and Ebstein anomaly of the tricuspid valve—a rare combination. A 7-week-old boy (Case 302, C76-26) had a small ASD II (4 × 2 mm), with TOF, that is, pentalogy of Fallot, plus an incompletely common AV canal. The mitral valve had congenital mitral stenosis with fusion of the papillary muscles, that is, parachute mitral valve. The mitral orifice consisted of the cleft in the anterior leaflet of the mitral valve. The tricuspid valve displayed Ebstein anomaly with abnormal chordae tendineae, obliteration of the interchordal spaces, muscularization of the anterior leaflet of the tricuspid valve, and severe tricuspid regurgitation. Thus, in addition to pentalogy of Fallot, this patient also had congenital mitral stenosis and severe congenital tricuspid regurgitation. The combination of parachute mitral valve and Ebstein anomaly of the tricuspid valve is rare. This patient may be considered to have a *double pentalogy:* (1) pentalogy of Fallot and (1) TOF, (2) ASD II, (3) incompletely common AV canal, (4) parachute mitral valve, and (5) Ebstein anomaly of the tricuspid valve, with 1 to 5 comprising the second pentalogy.

Congenital Lutembacher syndrome. An 11-week-old white girl (Case 312, A77-191) had an ASD II (valve incompetent patent foramen ovale [PFO] with a large left-to-right shunt at the atrial level) and a double-orifice mitral valve. The anterior orifice was smaller than the posterior orifice, and there was a bridge of fibrous tissue connecting the anterior and posterior mitral leaflets. Cardiac catheterization revealed a 3-mm diastolic gradient between the LA and the LV, confirming the presence of congenital mitral stenosis. Thus, this patient had both features of Lutembacher syndrome: an ASD II, and congenital mitral stenosis.

This patient also had a multiple muscular VSD (five) and a preductal coarctation of the aorta (3 mm in internal diameter).

Although most cases of Lutembacher syndrome appear to be due to *acquired* mitral stenosis (often rheumatic) plus a secundum ASD or a stretched PFO, this case indicates that Lutembacher syndrome can result entirely from *congenital* heart disease.

Concordant alignments between discordant atria and ventricles. This is Dr. Henry Wagner's amazing case (Case 313, C77-8, sex and age at death unknown to us) of double-outlet RV (DORV) {S,L,D} with AV alignment concordance (Fig. 9.24). The ASD II was large. The patient had mesocardia with a leftward pointing apex and right-sided JAA. There were crisscross AV relations, the mitral valve being superior relative to the tricuspid valve. (It is very rare for the tricuspid valve to be inferior to the mitral valve. Almost always, it is vice versa: tricuspid valve superior to the mitral valve.) Other findings included a small conoventricular type of VSD, a bilateral conus (subaortic and subpulmonary), subaortic stenosis, and preductal coarctation of the aorta.

But the most remarkable feature of this very rare case was the presence of concordant AV alignments and connections, despite the fact that the atria and the ventricles were discordant in terms of their segmental situs. The viscera and atria were in situs solitus, with the RA to the right and the LA to the left, that is, DORV {S,-,-}. L-loop or inverted ventricles were present, that is, DORV {S,L,-}. The morphologically RV was left-sided and left-handed. The morphologically LV was right-sided and right-handed.

But the AV alignments were concordant (not discordant, as expected): The right-sided RA was aligned with and ejected into the left-sided RV through the right-sided and inferior tricuspid valve. The left-sided LA was aligned with and ejected into the right-sided LV through the superior and left-sided mitral valve. The tricuspid valve opened inferiorly from right-to-left, and the mitral valve opened superiorly from left to right. Hence, crisscross AV relations were present, meaning that the AV inflow tracts from the atria into the ventricles were angulated relative to each other, rather than being approximately parallel to each other, which is normal (see Fig. 9.24).

How could situs solitus atria open into inverted (L-loop) ventricles in a concordant fashion—RA to RV and LA to LV? We think that the answer is that *both* the atrial segment and the ventricular segment were malpositioned. The presence of right-sided JAA indicates that the atria, although in situs solitus, were not entirely normally positioned. The ventricles were obviously malpositioned (L-loop ventricles).

When *both* the atrial and the ventricular segments are malpositioned, rare and surprising AV alignments and connections can occur. Usually, the atria are the "straight men"; they are normally positioned. Usually, it is only the ventricles that

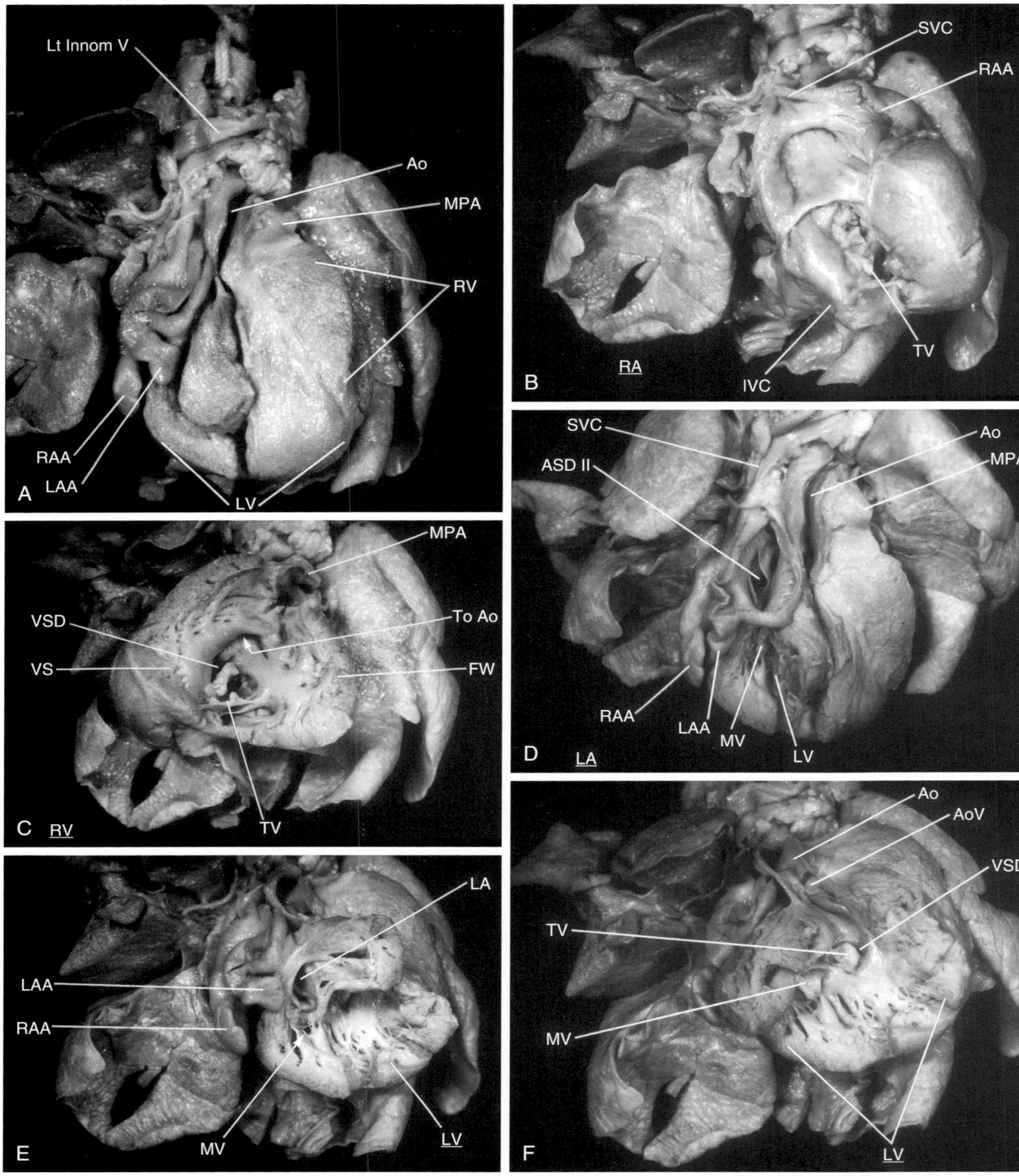

Fig. 9.24 Double-outlet right ventricle (DORV) with situs solitus of the viscera and atria, L-loop ventricles, and D-malposition of the great arteries, that is, DORV {S,L,D}, with right-sided juxtaposition of the atrial appendages (JAA), and concordant atrioventricular alignments and connections. (A) External frontal view. (B) Opened right atrium *(RA)* and tricuspid valve *(TV)*. (C) Opened left-sided morphologically right ventricle *(RV)*, giving origin to the widely patent outflow tract to the main pulmonary artery *(MPA)* and to the stenotic outflow tract leading to the ascending aorta *(Ao)*. (D) The opened left atrium *(LA)* and the large secundum atrial septal defect (ASD II). (E) Left-sided LA opening into the right-sided morphologically left ventricle *(LV)*. (F) Right-sided LV and the conoventricular type of ventral septal defect *(VSD)*. There was a bilateral muscular conus (subpulmonary and subaortic). The subaortic part of the conus has been opened, making it possible to see the stenotic aortic outflow tract arising from the left-sided RV. In A, one can see that the right atrial appendage *(RAA)* and the left atrial appendage *(LAA)* are juxtaposed. Both lie to the right of the vascular pedicle, Ao to the right and MPA to the left. Thus, this right-sided JAA consists of dextromalposition of the LAA in visceroatrial situs solitus. In other words, it is the LAA that is malpositioned relative to the vascular pedicle, resulting in right-sided JAA. But the really rare and amazing finding is the presence of atrioventricular (AV) alignment concordance with AV situs discordance. The RA is aligned with and opens into the RV through the very inferior TV (B–C).

Continued

Fig. 9.24 cont'd The LA is aligned with and opens into the LV through a superior mitral valve (MV) (D–F). This is a very rare form of crisscross AV relations, rare because the TV is inferior and the MV is superior. Thus, there is AV *alignment* concordance: right-sided RA to left-sided RV (B–C) and left-sided LA to right-sided LV (D–F). But the atria are in situs solitus (A, B, D) and L-loop ventricles are present (A, C, D–F). The RV is left-handed (C) and the LV is right-handed (F). Thus, there is AV *situs* discordance: solitus atria with L-loop ventricles. To the best of our present knowledge, whenever there is incongruence or disharmony between AV alignment and situs concordance or discordance, there always has been JAA. We think that JAA is important in this respect because both the atrial segment and the ventricular segment of the heart are malpositioned, rarely making it possible for AV alignment and AV situs concordance and/or discordance to be opposites. When only one cardiac segment is malpositioned—typically the ventricular segment, and when one atrium opens into one ventricle, AV alignment and situs concordance or discordance are the same, not opposites. This is Dr. Henry Wagner's case from Children's Hospital in Buffalo, New York. We shall be forever indebted to him for having been so kind as to let us study and learn from this very rare case. *AoV,* aortic valve; *IVC,* inferior vena cava; *FW,* free well; *Lt Innom V,* left innominate vein; *To Ao,* to aorta; *SVC,* superior vena cava; *VS,* ventricular septum. (From Van Praagh R, David I, Gordon D, Wright GB, Van Praagh S. Ventricular diagnosis and VSD. In: Godman M, ed. *Paediatric Cardiology.* 1980, Edinburgh: Churchill Livingtone;1981:153, reproduced with permission.)

are malpositioned, the ventricles being "professional contortionists." Usually, therefore, when the AV segmental anatomy is {S,L,-}, the AV alignments and connections are discordant (RA to LV and LA to RV) because *only* the ventricles are positioned abnormally. But when *both* the atrial and the ventricular segments are positionally abnormal, even though the AV segmental anatomy is {S,L,-}, the AV alignments and connections can be concordant, even though the situs (pattern of anatomic organization) of the atrial and ventricular segments is discordant.

The segmental anatomy of the conotruncal (infundibuloarterial) segment was D-malposition (aortic valve to the right of the pulmonary valve). Hence, the segmental anatomy was {S,L,D}. The ventriculoarterial alignments were those of DORV. Consequently, the segmental anatomy of this rare and fascinating case was DORV {S,L,D}—both great arteries arising above the left-sided RV.

As this rare case illustrates, there are two different kinds of concordance and discordance:

1. **alignment concordance and discordance** (the atrium is aligned with and opens into which ventricle?); and
2. **situs concordance and discordance** (what is the visceroatrial situs, and what is the ventricular situs or loop?).

Almost always, these two different types of concordance and discordance are the same, or congruent. For example, in typical congenitally physiologically corrected TGA, that is, TGA {S,L,L}, the AV alignments are discordant (RA to LV and LA to RV) and the pattern of AV situs is discordant {S,L,-}. Only rarely are AV alignment concordance/discordance and AV situs concordance/discordance opposites, or incongruent, as in this rare and instructive case of DORV {S,L,D} with AV alignment concordance and AV situs discordance (see Fig. 9.24).

Because AV segmental situs anatomy such as {S,D,-} and {S,L,-} does not predict AV alignments with 100% accuracy (because they are two different variables), whenever the AV alignments are different from what is usual, they must be specified. For example, typical congenitally physiologically corrected transposition may be represented as TGA {S,L,L}. If not otherwise specified, one may assume that the AV alignments are discordant: RA to LV and LA to RV. However, when this is not the case, the AV alignments and connections must be specified for clarity; that is, TGA {S,L,L} with double-inlet LV, with straddling tricuspid valve, with tricuspid atresia, with double-inlet RV, and so on.

Why is this necessary? Because, as this rare case of DORV {S,L,D} with AV alignment concordance but with AV situs discordance so clearly illustrates, AV alignment concordance/discordance and AV situs concordance/discordance are really two different variables that may be the same, or different.

Anomalous vein connecting umbilical vein with coronary sinus. A 10-day-old white boy (Case 364, A81-76) displayed a rare anomaly of systemic venous return. In addition to an ASD II (deficient septum primum), this patient had an anomalous vein connecting the umbilical vein with the coronary sinus via the right lobe of the liver. This anomalous vein also received a small hepatic vein. This patient was postmature (42 weeks gestation) and suffered from persistent fetal circulation. The pulmonary resistance was very elevated (systemic or suprasystemic). There was marked pulmonary arterial hypertension. The large PDA was closing. Congestive heart failure developed and the patient died.

This anomalous systemic vein connecting the umbilical vein with the coronary sinus via the right lobe of the liver was anatomically abnormal but physiologically normal in the sense that the umbilical venous blood returned normally to the RA.

Congenital mitral stenosis with absence of posteromedial papillary muscle of the LV: a rare form of parachute mitral valve. In typical parachute mitral valve with a divided AV canal (not with common AV canal), the anterolateral papillary muscle group is absent. The large posteromedial papillary muscle group receives all of the insertions of the chordae tendineae. However, in a 3-month-old white girl (Case 376, A82-26), a rare form of parachute mitral valve was found: the posteromedial papillary muscle group was absent, and the anterolateral group was well developed and received all of the mitral chordae tendinae. Hence, the papillary muscle architecture of this patient was the opposite of that which is usually seen in typical parachute mitral valve with a divided AV canal.

Interestingly, when the common AV canal is present, potentially parachute mitral valve[5] (after surgical repair of the AV septal defect) is characterized by the same left ventricular papillary muscle architecture as was seen in this patient without a common AV canal: absence of the posteromedial papillary muscle and a large anterolateral papillary muscle of the LV receiving all of the mitral chordae tendinae.

This patient also had *right-sided JAA*[6] {S,D,S}, which is characterized by left-sided obstructive lesions such as congenital mitral stenosis; whereas *left-sided JAA*[1,7] is frequently associated with right-sided obstructive anomalies such as tricuspid atresia or severe stenosis.

ASD II with primary pulmonary hypertension. A 2 7/12-year-old white boy (Case 391; A82-145) with pectus excavatum presented with failure to thrive and was found to have severe pulmonary hypertension of unknown cause. He developed congestive heart failure, pleural effusions (right, 50 mL and left, 10 mL), bilateral pulmonary congestion and hemorrhages, and ascites (55 mL) that led to death. Autopsy revealed a secundum ASD consisting of three fenestrations of the septum primum, one measuring 7 × 5 mm and the other two having diameters of 1 to 2 mm. The surprising findings were those indicative of primary pulmonary hypertension: decreased intra-acinar arteries and arterioles, increased connective tissue around larger vessels, medial hypertrophy, intimal proliferation, angiomatoid and plexiform lesions, periarteritis, and large vessel necrotizing arteritis.

Raghib Syndrome Without a Large Low Posterior Interatrial Communication

When a persistent LSVC opens into the LA because of a coronary sinus septal defect, almost always there is a large low posterior opening in the atrial septum that has been interpreted as an enlarged right atrial ostium of the unroofed coronary sinus; this combination of anomalies is known as the Raghib syndrome. However, in Case 397 (C82-96), a boy with a large ASD II (deficiency of the septum primum) had a persistent LSVC that opened into the LA because of a large coronary sinus septal defect. The fascinating finding was that this 19-week fetus did *not* have an enlarged right atrial ostium of the coronary sinus. Instead, this ostium was of normal size.

We are aware of no developmental hypothesis to explain this observation. Suffice it to say that it is rarely possible for a persistent LSVC to drain to the LA, apparently because of a coronary sinus septal defect, without a large low posterior interatrial communication.

It may be relevant to record that this fetus had a 42-year-old mother and that this fetus had trisomy-13 with polydactyly (six digits on both hands), a very small membranous VSD, and bilaterally trilobated lungs (with a normally formed spleen).

So, the answer to the question, Does the Raghib syndrome always have a large low posterior interatrial communication? is almost always, but not always, as this rare case demonstrates.

Does a rare form of cor triatriatum, consisting of a prominent interseptovalvular space, really exist? There has been considerable uncertainty about this, which is why this "theoretical" form of cor triatriatum is usually omitted from standard textbook accounts. The interseptovalvular space, which is well seen in the human embryo (please see Chapter 2), is the space between the septum primum to the left and the left venous valve to the right. Usually this space is largely or totally obliterated.

But rarely, the interseptovalvular space can persist, as in Case 403 (C82-350). The patient was a 55-year-old white man with a large ASD II, TGA {S,L,L}, and tricuspid atresia (left-sided). He also had severe mitral regurgitation (right-sided), atrial flutter, chronic congestive heart failure, and a systemic level of pulmonary hypertension without pulmonary regurgitation. The immediate cause of death was aspiration.

In addition to the foregoing, autopsy also revealed atherosclerosis of the pulmonary arterial tree (Heath-Edwards grade 3 changes), multiple fenestrations of the right-sided mitral valve (a rare finding), and evidence of multiple old brain abscesses.

This patient had cor triatriatum (a heart with three atria) in the following sense. The morphologically RA was right-sided. The morphologically LA was left-sided. There was a third space at the atrial level, between the right-sided RA and the left-sided LA. This third atrial space was bounded by the septum primum to the left and by a prominent left venous valve to the right, that is, the interoseptovalvular space. The ISVS (interseptovalvular space) received no pulmonary or systemic vein and hence was of no clinical or pathophysiologic significance.

The point of knowing about this rare form of cor triatriatum is understanding, that is to know what one is dealing with and *not* to undertake any unnecessary interventional or surgical steps.

Truncus arteriosus type B1,[8] that is, with intact ventricular septum (type B) and with aortopulmonary septal remnant (type 1). Case 407 (C82-471) had a secundum ASD because of the presence of a valve-incompetent PVO (the ASD measuring 5 × 2 to 3 mm). This was a consult that was received in 1982; unfortunately we do not know the sex of the patient or the age at death. This was the first case of truncus arteriosus type B1[8,9] that I had ever seen. There was no VSD; the membranous septum was large and intact. The aortopulmonary window component was small because the aortopulmonary septal remnant was quite well developed. The truncal valve was quadricuspid, the semilunar valves were in common, and the pulmonary valve leaflets were myxomatous. In 1982, we were excited to have discovered truncus arteriosus type B1. Up to that time, types B2 and B4[8,9] had been reported but not type B1.

Incompletely common AV canal with imperforate Ebstein anomaly. Case 440 was a consult that we received in 1984 (C84-34). Unfortunately, the patient's sex, race, and age at death are unknown to us. There was a large ASD II, with only a few strands of septum primum being present. This patient had the very rare combination of incompletely common AV canal (with an ostium primum type of ASD, an incompletely cleft anterior leaflet of the mitral valve, and an intact ventricular septum) and an imperforate Ebstein anomaly of the tricuspid valve. This patient also had severe valvar pulmonary stenosis and a persistent LSVC to the coronary sinus to the RA.

The incomplete form of common AV canal with Ebstein malformation is a rare combination of anomalies that was also found in a 2-month-old white girl (Case 506, C88-178, a consult from Dr. Dominique Metras of Marseilles, France). This patient had an unusual form of tricuspid atresia type Ib, the severe subpulmonary stenosis being produced by a tiny conoventricular type of VSD. In addition to the imperforate Ebstein anomaly, there was partial absence of the tricuspid valve leaflets. The septal leaflet was absent, and the posterior leaflet was almost totally absent. The anterior tricuspid leaflet was deep, curtain-like, and totally obstructive. There was Uhl disease of the right ventricular free wall. The LV had a bizarre "wrap-around" shape because it wrapped around the hypoplastic and dysplastic RV. Ebstein malformation is an anomaly not only of the tricuspid valve but also of the RV.

Right aortic arch without mirror-image branching of the brachiocephalic arteries. How is this possible? This occurs when both common carotid arteries arise from the right aortic arch but both subclavian arteries originate from the descending thoracic aorta (Case 443, A85-6, a 1-day-old white boy).

Congenital stenosis of the IVC at its junction with the RA. A 6-day-old white boy (Case 501, A88-72) with a secundum ASD (a sprung PFO with an aneurysm of the septum primum bulging into the RA) and aortic valvar atresia with an intact ventricular septum had large coronary-to-left ventricular sinusoids. There was a right coronary artery-to-left ventricular sinusoid inferiorly that measured 2 to 3 mm in diameter. A left anterior descending coronary artery–to–left ventricular sinusoid was 2 mm in diameter. There was also a sinusoid between the left circumflex coronary artery and the LV. These coronary arteries also displayed the typical coronary arteriopathy at their junction with these large sinusoids: coronary mural thickening and luminal narrowing.

Probably the most unusual finding in this case was severe congenital stenosis of the IVC at its junction with the RA. The lumen of the IVC at the IVC-RA junction measured less than 1 mm in diameter, which is an extraordinarily rare finding.

Stenosis of the right atrial ostium of the coronary sinus with a decompressing "snowman" pathway. A 3-month-old white boy (Case 525, A90-64) with a large secundum ASD had TGA {S,D,D} with a subpulmonary conoventricular type of VSD. However, the rare finding was marked stenosis of the right atrial ostium of the coronary sinus, with dilatation of the coronary sinus. A small persistent LSVC connected the obstructed coronary sinus to the left innominate vein and then to the right SVC and RA, constituting a compressing snowman type of venous pathway reminiscent of the supracardiac form of TAPVC but without TAPVC. The pulmonary veins were normally connected. This patient also had double-orifice mitral valve (DOMV) with a large central tongue of fibrous tissue resulting in an unusual form of congenital mitral stenosis.

Triple-outlet RV (TORV). How is it possible to have *triple-outlet* RV? The answer is in conjoined twins. This very rare anomaly was found in Case 556 (C91-146), a female white fetus (gestational age unknown to us) with a secundum type of ASD (multiple fenestrations in the septum primum). These conjoined twins had two heads, but only one body with two feet and two arms. The Latin term for this is *dicephalus dipus dibrachius* (two heads, two feet, two arms). The right twin had DORV {S,D,D} with pulmonary outflow tract stenosis and interrupted aortic arch type B. The left twin had normal segmental anatomy {S,D,S}. The two SVCs both connected with the RA. There was only one IVC that also connected with the RA.

Two coni arose above the one right ventricular sinus. The right conus gave rise to both great arteries of the right-sided twin, resulting in the right-sided twin's DORV {S,D,D}. The left-sided conus gave origin to the normally related and connected pulmonary artery of the left-sided twin. The aorta of the left-sided twin was normally related and connected with the LV, with aortic-mitral fibrous continuity.

The LV supplied only the left-sided twin. The RV supplied the head and neck of the right-sided twin and the pulmonary artery of the left-sided twin.

Thus, the TORV consisted of both great arteries of the right-sided twin, who had DORV {S,D,D}, and the pulmonary artery of the left-sided twin, who had {S,D,S}. To the best of our present knowledge, it is impossible for one individual (homo sapiens sapiens) to have TORV. In humans, this can occur only in conjoined twins.

However, TORV perhaps may occur in the higher reptilia such as alligators and crocodiles, because three great arteries normally occur in these life forms. They normally have a right ventricular pulmonary artery, a right ventricular aorta, and a left ventricular aorta. We are not aware that TORV has been documented in higher reptiles.

Familial TOF and truncus arteriosus. A 15-month-old white girl with a large ASD II (Case 563, A92-31) had TOF {S,D,S} (or pentalogy of Fallot) with pulmonary infundibular and valvar atresia with multiple aortopulmonary collateral arteries (MAPCAs). An older sibling of this patient had truncus arteriosus. Both patients were the products of a consanguineous (first-cousin) marriage.

This type of familial congenital heart disease—tetralogy and truncus in siblings—supports the concept that tetralogy with pulmonary outflow tract atresia and truncus arteriosus are closely related anomalies anatomically, embryologically, and genetically.[8-11]

This patient also illustrated a very practical surgical lesson. At 15 months of age, it was decided that this patient needed a change of her RV-to–pulmonary artery conduit because of the development of a 65–mm Hg gradient across the conduit. Most of the conduit was removed, except for its right ventricular origin and its pulmonary artery insertion. The patient could not be weaned from cardiopulmonary bypass, leading to death. Autopsy revealed severe obstructions at the conduit-to–right pulmonary artery junction and at the conduit-to–left pulmonary artery junction. The therapeutic lesson of this case was to replace the whole conduit, not just the middle part of it, even when the conduit narrowing may appear to be maximal in its central portion, rather than at its proximal or distal end. Conduit neopseudointimal lining or peel can detach from the conduit and embolize, resulting in a serious or fatal pulmonary embolus. Conduit "peel" is well named: it can and does and should never be "trusted." The treacherous nature of conduit peel should be borne in mind during and after interventional conduit dilations and stenting.

Absence of the main pulmonary artery, right pulmonary artery, left pulmonary artery, and ductus arteriosus does occur. A 7-hour-old white girl with a small secundum ASD caused by an abnormally short and thin septum primum (Case 571, A92-80) had multiple congenital anomalies and TOF {S,D,S} (or pentalogy of Fallot, a term that we really do not use very much, although everyone knows what it means) with pulmonary outflow tract atresia and absence of the main pulmonary artery, right pulmonary artery, left pulmonary artery, and ductus arteriosus. This patient had absence of the left lung and left pulmonary vein. The persistent LSVC connected with the coronary sinus and emptied into the RA. The left innominate vein was absent, which is not surprising because there were bilateral SVCs. A solitary collateral artery from the descending thoracic aorta supplied the right lung.

Why is this case noteworthy? One reason is that it proves that Collett and Edwards[12] truncus arteriosus type IV does indeed exist. There has been much uncertainty about this question. Indeed, Dr. Jesse Edwards renounced his truncus arteriosus communis type IV, not because it was illogical, but because he was not certain that this anomaly (no matter what one may prefer to call it) in fact exists. We shared Dr. Edwards' concern about the possible nonexistence of his type IV truncus arteriosus communis. As this case proves, although exceedingly rare, this anomaly does indeed exist.

Additional anomalies included absence of the right coronary arterial ostium, that is, a single left coronary artery; anophthalmia, bilateral (no eyes); dysmorphic Potter syndrome–like facies with a broad flat nose and high nasal bridge; flat malformed helices of the ears with paucity or absence of helical cartilage; renal dysplasia; persistent urogenital sinus; ureterovesicle stenosis; and uterine atresia with atresia of the Fallopian tubes.

TOF {I,D,S}. A 6-month-old Asian girl (Case 573, A92-94) with a secundum ASD (enlarged ostium secundum above the septum primum measuring 7 × 4 mm, and a fenestration within the septum primum measuring 6 × 4 mm) had a rare form of tetralogy (or pentalogy) of Fallot with interesting and unusual segmental anatomy: visceroatrial situs inversus *{I, -,-}*, with discordant D-loop ventricles {I,*D*,-} and concordant solitus normally related great arteries {I,D,*S*} that were also afflicted with TOF with infundibular and valvar pulmonary atresia. The circulations (pulmonary and aortic) were physiologically uncorrected ("complete" transposition-like) because of the presence of one intersegmental discordance (AV). This physiologic uncorrection of the circulations was further exacerbated by the coexistence of pulmonary infundibular and valvar atresia. The main pulmonary artery was absent, but the right and left pulmonary artery branches were in continuity. The aortic arch was left-sided (abnormal for visceroatrial situs inversus) and there was a right-sided PDA or ductus-like collateral. A portion of the anterolateral papillary muscle of the LV arose from the left ventricular septal surface and was associated with an anterolateral commissural cleft of the mitral valve with mitral regurgitation. The ostium of the left coronary artery was absent, resulting in a single right coronary artery.

Therapeutically, at 4 days of age a modified right Blalock-Taussig anastomosis was successfully performed. At 6 months of age, a cardiac catheterization was complicated by the rupture of a balloon at the catheter tip, releasing carbon dioxide into the LV. Hypotension and complete heart block followed, leading to death despite all resuscitative efforts. Autopsy confirmed the previously mentioned diagnoses and revealed the presence of a right-sided spleen (usual for visceroatrial situs inversus). Histologic examination revealed minor ventricular myocardial contraction band necrosis.

What are the most important lessons of this case? First, it is important to know that TOF can have rare segmental anatomy. Tetralogy is not always TOF {S,D,S} or TOF {I,L,I}. Like TGA, normally related great arteries complicated by TOF can occur with both concordant and discordant AV alignments. Second, it is important to realize that the intracardiac rupture of a balloon, even though filled with carbon dioxide, is not necessarily an innocuous event.

Pulmonary valvar atresia with a small membranous VSD, which is not TOF, does exist. When the great arteries are essentially normally related, and there also is pulmonary valvar atresia and a VSD, nearly always the patient has the worst form of TOF (tetralogy with pulmonary atresia). Rarely, the patient can have pulmonary valvar atresia (or stenosis), with a normally formed subpulmonary conus, without the anterosuperior conal septal malalignment that characterizes both TOF and the Eisenmenger complex. A 2-month-old Japanese boy (Case 582, C92-356) illustrated this point. The patient had valvar pulmonary atresia {S,D,S} with a normal subpulmonary conus and a small high subaortic membranous VSD.

This patient also had a prominent *left* venous valve forming a *rete Chiari* within the RA. Almost always it is the *right* venous valve that forms a rete Chiari. The unusually large left venous valve also resulted in a prominent *interseptovalvular space,* that is, an unusually well-demarcated space between the septum primum to the left and the left venous valve to the right. This unusually well-seen interseptovalvalar space can also create the impression of a rare form of *cor triatriatum* but without pulmonary (or systemic) venous obstruction because no pulmonary or caval vein drains into the interseptovalvular space.

But the salient lesson of this case is that pulmonary valvar atresia with a VSD is not always a tetralogy-atresia.

Asplenia with interrupted IVC. Almost always the IVC is intact (not interrupted) in visceral heterotaxy with asplenia. By contrast, interruption of the IVC is characteristic of visceral heterotaxy with polysplenia (see Chapter 29). Rarely, however, interruption of the IVC can occur in the asplenia syndrome, as in Case 595 (C93-135), a 5-day-old boy with dextrocardia and DORV {A(I),D,D} with pulmonary atresia. {A(I),D,D} briefly indicates the segmental anatomy. There was situs ambiguus of the viscera, which is typical of the asplenia syndrome, that is {*A*,-,-}, the atria probably being in situs inversus, that is {A(*I*),-,-}. There were D-loop ventricles, that is {A(I),*D*,-}; hence, there was probably AV discordance. The great arteries were in D-malposition, that is {A(I),D,*D*}. The ventriculoarterial alignments were those of DORV. Hence, the segmental anatomic set was DORV {A(I),D,D}. DORV is typical of the asplenia syndrome. DORV is a short form for "origin of both great arteries above the right ventricle," whether both great arteries are patent or not. In this patient, there was pulmonary outflow tract atresia, also frequent with the asplenia syndrome. So, DORV with pulmonary atresia really is not a contradiction in terms, even though that may be one's initial impression, because of what DORV really means.

This patient had an enlarged azygos vein connecting with the right SVC. The enlarged azygos vein, typically associated with interruption of the IVC, is often called an *azygos extension*. This designation may suggest to the uninitiated that there is something unusual about such an azygos extension. In fact, an azygos vein is a normal part of the systemic venous return. The only unusual feature of an azygos extension is its large size. With interruption of the IVC from the renal veins to the hepatic veins, the azygos vein must be much larger than it normally is in order to convey the systemic venous return from the lower body to a SVC and then to the RA.

The suprahepatic segment of the IVC, which is present in interruption of the IVC, connected with the left-sided atrium, strongly suggesting that the morphologically RA was left-sided. The connection of the IVC is one of the most highly reliable diagnostic markers of the RA because the RA consists in part of the systemic venous confluence. This connection of the suprahepatic segment of the IVC with the left-sided atrium is one of the reasons that we thought that the RA was left-sided and hence that there probably was situs inversus of the atria. We say "probably" because of the coexistence of visceral heterotaxy.

Another highly reliable diagnostic marker of the RA is the ostium of the coronary sinus. However, this structure is often absent in the asplenia syndrome, as it was in this patient.

The pulmonary veins often are of no help in identifying the atria in the heterotaxy syndrome with asplenia because they frequently have a totally anomalous connection, as they had in this patient: TAPVC below the diaphragm with obstruction.

The small right-sided PDA was almost closed, this being the cause of the patient's death at 5 days of age.

This unusual case indicates that, rarely, interruption of the IVC can occur in association with the asplenia syndrome.[13]

Primary hypoplasia of the RV. Primary right ventricular hypoplasia is an unfamiliar diagnosis, perhaps because right ventricular hypoplasia usually is (or appears to be) secondary to pulmonary valvar stenosis or atresia, tricuspid stenosis or atresia, or some combination of the foregoing. Occasionally, however, primary right ventricular hypoplasia occurs, that is, right ventricular hypoplasia without tricuspid or pulmonary valvar stenosis or atresia. This unusual finding was observed in Case 592, a 3-month-old white boy with multiple secundum ASDs: an enlarged ostium secundum above the free edge of septum primum (5 mm in diameter) and three fenestrations within the septum primum (4, 3, and 2 mm in diameter). This patient with a small RV also had right ventricular endocardial sclerosis for reasons unknown. We make the diagnosis of endocardial *sclerosis* (as opposed to endocardial *fibroelastosis*), when there is mild to moderate thickening and whitening. (We make the diagnosis of endocardial fibroelastosis when the thickening and whitening is marked, clear-cut, and striking.) This patient did not have Uhl disease; there was not a paucity or absence of right ventricular free wall myocardium. Instead, the RV was curiously small, with mild endocardial thickening and whitening, for no obvious reason. Hence, we regarded the RV hypoplasia as primary (i.e., idiopathic, not secondary to any known cause).

From the management viewpoint, this patient, who had normal segmental anatomy, that is, {S,D,S}, was treated with a modified right Blalock-Taussig anastomosis (3.5 mm in diameter) at 5 days of age. Postoperatively, he developed supraventricular tachycardia. This patient had no obstructive right heart lesion, except perhaps the small RV. Thinking that the modified right Blalock-Taussig anastomosis was excessive, it was decided to perform a bidirectional Glenn anastomosis, with occlusion of the Blalock Taussig anastomosis, at 2¾ months of age. Postoperatively, there was SVC obstruction followed by thrombosis, leading to death.

This unusual case of primary right ventricular hypoplasia raised a number of difficult management issues:

1. When there is no obstructive right heart lesion and no VSD and a secundum ASD permitting right-to-left shunting apparently because of a small RV, a modified Blalock-Taussig anastomosis in the first week of life may not be indicated.
2. How early can one do a bidirectional Glenn procedure? We usually say about 6 months of age, or perhaps a bit earlier. But 2¾ months of age may well have been too early.
3. Suffice it to say that the management of primary right ventricular hypoplasia with a secundum ASD is much more difficult than one might at first appreciate. "Masterful inactivity" may be the optimal therapeutic plan.

I will never forget the case of a colleague from the Johns Hopkins Hospital who had a patient in her 20s with this rare and poorly understood diagnosis. She was mildly cyanotic because of right-to-left atrial shunting. But she managed this problem with "creative makeup." Finally, she and her physicians wanted to fix her, to make her normal. So they surgically closed her large secundum ASD. The result was disastrous. She went into severe right heart failure and almost died. Fortunately, her surgeon reoperated and removed the ASD patch, and the patient recovered and resumed her mildly cyanotic but generally quite satisfactory life.

Now, I know very well that one or two cases prove nothing. I agree that "one mouse is no mouse." But still, when dealing with a patient with the rare and poorly understood diagnosis or primary right ventricular hypoplasia, remembering this cautionary tale may help save the patient's life. The management of this rare entity is much more subtle and difficult that it may at first appear.

The therapeutic problem appears to be as follows:

1. There is no cure for primary right ventricular hypoplasia (at the present time).
2. Palliation, such as a modified Blalock-Taussig anastomosis or a bidirectional Glenn procedure, may well not succeed, as our patient illustrates.
3. Closure of the secundum ASD may not be tolerated. If a patient shunts right to left through a secundum ASD in association with primary right ventricular hypoplasia, such a patient may *have* to shunt right to left to maintain adequate systemic cardiac output and closure of the secundum ASD may be contraindicated.

Needless to say, I very much hope that this therapeutic problem will be recognized and solved. But for now, sailor beware.

Primary endocardial fibroelastosis (EFE) of the RV. Right ventricular EFE with an intact ventricular septum almost always is secondary to pulmonary valvar atresia or severe stenosis. Primary EFE of the RV, not secondary to pulmonary valve obstruction or any other identified disease process, is very rare indeed. This disease was found in an 18-day-old boy (Case 612, A95-83). He had a moderately large secundum ASD (12 × 6 mm). The patient had right ventricular endomyocardial disease with marked EFE of the RV and mild endocardial sclerosis of the LV. The segment anatomy was normal, that is {S,D,S}, the pulmonary valve was unremarkable, and a very careful autopsy revealed no evidence of pheochromocytoma or other significant pathologic condition. Thus, this biventricular endomyocardial disease was, and is, an enigma.

Truncus arteriosus with single LV. A 3-week-old boy (Case 613, C95-364) with a large secundum ASD (18 × 9 mm with multiple fenestrations in a deficient septum primum) had truncus arteriosus type A2 (type A = VSD or bulboventricular foramen present; type 2 = no aortopulmonary septal remnant) with normal segmental anatomy ({S,D,S}), dextrocardia, left-sided JAA, extreme tricuspid stenosis (1 mm in diameter), double-inlet LV, single LV (right ventricular sinus absent), infundibular outlet chamber, and congenital absence of the ductus arteriosus. Truncus arteriosus and single LV with an infundibular outlet chamber constitute a rare combination of congenital heart disease.

Left-sided JAA syndrome. A 28-year-old-man (Case 624, MR 33) with a very large secundum type of ASD (multiple fenestrations in the septum primum resulting in a functionally common atrium) displayed the syndrome of left-sided JAA[1,7]: tricuspid atresia, large ASD II, VSD (high, large, conoventricular type), TGA {S,D,D}, pulmonary stenosis (subvalvar and valvar), and dextrocardia. Many still do not know that there is a left-sided JAA syndrome[1,7] and a right-sided JAA syndrome.[6] The left-sided JAA syndrome[1,7] is characterized by right heart obstructive lesions such as tricuspid atresia, as in this patient. Conversely the right-sided JAA syndrome frequently has obstructive left heart anomalies such as congenital mitral stenosis.[6] This 28-year-old man is one of the oldest patients known with the left-sided JAA syndrome.

Complete form of common AV canal with imperforate Ebstein anomaly, double-orifice of potential mitral valve, and incomplete cleft of the potential mitral valve. An 18-hour-old white girl (Case 630, MR 45) with Down syndrome had a large ASD II because of a defective septum primum. In addition to the previously mentioned anomalies, she had a small VSD of the AV canal type beneath the posteroinferior leaflet of the common AV valve. This case illustrates that completely common AV canal can be much more complex than most classifications suggest.

Infantile Marfan syndrome. Case 639 (C94-26) was a 3-month-old boy with infantile Marfan syndrome.[14] In addition to a secundum type of ASD (two fenestrations in the septum primum, 7 × 4 mm and 4 × 2 mm), this patient had massive cardiomegaly (72 g/28 to 38 g, which is normal). There was hypertrophy and enlargement of all cardiac chambers. The tricuspid valve had a circumference of 79 mm/28 to 32 mm (normal). The mitral valve had a circumference of 73 mm/29 to 37 mm (in normal controls). The pulmonary valvar annulus was very dilated (19 mm in diameter), as was the aortic valvar annulus (13.5 to 15 mm in diameter). There was myxomatous thickening and redundancy of the mitral and tricuspid leaflets, with marked elongation of the chordae tendineae. There was prominent dilatation of the aortic and pulmonary roots. The heart of a typical patient with infantile Marfan syndrome (not Case 639) is presented in Fig. 9.25,[14] illustrating many of the features mentioned previously.

The histology of the ascending aorta revealed severe disruption of the collagen and elastic fibers, with disarray and fragmentation plus increased interstitial ground substance (Fig. 9.26).[14]

In our clinical and postmortem series of 9 patients with infantile Marfan syndrome,[14] the mean age at death was 2.7 months. Hence, this patient who died at 3 months was typical. Mitral valve prolapse was present in all, with mitral regurgitation in 8 of 9 (89%). Tricuspid valve prolapse was present in 8 (89%), with tricuspid regurgitation in 6 of 9 (67%). Marked aortic root dilatation was present in all patients and it was progressive. Aortic regurgitation was documented in 4 of 7 patients (57%). Dilatation of the pulmonary arterial root and pulmonary regurgitation were found in 3 of 7 patients (43%). Severe heart failure was present in 7 of these 9 patients (78%).

In our paper by Geva et al[14] that was published in 1990 describing the infantile Marfan syndrome, we found 86 previously published patients with this syndrome, and their salient features are summarized in Table 9.5.

Infantile Marfan syndrome, as in Case 639, is characterized by clinical and morphologic features that are distinctly different from those of the "classic" form of Marfan syndrome as seen in adolescents and adults (Table 9.6).

Marfan syndrome diagnosed during the first year of life appears to be associated with a poor prognosis (see Tables 9.5 and 9.6). Nearly all of the fatalities were related to severe, intractable congestive heart failure associated with mitral or tricuspid regurgitation.[14] Mitral valve replacement in 22% of our patients often resulted in mortality because of the patient's young age and small size. The mean age at death in infantile Marfan syndrome was 1.4 years, whereas the average age at death in the "classic" adolescence and adult form of Marfan syndrome was 32 to 35 years (see Table 9.6). In the adolescent-adult form, most of the fatalities resulted from aortic dissection or rupture (see Table 9.6).

Why does the infantile form of Marfan syndrome have such a poor prognosis? The very high rate of sporadic cases is thought to be due to new mutations with more severe manifestations.[14] The volume overload associated with mitral and/or tricuspid regurgitation, often also associated with aortic or pulmonary regurgitation, is poorly tolerated in early infancy. Valve replacement during the first year of life is often associated with a high mortality rate. Pulmonary involvement—such as emphysema or obstructive lung disease because of severe kyphoscoliosis—may worsen congestive heart failure, as occurred in 3 of our 9 patients.[14]

Therapeutic options are difficult. Valve reconstruction may be preferable to valve replacement in the first year of life. The role of beta blockers to slow or prevent progressive aortic regurgitation remains uncertain, because this form of therapy is contraindicated in patients with severe congestive heart failure, which was the main cause of death in infantile Marfan syndrome.[14]

In 1896, Marfan[15] published a case report concerning his patient Gabrielle P., a 5½-year-old girl, with (as the title of the paper says) a congenital malformation of the four limbs, more pronounced at their extremities, characterized by elongation of the bones, with a certain degree of narrowing. Marfan called this anomaly, in succinct Latin, *dolichostenomelia* (meaning long narrow extremities). Marfan did not mention cardiovascular or ocular abnormalities in his patient, leading some later observers[16,17] to suggest that his patient may in fact have had contractura, arachnodactyly. Gabrielle P.[15] certainly did not

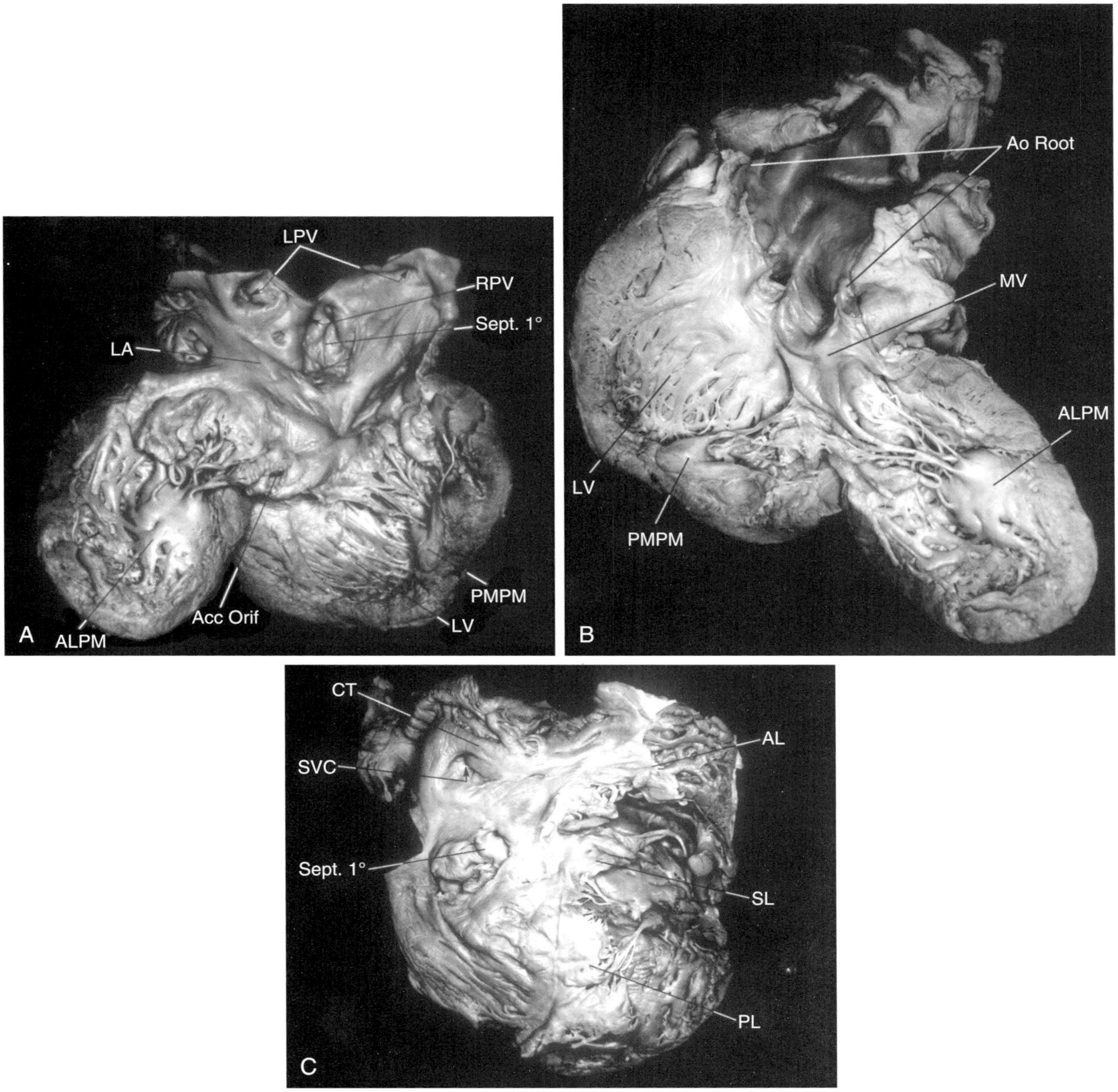

Fig. 9.25 Infantile Marfan syndrome can be associated with a secundum atrial septal defect (ASD), as occurred in our Case 639, a 3-month-old boy who had two perforations of septum primum (7 × 4 and 4 × 2 mm). However, infantile Marfan syndrome often does *not* have a secundum ASD, even though there is severe mitral regurgitation, a markedly enlarged left atrium *(LA)*, and a redundant septum primum, as in this 4-month-old girl who died from intractable congestive heart failure. Diagnosed as having infantile Marfan syndrome at birth, she had arachnodactyly, contractures, kyphoscoliosis, joint hyperelasticity, and a high-arched palate. (A) Opened LA, mitral valve *(MV)*, and the left ventricular *(LV)* inflow tract. Septum primum *(Sept 1°)* is redundant, but no secundum ASD was present. The leaflets of the MV are thickened, redundant, and herniate toward the LA, giving rise to the typical "hemorrhoidal" appearance of the regurgitant MV. Note the small accessory orifice *(Acc Orif)* in the anterior mitral leaflet. The LV is hypertrophied and enlarged, and the anterolateral papillary muscle *(ALPM)* is much more prominent than is the posteromedial papillary muscle *(PMPM)*. (B) Opened left ventricular outflow tract (LV), the outflow tract aspect of the mitral valve (MV), the markedly dilated aortic root *(Ao Root)* and sinuses of Valsalva, and the very dilated ascending aorta that tapers in diameter as one progresses distally. Note the elongated and redundant chordae tendineae of the markedly incompetent mitral valve. (C) Opened right atrium, tricuspid valve, and right ventricular inflow tract. The tricuspid valve's anterior leaflet *(AL)*, posterior leaflet *(PL)*, and septal leaflet *(SL)* are thickened, redundant, and protrude toward the markedly dilated right atrium, and the tricuspid chordae tendineae are elongated, all indicating tricuspid regurgitation. *CT,* Crista terminalis; *LPV,* left pulmonary veins; *RPV,* right pulmonary veins; *SVC,* superior vena cava. (From Geva T, Sanders SP, Diogenes MS, Rockenmacher S, Van Praagh R. Two-dimensional and Doppler echocardiographic and pathologic characteristics of the infantile Marfan syndrome. *Am J Cardiol.* 1990;65:1230, reproduced with permission.)

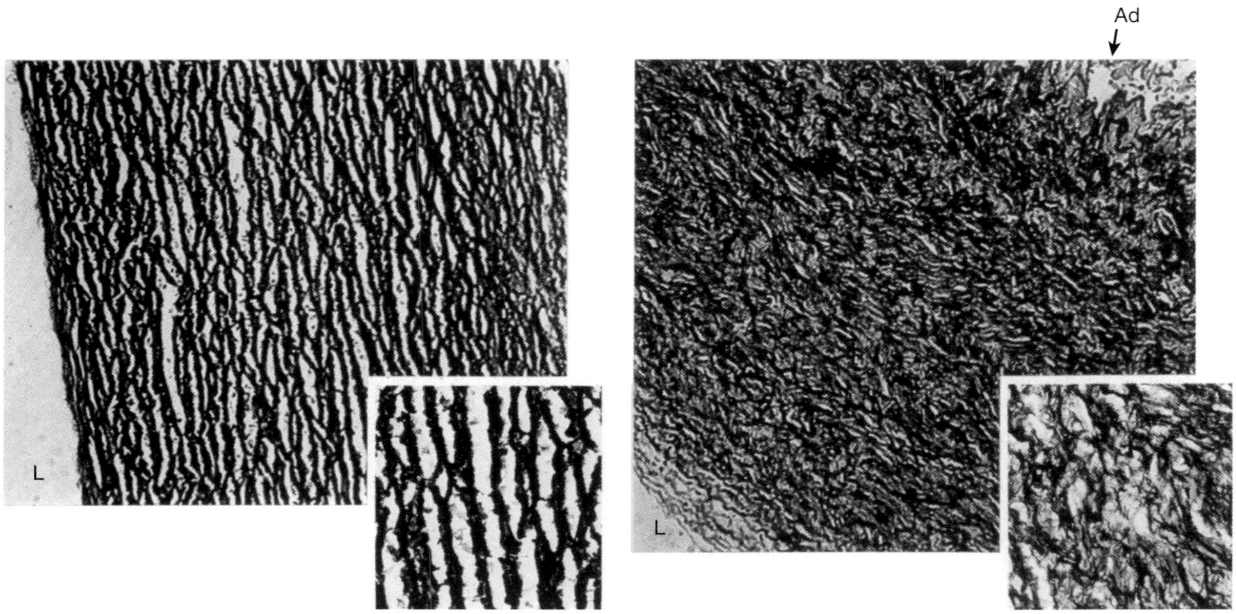

Fig. 9.26 **Histologic Characteristics of Infantile Marfan Syndrome.** *Left,* Section of ascending aorta at the level of the sinuses of Valsalva from age-matched normal control. *Right,* Section of ascending aorta at the level of the sinuses of Valsalva from a 10-month-old girl with infantile Marfan syndrome. Note the fragmented and disarrayed elastic fibers with increased interfiber ground substance compared with normal control (×100). *Insets,* High-power magnification (×400) shows details of elastic fibers (Verhoeff-Van Giesen stain for elastic fibers). *Ad,* Adventitia; *L,* lumen. (From Geva T, Sanders SP, Diogenes MS, Rockenmacher S, Van Praagh R. Two-dimensional and Doppler echocardiographic and pathologic characteristics of the infantile Marfan syndrome. *Am J Cardiol.* 1990;65:1230, reproduced with permission.)

TABLE 9.5 Summary of 86 Published Cases of Infantile Marfan Syndrome[14]

Male-to-female ratio: 2:3		
Positive family history: 18/59 (30%)		
Age at diagnosis: Mean, 3.2 months, range, birth to 12 months		
Characteristic musculoskeletal involvement: 80/80 (100%)		
Ocular abnormalities: 53/64 (83%)		
Cardiovascular involvement		
Mitral valve prolapse	64/67	96%
Mitral regurgitation	56/67	84%
Aortic root dilatation	62/72	86%
Aortic regurgitation	14/53	26%
Tricuspid valve prolapse	19/42	45%
Tricuspid regurgitation	12/51	24%
Pulmonary root dilation	12/50	24%
Congestive heart failure	39/53	74%
Surgical intervention	11/53	21%
Mortality rate	46/63	73%
Age at death, mean: 16.3 months, range: birth to 14 years		

have the infantile form of Marfan syndrome, but she may have had the adolescent-adult or classic form of Marfan syndrome; at 5½ years of age she may have been too young for cardiovascular involvement to have appeared. Therefore, I would suggest that we should not conclude that Marfan did not describe Marfan syndrome because we do not know for sure; I agree that there are grounds for doubt.[16,17]

Sixteen years later, in 1912, the German pediatrician Salle[18] described the first indubitable case of Marfan syndrome of dolichostenomelia with cardiac involvement. His patient died at 2½ months of age with failure to thrive and progressive dyspnea. Autopsy revealed massive cardiac enlargement with redundant and thickened mitral and tricuspid valve leaflets. Salle's case[18] appeared to be the first report of Marfan syndrome with cardiovascular involvement and the first documentation of the infantile type.

Subsequent reports focused on the classic adolescence-adult type of Marfan syndrome, with only a few studies in the pediatric age group.[19-21] Infants under 1 year of age were reported as individual cases or were included in series of patients of widely differing ages. Hence it was Geva et al[14] in 1990 who clearly delineated the existence of the infantile form of Marfan syndrome and highlighted the important differences between the infantile form and the adolescent-adult form of this connective tissue disorder.

In terms of cause, the Marfan syndrome of arachnodactyly, hyperextensibility, lens subluxation, and aortic dilatation is characterized by autosomal dominant inheritance with wide variability of expression. This disorder can occur without pronounced arachnodactyly and without ectopia lentis. Mucopolysaccharide accumulation has been noted in cells of the aorta, and cultured fibroblasts show cytoplasmic metachromatic inclusions.[22]

In 1992, Tsipouras et al[23] from the International Marfan Syndrome Collaborative Study reported genetic linkage of the Marfan phenotype to the fibrillin genes on chromosomes 15

TABLE 9.6 Comparison Between Infantile Marfan Syndrome and the Adolescent-Adult Form of Marfan Syndrome[14]

Salient Features	Infantile Marfan Syndrome	Adolescent-Adult Marfan Syndrome
Age at death (mean)	16.3 months	33.5 years
Main cause of death	Congestive heart failure associated with mitral and tricuspid regurgitation	Aortic dissection or rupture
Family history of Marfan syndrome	Negative in 70%–100% of cases	Negative in about 15% of cases
Musculoskeletal involvement	Joint contractures in about 67% of cases	Typically does not include joint contractures
Ocular involvement	In 67%–83% of cases	In 70% of cases
Mitral valve prolapse	100%	62%–91%
Mitral regurgitation, moderate to severe	89%	13%
Aortic root dilatation	100%	60%–85%
Aortic valvar regurgitation	11%	73%
Tricuspid regurgitation	67%	Uncommon
Pulmonary valvar regurgitation	22%	Uncommon

and 5. Impaired aortic distensibility in children with Marfan syndrome was documented by Savolainen et al[24] in 1992.

Summary. As can now be more fully understood, the ostium secundum type of ASD frequently is associated with other forms of congenital heart disease, with or without additional noncardiovascular disease, that often constitute the patient's main clinical and therapeutic problem (see Table 9.4). Moreover, these anomalies can be rare and fascinating, such as those that have been mentioned:

1. isolated ostium primum type of ASD, without a cleft in the anterior leaflet of the mitral valve;
2. totally anomalous pulmonary venous connection with physiologically normal pulmonary venous drainage;
3. umbilical vein running anterosuperiorly to the liver to connect with the IVC;
4. tracheal atresia with bronchoesophageal fistulae;
5. the combination of parachute mitral valve and Ebstein anomaly of the tricuspid valve;
6. congenital Lutembacher syndrome;
7. concordant AV alignments between solitus atria and L-loop (inverted) ventricles;
8. anomalous connection of umbilical vein with coronary sinus;
9. parachute mitral valve with absence of posteromedial papillary muscle of the LV;
10. secundum ASD with primary pulmonary hypertension;
11 Raghib syndrome without a large low posterior interatrial communication;
12. prominent interseptovalvular space, a rare form of cor triatriatum without pulmonary venous obstruction;
13. truncus arteriosus with intact ventricular septum;
14. incomplete form of common AV canal with imperforate Ebstein anomaly;
15. right aortic arch without mirror-image branching of brachiocephalic arteries;
16. severe congenital stenosis of the IVC at its junction with the RA;
17. stenosis of the right atrial ostium of the coronary sinus, with decompressing "snowman" systemic venous pathway, with normally connected pulmonary veins;
18. TORV in conjoined twins;
19. familial TOF and truncus arteriosus;
20. absence of the main pulmonary artery, right pulmonary artery, left pulmonary artery, and ductus arteriosus;
21. TOF {I,D,S};
22. pulmonary valvar atresia with small membranous VSD (not TOF);
23. asplenia syndrome with interrupted IVC;
24. primary hypoplasia of the RV and management problems associated therewith;
25. primary EFE of the RV;
26. truncus arteriosus with single LV;
27. the syndrome of left-sided JAA;
28. complete form of common AV canal with imperforate Ebstein anomaly of potential tricuspid valve, and double-orifice with incomplete cleft of potential mitral valve; and
29. infantile Marfan syndrome.

The Pathologic Anatomy of Secundum Atrial Septal Defects

What is the pathologic anatomy of the ostium secundum type of ASD itself? Let's just look at the defect (s) itself (themselves). What does one find? Earlier in this chapter I said that secundum ASD may be due to four different kinds of anomaly:

1. **defects of the septum primum**, this is, the flap valve of the foramen ovale, which is the "door" of the normally unidirectional atrial septal valve in utero that permits right-to-left blood flow and prevents left-to-right blood flow;
2. **defects of the superior limbic band of septum secundum,** which is the "door jamb" of the atrial septal valve in utero;
3. **defects of both septum primum (the valve occluder) and the superior limbic band of septum secundum** (the valve ring, against which the occluder normally closes); and
4. **defects of neither septum primum nor the superior limbic band of septum secundum,** such as when the RA of a structurally normal heart is distended by the torrential systemic venous return coming down the SVC when an unoccluded vein of Galen arteriovenous shunt is present in the head.

By describing the atrial septum as an intrauterine monocusp valve, it should be understood that the monocusp or occluder is the septum primum, the valve ring against which the monocusp closes is the superior limbic band of septum secundum, and the hinge at the base of the monocusp valve is the inferior limbic band of septum secundum and the more posteriorly located IVC. So the question we are going to try to answer quantitatively really is, What can go wrong with the atrial septal monocusp valve, which normally closes postnatally?

The four logical possibilities mentioned earlier are merely a beginning. The real questions are, What does one in fact find? and How large are these defects?

Deficiency of septum primum was by far the most common anatomic cause of secundum ASD. In many cases, the septum primum was underdeveloped, that is, too small to occlude the interatrial foramen.

Fenestrations or perforations were described within the septum primum in 143 of these 640 postmortem cases (22%). (I regard this as a minimum number. Many fenestrations may not have been described.) Fenestrations were usually multiple and small, but they could be numerous and large—resulting in a spider-web septum primum. When the fenestrations were small (1 to 3 mm in diameter), they were often described as *cribriform* [cribrum = sieve, Latin].

Septum primum was absent or very deficient in 53 of these 640 patients (8%), resulting in a huge secundum ASD, also often called a common atrium ["common" meaning not divided].

The **size** of the secundum ASD was not always described or measured. The ASD II was described in 498 cases. It was considered to be large in 279 patients (56%), and small in 219 cases (44%). When a defect was described as "moderately large," I recorded it as large. Sometimes the size of a secundum ASD was descried as "moderate." Thinking that the prosector meant that the defect was neither small nor huge, I recorded such defects as "large" (as opposed to "small").

But one may well ask, What do these descriptions mean? What does a "small" ASD II really mean? Similarly, what is a "large" ASD II? In an attempt to answer these questions quantitatively, which is important in device closure of ASD II, see Measurements (later).

First, however, I should describe the other anatomic types of secundum ASD that were found in this series.

A valve-incompetent PFO was described in 50 of the 219 patients with a small ASD II (23%).

Herniation or prolapse of septum primum into the RA (as with mitral atresia) or into the LA (as with tricuspid atresia) was found in 10 of the 219 patients with a small ASD II (5%). The process of herniation or prolapse of the septum primum often was associated with an aneurysm of the septum primum.

Septum primum malposition defect was found in 8 of these 640 cases (1.25%). This infrequent and newly recognized[3] anatomic type of ASD (see Fig. 9.11) was also described in our autopsy protocols as **superior malalignment of the septum primum.** The septum primum was normally hinged inferiorly to the inferior limbic band of septum secundum and to the IVC. But superiorly, the septum primum was fixed in an "open" position, being deviated far to the left of the superior limbic band of septum secundum. Neither the septum primum nor the septum secundum's superior limbic band appeared to be deficient in the cases with aortic atresia. Instead, the septum primum was fixed in an open position, permitting left-to-right or right-to-left shunting between the unapposed occluder (septum I) and the valve ring (superior limbic band of septum II). Stuck in an "open" position, the septum primum also could obstruct the approaches to the subjacent mitral valve, resulting in a supramitral stenosing membrane. The small and restrictive defect between the leftwardly malpositioned septum primum and the posterior left atrial free wall we called a **septum primum malposition defect, which we saw with polyspenia, but not with aortic atresia.**

The ostium secundum type of ASD is the large space between the normally located superior limbic band of the septum secundum to the right and the deviated septum primum to the left. The leftwardly deviated septum primum may lie between the right and left pulmonary veins, resulting in so-called **ipsilateral pulmonary veins,** often associated with polysplenia, or the leftwardly malpositioned septum primum may lie to the left of all of the pulmonary veins, resulting in **TAPVD,** ironically with normal pulmonary venous connections. The anomalous pulmonary venous drainage (partial or total) is caused by malposition of the septum primum, not by anomalous connection of some or all of the pulmonary veins, as used to be thought.

Because **leftward or rightward malalignment of the superior portion of the septum primum,** with or without a septum primum malposition defect, is such an unfamiliar type of ASD II, these 8 cases are summarized in detail (Table 9.7).

Secundum ASD associated with malposition of the superior portion of septum primum—abnormally leftward or abnormally rightward—relative to the superior limbic band of septum secundum thus occurred in several different settings (see Table 9.7):

1. **With visceral heterotaxy and polysplenia (Cases 261 and 609).** This anomaly was first noted and described, to my knowledge, by Stella Van Praagh, MD.[3]
2. **With the HLHS (Cases 292 and 601).** This malformation was first pointed out, to my knowledge, by Dr. Paul Weinberg in the mid-1970s when he was a fellow in cardiac pathology in the Cardiac Registry of Children's Hospital, Boston.
3. **With multiple congenital anomalies.** Case 308 had Noonan syndrome, and Case 603 had trisomy 13 (see Table 9.7).
4. **With TGA and with DORV.** (Cases 293 and 543, respectively, Table 9.7).

This unfamiliar anatomic type of secundum ASD is noteworthy because of the interatrial communication appears to be caused by malposition of the superior portion of the septum primum, rather than by deficiency or absence of septum primum, septum secundum, or both. Displacement (rather than deficiency) of the occluder (septum primum) is a new and recently recognized anatomic cause of secundum ASD.

There are two different kinds of malposition of septum primum: (1) with visceral heterotaxy, usually with polysplenia; and (2) without visceral heterotaxy, that is, with the HLHS.

1. When the septum primum malposition with visceral heterotaxy (usually with polyspenia) is present, the septum primum can lie between the right and left pulmonary veins,

TABLE 9.7 Atrial Septal Defect II With Leftward or Rightward Malposition of Septum Primum

Case No.	Gender	Age at Death	Description	Associated Abnormalities
261	Male	6½ months	Leftwardly malaligned septum I, with fenestrations and superior defect in septum I. All pulmonary veins drain into RA (TAPVD) because of leftward malalignment of sept I to left of left pulmonary veins	Polysplenia syndrome {S,D,S}, multiple fissures in left-sided spleen, bilaterally bilobed lungs, interrupted IVC, common GI mesentery, bilateral SVC, bilateral azygos veins, LSVC to CoS to RA, small membranous VSD, anomalous muscle bundles of RV with obstruction at mid-RV resulting in systemic and pulmonary venous hypertension, *Escherichia coli* sepsis
292	Female	5 days	ASD II because of leftward malalignment of superior portion of septum I relative to superior limbic band of septum II: septum I 3–4 mm to left of septum II	Hypoplastic left heart syndrome with multiple congenital anomalies: aortic atresia (valvar), mitral atresia, VSD (small, membranous), PDA, aberrant left subclavian artery, absence of lung fissures, bilateral hypoplasia of kidneys
293	Female	2 days and 20 hours	ASD II because of leftward deviation of superior portion of septum I relative to superior limbic band of septum II	TGA {S,L,L}, hypoplasia of RV (L), hypoplasia of TV (L), VSD (CV, slit-like), aortic valve bicuspid and hypoplastic, preductal coarctation of aorta, closing PDA
308	Female	4 months	ASD II with multiple fenestrations of septum I and abnormal attachment of septum I to roof of LA to the left of superior limbic band of septum II	Multiple congenital anomalies: Noonan syndrome with hypertrophic cardiomyopathy, RVOTO because of septal band hypertrophy, thick-walled and small-chambered LV, eccentric coronary ostia, coarctation of aorta (juxtaductal), valvar pulmonary stenosis
543	Female	12 days	ASD II with leftward displacement of superior portion of septum I relative to septum II	DORV {S,D,A}, left-sided juxtaposition of the atrial appendages, persistent LSVC to CoS to RA, myxomatous TV and MV, VSD (CV), severe PS (subvalvar), bicuspid PV
601	Female	11 days	Large ASD II with abnormal leftward malalignment and horizontal lie of septum I. Inferior limbic band of septum II is a rare dysmorphic mass: 9 mm long, 7 mm wide, 11 mm high	Mitral atresia {S,D,S}, multiple VSDs: CV (6 mm) and mid-muscular (4 mm). LV small-chambered, subaortic stenosis, preductal coarctation (1 mm), closing PDA, TV with multiple blood cysts, myxomatous, dysmorphic with congenital tricuspid regurgitation Dysplastic ventricular myocardial architecture of RV and LV
603	Male	6 days	ASD II because of leftward displacement of superior portion of otherwise well-developed septum I relative to superior limbic band of septum II. Septum I does not coapt with septum II because of leftward malalignment of sept I	Multiple congenital anomalies: trisomy 13 (karotype proved) Bilateral SVC, LSVC to CoS, to RA Bicommissural AoV with poorly formed RC/LC commissure Preductal coarctation of Ao, PDA closing
609	Female	5 years	ASD II because of markedly deficient septum I Septum I attaches into left-sided RA; that is, rare form of septum I malposition is present—malaligned into RA (there are two types of septum I malposition: malposition into the LA, the common form; and malposition into the RA, the rarer form, as in this patient; both types of septum I malposition are associated with secundum ASD)	Polysplenia with visceral heterotaxy, DORV {I,L,L}, interrupted IVC Right azygos vein to RSVC TAPVD to RA(L) Partially unroofed CoS communicates with both atria Hypoplasia of LV(R) CCAVC Pulmonary stenosis (valvar) Right aortic arch Liver predominantly left-sided Multiple right-sided splenuli Cecum right-sided (heterotaxy) SubPA conus Infantile type of DORV with hypoplastic LV(R)

Ao, Aorta; *ASD II,* ostium secundum type of atrial septal defect; *AoV,* aortic valve; *CCAVC,* completely common atrioventricular canal; *CoS,* coronary sinus; *CV,* conoventricular; *DORV* {I,L,L}, double-outlet right ventricle with situs inversus of the atria, L-loop ventricles, and L-malposition of the great arteries; *DORV {S,D,A},* double-outlet right ventricle with situs solitus of the atria, D-loop ventricles, and A-malposition of the great arteries; *GI,* gastrointestinal; *IVC,* inferior vena cava; *L,* left; *LA,* morphologically left atrium; *LSVC,* left superior vena cava; *LV,* morphologically left ventricle, *LV(R),* morphologically left ventricle, right-sided; *MV,* mitral valve; *PA,* pulmonary arteries; *PDA,* patent ductus arteriosus; *PS,* pulmonary stenosis; *PV,* pulmonary valve; *RA,* morphologically right atrium; *RA(L),* morphologically right atrium, left-sided; *RC/LC,* right coronary/left coronary; *RSVC,* right superior vena cava; *RV,* morphologically right ventricle; *RV(L),* morphologically right ventricle, left-sided; *RVOTO,* right ventricular outflow tract obstruction; *{S,D,S},* situs solitus of the atria, D-loop ventricles, and solitus normally related great arteries; *septum I,* septum primum; *septum II,* septum secundum; *SubPA,* subpulmonary arterial; *SVC,* superior vena cava; *TAPVD,* totally anomalous pulmonary venous drainage; *TGA {S,L,L},* transposition of the great arteries with solitus atria, L-loop ventricles, and L-transposition of the great arteries; *TV,* tricuspid valve; *TV(L),* tricuspid valve, left-sided; *VSD,* ventricular septal defect; VSDs, ventricular septal defects.

resulting in ipsilateral pulmonary veins. Or the septum primum can lie entirely on the "wrong" side of all the pulmonary veins (to the left in atrial situs solitus or to the right in atrial situs inversus), resulting in TAPVD. A septum primum malposition defect usually is present, consisting of one or more small openings between the malpositioned septum primum and the posterior left atrial free wall. The superior limbic band of septum secundum may be very hypoplastic or absent, making it possible to see septum primum with unusual clarity from the right atrial aspect. When the malposed septum primum lies far to the left within the LA, the malposed septum primum can function as a stenotic supramitral membrane. This can occur when the malposed septum primum is not (or minimally) fenestrated and when the septum primum malposition defects at the junction of the septum primum and the left atrial free wall are restrictively small. In the present study of ASDs, malposition of septum primum with visceral heterotaxy and polysplenia is exemplified by Cases 261 and 609 (see Table 9.7).

2. When septum primum malposition *without* visceral heterotaxy (e.g., with aortic atresia) is present, only the superior portion of the septum primum bulges into the LA. Because the leftwardly malpositioned superior portion of the septum primum does not coapt with the superior limbic band of septum secundum, a large secundum type of ASD results. The space above the superior margin of septum primum is wide open and far to the left of the superior limbic band of septum secundum. Because septum primum does not lie between the right and left pulmonary veins or on the "wrong" side of all the pulmonary veins, partially or totally anomalous pulmonary venous drainage into the RA does not occur. A septum primum malposition defect (hole or holes) between the malpositioned septum primum and the left atrial free wall also does not occur. Thus, the septum primum is much less malpositioned without visceral heterotaxy than with visceral heterotaxy. Malposition of the superior portion of the septum primum without visceral heterotaxy is exemplified by Cases 292, 293, 308, 543, 601, and 603 (see Table 9.7).

Absence or underdevelopment of the superior limbic band of septum secundum was the anatomic cause of a secundum ASD in 4 of these patients (Cases 268, 269, 390, and 461). It will be recalled that the superior limbic band of septum secundum is the valve "ring" against which the monocusp occluder normally coapts. When the superior limbic band of septum secundum is absent or very poorly developed, the monocusp occluder (septum primum) does not have a valve "ring" against which to close. Consequently, the unidirectional flap valve of the intrauterine individual (i.e., the atrial septum of the normal postnatal individual) is unable to prevent left-to-right shunting above the occluder (septum primum), resulting in a secundum ASD. Because this anatomic type of secundum ASD, caused by an absent or underdeveloped superior limbic band of septum secundum, but with a well-developed septum primum, is unfamiliar and poorly understood, these 4 patients are summarized in detail (Table 9.8).

Deficiency of the septum primum and of the superior limbic band of the septum secundum was found in two patients with ASD II (Cases 299 and 519). This was a decidedly infrequent anatomic type of ASD II: 2 of 640 cases (0.3%). In view of their rarity, these two patients are summarized in Table 9.9.

DEVICE CLOSURE OF SECUNDUM ATRIAL SEPTUM DEFECTS

An understanding of the various anatomic types of ASD II is very important relative to device closure by interventional cardiologists. (As always, a good understanding of the pathologic anatomy remains of vital importance for cardiac surgeons.) But let us concentrate for a few moments on the problems associated with device closure of secundum ASDs.

1. **A good rim.** Devices need a good rim all around the defect. Consequently, patients with absence or marked underdevelopment of the superior limbic band of septum secundum are not good candidates for device closure, because they do not have a good rim superiorly and anteriorly (see Tables 9.8 and 9.9). Fortunately, this problem of a deficient anterosuperior rim does not appear to be frequent: 6 in 640 cases (0.9%).

Can the posteroinferior rim be deficient, that is, a deficient inferior limbic band of septum secundum? Yes, for example, when a common AV canal is associated with a secundum ASD, as in Case 519 (see Table 9.9). However, one would probably not elect device closure in a patient with the asplenia syndrome. In isolated ASD II, deficiency of the inferior limbic band of septum secundum usually is not a problem.

2. **A normally located septum primum or its remnants.** This is a second desirable feature for successful device closure of a secundum ASD. In other words, with marked malposition of the anterosuperior portion of the septum primum, particularly if the septum primum is fixed in a very abnormal position, far removed from the superior limbic band of septum secundum, such patients appear *not* to be good candidates for ASD device closure from an anatomic standpoint (see Table 9.7). From the therapeutic viewpoint, fortunately such patients appear to be infrequent: 8 in 640 (1.25%).
3. **Size.** This is a third very important consideration concerning device closure of secundum ASDs. How big is the hole?

Unfortunately, not all cases in this postmortem series had accurate measurements of the dimensions of the defect recorded; however, many did. I shall now endeavor to summarize these measurements.

Each case will be represented by its greatest dimension. For example, if the ASD II measured 10 × 7 mm, this case will be regarded as having a defect 10 mm in diameter. The device will, of course, need to have a diameter greater than 10 mm to occlude the defect successfully, as all interventionists understand. The data concerning the greatest dimension of 225 measured cases of ASD II are summarized in Table 9.10.

Familial ASD II. One patient (Case 383) had familial secundum ASD. The patient was a white boy who died at 1 day of age. His mother also had an ASD II. This neonatal boy had a large ASD II measuring 6 × 4 mm. He was premature (32

TABLE 9.8 Atrial Septal Defect II With Absence or Marked Underdevelopment of the Superior Limbic Band of Septum Secundum

Case No.	Gender	Age at Death	Description	Associated Anomalies
268	Male	2 days	Absence of superior limbic band of septum secundum resulting in ASD II	Hypoplastic left heart syndrome: aortic atresia (valvar), endocardial fibroelastosis of left ventricle, coarctation of the aorta (juxtaductal, mild)
269	Male	2 days	Underdevelopment of superior limbic band of septum secundum resulting in small ASD II. Septum primum well developed	Aortic valvar stenosis, extreme (1-mm opening, AoV unicuspid); EFE of the LV, PDA closing
390	Female	2½ years	Very deficient superior limbic band of septum secundum, resulting in valve incompetent patent foramen ovale (small ASD II)	Left-sided juxtaposition of the atrial appendages, tricuspid atresia TGA {S,D,D}, multiple VSDs (large conoventricular and multiple slit-like muscular defects), severe PS, right aortic arch
461	Male	6 11/12 years	Superior limbic band of septum secundum is absent ASD II above well-formed septum primum Multiple small fenestrations of septum primum	Multiple congenital anomalies: heterotaxy with polysplenia syndrome and caudal regression syndrome (underdevelopment of both legs) DORV {A(S),S,D(S)} Bilobed spleen, LUQ symmetrical liver with right-sided gallbladder Interrupted IVC with azygos vein to RSVC LSVC to CoS to RA Bilateral unilobed lung CCAVC, type C, balanced DORV with sub-PA conus with AoV-CAVV fibrous continuity (infantile type of DORV with sub-PA conus) Preductal coarctation of Ao

Ao, Aorta; *AoV*, aortic valve; *ASD II*, ostium secundum type of atrial septal defect; *CAVV*, common atrioventricular valve; *CCAVC*, completely common atrioventricular canal; *CoS*, coronary sinus; *DORV {A(S),S,D(S)}*, double-outlet right ventricle with the segmental anatomic set of situs ambiguus of the viscera (with situs solitus of the atria), D-loop ventricles, and D-malposition of the great arteries (but resembling solitus normally related great arteries, i.e., having a subpulmonary conus with aortic valve-common atrioventricular valve direct fibrous continuity); *EFE*, endocardial fibroelastosis; *IVC*, inferior vena cava; LSVC, left superior vena cava; *LUQ*, left upper quadrant; *LV*, morphologically left ventricle; *PA*, pulmonary artery; *PDA*, patent ductus arteriosus; *PS*, pulmonary stenosis; *RSVC*, right superior vena cava; *TGA* {S,D,D}, transposition of the great arteries with solitus atria, D-loop ventricles, and D-transposition; *VSDs*, ventricular septal defects.

TABLE 9.9 Atrial Septal Defect II With Deficiency of Both Septum Primum and Septum Secundum

Case No.	Gender	Age at Death	Description	Associated Anomalies
299	Female	4¼ hours	Absence of superior limbic band of septum secundum and deficiency of septum primum, resulting in a large ASD II	Multiple congenital anomalies: left-sided juxtaposition of the atrial appendages, congenital tricuspid hypoplasia (stenosis), right ventricular hypoplasia, conoventricular type of VSD, posterior malalignment of conal septum with PAt, mesocardia, dysmorphic features (small head, flat nose, low-set ears, increased intercanthal distance), clubbed feet, hypospadias, anal atresia, cystic left kidney, common gastrointestinal mesentery, thoracic hemivertebrae, absent sacrum
519	Male	4 days	Markedly hypoplastic superior limbic band of septum secundum and very deficient septum primum, resulting in a large ASD II	Asplenia syndrome, mesocardia with ventricular apex pointing rightward, DORV {A(I),D,D}, subpulmonary conus with AoV-CAVV fibrous continuity, CCAVC (A) opening predominantly into the LV, hypoplasia of RV sinus, posterior malalignment of conal septum, valvar aortic stenosis, hypoplasia of ascending Ao and of aortic arch, multiple VSDs, unroofed coronary sinus (absent CoS ostium and absence of CoS septum)

Ao, Aorta; *AoV*, aortic valve; *CAVV*, common atrioventricular valve; *CCAVC (A)*, completely common atrioventricular canal, type A; *CoS*, coronary sinus; *DORV {A(I),D,D}*, double-outlet right ventricle with situs ambiguus of the viscera, situs inversus of the atria, D-loop ventricles, and D-malposition of the great arteries; *LV*, morphologically left ventricle; *PAt*, pulmonary atresia; *RV*, morphologically right ventricle; *VSD*(s), ventricular septal defect(s).

weeks estimated gestational age). The cause of death was not the secundum ASD, but sepsis caused by group B beta hemolytic streptococcal infection with congenital pneumonia. He also had respiratory distress syndrome with hyaline membrane formation.

Summary of the Anatomic Types of Secundum Atrial Septal Defect

The four anatomic types and subtypes of ostium secundum ASD that were found in this series of 640 postmortem cases are summarized in Table 9.11.

TABLE 9.10 Data Concerning the Greatest Dimension in Atrial Septal Defect II (n = 225)

	Millimeters
Mean	11.3
Standard deviation	±8.5
Range	2–50
Median	10

TABLE 9.11 Anatomic Types of Secundum Atrial Septal Defect Found in 640 Postmortem Cases

Anatomic Type	No. of Cases	% of Series
1. Deficiency of septum primum	626	97.8
a. With fenestrations, 143 (22.3%)		
b. Absence of sept I, 53 (8.3%)		
c. Valve incompetent PFO, 50 (7.8%)		
d. Herniation of sept I, 10 (1.6%)		
2. Septum primum malposition	8	1.3
3. Absence/hypoplasia of sept II	4	0.6
4. Deficiency of sept II and sept I	2	0.3

PFO, Patent foramen ovale; *sept I,* septum primum; *sept II,* septum secundum.

Representative examples of ostium secundum ASD that were found in this series of 640 postmortem patients are presented photographically in Fig. 9.27.

LITERATURE

Now let us turn to the literature[1-363] because this is fascinating resource that amplifies what we have been able to learn by the study of our own data. Most of these references[25-363] are arranged approximately chronologically, from the earliest to the latest, so that the interested reader can follow the growth and development over time of our understanding of interatrial communications. Although no one can read and record everything, I wish to begin by acknowledging the limitations of time and strength and by apologizing to those authors whose work has been inadvertently omitted here.

Who First Described the Ostium Secundum Type of Atrial Septal Defect?

Insofar as is known at present, the answer is **Leonard Da Vinci,** in 1513.[25] This discovery appears to have been made by Dr. William J Rashkind, the father of interventional cardiology and published by him in 1982.[25] Concerning Leonardo's "sketch of heart auricles" that now resides in the Royal Library of Windsor Castle in England, Rashkind wrote[25]: "This sketch was published by Leonardo Da Vinci in 1513, and the inscription reads: 'I have found from a, left auricle to b, right auricle, a perforating channel from a to b, which I note here to see whether this occurs in other auricles of other hearts.' "

Note that Leonardo Da Vinci describes this secundum ASD or PFO as a *channel,* that is, as having right-left length. This three-dimensional understanding has recently been rediscovered by Marshall and Lock.[274] As his surname indicates, Leonardo (1452–1519) was from Vinci in the valley of the Arno river south of Florence (Firenze), Italy. An artist, inventor, engineer, and anatomist, Leonardo Da Vinci attempted to understand the fundamentals of human anatomy and physiology and was the first to illustrate the anatomic structures of the human heart.

The second known description of PFO is that of **LeCat** in 1747. He found a PFO in no men, in 1 adolescent boy (15 years of age), and in 7 of 20 women (35%). These very early findings may be viewed as presaging the female preponderance in isolated secundum ASD.

The third known case of this type of interatrial communication was published in 1761 by **Morgagni**. His patient was a 15-day-old infant who had total absence of the valve of the foramen ovale, that is, a relatively very large secundum ASD or common atrium. Giovanni Battista Morgagni (1682–1771) was *the founder of pathologic anatomy*. Born at Forli in Italy, he studied medicine under Antonio Maria Valsalva (1662–1723) and Ippolito Francesco Albertini (1662–1738) in Bologna. Morgagni was appointed first professor of anatomy at Padua in 1715, where he served for 59 years. His most important work, *De Sedibus et Causis Morborum per Anatomen Indagatis*[27] *(Concerning the Seats and Causes of Disease Investigated by Anatomy, Latin),* was based on more than 600 postmortem examinations. Published in 1761, this work was written in the form of 70 letters to an anonymous friend and colleague. Thus pathology developed from anatomy with the work of Morgagni.

The next really big step in the ASD story did not occur for almost 200 years: the development of open-heart surgery, first with hypothermia and soon thereafter with cardiopulmonary bypass. In 1953, Lewis and Taufic[28] reported successful closure of a secundum ASD in a 5-year-old girl with the aid of hypothermia. After 2 hours and 10 minutes of surface cooling, her rectal temperature had dropped to 28° C. Using inflow occlusion for 5.5 minutes, a secundum ASD of 2 cm in diameter was closed under direct vision. The operative time was 58 minutes. The patient was discharged well on the 11th postoperative day. The operation of Lewis and Taufic[28] in 1953 was the first open-heart direct-vision surgical repair performed in a human.

The next year, Dr. John H Gibbon, Jr.[29] reported the application of a mechanical heart and lung apparatus of his own design to repair a secundum ASD in an 18-year-old girl. Performed on May 6, 1953, this surgical triumph was not reported until early 1954 in *Minnesota Medicine.*[29] The heart-lung machine had been "born," and with it modern cardiac surgery became possible. Gibbon used a transverse submammary incision form one axilla to the other. He closed the secundum ASD directly with a continuous silk suture. The patient was well postoperatively, and cardiac catheterization showed that the ASD was closed.

Successful surgery made accurate diagnosis (pediatric and adult cardiology and cardiovascular radiology) and detailed the morphologic understanding (pathology) necessary. These fields then developed rapidly, as the subsequent bibliography shows.[30-363] As Dr. Aldo Castaneda has often told me, the surgeons really led the way; this is true.

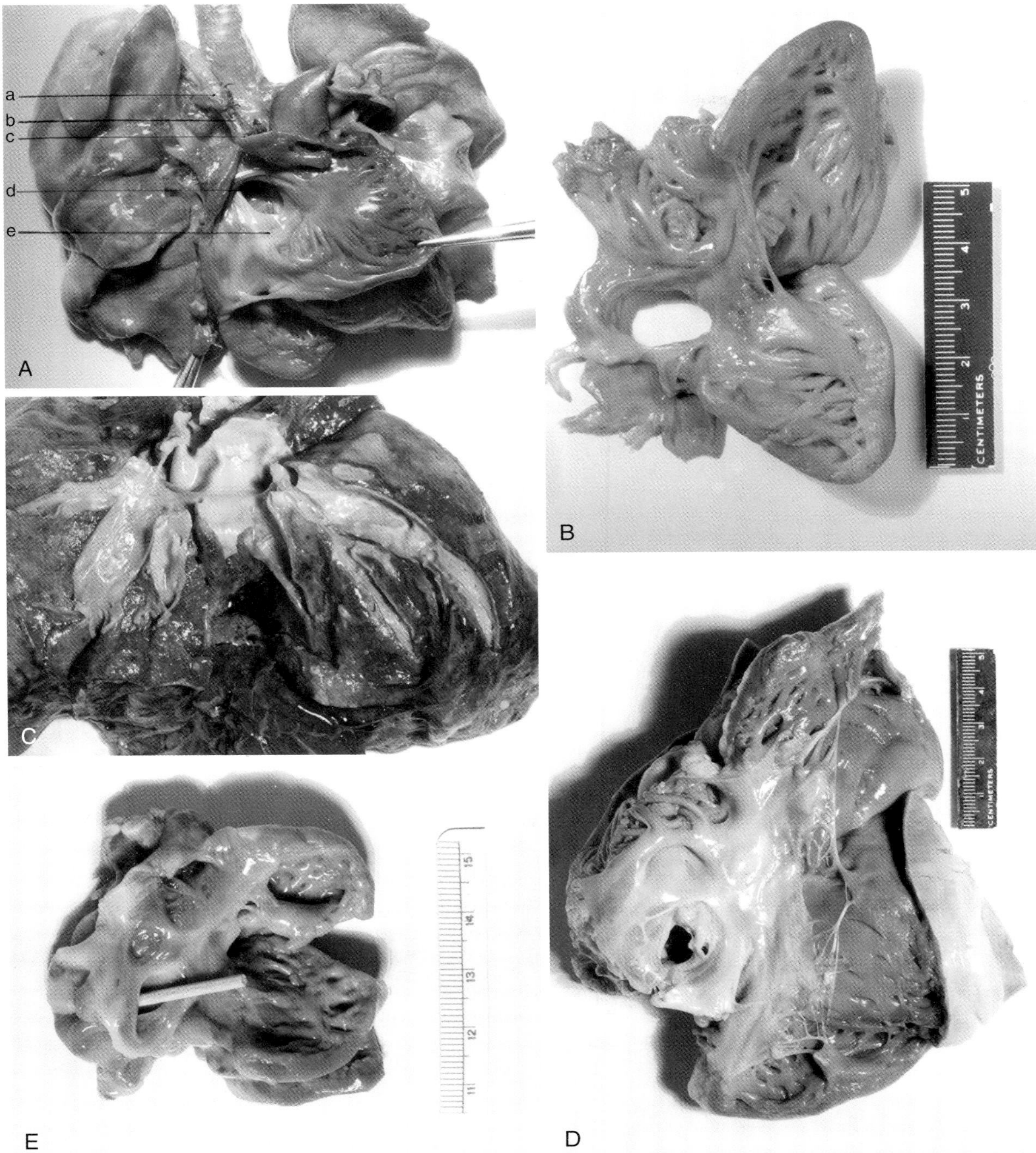

Fig. 9.27 Representative Ostium Secundum Atrial Septal Defects (All Photos Taken at the Time of Autopsy).

Continued

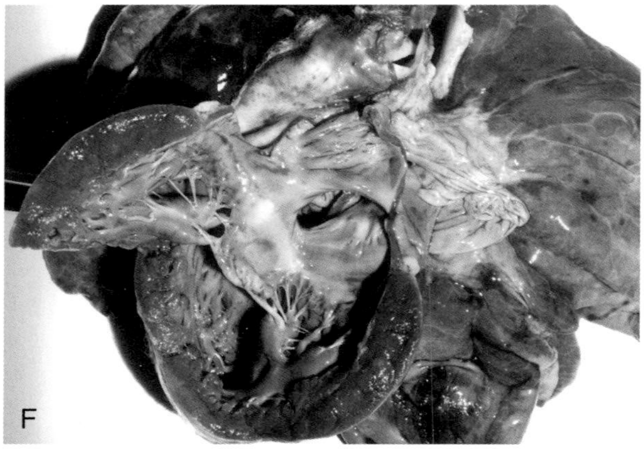

F

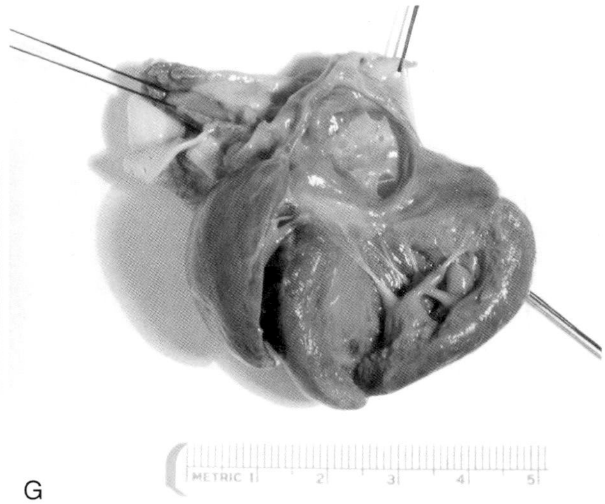

G

Fig. 9.27, cont'd (A) Opened right atrium of 5-month-old white boy with tricuspid atresia (type Ib) who died in 1960 18 hours after a classical Glenn anastomosis of the right pulmonary artery to the right superior vena cava. At autopsy, the Glenn anastomosis appeared restrictive. Note the deficient septum primum resulting in a secundum atrial septal defect (ASD). The opened right atrium is hypertrophied and enlarged. *a,* Right pulmonary artery; *b,* superior vena cava; *c,* suture occlusion of the superior vena caval–right atrial junction; *d,* large secundum atrial septal defect; *e,* tricuspid atresia. (B) Opened right atrium, tricuspid valve, and right ventricle of a 7-day-old white boy with hypoplastic left heart syndrome (hypoplastic mitral valve, left ventricle, aortic valve, ascending aorta, and aortic arch). The patient had hypertrophy and enlargement of the right atrium and right ventricle. The main pulmonary artery and branches were enlarged. An enlarged patent ductus arteriosus flowed directly into the top of the descending thoracic aorta. Thus, the left heart structures were hypoplastic, whereas the right heart structures were considerably enlarged. The patient also had a small ventricular septal defect (VSD) (3 mm in diameter). The secundum ASD is large (12 mm in maximal dimension). Septum primum is absent and septum secundum (superior limbic band) is poorly formed. The right atrium and right ventricle are hypertrophied and enlarged. This patient died in 1961 primarily from the hypoplastic left heart syndrome. (C) Note the dilatation and atheromatous plaques of the opened pulmonary arteries of this 15 8/12-year-old girl who died in 1965, 5 years after her secundum ASD had been well closed surgically. Pulmonary angiocardiography had shown dilatation, tortuosity, and pruning, indicating severe pulmonary vascular obstruction (PVO). This patient also had a VSD, mild pulmonary valvar stenosis, mitral regurgitation, and an aberrant right subclavian artery. At 10 years of age (in 1960) she underwent surgical ASD closure, mitral annuloplasty, and pulmonary valvotomy. Lung biopsy revealed severe PVO with grades 3 and 4 Heath-Edwards changes. Pulmonary hypertension was severe (106/24 mm Hg) and was associated with tricuspid regurgitation. Gradually, congestive heart failure appeared. At 15 years of age, she underwent surgical VSD closure, mitral valve replacement with a ball-valve prosthesis, and tricuspid annuloplasty. Postoperatively she convulsed, developed ventricular fibrillation, and resuscitation was unsuccessful. This case clearly indicates why early, accurate and complete diagnosis, followed by successful therapy are so important to avoid PVO disease that makes patients inoperable or untreatable, at least for curative (as opposed to palliative) procedures. This case also illustrates another very important point, namely, that secundum ASDs often are associated with other very serious forms of congenital heart disease. This is the "rule" in pediatric cardiology and cardiac surgery, not the exception. (D) Opened right atrium, tricuspid valve, and right ventricle of an 11 7/12-year-old white boy who died in 1965. He had a large secundum ASD (25 × 20 mm) with marked deficiency and small fenestrations of septum primum and right ventricular hypertrophy and enlargement. The immediate cause of death was staphylococcal sepsis with acute staphylococcal pneumonia, meningitis, otitis media, and right-sided cerebellar abscess. He also suffered from multiple congenital anomalies, including brachydactyly, bony fusion of phalanges of the fingers, fusion of cervical vertebrae from C2 to C8, hypospadias, and cerebral malformation with intellectual disability. The large secundum ASD may have predisposed to staphylococcal pneumonia, but this patient also had many other serious medical problems.(E) Opened right atrium, tricuspid valve, and right ventricle of a 2-day-old white girl with a relatively large secundum ASD (5 mm in diameter) caused by marked deficiency of septum primum (seen beneath the probe passing through the ASD). This patient also had tetralogy of Fallot with the secundum ASD, this combination often is called the pentalogy of Fallot. This patient also had Cantrell syndrome with large anterior diaphragmatic hernia, thoracoabdominal ectopia cordis, omphalocele, heart adherent to omphalocele sac, malrotation of the gut, and congenital absence of the gallbladder. The omphalocele was repaired (in 1952), and the patient died postoperatively. The large secundum ASD was thought not to be important as a cause of death in this neonate. (F) Opened left atrium, mitral valve, and left ventricle of a 2 2/12-year-old white girl with a huge secundum ASD (20 × 10 mm) that "easily admits two fingers," as the prosector wrote. No septum primum was found. This patient had tricuspid atresia type Ib (with normally related great arteries and with small VSD resulting in pulmonary outflow tract stenosis). In 1953, the patient was treated with a classic Blalock-Taussig anastomosis. Postoperatively, acute congestive heart failure developed, leading to death. The large secundum ASD was thought not to be important as a cause of death. Indeed, it was thought that a large ASD may have been hemodynamically beneficial in association with tricuspid atresia by removing all restriction to right-to-left blood flow at the level of the atrium septum. The left atrium and left ventricle are both hypertrophied and enlarged. This case illustrates the counterintuitive principle that, **depending on what associated cardiac malformations are present, a large secundum ASD is not always bad; in fact, it can be hemodynamically helpful preoperatively,** as in physiologically uncorrected transposition of the great arteries {S,D,D} with intact ventricular septum and closing or closed ductus arteriosus; a large secundum ASD promotes venoarterial mixing at the atrial level preoperatively. (G) Opened left atrium, mitral valve, and left ventricle of a 14-day-old white boy. Note the small ostium secundum superiorly, above septum primum, and the small fenestration inferiorly, within septum primum. This patient also had pulmonary valvar atresia with intact ventricular septum, a bicuspid aortic valve, and a probe-patent ductus arteriosus that was closing. This patient illustrates the same counterintuitive principle: **the secundum ASDs were not large enough; that is, they were too small.** Given the coexistence of pulmonary atresia with intact ventricular septum, all of the systemic venous return had to shunt from right atrium to left atrium above and through this restrictive septum primum. The fact that the ductus arteriosus was closing also appears to have been an important immediate cause of this boy's death in 1957.

It is also interesting to note that the ASD story is synonymous with the early history of modern medicine, and modern cardiology and cardiac surgery: Leonardo Da Vinci[25] in 1513 (part of the birth of modern medicine in the 16th century); Morgagni[27] in 1761 (the appearance of pathology in the 18th century); and Lewis and Taufic[28] in 1953 and Gibbon[29] in 1954 (the development of open-heart surgery and the successful repair of secundum ASD in the mid-20th century).

Much has happened since 1953 and 1954, as the literature documents.[30-363] To discuss all of this in detail would require a book-length manuscript. Instead, I shall make only a few relatively brief summary comments. The literature is referenced *in extenso* to facilitate investigation of any aspect of this subject.

PATHOLOGIC ANATOMY

Hemodynamic Changes of the Atrioventricular Valves

What Dr. Maurice Lev called hemodynamic changes of the AV valves in association with secundum ASD were noted early (in 1968).[44,55] These changes consisted of endocardial thickening and fibrosis (endocardial sclerosis) involving the leaflets and chordae tendinae of the mitral and tricuspid valves. This endocardial sclerosis of the AV valves proved to be clinically and surgically important, with calcification of the tricuspid valve[60] and *prolapse of the posterior leaflet of the mitral valve*[6,107] being reported in association with secundum ASD. Others called these changes *balloon mitral valve,*[88] *mitral regurgitation,*[92,124] or simply a *mitral valve lesion.*[147]

Attention is focused on the mitral valve lesion (and on the tricuspid valve lesion) that can be associated with ASD II, because many are not aware of this association.

Measurements of the Atrial Septal Defect II

The size of the secundum ASD, its location, whether it is single or multiple, and the nature of its rims have become important diagnostic details, particularly since the advent of percutaneous transcatheter device closure of ASD II.[a]

In 1993, Radzik et al[223] proposed the following:

1. When the ASD is less than 3 mm in diameter, such patients do not need to be followed because 100% will be closed by 18 months of age.
2. When the ASD is 8 mm or greater in diameter, there is little chance of spontaneous closure and therefore surgery (or transcatheter intervention) should be considered.
3. When the ASD is between 3 and 8 mm in diameter the patient should be evaluated between 12 and 15 months of age, when more than 80% of ASD II defects will have closed spontaneously.

In 1999, the same group[263] from Hopital Ste Justine in Montreal, Canada published the outcome of their patients with ASD II that had been considered too small for surgical closure. Their conclusions were as follows:

1. Secundum ASDs can close spontaneously beyond the age of 5 years.
2. In a minority of cases, the size of the ASD can increase.
3. Spontaneous closure of secundum ASD occurred in 17 of 30 patients (57%) at a mean age of 8.4 years.

Chan and Godman (1993)[228] concluded that half of secundum ASDs are closable by means of a clamshell device. This, of course, means that these investigators thought that half of secundum ASDs are *not* closable by this device. Ferreira, Ho, and Anderson (1992)[239] thought that 68% of secundum ASDs (within the fossa ovalis) are ideal for transcatheter device closure, that 3% are probably suitable, but that 29% are not suitable for such closure.

In 2002, McMahon et al[317] published a study of 104 cases of secundum ASD. These investigators focused on the natural history of the growth of secundum ASDs and the implications of these data for transcatheter closure. They defined a *small ASD II* as having a diameter greater than 3 but less than 6 mm, a *moderate ASD II* as having a diameter of 6 to less than 12 mm, and a *large ASD II* as having a diameter of 12 mm or greater. ASDs that have grown to 20 mm or greater in diameter were defined as having outgrown device closure. These workers found that secundum ASD diameter increased in 68 of 104 cases (65%), there being a greater than 50% increase in 31 of 104 patients (30%). Spontaneous closure occurred in 4 of 104 cases (4%). An insufficient rim was found in 20%. These authors concluded that two-thirds of secundum ASDs may enlarge with time, and that ASD II can outgrow closure with specific devices such as CardioSEAL or STARflex.

If one accepts the criteria of McMahon et al,[317] how large were the secundum ASDs in our series of 225 patients in which they were carefully measured and recorded at postmortem examination? It will be recalled from Table 9.10 that the secundum ASDs in our series had a mean diameter of 11.3 ± 8.5 mm, ranging from 2 to 50 mm, with a median diameter of 10 mm. Hence, the mean (11.3 mm) and median (10 mm) of our cases fell into the high moderate range (>6 to <12 mm) of McMahon et al.[317] However in order to get a more detailed assessment of the sizes of the secundum ASDs in our series, we must examine our raw data (Table 9.12). These data also may be of interest to interventionists who require devices of various sizes to occlude secundum ASDs using the percutaneous transcatheter method of defect closure.

The findings presented in Table 9.12 are summarized for the reader's convenience in Table 9.13.

Categories such as small, moderate, and large are, of course, somewhat arbitrary (but useful). One of our mental reservations concerning these size categories is that they should be indexed to the patient's body surface area (or body mass). To our knowledge, this has not as yet been done. Nonetheless, unindexed diameter data are useful for device selection.

In 2002, Du et al[329] published a study of transcatheter closure of secundum ASDs using the Amplatzer Septal Occluder in which they compared the results in patients with sufficient rims versus deficient rims. They defined a *sufficient rim* as greater than 5 mm and a *deficient rim* as less than 5 mm in height.

In patients with sufficient rims around their secundum ASD, the immediate complete closure rate is 92%; whereas in patients with deficient rims, the immediate complete closure rate was

[a]References 128, 144, 223, 239, 263, 264, 329.

TABLE 9.12 Sizes of Secundum Atrial Septal Defects (n = 225)

Size of Defect	Diameter (mm)	No. of Cases	% of Series
Small (<6 mm)[317]	2	12	5.3
	3	13	5.8
	4	11	4.9
	5	19	8.4
Moderate (>6 to <12 mm)[317]	6	15	6.7
	7	15	6.7
	8	17	7.6
	9	5	2.2
	10	32	14.2
	11	4	1.8
Large (>12 mm)[317]	12	14	6.2
	13	6	2.7
	14	3	1.3
	15	18	8.0
	16	2	0.9
	18	1	0.4
Too large for device closure (≥20 mm)[317]	20	18	8.0
	22	1	0.4
	23	1	0.4
	25	6	2.7
	27	1	0.4
	30	2	0.9
	33	1	0.4
	35	2	0.9
	38	1	0.4
	40	2	0.9
	45	2	0.9
	50	1	0.4

TABLE 9.13 Summary of Sizes of Secundum Atrial Septal Defect (n = 225)

Size of Defect	Diameter (mm)	No. of Cases	% of Series
Small[317]	<6	55	24.4
Moderate[317]	≥6 to <12	88	39.1
Large* [317]	≥12	82	36.4

*Too large for device closure according to McMahon et al[317]: 38 cases (16.9%).

74% ($p < .05$). However, even with deficient rims, the complete closure rate at 24 hours was 91% and at 6 months was 100%. With sufficient rims, the complete closure rate at 24 hours was 94% and at 6 months was 93%.

Du et al[329] concluded that the Amplatzer Septal Occluder is feasible even when there is a small anterior, inferior, or posterior rim.

This study[329] is noteworthy for pathologists: We usually measured the size of the ASD and carefully note the number and location of the defect(s). But we do not usually measure the height and width of the superior, anterior, and inferior rims of the ASD II, which now is very important information on device closure. However, it may come as no surprise that some prescient investigators have already done this:

Atkins et al[144] in 1982 published what they called the **ratio of the foramen ovale to the atrial septum area.** Their salient findings were as follows:

Normal = 0.19 ± 0.07
Tricuspid atresia = 0.43 ± 0.01
Pulmonary atresia = 0.38 ± 0.01
Coarctation of the aorta = 0.15 ± 0.07
Aortic stenosis = 0.11 ± 0.06
ASD II = 0.37 ± 0.08

These authors[144] suggested that secundum ASDs "may be a consequence of increased transatrial blood flow." This is an intriguing idea. Their hypothesis was that ASD II is not caused by deficiency of septum I, or septum II, or both. Instead, they are proposing that ASD II is caused by increased right-to-left blood flow in utero, resulting in a ratio of the foramen ovale to the atrial septum area that is significantly larger than normal, that is, a larger orifice with a smaller rim. Consequently the normal-sized valve occluder (septum primum) cannot close the enlarged valve orifice.

Their ratios are noteworthy. In tricuspid atresia that has 100% right-to-left shunt at the atrial level, the ratio of 0.43 is 2.26 times normal, that is, an increase of 126% compared with normal. Similarly, the ratio with pulmonary atresia of 0.38 is 2 times normal, 100% greater than normal. Again, with pulmonary atresia and an intact ventricular septum, there is essentially a 100% right-to-left shunt at the atrial level. But, with coarctation of the aorta (0.15) and aortic valvar stenosis (0.11), elevated left heart pressures would tend to produce premature narrowing (or even closure) of the foramen ovale. The foramen ovale–to–atrial septum area ratio is only 0.78 (78.9% of normal) with coarctation and is only 0.57 of normal (57.9% of normal) with aortic valve stenosis. With secundum ASD, the ratio is 1.94 of normal (94.7% greater than normal).

I tend to think that the foramen ovale–to–atrial septum area ratio is increased or decreased in the previously mentioned conditions, just as the authors[144] say, and that the transatrial blood flow is increased or decreased, just as they say. However, I would be hesitant to impute causality to these hemodynamic changes, important as they certainly are. My question would be why the increased (or decreased) transatrial blood flow occurs. I think that causality involves both form (morphology) and function (hemodynamics), rather than either one alone. Nonetheless, the foramen ovale–to–atrial septum area ratio is a useful quantitative approach to both the size of the interatrial communication and the size of the rim in secundum ASD. Some ASD II defects may well be due to too large an interatrial communication rather than a too small septum primum, and such cases are usually not correctly understood at the present time. We think that this situation often pertains in the polysplenia syndrome and left-sided JAA. In both situations, the rim (septum secundum) can be very poorly developed, resulting in a secundum ASD, even when the septum primum (the occluder) is well developed.

Conduction System Abnormalities

In 1970, Bizarro et al[61] reported familial secundum ASD with prolonged AV conduction. This syndrome had an autosomal dominant pattern of inheritance. In 1974, Bjornstad[94] reported another family with secundum ASD, prolonged PR interval, and autosomal dominant inheritance.

In 1975, Emanuel et al[102] documented a new syndrome in three families consisting of ASD II with autosomal dominant inheritance and left axis deviation in the electrocardiogram (ECG), often with progressive conduction system disease and risk for sudden death. They proposed that if a patient with secundum ASD also had left axis deviation or a prolonged PR interval in the ECG, the patient's relatives should be examined, looking for this syndrome.

In 1977, Pease et al[114] reported familial secundum ASD with prolonged AV conduction (i.e., a prolonged PR interval). They thought that the inheritance was polygenic. In 1978, Maron et al[132] reported the association of ASD II with AV nodal dysfunction. These authors agreed that this is a genetically transmitted syndrome. In 1982, Sobrino et al[145] again documented the association of secundum ASD and AV nodal dysfunction.

Natural History of Secundum Atrial Septal Defect

Dr. Maurice Campbell, a great natural historian, published a paper in 1970 concerning the natural history of secundum ASD.[58] The mortality statistics were as follows:

1. By 27 years of age, 25% were dead.
2. By 36 years of age, 50% were dead.
3. By 50 years of age, 75% were dead.
4. By 60 years of age, 90% were dead.

The mean and median ages at death were 37 years of age.

The natural history of secundum ASD is why early accurate diagnosis and early effective closure of secundum ASD are so important.

Familial Secundum Atrial Septal Defect

In 1999, Benson et al[294] reported 3 families with secundum ASD. The mode of inheritance in each family was autosomal dominant. In 1 family, the genetic abnormality mapped to chromosome 5p, but did not in the other 2 families. In 20 family members, a secundum ASD was present in 9 (*penetrance* = 45%). Of these 20 individuals, 8 were clinically normal (40%) but other forms of congenital heart disease were found in 3 of 20 (15%): aortic valve stenosis, atrial septal aneurysm, and persistent LSVC, respectively. Thus, *expression* was variable (secundum ASD, normal or other congenital heart disease).

Thus, Benson et al[294] concluded that familial secundum ASD is a genetically heterogenous disorder (one disease maps to chromosome 5p, but others do not), with low disease penetrance (45%), and variable expression (ASD II, or other congenital heart disease, or normal). They proposed that when congenital heart disease is present in more than one family member, all relatives should be evaluated.

In 2003, Elliott et al[343] reported that mutations in cardiac homeobox gene *NKX2-5* can infrequently be associated with *sporadic* cases of secundum ASD and the **HLHS.**

Patent Foramen Ovale

PFO is far more important than one might initially suppose because it permits paradoxical (i.e., right-to-left) embolization with the attendant risks for stroke, renal infarction, or other systemic embolization. This realization led to the question: How common is PFO in the normal population? In an autopsy study of 965 normal hearts during the first 10 decades of life (i.e., 100 years of age or less), Hagen, Scholz, and Edwards[155] found a PFO in 27.3%.

In 1995, using contrast transesophageal echocardiography in 1000 consecutive patients, Fisher et al[238] found a much lower incidence of PFO: 9.2%. I suspect that the pathologist's 1-mm probe may well be more accurate than demonstrable right-to-left shunt during echocardiographic examination. My interpretation is that the incidence of PFO in the normal population ≈ 27%.[155] But the incidence of demonstrable right-to-left atrial shunting in the normal population ≈ 9%.[238]

In 1990, Zabalgoitia-Reyes et al[202] proposed that in patients with *atrial septal aneurysm,* paradoxical embolization is the cause of transient ischemic attacks and strokes. They noted that they had not found thrombus in or around the atrial septal sac/aneurysm. However, in support of this hypothesis, they observed that right-to-left shunt was present in 85% of patients who had suffered paradoxical embolism.

But what is an atrial septal *aneurysm*? It is the septum primum—the flap valve of the foramen ovale.

Why does an atrial septal aneurysm support the concept of right-to-left atrial shunting and paradoxical embolization? Because the septum primum bows like a spinnaker into the left atrial cavity, clearly indicating that the direction of interatrial shunting is from right to left. When the direction of interatrial blood flow is from left to right, the atrial septal aneurysm bulges into the right atrial cavity. An atrial septal aneurysm indicates that the septum primum is restrictive. Consequently, an atrial septal aneurysm often is associated with a small secundum ASD or with no secundum ASD, just with a PFO.

The potentially great clinical importance of a PFO—without an ASD II—is indicated by the report of Etchells et al.[220] A 22-year-old young woman was involved in a car accident and sustained bilateral tibial fractures. She died of paradoxical fat embolism to the lungs and brain, with autopsy revealing a PFO 1 cm in diameter.

A PFO with a septum primum aneurysm is a risk factor, not only for paradoxical embolism, but also for refractory hypoxemia during pulmonary embolism.[256] Nitric oxide administration may reverse the shunt, making it left to right.[256]

The incidence of PFO in patients with sleep apnea is 69%,[260] much higher than in the general population. Thus, Shanoudy et al[260] estimate that right-to-left shunting through a PFO may contribute to hypoxemia in up to one-third of sleep apnea patients.

A PFO is important in neurologic decompression illness in divers. Walsh et al[265] reported transcatheter closure of PFO using the Amplatzer Septal Occluder to prevent recurrence of the devastating neurological complications of "the bends."

Are recurrent cerebrovascular events associated with a PFO alone, with a PFO and an atrial septal aneurysm, or with an atrial septal aneurysm only? Mas et al[311] tried to answer these questions in 2001.

In a group of 581 patients, all receiving aspirin (300 mg/day) for secondary prevention, after an interval of 4 years, the risks for recurrent stroke were as follows:

1. PFO alone, 2.3%;
2. PFO and atrial septal aneurysm, 15.2%;
3. atrial septal aneurysm alone, 0%; and
4. neither of these anomalies, 4.2%.

These investigators[311] concluded that the combination of PFO and atrial septal aneurysm significantly increased the risk for recurrent stroke, but that neither of these anomalies alone increased the risk for recurrent stroke.

Do these results[311] make sense? I think so. When there is a PFO but with no septum primum aneurysm, the lack of aneurysm suggests little or no right-to-left atrial shunt. But when there is an atrial septum aneurysm but no PFO, there cannot be a right-to-left shunt. It is clearly the combination (PFO plus aneurysm) that is dangerous. However, if there is an ASD II with a deficient septum primum, there can be no aneurysms; but the situation permitting paradoxical embolism should be just as dangerous as when an aneurysm is present.

Caught in the act! Finally, a right-to-left migrating thrombus got caught in the act.[284] Very fortunately and most unusually, the thrombus got trapped in the PFO. At surgery, a 36-year-old woman was found to have a thrombus of 10 cm (3.9 in) in length that was extracted. The PFO was closed, and a filter was inserted into the IVC.

Right-to-Left Shunt With a Secundum Atrial Septal Defect, Without Right-Sided Hypertension

When a secundum ASD is associated with normal right atrial, right ventricular, and pulmonary arterial pressures and structure, one expects that the direction of the interatrial shunt will be left to right, and usually that is the case. However, there are numerous reports in the literature in which the interatrial shunt was right to left, despite normal right-sided pressures.[b]

In 1991, Langholz et al[210] published a paper on this subject suggesting that there are at least three possible mechanisms that may explain this phenomenon:

1. transient spontaneous pressure reversal with each cardiac cycle;
2. sustained elevation of right atrial pressure above left atrial pressure by respiratory maneuvers; and
3. large right atrial mass redirecting interatrial blood flow.

There may be other mechanisms, in addition to the foregoing:

(1) a prominent right venous valve, baffling the IVC return through the ASD II into the LA; and

(2) the IVC normally overrides the superior limbic band of the septum secundum. This is why the superior limbic band is called the crista dividens (the dividing crest) of the intrauterine circulation. Approximately 60% of the IVC return flows into the LA and LV, carrying the more highly oxygenated blood from the placenta to the embryonic and fetal brain (the *via sinistra,* or left road, Latin), whereas the remaining approximately 40% of the IVC return mixes with the less oxygenated SVC return, flowing into the RV, through the pulmonary artery, and through the patent ductus to supply the lower thorax, the abdomen, and the lower extremities (the *via dextra,* or right road [Latin], of the normal intrauterine circulation). In other words, it is normal in utero for much of the IVC blood to flow into the left heart. That is one of the things that functional and anatomic closure of the foramen ovale postnatally is supposed to prevent, thereby redirecting all of the IVC blood flow into the right heart after birth. But when a secundum ASD is present, this normal postnatal redirection of the IVC blood flow may well not occur; hence, the phenomenon mentioned previously. This IVC-to-left atrial postnatal blood flow may be regarded as another aspect of *persistent fetal circulation.* Usually, of course, the normal drop in pulmonary arteriolar resistance, ductal closure, and deceleration of right ventricular growth lead to right heart pressures, flows, and compliances that favor left-to-right atrial shunting, despite the fact that the IVC opens partly into the LA. By contrast, the SVC opens only into the RA.

[b]References 34, 85, 87, 151, 178, 195, 205, 210, 218, 345.

Syndromes With Secundum Atrial Septal Defect

There are at least two noteworthy syndromes cited in the literature in which an ostium secundum type of ASD is an integral part:

1. the Holt-Oram syndrome,[38,66,106,207,268] and
2. the Ellis-van Creveld syndrome.[323]

DIAGNOSIS OF SECUNDUM ATRIAL SEPTAL DEFECT

Much has been written concerning the diagnosis, physiology, and natural history of ASD II.[c]

This fascinating tale, told in chronological sequence by these references, has many highlights, including the following:

1. the description by Bierman and Williams[118] in 1979 of subxiphoid two-dimensional echocardiographic diagnosis of abnormalities of the interatrial septum in neonates and infants;
2. the description by Magni, Cao, Sugeng, et al[254] of three-dimensional echocardiography for the diagnosis and description of ASDsand the understanding by Walker, Moran, Gauvreau, and Colan, et al[352] of the ventricular pathophysiology that is associated with secundum ASD. In 2004, based on a series of 34 patients, Walker, Moran, Gauvreau, and Colan[352] found that in patients with secundum ASD, right ventricular volume overload is associated with left ventricular distortion and dysfunction. Ejection fraction and left ventricular end-diastolic volume are both significantly decreased before device closure, and both normalized post–ASD II device closure. These investigators[352] concluded that left ventricular dysfunction and right ventricular volume overload are both secondary to

[c]References 32-35, 37, 38, 41, 42, 45, 46, 49, 50, 52-54, 56-58, 62, 64-72, 74-83, 85, 87, 90, 91, 96, 97, 99-102, 104, 106, 108-111, 115-118, 120, 123, 125-127, 129, 131, 133, 134, 139, 140, 146, 148, 150-154, 157-162, 164-173, 175-180, 182-184, 186, 188, 189, 193, 195, 197-199, 205-207, 210, 211, 217-219, 221, 223, 227-229, 233-235, 245, 250, 254, 255, 262, 263, 268, 270, 271, 313, 316, 317, 323, 336, 345, 352.

altered left ventricular chamber geometry and decreased left ventricular myofiber preload. This biventricular pathophysiology is immediately reversible by ASD device closure and is independent of heart rate and afterload

SURGERY FOR SECUNDUM ATRIAL SEPTAL DEFECT

Repair of the secundum ASD was one of the earliest successes of open-heart surgery.[d]

As mentioned earlier, surgical closure of secundum ASD began in 1953,[28] even before the heart-lung machine had been introduced by Gibbon,[29] when Lewis and Taufic[28] closed a 2-cm ASD II in a 5-year-old girl under direct vision using hypothermia and inflow occlusion.

By the turn of the century, a minimal access approach for the repair of secundum ASDs had been used successfully by Bichell et al[273] in a series of 135 patients. The principal advantages of the minimal access approach are that it is less traumatic and cosmetically superior because complete sternotomy is not done. Houyel et al[279] recommended the use of right posterolateral thoracotomy for open-heart surgery in infants, again for superior cosmetic results, particularly in girls. These authors noted that a persistent LSVC is a contraindication for the right posterolateral thoracotomy approach to secundum ASD and other types of congenital heart disease.

In 2001, a totally endoscopic computer-enhanced method of secundum ASD closure was reported in a series of 6 patients by Torracca et al.[304] Using telemanipulated robotic systems, these authors reported excellent results and rapid recovery, with all patients returning to normal function in the first postoperative week. Similar results were also reported by Argenziano et al[335] in 2003.

TRANSCATHETER INTERVENTION FOR DEVICE CLOSURE OF ATRIAL SEPTAL DEFECT II

Attempts have been made since 1975 (perhaps earlier) to occlude the secundum ASDs by means of percutaneous transcatheter devices. The earliest of which I am aware was reported in the *Hospital Tribune* on May 19, 1975.[95] The article in this medical newspaper (not a scientific journal) recounted the most interesting news that Dr. Terry King and Dr. Noel Mills of the Ochsner Medical Foundation in New Orleans had successfully closed a secundum ASD using a Dacron umbrella that was delivered by a cardiac catheter. Since that time, many reports have appeared concerning device closure of ASD II.[e]

It may be said, with tongue only slightly in cheek, that there has been an undeclared war between cardiologists (i.e., interventionist) and cardiac surgeons concerning who is going to be the therapist for patients with secundum ASD. Who's winning? In 2005, the interventionist approach appeared to be ahead, but as in most contests, there is something to be said in favor of both sides. Formigari et al[285]—the authors being both cardiologists and cardiac surgeons—reported in 2001 their experience with 171 children. They compared three types of therapy: device closure in 52, minimally invasive surgical repair in 72, and conventional median sternotomy surgical repair in 50 patients. The salient findings were as follows:

Death = 0
Residual left-to-right shunts = 0
Complication rates
  Device = 3.8% ($p < .01$)
  Minimally invasive = 12.6%
  Median sternotomy = 12.0%
Mean hospital stay
  Device = 2.1 ± 0.5 days ($p < .01$)
  Minimally invasive = 2.8 ± 1.0 days
  Median sternotomy = 6.5 ± 2.1 days
Skin-to-skin time
  Device = 118 ± 58 minutes ($p < .001$)
  Minimally invasive = 196 ± 43 minutes
  Median sternotomy = 163 ± 46 minutes
Expense (published)
Device = 13,000 lire
Minimally invasive = 12,500 lire
Median sternotomy = 15, 000 lire

Thus, these authors[285] concluded that device closure was significantly superior to either form of surgical repair in terms of rate of complications, length of hospital stay, and operative skin-to-skin time, and that there was no significant difference in expense among these three management strategies.

Berger, Vogel, Alexi-Meskishvili, and Lange[292] in 1999 compared the results and complications of surgical versus Amplatzer device closure of secundum ASDs. They found that the mean hospital stay for surgical patients was 8 days, versus 3 days for device patients. Therefore, they preferred Amplatzer device closure.

However, this same group[293] found that surgical closure remains mandatory in certain types of patients:

1. Atrial septal aneurysms with PFO always could be closed by a transcatheter device (n = 18).
2. However, when an atrial septal aneurysm was associated with a secundum ASD, 5 were closed by device, but 4 required surgery.
3. When the atrial septal aneurysm (septum primum) had two perforations, device closure was used in all 10 such patients, but there was residual shunt in 4.
4. When the septum primum had multiple perforations, all 13 such patients required surgical closure.

As pointed out by Hekmat, Mehlhorn, and de Vivie,[259] when the secundum ASD is large, a transcatheter device may fail to occlude the defect, necessitating surgical closure.

[d]References 28, 29, 36, 40, 43, 47, 48, 51, 59, 63, 73, 84, 93, 98, 103, 112, 113, 119, 122, 136, 143, 156, 187, 191, 192, 204, 215, 222, 224, 231, 232, 240, 242, 243, 248, 253, 257-259, 261, 267, 273, 279, 283, 287, 291, 297-299, 304, 309, 310, 312, 313, 320, 322, 324, 328, 335, 337-340, 351, 353.
[e]References 190, 200, 201, 208, 213, 214, 216, 225, 226, 237, 244, 247, 251, 252, 259, 266, 269, 272, 275, 276, 281, 282, 285, 286, 289, 290, 292, 295, 296, 301-303, 305, 307, 308, 317, 318-322, 324-327, 329, 330, 332-334, 341, 342, 344, 347-351, 354-357.

Thus, in 2005, closure of secundum ASDs is a *cooperative* venture in which the cardiologist/interventionist and the surgeon play mutually complementary roles.

Much more follow-up is needed concerning transcatheter devices. We still have much to learn. For example, in 2004, Anzai et al[349] published a study concerning the incidence of thrombus formation on the CardioSEAL and Amplatzer devices. Their salient findings were that in the first month postimplantation, thrombi occurred on 5 of 23 CardioSEAL devices (22%) and on 0 of 27 Amplatzer devices ($p = .02$). One CardioSEAL device was surgically explanted because of an increase in thrombus size. However, no thromboemboli occurred.

In 2004, Suda et al[357] found that of 162 patients in whom the Amplatzer device was used to close a secundum ASD, AV block occurred in 10 (6.2%). In all 10 patients, the AV block subsequently resolved or improved and the authors had observed no recurrences of AV block up to the time of publication.

Sudden unexpected death[275] also has been reported after device closure of secundum ASDs. But this is fortunately a rare event.

As this chapter is being completed, which way is the wind blowing in the literature? I will attempt to answer this question, fully realizing that conclusions may change in the future.

Is there a condition that is the opposite of secundum ASD? Yes, it is **premature narrowing or closure of the foramen ovale** in the fetus. The diagnosis and management of this entity were discussed in 2004 by Donofrio et al.[358]

What is it that causes paradoxical systemic embolization? Is it the atrial septal aneurysm, or is it the PFO? In the echocardiograms of 106 neonatal infants, Guntheroth et al[359] found an atrial septal aneurysm in 4%. These authors concluded that in neonates, atrial septal (septum primum) aneurysm is caused by the inadequate size of the PFO, that is, the septum primum (atrial septum) is restrictive and hence balloons like a spinnaker into the left atrial cavity. "There is no convincing evidence that an ASD alone causes strokes in adults; the confounder is probably atrial fibrillation." I think that this conclusion is essentially correct. However, it should be understood that atrial septal aneurysm/aneurysm of the septum primum also does not cause strokes in adults. The aneurysm indicates the presence of right-to-left atrial shunting, and it is this shunt (not the aneurysm per se) that causes the strokes. No doubt this is what these authors meant.[359]

The device "wars" of course continue. Butera et al[360] in 2004 compared the currently two leading contenders, CardioSEAL or STARflex (CS/SF) versus the Amplatzer. Their salient findings concerning secundum ASDs 18 mm or less in diameter were that the Amplatzer was quicker to implant and that the rate of complete occlusion was higher:

Procedure Time
- Amplatzer: 61 + 21 minutes ($p < .0003$)
- CS/SF: 75 + 32 minutes

Residual Shunt

At Procedure
- Amplatzer: 11/153 (7.2%)
- CS/SF: 48/21 (39.7%)

At Discharge
- Amplatzer: 5/153 (3.3%)
- CS/SF: 26/121 (21.5%)

At 6 months
- Amplatzer: 0/153 (0%)
- CS/SF: 12/121 (9.9%)

At 12 months
- Amplatzer: 0/120 (0%)
- CS/SF: 8/105 (7.6%)

At 2 Years
- Amplatzer: 0/85 (0%)
- CS/SF: 4/90 (4.4%)

Thus, residual shunt was more frequent with the CardioSEAL/STARflex device than with the Amplatzer occluder ($p < .0001$). (What I am writing here is based objectively on the data available to me, free of institutional bias.)

In 2004, Wang et al[361] reported their experience with the Amplatzer occluder in a series of 197 cases implanted from March 1999 to February 2003. A deficient rim (<5 mm) was present in 114 patients (58%). Salient findings:

Successful deployment: 191 (97%)

Failed deployment: 6 (3%)

Severe complications included transient complete AV block, 1 (0.5%); pericardial tamponade treated with drainage, 1 (0.5%); dislodgement of the device, successfully managed with emergency operation, 1 (0.5%); embolism to a fingertip, 1 (0.5%); and residual shunt—1 day, 19%; 6 months, 6%; 12 months, 5%; and 24 months, 4%. These investigators concluded that the Amplatzer Septal Occluder is safe and effective, even when one rim of the secundum ASD is deficient (<5 mm). In particular, they found that deficiency of the anterosuperior rim does not influence the success rate of closure.

The surgery versus Amplatzer "competition" continues: Bialkowski et al[362] in 2004 concluded that Amplatzer device closure of secundum ASDs has several advantages: few complications, shorter hospitalization, and reduced need for blood products. However, the advantage of surgical closure of secundum ASD is that any defect can be closed completely, regardless of its size, location, or number.

Cryptogenic Stroke and Migraine

In 2005, Tobis and Azarbal[363] considered the question, Does PFO (or secundum ASD) promote cryptogenic stroke and migraine headache? Their answer to both was a resounding yes. Interestingly, they did not even consider whether there was an atrial septal aneurysm (aneurysm of septum primum), as previous investigators[202] had done. Noting that there are approximately 700,000 strokes per annum in the United States in 2005, Tobis and Azarbal[363] wrote that about 80% are ischemic and 20% are hemorrhagic. Of the ischemic strokes, approximately 20% are cryptogenic. Thus, strokes caused by paradoxical embolism through a PFO in the United States are estimated to equal between 30,000 and 60,000 per annum.

The prevalence of PFO in the cryptogenic stroke population equals 40% to 50%, compared to that in the general population of about 20%.[363] Scuba divers with PFO are more susceptible to decompression illness than are those without a PFO.

Platypnea-orthodeoxia is a condition of dyspnea and desaturation that occurs when the individual is standing up, but not when lying down. Platypnea is the opposite of orthopnea. *Orthopnea* means dyspnea that is relieved by upright posture. Platypnea is dyspnea that is relieved by horizontal posture. *Orthodeoxia* means unsaturation that occurs with vertical posture (but not with horizontal posture). Hence, platypnea-orthodeoxia denotes dyspnea and hypoxia when upright, but not when recumbent. Such patients are symptomatic because their systemic saturations fall into the low 80% range. When the PFO is closed, the condition of vertical or standing dyspnea and desaturation is alleviated.[363]

PFO is a surgical risk factor for orthodeoxia: paradoxical fat emboli in orthopedic surgery and paradoxical air emboli in cardiac surgery and neurosurgery.[363]

Aging is a risk factor for paradoxical embolism through a PFO:

> *As you get older you probably have more venous emboli and your right atrial pressure goes up, raising the risk for PFO-mediated embolic events to the point at which, in the elderly, that risk may be just as important as underlying atherosclerotic disease. . . . Perhaps all elderly patients with stroke should be getting their PFOs closed in addition to getting their carotid arteries cleaned out.*[363]

As the authors agree, this proposal needs to be evaluated by a multicenter randomized trial.

In their 141 patients (2001 to 2004), there was a PFO in 104 and an ASD II in 37.[363] PFO device closure was successful in all. Complications included 1 new fenestration/tear shunt and 1 pericardial effusion (0.06% each), the effusion being interpreted as a possible nickel allergy. In their ASD patients, 2 had an insufficient rim (5.4%) and were sent for surgical closure. One ASD device closure patient had a small residual shunt (2.7%). Complications included 2 patients with groin bleeding (5.4%). One device was explanted because of thrombus. In view of a higher incidence of thrombus with the CardioSEAL device, these interventionists[363] report that they have stopped using it and now use the Amplatzer exclusively. Over the 4 years of this study, after PFO and secundum ASD device closure, they have had no recurrence of stroke or transient ischemic attack (TIA).

Migraine

Estimated to involve 12% of the population, approximately 27 million people in the United States suffer from migraine at the present time.[363] Migraine is three times as common in women as men: PFO occurs in about 50% of migraine patients with a visual aura, compared with a prevalence of approximately 20% in the general population. Migraine *without* visual aura also has a prevalence of PFO of about 20%. Thus, migraine with visual aura and migraine without visual aura are thought to be significantly different disorders.

Patients with migraine have 13 times the incidence of brain lesions demonstrated by magnetic resonance imaging (MRI) than do individuals without migraine. Positron emission tomography (PET) studies show no vasodilatation with migraine, indicating that the older understanding of migraine needs revision.

In migraine patients with aura, device closure of PFO/ASD resulted in no more migraine in 18 of 24 patients (75%), with significant improvement in the remainder.[363] Migraine-associated stroke is caused by paradoxical embolism through a PFO/ASD, not by vasospasm as used to be thought.[363] Consequently, these workers suggest that PFO device closure will reduce the risks both for stroke and migraine.[363]

The previous account of PFO and secundum ASD illustrates that these forms of congenital heart disease are of major importance to people of all ages.

Is there a situation, an anomaly, that seldom, if ever, has an ASD? The answer is yes, the **HLHS. Our hypothesis is that this is what the HLHS is, at least in part: a subnormal right-to-left interatrial communication during embryonic and fetal life, and the resulting sequelae.** However, the HLHS is often more than a restrictive atrial septum, a septum primum that does not open widely enough. Severe aortic stenosis or atresia and severe mitral stenosis or atresia are often additional important factors contributing to the morphogenesis of the HLHS. Nonetheless, it is a striking fact that the HLHS seldom if ever has a secundum type of ASD. In the HLHS, it often looks as though the septum primum cannot open widely enough to provide a nonrestrictive *via sinistra* into the left heart, thereby leading to hypoplasia of the left heart structures. In the HLHS, not only is the septum primum completely formed (not deficient and without holes), but also it does not deviate much in a leftward direction. The septum primum does not open well in a leftward direction, away from the septum secundum, into the LA. Instead, the septum primum opens only minimally or subnormally into the LA.

Is this why the septum primum undergoes such extensive fenestration early in embryonic life (see Figs. 9.14 to 9.17, inclusive), so that the septum primum does not obstruct the essential inflow of blood into the very important left heart? Is this why, later in development, the holes in the septum primum are filled in (see Fig. 9.18 to 9.22, inclusive), so as to make possible effective septation of the heart postnatally into double left-sided and right-sided hearts? Although I cannot answer these questions definitively, they are worthy of consideration.

Hence, it is suggested that the typically "well formed" atrial septum of the HLHS may in fact be restrictive to right-to-left atrial blood flow in utero, contributing to hypoplasia (smallness) of the left heart structures. In this sense, what does *not* occur (secundum ASD with the HLHS) may well be as significant as what *does* occur (secundum ASD with both left-sided and right-sided cardiac structures well developed). Thus, the prenatal interatrial conduit and valve that normally becomes the postnatal interatrial septum is prone to both prenatal and postnatal malfunction. The interatrial mechanism, like the ductus arteriosus, has opposite prenatal and postnatal functions. This dual function may predispose to ASDs.

SUMMARY

This chapter contains a new original study of 640 postmortem patients with an ostium secundum type of ASD. As we have seen here and in other chapters, any significant flaw in the growth and development of

1. septum primum (ostium secundum type of ASD),
2. septum secundum (ostium secundum type of ASD),
3. the AV septum (ostium primum type of ASD, i.e., incomplete form of common atrioventricular canal), and
4. the partition between the SVC and the RA anteriorly and the RPVs posteriorly (sinus venosus defect) can result in interatrial communications with serious and potentially fatal pathophysiologic consequences.

REFERENCES

1. Melhuish BPP, Van Praagh R. Juxtaposition of the atrial appendages, a sign of severe cyanotic congenital heart disease. *Br Heart J*. 1968;30:269.
2. Keane JF, McLennan JE, Chi JG, et al. Congenital heart disease in a tetra-X woman. *Chest*. 1974;66:726.
3. Van Praagh S, Carrera ME, Sanders SP, Mayer JE, Van Praagh R. Partial or total direct pulmonary venous drainage to right atrium due to malposition of septum primum: anatomic and echocardiographic findings and surgical treatment—a study based on 36 cases. *Chest*. 1995;107:1488.
4. Hendrix MJC. *An Investigation of the Atrial Septation in the Chick and Human Heart: An Electron and Light Microscopic Study, Ph.D. Dissertation Directed by Dennis E Morse, PhD (External Advisor), Assistant Professor of Anatomy, Medical College of Ohio and Richard S. Snell, MD, PhD (Internal Advisor), Professor and Chairman*. Washington, DC: Department of Anatomy, The George Washington University Medical Center; 1977.
5. David I, Castaneda AR, Van Praagh R. Potentially parachute mitral valve in common atrioventricular canal: pathologic anatomy and surgical importance. *J Thorac Cardiovasc Surg*. 1982;84:178.
6. Van Praagh S, O'Sullivan J, Brili S, Van Praagh R. Juxtaposition of the morphologically right atrial appendage in solitus and inversus atria: a study of 35 postmortem case. *Am Heart J*. 1996;132:382.
7. Van Praagh S, O'Sullivan J, Brili S, Van Praagh R. Juxtaposition of the morphologically left atrial appendage in solitus and inversus atria: a study of 18 postmortem cases. *Am Heart J*. 1996;132:391.
8. Van Praagh R, Van Praagh S. The anatomy of common aorticopulmonary trunk (truncus arteriosus communis) and its embryologic implications, a study of 57 necropsied cases. *Am J Cardiol*. 1965;16:406.
9. Calder L, Van Praagh R, Van Praagh S, et al. Truncus arteriosus communis: clinical, angiographic and pathologic findings in 100 patients. *Am Heart J*. 1976;92:23.
10. Vizcaino A, Campbell J, Litovsky S, Van Praagh R. Single origin of right and left pulmonary artery branches from ascending aorta with nonbranching main pulmonary artery: relevance to a new understanding of truncus arteriosus. *Pediatr Cardiol*. 2002;23:230.
11. Aru GM, Juraszek A, Moskowitz I, Van Praagh R. Tetralogy of Fallot with congenital aortic valvar stenosis: the tetralogy-truncus interrelationship. *Pediatr Cardiol*. 2006;27:354.
12. Collett RW, Edwards JE. Persistent truncus arteriosus: a classification according to anatomic types. *Surg Clin North Am*. 1949;29:1245.
13. Ruscazio M, Van Praagh S, Marrass AR, Catani G, Iliceto S, Van Praagh R. Interrupted inferior vena cava in asplenia syndrome and a review of the hereditary patterns of visceral situs abnormalities. *Am J Cardiol*. 1998;81:111.
14. Geva T, Sanders SP, Diogenes M, Rockenmacher S, Van Praagh R. Two-dimensional and Doppler echocardiographic and pathologic characteristics of the infantile Marfan syndrome. *Am J Cardiol*. 1990;65:1230.
15. Marfan A-B. Un cas de deformation congenitale des quatre members, plus prononcee aux extremites, caracterisee par l'allongement des os avec un certain degre d'amincissement. *Bull Mem Soc Med Hop Paris*. 1896;13:220.
16. Beals RK, Hecht F. Congenital contractural arachnodactyly. *J Bone Joint Surg*. 1971;53-A:987.
17. Hecht F, Beals RK. "New" syndrome of congenital contractural arachnodactyly originally described by Marfan in 1896. *Pediatrics*. 1971;49:574.
18. Salle V. Uber einen Fall von angeborener abnormer Grobe der Extremitaten mit einem Akromegalie erinnernden symptomenkomplex. *Jahrbuch Kunderheilkunde*. 1912;75:540.
19. Geva T, Hegesh J, Frand M. The clinical course and echocardiographic features of Marfan's syndrome in childhood. *Am J Dis Child*. 1987;141:1179.
20. Sisk HE, Zahka KG, Pyeritz RE. The Marfan syndrome in early childhood: analysis of 15 patients diagnosed at less than 4 years of age. *Am J Cardiol*. 1983;52:353.
21. Phornphutkul C, Rosenthal A, Nadas AS. Cardiac manifestations of Marfan syndrome in infancy and childhood. *Circulation*. 1973;47:587.
22. Jones KL. In: *Smith's Recognizable Patterns of Human Malformation*. 4th ed. Philadelphia: W.B. Saunders; 1988:422.
23. Tsipouras P, Del Mastro R, Safarazi M, et al. Ramirez F and the International Marfan Syndrome Collaborative Study: genetic linkage of the Marfan syndrome, ectopia lentis, and congenital contractural arachnodactyly to the fibrillin genes on chromosomes 15 and 5. *N Engl J Med*. 1992;326:905.
24. Savolainen A, Keto P, Hekali P, et al. Aortic distensibility in children with the Marfan syndrome. *Am J Cardiol*. 1992;70:691.
25. Da Vinci L. 1513, republished in 1911-1916. Sketch of heart auricles, Quadernia Anatomia III, in Fogli della Royal Library di Windsor, CL Vangensten. In: Fonahn A, Hopstock H, eds. *J Dibwad, Christiana, Later Republished in Congenital Heart Disease, WJ Rashkind*. Pennsylvania: Hutchinson Ross Publishing Co, Stroudsburg; 1982:102.
26. LeCat CN. In: Rashkind WJ, ed. *Concerning the Foramen Ovale Being Found Open in the Heart of Adults, Philsoph Trans 1747; 9:134, Later Republished in Congenital Heart Disease*. Pennsylvania: Hutchinson Ross Publishing Co, Stroudsburg; 1982:108 (translated from French).
27. Morgagni GB. *De Sedibus et Causis Morborum per Anatomen Indagatis*. Book III (The Seats and Causes of Disease Investigated by Anatomy, Latin); 1761.
28. Lewis FJ, Taufic M. Closure of atrial septal defects with the aid of hypothermia; experimental accomplishments and the report of one successful case. *Surgery*. 1953;33:52.
29. Gibbon JH. Application of a mechanical heart and lung apparatus to cardiac surgery. *Minn Med*. 1954;37:171.
30. Lewis FJ. High defects in the atrial septum. *J Thorac Surg*. 1958;36:1.
31. Bedford DE. The anatomic types of atrial septal defect. Their incidence and clinical diagnosis. *Am J Cardiol*. 1960;6:568.
32. Zaver AG, Nadas AS. Atrial septal defect—secundum type. *Circulation*. 1965;32(suppl 3):24.
33. Cayler GG. Spontaneous functional closure of symptomatic atrial septal defects. *N Engl J Med*. 1967;276:65.

34. Winters WL, Cortes F, McDonough M, et al. Venoarterial shunting from inferior vena cava to left atrium in atrial septal defects with normal right heart pressures. Report of two cases. *Am J Cardiol.* 1967;19:293.
35. Hartman AF, Elliott LP. Spontaneous physiologic closure of an septal defect after infancy. *Am J Cardiol.* 1967;19:290.
36. Daicoff GR, Brandenburg RO, Kirklin JW. Results of operation for atrial septal defect in patients forty-five years of age and older. *Circulation.* 1967;35:I–143.
37. Khoury GH, Hawes CR. Atrial septal defect associated with pulmonary hypertension in children living at high altitude. *J Pediatr.* 1967;70:432.
38. Starke H, Schimke RN, Dunn M. Upper limb cardiovascular syndrome, a family study. *Am J Cardiol.* 1967;19:588.
39. Nora JJ, McNamara DG, Fraser FC. Hereditary factors in atrial septal defect. *Circulation.* 1967;35:448.
40. Cohn LH, Morrow AG, Braunwald E. Operative treatment of atrial septal defect: clinical and hemodynamic assessments in 175 patients. *Br Heart J.* 1967;29:725.
41. Pagtakhan RD, Hartmann AF, Goldring D, Kissane J. The valve-incompetent foramen ovale. A report of seven infants with left-to-right shunt. *J Pediatr.* 1967;71:848.
42. Just H, Mattingly TW. Interatrial septal defect and pericardial disease. Coincidence or causal relationship. *Am Heart J.* 1968;76:157.
43. Wolf PS, Vogel JHK, Pryor R, Blount SG. Atrial septal defect in patients over 45 years of age. Merits of surgical versus medical therapy. *Br Heart J.* 1968;30:115.
44. Okada R, Glagov S, Lev M. Different effects of increased volume and increased pressure on endocardial structure in hearts with atrial septal defect. *Am Heart J.* 1968;75:474.
45. Craig RJ, Selzer A. Natural history and prognosis of atrial septal defect. *Circulation.* 1968;37:805.
46. Levin AR, Spach MS, Boineau JP, Canent RV, Capp MP, Jewett PH. Atrial pressure-flow dynamics in atrial septal defects (secundum type). *Circulation.* 1968;37:476.
47. Gault JH, Morrow AG, Gay WA, Ross J. Atrial septal defect in patients over the age of forty years. Clinical and hemodynamic studies and the effects of operation. *Circulation.* 1968;37:261.
48. Chen S-C, Arcilla RA, Moulder PV, Cassells DE. Postoperative conduction disturbances in atrial septal defect. *Am J Cardiol.* 1968;22:636.
49. Cumming GR. Functional closure of atrial septal defects. *Am J Cardiol.* 1968;22:888.
50. Ressl J, Kubis M, Lukl P, Vykydal J, Weinberg J. Resting hyperventilation in adults with atrial septal defect. *Br Heart J.* 1969;31:118.
51. Tikoff G, Keith TB, Nelson RM, Kuida H. Clinical and hemodynamic observations after surgical closure of large atrial septal defect complicated by heart failure. *Am J Cardiol.* 1969;23:810.
52. Sanchez J, Rodriguez-Torres R, Lin J-S, Goldstein S, Kavety V. Diagnostic value of the first heart sound in children with atrial septal defect. *Am Heart J.* 1969;78:467.
53. Chen S-C, Arcilla RA, Cassels DE, Thilenius OG, Renniger K. Abnormal initial QRS vectors in atrial septal defect. *Am J Cardiol.* 1969;24:346.
54. Sealy WC, Farmer JC, Young WG, Brown IW. Atrial dysrhythmia and atrial secundum defects. *J Thorac Cardiovasc Surg.* 1969;57:245.
55. Okada R, Glagov S, Lev M. Relation of shunt flow and right ventricular pressure to heart valve structure in atrial septal defect. *Am Heart J.* 1969;78:781.
56. Benchimol A, Barreto EC, Gartlan JL. Right atrial flow velocity in patients with atrial septal defect. *Am J Cardiol.* 1970;25:381.
57. Saksena FB, Aldridge HE. Atrial septal defect in the older patient. A clinical and hemodynamic study in patients operated on after age 35. *Circulation.* 1970;42:1009.
58. Campbell M. Natural history of atrial septal defect. *Br Heart J.* 1970;32:820.
59. Davies H, Oliver GC, Rappaport WJ, Gazetopoulos N. Abnormal left heart function after operation for atrial septal defect. *Br Heart J.* 1970;32:747.
60. Cooksey JD, Parker BM, Weldon CS. Atrial septal defect and calcification of the tricuspid valve. *Br Heart J.* 1970;32:409.
61. Bizarro RO, Callahan JA, Feldt RH, Kurland LT, Gordon H, Brandenburg RO. Familial atrial septal defect with prolonged atrioventricular conduction, a syndrome showing the autosomal dominant pattern of inheritance. *Circulation.* 1970;41:677.
62. Feldt RH, Avasthey P, Yoshimasu F, Kurland LT, Titus JL. Incidence of congenital heart disease in children born to residents of Olmsted County, Minnesota, 1950-1969. *Mayo Clin Proc.* 1971;46:794.
63. Ayla E, Headley Brown A, Braimbridge MV. Surgery for atrial septal defect in patients over 60 years of age. Report of surgical correction in 12 patients. *J Thorac Cardiovasc Surg.* 1971;62:788.
64. Banas JS, Meister SG, Gazzaniga AB, O'Connor NE, Haynes FW, Dalen JE. A simple technique for detecting small defects of the atrial septum. *Am J Cardiol.* 1971;28:467.
65. Blumenschein SD, Barr RC, Spach MS, Gentzler RC. Quantitative Frank vectocardiograms of normal children and a comparison to those of patients with atrial defects. *Am Heart J.* 1972;83:332.
66. Rainer WG, Sadler TR, Dirks DW, Swan H. Holt-Oram syndrome. Surgical implications. *J Thorac Cardiovasc Surg.* 1972;63:478.
67. Richer TJ, Gallen WJ, Friedberg DZ. Familial atrial septal defect in a single generation. *Br Heart J.* 1972;34:198.
68. Davia JE, Cheitlin MD, Bedynek JL. Sinus venosus atrial septal defect: analysis of fifty cases. *Am Heart J.* 1972;85:177.
69. Dimich I, Steinfeld L, Park SC. Symptomatic atrial septal defect in infants. *Am Heart J.* 1973;85:601.
70. Kamigaki M, Goldschlager N. Echocardiographic analysis of mitral valve motion in atrial septal defect. *Am J Cardiol.* 1972;30:343.
71. Hoffman JIE, Rudolph AM, Danilowicz D. Left to right atrial shunts in infants. *Am J Cardiol.* 1972;30:868.
72. Young D. Later results of closure of secundum atrial septal defect in children. *Am J Cardiol.* 1973;31:14.
73. Dave KS, Pakrashi BC, Wooler GH, Ionescu MI. Atrial septal defect in adults. Clinical and hemodynamic results of surgery. *Am J Cardiol.* 1973;31:7.
74. Goldschlager A, Goldschlager N, Brewster H, Kaplan J. Catheter entrapment in a Chiari network involving an atrial septal defect. *Chest.* 1972;62:345.
75. El-Said G, Ruzyllo W, Williams RL, McNamara DG. Atrial pressure gradients in isolated secundum atrial septal defect and partial anomalous pulmonary venous return. *Chest.* 1973;63:559.
76. Hunt CE, Lucas RV. Symptomatic atrial septal defect in infancy. *Circulation.* 1973;37:1042.
77. Kalmanson D, Veyrat C, Derai C, Savier C-H, Berkman M, Chiche P. Non-invasive technique for diagnosing atrial septal defect and assessing shunt volume using directional Doppler ultrasound. Correlations with phasic flow velocity patterns of the shunt. *Br Heart J.* 1972;34:981.

78. Anderson PAW, Rogers MC, Canent RV, Spach MS. Atrioventricular conduction in secundum atrial septal defects. *Circulation.* 1973;48:27.
79. Rees A, Farru O, Rodriguez R. Phonocardiographic, radiological, and hemodynamic correlation in atrial septal defect. *Br Heart J.* 1972;34:781.
80. Thomas HM, Spicer MJ, Nelson WP. Evaluation of P wave axis in distinguishing anatomical site of atrial septal defect. *Br Heart J.* 1973;35:738.
81. Somerville J, Khaliq SU, Brewer AC, Heath D. Clinical pathologic conference. *Am Heart J.* 1973;86:822.
82. Yokoyama M. The pressure difference across the pulmonary artery valve in cases with atrial septal defect. *Bull Heart Inst Japan.* 1973;14:19. 1972.
83. Mody MR. Serial hemodynamic observations in secundum atrial septal defect with special reference to spontaneous closure. *Am J Cardiol.* 1973;32:978.
84. Pieroni DR, Strife JL, Donahoo JS, Krovetz LJ. Postoperative assessment of residual defects following cardiac surgery in infants and children. III. Atrial septal defects. *Hopkins Med J.* 1973;133:287.
85. Rasmussen K, Simonsen S, Storstein O. Quantitative aspects of right-to-left shunting in uncomplicated atrial septal defects. *Br Heart J.* 1973;35:894.
86. Betriu A, Felderhof CH, McLoughlin MJ, Wigle ED. Prolapse of the posterior leaflet of the mitral valve (PPLMV) associated with secundum atrial septal defect. *Am J Cardiol.* 1974;7:11.
87. Maillis MS, Cheng TO, Meyer JF, Crawley IS, Lindsay J. Cyanosis in patients with atrial septal defect due to systemic venous drainage into the left atrium. *Am J Cardiol.* 1974; 33:674.
88. Victorica BE, Elliott LP, Gessner IH. Ostium secundum atrial septal defect associated with balloon mitral valve in children. *Am J Cardiol.* 1974;33:668.
89. Tandon R, Edwards JE. Atrial septal defect in infancy. Common association with other anomalies. *Circulation.* 1974;49:1005.
90. Giles TD, Burch GE. The atrial vectorcardiogram in adults with atrial septal defect. *Chest.* 1974;65:294.
91. Hawker RE, Freedom RM, Krovetz LJ. Preferential shunting of venous return from normally connected left pulmonary veins in secundum atrial septal defect. *Am J Cardiol.* 1974;34:339.
92. Hynes KM, Frye RL, Brandenburg RO, McGoon DC, Titus JL, Guiliani ER. Atrial septal defect (secundum) associated with mitral regurgitation. *Am J Cardiol.* 1974;34:333.
93. Murthy LNS, Griffin SG. Closure of atrial septal defect (secundum) under hypothermia. *Br Heart J.* 1974;36:1036.
94. Bjornstad PG. Secundum type atrial septal defect with prolonged PR interval and autosomal dominant mode of inheritance. *Br Heart J.* 1974;36:1149.
95. (No author given). Atrial septal defect repaired nonoperatively. *Hosp Trib.* 1975;9:1(May 19).
96. Tau K-T, Takao A, Hashimoto A, Sato T. Electrocardiogram of secundum type atrial septal defect simulating endocardial cushion defect. *Br Heart J.* 1975;37:209.
97. Jeresaty RM. Mitral valve prolapse-click syndrome in atrial septal defect. *Chest.* 1975;67:132.
98. Neal WA, Moller JH, Varco RL, Anderson RC. Operative repair of atrial septal defect without cardiac catheterization. *J Pediatr.* 1975;86:189.
99. Phillips SJ, Okies JE, Henken D, Sunderland CO, Starr A. Complex of secundum atrial septal defect and congestive heart failure in infants. *J Thorac Cardiovasc Surg.* 1975;70:696.
100. Popio KA, Gorlin R, Teichholz LE, Cohn PF, Bechtel D, Herman MV. Abnormalities of left ventricular function and geometry in adults with an atrial septal defect. Ventriculographic, hemodynamic, and echocardiographic studies. *Am J Cardiol.* 1975;36:302.
101. Shettigar UR, Hultgren HN, Berndt T, Wasnich RD. Occult atrial septal defect in adults. *Chest.* 1975;68:307.
102. Emanuel R, O'Brien K, Somerville J, Jefferson K, Hegde M. Association of secundum atrial septal defect with abnormalities of atrioventricular conduction or left axis deviation. Genetic study of 10 families. *Br Heart J.* 1975;37:1085.
103. Spangler JG, Feldt RH, Danielson GK. Secundum atrial septal defect encountered in infancy. *J Thorac Cardiovasc Surg.* 1976;71:398.
104. Baquero V, Leachman RD, Angelini P, Lufschanowski R. Left ventricular and mitral valve abnormalities in association with interatrial septal defect. *Arch Venez Cardiol.* 1976;3:25.
105. Barrera J, Gamino F, Tain J. Ostium secundum (OS) and mitral valvular cleft. *Arch Venez Cardiol.* 1976;3:25.
106. Mitsuoka H, Chughtai S, Cutarelli R, Beg RA, Naraghipour H, Kay EB. Holt-Oram syndrome associated with combined ostium primum and secundum atrial septal defects; successful surgical closure. *Am J Cardiol.* 1975;36:967.
107. Leachman RD, Cokkinos DV, Cooley DA. Association of ostium secundum atrial septal defects with mitral valve prolapse. *Am J Cardiol.* 1976;38:167.
108. Kambe T, Hibi N, Ito H, et al. Clinical study on the flow murmurs at the defect area of atrial septal defect by means of intracardiac phonocardiography. *Am Heart J.* 1976;91:35.
109. Vedoya RC, Kaplan MV, de la Fuente LM, Favaloro RO. Comunicacion interauricular en el adulto. *Rev Argent Cardiol.* 1975;43:398.
110. Hairston P, Parker EF, Arrants JE, Bradham RR, Lee WH. The adult atrial septal defect: results of surgical repair. *Ann Surg.* 1974;179:799.
111. Andersen M, Lyngborg K, Moller I, Wennevold A. The natural history of small atrial septal defects: long-term follow-up with serial heart catheterizations. *Am Heart J.* 1976;92:302.
112. Nasrallah AT, Hall RJ, Garcia E, Leachman RD, Cooley DA. Surgical repair of atrial septal defect in patients over 60 years of age. Long-term results. *Circulation.* 1976;53:329.
113. Forfang K, Simonsen S, Anderson A, Efskin L. Atrial septal defect of secundum type in the middle-aged. Clinical results of surgery and correlations between symptoms and hemodynamics. *Am Heart J.* 1977;94:44.
114. Pease WE, Nordenberg A, Ladda RL. Familial atrial septal defect with prolonged atrioventricular conduction. *Circulation.* 1977;53:759.
115. Fukumoto T, Ito M, Arita M, Tetsuo M, Fujino T, Mashiba H. Right parasternal lift in atrial septal defect. *Am Heart J.* 1977;94:699.
116. O'Toole JD, Reddy PS, Curtiss EI, Shaver JA. The mechanism of splitting of the second heart sound in atrial septal defect. *Circulation.* 1977;56:1047.
117. Ciafone RA, Aroesty JM, Weintraub RM, LaRaia PJ, Paulin S. Cyanosis in uncomplicated atrial septal defect with normal right cardiac and pulmonary arterial pressures. *Chest.* 1978c;74:596.
118. Bierman FZ, Williams RG. Subxiphoid two-dimensional imaging of the interatrial septum in infants and neonates with congenital heart disease. *Circulation.* 1979;60:80.
119. Shigenobu M, Kay JH, Mendez M, Zubiate P, Vanstrom N, Yokoyama T. Surgery for mitral and tricuspid insufficiency as-

sociated with secundum atrial septal defect. *J Thorac Cardiovasc Surg*. 1978;75:290.
120. De Maria AN, Oliver LE, Borgren HG, George L, Mason DT. Apparent reduction of aortic and left heart chamber size in atrial septal defect. *Am J Cardiol*. 1978;42:545.
121. Fenoglio JJ, Pham TD, Hordof A, Edie RN, Wit AL. Right atrial ultrastructure in congenital heart disease. II. Atrial septal defect: effects of volume overload. *Am J Cardiol*. 1979c;43:820.
122. Furuta S, Wanibuchi Y, Yokote Y, Natsume T, Machii K. A proposal of ASD (secundum type) and MR (mitral regurgitation) complex and surgical techniques for the MR in this complex. *VIII World Congress of Cardiol*. 1978; I:245 (abstracts).
123. Somerville J, Kaku S, Saravalli O. Prolapsed mitral cusps in atrial septal defect. An erroneous radiological interpretation. *Br Heart J*. 1978;40:58.
124. Boucher CA, Liberthson RR, Buckley MJ. Secundum atrial septal defect and significant mitral regurgitation. Incidence, management and morphologic basis. *Chest*. 1979;75:697.
125. Pearlman AS, Borer JS, Clarke CE, et al. Abnormal right ventricular size and ventricular septal motion after atrial septal defect closure. Etiology and functional significance. *Am J Cardiol*. 1978;41:295.
126. Fraker TD, Harris PJ, Behar VS, Kisslo JA. Detection and exclusion of interatrial shunts by two-dimensional echocardiography and peripheral venous injection. *Circulation*. 1979;59:379.
127. Kronik G, Slany J, Moesslacher H. Contrast M-mode echocardiography in diagnosis of atrial septal defect in acyanotic patients. *Circulation*. 1979;59:372.
128. King TD, Thompson SL, Mills NL. Measurement of atrial septal defect during cardiac catheterization. Experimental and clinical results. *Am J Cardiol*. 1978;41:537.
129. Wanderman KL, Ovsyshcher I, Gueron M. Left ventricular performance in patients with atrial septal defect: evaluation with noninvasive methods. *Am J Cardiol*. 1978;41:487.
130. Sahn DJ, Allen HD, Anderson R, Goldberg SJ. Echocardiographic diagnosis of atrial septal aneurysm in an infant with hypoplastic right heart syndrome. *Chest*. 1978;73:227.
131. Sutton MGSJ, Tajik AJ, Mercier L-A, Seward JB, Guiliani ER, Ritman EL. Assessment of left ventricular function in secundum atrial septal defect by computer analysis of the M-mode echocardiogram. *Circulation*. 1979;60:1082.
132. Maron BJ, Borer JS, Lan SH, Damato AN, Scott LP, Epstein SE. Association of secundum atrial septal defect and atrioventricular nodal dysfunction. A genetically transmitted syndrome. *Br Heart J*. 1978;40:1293.
133. Giardina ACV, Raptoulis AS, Engle MA, Levin AR. Spontaneous closure of atrial septal defect with cardiac failure in infancy. *Chest*. 1979;75:395.
134. Mirro MJ, Rogers EW, Weyman AE, Feigenbaum H. Angular displacement of the papillary muscles during the cardiac cycle. *Circulation*. 1979;60:327.
135. Sweeney LJ, Rosenquist GC. The normal anatomy of the atrial septum in the human heart. *Am Heart J*. 1979;98:194.
136. Schreiber TL, Feigenbaum H, Weyman AE. Effect of atrial septal defect repair on left ventricular geometry and degree of mitral valve prolapse. *Circulation*. 1980;61:888.
137. Steinbauer-Rosenthal I. Echocardiographic assessment of atrial septal effect size. *Herz*. 1980;5:223.
138. Gondi B, Nanda NC. Two-dimensional echocardiographic features of atrial septal aneurysms. *Circulation*. 1981;63:452.
139. Hung J, Uren RF, Richmond DR, Kelly DT. The mechanism of abnormal septal motion in atrial septal defect: pre-and postoperative study by radionuclide ventriculography in adults. *Circulation*. 1981;63:142.
140. Liberthson RR, Boucher CA, Strauss HW, Dinsmore RE, McKusick KA, Pohost GM. Right ventricular function in adult atrial septal defect. Preoperative and postoperative assessment and clinical implications. *Am J Cardiol*. 1981;47:56.
141. Hutchins GM, Moore GW, Jones JF, Miller ST. Postnatal endocardial fibroelastosis of the valve of the foramen ovale. *Am J Cardiol*. 1981;47:90.
142. Awan IH, Rice R, Moodie DS. Spontaneous closure of atrial septal defect with interatrial aneurysm formation. Documentation by noninvasive studies, including digital subtraction angiography. *Pediatr Cardiol*. 1982;3:143.
143. Valdes-Cruz LM, Pieroni DR, Jones M, et al. Residual shunting in the early postoperative period after closure of atrial septal defect. Echocardiographic comparison of patch materials. *J Thorac Cardiovasc Surg*. 1982;84:73.
144. Atkins DL, Clark EB, Marvin WJ. Foramen ovale/atrial septum area ratio: a marker of transatrial blood flow. *Circulation*. 1982;66:281.
145. Sobrino J-A, de Lombera F, del Rio A, et al. Atrioventricular nodal dysfunction in patients with atrial septal defect. *Chest*. 1982;81:477.
146. Hurwitz RA, Treves S, Keane JF, Girod DA, Caldwell RL. Current value of radionuclide angiocardiography for shunt quantification and management in patients with secundum atrial septal defect. *Am Heart J*. 1982;103:421.
147. Nagata S, Nimura Y, Sakakibara H, et al. Mitral valve lesion associated with secundum atrial septal defect. Analysis by real time two-dimensional echocardiography. *Br Heart J*. 1983;49:51.
148. Haworth SG. Pulmonary vascular disease in secundum atrial septal defect in childhood. *Am J Cardiol*. 1983;51:265.
149. Macdonald IL, McMurty TJ, Dodek A. Atrial septal defect in adult identical twins: a variation in theme. *Clin Cardiol*. 1983;6:507.
150. Cockerham JT, Martin TC, Gutierrez FR, Hartman AF, Goldring D, Strauss AW. Spontaneous closure of secundum atrial septal defect in infants and young children. *Am J Cardiol*. 1983;52:1267.
151. Ikaheimo MJ, Pokela RE, Karkola PJ, Takkunen JT. Cyanotic ostium secundum atrial septal defect without pulmonary hypertension and clinical signs of heart disease. Report of two cases. *Chest*. 1983;84:598.
152. Ghisla RP, Hannon DW, Meyer RA, Kaplan S. Spontaneous closure of isolated atrial septal defect in infants. *Circulation*. 1983;III-260.
153. Stevenson JG, Kawabori I. Sequential 2D echo/Doppler: improved noninvasive diagnosis of atrial septal defect. *Circulation*. 1983;68:III–110.
154. Perloff JK. Ostium secundum atrial septal defect—survival for 87 and 94 years. *Am J Cardiol*. 1984;53:389.
155. Hagen PT, Scholz DG, Edwards WD. Incidence and size of patent foramen ovale during the first 10 decades of life: an autopsy study of 965 normal hearts. *Mayo Clin Proc*. 1984;59:17.
156. Sondergard T, Paulsen PK. Some immediate hemodynamic consequences of closure of atrial septal defects of the secundum type. *Circulation*. 1984;69:905.
157. Freed MD, Nadas AS, Norwood WI, Castaneda AR. Is routine preoperative cardiac catheterization necessary before repair of secundum and sinus venosus atrial septal defects? *J Am Coll Cardiol*. 1984;4:333.

158. Iliceto S, Antonelli G, Sorino M, Ricci A. Detection of atrial septal defect by right sternal border echocardiography. *Am J Cardiol.* 1984;54:376.
159. Ruschhaupt DG, Khoury L, Thilenius OG, Replogle RL, Arcilla RA. Electrophysiologic abnormalities of children with ostium secundum atrial septal defect. *Am J Cardiol.* 1984;53:1643.
160. Ginzton LE, French W, Mena I. Combined contrast echocardiographic and radionuclide diagnosis of atrial septal defect: accuracy of the technique and analysis of erroneous diagnoses. *Am J Cardiol.* 1984;53:1639.
161. Green CE, Gottdiener JS, Goldstein HA. Atrial septal defect. *Semin Roentgenol.* 1985;20:214.
162. Suzuki Y, Kambara H, Kadota K, et al. Detection of intracardiac shunt flow in atrial septal defect using a real-time two-dimensional color-coded Doppler flow imaging system and comparison with contrast two-dimensional echocardiography. *Am J Cardiol.* 1985;56:347.
163. Topaz O, Feigl A, Edwards JE. Aneurysm of the fossa ovalis in infants: a pathologic study. *Pediatr Cardiol.* 1985;6:65.
164. Forfar JC, Godman MJ. Functional and anatomical correlates in atrial septal defect, an echocardiographic analysis. *Br Heart J.* 1985;54:193.
165. Joffe HS. Effect of age on pressure-flow dynamics in secundum atrial septal defect. *Br Heart J.* 1984;51:469.
166. Bolens M, Friedli B. Sinus node function and conduction system before and after surgery for secundum atrial septal defect: an electrophysiological study. *Am J Cardiol.* 1984;53:1415.
167. Sanders SP. Echocardiography and related techniques in the diagnosis of congenital heart defects. Part I: veins, atria and interatrial septum. *Echocardiography.* 1984;1:185.
168. Karpawich PP, Antillon JR, Cappola PR, Agarwal KC. Pre- and postoperative electrophysiologic assessment of children with secundum atrial septal defect. *Am J Cardiol.* 1985;55:519.
169. Ghisla RP, Hannon DW, Meyer RA, Kaplan S. Spontaneous closure of isolated secundum atrial septal defects in infants: an echocardiographic study. *Am Heart J.* 1985;109:1327.
170. Hanley PC, Tajik AJ, Hynes JK, et al. Diagnosis and classification of atrial septal aneurysm by two-dimensional echocardiography: report of 80 consecutive cases. *J Am Coll Cardiol.* 1985;6:1370.
171. Schofield PM, Barber PV, Kingston T. Preoperative and postoperative pulmonary function tests in patients with atrial septal defect and their relation to pulmonary artery pressure and pulmonary:systemic flow ratio. *Br Heart J.* 1985;54:577.
172. Soto B, Banuelos C, Ceballos R. Angiographic recognition of atrial septal defect. *Rev Latina Cardiol Inf.* 1985;1:181.
173. Yamaki S, Horiuchi T, Miura M, et al. Pulmonary vascular disease in secundum atrial septal defect with pulmonary hypertension. *Chest.* 1986;89:695.
174. Schamroth CL, Sareli P, Pocock WA, et al. Pulmonary arterial thrombosis in secundum atrial septal defect. *Am J Cardiol.* 1987;60:1152.
175. Steele PM, Fuster V, Cohen M, Ritter DG, McGoon DC. Isolated atrial septal defect with pulmonary vascular obstruction disease—long-term follow-up and prediction of outcome after surgical correction. *Circulation.* 1987;76:1037.
176. Wolf WJ, Casta A, Sapire DW. Atrial septal aneurysm in infants and children. *Am Heart J.* 1987;113:1149.
177. Fuzakawa M, Fukushige J, Ueda K. Atrial septal defects in neonates with reference to spontaneous closure. *Am Heart J.* 1988;116:123.
178. Thomas JD, Tabakin BS, Ittleman FP. Atrial septal defect with right to left shunt despite normal pulmonary artery pressure. *J Am Coll Cardiol.* 1987;9:221.
179. Yamaki S, Horiuchi T, Miura M, Haneda K, Ishizawa E, Suzuki Y. Secundum atrial septal defect with severe pulmonary hypertension. Open lung biopsy diagnosis of operative indication. *Chest.* 1987;91:33.
180. Zhon T-F, Guntheroth WG. Valve-incompetence foramen ovale in premature infants with ductus arteriosus: a Doppler echocardiographic study. *J Am Coll Cardiol.* 1987;10:193.
181. Vincent RN, Saurette RH, Pelech AN, Collins GF. Interventricular septal motion and left ventricular function in patients with atrial septal defect. *Pediatr Cardiol.* 1988;9:143.
182. Rice MJ, McDonald RW, Reller MD. Fetal atrial septal aneurysms, a cause of fetal arrhythmias. *J Am Coll Cardiol.* 1988;12:1292.
183. Hanseus K, Bjorkhem G, Lundstrom N-R, Soeroso S. Cross-sectional echocardiographic measurement of right atrial and right ventricular size in children with atrial septal defect before and after surgery. *Pediatr Cardiol.* 1988;9:231.
184. Pollick C, Sullivan H, Cujec B, Wilansky S. Doppler color-flow imaging assessment of shunt size in atrial septal defect. *Circulation.* 1988;78:522.
185. Mugge A, Daniel WG, Klopper JW, Lichtlen PR. Visualization of patent foramen ovale by transesophageal color-coded Doppler echocardiography. *Am J Cardiol.* 1988;62:837.
186. Finley JP, Nugent ST, Hellenbrand W, Craig M, Gillis DA. Sinus arrhythmia in children with atrial septal defect: an analysis of heart rate variability before and after surgical repair. *Br Heart J.* 1989;61:280.
187. Corone P, Davido A, Hallali P, Poivre B. Troubles du rythme observes chez les malades operes d'une communication interauriculaire. *Coeur.* 1988;19:340.
188. Corone P, Davido A, Hallali P, Capderon A, Poivre B. Evolution des pressions arterielles pulmonaires des communications interauriculaires. *Coeur.* 1988;19:284.
189. Guerin F, Gamerman G, Toussaint M, et al. Communications interauriculaires avec grande hypertension arterielle pulmonaire. A propos de 31 cas. *Coeur.* 1988;19:269.
190. Lock JE, Rome JJ, Davis R. et al: Transcatheter closure of atrial septal defects, experimental studies. *Circulation.* 1989;79:1091.
191. Hossack KF, Tewksbury JC, Reid LM. Successful repair of an atrial septal defect associated with right to left shunting. *Br Heart J.* 1989;62:69.
192. Pryor RE, Giannetto L, Bashore TM. Surgical repair of atrial septal defect in an 89-year-old man: progressive shunt due to concomitant aortic stenosis. *Am Heart J.* 1989;118:423.
193. Moosvi AR, Alam M, Gheorghiade M. The effect of a pericardial effusion on the shunt across an atrial septal defect. *Am Heart J.* 1989;118:627.
194. Brand A, Keren A, Branski D, Abrahamov A, Stern S. Natural course of atrial septal aneurysm in children and the potential for spontaneous closure of associated septal defect. *Am J Cardiol.* 1989;64:996.
195. Remy-Jardin M, Remy J, Wallaert B. Right-to-left shunting through a patent foramen ovale without pulmonary hypertension. Transient improvement after balloon catheter closure. *Chest.* 1990;97:1250.
196. Schwinger ME, Gindea AJ, Freedberg RS, Kronzon I. The anatomy of the interatrial septum: a transesophageal echocardiographic study. *Am Heart J.* 1990;119:1401.
197. Morimoto K, Matsuzaki M, Tohma Y, et al. Diagnosis and quantitative evaluation of secundum-type atrial septal defect by transesophageal Doppler echocardiography. *Am J Cardiol.* 1990;66:85.

198. Hellenbrand WE, Fahey JT, McGowan FX, Weltin GG, Kleinman CS. Transesophageal echocardiographic guidance of transcatheter closure of atrial septal defect. *Am J Cardiol.* 1990;66:207.
199. Smith AJ, Panidis IP, Berger S, Gonzales R. Large atrial septal aneurysm mimicking a cystic right atrial mass. *Am Heart J.* 1990;120:714.
200. Rome JJ, Keane JF, Perry SB, Spevak PJ, Lock JE. Double-umbrella closure of atrial defects. Initial clinical applications. *Circulation.* 1990;82:751.
201. Rocchini AP. Transcatheter closure of atrial septal defect: past, present, and future. *Circulation.* 1990;82:1044.
202. Zabalgoitia-Reyes M, Herrera C, Gandhi DK, Mehlman DJ, McPherson DD, Talano JV. A possible mechanism for neurologic ischemic events in patients with atrial septal aneurysm. *Am J Cardiol.* 1990;66:761.
203. Belkin RN, Kisslo J. Atrial septal aneurysm: recognition and clinical relevance. *Am Heart J.* 1990;120:948.
204. Murphy JG, Gersh BJ, McGoon MD, et al. Long-term outcome after surgical repair of isolated atrial septal defect. Follow-up at 27 to 32 years. *N Engl J Med.* 1990;323:1645.
205. Chong YM, So LY, Fok TF, Gerlis LM. Cyanotic atrial septal defect in a premature infant. *Pediatr Cardiol.* 1991;12:63.
206. Hiraishi S, Agata Y, Saito K, et al. Interatrial shunt flow profiles in newborn infants: a colour flow and pulsed Doppler echocardiographic study. *Br Heart J.* 1991;65:41.
207. Frontera-Izquierdo P, Cabezuelo-Huerta G. Severe Holt-Oram syndrome with pulmonary hypertension. *Am Heart J.* 1991;122:250.
208. Rao PS, Sideris EB, Chopra PS. Catheter closure of atrial septal defect: successful use in a 3.6 kg infant. *Am Heart J.* 1991;121:1826.
209. Bharati S, Patel AG, Varga P, Husain AN, Lev M. In utero echocardiographic diagnosis of premature closure of the foramen ovale with mitral regurgitation and large left atrium. *Am Heart J.* 1991;122:597.
210. Langholz D, Louie EK, Konstadt SN, Rao TLK, Scanlon PJ. Transesophageal echocardiographic demonstration of distinct mechanisms for right to left shunting across a patent foramen ovale in the absence of pulmonary hypertension. *J Am Coll Cardiol.* 1991;18:112.
211. Okamoto M, Tsubokura T, Kawagoe T, et al. Mitral stenosis with unusual atrial shunt diagnosed by bipolar transesophageal Doppler echocardiography. *Am Heart J.* 1991;122:1498.
212. Siostrzonek P, Zangeneh M, Gossinger H, et al. Comparison of transesophageal and transthoracic contrast echocardiography for detection of a patent foramen ovale. *Am J Cardiol.* 1991;68:1247.
213. Redington A, Rigby M. Transcatheter closure of interatrial communications with a modified umbrella device. *Cardiol Young.* 1993;3:I–92 (abstract 302).
214. Worms AM, Bourlon F, Hausdorf G, et al. Atrial septal defect occlusion with the buttoned device—early multicenter European clinical trial results. *Cardiol Young.* 1993;3:I–82.
215. Mauri L, Vignati G, Austoni P, et al. Outcome of atrial septal defect corrected after the fifth decade of life. *Cardiol Young.* 1993;3:I–46.
216. Rao PS, Sideris EB, Beekman RH, Lloyd TR. Results of Food and Drug Administration trial of atrial septal defect occlusion with a buttoned device. *Cardiol Young.* 1993;3:I–38 (abstract 112).
217. Mehta RH, Helmcke F, Nanda NC, et al. Uses and limitations of transthoracic echocardiography in the assessment of atrial septal defect in the adult. *Am J Cardiol.* 1991;657:288.
218. Sorrentino M, Resnekov L. Patent foramen ovale associated with platypnea and orthodeoxia. *Chest.* 1991;100:1157.
219. Jin Z, Briedigkeit W, Schirmer H, Kampmann C, et al. Echocardiographic right ventricular volumes and mass in normal children and those with atrial septal defects pre- and post-closure. *Cardiol Young.* 1993;3:I–141 (abstract 498).
220. Etchells E, Wong DT, Davidson G, Houston PL. Fatal cerebral fat embolism associated with a patent foramen ovale. *Chest.* 1993;104:962.
221. Fujiwara K, Naito Y, Higashine S-i, et al. Left main coronary trunk compression by dilated main pulmonary artery in atrial septal defect. *J Thorac Cardiovasc Surg.* 1992;104:449.
222. Dietl CA, Torres AR, Favaloro RG. Right submammarian thoracotomy in female patients with atrial septal defects and anomalous pulmonary venous connections. Comparison between the transpectoral and subpectoral approaches. *J Thorac Cardiovasc Surg.* 1992;104:723.
223. Radzik D, Davignon A, van Doesburg N, et al. Predictive factors for spontaneous closure of atrial septal defects diagnosed in the first 3 months of life. *J Am Coll Cardiol.* 1993;22:851.
224. Meijboom F, Hess J, Szatmari A, et al. Long-term follow-up (9 to 20 years) after surgical closure of atrial septal defect at a young age. *Am J Cardiol.* 1993;72:1431.
225. Boutin C, Musewe NN, Smallhorn JF, Dyck JD, Kobayashi T, Benson LN. Echocardiographic follow-up of atrial septal defect after catheter closure by double-umbrella device. *Circulation.* 1993;88:621.
226. Lloyd TR, Rao PS, Beekman RH, Mendelsohn AM, Sideris EB. Atrial septal defect occlusion with the buttoned device (a multi-institutional US trial). *Am J Cardiol.* 1994;73:286.
227. Lin S-L, Ting C-T, Hsu T-L, et al. Transesophageal echocardiographic detection of atrial septal defect in adults. *Am J Cardiol.* 1992;69:280.
228. Chan KC, Godman MJ. Morphological variations of fossa ovalis atrial septal defects (secundum): feasibility for transcutaneous closure with the clam-shell device. *Br Heart J.* 1993;69:52.
229. Siderys H, Bittles ML, Niemeir M, Genovely HC. Severe hypoxia related to uncomplicated atrial septal defect. *Tex Heart Inst J.* 1993;20:123.
230. Wilmshurst PT, Treacher DF, Crowther A, Smith SE. Effects of a patent foramen ovale on arterial saturation during exercise and on cardiovascular responses to deep breathing, Valsalva maneuver, and passive tilt: relation to history of decompression illness in divers. *Br Heart J.* 1994;71:229.
231. Shah D, Azhar M, Oakley CM, Cleland JGF, Nihoyannopoulos P. Natural history of secundum atrial septal defect in adults after medical or surgical treatment: a historical prospective study. *Br Heart J.* 1994;71:224.
232. Ward C. Secundum atrial septal defect: routine surgical treatment is not of proven benefit. *Br Heart J.* 1994;71:219.
233. Ricou FJ, Reynard CA, Lerch R. Transesophageal echocardiography in the diagnosis of inferior caval secundum atrial septum defect. *Am Heart J.* 1994;128:196.
234. Bonchek LI, Burlingame MW, Worley SJ, Vazales BE, Lundy EF. Cox/maze procedure for atrial septal defect with atrial fibrillation: management strategies. *Ann Thorac Surg.* 1993;55:607.
235. Evans N, Iyer P. Incompetence of the foramen ovale in preterm infants supported by mechanical ventilation. *J Pediatr.* 1994;125:786.
236. Shirani J, Zafari AM, Roberts WC. Morphologic features of fossa ovalis membrane aneurysm in the adult and its clinical significance. *J Am Coll Cardiol.* 1995;26:466.

237. Redington AN, Rigby ML. Transcatheter closure of interatrial communications with a modified umbrella device. *Br Heart J.* 1994;72:372.
238. Fisher DC, Fisher EA, Budd JH, Rosen SE, Goldman ME. The incidence of patent foramen ovale in 1,000 consecutive patients, a contrast transesophageal echocardiographic study. *Chest.* 1995;107:1504.
239. Ferreira SM, Ho SY, Anderson RH. Morphological study of defects of the atrial septum within the oval fossa: implications for transcatheter closure of left-to-right shunt. *Br Heart J.* 1992;67:316.
240. Horvath KA, Burke RP, Collins JJ, Cohn LH. Surgical treatment of adult atrial septal defect: early and long-term results. *J Am Coll Cardiol.* 1992;20:1156.
241. Mugge A, Daniel WG, Angermann C, et al. Atrial septal aneurysm in adult patients, a multicenter study using transthoracic and transesophageal echocardiography. *Circulation.* 1995;91:2785.
242. Perloff JK. Surgical closure of atrial septal defects in adults. *New Engl J Med.* 1995;333:513.
243. Konstantinides S, Geibel A, Olschweski M, et al. A comparison of surgical and medical therapy for atrial septal defect in adults. *N Engl J Med.* 1995;333:469.
244. Schenck MH, Sterba R, Foreman CK, Latson LA. Improvement in noninvasive electrophysiologic findings in children after transcatheter atrial septal defect closure. *Am J Cardiol.* 1995;76:695.
245. Brili S, McClemens B, Castellanos S, et al. Significance of an atrial septal aneurysm in the presence of an ostium secundum atrial septal defect. A transesophageal echocardiographic study. *Cardiology.* 1995;86:421.
246. Basson CT, Lin R, Bachinsky D, Seidman JG, Seidman CE. Refined genetic and physical mapping studies to identify the Holt-Oram syndrome gene. *Circulation.* 1995;92(suppl I):517.
247. Sideris EB, Leung M, Yoon JH, et al. Occlusion of large atrial septal defects with a centering buttoned device: early clinical experience. *Am Heart J.* 1996;131:356.
248. Gatzoulis MA, Redington AN, Somerville J, Shore DF. Should atrial septal defects in adults be close? *Ann Thorac Surg.* 1996;61:657.
249. Stone DA, Godard J, Corretti MC, Kittner SJ, et al. Patent foramen ovale: association between the degree of shunt by contrast transesophageal echocardiography and the risk of future ischemic neurologic events. *Am Heart J.* 1996;131:158.
250. Heller J, Hagege AA, Besse B, Desnos M, Marie F-N, Guerot C. "Crochetage" (notch) on R wave in inferior limb leads: a new independent electrocardiographic sign of atrial septal defect. *J Am Coll Cardiol.* 1996;27:877.
251. Agarwal SK, Ghosh PK, Mittal PK. Failure of devices used for closure of atrial septal defects: mechanisms and management. *J Thorac Cardiovasc Surg.* 1996;112:21.
252. Ende DJ, Chopra PS, Rao S. Transcatheter closure of atrial septal defect or patent foramen ovale with the buttoned device for prevention of recurrence of paradoxic embolism. *Am J Cardiol.* 1996;78:233.
253. Grinda J-M, Folliguet TA, Dervanian P, Mace L, Legault B, Neveux J-Y. Right anterolateral thoracotomy for repair of atrial septal defect. *Ann Thorac Surg.* 1996;62:175.
254. Magni G, Cao Q-L, Sugeng L, et al. Volume-rendered, three-dimensional echocardiographic determination of the size, shape and position of atrial septal defects; validation in an in vitro model. *Am Heart J.* 1996;132:376.
255. Eidem BW, O'Leary PW, Tei C, Seward JB. Adverse effect of chronic volume overload on right ventricular function in patients with atrial septal defect: assessment using a new simple Doppler index. *Pediatrics.* 1996;98(suppl):527.
256. Estagnasie P, Djedaini K, LeBourdelles G, Coste F, Dreyfuss D. Atrial septal aneurysm plus a patent foramen ovale, a predisposing factor for paradoxical embolism and refractory hypoxemia during pulmonary embolism. *Chest.* 1996;110:846.
257. Aksnes J, Lindberg HL, Ihlen H. Surgical elimination of an atrial septal aneurysm causing cerebral embolism. *Ann Thorac Surg.* 1996;62:1190.
258. Helber U, Baumann R, Seboldt H, Reinhard U, Hoffmeister HM. Atrial septal defect in adults: cardiopulmonary exercise capacity before and 4 months and 10 years after defect closure. *J Am Coll Cardiol.* 1997;29:1345.
259. Hekmat K, Mehlhorn U, de Vivie ER. Surgical repair of a large residual atrial septal defect after transcatheter closure. *Ann Thorac Surg.* 1997;63:1456.
260. Shanoudy H, Soliman A, Raggi P, Liu JW, Russell DC, Jarmukli NF. Prevalence of patent foramen ovale and its contribution to hypoxemia in patients with obstructive sleep apnea. *Chest.* 1998;113:91.
261. Kobayashi J, Yamamoto F, Nakano K, Sasako Y, Kitamura S, Kosakai Y. Maze procedure for atrial fibrillation associated with atrial septal defect. *Circulation.* 1998;98:II–399.
262. Vogel M, Berger F, Kramer A, Alexi-Meshkishvili V, Lange PE. Incidence of secondary pulmonary hypertension in adults with atrial septal or sinus venosus defects. *Heart.* 1999;82:30.
263. Brassard M, Fouron J-C, van Doesburg NH, Mercier L-A, DeGuise P. Outcome of children with atrial septal defect considered too small for surgical closure. *Am J Cardiol.* 1999;83:1552.
264. Dall'Agata A, McGhie J, Taams MA, et al. Secundum atrial septal defect is a dynamic three-dimensional entity. *Am Heart J.* 1999;137:1075.
265. Walsh KP, Wilmshurst PT, Morrison WL. Transcatheter closure of patent foramen ovale using the Amplatzer septal occluder to prevent recurrence of neurological decompression illness in divers. *Heart.* 1999;81:257.
266. Rigby ML. The era of transcatheter closure of atrial septal defects. *Heart.* 1999;81:227.
267. Gatzoulis MA, Freeman MA, Siu SC, Webb GD, Harris L. Atrial arrhythmia after surgical closure of atrial septal defects. *N Engl J Med.* 1999;340:839.
268. Bohm M. Holt-Oram syndrome. *Circulation.* 1998;98:2636.
269. Zamora R, Rao PS, Lloyd TR, Beckman RH, Sideris EB. Intermediate-term results of phase I Food and Drug Administration trials of button device. Occlusion of secundum atrial septal defects. *J Am Coll Cardiol.* 1998;31:674.
270. Sulc J, Andrle V, Hruda J, Hucin B, Samanek M, Zapletal A. Pulmonary function in children with atrial septal defect before and after heart surgery. *Heart.* 1998;80:484.
271. Yeager SB, Keane JF. Fate of moderate and large secundum type atrial septal defect associated with isolated coarctation in infants. *Am J Cardiol.* 1999;84:362.
272. La Rosee K, Deutsch HJ, Schnabel P, et al. Thrombus formation after transcatheter closure of atrial septal defect. *Am J Cardiol.* 1999;84:356.
273. Bichell DP, Geva T, Bacha EA, Mayer JE, Jonas RA, del Nido PJ. Minimal access approach for the repair of atrial septal defect: the initial 135 patients. *Ann Thorac Surg.* 2000;70:115.
274. Marshall AC, Lock JE. Structural and compliant anatomy of the patent foramen ovale in patients undergoing transcatheter closure. *Am Heart J.* 2000;140:303.

275. Perry YY, Treidman JK, Gauvreau K, Lock JE, Jenkins KJ. Sudden death in patients after transcatheter device implantation for congenital heart disease. *Am J Cardiol.* 2000;85:992.
276. Chan KC, Godman MJ, Walsh K, Wilson N, Redington A, Gibbs JL. Transcatheter closure of atrial septal defect and interatrial communications with a new self expanding nitinol double disc device (Amplatzer septal occluder: multicenter UK experience). *Heart.* 1999;82:300.
277. Hung J, Landzberg MJ, Jenkins KJ, et al. Closure of patent foramen ovale for paradoxical emboli: intermediate-term risk of recurrent neurological events following transcatheter device placement. *J Am Coll Cardiol.* 2000;35:1311.
278. Lock JE. Patent foramen ovale is indicted, but the case hasn't gone to trial. *Circulation.* 2000;101:838.
279. Houyel L, Petit J, Planche C, et al. Thoracotomie postero-lateral droite pour la chirurgie a coeur ouvert chez l'enfant. Indications et resultats. *Arch Mal Coeur Vaiss.* 1999;92:641.
280. Akter M, Lajos TZ. Pitfalls of undetected patent foramen ovale in off-pump cases. *Ann Thorac Surg.* 1999;67:546.
281. Dhillon R, Thanopoulos B, Tsaousis G, et al. Transcatheter closure of atrial septal defects in adults with the Amplatzer septal occluder. *Heart.* 1999;82:559.
282. Magni G, Hijazi ZM, Pandian NG, et al. Two- and three-dimensional transesophageal echocardiography in patient selection and assessment of atrial septal closure by the new DAS-angel wings device. Initial clinical experience. *Circulation.* 1997;96:1722.
283. Rhee EK, Evangelista JK, Nigrin DJ, Erikson LC. Impact of anatomic closure on somatic growth among small, asymptomatic children with secundum atrial septal defect. *Am J Cardiol.* 2000;85:1472.
284. Kessel-Schaefer A, Lefkovitz M, Zellweger MJ, et al. Migrating thrombus trapped in a patent foramen. *Circulation.* 2001;103:1928.
285. Formigari R, Di Donato RM, Mazzera E, et al. Minimally invasive or interventional repair of atrial septal defects in children: experience in 171 cases and comparison with conventional strategies. *J Am Coll Cardiol.* 2001;37:1707.
286. Taeed R, Shim D, Kimball TR, et al. One-year follow-up of the Amplatzer device to close atrial septal defects. *Am J Cardiol.* 2001;87:116.
287. Jemielity M, Dyszkiewicz W, Paluszkiewicz L, et al. Do patients over 40 years of age benefit from surgical closure of atrial septal defects? *Heart.* 2001;85:300.
288. Alp N, Clarke N, Banning AP. How should patients with patent foramen ovale be managed? *Heart.* 2001;85:242.
289. Sievert H, Babic UU, Hausdorf G, et al. Transcatheter closure of atrial septal defect and patent foramen ovale with the ASDOS device (a multi-institutional European trial). *Am J Cardiol.* 1998;82:1405.
290. Hoepp HW, Deutsch HJ, La Rosee K, et al. Transcatheter closure of atrial septal defects and patent foramen ovale in adults: optimal anatomic adaptation of occlusion device. *Am Heart J.* 1999;138:941.
291. Byrne JG, Adams DH, Mitchell ME, Cohn LH. Minimally invasive direct access for repair of atrial septal defects in adults. *Am J Cardiol.* 1999;84:919.
292. Berger F, Vogel M, Alexi-Meskishvili V, Lange PE. Comparison of results and complications of surgical and Amplatzer device closure of atrial septal defects. *J Thorac Cardiovasc Surg.* 1999;118:674.
293. Ewart P, Berger F, Vogel M, Dahnert I, Alex-Meshkisvili V, Lange PE. Morphology of perforated atrial septal aneurysm suitable for closure by transcatheter device placement. *Heart.* 2000;84:327.
294. Benson DW, Sharkey A, Fatkin D, et al. Reduced penetrance, variable expressivity, and genetic heterogeneity of familiar atrial septal defects. *Circulation.* 1998;97:2043.
295. Veldtman GR, Razack V, Siu S, et al. Right ventricular form and function after percutaneous atrial septal device closure. *J Am Coll Cardiol.* 1998;37:2108.
296. Thanopoulos VD, Laskari CV, Tsaousis GS, et al. Closure of atrial septal defects with the Amplatzer occlusion device: preliminary results. *J Am Coll Cardiol.* 1998;31:1110.
297. Black MD, Freedom RM. Minimally invasive repair of atrial septal defects. *Ann Thorac Surg.* 1998;65:765.
298. Barbero-Marcial M, Tanamati C, Jatene MB, Atik E, Jatene AD. Transxiphoid approach without median sternotomy for the repair of atrial septal defects. *Ann Thorac Surg.* 1998;65:771.
299. Berdat PA, Chatterjee T, Pfammatter J-P, et al. Surgical management of complications after transcatheter closure of an atrial septal defect or patent foramen ovale. *J Thorac Cardiovasc Surg.* 2000;120:1034.
300. Lethen H, Flachskampf FA, Schneider R, et al. Frequency of deep vein thrombosis in patients with patent foramen ovale and ischemic stroke or transient ischemic attack. *Am J Cardiol.* 1997;80:1066.
301. Losay J, Petit J, Lambert V, Esna G, et al. Percutaneous closure with Amplatzer device is a safe and efficient alternative to surgery in adults with large atrial septal defects. *Am Heart J.* 2001;142:544.
302. El-Said HG, Bezold LI, Grifka RG, et al. Sizing of atrial septal defects to predict successful closure with transcatheter Cardio-SEAL device. *Tex Heart Inst J.* 2001;28:177.
303. Cao Q-L, Du Z-D, Joseph A, et al. Immediate and six-month results of the profile of the Amplatzer septal occluder as assessed by transesophageal echocardiography. *Am J Cardiol.* 2001;88:754.
304. Torracca L, Ismeno G, Alfieri O. Totally endoscopic computer-enhanced atrial septal defect closure in six patients. *Ann Thorac Surg.* 2001;72:1354.
305. Kort HW, Balzer DT, Johnson MC. Resolution of right heart enlargement after closure of secundum atrial septal defect with transcatheter technique. *J Am Coll Cardiol.* 2001;38:1528.
306. Rhodes JF, Lane GK, Beachler LA, Latson LA. Transcatheter patent foramen ovale closure for adults with platypnea/desaturation. *Circulation.* 2001;104(suppl II):593.
307. Sievert H, Wilson N, Trepels T, et al. Catheter closure of patent foramen ovale: world experience with the new HELEX occluder. *Circulation.* 2001;104(suppl II):593.
308. Sievert H, Trepels T, Bilinger K, Zodan E, et al. Catheter closure of atrial septal defects in adults with the Amplatzer occluder: acute and follow-up results in 178 consecutive patients. *Circulation.* 2001;104(suppl II):593.
309. Ghosh S, Chatterjee S, Black E, Firmin RK. Do adults benefit from surgical closure of atrial septal defects? *Circulation.* 2001;104(suppl II):558.
310. Attie R, Rosas M, Granados N, Zabal C, Buendia A, Calderon J. Surgical treatment for secundum atrial septal defects in patients >40 years old, a randomized clinical trial. *J Am Coll Cardiol.* 2001;38:2035.

311. Mas J-L, Arquizan C, Lamy C, et al. Recurrent cerebrovascular events associated with patent foramen, atrial septal aneurysm, or both. *N Engl J Med*. 2001;345:1740.
312. Yoshimura N, Yamaguchi M, Oshima Y, Oka S, Ootaki Y, Yoshida M. Repair of atrial septal defect through a right posterolateral thoracotomy: a cosmetic approach for female patients. *Ann Thorac Surg*. 2001;72:2103.
313. Oliver JM, Gallego P, Gonzalez A, Benito F, Mesa JM, Sobrino JA. Predisposing conditions for atrial fibrillation in atrial septal defect with and without operative closure. *Am J Cardiol*. 2002;89:39.
314. Connuck D, Sun JP, Super DM, et al. Incidence of patent ductus arteriosus and patent foramen ovale in normal infants. *Am J Cardiol*. 2002;89:244.
315. Meier B. Patent foramen ovale—beauty spot or health threat? *Cardiol Rounds*. 2001;5:1.
316. Sariosmanoglu N, Hazan E, Metin K, Kazaz H, Oto O. Intrapericaridal diaphragmatic hernia and atrial septal defect in adults. *J Thorac Cardiovasc Surg*. 2002;123:353.
317. McMahon CJ, Feltes TF, Fraley JK, et al. Natural history of growth of secundum atrial septal defects and implications for transcatheter closure. *Heart*. 2002;87:256.
318. Chessa M, Carminati M, Butera G, et al. Early and late complications associated with transcatheter occlusion of secundum atrial septal defect. *J Am Coll Cardiol*. 2002;39:1061.
319. Sideris EB, Toumanides S, Macuil B, et al. Transcatheter patch correction of secundum atrial septal defects. *Am J Cardiol*. 2002;89:1082.
320. Du Z-D, Hijazi ZM, Kleinman CS, Silverman NH. Larntz K for the Amplatzer investigators: comparison between transcatheter and surgical closure of secundum atrial septal defect in children and adults. Results of a multicenter nonrandomized trial. *J Am Coll Cardiol*. 2002;39:1836.
321. Bruch L, Parsi A, Grad MO, et al. Transcatheter closure of interatrial communications for secondary prevention of paradoxical embolism. Single-center experience. *Circulation*. 2002;105:2845.
322. Hughes ML, Maskell G, Goh TH, Wilkinson JL. Prospective comparison of costs and short-term health outcomes of surgical versus device closure of atrial septal defect in children. *Heart*. 2002;88:67.
323. Sajeev CS, Roy TNS, Venugopal K. Common atrium in a child with Ellis-Van Creveld syndrome. *Heart*. 2002;88:142.
324. Humpl T, Campbell R, Stephens D, et al. Levels of exhaled nitric oxide before and after surgical and transcatheter device closure of atrial septal defects in children. *J Thorac Cardiovasc Surg*. 2002;124:806.
325. Martin F, Sanchez PL, Doherty E, et al. Percutaneous transcatheter closure of patent foramen ovale in patients with paradoxical embolism. *Circulation*. 2002;106:1121.
326. Brochu M-C, Baril J-F, Dore A, Juneau M, DeGuise P, Mercier L-A. Improvement in exercise capacity in asymptomatic and mildly symptomatic adults after atrial septal defect percutaneous closure. *Circulation*. 2002;106:1821.
327. Suarez de Lezo J, Medina A, Romero M, et al. Effectiveness of percutaneous device occlusion for atrial septal defect in adult patients with pulmonary hypertension. *Am Heart J*. 2002;144:877.
328. Ghosh S, Chatterjee S, Black E, Firmin RK. Surgical closure of atrial septal defects in adults: effect of age at operation on outcome. *Heart*. 2000;88:485.
329. Du Z-D, Koenig P, Cao Q-L, Waight D, Heitschmidt M, Hijazi ZM. Comparison of transcatheter closure of secundum atrial septal defect using the Amplatzer septal occluder associated with deficient versus sufficient rims. *Am J Cardiol*. 2002;90:865.
330. Mullen MJ, Dias BF, Walker F, Siu SC, Benson LN, McLaughlin PR. Intracardiac echocardiographic guided device closure of atrial septal defects. *J Am Coll Cardiol*. 2002;41:285.
331. Meier B, Lock JE. Contemporary management of patent foramen ovale. *Circulation*. 2003;107:5.
332. Fischer G, Stieh J, Morf G, Kramer HH. Experience with transcatheter closure of secundum atrial septal defects using the Amplatzer septal occluder: a single centre study in 236 consecutive patients. *Heart*. 2003;89:199.
333. Bichell DP, Pelletier G. Atrial septal defect and cor triatriatum. In: Sellke FW, del Nido PJ, Swanson SJ, eds. *Sabiston & Spencer Surgery of the Chest*. 7th ed. Philadelphia: Elsevier Saunders; 2005:1935 (Chapter 109).
334. Mignosa C, Vincenzo D, Ferlazzo G, Bianca I, Salvo D, Chylothorax. An unusual manifestation of a large atrial septal defect. *J Thorac Cardiovasc Surg*. 2001;122:1252.
335. Argenziano M, Oz MC, Kohmoto T, et al. Totally endoscopic atrial septal defect repair with robotic assistance. *Circulation*. 2003;108:[suppl II] II–191.
336. Homma S, Sacco RL, DiTullio MR, Sciacca RR. Mohr JP for the PICSS investigators (PICSS=patent foramen ovale in cryptogenic stroke study): atrial anatomy in non-cardioembolic stroke patients. Effect of medical therapy. *J Am Coll Cardiol*. 2003;42:1066.
337. Ryan WH, Cheirif J, Dewey TM, Prince SL, Mack MJ. Safety and efficacy of minimally invasive atrial septal defect closure. *Ann Thorac Surg*. 2003;75:1532.
338. Doll N, Walther T, Falk V, et al. Secundum ASD closure using a right lateral minithoracotomy: five-year experience in 122 patients. *Ann Thorac Surg*. 2003;75:1527.
339. Hopkins RA. Invited commentary [re reference 338]. *Ann Thorac Surg*. 2003;75:1530.
340. Alexi-Meskishvili VV, Konstantinov IE. Surgery for atrial septal defect: from the first experiments to clinical practice. *Ann Thorac Surg*. 2003;76:322.
341. Bartel T, Konorza T, Arjumand J, et al. Intracardiac echocardiography is superior to conventional monitoring for guiding device closure of interatrial communications. *Circulation*. 2003;107:795.
342. Mills NL, King TD. Late follow-up of nonoperative closure of secundum atrial septal defects using the King-Mills double-umbrella device. *Am J Cardiol*. 2003;92:353.
343. Elliott DA, Kirk EP, Yeoh T, Chandar S, et al. Cardiac homeobox gene NKX2-5 mutations and congenital heart disease. Associations with atrial septal defect and hypoplastic left heart syndrome. *J Am Coll Cardiol*. 2003;41:2072.
344. Pratali S, Mecozzi G, Milano A, Baglini R, Bortolotti U. Prevention of embolization of a displaced atrial septal occluder. *Tex Heart Inst J*. 2003;30:88.
345. Chidambaram M, Mink S, Sharma S. Atrial septal aneurysm with right-to-left interatrial shunting. *Tex Heart Inst J*. 2003;30:68.
346. Stumper O, Gewillig M, Vettukattil J, et al. Modified technique of stent fenestration of the atrial septum. *Heart*. 2003;89:1227.
347. Schwerzmann M, Windecker S, Wahl A, et al. Percutaneous closure of patent foramen ovale: impact of device design on safety and efficacy. *Heart*. 2004;90:186.

348. Boccalandro F, Baptista E, Muench A, Carter C, Smalling RW. Comparison of intracardiac echocardiography versus transesopagheal echocardiography guidance for percutaneous transcatheter closure of atrial septal defect. *Am J Cardiol.* 2004;93:437.
349. Anzai H, Child J, Natterson B, et al. Incidence of thrombus formation on the CardioSEAL and the Amplatzer interatrial closure devices. *Am J Cardiol.* 2004;93:426.
350. Hildick-Smith DJR, O'Sullivan M, Wisbey CR, Mackay JH, Lee EM, Shapiro LM. Amplatzer device closure of atrial septal defects in mature adults: analysis of 76 cases. *Heart.* 2004;90:334.
351. Morgan JA, Peacock JC, Kohmoto T, et al. Robotic techniques improve quality of life in patients undergoing atrial septal defect repair. *Ann Thorac Surg.* 2004;77:1328.
352. Walker RE, Moran AM, Gauvreau K, Colan SD. Evidence of adverse ventricular interdependence in patients with atrial septal defects. *Am J Cardiol.* 2004;93:1374.
353. Hopkins RA, Bert AA, Bucholz B, Guarino K, Meyers M. Surgical patch closure of atrial septal defects. *Ann Thorac Surg.* 2004;77:2144.
354. Giardini A, Donti A, Specchia S, et al. Recovery kinetics of oxygen uptake is prolonged in adults with an atrial septal defect and improved after transcatheter closure. *Am Heart J.* 2004;147:910.
355. Webb GD, Horlick EM. Lessons from cardiopulmonary testing after device closure of secundum atrial septal defects. A tale of two ventricles. *J Am Coll Cardiol.* 2004;43:1892.
356. Giardini A, Donti A, Formigari R, et al. Determinants of cardiopulmonary functional improvement after transcatheter atrial septal defect closure in asymptomatic adults. *J Am Coll Cardiol.* 2004;43:1886.
357. Suda K, Raboisson M-J, Piette D, Dahdah NS, Miro J. Reversible atrioventricular block associated with closure of atrial septal defects using the Amplatzer device. *J Am Coll Cardiol.* 2004;43:1677.
358. Donofrio MT, Bremer YA, Moskowitz WB. Diagnosis and management of restricted or closed foramen ovale in fetuses with congenital heart disease. *Am J Cardiol.* 2004;94:1348.
359. Guntheroth WG, Schwaegler R, Trent E. Comparative roles of the atrial septal aneurysm versus patent foramen ovale in systemic embolization with inferences from neonatal studies. *Am J Cardiol.* 2004;94:1341.
360. Butera G, Carminati M, Chessa M, Piazza L, Giamberti A, Frigiola A. CardioSEAL/STARflex versus Amplatzer devices for percutaneous closure of small to moderate (up to 18 mm) atrial septal defects. *Am Heart J.* 2004;148:507.
361. Wang J-K, Tsai S-K, Wu M-H, Lin M-T, Lue H-C. Short-and intermediate-term results of transcatheter closure of atrial septal defect with the Amplatzer septal occluder. *Am Heart J.* 2004;148:511.
362. Bialkowski J, Karwot B, Szkutnik M, Banaszak P, Kusa J, Skalski J. Closure of atrial septal defects in children. Surgery versus Amplatzer device implantation. *Tex Heart Inst J.* 2004;31:220.
363. Tobis JM, Azarbal B. Does patent foramen ovale promote cryptogenic stroke and migraine headache? *Tex Heart Inst J.* 2005;32:362.
364. Van Praagh S, Carrera ME, Sanders SP, Mayer JE, Van Praagh R. Sinus venosus defects: unroofing of the right pulmonary veins—anatomic and echocardiographic findings and surgical treatment. *Am Heart J.* 1994;128:365.
365. Pessotto R, Padalino M, Rubino M, Kadoba K, Buchler JR, Van Praagh R. Straddling tricuspid valve as a sign of ventriculoatrial malalignment: a morphometric study of 19 postmortem cases. *Am Heart J.* 1994;138:1184.

10

Juxtaposition of the Atrial Appendages

The anomaly now known as juxtaposition of the atrial appendages (JAA) was first described, to the best of our knowledge, by Thore[1] in 1843 in an 11-day-old boy with left-sided JAA. Thore[1] wrote that this neonate had "une anomalie du coeur" (an anomaly of the heart), which he described but did not name.

The first paper concerning this malformation in the English literature was that of Birmingham[2] in 1893. His patient was a 20-year-old woman, a "dealer in fish," who also had left-sided JAA with double-outlet right ventricle (DORV) {S,D,L}, dextrocardia, a large secundum atrial septal defect (ASD) (septum primum was absent), a persistent left superior vena cava to the coronary sinus that drained into the right atrium, a conoventricular type of ventricular septal defect, a bilateral conus (subaortic and subpulmonary), pulmonary outflow tract stenosis (infundibular and valvar), and a right aortic arch. She also had bilateral pulmonary tuberculosis. Understandably, Birmingham[2] called this *an extreme anomaly of the heart and great vessels.*

In the first half of the 20th century, multiple case reports appeared in the literature concerning left-sided JAA (Table 10.1).[3-12]

The complexity of the congenital heart disease associated with left-sided JAA is very impressive (see Table 10.1), leading to at least two questions: Is there any pattern here? Developmentally, what does JAA mean? These are the questions that we and others would subsequently explore. As pointed out by Harris and Farber[9] in 1939, Kettler[6] in 1933 proposed that what would subsequently be called JAA was caused by "insufficient torsion of the cardiac loop so that the bulbous portion fails to migrate to the left and join correctly with the remainder of the heart." Many other works have also contributed to our present understanding of JAA.[13-40]

There is much that could be said about Table 10.1. First, this is a meta-analysis, an analysis based on the literature, not on first-hand examination of these heart specimens. Although I did my best to be accurate, I am not entirely confident about some of these cases. Taussig's case[10] (see Table 10.1) is diagrammed, but the description is scanty.

Were the great arteries in Huebschmann's case[5] (see Table 10.1) really normally related? The main pulmonary artery arose posteriorly and slightly to the right of the aorta, which certainly does not sound like normally related great arteries. However, there was a small and stenotic subpulmonary conus from which the pulmonary artery arose, the aorta originated above the left ventricle (LV), and there was aortic-mitral fibrous continuity (see Table 10.1).[5] Hence, the internal relationships between the great arteries and the conus, between the great arteries and the LV, and between the great arteries and the atrioventricular (AV) canal all appear to have been normal; hence, our conclusion that the segmental anatomy was {S,D,S}, despite the abnormal relationships between the great arteries and external spatial coordinates (anterior-posterior and right-left).

Huebschmann's case[5] (see Table 10.1) leads to the question: **Is it possible for normally related great arteries to have an anterior aortic valve and a posterior pulmonary valve?** Surprising to relate, the answer is yes, as we learned in our first study of JAA that was published in 1968 (Fig. 10.1).[21] Although the *internal* relations of the great arteries are normal, as in Huebschmann's case (see Table 10.1),[5] the *external* relationships of the great arteries relative to fixed external spatial coordinates (such as anterior-posterior and right-left) can be very abnormal when the ventricles—from which the great arteries arise—are significantly malpositioned. In our patient (Case 21),[21] there was isolated ventricular inversion, that is, {S,L,S} (see Fig. 10.1).

Thus, this is why I diagnosed Huebschmann's case[5] as I did (see Table 10.1); but because this is a meta-analysis, I also want to acknowledge that my diagnosis of this case[5] could be erroneous. Nonetheless, it is helpful to understand that normally related great arteries rarely can have very abnormal spatial relationships relative to fixed external spatial coordinates when the ventricles are very malpositioned. Concerning whether the great arteries are normally or abnormally related, the relationships that matter are the *internal* intracardiac ones, not the *external* spatial relationship ones—particularly when the ventricles are malpositioned.

In 1954, Dixon[13] introduced the term *juxtaposition of the atrial appendages,* which subsequently has been widely used. In 1963, Ellis and Jameson[19] proposed the designation *congenital levoposition of the right atrial appendage.* In 1976, Park et al[29] introduced the term *congenital levojuxtaposition of the right atrial appendage.*

In 1996, Stella Van Praagh et al introduced the following designations:

1. juxtaposition of the morphologically right atrial appendage in solitus and inversus atria[39]; and
2. juxtaposition of the morphologically left atrial appendage in solitus and inversus atria[40]

TABLE 10.1 Early Case Reports Concerning Left-Sided Juxtaposition of the Atrial Appendages (1909–1950)

Author(s)	Year	Sex	Age	Diagnosis
Wenner[3]	1909	F	10½ y	Dextrocardia; DORV {S,D,D}; ASD II; LSVC to RA (not via coronary sinus); AV valve with direct insertion into small RV (no chordae tendinae); left AV valve larger, tricuspid, inserting into large LV; bilateral conus (subaortic and subpulmonary); pulmonary outflow tract stenosis, infundibular and valvar (bicuspid pulmonary valve); high conoventricular VSD and low muscular VSDs; left aortic arch; left probe patent ductus arteriosus
Dünner[4]	1914	NK	10 wk	TGA {S,D,D}; two ASDs: PFO and fenestrations in septum I; RA-to-LV communication; double-inlet left ventricle; large LV and small RV: functionally or anatomically single LV; bilateral conus without PS; low tunnel-like VSD leading to small RV; three coronary ostia, one from each sinus of Valsalva; large left-sided PDA
Huebschmann[5]	1921	M	5½ mo	Dextrocardia or mesocardia, apex pointing rightward; {S,D,S}; tricuspid atresia; ASD II; Ao from LV with AoV-MV fibrous continuity; small subpulmonary conus with PS, infundibular and valvar (bicuspid PV); small VSD (or BVF) from large LV to subpulmonary conus; MPA arises posteriorly and slightly to the right of the Ao; left aortic arch with right-sided closing PDA
Kettler[6]	1933	M	15 mo	Left-sided heart with rightward pointing ventricular apex; DORV {S,D,D}; tricuspid atresia; absent RSVC, but with right-sided SA node; LSVC to CoS to RA; bilateral conus (sub-Ao and sub-PA) with PS
Ngai[7]	1935	F	100 days	Died in a blue spell. Cardiomegaly (3× normal size); dextrocardia; DORV {S,D,A}; ASD II; large LV; small RV; concordant AV alignments (MV into LV, TV into RV); sinistroposition of right atrial appendage; bilateral conus with no outflow tract obstruction; absent left coronary ostium; right aortic arch; small right-sided PDA; lobar pneumonia of azygos lobe
Bredt[8]	1936	F	5¾ mo	Case 1 (Museum specimen #9): TGA {S,D,D}; small RV and large LV; VSD; bilateral conus; pulmonary atresia. (Case 2 is Dünner's case 4.)
Harris and Farber[9]	1939	M	1 y	Case 12: DORV {S,D,D}; ASD II; LVH and E; RV thick-walled, small-chambered, RV sinus small or possibly absent; VSD; bilateral conus; pulmonary outflow tract atresia; absent left coronary ostium, that is, single right coronary artery; small PDA
Taussig[10]	1947	F	25 y	Case 40, Chapter 33, Fig. 171: Dextrocardia; TGA {I,L,L} (may have had visceral heterotaxy with polysplenia; left-sided JAA with situs inversus of atria, that is, levomalposition of *left* atrial appendage (not levomalposition of *right* atrial appendage, as in all previous cases); common atrium; ipsilateral pulmonary veins (right-sided pulmonary veins to right of atrial septal remnant, left-sided pulmonary veins to left of atrial septal remnant); interrupted inferior vena cava; common AV valve and common AV canal; single LV (absence of RV sinus) with common inlet LV; bilateral conus; PS, severe; left aortic arch (abnormal in visceroarterial situs inversus)
Miskall and Fraser[11]	1948	F	11 mo	TGA {S,D,D} with intact ventricular septum; ASD II (1.0 × 0.5 cm); no outflow tract obstruction; meningocele at bifid T8 vertebra, operated on successfully at 5th day of life. Death from pneumonia of left lower lobe
Rogers, Cordes, and Edwards[12]	1950	M	12 y	TGA {S,D,D}; tricuspid atresia; ASD II, valve incompetent patent foramen ovale with fenestrated septum primum; bilateral conus; PS, severe, subvalvar and valvar with bicuspid pulmonary valve

Ao, Aorta; *AoV*, aortic valve; *ASD* II, secundum atrial septal defect; *AV*, atrioventricular; *BVF*, bulboventricular foramen; *CoS*, coronary sinus; *DORV*, double-outlet right ventricle; *F*, female; {I,L,L}, the set of inversus atria, L-loop ventricles, and L-transposition/malposition of the great arteries in which the aortic valve is to the left (levo or L) relative to the pulmonary valve; *JAA*, juxtaposition of the atrial appendages; *LSVC*, left superior vena cava; *LV*, morphologically left ventricle; *LVH & E*, left ventricular hypertrophy and enlargement; *M*, male; mo, months; *MPA*, main pulmonary artery; *MV*, mitral valve; *NK*, not known; *PA*, pulmonary artery; *PDA*, patent ductus arteriosus; *PFO*, patent foramen ovale; *PV*, pulmonary valve; *RA*, morphologically right atrium; *RSVC*, right superior vena cava; *RV*, morphologically right ventricle; *SA*, sinoatrial; septum I, septum primum; {S,D,A}, the set of solitus atria, D-loop ventricles, and A-malposition/transposition of the great arteries in which the aorta is directly anterior (antero—or A) relative to the pulmonary valve; {S,D,D}, the set of solitus atria, D-loop ventricles, and D-transposition/malposition of the great arteries in which the aortic valve is to the right (dextro or D) relative to the pulmonary valve; {S,D,S}, the set of solitus atria, D-loop ventricles, and solitus normally related great arteries in which typically the aortic valve is posterior, inferior, and to the right relative to the pulmonary valve (unless the semilunar interrelationship has been modified by malposition of the heart); *TGA*, transposition of the great arteries; *TV*, tricuspid valve; *T8*, eighth thoracic vertebra; *VSD*, ventricular septal defect; *y*, years.

The reasons for the introduction of these modified designations were twofold:

1. JAA should be described not only positionally, but also morphologically. In congenital heart disease, this is true of all parts of the heart; that is, this is a basic principle.
2. Juxtaposition of the atrial appendages with malposition of the right atrial appendage (JRAA)[39] and juxtaposition of the atrial appendages with malposition of the left atrial appendage (JLAA)[40] are two very different and largely opposite syndromes, as will be seen.

DEFINITION

Juxtaposition of the atrial appendages means that both atrial appendages lie side by side, rather than being separated by the great arteries as they normally are (*juxta*, near and *positio*, place,

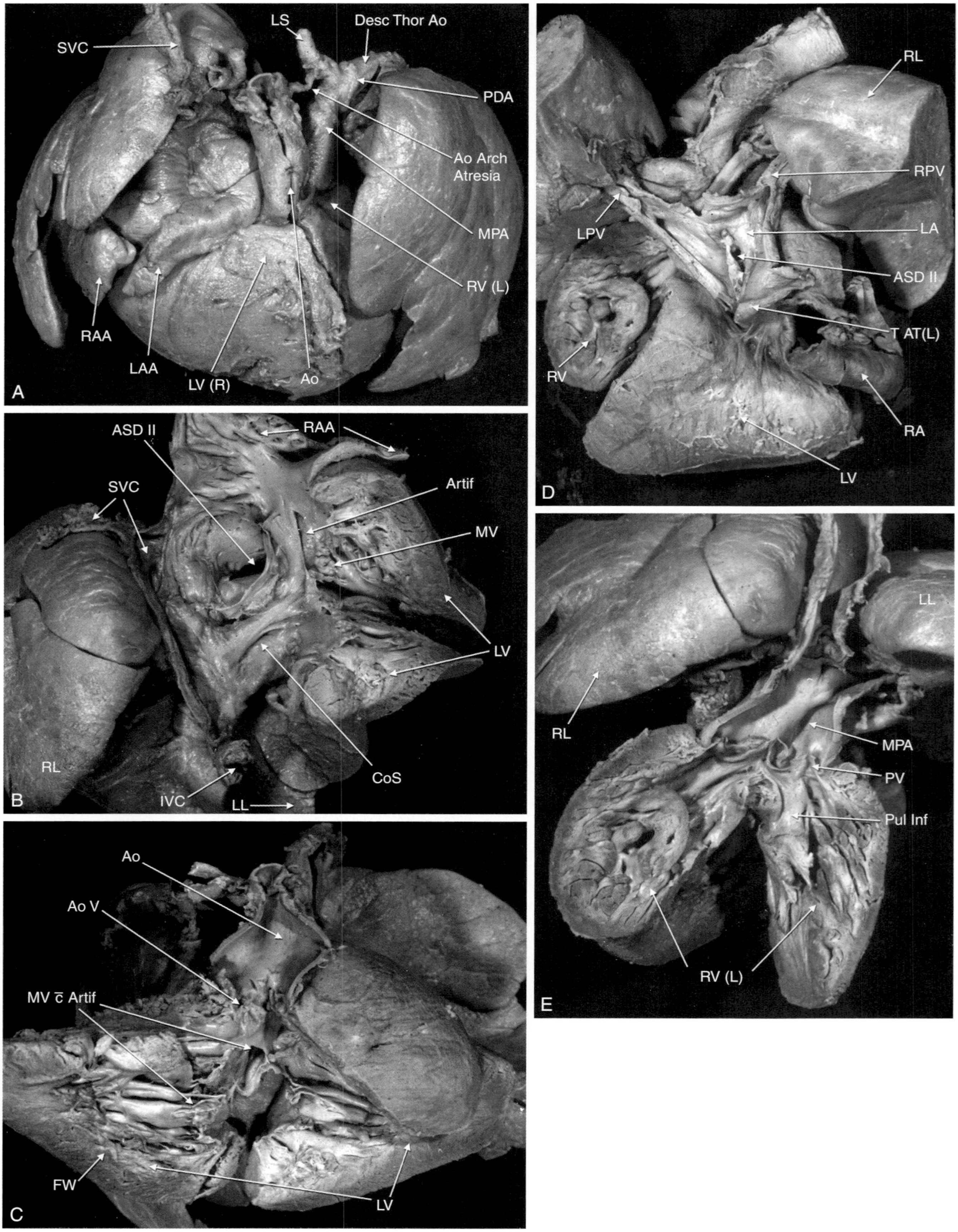

SVC
LS
Desc Thor Ao
PDA
Ao Arch
Atresia
MPA
RV (L)
RAA
LAA
LV (R)
Ao
A
ASD II
RAA
SVC
Artif
MV
LV
CoS
RL
IVC
LL
B
Ao
Ao V
MV c̄ Artif
FW
LV
C
RL
RPV
LPV
LA
ASD II
T AT(L)
RV
RA
LV
D
LL
RL
MPA
PV
Pul Inf
RV (L)
E

Fig. 10.1 (A) Right-sided juxtaposition of the atrial appendages (JAA), anterosuperior view. Both the right atrial appendage *(RAA)* and the left atrial appendage *(LAA)* lie side by side to the right of the ascending aorta *(Ao)* and the main pulmonary artery *(MPA)*. The RAA lies to the right of the LAA, indicating situs solitus of the viscera and atria. It is the LAA that is malpositioned; that is, the LAA should lie to the left of the great arteries. Hence, these are solitus atria with right-sided JAA because of malposition of the LAA. This 3-day-old girl had isolated ventricular inversion, that is, {S,L,S}. Note that the morphologically right ventricle *(RV)* is left-sided, *RV (L)*, relative to the morphologically left ventricle *(LV)* that is right-sided, *LV (R)*. This patient had mesocardia. Externally, the great arteries do not look solitus normally related, which they are (see C and E); the ascending Ao is anterior and to the right of the MPA. Note that there is atresia of the transverse aortic arch *(Ao Arch Atresia)*, correctly suggesting that there is aortic outflow tract stenosis; and a patent ductus arteriosus leads to the descending thoracic aorta *(Desc Thor Ao)*. The right superior vena cava *(SVC)* and the left subclavian artery *(LS)* are also seen. (B) A right lateral view of the opened RA shows the RAA, a large secundum type of ASD *(ASD II)*, the inferior vena cava *(IVC)*, the SVC, the ostium of the coronary sinus *(CoS)*, and the right-sided mitral valve *(MV)* opening into the inflow tract of the LV. *Artif*, Artifact. (C) The outflow tract of the right-sided LV leading into the ascending Ao. There is direct fibrous continuity between the aortic valve *(AoV)* and the right-sided artifacted MV. There is fibrous subaortic stenosis. *FW*, Left ventricular free wall. (D) Posterior view of the morphologically left atrium *(LA)*, revealing left-sided tricuspid atresia, *T At (L)*. The left pulmonary veins *(LPV)* and the right pulmonary veins *(RPV)* are normally connected. *LL*, Left lung; *RL*, right lung. (E) The opened left-sided RV (L), beneath the left-sided tricuspid atresia, TAt (L), has a small chamber. Note the presence of a muscular subpulmonary infundibulum *(Pul Inf)*, the well-formed pulmonary valve (PV), and the opened MPA. A ventricular septal defect was present (not seen). Thus, normally related great arteries (with ventriculoarterial concordance, a subpulmonary conus and aortic-mitral fibrous continuity) can be associated with right-sided JAA with malposition of the LAA (JLAA). Solitus normally related great arteries can have very abnormal relationships relative to fixed external spatial coordinates (anteroposterior, right-left) if the ventricles from which the great arteries arise are very malpositioned, as they are in this patient with isolated ventricular inversion {S,L,S}. This is a good example of the **juxtaposition of the left atrial appendage syndrome**.[40] Typical features include obstruction of the left-sided atrioventricular orifice (i.e., left-sided T At, D); small left-sided ventricle (i.e., small left-sided RV, E); and normally related great arteries (C and E). The ventricles and great arteries are *left shifted* relative to the *solitus* atria and relative to the atrioventricular valves (as in Fig. 10.3, diagram 3). (Reproduced with permission from Melhuish BPP, Van Praagh R. Juxtaposition of the atrial appendages, a sign of severe cyanotic congenital heart disease. *Br Heart J*. 1968;30:269.)

Latin). In addition to being apposed, the malpositioned atrial appendage is often superior to or even on top of the normally located atrial appendage (Fig. 10.2).[39]

MATERIAL

This chapter is based on 74 postmortem cases of JAA: 15 cases from the Congenital Heart Disease Research and Training Center, Hektoen Institute for Medical Research, Chicago, Illinois[21]; 6 cases from the Hospital for Sick Children, Toronto, Ontario, Canada[21]; and 53 cases from the Cardiac Registry of Children's Hospital Boston.[39,40]

CLASSIFICATION

Positional Classification

Until 1994, JAA was classified positionally:

1. **left JAA**, meaning that both atrial appendages lie to the left of the vascular pedicle (aorta and pulmonary artery) (see Fig. 10.2)[39]; and
2. **right JAA,** indicating that both atrial appendages lie to the right of the vascular pedicle (see Fig. 10.1).[21]

Morphologic and positional classification[39,40] asks three questions of the diagnostician:

1. **Morphologically, which appendage is malpositioned relative to the great arteries?** Is it the morphologically right atrial appendage that is on the wrong side of the vascular pedicle, as in Fig. 10.2? Or is it the morphologically left atrial appendage that is on the wrong side of the vascular pedicle, as in Fig. 10.1?
2. **Positionally what is the sidedness of the abnormally located atrial appendage** that results in JAA? Is it malpositioned to the left of the great arteries? Or is it malpositioned to the right of the great arteries?
3. **What is the atrial situs of the patient?** Is it situs solitus (usual or normal pattern of atrial organization)? Or is it situs inversus (the mirror-image pattern of atrial organization)? As will be seen, the type of atrial situs helps to make the JAA understandable.

Anatomic Types of Juxtaposition of the Atrial Appendages

There are four morphologic and positional anatomic types of JAA (Fig. 10.3):

1. Malposition of the morphologically right atrial appendage (RAA) to the left of the vascular pedicle in atrial situs solitus (see Fig. 10.2).[39] This is the classic type of malposition of the RAA to the left of the vascular pedicle, resulting in typical left-sided JAA, that occurred in 34 of our 35 cases with malposition of the RAA (97%).[39]
2. Malposition of the RAA to the right of the vascular pedicle in atrial situs inversus (Fig. 10.4).[39] This is the rare form of malposition of the RAA, resulting in right-sided JAA, that we observed in only 1 of these 35 patients (3%).[39]
3. Malposition of the left atrial appendage (LAA) to the right of the vascular pedicle in atrial situs solitus (Fig. 10.5).[40] This was the more frequent form of malposition of the LAA, which resulted in right-sided JAA, and was found in 16 of these 18 cases (89%).[40]
4. Malposition of the LAA to the left of the vascular pedicle in atrial situs inversus (Fig. 10.6).[40] This was the rare form of malposition of the LAA, found in only 2 of these 18 cases (11%).[40]

Thus, each atrial appendage was malpositioned in only one way in each type of atrial situs (see Fig. 10.3):

1. In visceroatrial situs solitus, the RAA can be malpositioned in only one way: to the left of the vascular pedicle (see Fig. 10.2).
2. In visceroatrial situs inversus, the left-sided RAA can be malpositioned in only one way: to the right of the vascular pedicle (see Fig. 10.4).

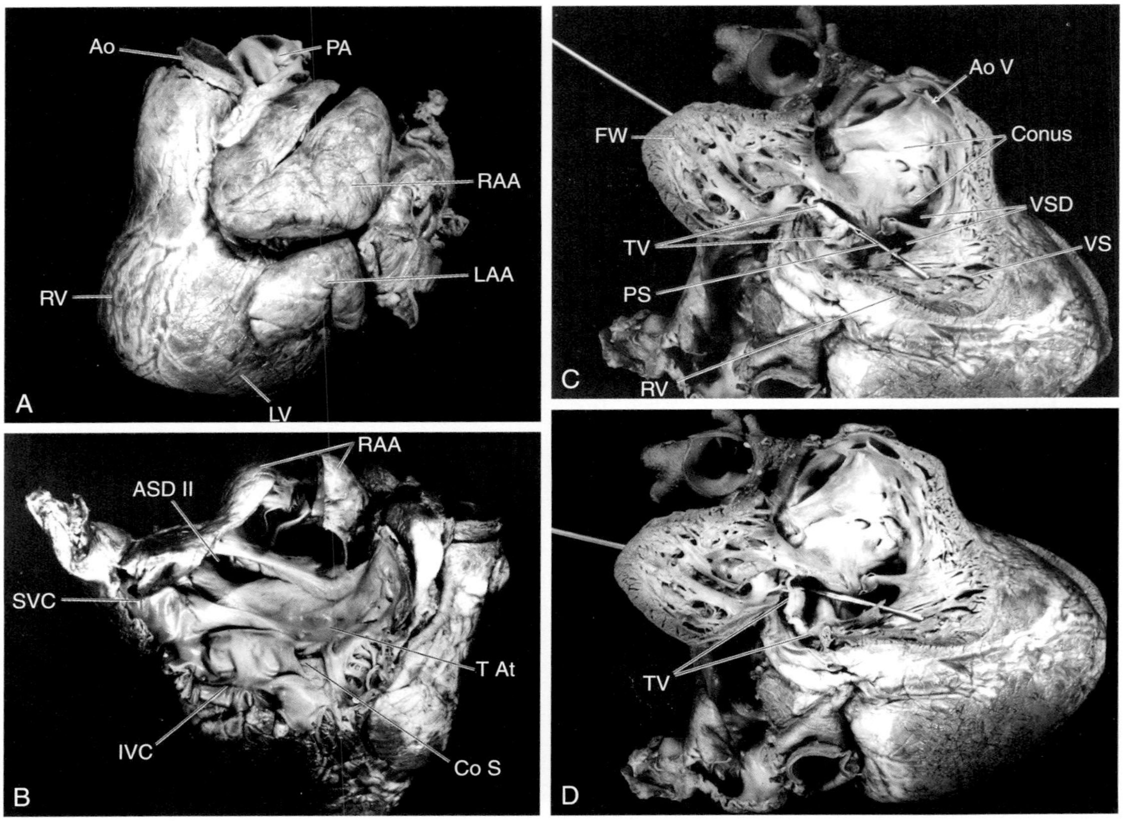

Fig. 10.2 (A) Left-sided juxtaposition of the atrial appendages (JAA) with malposition of the right atrial appendage *(RAA)* to the left of both the aorta *(Ao)* and the pulmonary artery *(PA)*, anteroposterior view. The malposed RAA is not only beside the left atrial appendage *(LAA)*, the RAA is also above the LAA. In JAA, the malposed atrial appendage is typically superior to the nonmalposed atrial appendage ("nonmalposed" because this appendage often is not normally located). The right atrium (RA) does not contribute to the right heart border in this anteroposterior view. The small PA and the large Ao accurately suggest pulmonary outflow tract stenosis and a widely patent aortic outflow tract, respectively. This 14-month-old girl had mesocardia, not dextrocardia as the rightwardly pointing ventricular apex suggests. (B) The opened RA revealed tricuspid atresia *(T At)* and a secundum atrial septal defect *(ASD II)*. The large RAA passes from right to left behind the great arteries. The RAA passes through the transverse sinus portion of the pericardial space to form a large convexity on the left upper heart border above the smaller convexity of the LAA, seen in A. In B, note that the large opening into the RAA lies anteriorly and superiorly to the ASD II. The inferior vena cava *(IVC)*, the superior vena cava *(SVC)*, and the coronary sinus *(Co S)* all return normally to the RA. (C) The opened RV is small, as expected with T At. Both great arteries originate above the right ventricle *(RV)*. This patient has double-outlet right ventricle (DORV) {S,D,D}. A conoventricular type of ventricular septal defect *(VSD)* is seen beneath the well-developed subaortic conus above and the ventricular septal crest below. The aortic outflow tract is confirmed to be widely patent. The pulmonary outflow tract is stenotic, as predicted by the small size of the PA seen in A. A probe is passed through this stenotic pulmonary outflow tract *(PS)*. The nature of this PS is rare and fascinating. In this case of T At (seen in B), the pulmonary outflow tract stenosis (seen in C) is importantly contributed to by a flap of obstructing tricuspid valve tissue *(TV)*. T At, as seen from the RA (B), associated with obstructive TV tissue in the RV (C) is rare in our experience. In D, the remnant of tricuspid valve tissue is displaced more to the right, to display the TV tissue and the stenotic pulmonary outflow tract (indicated by the *probe*) more clearly. This patient displays the **juxtaposition of the right atrial appendage syndrome**[39]: obstruction of the right-sided atrioventricular orifice (i.e., T At); small right-sided ventricle (i.e., small RV); and a major conotruncal malformation (i.e., DORV {S,D,D} with bilateral conus, PS, and VSD). The ventricles and great arteries are *right shifted* relative to the *solitus* atria and the *solitus* atrioventricular (AV) valves (as in Fig. 10.3, diagram 1). The situs of the AV valves typically is the same as that of the ventricles, solitus with D-loop ventricles and inversus with L-loop ventricles. *AoV*, Aortic valve; *FW*, free wall; *LV*, left ventricle; *VS*, ventricular septum. (Reproduced with permission from Van Praagh S, O'Sullivan J, Brili S, Van Praagh R. Juxtaposition of the morphologically right atrial appendage in solitus and inversus atria: A study of 35 postmortem cases. *Am Heart J*. 1996;132;382.)

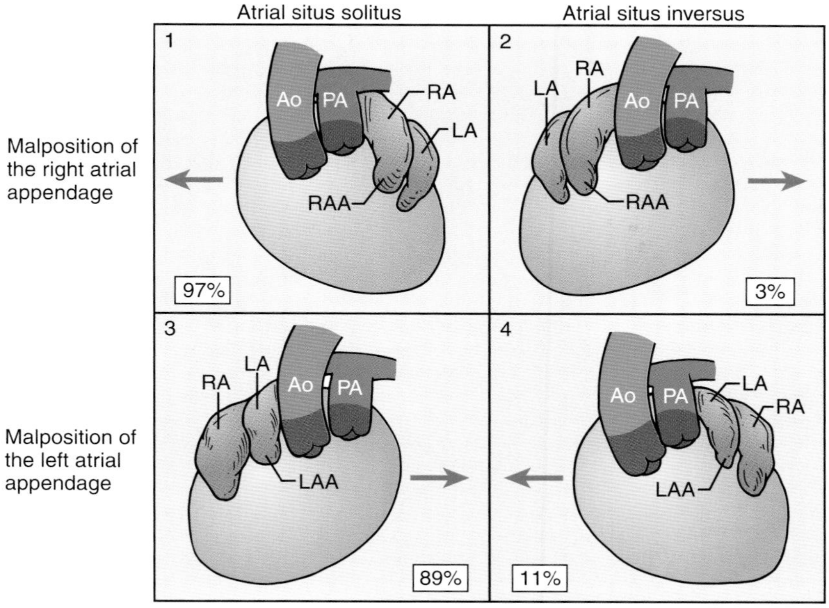

Fig. 10.3 Diagrams of the Four Anatomic Types of Juxtaposition of the Atrial Appendages (JAA). JAA with malposition of the morphologically right atrial appendage (JRAA) almost always had situs solitus of the viscera and atria with the right atrial appendage *(RAA)* lying to the right of the left atrial appendage *(LAA)*, with both atrial appendages lying to the left of both great arteries (97%).[39] However, in a few cases with JRAA, there was situs inversus of the viscera and atria, and in all of these patients both atrial appendages lay to the right of both great arteries (3%).[39] The *arrows* indicate the direction of malposition of the ventricular and infundibuloarterial segments relative to the atrial and the atrioventricular (AV) canal segments. In diagram *1*, there is *right shift* of the bulboventricular loop relative to the atria and the AV canal. In diagram *2*, there is *left shift* of the ventricles and great arteries relative to the atria and the AV valves. JRAA often had the JRAA syndrome (see Table 10.2). JAA with malposition of the morphologically left atrial appendage (JLAA) also usually had situs solitus of the viscera and atria (89%, in diagram *3*), but a minority had situs inversus of the viscera and atria (11%, in diagram *4*).[40] The directions of malposition of the bulboventricular loop relative to the atria and the AV canal (right shift or left shift) are indicated by *arrows*. Patients with JLAA often had the JLAA syndrome (see Table 10.2).[40] Analysis of JAA in terms of which atrial appendage is malpositioned relative to the vascular pedicle is helpful because such *morphologic* analysis correlates with the previously mentioned JRAA (diagrams *1* and *2*) and JLAA (diagrams *3* and *4*) syndromes (see Table 10.2).[39,40] *Positional* analysis of JAA is also illuminating. Right shift of the ventricles and great arteries relative to the atria and AV valves (diagrams *1* and *4*) results in (or is associated with) left-sided JAA both in visceroatrial situs solitus (diagram *1*) and in visceroatrial situs inversus (diagram *4*). But in situs solitus, malposition of the RAA occurs, whereas in situs inversus, malposition of the LAA occurs (compare diagrams *1* and *4*). So the JRAA syndrome applies in situs solitus, and the JLAA syndrome applies in situs inversus. Conversely, left shift of the ventricles and great arteries relative to the atria and the AV valves leads to right-sided JAA both in situs solitus (diagram *3*) and in situs inversus (diagram *2*), but the JLAA syndrome applies in situs solitus, and the JRAA syndrome is relevant in situs inversus. Thus, JAA should be understood both positionally and morphologically.[39,40] *Ao,* Aorta; *LA,* morphologically left atrium; *LAA,* morphologically left atrial appendage; *PA,* pulmonary artery; *RA,* morphologically right atrium. (From Van Praagh S, O'Sullivan J, Brili S, Van Praagh R. Juxtaposition of the morphologically right atrial appendage in solitus and inversus atria: A study of 35 postmortem cases. *Am Heart J.* 1996;132:382-390; and Van Praagh S, O'Sullivan J, Brili S, Van Praagh R. Juxtaposition of the morphologically left atrial appendage in solitus and inversus atria: A study of 18 postmortem cases. *Am Heart J.* 1996;132:391–402; with permission.)

The same is true of the LAA:

1. In visceroatrial situs solitus, the LAA can be malpositioned in only one way: to the right of the vascular pedicle (see Fig. 10.1 and 10.5).
2. In visceroatrial situs inversus, the LAA can be malpositioned in only one way: to the left of the vascular pedicle (see Fig. 10.6).

The foregoing is why there are four anatomic types of JAA, based on their morphologic and positional anatomy (see Fig. 10.3). The frequencies of these four anatomic types are also included in this diagram (see Fig. 10.3), based on our two most recent studies.[39,40]

One may ask why did we not include atrial situs ambiguus with visceroatrial heterotaxy and asplenia in the morphologic and positional classification of JAA (see Fig. 10.3). The answer is that we did not find any such cases in our data.[39,40] In addition, from a logical standpoint, atrial situs ambiguus is either undiagnosed or undiagnosable atrial situs solitus or atrial situs inversus. Consequently, no type of atrial situs has been omitted from Fig. 10.3 because atrial situs ambiguus is not a specific,

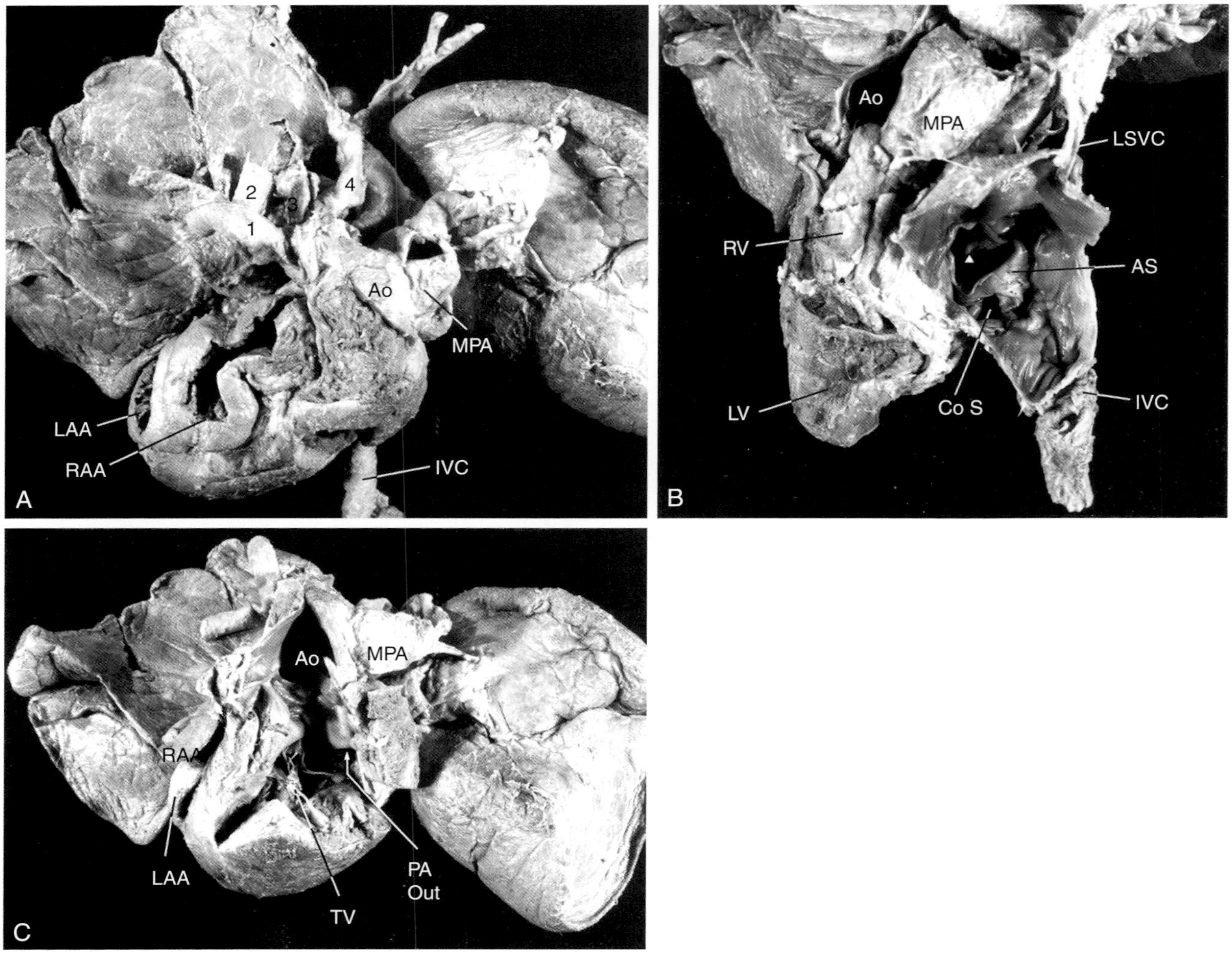

Fig. 10.4 (A) Right-sided juxtaposition of the atrial appendages (JAA) with malposition of the right atrial appendage *(RAA)* in atrial situs inversus, anterior view. The RAA is juxtaposed and superior to the nonmalposed left atrial appendage *(LAA)*. This 7-month-old girl had double-outlet right ventricle (DORV) {I,D,D} with dextrocardia, visceral heterotaxy, and asplenia. This was the first photographically documented case of JAA with malposition of the RAA in atrial situs inversus.[39] The ascending aorta *(Ao)* lies to the right of the dilated main pulmonary artery *(MPA)*. *IVC,* Left-sided inferior vena cava that returned to the left-sided right atrium (RA); *1,* left common carotid artery; *2,* right common carotid artery; *3,* aberrant right subclavian artery, anastomosed to the right pulmonary artery; *4,* left subclavian artery. Anastomosis of the ascending Ao to the MPA resulted in marked dilatation of the MPA. (B). Interior of the left-sided morphologically RA showing that the IVC returns to this atrium, as do the left superior vena cava *(LSVC)* and the coronary sinus *(CoS)*. The ostium of the CoS is enlarged because it receives a persistent right SVC. A large ostium secundum type of atrial septal defect *(solid white triangle)* is seen above a deficient septum primum *(AS)*. The morphologically RV is hypoplastic and superior to the morphologically left ventricle *(LV)*. The ascending Ao is anterior to the dilated MPA.(C) Interior of the underdeveloped and right-handed RV, showing the widely patent outflow tract to the anterior and right-sided Ao, and the stenotic outflow tract leading to the pulmonary artery *(PA Out)*. This patient had a bilateral conus (subaortic and subpulmonary). The pulmonary infundibular stenosis was produced both by the hypertrophied infundibular septum and by the hypertrophied subpulmonary infundibular free wall. The broad triangular RAA is seen sitting on top of the finger-like LAA. The tricuspid valve *(TV)* lies to the right of both great arterial outflow tracts, typical of a right-handed D-loop RV. There were concordant atrioventricular alignments (RA opening into RV, and LA opening into LV), despite the discordant atrial and ventricular situs: DORV {I,D,D}. Incongruence of alignment and situs concordance or discordance is one of the features of right-sided JAA. Note that the JRAA syndrome is present: small right-sided RV, and complex conotruncal anomaly (DORV {I,D,D} with bilateral conus and severe pulmonary outflow tract stenosis). There is *left shift* of the ventricles and great arteries relative to the *inverted* atria (as in Fig. 10.3, diagram 2), which explains why there is JAA, why the JAA is right-sided, and why it is the RAA that is malpositioned relative to the great arteries.Despite the fact that this patient had visceral heterotaxy with asplenia, the visceral situs was not undiagnosable or isomeric, as is indicated by the left-sided IVC. The atria and the atrial appendages were clearly inverted ("right isomerism" not being present). In the classification of the anatomic types of JAA (see Fig. 10.3), situs ambiguus (heterotaxy, or "isomerism") was not included for several reasons: (1) Situs ambiguus is not a specific anatomic type of situs; instead, it is undiagnosed (or undiagnosable, or scrambled) situs solitus or situs inversus. (2) The concept of atrial, or atrial appendage, isomerism is an error (see Chapter 29). (3) The anatomic classification of JAA (and of all other anomalies) should be as simple as possible, consistent with accuracy (Occam's razor, or the principle of economy or parsimony). (Reproduced with permission from Van Praagh S, O'Sullivan J, Brili S, Van Praagh R. Juxtaposition of the morphologically right atrial appendage in solitus and inversus atria: A study of 35 postmortem cases. *Am Heart J.* 1996;132;382.)

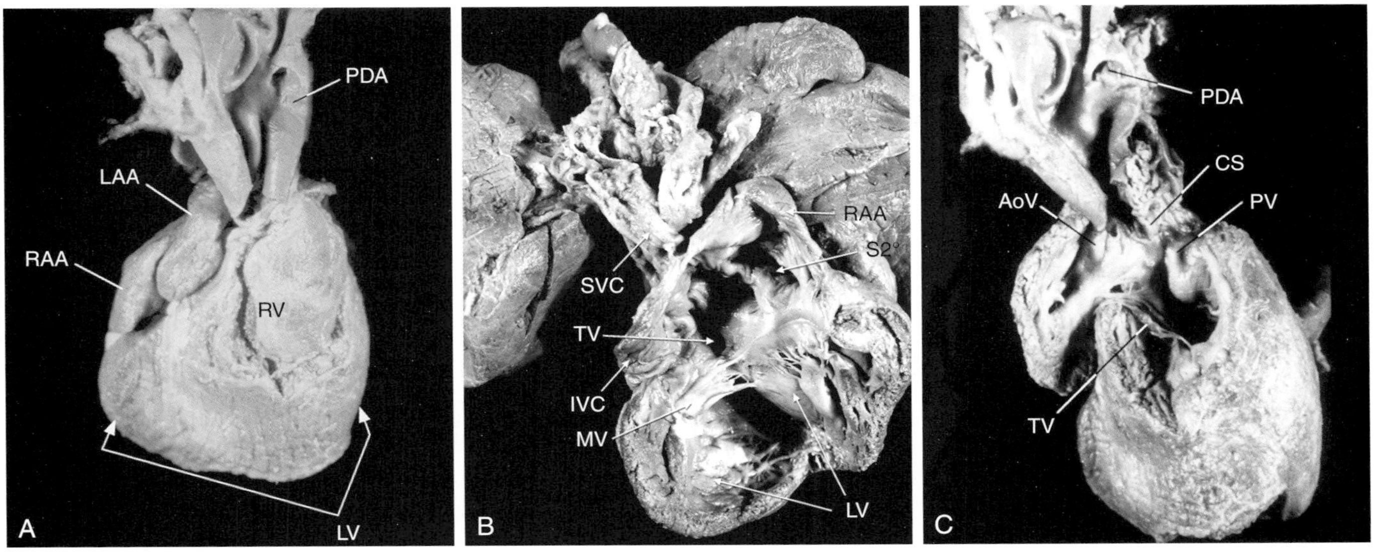

Fig. 10.5 (A) Right-sided juxtaposition of the atrial appendages (JAA), in visceroatrial situs solitus, with malposition of the left atrial appendage *(LAA)* relative to the great arteries, similar to Fig. 10.3, diagram 3. Anteroposterior view showing that the LAA is beside and superior to the right atrial appendage *(RAA)*. The morphologically right ventricle *(RV)* is relatively small and superior to the morphologically left ventricle *(LV)*. The aortic orifice of a large patent ductus arteriosus *(PDA)* is also seen. (B) Posterior view of opened atria, mitral valve *(MV)*, and LV. The septum primum is absent. The common atrium is present. It is possible to see into the RAA and the LAA. The inferior vena cava *(IVC)* and the superior vena cava *(SVC)* connect normally with the right atrium (RA). The RA is aligned with an opens into the large LV via a large MV. The left atrium (LA) is aligned with an opens into a small RV (not seen in this view) via a stenotic tricuspid valve *(solid white arrowhead)*. Thus, there is atrioventricular (AV) alignment discordance. (C) Interior of hypoplastic right-handed RV is seen. The inlet of the RV and the stenotic tricuspid valve *(TV)* lie to the right of the RV outflow tract, the RV being right-handed. Both the aortic valve *(AoV)* and the pulmonary valve *(PV)* arise above the RV; that is, double-outlet right ventricle (DORV) is present. The conal septum (CS) is extremely hypoplastic; pulmonary outflow tract stenosis is present; and there is AoV-TV direct fibrous continuity. The AoV lies to the right of the PV, and a stenotic muscular subpulmonary conus (with no subaortic conal free wall conus) is present. In summary, this 4-day-old boy with mesocardia had DORV {S,D,D} with AV alignment discordance. There was incongruence of AV alignment and situs concordance or discordance: discordant AV alignments with concordant AV situs. This patient also had visceral heterotaxy with hyposplenia (spleen smaller than normal, i.e., hypoplastic, as is often found with polysplenia which also has multiple small splenuli). The ventricles and great arteries are *left shifted* relative to the *solitus* atria and the atrioventricular valves (see Fig. 10.3, diagram 3). S2° septum secundum. (Reproduced with permission from Van Praagh S, O'Sullivan J, Brili S, Van Praagh R. Juxtaposition of the morphologically left atrial appendage in solitus and inversus atria: A study of 18 post-mortem cases. *Am Heart J.* 1996;132:391.)

third anatomic type of atrial situs, to the best of our present understanding.

How can one understand the frequencies of each anatomic type of JAA (see Fig. 10.3)?

Q. Why is JAA, involving malposition of the RAA, typically left-sided JAA (97%) rather than right-sided JAA (3%)?

A. Because atrial situs solitus is so much more common than atrial situs inversus. Atrial situs solitus is estimated to be 5000 to 15,000 times more frequent than atrial situs inversus. (See Chapter 3 for discussion of dextrocardia and other cardiac malpositions.)

Q. Why is JAA involving malposition of the LAA so much more frequently right-sided (89%) than left-sided (11%)?

A. Again, because atrial situs solitus is so much more frequent than atrial situs inversus.

Q. Is it possible to diagnose the atrial situs when visceral heterotaxy with asplenia coexists?

A. Yes. In some cases this can be done with confidence (see Fig. 10.3) (see Chapter 29).

Q. Why is it clinically and surgically important to diagnose the morphologic anatomic identity of the malpositioned atrial appendage in JAA?

A. Because JAA involving malposition of the RAA (left-sided malposition in situs solitus and right-sided malposition in situs inversus) and JAA involving malposition of the LAA (right-sided in situs solitus and left-sided in situs inversus) constitute distinctive and largely opposite syndromes (Table 10.2).[39,40]

The Syndrome of JAA With Malposition of the RAA[39]

The syndrome of JAAs with malposition of the RAA (JRAA) to the left or right of the vascular pedicle is characterized by multilevel right heart obstruction (see Table 10.2). Specifically there was right atrial outflow obstruction, that is, tricuspid atresia or stenosis, or hypoplasia in 21 of 35 cases (60%); right ventricular

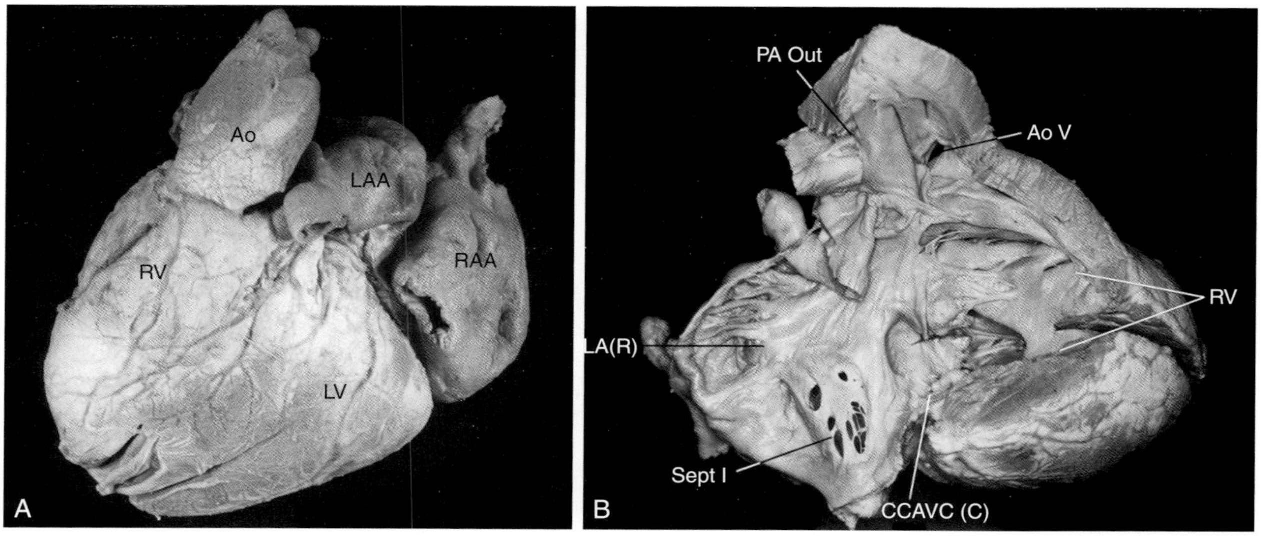

Fig. 10.6 (A) Left-sided juxtaposition of the atrial appendages (JAA) in visceroatrial situs inversus with malposition of the morphologically left atrial appendage *(LAA)* to the left of both great arteries, anterior view, similar to Fig. 10.3, diagram 4. The LAA is beside and superior to the morphologically right atrial appendage (RAA). The morphologically right ventricle *(RV)* is right-sided and superior relative to the morphologically left ventricle *(LV)*. This 2 9/12-year-old boy had dextrocardia. (B) Opened morphologically left atrium, right-sided, that is, LA (R), and opened RV, right-sided. The septum primum *(Sept I)* lies to the right of the superior limbic band of septum secundum (unlabeled), as is characteristic of atrial situs inversus. Sept I is deficient, resulting in an abnormally large ostium secundum above the septum primum and below the superior limbic band of septum secundum. The septum primum also displays multiple (at least 7) fenestrations. Hence, this patient has multiple ostium secundum type atrial septal defects (a valve incompetent patent foramen ovale with an excessively large ostium secundum, plus multiple fenestrations in the deficient septum primum). This patient also has a completely common atrioventricular canal, type C, that is, *CCAVC (C)*. Both great arteries arise from a bilateral conus (subaortic and subpulmonary) above the RV. The aortic valve *(AoV)* is well seen because the aortic outflow tract is widely patent, whereas the pulmonary valve is not well visualized because the pulmonary outflow tract *(PA Out)* is tightly stenotic. To summarize, this patient has left-sided JAA in visceroatrial situs inversus with malposition of the LAA relative to the great arteries (as in Fig. 10.3, diagram 4), and double-outlet right ventricle (DORV) {I,D,D} with multiple secundum ASDs, CCAVC type C, small right-sided RV, bilateral conus, and severe pulmonary outflow tract stenosis. The D-loop ventricles and great arteries are *right shifted* relative to the *inversus* atria (see Fig. 10.3, diagram 4). (Reproduced with permission from Van Praagh S, O'Sullivan J, Brili S, Van Praagh R. Juxtaposition of the morphologically left atrial appendage in solitus and inversus atria: A study of 18 postmortem cases. *Am Heart J.* 1996;132:391.)

TABLE 10.2 **JAA With Malposition of the RAA Compared With JAA With Malposition of the LAA**[39,40]

	MRAA (N = 35)		MLAA (N = 18)		
Associated Malformations	**No.**	**%**	**No.**	**%**	***p* Value**
1. Right atrial outlet obstruction (tricuspid atresia, stenosis, hypoplasia)	21	60	0	0	<.001
2. RV hypoplasia or absence	26	74	5*	28	<.01
3. Left atrial outlet obstruction (mitral atresia, stenosis, hypoplasia or left-sided tricuspid stenosis)	0	0	12	69	<.001
4. Common atrioventricular valve	0	0	5	28	<.01
5. Abnormal conus with TGA, DORV, or ACM	35	100	4	22	<.01
6. Aortic or subaortic stenosis or atresia	1	3	7	39	<.01
7. Heterotaxy with asplenia, polysplenia, or hyposplenia	1	3	5	28	<.05

*Double-inlet LV was present in 3 of these 5 cases, and in all 5 the hypoplastic or absent RV sinus was associated with stenosis of the left, not the right, atrial outlet. These cases were hemodynamically and anatomically very different from cases with RV hypoplasia or absence and JAA with malposition of the RAA.

ACM, Anatomically right ventricle; *JAA*, juxtaposition of the atrial appendages; *LAA*, morphologically left atrial appendage; *LV*, morphologically left ventricle; *MLAA*, morphologically left atrial appendage; *MRAA*, morphologically right atrial appendage; *RAA*, (morphologically) right atrial appendage; *RV*, (morphologically) right ventricle; *TGA*, transposition of the great arteries.

Fig. 10.7 cont'd *(VS)*, and the leftward ventricular free wall *(FW)*. This is a left-handed (inverted) RV, typical of L-loop ventricles. The widely patent outflow tract to the leftward MPA and the narrowed outflow tract leading to the rightward aorta *(To Ao)* are seen. There is a bilateral conus, both subpulmonary (not stenotic) and subaortic (stenotic), with no semilunar-atrioventricular fibrous continuity. The aortic outflow tract stenosis occurs between the conal septum to the left and the subaortic conal free wall to the right. Both great arteries arise above the RV; that is, double-outlet right ventricle (DORV) is present: DORV {S,L,D}. The ventricular septal defect *(VSD)* is subaortic. (D) The opened morphologically left atrium *(LA)* is viewed from the front and above. A secundum type of atrial septal defect *(ASD II)* is seen. The left-sided LA is aligned with and opens into a right-sided LV via the mitral valve *(MV)*. Note the smaller ascending Ao and the larger MPA arising to the left of the LA. (E) The left-sided LA opens into a right-sided LV via quite a high MV. (F) The LV is right-handed, typical of L-loop ventricles (the LV septal surface is leftward and the LV free wall is rightward). The VSD is partially plugged by left-sided TV tissue. The muscular subaortic conus and aortic valve *(AoV)* have been opened to facilitate photography. The only outlet from the LV was the VSD. To summarize, this was a patient with right-sided JAA in visceroatrial situs solitus with malposition of the LAA relative to the great arteries. In addition, this patient had DORV {S,L,D} with atrioventricular (AV) alignment concordance, crisscross AV relations with inferior TV and superior MV, ASD II, subaortic VSD, bilateral conus, aortic outflow tract stenosis, and mild to moderate hypoplasia of the ascending Ao and aortic arch. Rare features include incongruence of AV alignments (concordant) and AV situs (discordant); and crisscross AV relations with inferior TV and superior MV. The ventricles and great arteries are *left-shifted* relative to the *solitus* atria (see Fig. 10.3, diagram 3). (This anomaly was originally published in 1970 by Wagner, Alday, and Vlad[22] as their Case 6.) (Reproduced with permission from Van Praagh R, David I, Gordon D, Wright GB, Van Praagh S. Ventricular diagnosis and designation. In: Godman MJ, ed. *Pediatric Cardiology*. Vol. 4. London: World Congress London; 1980; Edinburgh: Churchill Livingstone, 1981;153.)

This rare patient (see Fig. 10.4) was the first reported case of JAA with right-sided malposition of the RAA in atrial situs inversus.[39]

Incongruence of AV alignment concordance or discordance relative to AV situs concordance or *LA* appendage (LLA) discordance almost always has occurred with JAA associated with malposition of the *LAA*,[22,36,40-42] and seldom with JAA and malposition of the *RA* appendage (RAA).[32] Why this difference? We do not know. It should be added that JAA with incongruence of AV alignments and situs is rare, the numbers are small, and judgment should therefore be deferred, awaiting more data.

Ventricular Septum. In JAA with malposition of the RAA, a ventral septal defect (VSD) was present in 32 of 35 patients (91%). The anatomic types of VSD that were present are summarized in Table 10.3.

Conoventricular VSD was by far the most common type. Including membranous VSDs and bulboventricular foramina (with a single LV, infundibular outlet chamber, and absence of the right ventricular sinus), conoventricular defects were found in 24 of 32 patients (75%).

However, a bulboventricular foramen customarily is not regarded as a VSD because "ventricular septal defect" is short for *interventricular* septal defect. Logically, one cannot have an interventricular septal defect if there is only one ventricular sinus, as typically is the case with a single LV, infundibular outlet chamber, and absence of the RV sinus.

Although I agree with the logic of this view, it should also be understood that the morphologic anatomy of a bulboventricular foramen per se (independent of what lies on either side of the defect) typically is the same as that of a conoventricular VSD: Above, the foramen is limited by the bulbar or conal septum. Below, the foramen is limited by the septal band and ventricular septum, or their remnants.

If one would prefer to remove the cases with a bulboventricular foramen from Table 1.3, the total number of VSDs becomes 28 and the number with conoventricular VSDs is 20 (71%). An intact ventricular septum was found in only 3 of 35 cases (9%).

TABLE 10.3 Anatomic types of Ventricular Septal Defect with JAA and Malposition of the RAA (n = 32)

Types of VSD	No.	%
1. Membranous*	4	12.5
2. Conoventricular with anterior CS malalignment	3	9
3. Conoventricular with posterior CS malalignment	11	34
4. Conoventricular and midmuscular	1	3
5. Conoventricular and AV canal type	1	3
6. Midmuscular	4	12.5
7. AV canal type	4	12.5
8. Bulboventricular foramen	4	12.5

*A membranous VSD is a small conoventricular defect (between the conal septum above and the ventricular septum and septal band below), in the region of the interventricular portion of the membranous septum, without significant malalignment of the conal septum.

AV, Atrioventricular; *CS*, conal septum (subsemilunar portion); *JAA*, juxtaposition of the atrial appendages; *RAA*, morphologically right atrial appendage; *VSD*, ventricular septal defect.

Ventriculoarterial Alignments. Ventriculoarterial alignments were abnormal in all (35/35 cases, 100%):

1. TGA, 18 (51%);
2. TGA with pulmonary outflow tract atresia, 4 (11%);
3. DORV, 10 (29%);
4 anatomically corrected malposition of the great arteries, 2 (6%); and
5. DOLV, 1 (3%).

Are the ventriculoarterial alignments always abnormal with JRAA?[39] I think that the answer may be no, because in our 1968 study of JAA[21] there were 2 cases in which the great arteries appeared to have been solitus normally related (Table III,[21] Case 25 = {S,D,S} and Case 38 = {S,L,S}). Nonetheless, the suggestion that the great arteries with JRAA rarely can be normally related is based on meta-analysis, not on personal study, and may be erroneous.

Conus. The conus arteriosus or subsemilunar infundibulum was bilateral (subaortic and subpulmonary) in 21 of 35 cases (60%), and subaortic (only) in 14 of 35 (40%).

Great Arterial Outflow Tracts. Pulmonary outflow tract stenosis was present in 14 of 35 patients (40%). Pulmonary outflow tract atresia was found in 6 of 35 cases (17%).

Aortic outflow tract stenosis (restrictive bulboventricular foramen or small midmuscular ventricular septal defect) with preductal coarctation of the aorta occurred in 3 of 35 patients (9%).

No outflow tract obstruction (aortic or pulmonary) was observed in 13 or 35 cases (37%).

Four Rare Cases. In this series of 35 postmortem patients with JAA related to malposition of the RAA,[39] we encountered 4 rare cases:

1. dextrocardia with TGA {S,D,D}, tricuspid atresia, and cor triatriatum (Fig. 10.8);
2. tricuspid atresia with tricuspid leaflet tissue below the atretic tricuspid orifice, with the tricuspid leaflet tissue contributing to pulmonary outflow tract stenosis (see Fig. 10.2);
3. DOLV {S,D,L} (Fig. 10.9); and
4. DORV {I,D,D} with AV alignment concordance and asplenia (see Fig. 10.4).

Summary of JRAA

The syndrome of JAAs with malposition of the morphologically JRAA is characterized by multilevel right heart anomalies.[39] Salient features include (see Table 10.2) right atrial outlet obstruction, that is, tricuspid atresia, stenosis, or hypoplasia in 60% of patients; right ventricular sinus hypoplasia or absence in 74%; and an abnormally formed conus arteriosus with abnormal ventriculoarterial alignments—TGA, or DORV, or DOLV, or anatomically corrected malposition of the great arteries—in 100% of these patients.[39]

Discussion of JRAA

1. The morphologic anatomic identity of the malposed atrial appendage is helpful in predicting associated malformations.
2. JRAA can be diagnosed accurately by angiocardiography, two-dimensional or three-dimensional echocardiography, or magnetic resonance imaging (MRI).
3. There are two different syndromes of JAA, JRAA, and JLAA, that were delineated for the first time in 1996.[39,40]
4. Understanding of these two largely opposite syndromes (see Table 10.2) is helpful for accurate diagnosis, interventional atrial procedures, and surgical atrial operations.
5. There are two different anatomic types of JRAA: (1) in visceroarterial situs solitus, JRAA to the left of the vascular pedicle (see Figs. 10.2, 10.3, 10.8, and 10.9) and (2) in atrial situs inversus, JRAA to the right of the vascular pedicle (see Figs. 10.3 and 10.4).
6. JAA in atrial situs inversus was documented for the first time in atrial situs inversus in 1996 (see Fig. 10.4).[39]
7. This case (see Fig. 10.4) also taught us that one of our previous conclusions was wrong. In 1968, we concluded that left-sided JAA always had D-loop ventricles and that right-sided JAA always had L-loop ventricles.[21]

However, with more data, we learned that right-sided JAA could have D-loop ventricles.[39] For example, the patients shown in Fig. 10.4 with right-sided JAA had DORV {I,D,D}, that is, right-sided JAA with D-loop (not L-loop) ventricles.[39]

8. The superior atrial appendages was always the malpositioned atrial appendage.
9. A normal type of conal connector (subpulmonary, with aortic-AV fibrous continuity) and normal ventriculoarterial alignments (RV to pulmonary artery and LV to aorta) appeared to be rare or perhaps nonexistent with JRAA to the left of the vascular pedicle in atrial situs solitus (see Fig. 10.3, diagram 1) and to the right of the vascular pedicle in atrial situs inversus (see Fig. 10.3, diagram 2). With JAA involving the RAA, an abnormally formed conal connector (bilateral or subaortic) and abnormal ventriculoarterial alignments (TGA, or DORV, or double-outlet LV, or anatomically corrected malposition of the great arteries) are the rule.
10. With JRAA, the exit of the RA is usually hypoplastic, stenotic, or atretic and the subjacent ventricular sinus is typically hypoplastic or absent.
11. Regarding the morphogenesis of JRAA (we will return to this topic in greater detail subsequently), two important factors were thought to be:
    a. hypoplasia of the RV sinus; and
    b. the abnormally formed conus (subaortic or bilateral).[39]
12. There are two anatomic types of left-sided JAA:
    a. with solitus atria (97% of such cases, Fig. 10.3, diagram 1); and
    b. with inversus atria (11% of such cases, Fig. 10.3, diagram 4)[39]
13. There are two anatomic types of right-sided JAA:
    a. with solitus atria (89% of such cases, Fig. 10.3, diagram 3); and
    b. with inversus atria (3% of such cases, Fig. 10.3, diagram 2).[40]

The Syndrome of JAA With Malposition of the LAA. The syndrome of JAA with malposition of the LAA[40] relative to the vascular pedicle (JLAA) is essentially the opposite of the syndrome of JAA with malposition of the RA appendage (JRAA) (see Table 10.2).

The salient features of JAA with malposition of the LAA are summarized in Table 10.2: left atrial outlet obstruction (mitral atresia, stenosis, hypoplasia, or left-sided tricuspid stenosis) in 69% of these patients; common AV valve in 28%; aortic inflow tract stenosis or atresia in 39%; and visceral heterotaxy with asplenia, polysplenia, or hyposplenia in 28%. All of the foregoing features are statistically significantly different from the findings in JAA with malposition of the RAA (see Table 10.2).

JAA with malposition of the LAA is a syndrome of multilevel left heart obstruction, very different from JAA with malposition of the RAA that is a syndrome of multilevel right heart obstruction (see Table 10.2).[39,40]

Now let's examine the syndrome of JAA with malposition of the LAA in greater detail:

Sex: Males-to-females = 8 of 10 (0.8).

Age at Death: Median, 36 days; and range, 1 hour to 4 years.

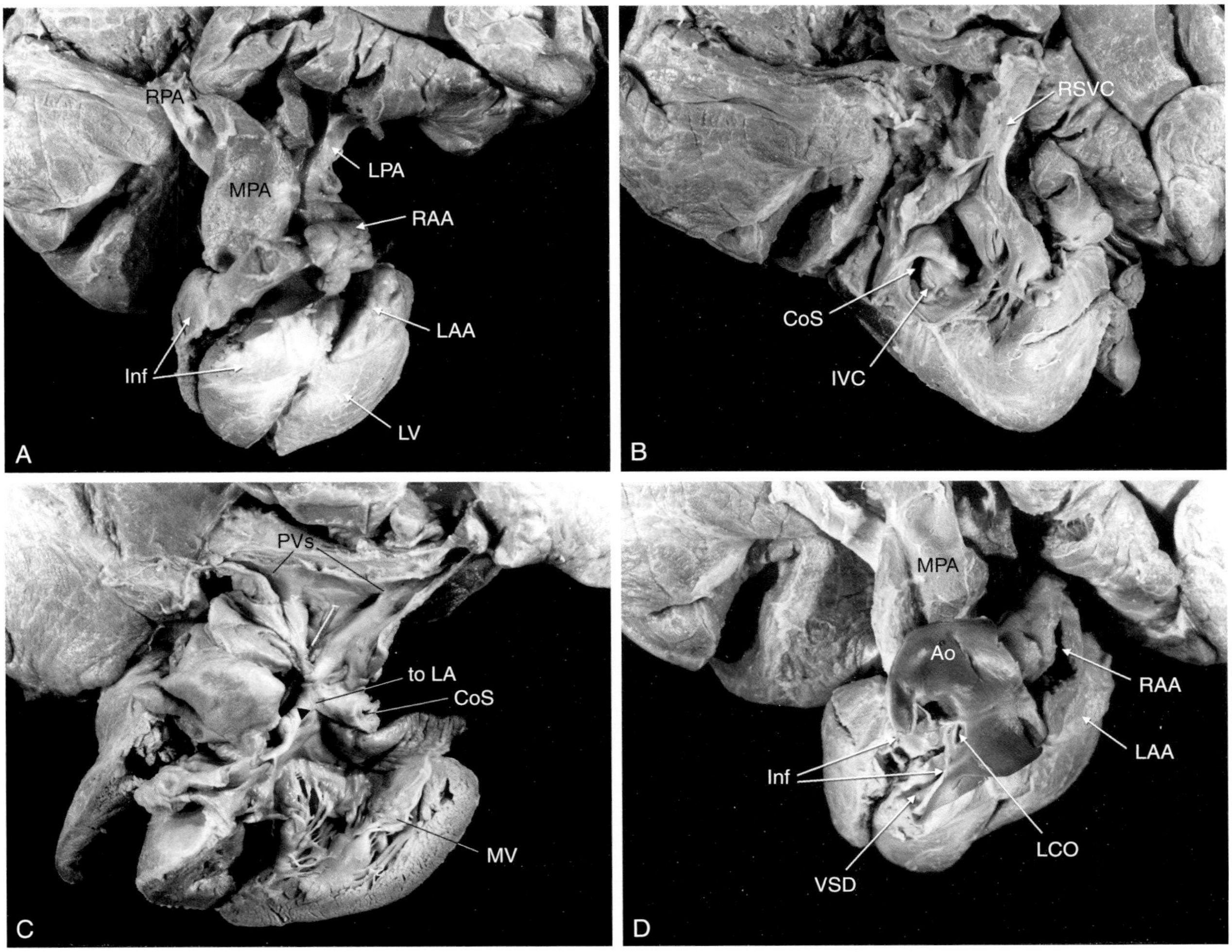

Fig. 10.8 (A) Left-sided juxtaposition of the atrial appendages (JAA) with situs solitus of the viscera and atria, anterior view. The malpositioned morphologically right atrial appendage *(RAA)* lies to the left of both great arteries. The RAA is to the right and superior relative to the morphologically left atrial appendage *(LAA)*. The infundibulum *(Inf)* is right sided and superior relative to the large morphologically left ventricle *(LV)*. No right ventricular sinus is externally obvious beneath the Inf. A small ascending aorta (Ao) arises anteriorly and to the right of the dilated main pulmonary artery *(MPA)*. The right pulmonary artery (RPA) and the left pulmonary artery *(LPA)* are also dilated. This unoperated 4-month-old boy with dextrocardia died in 1957. (B) Opened morphologically right atrium (RA), right lateral view, revealing tricuspid atresia (T At) *(black open triangle)*. The inferior vena cava *(IVC)* and the right superior vena cava *(RSVC)* connect normally with the RA. The ostium of the coronary sinus *(CoS)* is enlarged because the CoS receives a persistent left SVC. The *solid white triangle* marks the opening into the malpositioned RAA. (C) Interior of the morphologically left atrium *(LA)*, mitral valve *(MV)*, and LV. The very rare finding of cor triatriatum, in association with T At, is seen. The pulmonary veins *(PVs)* connect normally with a highly obstructed common pulmonary vein chamber. The subdividing diaphragm in the LA had two very stenotic exits, one into the RA indicated by the *probe* and the other toward the downstream portion of the LA and the MV (to LA, this stenotic orifice having been opened during original dissection). The absence of pulmonary outflow tract obstruction as the MPA exited the LV and the presence of highly stenotic cor triatriatum explain the dilatation of the MPA and its branches (seen in A). A large secundum type of atrial septal defect (ASD II) opened from the RA into the lower unobstructed portion of the LA. The upper margin of the septum primum is very thickened *(black solid arrow head)*. This thickening was attributed to hemodynamic change, the entire cardiac output having to pass through this ASD II. The thickened upper margin of septum primum forms the lower rim of the ASD II. (D) The interior of the small infundibular chamber (Inf) from which the small D-transposed aorta (Ao) originates. The conoventricular ventricular septal defect *(VSD)* between the conal septum above and the ventricular septal remnant below was restrictively small and constituted subaortic stenosis from the hemodynamic standpoint (in association with TAt), explaining the hypoplasia of the D-transposed ascending Ao and aortic arch. The ostium of the left coronary artery *(LCO)*, the left-sided juxtaposed RAA and LAA, and the dilated posterior MPA are also seen. In summary, this patient with TGA {S,D,D} had right shift of the bulboventricular D-loop and transposed great arteries relative to the solitus atria and atrioventricular canal, resulting in left-sided JAA with malposition of the RAA relative to the great arteries (as in Fig. 10.3, diagram 1). This patient also had JAA with malposition of the RAA syndrome with tricuspid atresia and marked underdevelopment of the RV sinus (inflow tract). An ASD II and a restrictive VSD constituting subaortic stenosis were also present. The very rare finding in this patient was the coexistence of tightly stenotic cor triatriatum and tricuspid atresia. (From Van Praagh S, O'Sullivan J, Brili S, Van Praagh R. Juxtaposition of the morphologically right atrial appendage in solitus and inversus atria: A study of 35 postmortem cases. *Am Heart J.* 1996;132;382; reproduced with permission.)

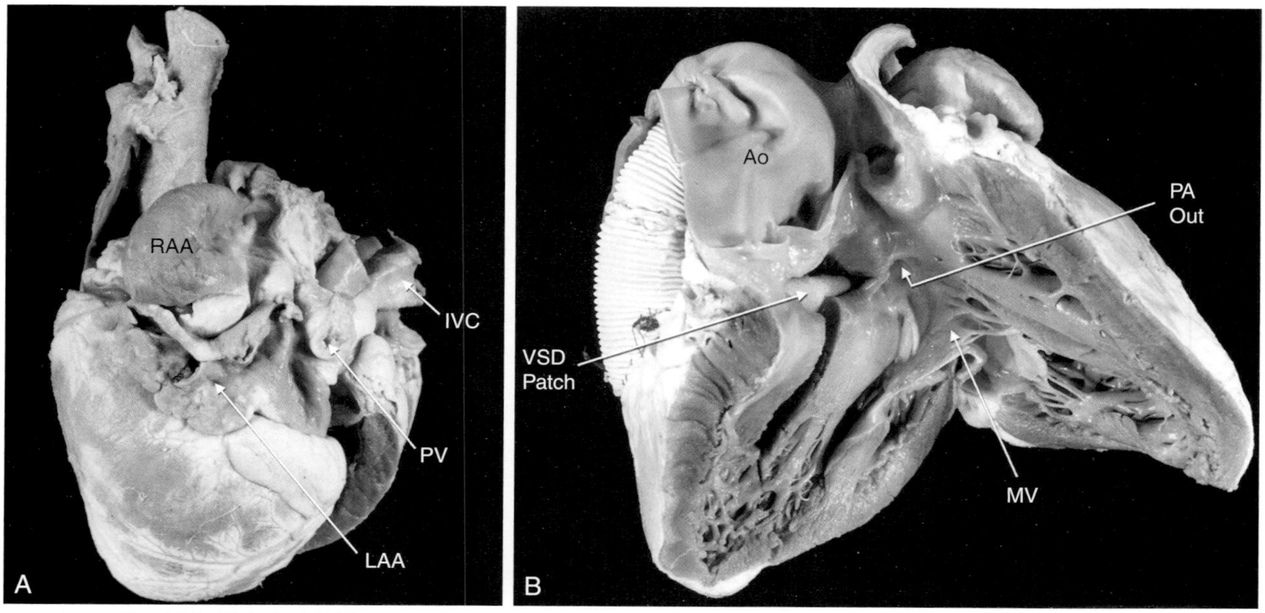

Fig. 10.9 (A) Left-sided juxtaposition of the atrial appendages (JAA) with solitus atria and malposition of the morphologically right atrial appendage *(RAA)* to the left of the great arteries, left lateral view. The RAA is to the right and superior relative to the morphologically left atrial appendage *(LAA)*. A large morphologically left ventricle (LV), the ascending aorta *(Ao)* immediately to the right of the RAA, the normally connected inferior vena cava *(IVC)*, and the left pulmonary vein *(PV)* are also seen. (B) The opened LV, left anterior oblique view, revealed the presence of double-outlet left ventricle (DOLV). The outflow tract from the LV to the aorta *(Ao)* is widely patent. Posteriorly and to the right, the outflow tract from the LV to the pulmonary artery (PA) is tightly stenotic between the hypoplastic and posteriorly malaligned conal septum superiorly and the mitral valve *(MV)* inferiorly *(PA Out)*. This 12-year-old boy had DOLV {S,D,L}. The ventricular septal defect *(VSD)* has been closed with a prosthetic patch (VSD Patch). Anteriorly, a valve-bearing conduit (unlabeled) connected the right ventricle with the PA. To summarize, this patient had right shift of the ventricles and great arteries relative to solitus atria, resulting in left-sided JAA with malposition of the RAA relative to the great arteries (as in Fig. 10.3, diagram 1) and associated with DOLV {S,D,L}, subaortic VSD, and pulmonary outflow tract stenosis. (From Van Praagh S, O'Sullivan J, Brili S, Van Praagh R. Juxtaposition of the morphologically right atrial appendage in solitus and inversus atria: A study of 35 postmortem cases. *Am Heart J.* 1996;132:382; reproduced with permission.)

Dextrocardia: 2 of 18 patients (11.11%). Dextrocardia occurred only with atrial situs inversus. There was no significant difference on comparison of the frequency of dextrocardia with JLAA (11.11%) and dextrocardia with JRAA (14.28%).

Mesocardia: 1 of 18 patients (5.55%). Mesocardia was more common with JRAA (7/35 patients, 14.28%), but this proved to be not a statistically significant difference: $p = .14$, Fisher exact test.

Absence of Eustachian and Thebesian Valves: The Eustachian valve of the inferior vena cava and the Thebesian valve of the coronary sinus were absent in 7 of 18 patients with JLAA (39%) and in 24 of 33 patients with JRAA (73%). This was a statistically significant difference ($p < .025$). Biologically, I am not sure what this statistical difference means, if anything. It is recorded here as an anatomic finding of uncertain biological significance, for future consideration.

Atrioventricular Valves: The differences between JLAA and JRAA are clearcut, statistically highly significant, and biologically very important (see Table 10.2). JLAA had a high frequency of left atrial outlet obstruction (i.e., mitral atresia, stenosis, hypoplasia, or left-sided tricuspid stenosis) in 12 of 18 patients (69%), whereas left atrial outlet obstruction was found in 0 of 35 patients with JRAA (0%), $p < .001$ (see Table 10.2).

A common AV valve was present in 5 of 18 patients with JLAA (28%), but in 0 of 35 patients with JRAA (0%), $p < .01$ (see Table 10.2).

The AV canal was divided (not in common) in 11 of these 18 patients with JLAA (61%). In 10 of these 11 cases with a divided AV canal (90%), the mitral valve, or in 1 case a left-sided tricuspid valve, was hypoplastic, stenotic, or atretic.

When a common AV canal was present (in 7/18 patients, 39%), the common AV valve was aligned predominantly or entirely with the morphologically RV when D-loop ventricles were present or with the right-sided morphologically LV when L-loop ventricles were present.

Only 1 of these 18 patients with JLAA (5.55%) had a normal mitral valve with a nonrestrictive left atrial outlet.

Atrioventricular (AV) Junction: One patient, a 4-day-old boy, had right-sided JAA with malposition of the LAA (JLAA). There was DORV. The segmental anatomic set was {S,D,D}. So the diagnosis, in part, was DORV {S,D,D}. Thus, there was AV situs concordance: solitus atria and solitus or D-loop ventricles. But the fascinating and rare finding was that there was AV alignment discordance: The morphologically RA opened into the morphologically LV, and the morphologically LA opened into the morphologically RV. This heart specimen is presented photographically in Fig. 10.5.[40] Thus, this patient with JLAA had incongruence between the atrial and ventricular situs (both concordant) and the AV alignments (both discordant).[40]

Ventricular Septum: In these 18 patients with JAA who had malposition of the LAA relative to the vascular pedicle (see Fig. 10.3), briefly called JLAA, the ventricular septum was intact in 4 of 18 cases (22%). A VSD was present in 14 of 18 patients (78%). A VSD was present in 91% of patients with JRAA. Using the Fisher exact test, this difference was found to be not statistically significant ($p = .13$). The anatomic types of VSD associated with JLAA were as follows:

- membranous, 1 of 14 (7.1%);
- conoventricular, with conal septal malalignment or absence, 4 of 14 (28.6%);
- bulboventricular foramen, 2 of 14 (14.3%);
- AV canal type, 5 of 14 (35.7%); and
- mid muscular, 2 of 14 (14.3%).

Left Ventricular Outflow Tract: Aortic or subaortic atresia or stenosis was present in 7 of 18 patients with JLAA (39%), but occurred in only 1 of 35 cases of JRAA (3%), $p < .01$.

Thus, we found that JLAA is a largely unrecognized form of the **hypoplastic left heart syndrome** with multilevel left heart obstruction.[40]

Not only is the sidedness of the obstruction in JLAA the opposite of that which typifies JRAA (left-sided, as opposed to right-sided, see Table 10.2), but there are other major differences.

Infundibulum and Great Arteries: The great arteries were solitus normally related in 9 of these 18 cases of JLAA (50%), but in 0 of the 35 patients with JRAA (0%), $p = .0001$ (Fisher exact test). The segmental anatomy was normal, that is, {S,D,S}, in 8 of these 18 JLAA patients (44.44%) and {S,L,S} in 1 of 18 (5.55%).

The patient with {S,L,S} had isolated inversion of the ventricular part of the heart (Fig. 10.10) In addition, this {S,L,S} patient had single LV because of absence of the right ventricular sinus or inflow tract, with an infundibular outlet chamber, and the heterotaxy syndrome with asplenia. It is notably rare to have solitus normally related great arteries in association with asplenia, or with single LV.

In the 50% of patients with JLAA and abnormally related great arteries, what were the ventriculoarterial alignments? The abnormal ventriculoarterial alignments were DORV in 8 of 18 patients (40%), and TGA in 1 of 18 (6%).

The cases of DORV were noteworthy. Half of them had DORV {S,D,D} *with a subpulmonary conus and aortic-tricuspid or aortic-common AV valve direct fibrous continuity.* This is Dr. Richard D. Rowe's **infantile type of DORV,** found in 4 of these 18 patients with JLAA (22%). DORV with a unilateral conus (subpulmonary with aortic-AV valve fibrous continuity or subaortic with pulmonary-AV fibrous continuity) occurs frequently with the hypoplastic left heart syndrome, as these cases with JLAA illustrate. The other 4 patients (22%) had DORV {S,D,D} with a bilateral conus (subaortic and subpulmonary, with no semilunar-AV fibrous continuity). The patient with TGA had TGA {S,D,D} (1 of 18 patients, 5.55%).

Thus far, based on our 1996 studies,[39,40] we have been able to establish that there are two JAA syndromes, a JRAA syndrome[39] and a JLAA syndrome.[40] Further, it has been shown that these syndromes are largely opposites and they have been compared statistically (see Table 10.2).

But how do hearts with JAA compare with hearts that do not have JAA? This we will now attempt to do, based on our 1968 study.[21]

JAA Versus Non-JAA. Are there any statistically significant differences between conotruncal malformations with JAA and conotruncal malformations without JAA? In an effort to answer this question, we compared 42 postmortem heart specimens with JAA with 100 randomly selected postmortem control heart specimens with conotruncal malformations but without JAA.[21] Of these 42 cases of JAA, 21 were personally studied and 21 were gathered from the literature.[21] Of these 42 cases of JAA, 39 had left-sided JRAA (92.9%) and only 3 had right-sided JLAA (7.1%). Hence, this study was essentially a comparison of the common type of JAA, that is, left-sided JAA with JRAA in visceroatrial situs solitus with conotruncal malformations without JAA. One patient from the literature had visceroarterial situs inversus, or situs ambiguus (we were not sure which). It should be added that these 100 control cases were called "transpositions," consistent with the custom at that time; however, 7 had DORV. (Transposition is now defined precisely as ventriculoarterial discordance. But in 1968, TGA was defined more broadly, following Abbott,[47] as any abnormality in the relationship between the semilunar valves themselves, or between the semilunar valves and the ventricles, ventricular septum, or AV valves.)

The salient findings of this comparative study of JAA hearts (mostly JRAA) and non-JAA hearts are presented in Table 10.4.

Table 10.4 summarizes the salient significant findings on comparison of hearts with JAA (mostly due to malposition of the RAA) and hearts with conotruncal malformations (transposition and DORV) but without JAA.[21] When a patient had JRAA in addition to a conotruncal malformation (TGA or DORV), he or she was more likely to have dextrocardia, anatomically corrected malposition of the great arteries, a secundum ASD, tricuspid atresia or severe stenosis, a VSD, a small or absent right ventricular sinus, a bilateral (subaortic and subpulmonary) conus, pulmonary outflow tract obstruction (stenosis or atresia), and/or aortic outflow tract obstruction than is a patient with a conotruncal anomaly but without JAA (see Table 10.4).

It is noteworthy that with JRAA, a small or absent right ventricular sinus (71%, see Table 10.4) was more common than tricuspid atresia or severe stenosis (40%, see Table 10.4). This observation suggests that underdevelopment of the RV sinus may be the morphogenetic cause of tricuspid atresia, rather than vice versa (which is how we usually think about this anomaly). Underdevelopment of the RV sinus was almost twice as common as tricuspid atresia. More precisely: underdevelopment of the RV sinus/tricuspid atresia or stenosis = 1.8/1.

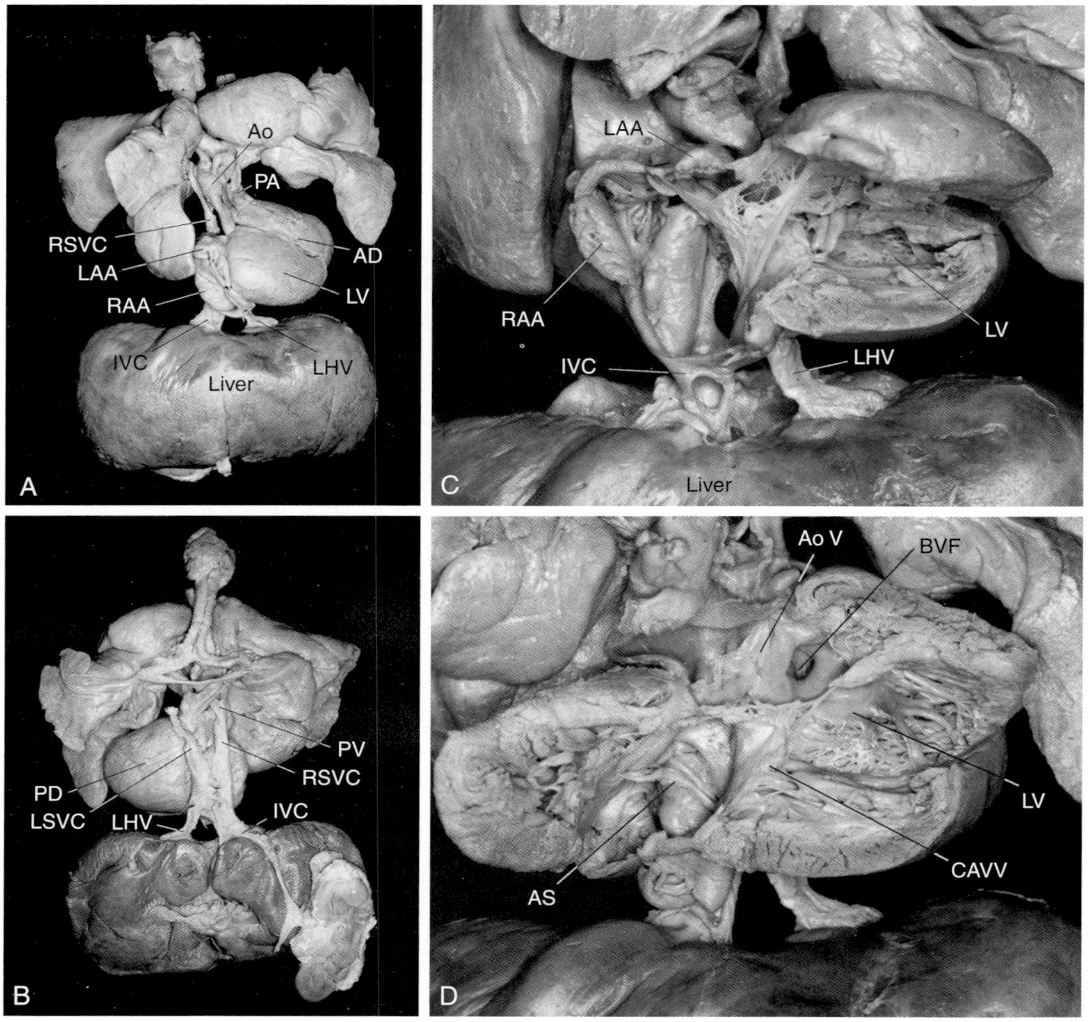

Fig. 10.10 Right-sided juxtaposition of the atrial appendages (JAA), anterior view of heart, lungs, and liver. This 20-day-old girl had a visceral heterotaxy, asplenia, bilaterally trilobed lungs, and an abnormally symmetrical liver. Solitus atria, ventricular L-loop, and solitus normally related great arteries were present; that is, the segmental anatomy was {S,L,S} indicating the presence of isolated inversion of the ventricular part of the heart. The right ventricular sinus (inflow tract) was absent, resulting in single left ventricle *(LV),* with an infundibular outflow chamber. As is frequent with the asplenia syndrome, this patient had a common atrioventricular canal, resulting in common-inlet LV (not double-inlet LV). (A) Right-sided JAA is seen with the morphologically left atrial appendage *(LAA)* malpositioned relative to the great arteries. The LAA sits right on top of the morphologically right atrial appendage *(RAA).* In JAA, the superior atrial appendage is virtually always the malpositioned appendage. Right-sided JAA with solitus atria indicates left shift of the ventricles and great arteries relative to the atria (as in Fig. 10.3, diagram 3). The inferior vena cava *(IVC)* and the right superior vena cava *(RSVC)* connect with the morphologically right atrium (RA). The left hepatic vein *(LHV)* connects with the morphologically left atrium (LA). This main pulmonary artery *(PA)* is anterior, superior, and to the left of the ascending aorta *(Ao),* typical of solitus normally related great arteries. The anterior descending coronary artery *(AD)* runs almost horizontally between the single LV below and the infundibular outlet chamber above from which the PA arises. (B) Posterior view of the heart, lungs, and liver. All of the pulmonary veins (PVs) connect by a single orifice with the RSVC, this being a frequent type of totally anomalous pulmonary venous connection with asplenia. The left superior vena cava *(LSVC)* and the LHV both connect with the LA. The IVC is seen to be intact (not interrupted), which also is typical of asplenia. The posterior descending coronary artery *(PD)* runs in an abnormally horizontal course, typical of single LV (below the PD) and an infundibular outlet chamber (above the PD). The similarly abnormally horizontal plane of the AD was seen in A. (C) Right lateral view of the opened atria and the single LV. Note the broad inferior RAA and the narrow superior LAA. The septum primum between the atria has multiple fenestrations; that is, a secundum atrial septal defect (ASD II) is present in addition to a common atrioventricular (AV) canal. The anteroinferior margin of septum primum is nude or bare (devoid of attaching AV valve tissue), which is typical of a common AV canal. Common inlet into the single LV is seen. (D) Interior view of the right-sided single LV. There is a large atrioventricular septal defect between the atrial septum *(AS)* and the common atrioventricular valve *(CAVV).* There is direct fibrous continuity between the aortic valve *(AoV)* and the anterosuperior leaflet of the CAVV, typical of normally related great arteries. The bulboventricular foramen (BVF) is superior and left sided, leading into the infundibular outlet chamber from which the PA originates. The AoV arises entirely above the LV. The smooth left ventricular septal surface is superior and left sided, anterior and inferior to the BVF, whereas the finely trabeculated LV free wall is right sided. Hence, the single LV is right handed (inverted). The infundibular outflow chamber is left handed and left sided relative to the single LV. In summary, this is right-sided JAA with solitus atria and a malpositioned LAA relative to the vascular pedicle, reflecting leftward malposition (left shift) of the ventriculoarterial segments relative to the solitus atria. This patient also had visceral heterotaxy, asplenia, bilateral SVCs with the LSVC and the LHV connecting with the LA, totally anomalous pulmonary venous connection to the RSVC, {S,L,S}, ASD II, common AV canal, common-inlet LV, and absent RV sinus resulting in single LV with infundibular outlet chamber. (From Van Praagh S, O'Sullivan J, Brili S, Van Praagh R. Juxtaposition of the morphologically left atrial appendage in solitus and inversus atria: A study of 18 postmortem cases. *Am Heart J.* 1996;132:391; reproduced with permission.)

TABLE 10.4 Comparison of Significant Differences Between JAA Hearts and Non-JAA Hearts[21]

	JAA Hearts (%)	Non JAA Hearts (%)	*p* Value
Dextrocardia	21	12	<.025
Anatomically corrected malposition of the GAs	9.5	0	<.005
Patent foramen ovale	16.7	61	<.001
Secundum ASD	71	23	<.001
Tricuspid atresia and severe stenosis	40	4	<.001
Ventricular septal defect	88	57	<.001
Small or absent RV sinus	71	20	<.001
Bilateral conus	77	25	<.001
Subaortic conus	14.3	75	<.001
Pulmonary outflow tract obstruction	52	19	<.001
Aortic outflow tract obstruction	38	8	<.001

ASD, Atrial septal defect; *GAs*, great arteries; *JAA*, juxtaposition of the atrial appendages; *RV*, morphologically right ventricle.

Atrioventricular Malalignment in JAA

Malposition of the atria relative to the ventricles is a salient feature of the pathologic anatomy of JAA. The fact that both the atrial and the ventricular segments of the heart are frequently malpositioned in JAA has been commented on frequently heretofore in an effort to make the occasional incongruity of AV alignment and situs concordance or discordance comprehensible. For example, how is it possible to have DORV {S,L,D} with AV alignment *concordance,* despite the fact that there is AV situs discordance (DORV {**S,L**,D} (see Fig. 10.7)? How is it possible to have DORV {**I,D**,D} with AV alignment *concordance* (see Fig. 10.4)? Or, how is it possible to have DORV {**S,D**,D} with AV alignment *discordance* (see Fig. 10.5)?

In JAA, AV malpositioning is not confined to these unusual cases of AV alignment versus situs incongruity (see Figs. 10.4, 10.5, and 10.7).[22,39,41-45] Instead, striking malpositioning of the atria relative to the ventricles is frequent in JAA, as is indicated quantitatively by the **atrioventricular septal angles.**[21]

It was possible to measure the plane of the atrial septum and the plane of the ventricular septum as projected on the horizontal plane in 18 of 21 postmortem heart specimens with JAA (mostly JRAA).[21] This was similar to a four-chamber long-axis echocardiography view. The normal atrial septal angle relative to the sagittal plane was approximately 30 degrees to the left. The normal ventricular septal angle relative to the sagittal plane was approximately 40 degrees to the left. The normal atrioventricular septal angle was approximately 10 degrees (40 degrees minus 30 degrees = 10 degrees).

The AV septal angles projected on the horizontal plane in these 18 cases of JAA were mean = 78.06 degrees, standard deviation = 51.48 degrees, range = 0 to 155 degrees, and median = 67.5 degrees. Of these 18 cases, the horizontal plane AV septal angle was normal in only 2 heart specimens: 0 degrees and 5 degrees. Suffice it to say, these AV septal angles were almost always very much greater than normal (normal ≤10 degrees), indicating marked malpositioning of the atrial and ventricular segments of the heart relative to each other.[21]

In terms of **clinical diagnostic imaging** using two-dimensional or three-dimensional echocardiography or MRI, very informative measurements could be made in the four-chamber long-axis view, and in the short-axis view, measuring not only the planes of the atrial and ventricular septa, and the angles between the septa. In addition, one could measure the displacement and the rotations of the atrial and the ventricular septa relative to each other. There is a book waiting to be written on the normal and abnormal geometry of the human heart as assessed by in vivo imaging.

Morphogenesis of JAA

The morphogenesis of JAA with malposition of the RAAs to the left of the great arteries in visceroatrial situs solitus (see Fig. 10.3, diagram 1) is illuminated by a consideration of normal cardiac development. Early after D-loop formation, JRAA is normal (Fig. 10.11). The right and left atria both lie to the left of the conotruncus in the normal human embryo at 23 days of age (horizon 11,[48] 17 somites, crown-rump length 4.3 mm; see Fig. 10.11A–B). However, by 27 days of age (horizon 13,[48] 4 mm; see Fig. 10.12A), the RAA normally lies at least partially to the right of the conotruncus.

Why this change between 23 and 27 days of age? What is happening? Well, the atria are expanding, and the ventricular part of the heart is gradually swinging from right to left. By 27 days of age, JRAA is largely "cured" (compare Fig. 10.12 with Fig. 10.11). However, the right-to-left swing of the developing ventricles still remains to be accomplished. At 27 days, the ventricular apex still points rightward (see Fig. 10.12A) and the RV still lies posterior (or dorsal) relative to the LV (see Fig. 10.12C). Hence, dextrocardia is normal at 27 days of intrauterine life. When the right-to-left swing of the ventricles has been accomplished (normally by 36 to 38 days of age), with a leftward pointing ventricular apex and an RV that is anterior (ventral) to the LV, the conotruncus normally lies even further to the left, between the atrial appendages.

Thus, JRAA represents retention of the normal early embryonic state seen at 23 days of age in which the conotruncus lies to the right of the RA (see Fig. 10.11). Horizontal plane sections are remarkable at this stage. The conotruncus is not right and anterior (ventral) relative to the RA. Instead, the conotruncus is right and lateral to the RA; that is, the conotruncus is to the right and beside the RA—directly to the right.

So the question becomes: **What are the factors that hold the conotruncus abnormally to the right relative to the atria?** In these 21 postmortem cases that we examined and measured personally, factors thought to be important in the morphogenesis of JRAA were as follows[21]:

1. **A bilateral conus** (both subaortic and subpulmonary) was present in 16 of 21 cases (76%). A bilateral conus separates the semilunar valves from the AV valves and prevents semilunar-AV fibrous continuity. A bilateral conus is frequently found with typical DORV, that is, DORV without hypoplastic left heart. A bilateral conus also may be regarded as failure of remodeling of the lesser curvature of the D-bulboventricular loop. Normally,

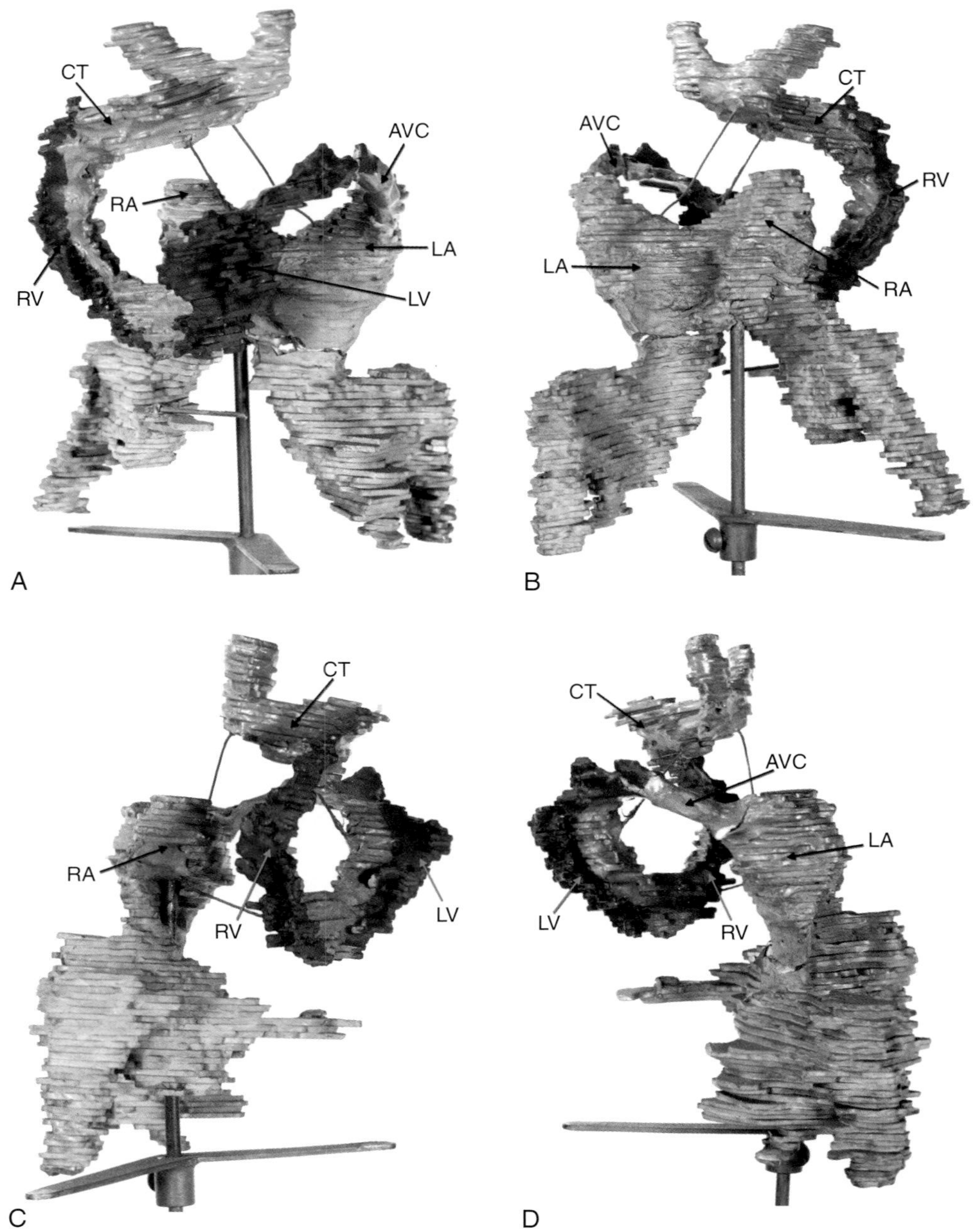

Fig. 10.11 Model of the cardiac lumen of human embryo Carnegie number 470, Streeter's horizon 11, 17 somites, 4.3-mm crown-rump length, estimated age since ovulation 23 days. The relations of left-sided juxtaposition of the atrial appendages are present. (A) Anterior (ventral) view; (B) posterior (dorsal) view; (C) right lateral view; and (D) left lateral view. This reconstruction of the cardiovascular lumen is like a perfect frozen angiocardiogram in which all chambers and vessels can be seen simultaneously from four different perspectives. The atria are in situs solitus, with the morphologically right atrium (RA) lying to the right of the morphologically left atrium *(LA)*. A ventricular D-loop is present, the morphologically right ventricle *(RV)* lying to the right of the morphologically left ventricle *(LV)*. The lumen of the RA lies entirely to the left of the lumen of the RV and the conotruncus *(CT)*. The CT is the developing conus (or infundibulum) and truncus (or great arteries). Thus, both the RA and the LA normally lie to the left of the CT at 23 days of age. The right and left omphalomesenteric veins below the atria, and the first pair of aortic arches at the distal end of the conotruncus are unlabeled. The trabecular zones of the LV and the RV are painted green (which looks dark in these black and white photos). In C and D, note that the RV is posterior (dorsal) relative to the LV. In A the developing ventricular apex (between the dark LV and RV) is pointing rightward; that is, dextrocardia is normal at 23 days. Note also that the circulation is in series at this stage, going from RA to LA (as in tricuspid atresia). From the LA, all of the blood passes via the atrioventricular canal *(AVC)* into the LV (as in double-inlet or common-inlet LV). From the LV, all of the blood passes into the RV (as in double-outlet RV). From the RV, all of the blood then passes via the conotruncus to the body.Why does the bulboventricular (conoventricular) part of the heart form a loop in air-breathing animals with systemic and pulmonary circulations? (Bulboventricular looping typically does not occur in water—"breathing" animals (fish) that are without separate systemic and pulmonary circulations.) Note how far apart the developing semilunar valves (CT) are from the developing AV valves (AVC) at 23 days of age. For aortic-mitral fibrous continuity to occur to achieve normally related great arteries with separate systemic and pulmonary circulations, bulboventricular looping is one of the morphogenetic steps necessary to achieve aortic-mitral approximation. Another necessary morphogenetic process to achieve aortic-mitral approximation is remodeling of the lesser curvature of the bulboventricular loop, that is, resorption of the subaortic conal free wall that is thought to occur by apoptosis (programmed cell death).The understanding that is implicit in Fig 10.11 explains why typical left-sided JAA is so often associated with complex congenital heart disease, including significantly increased frequencies of tricuspid atresia or severe tricuspid stenosis, secundum atrial septal defect, ventricular septal defect, small right ventricular sinus, dextrocardia or mesocardia, conal maldevelopment (bilateral or subaortic), and abnormally related great arteries (double-outlet RV and transposition of the great arteries [TGA]). Left-sided JAA is part of the normal 23-day-old human embryonic scene, and so are all of the other features mentioned above (except for TGA). If these anatomic features persist postnatally, they are regarded as congenital malformations. *Diagnostically,* left-sided JAA should be regarded as a "red flag," suggesting that other anatomic features, normal at 23 days of development, should be searched for and ruled out. (From Melhuish BPP, Van Praagh R. Juxtaposition of the atrial appendages, a sign of severe cyanotic congenital heart disease. *Br Heart J.* 1968;30:269 reproduced with permission.)

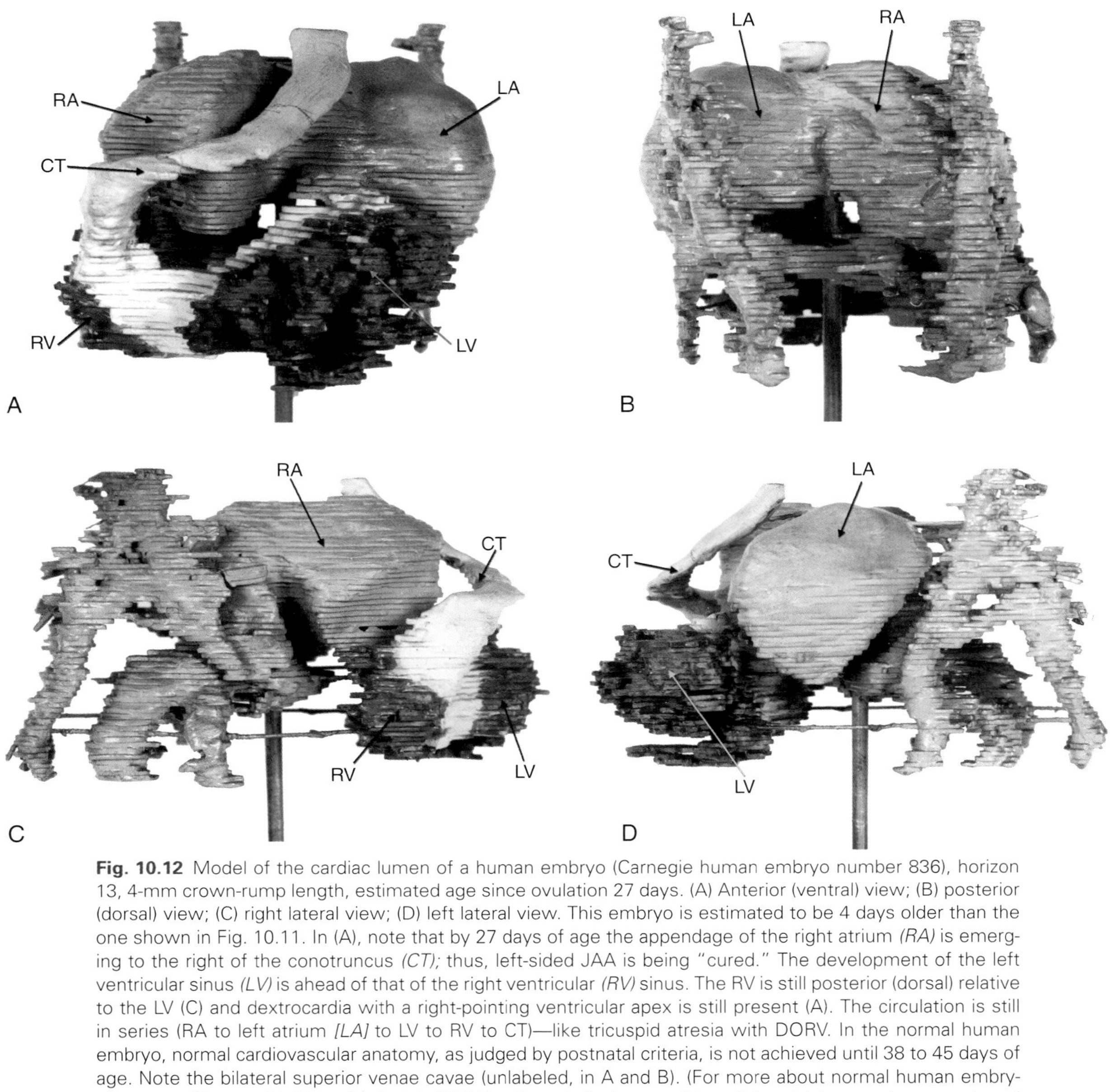

Fig. 10.12 Model of the cardiac lumen of a human embryo (Carnegie human embryo number 836), horizon 13, 4-mm crown-rump length, estimated age since ovulation 27 days. (A) Anterior (ventral) view; (B) posterior (dorsal) view; (C) right lateral view; (D) left lateral view. This embryo is estimated to be 4 days older than the one shown in Fig. 10.11. In (A), note that by 27 days of age the appendage of the right atrium *(RA)* is emerging to the right of the conotruncus *(CT)*; thus, left-sided JAA is being "cured." The development of the left ventricular sinus *(LV)* is ahead of that of the right ventricular *(RV)* sinus. The RV is still posterior (dorsal) relative to the LV (C) and dextrocardia with a right-pointing ventricular apex is still present (A). The circulation is still in series (RA to left atrium *[LA]* to LV to RV to CT)—like tricuspid atresia with DORV. In the normal human embryo, normal cardiovascular anatomy, as judged by postnatal criteria, is not achieved until 38 to 45 days of age. Note the bilateral superior venae cavae (unlabeled, in A and B). (For more about normal human embryology, see Chapter 2.) (From Melhuish BPP, Van Praagh R. Juxtaposition of the atrial appendages, a sign of severe cyanotic congenital heart disease. *Br Heart J*. 1968;30:269; with permission.)

the subaortic conal free wall undergoes resorption (probably by apoptosis or programmed cell death), facilitating normal aortic-mitral approximation and fibrous continuity. In typical TGA, the subpulmonary conal free wall undergoes resorption, facilitating pulmonary-mitral approximation and fibrous continuity. But with a bilateral conus, there is little or no subsemilunar conal free wall resorption and hence no remodeling and shortening of the lesser curvature of the bulboventricular loop. Hence, the conotruncus is held to the right, predisposing to JRAA, rather than migrating leftward.

2. **Failure of leftward rotation of the ventricular apex,** as indicated by measurement of the plane of the ventricular septum in the horizontal plane, was present in 16 of 21 cases (76%). Because the conotruncus arises from the underlying ventricles, failure of leftward swing of the ventricles holds the conotruncus abnormally to the right, predisposing to JRAA.
3. **A small right ventricular sinus** was found in 13 of these 21 cases (62%). Why is a small RV thought to be a factor that predisposes to JRAA? Because development of the RV is thought to be important in the right-to-left apical swing of the ventricular part of the heat.
4. **Tilt of the ventricles** displacing the great arteries to the right, documented by measuring the ventricular septal angle in the frontal plane, was found in 8 of 14 cases (57%).
5. **Abnormal atrial location,** documented by measuring the atrial septal angle in the horizontal plane, occurred in 12 of 19 cases (63%).

All five factors occurred in 3 of 21 cases (14%). Four factors were found in 6 of 21 (29%). Three factors occurred in 4 of 21 (19%). Two factors were found in 6 cases (29%). One factor only occurred in 2 cases (10%): a bilateral conus in 1 and failure of ventricular apical rotation in 1.

The foregoing is our best present understanding of the **morphogenesis of JRAA**—to the left of the conotruncus in visceroatrial situs solitus (see Fig. 10.3, diagram 1) and to the right of the conotruncus in visceroatrial situs inversus (see Fig. 10.3, diagram 2). The various developmental and anatomic factors mentioned earlier contribute to malalignment of the highly mobile bulboventricular loop relative to the comparatively fixed atria and AV canal.

For example, in typical JRAA in visceroatrial situs solitus with malposition of the RAA to the left of the great arteries (see Fig. 10.3, diagram 1), **the entire D-bulboventricular loop is malpositioned too far to the right relative to the atria and the AV canal.** The results of this rightward malposition of the ventriculoinfundibulo-arterial part of the heart, including the following:

1. **Ventriculoatrial malalignment.** The right AV junction is constricted as the ventricular septum gets abnormally close to lying beneath the right lateral portion of the right atrial free wall (Fig. 10.13B, compare with Fig. 10.13A, which is normal). This constriction or narrowing of right atrial-to-right ventricular inflow tract results in tricuspid hypoplasia, tricuspid stenosis, or tricuspid atresia and hypoplasia or absence of the right ventricular sinus (inflow tract), all typical features of the JRAA syndrome.
2. **Atrioarterial malalignment.** Rightward malposition of the ventriculoinfundibulo-arterial part of the heart (the bulboventricular loop) also results in the great arteries lying too far to the right relative to the atria and their appendages. Consequently, both the RAA and LAA lie side by side (juxtaposed),

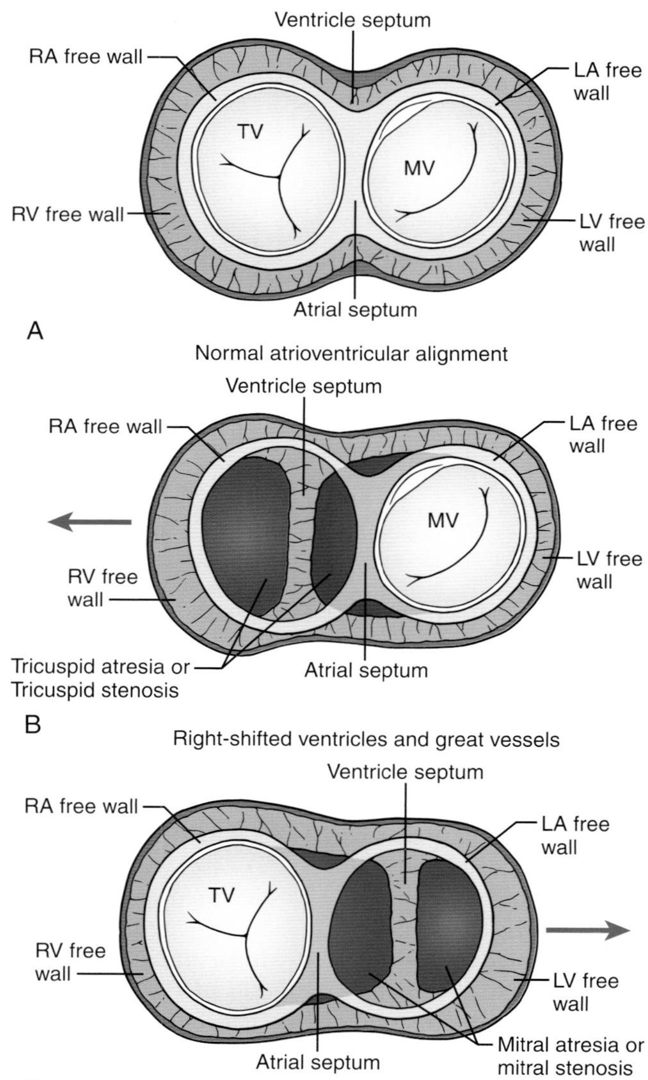

Fig. 10.13 Normal and right-shifted or left-shifted ventriculoatrial alignments, schematic short-axis views.(A) Normally, the ventricular free walls and the ventricular septum underlie the atrial free walls and the atrial septum, respectively, almost perfectly. The ventricular septum and the atrial septum lie in almost the same short axis plane, the ventricular septum slightly to the right of the atrial septum (the normal ventriculoatrial septal angle[55]: mean = 5 degrees ± 2 degrees, median = 6 degrees, and range = 1 to 7 degrees). This normal very small ventriculoatrial right shift is not depicted in A; but it is nonetheless important because it makes possible the left ventricular–to–right atrial shunt (the Gerbode shunt). *LA,* Morphologically left atrium; *LV,* morphologically left ventricle; *MV,* mitral valve; *RA,* morphologically right atrium; *RV,* morphologically right ventricle; *TV,* tricuspid valve. (B) Right-shifted ventricles and ventricular septum relative to the atria, the atrial septum, and the atrioventricular canal, schematic short-axis view.

Continued

Fig. 10.13 cont'd Note that the ventricular septum is displaced well to the right of the atrial septum. We hypothesize that the right-shifted ventricular septum helps to explain the high incidence of tricuspid atresia or congenital tricuspid stenosis with right-shift of a D-bulboventricular loop. The right-shifted ventricular septum is located where the tricuspid valve normally opens in the RV (compare with A). Note how small the RV cavity is (to the right of the right-shifted ventricular septum). The *arrow* indicates the anatomic direction of shift or malposition of the ventricles, infundibulum and great arteries relative to the atria, the atrial appendages, and the atrioventricular valves. Right-shift of the ventriculoarterial segments of the heart explains why both great arteries lie to the right of both atrial appendages, resulting in typical left-sided JAA with malposition of the right atrial appendage (as in Fig. 10.3, diagram 1). "Right-shift" of the ventriculoarterial parts of the heart are intended as a statement of anatomic fact, not as an hypothesis concerning embryonic morphogenetic movement. For example, we think that right-shifted ventricles and great arteries, from the embryologic standpoint, very probably result from a failure of the normal leftward movement of these structures. (C) Left-shifted ventricles and great arteries relative to the atria and atrioventricular canal, schematic short-axis view. Note that the ventricular septum is shifted far to the left relative to the atrial septum. Indeed, the left-shifted ventricular septum is located where the mitral valve normally opens into the left ventricle (compare with A). Note how small the LV cavity is (to the left of the left-shifted ventricular septum). Anatomic left shift of the ventricles and great arteries results in right-sided JAA with malposition of the left atrial appendage, as in Fig. 10.3, diagram 3. In summary, right-shift and left-shift of the ventricles and great arteries relative to the atria, the atrial appendages, and the atrioventricular valves appear to explain not only left-sided and right-sided juxtaposition of the atrial appendages, but also the syndrome associated with malposition of the right atrial appendage (hypoplastic right heart syndrome) and the syndrome associated with malposition of the left atrial appendage (hypoplastic left heart syndrome). Diagnostically, when juxtaposition of the atrial appendages is present, determine which atrial appendage is malposed relative to the great arteries (see Fig. 10.3). Then search specifically for the frequently associated syndrome. (From Pessotto R, Padalino M, Rubino M, Kadoba K, Büchler JR, Van Praagh R. Straddling tricuspid valve as a sign of ventriculoatrial malalignment: A morphometric study of 19 postmortem cases. *Am Heart J.* 1999;138:1184-95; with permission.)

with the RAA lying to the left of the great arteries, instead of lying to the right of the vascular pedicle as occurs normally.

Thus, JAA with malposition of the RAA to the left of the great arteries in visceroatrial situs solitus (see Fig. 10.3, diagram 1), JRAA is a clearcut externally visible indicator of rightward malposition of the ventriculoinfundibulo-arterial part of the heart relative to the atria and the AV canal. This externally visible atrioarterial malalignment (JRAA) indicates the increased probability of externally invisible AV malalignment, that is, the multilevel right heart obstructive syndrome of JRAA (see Table 10.2).

It should be emphasized that JAA is not an anomaly of the atrial appendages or of the atria per se. The atrial appendages are "the sinned against"; they are not "the sinners". The atrial appendages *reflect* the abnormality; they are *not the site* of the anomaly. The atrial appendages are "innocent bystanders." The malpositioned and malaligned bulboventricular loop is the "real villain," that is, the site of the anomaly/anomalies.

Summary. What is JRAA? It is rightward malposition of the bulboventricular loop relative to the atria and AV canal in patients with visceroarterial situs solitus and the sequelae of this rightward malposition (see Fig. 10.3, diagram 1); and it is leftward malposition of the bulboventricular loop relative to the atria and AV canal in visceroarterial situs inversus and the sequelae of this leftward malposition (see Fig. 10.3, diagram 2).

What is the morphogenesis of JAA with malposition of the LAA relative to the great arteries, that is, JLAA (see Fig. 10.3, diagrams 3 and 4)? The salient anatomic features of JLAA are summarized in Table 10.2 and are presented photographically in Figs. 10.1, 10.5, 10.6, 10.10, 10.14, and 10.15. Our conclusions concerning morphogenesis are that JLAA results from malposition of the ventriculoinfundibulo-arterial part of the heart relative to the atria and the AV canal, in a direction opposite to that seen in JRAA. In Figs. 10.3 and 10.13, arrows indicate the direction of malposition of the bulboventricular loop.

In JLAA to the right of the great arteries in patients with visceroatrial situs solitus, the bulboventricular loop is malpositioned to the left (see Fig. 10.13C). Hence, the ventricular septum tends to underlie the left lateral free wall of the LA, constricting the left atrial outlet and resulting in mitral hypoplasia or mitral stenosis, mitral atresia, and left ventricular underdevelopment or absence (see Fig. 10.13C)—these being the anatomic features typical of the JLAA syndrome (see Table 10.2). Leftward malposition of the ventriculoarterial part of the heart also results in JLAA to the right of the great arteries (see Fig. 10.3, diagram 3).

Note that in patients with visceroatrial situs solitus, *rightward* malposition of the ventriculoarterial part of the heart results in JRAA to the left of the great arteries (rightward pointing arrow, Figs. 10.3 diagram 1 and 10.13B), while *leftward* malposition of the ventriculoarterial part of the heart results in JLAA to the right of the great arteries (leftward pointing arrow, Fig. 10.3, diagram 3 and 10.13C).

In patients with visceroatrial situs inversus, as one might expect, the directions of ventriculoarterial malposition are the opposites of those in patients with visceroarterial situs solitus (note the directions of the arrows in Fig. 10.3, diagram 2 compared with Fig. 10.3, diagram 1 and Fig. 10.3, diagram 4 compared with Fig. 10.3, diagram 3).

In patients with visceroatrial situs inversus, rightward ventriculoarterial malposition results in JLAA to the left of the great arteries (see Fig. 10.3, diagram 4).

Morphogenetic Summary

JAA reflects malposition of the ventriculoinfundibulo-arterial segments of the heart relative to the atrial and AV canal segments. It will be recalled that the ventriculoinfundibulo-arterial part of the heart is a "professional contortionist," whereas the atria and the AV canal are relatively fixed in position by the venae cavae and the pulmonary veins. However as we have seen, the atria also can be malpositioned in JAA. But the primary site of the abnormality usually appears to be at the level of the bulboventricular loop, not the atria or the AV canal.

These ventriculoinfundibulo-arterial malpositions relative to the atria and the AV canal appear to explain not only the malpositions of the RAA and LAA relative to the great arteries (see Fig. 10.3), but also the JRAA and the JLAA syndromes (see Table 10.2). JAA is not only a malalignment of the atrial appendages relative to the great arteries but is also a malalignment of the ventricles and ventricular septum relative to the atrial and the

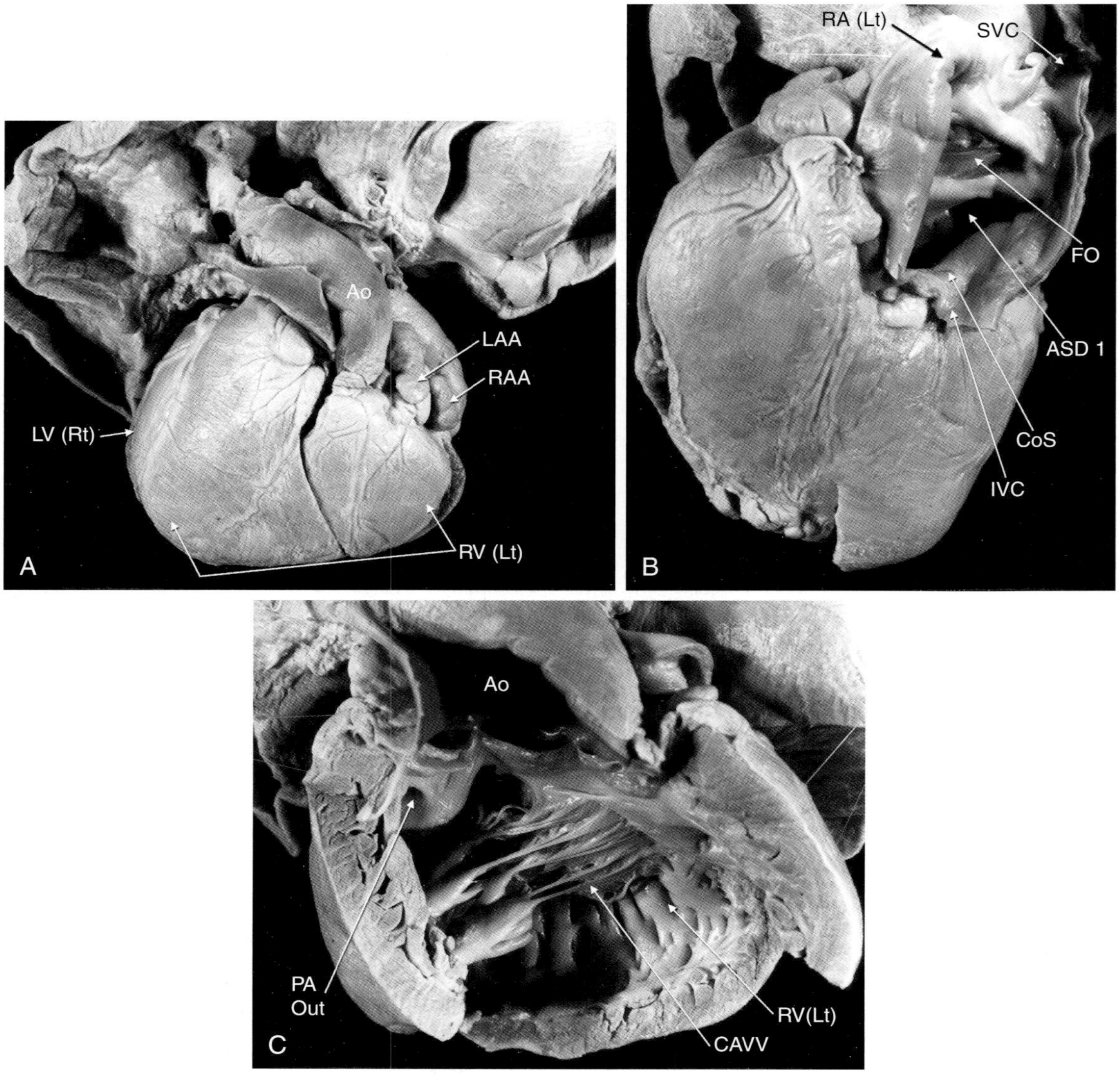

Fig. 10.14 (A) Left-sided juxtaposition of the atrial appendages (JAA) with atrial situs inversus, anterior view. The morphologically left atrial appendage *(LAA)* is malpositioned to the left relative to the great arteries; that is, the LAA should lie to the right of the great arteries. The LAA is not only juxtaposed relative to the morphologically right atrial appendage *(RAA)*. The LAA is also superior relative to the RAA. This patient also had polysplenia, dextrocardia, and double-outlet right ventricle (DORV) {I,L,L}. The large morphologically right ventricle is anterior and left-sided, that is, *RV (Lt)*. The morphologically left ventricle is small, right-sided, and posterior, that is, *LV (Rt)*. The ventricular apex points rightward. The large ascending aorta *(Ao)* is left-sided and posterior relative to the smaller main pulmonary artery (MPA) that lies to the right and anterior relative to the Ao (the MPA is not labeled). (B) The left-sided morphologically right atrium, that is, *RA (Lt)*, left lateral view. The inferior vena cava *(IVC)*, the superior vena cava *(SVC)*, and the coronary sinus *(CoS)* all connect with the left-sided RA. The right atrial aspect of the foramen ovale *(FO)* can be seen above the ostium primum type of atrial septal defect *(ASD 1°)*. Examination at the ventricular level revealed that a complete common AV canal was present, including ventricular septal defect of the AV canal type that was confluent with the ASD 1°. Examination at the ventricular level revealed that completely common AV canal was present, including a ventricular septal defect of the AV canal type that was confluent with the ASD 1°. The common AV valve opened predominantly into the large left-sided RV (seen in C) and only minimally into the small right-sided, and posterior LV. In this sense, common AV canal with "mitral stenosis" was considered to be present because the common AV valve opened only minimally into the LV (R). (C) View of the interior of the RV (Lt). The RV septal surface lies to viewer's right; and the RV free wall lies to the viewer's left. This left-sided RV is left-handed, typical of L-loop or inverted ventricles. Both great arteries arise above this left-sided RV; that is, double-outlet right ventricle (DORV) is present. The outflow tract from the RV (Lt) to the Ao is widely patent, whereas the pulmonary outflow tract *(PA Out)* is stenotic (PS) *(arrow)*. The presence of PS explains why the MPA appears so much smaller than the ascending Ao (in A). There is a muscular subpulmonary conus, with direct fibrous continuity between the aortic valve (AoV) and the anterior leaflet of the common atrioventricular valve *(CAVV)*. The stenotic PA Out is anterior and to the right relative to the aortic valve, similar to what one sees with inverted normally related great arteries. This is why the relationship between the great arteries (in A) suggests inverted tetralogy of Fallot. However, the ventriculoarterial alignments are those of DORV, as is seen in C. To summarize, this is a patient with polysplenia, dextrocardia, left-sided JAA, inverted atria, and malposition of the LAA to the left of the great arteries (similar to Fig. 10.3, diagram 4). Anatomically, there is right shift of the ventricles and great arteries relative to the atria and the atrioventricular canal (the *arrow* in Fig. 10.3, diagram 4). There is DORV {I,L,L} with common AV canal, a subpulmonary conus with AoV-CAVV direct fibrous continuity and right pulmonary outflow tract stenosis.
Noteworthy features of these cases include:
1. Left-sided JAA does not always have solitus atria.
2. Visceral heterotaxy with polysplenia almost always has a diagnosable atrial situs (not left atrial isomerism or left atrial appendage isomerism).
3. DORV does not always have a bilateral conus that prevents semilunar-atrioventricular fibrous continuity. The conus in DORV can be unilateral, subpulmonary only (with AoV-AVV [atrioventricular valve] fibrous continuity in this patient), or subaortic only (with pulmonary valve—atrioventricular valve fibrous continuity).

Continued

Fig. 10.14 cont'd 4. The segmental anatomy in this case could be expressed as DORV {I,L,*"I"*}. In other words, the great arteries in this case are very like inverted normally related great arteries, that is, {I, L, *I*}—very like inverted tetralogy of Fallot. However, the ventriculoarterial alignments are those of DORV. The AoV arises entirely above the large RV, not at all above the small LV; hence the quotation marks in DORV {I,L,*"I"*}. We prefer DORV {I,L,*L*}, adding that a subpulmonary conus with AoV-CAVV fibrous continuity is present.
5. This patient displays the **JAA with malposition of the LAA syndrome.**[40] The malposed LAA is left-sided. In this syndrome, the mitral valve and the LV are hypoplastic. In this patient, there was common-inlet RV (Lt). The CAVV opened almost not at all into the hypoplastic LV (R); in this sense, there was common AV canal with "MS" (mitral stenosis). Also, the LV (Rt) was hypoplastic.
6. This patient had what Dr. Richard D. Rowe called the ***infantile type of DORV,*** that is, DORV with a large RV and with mitral stenosis or atresia and a small LV. These are the cases of DORV that often have a unilateral (not a bilateral) conus: ***DORV with hypoplastic left heart*** (mitral stenosis or atresia, with a hypoplastic morphologically LV, right-sided in this patient with L-loop ventricles). In DORV with hypoplastic left heart, a unilateral conus should be expected. **DORV with the hypoplastic left heart syndrome (HLHS) and a unilateral conus is as specific an anatomic type of DORV as is DORV with bilaterally well-developed ventricles in which a bilateral conus is the rule.**
Why "infantile" type of DORV? Because Dr. Rowe understood that with the HLHS, such patients with DORV, tend to have a very unfavorable natural history, often dying in infancy. (From Van Praagh S, O'Sullivan J, Brili S, Van Praagh R. Juxtaposition of the morphologically left atrial appendage in solitus and inversus atria: A study of 18 postmortem cases. *Am Heart J.* 1996;132:391; reproduced with permission.)

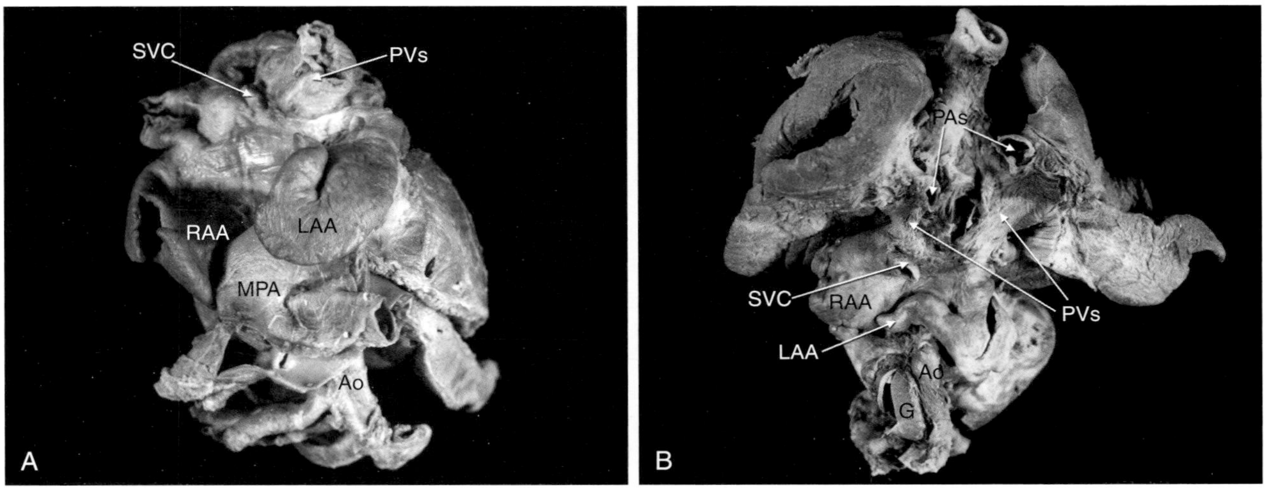

Fig. 10.15 Malposition of the Left Atrial Appendage ***(LAA),*** **Without Juxtaposition of the Atrial Appendages (JAA).** (A) Superior view of the heart of a 6-week-old girl with transposition of the great arteries {S,D,D} and mitral atresia or left atrial outlet atresia with a large left ventricle. The transposed aorta *(Ao)* and main pulmonary artery *(MPA)* have been retracted anteriorly to expose the malposed LAA that points posteriorly. The LAA does not protrude to the right of the MPA, and the LAA does not lie side-by-side relative to the morphologically right atrial appendage *(RAA)*. The superior vena cava *(SVC)* and the pulmonary veins *(PVs)* are labeled for spatial orientation. (B) Superior view of the heart of a 6.5-week-old boy with normal segmental anatomy, that is, {S,D,S}, but with aortic atresia and mitral stenosis. The LAA passes from left to right behind the ascending aorta (Ao). The LAA lies beside the RAA, but the LAA does not protrude anteriorly to the right of the great arteries. So, this anomaly is a ***partial form of right-sided JAA with malposition of the LAA and solitus atria.*** This patient had a modified Norwood procedure. A Gore-Tex conduit *(G)* connects the innominate artery with the right pulmonary artery. The MPA was transected, its distal end was occluded, and the proximal MPA was anastomosed to the ascending aorta. Postmortem, the pulmonary arteries *(PAs)* were transected to permit anterior retraction of the great arteries to expose the malposed LAA. To summarize, these 2 cases show malposition of the LAA, without right-sided JAA in A, and with partial right-sided JAA in B. We hypothesize that left shift of the ventriculoarterial part of the heart relative to the atria and AV canal occurred, as in Fig. 10.3, diagram 3, but without enough left shift to bring the LAA clearly to the right of the great arteries. Consequently, these partial or incomplete forms of right-sided JAA are characterized by a malposed LAA that is mostly posterior to the great arteries, rather than to the right of them. Nonetheless, both patients have the JAA with malposition of the LAA syndrome, that is, hypoplastic left heart: mitral atresia in A, and aortic atresia with mitral stenosis in B.

AV canal (see Fig. 10.13B–C); hence the JRAA syndrome and the JLAA syndrome (see Table 10.2).

For simplicity of expression, let us assume that situs solitus of the viscera and atria are present.

A right-shifted bulboventricular loop relative to the atrial appendages and the AV canal results in left-sided JAAs (see Fig. 10.3, diagram 1), malposition of the RAA (see Fig. 10.3, diagram 1), and the hypoplastic right heart syndrome with tricuspid atresia, stenosis, or hypoplasia (see Fig. 10.13B and Table 10.2).

A left-shifted bulboventricular loop relative to the atrial appendages and the AV canal results in right-sided JAAs (see Fig. 10.3, diagram 3), malposition of the LAA (see Fig. 10.3, diagram 3), and the hypoplastic left heart syndrome (see Fig. 10.13C and Table 10.2).

When the visceroatrial situs inversus is present, the results of ventriculoinfundibulo-arterial malposition in terms of which atrial appendage is malpositioned are the opposite of the foregoing.

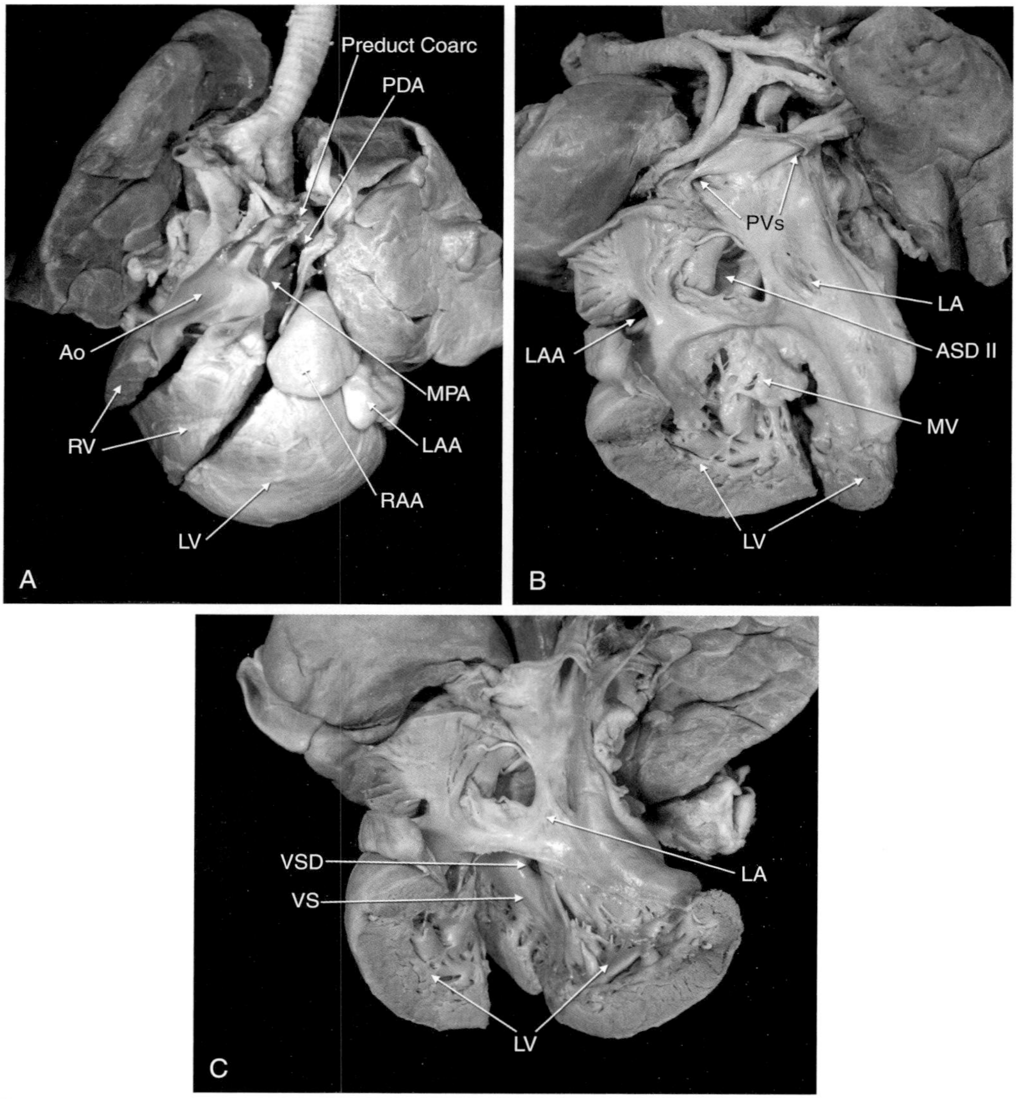

Fig. 10.16 Left-sided juxtaposition of the atrial appendages with solitus atria and malposition of the morphologically right atrial appendage *(RAA)* relative to the great arteries. (A) External frontal view of the heart and lungs of this 9-month-old boy. The patient had transposition of the great arteries (TGA) {S,D,D} with a thick-walled and small-chambered morphologically right ventricle *(RV)*. There was muscular subaortic stenosis, preductal coarctation *(Preduct Coarc)* of the aorta *(Ao)*, and a patent ductus arteriosus *(PDA)*. *LAA,* Left atrial appendage; *LV,* morphologically left ventricle; *MPA,* main pulmonary artery. (B) Opened left atrium *(LA)*, mitral valve *(MV)*, and LV. A large ostium secundum type of atrial septal defect *(ASD II)* is seen. *PVs,* pulmonary veins. (C) Removal of the mitral valve attempts to show the 130-degree angulation between the atrial and the ventricular septa. The atrial septum lay 60 degrees to the left of the sagittal plane (normal ≈ 30 degrees to the left), while the ventricular septum lay 70 degrees to the right of the sagittal plane (normal ≈ 40 degrees to the left). The ventricular septal defect *(VSD)* is also seen. In summary, this patient had TGA {S,D,D}, left-sided juxtaposition of the atrial appendages, malposition of the RAA, thick-walled and small-chambered RV, bilateral conus, subaortic stenosis, preductal coarctation o the aorta, patent ductus arteriosus, leftward displacement of the atrial septum (60 degrees left), marked rightward malposition of the ventricular septum (70 degrees right), huge ventriculoatrial septal angle (130 degrees) (normal ≈10 degrees). This case indicates that not only was there right shift of the ventriculoarterial segments of the heart, but also there was very abnormal ventriculoatrial angulation (ventriculoatrial septal angle = 130 degrees.) The malposition of the ventricles and great arteries relative to the atria and the atrioventricular valves that results in juxtaposition of the atrial appendages is characterized (1) by ***right shift or left shift*** of the ventricles and great arteries relative to the atria, the atrial appendages, and the atrioventricular valves and (2) by ***abnormal angulation*** of the ventricles and the atria in space relative to the sagittal plane and relative to each other. (From Melhuish BPP, Van Praagh R. Juxtaposition of the atrial appendages, a sign of severe cyanotic congenital heart disease. *Br Heart J.* 1968;30:269; reproduced with permission.)

A right-shifted bulboventricular loop results in left-sided JAAs (see Fig. 10.3, diagram 4), but it is the LAA that is malpositioned relative to the great arteries (see Fig. 10.3, diagram 4), and the result is constriction of the outlet of the LA (see Table 10.2).

A left-shifted bulboventricular loop (see Fig. 10.3, diagram 2) results in right-sided JAAs, but with malposition of the RAA and with the syndrome of juxtaposition of the RAA (see Table 10.2), that is, typically the hypoplastic right heart syndrome.

To summarize this section concerning morphogenesis, JAA is a sign of significant ventriculoatrial malalignment (see Fig. 10.3 and 10.13) and of the important malformations that are often associated with it (see Table 10.2).

Distinctive Anatomic Features of JAA. Distinctive anatomic features of JAA are shown in the following figures. Fig. 10.16[21] shows a fairly typical case of JRAA to the left of the great arteries. Why typical? Note that this 9-month-old boy had TGA {S,D,D} with a large secundum type of ASD, a conoventricular type of VSD, a small-chambered and thick-walled RV, and a bilateral conus (subaortic and subpulmonary) with no semilunar-AV fibrous continuity.

More interesting (see Fig. 10.16), the plane of the atrial septum was abnormally leftward, that is, 60 degrees to the left of the sagittal plane as projected on the horizontal plane,[21] the normal atrial septal angle being approximately 30 degrees to the left. The ventricular septal angle was also very abnormal, at 70 degrees to the right of the sagittal plane (as projected on the horizontal plane),[21] the normal ventricular septal angle being approximately 40 degrees to the left. The ventriculoatrial septal angle, instead of being normal (about 10 degrees), was huge, that is, 130 degrees: from 60 degrees left (the atrial septal angle) to 70 degrees right (the ventricular septal angle). In an attempt to show this huge ventriculoatrial septal angle photographically, we excised the anterior mitral leaflet so as to permit visualization of the left ventricular septal surface (see Fig. 10.16C). Very abnormal ventriculoatrial septal angles are typical of JAA because these abnormal angles reflect and quantitate the ventriculoatrial malposition that is the essence of JAA.

It is also noteworthy that the ventricular apex pointed rightward (see Fig. 10.16A). However, this patient's plain posteroanterior chest x-ray did not show dextrocardia. Why not? We think that the reasons were (1) the morphologically RV was small (typical of the JRAA syndrome)[39] and the morphologically LV was large (see Fig. 10.16A).

Thus, **dextrocardia** is not defined as a rightwardly pointing ventricular apex, but as a heart that is predominantly in the right hemithorax (no matter which way the ventricular apex points).

Features less typical of the JRAA syndrome[39] seen in this heart (see Fig. 10.16A) were aortic outflow tract (infundibular) stenosis, preductal coarctation of the aorta, and a patent ductus arteriosus.

In Fig. 10.17,[21] one sees the heart and lungs of a 10-month-old boy with left-sided JRAA. This patient had TGA {S,D,D} with severe tricuspid stenosis (see Fig. 10.17B–C). The widely patent mitral valve and the stenotic tricuspid valve both open into the hypertrophied and enlarged LV (see Fig. 10.17C); that is, double-inlet LV is present. The stenotic tricuspid valve opens into the LV above the VSD (see Fig. 10.17C). Although the subaortic infundibulum is well developed (typical of TGA), the right ventricular sinus (body or inflow tract) is very underdeveloped, resulting in a very small RV (typical of the JRAA syndrome) (see Table 10.2).[39] A bilateral conus was present with a poorly developed subpulmonary component with subpulmonary stenosis (see Fig. 10.17C).

In this patient (see Fig. 10.17), the atrial septal angle was abnormally leftward, at 75 degrees to the left of the sagittal plane (normal ≈30 degrees left), while the ventricular septal angle was 50 degrees to the right of the sagittal plane, resulting in a huge ventriculoatrial septal angle of 125 degrees (75 degrees + 50 degrees) (normal ventriculoatrial septal angle ≈ 10 degrees). This very abnormal ventriculoatrial septal angle (125 degrees) reflects and expresses quantitatively the ventriculoatrial malalignment that is typical of JAA.

Fig. 10.18[21] presents the heart of a 4½-month-old girl with left-sided JRAA. She had DORV {S,D,D} with bilateral conus, pulmonary stenosis (infundibular and valvar, see Fig. 10.18C), and a muscular VSD beneath the right posterior division of the septal band (see Fig. 10.18B).

Clinical and Surgical Relevance of Juxtaposition of the Atrial Appendages

JAA can be diagnosed accurately by angiocardiography, echocardiography, and MRI (Fig. 10.19).[49] Left-sided JRAA in situs solitus often is associated with a flat (nonprotruberant) right heart border in the plain anteroposterior chest x-ray, because the RAA is not right-sided. Instead, as we have seen, the RAA passes from right to left, through the transverse sinus, behind the great arteries, and emerges on the left upper heart border beside and above the LAA. Typically the convex RAA is located to the right and superiorly relative to the LAA. Often, the two convexities of these left-sided juxtaposed appendages can be seen as double convexities of the left upper heart border on the plain posteroanterior chest x-ray film.

As we have seen, left-sided JRAA often is associated with TGA. The presence of TGA in turn may make **balloon atrial septostomy** a desirable interventional procedure, in order to increase interatrial mixing of the systemic and pulmonary venous blood streams before a surgical procedure (atrial or arterial switch). However, as was reported by Tyrrell and Moes[50] in 1971, balloon atrial septostomy in the presence of left-sided JRAA can be much more difficult than usual.

Why? Because the balloon-tipped catheter tends to slip out into the malpositioned RAA as it passes behind the transposed pulmonary artery. Again, why? Because the atrial septum is often not located normally with left-sided JAA. Instead, the atrial septum often occupies an almost coronal (right-left) plane. In order to get the balloon to enter the LA, the catheter tip has to be directed almost straight posteriorly—rather than in the usual right-left direction. Thus, the abnormal plane of the atrial septum, as indicated by the abnormally large atrial septal angles (relative to the sagittal plane) noted heretofore, explain why it can be so difficult to perform a successful balloon atrial septostomy (BAS) in a patient with TGA and left-sided JRAA, unless the abnormally coronal plane of the atrial septum is understood. Once the interventional cardiologist knows where the atrial septum is located in JRAA, BAS becomes relatively easy to perform successfully.

An understanding of the altered atrial anatomy in typical left-sided JRAA also can be important surgically. If a cardiac surgeon wishes to perform an atrial switch operation—either a **Mustard procedure**[51,52] or a **Senning operation,**[53] he or she

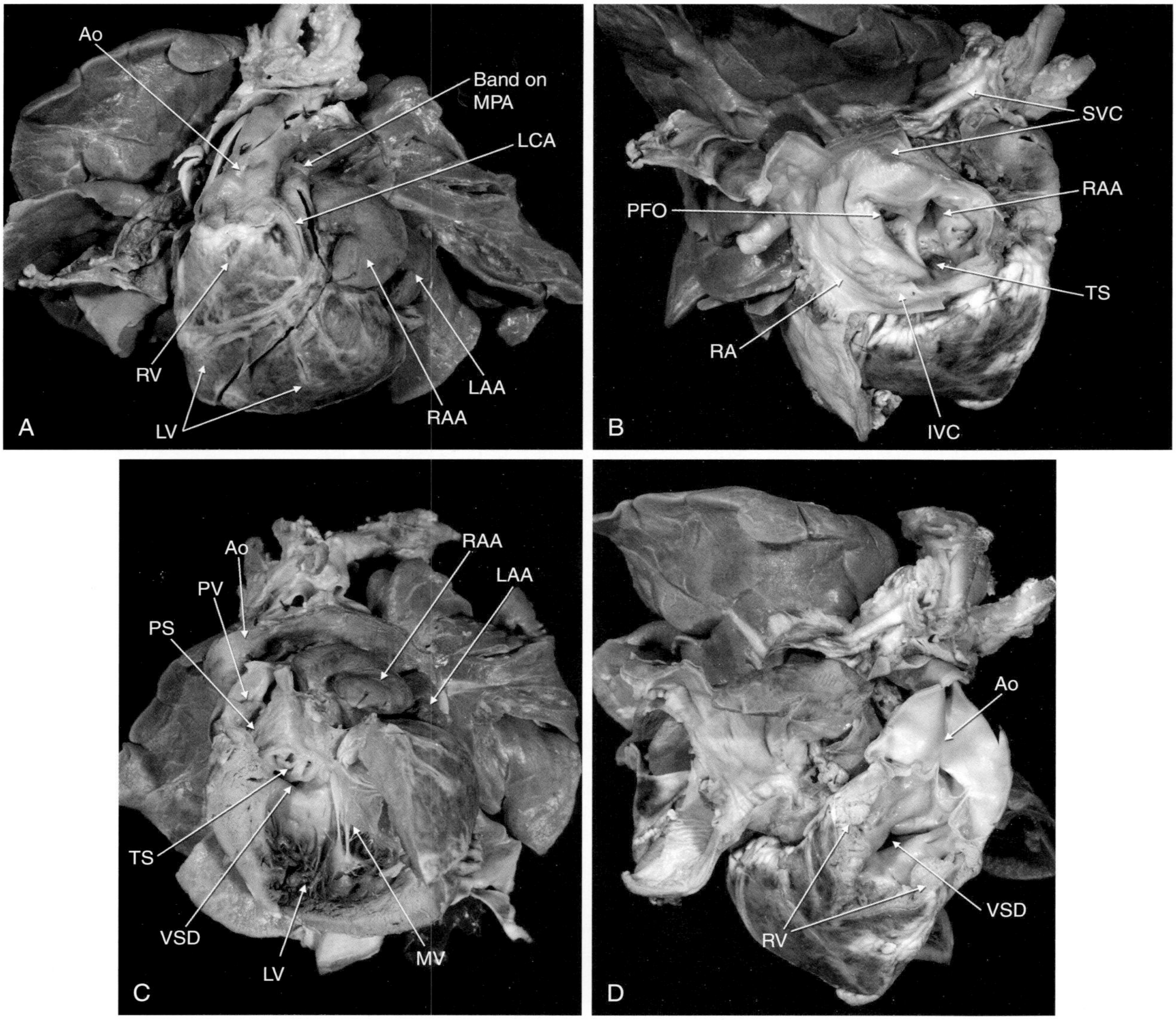

Fig. 10.17 (A) Left-sided juxtaposition of the atrial appendages (JAA), with solitus atria with malposition of the right atrial appendage *(RAA)* relative to the great arteries, anterior view of the heart and lungs. (B) Interior of morphologically right atrium *(RA)*. (C) Interior of morphologically left ventricle *(LV)*. (D) Interior of very small right ventricle *(RV)* and transposed aorta *(Ao)*. This 10-month-old boy had TGA {S,D,D} with single LV (C), absent RV sinus or inflow tract (D), double-inlet LV with severe tricuspid stenosis *(TS)* (B–C), and a subaortic infundibular outlet chamber (D). There was a bilateral conus, with a better developed subaortic component (D) and a less well-developed subpulmonary component (C). The stenotic tricuspid valve opens into the single LV above the ventricular septal defect *(VSD)*, better called the bulboventricular foramen. The small RV (A and D) is really the subaortic infundibular outlet chamber, because the RV sinus (or body, or inflow) is absent. There was subpulmonary stenosis *(PS)* (C); despite this, a band had been placed around this patient's main pulmonary artery *(MPA)* (A). The atrial septum is displaced abnormally far to the left (75 degrees to the left of the sagittal plane, normal ≈ 30 degrees left) (B). The left ventricular septal surface, which is beneath the bulboventricular foramen (VSD) and the stenotic tricuspid valve (TS) in C, lies 50 degrees to the right of the sagittal plane (normal ≈ 40 degrees to the left of the sagittal plane). Thus, the ventriculoatrial septal angle = 125 degrees (the normal ≈ 10 degrees). There is anatomic right shift of the ventriculoarterial parts of the heart resulting in left-sided JAA with malposition of the RAA (as in Fig. 10.3, diagram 1). In addition to ventriculoarterial right-shift, there is abnormal leftward angulation of the atria and abnormal rightward angulation of the ventricular part of the heart. The JAA with malposition of the RAA syndrome (i.e., the hypoplastic right heart syndrome) is present: severe tricuspid stenosis and absence of the RV sinus (inflow tract). *IVC,* Inferior vena cava; *LAA,* left atrial appendage; *LCA,* left coronary artery; *MV,* mitral valve; *PFO,* patent foramen ovale; *PV,* pulmonary valve; *SVC,* superior vena cava. In conclusion, JAA indicates the presence of a major malposition of the ventriculoarterial part of the heart relative to the atria, the atrial appendages, and the atrioventricular valves characterized by relative ventriculoarterial right shift or left shift (see Figs. 10.3 and 10.13), and by abnormal spatial orientations of both the atrial and the ventricular segments of the heart (abnormal atrial and ventricular septal angles relative to the sagittal plane). (From Melhuish BPP, Van Praagh R. Juxtaposition of the atrial appendages, a sign of severe cyanotic congenital heart disease. *Br Heart J.* 1968;30:269; reproduced with permission.)

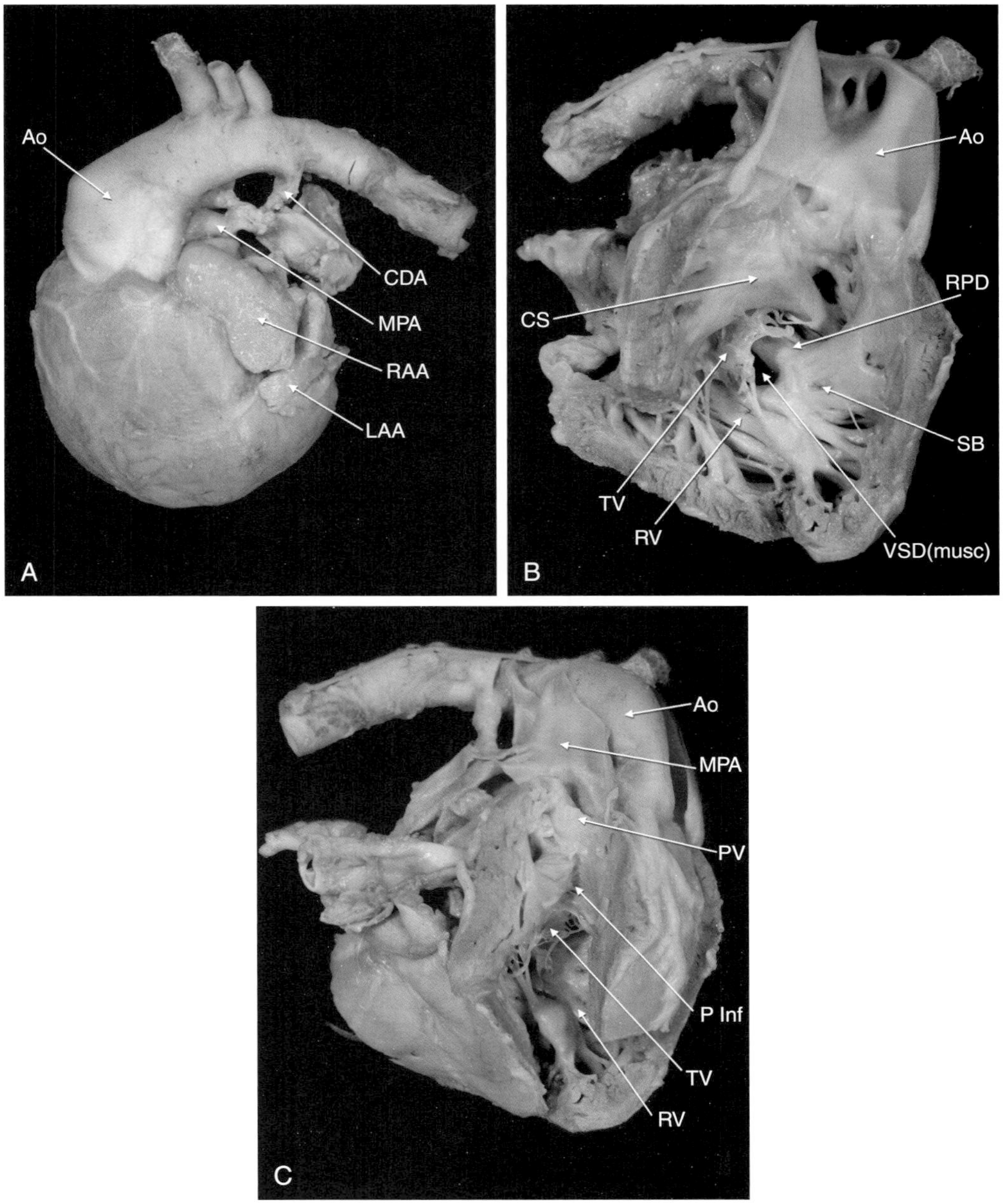

Fig. 10.18 (A) Left-sided juxtaposition of the atrial appendages (JAA), with solitus atria and malposed right atrial appendage *(RAA)* relative to the great arteries, external frontal view. (B) Opened morphologically right ventricle *(RV)* and widely patent outflow tract to D-malposed aorta *(Ao)*. (C) Opened RV and stenotic outflow tract to main pulmonary artery *(MPA)*. Thus, double-outlet right ventricle (DORV) is present. This 4½-month-old girl had DORV {S,D,D} with a bilateral conus, no aortic outflow tract obstruction and pulmonary outflow tract stenosis (PS) at the level of the pulmonary infundibulum *(P Inf)* and pulmonary valve *(PV)*. Only a muscular ventricular septal defect, *VSD(musc)*, was present beneath the right posterior division *(RPD)* of the septal band *(SB)* (B). There was no high conoventricular VSD beneath the conal septum *(CS)*. Note how small the MPA is compared with the ascending Ao (in A), indicating the severity of the PS. The ductus arteriosus was functionally closed *(CDA)* but not ligamentous. There was right shift of the ventriculoarterial part of the heart relative to the atria and the atrial appendages, resulting in left-sided JAA with malposition of the RAA. The atria appeared abnormally leftward in location (A), but it was not possible to measure the atrial septal angle accurately in this specimen. The ventricular septal angle was 25 degrees to the right of the sagittal plane, indicating that the ventricular part of the heart was abnormally rightward (65 degrees too far to the right). *LAA,* Left atrial appendage; *TV,* tricuspid valve. (From Melhuish BPP, Van Praagh R. Juxtaposition of the atrial appendages, a sign of severe cyanotic congenital heart disease. *Br Heart J.* 1968;30:269; reproduced with permission.)

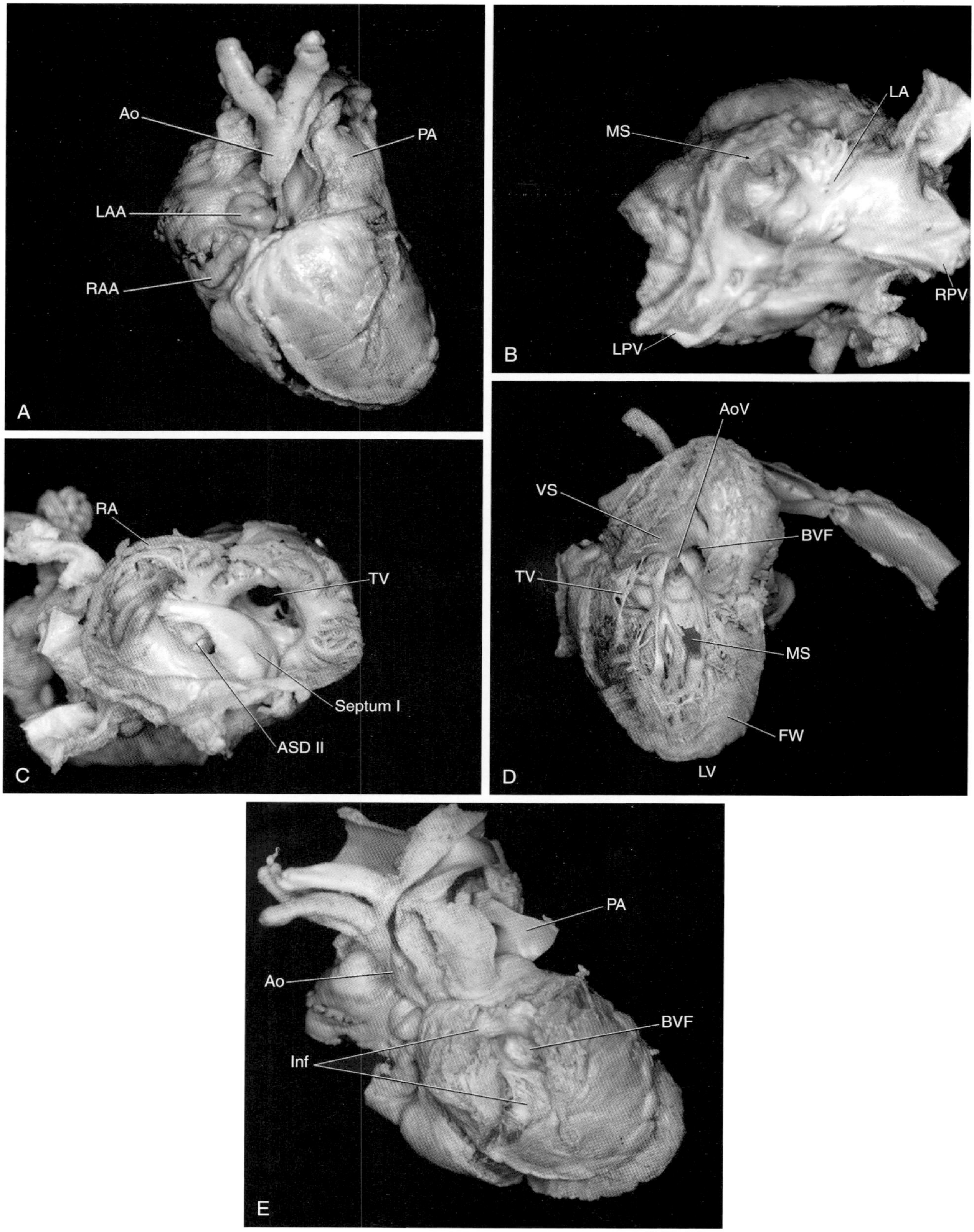

Fig. 10.19 (A) Right-sided juxtaposition of the atrial appendages (JAA) with solitus atria, D-loop ventricles, and solitus normally related great arteries, that is, {S,D,S}, anterior view. The left atrial appendage *(LAA)* is malpositioned to the right of both the ascending aorta *(Ao)* and the main pulmonary artery *(PA)*. The LAA is immediately beside and above the right atrial appendage *(RAA)*. (B) Interior of the single morphologically left ventricle *(LV)* with double-inlet LV. The mitral valve is stenotic *(MS)*, and there is direct fibrous continuity between the aortic valve *(AoV)* and the mitral valve, typical of normally related great arteries. The large tricuspid valve *(TV)* inserted into the papillary musculature of the single LV and into the crest of the ventricular septal remnant *(VS)*. The bulboventricular foramen *(BVF)* leads into the subpulmonary infundibular outflow chamber. The right ventricular sinus (body or inflow tract) is absent, resulting in single LV. The LV free wall *(FW)* is posterior inferior and left-sided, whereas the ventricular septal defect

Continued

Fig. 10.19 cont'd (VSD) remnant is anterior, superior, and right-sided. (D) The interior of the right-sided morphologically right atrium *(RA)* reveals an aneurismal septum primum *(Septum I)*, bulging into the RA cavity reflecting the severely stenotic MS. The secundum atrial septal defect *(ASD II)* above the Septum I has been enlarged surgically. The large right-sided TV is seen from above. In summary, this is a Holmes heart, that is, single LV with infundibular outlet chamber and solitus normally related great arteries, or {S,D,S} with congenital mitral stenosis, double-inlet LV, and rightward bulging aneurysm of septum primum. The rare finding is right-sided JAA with malposition of the LAA, reflecting left shift of the ventriculoarterial part of the heart relative to the atria and the AV canal (similar to Fig. 10.3, diagram 3). *LA,* Left atrium; *LPV,* left pulmonary vein; *RPV,* right pulmonary vein. (From Van Praagh S, O'Sullivan J, Brili S, Van Praagh R. Juxtaposition of the morphologically left atrial appendage in solitus and inversus atria: A study of 18 postmortem cases. *Am Heart J.* 1996;132:391; reproduced with permission.)

will find that the RA is disadvantageously small, or at least it seems too small. Why? Because the RA is "running away" from the surgeon, as it passes from right to left behind the great arteries. The smallness of the RA that is surgically accessible from the right side makes atrial switch operations technically more difficult to perform than they usually are.[51-53]

Left-sided JRAA frequently is associated with tricuspid atresia or stenosis, which, from a surgical standpoint, brings up the possibility of a **Fontan procedure.**[37,38,54] The pathologic anatomy of JRAA with TGA {S,D,D} appears to favor a direct right atrial–to–pulmonary artery anastomosis as part of a Fontan type of procedure because the RAA passes immediately behind the transposed main pulmonary artery. However, a surgical consensus still has not been reached concerning how best to do a Fontan type procedure. I am not trying to advocate any particularly surgical technique. Instead, I seek only to note the immediate approximation of the anterosuperior wall of the juxtaposed RAA and the posterior wall of the main pulmonary artery and the pulmonary arterial bifurcation—an approximation that perhaps could be exploited surgically. Our cardiologist and cardiac surgical colleagues will of course decide whether or not they wish to use this right atriopulmonary arterial approximation that is part of the pathologic anatomy of the most common form of JAAs (i.e., JRAA).

SUMMARY

So, what really is JAAs? Our best present understanding may be summarized as follows. JAAs indicates the presence of a major malposition of the ventricles, infundibulum, and great arteries relative to the atria, the atrial appendages, and the AV valves, characterized by:

1. right shift or left shift of the ventriculoarterial part of the heart relative to the atria, the atrial appendages, and the AV valves (see Figs. 10.3 and 10.13);
2. abnormal spatial orientation of the atria and the ventricles relative to fixed external coordinates such as the sagittal plane, and relative to each other (see Figs. 10.16, 10.17, 10.18); and
3. frequently associated syndromes (see Table 10.2):
   a. when the morphologically RAA is malpositioned relative to the great arteries, hypoplastic right heart is often present; and
   b. when the morphologically LAA is malpositioned relative to the great arteries, hypoplastic left heart frequently coexists.

Diagnostically, when JAA is present it is helpful to determine which atrial appendage is malposed relative to the great arteries. Is it the morphologically RAA that is malposed (see Figs. 10.2, 10.4, 10.8, 10.9, 10.11, and 10.16 to 10.18)? Or is it the morphologically LAA that is malposed (see Figs. 10.1, 10.5, 10.6, 10.7, 10.10, 10.14, 10.15, and 10.19)? Once the morphologic anatomic identity of the malposed appendage has been diagnosed, one may search specifically for the frequently associated syndrome.

There are **four anatomic types of JAAs,** two in atrial situs solitus and two in atrial situs inversus (see Fig. 10.3):

1. When the atria are in situs solitus, right shift of the ventricles and great arteries relative to the atria and the AV valves results in (or is associated with) left-sided juxtaposition, with malposition of the right atrial appendage relative to the great arteries (see diagram 1).
2. When the atria are in situs solitus, left shift of the ventricles and great arteries relative to the atria and the AV valves results in (or is associated with) right-sided juxtaposition, with malposition of the LAA relative to the great arteries (see diagram 3).
3. When the atria are in situs inversus, left-shift of the ventricle and great arteries relative to the atria and the AV valves results in (or is associated with) right-sided juxtaposition, with malposition of the RAA relative to the great arteries (see diagram 2).
4. When the atria are in situs inversus, right shift of the ventricles and the great arteries relative to the atria and the AV valves results in (or is associated with) left-sided juxtaposition, with malposition of the LAA (see diagram 4).

In Fig. 10.3, note that diagrams 1 and 2 are mirror images in terms of the direction of ventriculoarterial shift and the sidedness of the juxtaposition. Diagrams 1 and 2 also show the two anatomic types of juxtaposition with malposition of the right atrial appendage relative to the great arteries: one in situs solitus, to the left of the great arteries; and one in situs inversus, to the right of the great arteries.

In Fig. 10.3, diagrams 3 and 4 are also mirror images in terms of the direction of ventriculoarterial shift and the sidedness of the juxtaposition. There are two anatomic types of juxtaposition with malposition of the LAA: one in situs solitus, to the right of the great arteries, and one in situs inversus, to the left of the great arteries.

In the interest of maximal possible simplicity, many other important anatomic variables have been omitted intentionally from this classification of JAAs: visceral heterotaxy, the state of the spleen, the location of the heart (e.g., dextrocardia or mesocardia), the status of the AV valves, the type of ventricular loop (D- or L-), and other important associated malformations (e.g., single ventricle, pulmonary outflow tract stenosis, or atresia). However, all of these important variables are included in each case that is presented in the figures.

The salient conclusion from the present study is that JAA indicates the presence of a major malposition of the ventricles and great arteries relative to the atria, the atrial appendages, and the AV valves. The ventriculoarterial malpositions that result in JAAs are major and complex, but readily comprehensible and diagnosable. The two opposite syndromes, which frequently are associated with juxtaposition depending on which atrial appendage is malposed relative to the great arteries, help to make the important associated malformations comprehensible and predictable.

Conclusions

Here is what one needs to know about JAA:

Typical JAA is caused by underdevelopment of ventricular loop formation (hypolooping). D-looping occurs in two steps:

- looping to the right, often resulting in dextrocardia; and
- then the ventricular apex normally swings to the left, resulting in mesocardia or normal levocardia.

If step two does not occur, then both ventricles are abnormally rightward. Judged to be the normally located atrioventricular ostia, the ventricular septum is in the middle of the tricuspid orifice (Fig. 10.13B). Similarly in Fig. 10.13, both great arteries that arise from the right shifted ventricles are shown to arise to the right at both atrial appendages.

Left-sided JAA = right-shifted ventricles. Left-side JAA also indicates that the whole left ventricular loop may be sick. The following congenital candidate anomalies *with JAA* were all statistically significantly more frequent than were congenital cardiac anomalies *without JAA* (Table 10.4): dextrocardia, anatomically corrected malposition of the great arteries, patent foramen ovale, secundum ASD, tricuspid atresia and severe stenosis, ventricular septal defect, small or absent RV sinus, bilateral conus, subaortic conus; pulmonary outflow tract obstruction, and aortic outflow tract obstruction.

REFERENCES

1. Thore M. Note sur une anomalie du coeur chez un enfant nouveau-né. *Arch Gén Méd.* 1843;1:199.
2. Birmingham A. Extreme anomaly of the heart and great vessels. *J Anat Physiol.* 1893;27:139.
3. Wenner O. Beiträge zur Lehre des Herzmissbildungen. *Virchows Arch Pathol Anat Physiol Klin Med.* 1909;196:127.
4. Dünner L. Zur Klinik und pathologischen Anatomie der angeborenen Herzfehler. *Z Klin Med.* 1914;80:217.
5. Huebschmann P. Zwei Fälle von seltener Herzmissbildung (sogenannter Trikuspidalverschluss). *Verh Deutsch Ges Path.* 1921;18:174.
6. Kettler L. Ein besonders gearteter Fall von Transposition der grossen Gefässe. *Virchows Arch.* 1933;287:10.
7. Ngai SK. Congenital anomaly of the heart, report of a case with embryological discussion. *Am J Pathol.* 1935;11:309.
8. Bredt H. Formdeutung und entstehung des missgebildeten menschlichen herzens. I-V. *Virchows Arch.* 1936;296:114.
9. Harris JS, Farber S. Transposition of the great cardiac vessels with special reference to the phylogenetic theory of Spitzer. *Arch Pathol.* 1939;28:427.
10. Taussig HB. *Congenital Malformations of the Heart.* New York: The Commonwealth Fund; 1947:510.
11. Miskall EW, Fraser JA. Complete transposition of the great cardiac vessels. *Ohio State Med J.* 1948;44:709.
12. Rogers HM, Cordes JH, Edwards JE. Congenital tricuspid atresia in a boy twelve years of age. *Am J Dis Child.* 1950;80:427.
13. Dixon ASJ. Juxtaposition of the atrial appendages: two cases of an unusual congenital cardiac deformity. *Br Heart J.* 1954;16:153.
14. Edwards JE, Dry TJ, Parker RL, Burchell HB, Wood EH, Bulbulian AH. *An Atlas of Congenital Anomalies of the Heart and Great Vessels.* Springfield, Illinois: Thomas; 1954:100–101.
15. Smyth NPD. Lateroposition of the atrial appendages. a case of levoposition of the appendages. *AMA Arch Pathol.* 1955;60:259.
16. Polanco GB, Powell AM. Unusual combination of cardiac anomalies in a case of isolated dextrocardia. *Am Heart J.* 1955;49:102.
17. Stewart AM, Wynn-Williams A. Combined tricuspid and pulmonary atresia with juxtaposition of the auricles. *Br J Radiol.* 1956;29:326.
18. Fragoyannis SG, Nickerson D. An unusual congenital anomaly, tricuspid atresia, aortic atresia, and juxtaposition of atrial appendages. *Am J Cardiol.* 1960;6:678.
19. Ellis K, Jameson AG. Congenital levoposition of the right atrial appendage. *Am J Roentgen Rad Therap Nuclear Med.* 1963;89:984.
20. Edwards JE, Carey LS, Neufeld HN, Lester RG. Congenital heart disease. *Correlation of Pathologic Anatomy and Angiocardiography.* Philadelphia: Saunders Co; 1963:353.
21. Melhuish BPP, Van Praagh R. Juxtaposition of the atrial appendages, a sign of severe cyanotic congenital heart disease. *Br Heart J.* 1968;30:269.
22. Wagner HR, Alday LE, Vlad P. Juxtaposition of the atrial appendages, a report of six necropsied cases. *Circulation.* 1970;42:157.
23. Becker AE, Becker MJ. Juxtaposition of atrial appendages associated with normally oriented ventricle and great arteries. *Circulation.* 1970;41:685.
24. Charuzi Y, Spanos RK, Amplatz K, Edwards JE. Juxtaposition of the atrial appendages. *Circulation.* 1973;47:620.
25. Hunter AS, Henderson CB, Urquhart W, Farmer MB. Left-sided juxtaposition of the atrial appendages. Report of 4 cases diagnosed by cardiac catheterization and angiocardiography. *Br Heart J.* 1973;35:1184.
26. Deutsch V, Shem-Tov A, Yahini JH, Neufeld HN. Juxtaposition of atrial appendages: angiocardiographic observations. *Am J Cardiol.* 1974;34:240.
27. Rosenquist GC, Stark J, Taylor JFN. Juxtaposition of the atrial appendages. *Ann Thorac Surg.* 1974;18:456.
28. Mathew R, Replogle R, Thilenius OG, Arcilla RA. Right juxtaposition of the atrial appendages. *Chest.* 1975;57:483.
29. Park MK, Chang CHJ, Vaseenon T. Congenital levojuxtaposition of the right atrial appendage. Association with persistent truncus arteriosus, type 4. *Chest.* 1976;69:550.
30. Anderson RH, Smith A, Wilkinson JL. Right juxtaposition of the auricular appendages. *Eur J Cardiol.* 1976;4:495.

31. Allwork SP, Urban AE, Anderson RH. Left juxtaposition of the auricles with l-position of the aorta, report of 6 cases. *Br Heart J.* 1977;39:299.
32. Otero-Coto E, Wilkinson JL, Dickinson DF, Rufilanchas JJ, Márquez J. Gross distortion of atrioventricular and ventriculoarterial relations associated with left juxtaposition of atrial appendages. Bizarre form of atrioventricular criss-cross. *Br Heart J.* 1979;41:486.
33. Maître Azcárate MJ, Quero Jiménez M, Cabrera Duro A, Berrazeuta JR, Otero Coto E. Juxtaposition of the atrial appendages. Pathologic-anatomic findings in 15 cases and review of the literature. *Herz.* 1980;5:339.
34. Rice MJ, Seward JB, Hagler DJ, Edwards WD, Julsrud PR, Tajik AJ. Left juxtaposed atrial appendages: diagnostic two-dimensional echocardiographic features. *J Am Coll Cardiol.* 1983;1:1330.
35. Chin AJ, Bierman FZ, Williams RG, Sanders SP, Lang P. 2-dimensional echocardiographic appearance of complete left-sided juxtaposition of the atrial appendages. *Am J Cardiol.* 1983;52:346.
36. Seo JW, Choe GY, Chi JG. An unusual ventricular loop associated with right juxtaposition of the atrial appendages. *Int J Cardiol.* 1989;25:219.
37. Anjos RT, Ho SY, Anderson RH. Surgical implications of juxtaposition of the atrial appendages. A review of forty-nine autopsied hearts. *J Thorac Cardiovasc Surg.* 1990;99:897.
38. Leu M-R, Chiu I-S, Hung C-R, Wu M-H. Surgical implications of juxtaposed atrial appendages and the associated anomalies. *Ann Thorac Surg.* 1992;54:134.
39. Van Praagh S, O'Sullivan J, Brili S, Van Praagh R. Juxtaposition of the morphologically right atrial appendage in solitus and inversus atria: a study of 35 postmortem cases. *Am Heart J.* 1996;132:382.
40. Van Praagh S, O'Sullivan J, Brili S, Van Praagh R. Juxtaposition of the morphologically left atrial appendage in solitus and inversus atria: a study of 18 postmortem cases. *Am Heart J.* 132:391.
41. Van Praagh R, David I, Gordon D, Wright GB, Van Praagh S. Ventricular diagnosis and designation. In: Godman MJ, ed. *Pediatric Cardiology.* World Congress London 1980; Vol. 4. Edinburgh: Churchill Livingstone; 1981:153.
42. Anderson RH, Smith A, Wilkinson JL. Disharmony between atrioventricular connections and segmental combination, unusual variants of "crisscross" hearts. *J Am Coll Cardiol.* 1987;10:1273.
43. Van Praagh R. When concordant or discordant atrioventricular alignments predict the ventricular situs wrongly. I. Solitus atria, concordant alignments, and L-loop ventricles. II. Solitus atria, discordant alignments, and D-loop ventricles. *J Am Coll Cardiol.* 1987;10:1278.
44. Weinberg PM, Van Praagh R, Wagner HR, Cuaso CC. *New Form of Criss-Cross Atrioventricular Relation: An Expanded View of the Meaning of D- and L-Loops.* London: World Congress of Paediat Cardiol; 1980; abstract 319.
45. Geva T, Sanders SP, Ayres NA, O'Laughlin MP, Parness IA. Two-dimensional echocardiographic anatomy of atrioventricular alignment discordance with situs concordance. *Am Heart J.* 1993;125:459.
46. Foran RB, Belcourt C, Nanton MA, et al. Isolated infundibuloarterial inversion {S,D,I}: a newly recognized form of congenital heart disease. *Am Heart J.* 1988;116:1337.
47. Abbott ME. Transposition or reversed torsion of the arterial trunks. In: Osler W and McCrae T, eds. *Modern Medicine.* Vol. 4. Philadelphia, Lea & Febiger Co. 1913:716.
48. Streeter GL. *Developmental Horizons in Human Embryos, Age Groups XI to XXIII.* Vol. II. Washington DC: Carnegie Inst; 1951; Embryology Reprint.
49. Freedom RM, Mawson JB, Yoo S-J, Benson LN. Juxtaposition of atrial appendages and abnormalities of the right atrial wall, congenital heart disease. Textbook of Angiocardiography. Armonk, NY: Futura Publishing Co, Inc; 1997:339.
50. Tyrrell MJ, Moes CAF. Congenital levoposition of the right atrial appendage. *Am J Dis Child.* 1971;121:508.
51. Urban AE, Stark J, Waterston DJ. Mustard's operation for transposition of the great arteries complicated by juxtaposition of the atrial appendages. *Ann Thorac Surg.* 1976;21:304.
52. Wood AE, Freedom RM, Williams WG, Trusler GA. The Mustard procedure in transposition of the great arteries associated with juxtaposition of the atrial appendages with and without dextrocardia. *J Thorac Cardiovasc Surg.* 1983;85:451.
53. Dihmis WC, Eldrige J, Jordan SC, Wisheart JD. Modification of the Senning repair in a case of transposition of the great arteries with juxtaposition of the atrial appendages. *Eur J Cardio Thorac Surg.* 1995;9:50.
54. Thoele DG, Ursell PC, Ho SY, et al. Atrial morphologic features in tricuspid atresia. *J Thorac Cardiovasc Surg.* 1991;102:606.
55. Pessotto R, Padalino M, Rubino M, Kadoba K, Büchler JR, Van Praagh R. Straddling tricuspid valve as a sign of ventriculoatrial malalignment: a morphometric study of 19 postmortem cases. *Am Heart J.* 1999;138:1184.

11

Common Atrioventricular Canal

Definition. The anomaly known as common atrioventricular canal (or atrioventricular septal defect) is characterized anatomically by incomplete separation of the atrioventricular canal into mitral and tricuspid canals. Hence, the atrioventricular canal is incompletely subdivided, or in common.

The morphology and classification of these malformations are described in detail below. But first we should mention the history and terminology of these anomalies.

History and terminology. Common atrioventricular canal has been known for more than a century. In 1899, Griffith[1] presented an "example of a large opening between the two auricles of the heart, unconnected with the fossa ovalis." This was an ostium primum type of atrial septal defect, a partial form of common atrioventricular canal. Griffith[1] wrote that a Dr. Norman Moore had presented such a case to the Pathology Society of London in 1881.

In 1936, Maude Abbott[2] of McGill University in Montreal, Canada, described the "ostium primum atrial septal defect" and the "common atrioventricular canal defect." Following World War II, in 1948, Rogers and Edwards[3] at the Mayo Clinic in Rochester, Minnesota, recognized that incomplete division of the atrioventricular canal resulted in patency of the interatrial foramen primum, also known as *persistent common atrioventricular ostium*. They reported five cases and reviewed the literature. The older Latin name of this malformation had been *atrioventricularis communis*, persistent common atrioventricular ostium being an English translation. By 1956 and 1958, Wakai and Edwards[4,5] had described and classified *persistent common atrioventricular canal* into *complete*, *partial*, and *transitional* forms.[6]

As is shown under Morphology and Classification, the *complete* form of common atrioventricular canal has a complete atrioventricular septal defect and a common atrioventricular valve. The *partial* form typically has an ostium primum type of atrial septal defect—which is a partial atrioventricular septal defect—and a cleft anterior leaflet of the mitral valve, but no ventricular septal defect. The *transitional* form characteristically is like the partial form of common atrioventricular canal, except that in addition there are one or more small ventricular septal defects beneath the anterior and/or posterior endocardial cushion components of the cleft anterior leaflet of the mitral valve. Hence, the *transitional* form is an "almost" incomplete form, except that it also has one or more tiny ventricular septal defects.

Thus, by the mid to late 1950s, Dr. Jesse Edwards and his colleagues[4-6] had made a very good start toward the description and classification of the anomalies that they called common atrioventricular canal.

At about the same time in London, England, Bedford and his colleagues—one of whom was Dr. Walter Somerville—coined the term *atrioventricular defect* for these anomalies, as was later recounted by Dr. Jane Somerville[7] in 1968. Hence, it is not too surprising that the British pediatric cardiology community tended to prefer the designation *atrioventricular defect,* which was used by Piccoli et al[8] in 1979.

However, by 1982, our British colleagues[9,10] had concluded that Bedford and Somerville's term *atrioventricular defect* should be modified to *atrioventricular septal defect,* perhaps in order to make it more specific, and this remains their preference to this day.

It is noteworthy that the designation *atrioventricular (AV) septal defect* is an example of medical *synecdoche*. Linguistically, synecdoche is a figure of speech in which a part is used to represent a whole, or vice versa. AV septal defect, which is part of common AV canal, is used to represent the whole anomaly, which typically has both septal and leaflet malformations.

Another widely used term for common atrioventricular canal is *endocardial cushion defect*. This designation is somewhat passé now, probably because it is so very nonspecific. Almost any anomaly of the atrioventricular valves can be regarded as an endocardial cushion defect. Tricuspid atresia, stenosis, regurgitation, and Ebstein's anomaly may all be regarded as different kinds of endocardial cushion defect. So, too, can mitral atresia, stenosis, and regurgitation. But none of the aforementioned malformations has of necessity common atrioventricular canal. Thus, although common atrioventricular canal is an endocardial cushion defect, the latter term is far too broad and nonspecific to denote the anomalies that we are considering precisely.

We prefer the term *common atrioventricular (AV) canal* for several reasons. This designation includes both the septal defect component and the leaflet malformation component of this anomaly. In other words, common AV canal includes much more than an AV septal defect. Surgically, the leaflet malformations are the more difficult part of common AV canal.

Proponents of the AV septal defect terminology agree with the foregoing, of course, and they consequently are now talking and writing about *AV septal defect with a common AV valve,* and *AV septal defect with two AV valves,*[11] a considerable improvement, we think.

Bharati, Lev, and their colleagues have always preferred *common atrioventricular orifice,*[12] which is very close to Edwards' common atrioventricular canal.

In addition to the brevity, accuracy, and inclusiveness (septal and leaflet anomalies) of Edwards' designation, we think it appropriate to honor the pioneer who first described and classified these anomalies[3-6] by using his terminology. If there were something wrong with this designation *common AV canal,* then it should be changed. But this is not the case: it is brief, anatomically accurate, and all-inclusive—embracing both the septal and the leaflet malformations.

What about *common AV canal defect?*[13] This, too, is very close to Dr. Jesse Edwards' original designation. We think that *defect* is redundant: common AV canal is obviously a defect. No one thinks we are talking about human embryos, in which a common AV canal is normal prior to Streeter's horizon XVII, that is, prior to 34 to 36 days of gestational age. Earlier than horizon XVII in humans, common AV canal is not a defect; it is normal. But thereafter, common AV canal is a defect, as is generally understood. Thus, the term *AV canal defect* is certainly not wrong. However, our preference is to avoid redundancy in medical terminology whenever possible.

It should also be understood that not all partial forms of common AV canal have an AV septal defect. For example, isolated cleft of the mitral valve can have a cleft of the AV canal type, but without an AV septal defect. This means that *AV septal defect* is not a fully satisfactory common denominator for the entire spectrum of common AV canal.

From a developmental viewpoint, *common AV canal* really means that the superior and inferior endocardial cushions of the AV canal are *not completely fused in the normal way.* It must be remembered that the concept of common AV canal includes both the septal defect and the leaflet defect components. Consequently, *isolated cleft of the mitral valve of the AV canal type* represents a partial form of this anomaly in the sense that the superior and inferior endocardial cushions are not completely fused in the normal way.

From the anatomic standpoint, however, *isolated cleft of the mitral valve of the AV canal type* is *not* a partial form of common AV canal in the sense that the AV canal is completely divided into mitral and tricuspid canals.

Conversely, not all AV septal defects[14] have common AV canal. For example, left ventricular-to-right atrial shunting (Gerbode defect) has a hole in the AV portion of the membranous septum. This is why left ventricular-to-right atrial shunt has been called an AV septal defect.[14] But this type of AV septal defect is very different from that seen in common AV canal.

In somewhat greater detail, although the so-called **Gerbode defect** has been regarded as a defect in the AV portion of pars membranacea septi,[14] in our experience this membranous ventricular septal defect (VSD) really does not extend above the tricuspid annulus. The Gerbode defect does not have an ostium primum defect component. Instead, the blood shunts through and between the tricuspid valve leaflets and their chordal attachments at the anteriosuperior commissure of the tricuspid valve. Not all membranous VSDs have left ventricular-to-right atrial shunting. Those that do (Gerbode defects) have an incompletely occlusive anterosuperior commissure of the tricuspid valve. The tricuspid component of the Gerbode defect is indeed *above* the membranous VSD component. This is why Gerbode defects have been described as having an *atrio*ventricular septal defect. However, this atrioventricular septal defect is very different from that seen in common AV canal, as mentioned. In the typical membranous VSD, the anterior leaflet of the tricuspid valve closes the anterosuperior commissure. This portion of the anterior tricuspid leaflet bulges upward, forming a tricuspid pouch—produced by the left-to-right jet of blood striking the ventricular side of the anterior tricuspid leaflet.

Thus, the real difference between a typical membranous VSD and a Gerbode defect is not the nature of the septal defect. Both have membranous VSDs. But, in addition, the Gerbode defect has an incompetent (regurgitant) anterosuperior commissure of the tricuspid valve. Consequently, we think that the Gerbode defect should **not** be regarded as an AV septal defect.

To summarize, the foregoing are the reasons why we think that it is very difficult to improve on *common atrioventricular canal* as the name for the fascinating malformations that we are about to consider. To the best of our present knowledge, the term and concept of *common AV canal* is the only one that includes all forms of this anomaly, and excludes all malformations that are not part of the spectrum of common AV canal.

We also fully understand and respect the preferences of others: AV septal defect is an important part of common AV canal. The complete form of common AV canal certainly does have a common AV orifice. And common AV canal is indeed an endocardial cushion defect. All of the foregoing terms should be understood.

However, the main focus of this chapter—and of this book—is not terminology, but data. This chapter presents a detailed study of 443 postmortem cases of complete and partial forms of common AV canal. But first we must consider morphology and classification in greater detail.

MORPHOLOGY AND CLASSIFICATION

1. **The complete form**[6] of common AV canal typically has a complete AV septal defect, that is, an ostium primum type of atrial septal defect lying above and behind the leaflets of a common AV valve, which is confluent with a VSD of the AV canal or inlet type lying below and in front of the leaflets of the common AV valve (Fig. 11.1).
2. **The partial form**[6] of common AV canal typically has a partial AV septal defect, usually an ostium primum type of atrial septal defect (ASD), with no VSD of the AV canal type, and with a cleft in the anterior leaflet of the mitral valve.
3. **The transitional form**[6] of common AV canal is like the partial form, except that it has a few small interstices between the fibrous attachments of the leaflets of the mitral and tricuspid valves to the crest of the muscular ventricular septum. These few small interstices result in a very small restrictive ventricular septal defect(s) of the AV canal type. As mentioned, the transitional form of common AV canal lies between the complete and partial forms. The VSD of the AV canal type has been obliterated almost totally, so that the development of the AV canal has proceeded almost to the partial common AV canal stage; hence the transitional form is *almost* a partial common AV canal—except for the coexistence of a few small, slit-like VSDs.
4. **The intermediate form**[15] of common AV canal indicates the rare type in which the superior (anterior) and inferior

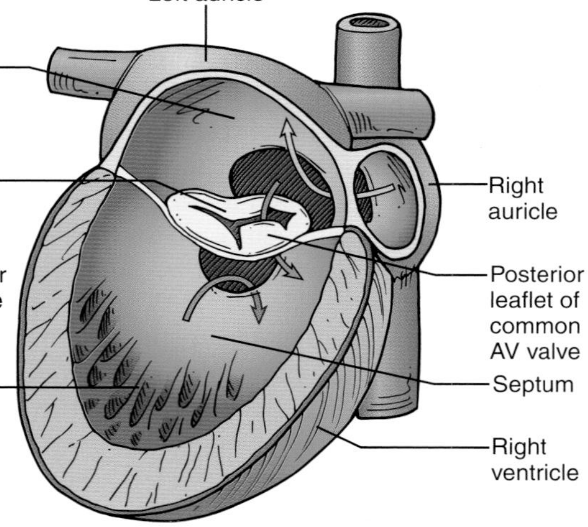

Fig. 11.1 Complete type of common atrioventricular canal. The posterior wall of the left atrium and the posterolateral wall of the left ventricle have been removed. The heart is seen from a left and posterior viewpoint. Note the anterior surface of the left ventricle for orientation. The atrioventricular *(AV)* canal extends from the atrial septum above to the ventricular septum below, and from the origin of the right lateral leaflets to the origin of the left lateral leaflet of the common AV valve. Medially at the septa, the AV canal consists of three components: (1) the lower atrial septum, (2) the AV valve, and (3) the upper ventricular septum. The AV canal is completely in common or undivided. The defect in the lower atrial septum is known as an ostium primum type of atrial septal defect (marked by a yellow arrow from right atrium to left atrium). The AV valve is in common or undivided (shown by the green atrioventricular arrow). The common AV valve consists of five leaflets: a bridging anterosuperior leaflet, a bridging posteroinferior leaflet, two right lateral leaflets, and one left lateral leaflet. The upper ventricular septum is also in common or undivided (shown by the purple arrow from the LV to the RV). This opening is known as a ventricular septal defect of the AV canal type. The ostium primum type of ASD is confluent with the AV valve from above. The VSD of the AV canal type is confluent with the AV valve from below. The ostium primum type of ASD and the VSD of the AV canal type are confluent with each other through the opening of the common AV valve during atrial systole (ventricular diastole), but usually not during ventricular systole (atrial diastole), if the common AV valve is competent. The confluent ASD primum plus VSD of the AV canal type are collectively known as an atrioventricular septal defect, that is, a defect in the septum of the AV canal. An atrioventricular septal defect typically is not present in partial forms of common AV canal, that is, with an ASD primum only, but with no VSD; or with a VSD of the AV canal type only, but with no ASD primum. Partial forms of common AV canal typically have a partial AV septal defect, but not always (e.g., isolated cleft of the mitral valve of the AV canal type). An AV septal defect is seen in the complete type of common AV canal, as shown here, and also in the transitional and intermediate types. *Auricle* is now called *atrium*. *Ant,* Anterior; *ASD,* atrial septal defect; *AV,* atrioventricular; *Lt,* left; *LV,* left ventricle; *Rt,* right; *RV,* right ventricle; *VSD,* ventricular septal defect. (From Rogers HM, Edward JE: Incomplete division of the AV canal with patent interatrial foramen primum [persistent common AV ostium]; report of five cases and review of the literature. *Am Heart J* 36:28, 1948, with permission.)

(posterior) leaflets of the common AV valve (Fig.11.1) have fused in the midline, dividing the common AV valve into left-sided and right-sided AV valves. In addition to a large ostium primum type of ASD, the rare feature is the coexistence of what can be a large VSD of the AV canal type. As Dr. Dwight McGoon commented to me as we were both examining heart specimens of the intermediate type at one of Dr. Maurice Lev's exhibits at a meeting of the American Heart Association, "The VSD is big enough to drive a Mack truck through." Usually, when the superior and inferior leaflets of the common AV valve have fused in the midline, the VSD component is absent (as in the partial form of common AV canal), or very small (as in the transitional form). This is why the intermediate form is rare.

5. **The left ventricular type**[12,15] of common AV canal indicates that the common AV valve opens predominantly into the morphologically left ventricle (LV). This in turn indicates that the morphologically right ventricle (RV) is hypoplastic or absent, which is why the common AV valve opens predominantly or entirely into the LV. This is also known as the **LV dominant type** of common AV canal.
6. **The right ventricular type**[12,15] of common AV canal means that the common AV valve opens predominantly or entirely into the RV—because the LV is hypoplastic or absent. This is also known as the **RV dominant type** of common AV canal.
7. **The balanced form**[12,15] of common AV canal indicates that the common AV valve opens approximately equally into the RV and the LV. This in turn means that both the RV and the LV are well developed. When the AV canal is described as **unbalanced to the left,**[12,15] this means that the common AV valve opens predominantly into the LV. Hence, unbalanced to the left is synonymous with the LV type of common AV canal.

Similarly, when the AV canal is described as **unbalanced to the right,**[12,15] this means that the common AV valve opens predominantly into the RV. Consequently, unbalanced to the right is synonymous with the RV type of common AV canal.

The LV type of common AV canal, or AV canal unbalanced to the left, indicates that the common AV valve is predominantly left-sided with D-loop ventricles, but predominantly right-sided with L-loop ventricles—because the LV is left-sided with a D-loop and right-sided with an L-loop.

Similarly, the RV type of common AV canal, or a common AV canal unbalanced to the right, means that the common AV valve is right-sided with D-loop ventricles (because the RV is right-sided), but left-sided with L-loop ventricles (because the RV is left-sided).

Hence, the right-sided and left-sided types of common AV canal are used *morphologically,* not positionally. The morphologically RV may be right-sided (D-loop ventricles) or left-sided (L-loop ventricles), and the morphologically LV may be left-sided (D-loop ventricles) or right-sided (L-loop ventricles).

It is also noteworthy that it is not the common AV valve or the common AV canal that is unbalanced. Instead, it is the development of the ventricles that is unbalanced. Hence, in so-called unbalanced common AV canal, one may say (with a wink) that it is not the AV canal that needs to see the psychiatrist. It's the ventricles.

It should be pointed out that the right ventricular type and the left ventricular type of unbalanced common AV canal were two of Dr. Maurice Lev's[12] most important contributions to the understanding of common AV canal. Another was the description of the intermediate type of common AV canal.[15] In both of these achievements, Dr. Saroja Bharati[12,15] played a significant role.

In the complete form of common AV canal, the **Rastelli classification**[16] is widely used and hence merits description:

In **type A,** the superior (anterior) leaflet of the common AV valve is divided and attached to the crest of the muscular ventricular septum (Fig. 11.2).

In **type B,** the superior leaflet of the common AV valve is partially divided and is not attached to the ventricular septal crest. Instead, the superior leaflet is attached to the anterior papillary muscle of the right ventricle (Fig. 11.3). Rastelli et al[16] said that the superior leaflet attaches to a papillary muscle that arises from the right ventricular septal surface. In the rare type B, this is how it looks—because the moderator band is so short. Consequently, the anterior papillary muscle of the RV appears to originate directly from the RV septal surface.

In **type C,** the superior leaflet of the common AV valve is undivided and unattached to the ventricular septal crest (Fig. 11.4).

Type A Completely Common AV Canal

In somewhat greater detail, let us carefully examine completely common AV canal *type A* (Fig. 11.2). In Rastelli's drawing (Fig. 11.2A), note that above the ventricular septum, the superior (anterior) leaflet of the common AV valve is divided into two components (A,A), which are attached to the crest of the muscular ventricular septum by numerous short chordae tendineae. The inferior (posterior) leaflet of the common AV valve is also attached to the crest of the muscular ventricular septum by numerous short chordae tendineae. Despite these chordal attachments, a VSD of the AV canal type exists through the chordae tendineae. The components of the mitral valve (MV) and tricuspid valve (TV) are readily recognizable, even though the AV valve is in common (undivided, or unfused in the midline). Note the left-sided and right-sided lateral leaflets (L) of the common AV valve, that lie between the superior (A, A) and the inferior (P) leaflets. The potentially TV opens into the morphologically right ventricle (RV) and the potentially MV opens into the morphologically left ventricle (largely unseen).

Fig. 11.2B shows a photograph of the complete form of common AV canal type A that is very comparable to Rastelli's drawing (Fig. 11.2A). Note the atrioventricular septal defect (D) that lies between the "scooped-out" or concave crest of the muscular ventricular septum anteroinferiorly and the nude margin of the atrial septum posterosuperiorly. The superior leaflet of the common AV valve (S, S) is divided and attached to the crest of the muscular ventricular septum by short chordae tendineae.

How can one be sure that common AV canal is present, given only the right atrial (i.e., surgical) view? Because the anteroinferior rim of the atrial septum is nude or bare. Anteroinferiorly, the atrial septum does not have its tricuspid valve "pants" on: it is naked. Once you see the bare anteroinferior margin of the atrial septum, you know that common AV canal is present. In front of and below this bare rim of the atrial septum lies the AV septal defect, that is, the defect in the septum of the AV canal.

So now you say to yourself, "Okay, a common AV canal is present." The next question is: "Is it a complete type or a partial type of common AV canal?" Can you make this diagnosis from the right atrial view? The answer is yes. Is there a VSD component? If so, this is a complete type of common AV canal—or a complete AV septal defect. Look at the superior leaflet (Fig. 11.2B). You can easily see that a VSD component is present between the short chordae tendineae attaching the superior leaflet to the ventricular septal crest. This VSD component extends in front of or below the divided superior leaflet of the common AV valve. So this definitely is a complete form of common AV canal. And it's a Rastelli type A, because the superior leaflet is divided and attached to the crest of the muscular ventricular septum. The large space behind and above the leaflets of the common AV valve is the ostium primum component of this complete atrioventricular septal defect. Note that the ostium primum type of atrial septal defect and the VSD of the AV canal or inlet type are confluent, which is typical of complete forms of common AV canal.

Is there a VSD beneath the inferior leaflet (I, Fig. 11.2B)? There may or may not be. Often there isn't.

Note also the small ostium secundum type of atrial septal defect, the normal opening of the coronary sinus, and the right atrial and right ventricular hypertrophy and enlargement (Fig. 11.2B).

Hence, it is readily possible for a surgeon to make a highly accurate diagnosis of completely common AV canal type A, given only a right atrial view (Fig. 11.2A).

The left ventricular views in completely common AV canal type A (Figs. 11.2C and D) are also highly informative. These views can be well imaged with two-dimensional and three-dimensional echocardiography and with magnetic resonance imaging (MRI). Again one can see that the divided superior leaflet is attached to the scooped-out crest of the muscular ventricular septum by a thicket of short chordae tendineae. There is a VSD component beneath (in front of, or anterior to) the superior leaflet in both cases (Figs. 11.2C and D). There is a VSD component beneath the inferior leaflet in Fig. 11.2D, but not in Fig. 11.2C.

Note that the inferior leaflet is much closer to the ventricular septal crest than is the superior leaflet. We think that this fact may well be of morphogenetic importance, as is explained subsequently.

It is noteworthy that the left ventricular inlet dimension (from the inferior leaflet component to the left ventricular apex) is much shorter than is the left ventricular outlet dimension (from the left ventricular apex to the aortic valve). This is particularly well seen in Fig. 11.2D, where the ratio of the left ventricular inlet dimension to the left ventricular outlet dimension equals approximately 0.6. Normally, the left ventricular inlet/outlet dimension ratio is approximately 1.0. This marked shortening of the left ventricular inlet dimension relative to the left ventricular outlet dimension is characteristic of common AV canal, both complete and incomplete. This typical shortening of the left ventricular inlet dimension contributes to the aforementioned "scooped-out" appearance, and reflects failure of formation of the septum of the AV canal, which contributes to the inlet part of the normal definitive interventricular septum.

The outlet portion of the septum also is not normal. Although approximately normal in apex-base length, the outlet part of the

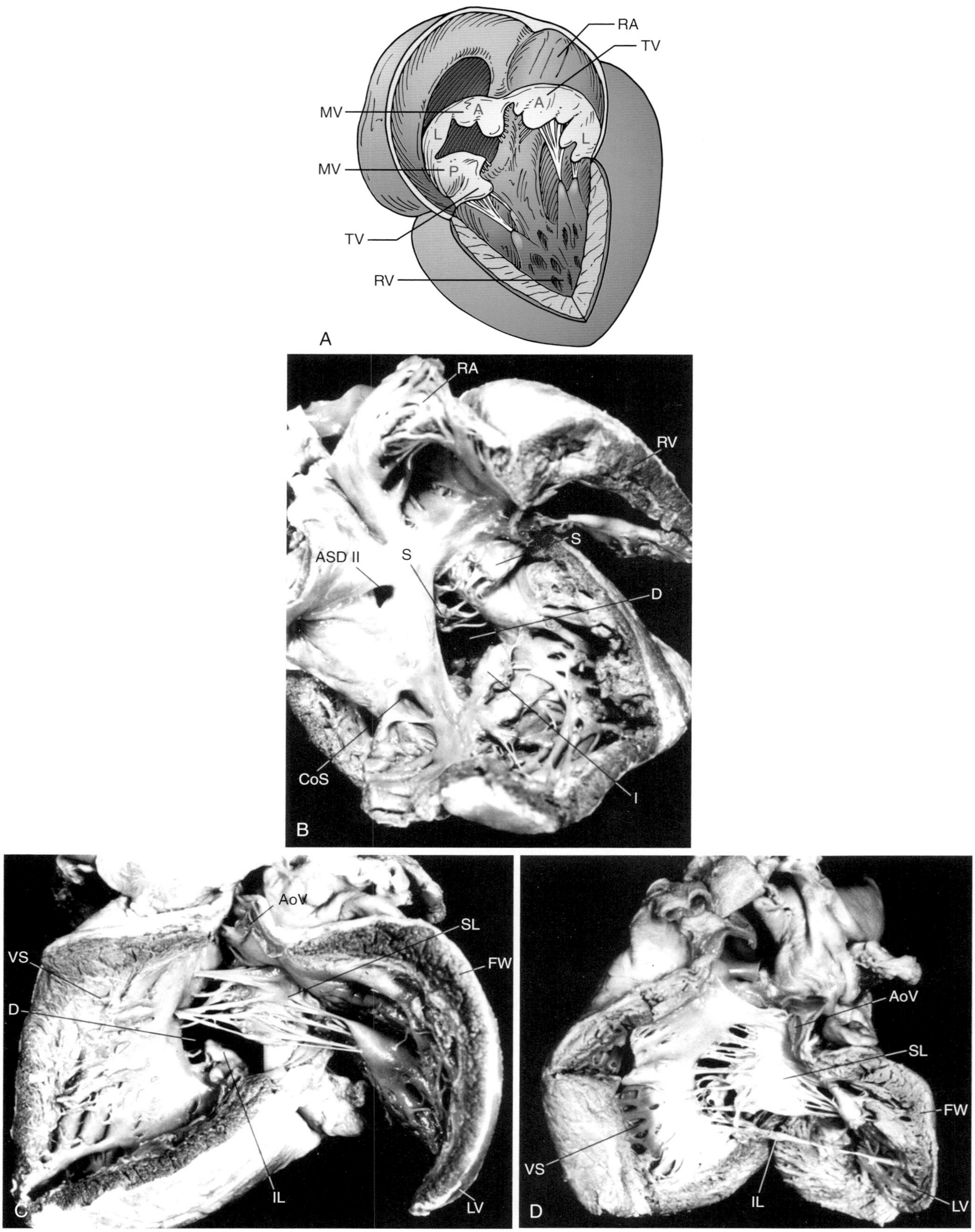
RA
TV
MV
MV
TV
RV
A
RA
RV
S
ASD II
S
D
CoS
I
B
AoV
SL
FW
VS
D
IL
LV
C
AoV
SL
FW
VS
IL
LV
D

Continued

Fig. 11.2 The complete form of common atrioventricular (AV) canal, type A. (A) The anterior (superior) leaflet of the common AV valve is divided into two components (A,A) and is attached to the crest of the "scooped-out" muscular ventricular septum by numerous short chordae tendineae. The posterior (inferior) leaflet *(P)* of the common AV valve is also attached to the crest of the muscular ventricular septum by short chordae tendineae. Despite the chordal attachments, a ventricular septal defect of the AV canal type exists through the chordae tendineae. Note also the left lateral leaflet *(L)* of the common AV valve. The components of the mitral valve *(MV)* and tricuspid valve *(TV)* are readily recognizable, even though the AV valve is in common (undivided). The potential TV opens into the morphologically right ventricle *(RV)* and the potential MV opens into the morphologically left ventricle (largely unseen). *RA,* Morphologically right atrium. (B) Complete form of common AV canal type A, showing the opened RA and RV. There is an AV septal defect that consists of an ostium primum type of atrial septal defect *(ASD I)* posterior and superior to the superior *(S)* and the inferior *(I)* leaflets of the common AV valve, plus a VSD of the AV canal type anterior and inferior to these leaflets (S and I). The ASD I and the VSD of the AV canal type are confluent during atrial systole, when the leaflets of the common AV valve are open, but not during ventricular systole, when the leaflets are closed—if there is no significant regurgitation of the common AV valve. The superior leaflet is divided into two parts (S,S) and is attached by chordae tendineae to the ventricular septal crest. The margins of the AV septal defect (the defect in the septum of the AV canal) are the crest of the muscular ventricular septum, which is "scooped out" (convex) in an anteroinferior direction, and the anteroinferior margin of the atrial septum, which is mildly convex in a posterosuperior direction. Note the nude anteroinferior rim of the atrial septum, which does not have its tricuspid valve "pants" on. (Normally, the anteroinferior part of the atrial septum is attached to the septal leaflet of the tricuspid valve.) Diagnostically, when you find that the anteroinferior rim of the atrial septum is nude (no tricuspid valve attachment), you know that common AV canal must be present. The next diagnostic question should be, Is this a complete type of common AV canal, or is it incomplete? In other words, is a VSD of the AV canal type present or not? Then you search beneath the superior *(S)* and the inferior *(I)* leaflets of the common AV valve to answer this question. Note that a small ostium secundum type of atrial septal defect (ASD II) is also present, and that the ostium of the coronary sinus *(CoS)* opens normally into the RA, which it often does not do with common AV canal. (C) Complete form of common AV canal, type A, left ventricular view. The superior leaflet component *(SL)* and the inferior leaflet component *(IL)* of the common AV valve both attach via multiple chordae tendineae to the "scooped-out" crest of the muscular ventricular septum. That a VSD component of the AV septal defect *(D)* is present is clear: note the patent spaces between the chordal attachments of both SL and the IL, and the space between the SL and the IL that extends down to the ventricular septal crest. Why does the ventricular septum look so "scooped out"? Because the septum of the AV canal is completely missing between the ventricular septum anteriorly and the atrial septum posteriorly (unseen), resulting in a complete AV septal defect. There is direct fibrous continuity between the aortic valve *(AoV)* superiorly and the SL of the common AV valve inferiorly, which is typical of normally related great arteries which has absence of the subaortic conal free wall—thereby permitting AoV-SL fibrous continuity. During atrial systole, the SL forms a high horizontal floor to the subaortic left ventricular outflow tract. This high horizontal floor results in the goose-neck appearance during atrial systole in imaging studies. The chordal insertions from SL into the ventricular septum *(VS)* just below the AoV can result in left ventricular outflow tract stenosis. Another factor contributing to this obstruction is the shallowness of the subaortic left ventricular septal surface in a superoinferior direction, because of the pronounced "scooping out" (deficiency) of the ventricular septum just below the AoV. Note also that the left ventricular inlet length/left ventricular outlet length ratio is reduced to 0.7 (normal = 1). The LV inlet length (from the IL to the LV apex) is much shorter than the LV outlet length (from the LV apex to the AoV) because the absent canal septum (hence the "scooped-out" appearance) contributes to the ventricular inlet septum, but not to the ventricular outlet septum. This is why VSDs of the AV canal type are also known as inlet VSDs. Hence, a reduced or subnormal LV inlet/outlet ratio is typical of common AV canal because of its AV septal defect component. *FW,* Free wall. (D) Completely common AV canal type A, LV view. Note how much closer the IL is to the crest of the VS than the SL is. This is also evident in C. This observation is relevant to the morphogenesis of normal and abnormal development of the AV canal (please see text). Normally, the next morphogenetic step is for endocardial cushion fibroblasts to fill in these interchordal spaces, converting a complete form of common AV canal into a partial form.

septum is much shallower in superior-inferior dimension than normal.

The "goose-neck" appearance seen angiocardiographically (and with other imaging modalities) during atrial systole and ventricular diastole is related in part to the high horizontal "floor" of the subaortic left ventricular outflow tract during atrial systole, which results in the goose-neck appearance. The superior leaflet component of the anterior mitral leaflet makes an angle of approximately 90° with the left ventricular septal surface. And the anterosuperior leaflet of the common AV valve inserts into the ventricular septum very high (very superiorly). Consequently, the subaortic left ventricular outflow tract is very shallow—very lacking in superoinferior depth.

Normally, with division of the atrioventricular canal into mitral and tricuspid valves, the angle formed by the anterior leaflet of the mitral valve and the left ventricular septal surface is much smaller, often about 45°. And the superoinferior dimension of the subaortic LV outflow tract is much deeper. The "floor" of the LV outflow tract is greatly lowered, increasing the superoinferior dimension of the LV outflow tract, thereby "degoosing" the goose-neck appearance.

This is why the normal subaortic LV outflow tract does not at all resemble a goose-neck appearance. Why not? Because the superoinferior dimension of the normal subaortic LV outflow tract is so much greater—so much deeper. Why? Normally, the superior and inferior leaflets of the common AV valve attach to each other—thereby closing the cleft, instead of attaching high up to the LV septal surface. By attaching to each other and closing the cleft in the anterior leaflet of the mitral valve, the superior and inferior leaflets of the common AV valve greatly lower the floor of the subaortic LV outflow tract. The process of superior cushion–inferior cushion fusion (cleft closure) also greatly reduces the angle between the endocardial cushions and the LV septal surface from about 90° in common AV canal to about 45° normally after cleft closure.

Thus, cleft closure is important not only for the formation of the anterior mitral leaflet, but also for the creation of a deep and nonstenotic subaortic LV outflow tract. Discrete fibrous subaortic stenosis is caused by residual, unremodeled endocardial cushion fibrous tissue (see the section on fibrous subaortic stenosis later in this chapter).

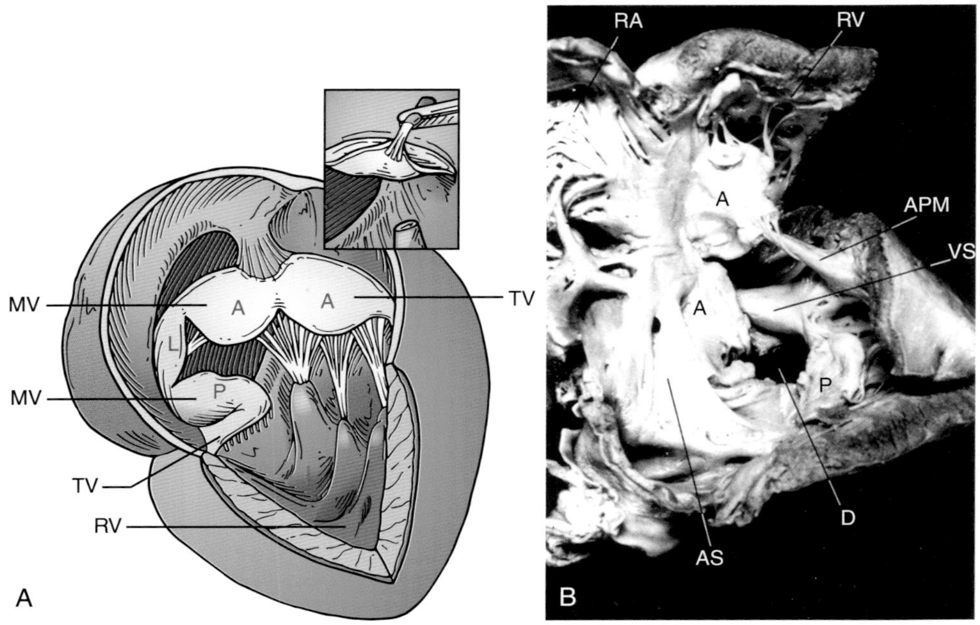

Fig. 11.3 (A) Complete form of common of atrioventricular (AV) canal, type B. The anterosuperior leaflet of the common AV valve is partially divided (A,A), but is not attached to the crest of the ventricular septum, as the inset confirms. Instead, the anterior leaflet attaches to a right ventricular papillary muscle. The posterior leaflet *(P)* and the left lateral leaflet *(L)* of the common AV valve are also shown. Normally, when the leftward *A* and the leftward part of P fuse, the composite anterior leaflet of the mitral valve *(MV)* is formed. L becomes the posterior leaflet of the MV. The rightward A becomes the anterior leaflet of the tricuspid valve *(TV)*. The rightward part of P forms the septal leaflet of the TV. The right lateral leaflet of the common AV valve is not shown; this leaflet normally forms the posterior leaflet of the TV (not shown). An AV septal defect is present consisting of an ostium primum type of ASD above the common AV valve, which is confluent with a VSD of the AV canal type below the common AV valve. *RV*, Right ventricle (From Rastelli GC, Kirklin JW, Titus JL: Anatomic observations on complete form of persistent common AV canal with special reference to the AV valves. *Mayo Clin Proc* 41:296, 1966, with permission.) (B) Complete form of common AV canal, type B, opened right atrium *(RA)* and right ventricle *(RV)*. The superior (anterior) leaflet (A,A) is partly divided (not all the way to the leaflet origin) to the right of the plane of the ventricular septum *(VS)*. The superior leaflet (A,A) does not insert by multiple chordae into the crest of the VS, but instead attaches to the anterior papillary muscle *(APM)* of the RV. The moderator band characteristically is very short; hence the APM appears to originate directly from the RV septal surface. In the atrial septum *(AS)* there is a small ostium secundum type of ASD. A complete AV septal defect *(D)* lies between the AS and the VS. The posterior leaflet of the common AV valve normally would form the septal leaflet of the TV.

The ventricular systolic image with common AV canal is **"the scallops."** The thicket of chordae tendineae in type A completely common AV canal creates a scalloped appearance in front of the anterior leaflet of the common AV valve during ventricular systole.

In Fig. 11.2C, it is noteworthy that subaortic insertions of short chordae tendineae can create, or contribute to, **subaortic left ventricular outflow tract stenosis** in type A completely common AV canal—and also in partially common AV canal in which these chordal insertions are dense enough to obliterate the VSD.

Why does **the electrocardiogram in common AV canal** typically have a counterclockwise and superior frontal QRS loop? Because the atrioventricular bundle of His has to enter the ventricular septum in a very low or inferior position—because of the relatively huge hole in the center of the heart, the AV septal defect. The accession wave of ventricular depolarization must therefore travel from inferiorly to superiorly as it progresses from the ventricular septum to the ventricular free walls. If the heart is pointing leftward (levocardia), and if the common AV canal is balanced (both ventricles well developed), then depolarization typically inscribes a counterclockwise and superior frontal QRS loop. It's like left anterior hemiblock that can be produced experimentally in the dog lab. The accession wave travels from inferiorly to superiorly, creating a counterclockwise QRS loop as projected on the frontal plane.

The foregoing was realized many years ago at the Mayo Clinic by a young physician from Mexico City, Dr. Toscano-Barbosa, one of Professor Sodi-Pallares' bright young men. The foregoing realization made it possible to diagnose common AV canal with the help of scalar electrocardiography, prior to the advent of good angiocardiography.

When you look at the opened left ventricle (Figs. 11.2C and D) from a *developmental perspective*, what do you see? I'll try to tell you some of the things that I see. Dr. David Kurnit put it

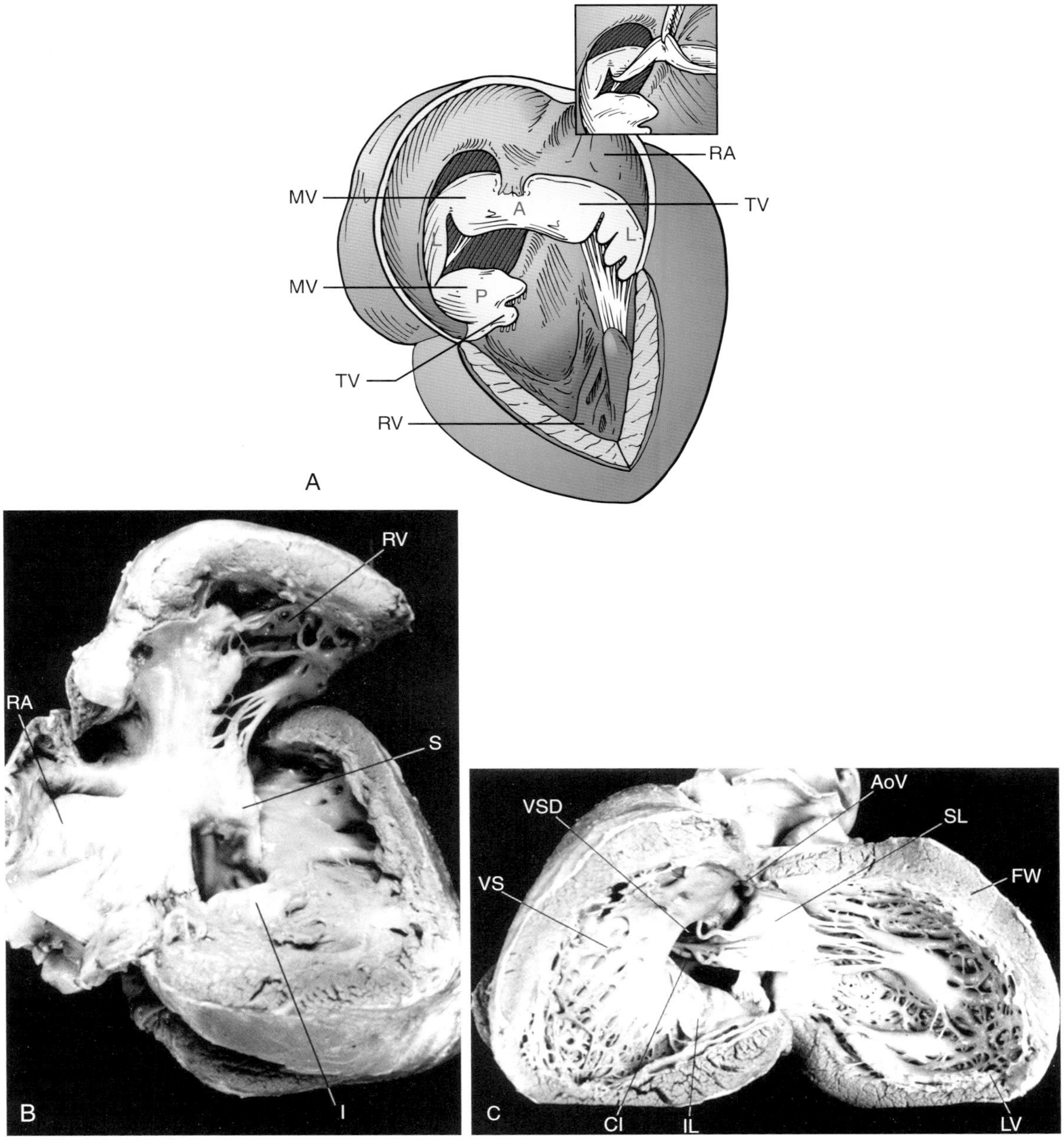

Fig. 11.4 (A) Complete form of common atrioventricular (AV) canal, type C, right atrial view. The anterosuperior leaflet *(A)* of the common AV valve is undivided and unattached to the crest of the muscular ventricular septum, as the inset confirms. The posteroinferior *(P)*, left lateral *(L)*, and right lateral *(L)* leaflets are also shown. A complete AV septal defect is present between the atrial and the ventricular septa. The leaflets of the potential mitral valve *(MV)* and tricuspid valve *(TV)* are seen. *RV*, Right ventricle. (B) Complete form of common AV canal, type C, right lateral view of opened right atrium *(RA)* and right ventricle *(RV)*. The superior leaflet *(S)* of the common AV valve is undivided and unattached to the crest of the "scooped-out" ventricular septum. The inferior leaflet *(I)* of the common AV valve contributes to the formation of the potentially septal leaflet of the tricuspid valve. A complete AV septal defect is present between the atrial septum posteriorly and the ventricular septum anteriorly. The heart is shown in a horizontal position, characteristic of fetuses, infants, and children, in which the diaphragm would be approximately parallel to the bottom of the photograph. In adolescents and adults, when the thorax elongates, the heart assumes a semivertical or vertical position: rotate the photograph 45° clockwise. Then the superior leaflet (S) becomes anterior, the inferior leaflet (I) posterior, the ventricular septum inferior, and the atrial septum superior. Thus, whether the anterosuperior bridging leaflet is anterior or superior depends on the heart position (horizontal or vertical), which in turn depends on the patient's age. (C) Complete form of common AV canal, type C, left ventricular *(LV)* view. Better than in (B), one can see that the superior leaflet *(SL)* is undivided and that its free margin does not attach to the crest of the muscular ventricular septum *(VS)*. However, a lone chorda does attach to the ventricular septal crest superiorly; but because this chorda does not come from the free margin of the SL, this case is classified as a type C (not as a type A). Note: the ventricular septal defect *(VSD)* component of this AV septal

Continued

Fig. 11.4 cont'd defect; the "scooped-out" crest of the VS; the direct fibrous continuity between the aortic valve *(AoV)* and the SL, characteristic of normally related great arteries; that the SL is larger than the inferior leaflet *(IL)*; that the SL inserts only into the anterolateral papillary muscle of the LV (the upper one); that the IL inserts only into the posteromedial papillary muscle of the LV (the lower one); that the anterolateral papillary muscle is larger than the posteromedial, reflecting the fact that the SL is larger than the IL; and that the LV inlet length is distinctly shorter than the LV outlet length, the LV inlet/outlet ratio = 0.75 (1 = normal). *FW,* free wall.

to me very nicely years ago: "The fibroblasts of the endocardial cushions of the AV canal take random walks in space, looking for something to attach to." When they contact the crest of the muscular ventricular septum, short chordae tendineae are formed, which are characteristics of type A completely common AV canal. This is really a normal stage in the morphogenesis of the AV canal which, for reasons still not completely understood (but probably genetic), becomes arrested at this stage of development in the complete form of common AV canal, type A.

Normally, the spaces between these short chordae tendineae then get filled in with fibrous tissue, converting a type A completely common AV canal into a partially common AV canal with no VSD, a cleft mitral valve, and an ostium primum type of atrial septal defect.

Thus, the short chordae tendineae, particularly well seen in Fig. 11.2D, are one of the stages in the normal morphogenesis of the AV canal. As will be seen, other types of common AV canal represent other normal stages in the morphogenesis of the AV septum and of the AV valves. Hence, the spectrum of common AV canal may be viewed as a series of natural experiments illustrating the various stages in the normal development of the AV canal region—a topic to which we shall return.

Type A completely common AV canal often shows you very clearly where the normal definitive mitral and tricuspid valve leaflets come from (Fig. 11.5). In this diagram, the common AV valve is viewed from above. Note the superior cushion component (SCC) and the inferior cushion component (ICC) that together normally form the anterior leaflet of the mitral valve. The superior cushion component and the inferior cushion component are separated by a cleft. The cleft does not run horizontally toward the left ventricular septal surface. Instead, it slants superiorly.

Note that the anterior leaflet of the normal mitral valve is composed of two endocardial cushions (the superior and the inferior). The other AV leaflets are formed essentially by one endocardial cushion only.

Why is this anterior mitral leaflet normally a doublet, whereas the other AV valve leaflets are singletons? Our hypothesis is that in order to form a deep semicircular anterior mitral leaflet to occlude the approximately *circular* systemic AV orifice, the contributions of two endocardial cushions are needed. By contrast, the pulmonic AV orifice (tricuspid) is semicircular (not round) prenatally and is crescentic postnatally. Consequently, a deep semicircular septal leaflet is not needed in the tricuspid valve in order to achieve valvar competence.

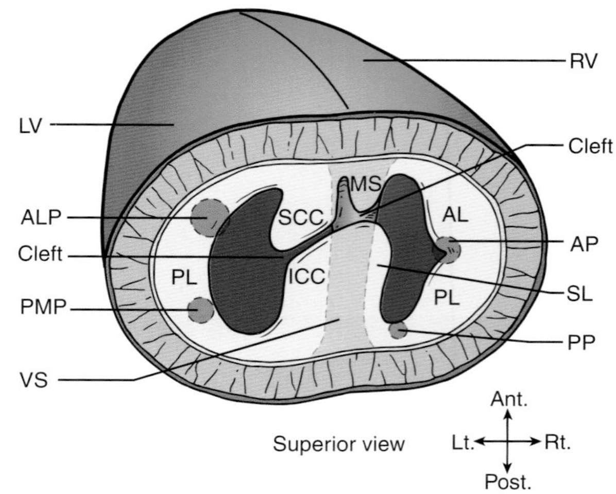

Fig. 11.5 Where do the mitral and tricuspid valve leaflets come from? Common atrioventricular (AV) canal type A is very illuminating in this regard. The AV canal is surrounded by endocardial cushion tissue indicated by cross-hatching. Conventionally, the anterior (A) or superior cushion is said to extend from the anterolateral papillary muscle *(ALP)* of the left ventricle *(LV)* to the anterior papillary muscle *(AP)* of the right ventricle *(RV)*. The posterior (P) or inferior endocardial cushion is said to lie between the posteromedial papillary muscle *(PMP)* of the LV and the posterior papillary muscle *(PP)* of the RV. The left (L) lateral endocardial cushion extends between the ALP and the PMP of the LV. The right (R) lateral endocardial cushion lies between the AP and PP muscles of the RV. These conventional designations of the endocardial cushions are convenient for describing the ring of endocardial cushion tissue that internally lines the AV canal. *What does the anterosuperior endocardial cushion give rise to?* The superior cushion component *(SCC)* of the anterior mitral leaflet above the cleft; the membranous septum *(MS)*; and the anterior leaflet *(AL)* of the tricuspid valve. *What does the posteroinferior endocardial cushion contribute to?* The inferior cushion component *(ICC)* of the anterior mitral leaflet below the cleft and the septal leaflet *(SL)* of the tricuspid valve. *What does the left lateral endocardial cushion give rise to?* The posterior leaflet *(PL)* or mural leaflet of the mitral valve between the ALP and the PMP muscles of the LV. *What does the right lateral endocardial cushion of the AV canal give origin to?* To the posterior leaflet (PL) of the tricuspid valve. Thus, common AV canal type A, diagrammed above, is very informative concerning the origins of the leaflets of the definitive normal AV valves. *VS,* ventricular septum.

In fact, this hypothesis is tested and substantiated by the findings in common AV canal. A normally formed two-component anterior mitral leaflet is not present in common AV canal because of the cleft, that is, the failure of the superior and inferior endocardial cushions to fuse and zipper closed the cleft from medially (at the ventricular septum, VS in Fig. 11.5) to laterally at the free margin of the anterior mitral leaflet. Failure of the normal zippering fusion results in the persistence of a cleft that is often associated with significant mitral regurgitation, as will be seen under Findings later in this chapter.

In Fig. 11.5, note also that the membranous septum (MS) is formed from the superior endocardial cushion. The tricuspid valve also often has a small cleft between the superior and the inferior endocardial cushions. This tricuspid cleft (Fig. 11.5) is seldom of major hemodynamic significance and hence is often ignored.

The anterolateral papillary muscle of the left ventricle (ALP, Fig. 11.2) usually is larger than the posteromedial papillary muscle (PMP, Fig. 11.2), reflecting the fact that the superior leaflet of the common AV valve typically is larger than the inferior leaflet.

When ***potentially parachute mitral valve***[17] occurs in the setting of common AV canal, typically the anterolateral papillary muscle of the left ventricle is large and receives all of the primary chordae tendineae of the abnormal mitral valve, whereas the posteromedial papillary muscle of the left ventricle is hypoplastic or absent. By *potentially* parachute mitral valve we mean that a parachute mitral valve would be present postoperatively because there is only a single focus of chordal insertion in the morphologically left ventricle.

When the AV canal is normally divided into mitral and tricuspid valves, parachute mitral valve typically has the opposite papillary muscle anatomy: a large posteromedial papillary muscle and a small or absent anterolateral papillary muscle.[18]

The size of the posterior or mural leaflet of the mitral valve depends on the distance between the anterolateral and posteromedial papillary muscles (Fig 11.5). In potentially parachute mitral valve, there is no discrete posterior or mural leaflet of the mitral valve, and the interchordal spaces are often poorly formed or absent. Hence the cleft typically is the major component of the mitral orifice and hence should *not* be sutured closed, in order to avoid or minimize iatrogenic mitral stenosis postoperatively.

Note also that normal aortic-mitral fibrous continuity with normally related great arteries is really aortic-to-superior endocardial cushion direct fibrous continuity (Fig. 11.2D).

The tricuspid cleft is about two-thirds of the way up as one proceeds from inferiorly to superiorly; that is, the tricuspid cleft lies below (or inferior to) the superior commissure of the tricuspid valve between the anterior leaflet (AL) and the septal leaflet (SL) (Fig. 11.5).

The septal leaflet of the tricuspid valve (SL, Fig. 11.5) consists mostly of inferior endocardial cushion tissue—below the tricuspid cleft. Above the cleft lies the membranous septum (MS, Fig. 11.5), which consists of superior endocardial cushion tissue. In the normal definitive tricuspid valve, the membranous septum may or may not be covered by tricuspid septal leaflet tissue. Thus, although the septal leaflet of the tricuspid valve normally consists mostly of inferior endocardial cushion or leaflet tissue—below the tricuspid cleft or fusion line (Fig. 11.5), the septal leaflet of the tricuspid valve may or may not have a contribution from the superior endocardial cushion—above the tricuspid cleft in completely common AV canal type A (Fig. 11.5), or when development is normal—above the tricuspid fusion line (closed cleft).

Thus, careful study of the common AV valve in type A from above helps one to understand where all of the components of the normal mitral and tricuspid valve leaflets come from (Fig. 11.5).

Grammatical Note: Please observe that we are talking about *completely* common AV canal, not *complete* common AV canal, and *partially* common AV canal, not *partial* common AV canal. Why? Because, as your elementary school grammar teacher no doubt taught you, an adverb (completely, or partially) is required to modify an adjective (common). One adjective cannot modify another adjective.

Since it has been a long time since most of us were in elementary school, let's briefly review the grammar: completely (adverb) common (adjective) atrioventricular (adjective) canal (noun). The adverb *completely* modifies the adjective *common*. The adjectives *common* and *atrioventricular* both modify the noun *canal*. The meaning is not whether the canal is complete or partial. Instead, the meaning is whether the canal is completely common, or only partly common, that is, completely undivided, or only partly undivided.

By contrast, *complete* and *partial*—the adjectives—are grammatically correct in *complete* AV defect and *partial* AV defect, because both adjectives are modifying the noun *defect*.

However, grammatically it should be *morphologically* right ventricle, not *morphologic* right ventricle, and *morphologically* left ventricle, not *morphologic* left ventricle. Why? Because the adverb (morphologically) is required to modify the adjective (right, or left). The question is: Is this ventricle morphologically right, or morphologically left? The meaning is not: Is this structure a morphologic ventricle—as opposed, for example, to a morphologic atrium?

The foregoing note concerning adjectives and adverbs is written in the hope that it may help to improve our terminology.

Type B Completely Common AV Canal

Let us now consider type B completely common AV canal in greater detail. The superior (anterior) leaflet is divided partially (Fig. 11.3), not completely as in type A (Fig. 11.2). Also note that the partial division of the superior leaflet in type B occurs above the right ventricular cavity (Fig. 11.3)—further to the right than the complete division of the superior leaflet in type A that occurs above the ventricular septum (Fig. 11.2). Perhaps this is why the margins of the incomplete division of the superior leaflet are not tethered to the crest of the ventricular septum in type B (Fig. 11.3), as they are in type A (Fig. 11.2).

In the diagram of Rastelli et al[16] (Fig. 11.3a), the inset confirms that there are no attachments between the partly divided superior leaflet (A,A) and the ventricular septal crest. Normally, when the leftward A and the leftward part of P fuse, the composite anterior leaflet of the MV is formed. L becomes the posterior leaflet of the mitral valve. The rightward A becomes the anterior leaflet of the TV. The rightward portion of P forms the septal leaflet of the TV. The posterior leaflet of the potential tricuspid valve is not shown in Fig. 11.3A. Note that an ostium primum type of atrial septal defect (above the leaflets of the common AV valve) is confluent with a ventricular defect of the AV canal type (below the leaflets of the common AV valve); hence a complete

AV septal defect is present, indicating that this is a complete form of common AV canal.

As indicated above, we found that Rastelli's right ventricular muscle that originates from the right ventricular septal surface is indeed the anterior papillary muscle of the right ventricle which is associated with a very short moderator band (Fig. 11.3B). This creates the impression that the anterior papillary muscle is originating directly from the right ventricular septal surface. As will be confirmed in the Findings section, type B completely common AV canal is rare.

Type C Completely Common AV Canal

Let us now have a somewhat more detailed look at the pathologic anatomy of type C completely common AV canal (Fig. 11.4). As the inset in Rastelli's[16] drawing shows, there were no fibrous attachments between the superior (anterior) leaflet of the common AV valve (A, Fig. 11.4A) and the underlying ventricular septum. In type C, the superior leaflet is a free-floating, bridging leaflet: it is like a bridge arching unsupported over the ventricular septum.

In the photograph of a heart specimen of type C (Fig. 11.4C), note that there is one lone chorda tendinea running from the central surface of the superior leaflet to the ventricular septal crest. Nonetheless, this case was still classified as a type C because the superior leaflet was undivided, and no chordae ran from the *free margin* of the superior leaflet to insert into the ventricular septal crest.

In the opened view of the left ventricle (Fig. 11.4C), note that the anterolateral papillary muscle (the upper one) is distinctly larger than the posteromedial (the lower one), which may be due to the fact that the superior leaflet of the common AV valve (SL, Fig. 11.4C) is much larger than the inferior leaflet (IL, Fig. 11.4C). The superior leaflet of the common AV valve inserts only into the anterolateral papillary muscle of the left ventricle, and the inferior leaflet inserts only into the posteromedial papillary muscle, these being the usual leaflet attachments in the complete form of common AV canal—but by no means the only ones that occur, as we shall see.

Also noteworthy in Fig. 11.4C: the "scooped-out" (concave) crest of the muscular ventricular septum; the reduced left ventricular inlet length/outlet length ratio (0.83), the normal being approximately 1.0; and the aortic valve-to-superior leaflet direct fibrous continuity, typical of normally related great arteries. Note also that the inferior leaflet of the common AV valve is much closer to the crest of the muscular ventricular septum that is the superior leaflet: this is a point of morphogenetic significance, to which we shall return.

In Fig. 11.4B, one can see the *ostium primum defect* well. This brings up the question: *Is an ostium primum defect really an atrial septal defect?* The answer, we think, is both yes and no. Yes, it has long been regarded as an atrial septal defect because the defect lies above the leaflets of the AV valve(s) (Fig. 11.4B). No, because an ostium primum defect is really a defect in the septum of the AV canal; that is, it is a partial AV septal defect. The AV septum lies in front of (or below) the atrial septum, and behind (or above) the ventricular septum (Fig. 11.4B). This is why the AV septum used to be known as the *septum intermedium*—because it is intermediate between the atrial septum behind (or above) and the ventricular septum in front (or below). Hence, accurately speaking, an ostium primum defect is not really an atrial septal defect. Instead, it is a partial atrioventricular septal defect. This is why we prefer to speak of an *ostium primum defect* (not an ostium primum type of atrial septal defect).

However, the term *ostium primum type of atrial septal defect (ASD I)* is deeply ingrained by common usage. The question becomes: Is this time-honored designation really wrong? We think the answer is no, in the following sense. From an anatomic standpoint, there are three main developmental components to the anatomic atrial septum: septum primum, septum secundum, and the interatrial part of the atrioventricular septum. When the latter is absent, the ostium that results resembles the first opening between the atria, prior to the development of the atrial septum in the embryo. Hence, this defect has been called an ostium primum type of ASD—because it is reminiscent of the first hole (ostium primum), the original interatrial foramen prior to atrial septation.

So, whenever we use the term *ASD I*, we do so with the understanding that it is a partial AV septal defect, the presence of which results anatomically in a typical low defect in the interatrial septum.

Is the atrioventricular septum in front of the atrial septum, or below it (Fig. 11.4B)? Is the atrioventricular septum behind the ventricular septum, or above it (Fig. 11.4B)? The answer depends on the position of the heart. In the fetus, the newborn, and young children, the cardiac position typically is horizontal, with the atria behind and the ventricles in front. Hence in the infant and child, the AV septum lies *in front of* the atrial septum and *behind* the ventricular septum (Fig. 11.4B).

However, with growth—when one becomes an adolescent or an adult—the heart position becomes semivertical or vertical. The ventricular apex no longer points anteriorly and to the left; instead, it points inferiorly and to the left. This is how the atria come to be above the ventricles. Hence, in an adolescent or an adult, and AV septal defect lies *below* the atria and *above* the ventricles. Similarly, the *superior* bridging leaflet of an infant or child with type C completely common AV canal becomes the *anterior* bridging leaflet of an adult patient. The *inferior* leaflet of the infant and child becomes the *posterior* leaflet of the adolescent and adult (Fig. 11.4). Hence, *heart position* is an important consideration for accurate cardiac description.

Partial Forms of Common AV Canal

The most frequent partial form of common AV canal is *ostium primum atrial septal defect with cleft mitral valve* (Fig. 11.6). The VSD of the AV canal type has been obliterated, but the ventricular septum is still "scooped-out" or deficient superiorly (Fig. 11.6B).

Let us examine such a case in somewhat greater detail, beginning on the right side. A large ostium primum type of atrial septal defect is seen between the intact atrial septum above and behind, and the intact ventricular septum below and in front

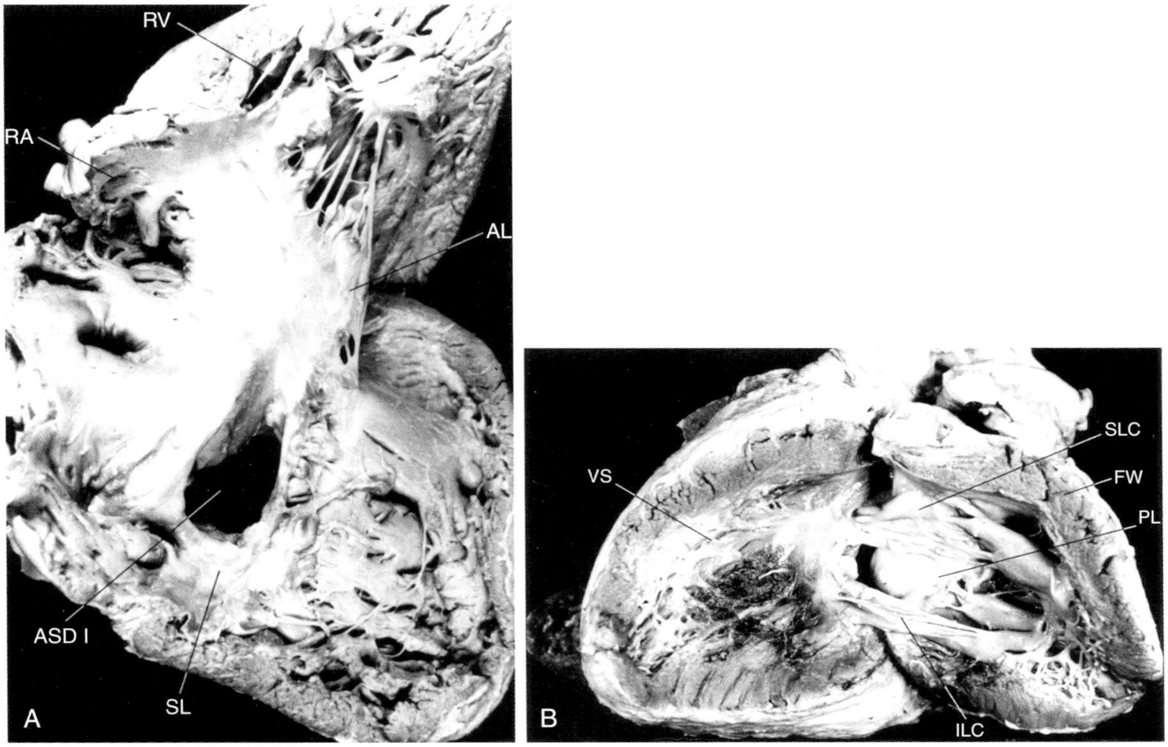

Fig. 11.6 Partial form of common atrioventricular (AV) canal with an ostium primum type of atrial septal defect *(ASD I)*, no ventricular septal defect (VSD) of the AV canal type, and a cleft mitral valve. (A) Right lateral view of opened right atrium *(RA)* and right ventricle *(RV)*. The ASD I is a partial AV septal defect extending from the bare lower rim of the atrial septum posterosuperiorly to the septal leaflet *(SL)* of the tricuspid valve *(TV)* anteroinferiorly. The anterior leaflet *(AL)* and the SL of the TV are fused at the superior commissure. There is no VSD beneath the SL of the TV. (B) Partial form of common AV canal, left ventricular (LV) view of another case (not the same patient as in A). There is a relatively large gap (more than a cleft) between the superior leaflet component *(SLC)* and the inferior leaflet component *(ILC)* of the unfused and tissue deficient anterior leaflet of the mitral valve. The thickening and rolling of the leaflet margins about the huge cleft (gap) in the anterior leaflet of the MV indicate severe mitral regurgitation. The posterior leaflet *(PL)* of the MV is attached to a third papillary muscle between the anterolateral papillary muscle above and the posteromedial papillary muscle below. There is no VSD; the ventricular septum *(VS)* is "scooped out," that is, tissue deficient superiorly; and the LV inlet/outlet ratio is very subnormal (0.63, normal = 1.0). *FW*, Free wall.

(Fig. 11.6A). The septal leaflet of the tricuspid valve is firmly adherent to the crest of the ventricular septum, and both the anterior and the posterior leaflets of the tricuspid valve appear unremarkable.

The bare or nude anteroinferior margin of the atrial septum, which does not have its tricuspid valve "pants" on, is the posterosuperior margin of the partial AV septal defect (the ostium primum defect) (Fig. 11.6A). This nude anteroinferior margin of the atrial septum is a highly reliable marker that a common AV canal (an AV septal defect) is present.

Is this a complete or a partial form of common AV canal? Look under the septal leaflet of the tricuspid valve. Absence of a VSD of the AV canal type beneath the septal leaflet of the tricuspid valve indicates that a partial form of common AV canal (a partial AV septal defect) is present. The tricuspid valve's septal leaflet forms the anteroinferior margin of this partial AV septal defect. (When the AV septal defect is complete, the anteroinferior margin of the defect is the muscular crest of the ventricular septum, as in Figs. 11.2 to 11.4).

An *ostium primum type of defect* is the only type of interatrial communication that typically is confluent with the septal leaflet of the tricuspid valve (Fig. 11.6A). The *ostium secundum type of atrial septal defect* (Fig. 11.3B) is located in the central portion of the atrial septum, and is not confluent with the septal leaflet of the tricuspid valve.

Is this tricuspid valve cleft (Fig. 11.6A)? No. There is no gap between the septal and the anterior leaflets of the tricuspid valve in this case, as there can be in other cases.

As Dr. Jesse Edwards[6] pointed out, in the partial form of common AV canal, the superior (anterior) and the inferior (posterior) leaflets of the common AV valve have fused in the midline and have obliterated the VSD.

Now let us examine the opened left ventricle of this case (Fig. 11.6B). Note that the superior leaflet component (SLC) of what normally becomes the anterior mitral leaflet inserts exclusively into the anterolateral papillary muscle (the upper one, Fig. 11.6B). The inferior leaflet component (ILC) of what normally becomes the anterior leaflet of the mitral valve inserts exclusively into the inferior papillary muscle (the lower one, Fig. 11.6B). The posterior leaflet (PL) or mural leaflet inserts into a third papillary muscle that we call the middle papillary muscle.

The middle papillary muscle of the left ventricle lies between the anterolateral papillary muscle above and the posteromedial papillary muscle below (Fig. 11.6B). The middle papillary muscle normally is attached by chordae tendineae to the posterior (mural) leaflet only. In one form of double-orifice mitral valve, chordae tendineae run from the middle papillary muscle to both the posterior and the anterior mitral leaflets, thereby subdividing the mitral orifice into two approximately equal-sized openings.[19]

The middle papillary muscle is noteworthy for two reasons:

1. It is a normal left ventricular structure.
2. Its existence is largely unknown.

The conventional description is that there are two papillary muscles in the left ventricle: the anterolateral and the posteromedial. In fact, there are three papillary muscles in the left ventricle: the anterolateral, the posteromedial, and the middle (Fig. 11.6B). However, the middle papillary muscle can be fused with the anterolateral or the posteromedial papillary muscle, obscuring the independent existence of the middle papillary muscle. This may well be why people often speak of the anterolateral or the posteromedial papillary muscle *group*. For example, the anterolateral papillary muscle *group* suggests that more than the anterolateral papillary muscle is present. The additional papillary musculature can be the middle papillary muscle—when the anterolateral and the middle papillary muscles are confluent.

The middle papillary muscle is seen with unusual clarity in Fig. 11.6B because of the coexistence of incompletely common AV canal with a large gap (more than a cleft) in the anterior mitral leaflet. This tissue-deficient gap in the anterior mitral leaflet resulted in severe congenital mitral regurgitation. Note the thickening and rolling of the free margins of the superior and inferior leaflet components of the anterior mitral leaflet above and below this very large cleft or gap. This thickening or rolling of the leaflet free margins indicates the presence of congenital mitral regurgitation (Fig. 11.6B).

A partial cleft in the anterior mitral leaflet is presented in Fig. 11.7. The patient was a 35-year-old woman with Down syndrome who had an ostium primum type of atrial septal defect, a partially cleft anterior leaflet of the mitral valve, and no ventricular septal defect. Note that the superior component (SC) and the inferior component (IC) are fused paraseptally (F). The cleft is partial because it does not extend all the way from the free margin of what should normally have been the anterior mitral leaflet to the left ventricular septal surface. This heart specimen illustrates with unusual clarity that the anterior leaflet of the mitral valve normally is a composite structure, and how the zippering closed of the cleft normally occurs, beginning at the left ventricular septal surface medially, and proceeding laterally to the free margins of the superior and inferior components of the definitive (fused) anterior leaflet of the mitral valve (Fig. 11.7).

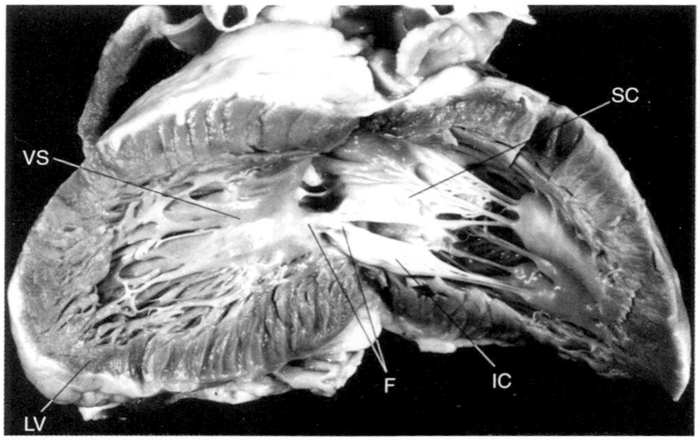

Fig. 11.7 Partial cleft of the anterior leaflet of the mitral valve, left ventricular *(LV)* view. The patient was a 35-year-old woman with Down syndrome, an ostium primum atrial septal defect, and a partially cleft anterior leaflet of the mitral valve. The cleft is partial because it does not extend from what normally is the free margin of the anterior mitral leaflet all the way to the left ventricular septal surface *(VS)*. The superior component *(SC)* and the inferior component *(IC)* of what normally is the anterior mitral leaflet are fused paraseptally *(F)*. The anterior mitral leaflet is a composite structure. Normally, the AML = SC + IC. Cleft closure normally occurs from medially (paraseptally) to laterally (at the free margin of the AML).

Are we looking at a cleft, or at a commissure (Fig. 11.7)? At a cleft. Why? Because the anterior mitral leaflet (AML) normally is composed of the superior endocardial cushion component (SC) and the inferior endocardial cushion component (IC), as partial fusion of the cleft proves (Fig. 11.7): briefly, AML = SC + IC.[20] The heart specimen shown in Fig. 11.7 is a very fortunate natural experiment: It shows the normal process of cleft closure, only partly completed, indicating that this is how the anterior mitral leaflet normally forms, and also showing what happens when fusion of the superior and inferior endocardial cushions fails to occur: a cleft results.[20]

Note also that the superior component and the inferior component of the anterior mitral leaflet are pulled *away* from each other during ventricular systole, because the superior component is attached to the anterolateral papillary muscle *(the upper one)* and the inferior component is attached to the posteromedial papillary muscle *(the lower one)* (Fig. 11.7). Thus, the leaflets bounding a cleft are pulled away from each other during ventricular systole, a feature that may predispose to mitral regurgitation.

By contrast, at a commissure—such as the anterolateral or posteromedial commissure of the normal mitral valve—the leaflets on either side of the commissure are pulled together, helping to prevent mitral regurgitation, because both leaflets are attached to the same papillary muscle group. This is what *commissure* literally means. Commissure comes to us from *commissura* (Latin), which is derived from *commissus,* the past participle of *committere,* which means to bring together: *com-* or *cum-*, together or with, + *mittere*, to send. Hence etymologically, commissure means "to send together." That is what happens to the AV valve leaflets at a commissure between leaflets. By contrast, a cleft is a defect within a leaflet, where the leaflet

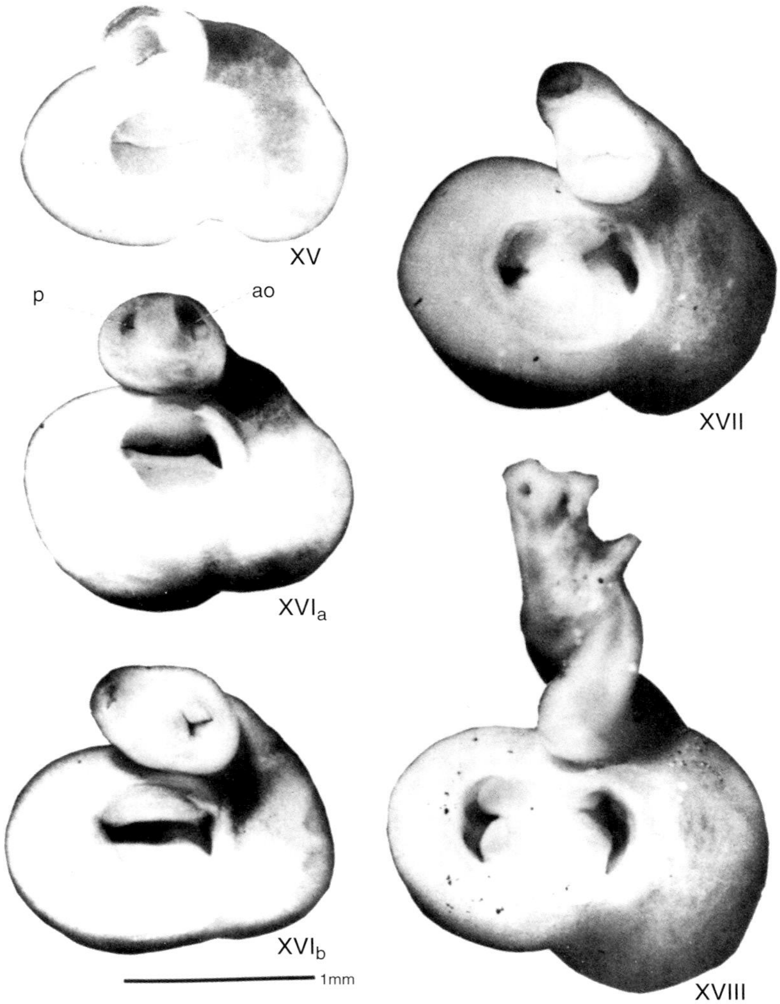

Fig. 11.8 Septation of the atrioventricular (AV) canal in human embryos from Streeter's horizon (stage) XV (30 to 32 days of age) to Streeter's horizon XVIII (36 to 38 days of age). The atria have been removed to permit visualization of the AV valve(s). The truncus arteriosus or great arteries have been removed to facilitate viewing of the semilunar valve(s). The hearts are viewed from behind (dorsally) and slightly from above (somewhat cranially); the superior surfaces face the top of the photograph; the inferior surfaces face the bottom of the photograph; and the right and left sides of these embryonic hearts are on the viewer's right right-hand side and left-hand side, respectively. The AV canal normally remains in common (undivided) until horizon XVII (34 to 36 days of age following ovulation), when the superior and inferior endocardial cushions of the AV canal fuse, which is part of the process of dividing the common AV canal into mitral and tricuspid canals. Late in horizon XVI, that is, in horizon XVIb (33 to 34 days of age), the common AV valve opens predominantly into the left ventricle and only slightly into the right ventricle. Even by horizon XVIII (36 to 38 days of age), the anterior leaflet of the mitral valve of this embryo remains cleft. Note also the associated morphogenetic movements of the developing pulmonary valve *(p)* and aortic valve *(ao)*. The aortic valve moves almost not at all, except that it turns to keep on facing the anteriorly moving pulmonary valve. In horizon XV (30 to 32 days), the pulmonary part of the undivided truncal valve is posterior and to the left of the aortic part of the truncal valve, similar to the semilunar interrelationship in D-transposition of the great arteries. Early in horizon XVI, that is, XVIa (32 to 33 days of age), the pulmonary valve (p) has moved anteriorly on the left and is now side-by-side relative to the aortic valve (ao), similar to the semilunar interrelationship in the Taussig-Bing type of double-outlet right ventricle. In the second half of horizon XVI, that is, XVIb (33 to 34 days of age), the pulmonary valve is now mildly anterior and left-sided relative to the aortic valve, similar to the semilunar relationship seen in tetralogy of Fallot with type C completely common AV canal. By horizon XVII (34 to 36 days of age), the common AV valve is divided into mitral and tricuspid valves, and the semilunar interrelationship is as in solitus normally related to great arteries. Maldevelopment of the AV canal and of the conotruncus often appear to be linked, as in the heterotaxy syndrome with asplenia, in which the findings resemble those normally found in horizons XV and XVI (30 to 34 days of age). However, the linkage between AV canal and conotruncal development often appears to be broken in the heterotaxy syndrome with polysplenia: the great arteries typically are normally

Continued

Fig. 11.8 cont'd related, or nearly normally related as in tetralogy of Fallot. But common AV canal, which may be of the partial type, is present. Thus, our hypothesis is that the heterotaxy syndrome with asplenia represents an earlier developmental arrest, resembling normal developmental stages XV and XVIa (30 to 33 days); whereas heterotaxy with polysplenia represents a slightly later developmental arrest, resembling normal horizon XVIb and perhaps early horizon XVII (33 days to early day 34 in normal development). It is understood that development in the heterotaxy syndromes with asplenia or polysplenia is not normal, and hence the above-mentioned timing based on normal development may well not be accurate. (From Asami I: Beitrag zur Entwicklung des Kammerseptums in menschlichen Herzen mit besonderer Berücksichtigung der sog Bulbusdrehung. *Z Anat Entwickl-Gesch* 128:1, 1969; and from Asami I: Partitioning of the arterial end of the embryonic heart. In: Van Praagh R, Takao A [eds], *Etiology and Morphogenesis of Congenital Heart Disease*. Futura, Mount Kisco, NY, 1980, p 51, with permission.)

components are pulled apart—in diverging directions during ventricular systole, not in a converging direction as occurs at a commissure.

Consequently, in the complete and partial forms of common AV canal, we think that the left-sided AV valve is a malformed mitral valve, not a trileaflet or tricuspid nonmitral valve.

Where does the idea that the mitral cleft is really a commissure come from? This line of thought runs essentially as follows: Let's look at the left-sided AV valve, particularly in the incomplete form of common AV valve. Anatomically, we see three leaflets (Fig. 11.6B). We don't really know anything about embryology. We are not going to be misled by embryologic theories. We are going to stick with the pathologic anatomy that we can see and know for sure. In incompletely common AV canal, we see three leaflets. Hence, the so-called cleft we regard as a commissure in a trileaflet left-sided AV valve.

What's wrong with this view? Why is it wrong? Why not rely on what we can see with our own eyes, and forget embryologic theories?

The problem with the aforementioned view is that the embryology of the AV canal region is well documented and well known (Figs. 11.8 and 11.9).[21-24] In the normal human embryo, the AV canal is in common during Streeter's horizon (stage) XV (estimated gestational age 30 to 32 days) and horizon XVI (estimated gestational age 32 to 34 days), as is shown by Asami's microdissections (Fig. 11.8).[21,22] In horizon XVII (estimated gestational age 34 to 36 days), the superior and inferior endocardial cushions of the AV canal normally fuse (Fig. 11.8), dividing the common AV canal into mitral and tricuspid canals. The same process of dividing the common AV canal into mitral and tricuspid canals also normally occurs in the rat between 13.75 and 14.5 days of gestational age (Fig. 11.9).[21,22]

In the human embryo, the mitral valve appears somewhat cleft even during horizon XVIII (estimated gestational age 36 to 38 days) (Fig. 11.8).[21,22] In the rat, the mitral cleft is clearly visible by 13.75 days, but has been fused closed by 14.5 days (Fig. 11.9).[21,22]

Hence, the embryology of septation of the common AV canal and of cleft closure of the mitral valve has been well documented in human and in comparative mammalian embryos, and is now well established and not controversial. We still have a lot to learn concerning exactly how these fusional processes occur, plus how and why they may go awry. But the phenomenology—what happens normally, and what can happen abnormally—is not hypothetical.[21-24]

The foregoing is why it can no longer be claimed that we know nothing about the relevant embryology and therefore that we must rely only on what our eyes can see of the pathologic anatomy. This attitude is what the late Dr. Tomas Pexeider called "declaring war on embryology." He regarded this as a very misguided approach, and we agree. The function of embryology is to make pathologic anatomy readily and accurately comprehensible. The dream of our field has long been to build an accurate bridge from the genome to the operating room. Embryology is an essential part of this bridge. Embryology is to pathology as vectorcardiography is to electrocardiography: both embryology and vectorcardiography are means of understanding.

Surgically, one can justify a failure to suture closed the cleft in the anterior leaflet of the mitral valve in the incomplete form of common AV canal, particularly if the cleft is not regurgitating at the time of surgery, by claiming that the left-sided AV valve is really a trileaflet valve and not a malformed mitral valve. One could even assert that one should not suture the "cleft" closed, because it is really a commissure. However, our surgical colleagues at Children's Hospital Boston have found that if one does not suture the cleft at the time of initial reparative surgery because it is not regurgitating, later on one often wishes one had closed the cleft—because the development of late mitral regurgitation in this situation is frequent. We are not surprised at this course of events because the view that the mitral cleft is really a commissure is anatomically and embryologically incorrect, for the reasons presented heretofore (Figs. 11.6 to 11.9).[21-24]

EMBRYOLOGY

The normal morphogenesis of the atrioventricular canal in man and in the rat has been illustrated by the elegant microdissections of Asami (Figs. 11.8 and 11.9).[21,22]

An understanding of the normal and abnormal morphogenesis of the atrioventricular canal can be augmented by a consideration of the spatial geometry of the superior and inferior endocardial cushions (Fig. 11.10).[25]

The superior and inferior endocardial cushions (leaflets) of the common AV valve form an anteriorly pointing V-shaped wedge (Figs. 11.2C and D, 11.4C, 11.6B, and 11.7). The superior and inferior endocardial cushions are not oriented superoinferiorly, like two little bricks standing on their ends, as they are often portrayed (Fig. 11.1).

The inferior endocardial cushion is much closer to the crest of the muscular interventricular septum than is the superior endocardial cushion (Figs. 11.2C and D, 11.4C).

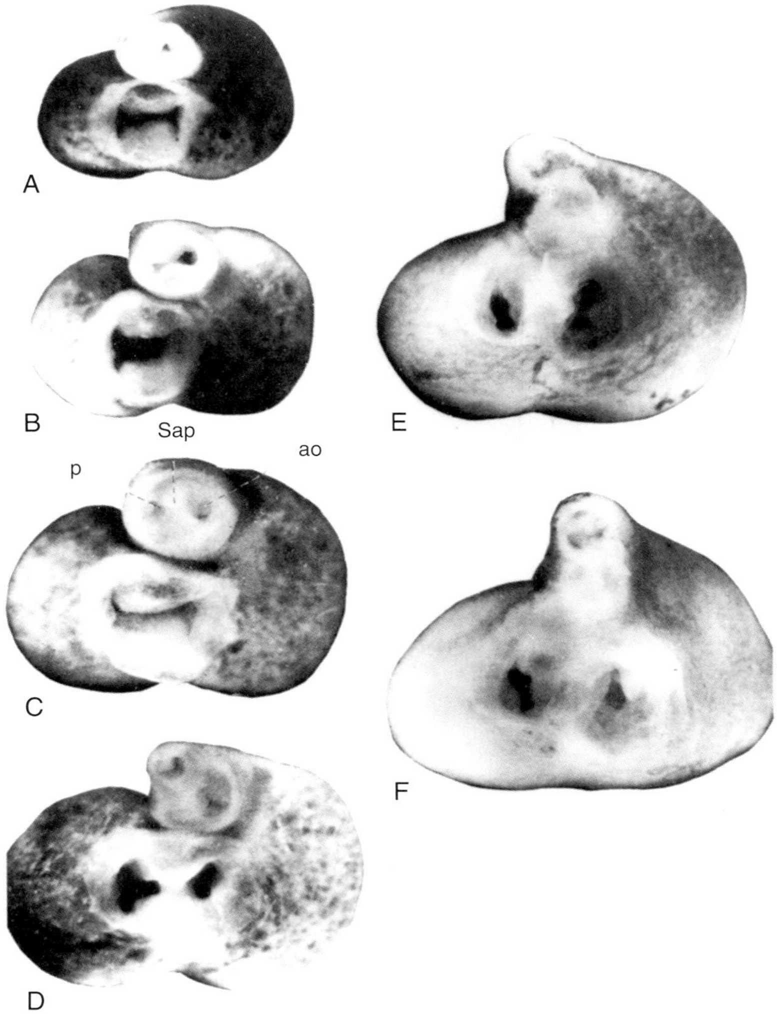

Fig. 11.9 Septation of the AV canal and morphogenetic movements of the conotruncus in the rat, dorsal view, same orientation as in Fig. 11.8. (A) 12.5 days of age; (B) 12.75 days; (C) 13 days; (D) 13.75 days; (E) 14.5 days; (F) 15.5 days. When the pulmonary valve *(p)* has moved from posteriorly to anteriorly to the left of the aortic valve *(ao)*, the pulmonary valve riding atop the developing subpulmonary conus and achieving normally related great arteries, only then do the superior and inferior endocardial cushions of the AV canal fuse, dividing the common AV canal into mitral and tricuspid canals. This linked development of the AV canal and conotruncus normally is accomplished in the rat embryo by 13.75 days (D). Although septation of the common AV canal has begun, the anterior leaflet of the mitral valve is still cleft. However, by 14.5 days of age (E), the mitral cleft has disappeared. *Sap,* Aortopulmonary septum. (From Asami I: Beitrag zur Entwicklung des Kammerseptums in menschlicken Herzen mit besonderer Berücksichtigung der sog Bulbusdrehung. *Z Anat Entwickl-Gesch* 128:1, 1969; and Asami I: Partitioning of the arterial end of the embryonic heart. In: Van Praagh R, Takao A [eds], *Etiology and Morphogenesis of Congenital Heart Disease.* Futura, Mount Kisco, NY, 1980, p 51, with permission.)

Let us call the distance between the inferior cushion and the ventricular septal crest χ (Fig. 11.10). The distance between the superior endocardial cushion and the ventricular septal crest may then be approximately 2χ to 3χ (Fig. 11.10).

The distance between the superior and inferior endocardial cushions and the lower margin of the atrial septum posterosuperiorly is much greater than either χ or 2χ to 3χ. Let us call this distance between the endocardial cushions and the atrial septum approximately 5χ to 10χ.

Now let us consider the above-mentioned spatial geometry and its influence on the normal and abnormal morphogensis of the AV canal (Fig. 11.10):

1. When the fibroblasts of the endocardial cushions of the AV canal take their random "walks" in space, these fibroblasts first encounter the crest of the muscular ventricular septum beneath the inferior endocardial cushion—because this is the shortest distance (χ) between the endocardial cushions and either septum. So, obliteration of the VSD beneath the inferior endocardial cushion is the first step in the formation of the AV septum. This spatial geometry also explains why many cases of completely common AV canal have no VSD component beneath the inferior leaflet of the common AV valve—only beneath the superior leaflet.

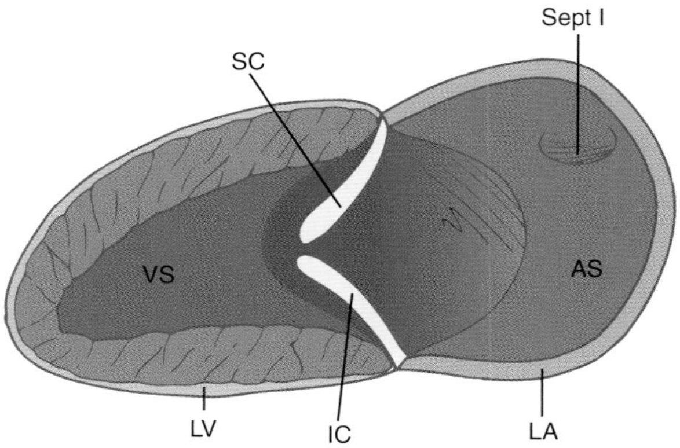

Fig. 11.10 Spatial geometry and the morphogenesis of common atrioventricular (AV) canal: diagram of the complete form of common AV canal, viewed from the left. Note that the inferior endocardial cushion *(IC)* of the AV canal is closer to the crest of the muscular ventricular septum *(VS)* than is the superior endocardial cushion *(SC)*. Both endocardial cushions are much closer to the crest of the VS than they are to the anteroinferior rim of the atrial septum *(AS)*. Our hypothesis is that these spatial geometric considerations are important determinants of the normal sequence of morphogenesis and the classification of common AV canal: (1) Because IC is closest to the VS, the VSD beneath the IC is obliterated first. (2) Because the SC is farther away from the VS, the VSD beneath the SC is obliterated as the second step in normal morphogenesis. In this way, the complete form of common AV canal is converted to the most frequent partial form of common AV canal. (3) Because the SC and the IC are so much farther away from the AS than from the VS, closure of the ostium primum type of atrial septal defect and closure of the cleft in the anterior leaflet of the mitral valve together constitute the third and last step in the normal morphogenesis of the septation of the AV canal and the formation of the mitral valve. Closure of the VSD component of the AV septal defect may well stabilize the SC and IC relative to each other, facilitating cleft closure from medially to laterally, despite the fact that the SC and the IC are moving back and forth 140 to 160 times/minute because of the heartbeat. *LA,* Left atrium; *LV,* left ventricle; *Sept 1,* septum primum; AV septal defect shown in black. (From Van Praagh S, Antoniadis S, Otero-Coto E, Leidenfrost RD, Van Praagh R: Common AV canal with and without conotruncal malformations: an anatomic study of 251 postmortem cases. In: Nora JJ, Takao A [eds], *Congenital Heart Disease: Causes and Processes.* Futura, Mount Kisco, NY, 1984, p 599.)

2. Fibroblasts from the superior endocardial cushion of the AV canal then encounter the muscular ventricular septal crest and obliterate this greater space (2χ to 3χ). This second step completes the closure of the VSD of the AV canal type. A completely common AV canal has now been converted into a partially common AV canal—with an ostium primum type of atrial septal defect, a cleft anterior leaflet of the mitral valve, and an intact ventricular septum. In other words, a complete AV septal defect has now become a partial AV septal defect with a cleft anterior mitral leaflet.
3. Step 3 in the normal morphogenesis of the AV canal has two parts that appear to occur approximately simultaneously: (a) cleft closure, and (b) closure of the ostium primum type of atrial septal defect. Let us consider each part of step 3 in turn.
   a. Why does cleft closure occur now? It must be remembered that the superior and inferior endocardial cushions (leaflets) are moving back and forth between 130 and 150 times per minute because of the heartbeat. How can the cleft possibly close when the superior and inferior cushion components are moving back and forth an average of 140 beats/minute? Our hypothesis is that once the VSD has been closed by fibrous tissue, then the superior and inferior endocardial cushion components have been anchored and stabilized relative to each other. Although both cushions move rapidly back and forth because of the heartbeat, they now are anchored medially at the septum, and consequently the superior and inferior leaflet components move very little relative to each other. This minimal movement of the superior and inferior cushions relative to each other permits the medial-to-lateral "zippering" process of cleft fusion to occur. Since cleft closure appears to depend on the great reduction or elimination of significant movement of the superior and inferior cushions relative to each other, closure or near closure of the AV septal defect may occur *before* cleft closure; that is, in addition to the closure of the VSD component, closure of much if not all of the ASD component may well be necessary to stabilize the superior and inferior cushions relative to each other. Note that in man (Fig.11.8) and in the rat (Fig. 11.9), the mitral cleft persists after fusion of the superior and inferior endocardial cushions of the AV canal. If indeed mitral cleft closure is the last act in this drama, as Figs. 11.8 and 11.9 suggest, such timing would help to explain the existence of isolated cleft of the mitral valve of the AV canal type, that is, isolated cleft of the anterior leaflet of the mitral valve with no septal defect. This is a topic to which we shall return.
   b. At approximately the same time, the relatively large ostium primum type of atrial septal defect (5χ to 10χ) is being closed as the posteriorly growing fibroblasts from the endocardial AV cushions encounter and fuse with the anterorinferior margin of the atrial septum. Why is closure of the ostium primum part of step 3 perhaps the last part of the septational process? Again, we think that spatial geometry is key (Fig. 11.10): the anteriorly pointing V-shaped wedge of the endocardial cushions of the AV canal is much farther away from the atrial septum than from the ventricular septum.

To summarize, the three normal morphogentic steps in the development of the AV canal—that become arrested in persistent common AV canal—are as follows (Figs. 11.8, 11.9, and 11.10):

1. inferior VSD closure; then
2. superior VSD closure; then
3. ostium primum ASD closure and mitral cleft closure (approximately simultaneously).

It should be added that this usual morphogenetic sequence can occasionally get out of order, as in VSD of the AV canal type, with or without straddling tricuspid valve. Usually, closure of the AV canal type of VSD is the first step in the morphogenetic sequence. But in VSD of the AV canal type with or without straddling tricuspid valve, step one in the usual morphogenetic sequence fails to occur, while the subsequent steps are accomplished normally (normal AV valves and no ostium primum type of atrial septal defect). Hence, although the aforementioned morphogenetic sequence is the usual progression of developmental events, it is by no means invariable.

It is fascinating to note that the foregoing *morphogentic sequence* helps to explain the pathologic anatomic classification of common AV canal:

1. In the complete form of common AV canal, step one (inferior VSD closure) may or may not have occurred.
2. When steps one and two have been accomplished (complete VSD closure), then the most frequent form of partially common AV canal has been reached (ostium primum ASD with cleft mitral valve).
3. Both parts of morphogenetic step three may not be completed, resulting in isolated mitral cleft (of the AV canal type—other types do exist); or resulting in isolated ostium primum ASD (without cleft mitral valve and with intact ventricular septum). The latter is very rare.

It is also interesting to understand that the *Rastelli classification*[16] of the complete type of common AV canal is backwards from a developmental standpoint:

Type C is the most primitive, with its undivided and unattached anterosuperior leaflet (Fig. 11.4).

Type B is slightly more advanced, the anterosuperior leaflet being partly divided, but unattached to the ventricular septum (Fig.11.3).

Type A is even more advanced, the anterosuperior leaflet being divided and attached by short chordae tendineae to the ventricular septal crest (Fig. 11.2).

Ironically, Rastelli, Kirklin, and Titus[16] did not intend to classify the complete form of common AV canal into types A, B, and C. Instead, their photographic figures 2 and 4 were labeled A, B, and C. And so, inadvertently, the medical artist who labeled these photographs made history because subsequently, these were known as types A, B, and C of the complete form of common AV canal.

ETIOLOGY

An increase in cell-surface adhesiveness[26,27] has been proposed as a possible etiologic factor in the common AV canal that occurs with Down syndrome. The idea essentially is that when the endocardial cushion fibroblasts take their random "walks" in space, if they have an increase in cell surface adhesiveness, these fibroblasts will tend to stick together too much, will migrate out subnormally, and hence will fail to form a normal AV septum and will also fail to close the cleft between the superior endocardial cushion component and the inferior endocardial cushion component of what should normally develop into the anterior leaflet of the mitral valve.

Cardiac morphogenesis appears to be strongly influenced by genetics and also by chance. The stochastic (probabilistic) single-gene hypothesis[28] now appears more appealing than does the multifactorial polygenic hypothesis. Identical twins with Down syndrome, but discordant for congenital heart disease, are more the rule than the exception. This suggests that although genetic factors are very important, random (chance, or stochastic) events also appear to play a significant role in determining the organic phenotype.[28]

The importance of genetics is emphasized by the work of Korenberg and colleagues.[29,30] These investigators think that the Down syndrome congenital heart disease genes are located in a small region at the distal end of chromosome 21, from q22.1 to q22.3.

Is the foregoing relevant to the etiology of common AV canal? The answer is yes, because common AV canal is by far the most frequent form of congenital heart disease associated with *Down syndrome*.[31] In 100 randomly selected cases of Down syndrome with congenital heart disease, common AV canal occurred in 63%: The complete form of common AV canal was found in 52% (type A in 29% and type C in 23%) and a partial form of common AV canal was present in 11%.[31]

Comparison of common AV canal with Down syndrome versus common AV canal without Down syndrome revealed several statistically highly significant differences:[31]

1. The complete form of common AV canal was much more frequent in patients with Down syndrome (83%) than in patients without Down syndrome (45%) ($p < .001$).
2. Conversely, the partial form of common AV canal was much more frequent in patients without Down syndrome (55%) than in patients with Down syndrome (17%) ($p < .001$).
3. Type A completely common AV canal was more frequent in patients without Down syndrome (83%) than in those with Down syndrome (56%) ($p < .005$).
4. Type C completely common AV canal was much more frequent in patients with Down syndrome (44%) than in those without Down syndrome (17%) ($p < .005$).
5. Hypoplastic left ventricle (i.e., the hypoplastic left heart syndrome) was more frequent in patients without Down syndrome (19%) than in those with Down syndrome (8%) ($p < .01$).
6. Left ventricular outflow tract obstruction was more frequent in individuals without Down syndrome (35%) than in those with Down syndrome (6%) ($p < .001$).

Thus, common AV canal with Down syndrome was more primitive than common AV canal without Down syndrome. Down syndrome cases had significantly higher prevalences of complete (as opposed to partial) canals, and type C (as opposed to type A).

There are two major groups of common AV canal:

1. **nonsyndromic common AV canal,** that is, not associated with any identified syndrome; and
2. **syndromic common AV canal,** that is, an integral part of an identified syndrome such as **Down syndrome** or the **heterotaxy syndromes** with asplenia, with polysplenia, and with a normally formed but right-sided spleen.

Regarding syndromic common AV canal, we have never seen **Down syndrome** in association with situs inversus totalis, nor with the heterotaxy syndromes with asplenia or polysplenia. Trisomy 21 has many pernicious effects, but there is at least one good thing about it: Trisomy 21 appears to guarantee situs solitus (the normal pattern of anatomic organization) at all segmental levels—visceroatrial situs, AV valves, ventricles, infundibulum (conus), and great arteries. The segmental situs set is always {S,D,S}: situs solitus of viscera and atria (S), D-loop ventricles (D), and solitus normally related great arteries (S).

To the best of our present knowledge, this means that Down syndrome never has atrial inversion or atrial situs ambiguus, ventricular inversion (L-loop formation), or a well-developed subaortic conus with transposition of the great arteries or double-outlet right ventricle. (We are continuing to search for exceptions to this generalization.) Down syndrome can have underdevelopment of the subpulmonary conus and its sequelae, that is, tetralogy of Fallot, and a lot of aortic overriding can lead to the diagnosis of double-outlet right ventricle. But double-outlet right ventricle with a well-developed muscular subaortic conus or a well-developed bilateral conus (subaortic and subpulmonary) we have never seen with Down syndrome. In other words, the conus is always subpulmonary—normally developed or underdeveloped (tetralogy of Fallot).

Other trisomies, such as 13-15 and 17-18, also seem always to have situs solitus at all segmental levels.

The other major form of syndromic common AV canal, that is, the heterotaxy syndromes with asplenia and polysplenia, is the exact opposite. Segmental situs discordance is the rule: they are a segmental situs salad or potpourri. One should expect anything: the atrial situs may be solitus, inversus, or ambiguus (undiagnosed).

Atrial isomerism—right isomerism or left isomerism—is an erroneous concept. Accurately speaking, atrial isomerism does not exist. See Chapter 29 for more details. D-loop ventricles or L-loop ventricles may be present. The conus may be subpulmonary, subaortic, or bilateral. The great arteries may be normally related or transposed, or double-outlet right ventricle may be present.

These anatomic findings suggest that trisomies such as Down syndrome may result in a ***genetic "overdosage."*** Despite their obviously deleterious effects, chromosomal trisomies appear to guarantee normal segmental situs at all levels. In other words, trisomies are characterized by visceroatrial situs solitus, segmental situs concordance at all levels, and concordant atrioventricular and ventriculoarterial alignments. Such genetic "overdosage" appears to guarantee situs solitus totalis.

By contrast, the heterotaxy syndromes may well be characterized by **genetic "underdosage,"** that is, lack of the genetic information that should specify situs solitus at all segmental levels. The result of such lack of apparent genetic control of segmental situs is the aforementioned ***segmental situs discordances*** that result in what we call complex congenital heart disease.

Lack of genetic information (perhaps at the level of genes or gene regulators) appears to be the fundamental problem in ***Kartagener syndrome,*** which is characterized by situs inversus totalis, sinusitis, and bronchiectasis. The bronchiectasis part of this triad is now known to be due to lack of dynein side arms in the nasal sinus and tracheobronchial cilia, which consequently do not beat properly and hence do not cleanse the nasal sinuses and the tracheobronchial tree in the normal way. Men with Kartagener syndrome may be infertile, because their sperm tails also lack dynein, and consequently their sperm do not swim normally.

Lack of a specific protein such as dynein is strong presumptive evidence that this protein is not being coded for. In turn, this strongly suggests a lack of genetic information. Lack of genetic information, resulting in segmental situs deregulation, suggests that segmental situs may be random, or occurring by chance. This is the ***Layton hypothesis***.[32,33] Dr. William M. Layton developed this hypothesis while working with the *iv/iv* mouse model. Indeed, Dr. Layton[32] was really the discoverer of the congenital heart disease in the *iv/iv* mouse model that has proved so helpful in clarifying the molecular genetics of laterality defects.

iv is the gene symbol for situs inversus. As it turned out, the so-called *iv/iv* mouse model is really a model not of situs inversus totalis, but of visceral heterotaxy with situs ambiguus, many of these animals having polysplenia, and a few having asplenia. Phenotypically, some also had situs inversus.

In approximately 3000 experiments with the *iv/iv* mouse model, Layton found that D-loop ventricles and L-loop ventricles were very nearly 50/50: half D-loops, half L-loops (i.e., randomized). This suggested that cardiac loop formation was occurring by chance, like a coin flip (with a true coin). The only model of inheritance that these data appeared to fit was a chance or stochastic model.[32,33] Hence, the data suggested a true or apparent lack of genetic information. The Layton hypothesis[32,33] is what we mean by genetic "underdosage."

Perhaps I should add that I served as the murine "cardiologist" in these early experiments with the *iv/iv* mouse model.[34] My job was to help make the diagnosis, for example, transposition of the great arteries (in about 20%) and double-outlet right ventricle (in about 22%).

Consequently, our impression is that both syndromic forms of common AV canal have a strong genetic component in their etiology, but that these genetic components are very different ("overdosage" versus "underdosage"), as are the anatomic findings. Much more remains to be learned about the specific genetic aspects of both forms of syndromic common AV canal.

Are the heterotaxy syndromes with asplenia and polysplenia totally chaotic? Are there no patterns amid these segmental situs mismatches? Comparison of 95 postmortem patients with the *asplenia syndrome* versus 67 postmortem patients with the *polysplenia syndrome* revealed several statistically highly significant differences between these two different heterotaxy syndromes:[20]

1. Common AV canal was more than twice as frequent with asplenia (96%) as with polysplenia (45%) ($p < .0001$).
2. The complete form of common AV canal occurred much more frequently with asplenia (81%) than with polysplenia (33%) ($p < .0001$).
3. Normally divided AV canal with normally formed AV valves were much more frequent with polysplenia (55%) than with asplenia (4%) ($p < .0001$).

PARACHUTE MITRAL VALVE

Potentially parachute mitral valve in common AV canal requires a more detailed presentation in order to be well understood.[17] First, what is meant by *potentially* parachute mitral valve in the setting of common AV canal? *Potentially* means following surgical repair, that is, following surgical division of the common AV canal into mitral and tricuspid canals in the complete form of common AV canal by closure of the AV septal defect,

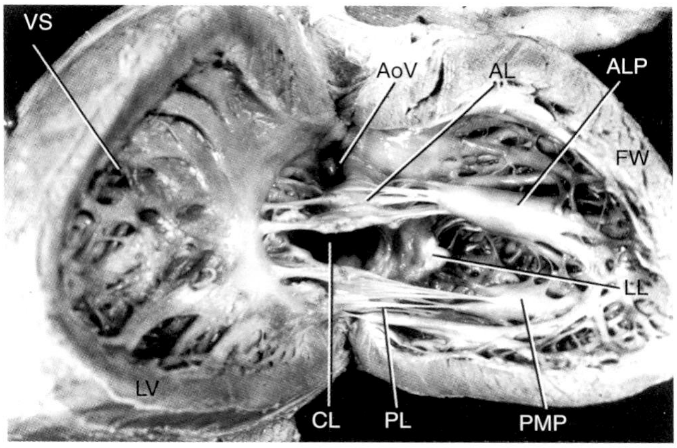

Fig. 11.11 Incomplete form of common atrioventricular canal (CAVC), that is, ostium primum type of atrial septal defect (ASD I) with cleft anterior leaflet of mitral valve. Note the typical cleft *(CL)* between the anterior leaflet component *(AL)* and the posterior leaflet component *(PL)* of what should normally be the anterior (noncleft) leaflet of the mitral valve. The AL component, derived from the anterior (superior) endocardial cushion of the AV canal, typically inserts only into the anterolateral (superior) papillary muscle group of the left ventricle *(ALP)*. The PL component, derived from the posterior (inferior) endocardial cushion of the common AV canal, typically inserts only into the posteromedial (inferior) papillary muscle group of the left ventricle *(PMP)*. The left lateral (mural) leaflet of mitral valve (LL) lies between the ALP and the PMP muscles of the left ventricle. Usually, the ALP and the PMP muscles constitute the two foci of chordal insertion of the left ventricle. *AoV,* Aortic valve; *FW,* free wall; *LV,* morphologically left ventricle; *VS,* ventricular septum. (From David I, Castañeda AR, Van Praagh R: Potentially parachute mitral valve in common atrioventricular canal, pathological anatomy and surgical importance. *J Thorac Cardiovasc Surg* 84:178, 1982; with permission.)

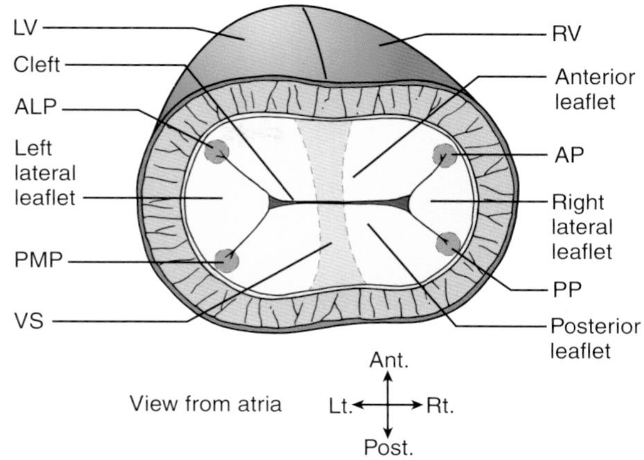

Fig. 11.12 Diagrammatic view of common atrioventricular (AV) canal *without* potentially parachute mitral valve, that is, with two widely spaced foci of chordal insertion, as seen from the atria—similar to the surgical view. The anterolateral papillary muscle *(ALP)* and the posteromedial papillary muscle *(PMP)* are widely spaced. Consequently there is a good-sized left lateral or mural leaflet *(Lt. Lat. Leaflet)* of the potentially mitral valve postoperatively. *AP,* Anterior papillary muscle group of the morphologically right ventricle *(RV)*; *LV,* morphologically left ventricle; *PP,* posterior papillary muscle of the RV; *VS,* ventricular septum. (From David I, Castañeda AR, Van Praagh R: Potentially parachute mitral valve in common atrioventricular canal, pathological anatomy and surgical importance. *J Thorac Cardiovasc Surg* 84:178, 1982; with permission.)

and following surgical reconstruction of the AV valves. Prior to surgical repair, in completely common AV canal, one cannot accurately speak of parachute mitral valve or double-orifice mitral valve—because there is no mitral valve, only a common AV valve. However, in the partial form of common AV canal, there is a malformed (cleft) mitral valve and hence the qualifier *potentially* is unnecessary.

What is "normal," that is, usual, in common AV canal? In the left ventricle, both in the complete and partial forms of common AV canal, there usually are two main foci of chordal insertion (Fig. 11.11): the anterolateral papillary muscle, the upper one; and the posteromedial papillary muscle, the lower one.

The superior (anterior) leaflet of the common AV valve or the mitral valve usually inserts only into the superior (anterolateral) papillary muscle (Fig. 11.11).

The inferior (posterior) leaflet of the common AV valve or the mitral valve usually inserts only into the inferior (posteromedial) papillary muscle group (Fig. 11.11).

Note that these two main foci of chordal insertion—the anterolateral and posteromedial papillary muscles—are widely separated. Consequently, the left lateral leaflet of the common AV valve—that will form the posterior or mural leaflet of the mitral valve postoperatively—lies between the anterolateral and the posteromedial papillary muscles of the left ventricle (Fig. 11.11).

The essential features of the potentially normal mitral valve are shown diagrammatically as seen from above in Fig. 11.12. The most important details are the two widely spaced papillary muscles (anterolateral and posteromedial), which makes possible the existence of a posterior or mural leaflet of the mitral valve, which is derived from the left lateral leaflet of the common AV valve. As mentioned, note that the superior (anterior) leaflet of the common AV valve inserts only into the anterolateral papillary muscle; the inferior (posterior) leaflet inserts only into the posteromedial papillary muscle; the posterior or mural leaflet (derived from the left lateral leaflet of the common AV valve) inserts into both papillary muscles; and there are no accessory orifices in any of the leaflets of the common AV valve.

Potentially parachute mitral valve in completely common AV canal type A is presented in Fig. 11.13. Note that both the superior (anterior) leaflet and the inferior (posterior) leaflet of the common AV valve insert only into the anterolateral papillary muscle. There is only one focus of chordal insertion in this left ventricle (the anterolateral papillary muscle), not the normal two foci of chordal insertion (the anterolateral and the posteromedial papillary muscles).

Note that there may well be a hypoplastic posteromedial papillary muscle in this left ventricle (?PMP, Fig. 11.13). However, this does not matter. What matters is how many foci of chordal insertion are present—not how many papillary muscles are present. Also, we are talking about the number of foci of chordal insertion of *primary* chordae tendineae—those that control the free margins of the superior and inferior leaflets of the common AV valve.

To summarize, this is regarded as a case of potentially parachute mitral valve (Fig. 11.13) because there is only a single focus of chordal insertion of the primary chordae tendineae that control both the superior and the inferior leaflet margins of the common AV valve.

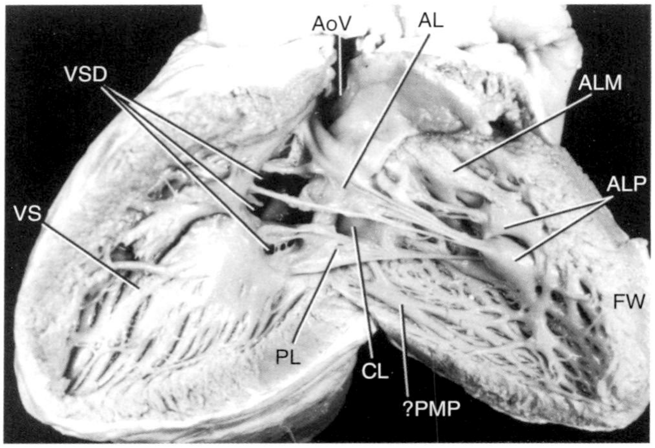

Fig. 11.13 Complete form of common AV canal, type A, with potentially parachute mitral valve, opened left ventricular view. All of the primary chordae tendineae from both the anterior leaflet component *(AL)* and the posterior leaflet component *(PL)* of the cleft *(CL)* anterior leaflet of the potentially mitral valve insert only into the anterolateral papillary muscle group *(ALP)*. Although a small posteromedial papillary muscle may be present *(?PMP)*, it does not receive primary chordal insertions of the PL component of the anterior mitral leaflet. Potentially parachute mitral valve is present because there is only one focus of left ventricular chordal insertion, not two (cf. Figs. 11.11 and 11.12). With only one focus of chordal insertion, there can be no left lateral (mural, or posterior) leaflet of the potentially parachute mitral valve postoperatively (cf. Figs. 11.11 and 11.12). Because the CL is the main orifice of the potentially parachute mitral valve, the cleft must not be sutured closed in order not to create iatrogenic mitral stenosis postoperatively. *ALM,* Anterolateral muscle of the left ventricle, also known as the muscle of Moulaert; *AoV,* aortic valve; *FW,* free wall; *VS,* ventricular septum; *VSD,* ventricular septal defects. (From David I, Castañeda AR, Van Praagh R: Potentially parachute mitral valve in common atrioventricular canal, pathological anatomy and surgical importance. *J Thorac Cardiovasc Surg* 84:178, 1982; with permission.)

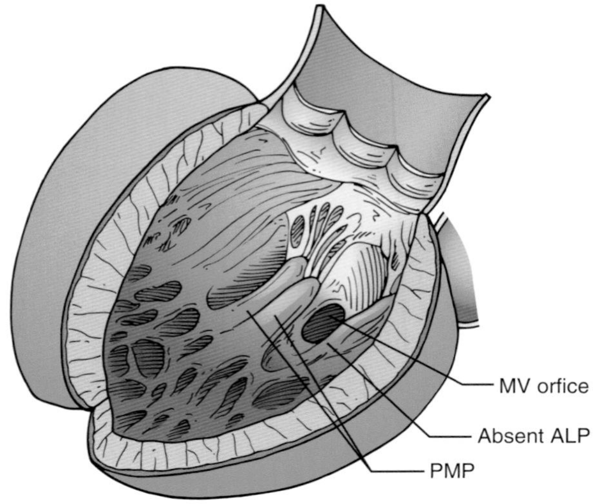

Fig. 11.14 Typical parachute mitral valve *(MV)* with divided (as opposed to common) atrioventricular (AV) canal. Note that the posteromedial papillary muscle group *(PMP)* is present and hypertrophied, whereas the anterolateral papillary muscle group *(ALP)* is absent. The papillary muscles typically are the *opposite* with common AV canal and potentially parachute mitral valve. With divided AV canal, parachute MV typically is severely stenotic, as in this figure. But with common AV canal, potentially parachute MV often is not demonstrably stenotic preoperatively (cf. Fig. 11.13). (From Ruckman RN, Van Praagh R: Anatomic types of congenital mitral stenosis. Report of 49 autopsy cases with consideration of diagnosis and surgical implications. *Am J Cardiol* 42:592, 1978; with permission.)

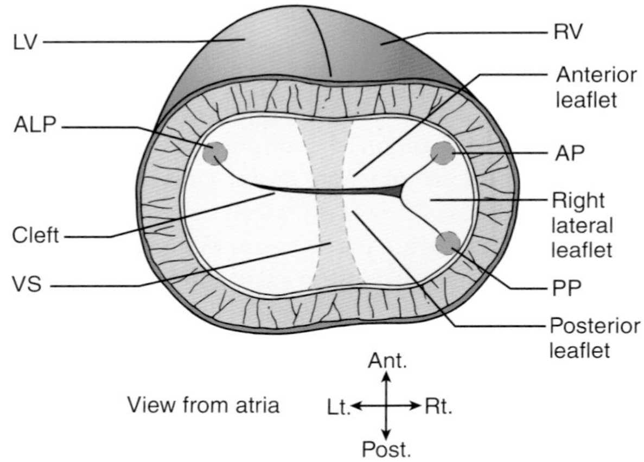

Fig. 11.15 Diagram of potentially parachute mitral valve (MV) with completely common atrioventricular (AV) canal type A, viewed from the atria. This is the same patient as is shown photographically in Fig. 11.13. Note that there is only one focus of left ventricular chordal insertion, the anterolateral papillary muscle group *(ALP)*. The orifice of the potential MV postoperatively is the cleft of the common AV valve. *LV,* left ventricle; *VS,* ventricular septum; *RV,* right ventricle; *AP,* anterior papillary muscle; *PP,* posterior papillary muscle. (From David I, Castañeda AR, Van Praagh R: Potentially parachute mitral valve in common atrioventricular canal, pathological anatomy and surgical importance. *J Thorac Cardiovasc Surg* 84:178, 1982; with permission.)

In common AV canal with potentially parachute mitral valve, the single focus of left ventricular chordal insertion typically is the anterolateral papillary muscle, the posteromedial papillary muscle being hypoplastic or absent, as in this patient (Fig. 11.13).

As mentioned heretofore, the anomalies of the papillary muscles of the left ventricle in common AV canal with potentially parachute mitral valve (Figs. 11.11 to 11.13) are the *opposite* of those found in typical cases of parachute mitral valve with a normally divided AV canal in which the posteromedial papillary muscle of the left ventricle is present and hypertrophied, while the anterolateral papillary muscle of the left ventricle is hypoplastic or absent (Fig. 11.14).

The salient features of common AV canal with a single left ventricular focus of primary chordal insertion is shown diagrammatically in Fig. 11.15. This is a diagram of the case shown in Fig. 11.13. Note that the diagram shows that both the superior and the inferior leaflets insert only into the anterolateral papillary muscle. There is no functional posteromedial papillary muscle receiving the primary chordae tendineae from the inferior leaflet.

Since there is only one functional papillary muscle group in this left ventricle, there can be no posterior or mural leaflet of the mitral valve. There can be no interpapillary muscle distance—an important component of the normal mitral orifice.[18] Consequently, from a surgical standpoint, *one must not suture closed the mitral cleft* because the cleft is the major part of the postoperative mitral orifice. Surgical closure of the cleft of the potential mitral valve, when there is only one functional left

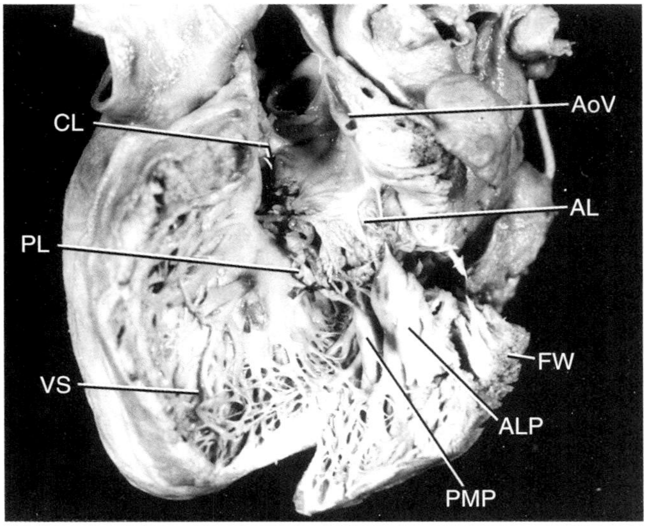

Fig. 11.16 Potentially parachute mitral valve in common atrioventricular (AV) canal with two juxtaposed papillary muscle groups. Note that the anterolateral papillary muscle group *(APL)* and the posteromedial papillary muscle group *(PMP)* are very close together (touching each other). The single focus of left ventricular chordal insertion consists of this clump of unseparated papillary musculature. Other abbreviations as previously noted. (From David I, Castañeda AR, Van Praagh R: Potentially parachute mitral valve in common atrioventricular canal, pathological anatomy and surgical importance. *J Thorac Cardiovasc Surg* 84:178, 1982; with permission.)

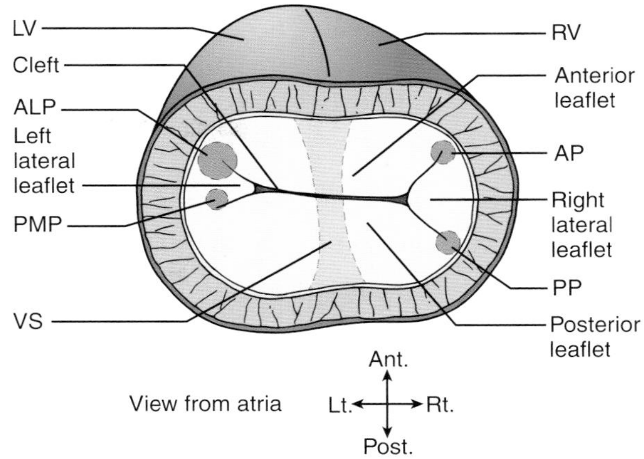

Fig. 11.17 Diagram of potentially parachute mitral valve in common atrioventricular (AV) canal with two juxtaposed papillary muscle groups and one mitral orifice. The larger anterolateral papillary muscle *(ALP)* and the smaller posteromedial papillary muscle *(PMP)* are very close together (touching). This is a diagram of the heart shown in Fig. 11.16. *AP*, anterior papillary muscle of the right ventricle; *LV*, left ventricle; *PP*, posterior papillary muscle of the right ventricle; *RV*, right ventricle; *VS*, ventricular septum. (From David I, Castañeda AR, Van Praagh R: Potentially parachute mitral valve in common atrioventricular canal, pathological anatomy and surgical importance. *J Thorac Cardiovasc Surg* 84:178, 1982; with permission.)

ventricular papillary muscle, results in *iatrogenic mitral stenosis* postoperatively and can lead to the death of such patients. This is why a clear understanding of potentially parachute mitral valve is so important both diagnostically and surgically.

The anatomy of potentially parachute mitral valve can be even more misleading diagnostically. Two papillary muscles can be present, the anterolateral large and the posteromedial small and juxtaposed to the larger one (Fig. 11.16). Despite the presence of two papillary muscles, admittedly not well spaced, most of the chordae inserted into the larger anterolateral group, and the potential posterior or mural leaflet of the mitral valve was very small—because of the markedly reduced interpapillary muscle distance (Fig. 11.17). This may be regarded as a forme fruste of potentially parachute mitral valve in the setting of common AV canal (Figs. 11.16 and 11.17). Although a forme fruste anatomically, this case functions like congenital mitral stenosis postoperatively unless handled expertly by the cardiac surgeon.

Finally, potentially parachute mitral valve in common AV canal can be even more misleading diagnostically. It is even possible to have potentially parachute mitral valve with two well-developed left ventricular papillary muscles—if all of the primary chordae tendineae insert only into the anterolateral papillary muscle (Fig. 11.18). This fortunately rare anatomic type of potentially parachute mitral valve is shown diagrammatically in Fig. 11.19.

Would it be possible to diagnose such a case accurately preoperatively (Figs. 11.18 and 11.19)? We think that the presence of two large left ventricular papillary muscles could be very confusing diagnostically. This, in turn, is why the final diagnosis may well have to be made by the well-educated cardiac surgeon, under direct vision.

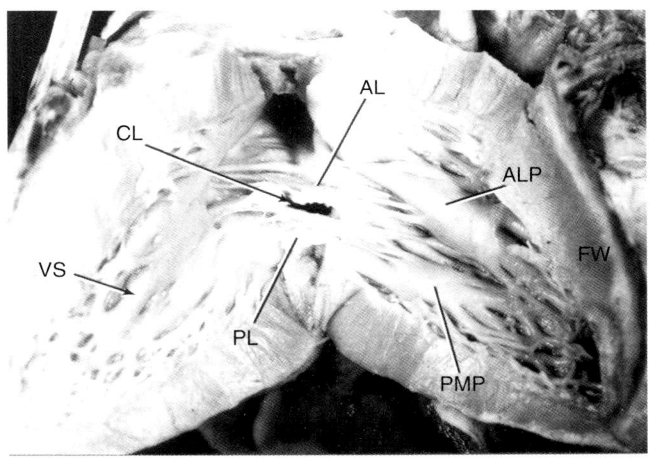

Fig. 11.18 Potentially parachute mitral valve in common atrioventricular (AV) canal with two papillary muscle groups and one mitral orifice. In this opened left ventricle, note that there are two well developed and well separated papillary muscle groups, the anterolateral *(ALP)* and the posteromedial *(PMP)*. However, the chordae tendineae from both the anterior (superior) leaflet *(AL)* above the cleft *(CL)* and from the posterior (inferior) leaflet *(PL)* below the cleft insert into the ALP muscle group. Why the free margin of the PL did not insert with primary chordae tendineae into the PMP muscle group is unknown. *FW*, Free wall; *VS*, ventricular septum. (From David I, Castañeda AR, Van Praagh R: Potentially parachute mitral valve in common atrioventricular canal, pathological anatomy and surgical importance. *J Thorac Cardiovasc Surg* 84:178, 1982; with permission.)

This, too, is why we have been saying that potentially parachute mitral valve in common AV canal is not just a question of the number of left ventricular papillary muscles. It is really a question of the number of *functional* left ventricular papillary muscles that receive primary chordae tendineae. In other words, it is a question of *the number of left ventricular foci of primary chordal insertion.* Unfortunately, the diagnosis of potentially

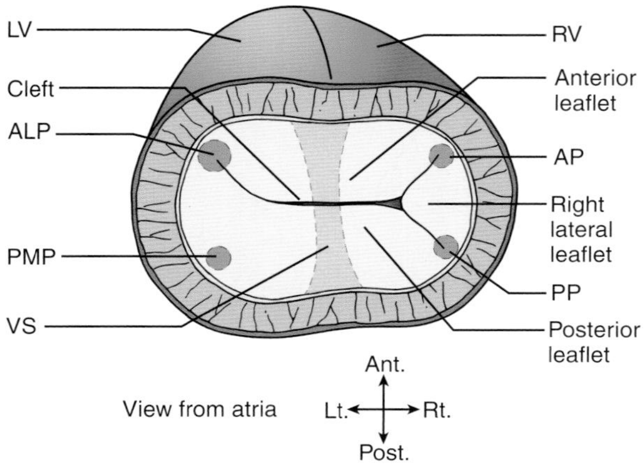

Fig. 11.19 Diagram of potentially parachute mitral valve in common atrioventricular (AV) canal with two papillary muscle groups and one potentially mitral orifice, viewed from the atrial (surgical) aspect. This is a diagram of the heart specimen shown in Fig. 11.18. Note that the anterolateral papillary muscle *(ALP)* and the posteromedial papillary muscle *(PMP)* are both present, well developed, and well separated. Nonetheless, both the anterior and the posterior leaflets insert chordae tendineae only into the ALP muscle group, thereby creating a potentially parachute mitral valve. The mitral orifice is the cleft and there is no posterior mitral leaflet. This is why we *define potentially parachute mitral valve with common AV canal* as a single focus of left ventricular insertion of primary chordae tendineae, that is, of the chordae that control the margins of the cleft. We do not define potentially parachute mitral valve in terms of the number of left ventricular papillary muscles, because this can be diagnostically misleading, as these cases (Figs. 11.16 to 11.19) illustrate. *AP*, anterior papillary muscle of the right ventricle; *LV*, left ventricle; *PP*, posterior papillary muscle of the right ventricle; *RV*, right ventricle; *VS*, ventricular septum. (From David I, Castañeda AR, Van Praagh R: Potentially parachute mitral valve in common atrioventricular canal, pathological anatomy and surgical importance. *J Thorac Cardiovasc Surg* 84:178, 1982; with permission.)

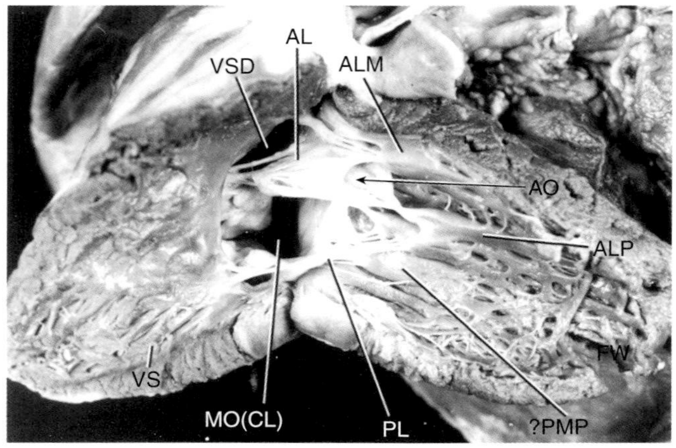

Fig. 11.20 Potentially parachute mitral valve with common atrioventricular (AV) canal and with an accessory orifice in the anterosuperior leaflet. In this opened left ventricle, note that the primary chordae tendineae of the anterosuperior leaflet *(AL)* and of the posterioinferior leaflet *(PL)* both insert into the anterolateral papillary muscle group *(ALP)*. There may be a posteromedial papillary muscle group present *(?PMP)*; but it does not receive the primary chordae tendineae of the PL that instead insert into the ALP. The primary chordae from the AL—from the superior margin of the cleft *(CL)*—also insert into the ALP muscle group. Hence, a potential parachute mitral valve is present, with one left ventricular focus of insertion of primary chordae tendineae into the ALP muscle group. In the AL, there is an accessory orifice *(AO)*. The superior chordae of this accessory orifice insert into the anterolateral muscle *(ALM)* or muscle of Moulaert. The inferior chordae from this accessory orifice insert into the ALP muscle group. Postoperatively, this patient would have not only a parachute mitral valve, but also a double-orifice mitral valve, that is, a parachute and double-orifice mitral valve. The cleft is the main orifice—*MO (CL)*—of this double-orifice parachute mitral valve. *VSD*, ventricular septal defect. (From David I, Castañeda AR, Van Praagh R: Potentially parachute mitral valve in common atrioventricular canal, pathological anatomy and surgical importance. *J Thorac Cardiovasc Surg* 84:178, 1982; with permission.)

parachute mitral valve is not just a question of counting left ventricular papillary muscles. Obviously, if there is only one left ventricular papillary muscle—the anterolateral—one should certainly make this diagnosis. However, the real problem is that this diagnosis is more subtle: potentially parachute mitral valve can be present with two papillary muscle groups (Figs. 11.16 to 11.19). Can we resolve and accurately visualize the chordae tendineae by imaging, and thus make this diagnosis preoperatively? That is the diagnostic challenge.

DOUBLE-ORIFICE MITRAL VALVE

Potentially double-orifice mitral valve also occurs with common AV canal[17] and hence needs to be understood. In the study of Baño et al[19] concerning double-orifice mitral valve with a divided AV canal and separate mitral and tricuspid valves, we learned how very important the tensor apparatus is in this anomaly. The same principles apply in potentially double-orifice mitral valve in common AV canal.

Double-Orifice Mitral Valve Principles

AV valve tissue is reminiscent of the law of conservation of mass and energy in the sense that there is only so much "stuff": it is either "mass" or "energy," but it cannot be both at the same time. By analogy, AV valve tissue can be either leaflet, or chorda tendinea, but cannot be both at the same place. The meaning of this metaphor will become clear on studying Fig. 11.20.

Potentially parachute mitral valve is present in this case of completely common AV canal because both the superior leaflet (AL) and the inferior leaflet (PL) send primary chordal insertions only to the anterolateral papillary muscle (ALP) of the left ventricle. A rudimentary posteromedial papillary muscle also appears to be present (?PMP), but it receives no primary chordae tendineae from the free margins of the inferior leaflet of the common AV valve. The inferior (or posterior) leaflet displays *crossing chordae:* the chordae tendineae of the inferior leaflet cross over from inferiorly to superiorly and insert only into the superior (anterolateral) papillary muscle—instead of inserting into the inferior (posteromedial) papillary muscle, which would be "normal" or usual for common AV canal (Fig. 11.11). Crossing chordae tendineae (from inferiorly to superiorly) are typical of potentially parachute mitral valve.

However, please note that this patient does not have a single focus of left ventricular chordal insertion (Fig. 11.20). It is true that there is only a single focus of *primary* chordal insertion (into the anterolateral papillary muscle); hence potentially parachute mitral valve is indeed present.

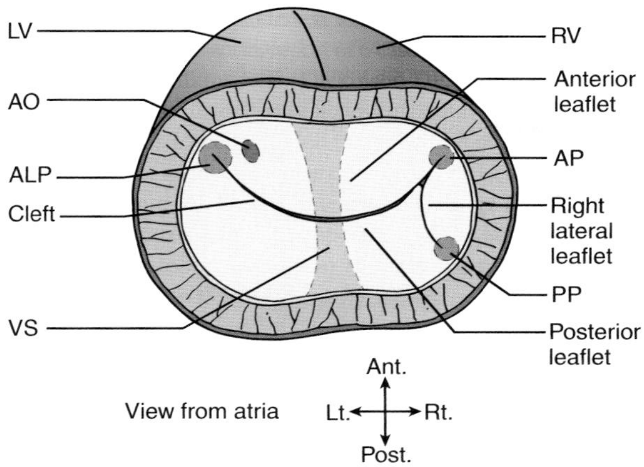

Fig. 11.21 Potentially parachute mitral valve in common atrioventricular (AV) canal with an accessory orifice *(AO)* in the anterosuperior leaflet. This is a diagram of the heart specimen shown in Fig. 11.20. *ALP,* anterolateral papillary muscle of the left ventricle; *AO,* accessory orifice; *AP,* anterior papillary muscle of the right ventricle; *LV,* left ventricle; *PP,* posterior papillary muscle of the right ventricle; *RV,* right ventricle; *VS,* ventricular septum. (From David I, Castañeda AR, Van Praagh R: Potentially parachute mitral valve in common atrioventricular canal, pathological anatomy and surgical importance. *J Thorac Cardiovasc Surg* 84:178, 1982; with permission.)

But there is a secondary focus of chordal insertion (Fig. 11.20): from the superior leaflet (AL) into the anterolateral muscle (ALM) of the left ventricle (also known as the muscle of Moulaert).[35]

So now the superior leaflet has a "problem": it has two foci of left ventricular chordal insertion—the usual one into the anterolateral papillary muscle, and an unusual one into the muscle of Moulaert (ALM).

So what does the superior leaflet do (Fig. 11.20)? Its substance is used to make these two chordal insertions. Consequently, the superior leaflet cannot make leaflet tissue at the same site. (Remember the rule: chordae, or leaflet, but not both at the same site, apparently because the amount of endocardial cushion tissue is limited.) Since the superior endocardial cushion tissue has been used to make closely adjacent chordae tendineae, consequently there is no leaflet tissue between these two foci of chordal insertion. The result is an accessory orifice in the superior leaflet (Figs. 11.20 and 11.21).

It must be emphasized that the aforementioned analogy or metaphor is presented in order to make this potentially double-orifice mitral valve in common AV canal comprehensible. The real morphogenesis of such an accessory orifice may be different from the foregoing explanatory analogy or metaphor.

However, it is anatomically factual that the main orifice of this potentially parachute mitral valve is the cleft orifice; and that there is an accessory orifice within the superior leaflet, between closely adjacent chordal insertions (Figs. 11.20 and 11.21).

Is it possible for there to be an accessory orifice in the inferior leaflet of the common AV valve, resulting in a different anatomic type of potentially double-orifice mitral valve? The answer, of course, is yes (Figs. 11.22 and 11.23). (In congenital heart disease, almost anything that one can imagine in fact does occur; hence the fascination of our field, which certainly isn't boring.) How does it work?

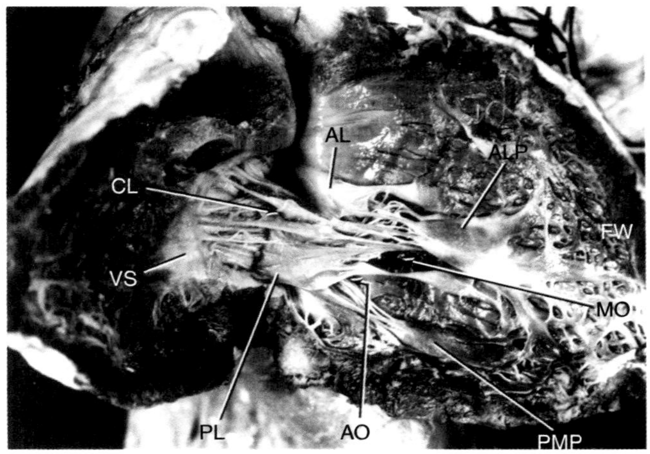

Fig. 11.22 Potentially parachute mitral valve in common atrioventricular (AV) canal with an accessory orifice in the posteroinferior leaflet. In this opened left ventricle, note that the cleft *(CL)* between the anterior leaflet *(AL)* and the posterior leaflet *(PL)* has been sutured closed, greatly narrowing the main orifice *(MO)*. The accessory orifice *(AO)* in the posterior leaflet sends some chordae tendineae to a small posteromedial papillary muscle *(PMP)* and other chordae tendineae to the larger anterolateral papillary muscle group *(ALP)*. *VS,* Ventricular septum; *FW,* free wall. (From David I, Castañeda AR, Van Praagh R: Potentially parachute mitral valve in common atrioventricular canal, pathological anatomy and surgical importance. *J Thorac Cardiovasc Surg* 84:178, 1982; with permission.)

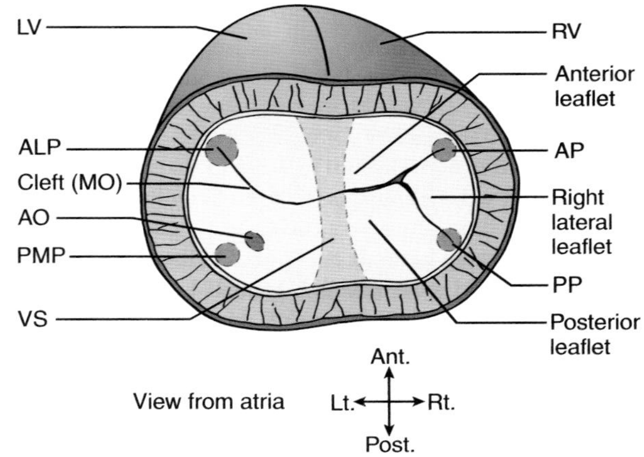

Fig. 11.23 Potentially parachute mitral valve in common atrioventricular (AV) canal with an accessory orifice in the posteroinferior leaflet of the common AV valve, diagram of the heart presented in Fig. 11.22. This case is an example of potentially parachute mitral valve with two papillary muscles and two orifices. *ALP,* anterolateral papillary muscle of the left ventricle; *AO,* accessory orifice; *AP,* anterior papillary muscle of the right ventricle; *LV,* left ventricle; *PP,* posterior papillary muscle of the right ventricle; *RV,* right ventricle; *VS,* ventricular septum. (From David I, Castañeda AR, Van Praagh R: Potentially parachute mitral valve in common atrioventricular canal, pathological anatomy and surgical importance. *J Thorac Cardiovasc Surg* 84:178, 1982.)

Examine Fig. 11.22 carefully. The main cleft orifice (CL) of this potentially double-orifice mitral valve looks quite small—because it was sutured closed surgically, greatly narrowing its main orifice (MO). The inferior leaflet (PL) sends a few small chordae to insert into a small posteromedial papillary muscle. However, most of the chordae of the inferior leaflet insert via crossing chordae into the superior (anterolateral) papillary muscle. So, now it is the inferior leaflet of the potentially parachute mitral valve that has an unusual "problem": two foci of chordal insertion.

Remembering our analogy with the law of mass and energy, we have two closely adjacent foci of chordal insertion involving the inferior leaflet (Fig. 11.22). Since the endocardial cushion tissue has been used up making chordae tendineae, it is not surprising that there is no leaflet tissue at the same site. Hence, there is an accessory orifice in the inferior leaflet between these closely adjacent chordae tendineae (Figs. 11.22 and 11.23).

Concerning the morphogenesis of potentially double-orifice mitral valve, there is the aforementioned "competition" between chordae and leaflets: one, or the other, but not both at the same site. Another way of expressing the same idea is as follows:

There is an inverse relationship between leaflet tissue and chordae tendineae. Think of the normal anterior leaflet of the mitral valve. It is semicircular in shape. Toward its center, leaflet tissue is maximal and chordae are minimal. Then, as one approaches either commissure, the leaflet tissue becomes less and less, while the chordae become more and more prominent.

Now think of the normal posterior leaflet of the mitral valve with its lateral, middle, and medial scallops. In the center of each scallop, the leaflet tissue is predominant and the chordae tendineae are less prominent. But between the scallops, the reverse situation is present: the chordae are predominant, and the leaflet tissue is minimized.

Hence, the inverse relationship between leaflet tissue and chordae tendineae is seen both in the normal anterior and posterior leaflets, and at the commissures.

Accessory orifices in AV valve leaflets (mitral, tricuspid, and common) appear to reflect this inverse relationship between leaflets and chordae, in which chordae are prominent, and the leaflet tissue between or among the chordae is minimal, that is, absent.

There may also be a simple mechanical explanation for accessory orifices: When there is a ring of chordae tendineae inserting into the ventricular surface of mitral leaflet tissue, the chordae pull on the endocardial cushion tissue with each ventricular systole. Traction by chordal rings may help to produce holes (accessory orifices) in AV leaflets.

Whatever the correct morphogenesis of potentially double-orifice mitral valve may ultimately prove to be, whenever you find a superior or an inferior leaflet of a common AV valve with two adjacent foci of chordal insertions, or with an abnormal chordal ring, you should also expect to find an accessory orifice between the two chordal foci, or within the chordal ring. One chordal focus is from the free margins of the leaflet: these are the primary chordae. The other chordal focus arises from the ventricular surface of the superior or inferior leaflet, away from the leaflet's free margins. These chordae may be called secondary chordae.

Consequently, the accessory orifices of a potentially parachute mitral valve often lie between the primary and secondary chordal insertions (Figs. 11.20 to 11.23).

The diagnostic implications of the foregoing include the following:

1. In common AV canal with potentially parachute mitral valve, although there is only one focus of primary chordal insertion, there may be an additional focus of secondary chordal insertion.
2. Between the primary and secondary foci of chordal insertion, a careful imaging search should be made for an accessory orifice, in order to establish or exclude the diagnosis of potentially parachute mitral valve with a primary (cleft) orifice, and with an additional accessory orifice in either the superior or inferior leaflet of the common AV valve.
3. The focus of diagnostic imaging should be primarily on the tensor apparatus—not just on the number of papillary muscles, but also on the number and type (primary or secondary) of chordal insertions.
4. Diagnostic attention should also be focused on the superior, inferior, and lateral leaflets of the common AV valve. One should use the tensor apparatus to understand and to explain the leaflet findings.

In other words, potentially double-orifice mitral valve is not just about double-orifice mitral valve. It is really about tensor apparatus abnormalities. The same principle also applies to potentially parachute mitral valve, with which double-orifice mitral valve may coexist. The key to diagnostic understanding is not just the leaflets: it really is the tensor apparatus.

FINDINGS

Complete Forms of Common AV Canal

Frequency: This study is based on 266 postmortem cases of completely common AV canal.

Percentage of Congenital Heart Disease: 266/3216 cases, that is, 8.27% of all patients with congenital heart disease (95% confidence interval [CI] 7.32% to 9.22%).

Gender: Males/females approximately equal, 126/130 (0.97/1). The gender was not known in 10 cases.

Age at Death: The mean age at death was 926 days (2.54 years) ± 2062 days (5.6 years), ranging from 0 (fetal demise) to 40.8 years. The median age of death was 120 days (4 months).

Associated Anomalies

Associated anomalies were frequent and important:

1. Down syndrome was the most frequent associated anomaly: 82/266 cases (30.8%).
   a. Down syndrome was associated with multiple congenital anomalies in 4/82 patients (4.9%).
   b. Down syndrome occurred with Hirschprung disease in 1/82 (1.2%).
   c. A Down mosaic was found in 1/82 (1.2%).
   d. Familial Down syndrome occurred in 1/82 (1.2%).
2. The heterotaxy syndrome with asplenia was the second most frequent associated anomaly: 51/266 cases (19.2%).
   a. The asplenia syndrome with additional multiple congenital anomalies occurred in 2/51 patients (3.9%).
   b. Familial asplenia syndrome was found in 2/51 (3.9%).
   c. Asplenia syndrome was observed in one of twins: 1/51 (2.0%).
3. Multiple congenital anomalies was the third most frequent type of associated anomalies: 21/266 (7.9%). Trisomy 13 occurred in 1/21 (4.8%).

4. The heterotaxy syndrome with polysplenia was found in 16/266 patients (6.0%). Of these 16 cases of the polysplenia syndrome, 1 had congenital heart block (6.25%) and 1 had additional multiple congenital anomalies (6.25%).
5. Familial congenital heart disease was encountered in 2/266 cases (0.75%).
6. Conjoined twins were observed twice: 2/266 (0.75%). Both were thoracopagus.
7. One patient (1/266, 0.38%) had, to the best of our knowledge, a previously unknown group of associated malformations: Noonan syndrome with Meckel diverticulum, microcardia, heterotaxy with a normally formed spleen and an accessory spleen, left ventricular type of completely common AV canal with tricuspid stenosis postoperatively, infant of a diabetic mother, isolated ventricular inversion {S,L,S}, familial Holt-Oram syndrome, and Ellis-van Creveld syndrome.

Heart Position

Levocardia in 221/266 cases (83%); dextrocardia in 40/266 patients (15%); and mesocardia in 5/266 cases (2%).

When levocardia (a left-sided heart) was present, the segmental anatomy of the heart was usually normal, that is, {S,D,S} in 166/221 cases (75%).

When levocardia was present, complex congenital heart disease (abnormal segmental anatomy) was present in 55/221 cases (25%).

In contrast, when dextrocardia (a right-sided heart) was present, the segmental anatomy was always abnormal: 40/40 cases, 100% ($p < .0001$).

When mesocardia (a centrally located heart) occurred, the segmental anatomy and alignments were normal, that is, {S,D,S}, in 3/5 patients (60%), and were abnormal in 2/5 cases (40%).

Is the sidedness of the heart (levocardia, or dextrocardia, or mesocardia) related to the type of ventricular loop that is present?

When dextrocardia was present, L-loop ventricles were present in 27 of 40 patients (67.5%), while D-loop ventricles were found in 13 of 40 (32.5%).

By contrast, when levocardia or mesocardia was present, L-loop ventricles occurred in only 10 of 226 cases (4.42%), while D-loop ventricles were found in 216 of 226 cases (95.58%).

Thus, L-loop ventricles were associated with dextrocardia (67.5%) and D-loop ventricles were associated with levocardia and mesocardia (95.58%) ($p < .0001$). From a developmental viewpoint, L-loop ventricles "should" have dextrocardia and D-loop ventricles "should" have levocardia (see Chapter 2)—and this is what was found in this study of the complete form of common AV canal.

Is the sidedness of the heart (levocardia, or dextrocardia, or mesocardia) related to the type of visceroatrial situs that is present?

With levocardia, the types of visceroatrial situs were:
situs solitus in 190 of 221, 86%;
situs inversus in 3 of 221, 1%;
situs ambiguus in 11 of 221, 5%;
situs ambiguus, probably solitus, in 8 of 221, 4%; and
situs ambiguus, probably inversus, in 9 of 221, 4%.

Thus, solitus atria [including S + A (S)] occurred in 198 of 221 patients (90%). Inversus atria [including I + A (I)] were found in 12 of 221 cases (5%). Situs ambiguus atrialis (undiagnosed atrial situs) occurred in 11/221 cases (5%).

TABLE 11.1 Ventriculoarterial Alignments

	Levocardia ($n = 221$)	Dextrocardia ($n = 40$)	p-Value
Solitus normal	168 (76.02%)	3 (7.5%)	<.0001
Inversus normal	3 (1.36%)	4 (10%)	NS
TGA	16 (7.24%)	7 (17.5%)	NS
DORV	33 (14.93%)	25 (62.5%)	<.0001
DOLV	1 (0.45%)	0 (0%)	
ACM	0 (0%)	1 (2.5%)	
Truncus	2 (0.90%)	0 (0%)	

ACM, Anatomically corrected malposition of the great arteries; *DOLV*, double-outlet left ventricle; *DORV*, double-outlet right ventricle; *NS*, not significant; *TGA*, transposition of the great arteries.

With dextrocardia, the types of visceroatrial situs were:
situs solitus in 12 of 40, 30%;
situs inversus in 11 of 40, 27.5%;
situs ambiguus, probably situs solitus, in 2/40, 5%;
situs ambiguus, probably situs inversus, in 14/40, 35%; and
situs ambiguus, 1 of 40, 2.5%

Thus, the atrial situs was:
solitus in 14 of 40, 35%;
inversus in 25 of 40, 62.5%; and
ambiguus in 1 of 40, 2.5%.

Conclusions

1. Situs solitus of the viscera and atria was much more frequent with levocardia (198/221, 90%) than with dextrocardia (14/40, 35%) ($p < .0001$).
2. Situs inversus of the viscera and atria was much more frequent with dextrocardia (25/40, 62.5%) than with levocardia (12/221, 5%) ($p < .0001$).
3. Situs ambiguus of the viscera and atria was somewhat more common with levocardia (11/221, 5%) than with dextrocardia (1/40, 2.5%) (p = not significant [NS]) (Fisher's exact test).

Summary. Thus, cardiac position (levocardia or dextrocardia) was significantly related (1) to the type of visceroatrial situs and (2) to the type of ventricular loop, as above.

Types of Ventricular Loop

In these 266 cases of the complete form of common AV canal, D-loop ventricles were present in 229 patients (86%) and L-loop ventricles were found in 37 cases (14%).

Types of AV Alignment

In these 266 cases, AV concordance was present in 220 (83%), AV discordance was observed in 33 (12%), and the AV alignment was indeterminate in 13 patients with visceral heterotaxy (5%). When the AV alignment was in determinate, the atrial and ventricular segmental anatomy was {A,D,-} in 10 patients and {A,L,-} in 3.

VENTRICULOARTERIAL ALIGNMENTS

The types of ventriculoarterial alignment in levocardia (n = 221) and in dextrocardia (n = 40) are presented in Table 11.1.

TABLE 11.2 Anatomic Types of Conus in 266 Cases of Completely Common AV Canal

Type of Conus	No. of Cases	% of Series
1. Subpulmonary	199	74.81
2. Subaortic	20	7.52
3. Bilateral (subaortic and subpulmonary)	45	16.92
4. Bilaterally deficient (neither subaortic nor subpulmonary)	2	0.75

Mesocardia was present in 5 cases. Solitus normally related great arteries were present in 3 cases (60%), and double-outlet right ventricle was found in 2 cases (40%).

Conclusions

1. Solitus normally related great arteries were significantly more frequent in completely common AV canal with levocardia (76%) than with dextrocardia (7.5%) ($p < .0001$, Table 11.1).
2. Double-outlet right ventricle was significantly more common in completely common AV canal with dextrocardia (62.5%) than with levocardia (15%) ($p < .0001$, Table 11.1).
3. Other VA (ventriculoarterial) alignments were not significantly different with levocardia and with dextrocardia (Table 11.1).

CONUS

The anatomic status of the conus arteriosus or infundibulum, which is the connector between the ventricular sinuses and the great arteries, is presented in Table 11.2.

Thus, a normal type of conus (subpulmonary, with aortic-mitral fibrous continuity) was present in almost three-quarters of the cases (74.81%, Table 11.2). Second in frequency was a bilateral conus (both subaortic and subpulmonary, preventing semilunar-atrioventricular fibrous continuity) in 16.92% (Table 11.2). Third in frequency was a subaortic conus (with pulmonary-atrioventricular fibrous continuity) in 7.52% (Table 11.2). Least frequent was a bilaterally deficient conus in 0.75% (Table 11.2), "bilaterally deficient" meaning that there were both aortic-atrioventricular and pulmonary-atrioventricular fibrous continuity—permitted by the bilateral muscular deficiency of the conus.

Perhaps even more interesting were the correlations between the anatomic types of conus on the one hand (subpulmonary, subaortic, bilateral, and bilaterally deficient) and the types of ventriculoarterial alignment on the other (normally related great arteries, transposition of the great arteries, double-outlet right ventricle, etc.). These correlations were as follows:

1. **A subpulmonary conus** was usually associated, as expected, with normally related great arteries (180/199 cases, 90.45%). Seven of these 180 cases had inverted normally related great arteries. However, double-outlet right ventricle (DORV) was found in 19 cases (9.55%); this was a surprise.

One is used to thinking of DORV as being associated with a bilateral conus (not with a subpulmonary conus). What do we think of this finding of a subpulmonary conus associated with DORV in almost 10% of the cases with the complete form of common AV canal? Many of these cases of DORV with a subpulmonary conus had the polysplenia syndrome. For reasons that are still unknown, cases with visceral heterotaxy and polysplenia never have had a well-developed muscular subaortic conus, in our experience, whereas patients with visceral heterotaxy and the asplenia syndrome almost always have had a well-developed subaortic conus, or a bilateral conus. Consequently, DORV with a subpulmonary conus is quite typical of the heterotaxy syndrome with polysplenia.

The other situation in which DORV typically has a unilateral conus (as opposed to a bilateral conus) is with what Dr. Richard D. Rowe used to call the **infantile type of DORV** ("infantile" because it has such an unfavorable natural history), that is, DORV with the hypoplastic left heart syndrome (e.g., with mitral atresia or severe congenital mitral stenosis). In DORV with the hypoplastic left heart syndrome, the unilateral conus can be supulmonary (only), with aortic-atrioventricular fibrous continuity, or subaortic (only), with pulmonary-atrioventricular fibrous continuity.

Thus, DORV with a subpulmonary conus should suggest two diagnostic possibilities: (1) the heterotaxy syndrome with polysplenia; and (2) DORV with the hypoplastic left heart syndrome.

One patient had truncus arteriosus, which we think is typically associated with an atretic subpulmonary conus.[36]

2. **A subaortic conus** was often associated with transposition of the great arteries (TGA), just as one would expect (14/20, 70%). However, DORV coexisted with a subaortic conus in 6/20 patients (30%). These findings serve as a reminder that a subaortic conus is certainly not associated exclusively with TGA. Again, DORV does not have to have a bilateral conus; the conus can be subaortic (only).
3. **A bilateral conus,** again as expected, was usually associated with DORV (35/45, 77.77%). TGA was associated with a bilateral conus in 7 of 45 patients (15.55%), also not surprising. But to find 2 of these 45 patients (4.44%) with a bilateral conus and normally related great arteries—this raised our eyebrows.

Morphogenetically, how can one understand **normally related great arteries with a bilateral (subpulmonary and subaortic) muscular conus (with no semilunar-AV fibrous continuity)?** Our best hypothesis is as follows. A bilateral conus is how it starts, early in embryogenesis. Then what normally happens is that the subpulmonary part of the conus grows and develops, whereas the subaortic infundibular free wall normally undergoes absorption—probably due to apoptosis (programmed cell death), thereby permitting the normal aortic-mitral fibrous contiguity and continuity. However, if subaortic conal free wall resorption is subnormal, some subaortic conal free wall can persist, resulting in normally related great arteries with a small tongue of subaortic conal free wall musculature separating the aortic and mitral valves. So, a bilateral conus can coexist with normally related great arteries if (1) the subpulmonary part of the conus is well developed, and (2) if a relatively small amount of subaortic conal free wall musculature persists and develops—but not enough subaortic conal free wall musculature to disrupt significantly the normal aortic-mitral and aortic-left ventricular approximations.

We obviously hope that our morphogenetic hypothesis is correct. But in any case, it is important to know that rarely, normally related great arteries can have a bilateral conus.

Finally, there was one patient with **anatomically corrected malposition (ACM) of the great arteries** with a bilateral conus (1/45, 2.22%). Is this surprising? No, just rare.[37] ACM means that despite the malposition of the great arteries, nonetheless the great arteries originate above the anatomically correct ventricles—aorta above the morphologically left ventricle, and pulmonary artery above the morphologically right ventricle.[37] In our 1967 paper that established the existence of anatomically corrected malposition of the great arteries, all three cases had a bilateral conus (with subaortic and subpulmonary conal musculature) and therefore with no semilunar-atrioventricular fibrous continuity.[37]

4. **A bilaterally deficient conus** was found in 2 of these 266 patients with the complete form of common AV canal (0.75%). One had TGA, and the other had DORV. Interestingly, neither had double-outlet left ventricle—that one often associates with a bilaterally deficient conus.

Segmental Sets or Combinations

In addition to the foregoing segment-by-segment analysis, what we now need is segment-by-segment synthesis. What segmental combinations (or sets) occurred? Only when one knows what the segmental combinations were is it possible to understand clearly the various types of heart in which the complete form of common AV canal occurred. For clarity and brevity, the segmental sets are presented in Table 11.3. This is a form of multivariable analysis: the study of three segments at a time, in triplets—{atria, ventricles, great arteries}—as they actually occur in life. The foregoing may be called **segmental set or combination analysis.**

Table 11.3 answers the question, *What was the segmental anatomy?*

Of these 32 different segmental combinations with completely common AV canal (Table 11.3), the first eight combinations have normally related great arteries, either solitus normally related, that is, {-,-,S}, or inversus normally related, that is, {-,-,I}. Thus, normally related great arteries comprised 68% of this series.

1. The normal segmental combination, {S,D,S}, was, of course, by far the most common segmental situs set (65%).
2. The inverted normal segmental combination, {I,L,I}, was noteworthy for its rarity (0.38%). This patient also had asplenia, so that the visceroatrial situs inversus was not "pure," but was admixed with visceral heterotaxy.
3. The second segmental combination, {S,D,I}, was also rare (0.38%). It consists of situs solitus of the viscera and atria {S,-,-}, D-loop ventricles {-,D,-}, and inverted normally related great arteries {-,-,I}. As the segmental set suggests, there were AV concordance and VA concordance. In words, {S,D,I} is known as ***isolated infundibuloarterial inversion.***[38] Only the infundibulum and the great arteries were inverted {-,-I}, whereas the atria and the ventricles were not inverted {S,D,-}. Because of the AV and VA concordances, the circulations can be physiologically normal (corrected), unless associated malformations such as tetralogy of Fallot[38] vitiate the potential physiologic correction. A tetralogy of Fallot type of conotruncal anomaly was not present in this 63-day-old female infant with a type A completely common AV canal and a relatively small left ventricle.
4. The fourth segmental combination (Table 11.3), {I,D,I}, is also rare (0.75% of the series) and consists of situs inversus of the viscera and atria, D-loop ventricles, and inverted normally related great arteries. Because there is atrioventricular discordance {I,D,-}, but with VA concordance {-,D,I}, the systemic and pulmonary circulations are physiologically uncorrected

TABLE 11.3 Segmental Combinations in Complete Form of Common AV Canal ($n = 266$)

	Segmental Combination or Set	No. of Cases	% of Series
1.	{S,D,S}	173	65.04
2.	{S,D,I}	1	0.38
3.	{I,L,I}	1	0.38
4.	{I,D,I}	2	0.75
5.	{A (S),D,S}	1	0.38
6.	{A,D,S}	1	0.38
7.	{A (S),L,I}	1	0.38
8.	{A,L,I}	1	0.38
9.	{A (I),L,I}	1	0.38
10.	TGA {S,D,D}	4	1.50
11.	TGA {S,L,L}	3	1.13
12.	TGA {I,D,D}	1	0.38
13.	TGA {I,D,L}	1	0.38
14.	TGA {A (S),L,L}	3	1.13
15.	TGA {A (I),L,L}	1	0.38
16.	TGA {A (I),D,D}	4	1.50
17.	TGA {A,D,D}	2	0.75
18.	TGA {A,L,L}	1	0.38
19.	TGA {A,L,D}	1	0.38
20.	DORV {S,D,D}	17	6.39
21.	DORV {S,L,L}	4	1.50
22.	DORV {S,L,D}	1	0.38
23.	DORV {I,L,L}	7	2.63
24.	DORV {I,D,D}	2	0.75
25.	DORV {A (S),D,D}	4	1.50
26.	DORV {A (S),L,L}	2	0.75
27.	DORV {A (I),L,L}	7	2.63
28.	DORV {A (I),L,D}	2	0.75
29.	DORV {A (I), D,D}	9	3.38
30.	DORV {A,D,D}	6	2.26
31.	DOLV {S,D,D}	1	0.38
32.	ACM {A,D,L}	1	0.38

For explanation, please see the text.

(one segmental alignment discordance, at the level of the AV junction). The segmental combination {I,D,I} may be called **isolated ventricular noninversion.** Only the ventricles were not inverted, that is, {-D,-}, whereas both the atria and the infundibuloarterial part of the heart were inverted, that is, {I,-,I}. As in all forms of **AV discordance with VA concordance,**[39] an atrial switch procedure (Senning or Mustard) is needed to correct the circulations physiologically.

It is noteworthy that in the study by Pasquini et al,[39] {I,D,I} was the only type of AV discordance with VA concordance that we did not know to have been documented (Fig. 11.24). So now it may be said that all six theoretically predictable types of AV discordance with VA concordance have been documented (Fig. 11.24):

1. {S,L,S}, that is, isolated ventricular inversion;
2. ACM {S,L,D}, that is, anatomically corrected malposition of the great arteries with solitus atria, L-loop ventricles (and hence AV discordance), and D-malposition of the great arteries (and thus VA concordance by the definition of ACM);
3. {S,L,I}, that is, solitus atria, L-loop ventricles (and hence AV discordance), and inverted normally related great arteries (and consequently VA concordance by the definition of normally related great arteries);
4. {I,D,I}, that is, inversus atria, D-loop ventricles (and thus AV disconcordance), and inverted normally related great arteries (with VA concordance in view of the definition of inverted normally related to great arteries);
5. ACM {I,D,L}, that is, anatomically corrected malposition of the great arteries with the segmental anatomic combination of inversus atria, D-loop ventricles (and hence AV discordance), and L-malposition of the great arteries (with VA concordance because of the definition of ACM); and
6. {I,D,S}, that is, situs inversus of the viscera and atria, D-loop ventricles (and thus AV discordance), and solitus normally related great arteries (and consequently VA concordance).

To our knowledge, this is the first time that {I,D,I}—isolated ventricular noninversion—has been reported.

5. and 6. {A(S),D,S}and {A,D,S} are also rare (each 0.38% of this series) and noteworthy. Infrequently, it is possible to have the heterotaxy syndrome with situs ambiguus of the viscera, but situs solitus of the atria, that is, {A(S),-,-}, and with D-loop ventricles and solitus normally related great arteries. Hence, the segmental was {A(S), D,S}. When we were unable to diagnose the atrial situs with confidence, we made the diagnosis of visceroatrial situs ambiguus, as in {A,D,S}.

To summarize this point, when we are able to diagnose the atrial situs, we note this fact, for example, as follows: {A(S),D,S} (Table 11.3). This notation indicates that visceroatrial situs ambiguus is present, but that we think that the atrial situs is situs solitus. Both {A(S),D,S} and {A,D,S} had the *heterotaxy syndrome with polysplenia,* and interruption of the inferior vena cava with a prominent azygos vein to a superior vena cava. When the segmental set is {A,(S)D,S}, there is AV concordance. But when the segmental combination is {A,D,S}, indicating that the atrial situs is not diagnosed, then the AV alignment (concordant/discordant) also remains undiagnosed.

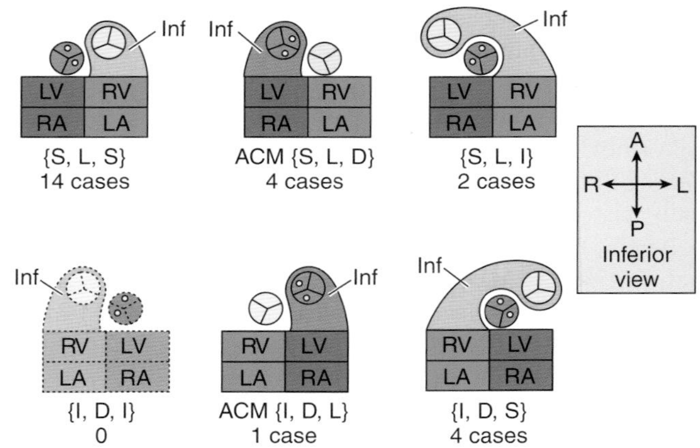

Fig. 11.24 Anatomic types of atrioventricular *(AV)* discordance with ventriculoarterial *(VA)* concordance. The heart diagrams are viewed from below, similar to a subxiphoid 2-dimensional echocardiogram. *A,* Anterior; *P,* posterior; *R,* right; *L,* left; *Inf,* infundibulum (conus); *LA,* morphologically left atrium; *LV,* morphologically left ventricle; *RA,* morphologically right atrium; *RV,* morphologically right ventricle. The aortic valve is indicated by coronary ostia, and the pulmonary valve by absence of coronary ostia. Braces {} mean "the set (or combination) of." The set of {atria, ventricles, great arteries} is shown. The atria may be in situs solitus, as in the top row: {S,-,-}, or in situs inversus, as in the bottom row: {I,-,-}. The ventricles may have D-loop situs with RV to the right and right-handed: {-,D,-}; or the ventricles may have L-loop situs with RV to the left and left-handed: {-,L,-}. The great arteries may be solitus normally related: {-,-,S}; or the great arteries may be inversus normally related: {-,-,I}. If anatomically corrected malposition (ACM) of the great arteries is present, then VA alignment concordance is present, but the infundibular connector is abnormal (subaortic, or subaortic and subpulmonary), rather than normal (subpulmonary)—as it is with solitus and inversus normally related great arteries. When the great arteries are normally related, the VA alignments and connections (type of conal connector) are both normal. With ACM, the VA alignments are concordant (but not fully normal), and the VA connections (anatomic type of conal or infundibular connector) are abnormal. With ACM, the direction of ventricular looping and the direction of infundibuloarterial twisting always are opposites (to the best of our present knowledge). (From Pasquini L, Sanders SP, Parness I, Colan S, Keane JF, Mayer JE, Kratz C, Foran RB, Marino B, Van Praagh S, Van Praagh R: Echocardiographic and anatomic findings in atrioventricular discordance with ventriculoarterial concordance. *Am J Cardiol* 62:1256, 1988; with permission.)

7. and 8. {A,(S),L,I} with polysplenia, and {A,L,I}with asplenia (sister also with asplenia) were both infrequent (1 case each, 0.38%, Table 11.3). These similar segmental combinations are noteworthy. In the patient with polysplenia, we were able to make the diagnosis of atrial situs solitus, that is, {A(S),L,I}. However, in the patient with familial asplenia, we were not able to diagnose the atrial situs, as the segmental combination indicates: {A,L,I}.

In the patient with {A,(S),L,I}, there was AV discordance: {-(S),L,-}. In this polysplenic patient with discordant L-loop ventricles, the usual corrected transposition was *not* present; that is, this patient did not have the more usual segmental combination of TGA {S,L,L}. Instead, this patient had the much more rare segmental combination of {A,(S),L,*I*}. Why? No one fully understands this at the present time. But remember that with the polysplenia syndrome, solitus or inversus *normally related great arteries* is the rule. We have never seen a well-developed muscular subaortic conus, typical of TGA {S,L,L}, in the heterotaxy syndrome with polysplenia.

The patient with {A,L,I} and familial asplenia was similarly unusual. DORV or TGA is the rule with asplenia. But this rare case had inverted normally related great arteries.

9. {A(I),L,I} with polysplenia occurred in only 1 patient (0.38%), serving to emphasize how rare hearts resembling situs inversus totalis are. This case, as in the patient mentioned above with {I,L,I} and the asplenia syndrome (category 3, Table 11.3), did not have so-called pure situs inversus. Instead, both patients had some degree of visceroatrial heterotaxy; however, the patient mentioned in category 3 of Table 11.3 was phenotypically {I,L,I}.

This mixing or blending of visceroatrial situs inversus on the one hand and visceral heterotaxy with situs ambiguus on the other makes us think that **there really may be only two basic types of visceroatrial situs: (1) normal (situs solitus); and (2) abnormal (situs inversus and situs ambiguus), that share overlapping phenotypes.** We hope that molecular genetics will be able to resolve this question.

10.–19. Ten different phenotypes of TGA were found (Table 11.3) in 21 patients, accounting for 8% of this series. Note how infrequent typical D-TGA was: TGA{S,D,D} in only 4 patients (1.5% of this series of 266 cases of the complete form of common AV canal). Similarly, classical corrected L-TGA was even less frequent: TGA{S,L,L} in 3 patients (1.13%, Table 11.3).

20.–30. Eleven different segmental combinations of DORV were found in 61 patients (23%, Table 11.3).

31. and 32. Double-outlet left ventricle (DOLV) and anatomically corrected malposition of the great arteries (ACM) were both represented by 1 case each (0.38% each, Table 11.3).

Segmental combination analysis is helpful and convenient because it makes it possible to see clearly the many different types of heart in which completely common AV canal occurred. In this way, the segmental anatomic combinations are conveyed quickly, briefly, and precisely, no matter how complex they may be (Table 11.3).

The Common AV Valve and the AV Septal Defect

The salient features of the complete form common AV canal are presented in Table 11.4.

Type A (Fig. 11.2) completely common AV canal (43%) was only slightly more common than **type C** (Fig 11.4) (41%), whereas **type B** (Fig. 11.3) was rare (1%) (Table 11.4).

A sizeable minority of cases (15%) was not assigned a Rastelli type for a variety of reasons (e.g., surgery, artifact, or inapplicability).

Inapplicability? Yes. For the Rastelli classification to apply, a relatively well developed and normally positioned ventricular septum must be present. The Rastelli classification of the complete form of common AV canal breaks down when a relatively well developed and approximately normally positioned ventricular septum is not present. Examples of inapplicability include common AV valve with common-inlet RV, or common-inlet LV, or tricuspid atresia, or mitral atresia, or single LV, or single RV.

TABLE 11.4 Salient Anatomic Features of Completely Common AV Canal (*n* = 266)

Anatomy	No. of Cases	% of Series	95% CI
Type A	115	43.23	37–49
Type B	3	1.13	0–2
Type C	108	40.60	35–47
Not typed	40	15.04	
RV type	55	20.68	16–26
LV type	21	7.89	5–11
Regurgitation of CAVV	13	4.89	
Potentially parachute MV	10	3.76	
Double-orifice MV	7	2.63	
Ebstein's anomaly of TV component of CAVV	3	1.13	
Congenital MS	3	1.13	
Mitral atresia	3	1.13	
Double-orifice TV	2	0.75	
Tricuspid atresia	1	0.38	
Tricuspid stenosis	1	0.38	
Mitral regurgitation	1	0.38	
Muscular MV	1	0.38	
Muscular "island" in superior leaflet	1	0.38	

CAVV, Common atrioventricular valve; *CI*, confidence interval; *MS*, mitral stenosis, i.e., congenital stenosis of mitral component of CAVV; *MV*, mitral valve, i.e., mitral component of CAVV; *TV*, tricuspid valve, i.e., tricuspid component of CAVV.

The right ventricular type of completely common AV canal (21%) (the situation in which the common AV valve opens predominantly into the morphologically RV, because the morphologically LV is underdeveloped or absent) was almost three times as common as the **left ventricular type** (8%) (the situation in which the common AV valve opens predominantly into the morphologically LV, because the sinus, body, or inflow tract of the morphologically right ventricular sinus is hypoplastic or absent).

The foregoing data focus on the contributions to the classification of completely common AV canal of Rastelli and his colleagues,[16] Edwards and his associates,[3-6] and Bharati and Lev.[12,15,16] Infrequently, however, we encountered other anatomic findings of considerable diagnostic and surgical importance that often are not mentioned in association with completely common AV canal (Table 11.4):

Significant regurgitation of the common AV valve was encountered in 13 patients (5%).

Potentially parachute mitral valve, mentioned previously, was found in 10 patients (4%) (Figs. 11.13, 11.15, and 11.16).[18]

Double-orifice mitral valve was present in 7 cases (3%) (Figs. 11.20 and 11.22).[17]

Ebstein's malformation of the tricuspid component of the common AV valve was found in 3 patients (1%).[25]

Mitral stenosis, that is, congenital stenosis of the mitral component of the common AV valve, was present in 3 cases (1%).

Mitral atresia, that is, atresia of the mitral component of the common AV valve, was found in 3 patients (1%).

How does "mitral atresia" occur in the setting of common AV canal? If the common AV valve opens essentially only into the RV, and if the leftward or mitral component of the common AV valve becomes adherent to the crest of the muscular ventricular septum, then no blood can pass directly from the left atrium into the left ventricle. Because there is no left-sided atrioventricular inlet, all of the left atrial (LA) blood has to shunt from left-to-right into the right atrium (RA) via the ostium primum type of atrial septal defect and thence into the RV. Blood can enter the small LV only by right-to-left shunting at the ventricular level. Hence, absence of a direct left atrial–to–left ventricular communication is what we mean by mitral atresia with common AV canal.

Double-orifice tricuspid valve, that is, two orifices in the tricuspid component of the common AV valve, was observed in 2 cases (0.75%).

Tricuspid atresia, that is, atresia of the tricuspid component of the common AV valve, was found in 1 patient (0.38%). This type of tricuspid atresia is characterized by adherence of the tricuspid component of the common AV valve to the crest of the ventricular septum, preventing direct communication between the RA and the RV. Hence, the blood has to shunt right-to-left at the atrial level (RA to LA), and left-to-right at the ventricular level (LV to RV).

Tricuspid stenosis, that is, congenital stenosis of the tricuspid component of the common AV valve, was found in 1 case (0.38%).

Congenital mitral regurgitation, that is, regurgitation of the mitral component of the common AV valve, was present in 1 patient (0.38%).

A muscular mitral valve component of the common AV valve was observed in 1 patient (0.38%). Another had an "island" of muscular tissue in the superior leaflet of the common AV valve.

The observation that the mitral component of the common AV valve can be muscular is both fascinating and perplexing. This observation suggests that the mitral valve is, in part, myogenic. Hence, these fascinating cases pose the question: Are the endocardial cushions derived in part from the myocardium (as well as from the endocardium)?

Additional Interatrial Communications

In addition to an ostium primum type of atrial septal defect (an incomplete AV septal defect), many of these 266 cases of completely common AV canal had additional interatrial communications:

1. **A secundum type of atrial septal defect** (i.e., an ostium secundum type of atrial septal defect) was present in 120 patients (45.11%) (95% CI 39% to 51%).
2. **A common atrium** (an essentially absent interatrial septum) was found in 47 cases (17.67%) (95% CI 13% to 22%). Dr. Jesse Edwards used to say that common atrium is the forgotten type of common AV canal. We would agree and would add that there are several different settings in which common atrium occurs:
   a. with common AV canal, complete or partial, in visceroatrial situs solitus;
   b. with the Ellis-van Creveld syndrome, in which the common atrium is associated with a divided AV canal (separate mitral and tricuspid valves), but the mitral valve may have a cleft anterior leaflet of the AV canal type, and a persistent left superior vena cava may be unroofed into the LA;
   c. with visceral heterotaxy and polysplenia, with two AV valves, and often with a cleft anterior mitral leaflet of the AV canal type; and
   d. with visceral heterotaxy and asplenia, typically with a common AV valve.
3. **Coronary sinus septal defect** (unroofing of the coronary sinus into the LA) was found in 1 patient (0.38%). Although a coronary sinus septal defect is not an atrial septal defect, it acts like one physiologically. Typically, bright red blood from the left atrium passes through the defect in the posterior wall of the LA and the anterior wall of the coronary sinus. In this way, the left atrial blood enters the coronary sinus and passes into the RA through an only mildly enlarged right atrial coronary sinus ostium; hence, an ASD-like left-to-right shunt is present. If the surgeon has the patient on cardiopulmonary bypass when the right atrial septal surface is inspected, he or she may well not see the tell-tale bright red blood issuing from the mouth of the coronary sinus. The surgeon may then conclude (correctly) that the patient does not have an atrial septal defect, but may not suspect the presence of a coronary sinus septal defect that cannot be seen from the right atrial perspective. Preoperative or intraoperative diagnostic evaluation—such as transesophageal echocardiography with color-flow Doppler interrogation—should prevent misdiagnosis. (Parenthetically, although the right atrial ostium of the coronary sinus is only slightly enlarged with typical coronary sinus septal defect, the coronary sinus ostial enlargement with totally anomalous pulmonary venous connection to the coronary sinus is not subtle: it's huge.[40] This difference is helpful in the differential diagnosis of atrial level left-to-right shunts without an atrial septal defect.)
4. **The Raghib syndrome**[41] was present in 1 patient (0.38%). This syndrome is characterized by a large low posterior opening in the atrial septum (interpreted as an enlarged right atrial ostium of the coronary sinus), with extensive unroofing of a persistent left superior vena cava to coronary sinus into the LA (see Chapter 5).
5. **The primum atrial septal defect was tiny** in 1 of these 266 cases of completely common AV canal (0.38%). This patient was a 6-year-old boy with visceral heterotaxy, polysplenia, and DORV {A(S),D,D} with a subpulmonary conus. In addition to a tiny ostium primum type of ASD, he also had a moderate sized secundum ASD. He had aortic outflow tract stenosis, had preductal coarctation of the aorta, and was status post–subclavian flap aortoplasty for coarctation of the aorta.

6. **Leftward deviation of septum primum** was found in 3 cases (1.13%).
7. **Septum primum attached to the right of septum secundum** in 1 patient who was thought to have visceroatrial situs solitus. This 3-day-old female infant had DORV {S,D,D}, asplenia, bilateral conus, subpulmonary stenosis, unicommissural pulmonary valve, and hypoplastic pulmonary arteries.

Why did we think this asplenic patient had atrial situs solitus? Because the inferior vena cava was right-sided; the superior vena cava was right-sided; there was no left superior vena cava; and the left hepatic veins connected with an unroofed coronary sinus. There was totally anomalous pulmonary venous connection below the diaphragm. The right atrial appendage was enlarged, and the left atrial appendage was small. However, the right lung was bilobed and the left lung was trilobed, suggesting situs inversus of the lungs.

Whenever the right-left relationship of septum primum relative to septum secundum has been surprising, as in this case, visceral heterotaxy has always been present. We have concluded that septum primum occasionally can lie on the right atrial sided of septum secundum in the heterotaxy syndromes. Why? Perhaps because the superior limbic band of septum secundum is often poorly developed in the heterotaxy syndromes, and consequently septum primum may not attach normally to septum secundum. This is our best present hypothesis to explain surprising septum primum/septum secundum right-left relationships, as in this case.

An alternative hypothesis, that we doubt, is that our diagnosis of the atrial situs in such heterotaxic cases is wrong.

To summarize this intriguing observation in a factual, nonspeculative way: Occasionally in the heterotaxy syndrome (with asplenia or polysplenia), septum primum can be on the apparently right atrial side of septum secundum—instead of vice versa, which is normal.

THE VENTRICULAR SEPTAL DEFECTS

1. **An isolated VSD of the atrioventricular canal (AVC) type** was found in 233 of these 266 cases of completely common AV canal (88%) (95% CI 84% to 92%). The "scooped-out" crest of the muscular ventricular septum forms the anteroinferior rim of the VSD below the plane of the AV valve leaflets (Figs. 11.2 to 11.4). Above the plane of the AV valve leaflets, the superoposterior rim of the ostium primum type of atrial septal defect (ASD I) is formed by the anteroinferior margin of the atrial septum, that is, the so-called inferior limbic band of septum secundum. Hence, the AV septal defect in completely common AV canal is formed by the VSD of the AV canal type plus the ASD I, these defects being confluent (Figs. 11.2 to 11.4).

We prefer not to call a VSD of the AV canal type an "inlet VSD" because one can also have a muscular VSD in the inlet portion of the muscular ventricular septum. In other words, there are two very different anatomic types of "inlet" VSD, whereas VSD of the AV canal type is specific and therefore clear.

In somewhat greater detail, what is the difference between a VSD of the AV canal type and a muscular inlet VSD? A VSD of the AV canal type is confluent with the tricuspid valve or with the common AV valve, whereas a muscular inlet VSD is not confluent with the tricuspid valve or with the common AV valve—because the muscular inlet VSD is separated from the tricuspid valve or the common AV valve by septal myocardium. Thus, there are two very different anatomic types of "inlet" VSD, which the above-mentioned terminology helpfully distinguishes.

2. **VSD of the AV canal type confluent with a conoventricular VSD** was present in 17 of these 266 cases of completely common AV canal (6%) (95% CI 3% to 9%). A conoventricular VSD is one that extends superiorly beneath the conal septum, as in the tetralogy of Fallot in which the conal septum is malaligned anterosuperiorly.
3. **VSD of the AV canal type plus muscular VSD** was found in 16 patients (6%) (95% CI 3% to 9%).

Regarding the first type of VSD mentioned above, isolated VSD of the AV canal type means (1) that there is no anterosuperior extension beneath the conal septum (no conoventricular VSD component) and (2) that there is no additional muscular VSD(s). Thus, an isolated VSD of the AV canal type is purely an "inlet" VSD, with no "outlet" component (no conoventricular VSD component), and with no additional muscular VSD(s).

Hence, in this series of 266 cases of the complete form of common AV canal (complete AV septal defect), all had a VSD of the AV canal type (100%), 6% had outlet extension of the VSD, and 6% had additional muscular VSD(s).

The Right Ventricle

1. **Hypoplasia of the morphologically RV sinus** was present in 40 of these 266 patients with completely common AV canal (15%) (95% CI 10% to 19%).
2. **Absence of the RV sinus**, resulting in single LV with common-inlet LV was found in 2 patients (0.75%).
3. **Common AV canal with tricuspid atresia** was observed in 1 case (0.38%).
4. **Superoinferior ventricles** with RV superior, LV inferior, and ventricular septum approximately horizontal were present in 4 patients (1.5%).
5. **Double-chambered RV**, also known as anomalous muscle bundles of the RV, was observed in 1 patient (0.38%).

Thus, the RV sinus (body or inflow tract) was hypoplastic or absent in 42 patients (16%). Consequently, the RV was well developed in the great majority of these patients with completely common AV canal (84%).

The Left Ventricle

1. **The morphologically LV was hypoplastic** in 66 of these 266 cases of completely common AV canal (25%) (95% CI 20% to 30%).
2. **Potentially parachute mitral valve** was found in 5 patients (1.88%). They all had only one focus of insertion of the primary chordae tendineae: into the anterolateral papillary muscle group of the LV, not into the posteromedial papillary muscle group (Fig. 11.13).
3. **A small diverticulum of the LV** was present in 1 case (0.38%).

4. **Criss-cross AV relations** were observed in 1 patient (0.38%).

In conclusion, LV sinus hypoplasia (66/266 patients, 25%) was significantly more frequent than RV sinus hypoplasia, or atresia, or absence (43/266 patients, 16%) in the complete form of common AV canal ($p < .01$).

THE PULMONARY OUTFLOW TRACT

1. **Pulmonary outflow tract stenosis** was found in 71 of these 266 cases of the complete form of common AV canal (27%) (95 CI 21% to 32%).
2. **Pulmonary outflow tract atresia** occurred in 22 of the 266 patients (8%) (95% CI 5% to 12%).
3. **Tetralogy of Fallot** was present in 18 of these 266 patients (7%) (95% CI 4% to 10%). Inverted tetralogy of Fallot (TOF) was found in 1 case, a 2{11/12}-year-old girl with polysplenia and TOF {A(S),L,I}, interruption of the inferior vena cava, prominent azygos vein to the right superior vena cava, suprahepatic segment of the inferior vena cava connecting with the RA, and coronary sinus opening into the LA.
4. **Truncus arteriosus type A2**[36] was present in 1 of these 266 cases of completely common AV canal (0.38%).

The Aortic Outflow Tract

1. **Aortic outflow tract stenosis** was found in 47 of 266 cases of the complete form of common AV canal (18%) (95% CI 13% to 22%).
2. **Subaortic stenosis produced by the anterolateral muscle of the left ventricle**, also known as the muscle of Moulaert,[35] was found in 3 cases (1.13%).

Hence, aortic outflow tract obstruction was present in a total of 50 of 266 cases (19%).

In conclusion, pulmonary outflow tract obstruction (93/266 cases, 35%) was significantly more frequent than aortic outflow tract obstruction (50/266, 19%) in the complete form of common AV canal ($p < .0001$).

The Pulmonary Valve

1. **Pulmonary valvar stenosis** was present in 46 of 266 cases of completely common AV valve (17%).
2. **Pulmonary valvar atresia** (congenital) occurred in 28 of the 266 cases (11%).
3. **Acquired pulmonary atresia** was observed in 2 patients (0.75%). Acquired means that the atresia was not present at birth, but was acquired postnatally.
4. **Bicuspid pulmonary valve** was found in 39 of 266 cases (15%).
5. **Unicuspid (unicommissural) pulmonary valve** occurred in 7 of 266 patients (3%).
6. **Hypoplasia of the pulmonary valve** was observed in 6 cases (2%).
7. **A domed pulmonary valve** was described in 4 patients (1.5%).
8. **A myxomatous pulmonary valve** was found in 2 cases (0.75%).

Thus, pulmonary valvar obstruction was present in 76 patients (29%) (95% CI 23% to 34%): (a) valvar pulmonary stenosis in 46 of 266 patients (17.29%); and (b) valvar pulmonary atresia in 30 of 266 patients (11.28%).

The Aortic Valve

1. **Aortic valvar stenosis** was present in 5 of 266 cases of completely common AV canal (2%).
2. **Aortic valvar atresia** was found in 1 patient (0.38%).
3. **Aortic valvar regurgitation** occurred in 2 of the 266 cases (0.75%).
4. **Bicuspid (bicommissural) aortic valve** was found in 12 of 266 patients (5%).
5. **Unicuspid (unicommissural) aortic valve** was observed in 1 of 266 patients (0.38%).
6. Other interesting findings included:
   a. hypoplastic noncoronary leaflet in 1 of 266 patients (0.38%);
   b. fenestrated aortic valve in 2 cases (0.75%); and
   c. perforated aortic valve in 1 patient (0.38%).

Thus, **aortic valvar obstruction** occurred in 6 of 266 patients (2%) (95% CI 0.47% to 4%):

a. aortic valvar stenosis in 5 (1.88%) and
b. aortic valvar atresia in 1 (0.38%).

In conclusion, pulmonary valvar obstruction (29%) was significantly more frequent than aortic valvar obstruction (2%) in this series of 266 cases of completely common AV canal ($p < .0001$).

Pulmonary Arteries

1. **Hypoplasia** of the main pulmonary artery and branches was present in 62 of 266 patients (23%).
2. **Atresia** of the main pulmonary artery was found in 6 of the 266 cases (1.5%). In one patient with atresia of the main pulmonary artery, there were **double ductus arteriosi.** A right patent ductus arteriosus supplied the right pulmonary artery, and a left patent ductus arteriosus connected with the left pulmonary artery. This 28-day-old baby boy had a left aortic arch, dextrocardia, and a rare segmental combination: {I,D,I}. This segmental set may be called **isolated ventricular noninversion** because the other two main cardiac segments—the atria and the great arteries—are both inverted. From the hemodynamic perspective, this patient ideally should have an atrial switch operation (a Senning or a Mustard procedure), because the segmental combination has one alignment discordance at the level of the AV junction: {I,D,I}. There is AV discordance, with VA concordance.

Because of the associated atresia of the main pulmonary artery, ideally such a patient should also have reconstruction of the right ventricular outflow tract to both pulmonary artery branches, plus ligation of both ductus arteriosi.

(**Language Note:** The plural of patent ductus arteriosus is patent ductus arteriosi. Why? Because ductus is a fourth declension masculine Latin noun. If ductus were a second declension Latin noun, then the plural would be ducti arteriosi. But it's not.)

3. **Absence** of the main pulmonary artery was observed in 4 of 266 cases (1.5%).

Thus, the pulmonary arteries were hypoplastic, atretic, or absent in 72 of 266 cases of completely common AV canal (27%) (95% CI 22% to 32%).

Other relevant findings included the following:

a. atheromatous pulmonary arteries, indicating pulmonary vascular obstructive disease in 5 of 266 cases (2%);
b. dilation of the pulmonary arteries in 86 of 266 cases (32%);
c. pulmonary artery sling (origin of the left pulmonary artery from the proximal right pulmonary artery, with the anomalously arising left pulmonary artery then coursing leftward and passing between the trachea anteriorly and the esophagus posteriorly to reach the left lung) in 1 of 266 cases (0.38%);
d. rupture of the pulmonary artery in 1 case (0.38%);
e. stenosis of the pulmonary artery branches in 1 case (0.38%); and
f. nonconfluent pulmonary artery branches in 1 case (0.38%).

Coronary Arteries

1. **Absent right coronary artery (RCA) ostium,** resulting in a "single" left coronary artery (LCA), was found in 13 of 266 cases of completely common AV canal (5%).
2. **Absent LCA ostium,** resulting in a "single" RCA, occurred in 5 of 266 cases (2%).
3. Two other patients were described as having a single coronary ostium, but not otherwise specified.

"Single" coronary artery, that is, absence of one coronary arterial ostium, was observed in 20 of 266 cases (8%) (95% CI 4% to 11%), as above. Quotation marks around "single" indicate that it's not entirely correct. When one coronary arterial ostium is absent, the result is not really a single coronary artery. Most of the coronary artery, whose ostium is absent, is in fact present. Just the ostium and the most proximal portion of LCA, or RCA, are truly absent. In other words, most of the LCA typically is present even when its ostium does not form. Similarly, most of the RCA typically is present, even when its ostium is absent.

The concept of a single coronary artery—single LCA or single RCA—was born in the cath and angio lab. That's how it looks on aortic root coronary arteriography. Only one coronary artery is seen. But that's not how it looks to the pathologist, or to the surgeon. We hope that improving two-dimensional echocardiography and MRI will soon make it possible to visualize the patent coronary artery just beyond its atretic ostium.

Other coronary artery findings include the following:

a. two left anterior descending (LAD) coronary arteries arising from separate ostia, in 2 cases (0.75%);
b. a circle of Vieussens connecting the RCA and the LCA via a conus coronary artery, in 1 case (0.38%);
c. hypoplasia of an inverted RCA ostium, in 1 patient (0.38%);
d. LAD arising from the RCA ostium, in 1 case (0.38%);
e. small high origin of the RCA, in 1 patient (0.38%); and
f. stenotic intramural proximal RCA, in 1 case (0.38%).

The coronary arteries appeared normal in 241 of 266 cases of the complete type of common AV canal (90.6%). However, a coronary artery anomaly was present in just under 10% of patients with the complete form of common AV canal: in 25 of 266 cases (9.4%).

Aortic Arch

Of these 266 cases of the complete type of common AV canal, the sidedness of the aortic arch was known in 240:

1. A **left aortic arch** was present in 181 patients (75.42%).
2. A **right aortic arch** was found in 56 cases (23.33%).
3. A **double aortic arch** occurred in 3 patients (1.25%). The left aortic arch was dominant (larger) in two, and the right aortic arch was dominant in one.
4. A **left aortic arch occurred with a right abdominal aorta** in 2 of the 240 patients (0.83%).
5. **Hypoplasia** of the left aortic arch was found in 10 patients (4%) and of the right aortic arch in 1 (0.41%).
6. A **left aortic arch with a right ductus arteriosus** occurred in 1 patient (0.41%).

Comment. We were surprised to find that the complete form of common AV canal had such a high prevalence of right aortic arch (23%). This is almost as high as one might expect with tetralogy of Fallot. However, in tetralogy, the visceroatrial situs is almost always situs solitus. But in completely common AV canal, the visceroatrial situs certainly is not almost always situs solitus. So, we decided to examine the relationship between the types of visceroatrial situs on the one hand, and the sidedness of the aortic arch on the other.

Relationship Between the Types of Visceroatrial Situs and the Sidedness of the Aortic Arch. In this study of completely common AV canal, the findings were as follows:

1. In 180 cases of visceroatrial situs solitus, a left aortic arch was present in 160 patients (88.88%), and a right aortic arch was found in 20 cases (11.11%).
2. By contrast, in 12 cases of visceroatrial situs inversus, a left aortic arch was present in only 4 patients (33.33%), whereas a right aortic arch was found in 8 cases (66.66%).

Conclusions

1. A left aortic arch was usual in visceroatrial situs solitus (89%), but unusual in visceroatrial situs inversus (33%).
2. A right aortic arch was usual in visceroatrial situs inversus (67%), but unusual is visceroatrial situs solitus (11%).
3. These differences are statistically significant ($p < .0001$).
4. These findings are consistent with the view that the sidedness of the aortic arch (left or right) is related to the type of visceroatrial situs (solitus or inversus) that coexists. In this study of 266 cases of the complete form of common AV canal, non–solitus visceroatrial situs was present in 52 cases (20%). (Non–solitus visceroatrial situs includes situs ambiguus and situs inversus.) Situs solitus was found in 214 cases (80%).

Thus, in view of the high prevalence of non–solitus visceroatrial situs (20%) in these cases of completely common AV canal, the high prevalence of right aortic arch (23%) is less surprising than it initially seemed, in view of the link that exists between the sidedness of the aortic arch and the type of visceroatrial situs.

PARTIAL FORMS OF COMMON AV CANAL

This is a study of 93 postmortem cases of the partial forms of common AV canal (Figs. 11.6 and 11.7).

Prevalence. Of the 3216 postmortem cases of congenital heart disease that comprise this study as a whole, the 93 cases of partially common AV canal constitute only 2.89% (95% CI 2.31% to 3.47%).

Heart Position

1. **Levocardia** (left-sided heart) was present in 88 of 93 patients (95%).
2. **Dextrocardia** (right-sided heart) was found in 4 of 93 cases (4%).
3. **Mesocardia** (centrally located heart, neither predominantly left-sided nor right-sided) occurred in 1 patient (1%).

Conclusions

1. Levocardia was commoner with the partial form of common AV canal (88/93 patients, 95%) than with the complete form of common AV canal (221/266 cases, 83%) ($p < .01$).
2. Conversely, dextrocardia was commoner with the complete form of common AV canal (40/266 patients, 15%) than with the partial form of common AV canal (4/93 cases, 4%) ($p < .01$).
3. Mesocardia was approximately equally infrequent both with completely common AV canal (5/266 cases, 2%) and with partially common AV canal (1/93 patients, 1%) (p = NS).

The patients with **dextrocardia and partially common AV canal** had interesting segmental anatomy:

1. One patient had mirror-image dextrocardia {I,L,I}, in which one would expect a right-sided heart.
2. However, one other patient had normal segmental anatomy, that is, {S,D,S}. This is a rare finding known as **isolated dextrocardia.** Such cases are mysterious. No one really understands why patients with normal segmental anatomy rarely can have dextrocardia. The conventional "explanation" is that D-loop formation is a two-step process: First, the straight heart tube loops to the right, resulting in dextrocardia. Second, the apex of the D-looped ventricles swings horizontally from right to left during the fourth week of embryonic life, normally resulting in levocardia. If the right-to-left swing of the ventricular apex stops half way, then the result is mesocardia. All this is true enough. But the real question is: Why does this happen? Why does the right-to-left swing of the ventricular apex fail to occur—in patients without other cardiac or extracardia malformation? To our knowledge, no one knows.
3. A third patient with normal segmental anatomy had dextrocardia secondary to hypoplasia of the right lung in association with the scimitar syndrome.[42] All veins from the hypoplastic right lung connected with the inferior vena cava. This 2{3/12}-year-old girl with polysplenia had **secondary dextrocardia** (secondary to hypoplasia of the right lung).
4. The final patient with dextrocardia, a 16-day-old boy with asplenia, had double-outlet infundibular outlet chamber {I,D,D}. The inferior vena cava and superior vena cava were both left-sided. The right superior vena cava was atretic. The left-sided atrial appendage was broad and triangular, while the right-sided atrial appendage was small and finger-like. Hence, we thought that the atrial situs was inversus, that is, {I,-,-}. There was obstructive totally anomalous pulmonary venous connection to the left superior vena cava. The lungs were bilaterally trilobed. There were an ostium primum type of atrial septal defect and a secundum type of atrial septal defect, both large. D-loop ventricles were present, with AV discordance, that is, {I,D,-}. The right-sided AV valve displayed an imperforate Ebstein's anomaly. The left-sided AV valve had double-orifice mitral valve, mild mitral stenosis, and mild mitral regurgitation. The RV sinus was absent. A bulboventricular foramen led from the LV into the infundibular outlet chamber. There was a bilateral conus with no semilunar-AV fibrous continuity. There was obstruction of the subpulmonary infundibulum and of the pulmonary valve. Both great arteries originated from the infundibular outlet chamber, and the widely patent bicuspid aortic valve lay to the right of the atretic pulmonary valve. Hence, our brief description of the segmental anatomy was DOIOC {I,D,D} with asplenia. (DOIOC means double-outlet infundibular outlet chamber.)

To summarize, when the partial form of common AV canal was associated with dextrocardia, the cardiac anatomy could be normal (isolated dextrocardia), or normal but with the scimitar syndrome (secondary dextrocardia), or with mirror-image dextrocardia and polysplenia, or with asplenia and more complex dextrocardia. Hence, with dextrocardia, the cardiac anatomy spanned the entire spectrum from normal (apart from partially common AV canal) to the very complex. So, when next you encounter a case of dextrocardia, diagnostically you should be ready for anything. No assumptions are warranted.

Gender

The sex of the patient was known in 92 cases with partially common AV canal: males, 45 (49%), and females, 47 (51%). The male/female ratio was 0.96.

Age at Death

The age at death was known in 91 cases. The mean was 4.31 years ± 8.67 years, ranging from 0 (fetus) to 58 years. The median age at death was 228 days (0.62 years).

Comparison of the Partial and Complete Forms of Common AV Canal

1. **Prevalence.** In this entire series of 3216 postmortem cases of congenital heart disease, the complete form of common AV canal (266 cases, 8.27%) was more than twice as common as the partial form (2.89%): 2.86/1.
2. **Gender.** The male/female ratio in the complete form of common AV canal (0.97) was almost identical to that in the partial form (0.96).
3. **Associated anomalies.** Here there were significant differences.
   a. **Down syndrome** was less common with the partial forms of common AV canal (7/93, 7.53%) than with the complete form (82/266, 30.8%) ($p < .001$).

b. **The heterotaxy syndrome with asplenia** was less frequent with partially common AV canal (7/93, 7.53%) than with completely common AV canal (51/266, 19.2%) ($p < .01$).
c. **The heterotaxy syndrome with polysplenia** was approximately equally frequent with partially common AV canal (6/93, 6.45%) and with completely common AV canal (16/266, 6.0%) (p = NS).
d. **Multiple congenital anomalies** were somewhat more frequent with partial forms of common AV canal (13/93, 13.98%) than with complete forms (21/266, 7.9%), but this difference did not quite reach statistical significance ($p = .08$, NS).

SEGMENTAL ANATOMY

1. **Normal segmental anatomy**, that is, {S,D,S}, was the rule in association with partial forms of common AV canal (79/93 cases, 85%).
2. **Complex congenital heart disease** occurred in 14 of 93 patients (15%):
   1. {A(S),D,S} in 4 (4%);
   2. {I,L,I} in 1 (1%);
   3. TGA {S,D,D} in 1 (1%);
   4. DORV {S,D,D} in 3 (3%);
   5. DORV {S,L,L} in 1 (1%);
   6. DORV {I,D,D} in 1 (1%);
   7. DORV {A(I),D,D} in 1 (1%);
   8. DORV {A,D,D} in 1 (1%); and
   9. DOIOC {I,D,D} in 1 (1%).

Key to Foregoing Abbreviations

1. {A(S),D,S} means the segmental combination of situs ambiguus ({A,-,-}) of the viscera, that is, the heterotaxy syndrome with solitus atria ({A(S),-,-}), concordant D-loop ventricles ({A(S),D,-}), and solitus normally related great arteries ({A(S),D,S}) and hence VA concordance.
2. {I,L,I} is the mirror-image "normal" type of heart with situs inversus of the viscera and atria ({I,-,-}), concordant L-loop ventricles ({I,L,-}), and inverted normally related great arteries ({I,L,I}).
3. TGA {S,D,D} is the classical form of complete, physiologically uncorrected transposition of the great arteries (TGA{-,-,-}), with the segmental combination of visceroatrial situs solitus (TGA{S,-,-}), concordant D-loop ventricles (TGA{S,D,-}), and D-transposition of the great arteries (TGA{S,D,D}) with VA discordance (understood from the definition of TGA).
4. DORV {S,D,D} indicates double-outlet right ventricle (DORV{-,-,-}) with the segmental set of visceroatrial situs solitus (DORV{S,-,-}), concordant D-loop ventricles (DORV {S,D,-}), and D-malposition of the great arteries (DORV {S,D,D}).
5. DORV {S,L,L} denotes DORV with the segmental combination of visceroatrial situs solitus (DORV{S,-,-}), discordant L-loop ventricles (DORV{S,L,-}), and L-malposition of the great arteries (DORV{S,L,L}).
6. DORV {I,D,D} means DORV with the segmental set of visceroatrial situs inversus (DORV{I,-,-}), discordant D-loop ventricles (DORV{I,D,-}), and D-malposition of the great arteries (DORV{I,D,D}).
7. DORV {A(I),D,D} signifies DORV with the segmental combination of visceral situs ambiguus with heterotaxy (DORV{A,-,-}), with situs inversus of the atria (DORV{A(I),-,-}), discordant D-loop ventricles (DORV{A(I),D,-}), and D-malposition of the great arteries (DORV{A(I),D,D}).
8. DORV {A,D,D} means DORV with the segmental combination of visceroatrial situs ambiguus with heterotaxy (DORV{A,-,-}), D-loop ventricles (DORV{A,D,-}), with AV concordance or discordance unknown because of visceroatrial situs ambiguus, and D-malposition of the great arteries (DORV {A,D,D}).
9. DOIOC {I,D,D} denotes double-outlet infundibular outlet chamber (DOIOC{-,-,-}) with visceroatrial situs inversus (DOIOC{I,-,-}), discordant D-loop ventricles (DOIOC{I,D,-}), and D-malposition of the great arteries (DOIOC{I,D,D}).

In the aforementioned cases of complex congenital heart disease associated with partially common AV canal, it is noteworthy that DORV (7 cases) was much more frequent than TGA (1 case), in this small series.

Comparison of the Segmental Anatomy in the Partial and Complete Forms of Common AV Canal

1. Normal segmental anatomy, that is, {S,D,S}, was more frequent with partial forms of common AV canal (79/93 patients, 85%) than with complete forms of common AV canal (171/266, 64%) ($p < .001$).
2. TGA was more frequent with complete forms of common AV canal (21/266, 7.89%) than with partial forms (1/93, 1.08%) ($p < .025$, $\chi^2 = 5.57$).
3. DORV was more frequent with complete forms of common AV canal (63/266, 23.68%) than with partial forms (7/93, 7.53%) ($p < .001$).

So that the interested reader will be able to do a detailed comparison of the complex congenital heart disease associated with partial forms of common AV canal (presented above) and that associated with complete forms (not yet presented in detail), we will now consider the various different types of segmental anatomy found in association with complete forms of common AV canal. In the interests of brevity, we will now assume that the reader understands segmental terminology and notation (explained above).

Complex Congenital Heart Disease With Complete Forms of Common AV Canal: Segmental Combinations and Their Frequencies ($n = 266$)

1. **Tetralogy of Fallot {S,D,S}** in 1 (0.38%).
2. **Truncus arteriosus {S,D,S}** in 1 (0.38%).
3. **{S,D,I}** in 1 (0.38%). This is isolated infundibuloarterial inversion.[38]
4. **{I,L,I}** in 1 (0.38%). This is the mirror-image "normal" type of heart in situs inversus totalis.
5. **{I,D,I}** in 2 (0.75%). This is isolated ventricular noninversion.

6. **{A(S),D,S}** in 1 (0.38%). This is the solitus normal type of heart occurring with visceral situs ambiguus and heterotaxy.
7. **{A(I),L,I}** in 1 (0.38%). This is an inverted normal type of heart, occurring in the setting of visceral heterotaxy and situs ambiguus.
8. **{A,D,S}** in 1 (0.38%). This is a patient with visceroatrial heterotaxy and situs ambiguus, in which the situs (pattern of anatomic organization) of the ventricles, infundibulum, and great arteries is normal. The atrial situs is not diagnosed.
9. **{A,L,I}** in 1 (0.38%). This is a mirror-image of the previous case (item 8). Again the atrial situs is undiagnosed because of heterotaxy with visceroatrial situs ambiguus. But the ventricles, infundibulum, and great arteries are mirror-image "normal."
10. **{A(S),L,I}** in 1 (0.38%). This patient had visceral heterotaxy with visceral situs ambiguus, but the atria were in situs solitus. The ventricles and the great arteries were inverted "normal." Hence, this patient had ventriculoarterial inversion, noninverted atria, and visceral heterotaxy.

Note that in the 10 cardiac phenotypes presented thus far, the great arteries were always normally related, that is, solitus normally related or inverted normally related, with aortic-mitral direct fibrous continuity. The next group of hearts with completely common AV canal to be considered all have TGA:

11. **TGA{S,D,D}** in 3 (1.13%). This is classical complete physiologically uncorrected TGA.
12. **TGA{S,L,L}** in 3 (1.13%). This is classical congenitally physiologically corrected TGA.
13. **TGA{I,D,D}** in 1 (0.38%). This is congenitally physiologically corrected TGA in visceroatrial situs inversus.
14. **TGA{I,D,L}** in 1 (0.38%). This, again, is corrected TGA in situs inversus. The only anatomic difference between this patient and the one summarized in item 13 is that in the present case, the transposed aorta lay to the left of the transposed pulmonary valve, that is, TGA{I,D,L}; whereas the case summarized in item 13 had a rightward aortic valve relative to the pulmonary valve, that is, TGA{I,D,D}. Briefly, the present case has L-TGA, whereas the case summarized in item 13 has D-TGA.
15. **TGA{A(S),L,L}** in 3 (1.13%). This patient had heterotaxy with visceral situs ambiguus, but atrial situs solitus. The heart per se had congenitally physiologically corrected TGA.
16. **TGA{A(I),L,L}** in 1 (0.38%). This patient had visceral heterotaxy, but atrial inversion. The heart itself had classical complete physiologically uncorrected TGA of the type that occurs in situs inversus. As this case again illustrates, visceral heterotaxy with situs ambiguus is much more frequent in our database than is situs inversus of the viscera and atria.
17. **TGA{A(I),D,D}** in 4 (1.5%). These patients had heterotaxy with visceral situs ambiguus, but with atrial situs inversus. The heart had congenitally physiologically corrected TGA of the type that occurs in visceroatrial situs inversus (except that these patients did not have situs inversus viscerum).
18. **TGA{A,D,D}** in 3 (1.13%). In these patients, the atrial situs was not diagnosed, but D-loop ventricles and D-TGA were present.
19. **TGA{A,L,L}** in 1 (0.38%). This patient had a heart that was a partial mirror-image of those described in item 18. Again, the visceroatrial situs was undiagnosed because of heterotaxy, but L-loop ventricles and L-TGA coexisted.
20. **TGA{A,L,D}** in 1 (0.38%). The only difference in the segmental anatomy of this patient and that summarized in item 19 is that this one has D-TGA whereas the previous patient had L-TGA, which is more usual with L-loop ventricles.

Thus, 10 different TGA phenotypes were found with the complete form of common AV canal (items 11 to 20, inclusive). Next come the DORV phenotypes:

21. **DORV{S,D,D}** in 17 patients (6.39%).
22. **DORV{S,L,L}** in 4 (1.5%).
23. **DORV{S,L,D}** in 2 (0.75%). The only difference in the segmental set of these patients and those in item 22 is that the present cases have D-malposition of the great arteries, whereas those in item 22 have L-malposition.
24. **DORV{I,L,L}** in 7 (2.63%).
25. **DORV{I,D,D}** in 2 (.75%).
26. **DORV{A(S),D,D}** in 4 (1.5%).
27. **DORV{A(S),L,L}** in 2 (0.75).
28. **DORV{A(I),L,L}** in 7 (2.63%).
29. **DORV{A(I),L,D}** in 2 (0.75%).
30. **DORV{A(I),D,D}** in 9 (3.38%).
31. **DORV{A,D,D}** in 6 (2.26%).
32. **DORV {A,L,L}** in 1 (0.38%).

Thus, 12 anatomically different DORV segmental combinations were found in these 266 patients with completely common AV canal (items 21 to 32, inclusive). Two rare segmental combinations were also found:

33. **DOLV{S,D,D}** in 1 (0.38%). Double-outlet left ventricle (DOLV) is a very infrequent type of ventriculoarterial alignment.[43]
34. **ACM{A,D,L}** in 1 (0.38%). Anatomically corrected malposition (ACM) of the great arteries[37] is a rare form of congenital heart disease in which the ventricular loop bends in one direction, in this case to the right [ACM{S,D,L}], while the infundibuloarterial (conotruncal) part of the heart twists in the opposite direction, in this case to the left [ACM{S,D,L}. Almost always, the direction of ventricular looping and the direction of conotruncal twisting are the same. For example, both are to the right in typical TGA{S,D,D}. However, in ACM, the opposite directions of ventricular looping and conotruncal twisting place the very malposed great arteries above the anatomically correct ventricles: aorta above the morphologically left ventricle, and pulmonary artery above the morphologically right ventricle. As mentioned previously, because the malposed great arteries are located above the anatomically correct ventricles, this is why this rare anomaly is called anatomically corrected malposition of the great arteries.

To summarize, in these 266 cases of the complete forms of common AV canal, 34 different segmental combinations were found (as above).

Anatomic Types of Partial Form of Common AV Canal (*n* = 90)

1. The typical type of partially common AV canal, that is, an ostium primum type of atrial septal defect (ASDI) (also known as a partial AV septal defect), plus an AV canal type of cleft in the anterior leaflet of the mitral valve (MV), and an intact ventricular septum (meaning no ventricular septal defect, that is, no hole) was found in 51 of 90 cases (56.66%) (Figs. 11.6 and 11.7).
   Several points merit mention:
   1. Partial atrioventricular septal defect is not an anatomically specific designation: ASD I is one type of partial AV septal defect. VSD of the AV canal type (without an ASD I) is another anatomic type of partial AV septal defect. This is why we prefer the anatomically specific terms (ASD I, and VSD of the AV canal type) to the anatomically nonspecific designation (partial AV septal defect).
   2. In the typical type of partially common AV canal, there is no VSD (no hole); however, the ventricular septum is nonetheless deficient, with a "scooped-out" ventricular septal crest (Fig. 11.6).
   3. The so-called typical type of partially common AV canal (ASD I with cleft mitral valve) accounted for only slightly more than half of this series (57%). This means that so-called atypical types of partially common AV canal were frequent: 39 of 90 patients (43%). This observation leads to the question: What were the atypical types of partially common AV canal?

Atypical Anatomic Types of Partially Common AV Canal

1. Cleft MV, no ASD I, no VSD of AV canal type, but with conoventricular type of VSD, in 1/90 cases (1.11%). This is an isolated cleft of the mitral valve (of the AV canal type) plus a CV type of VSD.
2. Common atrium, cleft MV, no VSD, in 2/90 (2.22%). This is common atrium with cleft MV.
3. Common atrium, small AV canal type and muscular VSDs, cleft MV with congenital mitral stenosis, cleft tricuspid valve (TV), both mitral and tricuspid valves attached to ventricular septal crest, in 1/90 (1.11%). This is common atrium with cleft and stenotic MV, with small AV canal type and muscular VSDs. Cleft TV means that the anterior and septal leaflets are abnormally widely separated. Despite the coexistence of common atrium and a small VSD of the AV canal type, this case cannot be classified as a complete form of common AV canal because the common AV valve is divided into mitral and tricuspid valves. It was the existence of this type of case that prompted Bharati and Lev et al[15] to introduce the intermediate type of common AV canal. In the interests of clarity, we have stuck with the conventional classification of complete or partial forms of common AV canal. It should be understood that the intermediate type is a rare partial form of common AV canal.
4. ASD I, severe congenital mitral stenosis (MS), cleft TV, AV canal type VSD, in 2/90 cases (2.22%). Again, these patients do not have the complete form of common AV canal because the common AV valve is divided into mitral and tricuspid valves. Again, because of the coexistence of a complete AV septal defect with divided AV valves, these cases may be regarded as having the intermediate type[15] of common AV canal. It is also anatomically accurate to regard these cases as having a partial form (as opposed to a complete form) of common AV canal.

Classifying a spectrum is always somewhat difficult and arbitrary. The foregoing is written in the interests of widespread understanding. We are not trying to suggest that our classification is "better" than that of our friends Bharati et al.[15] Instead, our hope is that both approaches will be clearly understood. Hence, this is ASD I, VSD of AV canal type, with congenital MS.

5. ASD I, anterior leaflet of MV attached to the crest of ventricular septum, tricuspid regurgitation (TR), hypoplastic LV, in 1/90 (1.11%). This is ASD I, TR, and hypoplastic LV. This type is also known as the RV type of partially common AV canal, or the unbalanced type of common AV canal—unbalanced to the right.
6. ASD I, noncleft MV, intact ventricular septum, TR, in 1/90 (1.11%). This is isolated ASD I with TR.
7. ASD I, cleft MV, and small membranous VSD, in 1 (1.11%). This is typical ASD I with cleft MV plus a membranous VSD.
8. ASD I, congenital MS, double-orifice MV, TR, and hypoplastic LV in 1/90 cases (1.11%). This is another RV type of partially common AV canal with hypoplastic LV, congenital MS, and TR.
9. ASD I, cleft MV, intact ventricular septum, and hypoplastic LV, in 1/90 (1.11%). This is the *RV type of partially common AV canal with hypoplastic LV, otherwise uncomplicated.*
10. ASD I, tricuspid atresia, noncleft MV, AV canal type of VSD, in 2/90 (2.22%). This is partially common AV canal with tricuspid atresia, noncleft MV, and VSD of AV canal type.
11. ASD I, intact ventricular septum, parachute mitral valve with absent anterolateral papillary muscle, and hypoplastic LV, in 1/90 cases (1.11%). This is RV type of partially common AV canal with parachute MV and hypoplastic LV. It is noteworthy that the anterolateral papillary muscle was absent. In common AV canal, it is typical for the posteromedial papillary muscle to be absent when parachute MV coexists; in other words, only the anterolateral papillary muscle usually is present in common AV canal with potentially parachute MV.[17]
12. ASD I, cleft and myxomatous MV, myxomatous TV, with intact ventricular septum or membranous VSD, in 3/90 cases (3.33%). This is ASD I with cleft and myxomatous MV and myxomatous TV.
13. ASD I, cleft MV, perforate or imperforate Ebstein's anomaly of the TV, and CV VSD in 2 (2.22%). This is ASD I, cleft MV, Ebstein's anomaly of the TV ± TAt, and VSD of CV type.
14. ASD I, cleft MV, with congenital MS due to decreased interchordal spaces, in 2/90 cases (2.22%). This is ASD I, cleft MV, and congenital MS, not otherwise complicated (no LV hypoplasia, no TR, etc.).

15. Common atrium, cleft MV, parachute MV with MS in 1/90 (1.11%). This is common atrium with cleft MV, parachute MV, and congenital MS.
16. ASD I, cleft MV, tricuspid atresia, with VSDs (small membranous and 2 small midmuscular VSDs, or CV VSD), in 2/90 cases (2.22%). This is *ASD I, cleft MV, TAt, with VSDs.*
17. ASD I, cleft MV, parachute MV, ± VSDs (intact ventricular septum, or muscular VSDs, or membranous VSD, or CV VSD), in 5/90 (5.56%). This is *ASD I, cleft MV, parachute MV, ± VSDs of the non-AV canal type.*
18. ASD I, MAt, TR, and VSDs (CV VSD and 2 muscular VSDs), in 1 (1.11%). This is ASD I with MAt, TR, and VSDs.
19. Isolated cleft of the MV, without VSD or other anomaly, in 1 (1.11%).
20. ASD I, cleft and myxomatous MV, Ebstein's anomaly of the TV (perforate or imperforate), ± VSD, ± Uhl's disease, in 2 (2.22%).
21. Common atrium, RV type of partially common AV canal (left-sided RV), hypoplastic LV (right-sided), in (1.11%).
22. Common atrium or ASD I, double-orifice MV with congenital MS and MR, imperforate Ebstein's anomaly of the TV, and VSD (CV or AV canal type), in 3/90 (3.33%).
23. No ASD I, cleft MV, VSD of AVC type with membranous extension, in 1/90 (1.11%).
24. ASD I, myxomatous MV, congenital MS, in 1/90 (1.11%).

To summarize, these 39 patients (43% of the series) displayed 24 different phenotypes of atypical partially common AV canal. These 39 cases illustrate how inadequate the current classification of common AV canal really is. For example, it is not widely understood that incompletely common AV canal can have tricuspid atresia, or Ebstein's anomaly of the tricuspid valve (perforate or imperforate), or mitral atresia, or congenital mitral stenosis, or parachute mitral valve, or double-orifice mitral valve. All of these possibilities are of considerable surgical importance, and consequently they are also highly relevant to accurate preoperative diagnosis. The current understanding of partial forms of common AV canal is greatly oversimplified, which is a real liability in dealing surgically with these complex atypical cases. This is why the findings have been presented in detail above.

The Pulmonary Outflow Tract in Partially Common AV Canal

1. **Pulmonary outflow tract stenosis** was present in 12 of 90 cases (13.33%).
2. **Pulmonary outflow tract atresia** was found in 5 of 90 patients (5.55%).

Thus pulmonary outflow tract obstruction (stenosis or atresia) occurred in 17 of 90 cases (18.89%).

Pulmonary outflow tract obstruction was approximately twice as common with completely common AV canal (93/266, 35%) as with partially common AV canal (17/90, 19%) ($p < .005$).

COMPARISON OF PULMONARY VALVAR OBSTRUCTION

In partially common AV canal, valvar pulmonary stenosis was present in 12 of 90 cases (13.33%), while valvar pulmonary atresia was found in 5 of 90 patients (5.55%). Thus valvar pulmonary obstruction (stenosis and atresia) occurred in 17 of 90 patients (18.89%).

Comparison. Pulmonary valvar obstruction (stenosis and atresia) was more common with completely common AV canal (76 of 266 cases, 28.57%) than with partially common AV canal (17 of 90 patients, 18.88%), but this difference did not quite reach statistical significance ($p = .07$, NS).

The Aortic Outflow Tract in Partially Common AV Canal

1. **Subaortic stenosis**, produced by the anterior leaflet of the mitral valve, was present in 28 of 90 patients (31.1%).
2. Subaortic atresia was found in 1 of 90 patients (1.11%).

Hence, in this series of partially common AV canal, aortic outflow tract obstruction occurred in 29 of 90 cases (32.22%).

Comparison. Aortic outflow tract obstruction was more frequent with partially common AV canal (29/90, 32.22%) than with completely common AV canal (50/266, 18.80%) ($p < .01$). The significantly higher frequency of aortic outflow tract obstruction in partially common AV canal appeared to be due to the subaortic attachments of the cleft MV, that is, of the superior endocardial cushion component of the cleft anterior leaflet of the MV.

Aortic Valve

1. **Valvar aortic stenosis** was never diagnosed in partially common AV canal. However, the aortic valve was somewhat hypoplastic in 7/90 cases (7.77%).
2. **Valvar aortic atresia** was found in 1/90 patients (1.11%). Thus, aortic valvar obstruction with partially common AV canal was found in only 1 patient (1.11%).

Comparison. Aortic valvar obstruction was approximately the same in partially common AV canal (1/90, 1.11%) as in completely common AV canal (6/266, 2.26%).

Pulmonary Arteries

In 87 cases of partially common AV canal, the pulmonary arteries (main and branches) were hypoplastic ($n = 10$), or atretic ($n = 1$), or absent ($n = 1$) in 12 patients (13.79%). The pulmonary artery branches were nonconfluent in 1/87 cases (1.15%). Aortopulmonary window coexisted in 1 patient (1.15%).

Comparison. The pulmonary arteries were more frequently hypoplastic, atretic, or absent with completely common AV canal (72/264 patients, 27.27%) than with partially common AV canal (12/87 patients, 13.79%) ($p < .025$).

Coronary Arteries

1. **Absent left coronary arterial ostium** ("single" right coronary artery) occurred in 2 of 89 cases (2.25%).
2. **Absent right coronary arterial ostium** ("single" left coronary artery) was observed in 1 of 89 patients (1.12%).
3. **High origins of both coronary arteries** was found in 1 patient (1.12%).
4. **Hypoplasia of the ostium of the right coronary artery** was found in 1 (1.12%).

5. **The circumflex coronary artery originated from the right coronary artery,** and passed behind the aortic valve to reach the left AV groove in 1 patient (1.12%).
6. **The conal branch originated from the left coronary artery** in 1 patient (1.12%).

Comparison. "Single" coronary artery, that is, absence of a coronary arterial ostium, was somewhat more frequent with completely common AV canal (20/262, 7.6%) than with partially common AV canal (3/89, 3.4%), but this difference was not statistically significant ($p = .16$, NS).

Aortic Arch

1. **A left aortic arch** was present in 81 of 85 cases of partially common AV canal (95.29%).
2. **A right aortic arch** was found in 4 of 85 patients (4.71%).

Comparison. A right aortic arch was much more common with the complete form of common AV canal (56/240 cases, 23.33%) than with the partial form (4/85, 4.71%) ($p < .001$).

Aortic Isthmus

1. **A normal aortic isthmus** was present in 55 of 83 cases of partially common AV canal (66.27%).
2. **Hypoplasia of the aortic isthmus** was found in 14 of 83 patients (16.87%).
3. **Coarctation of the aorta** occurred in 16 of 83 patients (19.28%).

Comparison. In completely common AV canal, the aortic isthmus was normal in 195 of 249 patients (78.31%) and hypoplastic in 25 (10.04%).

Coarctation of the aorta was somewhat more frequent with partially common AV canal (16/83, 19.28%) than with completely common AV canal (30/249, 12.05%), but this difference was not statistically significant ($p = .10$, NS).

TRANSITIONAL FORM OF COMMON AV CANAL

We classified 9 cases as having the transitional form of common AV canal (9/3216 cases of congenital heart disease = 0.28%), meaning that they strongly resembled the typical incomplete form of common AV canal, that is, ostium primum type of atrial septal defect with cleft anterior leaflet of the mitral valve, except that they also had one or more small to tiny ventricular septal defects of the AV canal type. Hence, a transitional common AV canal is an almost incomplete common AV canal.

Gender: Males, 5; females, 4; male/female ratio = 1.25/1.

Age at death: The mean age at death was 645 ± 792 days (or 1.77 ± 2.17 years), ranging from 2 to 2213 days (or 2 days to 6.06 years). The median age at death was 201 days (or 6.7 months).

Heart position: Left-sided in all.

Segmental anatomy: Normal {S,D,S} in all.

Conus: Subpulmonary in all.

Atrial septum: ASD I in 8 of 9 (89%). A secundum type of ASD (ASD II) was present in 3 of 9 cases (33%): in 2, an ASD I and an ASD II coexisted; in 1, an ASD II was the only interatrial communication, and there was a wide cleft of the mitral valve.

Mitral valve: A cleft anterior leaflet of the MV in all. Mitral regurgitation was found in 4 of 9 cases (44%), with mitral hypoplasia and stenosis in 1 (11%).

Tricuspid valve: As mentioned, tricuspid atresia occurred with transitional common AV canal in 1 of 9 cases (11%). In this patient, the RV sinus was diminutive and a restrictive VSD of the AV canal type was present.

Double-orifice tricuspid valve with tricuspid regurgitation was found in 1 (11%).

Right ventricle: Right ventricular hypertrophy and enlargement were present in 8 of 9 cases (89%), the only exception being the above-mentioned patient with tricuspid atresia and a diminutive RV sinus.

Left ventricle: Hypoplasia of the left ventricle was found in 1 of 9 cases (11%). Otherwise, the LV was described as hypertrophied and enlarged in 2, enlarged in 3, normal in 2, and hypertrophied in 1.

Ventricular septum: The VSD of the AV canal type was described as tiny or small in 8 of 9 cases (89%). One patient with a cleft MV and mitral regurgitation had a small membranous VSD.

Parenthetically, one might wonder, Did we misclassify this case? After all, a membranous VSD is not a VSD of the AV canal type. True. However, a membranous VSD is a defect in the top—the most cephalad portion—of the septum of the AV canal. In this sense, a membranous VSD may be regarded as one type of AV septal defect, that is, a defect in the territory of the superior endocardial cushion of the AV canal. However, for more conventional diagnosticians who insist that the VSD should be of the AV canal type in transitional common AV canal, the latter patient may be regarded as an atypical partial form of common AV canal with an ASD I and an ASD II, cleft MV, and small membranous VSD. At least physiologically, this patient resembled a typical transitional AV canal.

We may have misclassified this case in the sense that when one insists that the tiny VSD(s) must be of the AV canal type, then there is no argument. Everyone then agrees that a transitional type of common AV canal is present. (If one prefers the latter stricter interpretation, then we have only 8 cases of transitional common AV canal, not 9.)

Pulmonary outflow tract: Unremarkable in all 9 cases.

Aortic outflow tract: Subaortic stenosis in 2 of 9 cases (22%), produced in part by a muscular ridge in 1 case, and by abnormal mitral valve attachments in the other case.

Other significant findings included mild coarctation of the aorta in 1 patient (11%), aberrant right subclavian artery in 2 of 9 (22%), patent ductus arteriosus in 3 (33%), Down syndrome in 2 (22%), Meckel's diverticulum in 1 (11%), and maternal pulmonary valvar stenosis, that is, familial congenital heart disease, in 1 patient (11%).

VENTRICULAR SEPTAL DEFECT OF THE AV CANAL TYPE

VSD of the AV canal type is another important partial form of common AV canal. As will be seen, this typically occurs without other evidence of common AV canal (typically without common AV valve, without cleft mitral valve, and without an ostium primum type of atrial septal defect). VSD of the AV canal type occurs with or without straddling tricuspid valve, and often is associated with other complex forms of congenital heart disease. VSD of the AV canal type is another "forgotten" partial form of common AV canal (common atrium being the other "forgotten" form).

The findings in 20 postmortem cses of VSD of the AV canal type may be summarized as follows:

Incidence: 20 of 3216 cases of autopsy-proved congenital heart disease (0.62%).

Gender: Males, 13; females, 6; not known, 1; male/female ratio = 2.2/1.

Age at death: Mean = 2861 ± 3665 days (7.8 ± 10.04 years); range, 8 days to 10,045 days (27.5 years); and median = 1499 days (4.11 years). The age at death was not known in 1 patient.

Heart position: levocardia in 19 of 20 (95%); and dextrocardia in 1 of 20 (5%).

Segmental anatomy: The segmental combinations or sets encountered in these 20 postmortem cases of VSD of the AV canal type were as follows:

1. {S,D,S}, the solitus normal segmental situs set, in only 4 (20%);
2. physiologically uncorrected TGA in 7 cases (35%): TGA {S,D,D} in 5, TGA {S,D,A} in 1, and TGA {S,D,L} in 1;
3. congenitally physiologically corrected TGA in 4 patients (20%): TGA {S,L,L} in 3, and TGA {S,L,D} in 1;
4. double-outlet right ventricle with concordant D-loop ventricles in 3 cases (15%): DORV {S,D,A} in 1, and DORV {S,D,L} in 2; and
5. double-outlet right ventricle with discordant L-loop ventricles, that is, DORV {S,L,L} and DORV {S,L,D}, in 2 (10%).

Thus, in this series of 20 cases of VSD of the AV canal type, complex congenital heart disease was present in 90%, with TGA (55%) being more frequent than DORV (25%).

The conus was subpulmonary in 5 of 20 cases (25%), subaortic in 12 (60%), and bilateral in 3 (15%).

A subpulmonary conus was associated with solitus normally related great arteries [{S,D,S}] in 4 cases, and with DORV [DORV {S,L,D}] in 1.

A subaortic conus was associated with TGA in 10 cases and with DORV in 2.

A bilateral (subaortic and subpulmonary) conus was associated with DORV in 2 cases and with TGA in 1.

Systemic veins: Normal in 17 of 20 (85%), with a persistent left superior vena cava to coronary sinus to right atrium in 3 (15%).

Pulmonary veins: Normal in all.

Atrial appendages: Juxtaposition of the atrial appendages was present in 4 of 20 patients (20%): left-sided juxtaposition of the atrial appendages, that is, malposition of the right atrial appendage to the left of the vascular pedicle in visceroatrial situs solitus, in 3 cases; and right-sided juxtaposition of the atrial appendages, that is, malposition of the left atrial appendage to the right of the vascular pedicle, in 1 case.

It is noteworthy that juxtaposition of the atrial appendages (JAA) often is associated with complex cyanotic congenital heart disease,[44] that left-sided JAA is associated with right heart hypoplasia and obstruction,[45] and that right-sided JAA is associated with left heart hypoplasia and obstruction.[46]

Atrial septum: In these patients with VSD of the AV canal type, an ostium primum type of atrial septal defect (ASD I) was never present. In the 19 cases in which the status of the atrial septum was known, the findings were as follows: (1) an ostium secundum type of atrial septal defect (ASD II) in 13 patients (68%); (2) a probe patent foramen ovale in 3 (16%); and (3) an intact atrial septum in 3 (16%).

Ventricular septum: A VSD of the AV canal type was present in all (by definition). The AV canal type of VSD was confluent with a conoventricular type of VSD in 1 case (5%) that also had conal septal malalignment. Another case of VSD of the AV canal type (5%) also had an aneurysm of the membranous septum.

Tricuspid valve: The TV was normal in only 4 of 20 cases (20%). Straddling TV[47] was present in 6 patients (30%). The TV attached to the crest of the ventricular septum in 2 additional cases (10%), but did not frankly straddle the ventricular septum. The TV was stenotic or hypoplastic in 3 cases (15%), one of which had straddling tricuspid valve. Tricuspid atresia was present in 2 patients (10%), one with D-loop ventricles (right-sided tricuspid atresia) and one with L-loop ventricles (left-sided tricuspid atresia). Tricuspid regurgitation was found in 1 (5%). Myxomatous change of the tricuspid valve leaflets was observed in 1 case (5%). Another patient had a TV with the morphology of a type C common AV valve, with mitral atresia, and without an ASD I (5%).

Mitral valve: The MV was normal in 11 of 20 cases (55%), which was significantly different from the incidence of normal TV (4/20, 20%) ($p < .025$). Mitral atresia was present in 3 patients (15%), 2 having left-sided mitral atresia (D-loop ventricles) and 1 having right-sided mitral atresia (L-loop ventricles). Mild MV straddling with mitral regurgitation was found in 1 patient (5%), which was significantly less than the incidence of straddling TV (6/20, 30%) ($p < .05$, Fisher's exact test). Myxomatous MV was found in 2 patients (10%). Congenital mitral stenosis was observed in 1 case (5%). Abnormal insertions of the MV into the ventricular septal crest were found in 1 patient (5%). Calcified vegetations, indicating old healed bacterial endocarditis, were found in the right-sided mitral valve of a 25-year old man with TGA {S,L,L}.

RIGHT VENTRICLE

Hypoplasia of the RV sinus was present in 10 of 20 cases (50%), and absence of the RV sinus resulting in single LV was found in 2 patients (10%). Thus, underdevelopment or absence of the RV sinus (body, or inflow tract) occurred in 12 of 20 cases (60%). Superinferior ventricles with crisscross AV relations occurred in 1 patient with underdevelopment of the RV sinus (5%). Double-chambered RV (anomalous muscle bundles of the RV) was found in another patient with hypoplasia of the RV sinus (5%).

Hypertrophy and enlargement of the RV were present in 5 cases (25%), while right ventricular hypertrophy (without enlargement) was observed in 3 patients (15%).

LEFT VENTRICLE

LV hypoplasia was present in only 2 of 20 patients (10%). There was no case of LV absence. The prevalence of LV hypoplasia was significantly less than was the prevalence of RV sinus hypoplasia or absence (12/20, 60%) ($p < .001$). Thus, VSD of the AV canal type was characterized by underdevelopment or absence of the RV sinus, which was significantly more frequent than was LV hypoplasia.

LV hypertrophy and enlargement were present in 10 of 20 cases (50%). A normal LV was found in 4 patients (20%), and a hypertrophied LV was described in another 4 cases (20%). Hence, a well-developed LV occurred in 90% of these cases of VSD of the AV canal type.

Double-inlet LV occurred n 2 cases with RV sinus hypoplasia (10%). Single LV (i.e., absence of the RV sinus) was found in 1 patient (5%).

Pulmonary Outflow Tract

An unobstructed pulmonary outflow tract was present in 10 of 20 patients (50%). Subpulmonary stenosis was found in 8 cases (40%) and pulmonary atresia occurred in 2 cases (10%).

Aortic Outflow Tract

An unobstructed aortic outflow tract was present in 15 patients (75%). Subaortic stenosis was found in 5 (25%).

Pulmonary Valve

A normal pulmonary valve was present in 11 of 20 patients (55%). Pulmonary valvar stenosis was found in 7 (35%): bicuspid in 4, thick and myxomatous in 2, and tricuspid in 1. Pulmonary atresia occurred in 2 patients (10%).

Aortic Valve

A normal aortic valve was present in 14 of 20 patients (70%). A hypoplastic aortic valve (not intrinsically stenotic) was found in 5 cases (25%), and mild valvar aortic stenosis with a bicuspid aortic valve occurred in 1 patient (5%).

Although pulmonary outflow tract obstruction (10 cases, 50%) was more frequent than aortic outflow tract obstruction (25%), this difference did not reach statistical significance ($p =$ .10, NS).

Coronary Arteries

In these 20 patients with a VSD of the AV canal type, the coronary arteries were unremarkable in 17 (85%). The coronary ostia were abnormal in 3 cases (15%):

1. Absence of the left coronary ostium, resulting in a "single" right coronary artery, was found in 1 patient (5%) with TGA {S,D,L}. Because D-loop ventricles were present, the abnormal left-sided coronary artery was a noninverted left coronary artery (LCA).
2. Hypoplasia of the left coronary ostium, with 2 large right coronary arteries, was present in 1 patient (5%) with DORV {S,D,A}. Because D-loop ventricles coexisted, the abnormal left-sided coronary artery was a noninverted LCA.
3. The left coronary ostium was above the intercoronary commissure in 1 patient (5%) with TGA {S,L,D}. Because L-loop ventricles were present, the abnormal left-sided coronary artery was an inverted right coronary artery (RCA). In other words, with L-loop ventricles, the RV is left-sided, and so too is the RCA which supplies the RV.

Aortic Arch

The sidedness of the aortic arch was known in 19 of these 20 patients:

1. A left aortic arch was present in 18 of 19 cases (95%).
2. A right aortic arch was found in 1 of 19 cases (5%). This patient had DORV {S,D,A}. Hence, this right aortic arch was not related to the visceroatrial situs, which was solitus.

Aortic Isthmus

The status of the aortic isthmus was known in 19 of these 20 patients:

1. The aortic isthmus was normal in only 13 of 19 patients (68%).
2. Coarctation of the aorta was present in 3 of 19 patients (16%), none of whom had aortic outflow tract obstruction.
3. Interruption of the aortic arch type A (distal to the left subclavian artery) was found in 2 of 19 patients (11%).
4. Hypoplasia of the aortic isthmus was present in 3 of 19 patients (16%), all of whom had subaortic stenosis.

Thus, obstruction of the aortic isthmus (coarctation, or interruption) was definitely present in 5 of 19 patients (26%). If one includes those cases with hypoplasia of the aortic isthmus secondary to subaortic stenosis, the prevalence of aortic isthmic obstruction rises to 8 of 19 cases (42%).

Brachiocephalic Arteries

1. Normal brachiocephalic arteries were present in only 13 of 19 patients (68%).
2. Mirror-image brachiocephalic arteries were associated with a right aortic arch in 1 of 19 patients (5%).
3. The vertebral artery arose from the aortic isthmus in 1 of 19 patients (5%).
4. An aberrant right subclavian artery was found in 1 patient (5%).
5. The left subclavian artery was located at the ductal entry in 1 case (5%).
6. A brachiocephalic artery was observed in 1 patient (5%). This artery gave rise to the innominate and to the left common carotid arteries. Hence, only 2 brachiocephalic arteries originated from the aortic arch, the other being the left subclavian artery.
7. Hypoplasia of the brachiocephalic arteries was described in 1 of 19 patients (5%).

Ductus Arteriosus

The status of the ductus arteriosus was known in 8 of these 20 patients with VSD of the AV canal type:

1. A closed ductus arteriosus was present in 8 of 18 patients (44%).

2. A patent ductus arteriosus (PDA) was found in 8 of 18 cases (44%).
3. Absence of the ductus arteriosus was noted in 1 patient (6%), a 23-year-old man with dextrocardia, TGA {S,D,L} with subpulmonary stenosis, and pulmonary valvar stenosis with a unicuspid pulmonary valve.
4. Ligation of the ductus arteriosus was found in 1 patient (6%).

Associated Anomalies

Of these 20 patients with VSD of the AV canal type, significant associated anomalies were present in 4 (20%).

1. Turner syndrome was present in 2 of 20 patients (10%), 1 of whom had a Turner mosaic.
2. Multiple congenital anomalies were found in 2 patients (10%), 1 of whom also had Turner syndrome.
3. A trisomy 8 mosaic was present in 1 patient (5%).

COMMON AV CANAL WITH SINGLE VENTRICLE

Common AV canal with functionally or anatomically single ventricle is another "forgotten" type of common AV canal, that seldom appears in classifications or accounts of common AV canal, and to which the aforementioned Rastelli classification often does not apply.

Functionally single ventricle means that, although two ventricular sinuses are present, one is so small as to be functionally useless. Consequently, from a hemodynamic or functional or surgical perspective, such patients really have only one functioning ventricle.

Anatomically single ventricle means that anatomically, only one ventricular sinus is present, that is, that the patient has either single LV because the RV sinus is absent, or single RV because the LV sinus is absent.

Why does the Rastelli classification often not apply when single ventricle coexists? Because a normally developed and normally located ventricular septum is not present. For example, in single RV with absence of the LV sinus, the ventricular sinus septum typically cannot be identified with certainty, and nothing that looks like a ventricular septum is present. Instead, one finds common-inlet RV, with the common AV valve opening into the single RV, or double-inlet RV when both AV valves open into the single RV.

With single LV because of absence of the RV sinus (body or inflow tract), the situation is similar. Nothing that looks like a ventricular septum is present because, although the LV septal surface is well developed, the RV sinus septal surface is absent—because the RV inflow tract has failed to evaginate or pouch out. Since the RV sinus has failed to develop, there is no RV sinus septal surface. Conversely, because the LV sinus has developed well, both the LV septal surface and the LV free-wall surface are well formed.

Consequently, one sees either common-inlet LV when a common AV valve opens into the single LV, or double-inlet LV when both AV valves open into the single LV.

With single LV, there is an identifiable ventricular septal crest between the single LV cavity and the cavity of the infundibular outlet chamber. The ventricular septal crest of the malformed ventricular septum (with a well-developed LV septal surface, but with no RV sinus septal surface below the top of the septal band) forms the floor or inferior margin of the bulboventricular foramen.

By contrast, in single RV (because of absence of the LV sinus), there is no demonstrable ventricular septal crest.

Hence, the Rastelli classification (Figs. 11.2 to 11.4) cannot apply to single RV. Even though a demonstrable ventricular septal crest is present in single LV, the Rastelli classification does not apply well because the ventricular septal remnant is so far to the side of the common AV valve: far to the right with a ventricular D-loop, or far to the left with a ventricular L-loop.

With single RV, because the ventricular septal remnant is not demonstrable, one cannot say whether a VSD is present or not. Hence, the distinction between the complete and partial forms of common AV canal cannot be made with single RV and common-inlet RV—because one cannot prove whether a VSD of the AV canal type is present or not, in turn because the crest of the malformed ventricular septum (with a well-developed RV septal surface, but with an absent LV septal surface) cannot be identified.

In other words, the Rastelli classification of completely common AV canal does not apply and is irrelevant when single RV (absent LV) coexists. Similarly, the Rastelli classification does not apply well and is essentially irrelevant when single LV (absent RV sinus) is present. Thus, the Rastelli classification applies well and is relevant when two well developed, or fairly well developed, ventricles are present. However, the Rastelli classification of completely common AV canal does not apply well and is not relevant to common AV canal when either ventricular sinus is markedly hypoplastic or absent, resulting in functionally or anatomically single ventricle, respectively.

The reason that the conventional Rastelli classification of common AV canal applies well to biventricular hearts, but not to univentricular hearts, is that the conventional classification of common AV canal depends on the coexistence of a relatively normally developed and normally located ventricular septum. In other words, the conventional classification of common AV canal is based not only on the status of the AV canal (in common, or divided), but also on the relationship between the AV valve and the ventricular septum (types A, B, C; balanced and unbalanced).

Classifying one variable (the status of the AV canal) in terms of another variable (the ventricular septum) is an error in logic (or mathematics). Each variable should be defined primarily in terms of itself. In other words, the state of the AV canal should be defined in terms of itself, not in terms of any other variable—such as the ventricular septum, or the atrial septum. This is why the conventional classification of common AV canal breaks down in the face of single ventricle. In other words, single ventricle exposes the artificiality or the weakness of the conventional classification of common AV canal, which really represents an error in logic, strictly speaking.

Are we suggesting any change in the classification of common AV canal? No. Instead, our hope is to make it clear why the conventional classification of common AV canal breaks down when single ventricle coexists. This insight deepens one's understanding of the classification of common AV canal. Why do we (often) classify one variable, at least in part, in terms of another variable? Although this practice is a violation of pure logic, it is also convenient and important, both clinically and surgically. This is why our aim is not to alter the classification of common AV canal, but instead to promote a deeper understanding of it.

The foregoing are some of the more important generalities concerning common AV canal with single ventricle. Now let's look at the data.

FINDINGS

Heterotaxy was present in 33 of these 56 cases of common AV canal with single ventricle (59%):

1. asplenia in 29 patients (52%);
2. polysplenia in 3 cases (5%); and
3. heterotaxy with a right-sided spleen in 1 patient (2%).

Multiple congenital anomalies were present in an additional 4 patients (7%).

Thus, 66% of these patients with common AV canal and functionally or anatomically single ventricle also had major extracardiac anomalies.

Prevalence: n = 56 of 3216 cases of congenital heart disease (1.7%).

Gender: Males/females = 27/29 (0.93).

Age at death (n = 52): Mean, 2{1/12} ± 5{8/12} years; range, 0 (fetus) to 35{8/12} years; and median, 24 days.

Heart position: Levocardia, 38 of 56 patients (68%); and dextrocardia, 18 of 56 cases (32%). Why is there such a high prevalence of dextrocardia? We think that the answer probably is: Because of the high frequency of heterotaxy (59%).

Types of Single Ventricle

1. Anatomically single LV (RV sinus absent, infundibular outlet chamber present) was found in 13 of 56 cases (23%). One of these patients had a persistent stratum spongiosum—also known as myocardial noncompaction—of the single LV.
2. Functionally single LV (RV sinus hypoplastic, infundibular outlet chamber present) occurred in 5 of 56 cases (9%).
3. Anatomically single RV (LV sinus absent) was found in 20 of 56 patients (36%).
4. Functionally single RV (LV sinus markedly hypoplastic) occurred in 18 of 56 cases (32%).

Comment. This is an amazingly high prevalence of anatomically or functionally single RV (68%) and a remarkably low prevalence of anatomically or functionally single LV (32%), compared with the findings in single ventricle as a whole. For example, in our 1979 study of anatomically single ventricle,[48] anatomically single LV occurred in 23 cases (74%) and anatomically single RV was found in only 8 cases (26%).

Statistical comparison reveals that anatomically single RV was somewhat more prevalent with common AV canal (36%) than in single ventricle as a whole (26%)[48] (p = .34, NS). However, anatomically single LV was much less prevalent with common AV canal (23%) than in single ventricle as a whole (74%) (p < .0001).

The real question is: Why? Considering both anatomically and functionally single ventricle, why was single RV so much more frequent with common AV canal (68%), thus making single LV relatively less frequent (32%)?

We think that the answer is that anatomically and functionally single RV is very characteristic of the asplenia syndrome, and that the high prevalence of single RV with common AV canal reflects the high prevalence of the asplenia syndrome (52%) in this population.

Indeed, whenever one sees the combination of common AV canal with functionally or anatomically single right ventricle, one's first diagnostic thoughts should be: Heterotaxy? Asplenia syndrome?

ATRIAL SEPTUM

The status of the atrial septum in 55 cases of common AV canal with single ventricle was as follows:

1. an ostium primum type of atrial septal defect (ASD I) in 38 of 55 patients (69%);
2. common atrium in 15 of 55 cases (27%);
3. an ostium secundum type of atrial septal defect (ASD II) associated with an ASD I in 23 of 55 patients (42%); and
4. an ASD II only (without ASD I or common atrium) was found in only 2 of 55 patients (4%).

Thus, an ASD I or common atrium occurred in 53 of 55 patients (96%).

VENTRICULAR SEPTUM

The status of the ventricular septum in 56 cases of common AV canal with single ventricle was as follows:

1. *The ventricular septum was intact*—no VSD or bulboventricular foramen—in 33 patients (59%). This included 1 patient with a functionally single RV and a diminutive LV, and another with an intact (closed) bulboventricular foramen.
2. *A VSD or bulboventricular foramen* was present in 23 patients (41%) with common AV canal and single ventricle.

Comment: What is a *bulboventricular foramen?* Briefly, it is the opening between the infundibular outlet chamber (also known as the bulbus cordis) and the single LV (which is derived from the ventricle of the bulboventricular loop). Hence, the bulboventricular foramen connects the bulbar and the ventricular portions of the bulboventricular loop.

What is the difference between a bulboventricular foramen on the one hand and a VSD on the other? This is the real question in the minds of many. First, it should be remembered that *ventricular septal defect* is really a short form for ***inter**ventricular septal defect.* The *inter-* has been clipped in modern usage for brevity and convenience. VSD means an opening between the ventricles, as *interventricular septal defect* makes clear. In other words, one cannot have a VSD unless both ventricles are present. When one ventricular sinus is absent, a VSD cannot be present, by definition. Hence, in the interests of anatomic accuracy, the opening between the single LV (which has a ventricular sinus) and the infundibulum (which does not have a ventricular sinus) is known as a bulboventricular (or outlet) foramen, because only one ventricular sinus is present (not two). Accurately speaking, this is why one cannot talk about an interventricular septal defect (i.e., a VSD) when only one ventricle is present.

What is a ventricle? The short answer to this question is: a ventricular sinus. The sinus is the inflow tract or pumping portion of a ventricle. The sinus is the *sine qua non* of a ventricle: no sinus, no ventricle.

For example, when the RV sinus is absent, the result is a single LV. Although the proximal connecting segment (the tricuspid valve) and the distal connecting segment (the infundibulum) are both present, the result is nonetheless a single LV because the RV pumping portion (the RV sinus) is absent. Absence of the main segment (the RV sinus) results in single ventricle even though the proximal and distal connecting segments are present.

The infundibular outlet chamber is not a "rudimentary RV;" instead, it is simply the infundibulum, that is, the distal or conal connecting segment of the absent RV sinus.

So the foregoing then is the distinction between *VSD* and *bulboventricular foramen,* plus the understanding behind this distinction.

Does the fact that the ventricular septum was intact in 59% of these cases of common AV canal with single ventricle mean that the partial (as opposed to complete) form of common AV canal was present in almost 60% of these patients? The answer is no. As was mentioned heretofore, when the ventricular septum is very malformed, as it is in single ventricle, one cannot reliably distinguish between the complete and partial forms of common AV canal, and the Rastelli classification of the complete form of common AV canal (types A, B and C) does not apply. The conventional classification of common AV canal breaks down.

We think that the concept of unbalanced common AV canal needs to be understood. It is not the AV canal *per se* that is *unbalanced* toward the RV or the LV. Instead, it is the ventricular development that is unbalanced. *Common AV canal unbalanced toward the RV*—and hence opening mostly into the RV—really means that the LV sinus is underdeveloped, or absent. This is why the common AV canal opens largely or entirely into the RV. It is the ventricular development (not the AV canal) that is unbalanced.

Conversely, *common AV canal unbalanced toward the LV*—and hence opening mostly into the LV—really means that the RV sinus is underdeveloped or absent. This is why the common AV canal opens mostly or entirely into the LV. Again, it is the ventricular development (not the AV canal) that appears to be unbalanced.

This is why we prefer to talk about the *LV type or the RV type of common AV canal*—to indicate that the LV or the RV, respectively, is receiving the majority of the common AV canal's inflow—without suggesting, we think erroneously, that the AV canal has shifted abnormally in a leftward or rightward direction.

With the foregoing understanding in mind, it may be said that common AV canals with single LV and with single RV represent the most extreme forms of "unbalanced" common AV canals.

The AV Valve(s)

The status of the AV valves in 55 cases of common AV canal with single ventricle was as follows:

1. *The RV type of common AV valve* was present in 25 patients (45%). Common-inlet RV was by far the most common finding in this study. The RV was hypertrophied and enlarged, while the LV was absent or diminutive.
2. *The RV type of common AV valve* with "mitral atresia" was found in 10 patients (18%). Typically this means that the left corner of the common AV valve was adherent to the crest of the malformed ventricular septum, blocking any direct inlet into a diminutive LV from the left atrium. This was the second most common type of common AV valve found in this study.
3. *The left ventricular type of common AV valve* occurred in 9 of these 55 patients (16%). Common-inlet LV was third in prevalence. One of these patients had *double orifice-common AV valve.* Another had significant regurgitation of the common AV valve.
4. *The left ventricular type of common AV valve* with "tricuspid atresia" was found in 8 patients (15%). Typically, the right corner of the common AV valve was adherent to the crest of the malformed ventricular septum, blocking any direct inlet from the right atrium into the diminutive RV. This anatomic type of common AV valve was fourth in frequency.
5. *Isolated ostium primum type of atrial septal defect* was found in 1 patient (2%) who also had a hypoplastic mitral valve, a normal tricuspid valve, and an intact ventricular septum. We regarded this rare case as a partial form of common AV canal with isolated ASD I because no other sign of common AV canal was present except the ASD I.
6. Another rare patient (2%) had an *ASD I, a VSD of the AV canal type, "tricuspid atresia" type 1B and a noncleft mitral valve* with a raphé between the anterior leaflet of the mitral valve and the left ventricular septal surface. This left ventricular type of common AV canal is a very rare form of partially common AV canal, not only because of the coexistence of tricuspid atresia but also because of the absence of a cleft in the anterior mitral leaflet—despite the coexistence of an ASD I and a VSD of the AV canal type. Note that with common AV canal and single ventricle, it is occasionally possible to make the diagnosis of the partial (as opposed to the complete) form of common AV canal when a ventricular septal remnant is discernible; that is, this distinction (complete versus partial) is not always impossible to make, as these rare partial forms of common AV canal illustrate.
7. *Cleft anterior leaflet or the mitral valve, with tricuspid atresia, but without an ASD I or a VSD of the AV canal type* was found in 1 patient (2%). We regard this as another rare partial form of common AV canal with single LV. Cleft anterior leaflet of the MV was the only sign of common AV canal.

But the question remains: Is a cleft of the anterior leaflet of the mitral valve, without other signs of common AV canal (i.e., a so-called *isolated cleft of the mitral valve*), a partial form of common AV canal, or is it not? This is a question to which we shall return.

SEGMENTAL ANATOMY

1. **Normal.** Only 12 of these 56 cases of common AV canal with single ventricle had normal segmental anatomy, that is, {S,D,S} (21%).
2. **Abnormal.** This means that 44 of these 56 patients had abnormal segment anatomy (79%), that is, complex congenital heart disease:
   1. Rare forms of normally related great arteries were found in 3 patients:
      a, {S,L,S}, that is, isolated ventricular inversion, in 1/56 (2%);
      b, {A (S), L,S}, that is, isolated ventricular inversion with visceral heterotaxy, in 1 (2%); and
      c, {A(I),L,I}, that is, a mirror-image normal type of heart in visceral heterotaxy (situs ambiguus), was present in 1 patient (2%).
   2. *A rare form of ventriculoarterial concordance with abnormally related great arteries,* that is, anatomically corrected malposition of the great arteries {A(I),D,L} was found in 1 patient (2%).
   3. *Double-outlet right ventricle* was by far the most common type of ventriculoarterial malalignment found in association with common AV canal and single ventricle, occurring in 30 of 56 patients (54%). Thirteen variations in segmental anatomy were found:
      a. DORV {S,D,D} in 5/56 cases (9%);
      b. DORV {S,L,L} in 1 (2%);
      c. DORV {I,L,L} in 2 (4%);
      d. DORV {I,D,D} in 1 (2%);
      e. DORV {A(S),D,D} in 5 (9%);
      f. DORV {A(S), D,L} in 1 (2%);
      g. DORV {A(S), L,L} in 2 (4%);
      h. DORV {A(I), L,L} in 1 (2%);
      i. DORV {A (I), L,A} in 1 (2%);
      j. DORV {A(I), D,D} in 4 (7%);
      k. DORV {A,D,D} in 3 (5%);
      l. DORV {A,D,L} in 1 (2%); and
      m. DORV {A,L,L} in 3 (5%).

As one can see at a glance from the foregoing, visceroarterial situs solitus (without heterotaxy) was present in only 6 of these 30 DORVs (20%). Situs inversus of the viscera and atria (without heterotaxy) was found in 3 of these 30 DORVs (10%). Visceral heterotaxy with situs ambiguus occurred in 21 of these 30 cases of DORV (70%). Hence, it is not surprising that such complex congenital heart disease is present.

Ventricular D-loops ($n = 20$) were twice as common as ventricular L-loops ($n = 10$).

   4. *Transposition of the great arteries* was present in 6 of these 54 patients with common AV canal and single ventricle (11%). Four different segment sets were found:
      a. TGA {S,D,D} in 3 of these 6 patients (50%);
      b. TGA {S,D,L} in 1 of 6 (17%);
      c. TGA {S,L,L} in 1 (17%); and
      d. TGA {A(S),D,D} in 1 (17%).

Thus, as one can readily see from the segmental anatomic analysis, visceroarterial situs solitus predominated (5/6 patients, 83%) with visceral heterotaxy occurring in only 1 (17%). Ventricular D-loops also predominated (in 5/6 patients, 83%).

Because of the coexistence of single ventricle in all cases, the concepts of AV concordance or discordance and the concepts of physiologically uncorrected (complete) and corrected TGA are physiologically meaningless. This is why we describe TGA anatomically (e.g., TGA {S,D,D}; or briefly D-TGA; and TGA {S,L,L}, or briefly, L-TGA), rather than physiologically, because the anatomic descriptions are clear, specific, and never change meaning or become meaningless.

   5. *Double-outlet infundibular outlet chamber* occurred in 2 of these 54 patients (4%): (a) DOIOC {S,D,D} in 1 patient (2%); and (b) DOIOC {S,D,L} in the other (2%).
   6. *Double-outlet left ventricle* was present in 1 of these 54 patients (2%) with single LV: DOLV {S,D,D}.

Conus

Because the development of the conal connector is one of the principal determinants of the ventriculoarterial alignments (the development of the ventricles, the ventricular septum, and the AV canal are the other major determinants), the anatomic status of the conus arteriosus (infundibulum) is of considerable interest. Four conal phenotypes were found, as follows:

1. *bilateral conus* (subpulmonary and subaortic conal musculature) in 30 of 56 patients (54%);
2. *subpulmonary conus* (but not subaortic) in 16 patients (29%);
3. *subaortic conus* (but not subpulmonary) in 9 cases (16%); and
4. *bilaterally deficient conus* (neither subpulmonary nor subaortic) in 1 patient (2%).

Note that these are the four logically predictable anatomic types of conus.

Although we are fond of saying that, in general, a subpulmonary conus is associated with normally related great arteries, that a subaortic conus is associated with transposition of the great arteries, that a bilateral conus is associated with double-outlet right ventricle, and that a bilaterally deficient conus is associated with double-outlet left ventricle, we know that this simple generalization is far from the whole story. Consequently, the question arises: *What types of ventriculoarterial alignment were associated with each type of conus in the present series?*

1. A *bilateral conus* was associated with *double-outlet right ventricle* in 22 of these 30 patients (73%). But a bilateral conus was also associated with *transposition of the great arteries* in 4 of 30 cases (13%), with *double-outlet infundibular outlet chamber* in 2 patients (7%), and with *anatomically corrected malposition of the great arteries* and with *double-outlet left ventricle* in 1 case each (3%). In the patient with double-outlet left ventricle, the bilateral conus was poorly developed.
2. A *subpulmonary conus* was associated with solitus normally related great arteries in 14 of 16 patients (87.5%), with inverted normally related great arteries in 1 (6%), and with double-outlet right ventricle with absent LV in 1 patient (6%).

The latter case merits comment. DORV with hypoplastic left heart is what the late Dr. Richard D. Rowe used to call the *infantile type of DORV* because it has such an unfavorable natural history. But another noteworthy feature of DORV with hypoplastic or aplastic LV, as in this case, is that such cases of DORV often have a unilateral conus (not a bilateral conus): a subpulmonary conus (as in the present patient), or a subaortic conus. With a subpulmonary conus there is aortic valve–AV valve fibrous continuity; and with a subaortic conus there is pulmonary valve–AV valve fibrous continuity. The infantile type of DORV, that is, DORV with a hypoplastic or absent LV and a unilateral (subpulmonary or subaortic) conus, is as specific a type of DORV, even though it is not widely understood, as is the Taussig Bing malformation.[49]

3. A *subaortic conus* was associated with TGA in 2 of 9 cases (22%), and with DORV in 7 of 9 patients (78%). Again, remember that DORV with a unilateral conus (in these cases subaortic) is typical of DORV with a hypoplastic or aplastic LV. Hence, in this setting of single ventricle, DORV with a unilateral conus—subpulmonary or subaortic—is to be expected.
4. *A bilaterally deficient conus* was present in 1 of these 56 patients (2%), and as expected,[43] DOLV was present. A bilaterally deficient conus permits both aortic valve–AV valve and pulmonary valve–AV valve direct fibrous continuity.

SYSTEMIC VEINS

You may be wondering "What about the systemic veins?" In patients with very severe congenital heart disease—such as common AV canal with single ventricle—such patients may be candidates for heart transplantation, or for heart and lung transplantation. Hence the status of the systemic (and the pulmonary) veins may be very important. First, let us consider the systemic veins.

1. *Normal.* The systemic veins were normal in only 15 of 55 patients (27%).
2. *Inverted normal.* The systemic veins were inverted or mirror-image normal in 4 of 55 patients (7%), 1 of whom had visceral heterotaxy and asplenia.
3. *Bilateral superior venae cavae.* Bilateral SVCs draining into the contralateral atria was by far the most frequent anomaly of the systemic veins, being found in 23 of 55 patients (42%). Of these 23 patients, heterotaxy with asplenia was present in 17 (74%), heterotaxy with polysplenia was found in 2 (9%), and heterotaxy with a normally formed spleen occurred in 1 (4%). Thus, heterotaxy was present in a total of 20 of these 23 patients with bilateral superior venae cavae (87%).

   Consequently, whenever you see bilateral superior venae cavae, one of your first diagnostic thoughts should be: Heterotaxy?

   Multiple congenital anomalies (without heterotaxy) were found in 1 patient with bilateral SVCs (4%).

   Visceroatrial situs solitus was present in only 2 of 23 patients with bilateral SVCs (9%).
4. *Absence of the coronary sinus* (i.e., inability to identify the coronary sinus) was observed in 10 of 55 patients with common AV canal and single ventricle (18%). Of these 10 patients with an unidentifiable coronary sinus, heterotaxy with asplenia was present in 7 (70%), multiple congenital anomalies were found in 1 (10%), and visceroarterial situs solitus occurred in only 2 (20%).
5. *Coronary sinus septal defect.* Unroofing of the coronary sinus was present in 8 of these 55 patients (15%). Of these 8 patients, heterotaxy with asplenia was present in 4 (50%) and heterotaxy with polysplenia was found in 1 (12.5%). Visceroarterial situs solitus occurred in only 3 (37.5%).
6. *Persistent left superior vena cava to coronary sinus to right atrium.* In this form of bilateral SVCs, all of the upper body's systemic venous blood returns to the right atrium (as opposed to contralateral atria) and consequently this pattern may be regarded as a variant of normal, at least hemodynamically, rather than as a significant malformation of the systemic veins. There were 6 of 55 patients with this finding (11%), 2 of whom (25%) had visceral heterotaxy with asplenia.
7. Persistent left superior vena cava to coronary sinus to right atrium with atretic right superior vena cava. This pattern was present in 1 of 55 patients (2%) and again was not hemodynamically abnormal.
8. *Left inferior vena cava with right superior vena cava.* This pattern was present in 3 of 55 patients with common AV canal and single ventricle (5%). Of these 3 patients, 2 had heterotaxy with asplenia and 1 had a common gastrointestinal mesentery.
9. *Left inferior vena cava draining into right superior vena cava.* This pattern was present in 2 of 55 patients with common AV canal and single ventricle (4%). Both had visceral heterotaxy, 1 with asplenia and 1 with polysplenia.
10. *Left superior vena cava to left atrium.* An LSVC drained into the LA in 1 of 55 patients (2%), this patient having visceral heterotaxy with asplenia.
11. *A left inferior vena cava connected with an unroofed coronary sinus and drained into the left atrium.* This rare pattern was found in 1 of 55 patients (2%). Again, this patient had visceral heterotaxy with asplenia. To the best of our present knowledge, we have never seen a case in which the IVC connected directly with the LA. However, as in this very rare case, it is possible for the IVC to connect with the coronary sinus, and if the coronary sinus is unroofed because of the coexistence of a coronary sinus septal defect, then the IVC can drain into the LA (even though the IVC does not connect directly with the LA).
12. *Abnormal hepatic vein draining into left atrium.* This pattern was seen in 1 of 55 patients (2%). This patient had visceroarterial situs solitus (not heterotaxy with situs ambiguus).

PULMONARY VEINS

1. *Normal.* The connection and drainage of the pulmonary veins were normal in 24 of 55 patients with common AV canal and single ventricle (44%). However, 4 of these 24 patients (17%) had visceral heterotaxy, 3 with asplenia and 1 with polysplenia.

2. *Inverted normal.* Of these 55 patients, inverted normally connected pulmonary veins were present in 3 (5%). However, 2 of these 3 patients had visceral heterotaxy, 1 with asplenia and the other with polysplenia. Thus, normally or inverted normally connected pulmonary veins were present in almost half of these patients (49%).
3. *Totally anomalous pulmonary venous connection to the right superior vena cava.* This was the most common anomaly of the pulmonary veins, present in 11 of 55 patients (20%). Of these 11 cases, heterotaxy with asplenia was present in 10 (91%); the other patient had a common gastrointestinal mesentery.
4. *Totally anomalous pulmonary venous connection to the left superior vena cava.* This was the second most common malformation of the pulmonary veins found in 7 of 55 patients (13%). Of these 7 patients, heterotaxy with asplenia was present in 5, heterotaxy with a normal spleen was found in 1, and in the final patient, asplenia was suspected but was not proved (autopsy limited to heart and lungs).
5. *Totally anomalous pulmonary venous connection with obstruction.* This anomaly was found in 3 of 55 patients (5%). Of these 3 patients, visceral heterotaxy with asplenia was present in 2, and multiple congenital anomalies were found in the third patient.
6. *Common pulmonary vein to left atrium.* This pattern was found in 1 of 55 patients (2%). This patient had visceral heterotaxy with asplenia. Although this anomaly resulted in no hemodynamic derangement, the common pulmonary vein remained discrete and was not incorporated normally into the left atrium.
7. *Totally anomalous pulmonary venous connection to the right atrium (left-sided).* This anomaly was found in 1 of 55 patients (2%). Again, this patient had visceral heterotaxy with asplenia.
8. *Totally anomalous pulmonary venous connection to the right-sided atrium in situs ambiguus.* This pattern was found in 3 of 55 patients (5%), all of whom had visceral heterotaxy with asplenia. These pulmonary veins connected to what we thought was the morphologically right atrium.[50] However, the diagnosis of atrial identity (RA or LA) is more difficult with visceral heterotaxy than it is with visceroatrial situs solitus or inversus.[50]
9. *Partially anomalous pulmonary venous connection to the right superior vena cava.* A small connection of the right pulmonary veins to the right SVC was found in 1 of these 55 patients (2%). The patient had visceral heterotaxy with asplenia.
10. *Mixed totally anomalous pulmonary venous connection.* The right pulmonary veins connected with the right SVC, and the left pulmonary veins connected with the right atrium in 1 of these 55 patients (2%) who had visceral heterotaxy with asplenia.

Lobation of Lungs

1. *Normal.* In only 12 of 44 patients (27%) was the lung lobation normal, and 3 of these 12 patients (25%) had visceral heterotaxy with asplenia.
2. *Inverted.* An inverted or mirror-image pattern of lung lobation was found in 3 of 44 patients (7%). Of these 3 patients, 1 had visceral heterotaxy with polysplenia, and the other had multiple congenital anomalies.
3. *Bilaterally trilobed.* This was by far the most common pattern of lobation in this series of common AV canal with anatomically or functionally single ventricle, occurring in 24 of 44 patients (55%). In these 24 patients, the visceral situs was as follows:
   a. heterotaxy with asplenia in 18 (75%);
   b. ? asplenia (strongly suspected but not proved) in 2 (8%);
   c. situs solitus in 2 (8%);
   d. visceral heterotaxy with polysplenia in 1 (4%); and
   e. common gastrointestinal mesentery (resembling heterotaxy) in 1 (4%).
4. *Bilaterally bilobed.* One of 44 patients (2%) displayed this pattern of lobation, and this patient had visceral heterotaxy with asplenia (rather than the expected polysplenia).
5. *Bilaterally quadrilobed.* Two of these 44 patients (5%) had this pattern of lung lobation and both had visceral heterotaxy with asplenia.
6. *Quadrilobed right lung and trilobed left lung.* Of these 44 patients, 1 (2%) displayed this unusual pattern of lung lobation. This patient had visceral heterotaxy with a normally formed but right-sided spleen.
7. *Unilobed right lung and bilobed left lung.* One of these 44 patients (2%) had this pattern of lung lobation and this patient had visceroatrial situs solitus.

THE ATRIA

In 54 cases of common AV canal with single ventricle, the atria were as follows:

1. right atrial hypertrophy and enlargement with a normal left atrium in 10 patients (19%);
2. common atrium in 10 patients (19%);
3. inverted atria in 7 cases (13%);
4. right atrial enlargement and left atrial enlargement in 7 patients (13%), with endocardial fibroelastosis (EFE) of the left atrium in 1;
5. right atrial hypertrophy and enlargement with left atrial hypoplasia in 5 patients (9%);
6. bilaterally rightish atrial appendages (also known as right atrial appendage isomerism) in 4 patients (7%);
7. situs solitus of the atrial appendages in 4 cases (7%);
8. right atrium present, but *left atrium absent* in 2 patients (4%);
9. right atrial hypertrophy and enlargement, and left atrial hypertrophy and enlargement in 2 cases (4%);
10. normal right atrium and left atrium in 2 patients (4%);
11. situs ambiguus of the atria (undiagnosed atrial situs) in 1 patient (2%);
12. left-sided juxtaposition of the atrial appendages[45] in 1 patient (2%); and
13. right-sided juxtaposition of the atrial appendages[46] in 1 case (2%).

Comment: Absence of the morphologically left atrium, which was observed in two of these patients (as above), is noteworthy because this is an essentially unknown malformation that, to the best of our present knowledge, has not been reported previously.

Pulmonary Outflow Tract

In 56 patients with common AV canal and single ventricle, the status of the pulmonary outflow tract was as follows:

1. *Subpulmonary stenosis* was present in 22 patients (39%). Two of these patients had inverted tetralogy of Fallot.
2. *Atresia* of the pulmonary outflow tract was found in 21 patients (37.5%).

Hence, obstruction (stenosis or atresia) of the pulmonary outflow tract was present in a total of 43 of these 56 patients (77%).

3. A *normal (unobstructed)* pulmonary outflow tract occurred in only 13 patients (23%).

Pulmonary Valve

In 55 patients, the status of the pulmonary valve was as follows:

1. atretic, in 21 patients (38%);
2. normal, in 12 (22%);
3. bicuspid with pulmonary valvar stenosis in 9 (16%);
4. bicuspid, without pulmonary valvar stenosis in 4 (7%);
5. hypoplastic but tricuspid and tricommissural in 4 (7%);
6. unicuspid and unicommissural, with pulmonary stenosis, in 3 (5%); and
7. pulmonary valvar stenosis (not further described) in 2 patients (4%).

Thus, pulmonary valvar obstruction (stenosis or atresia) was present in 35 of 55 patients (64%).

Aortic Outflow Tract

In 55 patients with common AV canal and single ventricle, the status of the aortic outflow tract was as follows:

1. normal (not obstructed) in 50 patients (91%);
2. atretic in 2 (4%);
3. subaortic stenosis (hypoplasia) in 1 (2%);
4. muscle of Moulaert (anterolateral muscle of the LV) present but nonobstructive, in 1 (2%); and
5. no left ventricular outflow tract, that is, double-outlet right ventricle with intact ventricular septum, in 1 patient (2%).

Thus, aortic outflow tract obstruction (stenosis or atresia) was present in only 3 of 55 patients (5%).

Aortic Valve

In 55 patients, the aortic valve was as follows:

1. normal in 47 patients (85%);
2. bicuspid but nonstenotic in 3 (5%);
3. aortic valvar atresia in 2 (4%);
4. abnormal right coronary leaflet in 1 (2%);
5. aortic valvar stenosis with tricuspid aortic valve, in 1 patient (2%); and
6. aortic valvar stenosis with bicuspid aortic valve, in 1 patient (2%).

Pulmonary Artery

The status of the main pulmonary artery and branches in 52 cases of common AV canal with single ventricle was as follows:

1. hypoplastic in 25 patients (48%);
2. normal in 12 (23%);
3. atresia of the main pulmonary artery in 7 (13%);
4. dilated in 4 (8%);
5. nonconfluent pulmonary artery branches in 2 (4%);
6. stenosis of the left pulmonary artery in 1 (2%); and
7. aortopulmonary window in 1 (2%).

Coronary Arteries

In 54 patients of common AV canal with single ventricle, the salient coronary artery findings were as follows:

1. normal in 35 patients (65%);
2. single right coronary artery, that is, absent left coronary arterial ostium, in 4 patients (7%);
3. single left coronary artery, that is, absent right coronary arterial ostium, in 3 cases (6%)—with the right coronary artery running across the right ventricular outflow tract in 1 patient;
4. absence of the left anterior descending coronary artery in 3 (6%);
5. hypoplastic left coronary artery with 2 ostia in 1 (2%);
6. absent left circumflex and posterior descending coronary arteries in 1 (2%);
7. left anterior descending coronary artery arising from the right coronary artery in 1 (2%);
8. right coronary artery originating above the intercoronary commissure in 1 (2%); and
9. other branching variations in 4 patients (7%).

Aortic Arch

In 53 patients with common AV canal and single ventricle, the aortic arch was left-sided in 31 patients (58%) and right-sided in 22 (42%).

From the diagnostic standpoint, what should a right aortic arch make you think of? In addition to tetralogy of Fallot, truncus arteriosus, and situs inversus totalis, you should add the heterotaxy syndrome with asplenia. In this series, the prevalence of right aortic arch (42%) is impressively high.

Aortic Isthmus

In 52 cases of common AV canal with single ventricle, the aortic isthmus was normal in 49 (94%). Coarctation of the aorta occurred in 3 patients (6%).

Brachiocephalic Arteries

The salient findings in 53 patients with common AV canal and single ventricle were as follows:

1. Normal brachiocephalic arteries were present in 27 patients (51%).
2. Mirror-image brachiocephalic arteries were found in 17 cases (32%).
3. The vertebral artery arose directly from the aorta in 2 patients (4%).
4. A brachiocephalic ("bovine") trunk was present in 2 cases (4%). This means that only two arteries originated from the

aortic arch: the brachiocephalic trunk (which in turn gave origin to the innominate artery and to the left common carotid artery) and the left subclavian artery.
5. An aberrant right subclavian artery was found in 1 case (2%).
6. The right subclavian artery and the right common carotid arteries had separate origins from the aortic arch, the innominate artery being absent, in 1 patient (2%).

Ductus Arteriosus

In 54 patients with common AV canal and single ventricle, the findings concerning the ductus arteriosus were as follows:
1. A closed ductus arteriosus was present in 18 patients (33%), 1 of whom was a 19-week male fetus.
2. A probe patent ductus arteriosus, probably functionally closing, was found in 14 patients (26%).
3. A patent ductus arteriosus was observed in 9 patients (17%).
4. Absence of the ductus arteriosus was noted in 8 patients (15%).
5. *Bilateral patent ductus arteriosi* were found in 3 patients (6%). Two were 1 day of age and the third was a 19-week fetus. Bilateral PDAs are rare and noteworthy.

ISOLATED CLEFT OF THE MITRAL VALVE

Is cleft of the anterior leaflet of the mitral valve, without other findings of common AV canal—known as isolated cleft of the mitral valve (ICMV)—a partial form of common AV canal, or is it not?

In a study of 41 cases (36 postmortem cases and 5 explanted hearts), we found[51] that there are two different types of cleft mitral valve:
1. the *AV canal type* of ICMV in 20 of 41 cases (49%); and
2. the *abnormal conus type* of ICMV in 21 of 41 cases (51%).

In the AV canal type of ICMV, the cleft "points" horizontally at the canal portion of the ventricular septum, and the left ventricular inlet/outlet ratio is abnormally small, typical of common AV canal: median = .75, mean = .76 ± .10, ranging from .59 to 1.0. The conotruncus is of the normal type: a subpulmonary conus with normally related great arteries.

In the abnormal conus type of ICMV, the mitral cleft is oriented approximately vertically, "pointing" at the abnormal conus that is associated with TGA or DORV. The LV septal inlet/outlet ratio typically is normal: mean = 1.0, mean = .96 ± .13, ranging from .53 to 1.1. If one excludes 2 cases with TGA/DORV and straddling tricuspid valve that had a VSD of the AV canal type with abnormally small LV inlet/outlet ratios (.53 and .71), then the values of this ratio are as follows: median = 1.0, mean = 1.0 ± .055, and range = .86 to 1.1.

The difference between the LV septal inlet/outlet ratio associated with AV canal clefts and with abnormal conus clefts is statistically highly significant ($p < .0001$).

So, is the cleft in the anterior leaflet of the mitral valve in isolated cleft of the mitral valve a partial form of common AV canal, or is it not? The answer is yes, and no: yes, if it is a canal cleft with an abnormally small LV inlet/outlet ratio; and no, if it is an abnormal conus cleft without a straddling tricuspid valve and with an LV inlet/outlet ratio of approximately 1.

Clinically and surgically, does this distinction matter between canal and abnormal conus types of isolated mitral cleft? The answer is yes, it matters very much. Canal clefts tend to develop progressive mitral regurgitation that typically can be eliminated or greatly reduced by surgical cleft closure—as long as parachute mitral valve, that precludes cleft closure, does not coexist. By contrast, abnormal conus clefts seldom are associated with significant and progressive mitral regurgitation. Instead, abnormal conus clefts are associated with left ventricular outflow tract obstruction because of the attachment of this type of cleft mitral valve close to the pulmonary valve in TGA or DORV. Suture closure of an abnormal conus type of mitral cleft does not reduce or eliminate the LV outflow tract obstruction. Thus, surgical cleft closure is very helpful in canal type mitral clefts, but not in conal anomaly type mitral clefts.

To our knowledge, this is the first time that these two very different anatomic types of isolated mitral cleft have been distinguished, and their relevance to surgical management has been delineated.[51]

Summary of Findings

The foregoing Findings section presents the salient pathologic anatomic data concerning the following:
1. complete forms of common AV canal, $n = 266$ cases;
2. partial forms of common AV canal, $n = 93$ cases;
3. transitional form of common AV canal, $n = 9$ cases;
4. common AV canal with single ventricle, $n = 56$ cases; and
5. isolated cleft of the mitral valve of the AV canal type, $n = 20$ cases.

DISCUSSION

Let us now turn briefly to the literature—a fascinating "gold mine" of information. At the outset of this chapter, under History and Terminology, some of the early history of common AV canal and many of the basic concepts were introduced.[1-51] What now follows are salient references, presented in approximately chronological order, that make it possible for the reader to trace the growth of understanding of common AV canal.[52-343]

Are Our Data Accurately Representative?

The data of the present study and the data of the Baltimore-Washington Infant Study—a large epidemiologic study conducted by Ferencz and her colleagues[311]—are virtually identical in the following respect: In the present study of 359 postmortem cases of common AV canal, the complete form was present in 266 patients (74.0%) and the partial form was found in 93 cases (25.9%); whereas in the 288 infants of the epidemiologic study,[311] the complete form of common AV canal was diagnosed in 212 patients (73.61%) and the partial form was found in 76 infants (26.39%). The fact that the Boston data and the Baltimore-Washington data[311] are virtually identical supports the conclusion that the data of the present study do indeed represent common AV canal accurately, despite the fact that ours is a pathology-based, single-institutional study. The representative nature of our data is thought to be related to the fact that our data have been collected for more than 50 years (since the late 1940s) and are based on referrals from the six New England states and elsewhere in the world.

Terminology

As perusal of the literature[1-343] indicates, these anomalies are no longer called *atrioventricularis communis persistens*, this being its old Latin name. Instead, they are now called *persistent common atrioventricular canal,* now usually shortened to *common atrioventricular canal;* or *atrioventricular canal defect;* or *endocardial cushion defect;* or *common atrioventricular orifice;* or *atrioventricular septal defect.*

Although various groups have different preferences, all of the aforementioned terms are generally understood and hence are satisfactory for accurately conveying information. Although we prefer *common AV canal*—because it was the original term,[3-6] because there is nothing wrong with this designation, and because it contains both the concept of an atrioventricular septal defect and the concept of the atrioventricular valvar leaflet anomalies—the designation *atrioventricular septal defect* could be made more satisfactory by also describing the atrioventricular valve leaflets, as some have already done:[325] for example, *AV septal defect with common AV valve;* or *AV septal defect with two AV valves and cleft mitral valve.*

However, one must never forget that language is "alive." It is always slowly changing. This is why the emphasis in this work is on pathologic anatomic data, not on terminology. Data are immortal, but terminology—like fashion—is prone to change. So, if the reader happens not to like some of our terminology, we hope that he/she will mentally substitute his/her favorite nomenclature and will concentrate on the anatomic data. It is the factual data (not the words) that really matter.

Nonetheless, one may still wonder, "How is it possible for a controversy to develop over whether to call these anomalies *common AV canal* or *AV septal defect?*" I think that the answer is to be found in an aphorism of the Italian philosopher Benedetto Croce (1866–1952): Everything is history.

In a certain profound sense this is true. We would say: Only if you know the history well enough, only then can you really understand.

Here is the real story behind the designation *AV septal defect* ("to the best of my present understanding" must always be understood).

In 1968, Dr. Jane Somerville and her colleagues (Emanuel et al)[67] stated that *AV defect* was introduced in 1957 by Bedford and his coworkers.[342] By "atrio-ventricular defects," Bedford et al[342] meant "persistent ostium primum; endocardial cushion defect; partial common atrioventricular canal" and "there may be a common atrio-ventricular (A-V) canal."

It is also noteworthy that one of Dr. Evan Bedford's coauthors was Dr. Walter Somerville, who was or would soon become the distinguished cardiologist husband of Dr. Jane Somerville. It is also relevant to note that Dr. Jane Somerville's MD thesis in 1966 was titled *Atrioventricular Defects.*[343]

But then something happened. Someone wanted to improve this blanket term by making it more specific. This must have been why the word *septal* was added, resulting in the designation *atrioventricular septal defect.* This "improvement" was both good and bad. The term did indeed become more specific, referring only to its septal defect component. But the disadvantage was that this designation now ignored the AV leaflet anomalies—which remain the major surgical problem posed by these malformations.

As suggested above, a more satisfactory modification of *atrioventricular defect* would be *atrioventricular septal and leaflet defect.* This additional small change makes the term both specific and inclusive (septal and leaflet anomalies). This is what was meant by Bedford's designation *atrioventricular defect*[342,343] and by Edwards' term *common atrioventricular canal.*[3-6]

The above-mentioned history now makes it clear why our British friends and colleagues prefer *atrioventricular defect* or *atrioventricular septal defect,* while our American friends and colleagues—particularly those trained by Dr. Jesse Edwards—prefer *common AV canal* or *AV canal defect.* Everything is history.

Complete and Partial. Falcão, Anderson, and their colleagues[307] realized in 1999 that there really is no justification for talking about "complete" and "partial" variants of AV septal defect (common AV canal) in the sense that there is no significant difference in the atrial or ventricular septa in the so-called "complete" and "partial" forms. Nonetheless, these distinctions are clinically and hemodynamically important, as these authors correctly state.[307] We reached very similar conclusions concerning common AV canal with single ventricle (as above): when the ventricular septum cannot be identified, one cannot say whether the common AV canal is "complete" or "partial."

Systemic and Pulmonary Veins. Utley, Noonan, and colleagues[96] have reported, in association with common AV canal, anomalous position of the atrial septum with anomalous systemic and pulmonary venous drainage.

Cor Triatriatum. Although not encountered in our series, cor triatriatum can occur in association with common AV canal.[132-134]

Common AV Canal Without Ostium Primum ASD. Rarely, it is possible for common AV canal to occur without an ostium primum type of atrial septal defect.[145,219] The two patients of Piccoli et al[145] had a common atrioventricular valve type C, but no primum ASD. The patient of Rowley and associates[219] also had a common AV valve, a VSD of the AV canal type, but an intact atrial septum. We regard this as a rare partial form of common AV canal.

Tricuspid Atresia or Severe Stenosis With Common AV Canal. This too is a rare but well-documented partial form of common AV canal.[94,250]

Ebstein's Anomaly With Common AV Canal. One might suppose that a patient could have either Ebstein's anomaly of the tricuspid valve, *or* common AV canal. But rarely is it possible for one patient to have both.[129,186]

Mitral Atresia With Common AV Canal. This infrequent variation was reported by Williams, Tandon, and Edwards[94] and by Alivizatos, Anderson, and colleagues.[198] In the latter case, the atrial septum was displaced to the left; the only outlet from the left atrium was the primum ASD; and the right atrium emptied through a common AV valve into two well-developed ventricles.

Parachute Mitral Valve With Common AV Canal. This surgically important anomaly has been well documented.[17,224] The presence of a potentially parachute mitral valve (following surgical septation) means (a) that the cleft should not be sutured closed, in order to avoid iatrogenic mitral stenosis postoperatively, and (b) that a single ventricle type of repair (as opposed to a biventricular repair) should be strongly considered—because of frequently associated left ventricular hypoplasia and left ventricular outflow tract obstruction.

Double-Orifice Mitral Valve With Common AV Canal. This anomaly[17,174,339] may or may not be of hemodynamic importance and hence of surgical significance. Nakano and colleagues[339] concluded that double-orifice mitral valve in the partial form of common AV canal is a predictor of mitral regurgitation and the need for reoperation—if the double orifice is not repaired at the primary surgical procedure. However, in the complete form of common AV canal, these investigators[339] concluded that potentially double-orifice mitral valve is not associated with significant mitral regurgitation and the need for reoperation. We tend to agree in general, except that occasionally, double-orifice mitral valve with completely common AV canal can be associated with severe mitral regurgitation,[17] requiring surgical repair.

Isolated Mitral Cleft. This malformation[51,201,283,291] has generated debate and controversy concerning whether it is, or is not, a partial form of common AV canal. We think that we have just solved this problem, as mentioned heretofore. The answer is both yes and no:[51] *yes,* when a normal subpulmonary type of conus is present with normally or nearly normally related great arteries (including tetralogy of Fallot), when the cleft is approximately horizontal and pointing at the AV canal region, and when the left ventricular inlet length/outlet length ratio is significantly <1; and *no,* when an abnormal type of conus (subaortic, or subaortic and subpulmonary) is present with TGA or DORV, when the cleft is approximately vertical and pointing at the abnormal type of conotruncus, and when the LV inlet/outlet ratio is ≈ 1.

Isolated ASD I. An isolated ostium primum type of atrial septal defect, that is, without a cleft mitral valve, has been reported.[223] In the series of 106 surgical cases treated by Pan-Chih and Chen-Chun[229] in Shanghai, 11 patients (10%) had an isolated ASD I (without a mitral valve cleft). This is a far higher prevalence of isolated ASD I in a Mongoloid population than we have encountered in Boston in a Caucasoid and Negroid population. This observation raises the possibility that there may be a racial difference in the prevalence of isolated ASD I. More data are needed to answer this question.

Where Is the Coronary Sinus? The frequently abnormal location of the coronary sinus ostium with common AV canal was reported by Yokoyama and coworkers[79] and Wilcox and colleagues.[246] In a series of 46 heart specimens, Yokoyama, Ando, et al[79] found that the coronary sinus opened into the right atrium in 22 (48%), into the left atrium in 18 (39%), and no definite coronary sinus ostium was found in 6 cases (13%).

Where Is the Conduction System? There are several studies of the conduction system in common AV canal.[73,148,151] As was shown by Ho and colleagues,[276] the atrioventricular node and the penetrating bundle of His are located at the intersection of the ventricular septum and the atrioventricular junction, no matter where the ostium of the coronary sinus may be.

Spontaneous Closure of a VSD of the AV Canal Type. This infrequent event has been reported by Papa and colleagues.[264]

The Muscle of Moulaert in Common AV Canal. The anterolateral muscle bundle of the left ventricle (the muscle of Moulaert)[35] may contribute to subaortic stenosis in common AV canal.[247]

Hypoplasia of the Left Ventricle. Hypoplasia of the LV[301,304] is the real problem in the right ventricular dominant type of common AV canal that is often said to be "unbalanced" to the right. Surgically, LV hypoplasia is a very important problem. Cohen and colleagues[301] concluded that when the area of the left AV valve/the area of the right AV valve is less than .67 with a large VSD, then a single ventricle type of surgical approach should be considered. van Son and associates[304] proposed that when the LV volume is ≥ 15 mL/m^2, then a biventricular repair is feasible.

Left Ventricular Outflow Tract Obstruction (LVOTO). Left ventricular outflow tract obstruction with common AV canal is a major surgical challenge.[266,272,289,303] DeLeon, Ilbawi, and colleagues[266] advocated resection if the obstruction is discrete, or a Konno procedure if there is a tunnel type of LVOTO or if the obstruction is due to malattachment of the mitral valve.

Starr and Hovaguimian[272] described a *mitral valve releasing procedure* that makes excellent sense anatomically: (1) The superior cushion component of the cleft anterior leaflet of the mitral valve is detached from the crest of the ventricular septum. (2) A triangular-shaped patch of pericardium (glutaraldehyde treated, autologous) is sutured to the scooped-out crest of the ventricular septum. (3) The freed margin of the anterior mitral leaflet is sutured to the pericardial patch with 6-0 dacron. (4) A second pericardial patch is used to close the primum ASD, and the cleft is sutured closed. The triangular-shaped pericardial patch between the ventricular septal crest and the detached mitral valve lowers the subaortic floor of the left ventricular outflow tract (LVOT), augmenting this region and unobstructing it. This procedure gets rid of the goose-neck appearance by lowering the floor of the LVOT: it "degooses" the goose neck.

Van Arsdell, Williams, Boutin, and colleagues[289] utilized fibrous tissue resection, myectomy, and leaflet augmentation in 18 of 19 patients (95%). They emphasized the complexity and palliative nature of LVOT surgery with common AV canal.

van Son et al[303] utilized patch augmentation of the ventricular septum, resuspension of the atrioventricular valves, and septal myectomy.

Mitral Regurgitation (MR). What do you do for severe MR with a tissue-deficient cleft—or gap—in the anterior mitral leaflet? As reported by van Son, Van Praagh, Falk, and Mohr,[300] mitral competence can be achieved by pericardial patch augmentation of the tissue-deficient anterior mitral leaflet. When faced with moderate to severe MR postoperatively, another approach published in 2001 by Macé and colleagues,[321] based on 10 cases not amenable to annuloplasty, is to anchor the mural leaflet of the mitral valve to the facing cleft, using a pledgeted mattress suture, with one or two flanking interrupted sutures.

As the authors say, this is a valve-sparing repair (i.e., better than mitral valve replacement). The authors also point out that in order to surgically create double-orifice mitral valve in this way, a relatively large mural leaflet and long chordae tendineae are necessary. Again, medium- and long-term follow-up data are necessary to permit reliable assessment of this surgical option.

Regurgitation of the Common AV Valve. Pericardial patch augmentation currently appears very promising.[332] In Lev's intermediate type of common AV canal, Bharati et al,[15] including Dr. John W. Kirklin, concluded that there was not enough tissue to fashion a mitral valve in 41% of their 81 postmortem cases. Hence, the surgical need for valve augmentation[332] is very real.

Regurgitation of the Tricuspid Component of a Common AV Valve. Again, pericardial patching has a role in surgical reconstruction.[295]

How Should the AV Septal Defect Component of Common AV Canal Be Repaired Surgically: One Patch, or Two Patches? The original repair described by Rastelli, Ongley, Kirklin, and McGoon in 1968[65] used one patch with incision and resuspension of the AV leaflets. For a long time this was the standard method. But by (or before) 1982, the double-patch technique had been introduced.[158] The VSD component and the ostium primum ASD component of the AV septal defect were patched separately. Typically, the VSD patch and the ASD primum patch were sewn to each other, through the undivided AV valve leaflets. Each technique—single patch or double patch—won proponents, as perusal of the literature shows. Both techniques seemed to work quite well.

Then, to the surprise of almost everyone, Wilcox et al[331] in 1997 and Nicholson et al[327] in 1999 described a simplified method of repair of the complete form of common AV canal. Using only one patch, the leaflets of the common AV valve were sutured directly to the ventricular septal crest, thereby obliterating the VSD component. The ASD primum component was closed with a single patch and the mitral cleft was sutured closed. The AV leaflets were not incised or resuspended. In Boston, this is known as the "Australian method" of repairing the complete form of common AV canal in honor of Nicholson, Nunn, and their colleagues.[327] How well does this simplified surgical procedure work? It's too early for us to have any definite opinion (as of 2002), but its proponents say that the results of the simplified single-patch technique are no different from those of the convention single- and double-patch techniques. We hope that further experience will confirm this favorable impression, but only time will tell.

Is Common AV Canal an Endocardial Cushion Defect? Do We Know Anything About Etiology? Although some of our friends and colleagues[147] have said that common AV canal (or AV septal defect) really is not an endocardial cushion defect, this view now appears to be incorrect. Not only is it an endocardial cushion defect, but also we are starting to understand what is wrong with the endocardial cushions of the AV canal that may result in persistent patency of the AV canal and AV leaflet malformations.

Common AV canal is by far the most frequent form of congenital heart disease in **Down syndrome.**[31] Zittergruen and colleagues[285] have shown that the nondisjoined chromosome is of maternal origin in 86% of Down syndrome patients, 14% being of paternal origin. Whether the nondisjunction was of maternal or paternal origin did not influence the prevalence of common AV canal. In maternally derived trisomies, nondisjunction occurred in meiosis I in 76.5%. However, in paternally derived trisomy 21, nondisjunction occurred in meiosis II in 76.9%.

In the AV cushions, endocardial cells normally transform into mesenchyme. As Wienecke, Markwald, and colleagues[286] have shown in a murine model, the protein responsible for this transformation is the mouse homologue of a myocardially derived 130 kiloDalton chick protein *ES/130*. Both in the chick and in the mouse, this protein is required for endothelium-to-mesenchyme transformation.[286]

In case you are wondering, "What is *mesenchyme*?"—mesenchyme (or mesenchymal) is derived from two Greek words: *meso*, middle, + *enchyma*, infusion. Thus, mesenchyma literally means flowing into the middle, or a middle infusion. *Mesenchyme* is defined in *Dorland's Illustrated Medical Dictionary,* 24th edition, page 902, as follows: "The meshwork of embryonic connective tissue in the mesoderm from which are formed the connective tissues of the body, and also the blood vessels and lymphatic vessels."

ES/130 is also expressed in the developing endocardial cushions of humans. Basson, the Seidmans, and their colleagues[287] have localized the human ES gene by FISH to human chromosome 20 p 1.2. These investigators found that human ES protein (hES) is expressed during cardiac septation. It is of interest to note that hES is different from the Holt-Oram gene, which typically may have an ostium secundum type of ASD (not an ostium primum type of ASD). The Holt-Oram gene has been localized to human chromosome 12, whereas the ES gene is on chromosome 20. Thus, different genes appear to underlie these priumum and secundum ASDs. The authors[287] suggest that aberrant expression of hES may produce human cardiovascular disease. Their commendable caution reflects the fact that it is very early days in human phenotype-genotype correlation.

Brown and colleagues[288] published data suggesting that congenital heart defects due to AV endocardial cushion abnormalities may arise because of failure of transforming growth factor beta (TGFβ) to appropriately initiate AV cushion endocardial cell activation. Or the abnormalities may be due to altered temporal or spatial expression of TGFβ after activation, resulting in incomplete or disorganized migration of mesenchymal cells. Brown et al[288] found that antibodies to the type II TGFβ receptor block the activation of endocardial cells and their migration during AV cushion transformation.

Thus, it is now very safe to say that both features of common AV canal—the AV septal defect and the leaflet anomalies—are endocardial cushion defects.[286-288]

Is Down Syndrome a Risk Factor in the Repair of Common AV Canal? No. Rizzoli, Mazzucco, and colleagues[279] from Verona found that Down syndrome was not a significant incremental risk factor.

Is there a good, modern consecutive echocardiographic study of all types of common AV canal? Yes. One of the best that we are aware of is that of Geva and his colleagues[310] (1996). These authors studied 206 consecutive cases and the salient findings were as follows:

- Completely common AV canal (68.4% of the series) was the most frequent form and it presented earliest (average = 1.6 ± 2.4 months).
- Partially common AV canal (20.4% of the series) presented later (9.2 ± 10 months).
- Transitional type of common AV canal (a few small restrictive VSDs of the AV canal type) accounted for 11.2% of the series.
- Down syndrome was present in 34% of this series. Completely common AV canal was present in 79% of these patients with trisomy 21.
- Significant associated malformations were present in almost half of these patients (46%): conotruncal anomalies (18%), secundum ASD (14.1%), anomalous pulmonary venous connection (11.2%), and heterotaxy syndrome with asplenia, or polysplenia (11.2%).
- "Unbalanced" AV canal occurred in 14.1%: RV dominant in 10.7%, and LV dominant in 3.4%.

The authors used a segment-by-segment approach to echocardiographic examination and diagnosis, and Doppler evaluation provided crucial hemodynamic information.

Is accurate echocardiographic diagnosis of common AV canal possible prenatally, including associated cardiac and extracardiac anomalies? Again the answer is yes. In a series of 301 fetuses, Huggon and colleagues[317] reported that the karyotype was known in 218. Down syndrome (trisomy 21) was present in 39%, and other chromosomal anomalies were found in an additional 10%. Hence, chromosomal anomalies were present in almost half of these fetuses (49%).

Visceral heterotaxy was present in 32%, with the asplenia syndrome ("right isomerism") in 12% and the polysplenia syndrome ("left isomerism") in 20%. Visceroatrial situs solitus was found in only two-thirds of the fetuses (67%), with situs inversus in 1%.

Thus, the problems of **fetal cardiology** include chromosomal abnormalities in about one-half of fetuses and visceral situs anomalies in one-third of fetuses.[317]

Common AV canal was isolated (nothing else wrong) in only 51%. Approximately half of the fetuses (49%) had something else wrong—in addition to common AV canal. Extracardiac anomalies were diagnosed in 13%. (This figure seems low, given the prevalence of heterotaxy as 32%.)

Termination of pregnancy was elected in 58.5%.

The Kaplan-Meier estimates for live birth were 82%, for survival beyond the neonatal period were 55%, and for survival to 3 years of age were 38%.

With common AV canal, is the frontal QRS loop of the ECG always counterclockwise and superior? No.[52,74,263] For example, when the LV is hypoplastic in the RV dominant type of common AV canal, the frontal QRS loop of the electrocardiogram may be clockwise and superior. Since the advent of echocardiography, the diagnostic importance of the ECG for suggesting the diagnosis of common AV canal is now less than it used to be.

Subacute Bacterial Endocarditis. Your patient with common AV canal has subacute bacterial endocarditis. A course of appropriate antibiotics has failed to clear the infection. What are you going to do? In 1982, Bove and colleagues[164] encountered this situation in an 18-year-old black woman. Bove performed the first successful repair of common AV canal with double valve (mitral and tricuspid valve) replacement.

Natural History. Without surgical treatment, how old can a person live with the complete form of common AV canal? In 1984, Zion et al[188] reported a 73-year-old man—the oldest known case reported up to that time. The diagnosis was made by echocardiography. This case is, of course, an extreme outlier. It will be recalled that in the present series of 266 postmortem cases of the complete form of common AV canal, the mean age to death was 2.54 ± 5.6 years, with a median of 4 months, and a range from 0 (fetal death) to 40.8 years.

Pulmonary Vascular Obstructive Disease. Especially in the complete form of common AV canal without pulmonary stenosis, pulmonary vascular obstructive disease (PVOD) can be a major problem in older patients.[117,226,267,328] But what does "older" mean? To avoid the risk of PVOD, Yamaki and colleagues[267] advocate repair in the complete form of common AV canal at less than 6 months of age. Suzuki and associates[328] found that type A completely common AV canal did worse than type C, and consequently they suggested that type A may be an independent risk factor for pulmonary vascular obstructive disease. This possibility requires further assessment.

Tetralogy of Fallot. Common AV canal with tetralogy of Fallot[222,243] merits comment from the surgical standpoint. First, for reasons unknown, one almost always is dealing with type C completely common AV canal. Then the problem presents itself: where to incise the anterosuperior leaflet (original single-patch technique), or where to suture the anterosuperior leaflet directly to the ventricular septal crest (new simplified single-patch technique)? In 1986, Vargas, Otero Coto, Mayer, Jonas, and Castaneda[222] realized that it is important to transect (or suture) the anterosuperior bridging leaflet further to the right than usual. Why? In order to give more tissue to the mitral valve postoperatively. This maneuver helps to avoid postoperative subaortic fibrous left ventricular outflow tract obstruction. In tetralogy, the overriding or dextroposed aortic valve is further to the right than normal, which in turn makes it easier than usual to get fibrous subaortic stenosis. Giving more leaflet tissue to the mitral valve relaxes and lowers the mitral floor of the subaortic left ventricular outflow tract, thereby avoiding postoperative subaortic fibrous stenosis.

Ilbawi and his colleagues[243] appear to have achieved the same effect by using a two-patch technique. The VSD patch amplifies the subaortic vestibule, thereby avoiding subaortic stenosis postoperatively.

So, however it is achieved, it is important to avoid postoperative subaortic stenosis in completely common AV canal type C with tetralogy of Fallot.

The data of Ilbawi et al[243] also make one other important point: avoid residual pulmonary stenosis postoperatively. The only patient in their series of 9 cases who died had residual pulmonary stenosis.

What Is the Fate of the Endocardial Cushions? Using an antifibronectin antibody to identify fibrous tissue and an antiactin antibody to identify myocardium, Chin and his colleagues[274] showed in the chick that the mitral valve is fibronectin rich but contains no actin, whereas the tricuspid valve is both fibronectin rich and actin rich. These observations support the conclusion that the **mitral valve** forms predominantly from the endocardial cushions, whereas the **tricuspid valve** forms from the endocardial cushions and from the myocardium.

These fascinating findings appear highly relevant to the understanding of **Ebstein's malformation.** The downwardly displaced septal leaflet represents a failure of delamination and ascent of this leaflet. The development of the septal leaflet of the tricuspid valve has an intimate relationship with the development of the right ventricular sinus septal surface myocardium. One often sees anterior and posterior tricuspid leaflets that are only partly demuscularized: RV myocardium toward the base of these leaflets, with fibrous free margins. We have seen one rare human case in which the tricuspid valve is entirely muscularized, with no demuscularization and hence no fibrous free margins of the tricuspid leaflets.

The findings of Chin, Choy, and colleagues[274] also strongly support the view that the mitral cleft is an endocardial cushion defect—because the mitral valve is derived from the endocardial cushions that are fibronectin (fibrous tissue) rich, but without actin (muscle tissue).

SUMMARY

In this chapter, we have focused not only on the pathologic anatomy of the common AV canal, but also on the pathologic anatomy of those many other details—from the systemic veins to the aortic isthmus—that are essential to complete an accurate diagnosis and to successful surgical management of such patients. One must understand not only the pathologic anatomy of the common AV canal, but also one must know everything of diagnostic and therapeutic significance about the hearts in which common AV canal occurs.

The salient anatomic types of common AV canal found in this study of 464 cases (Chapter 20) were as follows: complete, in 266 (57%); partial, in 93 (20%); transitional, in 9 (2%); VSD of the AV canal type, in 20 (4%); with single ventricle, in 56 (12%); and isolated cleft of the mitral valve of the AV canal type, in 20 cases (4%).

ACKNOWLEDGMENT

I would like to thank Silvio Litovsky, M.D., for his great help in analyzing the data on which this chapter is based.

REFERENCES

1. Griffith TW. Example of a large opening between the two auricles of the heart, unconnected with the fossa ovalis. *J Anat Physiol.* 1899;33:261.
2. Abbott ME. Defects of the interauricular septum and patent foramen ovale. In: *Atlas of Congenital Cardiac Disease.* New York: Abbott ME. American Heart Association; 1936.
3. Rogers HM, Edwards JE. Incomplete division of the atrioventricular canal with patent interatrial foramen primum (persistent common atrioventricular ostium): report of five cases and review of the literature. *Am Heart J.* 1948;36:28.
4. Wakai CS, Edwards JE. Development and pathologic considerations in persistent common atrioventricular canal. *Proc Mayo Clin.* 1956;31:487.
5. Wakai CS, Edwards JE. Pathology study of persistent common atrioventricular canal. *Am Heart J.* 1958;56:779.
6. Edwards JE. Congenital malformations of the heart and great vessels. A. Malformations of the atrial septal complex. In: Gould SE, ed. *Pathology of the Heart and Blood Vessels.* Springfield: Charles C. Thomas; 1968:262.
7. Somerville J, Jefferson K. Left ventricular angiocardiography in atrioventricular defects. *Br Heart J.* 1968;30:446.
8. Piccoli GP, Gerlis LM, Wilkinson JL, Lozsadi K, Macartney FJ, Anderson RH. Morphology and classification of atrioventricular defects. *Br Heart J.* 1979;42:621.
9. Smallhorn JF, Tommasini G, Anderson RH, Macartney FJ. Assessment of atrio-ventricular septal defects by two dimensional echocardiography. *Br Heart J.* 1982;47:109.
10. Allwork S. Anatomical-embryological correlates in atrioventricular septal defect. *Br Heart J.* 1982;47:419.
11. Suzuki K, Ho SY, Anderson RH, et al. Morphometric analysis of atrioventricular septal defect with common valve orifice. *J Am Coll Cardiol.* 1998;31:217.
12. Bharati S, Lev M. The spectrum of common atrioventricular orifice (canal). *Am Heart J.* 1973;86:553.
13. Kirklin JW, Barratt-Boyes BG. Atrioventricular canal defect. In: *Cardiac Surgery: Morphology, Diagnostic Criteria, Natural History, Techniques, Results, and Indications.* New York: Churchill Livingstone; 1993:693.
14. Taguchi K, Matsuura Y, Yoshizaki E, Tamura M. Surgery of atrioventricular septal defects with left ventricular-right atrial shunt. *J Thorac Cardiovasc Sur.* 1968;56:265.
15. Bharati S, Lev M, McAllister HA, Kirklin JW. Surgical anatomy of the atrioventricular valve in the intermediate type of common atrioventricular orifice. *J Thorac Cardiovas Surg.* 1980;79:884.
16. Rastelli GC, Kirklin JW, Titus JL. Anatomic observations on complete form of persistent common atrioventricular canal with special reference to atrioventricular valves. *Mayo Clin Proc.* 1966;41:296.
17. David I, Castañeda AR, Van Praagh R. Potentially parachute mitral valve in common atrioventricular canal: pathologic anatomy and surgical importance. *J Thorac Cardiovasc Surg.* 1982;84:178.
18. Ruckman RN, Van Praagh R. Anatomic types of congenital mitral stenosis: report of 49 autopsy cases with consideration of diagnosis and surgical implications. *Am J Cardiol.* 1978;42:592.

19. Baño-Rodrigo A, Van Praagh S, Trowitzsch E, Van Praagh R. Double-orifice mitral valve: a study of 27 postmortem cases with developmental, diagnostic, and surgical considerations. *Am J Cardiol.* 1988;61:152.
20. Van Praagh R, Litovsky S. Pathology and embryology of common atrioventricular canal. *Progress in Pediatr Cardiol.* 1999;10:115.
21. Asami I. Partitioning of the arterial end of the embryonic heart. In: Van Praagh R, Takao A, eds. *Etiology and Morphogenesis of Congenital Heart Disease.* Mount Kisco, NY: Futura Publishing Co; 1980:51.
22. Asami I. Beitrag zur Entwicklung des Kammerseptums in menschlichen Herzen mit besonderer Berücksichtigung der sog, *Bulbusdrehung. Z Anat Entwickl-Gesch.* 1969;128(1).
23. Van Mierop LHS, Alley RD, Kausel HW, Stranahan A. The anatomy and embryology of endocardial cushion defects. *J Thorac Cardiovas Surg.* 1962;43:71.
24. Netter FH. Embryology: development of the ventricles and cardiac septa and the atrioventricular canal. In: *The Ciba Collection of Medical Illustrations, Volume 5, A Compilation of Paintings on the Normal and Pathologic Anatomy and Physiology, Embryology, and Diseases of the Heart.* Summit NJ: Ciba Pharmaceutical Co; 1969. 120 and 121, respectively.
25. Van Praagh S, Antoniadis S, Otero-Coto E, Leidenfrost RD, Van Praagh R. Common atrioventricular canal with and without conotruncal malformations: an anatomic study of 251 postmortem cases. In: Nora JJ, Takao A, eds. *Congenital Heart Disease: Causes and Processes.* Mount Kisco, NY: Futura Publishing Co; 1984:599.
26. Kurnit DM, Aldridge JF, Matsuoka R, Matthysse S. Increased adhesiveness of trisomy 21 cells and AV canal malformations in Down syndrome: a stochastic model. *Am J Med Genet.* 1985;30:385.
27. Wright TC, Orkin RW, Destrempes M, Kurnit DM. Increased adhesiveness of Down syndrome fetal fibroblasts in vitro. *Proc Natl Acad Sci USA.* 1984;81:2426.
28. Kurnit DM, Layton WM, Matthysse S. Genetics, chance, and morphogenesis. *Am J Hum Genet.* 1987;41:979.
29. Korenberg JR, Bradley C Disteche CM. Down syndrome: molecular mapping of the congenital heart disease and duodenal stenosis. *Am J Hum Genet.* 1992;50:294.
30. Korenberg JR, Kurnit DM. Molecular and stochastic basis of congenital heart defects in Down syndrome. In: Marino B, Pueschel SM, eds. *Heart Disease in Persons with Down Syndrome.* Baltimore: Paul H. Brookes Publishing Co; 1996:21.
31. Van Praagh R, Papagiannis J, Bar-El YI, Schwint OA. The heart in Down syndrome: pathologic anatomy. In: Marino B, Peuschel SM, eds. *Heart Disease in Persons with Down Syndrome.* Baltimore: Paul H. Brookes Publishing Co; 1996:69.
32. Layton WM. Random determination of a developmental process. Reversal of normal visceral asymmetry in the mouse. *J Hered.* 1976;67:336.
33. Layton WM, Manasek FJ. Cardiac looping in early iv/iv mouse embryos. In: Van Praagh R, Takao A, eds. *Etiology and Morphogenesis of Congenital Heart Disease.* Mount Kisco, NY: Futura Publishing Co; 1980:109.
34. Van Praagh R, Layton WM, Van Praagh S. The morophogenesis of normal and abnormal relationships between the great arteries and the ventricles: pathologic and experimental data. In: Van Praagh R, Takao A, eds. *Etiology and Morphogenesis of Congenital Heart Disease.* Mount Kisco, NY. 1980:271.
35. Moulaert AJMG. *Ventricular septal defects and anomalies of the aortic arch.* Leiden: Drukkerij "Luctor et Emergo"; 1974 (MD thesis): 22, 25, 27, 34, 36, 38, 46, 48, 49, 53, 56, 59, 64, 72, 76, 78, 79, 82.
36. Van Praagh R, Van Praagh S. The anatomy of common aorticopulmonary trunk (truncus arteriosus commnis) and its embryologic implications, a study of 57 necropsied cases. *Am J Cardiol.* 1965;16:406.
37. Van Praagh R, Van Praagh S. Anatomically corrected transposition of the great arteries. *Br Heart J.* 1967;29:112.
38. Foran RB, Belcourt C, Nanton MA, et al. Isolated infundibuloarterial inversion {S,D,I}: a newly recognized form of congenital heart disease. *Am Heart J.* 1988;116:1337.
39. Pasquini L, Sanders SP, Parness I, et al. Echocardiographic and anatomic findings in atrioventricular discordance with ventriculoarterial concordance. *Am J Cardiol.* 1988;62:1256.
40. Van Praagh R, Harken AH, Delisle G, Ando M, Gross RE. Total anomalous pulmonary venous drainage to the coronary sinus: a revised procedure for its correction. *J Thorac Cardiovasc Surg.* 1972;64:132.
41. Raghib G, Ruttenberg HD, Anderson RC, Amplatz K, Adams Jr P, Edwards JE. Termination of left superior vena cava in left atrium, atrial septal defect, and absence of coronary sinus—a developmental complex. *Circulation.* 1965;31:906.
42. Neill CA, Ferencz C, Sabiston DC, Sheldon H. The familial occurrence of hypoplastric right lung with systemic arterial supply and venous drainage: "scimitar syndrome". *Bull Johns Hopkins Hosp.* 1960;107:1.
43. Van Praagh R, Weinberg PM, Srebro J. Double-outlet left ventricle. In: Adams FH, Emmanouilides GC, Riemenschneider TA, eds. *Moss' Heart Disease in Infants, Children, and Adolescents.* 4th ed. Baltimore: Williams and Wilkins; 1989:530.
44. Melhuish BPP, Van Praagh R. Juxtaposition of the atrial appendages, a sign of severe cyanotic congenital heart disease. *Br Heart J.* 1968;30:269.
45. Van Praagh S, O'Sullivan J, Brili S, Van Praagh R. Juxtaposition of the morphologically right atrial appendage in solitus and inversus atria: a study of 35 postmortem cases. *Am Heart J.* 1996;132:382.
46. Van Praagh S, O'Sullivan J, Brili S, Van Praagh R. Juxtaposition of the morphologically left atrial appendage in solitus and inversus atria: a study of 18 postmortem cases. *Am Heart J.* 1996;132:391.
47. Pessotto R, Padalino M, Rubino M, Kadoba K, Büchler JR, Van Praagh R. Straddling tricuspid valve as a sign of ventriculoatrial malalignment: a morphometric study of 19 postmortem cases. *Am Heart J.* 1999;138:1184.
48. Van Praagh R, Plett JA, Van Praagh S. Single ventricle: pathology, embryology, terminology, and classification. *Herz.* 1979;4:113.
49. Van Praagh R. What is the Taussig-Bing malformation? *Circulation.* 1968;38:445.
50. Rubino M, Van Praagh S, Kadoba K, Pessotto R, Van Praagh R. Systemic and pulmonary venous connections in visceral heterotaxy with asplenia: diagnostic and surgical considerations based on seventy-two autopsied cases. *J Thorac Surg.* 1995;110:641.
51. Van Praagh S, Porras D, Oppido G, Geva T, Van Praagh R. Cleft mitral valve, without ostium primum defect: anatomic data and surgical considerations based on 41 cases, *Ann Thorac Surg.* (in press).
52. Baum D, Roth GJ, Creighton SA. Right axis deviation, clockwise QRS loop and signs of left ventricular underdevelopment in a child with complete type of persistent common atrioventricular canal. *Circulation.* 1964;30:755.
53. Frater RWM. Persistent common atrioventricular canal, anatomy and function in relation to surgical repair. *Circulation.* 1965;32:120.
54. Somerville J, Resnekov L. The origin of an immediate diastolic murmur in atrioventricular defects. *Circulation.* 1965;32:797.

55. Rastelli GC, Ongley PA, Kirklin JW. Surgical correction of common atrium with anomalously connected persistent left superior vena cava: report of a case. *Mayo Clin Proc.* 1965;40:528.
56. Weyn AS, Bartle SH, Nolan TB, Dammann JF. Atrial septal defect, primum type. *Circulation.* 1965;32(suppl III:13).
57. Durrer D, Rose JP, van Dam RT. The genesis of the electrocardiogram of patients with ostium primum defects (ventral atrial septal defects). *Am Heart J.* 1966;71:642.
58. Somerville J. Clinical assessment of the function of the mitral valve in atrioventricular defects related to the anatomy. *Am Heart J.* 1966;71:701.
59. Hara M, Char F. Partial cleft of septal mitral leaflet associated with atrial septal defect of the secundum type. *Am J Cardiol.* 1966;17:282.
60. Thompson NB, Niguidula FN, Hohn A. Correction of complete atrioventricular canal defect in patients with previous pulmonary artery banding. *Am J Cardiol.* 1966;18:769.
61. Bourakovski VI, Bukharin VA, Romashov FN. Experience in the surgical treatment of patients with common atrioventricular canal. *Br Heart J.* 1967;29:96.
62. Somerville J, Agnew T, Stark J, et al. Banding of the pulmonary artery for common atrioventricular canal. *Br Heart J.* 1967;29:816.
63. Schlesinger Z, Deutsch V, Yahini JH, Neufeld HN. Deformed anterior mitral leaflet without mitral insufficiency in persistent common atrioventricular canal. Anatomic and angiocardiographic correlations. *Am Heart J.* 1967;73:742.
64. Gotsman MS, Beck W, Schrire V. Left ventricular cineangiocardiography in endocardial cushion defect. *Br Heart J.* 1968;30:182.
65. Rastelli GC, Ongley PA, Kirklin JW, McGoon DC. Surgical repair of the complete form of persistent common atrioventricular canal. *J Thorac Cardiovasc Surg.* 1968;55:299.
66. Taguchi K, Sasaki N, Okii Y, Matsuura Y, Hirao M. Surgical experience with persistent common atrioventricular canal in a series of eighty-two patients. Particular consideration on the correction of valve incompetence and deficiency of the ventricular septum. *J Thorac Cardiovasc Surg.* 1968;55:501.
67. Emanuel R, Nichols J, Anders JM, Moores EC, Somerville J. Atrioventricular defects, a study of 92 families. *Br Heart J.* 1968;30:645.
68. Rastelli GC, Rahimtoola SH, Ongley PA, McGoon DC. Common atrium: anatomy, hemodynamics, and surgery. *J Thorac Cardiovasc Surg.* 1968;55:834.
69. Griffiths SP, Ellis K, Burris JO, Blumenthal S, Bowman FO, Malm JR. Postoperative evaluation of mitral valve function in ostium primum defect with cleft mitral valve (partial form of atrioventricular canal). *Circulation.* 1969;40:21.
70. Shah CV, Patel MK, Hastreiter AR. Hemodynamics of complete atrioventricular canal and its evolution with age. *Am J Cardiol.* 1969;24:326.
71. Lillehei CW, Anderson RC, Ferlic RM, Bonnabeau RC. Persistent common atrioventricular canal. Recatheterization results in 37 patients following intracardiac repair. *J Thorac Cardiovasc Surg.* 1969;57:83.
72. Titus JL. Congenital malformations of the mitral and aortic valves and related structures. *Dis Chest.* 1969;55:358.
73. Feldt RH, Dushane JW, Titus JL. The atrioventricular conduction system in persistent common atrioventricular canal defect, correlations with electrocardiogram. *Circulation.* 1970;42:437.
74. Morgan BC, Ricketts HJ, Winterscheid LC. Inferior clockwise frontal plane forces in a child with endocardial cushion defect. *Am Heart J.* 1971;82:275.
75. Yokoyama M, Kudo T, Konno S, Sakakibara S. Selective left ventriculography in 61 cases with endocardial cushion defects. *Bull Heart Inst Japan.* 1971;13:44.
76. Eckberg DL, Ross J, Morgan JR. Acquired right bundle branch block and left anterior hemiblock in ostium primum atrial septal defect. *Circulation.* 1972;45:658.
77. Baron MG. Abnormalities of the mitral valve in endocardial cushion defects. *Circulation.* 1972;45:672.
78. Fellows K, Henschel WG, Keck EW, Lassrich A. Left ventricular angiocardiography in endocardial cushion defects: emphasis on the lateral projection. *Ann Radiol.* 1972;15:223.
79. Yokoyama M, Ando M, Takao A, Sakakibara S. The location of the coronary sinus orifice in endocardial cushion defects. *Am Heart J.* 1973;85:302.
80. Pacifico AD, Kirklin JW. Surgical repair of complete atrioventricular canal with anterior common leaflet attached to an anomalous right ventricular papillary muscle. *J Thor Cardiovas Surg.* 1973;65:727.
81. Danielson GK. Traitement chirurgical des formes complètes de canal atrioventriculaire. *Coeur.* 1973:487.
82. Binet JP. A propos de la ŕeparation du CAV (canal atrioventriculaire). *Coeur.* 1973:495.
83. Khaja F, Sanghvi VR, Parker JO. Persistent common atrioventricular canal and Down's syndrome with unusually prolonged survival. *Chest.* 1973;64:262.
84. Hung J-S, Ritter DG, Feldt RH, Kincaid OW. Electrocardiographic and angiographic features of common atrium. *Chest.* 1973;63:970.
85. Waldo AL, Kaiser GA, Bowman FO, Malm JR. Etiology of prolongation of the P-R interval in patients with an endocardial cushion defect. Further observations on internodal conduction and the polarity of the retrograde P wave. *Circulation.* 1973;48:19.
86. Tenckhoff L, Stamm SJ. An analysis of 35 cases of the complete form of persistent common atrioventricular canal. *Circulation.* 1973;38:416.
87. Danielson GK, McMullan MH, Kinsley RH, DuShane JW. Successful repair of complete atrioventricular canal associated with dextroversion, common atrium, and total anomalous systemic venous return. *J Thorac Cardiovasc Surg.* 1966;66:817.
88. Los JA, van Eijndthoven E. The fusion of the endocardial cushions in the heart of the chick embryo, a light-microscopical and electron-microscopical study. *Z Anat Entwickl-Gesch.* 1973;141:55.
89. McGoon DC. Complex congenital malformations: surgery for complete form of atrioventricular canal. In: Kirklin JW, ed. *Advances in Cardiovascular Surgery.* New York: Grune & Stratton; 1973:p45.
90. McGoon DC, McMullan MH, Mair DD, Danielson GK. Correction of complete atrioventricular canal in infants. *Mayo Clin Proc.* 1973;48:769.
91. Boineau JP, Moore EN, Patterson DF. Relationship between the ECG, ventricular activation, and the ventricular conduction system in ostium primum ASD. *Circulation.* 1973;48:556.
92. Turnoff HB, Kingsley B, Linhart JW. Echocardiographic features of endocardial cushion defect. *Am J Cardiol.* 1974;33:135.
93. Goodman DJ, Harrison DC, Cannom DS. Atrioventricular conduction in patients with incomplete endocardial cushion defect. *Circulation.* 1974;49:631.
94. Williams HJ, Tandon R, Edwards JE. Persistent ostium primum coexisting with mitral or tricuspid atresia. *Chest.* 1974;66:39.

95. Kudo T, Yokoyama M, Imai Y, Konno S, Sakakibara S. The tricuspid pouch in endocardial cushion defect. *Am Heart J.* 1974;87:544.
96. Utley JR, Noonan JA, Walters LR, Frist RA. Anomalous position of atrial septum with anomalous pulmonary and systemic venous drainage. Correction including ligation of persistent left superior vena cava. *J Thorac Cardiovasc Surg.* 1974;67:730.
97. Williams RG, Rudd M. Echocardiographic features of endocardial cushion defects. *Circulation.* 1974;49:418.
98. Lévy S, Blondeau P, Dubost C. Long-term follow-up after surgical correction of the partial form of common atrioventricular canal (ostium primum). *J Thorac Cardiovasc Surg.* 1974;67:353.
99. Sahn DJ, Terry RW, O'Rourke R, Leopold G, Friedman WF. Multiple crystal echocardiographic evaluation of endocardial cushion defect. *Circulation.* 1974;50:25.
100. Tandon R, Moller JH, Edwards JE. Unusual longevity in persistent common atrioventricular canal. *Circulation.* 1974;50:619.
101. Okamura K, Kudo T, Koyanagi H, Imai Y, Konno S. Evaluation of mitral regurgitation in endocardial cushion defect by selective left ventriculography with reference to surgical intervention on mitral valvular cleft. *Am Heart J.* 1974;88:579.
102. Eshaghpour E, Turnoff HB, Kingsley B, Kawai N, Linhart JW. Echocardiography in endocardial cushion defects: a preoperative and postoperative study. *Chest.* 1975;68:172.
103. Goodman DJ, Harrison DC, Schroeder JS. Ostium primum defect in the adult: postoperative follow-up studies. *Chest.* 1975;67:185.
104. Pieroni DR, Homcy E, Freedom RM. Echocardiography in atrioventricular canal defect, a clinical spectrum. *Am J Cardiol.* 1975;35:54.
105. Borkon AM, Pieroni DR, Varghese PJ, Ho CS, Rowe RD. The superior QRS axis in ostium primum ASD: a proposed mechanism. *Am Heart J.* 1975;90:215.
106. Quero Jiménez M, Ugarte Peña M, De Salamanca FE, Calabró R, Pérez Martinez V. Risultati anatomici ed implicazioni embriologiche. *La Settimana Med.* 1974;62:333.
107. Beppu S, Nimura Y, Nagata S, et al. Diagnosis of endocardial cushion defect with cross-sectional and M-mode scanning echocardiography. Differentiation from secundum atrial septal defect. *Br Heart J.* 1976;38:911.
108. Komatsu Y, Nagai Y, Shibuya M, Takao A, Hirosawa K. Echocardiographic analysis of intracardiac anatomy in endocardial cushion defect. *Am Heart J.* 1976;91:210.
109. Feldt RH, McGoon DC, Ongley PA, Rastelli GC, Titus JL, Van Mierop LHS. *Atrioventricular Canal Defects.* Philadelphia: W.B. Saunders Co; 1976.
110. Jacobsen JR, Gillette PC, Corbett BN, Rabinovtich M, McNamara DG. Intracardial electrography in endocardial cushion defects. *Circulation.* 1976;54:599.
111. Mills NL, Ochsner JL, King TD. Correction of type C complete atrioventricular canal, surgical considerations. *J Thorac Cardiovasc Surg.* 1976;71:20.
112. Ugarte M, Enríquez de Salamanca F, Quero M. Endocardial cushion defects, an anatomical study of 54 specimens. *Br Heart J.* 1976;38:674.
113. Spanos PK, Fiddler GI, Mair DD, McGoon DC. Repair of atrioventricular canal associated with membranous subaortic stenosis. *Mayo Clin Proc.* 1977;52:121.
114. Kahn DR, Levy J, France NE, Chung KJ, Dacumos GC. Recent results after repair of atrioventricular canal. *J Thorac Cardiovsac Surg.* 1977;73:413.
115. Mair DD, McGoon DC. Surgical correction of atrioventricular canal during the first year of life. *Am J Cardiol.* 1977;40:66.
116. Quero-Jiménez M, Ugarte Pena M, Enríquez de Salamanca F, Knapp K, Acerete F, Herraíz-Sarachaga I. Anatomie der atrioventrikularklappen bei endokardkissendefekten. *Diagnostische folgerungen Herz.* 1977;2:385.
117. Newfeld EA, Sher M, Paul MH, Nikaidoh H. Pulmonary vascular disease in complete atrioventricular canal defect. *Am J Cardiol.* 1977;39:721.
118. Bass JL, Bessinger B, Lawrence C. Echocardiographic differentiation of partial and complete atrioventricular canal. *Circulation.* 1978;57:1144.
119. Berger TJ, Kirklin JW, Blackstone EH, Pacifico AD, Kouchoukos NT. Primary repair of complete atrioventricular canal in patients less than 2 years old. *Am J Cardiol.* 1978;41:906.
120. Culpepper W, Kolff J, Lin C-Y, et al. Complete common atrioventricular canal in infancy, surgical repair and postoperative hemodyanamics. *Circulation.* 1978;58:550.
121. Losay J, Rosenthal A, Castañeda AR, Bernhard WH, Nadas AS. Repair of atrial septal defect primum—results, course, and prognosis. *J Thorac Cardiovasc Surg.* 1978;75:248.
122. Toussaint M, Planche C, Ribierre M. Le canal atrio-ventriculaire complet, étude anatomique de 31 cas de formes isolées. *Coeur.* 1978;9:1171.
123. Toussaint M, Planche C, Neveux JY, Ribierre M. Ventricule gauche à double entrée avec persistence du canal atrioventriculaire. *Coeur.* 1978;9:1192.
124. Thanopoulos BD, Fisher EA, DuBrow IW, Hastreiter AR. Right and left ventricular volume characteristics in common atrioventricular canal. *Circulation.* 1978;57:991.
125. Jarmakani JM, George B, Wheller J. Ventricular volume characteristics in infants and children with endocardial cushion defects. *Circulation.* 1978;58:153.
126. Jung JY, Almond CH, Lababidi Z, Politte LL, Watson LE. Cyanosis in a patient with combined ostium primum and secundum atrial septal defects and anomalous inferior vena cava with azygos continuation. Case report and surgical considerations. *J Thorac Cardiovasc Surg.* 1978;75:244.
127. Ebert PA, Goor DA. Complete atrioventricular canal malformation: further clarification of the anatomy of the common leaflet and its relationship to the VSD in surgical correction. *Ann Thorac Surg.* 1978;25:134.
128. Antar R, Krongrad E. Etiology of right bundle branch block pattern following surgical repair of atrioventricular cushion defects. *Chest.* 1978;73:642.
129. Caruso G, Losekoot TG, Becker AE. Ebstein's anomaly in persistent common atrioventricular canal. *Br Heart J.* 1978;40:1275.
130. Hagler DJ, Tajik AJ, Seward JB, Mair DD, Ritter DG. Real-time wide-angle sector echocardiography: atrioventricular canal defects. *Circulation.* 1979;59:140.
131. Epstein ML, Moller JH, Amplatz K, Nicoloff DM. Pulmonary artery banding in infants with complete atrioventricular canal. *J Thorac Cardiovasc Surg.* 1979;78:28.
132. Richardson JV, Jensen CB, Doty DB. Complete atrioventricular canal and cor triatriatum. *Cardiovasc Dis Bull Texas Heart Inst.* 1979;6:137.
133. Stewart S, Harris P, Manning J. Complete endocardial cushion defect, operative technique and results. *J Thorac Cardiovasc Surg.* 1979;78:914.
134. Thilenius OG, Vitullo D, Bharati S, et al. Endocardial cushion defect associated with cor triatriatum sinistrum or supravalve mitral ring. *Am J Cardiol.* 1979;44:1339.

135. Bloom KR, Freedom RM, Williams CM, Trusler GA, Rowe RD. Echocardiographic recognition of atrioventricular valve stenosis associated with endocardial cushion defect: pathologic and surgical correlates. *Am J Cardiol.* 1979;44:1326.
136. Macartney FJ, Rees PG, Daly K, et al. Angiocardiographic appearances of atrioventricular defects with particular reference to distinction of ostium primum atrial septal defect from common atrioventricular orifice. *Br Heart J.* 1979;42:640.
137. Mehta S, Hirschfeld S, Riggs T, Liebman J. Echocardiographic estimation of ventricular hypoplasia in complete atrioventricular canal. *Circulation.* 1979;59:888.
138. Thiene G, Frescura C, DiDonato R, Gallucci V. Complete atrioventricular canal associated with conotruncal malformations in 13 specimens. *Europ J Cardiol.* 1979;9:199.
139. Midgley FM, Galioto FM, Shapiro SR, Perry LW, Scott LP. Experience with repair of complete atrioventricular canal. *Ann Thor Surg.* 1980;30:151.
140. Pyeritz RE, Humphries JO. Partial endocardial cushion defect and persistence of the left superior vena cava draining into the left atrium in a 34-year-old man with features of the Kaufman and Marfan syndromes. *Johns Hopkins Med J.* 1980;146:28.
141. Sade RM, Riopel DA, Lorenzo R. Tetralogy of Fallot associated with complete atrioventricular canal. *Ann Thor Surg.* 1980;30:177.
142. Pacifico AD, Kirklin JW, Bargeron LM. Repair of complete atrioventricular canal associated with tetralogy of Fallot or double-outlet right ventricle: report of 10 patients. *Ann Thor Surg.* 1980;29:351.
143. Bharati S, Lev M, McAllister HA, Kirklin JW. Surgical anatomy of the atrioventricular valve in the intermediate type of common atrioventricular orifice. *J Thorac Cardiovasc Surg.* 1980;79:884.
144. Beppu S, Nimura Y, Sakakibara H, et al. Mitral cleft in ostium primum atrial septal defect assessed by cross-sectional echocardiography. *Circulation.* 1980;62:1099.
145. Piccoli GP, McKay R, Macartney FJ, Stark J, de Leval M. Surgical repair of common atrioventricular orifice without atrial septal defect in two patients. *Br Heart J.* 1980;43:102.
146. Bharati S, Kirklin JW, McAllister HA, Lev M. The surgical anatomy of common atrioventricular orifice associated with tetralogy of Fallot, double outlet right ventricle and complete regular transposition. *Circulation.* 1980;61:1142.
147. Wenink ACG. The ventricular septum in hearts with an atrioventricular defect. In: Oppenheimer-Dekker A, Moulaert AJ, eds. *The Ventricular Septum of the Heart, Wenink ACG, the Hague.* Martinus Nijhoff; 1981:131.
148. Thiene G, Wenink ACG, Frescura C, et al. Surgical anatomy and pathology of the conduction tissues in atrioventricular defects. *J Thorac Cardiovasc Surg.* 1981;82:928.
149. Goldfaden DM, Jones M, Morrow AG. Long-term results of repair of incomplete persistent atrioventricular canal. *J Thorac Cardiovasc Surg.* 1981;82:669.
150. Taylor NC, Somerville J. Fixed subaortic stenosis after repair of ostium primum defects. *Br Heart J.* 1981;45:689.
151. Dick M, Behrendt DM, Jochim KE, Castañeda AR. Electrophysiologic delineation of the intraventricular His bundle in two patients with endocardial cushion type of ventricular septal defect. *Circulation.* 1981;63:225.
152. DeTommasi SM, Daliento L, Ho SY, Macartney FJ, Anderson RH. Analysis of atrioventricular junction, ventricular mass, and ventriculoarterial junction in 43 specimens with atrial isomerism. *Br Heart J.* 1981;45:236.
153. Ben-Shachar G, Moller JH, Castañeda-Zuniga W, Edwards JE. Signs of membranous subaortic stenosis appearing after correction of persistent common atrioventricular canal. *Am J Cardiol.* 1981;48:340.
154. Waller BF, Sheikh MU, Roberts WC. Prolapsing atrioventricular valve in partial atrioventricular defect. *Am Heart J.* 1981;101:108.
155. Soto B, Bargeron LM, Pacifico AD, Vanini V, Kirklin JW. Angiography of atrioventricular canal defects. *Am J Cardiol.* 1981;48:492.
156. Becker AE, Anderson RH. Atrioventricular septal defects. In: *Pathology of Congenital Heart Disease.* London: Butterworths; 1981:77.
157. Hynes TK, Tajik AJ, Seward JB, et al. Partial atrioventricular canal defect in adults. *Circulation.* 1981;66:284.
158. Moreno-Cabral RJ, Shumway NE. Double-patch technique for correction of complete atrioventricular canal. *Ann Thor Surg.* 1982;33:88.
159. Smallhorn JF, Tommasini G, Anderson RH, Macartney FJ. Assessment of atrioventricular septal defects by two dimensional echocardiography. *Br Heart J.* 1982;47:109.
160. Allwork S. Anatomical-embryological correlates in atrioventricular septal defect. *Br Heart J.* 1982;47:419.
161. David I, Castañeda AR, Van Praagh R. Potentially parachute mitral valve in common atrioventricular canal, pathologic anatomy and surgical importance. *J Thorac Cardiovasc Surg.* 1982;84:178.
162. Wright JS, Newman DC. Complete and intermediate atrioventricular canal in infants less than a year old: observations of anatomical and pathological variants in left ventricular outflow tract. *Ann Thor Surg.* 1982;33:171.
163. Fernandez Aceytuno AM, Bethencourt Gonzales A, Macaya Miguel C, Tynan M, Anderson RH. Subxiphoid M-mode echocardiography in atrioventricular defects. *Ped Cardiol.* 1982;3:119.
164. Bove EL, Kavey R-EW, Sondheimer HM, Parker FB. Subacute bacterial endocarditis and complete endocardial cushion defect. *Ann Thor Surg.* 1982;34:466.
165. Bender HW, Hammon JW, Hubbard SG, Muirhead J, Graham TP. Repair of atrioventricular canal malformation in the first year of life. *J Thorac Cardiovasc Surg.* 1982;84:515.
166. Chin AJ, Keane JF, Norwood WI, Castañeda AR. Repair of complete common atrioventricular canal in infancy. *J Thorac Cardiovasc Surg.* 1982;84:437.
167. Becker AE, Anderson RH. Atrioventricular septal defects: what's in a name? *J Thorac Cardiovasc Surg.* 1982;83:461.
168. Piccoli GP, Ho SY, Wilkinson JL, Macartney FJ, Gerlis LM, Anderson RH. Left-sided obstructive lesions in atrioventricular septal defects, an anatomic study. *J Thorac Cardiovasc Surg.* 1982;83:453.
169. Mavroudis C, Weinstein G, Turley K, Ebert PA. Surgical management of complete atrioventricular canal. *J Thorac Cardiovasc Surg.* 1982;83:670.
170. Alfieri O, Plokker M. Repair of common atrioventricular canal associated with transposition of the great arteries and left ventricular outflow obstruction. *J Thorac Cardiovasc Surg.* 1982;84:872.
171. Studer M, Blackstone EH, Kirklin JW, et al. Determinants of early and late results of repair of atrioventricular septal (canal) defects. *J Thorac Cardiovasc Surg.* 1982;84:523.
172. DiSciascio G, Bargeron LM. The electrocardiogram in tetralogy of Fallot with complete atrioventricular canal. *Texas Heart Inst J.* 1982;9:163.

173. Lappen RS, Muster AJ, Idriss FS, et al. Masked subaortic stenosis in ostium primum atrial septal defect: recognition and treatment. *Am J Cardiol.* 1983;52:336.
174. Warnes C, Somerville J. Double mitral orifice in atrioventricular defects. *Br Heart J.* 1983;49:59.
175. Chin AJ, Bierman FZ, Sanders SP, Williams RG, Norwood WI, Castañeda AR. Subxyphoid 2-dimensional echocardiographic identification of left ventricular papillary muscle anomalies in complete common atrioventricular canal. *Am J Cardiol.* 1983;51:1695.
176. Abbruzzese PA, Livermore J, Sunderland CO, et al. Mitral repair in complete atrioventricular canal. Ease of correction in early infancy. *J Thorac Cardiovasc Surg.* 1983;85:388.
177. Emanuel R, Somerville J, Inns A, Withers R. Evidence of congenital heart disease in the offspring of parents with atrioventricular defects. *Br Heart J.* 1983;49:144.
178. Cloez JL, Ravault MC, Worms AM, Marcow F, Pernot C. Complete atrioventricular canal defect associated with congenitally corrected transposition of the great arteries: two-dimensional echocardiographic identification. *J Am Coll Cardiol.* 1983;1:1123.
179. Ibawi MN, Idriss FS, DeLeon SY, et al. Unusual mitral valve abnormalities complicating surgical repair of endocardial cushion defects. *J Thorac Cardiovasc Surg.* 1983;85:697.
180. Kawashima Y, Matsuda H, Hirose H, Nakano S, Shinazaki Y, Miyamoto K. Surgical treatment of complete atrioventricular canal defect with an endocardial cushion prosthesis. *Circulation.* 1983;68:II–139.
181. Silverman N, Levitsky S, Fisher E, DuBrow I, Hastreiter A, Scagliotti D. Efficacy of pulmonary artery banding in infants with complete atrioventricular canal. *Circulation.* 1983;68:II–148.
182. Williams WH, Guyton RA, Michalik RE, et al. Individualized surgical management of complete atrioventricular canal. *J Thorac Cardiovasc Surg.* 1983;86:838.
183. Ebels T, Meijboom EJ, Anderson RH, et al. Anatomic and functional "obstruction" of the outflow tract in atrioventricular septal defects with separate valve orifices ("ostium primum atrial septal defect"): an echocardiographic study. *Am J Cardiol.* 1984;54:843.
184. Gow RM, Freedom RM, Williams WG, Trusler GA, Rowe RD. Coarctation of the aorta or subaortic stenosis with atrioventricular septal defect. *Am J Cardiol.* 1984;53:1421.
185. Rizzoli G, Mazzucco A, Brumana T, et al. Operative risk of correction of atrioventricular septal defects. *Br Heart J.* 1984;52:258.
186. Roach RM, Tandon R, Moller JH, Edwards JE. Ebstein's anomaly of the tricuspid valve in persistent common atrioventricular canal. *Am J Cardiol.* 1984;53:640.
187. Uretzky G, Puga FJ, Danielson GK, et al. Complete atrioventricular canal associated with tetralogy of Fallot, morphologic and surgical considerations. *J Thorac Cardiovasc Surg.* 1984;87:756.
188. Zion MM, Rosenman D, Balkin J, Glaser J. Complete atrioventricular canal with survival to the eighth decade. *Chest.* 1984;85:437.
189. Bove EL, Sondheimer HM, Kavey R-EW, Byrum CJ, Blackman MS. Results with the two-patch technique for repair of complete atrioventricular septal defect. *Ann Thor Surg.* 1984;38:157.
190. Tennant SN, Hammond JW, Bender HN, Graham TP, Primm RK. Familial clustering of atrioventricular canal defects. *Am Heart J.* 1984;108:175.
191. Warnes CA, Shugol GI, Wallace RB, Roberts WC. Atrioventricular septal defect (primum atrial septal defect) with prolonged survival (despite severe mitral regurgitation and pulmonary hypertension) and associated cardiac calcification (mitral annulus, coronary artery and pulmonary trunk). *Am J Cardiol.* 1984;54:689.
192. Schwartz DC. Atrioventricular septal defects. *Sem Roentgenol.* 1985;20:226.
193. Otero-Coto W, Castañeda AR. Dysplasia of AV valve in complete AV canal with tetralogy of Fallot: surgical repair. *Pediatr Cardiol.* 1984;5:213.
194. Fisher EA, Doshi M, DuBrow IW, Silverman N, Levitsky S. Effect of palliative and corrective surgery on ventricular volumes in complete atrioventricular canal. *Pediat Cardiol.* 1984;5:159.
195. McGrath LB, Kirklin JW, Soto B, Bargeron LM. Secondary left atrioventricular valve replacement in atrioventricular septal (AV canal) defect: a method to avoid left ventricular outflow tract obstruction. *J Thorac Cardiovasc Surg.* 1985;89:632.
196. Jacobstein MD, Fletcher BD, Goldstein S, Riemenschneider TA. Evaluation of atrioventricular septal defect by magnetic resonance imaging. *Am J Cardiol.* 1985;55:1158.
197. Anderson RH, Zuberbuhler JR, Penkoske PA, Neches WH. Of clefts, commissures, and things. *J Thorac Cardiovasc Surg.* 1985;90:605.
198. Alivizatos P, Anderson RH, Macartney FJ, Zuberbuhler JR, Stark J. Atrioventricular septal defect with balanced ventricles and malaligned atrial septum: double-outlet right atrium, report of two cases. *J Thorac Cardiovasc Surg.* 1985;89:295.
199. Stewart S, Harris P, Manning J. Complete endocardial cushion defect: the late result of repair using the single-patch technique. *Ann Thor Surg.* 1985;39:234.
200. Portman MA, Beder SD, Ankeney JL, van Heecheren D, Liebman J, Riemenschneider TA. A 20-year review of ostium primum defect repair in children. *Am Heart J.* 1985;110:1054.
201. Penkoske PA, Neches WH, Anderson RH, Zuberbuhler JR. Further observations on the morphology of atrioventricular septal defects. *J Thorac Cardiovasc Surg.* 1985;90:611.
202. Kurnit DM, Aldridge JF, Matsuoka R, Matthysse S. Increased adhesiveness of trisomy 21 cells and atrioventricular canal malformations in Down syndrome: a stochastic model. *Am J Med Genetics.* 1985;30:385.
203. Román MI, Binello MM, Zarlenga B, et al. Echocardiographic method to evaluate the size of AVC defects, surgical importance. *Rev Latina de Cardiología y Cirugía Cardiovascular Infantil.* 1985;1:61.
204. de la Cruz MV, Valadez EF. Embriología del canal auriculoventricular y del septum auriculoventricular (normal). *Revista Latina de Cardiología y Cirugía Cardiovasc Infantil.* 1985;1:3.
205. de la Cruz MV, Fernández Valadez E. Embriología de la persistencia del canal auriculoventricular commún. *Rev Lat Cardiol y Cirugía Cardiovasc Infantil.* 1985;1:13.
206. De Biase L, DiCiommo L, Ballerini L, Bevilacqua M, Marcelletti C, Marino B. Prevalence of left-sided obstructive lesions in patients with atrioventricular canal without Down's syndrome. *J Thorac Cardiovasc Surg.* 1986;91:467.
207. Stewart S, Alexson C, Manning J. Partial atrioventricular canal defect: the early and late results of operation. *Ann Thorac Surg.* 1987;43:527.
208. Meijboom EJ, Ebels T, Anderson RH, et al. Left atrioventricular valve after surgical repair in atrioventricular septal defect with separate valve orifices ("ostium primum atrial septal defect"): an echo-Doppler study. *Am J Cardiol.* 1986;57:433.
209. Curcio CA, Cronje SH. Partial atrioventricular canal in an adult: mitral valve repair by reverse implantation of a Carpentier ring. *J Thorac Cardiovasc Surg.* 1987;94:444.

210. Quero Jiménez M, Arteaga Martínez M, eds. *Paediatric Cardiology, Atrioventricular Septal Defects*. Madrid: Ediciones Norma; 1988.
211. Barnett MG, Chopra PS, Young WP. Long-term follow-up of partial atrioventricular septal defect repair in adults. *Chest*. 1988;94:321.
212. Chang C-I, Becker AE. Surgical anatomy of left ventricular outflow tract obstruction in complete atrioventricular septal defect, a concept for operative repair. *J Thorac Cardiovasc Surg*. 1987;94:897.
213. Fournier A, Young M-L, Garcia OL, Tamer DF, Wolff GS. Electrophysiologic cardiac function before and after surgery in children with atrioventricular canal. *Am J Cardiol*. 1986;57:1137.
214. Lipshultz SE, Sanders SP, Mayer Jr JE, Colan SD, Lock JE. Are routine preoperative cardiac catheterization and angiocardiography necessary before repair of ostium primum atrial septal defect? *J Am Coll Cardiol*. 1988;11:373.
215. Machado MVL, Crawford DC, Anderson RH, Allan LD. Atrioventricular septal defect in prenatal life. *Br Heart J*. 1988;59:352.
216. Pillai R, Ho SY, Anderson RH, Lincoln C. Ostium primum atrioventricular septal defect: an anatomical surgical review. *Ann Thor Surg*. 1986;41:458.
217. LeBlanc JG, Williams WG, Freedom RM, Trusler GA. Results of total correction in complete atrioventricular septal defects with congenital or surgically induced right ventricular outflow tract obstruction. *Ann Thor Surg*. 1986;41:387.
218. Santos A, Boucek M, Ruttenberg H, Veasy G, Orsmond G, McGough E. Repair of atrioventricular septal defects in infancy. *J Thorac Cardiovasc Surg*. 1986;91:505.
219. Rowley KM, Kopf GS, Hellenbrand W, Kleinman CS, Downing SE. Atrioventricular canal with intact atrial septum. *Am Heart J*. 1988;115:902.
220. King RM, Puga FJ, Danielson GK, Schaff HV, Julsrud PR, Feldt RH. Prognostic factors and surgical treatment of partial atrioventricular canal. *Circulation*. 1986;74(suppl 1). I-42.
221. Ebels T, Ho SY, Anderson RH, Meijboom EJ, Eijgelaar A. The surgical anatomy of the left ventricular outflow tract in atrioventricular septal defect. *Ann Thor Surg*. 1986;41:483.
222. Vargas FJ, Otero Coto E, Mayer JE, Jonas RA, Castañeda AR. Complete atrioventricular canal and tetralogy of Fallot: surgical considerations. *Ann Thorac Surg*. 1986;42:258.
223. Guo-wei H, Mee RBB. Complete atrioventricular canal associated with tetralogy of Fallot or double-outlet right ventricle and right ventricular outflow tract obstruction: a report of successful surgical treatment. *Ann Thorac Surg*. 1986;41:612.
224. Tandon R, Moller JH, Edwards JE. Single papillary muscle of the left ventricle associated with persistent common atrioventricular canal: variant of parachute mitral valve. *Pediatr Cardiol*. 1986;7:111.
225. Gutgesell HP, Huhta JC. Cardiac septation in atrioventricular canal defect. *J Am Coll Cardiol*. 1986;8:1447.
226. Haworth SG. Pulmonary vascular bed in children with complete atrioventricular septal defect: relation between structural and hemodynamic abnormalities. *Am J Cardiol*. 1986;57:833.
227. Clapp SK, Perry BH, Farooki ZQ, et al. Surgical and medical results of complete atrioventricular canal: a ten year review. *Am J Cardiol*. 1987;59:454.
228. Pacifico AD, Ricchi A, Bargeron LM, Colvin EC, Kirklin JW, Kirklin JK. Corrective repair of complete atrioventricular canal defects and major associated cardiac anomalies. *Ann Thorac Surg*. 1988;46:645.
229. Pan-Chih, Chen-Chun. Surgical treatment of atrioventricular canal malformations. *Ann Thorac Surg*. 1987;43:150.
230. Mortera C, Rissech M, Payola M, Miro C. Cross sectional subcoastal echocardiography: atrioventricular septal defects and the short axis cut. *Br Heart J*. 1987;58:267.
231. Corno A, Marino B, Catena G, Marcelletti C. Atrioventricular septal defects with severe left ventricular hypoplasia, staged palliation. *J Thorac Cardiovasc Surg*. 1988;96:249.
232. Carvalho JS, Rigby ML, Shinebourne EA, Anderson RH. Cross sectional echocardiography for recognition of ventricular topology in atrioventricular septal defect. *Br Heart J*. 1989;61:285.
233. Wenink ACG, Ottenkamp J, Guit GL, Draulans-Noe Y, Doornbos J. Correlation of morphology of the left ventricular outflow tract with two-dimensional Doppler echocardiography and magnetic resonance imaging in atrioventricular septal defect. *J Am Coll Cardiol*. 1989;63:1137.
234. Ceithaml EL, Midgley FM, Perry LW. Long-term results after surgical repair of incomplete endocardial cushion defects. *Ann Thor Surg*. 1989;48:413.
235. Canter CE, Sekarski DC, Martin TC, Guitierrez FR, Spray TL. Intraoperative evaluation of atrioventricular septal defect repair by color flow mapping echocardiography. *Ann Thor Surg*. 1989;48:544.
236. Szulc M, Poon E, Cooper R, Kaplovitz H, Frenkel M, Tranbaugh R. Single papillary muscle and ostium primum defect. *Pediatr Cardiol*. 1990;11:96.
237. Marino B, Digilio MC, Giannotti A, Dallapiccola B. Atrioventricular canal associated with trisomy 9. *Chest*. 1989;96:1420.
238. Abbruzzese PA, Napoleone A, Bini RM, Annechino FP, Merlo M, Parenzan L. Late left atrioventricular valve insufficiency after repair of partial atrioventricular septal defects: anatomical and surgical determinants. *Ann Thor Surg*. 1990;49:111.
239. Parsons JM, Baker EJ, Anderson RH, Ladusans EJ, et al. Morphological evaluation of atrioventricular septal defects by magnetic resonance imaging. *Br Heart J* 1990;64:138.
240. Weintraub RG, Brawn WJ, Venables AW, Mee RBB. Two-patch repair of complete atrioventricular septal defect in the first year of life, results and sequential assessment of atrioventricular valve function. *J Thorac Cardiovasc Surg*. 1990;99:320.
241. Ebels T, Anderson RH, Devine WA, Debich DE, Penkoske PA, Zuberbuhler JR. Anomalies of the left atrioventricular valve and related ventricular septal morphology in atrioventricular septal defects. *J Thorac Cardiovasc Surg*. 1990;99:299.
242. Marino B, Guccione P, Marcelletti C, Dallapiccola B. Atrioventricular canal without Down syndrome associated with additional cardiac and noncardiac anomalies. *Am J Dis Child*. 1990;144:752.
243. Ilbawi M, Cua C, DeLeon S, et al. Repair of complete atrioventricular septal defect with tetralogy of Fallot. *Ann Thor Surg*. 1990;50:407.
244. Marino B, Marcelletti C, Giannotti A, Dallapiccola B. DiGeorge anomaly with atrioventricular canal. *Chest*. 1991;99:242.
245. Pozzi M, Remig J, Fimmers R, Urban AE. Atrioventricular septal defects, analysis of short- and medium-term results. *J Thorac Cardiovasc Surg*. 1991;101:138.
246. Wilcox BR, Anderson RH, Henry GW, Mattos SS. Unusual opening of coronary sinus in atrioventricular septal defects. *Ann Thor Surg*. 1990;50:767.
247. Draulans-Noë HAY, Wenink ACG. Anterolateral muscle bundle of the left ventricle in atrioventricular septal defect: left ventricular outflow tract and subaortic stenosis. *Pediatr Cardiol*. 1991;12:83.

248. Gembruch U, Knöpfle G, Chatterjee M, et al. Prenatal diagnosis of atrioventricular canal malformations with up-to-date echocardiographic technology: report of 14 cases. *Am Heart J.* 1991;121:1489.
249. Roberson DA, Muhiudeen IA, Silverman NH, Turley K, Haas GS, Cahalan MK. Intraoperative transesophageal echocardiography of atrioventricular septal defect. *J Am Coll Cardiol.* 1991;18:537.
250. Van Praagh S, Vangi V, Sul JH, et al. Tricuspid atresia or severe stenosis with partial common atrioventricular canal: anatomic data, clinical profile, and surgical considerations. *J Am Coll Cardiol.* 1991;17:932.
251. Capouya ER, Laks H. Atrioventricular canal defects. *Ann Thor Surg.* 1991;51:860.
252. Bailey SC, Watson DC. Atrioventricular septal defect repair in infants. *Ann Thor Surg.* 1991;52:33.
253. Espinosa-Caliani JS, Alvarez-Guisado L, Muños-Castellanos L, et al. Atrioventricular septal defect: quantitative anatomy of the right ventricle. *Pediatr Cardiol.* 1991;12:206.
254. Merrill WH, Hammon JW, Graham TP, Bender HW. Complete repair of atrioventricular septal defect. *Ann Thor Surg.* 1991;52:29.
255. Fyler DC. Endocardial cushion defects. In: Flyer DC, ed. *Nadas' Pediatric Cardiology*. Philadelphia: Hanley & Belfus, Inc; 1992:577.
256. Minich LA, Snider AR, Bove EL, Lupinetti FM, Vermilion RP. Echocardiographic evaluation of atrioventricular orifice anatomy in children with atrioventricular septal defect. *J Am Coll Cardiol.* 1992;19:149.
257. Metras D, Kreitmann B, Riberi A, Wernert F, Attali T, Garbi O. Complete atrioventricular canal, correction with one patch under the age of one year—mid-term and long-term results. *Cardiol Young.* 1993;3:I–48.
258. Spray TL, Canter C. Utility of intraoperative echocardiography in repair of atrioventricular septal defects in infancy. *Cardiol Young.* 1993;3:I–145.
259. Loebe M, Hetzer R, Alexi-Meskishvili V, et al. Repair of complete atrioventricular septal defect with two-patch technique in patients over two years of age. *Cardiol Young.* 1993;3:I–142.
260. Grossi EA, Glickstein J, Parish MA, et al. Primary correction of complete endocardial cushion defect during the first year of life. *Cardiol Young.* 1993;3:I–141.
261. Kirklin JW, Barratt-Boyes BG. Atrioventricular canal defect. In: Kirklin JW, Barratt Boyes BG, eds. *Cardiac Surgery—Morphology, Diagnostic Criteria, Natural History, Techniques, Results, and Indications.* New York: Churchill Livingstone; 1973:693.
262. Brandt B, Heintz S, Smith F. Mitral regurgitation following repair of complete atrioventricular septal defects. *Cardiol Young.* 1993;3:I–139.
263. Suzuki K, Murakami Y, Tatsuno K, et al. Atypical form of atrioventricular septal defect without left axis deviation: relation between morphology and unusual QRS axis. *Br Heart J.* 1993;70:180.
264. Papa M, Santoro F, Corno A. Spontaneous closure of inlet ventricular septal defect in an infant with Down's syndrome and aortic coarctation. *Chest.* 1993;104:620.
265. Capouya ER, Laks H, Drinkwater DC, Pearl JM, Milgalter E. Management of the left atrioventricular valve in the repair of complete atrioventricular septal defects. *J Thorac Cardiovasc Surg.* 1992;104:196.
266. DeLeon SY, Ilbawi MN, Wilson WR, et al. Surgical options in subaortic stenosis associated with endocardial cushion defects. *Ann Thorac Surg.* 1991;52:1076.
267. Yamaki S, Yasui H, Kado H, et al. Pulmonary vascular disease and operative indications in complete atrioventricular canal defect in early infancy. *J Thorac Cardiovas Surg.* 1993;106:398.
268. Hanley FL, Fenton KN, Jonas RA, et al. Surgical repair of complete atrioventricular canal defects in infancy, twenty-year trends. *J Thorac Cardiovasc Surg.* 1993;106:387.
269. Akiba T, Becker AE, Neirotti R, Tatsuno K. Valve morphology in complete atrioventricular septal defect: variability relevant to operation. *Ann Thor Surg.* 1993;56:295.
270. Ebels T, Anderson RH. The concept and definition of an "intermediate form" of atrioventricular septal defect. *J Thorac Cardiovasc Surg.* 1991;102:799.
271. Kumar A, Williams CA, Victorica BE. Familial atrioventricular septal defect: possible genetic mechanisms. *Br Heart J.* 1994;71:79.
272. Starr A, Hovaguimian H. Surgical repair of subaortic stenosis in atrioventricular canal defects. *J Thorac Cardiovasc Surg.* 1994;108:373.
273. Ashraf MH, Amin Z, Sharma R, Subramanian S. Atrioventricular canal defect: two-patch repair and tricuspidization of the mitral valve. *Ann Thor Surg.* 1993;55:347.
274. Chin C, Gandour-Edwards R, Oltjens S, Choy M. Fate of endocardial cushions. *Am J Cardiol.* 1992;70:563.
275. Reeder GS, Danielson GK, Seward JB, Driscoll DJ, Tajik AJ. Fixed subaortic stenosis in atrioventricular canal defect: a Doppler echocardiographic study. *J Am Coll Cardiol.* 1992;20:386.
276. Ho SY, Gerlis LM, Toms J, Lincoln C, Anderson RH. Morphology of the posterior junctional area in atrioventricular septal defects. *Ann Thor Surg.* 1992;54:264.
277. Bergin ML, Warnes CA, Tajik AJ, Danielson GK. Partial atrioventricular canal defect: long-term follow-up after initial repair in patients ≥ 40 years old. *J Am Coll Cardiol.* 1995;25:1189.
278. Manning PB, Mayer JE, Sanders SP, et al. Unique features and prognosis of primum ASD presenting in the first year of life. *Circulation.* 1994;90[part 2]: II–30.
279. Rizzoli G, Mazzucco A, Maizza F, et al. Does Down syndrome affect prognosis of surgically managed atrioventricular canal defects? *J Thorac Cardiovasc Surg.* 1992;104:945.
280. Gallo P, Formigari R, Hokayem NJ, Pizzuto F, et al. Left ventricular outflow tract obstruction in atrioventricular septal defects: a pathologic and morphometric evaluation. *Clin Cardiol.* 1991;14:513.
281. Marino B. Complete atrioventricular septal defect in patients with and without Down's syndrome. *Ann Thor Surg.* 1994;57:1687.
282. Castañeda AR, Jonas RA, Mayer JE, Hanley FL. Atrioventricular canal defect. In: Castañeda AR, Jonas RA, Mayer JE, eds. *Cardiac Surgery of the Neonate and Infant.* Hanley FL, Philadelphia: W.B. Saunders Co; 1994:167.
283. Sigfússon G, Ettedgul JA, Silverman NH, Anderson RH. Is a cleft in the anterior leaflet of an otherwise normal mitral valve an atrioventricular canal malformation? *J Am Coll Cardiol.* 1995;26:508.
284. Backer CL, Mavroudis C, Alboliras ET, Zales VR. Repair of complete atrioventricular canal defects: results with the two-patch technique. *Ann Thor Surg.* 1995;60:530.
285. Zittergruen MM, Murray JC, Lauer RM, Burns TL, Sheffield VC. Molecular analysis of nondisjunction in Down syndrome patients with and without atrioventricular septal defects. *Circulation.* 1995;92:2803.
286. Wienecke MM, Mjaatvedt CH, Capehart AA, Markwald RR, Krug EL. Identification of a murine homologue of chicken

ES/130: a protein which plays an integral role in endocardial cushion development. *Circulation*. 1995;92(Suppl I-116).
287. Basson CT, Schonberg-Fejzo M, MacRae CA, et al. Identification, chromosomal localization, and developmental cardiac expression of human ES/130. *Circulation*. 1995;92(Suppl I-117).
288. Brown CB, Boyen AS, Runyon RB, Barnett JV. Antibodies to the type II transforming growth factor ß receptor block cell activation and migration during atrioventricular cushion transformation. *Circulation*. 1995;92(Suppl I-118).
289. Van Arsdell GS, Williams WG, Boutin C, et al. Subaortic stenosis in the spectrum of atrioventricular septal defects. Solutions may be complex and palliative. *J Thorac Cardiovasc Surg*. 1995;110:1534.
290. Bando K, Turrentine MW, Sun K, et al. Surgical management of complete atrioventricular septal defects, a twenty-year experience. *J Thorac Cardiovasc Surg*. 1995;110:1543.
291. Kohl T, Silverman NH. Comparison of cleft and papillary muscle position in cleft mitral valve and atrioventricular septal defect. *Am J Cardiol*. 1996;77:164.
292. Burke RP, Horvath K, Landzberg M, Hyde P, Collins JJ, Cohn LH. Long-term follow-up after surgical repair of ostium primum atrial septal defects in adults. *J Am Coll Cardiol*. 1996;27:696.
293. Alexi-Meskishvili V, Ishino K, Dähnert I, et al. Correction of complete atrioventricular septal defects with the double-patch technique and cleft closure. *Ann Thor Surg*. 1996;62:519.
294. Tweddell JS, Litwin SB, Berger S, et al. Twenty-year experience with repair of complete atrioventricular septal defects. *Ann Thor Surg*. 1996;62:419.
295. Falk V, van Son JAM, Mohr FW. Pericardial patch augmentation of right atrioventricular valve in atrioventricular canal. *Ann Thor Surg*. 1996;62:288.
296. Meisner H, Guenther T. Atrioventricular septal defect. *Pediatr Cardiol*. 1998;19:276.
297. Van Praagh R, Papagiannis J, Bar-El YI, Schwint OA. The heart in Down syndrome: pathologic anatomy. In: Marino B, Pueschel SM, eds. *Heart Disease in Persons with Down Syndrome*. Baltimore: Paul H. Brookes Publishing Co; 1996:69.
298. Ferencz C, Neill CA, Boughman JA, Rubin JD, Brenner JI, Perry LW. Congenital cardiovascular malformations associated with chromosomal abnormalities: an epidemiologic study. *J Pediatr*. 1989;114:79.
299. Giamberti A, Marino B, diCarlo D, et al. Partial atrioventricular canal with congestive heart failure in the first year of life: surgical options. *Ann Thor Surg*. 1996;62:151.
300. van Son JAM, Van Praagh R, Falk V, Mohr FW. Pericardial patch augmentation of the tissue-deficient mitral valve in common atrioventricular canal. *J Thorac Cardiovasc Surg*. 1996;112:1117.
301. Cohen MS, Jacobs ML, Weinberg PM, Rychik J. Morphometric analysis of unbalanced common atrioventricular canal using two-dimensional echocardiography. *J Am Coll Cardiol*. 1996;28:1017.
302. Massetti M, Babatasi G, Neri E, Khayat A. Alternative technique for the ostium primum defect repair: a free wall flap of right atrium. *Ann Thor Surg*. 1997;63:1803.
303. van Son JAM, Schneider P, Falk V. Repair of subaortic stenosis in atrioventricular canal with absent or restrictive interventricular communication by patch augmentation of ventricular septum, resuspension of atrioventricular valves, and septal myectomy. *Mayo Clin Proc*. 1997;72:220.
304. van Son JAM, Phoon CK, Silverman NH, Haas GS. Predicting feasibility of biventricular repair of right-dominant unbalanced atrioventricular canal. *Ann Thor Surg*. 1997;63:1657.
305. Acar P, Laskari C, Rhodes J, Pandian N, Warner K, Marx G. Three-dimensional echocardiographic analysis of valve anatomy as a determinant of mitral regurgitation after surgery for atrioventricular septal defects. *Am J Cardiol*. 1999;83:745.
306. O'Blenes SB, Ross DB, Nanton MA, Murphy DA. Atrioventricular septal defect with tetralogy of Fallot: results of surgical correction. *Ann Thor Surg*. 1998;66:2078.
307. Falcâo S, Daliento L, Ho SY, Rigby ML, Anderson RH. Cross sectional echocardiographic assessment of the extent of the atrial septum relative to the atrioventricular junction in atrioventricular septal defect. *Heart*. 1999;81:199.
308. Suzuki K, Ho SY, Anderson RH, et al. Interventricular communication in complete atrioventricular septal defect. *Ann Thor Surg*. 1998;66:1389.
309. Hubert R, Korenberg JR. The genetics of Down syndrome congenital heart disease. In: Imai Y, Momma K, eds. *Proc Second World Congress Pediatr Cardiol & Cardiac Surgery*. Armonk NY: Futura Publishing Co, Inc; 1998.10.
310. Geva T, Ayres NA, Pignatelli RH, Gajarski RJ. Echocardiographic evaluation of common atrioventricular canal defects: a study of 206 consecutive patients. *Echocardiography*. 1996;13:387.
311. Atrioventricular septal defects with and without Down syndrome. In: Ferencz C, Loffredo CA, Correa-Villaseñor A, Wilson PD, eds. *Genetic and Environmental Risk Factors of Major Cardiovascular Malformations: The Baltimore-Washington Infant Study 1981-1989*. Armonk, NY: Futura Publishing Co Inc; 1997:103.
312. Weinberg PM. Morphology of congenital heart disease. In: *Atlas of Heart Diseases. Congenital Heart Disease*. Vol. XII. St. Louis: Mosby; 1997:4–8.
313. El-Najdawi EK, Driscoll DJ, Puga FJ, et al. Operation for partial atrioventricular septal defect: a forty-year review. *J Thorac Cardiovasc Surg*. 2000;119:880.
314. Gatzoulis MA, Hechter S, Webb GD, Williams WG. Surgery for partial atrioventricular septal defect in the adult. *Ann Thorac Surg*. 1999;67:504.
315. Tsang JC, Shum-Tim D, Tchervenkov CI, Jutras L, Sinclair B. Hemolytic anemia after atrioventricular septal defect repair without synthetic material. *Ann Thor Surg*. 1999;68:1838.
316. Kuralay E, Özal E, Demirkiliç U, Cingöz F, Tatar H. Left atrioventricular valve repair technique in partial atrioventricular septal defects. *Ann Thor Surg*. 1999;68:1746.
317. Huggon IC, Cook AC, Smeeton NC, Magee AG, Sharland GK. Atrioventricular septal defects diagnosed in fetal life: associated cardiac and extra-cardiac abnormalities and outcome. *J Am Coll Cardiol*. 2000;36:593.
318. Lange A, Mankad P, Walayat M, Palka P, Burns JE, Goodman MJ. Transthoracic three-dimensional echocardiography in the preoperative assessment of atrioventricular septal defect morphology. *Am J Cardiol*. 2000;85:630.
319. Shiokawa Y, Becker AE. The left ventricular outflow tract in atrioventricular septal defect revisited: surgical considerations regarding preservation of aortic valve integrity in the perspective of anatomic observations. *J Thorac Cardiovasc Surg*. 1997;114:586.
320. Lin AE, Ardinger HH, Ardinger RH, Cunniff C, Kelley RI. Cardiovascular malformations in Smith-Lemli-Opitz syndrome. *Am J Med Genet*. 1997;68:270.
321. Macé L, Dervanian P, Houyel L, et al. Surgically created double-orifice left atrioventricular valve: a valve-sparing repair in selected atrioventricular septal defects. *J Thorac Cardiovasc Surg*. 2001;121:352.

322. Najm HK, Williams WG, Chuaratanaphong S, Watzka SB, Coles JG, Freedom RM. Primum atrial septal defect in children: early results, risk factors, and freedom from reoperation. *Ann Thor Surg.* 1998;66:829.
323. Radermecker MA, Somerville J, Li W, Anderson RH, deLeval MR. Double orifice right atrioventricular valve in atrioventricular septal defect: morphology and extension of the concept of fusion of leaflets. *Ann Thor Surg.* 2001;71:358.
324. Moran AM, Daebritz S, Keane JF, Mayer JE. Surgical management of mitral regurgitation after repair of endocardial cushion defects, early and midterm results. *Circulation.* 2000;102(suppl III):III–160.
325. Suzuki K, Ho SY, Anderson RH, et al. Morphometric analysis of atrioventricular septal defect with common valve orifice. *J Am Coll Cardiol.* 1998;31:217.
326. Suzuki K, Tatsuno K, Kikuchi T, Mimori S. Predisposing factors of valve regurgitation in complete atrioventricular septal defect. *J Am Coll Cardiol.* 1998;32:1449.
327. Nicholson IA, Nunn GR, Sholler GF, Hawker RE, Cooper SG, Lau KC. Simplified single patch technique for the repair of atrioventricular septal defect. *J Thorac Cardiovasc Surg.* 1999;118:642.
328. Suzuki K, Yamaki S, Mimori S, et al. Pulmonary vascular disease in Down's syndrome with complete atrioventricular septal defect. *Am J Cardiol.* 2000;86:434.
329. Sittiwangkul R, Ma RY, McCrindle BW, Coles JG, Smallhorn JF. Echocardiographic assessment of obstructive lesions in atrioventricular septal defects. *J Am Coll Cardiol.* 2001;38:253.
330. Günther T, Mazzitelli D, Haehnel CJ, Holper K, Sebening F, Meisner H. Long-term results after repair of complete atrioventricular septal defects: analysis of risk factors. *Ann Thor Surg.* 1998;65:754.
331. Wilcox BR, Jones DR, Frantz EG, et al. Anatomically sound, simplified approach to repair of "complete" atrioventricular septal defect. *Ann Thor Surg.* 1997;64:487.
332. van Son JAM, Walther T, Mohr FW. Patch augmentation of regurgitant common atrioventricular valve in univentricular physiology. *Ann Thor Surg.* 1997;64:508.
333. Oshima Y, Yamaguchi M, Yoshimura N, Oka S, Ootaki Y. Anatomically corrective repair of complete atrioventricular septal defects and major cardiac anomalies. *Ann Thor Surg.* 2001;72:424.
334. Reddy VM, McElhinney DB, Brook MM, Parry AJ, Hanley FL. Atrioventricular valve function after single patch repair of complete atrioventricular septal defect in infancy: how early should repair be attempted? *J Thorac Cardiovasc Surg.* 1998;115:1032.
335. Rhodes J, Warner KG, Fulton DR, Romero BA, Schmid CH, Marx GR. Fate of mitral regurgitation following repair of atrioventricular septal defect. *Am J Cardiol.* 1997;80:1194.
336. Crawford FA, Stroud MR. Surgical repair of complete atrioventricular septal defect. *Ann Thor Surg.* 2001;72:1621.
337. Friedman WF, Silverman N. Congenital heart disease in infancy and childhood. In: Braunwald E, Zipes DP, Libby P, eds. *Heart Disease, a Textbook of Cardiovascular Medicine.* 6th ed. Philadelphia: WB Saunders Co; 2001:1527.
338. Feldt RH, Edwards WD, Porter C-BJ, Dearani JA, Seward JB, Puga FJ. Atrioventricular septal defects. In: Allen HD, Gutgesell HP, Clark EB, Driscoll DJ, eds. *Moss and Adams' Heart Disease in Infants, Children and Adolescents, Including the Fetus and Young Adults.* 6th ed. Philadelphia: Lippincott Williams & Wilkins; 2001:618.
339. Nakano T, Kado H, Shiokawa Y-i, Fukae K. Surgical results of double-orifice left atrioventricular valve associated with atrioventricular septal defects. *Ann Thor Surg.* 2002;73:69.
340. Bharati S, Lev M. Common atrioventricular orifice—complete type, common atrioventricular orifice—intermediate type, and atrial septal defect, primum. In: *The Pathology of Congenital Heart Disease, a Personal Experience with More than 6,300 Congenitally Malformed Hearts.* Vol. 553. Armonk NY: Futura Publishing Company, Inc; 1996. 587, and 467, respectively.
341. Castañeda AR, Jonas RA, Mayer JE, Hanley FL. Atrioventricular canal defect. In: *Cardiac Surgery of the Neonate and Infant.* Philadelphia: W.B. Saunders Co; 1994:167.
342. Bedford DE, Sellors TH, Somerville W, Belcher JF, Besterman EMM. Atrial septal defect and its surgical treatment. *Lancet.* 1957;1:1255.
343. Somerville J: *Atrioventricular Defects.* MD, London, Thesis.

12

Double-Outlet and Common-Outlet Right Atrium

Definition. The morphologically right atrium (RA) opens into both the morphologically right ventricle (RV) and the morphologically left ventricle (LV) via two atrioventricular (AV) valves resulting in double-outlet right atrium (DORA), or via a common AV valve resulting in common-outlet right atrium (CORA).

ANATOMIC TYPES OF DOUBLE-OUTLET RIGHT ATRIUM/COMMON-OUTLET RIGHT ATRIUM

Three anatomic types of DORA or CORA are known at the present time: (1) **leftward malalignment of the atrial septum** relative to the atrioventricular valve(s); (2) **rightward malalignment of the ventricular septum** relative to the atrial septum; and (3) **an accessory valve between the coronary sinus and the LV.**

DOUBLE-OUTLET RIGHT ATRIUM AND COMMON-OUTLET RIGHT ATRIUM WITH LEFTWARD MALALIGNMENT OF THE ATRIAL SEPTUM

The concepts of DORA and double-outlet left atrium (DOLA) were first proposed in 1977 by Van Mierop[1] in the setting of common atrioventricular (AV) canal, also known as endocardial cushion defect. His concept was that DORA is present when the RA opens in the RV and into the LV via a common AV valve. Van Mierop did not distinguish between DORA and CORA.[1]

Equally noteworthy is that left atrial outlet atresia is present, and that the only exit from the LA is an atrial septal defect (ASD) that can be hemodynamically restrictive, resulting in pulmonary venous obstruction. Also noteworthy is the fact that the ASD can be of the ostium primum type (consistent with common AV canal), or an ASD of the ostium secundum type, or even of the sinus venosus defect type. Van Mierop[1] did not present any cases of DORA (or of DOLA); instead, he coined these terms and defined these concepts.

We have regarded this anatomic type of DORA as **common AV canal with left atrial outlet atresia** (see Chapter 11).

By now it has become clear that this anatomic type of DORA is associated with (or perhaps caused by) leftward malposition of the atrial septum relative to the AV valve(s). This is why there can be LA outlet atresia with significant pulmonary venous obstruction, depending on the patency (or otherwise) of the atrial septum.

DORA with levomalposition of the atrial septum relative to the AV valves in visceroatrial situs solitus appears to be the most common form of this rarity.[2-10] To the best of our knowledge, Utley, Noonan, Walters, and Frist[2] first reported DORA with an anomalous position of the atrial septum that was displaced posteriorly and to the left of the mitral valve in a 2½-year-old boy (Fig. 12.1). The interatrial communication was small, was probably restrictive, and was interpreted as an ostium primum type of atrial septal defect. The mitral valve was thought not to be cleft, but angiocardiography revealed a goose-neck deformity suggestive of common AV canal. The *goose-neck deformity* is the diastolic angiocardiographic picture in common AV canal. Consequently, their patient[2] appears to have a rare partial form of common AV canal with a restrictively small ASD I, no mitral cleft, an intact ventricular septum, and a goose-neck deformity. No coronary sinus ostium was found in the right atrium. Instead, the coronary sinus, the left upper pulmonary vein, and a left superior vena cava were confluent with a common channel that opened into the roof of the left atrium. This patient had bilateral superior venae cavae with absence of the left innominate vein.

Was the left atrial appendage part of the left atrium? This important point in differential diagnosis remains unclear. If the left atrial appendage lay below the leftwardly displaced atrial septum, then cor triatriatum (see Chapter 8) was present, not DORA.

Did this patient have a levoatrial cardinal vein decompressing this obstructed LA? This interesting diagnostic possibility also remains unresolved.

With the aforementioned uncertainties borne in mind, I think it is reasonable to regard Utley's case[2] as the first known example of DORA with leftward displacement of the atrial septum. The malpositioned atrial septum was excised and replaced by a normally positioned pericardial patch, and the persistent left superior vena cava was ligated above the aberrant left upper pulmonary vein. It should be added that whether or not the correct diagnosis was DORA or cor triatriatum, the surgical management of Utley et al[2] was appropriate for both: excision of the obstructive and leftwardly malaligned atrial septum or intra-left-atrial membrane, and replacement with a normally located atrium septum.

In 1983, Corwin and his colleagues[3] reported the first indubitable case of DORA with leftward deviation of the lower portion of the atrial septum, again in a 2½-year-old boy. These investigators noted that the levomalpositioned atrial septum inserted into the left atrial wall to the left of and posterior to the mitral valve. The only outlet from the obstructed left atrium was via a small secundum atrial septal defect. These authors stated that the left atrial appendage was in the high-pressure left atrium

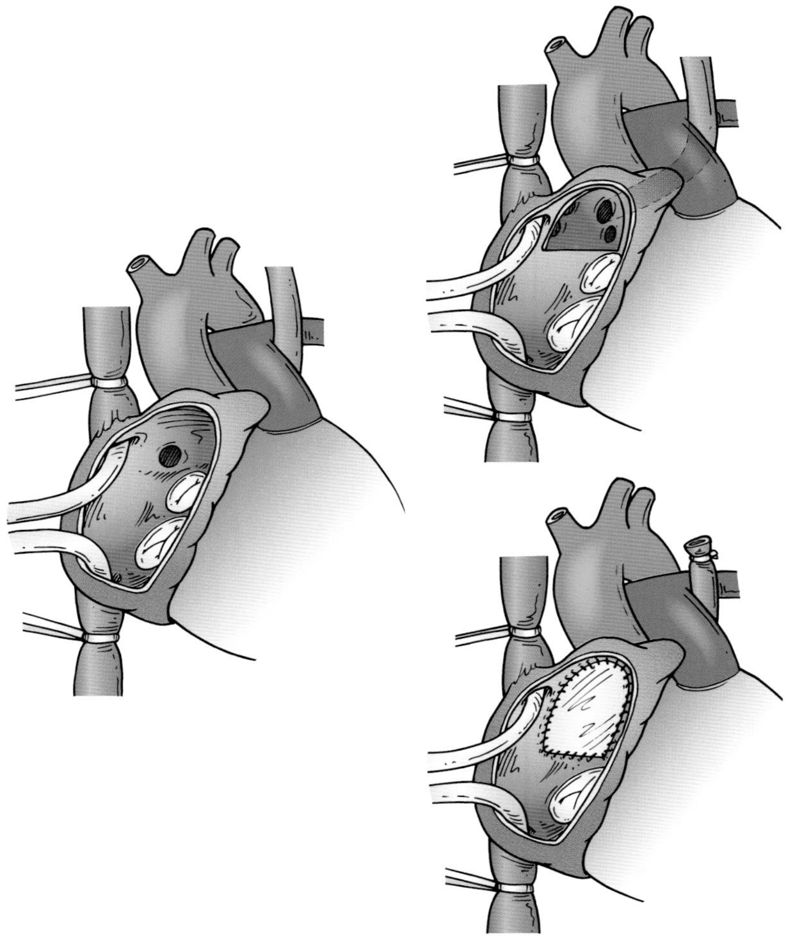

Fig. 12.1 Diagrams of the first known case of the leftward atrial septal malalignment type of DORA. *Left.* Both the mitral and the tricuspid valves fill from the right atrium. The atrial septum is displaced to the left and posteriorly relative to both atrioventricular valves. The atrial septum has a small inferior defect, identified by the authors as an ostium primum defect, well posterior to the mitral valve. Because there was left atrial outlet atresia—apparently related to the leftward and posterior atrial septal malalignment—this small low atrial septal defect was restrictive and was associated with pulmonary venous obstruction (physiologically like cor triatriatum). *Upper right.* Excision of the atrial septum revealed that a persistent left superior vena cava (LSVC) drained into the left atrium (LA). The authors stated that before the LSVC opened into the LA, the LSVC received the coronary sinus and the left superior pulmonary vein. The other three pulmonary veins connected normally with the LA. This patient had bilateral superior venae cavae and the left innominate vein was absent. The authors[2] did not describe whether or not the left atrial appendage communicated with the LA (that received the three normally connected pulmonary veins). I am assuming that the LA appendage did communicate with this LA; hence the diagnosis of DORA with leftward and posterior malalignment of the atrial septum. However, if the LA appendages did *not* communicate with this obstructed pulmonary vein chamber, then the correct diagnosis (that these authors[2] also considered) would have been common atrium (absence of the atrial septum) with cor triatriatum sinistrum. *Lower right.* The atrial septum was repositioned with a pericardial patch, directing the pulmonary venosus blood through the mitral valve. The LSVC was ligated above the entry of the left superior pulmonary vein. Significant systemic venous obstruction with swelling of the left arm and left face did not occur. Left ventricular cineangiocardiography preoperatively had shown a goose-neck deformity (the characteristic diastolic picture of common atrioventricular canal) with minimal mitral regurgitation. No cleft of the anterior leaflet of the mitral valve was found at surgery. Consequently, this historic patient is considered to have had a rare partial form of common AV canal (small restrictive ostium primum defect, no ventricular septal defect of the AV canal type, no cleft of the mitral valve, but with a goose-neck deformity) with marked leftward and posterior malalignment of the atrial septum relative to the AV valves, left atrial outlet atresia, and DORA. (Reproduced with permission from Utley JR, Noonan JA, Walters LR, Frist RA: Anomalous position of atrial septum with anomalous pulmonary and systemic venous drainage. Correction including ligation of persistent left superior vena cava, *J Thorac Cardiovasc Surg* 67:730, 1974.)

along with the pulmonary veins, thereby excluding the diagnosis of cor triatriatum sinistrum. The RA opened into the RV and the LV via a common AV valve. There was no ventricular septal defect (VSD).

Parenthetically, it is noteworthy that common AV canal was present in the form of a common AV valve. Also, both the mitral valve and the tricuspid valve were described as cleft. But no atrioventricular septal defect was present; that is, there was no ostium primum type of atrial septal defect, and there was VSD. This is just one example of why we prefer the diagnosis of common AV canal to that of AV septal defect. The concept of common AV canal is more inclusive: it embraces partial forms of common AV canal, even when an AV septal defect is not present.

It should be added that we like the diagnosis of *AV septal defect* when this anomaly is present, completely or in part. But we prefer the overall diagnosis of *common AV canal* because this diagnosis is more inclusive, more flexible, and more sensitive than AV septal defect, which is only one part of common AV canal, as the patient of Corwin, Singh, and Karlson[3] demonstrates.

Despite the absence of a VSD, this little boy had moderate pulmonary artery hypertension (57/19 mm Hg), congestive heart failure, and failure to thrive—all of which were thought to be related to the presence of significant pulmonary venous obstruction (left atrial outlet atresia with a small secundum ASD).

The patient[3] also had multiple congenital anomalies with dysmorphic facies: bilateral epicanthal folds, blepharophimosis (narrowing of the opening of the eyelids), mild ptosis of the eyelids, and a coloboma of the right iris.

Successful surgical management of this anatomic type of DORA involved excision of the levodeviated atrial septum, and its replacement with a normally located pericardial atrial septum.

Thus, in 1983, Corwin et al[3] confirmed the existence of DORA with marked leftward deviation of the atrial septum, left atrial outlet atresia, and pulmonary venous obstruction, and reported successful surgical management of this rare anomaly. Further confirmation and description subsequently occurred with the publications of Pérez-Martínez et al (1984),[4] Alivizatos et al (1985),[5] Westerman et al (1986),[6] Suzuki et al (1994),[9] and Radermecker et al (1995).[10] What else did we learn? Much, as is summarized below.

Such patients could present almost as teenagers, not just as very young children: a 12-year-old boy[4] and a 12-year-old girl.[5]

The right superior vena cava could be atretic, with a persistent left superior vena cava (LSVC), making it necessary surgically to tunnel the LSVC to the RA, as well as excising the levomalpositioned atrial septum and replacing it.[4]

In the 12-year-old girl,[5] the only outlet from the LA was a small ostium primum type of ASD (6 mm in diameter). The mean left atrial pressure was 25 mm Hg. At surgery, lung biopsy interpreted by Dr. Sheila Haworth showed large thick-walled pulmonary veins with pronounced intimal fibrosis. The small pulmonary arterial changes were much milder than the pulmonary venous histopathology: an increase in arterial medial muscularity, but without intimal proliferation (grade 1 Heath-Edwards changes in the small pulmonary arteries). Mr. Jaroslav ("Jarda") Stark found severe regurgitation through the mitral cleft into the RA (none into the left); hence he closed the cleft with sutures. He also excised the leftwardly deviated atrial septum and replaced it with a correctly positioned pericardial patch.

Westerman et al[6] documented the fact that the segmental anatomy in this anatomic type of DORA is not always normal, that is, {S,D,S}—as it had been in all previously published cases. In Westerman's 3-year-old male patient, the segmental anatomy was tetralogy of Fallot (TOF) {S,D,S}. TOF has nearly normally related great arteries, but not entirely normally related great arteries (see Chapter 20).

These authors[6] found that the RA opened through a common AV valve into both ventricles. Accurately speaking, this is **common-outlet right atrium,** not *double*-outlet right atrium, because a common AV valve connected the RA with both ventricles. Two AV valves were not present—only one, a common AV valve. This 3-year-old boy had no ostium primum type of atrial septal defect. There was left atrial outlet atresia, the only outlet from the LA being an ostium secundum type of atrial septal defect that was 1 cm in diameter. The atrial septum deviated to the left of the common AV valve, and the coronary sinus was noted to drain into the RA, which it did not do in the cases of Utley[2] and Pérez-Martínez.[4] Westerman's patient[6] also had a brain abscess. The common AV valve was type C of Rastelli, and there was an underlying VSD of the AV canal type.

Hence, this patient had an interesting form of partial common AV canal: no primum atrial septal defect, but with a VSD of the confluent AV canal and TOF types, with a type C common AV valve. We have noted repeatedly that when common AV canal is associated with tetralogy of Fallot, the primum ASD is often unusually small or absent, as in Westerman's patient,[6] resulting in an unusual form of partially common AV canal.

In addition to repairing the stenotic pulmonary outflow tract, these authors enlarged the restrictive atrial septal defect and used one patch to close the ASD and the VSD and to subdivide the common AV valve.

Thus, the report of Westerman, Norton, and Van Devanter[6] was important because it documented CORA opening into both ventricles, and because it showed that an important conotruncal malformation (TOF) can coexist with malalignment of the atrial septum to the left of the AV junction and valve(s).

The 18-month-old patient reported by Starc, Bierman, Bowman, Steeg, Wang, and Krongrad[7] (Case 3) had Down syndrome with completely common AV canal and CORA. The atrial septum deviated to the left and attached to the lateral wall of the LA above the plane of the AV groove. The left atrial appendage was part of the high-pressure left atrium (excluding the diagnostic possibility of cor triatriatum). A persistent left superior vena cava returned to the coronary sinus. The levomalposed atrial septum was excised and double-patch closure with repositioning was used to repair the complete form of common AV canal that was present. The thrust of this report by Starc et al[7] was that DORA or CORA and cor triatriatum are surgically correctable forms of pulmonary venous obstruction.

Ahmadi and colleagues[8] reported a 4-year-old boy with the Ellis-van Creveld syndrome. The atrial septum was deviated far to the left resulting in DORA, left atrial outlet atresia, and severe pulmonary venous obstruction. The primum ASD was described as small and the ventricular septum was intact. The mean left atrial pressure was 28 mm Hg, and the mean right atrial pressure was 6 mm Hg. Systemic arterial desaturation was noted (89%). The cleft anterior leaflet of the mitral valve permitted a Gerbode-like LV-to-RA shunt. A persistent left superior vena cava was present.

The authors made the most interesting observation that the left atrium *as a whole* was malpositioned. The LA was located to the left, above and posterior to the RA. In other words, this form of DORA or CORA that has been described as having leftward malposition of the atrium septum may well in fact have *malposition of the whole LA, or malposition of the atrial segment of the heart relative to the ventriculoarterial part of the heart (the bulboventricular loop).*

It is probably inevitable that this anatomic type of DORA/CORA would be described as having leftward malposition of the arterial septum relative to the AV valve(s)—because this is how it looks. But one should remember that cardiac septa usually are where they are because of what is happening on either side of the septa, or below the septa, or elsewhere. I am thinking of the location of the ventricular septum in single ventricle, and in straddling tricuspid and mitral valves, and of the configuration of the aortopulmonary septum in conotruncal malformations (see Chapters 17, 22, 23, 24, and 25). Suffice it to say that malposition of a cardiac septum typically does not indicate malseptation as a primary morphogenetic mechanism. Malposition of a cardiovascular septum is usually related to an abnormality somewhere else.

If the same principle applies to DORA and CORA, it may well be that *the atrial septum is in fact normally located and that the ventriculoarterial parts of the heart are malaligned—displaced to the right relative to the normally located atria and atrial septum.* Developmentally, the atria are relatively fixed in position by the great veins (the venae cavae) and the pulmonary veins; whereas the bulboventricular parts of the heart are "professional contortionists" and hence prone to malalignment (see Chapters 2, 3, and 4).

This hypothesis of rightward malalignment of the ventricles and the AV valves relative to the atria and the atrial septum is mentioned here in the interests of in-depth understanding. No change in terminology is being suggested. Leftward malposition of the atrial septum relative to the AV valve(s) should be understood as an anatomic description, not as an embryologic hypothesis or developmental mechanism.

Another problem merits mention: In this anatomic type of DORA or CORA with leftward malalignment of the atrial septum relative to the AV valve(s) and left atrial outlet atresia with pulmonary venous obstruction, **what is/are the AV valve/valves?** Does left atrial outlet atresia mean that mitral atresia is present? If so, then the AV valve or valves that underlie the RA and open into the RV and the LV are in fact the tricuspid valve that straddles the ventricular septum. If the straddling tricuspid valve, in this interpretation, attaches to the ventricular septum, the result is two AV valves that resemble the tricuspid valve (entering the RV) and the mitral valve (entering the LV). But if the straddling tricuspid valve, in this interpretation, does not become adherent to the ventricular septum, then it morphologically resembles a common AV valve.

So the problem in this anatomic type of DORA or CORA is: What is the AV valve (or valves)? Are we dealing with a common AV valve or a divided AV valve (tricuspid and mitral)? Or are we dealing with mitral atresia and a straddling tricuspid valve that may or may not be subdivided into two AV valves—one opening into the RV and the other opening into the LV?

I don't really know the answer to this question. However, I suspect that we are not really dealing with mitral atresia, that is, with atresia of the mitral valve *per se*. Note that the left ventricle typically is well developed in DORA and CORA, whereas in "real" mitral atresia, the LV typically is diminutive. This is why it is generally known as left atrial outlet atresia (due to malposition of the atrial septum), rather than as mitral atresia. However, as indicated above, we don't really know for sure. I think it is very important to realize what we know, and also what we don't know. There is so much that we really don't know for sure. Intellectual honesty requires that this be stated clearly. That said, I think we are dealing with left atrial outlet atresia (different from typical mitral atresia) and with a common AV valve or an AV valve that has divided into mitral and tricuspid valves. These two AV valves could also be called by other names, such as the RA-to-RV valve and the RA-to-LV valve. Instead, we usually call the AV valve entering the RV the *tricuspid* valve and the AV valve entering the LV the *mitral* valve.

To summarize, Ahmadi et al[8] observed that the *entire* LA is abnormally located relative to the RA in this anatomic type of DORA/CORA—a very important observation (as above). Surgically, these authors resected the malpositioned atrial septum, replaced it with an appropriately positioned Dacron atrial septum, and suture closed the mitral cleft.

Suzuki and colleagues[9] reported an 18-month-old boy with CORA. The common AV valve had a free floating anterior leaflet (type C of Rastelli). The marked leftward malalignment of the atrial septum relative to the common AV valve resulted not only in CORA, with the RA opening into both the RV and the LV, but also in left atrial outlet atresia with severe pulmonary venous obstruction and systemic pulmonary arterial hypertension. At 13 months of age, this patient with Down syndrome underwent palliative surgical management with atrial septal resection and inadequate banding of the main pulmonary artery (MPA). Complete repair was not attempted because of the coexistence of severe pulmonary vascular disease. The small pulmonary arteries showed not only medial hypertrophy, but also intimal proliferation or total luminal occlusion (grade 3 Heath-Edward changes). The pulmonary veins displayed medial hypertrophy. Adequate pulmonary artery banding was prevented by the development of cyanosis and bradycardia. Following what was thought to be inadequate MPA banding, the pressure in the MPA was 58/22 mm Hg and systemic arterial pressure was 75/44 mm Hg.

Thus, the patient of Suzuki et al[9] indicates that very severe occlusive disease of the small pulmonary arteries can occur by 12 months of age in a patient with Down syndrome, CORA, left atrial outlet atresia, and marked pulmonary venous obstruction produced by the malalignment of the atrial septum to the left of the common AV valve. The ASD was only 1 to 2 mm in diameter.

Radermecker, Chauvaud, and Carpentier[10] reported the oldest patient to date with this anatomic type of DORA: a 14-year-old girl. She had multiple congenital anomalies consisting of pectus excavatum and mild psychomotor impairment. Preoperatively she was misdiagnosed as having congenital mitral stenosis. At surgery, Carpentier and his colleagues[10] found that their patient had a partial form of common AV canal (Fig. 12.2). However, the ostium primum atrial septal defect was restrictively small (1 cm in diameter) and the atrial septum was displaced posteriorly and to the left of the left AV valve (a cleft mitral valve). Radermecker and his colleagues[10] prefer to regard this cleft as a commissure. They also prefer to call this the *left atrioventricular valve* (not the mitral valve) because this left AV valve is trifoliate: it has three leaflets, if one regards the cleft as a commissure. (With respect, we think the cleft is a cleft, not a commissure; see Chapter 11.) This patient also had a persistent left superior vena cava returning to the coronary sinus.

Surgically, the authors[10] resected the malpositioned atrial septum and replaced it with a normally located atrial septum using glutaraldehyde-treated pericardium.

Radermecker, Chauvaud, and Carpentier[10] stated: "We present a case to draw attention to this rare diagnosis (double-outlet right atrium) as an unusual cause of impediment to left AV valve inflow and to include it in the differential diagnosis of mitral stenosis with basically normal subvalvar apparatus."

Exactly right. The differential diagnosis of patients that appear physiologically to have congenital mitral stenosis should include the following:

- congenital mitral stenosis;
- Shone syndrome;
- cor triatriatum (sinistrum);
- double-outlet right atrium; and
- common-outlet right atrium.

There are, of course, additional conditions such as stenosis of individual pulmonary veins.

The problem that Radermecker and colleagues[10] were getting at, although they were perhaps too polite to say so, is that still many pediatric cardiologists, radiologists, and cardiac surgeons have never heard of DORA or CORA with leftward malposition of the atrial septum, left atrial outlet atresia, and pulmonary venous obstruction (Figs. 12.1 to 12.2).

Understanding the disorder is at least 50% of the cure, which is why pathology is so important. In our field, the disorder typically *is* the pathology—and its physiologic sequelae. The pathology is what we try to diagnose with accuracy. And the pathology is what we try to modify surgically and interventionally, in a physiologically advantageous way.

Next we are going to consider an even less well known form of double-outlet right atrium.

Double-Outlet Right Atrium With Rightward Malalignment of the Ventricular Septum

This is the straddling tricuspid valve type of DORA, except that the straddling tricuspid valve has become adherent to the crest of the muscular, rightwardly malaligned ventricular septum.

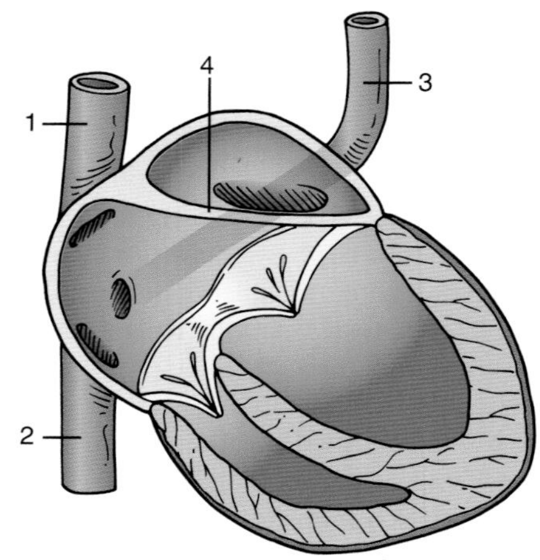

Fig. 12.2 Excellent diagram of DORA with marked leftward malalignment of the atrial septum *(4)*. A restrictively small ostium primum defect (approximately 1 cm in diameter in a 14-year-old girl) arched over the posterior leaflet of this cleft mitral valve, extending from the anterolateral to the posteromedial commissure of the mitral valve. The authors[10] described the arching inferior rim of the leftwardly malaligned atrial septum as an "incomplete supravalvular ring." This is how it looks. However, it should be understood that this incomplete supravalvular ring is the superior rim or roof of the small primum defect. (The authors were not dealing with a supramitral ring that is continuous with the mitral valve leaflet tissue, as in Shone syndrome.) The mitral cleft was suture closed because of mitral regurgitation. There was no ventricular septal defect of the AV canal type. The leftwardly malpositioned atrial septum was excised and replaced with a normally positioned atrial septum fashioned out of glutaraldehyde treated pericardium. *1,* superior vena cava; *2,* inferior vena cava; and *3,* persistent left superior vena cava. Thus, this is a rare partial or incomplete form of common AV canal first reported by Utley et al[2] in 1974 and later diagrammed by Van Mierop[1] in 1977, characterized by leftward and posterior malposition of the atrial septum relative to the AV orifices, left atrial outlet atresia (but not mitral atresia), restrictively small ostium primum defect, cleft anterior leaflet of the mitral valve, no ventricular septal defect, persistent left superior vena cava, and double-outlet right atrium. (Reproduced with permission from Radermecker MA, Chauvaud S, Carpentier A: Double-outlet right atrium with restrictive ostium primum and incomplete supravalvular ring presenting as congenital mitral valve stenosis, *J Thorac Cardiovasc Surg* 109:804, 1995.)

Consequently, the straddling tricuspid valve (TV) has become subdivided into two AV valves: the rightward that opens from the RA into the small RV; and the leftward TV that opens from the RA into the large LV. The adherence of the straddling TV to the underlying rightwardly malaligned ventricular septum has occluded the VSD of the AV canal (inlet) type that usually is associated with typical straddling TV. Consequently, there are three AV valves: the right-sided TV connecting the RA with the small RV; the left-sided TV connecting the RA with the large LV; and the mitral valve connecting the LA with the large LV. DORA and double-inlet left ventricle (DILV) may both be present. The mitral valve can be unobstructed, or stenotic, or atretic. If the mitral valve is atretic, then DILV is not present in this anatomic type of DORA.

Why is the ventricular septum malaligned to the right, and why is this rightward malalignment important? We think that the ventricular septum is malaligned to the right relative to the atrial septum (with D-loop ventricles) because the RV sinus (inflow tract) is underdeveloped or poorly expanded. So rightward malalignment of the ventricular septum appears to be of basic importance in this anatomic type of DORA, just as it is with typical straddling TV[11] (in which the TV does not adhere to the ventricular septum).

DORA with rightward malalignment of the ventricular septum was first reported by Büchler, Rabelo, Marino, David, and Van Praagh[12] at the World Congress of Paediatric Cardiology in London, England, in 1980 (Fig. 12.3). Another very similar example of DORA with rightward malposition of the ventricular septum was reported by Birincioğlu and colleagues in 1999 (Fig. 12.4).

The abstract of Büchler and colleagues[12] (see below) was mailed to Dr. Jane Somerville, Scientific Secretary of the World Congress of Paediatric Cardiology, on November 6, 1979, and was subsequently published in the abstract book of the 1980 World Congress (abstract 223). But because this abstract was not selected for platform presentation, no paper on this newly recognized entity was included in the subsequently published proceedings of this meeting.[13] Those who attended this memorable Congress were aware of this abstract,[12] for example, Pérez-Martínez et al,[4] but many other subsequent authors did not have access to Büchler's abstract.[12] Consequently we are publishing it here to make it generally available:

DOUBLE OUTLET RIGHT ATRIUM: AUTOPSIED CASE OF NEWLY RECOGNIZED ENTITY

J. Büchler, R. Rabelo, R. Marino, I. David, R. Van Praagh
Inst. Dante Pazzanese of Cardiologia, Sao Paulo, Hosp. Santa Rita, Minas Gerais, Brazil and Children's Hosp. Medical Center, Boston, U.S.A.

This is a presentation of the clinical, hemodynamic, angiocardiographic, and pathologic findings in the first autopsy-proven case of double outlet right atrium (DORA). The patient was a white boy, first observed to be cyanotic at 3 months of age, who did well clinically until 5 years of age when congestive heart failure supervened. Cardiac catheterization revealed bidirectional shunting at the atrial level. Pressures were normal. Angiocardiography disclosed a communication between the left ventricle (LV) and the right atrium (RA). DORA was found at open heart surgery. A regurgitant atrioventricular (AV) valve between the RA and the LV was occluded with a Dacron patch. A patent membrane-like AV valve between the RA and the small RV was replaced with a dura-mater prosthesis. The patient died intraoperatively. DORA was confirmed at autopsy. The RV inflow tract was underdeveloped, the posterior portion of the interventricular septum being displaced to the right relative to the atrial septum. There was no ventricular septal defect (VSD). The superior and slightly right-sided AV orifice containing the dura-mater prosthesis connecting the large RA with the small RV. The inferior and somewhat left-sided AV valve connected the RA with the large LV, this valve having abnormal LV attachments and hence being regurgitant. The mitral valve between the left atrium and the LV was normal. The patent foramen ovale was sutured closed and the heart was structurally otherwise normal. This anatomic type of DORA appears to be closely related to straddling tricuspid valve except that there was no VSD or the AV canal type and there were two "tricuspid" annuli. Other anatomic types of DORA exist.

Büchler's Case 12 (Fig. 12.3). Thanks to Dr. Jorge Büchler of São Paulo, Brazil, I had the privilege of examining this historic, formalin-fixed heart (C79-344) specimen on October 17, 1979. The external frontal view (Fig. 12.3A) showed situs solitus of the atria, D-loop ventricles, and solitus normally related great arteries; so the segmental anatomy was normal, {S,D,S}. Levocardia was present. The great arteries had been transected shortly above the semilunar valves. But the caliber of each was unremarkable. Consequently, both arterial outflow tracts seemed probably to be unobstructed.

The anterior descending coronary artery approximately bisected the anterior (ventral) surface of the ventricles (Fig. 12.3A), suggesting that the LV was large and that the RV was small. The LV free wall was thick (10 to 11 mm), whereas the RV free wall was thin (2 to 5 mm), accurately suggesting that the ventricular septum was intact. Inspection of the posterior external surface showed that the superior and inferior venae cavae and the pulmonary veins all appeared normally connected.

The interior of the morphologically RA (Fig. 12.3B) showed that the RA was hypertrophied and enlarged. The superior vena cava (SVC), inferior vena cava (IVC), and coronary sinus (CoS) all returned normally to the RA, and there was an unusually clearly marked right venous valve remnant to the right of the SVC and to the right of the IVC (the latter being known as the Eustachian valve). Remnants of the left venous valve were seen both above and below the fossa ovalis. Septum spurium (the superior commissure of the sinoatrial or venous valve) was also unusually clearly seen. The right atrial ostium of the CoS was normal in location and size. Evidence of surgical right atriotomy (blue ligatures in the RA free wall) was noted and the foramen ovale had been sutured closed.

An approximately circular prosthetic patch had been surgically placed to close the left-sided TV between the RA and the large LV. This prosthetic patch was posterior, inferior, and somewhat to the left of the right-sided TV between the RA and the small RV. Removal of this circular prosthetic patch revealed that the RA-to-LV valve was tricuspid (three leaflets) and large, measuring 17 mm in diameter in the fixed state (Fig. 12.3B).

The superior, smaller, and somewhat right-sided valve connecting the RA with the small RV sinus has been replaced surgically by a dura mater prosthesis. This is the right-sided tricuspid valve (Fig. 12.3B). The right atrioventricular orifice was subdivided by the right-sided and superior TV (RA-to-RV) and the left-sided and inferior TV (RA-to-LV). This large, subdivided, right atrioventricular orifice straddles the posterior portion of the rightwardly malaligned ventricular septum (VS) (Fig. 12.3B to D).

The RV was right-sided, superior, and small (Fig. 12.3E). It received the right-sided TV, but the RV sinus (body, or inflow tract) was very small. The RV consisted mostly of the infundibulum (conus arteriosus, or outflow tract). The infundibulum was well expanded (not obstructive) (Fig. 12.3E). The ventricular septum was intact. The pulmonary valve was tricuspid, tricommissural, and unremarkable.

Removal of the dura mater prosthesis from the orifice of the right-sided TV revealed a small amount of valve tissue. This small white "cauliflower" of valve tissue did not attach by

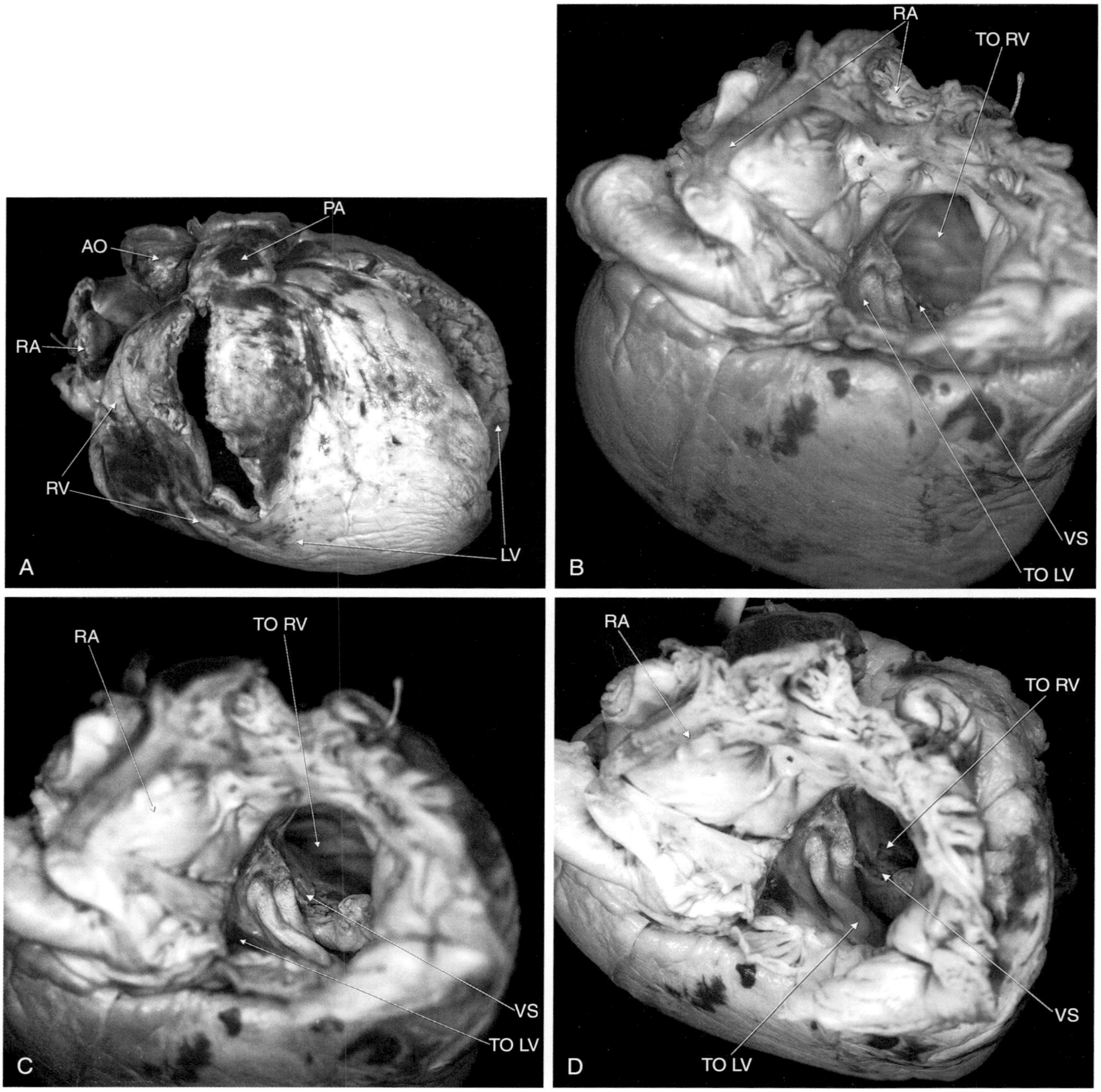

Fig. 12.3 This is the first known case of double-outlet right atrium with rightward malalignment of the ventricular septum relative to the atrial septum that was presented at the World Congress of Paediatric Cardiology in London in 1980,[12] but that has not previously been published photographically. (A) External frontal view of the formalin-fixed heart specimen. The morphologically right atrium *(RA)* is right-sided, indicating that this patient had situs solitus of the viscera and atria. The morphologically right ventricle *(RV)* is right-sided and the morphologically left ventricle *(LV)* is left-sided; hence D-loop ventricles are present. The great arteries appear to be solitus normally related: the main pulmonary artery *(PA)* appears to arise anteriorly, superiorly, and to the left relative to the origin of the ascending aorta *(AO)*. The anterior descending coronary artery (unlabeled) between the RV and the LV approximately bisects the anterior surface of the ventricular part of the heart. This external appearance suggests that the RV is unusually small, or that the LV is unusually large, or both. If the RV of this 5-year-old boy really is hypoplastic (abnormally small), this in turn suggests that the ventricular septum may be abnormally rightward relative to the atrial septum, as in straddling tricuspid valve.[11] (B) Looking into the RA, one can see that the muscular ventricular septum *(VS)* underlies the right atrioventricular orifice, as in straddling tricuspid valve with rightward malalignment of the VS related to smallness of the RV sinus (inflow tract). However, in this rare case, there was a right-sided tricuspid valve connecting the RA with the small RV *(TO RV)*. The patient's native dysplastic right-sided tricuspid valve (TV) was replaced with a dura mater prosthetic valve that has been removed to permit visualization of the RA-to-RV flow pathway via the right-sided TV. There was also a left-sided TV *(TO LV)* connecting the RA with the LV. The prosthetic patch occluding this RA-to-LV valve has been removed to permit visualization of what we have called the left-sided TV that connects the RA with the large LV. (C) A closer view of the RA-to-RV flow pathway and of the RA-to-LV flow pathway. A small remnant of the dysplastic right-sided and superior TV tissue can be seen adhering to the right side of the rightwardly malaligned VS. The top of the large left-sided and inferior TV is also seen. There was no ventricular septal defect. (D) A slightly different view from the RA. Note how displaced the VSD is: both to the right and superiorly, reminiscent of the very abnormal location of the ventricular septal remnant in patients with single LV, absent RV sinus (inflow tract), and double-inlet LV. But here, double-inlet LV is *not* present. Nonetheless, this degree of displacement of the ventricular septal remnant *(VS)* suggests that the RV sinus must be very small, i.e., that the small RV probably is mostly infundibular outlet chamber with only a small RV sinus (inflow tract) component.

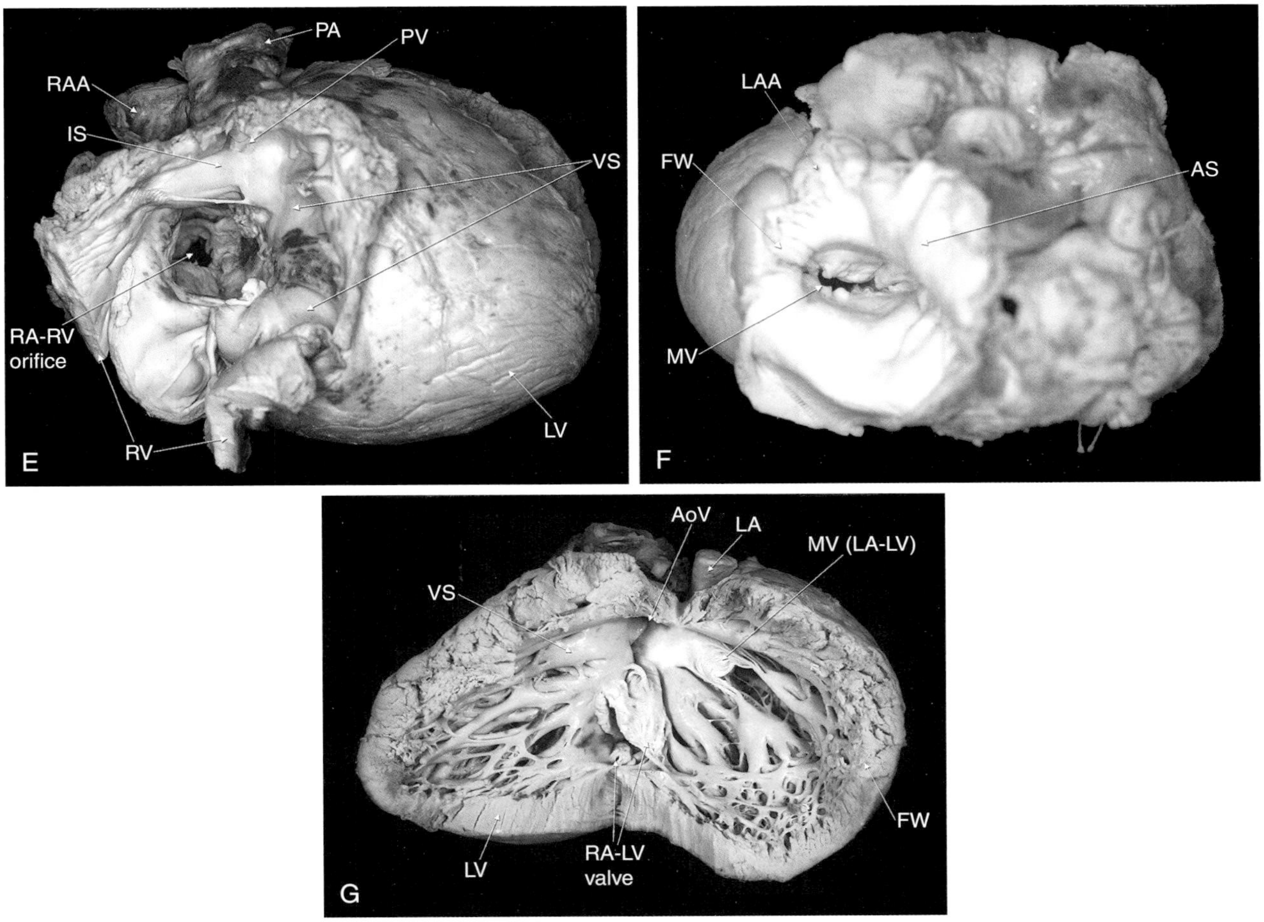

Fig. 12.3, cont'd (E) A frontal view of the small RV confirms the impressions gained from inspection from the RA. The RV sinus (inflow tract) is very small or hypoplastic (labeled *RV*). Remnants of the right-sided TV and the RA-to-RV orifice are seen. Absence of a ventricular septal defect is confirmed. The subpulmonary infundibulum (conus) is well developed, well expanded, and not obstructive. The infundibular septum *(IS)* underlies the well-developed pulmonary valve *(PV)*. The PA is of good size. The right atrial appendage *(RAA)* lies to the right of the PA. The right ventricular septal surface is shallow (compared with the left ventricular septal surface in G), consistent with marked underdevelopment of the RV sinus, which explains why the RV is so small compared with the LV (noted in A). (F) View of the interior of the morphologically left atrium (LA) showing the opened left atrial appendage *(LAA)*, the unremarkable atrial septum *(AS)* and the LA free wall *(FW)*, and the normal-appearing mitral valve *(MV)*. (G) Interior of the large morphologically LV showing the LV septal surface *(VS)* and the LV free wall surface *(FW)*, both of which are well developed, hypertrophied, and enlarged. Just as there is double-outlet right atrium (B, C, and D), so too there is double-inlet left ventricle. The left-sided TV or the RA-to-LV valve is malformed and regurgitant, permitting LV-to-RA shunting preoperatively. The septal leaflet of this central RA-to-LV valve is poorly formed, with little free valve tissue; hence the LV-to-RA regurgitation. The accessory orifice in this left-sided TV is not well seen. The left-sided TV inserts into the posteromedial papillary muscle group of the LV, whereas the mitral valve *(MV)*, i.e., the LA-to-LV valve, inserts into two well-separated heads of the anterolateral papillary muscle group of the LV. Consequently, the risks of parachute mitral valve, i.e., congenital mitral stenosis, were avoided in this case. Similarly, there was no subvalvar stenosis of the left-sided TV that also inserted into only one papillary muscle group. Absence of a ventricular septal defect (VSD) is again confirmed. There is direct fibrous continuity between the aortic valve *(AoV)* and the MV, typical of normally related great arteries. There is also direct fibrous continuity between the AoV and the left-sided TV (the RA-LV valve). Thus, this type of DORA with a small RV sinus and rightward malalignment of the VS relative to the atrial septum is thought to be closely related to typical straddling TV,[11] except that there is no VSD of the AV canal type because the straddling TV has become adherent to the underlying crest of the muscular VS. Consequently, this anatomic type of DORA has three AV valves (RA to small RV, RA to large LV, and LA to LV) and double-inlet LV.

chordae tendineae to RV papillary muscles. Indeed, no well-formed papillary musculature was found within this small RV. Instead, we found what appeared to be several vestigial, markedly hypoplastic right ventricular papillary muscles at the most rightward, posterior, and inferior corner of this hypoplastic RV sinus.

The conal septum and parietal band were well developed and normally located (Fig. 12.3E). The septal band was present. Thus, the subpulmonary infundibular outflow tract was well developed and not obstructive, whereas the right ventricular sinus and the right-sided tricuspid valve were both markedly underdeveloped and malformed (Fig. 12.3E).

The interior of the morphologically left atrium (LA) appeared unremarkable (Fig. 12.3F). The pulmonary veins all connected normally. Septum primum displayed a normal appearance on the left atrial septal surface. The left atrial appendage appeared unremarkable. From the left atrial aspect, the mitral valve appeared to be of good size (not stenotic) and otherwise normal.

The interior of the morphologically LV confirmed that it is very large, left-sided, and left-handed (Fig. 12.3G)—typical of

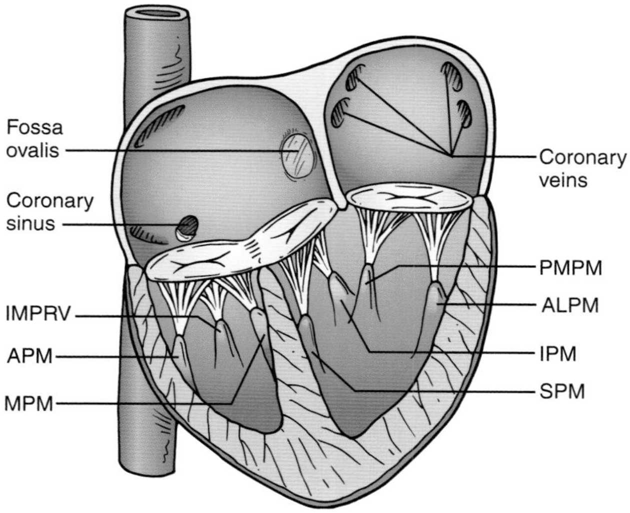

Fig. 12.4 Excellent frontal-plane diagram of the case of Birincioğlu et al[15] that was published in 1999, very similar to the case of Büchler et al[12] that was presented in 1980. Note that the ventricular septum is displaced well to the right of the atrial septum. Consequently, what normally would be the tricuspid valve straddles the ventricular septum and adheres to the muscular ventricular septal crest. Hence there is no ventricular septal defect.[11] The result is double-outlet right atrium: the RA opens through a right-sided tricuspid valve into a small right ventricle and through a left-sided tricuspid valve into a large left ventricle. The mitral valve also opens into the large left ventricle from the left atrium; consequently there is double-inlet left ventricle. It is noteworthy that double-inlet left ventricle is not synonymous with single left ventricle; although the right ventricular sinus (body or inflow tract) is small, it is not absent (as it is with single left ventricle). The right-sided tricuspid valve connects with the small right ventricle via the anterior papillary muscle *(APM)*, the inferior papillary muscle of the right ventricle (*IPMRV;* incorrectly labeled IMPRV), and the medial papillary muscle *(MPM)*. The left-sided tricuspid valve attaches into the large left ventricle by what the authors call the superior papillary muscle *(SPM)* and the inferior papillary muscle *(IPM)* of the left ventricle. The mitral valve connects with the large left ventricle via what the authors identify as the anterolateral papillary muscle *(ALPM)* and the posteromedial papillary muscle *(PMPM)* of the left ventricle. The superior vena cava, inferior vena cava, coronary sinus, and pulmonary veins all are normally connected and the atrial septum is intact *(Fossa ovalis)*. The right-sided tricuspid valve had four leaflets; the left-sided tricuspid valve had three leaflets; and the mitral valve had two leaflets. What we called the mitral valve the authors termed the mitral valve 1. What we called the leaflet-sided tricuspid valve the authors designed the mitral valve 2 or the central atrioventricular valve. We called this middle AV valve the left-sided tricuspid valve because of its relationship to straddling tricuspid valve.[11] (Reproduced with permission from Birincioğlu CL, Ulus AT, Bardakci H, Küçüker S, Kara F, Taşdemir O: Is there another type of biventricular atrioventricular connection? *Texas Heart Inst J* 26:252, 1999.)

solitus or D-loop ventricles in organizational pattern: The palm of only the left hand faced the left ventricular septal surface, and the dorsum of only the left hand was adjacent to the left ventricular free wall surface.

DILV was present. The mitral valve, which connected the LA with the LV, was left-sided and unremarkable in appearance; that is, it appeared neither stenotic nor regurgitant (Fig. 12.3G). The mitral valve inserted into two separate papillary muscles of the anterolateral papillary muscle group of the LV.

The left-sided tricuspid valve that connected the RA with the large LV lay to the right of a prominent muscular ridge that was located between the attachments of these two AV valves. This type of prominent posterior muscular ridge between the insertions of the AV valves is often present in DILV (see Chapter 17). This left-sided tricuspid valve had two ostia; that is, double-orifice of the left-sided tricuspid valve was present. In the approximate middle of the orifice of this left-sided tricuspid valve, leaflet tissue inserted into the left ventricular trabeculations, subdividing the orifice and resulting in double-orifice of this left-sided tricuspid valve.

The left-sided tricuspid valve was regurgitant. The leftward part of this valve did not have thickening and rolling of the leaflet margins and was not the site of the LV-to-RA regurgitation. Only the rightward portion of this left-sided tricuspid valve had thickening and rolling of the leaflet margins, pinpointing this as the site of the prominent LV-to-RA regurgitation. The septal leaflet of the left-sided tricuspid valve was plastered down onto the crest of the muscular ventricular septum—like icing on a cake. Consequently, the right-sided septal part of this left-sided tricuspid valve lacked free leaflet tissue. Consequently, prominent LV-to-RA regurgitation occurred through the rightward paraseptal portion of this left-sided tricuspid valve (Fig. 12.3G).

This plastering down of the rightward septal leaflet tissue of the left-sided tricuspid valve onto the crest of the muscular ventricular septum also appeared to explain (1) why there was no VSD of the AV canal type, as there usually is with straddling tricuspid valve,[11] and (2) why the straddling tricuspid valve was subdivided, resulting in DORA within RA-to-RV valve and an RA-to-LV valve (Fig. 12.3).

From the anatomic and morphogenetic standpoints, we think that DORA with rightward malalignment of the ventricular septum (Fig. 12.3) is closely related to straddling tricuspid valve,[11] except that in this anatomic type of DORA, the straddling tricuspid valve has become adherent to the crest of the underlying ventricular septum.

Another striking feature of DORA with rightward malalignment of the ventricular septum is that there are **three atrioventricular valves** (Fig. 12.3): (1) the right-sided tricuspid valve (RA-to-RV); (2) the left-sided tricuspid valve (RA-to-LV); and (3) the mitral valve (LA-to-LV). In the original case of Büchler et al,[12] the mitral valve was neither stenotic nor atretic.

Morphogenesis. As with **straddling tricuspid valve,**[11] in DORA with rightward malalignment of the ventricular septum (Figs. 12.3 and 12.4), we think that the "real villain" is underdevelopment of the RV sinus, which results in rightward malalignment of the ventricular septum relative to the atrial septum. More precisely, failure of normal expansible growth of the RV sinus (inflow tract) results in a failure of leftward movement of the muscular ventricular septum. Consequently, the muscular ventricular septum does not underlie the atrial septum, as it normally does, but instead underlies the normally located tricuspid valve. If the tricuspid valve then becomes adherent to the muscular ventricular septum, the result is DORA (Figs. 12.3 and 12.4).

DORA with rightward malalignment of the ventricular septum also appears to be closely related anatomically and developmentally to the **Lambert heart,**[14] the salient features of which are as follows:

1. There is a single LV, because the RV sinus (body or inflow tract) is absent. (In this anatomic type of DORA, the RV sinus appears to be very underdeveloped, but not absent [Figs. 12.3 and 12.4]).[12,13]
2. The infundibular outlet chamber is well developed.
3. In the Lambert heart,[14] the tricuspid valve opens predominantly or entirely into the infundibular outlet chamber, as in this anatomic type of DORA. In the usual case of single LV with infundibular outlet chamber and absence of the RV sinus, both the mitral valve and the tricuspid valve open into the single LV; that is, double-inlet LV is present. However, in the Lambert heart[14] variation of single LV and in DORA with rightward malalignment of the ventricular septum, the tricuspid valve opens into the very small RV.

Management. Today (2006) we would probably favor a modified Fontan type of procedure (a cavopulmonary anastomosis) for a patient with DORA and rightward malalignment of the ventricular septum. Why? Because the RV is very small—little more than an infundibular outlet chamber, with only a tiny RV sinus. Such a restrictively small RV is hemodynamically disadvantageous. Consequently, we would probably favor an RV bypass procedure of the Fontan type, with occlusion of both tricuspid valves (right-sided and left-sided).

However, we might attempt a biventricular repair if we thought the RV was big enough and if the function of the right-sided TV was judged to be good enough.

Long experience has taught me not to try to second guess our superb cardiologists and surgeons. However, at least one anatomic point merits mention. The infundibulum (conus arteriosus) is not a good pump. The RV sinus (body, or inflow tract) is. In this type of DORA, the "small RV" is mostly infundibulum or conus arteriosus—not good news hemodynamically.

In 1999, Birincioğlu and colleagues[15] presented another patient very similar to Büchler's case.[12] Their patient was a 9-year-old girl (Fig. 12.4)[15] who had one subdivided valve beneath the RA that connected with both the RV and the LV. The atrial and ventricular septa were intact. What we called the *right-sided tricuspid valve* Birincioğlu et al[15] called the *tricuspid valve.* What we called the *mitral valve* they called the *mitral valve 1.*[13] What we called the *left-sided tricuspid valve* they called the *mitral valve 2,* or a *central AV valve* (Fig. 12.4).[15]

These authors did not call their case DORA. They did not mention the relevance of straddling tricuspid valve. Understandably, these authors[13] were unaware of the previously presented case of Büchler and colleagues.[12] Consequently, Birincioğlu et al[15] thought that they were presenting a newly recognized anomaly. Theirs was a very good case report with an excellent diagram of complex and unfamiliar cardiac anatomy (Fig. 12.4).[15]

Their successful surgical management of this very rare and largely unknown form of congenital heart disease merits recounting.[15] They incised the atrial septum from the fossa ovalis down to the level of the AV junction. Then they refashioned the lower atrial septum with a Gore-Tex patch, placing the prosthetic atrial septum to the right of the central AV valve and to the right of the ostium of the coronary sinus.

Why did Birincioğlu and his colleagues[15] choose this form of repair? They wished "to avoid restricting the left ventricular blood supply when closing the central valve, which was also as large as the mitral valve." In other words, had they closed the central AV valve, they were afraid that they might produce a form of mitral stenosis—because the central valve was almost as large as the mitral valve (Fig. 12.5). By deviating the atrial septum to the right of the central AV valve and by leaving it patent, they preserved the size of the left ventricular inflow tract (avoiding possible iatrogenic mitral stenosis) and they excluded the right atrium from the left ventricle (avoiding significant systemic arterial desaturation). By placing the prosthetic atrial septum to the right of the coronary sinus ostium, they avoided potential iatrogenic AV conduction system problems, preserving sinus rhythm.

Double-Outlet Right Atrium With an Accessory Valve Between the Coronary Sinus and the Left Ventricle

An accessory valve between the coronary sinus and the left ventricle was reported in Chapter 6 concerning systemic venous anomalies (Fig 6.6). When the coronary sinus is large and this coronary sinus–to–left ventricular communication is located just inside the coronary sinus—only slightly to the left of the right atrial ostium of the coronary sinus—and opens into the LV behind (through, between, very close to) the posteromedial papillary muscle group of the LV, then it can look as though there is DORA: The tricuspid valve opens in the normal way from the RA into the RV. This small, occult, and perhaps functionally insignificant valve opens from the coronary sinus into the LV. And the mitral valve opens from the LA into the LV. Hence, there are *three* atrioventricular valves.

One can, of course, object (as we initially did) that this coronary sinus–to–left ventricular valve is not really exiting from the RA, but from just inside the coronary sinus. This is true. But again, when the coronary sinus is large for any reason, then it looks as though this diminutive coronary sinus–to–LV communication is exiting form the RA. So, in an effort not to be too much of a purist, not too much of a splitter—but more of a lumper—I thought I should mention this anomaly here because anatomically, it looks very much like DORA, and physiologically, it functions very much like DORA. But if you were to object that the coronary sinus is not really part of the RA, and hence the above-mentioned anomaly should not be regarded as a form of DORA, I might reply that the coronary sinus is derived from the left horn of the sinus venosus, and the sinus venosus is an important component of the RA.

You might reply, "True, but the coronary sinus is the *left* horn of the sinus venosus. It's the *right* horn of the sinus venosus that is part of the normal RA." At this point, I would run up a white flag. I would certainly not insist. Indeed, I would say that I agree with all that.

But I might add, "Have another look. When the communication is just to the left of the right atrial ostium of the coronary sinus, it looks like it's coming from the RA. The ostium of the coronary sinus is correctly regarded as part of the normal morphologically RA. Indeed, the ostium of the coronary sinus is one of the most highly reliable diagnostic markers of the RA. People are going to need to know about this."

So, this is the case for and against regarding this anomaly as a form of DORA. If you are a purist, you may want to exclude it. If you are more of a lumper, you may want to include it, but with aforementioned reservations being understood (which is where I come down).

The problem is that DORA is not one anatomic entity. Instead, it is multiple very different entities. But this is true of many of our other diagnostic categories (e.g., transposition of the great arteries, double-outlet right ventricle, etc.) The important thing is to understand the anatomy. What you call it is less important; but others must be able to understand what you mean, and accuracy is important.

Otero Coto, Quero Jimenez, and Deverall[16] published a paper in 1984 about hidden or supernumerary AV valves. Their Case 2 (Fig. 12.5)[16] had a small valve between the coronary sinus and the LV, very similar to the anomaly that we are now considering here. However, their patients all had tricuspid atresia and hence did not have DORA.[16]

Dr. Peter Vlad's Case. When he was Chief of the Department of Cardiology at Buffalo Children's Hospital in Buffalo, New York, Dr. Peter Vlad—of Keith, Rowe, and Vlad[17] fame—sent us a most fascinating case of this type (C78-322). Based on examination of the formalin-fixed heart specimen of this 15{9/12}-year-old young woman, our anatomic diagnoses were as follows:

- Completely common AV canal, type A of Rastelli
- Persistent LSVC to coronary sinus to RA
- Sinus venosus–to–left ventricular valve (DORA)
- Aneurysmal dilation of the coronary sinus
- Valved communication between coronary sinus and cavity of LV, opening behind posteromedial papillary muscle of LV
- Postoperative status, 6{9/12} years of age (10/28/1968): Exploratory cardiotomy with mitral and tricuspid annuloplasties
- Postoperative status, 7 years of age (2/21/1968): Patch closure of atrial and ventricular septal defects with mitral valve replacement (Starr-Edwards prosthesis)
- Onset of ventricular and atrial dysrythmias at 9 years of age (1971)
- Postoperative status, 14{11/12} years of age (1/5/1977): mitral valve replacement with Bjork-Shiley prosthesis
- Continuing low cardiac output leading to death at 15{9/12} years of age (10/11/1977)

We thought that this patient had DORA with DILV. (**Note:** DILV is not always associated with single left ventricle, i.e., absence of the right ventricular sinus or inflow tract.)

The coronary sinus was thought to be enlarged because of the persistent left superior vena cava that connected with it and drained into the right atrium.

In my consultation I stated that just where the left horn of the sinus venosus or the enlarged coronary sinus is about to enter the RA one sees in the floor of the coronary sinus at the coronary sinus–right atrial junction a small intact AV valve that leaves the RA and the floor of the coronary sinus and opens exclusively into the enormously hypertrophied and dilated left ventricle, right behind the Bjork-Shiley mitral valve prosthesis.

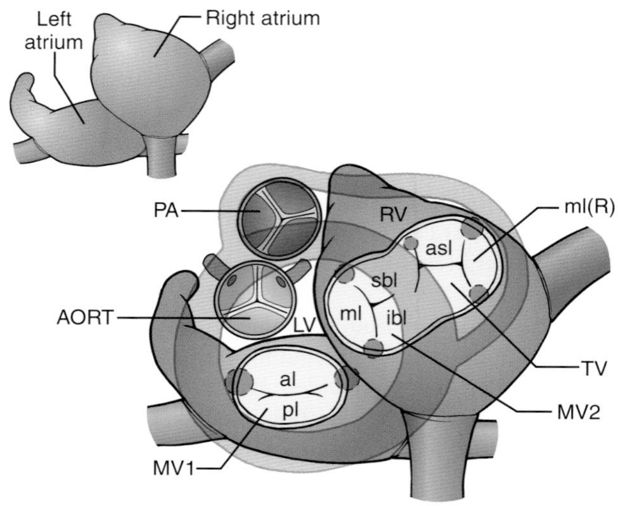

Fig. 12.5 Birincioğlu's case,[15] surgical view. *al,* Anterior leaflet of mitral valve (authors' mitral valve 1, *MV1*); *AORT,* aortic valve leaflets; *asl,* anterior superior leaflet of tricuspid valve *(TV)*; *ibl,* inferior bridging leaflet (posterior septal leaflet of left-sided tricuspid valve, authors' mitral valve 2, *MV2*); *LV,* morphologically left ventricle; *ml,* mural leaflet (posterior or mural leaflet of left-sided tricuspid valve, authors' *MV2*); *ml(R),* lateral leaflet of right ventricle (posterior leaflet of TV); septal leaflet of TV not labeled; *MV1,* mitral valve 1 (mitral valve); *PA,* pulmonary valve leaflets; *pl,* posterior leaflet of mitral valve; *RV,* morphologically right ventricle; *sbl,* superior bridging leaflet (anterior septal leaflet of left-sided TV). The authors[13] called the central AV valve mitral valve 2 because it was a second AV valve opening into the LV. The authors[13] used the terms *superior bridging leaflet* and *inferior bridging leaflet* because of the resemblance of the leaflets to those seen in common AV canal. (Reproduced with permission from Birincioğlu CL, Ulus AT, Bardakci H, Küçüker S, Kara F, Taşdemir O: Is there another type of biventricular atrioventricular connection? *Texas Heart Inst J* 26:252, 1999.)

This small valve showed no evidence of regurgitation. There is no thickening or rolling of its leaflet margins or chordae tendineae. Hence, this valve appears to be moderately hypoplastic and not regurgitant. (This is almost exactly how my consultation reads. I am not using quotation marks, because a few words have been added or omitted.)

In the fixed state, this accessory valve measured 17 mm in length and 8 mm in maximal width, as measured from the right atrial and coronary sinus aspect. The left ventricular orifice of this accessory valve measures only 8 × 6 mm. The effective orifice of this accessory valve is distinctly smaller than its right atrial/coronary sinus dimensions might suggest. Hence, this is quite a small valvar orifice.

This small coronary sinus–to–left ventricular valve lies directly behind or dorsal to the Bjork-Shiley prosthesis, and this valve is behind several prominent muscular trabeculae carneae of left ventricular morphological type. On first looking into the LV, one may well not see this small accessory valve because it lies right behind what has been called the median posterior ridge (that can be prominent in DILV, between the papillary muscle attachments of the two AV valves). The accessory valve is separated from the mitral part of the common AV orifice by a cuff of LV muscular tissue that is composed of approximately three

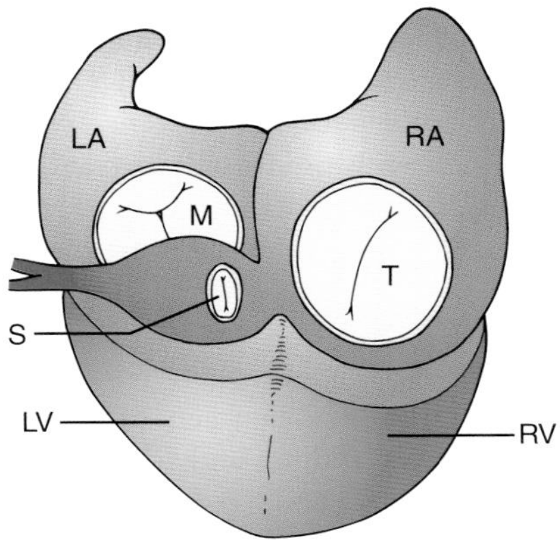

Fig. 12.6 Excellent diagram from Otero Coto et al[16] showing the essential feature of a third anatomic type of DORA. A small supernumerary valve *(S)* opens from the floor of a dilated coronary sinus into the morphologically left ventricle *(lv)*, posteroinferior to the mitral valve *(M)*. This coronary sinus–to–left ventricle valve looks as though it is arising from the right atrium *(ra)* because it is close to the right atrial ostium of the coronary sinus and because enlargement of the coronary sinus (CoS) makes it look as though the CoS is incorporated into the RA. In this case of Otero Coto et al[16] the tricuspid valve *(T)* was atretic (imperforate Ebstein's anomaly); hence this patient[16] did *not* have DORA. For more information concerning this rare form of DORA, see Chapter 6 concerning systemic venous anomalies: aneurysm of the left horn of sinus venosus with *two* coronary sinus–to–left ventricle valves (see Figs. 6.6 and 6.7). Such cases have **triple-outlet right atrium with four AV valves:** tricuspid valve, mitral valve, and two sinoventricular valves. (Reproduced with permission from Otero Coto E, Quero Jimenez M, Deverall PB: Rare anomalies of atrioventricular connection: hidden or supernumerary valves with imperforate right atrioventricular connection. *Int J Cardiol* 6:149, 1984.)

prominent left ventricular trabeculae carneae: a prominent lateral trabeculation, the median posterior ridge, and a prominent medial trabeculation. These muscular structures run in front of the accessory valve and separate it from the posterior part of the main ring of the common AV valve.

From the anatomic and morphogenetic viewpoints, we think that this valve is *not* a coronary sinus septal defect, that is, not a defect in the anterior wall of the coronary sinus and in the posterior wall of the left atrium.

Instead, this appears to be an even rarer malformation, namely a defect in the floor of the right atrial ostium of the coronary sinus that communicates not with the left atrium, but with the left ventricle. This accessory valve opens behind and a bit below what should have been the posterior (dorsal) leaflet of the mitral component of the common AV valve.

One may say that there are **two anatomic types of coronary sinus septal defect:**

1. **the anterior (ventral) type** that communications with the LA—this being the common type; and
2. **the inferior (caudal) type** that communicates with the LV—this being the rare type that we are reporting here (for the first time without tricuspid atresia,[16] to our knowledge). The diagram of Otero Coto and colleagues shows this coronary sinus–to–left ventricular valve very well (Fig. 12.6),[16] except that their patient also had tricuspid atresia.

OTHER CASES OF DORA

In our Cardiac Pathology Database, we have two other cases of DORA that merit inclusion here: A78-130 and C82-80. Both have a small RV sinus, rightward malalignment of the ventricular septum relative to the atrial septum, and a straddling tricuspid valve that is adherent to the ventricular septum—similar to Büchler's case (Fig. 12.3)[12] and Birincioğlu's case (Fig. 12.4).[15]

The first patient (A78-130) was a 2-day-old boy with transposition of the great arteries (TGA) with {S,D,D} segmental anatomy, that is, TGA {S,D,D}. The RV was mildly underdeveloped. The tricuspid valve straddled the ventricular septum and adhered to its crest, thereby obliterating the usual VSD of the AV canal type, and resulting in an intact ventricular septum and DORA. The patient was the infant of a diabetic mother (type 2, controlled by diet without exogenous insulin).

The right atrial appendage was unusually large and redundant, extending unusually far along the inferior surface of the heart. The left atrial appendage was also unusually long and "snakey." The right-sided tricuspid valve was somewhat small, but was an otherwise well-developed RA-to-RV valve. The left-sided "tricuspid" valve (RA-to-LV) was small, but with leaflets and papillary muscles of LV configuration. The mitral valve (LA-to-LV) was unremarkable, except that the posteromedial commissure was absent. There was pulmonary valve–mitral valve direct fibrous continuity. Although the ventricular septum was intact (no VSD), the muscularization of the base of the ventricular septum was deficient.

Despite an adequate balloon atrial septostomy, the patient was thought to have severe lung disease leading to increased cyanosis, hypotension, acidosis (pH = 6.9), elevated pCO_2, decreased urine output, and seizures leading to death at 2 days of age. Pulmonary histology showed that this patient had hyaline membrane disease that was thought to be the immediate cause of death.

This was the first time that we had encountered a patient with DORA with rightward malalignment of the ventricular septum plus a straddling and adherent tricuspid valve who also had TGA {S,D,D}.

The second patient (C82-80) was also a 2-day-old boy, a patient of Dr. Richard McFaul of Portland, Maine. This patient had the same type of DORA as the last patient and also had TGA {S,D,A}. (In A-TGA, the transposed aortic valve is directly anterior [antero- or A] relative to the transposed pulmonary valve.)

There was a large ostium secundum type of atrial septal defect. There was a right-sided tricuspid valve (RA-to-RV) and a left-sided "tricuspid" valve (RA-to-LV). There were two separate "tricuspid" annuli. The ventricular septum was intact but was deficient superiorly (or basally).

There was marked congenital mitral stenosis (of the LV-to-LV valve), a very significant finding—and the first time that we had encountered this.

There was myxomatous change of the leaflets of both the right-sided and left-sided tricuspid valves. Thus, all three AV valves were malformed. (We have no information concerning this patient's karyotype; polyvalvular disease can be associated with an abnormal karyotype.)

There was marked angulation of the muscular interventricular septum relative to the atrial septum. The ventriculoatrial septal angle equaled 80 degrees. The normal ventriculoatrial septal angle = 5° ± 2°.[11] A very abnormally large ventriculoatrial septal angle is characteristic of typical straddling tricuspid valve.[11]

In a series of 19 postmortem cases of straddling tricuspid valve, the ventriculoatrial septal angle averaged 61° ± 24°.[11] In 4 of these 19 patients (21%), the straddling tricuspid valve was adherent to the crest of the rightwardly malaligned ventricular septum, resulting in this anatomic type of DORA.[11]

In addition, this patient also had hypoplasia of the ascending aorta and aortic arch with preductal coarctation of the aorta, and a large patent ductus arteriosus that appeared functionally to be closing (a fatal combination of misfortunes).

SUMMARY

Three anatomy types of DORA are known at the present time:

1. DORA with marked leftward malalignment of the atrial septum relative to the AV valve(s), with left atrial outlet atresia and often with pulmonary venous obstruction (Figs. 12.1 to 12.2);[1-10]
2. DORA with rightward malalignment of the ventricular septum, small RV, and straddling and adherent tricuspid valve (Figs. 12.3 to 12.5);[11,12,15] and
3. DORA with coronary sinus–to–LV accessory valve (Fig. 12.6).

REFERENCES

1. Van Mierop LHS. Pathology and pathogenesis of endocardial cushion defects: surgical implications. In: Davila JC, ed. *Second Henry Ford Hospital International Symposium on Cardiac Surgery.* New York: Appleton-Century-Crofts; 1977:201.
2. Utley JR, Noonan JA, Walters LR, Frist RA. Anomalous position of atrial septum with anomalous pulmonary and systemic venous drainage. Correction including ligation of persistent left superior vena cava. *J Thorac Cardiovasc Surg.* 1974;67:730.
3. Corwin RD, Singh AK, Karlson KE. Double-outlet right atrium: a rare endocardial cushion defect. *Am Heart J.* 1983;106:1156.
4. Pérez-Martínez VM, García-Fernandez F, Oliver-Ruiz J, Nuñez-Gonzalez L. Double-outlet right atrium with two atrioventricular valves and left atrial outlet atresia. *J Am Coll Cardiol.* 1984;3:375.
5. Alivizatos P, Anderson RH, Macartney FJ, Zuberbuhler JR, Stark J. Atrioventricular septal defect with balanced ventricles and malaligned atrial septum: double-outlet right atrium. Report of two cases. *J Thorac Cardiovasc Surg.* 1985;89:295.
6. Westerman GR, Norton JB, Van Devanter SH. Double-outlet right atrium associated with tetralogy of Fallot and common atrioventricular valve. *J Thorac Cardiovasc Surg.* 1986;91:205.
7. Starc TJ, Bierman FZ, Bowman FO, Steeg CN, Wang NK, Krongrad E. Pulmonary venous obstruction and atrioventricular canal anomalies: role of cor triatriatum and double outlet right atrium. *Am J Cardiol.* 1987;9:830.
8. Ahmadi A, Mocellin R, Spillner G, Gildein HP. Atrioventricular septal defect with double-outlet right atrium. *Pediatr Cardiol.* 1989;10:170.
9. Suzuki K, Kikuchi T, Mimori S. Double outlet right atrium and complete atrioventricular septal defect with abnormal findings of the biopsied lung. *Cardiol Young.* 1994;4:402.
10. Radermecker MA, Chauvaud S, Carpentier A. Double-outlet right atrium with restrictive ostium primum and incomplete supravalvular ring presenting as congenital mitral valve stenosis. *J Thorac Cardiovasc Surg.* 1995;109:804.
11. Pessotto R, Padalino M, Rubino M, Kadoba K, Büchler JR, Van Praagh R. Straddling tricuspid valve as a sign of ventriculoatrial malalignment: a morphometric study of 19 postmortem cases. *Am Heart J.* 1999;138:1184.
12. Büchler JR, Rabelo R, Marino R, David I, Van Praagh R. *Double-outlet Right Atrium: Autopsied Case of Newly Recognized Entity.* London: World Congress of Paediatric Cardiology; 1980:223 (abstract).
13. Godman MJ, ed. *Paediatric Cardiology.* Vol. 4. World Congress London 1980, Edinburgh, London, Melbourne, New York: Churchill Livingstone; 1981.
14. Lambert EC. Single ventricle with a rudimentary outlet chamber, case report. *Bull Johns Hopkins Hosp.* 1951;88:231.
15. Birincioğlu CL, Ulus AT, Bardakci H, Küçüker S, Kara F, Taşdemir O. Is there another type of biventricular atrioventricular connection? *Tex Heart Inst J.* 1999;26:252.
16. Otero Coto E, Quero Jimenez M, Deverall PB. Rare anomalies of atrioventricular connection: hidden or supernumerary valves with imperforate right atrioventricular connection. *Int J Cardiol.* 1984;6:149.
17. Keith JD, Rowe RD, Vlad P. *Heart Disease in Infancy and Childhood.* New York: Macmillan Publishing Co, Inc; 1958, 1967, 1978.

13

Tricuspid Valve Anomalies

How many anatomically different kinds of malformation can befall the tricuspid valve? Our database suggests that the answer is at least 12 (Table 13.1).

We also encountered 41 cases of acquired tricuspid regurgitation (1.27%) and one patient with nonspecific tricuspid valvulitis (0.03%) that are not included in Table 13.1.

It is widely thought that congenital tricuspid regurgitation is very uncommon, except for patients with Ebstein's anomaly of the tricuspid valve.[1] Consequently, we were surprised to find that our database (Table 13.1) suggests that non-Ebstein congenital tricuspid regurgitation (80 cases, 2.49% of 3216 cases of congenital heart disease) may be about as common as Ebstein's malformation (78 cases, 2.43% of this series of autopsy-proved congenital cardiac malformations). In order to clarify this situation, we realized that we had to do a detailed study of Ebstein's malformation, and of non-Ebstein's congenital tricuspid regurgitation. At the outset, we knew, of course, that Ebstein's malformation does not always have tricuspid regurgitation. Ebstein's anomaly can also have congenital tricuspid stenosis, or tricuspid atresia (imperforate Ebstein's malformation). Thus, the 78 patients in Table 13.1 with Ebstein's anomaly should not be misunderstood as all having congenital tricuspid regurgitation.

EBSTEIN'S MALFORMATION

Ebstein's malformation of the tricuspid valve and right ventricular sinus (body, or inflow tract) turned out to be much more interesting and complex than is generally understood.

This fascinating anomaly was first described by Wilhelm Ebstein[2] (1836–1912) in 1866. Ebstein was a student of Rudolph Virchow (1821–1902) and Moritz Heinrich Romberg (1795–1873).[3] Virchow, of course, was an eminent German pathologic anatomist who, working in Berlin, established the cellular basis of pathology (*Die Cellular pathologie,* published in 1856). Thus, one may assume that Ebstein had received training in pathology, which helps to explain why at the age of only 30 years he was able to publish a definitive description of a newly discovered malformation of displacement of the tricuspid valve into the right ventricle, which is how Ebstein's anomaly is often briefly described. Later, Ebstein became a distinguished professor of medicine at Göttingen.[3-6]

Ebstein's famous patient,[2] Joseph Prescher, was a 19-year-old laborer with marked cyanosis. He had been short of breath, particularly with exertion, since childhood and had always been troubled with palpitations. Since the age of 17 he had been sick, but not bedridden. Eight days prior to admission to All Saints' Hospital in Breslau, Prussia (which is now Wroclaw, Poland), swelling of his lower legs had appeared. In hospital, he was treated with bed rest and morphine to quiet a troublesome cough. He seemed to be improving, but then suddenly collapsed and died. It is thought that the causes of his death were a cardiac arrhythmia and congestive heart failure, complicating Ebstein's anomaly.[4-7]

Wilhelm Ebstein did not take care of the patient clinically, but he did perform the autopsy. A physician colleague, Oskar Wyss, made two excellent drawings of the cardiac anomalies (Fig. 13.1).

Definition. Ebstein's anomaly of the tricuspid valve and right ventricle is characterized by the following features (Figs. 13.2, 13.3, and 13.4):

1. The *septal leaflet* is downwardly displaced; that is, its origin is variably below the right atrial–right ventricular junction. When discordant L-loop ventricles coexist with visceroatrial situs solitus, that is, when the segmental anatomy is {S,L,-},

TABLE 13.1 Anatomic Types of Tricuspid Malformation

Tricuspid Valve Anomaly	No. of Cases	Percent of Series (n = 3216)
1. Tricuspid regurgitation, congenital	80	2.49
2. Tricuspid atresia	94	2.92
3. Ebstein's malformation With tricuspid atresia (2)* With common AV canal (9)	78	2.43
4. Tricuspid stenosis, congenital	70	2.18
5. Double-orifice tricuspid valve	12	0.25
6. Myxomatous tricuspid valve	8	0.25
7. Hypoplasia of tricuspid valve leaflets	6	0.19
8. Tricuspid valve prolapse	4	0.12
9. Triple-orifice tricuspid valve	3	0.09
10. Congenitally unguarded tricuspid orifice†	2	0.06
11. Muscular tricuspid valve	1	0.03
12. Filigree (multiply fenestrated) tricuspid valve	1	0.03

*Also known as Ebstein's anomaly with imperforate tricuspid valve.
†Also known as absence of tricuspid leaflets.

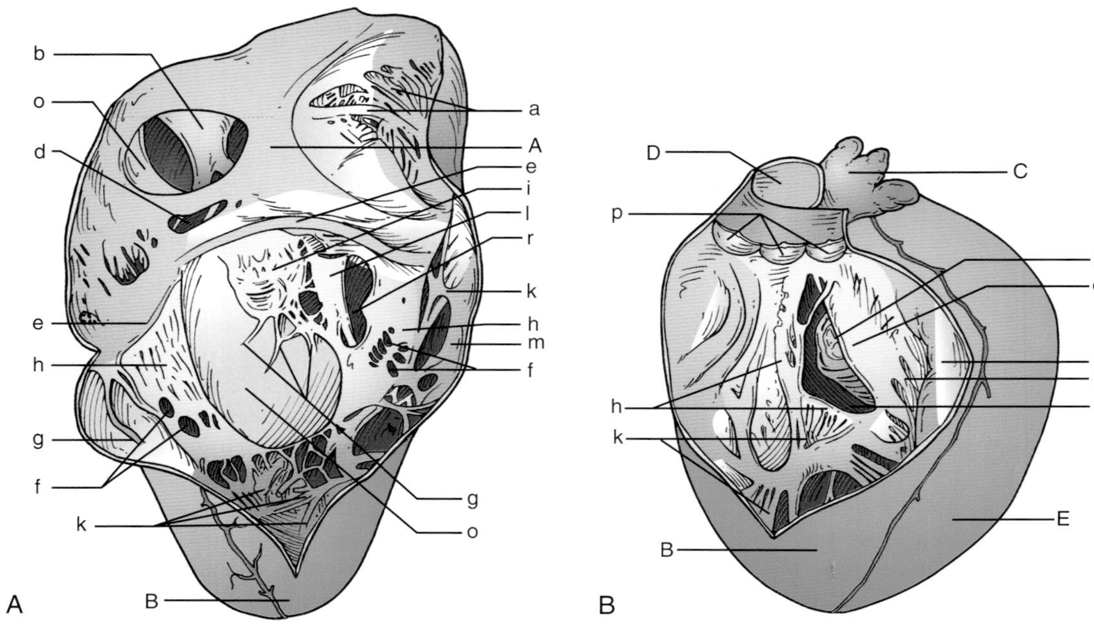

Fig. 13.1 Ebstein's original case.[2] (A) Opened right atrium, *A,* and right ventricular outflow tract, *B.* (B) Opened right ventricular outflow tract and proximal pulmonary artery. (Drawings by Dr. Oskar Wyss, friend of Ebstein.) These elegant drawings are much more interesting than is usually understood. The right atrium appears enlarged, but not hypertrophied. There is a secundum type of atrial septal defect because of an excessively large ostium secundum anterosuperior to septum primum, *b.* The ostium of the coronary sinus appears enlarged and lacking a thebesian valve, *d.* (So far, nothing is too surprising.) The right annulus fibrosus, or right atrioventricular junction, is labeled *e.* The septal leaflet of the tricuspid valve is labeled *i;* it is clearly deficient posteroinferiorly (not surprising). The posterior leaflet, *h',* has many obliterated interchordal spaces, and a few patent ones, *f* (also not surprising). The anterior tricuspid leaflet is labeled *h.* But note that the origin—neither of the septal leaflet (i), not of the posterior leaflet (h'), is downwardly displaced beneath the right atrioventricular junction *(e).* This is very surprising indeed. By modern standards, most observers would say that this is not Ebstein's anomaly. However, my view is that we should be kind. I think this is an error, "artistic license," if you wish. The anterior leaflet is shown arising from the right atrioventricular junction; this is correct. The right ventricular sinus septal surface, *o,* is shown as smooth or nontrabeculated; this is correct and proves that Ebstein's patient did indeed have Ebstein's malformation. The septal band, *l,* is just where it should be. Note how thin the right ventricular free wall is shown to be. If this detail is accurate, it is consistent with a Uhl's disease component, which also seems correct. Note that posteroinferior to the posterior leaflet (h'), the very thin right ventricular free wall bulges outward and is nontrabeculated; this is consistent with a subtricuspid aneurysm, which is characteristic of Ebstein's anomaly. Note also that the right ventricular free wall distal to the anterior leaflet *(h)* is trabeculated; this, too, is typical of Ebstein's anomaly. (B) The tricuspid valve opens upward toward the pulmonary valve *(p).* Many of the interchordal spaces are obliterated. (Both of these findings are typical.) The septal band *(o)* and the moderator band *(r)* are as expected. B is the exterior of the right ventricle and *E* is the exterior of the left ventricle. Note that the anterior descending coronary artery (unlabeled, between E and B) veers towards the right in the lower part of its course. This, too, is typical of Ebstein's. The larger left ventricle wraps around the smaller right ventricular apex, apparently because the right ventricular sinus (inflow tract) is not only dysplastic, but also somewhat hypoplastic—smaller than normal, which is reflected by the rightward course of the lower anterior descending coronary artery. (Reproduced with permission. Ebstein W. Ueber einen sehr seltenen Fall von Insufficienz der Valvula tricuspidalis, bedingt durch eine angeborene hochgradige Missbildung derselben. *Arch Anat Physiol Wiss Med* 1866;238.)

the septal leaflet of the left-sided tricuspid valve is displaced below the *left* atrial–right ventricular junction (Fig. 13.4).

2. The *anterior leaflet* is deep and curtain-like. It originates normally from the right atrioventricular junction; that is, typically its origin is not downwardly displaced. The tensor apparatus of the anterior leaflet has few (or occasionally no) interchordal spaces (Figs. 13.2, 13.3, and 13.4). (Normally, there are abundant, well-formed spaces between the chordae tendineae.) The lack of interchordal spaces—which are filled with fibrous leaflet tissue—makes it look as though the anterior leaflet is inserting directly in the papillary musculature or directly in the right ventricular free wall. However, transillumination of the anterior tricuspid leaflet makes it clear that the chordae tendineae are in fact present; but they are not immediately obvious—because what should normally be the interchordal spaces are filled with fibrous leaflet tissue. This is also why the anterior leaflet of the tricuspid valve in Ebstein's anomaly looks so deep, extending as it does from its origin at the right atrioventricular junction to its insertion into the small anterior papillary muscle of the right ventricle or directly into the right ventricular free wall. The lack of normally formed interchordal spaces also explains why this very deep anterior

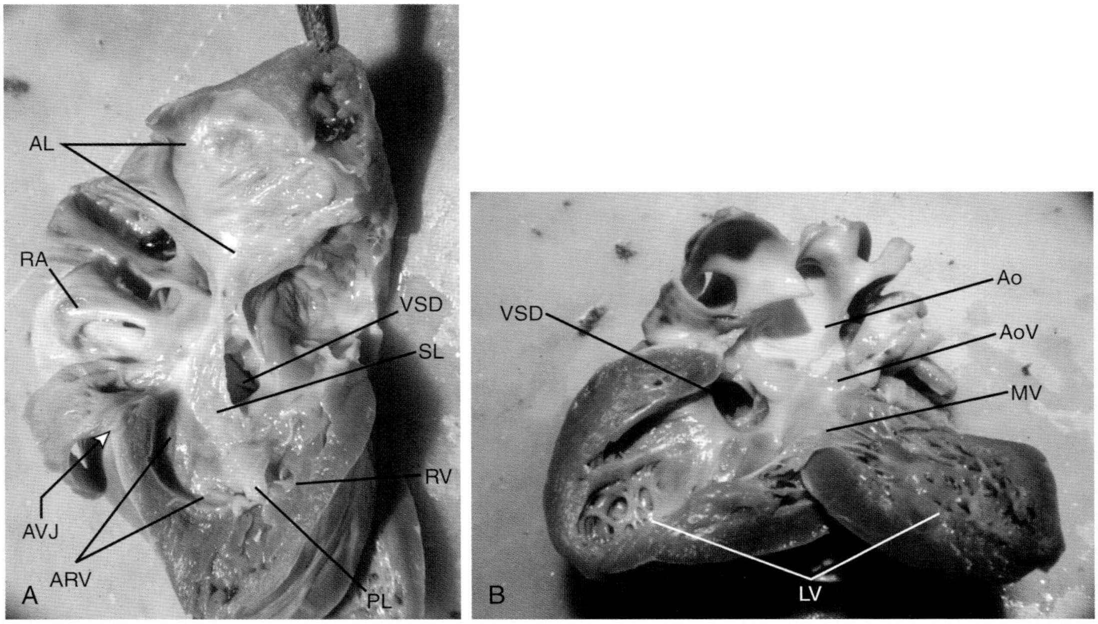

Fig. 13.2 Ebstein's anomaly with ventricular septal defect *(VSD)*. (A) Opened right atrium *(RA)* and right ventricle *(RV)*. (B) Opened left ventricle *(LV)* and aorta *(Ao)*. In (A), the septal leaflet *(SL)* of the tricuspid valve is displaced far below the right atrioventricular junction *(AVJ)*. The right ventricular septal surface above the septal leaflet in the atrialized right ventricle *(ARV)* is smooth (nontrabeculated). The anterior leaflet of the tricuspid valve is deep and curtain-like, with few if any interchordal spaces. Hence, the anterior leaflet appears to insert directly into the right ventricular free wall. The anterior leaflet originates from the right atrioventricular junction; its origin is not downwardly displaced. A patent foramen ovale and a conoventricular type of ventricular septal defect are also seen. (B) The opened left ventricle *(LV)* and mitral valve *(MV)* are unremarkable. There is aortic-mitral fibrous continuity *(AoV-MV)*, typical of normally related great arteries, and the subaortic ventricular septal defect *(VSD)* is well seen.

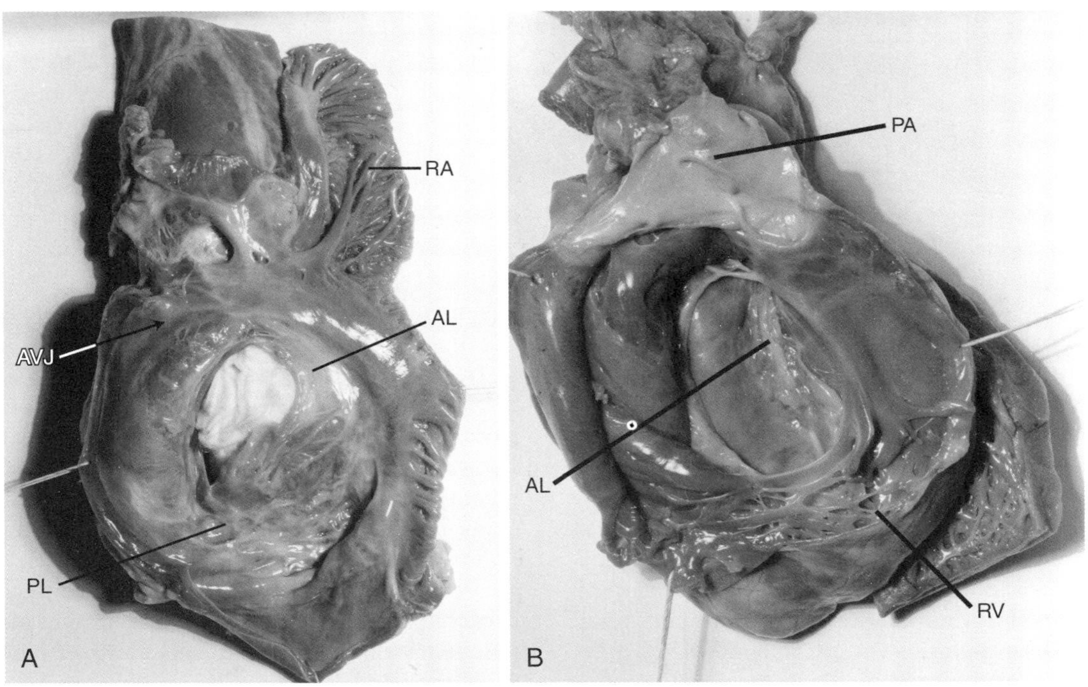

Fig. 13.3 Ebstein's anomaly with tricuspid insufficiency. (A) Opened right atrium *(RA)* and unopened tricuspid valve seen from above. (B) Opened right ventricle and pulmonary artery *(PA)* and unopened tricuspid valve seen from below. Case 6 was an $8\frac{3}{12}$-year-old girl. Cyanosis was noted at 4½ years. Congestive heart failure appeared at 6 years of age. She died during cardiac catheterization at $8\frac{3}{12}$ years, presumably from an arrhythmia, in 1951. Cardiomegaly was massive: 322 grams (normal = 160 grams, 101% greater than normal). A secundum atrial septal defect measured 3 × 10 mm. In (A), the deep curtain-like anterior leaflet *(AL)* originates normally from the right atrioventricular junction; whereas the deficient septal and posterior leaflets *(PL)* are downwardly displaced, far below the right atrioventricular junction *(AVJ)*. The anterior leaflet has very few patent interchordal spaces. In (B), note the thickening and rolling of the free margin of the anterior tricuspid leaflet *(AL)*, consistent with tricuspid regurgitation and the great paucity of interchordal spaces. These photos were taken at the time of autopsy.

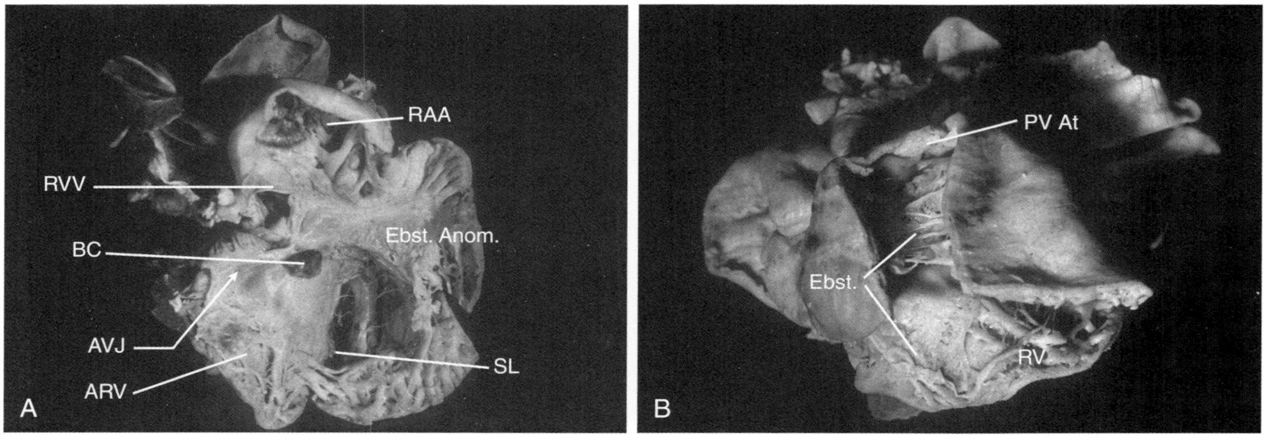

Fig. 13.4 Ebstein's anomaly *(Ebst. Anom.)* with pulmonary valvar atresia and intact ventricular septum. (A) The opened right atrium and right ventricular inflow tract, i.e., the atrialized right ventricle *(ARV)*—above the downwardly displaced septal leaflet *(SL)* of the tricuspid valve. There is a prominent blood cyst *(BC)* at the right atrioventricular junction *(AVJ)*, just above the smooth, nontrabeculated right ventricular septal surface. The septal leaflet *(SL)* is displaced down almost to the septal band. The right atrial appendage *(RAA)* is hypertrophied and enlarged, reflecting tricuspid regurgitation. The right venous valve *(RVV)*, also known as the Eustachian valve, is markedly enlarged, as is frequent with pulmonary valvar atresia and intact ventricular septum. (B) The broad insertion of the deep curtain-like anterior leaflet of the tricuspid valve into the thin right ventricular free wall. The paucity of interchordal spaces is noteworthy; the spaces that normally exist between the chordae tendineae are filled with fibrous, leaflet-like tissue. *PV At,* Pulmonary valvar atresia. The upper leader from the *Ebst.* label points to the anterior tricuspid leaflet, and the lower leader points to the septal and posterior tricuspid leaflets.

leaflet appears to "wave" at the imaging observer (for example, on two-dimensional echocardiography).

3. The *posterior leaflet* of the tricuspid valve in Ebstein's malformation typically arises from the right atrioventricular junction laterally, adjacent to the right ventricular free wall. But as the origin of the posterior leaflet approaches the right ventricular septal surface, its origin becomes progressively displaced below the right atrioventricular junction.
4. *Deficiency of leaflet tissue* is frequent with Ebstein's anomaly, often involving the septal leaflet, as in Ebstein's patient (Fig. 13.1A), and quite often also involving the posterior leaflet. Absence of tricuspid valve leaflet tissue, that is, a partial form of congenitally unguarded tricuspid orifice, means that the tricuspid valve's leaflets cannot effectively coapt, typically resulting in tricuspid regurgitation.
5. Downward displacement of the origin of the tricuspid valve septally and posteriorly subdivides the right ventricle into an *"atrialized" right ventricle* (above the tricuspid leaflets) and a *"ventricularized" right ventricle* (below the tricuspid leaflets). The "atrialized" right ventricle has atrial hemodynamics (e.g., right atrial pressures), whereas the "ventricularized" right ventricle typically has ventricular hemodynamics (e.g., right ventricular pressures).
6. *Deficiency or absence of right ventricular musculature* is an integral part of Ebstein's anomaly. The septal surface of the "atrialized" right ventricle (between the right atrioventricular junction above and the tricuspid leaflet tissue below) is typically smooth or nontrabeculated (Figs. 13.1A, 13.2A, 13.3A, and 13.4A). This usually is *not* because the tricuspid valve's septal leaflet has been plastered down on the right ventricular septal surface, thereby obscuring the coarse underlying trabeculae carneae of the right ventricular septal surface myocardium. Surprising though it may at first seem, the right ventricular septal surface myocardial above the downwardly displaced septal leaflet is really absent. One is looking at the featureless (smooth), normally hidden, left ventricular component of the interventricular septum. This surface is what electrophysiologists call "the barrier," the normal junction between the left ventricular component (which is present) and the right ventricular component (which is absent in typical Ebstein's malformation). This junction between the left and right ventricular components of the normal interventricular septum is well seen histologically in cross sections of the ventricular septum.

How far down may the septal leaflet of the tricuspid valve be displaced in Ebstein's anomaly? The degree of "downward displacement" below the right atrioventricular junction is variable. But when Ebstein's anomaly is severe: down to where the infundibulum begins. Where is that? The septal band and the moderator band demarcate the beginning of the infundibulum (or right ventricular outflow tract) (Fig. 13.5A). Thus, in a typical severe case of Ebstein's malformation, the septal leaflet may be displaced all the way down to the septal and moderator bands (also known as the septomarginal trabeculation). In less severe cases, the septal leaflet is displaced only part of the way down toward the septal and moderator bands.

In fact, **the very worst case** is far more extreme than displacement of the septal leaflet of the tricuspid valve down to the level of the septal and moderator bands. In the extreme case, often with pulmonary valvar atresia or severe stenosis and intact ventricular septum, a tricuspid leaflet remnant is found just below the pulmonary valve. At first glance, it looks as though

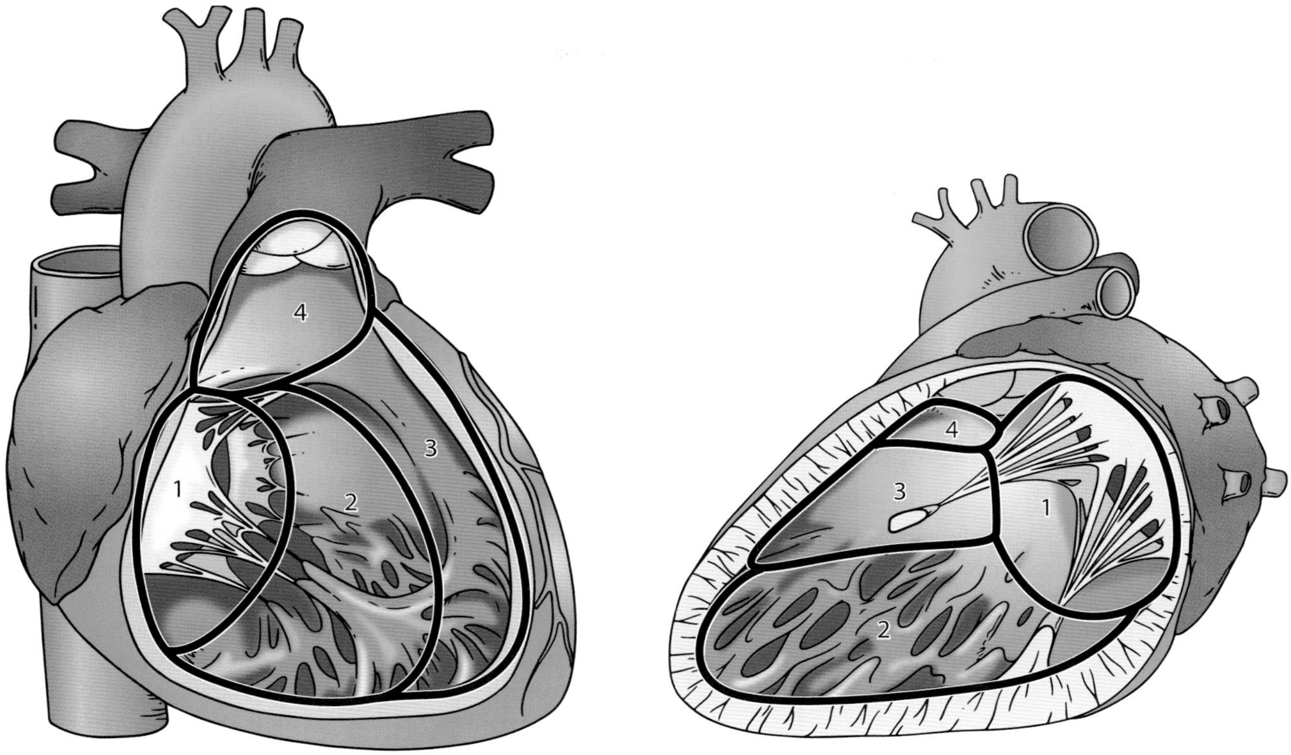

A B

Fig. 13.5 The four components that make up the normal morphologically right ventricle (A) and the normal morphologically left ventricle (B). In (A), *component 1* is the right atrioventricular junction, i.e., the tricuspid valve and the atrioventricular septum. *Component 2* is the right ventricular sinus, body, or inflow tract—the essence of the right ventricle. *Component 2* lies distal or downstream relative to *component 1*, but proximal or upstream relative to *components 3 and 4*. The normal right ventricular inflow tract equals *component 1* plus *component 2*. *Component 3* is the septal band and the moderator band. *Component 4* is the conal septum and the parietal band. The normal right ventricular outflow tract equals *component 3* plus *component 4*. All four components consist of septal and confluent free wall portions. Ebstein's anomaly typically involves malformation of *components 1* and *2*. However, malformation of the right ventricular outflow tract, particularly *component 4*, can also be involved. The four components that make up the normal left ventricle (B) typically are not involved in Ebstein's anomaly: *component 1* is the mitral valve and the atrioventricular septum. *Component 2* is the trabeculated left ventricular sinus septum. *Component 3* is the smooth upper component of the ventricular septum that carries the left bundle branches of the conduction system. *Component 3* on the left ventricular side is confluent with *component 3* on the right ventricular side that also carries the conduction system (the right bundle branch). On the left ventricular side, *component 4* is the distal conal septum. We regard left ventricular *component 3* as the proximal conal septum. Left ventricular *components 1* and *2* make up the normal left ventricular inflow tract. *Components 3 and 4* make up the normal left ventricular outflow tract. Typically, but far from always, only right ventricular *components 1* and *2* are involved in Ebstein's anomaly. When we talk about the conus or the infundibulum (not otherwise qualified), we mean component 4; this is the part that is abnormal in conotruncal malformations such as tetralogy of Fallot and transposition of the great arteries, etc.: the distal or subsemilunar conus/infundibulum. *Component 3* is the proximal part of the infundibulum that is involved in anomalous muscle bundles of the right ventricle. *Component 3* appears to be the "mother" of the right and left ventricular sinuses *(component 2)*. The trabeculated ventricular sinuses outpouch beneath *component 3*, forming the most effective pumping portions of both ventricles. *Component 3* and the ventricular sinuses never dissociate; for example, the right ventricular sinus and the septal band never dissociate: the RV sinus is always located just beneath the septal and moderator bands. By contrast, *component 4* and the ventricular sinuses do dissociate or separate from one another. *Component 4* can be located almost entirely above the right ventricle; or *component 4* can override the ventricular septum to any degree; *component 4* can be located almost entirely above the left ventricle. Why this dissociation? Because the subsemilunar conus "belongs to" the great arteries, i.e., the conotruncal segment, not to the ventricular sinuses. (Reproduced with permission from Van Praagh R, Geva T, Kreutzer J: Ventricular septal defects: how shall we describe, name and classify them? *J Am Coll Cardiol* 1989;14;1298.)

the patient has no tricuspid valve and *two pulmonary valves,* one above the other. The upper one is the real pulmonary valve. The lower one is a markedly displaced tricuspid valve leaflet remnant. It looks as though the tricuspid valve has been rotated down into the right ventricular cavity and then upward to just under the pulmonary valve. The axis of this apparent tricuspid valvar rotation is its anteroseptal commissure. This is the point around which the downward, anterior, and then the upward rotation of the tricuspid valve appears to have occurred.

It should be understood that our conventional description of *downward* displacement of the septal leaflet of the tricuspid valve (compared with its normal location) is exactly backwards, from a developmental or embryologic standpoint. In normal development, the septal leaflet delaminates or separates from the underlying ventricular septum and *ascends* toward the right atrioventricular junction.[8] This upward ascent of the septal leaflet of the tricuspid valve is normally associated with the laying down of right ventricular septal surface myocardium beneath the delaminated and ascending septal leaflet of the tricuspid valve.[8,9] This is why there is no right ventricular septal surface myocardium above the unascended septal leaflet of the tricuspid valve in Ebstein's anomaly. Thus, it should be understood that in typical Ebstein's malformation, the septal (and often the posterior) leaflets are not really downwardly displaced; instead, *they have failed to ascend.*

Deficiency of right ventricular myocardium in Ebstein's malformation is not confined to the septal surface (of the "atrialized" right ventricle). Right ventricular myocardial deficiency also typically involves the diaphragmatic surface of the "atrialized" right ventricular *free wall,* where it forms an *aneurysm* that can be progressive and that may be associated with a characteristic right intraventricular block pattern electrocardiographically.

Right ventricular free wall myocardial deficiency or absence can also involve the anterior wall, where it forms the picture known as *Uhl's disease*[10] *(parchment right ventricle).*

Thus, Ebstein's anomaly is a tricuspid valvar, an atrioventricular junctional, and a right ventricular (sinus) malformation. The infundibulum typically is not malformed, as in Ebstein's original patient[2] (Fig. 13.1B).

Ebstein's anomaly clearly indicates the important distinction between the right ventricle (i.e., the right ventricular sinus, body, or inflow tract) on the one hand, and the conus arteriosus (infundibulum or outflow tract) on the other. Ebstein's malformation is a dysplasia of the tricuspid portion of the atrioventricular canal (Fig. 13.5A, component 1) and of the right ventricular sinus (Fig. 13.5A, component 2), but typically not of the proximal or distal parts of the conus (Fig. 13.5A, components 3 and 4, respectively). Ebstein's anomaly also indicates the very close relationship that exists between the development of the right ventricle (i.e., the right ventricular sinus) and the tricuspid valve (and vice versa).

The tricuspid valve may be described as myogenic, whereas the mitral valve is fibrogenic. It is worth recalling that in many birds, the tricuspid valve consists of a muscular strap (a free wall "leaflet") with no septal leaflet.[11]

In this sense, birds normally have something akin to Ebstein's malformation in man. However, birds are much more left ventricular dominant than we are. Flying appears to be much harder work than walking. Consequently, the avian interventricular septum bulges into the right ventricular cavity much more than it does in man. Hence, the free-wall tricuspid leaflet in birds (corresponding to the anterior and posterior tricuspid leaflets in man) coapts against the ventricular septum, resulting in a competent "tricuspid" (i.e., right atrioventricular) valve. Hemodynamically, therefore, birds do not need a septal leaflet of the right atrioventricular valve, whereas humans usually do. (Anecdotally, some drug addicts have survived, despite loss of the septal leaflet of the tricuspid valve because of bacterial endocarditis. Nonetheless, a normal septal leaflet and a competent tricuspid valve are highly desirable hemodynamically for most humans, as Ebstein's anomaly indicates.)

The atrioventricular endocardial cushions, which may be regarded as fibrogenic, initially open only into the left ventricle and they form the mitral valve. Rarely, a primitive tricuspid valve can be an entirely muscular structure in human beings (Fig. 13.6). Normally, the tricuspid valve undergoes demuscularization, resulting in a fibrous tricuspid valve. But this process of tricuspid demuscularization is often incomplete, particularly high up, close to the origins of the anterior and posterior leaflets.

Thus, Ebstein's anomaly suggests that we do not fully understand the normal and abnormal morphogenesis of the atrioventricular canal or junction. In our considerations of the embryology of the malformation known as common atrioventricular canal (also known as atrioventricular septal defect), we usually assume that everything can be understood as various kinds of defects of the atrioventricular endocardial cushions. But Ebstein's anomaly is telling us that our conventional understanding of the morphogenesis of the atrioventricular canal region is oversimplified. There is more to it than just the atrioventricular endocardial cushions. The tricuspid valve has an

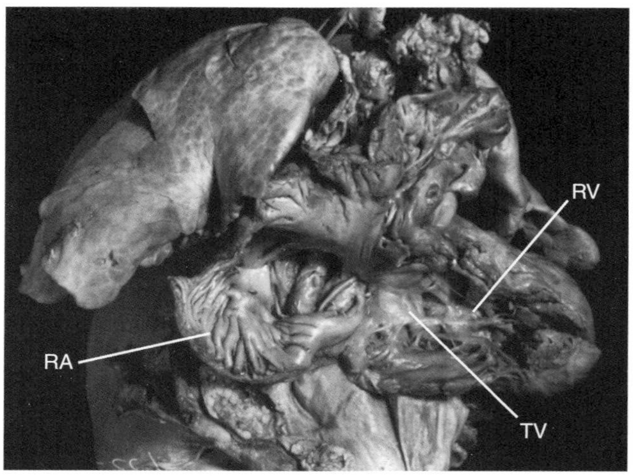

Fig. 13.6 Two-week-old boy with pulmonary valvar atresia, intact ventricular septum and ***muscular tricuspid valve*** *(TV);* i.e., the tricuspid leaflets have not undergone demuscularization. This patient's older brother also had pulmonary atresia (valvar) with intact ventricular septum and congenitally unguarded tricuspid orifice: the present patient (in the above figure) is part of *familial* pulmonary atresia with intact ventricular septum and right ventricular dysplasia. It is very rare to find all three tricuspid leaflets completely muscularized, as in this patient. *RA,* Right atrium; *RV,* right ventricle.

important myogenic component, as Ebstein's anomaly dramatically illustrates and as the rare anomaly of **muscular tricuspid valve** (Fig. 13.6) also indicates.

7. *From a functional standpoint,* Ebstein's anomaly can result in congenital tricuspid regurgitation (insufficiency), or congenital tricuspid stenosis, or tricuspid atresia (when the tricuspid valve is imperforate), as will be seen.
8. Ebstein's anomaly occurs in various *different settings or complexes,* as Dr. Maurice Lev would say. Ebstein's anomaly may or may not be an isolated malformation. These various different settings are of great clinical, diagnostic, and surgical importance, as will be seen.

STUDY OF EBSTEIN'S ANOMALY OF THE TRICUSPID VALVE AND RIGHT VENTRICLE

This study of the pathologic anatomy of all forms of Ebstein's malformation was based on 78 postmortem cases, which constituted 2.43% of the 3216 autopsied cases of congenital heart disease in this series as a whole (the database on which this book is based). (Note: 184 postmortem cases of *acquired* heart disease bring the total database to 3400 cases.)

Gender: males = 39; females = 35; and not known = 4. Thus the male/female ratio = 39/35 = 1.11/1. Hence, no significant gender preponderance was found.

Age at death ($n = 69$) or cardiac transplantation ($n = 4$): mean = 3.92 ± 6.77 years; range = 0 (abortus or stillborn) to 25 years; and median = 2.5 months (10 weeks). The median age at death was surprisingly young, indicating that Ebstein's anomaly with or without associated malformations in our pediatric population of patients was often a lethal, rapidly fatal anomaly.

Only 4 of 78 heart specimens were explants following cardiac transplantation (5%). Consequently, the above-mentioned statistics do indeed refer almost always (95%) to the age at death, not to the age at cardiac transplantation.

Is this a Children's Hospital Boston series of cases, that is, a single-institution series? No, in the sense that 27 of these 78 cases (35%) were consultations from other institutions from as far away as Marseille, France; but yes in the sense that all of these cases were studied in the Cardiac Registry of Children's Hospital Boston.

The anatomic settings in which Ebstein's anomaly occurred are summarized in Table 13.2.

As Table 13.2 indicates, Ebstein's anomaly occurs in (at least) four different settings:

1. **Ebstein's anomaly** (not otherwise qualified). We could not call it "isolated" Ebstein's malformation because, as will be seen, this—the most common form of Ebstein's (53%)—was often associated with additional anomalies (tricuspid regurgitation, stenosis, atresia, regurgitation and stenosis, secundum atrial septal defect, etc.).
2. **Ebstein's anomaly in the setting of pulmonary valvar atresia or severe stenosis with intact ventricular septum** occurred in 14 patients (18%, Table 13.2).
3. **Left-sided Ebstein's anomaly with discordant L-loop ventricles** was found in 14 patients (18% of this series, Table 13.2).
4. **Ebstein's anomaly with the incomplete form of common atrioventricular canal** was present in 9 patients (12%, Table 13.2).

Now let us consider each of these four groups in detail because, as will be seen, each is clinically and surgically very different from the others.

Ebstein's Anomaly With Tricuspid Regurgitation

Ebstein's anomaly of the tricuspid valve and right ventricle *with tricuspid regurgitation* was the single largest group in this study, although it comprised only 25 of 78 cases (32%) (Table 13.2). This is what most people mean when they speak of "typical" Ebstein's anomaly, even though this subset constituted only slightly less than one-third of all of our cases.

Gender: males, 10; females, 13; and unknown, 2. The male/female ratio in this subset was 0.77/1.

Age at death ($n = 24$): mean, 6.26 years ± 7.48 years; range, 0 to 20 years; and median, 1.67 years. There were 3 abortus, who were regarded as having a postnatal life = 0. The foregoing data refer only to ages at postnatal death.

Language note: *Abortus* is a fourth declension, masculine Latin noun: abortus, -ūs, meaning a miscarriage. Consequently, the correct plural of *abortus* is abortūs, or simply *abortus* (without the macron).

The foregoing concerns only the ages at *death;* that is, there were no cardiac transplants, leading to living patients, in this group.

Important associated findings: Clinically and surgically important findings that were associated with these 25 postmortem cases of Ebstein's anomaly of the tricuspid valve and right ventricle with tricuspid regurgitation are summarized in Table 13.3.

TABLE 13.2 Ebstein's Anomaly: The Anatomic Settings ($n = 78$)

Settings	No. of Cases	%* of Series
1. Ebstein's anomaly (not otherwise	41	53
qualified)	25	32
(a) With tricuspid regurgitation	11	14
(b) With tricuspid stenosis	2	3
(c) With tricuspid atresia	1	1
(d) With tricuspid regurgitation and	2	3
tricuspid stenosis		
(e) Without tricuspid regurgitation		
or tricuspid stenosis		
2. Ebstein's anomaly with pulmonary	14	18
atresia or severe stenosis and intact	12	15
ventricular septum	2	3
(a) With tricuspid regurgitation		
(b) With tricuspid stenosis		
3. Left-sided Ebstein's anomaly	14	18
(a) With tricuspid regurgitation	12	15
(b) With tricuspid stenosis	2	3
4. Ebstein's anomaly with incompletely	9	12
common atrioventricular canal	6	8
(a) With tricuspid atresia (4) or	3	4
tricuspid stenosis (2)		
(b) With tricuspid regurgitation		

*All percentages are rounded off to the nearest whole number.

TABLE 13.3 Ebstein's Anomaly With Tricuspid Regurgitation: Important Associated Findings (n = 25)

Associated Findings	No. of Cases	%* of Series
Secundum atrial septal defect	13	52
Cyanosis	7	28
Partial absence of tricuspid leaflets	6	24
Ventricular septal defect	6	24
Conoventricular	5	20
Muscular	3	12
Heart failure	6	24
Pulmonary stenosis, valvar	6	24
Sudden arrhythmic death	5	20
Biventricular pathology	4	16
History of paroxysmal atrial tachycardia/supraventricular tachycardia/Wolff-Parkinson-White syndrome	3	12
Uhl's disease of the right ventricle (parchment right ventricle)	2	8
Prominent right ventricular diaphragmatic aneurysm	3	12
Prominent Eustachian valve of the inferior vena cava	3	12
Multiple congenital anomalies (cardiovascular and noncardiovascular)	3	12
Chromosomal anomaly	2	8
Left superior vena cava to coronary sinus to right atrium	2	8
History of prior syncope	1	4
Tetralogy of Fallot {S,D,S}	1	4
Transposition of the great arteries {S,D,D}	1	4
Double-outlet right ventricle {S,D,D}	1	4
Congenital mitral stenosis	1	4
Subacute bacterial endocarditis of stenotic mitral valve	1	4
Double-orifice mitral valve	1	4
Mitral atresia with hypoplastic left heart syndrome	1	4
Dysplasia of left ventricle	1	4
Aortic stenosis, supravalvar	1	4
Aortic atresia, valvar	1	4
Pulmonary regurgitation	1	4
Myxomatous change of all four cardiac valve leaflets	1	4
Aneurysm of the right horn of the sinus venosus	1	4
Diverticulum of right atrioventricular junction	1	4

*All percentages are rounded off to the nearest whole number.

A secundum type of atrial septal defect was the most common associated malformation (13 cases, 52%, Table 13.3), as in Ebstein's original patient (Fig. 13.1A)[2] and as in **Case 1** of our series (Fig. 13.7A).

Partial absence of the tricuspid valve leaflets was one of the second most common associated anomalies (6 patients, 24%, Table 13.3). The septal leaflet of the tricuspid valve may be partially absent (Fig. 13.1A) or totally absent; and the posterior leaflet of the tricuspid valve can be deficient or absent, particularly adjacent to the septal surface of the atrialized right ventricle.

This deficiency or absence of the septal and posterior leaflets of the tricuspid valve is associated with downward displacement of these tricuspid leaflets, or leaflet remnants, toward the septal and moderator bands, and away from or beneath the right atrial–right ventricular junction. Downward displacement and leaflet deficiency or absence of the septal and posterior leaflets of the tricuspid valve are integral parts of Ebstein's anomaly.

Indeed, if the origins of the septal and posterior leaflets of the tricuspid valve are not downwardly displaced below the right atrioventricular junction, that is, if there is no atrialized right ventricle, then we do not make the diagnosis of Ebstein's anomaly. An Ebstein's-like anomaly may be present, but not typical Ebstein's malformation.

Deficiency or absence of the septal and posterior leaflets of the tricuspid valve in typical Ebstein's malformation often means that the deep curtain-like anterior leaflet has no leaflet against which it can coapt, resulting, as noted heretofore, in tricuspid regurgitation.

Although the origin of the anterior leaflet of the tricuspid valve typically is not downwardly displaced beneath the right atrioventricular junction, this leaflet is very abnormal in other respects: it is deep, curtain-like, myxomatous, and with reduction of interchordal spaces. The anterior papillary musculature is much smaller than normal. The insertion of the anterior leaflet can be broad, right into the right ventricular free wall (Figs. 13.2 and 13.3).

The normal origin of the anterior tricuspid leaflet and the very low origins of the septal and posterior leaflets means that the atrialized right ventricle is bizarrely asymmetrical: high laterally and low medially. Consequently, the annulus of the tricuspid leaflets in Ebstein's anomaly is much larger than normal and is at very different levels, which often predisposes to tricuspid regurgitation. So, too, does functional hypoplasia or absence of the septal and posterior leaflets.

The heart of an 8-month-old girl with typical Ebstein's malformation is shown in Fig. 13.2. Note the small secundum atrial septal defect or stretched patent foramen ovale (Figs. 13.2A and 13.7A); the downward displacement of the septal leaflet of the tricuspid valve (Fig. 13.2A); the atrialized right ventricle between the downwardly displaced septal leaflet below and the atrioventricular junction above (Fig. 13.2A); the smooth septal surface of the atrialized right ventricle—smooth because it is covered by no trabeculated right ventricular septal surface myocardium above the downwardly displaced septal leaflet of the tricuspid valve (Fig. 13.2A); and the very deep curtain-like anterior leaflet of the tricuspid valve (Fig. 13.2A).

The malformation of the anterior leaflet of the tricuspid valve is also functionally important. This large and deep anterior leaflet appears to insert directly into the right ventricular free wall (Figs. 13.2A, 13.4, and 13.7). Why? Because there are few or no interchordal spaces. Consequently, the chordae tendineae are not apparent. They are not free, readily visible structures. Although present, they are abnormally surrounded by leaflet tissue and hence at first glance appear to be absent. The surrounded chordae tendineae are thus disguised as leaflet tissue; but the chordae are revealed by careful inspection and by transillumination.

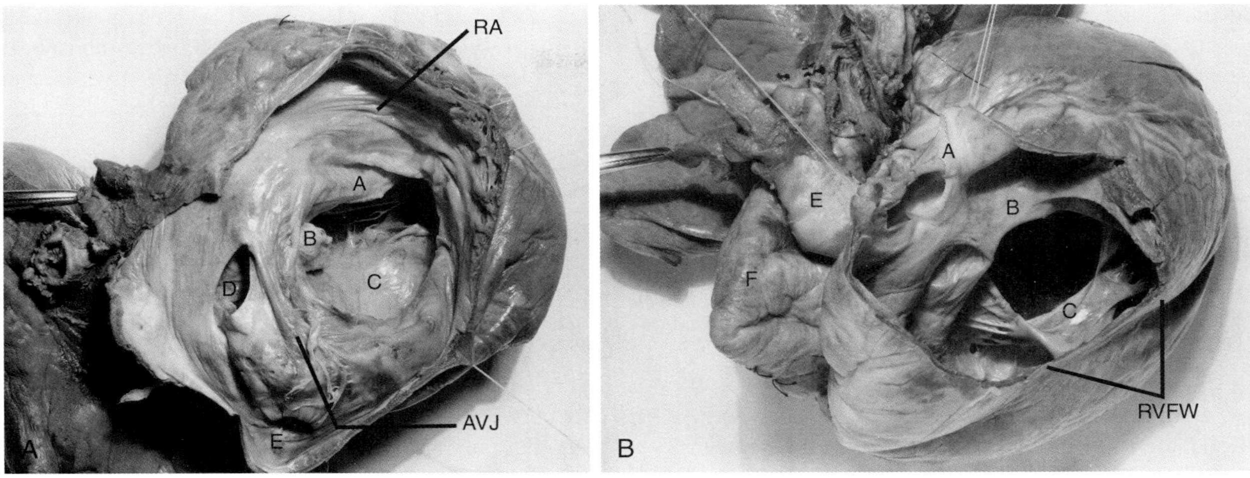

Fig. 13.7 Ebstein's anomaly with pulmonary valvar stenosis, tricuspid regurgitation, secundum atrial septal defect, large right-to-left shunt at the atrial level, and cyanosis since birth. The patient was an 11-year-old boy who received a classical Glenn anastomosis (right superior vena cava–to–right pulmonary artery) in 1962. The operation was complicated by bradycardia, cardiac dilatation, ventricular fibrillation, and intraoperative death. These are the cardiac photos that were taken at the time of autopsy. (A) The opened right atrium *(RA)* and atrialized right ventricle (the right ventricular inflow tract), viewed from above. The large secundum type of atrial septal defect *(D)* measured 22 × 12 mm. The anterior leaflet of the tricuspid valve *(A)* is deep and curtain-like, and its origin is from the right atrioventricular junction (not downwardly displaced). The septal leaflet of the tricuspid valve *(B)* is hypoplastic and downwardly displaced. The posterior leaflet *(C)* is markedly downwardly displaced beneath the right atrioventricular junction *(AVJ)*. The inferior vena cava *(E)* is also seen. Note that the tricuspid leaflets do not coapt, explaining the tricuspid regurgitation. (The right lateral atrioventricular junction has not been cut through.) (B) The ventricularized right ventricle (below the tricuspid valve) and the right ventricular outflow tract. *A* is the stenotic unopened pulmonary annulus. The septal band *(B)* and the moderator band are strikingly thin and attenuated. The posterior leaflet of the tricuspid valve *(C)* is markedly downwardly displaced, close to the right ventricular apex; some of the chordae tendineae of the posterior leaflet are seen, but the interchordal spaces are filled with fibrous leaflet-like tissue. Note how very thin the right ventricular free wall *(RVFW)* is, even of the ventricularized right ventricle; this is a Uhl's disease–like feature, often seen with Ebstein's anomaly of the tricuspid valve and right ventricle. The right atrium *(F)* is markedly hypertrophied and enlarged. *E* is the ascending aorta.

The right ventricular free wall papillary muscles are very small, numerous, and spread out. The papillary musculature is thus diffuse, instead of being normally concentrated to form the anterior papillary muscle of the right ventricle.

The lack of free chordae tendineae of the anterior (and posterior) leaflets of the tricuspid valve means that in Ebstein's anomaly, the *parietal* leaflet of the tricuspid valve (i.e., the anterior and the posterior leaflets) are tethered to the right ventricular parietal or free wall. The failure of formation of interchordal spaces explains why the chordae tendineae of the anterior and the posterior leaflets seem to be so short.

The "free" margin of the anterior and posterior tricuspid leaflets may be attached to the right ventricular free wall (Fig. 13.2A); that is, there really may be no *free* leaflet margins. Or, the free margins of the anterior and posterior leaflets may be much too close to the right ventricular free wall—tethered to the right ventricular free wall, but not fused with it.

Both situations are functional disasters. The fused or tethered free margins of the anterior and posterior leaflets cannot move normally toward and coapt with the septal leaflet (if functionally present) of the tricuspid valve.

Thus, the downward displacement of the deficient or absent *septal* and *posterior* leaflets, and the tethering or fusion of what normally should be the free margin of the *anterior* leaflet of the tricuspid valve combine to result in tricuspid regurgitation that is often severe in typical Ebstein's anomaly. Hence, all three leaflets (septal, posterior, and anterior) can be involved in the production of tricuspid regurgitation.

As mentioned heretofore, it should be reiterated that the origin of the anterior tricuspid leaflet is from the right atrioventricular junction; that is, the origin of the anterior leaflet of the tricuspid valve in Ebstein's' anomaly is *not* downwardly displaced in typical cases. But this, too, results in another geometric problem in typical Ebstein's malformation. The origin of the tricuspid valve, that is, the tricuspid "ring," is at very different levels, and is both deformed and enlarged. The origin of the anterior leaflet laterally is at the normal height, that is, at the right atrioventricular junction. But as one goes posteriorly, the origin of the posterior leaflet often dips down well below the right atrioventricular junction; or part of the posterior leaflet can be absent (the origin can be broken, or cease to exist, at this point). When one reaches the ventricular septum medially, the origin of the septal leaflet is often displaced markedly downward to the level of the septal and moderator bands, or the septal leaflet can be partially or totally absent (Fig. 13.1A).

Thus, the tricuspid valve in typical Ebstein's malformation is seated very abnormally into the right ventricle: Normally high laterally (anterior leaflet); very low or absent medially (septal leaflet); with the high and low levels of leaflet origin being joined posteriorly (posterior leaflet).

The abnormal locations of the origins of the septal and posterior leaflets of the tricuspid valve in Ebstein's anomaly indicate where the right ventricular sinus myocardium is (or is not).

Explanation: How far down is the septal leaflet of the tricuspid valve in Ebstein's anomaly? The septal leaflet is displaced down to where the right ventricular myocardium has formed. In severe cases, the septal leaflet is displaced all the way down to where the infundibulum begins, that is, down to the septal and moderator bands (that are proximal infundibular structures).

When there is partial absence of septal leaflet or posterior leaflet tissue, this means that both the right ventricular myocardium and the tricuspid leaflet tissue have focally failed to form. This closely interrelated developmental process involves the so-called delamination of the tricuspid leaflet tissue, and immediately below that the laying down of right ventricular sinus myocardium septally and posteroinferiorly.[8,9] The downwardly displaced septal and posterior tricuspid leaflet tissue in Ebstein's anomaly is an eye-catching marker of the *failure of ascent* of these tricuspid leaflets and of the related failure of right ventricular myocardial morphogenesis above these unascended tricuspid leaflets.

Sudden arrhythmic death was also relatively frequent in this subset: 5 of 25 patients (20%, Table 13.3). As mentioned above, this is what happened to Ebstein's patient: sudden, unexpected arrhythmic death.[2]

Ebstein's anomaly is a well-known and important cause of electrocardiographic and electrophysiologic abnormalities, including right ventricular conduction delay, P-R interval prolongation, and Wolff-Parkinson-White (WPW) syndrome (in 10% to 25% of patients).[12] Arrhythmias with Ebstein's malformation are common, increase with age, and include supraventricular tachycardia, atrial flutter, and atrial fibrillation.[13,14] When present, accessory conducting pathways are usually single (62%).[15] Such accessory pathways can be located in the right atrioventricular free wall, or they can be right septal in 34%, or atrioventricular nodal, or multiple in 29%.[15]

Ebstein's anomaly is an important cause not only of supraventricular tachyarrhythmias, but also of sudden, unexpected, arrhythmic death presumably related to ventricular tachycardia progressing to ventricular fibrillation (20%, Table 13.3).

The *lack* of a normally formed, fibrous, right atrioventricular junction that normally insulates and separates the right atrium from the ventricles—except at the penetrating atrioventricular bundle of His—is thought to provide an anatomic substrate that is vulnerable to ventricular preexcitation (WPW syndrome) and to catastrophic ventricular tachyarrhythmias. Hence, sudden unexpected arrhythmic death is an important part of the natural history of Ebstein's malformation of the tricuspid valve, *right atrioventricular junction,* and right ventricular sinus.

Ventricular septal defect was also a frequent abnormality associated with Ebstein's anomaly with tricuspid regurgitation: 6 of 25 patients (24%, Table 13.3) (Fig. 13.2B). High conoventricular ventricular septal defects (between the conal septum above and the ventricular septum below) were slightly more common (5) than muscular ventricular septal defects (3) (Table 13.3) that were often midmuscular—between the smooth non-trabeculated left ventricular septal surface superiorly and the finely trabeculated more apical left ventricular septal surface inferiorly.

Heart failure was a prominent clinical feature in 6 of these patients (24%) (Table 13.3). The mean age at death of these patients in which heart failure was reported was 6.96 years ± 8.24 years, ranging from 14 hours to 17 4/12 years. The median age at death was 4 2/12 years.

We regard the *median* age at death, as opposed to the *mean* age at death, as more accurately indicative of the true situation. The mean age at death was skewed to an older age by the presence of two teenagers in this series (16 2/12 years and 17 4/12 years). Thus, Ebstein's anomaly with tricuspid regurgitation and congestive heart failure is a serious situation, accurately reflected by the young median age at death (4 2/12 years).

One of our youngest patients with congestive heart failure was a 2-day-old female infant who presented with hydrops fetalis. She had congestive heart failure both prenatally and postnatally. Autopsy (in 1992) revealed ascites and bilateral pleural effusions. Her Ebstein's anomaly was characterized by a deep, curtain-like anterior leaflet with reduction of interchordal spaces, marked downward displacement of the origin of the septal leaflet (maximal downward displacement = 17 mm), and functional absence of the septal and posterior leaflets. The pulmonary leaflets were thickened and myxomatous, and had a blood cyst. Tricuspid regurgitation was very marked. Right atrial hypertrophy and enlargement were severe and a relatively large ostium secundum type of atrial septal defect (7 mm in diameter) coexisted. A prominent Eustachian valve of the inferior vena cava was also noted and was thought to be of no functional significance.

Thus, heart failure was even more important as an immediate cause of death (24%) than were arrhythmias (20%) (Table 13.3).

Cyanosis was reported in 7 of these 25 patients (28%, Table 13.3). This finding was eye-catching because one does not ordinarily think of Ebstein's anomaly as a form of cyanotic congenital heart disease; and usually it was not (72%, Table 13.3).

The ages at death of these patients with Ebstein's malformation, tricuspid regurgitation, and *cyanosis* were older than in the previous group with congestive heart failure. In the 7 patients with cyanosis, the ages at death were as follows: mean, 9.88 years ± 6.84 years; range, 4 months to 17 8/12 years; and median 11 years.

Why were these patients with Ebstein's anomaly and tricuspid regurgitation cyanotic? (Table 13.3.) There appeared to be four different groups:

1. *Isolated Ebstein's anomaly,* as in **Case 6** (Fig. 13.3A and B). This 8 3/12-year-old girl was found at autopsy to have marked cardiomegaly. Her heart weighed 322 grams, compared with normal controls for the age of 160 grams (2.01/1, or 101% greater than normal). Cyanosis had appeared at 4½ years of age because of right-to-left shunting through an ostium secundum atrial septal defect (a 10 × 3 mm defect). Congestive heart failure appeared at 6 years of age. The patient died at 8 3/12 years of age during cardiac catheterization (in 1951) from a ventricular tachyarrhythmia.

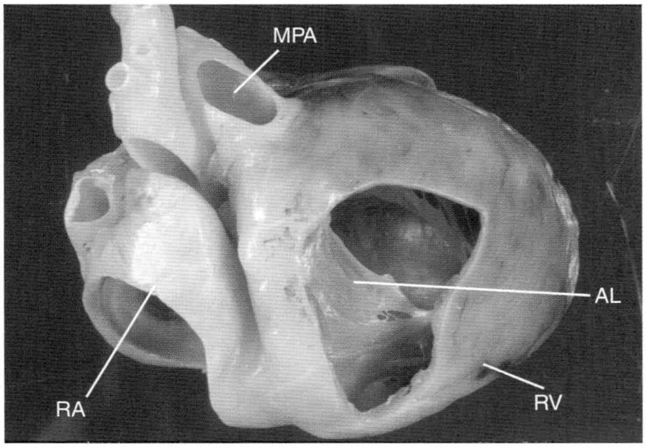

Fig. 13.8 This is the waxed-heart specimen of a 25-year-old man with Ebstein's anomaly and tricuspid regurgitation (our Case 19). Through the window that has been cut in the right ventricular free wall *(RV)*, one can see the deep curtain-like anterior leaflet *(AL)* of the tricuspid valve—typical of Ebstein's anomaly. The free margin of the anterior leaflet is *not* thickened or rolled, consistent with normal leaflet function. There are almost no interchordal spaces, because they are filled by leaflet-like fibrous tissue. Note how very thin the right ventricular free wall is. Despite this Uhl's disease–like component of this patient's Ebstein's anomaly, he had no hemodynamic problems. Instead, his problems were electrophysiologic: Wolff-Parkinson-White (WPW) syndrome, with a history of many episodes of paroxysmal atrial tachycardia and atrial flutter, for which he was treated with quinidine (in 1974). His WPW syndrome was complicated by ventricular fibrillation, leading to death. He was thought to have *no* tricuspid regurgitation or stenosis. He had **isolation of the left atrial** appendage: the cavity within the left atrial appendage did not communication with the main left atrial cavity. To our knowledge, isolation of the left atrial appendage is of no functional significance. *MPA,* Main pulmonary artery; *RA,* right atrium.

Thus, typical isolated Ebstein's anomaly (Fig. 13.8) can develop cyanosis when/if right-to-left shunting occurs at the atrial level through a secundum atrial septal defect or a stretched patent foramen ovale. This phenomenon also occurred in our **Case 24** (2 of 7 patients, 29%).

2. *Ebstein's anomaly with pulmonary stenosis*, as in our Case 1 (Fig. 13.7). This 11-year-old boy with Ebstein's malformation, tricuspid regurgitation, a secundum atrial septal defect, supravalvar pulmonary stenosis, and supravalvar aortic stenosis was cyanotic at birth. He developed intraoperative ventricular fibrillation leading to death in 1962. Chronic cyanosis was associated with marked clubbing (digital osteoarthropathy). Cyanosis *at birth* was thought to be due to the coexistence of congenital pulmonary stenosis, most marked at the top of the pulmonary sinuses of Valsalva, hence often called "supravalvar" pulmonary stenosis. This is really a form of pulmonary valvar stenosis, the tops of the pulmonary sinuses of Valsalva being part of the pulmonary valve (the so-called "annulus" or "ring," as opposed to the leaflets).
3. *Ebstein's anomaly with Uhl's disease*, that is, parchment right ventricle that is marked and widespread, often involving the anterior and the diaphragmatic portions of the right ventricular free wall, as in our Cases 47 and 75 (Table 13.3).

Case 47 was a $1\frac{8}{12}$-year-old boy with Ebstein's and severe tricuspid regurgitation. The right ventricular free wall was almost paper thin (2 mm). A secundum atrial septal defect measured 7×4 mm. In addition to Uhl's disease, this boy also had "supravalvar" pulmonary stenosis; the top of the pulmonary sinuses of Valsalva had an internal diameter of 9 mm, while the bottom of the pulmonary sinuses of Valsalva had an internal diameter of 12 mm. Right-to-left atrial shunting resulted in cyanosis and clubbing.

Case 75 was a $14\frac{1}{12}$-year-old girl who also had marked and widespread Uhl's disease. Her secundum atrial septal defect was small and her pulmonary valve leaflets and annulus were mildly hypoplastic, but not otherwise malformed. Right atrial hypertrophy and enlargement were moderately marked. Left atrial hypertrophy and enlargement were mild to moderate.

Left ventricular hypertrophy was very marked, so much so that this young woman had a form of hypertrophic cardiomyopathy of the left ventricle, but without asymmetric septal hypertrophy and without idiopathic hypertrophic subaortic stenosis. Given that this teenager had widespread Uhl's disease of the right ventricle, she had a functionally single left ventricle, which may explain her marked concentric left ventricular hypertrophy (hypothesis). It is also noteworthy that patients with Ebstein's anomaly can have significant *biventricular pathology*.

At $9\frac{9}{12}$ years of age, the patient underwent a classical Glenn anastomosis between the right superior vena cava and the right pulmonary artery. This anastomosis remained large and unobstructed.

After dancing, she suffered syncope because of documented ventricular fibrillation leading to death (in 1979). Subpleural venous lakes were found at autopsy in the right lung. Such pulmonary venous "lakes" are associated with systemic venous blood flow that goes directly to the lungs, bypassing the liver. Lack of hepatic venous blood flow to the lungs may lead to the formation of pulmonary venous lakes, perhaps because of the lack of a still mysterious "hepatic factor." Systemic venous blood going directly to the lungs (as in Glenn shunts or Fontan operations) also is nonpulsatile, which also may predispose to pulmonary venous lakes. Such lakes are not fully understood at the present time.

This case illustrates that typical Ebstein's with Uhl's disease is compatible with life into the teenage years. Note how thin the right ventricular free wall can be in patients with Ebstein's anomaly even when we did *not* make the diagnosis of Uhl's disease (Fig. 13.7). This is the heart of a 25-year-old man **(Case 19)** who died in 1974. He had WPW syndrome, with a history of many episodes of paroxysmal atrial tachycardia with atrial flutter. Treatment with quinidine was followed by ventricular fibrillation and death. Despite the thinness of his right ventricular free wall, his problems were electrophysiologic, not hemodynamic.

4. *Ebstein's anomaly with cyanotic congenital heart disease* (Table 13.3) was illustrated by **Case 43,** a 4-month-old boy with *tetralogy of Fallot* (Fig. 13.9), and by **Case 45,** a $16\frac{2}{12}$-year-old young woman with *D-transposition of the great arteries* (Fig. 13.10).

In somewhat greater detail, the patient with tetralogy of Fallot {S,D,S} also had a large secundum atrial septal defect (10×4 mm) and hence had *pentalogy of Fallot*. In addition to

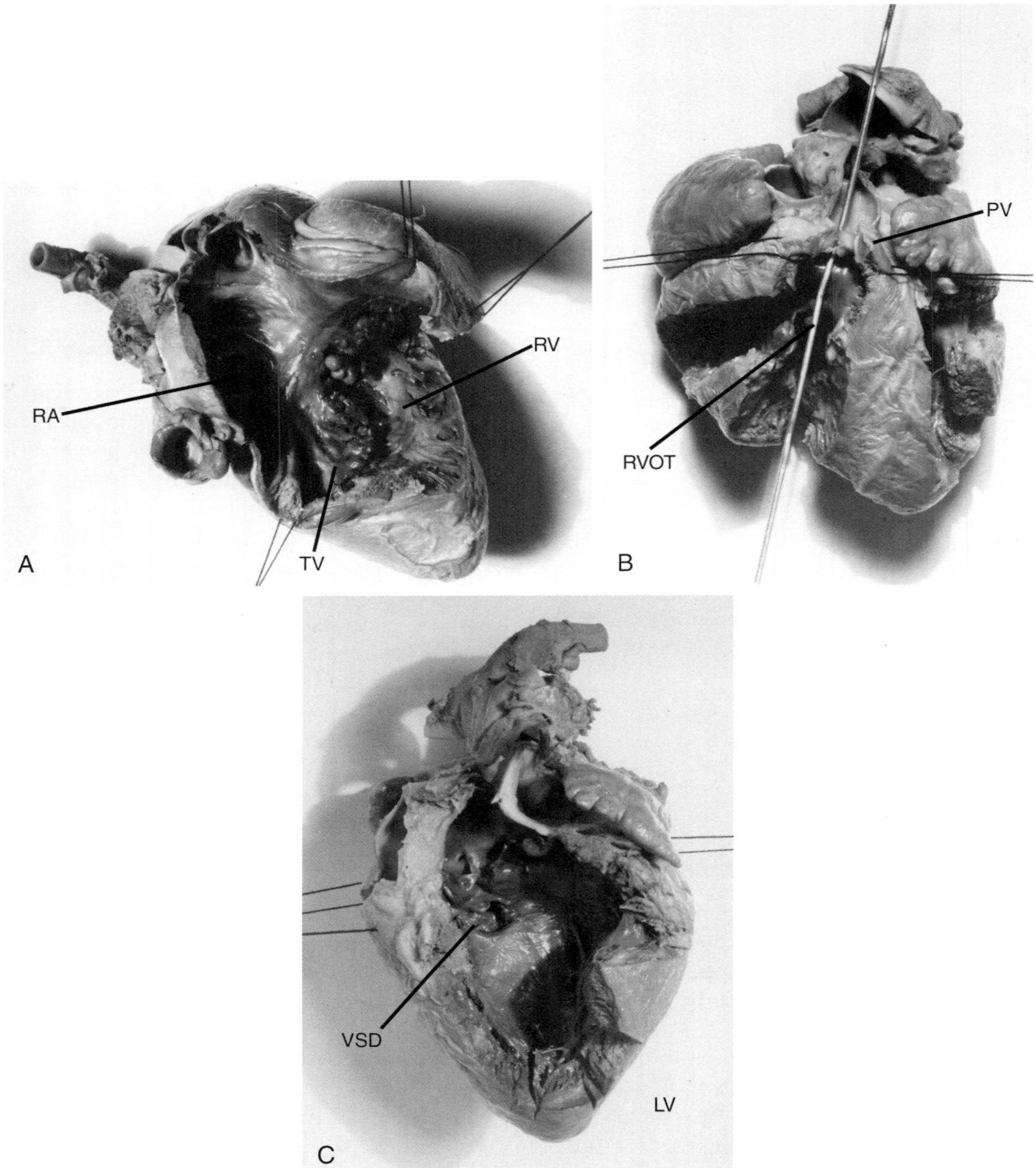

Fig. 13.9 This is the heart of Case 43, a 4-month-old boy with Ebstein's malformation of the tricuspid valve *(TV)* and tricuspid regurgitation, with pentalogy of Fallot {S,D,S} and multiple congenital anomalies. (A) The opened right atrium *(RA)* and right ventricular inflow tract *(RV)*. (B) The stenotic right ventricular outflow tract *(RVOT)*. (C) The opened left ventricle *(LV)* and the ventricular septal defect *(VSD)*. This patient with Ebstein's anomaly and tetralogy of Fallot had a large (10 × 4 mm) secundum atrial septal defect (hence pentalogy of Fallot), a persistent left superior vena cava to the coronary sinus to the right atrium, a thick bicuspid pulmonary valve *(PV)* 4 mm in diameter, congenital absence of the left kidney, bilateral undescended testes, absence of the distal portion of the vas deferens, lissencephaly (familial), subnormal brain weight (350/510 grams) and thrombosis of an end-to-end left Blalock-Taussig anastomosis (in 1961), which led to death 2 days postoperatively. These photos were taken at the time of autopsy.

Ebstein's anomaly with tricuspid regurgitation and a persistent left superior vena cava to the coronary sinus and thence to the right atrium, he also had *multiple congenital anomalies:* congenital absence of the left kidney; bilaterally undescended testes with absence of the distal vas deferens; and familial lissencephaly. The patient's brain weighed less than normal for his age (370/510 grams).

The pulmonary valve had thick myxomatous leaflets (1.5 mm); this valve was bicuspid and 4 mm in internal diameter.

The tricuspid valve displayed marked downward displacement of the septal and posterior leaflets (10 mm down, Fig. 13.9). The septal leaflet was very small, with warty growths at its margin, and was nonfunctional (noncoapting). The anterior tricuspid leaflet was curtain-like, with a wide attachment to the

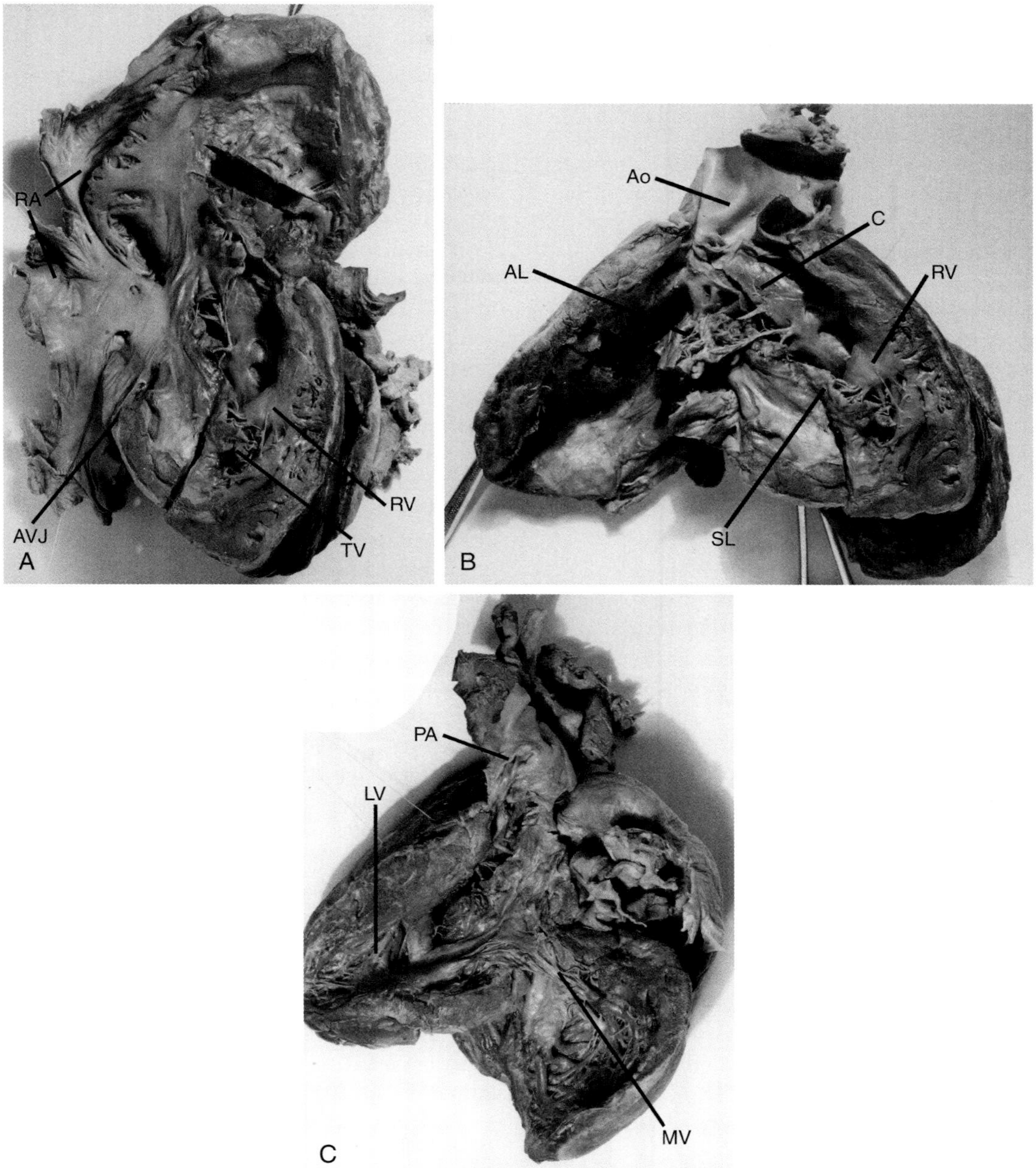

Fig. 13.10 This is the heart specimen of Case 45, a $16\frac{2}{12}$-year-old woman with Ebstein's anomaly, severe tricuspid regurgitation, transposition of the great arteries {S,D,D}, ventricular septal defect (conoventricular type), bicuspid pulmonary valve with pulmonary regurgitation, slit-like secundum atrial septal defect (8 × 2 mm), and enormous cardiomegaly (cardiothoracic ratio = 18/19.5 cm, or 92%). She had a long history of cyanosis and severe clubbing. One year prior to death, at 15 years of age, pedal edema and congestive heart failure appeared. Congestive heart failure progressed and she died, without surgical treatment, in 1959. (An atrial switch operation that surgeons were able to perform, i.e., the Mustard procedure, was not introduced until 1964.) (A) Opened right atrium *(RA)*, tricuspid valve *(TV)*, and right ventricular inflow tract *(RV)*. The septal and posterior leaflets of the TV are displaced well below the right atrioventricular junction *(AVJ)*. (B) Opened right ventricular outflow tract and D-transposed aorta *(Ao)*. The nondownwardly displaced anterior leaflet *(AL)* and downwardly displaced septal leaflet *(SL)* of the TV afflicted with typical Ebstein's anomaly is well seen. The subaortic conus arteriosus *(C)* separates the D-transposed aortic valve from the TV. The downwardly displaced SL of the TV separates the "atrialized" RV above the SL (to the viewer's left) from the "ventricularized" RV below the SL (to the viewer's right). (C) Opened mitral valve *(MV)*, left ventricle *(LV)*, and transposed pulmonary artery *(PA)*. These photos were taken at the time of autopsy.

right ventricular free wall, instead of a normal discrete focal attachment by chordae tendineae to a well-formed anterior papillary muscle (Fig. 13.9). The right ventricular free wall was 6 mm thick; that is, Uhl's disease was not present.

Our patient (Case 45) with Ebstein's anomaly and severe tricuspid regurgitation who also had transposition of the great arteries (TGA) {S,D,D}, a conoventricular type of ventricular septal defect, and a bicuspid pulmonary valve with pulmonary regurgitation (Fig. 13.10) was a remarkable example of the natural history of complex TGA. Briefly, she was a 16²⁄₁₂-year-old young woman with cyanosis and severe clubbing who had enormous cardiomegaly. Her heart almost completely filled her chest, her cardiothoracic ratio being 18/19.5 cm (92%). A secundum atrial septal defect was relatively small, just a slit (2 × 8 mm). Congestive heart failure with pedal edema appeared at 15 years of age, 1 year before she died (in 1959).

To summarize, cyanosis can be present in patients with Ebstein's anomaly and tricuspid regurgitation, 7/28 (28%), in at least four different settings:

(1) isolated Ebstein's malformation, 2/7 patients (29%);
(2) Ebstein's with pulmonary stenosis, 1/7 cases (14%);
(3) Ebstein's with Uhl's disease, 2/7 patients (29%); and
(4) Ebstein's with cyanotic congenital heart disease, that is, tetralogy of Fallot or D-transposition of the great arteries, 2/7 patients (29%).

Biventricular pathology can be prominent in patients with Ebstein's anomaly and tricuspid regurgitation, as in 4 of these 25 patients (16%, Table 13.3):

Case 75, a 14¹⁄₁₂-year-old girl with widespread Uhl's disease of the right ventricle and *marked concentric left ventricular hypertrophy,* has been mentioned heretofore.

Congenital mitral stenosis with absence of interchordal spaces was found in a 15-year-old boy **(Case 37).** He also had subacute bacterial endocarditis with vegetations on his stenotic mitral valve. This boy had the daunting combination of severe tricuspid regurgitation (Ebstein's anomaly), congenital mitral stenosis, a hypoplastic right ventricle, and pulmonary annular stenosis. He was treated with a Brock pulmonary valvotomy at 2 years of age, tricuspid valvuloplasty and pulmonary valvotomy at 8 years of age, and a Glenn anastomosis at 15 years of age (in 1965). He did not survive the latter procedure because of the coexistence of congenital mitral stenosis.

Familial biventricular myocardial dysplasia was found in a boy who died at 4 years of age **(Case 51).** In addition to Ebstein's malformation with tricuspid regurgitation and a small-chambered and dysplastic right ventricular sinus (typical of Ebstein's), he also had bizarre left ventricular myocardial architecture and *double-orifice mitral valve.* There was a small anterolateral accessory orifice and a larger posteromedial main orifice—typical of double-orifice mitral valve.[16] There was also a large conoventricular type of ventricular septal defect.

A final rare anomaly in this patient was an *aneurysm of the right horn of the sinus venosus* that underlay the right ventricular sinus and that communicated with the right atrium via two nonvalved openings. (Aneurysms of the sinus venosus are considered in detail in Chapter 6 concerning systemic venous anomalies.) Although most patients with Ebstein's malformation have what may be called *"isolated" Ebstein's anomaly,* occasionally we encountered patients such as this with multiple congenital cardiovascular anomalies, who may be regarded as having *nonisolated Ebstein's malformation.*

A 27-week-old aborted female fetus **(Case 60)** from Paris, France (Courtesy of Dr. Lucile Houyel) also had a rare form of nonisolated Ebstein's anomaly with tricuspid regurgitation. *Double-outlet right ventricle {S,D,D} was associated with the hypoplastic left heart syndrome.* The fetus had mitral atresia with a tiny left ventricle, and a relatively small muscular ventricular septal defect.

It should be understood that *double-outlet right ventricle (DORV) with hypoplastic left heart syndrome* is a special type of DORV that typically has a *unilateral* conus (a subpulmonary conus, with aortic valve–tricuspid valve fibrous continuity, or a subaortic conus with pulmonary valve–tricuspid valve fibrous continuity), rather than a bilateral conus (subaortic and subpulmonary, and consequently with no semilunar valve–atrioventricular valve direct fibrous continuity), which is usually present when DORV is associated with two well-developed ventricles. (For more information about DORV, see Chapter 23.)

Hence, in this patient, it was no surprise that there was a subpulmonary conus (only, not a bilateral conus) with aortic valve–to–tricuspid valve direct fibrous continuity. The rightward and posteroinferior aortic outflow tract was squeezed between the conal septum anteriorly and somewhat to the left and the tricuspid annulus and leaflets posteriorly and to the right. As usual, this posteroinferior outflow tract was stenotic. The tight subaortic outflow tract was associated with aortic valvar atresia. DORV with *aortic* valvar atresia is rare. Aortic valvar atresia almost always occurs with normally related great arteries. As is usual with aortic valvar atresia, the ascending aorta was markedly hypoplastic (1 mm in internal diameter). The unobstructed pulmonary outflow tract led to a good sized main pulmonary artery and a large patent ductus arteriosus.

The right ventricular sinus (body, or inflow tract) was underdeveloped, and the septal and posterior tricuspid leaflets were downwardly displaced, typical of Ebstein's anomaly.

Thus, biventricular pathology was present. A persistent left superior vena cava connected with the coronary sinus and flowed in the right atrium (not an unusual finding).

However, this feature had one other rare anomaly: *a diverticulum at the right atrioventricular junction* that communicated with the right atrium via a circular orifice in the leftward (medial) portion of the posterior leaflet of the tricuspid valve.

Thus, the pathology associated with Ebstein's anomaly can be biventricular, complex, and rare.

Finally, a 1-day-old female infant with Ebstein's anomaly and severe tricuspid regurgitation **(Case 64)** had a hypoplastic but patent right ventricular outflow tract to the pulmonary artery. However, at the time of study, echocardiography showed that there was no antegrade blood flow from the right ventricle into the pulmonary artery. The right ventricle and right atrium were severely dilated. The ductus arteriosus was patent, and a secundum atrial septal defect was present. *Moderate global left ventricular dysfunction* was observed echocardiographically. This newborn girl was in low cardiac output, had metabolic acidosis, and died on the first day of life.

This patient had no detectable *anatomic* abnormality of the left ventricle; hence, we did not include this case as an example of biventricular abnormality. This patient's left-sided abnormality was *physiologic* not anatomic. Nonetheless, we think that physiologic dysfunction can be as important as anatomic malformations. This is why Table 13.3 is titled (in part): "Important Associated Findings" (not "Important Associated Anomalies/Malformations"). In this way we were able to include important physiologic events such as sudden arrhythmic death, heart failure, and cyanosis. That said, this patient's echocardiographic study was performed when she was moribund and dying; hence the finding of left ventricular functional abnormality is not surprising. (Not many of our patients were studied echocardiographically while they were dying; but had they been, probably a high percentage would have revealed left-sided *functional* abnormality, as in this patient.)

To summarize, biventricular anomalies were found in 4 of these 25 patients with Ebstein's anomaly and tricuspid regurgitation (16%):

1. congenital mitral stenosis with absence of interchordal spaces plus subacute bacterial endocarditis and mitral vegetations in a 15-year-old boy (Case 37);
2. familial biventricular dysplasia with double-orifice mitral valve and a dysplastic left ventricle in a 4-year-old boy (Case 51);
3. hypoplastic left heart syndrome, that is, aortic atresia, mitral atresia, tiny left ventricle, and small muscular ventricular septal defect, in a 27-week-gestation female fetal abortus (Case 60); and
4. very marked left ventricular hypertrophy, resembling left ventricular hypertrophic cardiomyopathy, in a 14 1/12-year-old girl (Case 75).

Other Less Common Associated Findings. Table 13.3 provides our best attempt to answer many other clinically and surgically important questions regarding typical Ebstein's anomaly with tricuspid regurgitation.

How common was pulmonary outflow tract stenosis (excluding atresia)? 24%.

How often did we find a prominent right ventricular diaphragmatic aneurysm? 12%.

A prominent Eustachian valve of the inferior vena cava? 12%.

Multiple congenital anomalies (cardiovascular and noncardiovascular)? 12%.

Uhl's disease of the right ventricle (parchment right ventricle), involving the anterior and diaphragmatic surfaces of the right ventricular free wall? 12%.

Left superior vena cava to coronary sinus to right atrium? 8%.

Known history of supraventricular tachycardia, including paroxysmal atrial tachycardia and WPW syndrome? 12%.

History of syncope prior to death? Only 1 patient (4%).

Fifteen other important findings (mostly malformations) occurred in only 1 patient each, or 4% (Table 13.3).

Ebstein's Anomaly With Congenital Tricuspid Stenosis

Ebstein's anomaly with congenital tricuspid stenosis was the second most common type of "typical" Ebstein's malformation, being found in 11 of 78 postmortem cases (14%, Table 13.2).

By "typical" Ebstein's, we mean that other major forms of congenital heart disease were *not* present, such as pulmonary atresia with intact ventricular septum, typical congenitally corrected transposition of the great arteries {S,L,L}, or common atrioventricular canal (Table 13.2).

Gender: males, 5; and females, 6. The male/female ratio in this subset was 0.83/1.

Age at death: mean 4¾ months ± 7½ months, ranging from 2.5 days to 2 10/12 years in these 11 patients. The median age at death was 27 days.

It is noteworthy that the median age at death in Ebstein's anomaly with tricuspid stenosis (27 days) was much younger than with tricuspid regurgitation (1 8/12 years), consistent with the view that *Ebstein's anomaly with tricuspid stenosis is a more lethal subset than is Ebstein's anomaly with tricuspid regurgitation.*

Severity of tricuspid stenosis. At autopsy, the degree of tricuspid stenosis was regarded as severe in 6 of 11 (55%) (Cases 18, 22, 39, 57, 66, and 76) and as moderate in 5 (45%) (Cases 12, 24, 25, 70, and 71). In an effort to describe what these two different degrees of severity are like, I will present several of these patients in detail.

Severe Tricuspid Stenosis With Ebstein's Malformation. **Case 66** was a 9-day-old boy. The septal and posterior leaflets of the tricuspid valve were largely absent. Cauliflower-like excrescences of tricuspid valve tissue were found anterosuperiorly, just beneath the pulmonary valve. It looks as though there were two valves in the right ventricular outflow tract: the true pulmonary valves above (normally located), and a short distance below the dysplastic and very stenotic tricuspid valve, with an orifice of only 3 to 4 mm in diameter. There was one patent interchordal space (1 mm in width). All of the other interchordal spaces were closed by dysplastic leaflet tissue.

Thus, compared with a normal tricuspid valve, this highly stenotic Ebstein tricuspid valve was displaced inferiorly, anteriorly, and superiorly, so that it lay just below the pulmonary valve.

As mentioned earlier, we said that the septal and posterior leaflets of the tricuspid valve in severe Ebstein's anomaly can be displaced down to the septal and moderator bands, and that the anterior tricuspid leaflet originates from the right atrioventricular junction. *Please note that the case we are now describing is far worse.* There is only a small amount of tricuspid valve tissue at the anterosuperior commissural region of the tricuspid valve that is highly obstructive (stenotic), and that is associated with a major degree of absence of all three tricuspid leaflets.

The atrialized right ventricle was large, with diffuse white thickening of the endocardium. Septum primum was muscularized and bulged aneurysmally into the left atrium. There was a blood cyst of the rudimentary septal leaflet (Fig. 13.3A) and there was also a small blood cyst of the mitral valve, less than 1 mm in diameter.

Other cardiac anomalies included a high small membranous subaortic ventricular septal defect, a bicuspid aortic valve (because of rudimentary development of the intercoronary commissure), and a diminutive right coronary ostium (resulting functionally in a “single” left coronary artery). Thus, this was a case of nonisolated Ebstein’s anomaly with severe tricuspid stenosis.

In **Case 70,** an 11-month-old girl, again the dysplastic, severely stenotic tricuspid valve was located at what would normally be the anterosuperior commissure of the tricuspid valve. The stenotic tricuspid valve opened upward toward the pulmonary valve. The septal and posterior tricuspid leaflets were absent. Right-to-left shunting through a secundum atrial septal defect was associated with cyanosis (systemic arterial saturation 72% to 74%) and polycythemia (hemoglobin 20 gm% and hematocrit 60%).

At 4½ months of age, a right Blalock-Taussig (subclavian-pulmonary) anastomosis was performed (in 1983); the systemic arterial saturation improved somewhat (to 80%), but congestive heart failure appeared that gradually responded to decongestive therapy. This patient had the characteristic abnormal “wrap-around” left ventricular shape, caused by the large left ventricle wrapping around the small, dysplastic right ventricle. The left ventricular septal surface bulged with abnormal convexity into the left ventricular cavity.

Then acute meningitis *(Haemophilus influenzae)* occurred, with focal grand mal seizures. Subsequently, arrhythmias appeared, leading to hypotension and death.

In addition to the above-mentioned cardiovascular anomalies, autopsy revealed multiple infarcts of the brain. Hence, this case illustrates some of the important risks of right-to-left shunting at the atrial level caused by Ebstein’s anomaly with severe tricuspid stenosis associated with a secundum atrial septal defect.

Moderate Tricuspid Stenosis With Ebstein’s Malformation. **Case 12** was the explanted heart specimen from a boy who underwent cardiac transplantation at 2½ years of age in 1986. His anterior tricuspid leaflet was curtain-like, with extreme reduction of the interchordal spaces, and the septal and posterior leaflets were present but downwardly displaced. The tricuspid valve had a high small opening anterosuperiorly (3 mm in maximal dimension) and a larger inferior opening (16 × 5 mm).

Other cardiovascular anomalies included a subaortic membranous ventricular septal defect, a high large muscular ventricular septal defect (20 mm), a noncanal cleft of the mitral valve, pulmonary stenosis (5 mm) with a bicuspid pulmonary valve (poorly developed right septal-nonseptal commissure), and with the left bundle branches of the conduction system running freely—creating a space between the conduction system to the left and the rightwardly deviated ventricular septum. Thus, Ebstein’s anomaly with moderate tricuspid stenosis was associated with multiple other cardiac anomalies in this explanted heart specimen. Other important findings associated with Ebstein’s anomaly and congenital tricuspid stenosis are summarized in Table 13.4.

TABLE 13.4 Ebstein’s Anomaly With Tricuspid Stenosis: Important Associated Findings (*n* = 11)

Associated Findings	No. of Cases	%* of Series
Ventricular septal defect	7	64
Conoventricular	4	36
Muscular	3	27
Secundum atrial septal defect	5	45
Pulmonary stenosis	4	36
Uhl’s disease (parchment RV)	2	18
Congestive heart failure	2	18
Left superior vena cava to coronary sinus to right atrium	2	18
Prominent right venous valve remnants	2	18
Eustachian valve of IVC	1	9
Chiari’s network	1	9
Cleft of mitral valve (non-AV canal type)	1	9
Double-orifice tricuspid valve	1	9
Triple-orifice mitral valve	1	9
Polyvalvar disease (all myxomatous)	1	9
Aneurysm of right sinus horn	1	9
Down’s syndrome	1	9
DiGeorge syndrome with marked thymic hypoplasia	1	9
Multiple congenital anomalies (cardiac and noncardiac)	1	9
History of WPW syndrome	1	9
Moderator band of left ventricle	1	9
Hyposplenia without visceral heterotaxy	1	9
Abnormal left ventricular architecture (posteroinferior recess)	1	9
Absent left coronary ostium (“single” right coronary artery)	1	9
Hypoplastic right coronary ostium (functionally “single” left coronary artery)	1	9
Absent ductus arteriosus	1	9
Double-outlet left ventricle {S,D,D}	1	9
Blood cyst of septal leaflet remnant of tricuspid valve	1	9
Blood cyst of mitral valve	1	9
Bicuspid aortic valve	1	9
Cyanosis	1	9
Meningitis, acute	1	9
Central nervous system infarcts	1	9
Periventricular telencephalic leukoencephalopathy	1	9

AV, Atrioventricular; *RV,* right ventricle; *{S,D,D},* segmental anatomy of solitus atria, D-loop ventricles, and D-malposition of the great arteries; *WPW,* Wolff-Parkinson-White.
*All percentages are rounded off to the nearest whole number.

Ebstein’s Anomaly With Tricuspid Atresia (Imperforate Ebstein’s)

There were two patients with Ebstein’s anomaly of the tricuspid valve and right ventricle who had tricuspid atresia (Cases 5 and 64), comprising 3% of this series (Table 13.2). This malformation is also known as *imperforate Ebstein’s anomaly,* in order to indicate that it is anatomically and developmentally different from typical tricuspid atresia, although physiologically the same.

Atresia is derived from two Greek words: *a,* the privative prefix meaning the want or absence of; and *tresis,* meaning hole. Thus, *atresia* literally means “no hole.” Consequently, imperforate Ebstein’s and typical tricuspid atresia have no opening at the junction between the right atrium and the right ventricle and hence are functionally identical in this respect.

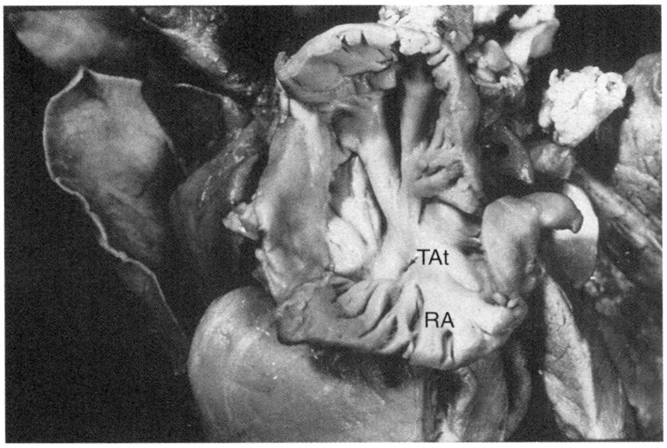

Fig. 13.11 Typical tricuspid atresia *(TAt)*. The morphologically right atrium *(RA)* has been opened, revealing that the floor of the RA is smooth, flat, and muscular, with no evidence of the tricuspid valve. Often there is a little dimple or fibrous depression in the floor of the RA: the leader from the label RA is pointing right at this dimple. This slight depression used to be regarded as a remnant of the atretic tricuspid valve; but now this dimple is thought to be the atrioventricular portion of the pars membranacea septi (the membranous septum). Typical tricuspid atresia is not related to Ebstein's anomaly. Typical tricuspid atresia is now understood to be a misnomer: the tricuspid valve is absent, not atretic (lacking an orifice). Typical tricuspid atresia is **lack of a right atrioventricular communication:** the RA does not open directly into either ventricle. Note also how hypertrophied the right atrial myocardium is. The atrial septum is well formed in this case. It has only recently been realized that the concept of tricuspid atresia is literally erroneous. However, the term *tricuspid atresia* is well entrenched and we are not trying to change it. The foregoing is written in the interests of deeper understanding. The updated concept should be absent right atrioventricular *communication,* not absent right atrioventricular *connection*—because the right atrium may physically connect with a ventricle, but without opening into it. It is absence of the communication or opening that is key. So this is what is meant by typical tricuspid atresia (so-called): absence of a right atrioventricular valvar opening.

But what are the anatomic and the embryologic differences?

In *typical tricuspid atresia,* the floor of the right atrium is relatively flat (Fig. 13.11). There is often a very small little dimple at the expected site of the tricuspid valve, which really is the atrioventricular portion of pars membranacea septi (the AV portion of the membranous septum). In typical tricuspid atresia, the tricuspid valve usually is absent, and the right ventricular sinus (body, or inflow tract) characteristically is small, tiny, or apparently absent, that is, unexpanded or atretic—with little or no lumen of the right ventricular sinus, body, or inflow tract.

In *Ebstein's anomaly with tricuspid atresia,* the floor of the atretic right atrium is not flat. Instead, there is a blind, downwardly depressed hole—reminiscent of a hole on a golf course (Fig. 13.12). The downward depression is the atrialized right ventricle. The atrialized right ventricle is blind (atretic), with no outlet, because the small opening at the anterosuperior commissure of the tricuspid valve is sealed closed (instead of having a small opening, as is typically found in Ebstein's with severe tricuspid stenosis). Also, the interchordal spaces are occluded with leaflet-like tissue. And all three leaflets—anterior, septal, and posterior—are fused. Consequently, there is no opening through this imperforate tricuspid valve (Fig. 13.13).

The anatomic differences between imperforate Ebstein's and typical tricuspid atresia may be summarized as follows:

1. In imperforate Ebstein's, the tricuspid valve leaflet tissue, although very abnormal, is present; whereas in typical tricuspid atresia, the tricuspid valve leaflet tissue is largely or totally absent.
2. In imperforate Ebstein's, the right ventricular inflow tract (the atrialized right ventricle) is present, forming a blind depression (like a hole on a putting green of a golf course); whereas in typical tricuspid atresia, the right ventricular sinus, body, or inflow tract is largely or perhaps totally absent (it may be present, but unexpanded).
3. Ventriculoatrial malalignment typically is not present (or not at all prominent) in imperforate Ebstein's, that is, the ventricular septum underlies the atrial septum (Fig. 13.12); whereas with typical tricuspid atresia (Fig. 13.14) and with straddling tricuspid valve (Fig. 13.12), the ventricular septum underlies the tricuspid valve (in straddling tricuspid valve), or the ventricular septum underlies the expected site of the tricuspid valve (in typical tricuspid atresia) (Fig. 13.14).

In typical tricuspid atresia, take a long straight needle and stick it straight down through the expected site of the atretic tricuspid valve. Then look at the ventricular part of the heart. Where did the needle come out? Typically, the point of the long straight needle emerges out of the posterior portion of the rightwardly deviated ventricular septum. This finding indicates that in typical tricuspid atresia, the posterior portion of the ventricular septum underlies the expected site of the tricuspid valve. The posterior portion of the ventricular septum is displaced to the right relative to the atrial septum.

Why? Our hypothesis is that when the right ventricular sinus (body or inflow tract) is underdeveloped, then the muscular ventricular septum is not moved normally to the left by expansile growth of the right ventricular sinus and consequently does not underlie the atrial septum, as the ventricular septum does normally, and as it does even with Ebstein's anomaly of the tricuspid valve and right ventricle with tricuspid atresia (imperforate Ebstein's anomaly) (Fig. 13.12, right). Thus, in typical tricuspid atresia there is an important rightward malalignment of the ventricular part of the heart relative to the atria that is not present in Ebstein's anomaly with tricuspid atresia (Fig. 13.14). In typical so-called tricuspid atresia, the floor of the right atrium is not only flat, it is also muscular. One does not see an atretic tricuspid valve, as one does in imperforate Ebstein's anomaly. Instead, one sees a flat muscular right atrial floor, with little or no evidence of a tricuspid valve. Typically, the tricuspid valve is largely or totally *absent,* not atretic. The right ventricular sinus (inflow tract) is also largely or totally absent in so-called typical tricuspid atresia. Note again the very close relationship between the development of the right ventricular sinus and the tricuspid valve. This interrelationship is also evident in typical Ebstein's anomaly, as noted heretofore.

Ironically, typical tricuspid atresia does not really have an atretic tricuspid valve—a tricuspid valve with no hole through it. Only imperforate Ebstein's anomaly really has tricuspid atresia. This insight is recorded here in the interests of understanding. I do not wish to change conventional terminology.

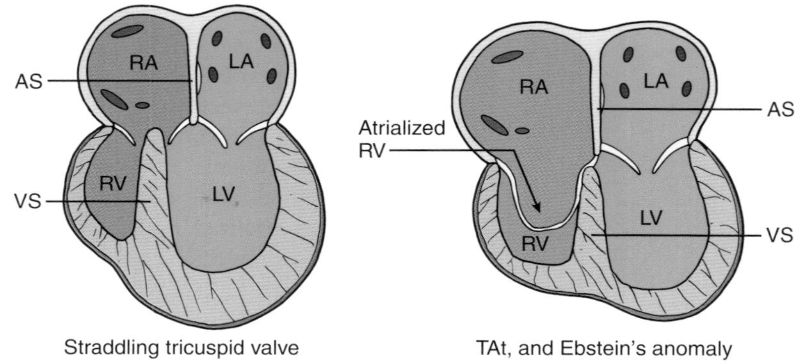

Fig. 13.12 *Right:* Imperforate Ebstein's anomaly, i.e., Ebstein's with tricuspid atresia. The floor of the right atrium *(RA)* is not flat, as in typical tricuspid atresia (Fig. 13.11). Instead, in atretic Ebstein's anomaly, the floor of the RA is a blind, downwardly depressed hole—like a hole on a golf course. The anterior or parietal leaflet of the tricuspid valve originates from the right atrioventricular junction; whereas the septal and posterior leaflets of the tricuspid valve originate below the right atrioventricular junction. The blind pocket above the atretic tricuspid valve is often called the "atrialized" right ventricle *(RV)* because, although this blind pocket is the right ventricular inflow tract (lying below the right atrioventricular junction), the pressures are the same as they are in the RA, because the tricuspid valve is downwardly displaced. The pressures in the RV below the atretic tricuspid valve are typical of the RV; hence this subtricuspid portion of the RV is known as the "ventricularized" RV. In the atrialized RV, the intracardiac electrocardiogram is typical of the RV, even though the pressures are characteristic of the RA. This discordance between the pressures and the intracardiac electrogram in the atrialized RV is diagnostically typical of Ebstein's anomaly. *Left:* straddling tricuspid valve. There is ventriculoatrial malalignment such that the ventricular septum *(VS)* underlies the tricuspid orifice. Consequently the tricuspid valve straddles the ventricular septum, typically through a ventricular septal defect of the atrioventricular canal type. Ventriculoatrial malalignment is not typical of Ebstein's anomaly. *Right:* The ventricular septum *(VS)* underlies the atrial septum *(AS)* in an approximately normal way; whereas, with straddling tricuspid valve *(Left),* the VS is malaligned well to the right of the AS (when D-loop ventricles are present). *LA,* Left atrium; *LV,* left ventricle. (From Edalji Kumar A, Gilbert C, Aerichide N, Van Praagh R: Ebstein's anomaly, Uhl's disease and absence of tricuspid leaflets: a new spectrum. *Am J Cardiol* 1970;25:111-112 and Van Praagh R, Ando M, Dugan WT: Anatomic types of tricuspid atresia: clinical and developmental implications. *Circulation* 1971;44:II-115; with permission.)

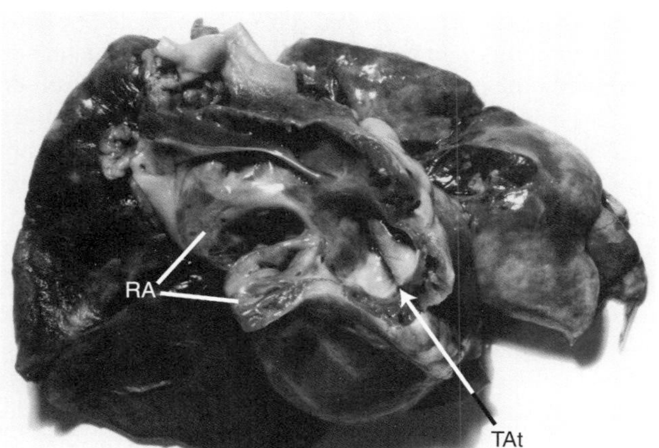

Fig. 13.13 Imperforate Ebstein's anomaly. The dilated right atrium and the downwardly displaced, atretic tricuspid valve are seen. The hepatic veins were dilated and centrilobular necrosis of the liver was present. Case 5 was a 1 10⁄12-year-old girl. In addition to an imperforate Ebstein anomaly, they also had a small muscular ventricular septal defect (3 mm in diameter) and a secundum atrial septal defect (6 × 4 mm). At 3 months of age, a left Blalock-Taussig anastomosis was performed, which gradually closed. Consequently, at 1 10⁄12 years of age (in 1966), she had a Waterston anastomosis (between the posterior surface of the ascending aorta and the anterior surface of the right pulmonary artery). Postoperatively, massive hemorrhage developed in the right lower lobe of the lung, leading to death.

Diagnostically, the blind atrialized right ventricle is typical of imperforate Ebstein's anomaly, but this diagnostic finding is not seen with typical tricuspid atresia because anatomically and developmentally, these are two very different malformations (as above).

Data concerning our two patients with imperforate Ebstein's anomaly follow:

Sex: both females.

Age at death: 1 10⁄12 years (Case 5) (Fig. 13.13) and 2½ years (Case 64).

Associated malformations: secundum atrial septal defect in 1 (6 × 4 mm); ventricular septal defect in both, muscular in Case 5 (3 mm), and membranous (conoventricular, subaortic) in Case 64. The latter patient also had conspicuous endocardial thickening of the atrialized right ventricle, right atrium, and left ventricle. Cyanosis appeared at 4 months of age and was associated with frequent squatting. (Note that *squatting* does not occur only with tetralogy of Fallot.)

Management: Case 5 was treated with a left Blalock-Taussig anastomosis at 3 months of age. Subsequently, this anastomosis closed, and consequently a Waterston anastomosis (between the posterior side of the ascending aorta and the anterior side of the right pulmonary artery) was done in 1966. Postoperatively, a massive right pulmonary hemorrhage developed, leading to death.

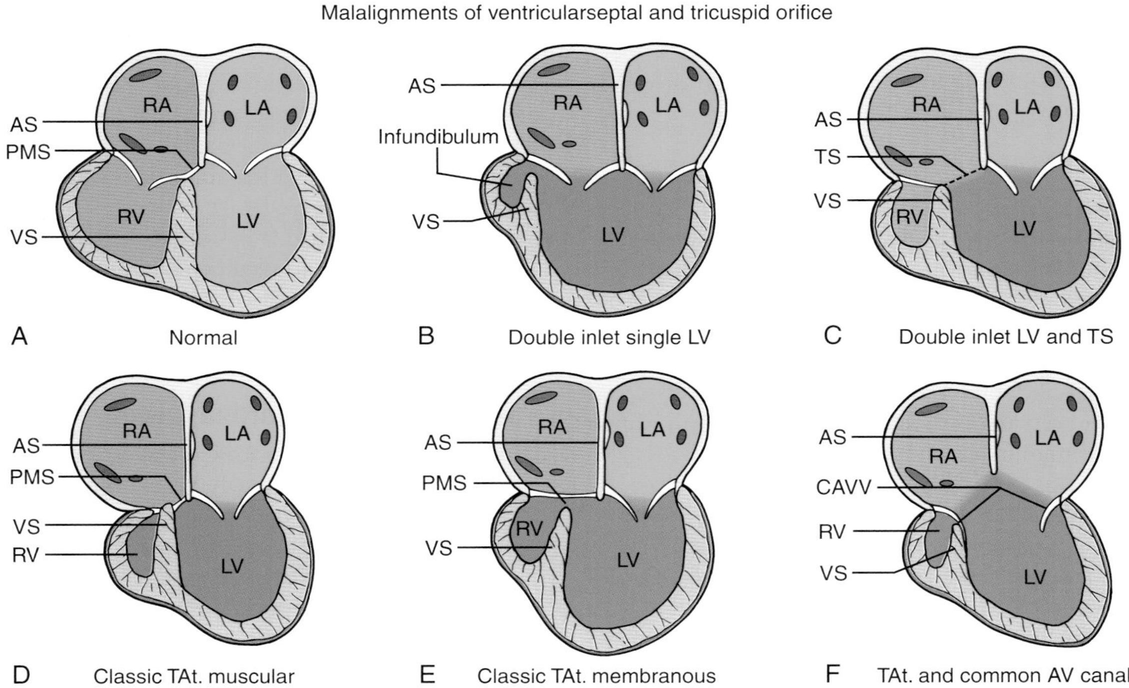

Fig. 13.14 Malalignments of the ventricular septum and the tricuspid orifice. (A) In the normal heart, the ventricular septum *(VS)* lies slightly to the right of the plane of the atrial septum *(AS)*. Consequently, the atrioventricular portion of the membranous septum (pars membranacea septi, *PMS*) normally separates the morphologically left ventricle *(LV)* from the morphologically right atrium *(RA)*. A defect in the atrioventricular portion of the PMS results in a left ventricular–to–right atrial shunt (a Gerbode shunt). (B) With single left ventricle *(LV)* caused by absence of the right ventricular *(RV)* sinus, double-inlet LV is typical. Why? Because absence of the RV sinus results in the ventricular septal remnant being displaced to the right—toward the absent RV sinus. Consequently, the ventricular septum is markedly malaligned relative to the atria and the atrioventricular valves. With a ventricular D-loop, the VS remnant and the infundibular outlet chamber lie to the right of the tricuspid valve; hence double-inlet LV is typical of single LV with an infundibular outlet chamber. (C) If the RV sinus is not absent, but just hypoplastic, the ventricular septum can be moved somewhat further to the left than it is in (B). Consequently, the result can be double-inlet left ventricle, but with congenital tricuspid stenosis *(TS)* due to crowding of the tricuspid valve, resulting in tricuspid hypoplasia. (D) In typical tricuspid atresia, the ventricular septal remnant often underlies the expected site of the tricuspid orifice. This type of ventriculoatrial malalignment, in which the ventricular septal remnant appears to obstruct the potential tricuspid orifice, may be important in the morphogenesis of typical tricuspid atresia. This is the usual muscular type of typical tricuspid atresia, meaning that the floor of the right atrium—in the expected site of the tricuspid valve and orifice—displays a flat muscular appearance, often with a fibrous dimple that is thought to be fibrous membranous septal tissue. (E) The typical or classical form of tricuspid atresia occasionally can be membranous (not muscular). The floor of the right atrium displays smooth, flat, fibrous tissue that we interpret as a larger than usual membranous septal component. Typical membranous tricuspid atresia transilluminates brilliantly, can occur quite frequently with left-sided juxtaposition of the atrial appendages (for reasons unknown), and this membranous right atrial floor does not resemble tricuspid leaflet tissue. (F) Tricuspid atresia *(TAt)* can occur with common atrioventricular canal with a common atrioventricular valve *(CAVV)* and an atrioventricular septal defect. When the right ventricular sinus *(RV)* is quite markedly underdeveloped, the ventricular septum *(VS)* can be displaced far to the right relative to the plane of the atrial septum *(AS)*. The CAVV can open entirely into the morphologically left ventricle *(LV)*, resulting in common-inlet LV. If the right corner of the common AV valve becomes attached to the ventricular septal crest, then the right atrium cannot open directly into the small right ventricle, resulting in a form of tricuspid atresia. This is what Dr. Maurice Lev and his colleagues called *the left ventricular type of common AV canal (or orifice)*, meaning that the common AV orifice and valve open entirely (or almost entirely) into a large LV, and little or not at all into the small RV. Hypothesis: Ventricular septal tricuspid valve malalignments appear to be an important mechanism leading to tricuspid valve anomalies. Often, the tricuspid valve appears to be the "victim," not the "villain"; i.e., tricuspid valve anomalies often appear be secondary to ventriculoatrial malalignment. For example, variable degrees of underdevelopment of the RV sinus (hypoplasia to asplasia) may play an important role in the pathogenesis of ventricular septal–to–tricuspid valvar malalignment mentioned above. Other similar anomalies include straddling tricuspid valve (Fig. 13.12, *Left*) and double-outlet right atrium.

In Case 64, a Waterston anastomosis was also performed (in 1968) and the patient died 3 weeks postoperatively.

Historical Note: It should be recalled that the Fontan procedure for the physiologic correction of tricuspid atresia was not published until 1971[17,18] and was not widely utilized surgically until later in the 1970s.

Ebstein's Anomaly With Tricuspid Stenosis and Tricuspid Regurgitation. Is it possible for Ebstein's anomaly of the tricuspid valve to have both severe tricuspid stenosis and severe tricuspid regurgitation? We found one such patient in this series of 78 postmortem cases (1%, Table 13.2). **Case 50** was a 48-hour-old black female who was thought to have both marked stenosis and marked regurgitation of her very abnormal tricuspid valve that had a curtain-like anterior leaflet, a downwardly displaced and very deficient septal leaflet, and an absent posterior leaflet. She also had a secundum atrial septal defect.

Ebstein's Anomaly With a Normally Functioning Tricuspid Valve. Fascinating to relate, it seems to be possible to have Ebstein's anomaly of the tricuspid valve and right ventricle *without* either tricuspid stenosis or tricuspid regurgitation, as is thought to have occurred in 2 patients (3%) in this series (Table 13.2). **Case 13** was an entirely asymptomatic 21⁸⁄₁₂-year-old young man, a ski instructor at North Conway, New Hampshire. He died a sudden, apparently arrhythmic death following a day of skiing, while taking off his ski boots, just before Christmas in 1978. The anterior leaflet of his tricuspid valve was deep and curtain-like, with obliteration of the interchordal spaces. The septal and posterior leaflets of the tricuspid valve were displaced inferiorly and anteriorly, toward the right ventricular apex. The orifice of the tricuspid valve pointed superiorly toward the pulmonary artery. The maximal dimension of the tricuspid orifice was 25 mm (0.98 inch). There was no thickening or rolling of the free margins of the tricuspid valve (as one ordinarily sees either with tricuspid stenosis and/or regurgitation). The right ventricular free wall was extremely thin (0.75 to 1 mm in thickness); that is, he also had Uhl's disease.

The mitral valve showed thickening of the raphé between the superior endocardial cushion component and the inferior endocardial cushion component of the anterior mitral leaflet. This linear ridge of thickening was thought to be of no functional significance. He also had a patent foramen ovale (but not a secundum atrial septal defect). The ski instructor had had an echocardiogram (we do not know what the interpretation was), but he never had a cardiac catheterization or an angiocardiogram. I saw this heart as a consultation in 1979.

What do I really think about this remarkable case? I thought that the tricuspid orifice was too small, that is, that congenital tricuspid stenosis was present. However, we had to accept the history that he had been apparently entirely asymptomatic and that there were no morphologic signs of tricuspid stenosis or regurgitation. As mentioned above, the tricuspid leaflet margins were thin and delicate without thickening or rolling. Although this young man was a *ski instructor*, as sports medicine specialists know, it is amazing how well the hearts of athletes can adjust to obstructive forms of congenital heart disease. Coarctation is another example. My skepticism notwithstanding, the history was that this young athlete was "entirely asymptomatic." Hence, his case is so recorded here.

Case 19 (Fig. 13.8) was a 25-year-old man with no hemodynamic symptoms whatsoever: no evidence of tricuspid regurgitation or tricuspid stenosis. However, he did have a history of many episodes of paroxysmal atrial tachycardia, WPW syndrome, and atrial flutter. The patient was treated with quinidine for his arrhythmias, which unfortunately led to ventricular fibrillation and death (in 1974).

This patient also had **isolation of the left atrial appendage.** The cavity of the left atrial appendage and of the main portion of the left atrium did not connect; that is, these two separate cavities were nonconfluent. To the best of our knowledge, this rare anomaly was of no clinical significance.

The Problem of Borderline Cases

Perhaps somewhat arbitrarily, we decided not to make the diagnosis of Ebstein's anomaly unless the septal leaflet of the tricuspid valve was downwardly displaced below the right atrioventricular junction. This is why we began this study thinking that we had 79 cases of Ebstein's anomaly, not the 78 cases (Table 13.2) that we ended up with. For example, a 32-hour-old newborn infant boy had a deep curtain-like anterior leaflet of the tricuspid valve, with extensive obliteration of the interchordal spaces. The septal leaflet of the tricuspid valve was bound down, with little functional free leaflet tissue; but *the origin of the septal leaflet was not downwardly displaced.* There was partial absence of tricuspid valve leaflet tissue beneath the anterosuperior commissure. Double-orifice of the tricuspid valve involved the posterior leaflet. All of the tricuspid leaflets were thick and myxomatous. Additional findings include marked pulmonary valve stenosis with a bicuspid pulmonary valve, an intact ventricular septum, and severe tricuspid regurgitation (confirmed by echocardiography and cardiac catheterization). The patient also had a history of fetal tachycardia (190 beats/min).

We concluded that this patient certainly had an *Ebstein-like* anomaly of the tricuspid valve; however, we did not make the diagnosis of Ebstein's anomaly (unqualified) because Ebstein's is generally understood to have downward displacement of the septal leaflet, and of at least part of the posterior leaflet of the tricuspid valve into the right ventricle, resulting in an atrialized right ventricle—which this patient did *not* have. Nonetheless, we now seek to focus attention and understanding on the arbitrary and artificial nature of classification, which is highlighted by borderline cases such as this. The abnormal septal leaflet underwent delamination and ascent up to the right atrioventricular junction.

All anomalies form a *spectrum*—from the most severe, to the mildest forms of disease. So that the accuracy of our diagnoses can be relied on, we have excluded borderline cases like this. But it must also be understood that such borderline cases—*Ebstein-like or "Ebsteinoid" cases*—do indeed exist, as is to be expected because all anomalies are parts of a spectrum of malformation.

Ebstein's Anomaly With Pulmonary Valvar Atresia or Severe Stenosis and Intact Ventricular Septum. This was the second largest group of Ebstein's patients (14 patients, 18%, Table 13.2). Most patients with Ebstein's anomaly and pulmonary atresia/severe stenosis with intact ventricular septum had tricuspid regurgitation (12 patients, 15%, Table 13.2), although a few had tricuspid stenosis (2 patients, 3%, Table 13.2). Of these 14 patients, 12 had pulmonary atresia (86%) and 2 had severe pulmonary valvar stenosis (14%).

(As will be seen, left-sided Ebstein's anomaly also was tied for second in prevalence, being found in 14 patients, or 18% of this series, Table 13.2.)

With Tricuspid Regurgitation

Of these 12 patients, the age death was known in 11.

Age at death: mean = 11.4 ± 15.3 days; the range was 0 (stillborn) to 45 days; and the median was 5 days.

In terms of natural history, the age at death of Ebstein's anomaly with pulmonary atresia or severe pulmonary stenosis, intact ventricular septum, and tricuspid regurgitation is much the youngest of any Ebstein's group encountered to date. The median ages at death were as follows:

1. series as a whole, 10 weeks;
2. Ebstein's with tricuspid regurgitation, 1 8/12 years;
3. Ebstein's with tricuspid stenosis, 27 days;
4. Ebstein's with tricuspid atresia (imperforate), $n = 2$, average = 2.16 years or 26 months; and
5. Ebstein's with pulmonary atresia or very severe stenosis, intact ventricular septum, and tricuspid regurgitation, 5 days.

These data suggest that pulmonary atresia with intact ventricular septum and tricuspid regurgitation may well be one of the most lethal forms of congenital heart disease.

Sex: Of these 12 patients, the gender was known in 11: males, 9; and females, 2. The male/female ratio was 9/2 (4.5/1). This is the first time in studying Ebstein's anomaly that we have encountered a strong gender preponderance, suggesting that perhaps this strong male preponderance may be related to pulmonary atresia with intact ventricular septum, rather than to Ebstein's anomaly (speculation).

Of these 12 patients, 2 (Cases 35 and 52) had very severe pulmonary valvar stenosis (17%) (Fig. 13.15), rather than pulmonary atresia (10 of 12, 83%). The anatomy of the Ebstein's anomaly of the tricuspid valve with tricuspid regurgitation was

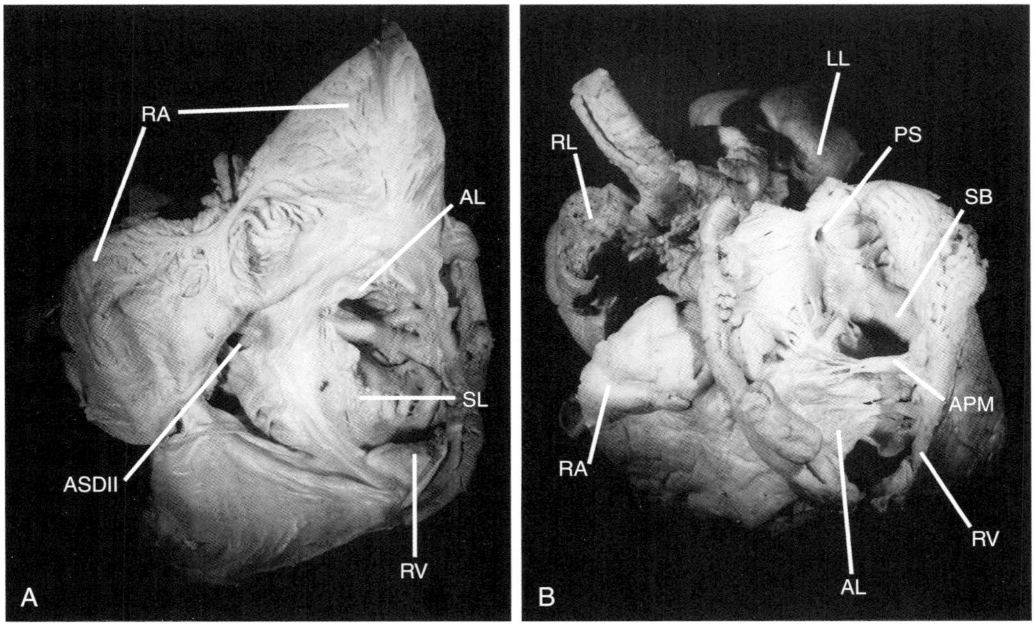

Fig. 13.15 Ebstein's anomaly with severe tricuspid regurgitation in a patient who also had severe (dome) pulmonary valvar stenosis (opening 2 mm in diameter) with intact ventricular septum. This 1-hour-old girl had severe respiratory distress and cyanosis at birth. When she had been intubated, the lungs could not be inflated, and she could not breathe on her down. Autopsy revealed **marked hypoplasia of both lungs, i.e., half the volume of normal control lungs.** Her very early death was thought to be primarily related to pulmonary failure, not cardiac insufficiency. The pulmonary veins bilaterally were markedly hypoplastic and could be probed only with difficulty. Her congenital heart disease was also very severe. (A) The opened right atrium *(RA),* tricuspid valve, and right ventricle *(RV).* (B) The opened tricuspid valve and RV. In (A), note the marked right atrial hypertrophy and enlargement. A secundum type of atrial septal defect *(ASDII),* measuring 8 × 6 mm, is seen above a deficient septum primum. The septal leaflet *(SL)* of the tricuspid valve is downwardly displaced and deficient, with a small blood cyst located above it (closer to the RA). The anterior leaflet *(AL)* of the tricuspid valve originates normally from the right atrioventricular junction. (B) The anterior leaflet *(AL)* of the tricuspid valve, with very few well-formed interchordal spaces. Consequently, the AL appears to insert broadly, with few intervening papillary muscles, directly into the right ventricular free wall—immediately inferior to the anterior papillary muscle *(APM)* of the right ventricle. The septal band *(SB)* and the infundibular wall are hypertrophied. The very tight (2 mm internal diameter) unopened dome pulmonary valvar stenosis *(PS)* is seen from below. Note the very hypoplastic left lung *(LL)* and right lung *(RL).*

similar to that in previous settings (Fig. 13.15). Other findings are summarized in Table 13.5.

Ebstein's Anomaly With Pulmonary Atresia, Intact Ventricular Septum, and Tricuspid Stenosis. Only two patients had Ebstein's anomaly, pulmonary atresia, intact ventricular septum, and tricuspid stenosis (3%, Table 13.2).

Case 59 was a 14 3/12-year-old girl at the time of her heart transplantation. The explanted heart specimen revealed severe congenital tricuspid stenosis, immediately beneath her atretic pulmonary valve. The opening in the stenotic tricuspid valve measured only 5 × 2 mm. In the right atrioventricular junctional region, there was no tricuspid valvar tissue. Tricuspid leaflet tissue was located only in an immediately subpulmonary site.

TABLE 13.5 Associated Abnormalities With Ebstein's Anomaly, Tricuspid Regurgitation, and Pulmonary Atresia or Severe Stenosis* With Intact Ventricular Septum (*n* = 12)

Associated Abnormalities	No. of Cases	% of This Group
Secundum atrial septal defect	8	67
Pulmonary hypoplasia, bilateral	2	17
Prominent Eustachian valve	1	8
Incomplete form of common AV canal with ASD I and cleft MV	1	8
Parachute mitral valve (all chordae tendineae to anterolateral papillary muscle)	1	8
Double-orifice mitral valve	1	8
Mitral regurgitation, severe	1	8
Uhl's disease (parchment right ventricle)	1	8
Atrial flutter	1	8
Right atrial aneurysm	1	8
Heart failure	1	8
Multiple congenital anomalies (i.e., cardiovascular and noncardiovascular: hypospadias)	1	8
Atresia of main pulmonary artery (cord-like)	1	8
Brachiocephalic artery†	1	8
"Single" coronary artery‡	1	8
Pulmonary atresia, valvar and infundibular	1	8
Partially anomalous pulmonary venous connection (all right PVs to RSVC)	1	8
Sinus venosus defect (between RSVC and right pulmonary veins, 6 × 4 mm)	1	8

ASD I, Ostium primum type of atrial septal defect; *AV*, atrioventricular; *MV*, mitral valve; *PV*, pulmonary valve; *RSVC*, right superior vena cava.
*Severe pulmonary valvar stenosis (*n* = 2, Cases 35 and 52).
†Innominate artery and left common carotid artery both arising from single brachiocephalic artery; typically only two brachiocephalic arteries arising from aortic arch, unless the right subclavian artery originates aberrantly.
‡Quotation marks indicate that the coronary arterial blood supply is not really single; two coronary arteries typically are present, but one coronary ostium is absent: "single" coronary artery usually really means single coronary ostium.

Case 74 was a 3¾-month-old girl (17 weeks). The expected main orifice of her tricuspid valve was atretic. However, she had several patent interchordal spaces on the diaphragmatic surface of the posterior leaflet (Fig. 13.16) and of the anterior leaflet; hence, she had severe congenital tricuspid stenosis. The tricuspid leaflets were thick and myxomatous with a blood cyst.

The right coronary arterial ostium was absent, resulting in a "single" left coronary artery. The left anterior descending coronary artery was markedly enlarged, with three sinusoidal connections between the left anterior descending coronary artery and the right ventricular apical region (Fig. 13.17). Sinusoids were also present between the right coronary artery and the right ventricular cavity on the diaphragmatic surface of the right ventricle. Widespread coronary arteriopathy was present.

Many of these features are characteristic of what has been called the **venous valve syndrome.**[19] We think that this syndrome is better understood as **the pulmonary atresia with intact ventricular septum syndrome.** Characteristic features include not only pulmonary atresia or very severe pulmonary valvar stenosis with intact ventricular septum, but also coronary-cameral sinusoids (Fig. 13.17), coronary arteriopathy with luminal narrowing or occlusion, prominent venous valve remnants (in particular a prominent Eustachian valve of the inferior vena cava), Uhl's disease, Ebstein's anomaly, and partial or total absence of the tricuspid valve leaflets (i.e., partially or totally unguarded tricuspid orifice). Thus, pulmonary atresia with an intact ventricular septum often involves much more than just these two features.

As we noted in 1970,[20] there appears to be an **anatomic and developmental relationship between Ebstein's anomaly, Uhl's disease, and absence of tricuspid valve leaflets.** As will be seen later, these three anomalies also occur together in the setting of **pulmonary atresia with intact ventricular septum.**

This is why we have been emphasizing from the beginning of this chapter that Ebstein's anomaly is about much more than

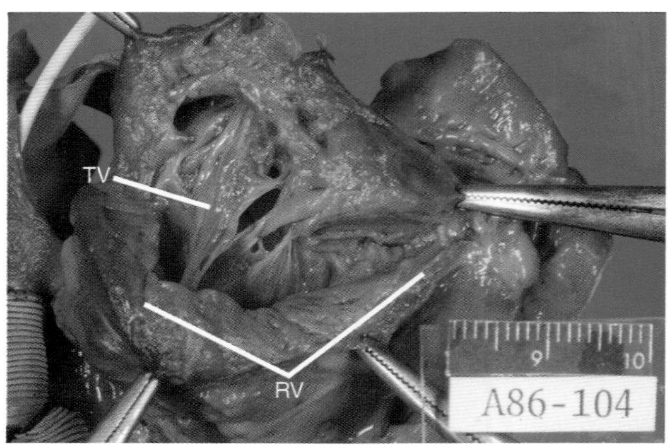

Fig. 13.16 This is the opened right ventricle *(RV)* of a 3¾-month-old (17 weeks) girl with pulmonary atresia, intact ventricular septum, and Ebstein's anomaly (Case 74). The main tricuspid orifice was atretic. However, several interchordal spaces were patent, as can be seen by examining the tricuspid leaflets *(TV)* from below. Hence, this was severe congenital tricuspid stenosis. The tricuspid leaflets were also thick and myxomatous, with a blood cyst (not seen). This photo was taken at autopsy. (The ruler is in millimeters.)

just a tricuspid valve anomaly. There is a major right ventricular myocardial component, involving the right ventricular septal surface with the downward displacement of the septal leaflet, creating the "atrialized" right ventricle; plus involvement of the right ventricular free wall surface with the aneurysm of the right ventricular diaphragmatic surface, or, if more extensive, Uhl's

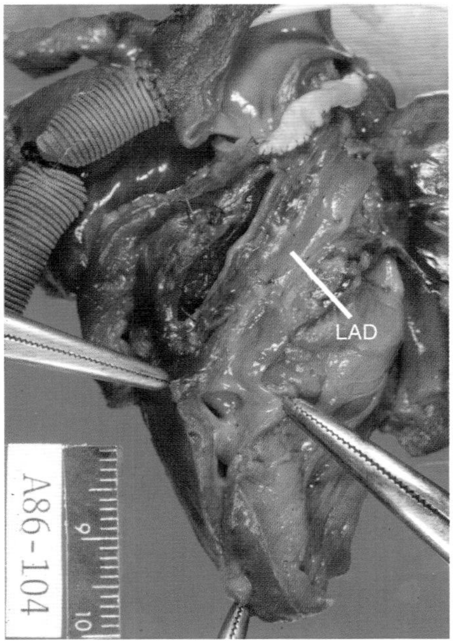

Fig. 13.17 This is the same patient as is shown in Fig. 13.16 (Case 74). The right coronary arterial ostium was absent, resulting in a "single" left coronary artery. This photo shows marked enlargement of the "single" left anterior descending *(LAD)* coronary artery. Between and below the forceps one can see the ostia of sinusoidal communications between the right ventricular apical region and the large left anterior descending coronary artery; there were 3 sinusoids connecting with the left anterior descending coronary artery. Sinusoids were also present between the right ventricular cavity and the right coronary artery on the diaphragmatic surface (not shown). Widespread coronary arteriopathy was also present: coronary mural thickening with luminal narrowing, which may be regarded as coronary artery "jet lesions" and their sequelae. The hypothesis concerning the coronary arteriopathy associated with sinusoids is as follows: Jets from a systemic or suprasystemic right ventricular cavity strike the coronary arteries, producing focal coronary arterial disease with mural thickening and luminal narrowing or occlusion. Sinusoids are typically associated with pulmonary atresia and intact ventricular septum, resulting in systemic or suprasystemic right ventricular pressures. But if Ebstein's anomaly is also associated with pulmonary atresia and intact ventricular septum, and if enough blood can get into the right ventricular cavity to lead to systemic or suprasytemic right ventricular pressure, then right ventricular–to–coronary arterial sinusoids can be associated with Ebstein's anomaly. However, it should be understood that coronary-cameral sinusoids typically are associated with high-grade semilunar valvar obstruction (e.g., pulmonary/aortic atresia) with intact ventricular septum and systemic/suprasystemic ventricular pressures. Hence, this is a rare and noteworthy case because sinusoids usually are *not* associated with Ebstein's anomaly—we think because usually, Ebstein's is not associated with system/suprasystemic right ventricular pressures, as it was in this case. If blood can get into the right ventricular cavity, and then has difficulty getting out, in this situation, right ventricular pressures can become systemic/suprasystemic. This is when sinusoids may occur (or persist) with Ebstein's, as in this rare case.

disease or parchment right ventricle involving much or most of the right ventricular free wall anteriorly.

Now, in the present group, we are seeing the association between the Ebstein's anomaly of the tricuspid valve and pulmonary valvar atresia or extreme stenosis, with intact ventricular septum, and also prominent venous valves.

How does this all make sense anatomically and developmentally? Ebstein's anomaly is often only a part of something larger—that may be regarded as the **tricuspid and right ventricular dysplasia syndrome** that can also be associated with **right ventricular outflow tract pathology** (pulmonary atresia or extremely stenosis) as well as **right ventricular inflow tract pathology**—prominent right and left venous valve remnants, Ebstein's anomaly of the tricuspid valve, right ventricular aneurysm inferiorly, or Uhl's disease (parchment right ventricle) globally.

The foregoing is not merely a developmental hypothesis. Instead, as we are seeing, these are the anatomic facts. These findings, of course, require a developmental explanation. My task here is to try to present the anatomic data as clearly as possible. Briefly, Ebstein's anomaly, not rarely, is part of something larger, the Ebstein tricuspid valvar and right ventricular dysplasia syndrome. What does "not rarely" mean? In the 50 cases of Ebstein's anomaly considered in detail thus far (Tables 13.3, 13.4, and 13.5), there have been 6 cases of Uhl's disease (12%), 3 patients with a prominent diaphragmatic right ventricular aneurysm (6%), and 5 cases with a prominent right venous valve remnant or Eustachian valve (10%). If one combines the case of Uhl's disease with those having a prominent aneurysm, the prevalence of striking right ventricular free wall thinning is 9 patients (18%). This may well be an underestimate because we have only counted cases in which these findings were *prominent*. (Our impression is that the majority of adult patients with Ebstein's anomaly have a diaphragmatic surface right ventricular free wall aneurysm that tends to become more and more prominent over time.)

Left-Sided Ebstein's Anomaly

Wherever the morphologically tricuspid valve and the morphologically right ventricular sinus, body, or inflow tract (the true morphologically right ventricle, as opposed to the conus or infundibulum) are located, one would anticipate that there, Ebstein's anomaly should also occur. Hence, one would expect to find left-sided Ebstein's anomaly in association with discordant L-loop ventricles, as in classical congenitally physiologically corrected transposition of the great arteries {S,L,L} and as in double-outlet right ventricle {S,L,L}. As will soon be seen, these expectations are correct. However, to the best of my knowledge, we have never seen Ebstein's anomaly with concordant L-loop ventricles, as in situs inversus totalis {I,L,I}. However, our failure to observe such a case may simply reflect the rarity of concordant L-loop ventricles. In principle, Ebstein's anomaly "should" also occur in this situation.

Age at death or cardiac transplantation (in 12 patients, unknown in 2): mean = $6\frac{3}{12} \pm 7\frac{11}{12}$ years; range from 0 (stillborn) to $19\frac{2}{12}$ years; and mean = $1\frac{8}{12}$ years.

Sex: males = 8; females = 4; unknown = 2. The male/female ratio was 2/1. Such a strong preponderance of one gender (males) was not found in our cases of Ebstein's anomaly without other major associated cardiovascular anomalies, suggesting that this strong male preponderance *may* be related to the coexistence of discordant L-loop ventricles and/or major conotruncal malformations (such as L-transposition or double-outlet right ventricle with L-malposition of the great arteries) (hypothesis). However, the series is very small (n = 12, in which the gender is known); hence no firm conclusion is drawn.

Findings

All 14 cases had Ebstein's anomaly of the left-sided tricuspid valve and morphologically right ventricular sinus (Figs. 13.18, 13.19, and 13.20). The downward displacement of the septal leaflet of the inverted (left-sided) tricuspid valve is well seen in Fig. 13.18 and in Fig. 13.20.

Transposition of the great arteries {S,L,L} (classical physiologically "corrected" transposition) was present in 12 of 14 patients (86%), whereas DORV was found in 2 (14%). The segmental anatomy was DORV {S,L,L} in one, and DORV {S,L,D} in the other. The patient with DORV {S,L,**L**} indicates that the aortic valve lay to the left (levo, or L) relative to the pulmonary valve; whereas DORV {S,L,**D**} means that the aortic valve lay to the right (dextro or D) relative to the pulmonary valve.

In TGA {**S,L,**L}, DORV {**S,L,**L}, and DORV {**S,L,**D}, the S,L part of the segmental anatomy indicates that visceroatrial situs solitus {S,-,-}—the usual or normal pattern of anatomic organization—coexisted with L-loop ventricles, {S,L,-}. Hence, discordant or inappropriate L-loop ventricles were present in patients with visceroatrial situs solitus. (In visceroatrial situs solitus, D-loop ventricles "should" be present, as in the solitus normal heart, {**S,D,**S}.)

Many of the important findings in these 14 patients with discordant L-loop ventricles in visceroatrial situs solitus are summarized in Table 13.6.

One of our patients with transposition of the great arteries {S,L,L} had the very rare findings of aortic valvar atresia with left-sided Uhl's disease, left-sided Ebstein's anomaly with extreme tricuspid regurgitation, and atresia of the right atrial ostium of the coronary sinus (Fig. 13.21, patient of Dr. Ghislaine Gilbert, Institut de Cardiologie de Montreal, Canada, our Case 53). Valvar aortic atresia occurs almost always with normally related great arteries, almost never with transposition of the great arteries. Uhl's disease almost always involves the ventricle of the pulmonary or lesser circulation, almost never the ventricle of the aortic or systemic circulation. So this is a very rare and noteworthy case (Fig. 13.21).

Ebstein's Anomaly With Common Atrioventricular Canal. Ebstein's anomaly with common atrioventricular (AV) canal (also known as atrioventricular septal defect) may sound like an

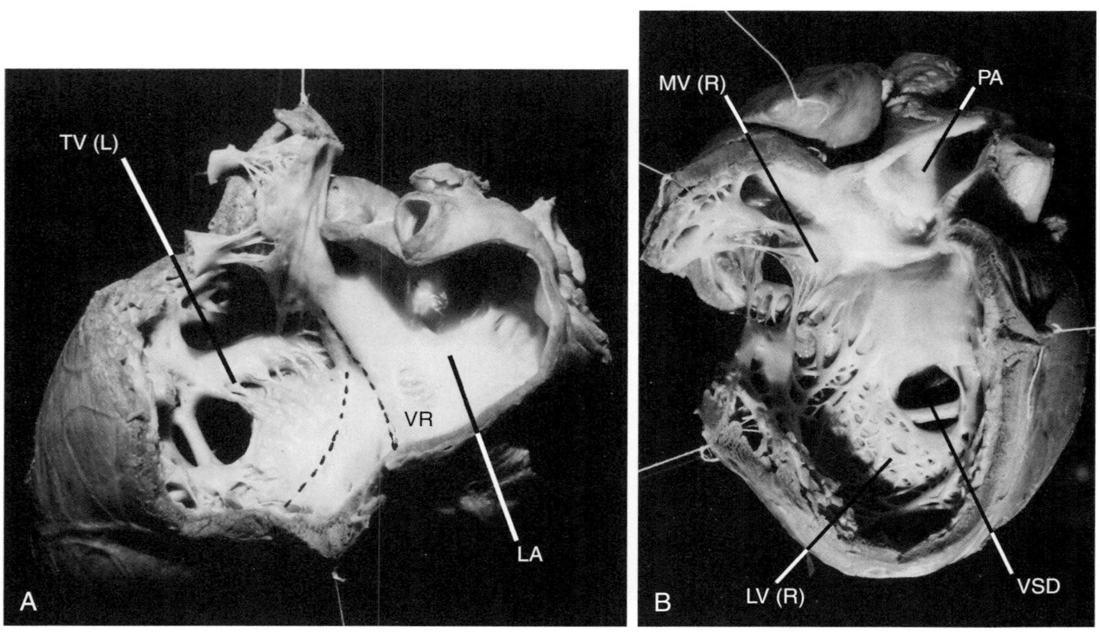

Fig. 13.18 This is the heart of a 4-month-old-girl (Case 44) with transposition of the great arteries {S,L,L}, a large muscular ventricular septal defect (18 × 14 mm), left-sided Ebstein's anomaly, left-sided tricuspid regurgitation, congenital complete heart block with a heart rate of 64 beats/minute, and congestive heart failure. Sudden and unexpected cardiac arrest at 5 months of age led to death in 1961. (A) The left-sided cardiac chambers are seen from above and behind, looking down on the left atrium *(LA)* and the left-sided tricuspid valve, *TV (L)*. *VR* indicates the location of what normally should have been the valve ring of the left-sided tricuspid valve at the left-sided atrioventricular junction. The *lower dotted line* (to the viewer's left) indicates the actual origin of the left-sided septal and posterior leaflets of the left-sided tricuspid valve. The difference between these two lines indicates the downward displacement of the origins of the septal and posterior leaflets of the left-sided tricuspid valve. (B) The opened right-sided mitral valve, *MV (R)*, the right-sided morphologically left ventricle, *LV (R)*, and the transposed pulmonary artery *(PA)*. The muscular ventricular septal defect is well seen. These photos were taken at the time of autopsy.

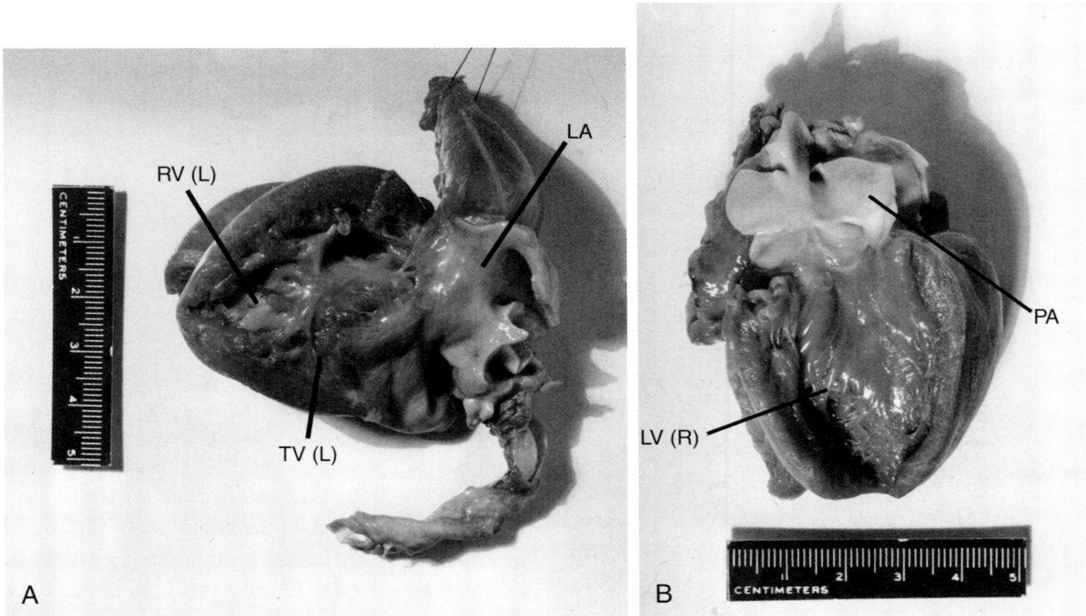

Fig. 13.19 Transposition of the great arteries {S,L,L} with left-sided Ebstein's anomaly, marked left-sided tricuspid regurgitation, and mild coarctation of the aorta in a 2-month-old boy. Cardiomegaly was marked, the heart weighing 61 grams (normal for the age =19 grams): 61/19 = 3.2/1, i.e., 221% greater than normal. This patient also had multiple congenital anomalies: bilateral hare lip, bilateral cleft palate, and Meckel's diverticulum. (A) Opened left-sided morphologically right ventricle, *RV (L)*, and L-transposed aorta *(Ao)*. The posterior tricuspid leaflet was rudimentary, *TV (L)*. (B) The opened right-sided morphologically left ventricle, *LV (R)*, and transposed pulmonary artery *(PA)*. The ventricular septum was intact. The atrial septum was normally formed with an obliquely probe patent foramen ovale. The ductus arteriosus was closed and the coarctation was mild (no measurement was recorded). Hence, from a physiologic standpoint, this patient's main cardiovascular disability was left-sided Ebstein's anomaly with severe tricuspid regurgitation (functionally tantamount to severe mitral regurgitation) that led to death at 2 months of age. These photographs were taken at the time of autopsy.

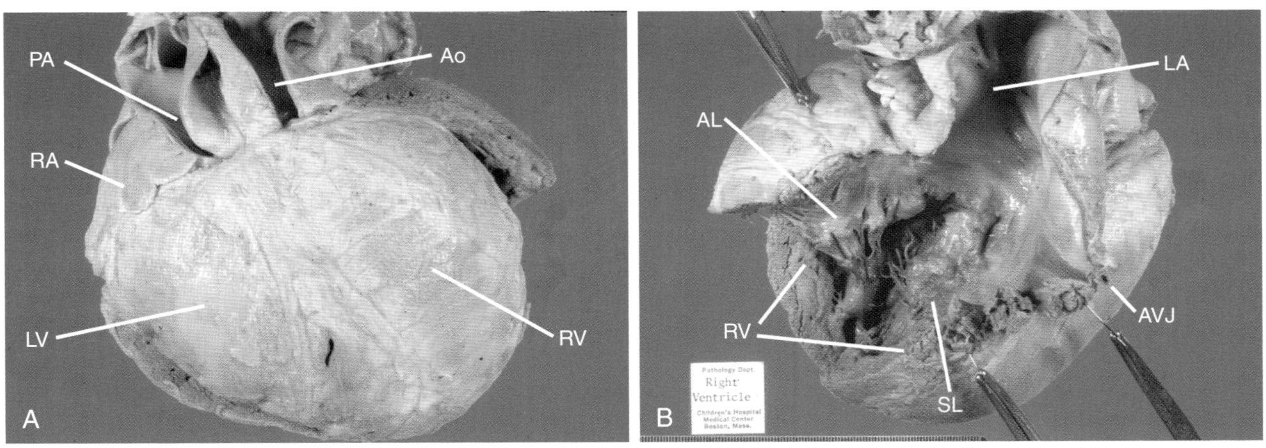

Fig. 13.20 This is the heart of a 15-year-old boy with TGA {S,L,L} with two well-developed ventricles, a conoventricular type of ventricular septal defect that was partially obstructed by tricuspid valve tissue, subpulmonary stenosis produced by excessive atrioventricular valvar tissue attached to the right-sided mitral valve (fibrous subpulmonary stenosis) and left-sided Ebstein's anomaly with moderate tricuspid regurgitation. He suffered a sudden, unexpected, probably arrhythmic death: he was feeling as well as usual; then he suddenly dropped dead after playing hockey. (A) External frontal view of the heart, typical of TGA {S,L,L}. The left-sided morphologically right ventricle *(RV)* is hypertrophied and enlarged. *Ao,* L-transposed ascending aorta; *LV,* morphologically left ventricle, right-sided; *PA,* transposed main pulmonary artery; *RA,* morphologically right atrium. (B) The opened left-sided left atrium *(LA)*, tricuspid valve with Ebstein's anomaly, and the markedly hypertrophied right ventricular inflow tract *(RV)*. The anterior leaflet *(AL)* of the tricuspid valve arises normally from the atrioventricular junction, but this leaflet is deep and curtain-like, with marked reduction of the interchordal spaces. The anterior leaflet appears to insert directly into the anterior papillary muscle of the right ventricle—without apparent chordae tendineae intervening between the leaflet and the papillary muscle because most of the interchordal spaces are filled with, and occluded by fibrous valve leaflet-like tissue. The septal leaflet *(SL)* is markedly hypoplastic, plastered down against the right ventricular septal surface, and this leaflet appears to be nonfunctional. The septal leaflet is mostly well below the atrioventricular junction *(AVJ)*. The posterior leaflet is vestigial and is also markedly downwardly displaced. The RV is left-sided and left-handed. These photos were taken at the time of this consultation (in 1974).

TABLE 13.6 Findings Associated With Left-Sided Ebstein's Anomaly (*n* = 14)*

Findings	No. of Patients	%† of Group
Ventricular septal defect	12	86
Conoventricular	9	64
Muscular	1	7
AV canal type	2	14
Tricuspid regurgitation (L)	12	86
Tricuspid stenosis (L)	2	14
Coarctation of the aorta	4	29
Pulmonary outflow tract atresia	4	29
Pulmonary outflow tract stenosis	2	14
Secundum atrial septal defect	2	14
Congenital complete heart block	2	14
Straddling mitral valve (R)	2	14
Coronary sinus ostial atresia	2	14
Aortic stenosis	2	14
Valvar	1	7
Subvalvar	1	7
Superoinferior ventricles	2	14
Aortic atresia, valvar	1	7
Uhl's disease of the RV (L)	1	7
Crisscross AV relations	1	7
Pulmonary hypoplasia, bilateral	1	7
Right coronary artery (L) running between Ao and PA	1	7
Dextrocardia	1	7
Straddling tricuspid valve (L)	1	7
Straddling of both AV valves	1	7
Double-orifice tricuspid valve	1	7
Mitral regurgitation (R)	1	7
Cleft of mitral valve (R), without MR	1	7
Double-outlet left atrium, with both orifices (to RV and to LV) stenotic	1	7
Multiple congenital anomalies	1	7
Hypoplastic aortic isthmus	1	7
Left superior vena cava to coronary sinus to right atrium	1	7
Congestive heart failure	1	7
Brain abscess	1	7
Heart transplantation	1	7

Ao, Aorta; *AV*, atrioventricular; *DORV*, double-outlet right ventricle; *(L)*, left-sided; *LV*, morphologically left ventricle; *MR*, mitral regurgitation; *PA*, main pulmonary artery; *(R)*, right-sided; *RV*, morphologically right ventricle; *TGA*, transposition of the great arteries.
**n* = 14: TGA {S,L,L} = 12; DORV {S,L,L} = 1; and DORV {S,L,D} = 1.
†All percentages are rounded off to the nearest whole number.

anatomic and developmental impossibility. One is tempted to think, "One can have common AV canal, *or* Ebstein's anomaly, but surely not both at the same time." Remarkably enough, they can coexist. Common AV canal is probably one of the least well known settings in which Ebstein's anomaly can occur (Table 13.2).

Ebstein's anomaly with common AV canal occurred in 9 cases (12% of the series as a whole); 6 patients had tricuspid atresia or stenosis (8%), while 3 had tricuspid regurgitation (4%) (Table 13.2).

Ebstein's Anomaly With Common AV Canal and Tricuspid Atresia or Stenosis

Age at death (*n* = 5; 1 unknown): mean = 2 months and 24 days ± 2 months and 23 days; range, from 18 hours to 6 months; and median = 2 months.

Gender: males, 3; females, 2; unknown, 1. The male/female ratio was 3/2 (1.5/1).

Findings: The segmental anatomy was normal, that is, {S,D,S} in 4 of these 6 patients (66.7%) (Figs. 13.22 and 13.23), but was abnormal in 2 patients with visceral heterotaxy and asplenia.

A 16-day-old boy **(Case 11)** with the asplenia syndrome had dextrocardia (a predominantly right-sided heart as seen in a posteroanterior chest X-ray), single left ventricle (absent right ventricular sinus) with infundibular outlet chamber and double-outlet infundibular outlet chamber (DOIOC). This designation, DOIOC, indicates that both great arteries arose above the infundibulum or conus, one might say *per force,* because the right ventricle (the right ventricular sinus or inflow tract) was absent. (*"Per force,"* above, is not entirely correct because rarely, both great arteries can originate above the *left* ventricle, resulting in double-outlet left ventricle, which is presented in Chapter 24.) However, the real point is that when the right ventricular sinus is absent (resulting in single left ventricle) and when a bilateral conus (subaortic and subpulmonary) is present, this combination of malformations usually results in double-outlet infundibular outlet chamber.

The segmental anatomy in this patient was DOIOC {A(I),D,D}. {A-,-.-} indicates that situs ambiguus of the viscera was present, typical of the asplenia syndrome. {-(I),-,-} denotes that we thought that the situs of the atria was inversus. {--,D,-} indicates that a discordant ventricular D-loop was present. {--,-,D} signifies that D-malposition of the great arteries (aortic valve to the right [dextro or D] relative to the pulmonary valve) was present. Hence, the tricuspid valve component of the common AV valve was to the right of the mitral valve (component) because the situs (pattern of anatomic organization) of the atrioventricular valves corresponds to that of the ventricle(s) of entry, not to that of the atrium (atria) of exit.

This 16-day-old boy had an incomplete form of common AV canal with an ostium primum type of atrial septal defect (an incomplete atrioventricular septal defect). We classified this as an *incomplete* form of common AV canal because of the coexistence of an imperforate Ebstein's anomaly of the tricuspid valve, that is, Ebstein's with tricuspid atresia. In other words, the AV valve was not in common: the mitral and tricuspid components of the common AV valve were not confluent or in common—because of the coexistence of tricuspid atresia. The tricuspid component of this atrioventricular valve was not confluent with the mitral component because the tricuspid component lacked a patent orifice.

However, it is noteworthy that a bulboventricular foramen was present, as is almost always the case with single left ventricle

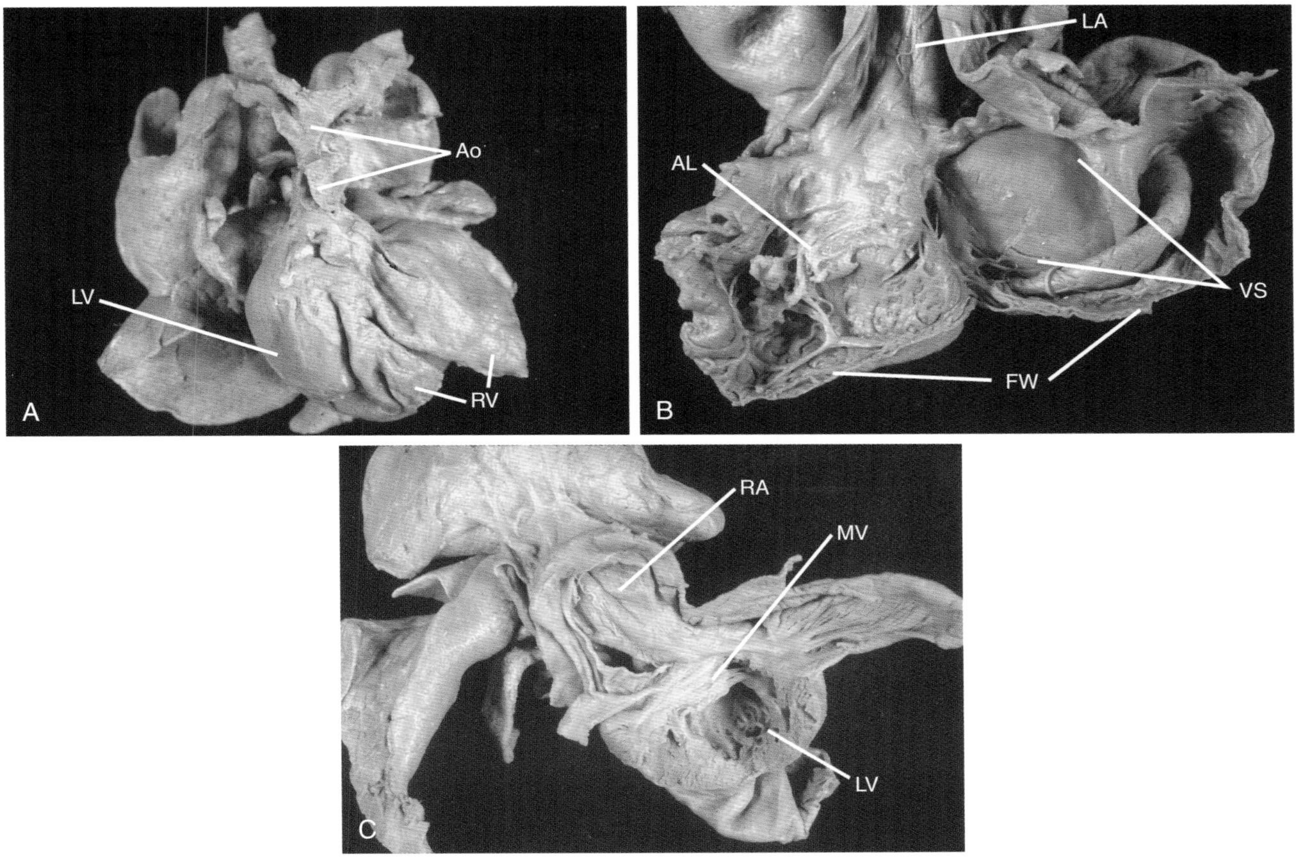

Fig. 13.21 This is the heart of a patient with transposition of the great arteries {S,L,L} with aortic valvar atresia, Uhl's disease of the left-sided morphologically right ventricle, Ebstein's anomaly of the left-sided tricuspid valve and right ventricle, extreme left-sided tricuspid regurgitation and atresia of the right atrial ostium of the coronary sinus. (A) External frontal view of the heart and lungs. Note that the free wall of the left-sided morphologically right ventricle *(RV)* appears thin and wrinkled. The ascending aorta *(Ao)* is very hypoplastic. The morphologically left ventricle *(LV)* is right-sided and well developed. (B) Interior view of the left-sided left atrium *(LA)* opening into the very dysplastic morphologically right ventricle (left-sided). The septal and posterior leaflets of the tricuspid valve are markedly hypoplastic, i.e., functionally absent. The anterior leaflet *(AL)* of the tricuspid valve is deep, curtain-like, and bound-down to the right ventricular free wall *(FW)*. Note how very thin and almost membranous much of the collapsed right ventricular free wall is. Not only is the right ventricular free wall very deficient in myocardium, but so too is the right ventricular septal surface *(VS)*. The right ventricular septal surface appears smooth or nontrabeculated—because there is no right ventricular septal myocardium covering the left ventricular component of the interventricular septum. This is what electrophysiologists sometimes call "the barrier": the normally invisible surface of the left ventricular component of the interventricular septum, which normally is covered by right ventricular septal myocardium (but is not in this rare case). Normally, the junction between the left ventricular and right ventricular myocardial components of the ventricular septum can only be seen histologically on transverse sections of the septum. (C) The opened right-sided right atrium, mitral valve, and morphologically left ventricle. Septum primum is deficient and is deflected into the right atrium; a secundum atrial septal defect was also present. This was a patient of Dr. Ghislaine Gilbert of the Institut de Cardiologie de Montréal (the Institute of Cardiology of Montreal), Canada, that we were privileged to study in consultation in 1976. These photographs were taken at the time of this consultation.

and an infundibular outflow chamber. It should be understood that a bulboventricular foramen is a ventricular-septal-defect-like communication between the single left ventricle and the infundibular outlet chamber. A bulboventricular foramen (BVF) is usually *not* called a ventricular septal defect (VSD) for the following reason. VSD is really a short form for *interventricular* septal defect (IVSD), meaning a defect between the ventricles (plural). But when there is only *one* ventricle, as with single LV, it is illogical and anatomically inaccurate to speak of a VSD, meaning *I*VSD. The infundibulum is not a ventricle, meaning ventricular sinus. Hence, BVF is anatomically accurate, whereas VSD is not. In this patient there was no ventricular septal defect of the atrioventricular canal type—only an ostium primum type of defect. Hence, the atrioventricular septal defect was partial (not complete); and the atrioventricular valve was not in common because of atresia of its tricuspid valve component. For these two reasons we made the diagnosis of partial (not complete) common AV canal.

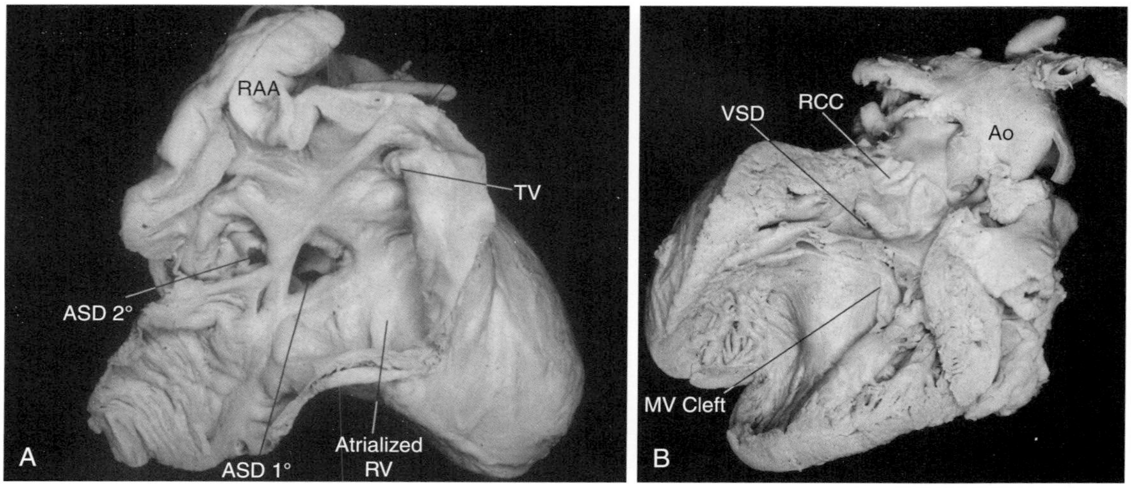

Fig. 13.22 Case 9 was a 2-month-old girl with normal {S,D,S} segmental anatomy; Ebstein's anomaly with extremely severe tricuspid stenosis (only a pinhole opening at the superior commissure of the tricuspid valve, i.e., nearly imperforate Ebstein's anomaly); a very small conoventricular type of ventricular septal defect, which contributed to severe subpulmonary stenosis; Uhl's disease of the right ventricular free wall (transilluminates brilliantly); and incompletely common atrioventricular canal with an ostium primum type of atrioventricular septal defect, no ventricular septal defect of the atrioventricular canal type, and a cleft anterior mitral leaflet. (A) Opened right atrium and right ventricular inflow tract. (B) Opened left ventricle and ascending aorta. In (A), note the ostium primum type of atrioventricular septal defect *(ASD 1°)*, the ostium secundum type of atrial septal defect *(ASD 2°)*, and the atrialized right ventricle *(RV)* or right ventricular inflow tract. The septal leaflet of the tricuspid valve was absent and the posterior leaflet was very deficient. A small amount of tricuspid valve leaflet tissue was present only at the superior commissure of the tricuspid valve *(TV)*, where it constituted very severe congenital tricuspid stenosis (almost imperforate Ebstein's anomaly). *RAA*, Right atrial appendage. (B) Note the cleft anterior leaflet of the mitral valve *(MV Cleft)*, no ventricular septal defect of the atrioventricular canal type, and only a very small ventricular septal defect *(VSD)* of the conoventricular type (between the conal septum above and the ventricular septum below). Note the wraparound shape of the left ventricle: the left ventricular septal surface wraps convexly around the small and dysplastic right ventricular inflow tract (the atrialized right ventricle). *Ao*, Ascending aorta; *RCC*, right coronary leaflet of the aortic valve. This case illustrates what may be regarded as the *tricuspid and right ventricular dysplasia syndrome* that combines features of the following entities (that may occur together or separately): Ebstein's anomaly of the tricuspid valve and right ventricle, Uhl's disease, severe tricuspid stenosis, and an incomplete form of common atrioventricular canal. (Consultation courtesy of Prof Dominique Metras, Marseille, France. Photographs in 1988 by Dr. Stella Van Praagh.)

Accurate diagnosis and classification requires careful consideration of *all aspects* of the anatomy, not of just one feature only. Common AV canal is really more than an atrioventricular septal defect—because of its atrioventricular *leaflet* component. Similarly, as in this patient, it is often possible to diagnose the situs of the atria, even when visceral heterotaxy and asplenia or polysplenia coexist. But is necessary to consider carefully not just one anatomic feature—such as the pattern of the pectinate musculature. Instead, in order to reach an accurate anatomic diagnosis, it is necessary to consider all relevant anatomic features (see Chapter 29). For example, in this patient, the atrial situs was diagnosed as situs inversus. This revealed that atrioventricular discordance was present, as the segmental anatomy indicates: DOIOC {A(I),D,D}.

The concept of isomerism (mirror-imagery) as applied to the atria (to the atria as a whole, or to the appendages only, or to the pectinate muscles only) is considered to be anatomically erroneous. Instead, visceral heterotaxy with asplenia, polysplenia, or a normally formed but often right-sided spleen is characterized by visceral anomalies of *asymmetry* (not anomalies of symmetry), and by malformations of midline-associated structures (the midline being the axis about which right-left asymmetry normally develops) (see Chapter 29).[21-23]

Case 11 had other noteworthy findings: double-orifice mitral valve; a large secundum atrial septal defect; pulmonary atresia (infundibular and valvar); a bicuspid aortic valve (underdevelopment of the right coronary/left coronary commissure); right-sided patent ductus arteriosus from the innominate artery to the proximal right pulmonary artery, with a left aortic arch; totally anomalous pulmonary venous connection to the left superior vena cava via a small orifice, resulting in supracardiac pulmonary venous obstruction; and atresia of the right superior vena cava below the level of the innominate vein.

Visceral heterotaxy with asplenia, Ebstein's anomaly, and tricuspid obstruction occurred in 3 of these 6 cases (50%): tricuspid atresia in 2 of 6 (Cases 11 and 17), and severe tricuspid stenosis in 1 of 6 (Case 21).

The segmental anatomy in all three cases of heterotaxy with asplenia and Ebstein's anomaly with tricuspid atresia (imperforate Ebstein's) or severe tricuspid stenosis was essentially the same: DOIOC {A(I),D,D}, Case 11; DORV {A(I),D,D}, Case 17; and DORV {A(I),D,D}, Case 21. If you

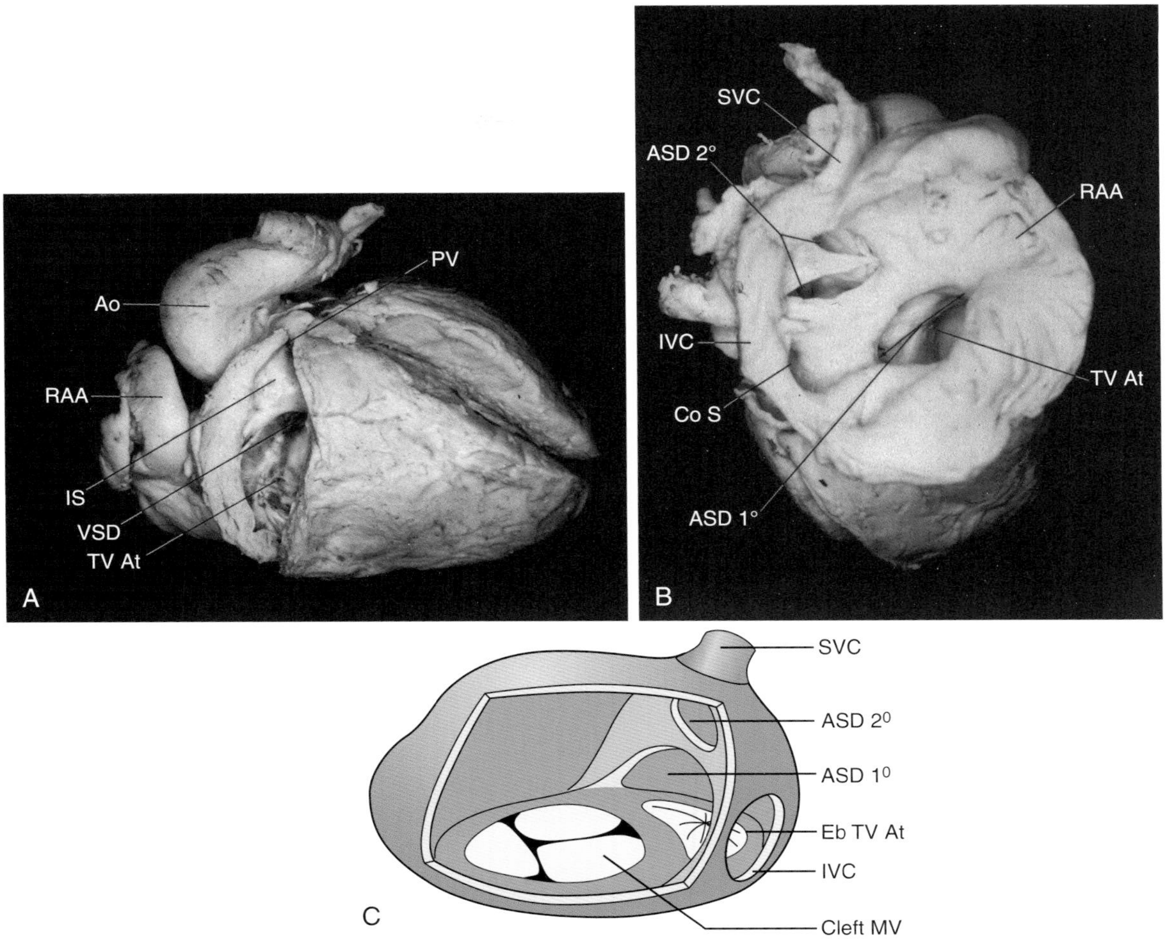

Fig. 13.23 Imperforate Ebstein's anomaly with very thin aneurysm of diaphragmatic surface of atrialized right ventricle, incomplete form of common atrioventricular canal (ostium primum type of atrioventricular septal defect, incomplete cleft of anterior mitral leaflet, no ventricular septal defect of the atrioventricular canal type), small subcristal ventricular septal defect of the conoventricular type, severe pulmonary valvar stenosis, normal segmental anatomy {S,D,S}, large ostium secundum type of atrial septal defect, and persistent left superior vena cava to coronary sinus to right atrium. (A) External frontal view of the heart. (B) Opened right atrium and atrialized right ventricle. (C) Diagram of this type of anomaly, viewed from posteriorly, looking through a "window" in the posterior left atrial free wall. In (A), note the normal segmental anatomy. The right atrial appendage *(RAA)* is right-sided, hypertrophied, and enlarged. The small right ventricle is also right sided. The great arteries are solitus normally related. The pulmonary artery is much smaller than the ascending aorta *(Ao)*. The tricuspid valvar atresia *(TV At)* is seen from the distal or downstream aspect. The conoventricular ventricular septal defect *(VSD)* is small, constituting subpulmonary stenosis. The infundibular septum *(IS)* is well seen. The pulmonary valve *(PV)* is tightly stenotic. Thus, there was both valvar and subvalvar pulmonary stenosis. In (B), one can see the atretic markedly downwardly displaced tricuspid valve *(TV At)*, the ostium primum incomplete atrioventricular septal defect *(ASD 1°)*, the enlarged right atrial ostium of the coronary sinus *(Co S)*, the secundum atrial septal defect due to deficiencies of septum primum, and the normally connected inferior vena cava *(IVC)* and superior vena cava *(SVC)*. (C) The Ebstein's anomaly with tricuspid atresia *(Eb TV At)*, the ASD 1°, the cleft anterior leaflet of the mitral valve *(MV)* (the cleft was incomplete in Case 10, but complete in Case 9), the ASD 2°, the IVC, and the SVC. This case was a consultation from Abidjan, Côte d'Ivoire (Ivory Coast). The patient's age and gender are not known by us. (Case courtesy of Dr. Dominique Metras. Photographs in 1984 by Dr. Stella Van Praagh.)

would prefer to simplify the segmental anatomy as much as possible, one could omit the A as unnecessary, since it is understood that all three patients had visceral heterotaxy with situs ambiguus (A) and asplenia. Focusing on the cardiac segmental anatomy only, all three asplenic patients had {I,D,D} segmental anatomy—which is what one sees in the infrequent form of congenital physiologically corrected transposition of the great arteries: TGA {I,D,D}. But all three had a bilateral conus (subaortic and subpulmonary), resulting in DORV in two, and in DOIOC in one.

Down syndrome was present in 1 of these 6 patients (Case 28), who had tricuspid atresia {S,D,S}.

Incompletely common atrioventricular canal was present in all 6 patients with Ebstein's anomaly and tricuspid stenosis or atresia (100%) (Figs. 13.22 and 13.23). Other salient findings are summarized in Table 13.7.

TABLE 13.7 Ebstein's Anomaly With Incompletely Common Atrioventricular Canal and Tricuspid Atresia or Severe Stenosis ($n = 6$)

Finding	No. of Cases	%* of Group
Tricuspid atresia (imperforate)	4	67
Tricuspid stenosis, extreme	2	33
Incompletely commonly AV canal	6	100
Secundum atrial septal defect	4	67
Double-orifice mitral valve	4	67
Heterotaxy syndrome with asplenia	3	50
Pulmonary outflow tract atresia	2	33
Uhl's disease of RV free wall	3	33
Posterior leaflet of TV partially absent	2	33
Double-outlet right ventricle {A(I),D,D}	2	33
Ventricular septal defect, conoventricular	2	33
Septal leaflet of TV absent	1	17
Bicuspid aortic valve	1	17
Single LV with IOC	1	17
Aneurysm of diaphragmatic RV	1	17
Atresia of RSVC below innominate vein	1	17
TAPVC to LSVC with stenosis	1	17
Right PDA with left aortic arch	1	17
Pulmonary stenosis, valvar	1	17
LSVC to CoS to RA	1	17
DOIOC {A(I),D,D}	1	17
Dextrocardia	1	17
Down syndrome	1	17
Anomalous muscle bundles of the RV	1	17
Multiple congenital anomalies (hydrocephalus)	1	17

{A(I),D,D}, The segmental anatomic set of visceral situs ambiguus (A), with situs inversus of the atria (I), ventricular D-loop (D), and D-malposition of the great arteries; *AV*, atrioventricular; *CoS*, coronary sinus; *DOIOC*, double-outlet infundibular outlet chamber; *IOC*, infundibular outlet chamber; *LSVC*, left superior vena cava; *LV*, morphologically left ventricle; *PDA*, patent ductus arteriosus; *RA*, morphologically right atrium; *RSVC*, right superior vena cava; *RV*, morphologically right ventricle; *TAPVC*, totally anomalous pulmonary venous connection; *TV*, tricuspid valve.
*All percentages are rounded off to the nearest whole number.

Ebstein's Anomaly With Incompletely Common Atrioventricular Canal and Tricuspid Regurgitation. Three patients had Ebstein's anomaly with incompletely common atrioventricular canal and tricuspid regurgitation (Table 13.2, 4%): Cases 15, 48, and 78.

Age at death: mean = 5.92 ± 8.77 months; range, 9 hours to 1 4/12 years; and median = 7 weeks.

Gender: males, 2; female, 1; male/female = 2/1.

Findings: All three patients had tricuspid regurgitation. The anterior leaflet of the tricuspid valve was deep, curtain-like, with obliteration of the interchordal spaces, very small anterior papillary muscle of the right ventricle, and with or without direct attachment of the anterior tricuspid leaflet to the right ventricular free wall. The posterior tricuspid leaflet was similar to the anterior leaflet. The septal leaflet of the tricuspid valve appeared downwardly displaced and very deficient or absent, functionally permitting severe tricuspid regurgitation. One newborn girl (Case 48) died at 9 hours of age from hydrops fetalis (massive prenatal and postnatal congestive heart failure).

TABLE 13.8 Ebstein's Anomaly With Incompletely Common Atrioventricular Canal and Congenital Tricuspid Regurgitation ($n = 3$)

Finding	No. of Cases	% of Group
Incompletely common AV canal	3	100
Congenital tricuspid regurgitation	3	100
Secundum atrial septal defect	2	67
Parachute mitral valve with MS	2	67
Congenital mitral regurgitation	1	33
Down syndrome	1	33
Hydrops fetalis	1	33
Double-orifice tricuspid valve	1	33
Tetralogy of Fallot (pentalogy)	1	33

AV, Atrioventricular; *MS*, congenital mitral stenosis.

All three of these patients also had the incomplete form of common AV canal with an ostium primum defect, a cleft anterior leaflet of the mitral valve, and no ventricular septal defect of the AV canal type. Hence, all of these patients had major anomalies of both the tricuspid and the mitral valves. Two patients had congenital mitral stenosis with parachute mitral valve, while the other had severe congenital mitral regurgitation.

One of these patients (Case 78) had tetralogy of Fallot {S,D,S}, a secundum atrial septal defect (hence pentalogy of Fallot), an incomplete form of common AV canal with an ostium primum defect, congenital mitral stenosis with parachute mitral valve (all chordae tendineae inserting into the posteromedial papillary muscle of the left ventricle, the anterolateral papillary muscle of the left ventricle being absent, the mitral cleft being the only orifice of the mitral valve), and severe tricuspid regurgitation with obliteration of the interchordal spaces and muscularization (or failure of demuscularization) of the anterior tricuspid leaflet.

The foregoing little boy, who died at 7 weeks of age (in 1976), had a **rare quartet of anomalies that, to best of our knowledge, is a previously undescribed constellation of malformations:**

1. tetralogy (pentalogy) of Fallot;
2. the incomplete form of common AV canal;
3. Ebstein's anomaly with severe tricuspid regurgitation; and
4. parachute mitral valve with marked congenital mitral stenosis.

The anomalies found in this group are summarized in Table 13.8.

It should be recalled that there was one other patient (Case 38), a 2-day-old boy, who had incompletely common AV canal with an ostium primum type of defect, a cleft anterior leaflet of the mitral valve, a parachute mitral valve with all chordae inserting into the anterolateral papillary muscle group of the left ventricle, with double-orifice of the mitral valve (a small accessory posteromedial orifice thought to be of little or no functional significance), severe mitral regurgitation with thickened and rolled margins of the main mitral orifice, Ebstein's anomaly with severe tricuspid regurgitation of the tricuspid valve (deep curtain-like anterior tricuspid leaflet, without papillary muscles, with marked reduction of interchordal spaces, and with absence of the septal and posterior tricuspid leaflets, accounting for the severe tricuspid regurgitation), Uhl's disease of the right ventricle with parchment-like thinning of the entire right ventricular free wall, a secundum type of atrial septal defect (multiple fenestrations of a very thin septum primum), partially anomalous pulmonary venous connection (right pulmonary veins connecting with the right superior vena cava), stenosis of the proximal left pulmonary artery, an aberrant right subclavian artery, a brachiocephalic artery (both the right common carotid and the left common carotid arteries originating from a single orifice), and multiple congenital anomalies (hypospadias, a noncardiovascular anomaly). This patient also had *valvar pulmonary atresia with an intact ventricular septum*. Hence, Case 38 was presented above as one of the 12 patients with Ebstein's anomaly, pulmonary atresia/severe stenosis with intact ventricular septum, and tricuspid regurgitation (Table 13.2).

In other words, Ebstein's anomaly with tricuspid atresia and the incomplete form of common AV canal did not have pulmonary atresia or severe stenosis with intact ventricular septum in three patients (Cases 15, 48, and 78), but did have pulmonary atresia with intact ventricular septum in one patient (Case 38) (Table 13.2).

Ebstein's anomaly with the incomplete form of common AV canal was the least frequent of the four main subsets of Ebstein's anomaly (9 patients, 12% of this series, Table 13.2). Consequently, this anatomic subset of Ebstein's malformation is not well known. Indeed, in December 1970, Dr. Stella Van Praagh and Dr. Masahiko Ando thought that our Case 28 might well be the first autopsy-proved case of the incomplete form of common AV canal with imperforate Ebstein's anomaly of the tricuspid valve. But further investigation revealed that the combination of Ebstein's anomaly and common AV canal had first been reported in 1956 by Kilby, DuShane, Wood, and Burchell[24] from the Mayo Clinic in Rochester, Minnesota.

Literature Review and Discussion Concerning Ebstein's Anomaly. In addition to the references that have been cited heretofore,[1-24] much more has been written about Ebstein's anomaly.[25-216] One of the more striking features of the literature concerning this anomaly is that it focuses very largely on Ebstein's anomaly with tricuspid regurgitation. While this is a very important subset, it constituted only 25 of our 78 autopsy proved cases, that is, only 32% of this series (Table 13.2). Seldom mentioned are patients with Ebstein's malformation and tricuspid stenosis (11 cases, 14%), or tricuspid atresia (2 cases, 3%), or with both significant tricuspid regurgitation and tricuspid stenosis (1 case, 1%), or those rare and fortunate individuals with neither significant tricuspid regurgitation nor tricuspid stenosis (2 cases, 3%) (Table 13.2). All of the foregoing patients had relatively isolated Ebstein's anomaly, that is, without other major forms of congenital heart disease (53%, Table 13.2).

Ebstein's malformation with other major forms of congenital heart disease constituted almost half of this series (48%, Table 13.2). These are the largely "forgotten" forms of Ebstein's anomaly (Table 13.2):

1. with pulmonary valvar atresia or severe stenosis and intact ventricular septum (14 cases, 18%);
2. left-sided Ebstein's anomaly with classical congenitally physiologically corrected transposition of the great arteries {S,L,L} or with double-outlet from the left-sided morphologically right ventricle {S,L,L} (14 cases, 18%); and
3. with the incomplete form of common AV canal (9 cases, 12%).

When describing Ebstein's malformation, the authors of excellent and prestigious textbooks often exclude Ebstein's anomaly with tricuspid stenosis, tricuspid atresia, pulmonary atresia with intact ventricular septum, left-sided Ebstein's malformation, and Ebstein's with common AV canal, consigning these types to other chapters. The effect is that many well-informed pediatric cardiologists and cardiac surgeons do not know that Ebstein's anomaly can complicate pulmonary atresia with intact ventricular septum and the incomplete forms of common AV canal. Left-sided Ebstein's with corrected L-transposition and double-outlet right ventricle with atrioventricular discordance is better known.

This is why Ebstein's anomaly is presented "whole" in this chapter, in all of its forms, so that the full spectrum of this malformation can be clearly seen, as it really occurs.

This understanding is very relevant to accurate diagnosis and successful surgical management because these four major subsets of Ebstein's anomaly are distinctive and very different from each other (Table 13.2).

Perhaps it should be added that congenital heart disease is classified in terms of its pathologic anatomy, not in terms of its clinical symptoms or physiology, and not in terms of its current interventional or surgical management, because all of the latter are variables in congenital heart disease. The pathologic anatomy is relatively constant in comparison with these other admittedly very important variables. Hence, classification is based on anatomy, but also with full awareness of the importance of symptoms, physiology, and therapeutics. The aforementioned anatomic method of classification is the essence of **the morphologic (anatomic) approach to the diagnosis of congenital heart disease.**

As a practical matter, our approach to diagnostic classification has always been inclusive, not exclusive. As far as Ebstein's anomaly is concerned, our suggestion is that this malformation should be *included* in whatever chapters, or sections, or papers to which it is diagnostically and therapeutically important. Specifically, Ebstein's malformation should be included in considerations of tricuspid atresia, tricuspid stenosis, tricuspid regurgitation, pulmonary atresia or severe stenosis with intact ventricular septum, discordant L-loop ventricles, common AV canal, and perhaps in other settings not found in our series. But in chapters, sections, or papers on Ebstein's anomaly, *all* of the major settings or subsets should also be included, so that all concerned will become familiar with the full spectrum of Ebstein's malformation, the relative frequencies of each (Table 13.2), and the associated cardiac anomalies that are typically found with each major Ebstein subset (Tables 13.3 to 13.8).

TABLE 13.9 Tricuspid Valve Function in Ebstein's Anomaly (n = 78)

Function	No. of Cases	% of Series*
Tricuspid regurgitation (TR)	52	67
Tricuspid stenosis (TS)	17	22
Tricuspid atresia (imperforate)	6	8
TR and TS	1	1
"Normal" function (no TR or TS)	2	3

*Percentages rounded off to nearest whole number.

Tricuspid Valve Function in Ebstein's Anomaly

Tricuspid valve function in these 78 postmortem cases of Ebstein's malformation is summarized in Table 13.9.

In this series as a whole, tricuspid regurgitation (67%) was much more common than tricuspid stenosis (22%) or tricuspid atresia (imperforate Ebstein's) (8%). Essentially normal function (no significant tricuspid regurgitation or stenosis) (3%) and noteworthy tricuspid regurgitation plus tricuspid stenosis (1%) were both infrequent (Table 13.9).

Tricuspid regurgitation was more common than tricuspid stenosis or tricuspid atresia, not only in the series as a whole (Table 13.9), but also in each of the four major Ebstein's subsets, except for Ebstein's anomaly with incompletely common atrioventricular canal (Table 13.2). In the latter infrequent and consequently unfamiliar Ebstein's subset (n = 9), only 3 patients had tricuspid regurgitation (4%), while 4 patients had tricuspid atresia (5%) and 2 had tricuspid stenosis (3%). Thus, 6 patients had tricuspid obstruction (atresia in 4 and stenosis in 2) (8%), while only 3 had tricuspid regurgitation (4%) (Table 13.2). Because the numbers are so small, no conclusion is drawn.

The Ebstein subset with an incomplete form of common AV canal was also interesting in terms of **associated anomalies.** *Congenital asplenia* was present in 3 of the 6 patients with tricuspid obstruction: 2 with tricuspid atresia and 1 with tricuspid stenosis (Cases 11 and 17, and Case 21, respectively). One patient with tricuspid atresia (Case 28) had *Down syndrome*, and another (Case 9) had *Uhl's disease.* One patient with Ebstein's, common AV canal, and tricuspid regurgitation (Case 78) also had coexisting *tetralogy of Fallot.*

Types of Literature

There are many different kinds of published studies concerning Ebstein's anomaly:

Pathologic anatomy. Investigations that focus importantly on the pathologic anatomy include the following references: 1, 2, 4, 8, 9, 20, 25, 28, 37, 38, 47, 55, 59, 61, 70, 75, 78, 79, 85, 86, 88, 90, 94, 101, 102, 111, 113, 114, 115, 118, 119, 126, 127, 138, 140, 141, 146, 155, 168, 175, 176, 177, 194, 197, 206.

Clinical profile and natural history. Studies that focus mainly on the clinical profile and natural history of prenatal and postnatal patients with Ebstein's anomaly include the following: 12, 13, 14, 24, 30, 35, 41, 44, 46, 49, 50, 51, 54, 62, 76, 83, 87, 100, 121, 122, 125, 132, 134, 135, 137, 141, 143, 145, 147, 149, 152, 154, 158, 161, 165, 172, 175, 187, 189, 195, 211.

Imaging studies. Investigations that focus on diagnostic imaging studies (angiocardiography, echocardiography, magnetic resonance imaging, and other modalities) are also very important: 1, 12, 38, 40, 52, 56, 58, 60, 61, 64, 66, 67, 74, 77, 83, 91, 93, 96, 107, 108, 112, 113, 115, 116, 124, 126, 131, 132, 134, 135, 137, 140, 144, 153, 156, 157, 159, 167, 168, 200, 207.

Electrophysiologic studies. Investigations of arrhythmias, their anatomic basis, and their management have also been of considerable importance in patients with Ebstein's anomaly: 15, 32, 36, 42, 43, 53, 55, 58, 68, 80, 91, 103, 114, 120, 123, 130, 145, 163, 177, 180, 182, 190, 191, 202, 204, 205, 210, 211, 216.

Pregnancy and delivery. The management and outcome of the pregnancy and delivery of mothers with Ebstein's anomaly have also been studied with care: 46, 143, 152, 211.

Who was Wilhelm Ebstein? A few papers have told his story: 3, 5, 6.

Etiology. What are the basic causes of Ebstein's anomaly? Several investigations have attempted to address this important question: 31, 41, 65, 71, 119, 120, 141, 155, 203. There appear to be genetic,[71] familial,[31,41] embryologic,[155] and teratogenic (i.e., lithium)[65,203] aspects to this question.

Cardiovascular support. The use of extracorporeal membrane oxygenation (ECMO)[136] as a postnatal rescue technique has been advocated. Balloon pulmonary valvuloplasty[138] has been helpful when significant pulmonary valvar stenosis coexists. The use of prolonged prostaglandin therapy (PGE) to keep the ductus arteriosus open has been advocated,[151] until the neonatal pulmonary resistance falls sufficiently to permit adequate pulmonary blood flow (Qp) at subsystemic right heart pressures. On the other hand, it has been pointed out that limiting ductal patency[196] can be very helpful in avoiding deleterious "circular" shunts that promote right heart failure. So the medical aspects of management can be delicate and difficult.[137,195,196]

Surgical management. How should patients with Ebstein's anomaly be managed surgically?

First, perhaps not everyone with Ebstein's anomaly requires cardiac surgery. For example, Seward and his colleagues[83] reported Ebstein's anomaly in an unoperated 85-year-old man, the longest known survival in the natural history of this malformation. But what happened to this man? He had tricuspid regurgitation leading to congestive heart failure and death. Despite his "great age," he might have lived a healthier and longer life had he not had the Ebstein-related tricuspid regurgitation that led to his death. Bearing in mind that the human longevity limit is about 120 years,[217] and 85 is no longer considered all that old.

Although patients with "mild" Ebstein's (i.e., with little tricuspid regurgitation, no arrhythmias, and no associated malformations) may never require surgery, many do. The worst group is those who present in utero. The dilemma of these patients is presented in several studies. These are the "presurgical" patients, too young (in utero) to be helped by currently available surgical procedures. For example, in the ultrasound (two-dimensional echocardiography) study by Hornberger, Sahn, Kleinman, Copel, and Reed (1991),[135] there were 26 fetuses, 17 with Ebstein's (63%) and 7 with tricuspid valve dysplasia with normally attached but poorly developed leaflets (27%). Two patients had congenitally unguarded tricuspid orifice (8%). All of these patients had massive right atrial dilation (100%).

Hydrops fetalis (massive congestive heart failure) was observed in 6 of 26 (23%). Atrial flutter was present in 5 (19%). Pulmonary outflow tract obstruction coexisted in 11 of 26 (42%): stenosis in 5 and atresia in 6.

The clinical course of 23 patients tells the story:[135] death in utero, 48%, and live born but died, 35%. Hence, the prenatal plus the neonatal death rate was 83%—a devastating natural history. Significant lung hypoplasia—probably secondary to massive cardiomegaly—was found in 10 of 19 autopsied cases (53%).

It is not widely understood that Ebstein's malformation is a much more malignant disease than are most other forms of congenital heart disease that we think of as being very bad (e.g., transposition of the great arteries), because Ebstein's anomaly is associated with a high intrauterine death rate, whereas transposition of the great arteries is not.

This grave conclusion was also reached by McElhinney, Salvin, Colan, Thiagarajan, Crawford, Marcus, del Nido, and Tworetzky (2005).[195] Fetal death occurred in 9 of 25 (36%). Of the prenatally diagnosed patients (excluding 8 abortions or terminations), only 7 of 25 survived beyond the neonatal period (28%); that is, the fetal plus neonatal mortality rate was 72%. Independent predictors of death (by multivariable logistic regression analysis) included the following:[195]

1. a right atrial (RA) area >1; and
2. absence of anterograde blood flow across the pulmonary valve.

(The RA area index = the ratio of the RA area/the area of the "ventricularized" right ventricle + the area of the left atrium + the area of the left ventricle.)

These authors[195] concluded that although outcomes in fetuses and neonates with Ebstein's anomaly have improved, survival at the severe end of the spectrum remains poor. As a novel approach to management, McElhinney and his colleagues[195] suggested the possibility of giving corticosteroids to ensure fetal pneumatocyte maturity, followed by elective mid-third trimester delivery and then intensive postnatal care.

Thus, at the present time, the surgeons are meeting only the "winners"—the survivors of the often devastating prenatal and neonatal periods.

So this, then, is the current surgical question: how best to treat those Ebstein patients who require (postnatal) surgery? (Prenatal surgery is, of course, the dream. But we're not there yet.)

Repair. Investigators who favored repair, that is, tricuspid annuloplasty and valvuloplasty typically with plication or exclusion or the atrialized right ventricle, include the following: 27, 45, 69, 73, 87, 97, 105, 106, 110, 129, 131, 142, 144, 150, 160, 166, 169, 173, 174, 178, 180–186, 188, 190, 192, 193, 198–201, 208, 212, 213.

Replacement. Investigators who favored tricuspid valve replacement include the following: 26, 29, 34, 39, 48, 57, 72, 81, 82, 89, 95, 98, 99, 104, 109, 110, 117, 128, 162, 171, 179, 199.

Fontan. Ebstein's anomaly with severe tricuspid stenosis has been treated with a Fontan procedure: 92, 148.

Creation of tricuspid atresia with central shunt. Another approach to the almost imperforate Ebstein's anomaly has been pericardial patch closure of the tricuspid orifice and aortopulmonary central shunt (Gore-Tex conduit, 4 mm in diameter).[142]

Which is the best surgical approach? As the aforementioned references indicate, there is still considerable disagreement concerning the best surgical approach to the management of Ebstein's anomaly. I am now more than old enough to know that a cardiologist-pathologist-embryologist (like me) should never try to tell a surgeon how to do the operation. However, a few anatomic hints may be helpful.

First, read all the references, think about them, and then make up your own mind, as a surgeon. What can you do technically? What do you feel about the various options? You should like the operation that you are going to do.

I favor repair (as opposed to tricuspid valve replacement). As Carpentier and his colleagues have repeatedly emphasized (correctly, I think), the surgical operation should be tailored to the patient's function and anatomic status.[129,160,185]

I like the posterior annular plication technique used by Hancock Friesen and her colleagues (2004).[193] It is elegant, it is simple, and it worked well. One ends up with a bicuspid right atrioventricular valve. However, this was a small series ($n = 7$) and the ages of the patients ranged from 3.6 to 63.8 years, the mean being 39 years. Hence, this was not a neonatal series, even in part. Mortality was 0 and long-term follow-up will be necessary.

The report by Chauvaud and colleagues (2006)[200] is another excellent example of where we are surgically at the present time. In a series of 26 consecutive patients, mean age 30 ± 16 years (a *postneonatal* series), the surgeon mobilized the anterior tricuspid leaflet, did a longitudinal placation of the atrialized right ventricle, reduced the size of the tricuspid annulus, closed the secundum atrial septal defect or patent foramen ovale, and performed a bidirectional Glenn procedure in 54% of cases (14/26) to reduce right ventricular preload. Chauvaud et al[200] thought that the indication for plication of the atrialized right ventricle is dyskinesis of this structure. In all cases (mortality = 0), the left ventricular ejection fraction and stroke volume index increased postoperatively.

But now let us consider the more difficult problem: *neonatal Ebstein's*. For example, Reemtsen, Fagan, Wells, and Starnes (2006)[201] published their experience with 16 neonates who all had profound heart failure. The indications for surgery were overt heart failure, cyanosis, acidosis, tricuspid regurgitation, depressed right ventricular function, and severe cardiomegaly.

The operative strategy[201] began with an assessment of the possibility of tricuspid valve repair, with or without right ventricular outflow tract reconstruction. If the tricuspid valve was thought to be repairable, this was done ($n = 3$, 19%).

If tricuspid valve repair did not seem feasible, then the tricuspid valve was oversewn with a pericardial patch; the tricuspid patch was fenestrated (in 10 of 13 patients) to decompress the right ventricle; reduction atrioplasty was performed; if extensive, the atrialized right ventricle was plicated; and a modified Blalock-Taussig shunt was established to guarantee adequate pulmonary blood flow. Heart transplantation was the initial therapeutic option in 1 patient (6%). Early (hospital) mortality was 31% (5 of 16 patients). Late deaths were 0 of 11 survivors.

In the discussion that followed Dr. Reemtsen's presentation,[201] Dr. Knott-Craig,[184] who has championed the repair of Ebstein's malformation to create a competent monocusp valve, noted that his mortality was less than 30%. (In fact it was 12.5%, 1/8.)[184]

Then Dr. Sano, who has advocated total right ventricular exclusion for isolated congestive right ventricular failure,[183] said that he excises the right ventricular free wall, instead of plicating it, in order to reduce the size of the right ventricle and the right atrium. He reported that immediately postoperatively, the cardiothoracic ratio was reduced to 52%; the left ventricular ejection fraction increased from 27% to 62%; and the cardiac index increased from 2.1 to 3.5. Dr. Sano's mortality with this operative approach has been zero (early = 0; late = 0).

The foregoing are just a few of the many promising surgical studies concerning the surgical therapy of Ebstein's anomaly. If time, strength, and space permitted, many other investigations would merit discussion. But this I must leave to the reader. I have only three general comments:

1. We should distinguish between studies of the surgical management of **neonatal Ebstein's anomaly,** and those that deal with **postneonatal Ebstein's malformation.** The difference in severity is huge.
2. We should be in favor of whatever works best. Although my present bias is in favor of repair rather than replacement, it must be understood that there are many examples of successful results following tricuspid valve replacement (see the above-cited references). At the present time, we simply do not know what the conclusions of the future will be. The optimal medical and surgical management of Ebstein's anomaly is still evolving. As my old friend and teacher, Dr. Maurice Lev, used to say, "It's a research problem." I agree and I would like to add that we are making progress. As mentioned heretofore, I think that repair of the tricuspid valve and of the atrialized right ventricle may well ultimately be accepted as preferable to tricuspid valve replacement; but only time will tell.
3. Most of the references concerning Ebstein's anomaly are presented in chronological order (from references 24 onward). This makes it readily possible to comprehend our growth in the understanding of this malformation. In-depth understanding, facilitated by a *historical approach,* is much better than memorizing a few rules or criteria.

NON-EBSTEIN TRICUSPID REGURGITATION

First, it is noteworthy that we have in our database approximately as many cases of congenital non-Ebstein tricuspid regurgitation (n = 80) as we have of all types of Ebstein's anomaly (n = 78, Table 13.1). So, non-Ebstein tricuspid regurgitation is *not* rare (80 of 3216 cases of congenital heart disease, i.e., 2.49%), at least when compared with Ebstein's anomaly.

But the question remains: **What is so-called congenital non-Ebstein tricuspid regurgitation?** Before doing this study, I really had no clear idea what the answers were. For me, this was a surprising *terra incognita*. In retrospect, the answers may seem obvious; but prospectively, they were not (Table 13.10).

Just a glance at Table 13.10 indicates that congenital *non-Ebstein* tricuspid regurgitation is more complicated and variable than *Ebstein* tricuspid regurgitation. Indeed, there were 16 different anatomic types of non-Ebstein congenital tricuspid regurgitation (Table 13.10). Let us look at each in turn.

TABLE 13.10 Congenital Non-Ebstein Tricuspid Regurgitation: Associated Findings

Associated Findings	No. of Cases (n = 80)	% of Series
1. With pulmonary atresia and intact ventricular septum	18	22.5
2. With double-inlet left ventricle	13	16.25
3. With hypoplastic left heart syndrome	12	15
4. With transposition of the great arteries {S,L,L}	9	11.25
5. With trisomies Trisomy 18, 3 Trisomy 13, 2	5	6.25
6. With Marfan syndrome	4	5
7. With Uhl's disease	3	3.75
8. With myxomatous tricuspid valve and polyvalvar disease	3	3.75
9. With transposition of the great arteries {S,D,D} and dysplastic tricuspid valve	3	3.75
10. With tricuspid valve prolapsed	2	2.5
11. With dysplastic right ventricle and tricuspid valve	2	2.5
12. With double-inlet and double-outlet right ventricle	2	2.5
13. With congenitally unguarded tricuspid orifice	1	1.25
14. With downward displacement of anterior tricuspid leaflet and blood cysts	1	1.25
15. With congenital mitral regurgitation and pulmonary vascular obstructive disease	1	1.25
16. With hypoplastic pulmonary artery branches and pulmonary artery hypertension	1	1.25

Tricuspid Regurgitation With Pulmonary Atresia and Intact Ventricular Septum

It will perhaps come as no surprise that tricuspid regurgitation (TR) with pulmonary atresia (or extremely severe pulmonary valvar stenosis) and intact ventricular septum (or with one or more very small ventricular septal defects) (Fig. 13.24) was the most common anatomic type of congenital TR without Ebstein's anomaly (Table 13.10). It should be recalled that Davignon, Greenwold, DuShane, and Edwards[218] described two anatomic types of pulmonary atresia with intact ventricular septum in 1961. When the tricuspid valve was competent, allowing little or no tricuspid regurgitation, then the right ventricular cavity was *small,* with a very thick-walled right ventricle. However, when the tricuspid valve was regurgitant or incompetent, then the right ventricular cavity was much *larger* (Fig. 13.25). A competent tricuspid valve permitted the right ventricle (RV) to do pressure work, but little or no flow work; hence the RV was thick-walled and small-chambered. By contrast, an incompetence or regurgitant tricuspid valve allowed the RV to do both pressure work and flow work (even though the flow was largely retrograde into the right atrium). Thus, severe tricuspid regurgitation was associated with an RV that was larger-chambered and thinner-walled. The importance of tricuspid regurgitation in association with pulmonary atresia and intact ventricular septum has been known for almost 50 years[218] (time of writing, 2007).

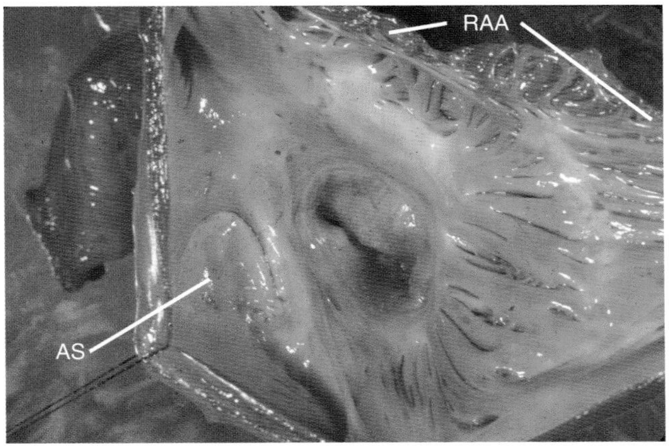

Fig. 13.24 Case 17 was 14-month-old boy with pulmonary atresia, intact ventricular septum, and massive tricuspid regurgitation. The tricuspid valve displayed thickened leaflets, fusion of chordae tendinae, and a markedly reduced number of chordae. The right atrium was hypertrophied and enlarged, with large focal areas of endocardial thickening and whitening (jet lesions). The right ventricular cavity size was considered to be moderate (neither very small, nor very large). An aberrant right subclavian artery was also present. Therapy included the injection of 10% formalin into the adventitia of the ductus arteriosus (in an effort to promote ductal patency) at 1 day of age (in 1976); surgical pulmonary valvotomy at 2 days of age using inflow occlusion; a Waterston anastomosis (ascending aorta to right pulmonary artery, side-to-side) at 3 weeks of age; and attempted repair of the atretic pulmonary valve and right ventricular outflow tract at 3½ weeks of age, leading to death 6 weeks postoperatively. View of the opened right atrium. Note that the tricuspid leaflets are bulging upward, toward the right atrium. The jet lesions on the interior of the right atrial free wall are large, but focal. Right atrial hypertrophy and enlargement are very marked. *AS*, Atrial septum; *RAA*, right atrial appendage or free wall. (Photograph taken at autopsy in 1977.)

Age at death (n = 18):
  mean = 191.153 ± 280.159 days (6.37 ± 9.34 months);
  range = 1.25 to 850 days (1.25 days to 2.33 years); and
  median = 43.5 days (1.45 months).

As you can see, the *mean* age at death in this anatomic type of non-Ebstein tricuspid regurgitation was young (6.37 ± 9.34 months). However, the *median* age at death, which more truly reflects the real situation, was even younger (1.45 months). Thus, pulmonary atresia with an intact ventricular septum and non-Ebstein tricuspid regurgitation was a rapidly fatal combination of anomalies.

Gender: males = 10, females = 8; male/female ratio = 1.25/1.0.

Death related closely in time to surgery: In these 18 patients, death was closely related in time to surgical intervention in 13 (72%). In another patient (Case 17, in 1977), death occurred 6 weeks postoperatively (more than 30 days postoperatively; so we did not regard it as "hospital" death, occurring soon after surgery). An additional case (Case 50, in 1969) died from severe intractable congestive heart failure and supraventricular tachyarrhythmia related to an excessively large Waterston anastomosis (5 × 4 mm). None of these fatalities occurred following a Fontan or Fontan-like procedure.

Anatomic variations: One of these patients (Case 37) had multiple very small ventricular septal defects (not an anatomically intact ventricular septum). Two of these patients had extremely severe pulmonary valvar stenosis (Cases 50 and 60), not a totally atretic pulmonary valve.

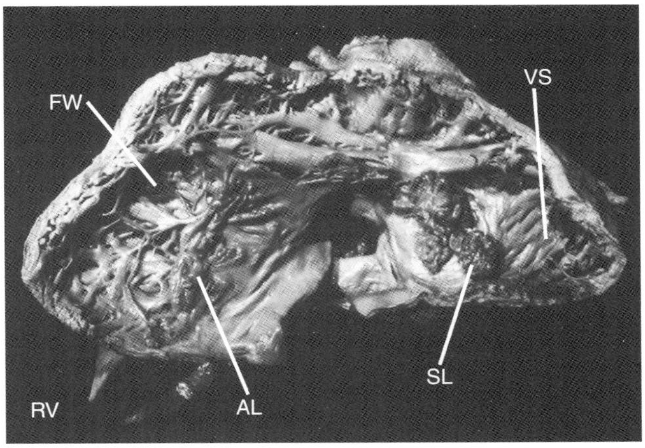

Fig. 13.25 Pulmonary atresia (valvar and subvalvar), intact ventricular septum, massive tricuspid regurgitation with hypertrophied and large-chambered right ventricle *(RV)*. The anterior leaflet *(AL)* is quite deep, curtain-like, and bound down by its chordae tendineae and papillary muscles. The septal leaflet *(SL)* is dysplastic, consisting of several masses of fibrous tissue that appear to be nonfunctional. The upper two masses of fibrous tissue are downwardly displaced only minimally; however, the most inferior mass of dysplastic septal leaflet fibrous tissue is definitely downwardly displaced. Consequently, we regarded this patient as having an Ebstein variant anomaly or an Ebstein-like malformation (but not typical Ebstein's anomaly). This is an excellent example of the large RV cavity that can be associated with pulmonary atresia, intact ventricular septum, tricuspid dysplasia, and severe congenital tricuspid regurgitation. *FW*, Free wall; *VS*, ventricular septum. (This patient was studied prior to our coming to Boston. Consequently, this case was not included in the present study. I can find no record of this patient's gender, or age at death.)

Non-Ebstein Tricuspid Regurgitation With Double-Inlet Left Ventricle

Congenital tricuspid regurgitation with double-inlet left ventricle was the second most common anatomic type of tricuspid regurgitation in patients who did not have Ebstein's anomaly: in 13 of 80 patients (16.25%) (Table 13.10).

Age at death: (n = 13):
  mean = 9.65 ± 9.66 years;
  range = 0 (18-week fetus) to 31 years; and
  median = 4.67 years (4⁸⁄₁₂ years).

Gender (n = 12): males = 6, females = 6; male/female ratio = 1.

The gender of the 18-week fetus was unknown to us.

Segmental anatomy (n = 13): Four different segmental anatomic sets* (or combinations) were found:

1. TGA {S,L,L} = 6 (46%) (Fig. 13.26);

**TGA {S,L,L}* means transposition of the great arteries with the segmental situs set of situs solitus of the viscera and atria, ventricular L-loop, and L-transposition of the great arteries.

TGA {S,D,D} means TGA with solitus atria, ventricular D-loop and D-TGA.

{S,D,S} denotes solitus atria, ventricular D-loop, and solitus normally related great arteries.

DORV {S,L,L} indicates double-outlet right ventricle with solitus atria, ventricular L-loop, and L-malposition of the great arteries. The atrioventricular alignments were double-inlet into the morphologically left ventricle in all (Table 13.10). The ventriculoarterial alignments are indicated by the segmental anatomy: L-TGA in 6, D-TGA in 3, solitus normally related great arteries in 3, and DORV with L-malposition of the great arteries in 1.

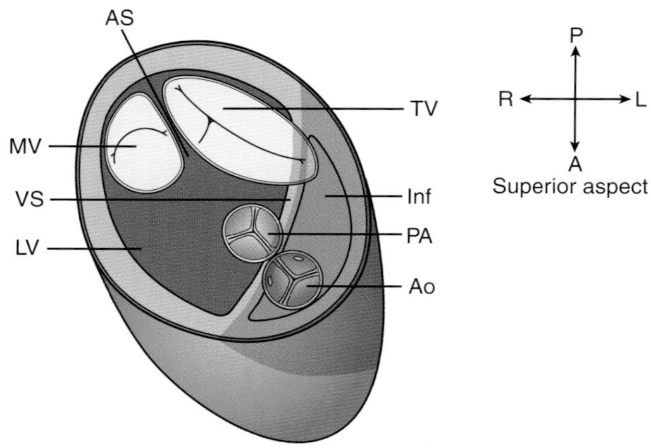

Fig. 13.26 The most common anatomic type of single left ventricle *(LV)* with an infundibular outlet chamber *(Inf)* and L-transposition of the great arteries. The aortic valve *(Ao)* is anterior and to the left of the pulmonary valve *(PA)*. The segmental anatomy is TGA {S,L,L}. The angulation of the atrial septum *(AS)* 30° to the left of the anteroposterior plane *(AP)* is typical of solitus atria. The morphologically right atrium (RA) (not drawn) lies to the right of the AS, and the morphologically left atrium (LA) (not drawn) lies to the left of the AS. Double-inlet LV is present because the RA opens through the right-sided mitral valve *(MV)* into the LV, and the LA opens through the left-sided tricuspid valve *(TV)* also into the right-sided LV and a little bit into the left-sided and anterior infundibular outlet chamber. The ventricular septal remnant *(VS)* is located anteriorly and to the left relative to the AS. Why? Because the right ventricular sinus (body, or inflow tract) is absent. The VS is displaced toward the location of the absent RV sinus. Absence of the RV sinus is why the LV is regarded as single (or unpaired), even though an infundibular outlet chamber (which is not a ventricle) is also present. Displacement of the VS to the left and anteriorly is also why there is double-inlet LV. Why is the TV regurgitant? Because of its abnormal insertions, both into the large LV and also into the Inf. Although the TV opens mostly into the right-sided LV, it also opens to a small degree into the left-sided and anterior Inf; consequently the left-sided TV straddles the VS. The abnormal bicameral insertion of the straddling TV appears to be the most important factor predisposing toward tricuspid regurgitation (left-sided). Note the thickening and rolling of the tricuspid leaflet margins (depicted diagrammatically). Geometrically, the AS lies 30° to the left of the anteroposterior (AP) plane. The VS is 20° to the right of the AP plane. The semilunar valves show 40° of rotation to the left of the AP plane. (Reproduced with permission from Van Praagh R, Ongley PA, Swan HJC: Anatomic types of single or common ventricle in man. Morphologic and geometric aspects of 60 necropsied cases. *Am J Cardiol* 1964;13:367.)

2. TGA {S,D,D} = 3 (23%);
3. {S,D,S} = 3 (23%) (Fig. 13.27); and
4. DORV {S,L,L} = 1 (8%).

State of the Right Ventricular Sinus

All 13 patients had double-inlet left ventricle because the RV sinus (body, or inflow tract) was either very underdeveloped ($n = 4$, 31%) or absent ($n = 9$, 69%). All had *functionally* single left ventricle because none had a physiologically adequate RV sinus (body, or inflow tract). Of these 13 patients, 9 (69%) had no anatomically demonstrable RV sinus. Hence, the RV sinus was considered to be absent, resulting in an *anatomically* single LV in these 9 patients. Thus, double-inlet LV indicated (1) that the atrioventricular canal was divided into two AV valves, that is, that the AV canal was not in common (undivided), and (2) that anatomically single LV (absent RV sinus) or functionally single LV (marked hypoplasia of the RV sinus) was present. From a physiologic and/or surgical standpoint, there is no practical difference between functionally and anatomically single LV. Both types of patients must be treated as having univentricular hearts (i.e., single LV), because the RV inflow tract (the main pumping portion of the RV) is functionally useless or absent.

Why was tricuspid regurgitation present in all? Typically, because the tricuspid valve was abnormally attached, opening into both the morphologically left ventricle (the LV) and into the infundibular outflow chamber (when the RV sinus was absent), or into the infundibular outlet chamber and into the diminutive RV sinus (when the latter was present). Consequently, the tricuspid valve typically straddled the ventricular septal remnant because of its bicameral insertions, resulting in tricuspid regurgitation that was *right-sided* relative to the mitral valve with a ventricular D-loop, or *left-sided* relative to the mitral valve when a ventricular L-loop was present (Figs. 13.26 and 13.27).

Let us examine this important question (why TR?) on a case-by-case basis.

Case 7: An 11-year-old girl, with normal segmental anatomy, that is, {S,D,S}, had double-inlet LV because the RV sinus was extremely underdeveloped, but not absent. She had congenital mitral stenosis (supravalvar and valvar). The tricuspid valve was straddling through a ventricular septal defect of the AV canal type with biventricular insertions into the large LV and the diminutive RV. The tricuspid leaflets were thickened and rolled, typical of tricuspid regurgitation. This patient also had severe pulmonary outflow tract stenosis involving marked narrowing of the subpulmonary os infundibuli. She died 3 days following a modified Fontan procedure.

Thus, the most important factor predisposing to tricuspid regurgitation appeared to be the abnormal tensor apparatus: the straddling tricuspid valve inserting into the large LV and the diminutive RV; the tricuspid valve straddled through a VSD of the AV canal type (typical of straddling tricuspid valve).[219] In association with marked underdevelopment of the RV sinus, there was marked ventriculoatrial malalignment, because the ventricular septal remnant was displaced in the direction of the small or absent right ventricular sinus—to the right with a ventricular D-loop, or to the left with a ventricular L-loop (Figs. 13.26 and 13.27). Congenital mitral stenosis was also present. Thus, *both* AV valves were dysfunctional.

From a physiologic and surgical standpoint, this patient did have a *functionally (if not anatomically) Holmes heart*, that is, a functionally single LV (because the RV sinus was uselessly small), with an infundibular outlet chamber and normally related great arteries. The presence of *double-inlet LV* helpfully indicates that a functionally single LV is present.

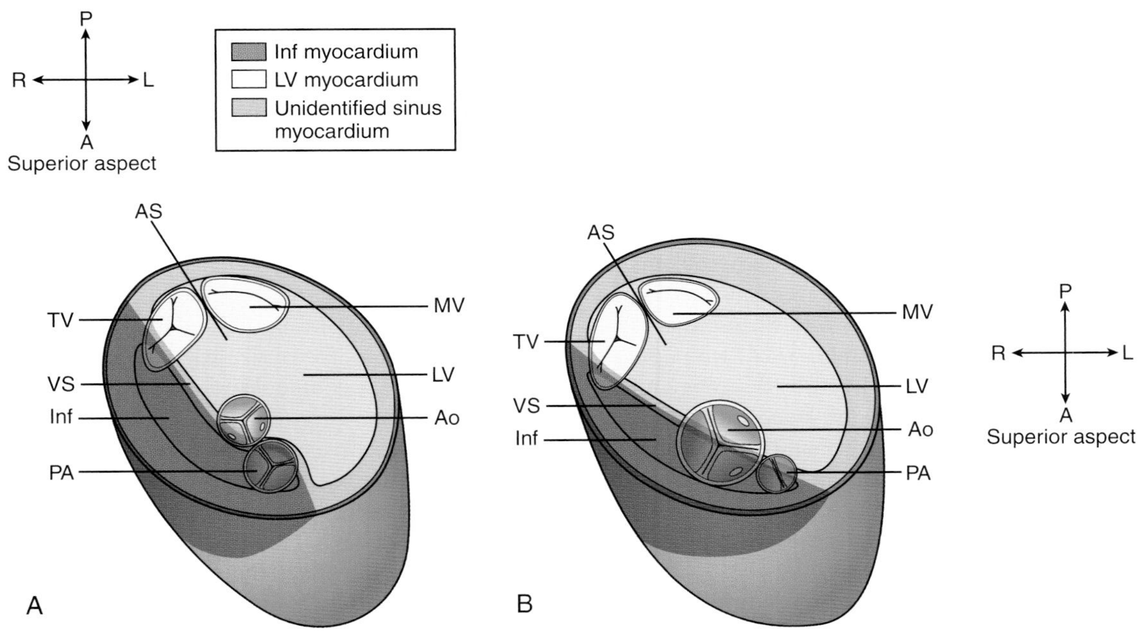

Fig. 13.27 Holmes hearts,[221] without pulmonary outflow tract stenosis (A), and with pulmonary outflow tract stenosis (B). Single left ventricle *(LV)* with infundibular outlet chamber *(Inf)* and normally related great arteries was first described in 1824 by W. F. Holmes,[221] the first Dean of Medicine at McGill University in Montreal, Canada. The right ventricular sinus (RV) is absent; hence the LV is single or unpaired. Absence of the RV inflow tract is also why there is double-inlet LV: there is no RV sinus for the tricuspid valve *(TV)* to open into. The ventricular septum is displaced to the right—in the direction of the absent RV inflow tract. Although the TV opens mostly into the LV because of the rightward displacement of the VS, the TV straddles the VS remnant to a small degree and opens into the infundibular outlet chamber. Tricuspid regurgitation is frequent, apparently because of the bicameral insertions of the TV associated with straddling of the TV. Tricuspid regurgitation is suggested diagrammatically by the thickening of the tricuspid leaflet margins and by the incomplete coaptation of the TV leaflets. In (B), pulmonary outflow tract stenosis is suggested by the relative smallness of the pulmonary artery *(PA)* compared with the aorta *(Ao)* and by the fact that the pulmonary valve is bicuspid. The distinctive and unusual feature of the Holmes heart is that the great arteries are normally related; single LV with infundibular outflow chamber is usually associated with abnormally related great arteries, such as transposition of the great arteries. The segmental anatomy in the Holmes heart[221] is {S,D,S}. In (A), the anatomic geometry is as follows: The atrial septum *(AS)* is angulated 30° to the left of the sagittal plane (if the AS is considered to be hinged posteriorly to the sagittal plane); this angulation is normal for solitus atria. The ventricular septal remnant *(VS)* is displaced far to the right of the AS, and the VS is 40° to the left of the sagittal plane (if the VSD is considered for the purposes of measurement to be hinged posteriorly to the sagittal plane). The semilunar valves display 150° dextrorotation relative to the sagittal plane, which is normal (for solitus normally related great arteries). In (B), the anatomic geometry is as follows: atrial septum, 30° to the left (normal); ventricular septum, marked rightward displacement and angulated 60° to the left; and the semilunar relationships as in tetralogy of Fallot (TOF), the aortic valve 100° dextrorotation (subnormal). Even though the dextrorotation of the aortic valve is subnormal (150° is normal), nonetheless this TOF-like semilunar interrelationship is considered to be within the normal range (but at the subnormal end of the range) because there is aortic valve–to–mitral valve direct fibrous continuity (typical of normally related great arteries). *MV,* Mitral valve. (Reproduced with permission from Van Praagh R, Ongley PA, Swan HJC: Anatomic types of single or common ventricle in man. Morphologic and geometric aspects of 60 necropsied cases. *Am J Cardiol* 1964;13:367 and from Van Praagh R, Plett JA, Van Praagh S: Single ventricle: pathology, embryology, terminology, and classification. *Herz* 1979;4:113.)

Case 8, a 4-year-old girl with normal segmental anatomy, that is, {S,D,S} and extreme hypoplasia of the RV sinus, also had a tricuspid valve that straddled through a VSD of the AV canal type. The tricuspid valve inserted into the infundibular outlet chamber and into the large left ventricle. The tricuspid valve leaflets were thickened, consistent with tricuspid regurgitation, and mitral regurgitation was also present. Double-inlet left ventricle indicated that from the functional standpoint, a Holmes heart was present. Again, both AV valves were dysfunctional (both regurgitant). This patient died after a Fontan takedown.

Case 10, a 21-year-old man, had TGA {S,D,D} (TGA {S,D,D} indicates that transposition of the great arteries is present with situs solitus of the viscera and atria, ventricular D-loop, and D-TGA), double-inlet left ventricle, marked hypoplasia of the RV sinus, and two ventricular septal defects (of the AV canal type and of the conoventricular type). The regurgitant tricuspid valve straddled through the VSD of the AV canal type. A persistent left superior vena cava drained into the coronary sinus and opened into the right atrium. Pulmonary stenosis (valvar and subvalvar) coexisted. The patient also had Leopard syndrome. Atrial flutter-fibrillation, congestive heart failure, and left ventricular dysfunction led to terminal ventricular fibrillation. Tricuspid regurgitation was moderate in severity and was only one of this young man's many cardiovascular problems.

Case 13, a $2\frac{5}{12}$-year-old boy, had TGA {S,L,L} (TGA {S,L,L} means transposition of the great arteries with situs solitus of the viscera and atria, ventricular L-loop, and L-TGA) with double-inlet into the right-sided LV, single LV (no RV sinus found), and infundibular outlet chamber. The left-sided tricuspid valve leaflets opened into the LV free wall, without well-formed chordae tendineae or papillary muscles. This myxomatous tricuspid valve was both regurgitant and stenotic. A blood cyst of the pulmonary valve resulted in pulmonary valvar stenosis. Congestive heart failure appeared at 3 months of age.

At 22 months of age, atrial septectomy was performed, followed by a modified Fontan procedure at $2\frac{5}{12}$ years. A subsequent Fontan takedown was followed by intraoperative death. This patient illustrated tricuspid regurgitation and stenosis occurring together, the left-sided tricuspid valve having congenital absence of tensor apparatus (no chordae tendineae and no papillary musculature). **Congenital absence of the tricuspid tensor apparatus (chordae tendineae and papillary muscles) is a rare and largely unknown anomaly.**

Case 15, a 31-year-old woman, had TGA {S,L,L} with double-inlet LV, single LV with infundibular outlet chamber, moderate fibrous subvalvar pulmonary stenosis, and straddling of the left-side tricuspid valve through the bulboventricular foramen into the infundibular outlet chamber. The tricuspid valve did not obstruct the bulboventricular foramen. *The left-sided tricuspid valve was basket-like* and was associated with only mild tricuspid regurgitation. The Eustachian valve of the inferior vena cava was prominent. Complete heart block appeared spontaneously postnatally. Ventricular premature beats and atrial flutter—fibrillation occurred later. There was one episode of syncope. A pacemaker was inserted at $22\frac{5}{12}$ years. The pacemaker generator was changed at $24\frac{8}{12}$ years. Another pacemaker was inserted at $30\frac{7}{12}$ years of age. Sudden death occurred 10 months later at age $31\frac{5}{12}$ years of age, thought to be secondary to a ventricular tachyarrhythmia.

This patient, with the most common form of single ventricle (i.e., single LV with an infundibular outlet chamber and TGA {S,L,L}) demonstrates a situation in which ectopy was predominant and led to death. Tricuspid regurgitation (left-sided) was only mild in severity and was regarded as of relatively minor clinical importance.

Case 27, a $3\frac{11}{12}$-year-old boy, had TGA {S,D,D}, double-inlet LV, single LV with infundibular outlet chamber, and thickening and rolling of the right-sided tricuspid valve indicating tricuspid regurgitation. At 1 month of age, he had banding of the main pulmonary artery. At 1 year, he had a modified right Blalock-Taussig anastomosis. By $3\frac{11}{12}$ years of age (in 1987), he underwent a Stansel procedure (anastomosis of the proximal main pulmonary artery to the ascending aorta to bypass developing subaortic stenosis at the bulboventricular foramen) and a modified Fontan procedure (anastomosis of the right atrium to the distal main pulmonary artery, to reestablish pulmonary arterial blood flow); he died intraoperatively.

This patient exemplifies the problem of achieving optimal pulmonary blood flow, and managing the development of subaortic stenosis in TGA {S,D,D} with single LV and double-inlet LV. Tricuspid regurgitation was present, but was not the main clinical problem.

Case 28, a 22-day-old boy, had TGA {S,L,L} with double-inlet LV, single LV and infundibular outlet chamber, and subaortic stenosis because of a restrictively small bulboventricular foramen. There was mild stenosis of the right atrial ostium of the superior vena cava. The leaflets of the left-sided tricuspid valve were thickened, nodular, regurgitant, and stenotic. The tricuspid chordae tendineae inserted directly into the left ventricular septal surface; the tricuspid valve had no papillary muscles. Death at 22 days of age occurred in 1967.

This patient illustrates **the general problem of all of these patients with double-inlet LV:** marked ventriculoatrial malalignment, resulting in abnormal tensor apparatus of the tricuspid valve—when the right ventricular inflow tract is diminutive or absent (absent in this patient) (Figs. 13.26 and 13.27). Tricuspid regurgitation (with or without tricuspid stenosis) is a sequela of ventriculoatrial malalignment and right ventricular sinus malformation. In other words, congenital tricuspid regurgitation (with or without congenital tricuspid stenosis) is not really a *primary* diagnosis; instead congenital TR (with or without tricuspid stenosis) is a *secondary* effect of the malformations of the tricuspid tensor apparatus, the small or absent RV sinus, the very abnormal location of the ventricular septal remnant, the abnormally hypertrophied and enlarged LV, and the associated ventriculoatrial malalignment.

Case 36, a $15\frac{7}{12}$-year-old boy with TGA {S,L,L}, had absence of the left-sided right ventricular sinus, single left ventricle (right-sided) with infundibular outlet chamber (left-sided), double-inlet left ventricle (right-sided), with straddling of the left-sided tricuspid valve, and tricuspid regurgitation (left-sided) with left atrial jet lesions.

This patient underwent banding of the main pulmonary artery at 18 months of age. At $4\frac{1}{12}$ years of age, he developed acquired complete heart block. In 1980, at $15\frac{7}{12}$ years of age, the patient had a Fontan type of procedure. His right-sided normally functioning mitral orifice was closed with a Dacron patch. The band of the main pulmonary artery was removed. The pulmonary valve was sutured closed. A 20 mm nonvalved conduit was placed from the right atrium to the distal main pulmonary artery. The patient died soon postoperatively.

Enthusiasm at our institution soon waned for the surgical creation of "tricuspid" atresia to facilitate a Fontan type of procedure, particularly when it involved patching closed the patient's only normally functioning atrioventricular valve, the only postoperatively patent atrioventricular valve being malfunctional (in this case, regurgitant).

Case 58, a $4\frac{8}{12}$-year-old boy, had TGA {S,D,D} with single left ventricle and infundibular outlet chamber. There was double-inlet left ventricle with tricuspid regurgitation. The tricuspid leaflets were thickened and rolled, whereas the mitral leaflets were unremarkable. The right superior vena cava was absent. A persistent left superior vena cava drained into the coronary sinus and thence into the right atrium, where a prominent Chiari's network (remnants of the right sinoatrial valvar leaflet) was present.

Case 65 was an 18-week-old fetus with complex congenital heart disease. We examined the heart of this patient as a consultation; we do not know the gender of this fetus.

The heart displayed double-outlet right ventricle {S,L,L} with mitral atresia (right-sided), a large and functionally single left ventricle (right-sided), an almost absent right ventricular sinus (left-sided), and a secundum type of atrial septal defect. The leaflets of the left-sided tricuspid valve were myxomatous, with attachments to the left ventricular free wall (right-sided), to the ventricular septal crest, and to the right ventricular free wall (left-sided). This left-sided tricuspid valve straddled the ventricular septum and severe tricuspid regurgitation was thought to have been present in utero because of noncoaptation of the leaflets.

In order to understand this case it is necessary to know that mitral atresia rarely can be associated with a *large* left ventricle. Usually with mitral atresia, the left ventricle is small to tiny. Mitral atresia with a large left ventricle also is typically associated with a small (or absent) right ventricular sinus. Hence, mitral atresia with a large left ventricle is an anatomically or functionally single left ventricle (depending on whether the right ventricular sinus is absent, or very small as it was in this patient) with an infundibular outlet chamber. Both great arteries originated above the diminutive right ventricle in this patient; hence the diagnosis of *DORV* {S,L,L}—with mitral atresia (right-sided), tricuspid regurgitation (left-sided), large left ventricle (right-sided), diminutive right ventricle (left-sided) and straddling tricuspid valve (left-sided). To the best of our present knowledge, mitral atresia with large (or single) left ventricle was first reported by Quero in 1972.[220]

Case 68 was a 12-year-old girl with dextrocardia, TGA {S,L,L}, single left ventricle with infundibular outlet chamber, double-inlet left ventricle, extreme mitral stenosis (right-sided) with parachute mitral valve and all chordae tendineae inserting into the anterolateral papillary muscle of the left ventricle, tricuspid regurgitation (left-sided) with marked left atrial hypertrophy, enlargement, and jet lesions. The regurgitant tricuspid valve was replaced with a Björk-Shiley valve in 1985 at another institution. Postoperatively, there was severe pulmonary outflow tract obstruction related to the tricuspid valve prosthesis. A modified Fontan procedure had also been performed.

Case 70 was a 9-month-old girl with a Holmes heart.[221] She had a single left ventricle with double-inlet left ventricle, an infundibular outlet chamber, normally related great arteries, normal segmental anatomy—{S,D,S}, tricuspid regurgitation, and subaortic stenosis (related to abnormal insertion of the septal leaflet of the tricuspid valve). The anterior papillary muscle was absent from the infundibular outlet chamber. The superior commissure of the tricuspid valve inserted abnormally into the conal septum.

Case 71 was a 19-year-old woman with TGA {S,L,L}, a single left ventricle with infundibular outlet chamber, double-inlet left ventricle, straddling of *both* atrioventricular valves with tricuspid regurgitation (left-sided) and mitral regurgitation (right-sided). Both AV valves inserted into the single left ventricle and into the infundibular outlet chamber. Both AV valves had thickening and rolling of the leaflet free margins. There was mild to moderate subaortic stenosis caused by narrowing of the bulboventricular foramen, with a fibrous rim of endocardial sclerosis surrounding the bulboventricular foramen. Subpulmonary stenosis was also present because the pulmonary outflow tract passed between the medial leaflets of both AV valves as they entered the left ventricle. Hence, this 19-year-old woman had the devastating combination of regurgitation of both atrioventricular valves and stenosis of both great arterial outflow tracts.

Non-Ebstein Regurgitation Associated With Hypoplastic Left Heart Syndrome

Although the two most common anatomic types of non-Ebstein tricuspid regurgitation are, on reflection, not too surprising (pulmonary atresia with intact ventricular septum in 22.5%, and double-inlet left ventricle in 16.25%, Table 13.10), the third most common anatomic type—with hypoplastic left heart syndrome in 15% (Table 13.10)—is not as intuitively obvious. One wonders, why may the hypoplastic left heart syndrome have tricuspid regurgitation? This is the question that we must now explore. To avoid vague generalizations let's examine these patients case by case.

Case 34 was an 8-month-old girl with double-outlet right ventricle {S,D,D} with a subpulmonary conus and aortic valve–tricuspid valve fibrous continuity, mitral atresia, a subaortic conoventricular type of ventricular septal defect, subaortic stenosis between the conal septum anterosuperiorly and the tricuspid valve posteroinferiorly. *There was tricuspid regurgitation with thickened and myxomatous tricuspid leaflets.* The aortic valve was bicuspid (bicommissural) because of absence of the right coronary–left coronary commissure, the aortic isthmus was hypoplastic, and the ductus arteriosus was patent. At 12 days of age, the main pulmonary artery was banded, the patent ductus arteriosus was ligated, and the hypoplastic aortic isthmus was amplified with a subclavian flap angioplasty. Congestive heart failure postoperatively was associated with ineffective main pulmonary artery banding. Consequently, at 1½ months of age (in 1983) the main pulmonary artery was rebanded and an atrial septectomy was performed. Sudden unexpected death occurred at home at 8 months of age. The immediate cause of death was thought probably to have been a ventricular arrhythmia.

Why did this patient have congenital, non-Ebstein, tricuspid regurgitation? We think that the answer may involve two factors: (1) the thick and myxomatous tricuspid valve leaflets; and (2) the coexistence of double-outlet right ventricle with aortic outflow tract stenosis, plus main pulmonary artery banding.

Again, it is noteworthy that this patient had a **specific type of DORV associated with hypoplastic left heart syndrome**, that is, DORV with a subpulmonary conus (only)—a unilateral (not a bilateral) conus, with aortic-tricuspid fibrous continuity, and aortic outflow tract stenosis between the conal septum anterosuperiorly and the tricuspid valve posteroinferiorly, with a somewhat hypoplastic and bicuspid aortic valve and a hypoplastic (low-flow) aortic isthmus.

Some of the problems associated with DORV plus hypoplastic left heart syndrome are illustrated by this case: an abnormal and myxomatous tricuspid valve and double-outlet right ventricle with obstruction of *both* great arterial outflow tracts (congenital aortic outflow tract narrowing, and banding of the main pulmonary artery).

Case 46 was a 1 8/12-year-old boy with mitral atresia {S,D,S}. Tricuspid regurgitation was observed both echocardiographically and angiocardiographically. A Norwood procedure was performed at 21 days of age (in 1986). The postoperative course was characterized by otitis media and upper respiratory tract infections. The clinical picture of congestive heart failure appeared. The modified Blalock-Taussig anastomosis was thought to be excessive. At autopsy, the tricuspid valve appeared to be morphologically unremarkable.

How should we interpret this case? Certainly the tricuspid regurgitation, although well documented, did not appear to be the patient's only hemodynamic problem. This may well be the type of patient that may have done better with a Sano shunt[222] from the right ventricular infundibulum to the pulmonary artery bifurcation, rather than having a modified Blalock-Taussig shunt as in the original Norwood procedure.[223]

This case also reminds one that **the tricuspid valve is not designed to occlude an approximately circular systemic atrioventricular orifice.** This task is well performed by the deep anterior leaflet of an uncleft mitral valve. The tricuspid valve is designed to occlude the elliptical pulmonary atrioventricular orifice, not the nearly circular systemic atrioventricular orifice; and the tricuspid valve is normally cleft (between the anterior and the septal tricuspid leaflets). So, when the tricuspid valve is required to serve as the systemic atrioventricular valve it is not surprising that it may prove to be regurgitant. The papillary muscles of the tricuspid valve also are not the large, well-balanced pair that the mitral valve normally has. The right ventricle has only one radiation of the conduction system: the right bundle branch is the superior radiation. The right ventricle normally does not have an inferior radiation of the conduction system, whereas the left ventricle normally does. The right ventricle normally is supplied mainly by only one coronary artery branch (the right coronary artery), whereas the left ventricle is normally supplied mainly by two coronary artery branches (the anterior descending and the circumflex branches).

Hence, there are a lot of anatomic reasons why the tricuspid valve and its tensor apparatus and ventricle may not perform as well as the mitral valve and its tensor apparatus and ventricle.

Nonetheless, it is still sobering to see that significant tricuspid regurgitation can and does occur through *a morphologically normal tricuspid valve* in the setting of typical hypoplastic left heart syndrome (as in this case of mitral atresia).

Case 48 was a 36-day-old black boy with aortic valvar atresia, mitral atresia, intact ventricular septum, a restrictive patent foramen ovale, and normal segmental anatomy, that is, {S,D,S}. At 14 days of age the patient underwent a Norwood procedure (in 1985). The postoperative course was characterized by supraventricular tachycardia, and mild coarctation of the aorta was noted at the distal end of the aortic arch reconstruction. Mild to moderate tricuspid regurgitation was observed both by angiography and by echocardiography. At autopsy, tricuspid regurgitation was thought to have been significant because the tricuspid leaflets were unable to coapt completely. Right ventricular hypertrophy and enlargement were very marked, as were right atrial hypertrophy and enlargement.

Thus, in this 36-day-old post-Norwood patient, significant tricuspid regurgitation was confirmed at autopsy because of incomplete tricuspid leaflet coaptation associated with very marked right ventricular hypertrophy and enlargement. This case again illustrates that the tricuspid valve is not designed to occlude the approximately circular systemic atrioventricular orifice that is associated with mitral and aortic valvar atresia.

Case 49 was at autopsy a 1 1/12-year-old-boy with aortic valve atresia {S,D,S} and intact ventricular septum. There was also fibrous subaortic stenosis produced by adherence of the anterior mitral leaflet to the left ventricular septal surface. A Norwood procedure was performed at 5 days of age (in 1985). Postoperatively, a residual coarctation was found at the distal end of the aortic arch reconstruction with a gradient of 70 mm Hg. Attempted balloon dilation of the coarctation site was ineffective. Sudden unexpected death occurred 12¾ months postoperatively. Autopsy revealed partial obstruction of the modified right Blalock-Taussig shunt. Thickening and rolling of the anterior tricuspid leaflet was also found, consistent with tricuspid regurgitation. However, tricuspid regurgitation was *not* regarded as the patient's most important disability. Instead, the coarctation of the aorta and the partially obstructed Blalock-Taussig shunt were thought to be the patient's main hemodynamic problems.

This patient illustrates the important point that tricuspid regurgitation is not necessarily the patient's most important hemodynamic problem; instead, tricuspid regurgitation may be only part of the hemodynamic handicap—and not necessarily the most important part. Hemodynamic problems are often multiple.

Case 51 was a 3½-year-old girl with aortic valve atresia, extreme mitral stenosis, intact ventricular septum, and {S,D,S} segmental anatomy who underwent a Norwood procedure in 1985 at 3½ days of age and who died intraoperatively. Autopsy revealed precoronary stenosis, that is, kinking of the neoaortic root such that the coronary ostia were nonpatulous. Echocardiography preoperatively had shown moderate tricuspid regurgitation, but at autopsy the tricuspid valve appeared morphologically normal. This case again illustrates that in hypoplastic left heart syndrome, tricuspid regurgitation can occur through an anatomically normal tricuspid valve.

Case 53 was a 43-day-old boy with aortic valvar atresia, mitral atresia, and {S,D,S} segmental anatomy who had tricuspid regurgitation with marked hypoplasia of the right ventricular papillary muscles, and very abnormal chordae tendineae. The chordae were reduced in number and were long and redundant. Thus, tricuspid regurgitation in this patient was related to very abnormal tricuspid tensor apparatus (papillary muscles and chordae tendineae).

This patient illustrates how difficult it is to generalize about the tricuspid regurgitation that may be associated with hypoplastic left heart syndrome. The tricuspid valve can be morphologically unremarkable (as above), or very abnormal (as in this patient).

This patient with hypoplastic left heart syndrome had additional cardiovascular abnormalities. There was atresia of the right atrial ostium of the coronary sinus. A small persistent left superior vena cava was confluent with the coronary sinus. Because the right atrial ostium of the coronary sinus was atretic, we thought that the blood flow in the coronary sinus may well have been retrograde—into the small left superior vena cava.

This patient died in 1984. One wonders, was there trisomy 18, or some other trisomy? We don't know the answers to these questions. (One may assume that if we do not mention an abnormal finding, either it was not present, or we do not know. All relevant findings of which we are aware are included here.)

Case 57 was a stillborn male fetus. (The intrauterine demise was natural, not induced by abortion.) This fetus had DORV {S,D,D}, that is, double-outlet right ventricle with solitus viscera and atria, D-loop ventricles, and D-malposition of the great arteries. The infundibulum was subpulmonary, with aortic valve-to-tricuspid valve direct fibrous continuity.

It should be recalled at this point that DORV with a unilateral (as opposed to bilateral) conus, either a subpulmonary infundibulum with aortic-tricuspid fibrous continuity or a subaortic conus with pulmonary-tricuspid fibrous continuity, is typical of DORV with hypoplastic left heart syndrome. So, one should be wondering at this point, What kind of hypoplastic left heart syndrome did this fetus have?

Septum primum was redundant and spinnaker-like, reducing the via sinistra into left atrium which was small. The mitral valve was hypoplastic and was abnormally attached both to the left ventricular septal surface and to the left ventricular free wall. Hypoplasia of the left ventricle was marked.

There was a patent foramen ovale, as was suggested above. Tricuspid regurgitation was severe. The anterior tricuspid valve was deep and curtain-like, tethered to the right ventricular free wall, and this leaflet was nonfunctional. The septal leaflet of the tricuspid valve was not downwardly displaced. Hence, Ebstein's malformation of the tricuspid valve was considered not to be present. The pulmonary valve was bicuspid (bicommissural). This fetus also had a small ventricular septal defect of the conoventricular type (between the conal septum above and the ventricular septum and septal band below).

Thus, this fetus died in utero because of the combination of hypoplastic left heart syndrome with severe tricuspid regurgitation through a dysplastic tricuspid valve with a tethered and nonfunctional anterior leaflet.

Case 62 was a 19-month-old boy whose hypoplastic left heart syndrome consisted of marked congenital mitral stenosis (thickening of leaflet tissue, with a small anterolateral papillary muscle, but not parachute mitral valve, and not Shone syndrome), mild valvar aortic stenosis with a hypoplastic and bicuspid (bicommissural) aortic valve, and preductal coarctation of the aorta. This patient also had pulmonary artery hypertension, severe congenital tricuspid regurgitation (with thickening, rolling, and redundancy of the anterior and septal leaflet), massive right ventricular hypertrophy and enlargement, and marked right atrial hypertrophy and enlargement. This patient, who died in 1992, had polyvalvar disease (mitral, aortic, and tricuspid). His karyotype is unknown; hence we cannot establish or exclude the possibility of a trisomy.

Case 72 was a 12-year-old boy with DORV {S,L,L}, that is, double-outlet right ventricle with situs solitus of the viscera and atria, a discordant ventricular L-loop, and L-malposition of the great arteries. His hypoplastic left heart syndrome consisted of membranous right-sided mitral atresia, very marked hypoplasia of the right-sided left ventricle (the left ventricular cavity was 1 to 2 peas in size, with endocardial fibroelastosis), with an intact ventricular septum. The patent foramen ovale was restrictive. Left-sided tricuspid regurgitation was marked, with thickening and rolling of all leaflet free margins. Congenital absence of pulmonary valve leaflets was associated with marked pulmonary outflow tract stenosis (3 to 4 mm in diameter). This patient had a functionally single right ventricle (because the diminutive left ventricle was functionally useless).

This patient, who died in 1978, illustrates that severe congenital *left-sided* tricuspid regurgitation can be associated with *right-sided* hypoplastic left heart syndrome in discordant L-loop ventricles.

Case 75 was a 5-day-old girl with mitral atresia, aortic atresia, intact ventricular septum, and {S,D,S}. She had a truly hypoplastic left heart syndrome with a tiny left ventricle that was both small-chambered and *thin-walled*.

It should be understood that many patients with so-called hypoplastic left heart syndrome may in fact *not* have a hypoplastic left ventricle. Consider aortic valvar atresia with intact ventricular septum and a patent mitral valve. The left ventricle typically is small-chambered, but it is also *thick-walled*. This is the so-called peach-stone left ventricle: the left ventricle resembles a thick-walled peach from which the peach stone has been removed. When pulmonary valvar atresia is associated with an intact ventricular septum and a patent tricuspid valve, the same analogy pertains: this is a peach-stone right ventricle, resembling a thick-walled peach from which the peach stone has been removed.

In both situations, the same question remains: Is the ventricle truly hypoplastic? Yes, the cavity is small because the ventricle can do little or no flow work (assuming that the atrioventricular valve is competent). But the wall is thick, because the ventricle can do pressure work. Are such ventricles really hypoplastic? Do they weigh significantly less than normal? This question has proved difficult to answer with certainty because each ventricle makes a contribution to the ventricular septum. To get an accurate weight of the left ventricle, one would have to weigh not only the left ventricular free wall, *but also the left ventricular component of the interventricular septum*. It is the latter—the ventricular septal component—that has proved difficult to weigh with precision. This understanding, or mental reservation, concerning hypoplastic left heart syndrome applies to this entire section concerning congenital tricuspid regurgitation with hypoplastic left heart syndrome. Patients with mitral and aortic valvar atresia and intact ventricular septum have truly hypoplastic left ventricles (like Case 75). However, patients with aortic atresia, intact ventricular septum, and patent mitral valves may or may not in fact have truly hypoplastic left ventricles.

To summarize, **there are two very different anatomic types of hypoplastic left heart syndrome:** (1) those with mitral and aortic valvar atresia and intact ventricular septum with very thin left ventricular free walls; and (2) those with aortic atresia with intact ventricular septum and patent mitral valve with thick left ventricular free walls, and often with endocardial fibroelastosis. We call these patent mitral valves "hypoplastic." Often they are as normal as they can be, but these mitral valves have to be small in order to open into these small left ventricular cavities.

So Case 75 had a truly hypoplastic left ventricle. The secundum atrial septal defect measured 5 × 8 mm. Echocardiography revealed moderate tricuspid regurgitation, confirmed at autopsy by thickened and myxomatous tricuspid leaflets. Dextrocardia was present. A ventricular malposition similar to crisscross atrioventricular relations was also found. Compared with normal, the ventricles were rotated 90°. The rotation was 90° in a counterclockwise direction as viewed from the atria, or 90° in a clockwise direction as seen from the ventricular apex. The ventricles were superoinferior with a horizontal ventricular septum, large right ventricle superiorly and small left ventricle inferiorly. The appearance of crisscross AV relations is better seen when both AV valves are patent. In typical crisscross AV relations, which this patient did not have, the ventricular malposition, as measured by the ventriculoatrial septal angle, often is greater than 90°.

Case 76 was a 17-day-old girl with membranous mitral atresia, subaortic narrowing, a bicuspid aortic valve with underdevelopment of the right coronary/left coronary commissure, tubular hypoplasia of the transverse aortic arch, preductal coarctation of the aorta, a large patent ductus arteriosus, a small secundum type of atrial septal defect consisting of multiple small restrictive foramina in septum primum, and tricuspid regurgitation with thickening and rolling of the free margins of the anterior and septal leaflets. Therapeutic interventions in 1993 included a balloon atrial septostomy and a Norwood procedure.

So, this is another patient with significant non-Ebstein tricuspid regurgitation associated with hypoplastic left heart syndrome.

Case 77 was a 1½-month-old girl with a small-chambered left ventricle, with a left ventricular free wall that was 4 to 6 mm thick. There was diffuse endocardial fibroelastosis of the left ventricular endocardium. Remarkably, the mitral valve was a normal miniature, and the aortic valve was also a normal miniature.

Consequently, we concluded that the patient had **primary hypoplasia of the left ventricle with endocardial fibroelastosis;** in other words, the left ventricular hypoplasia did not appear to be secondary to mitral or aortic valve pathology. In this sense, the left ventricular hypoplasia and the left ventricular endocardial fibroelastosis were both regarded as "primary," that is, idiopathic, of cause unknown—not apparently secondary to (or associated with) mitral and/or aortic obstructive pathology, as left ventricular hypoplasia usually is.

A secundum type of atrial septal defect (6 × 2 mm) was present. Right ventricular hypertrophy and enlargement were massive. Right atrial hypertrophy and enlargement were marked. Tricuspid regurgitation was described as moderate by two-dimensional echocardiography.

Autopsy revealed thickened, myxomatous nodules of the septal leaflet of the tricuspid valve. However, the anterior and posterior leaflets were morphologically unremarkable. The papillary muscles of the right ventricle were very small. Diffuse jet lesions were present of the right atrial endocardium.

In 1993 it was decided not to perform a Norwood procedure because of the presence of significant tricuspid regurgitation. Instead, the therapeutic plan was cardiac transplantation. However, this patient died waiting for a donor heart.

Non-Ebstein Tricuspid Regurgitation With Transposition of the Great Arteries {S,L,L}. TGA {S,L,L} is the classical form of congenital physiologically "corrected" transposition of the great arteries with visceroatrial situs solitus, discordant L-loop ventricles, and L-transposition of the great arteries with discordant atrioventricular (AV) and ventriculoarterial (VA) alignments (i.e., double discordance). We put physiologically "corrected" transposition in quotes because the potential physiologic corrections of the systemic venous and pulmonary venous circulations often are vitiated by associated malformations, as will be seen. Patients with single LV and infundibular outlet chamber with TGA {S,L,L} are not included here because they were presented in Group 2 above with double-inlet or common-inlet left ventricle (13 patients, 16.25%, Table 13.10).

Non-Ebstein tricuspid regurgitation with TGA {S,L,L} was fourth in frequency in this series of 80 postmortem cases, occurring in 9 patients (11.25%, Table 13.10).

Gender: males/females = 6/3 (2/1).

Age at death: mean = 9.75 ± 8.29 years; range from 3 months to 25.33 years; and median = 8.67 years.

Case 1 was a 3-month-old boy with TGA {S,L,L} and left-sided tricuspid regurgitation and double-orifice of the left-sided tricuspid valve. The patient also had WPW syndrome with paroxysmal atrial tachycardia (250/minute). Congestive heart failure appeared at 2 weeks of age. The respiratory rate was 60 to 80 breaths/minute.

The patient died at 3 months of age in 1961. Autopsy revealed massive left-sided cardiomegaly with very marked hypertrophy of the left-sided right ventricle and left atrium. There was a patent foramen ovale and an intact ventricular septum.

We concluded that the main immediate causes of this patient's death were the combination of the WPW syndrome with paroxysmal atrial tachycardia and left-sided tricuspid regurgitation associated with double-orifice of the left-sided tricuspid valve.

It should be understood that left-sided tricuspid regurgitation in TGA {S,L,L} is tantamount to mitral regurgitation in a segmentally normal heart, that is, {S,D,S}, because in TGA {S,L,L} the left-sided tricuspid valve is the systemic atrioventricular valve (not the pulmonary atrioventricular valve).

Case 6 was a 14-year-old girl with TGA {S,L,L}, a ventricular septal defect of the AV canal type, mild left-sided tricuspid regurgitation as judged by cardiac catheterization and angiocardiography and confirmed at autopsy by left atrial jet lesions, cleft right-sided mitral valve but without mitral regurgitation, abnormal insertions of the mitral valve into the crest of the ventricular septum, no ostium primum atrial septal defect, separate tricuspid and mitral annuli, subpulmonary stenosis produced by a spinnaker of accessory mitral valve tissue, spontaneous development of complete heat block, and premature ventricular contractions.

At 14 years of age in 1975 she underwent surgical closure of the ventricular septal defect, closure of a patent foramen ovale, and excision of subpulmonary stenosis. Postoperatively she developed ventricular fibrillation that led to sudden unexpected death. She also had kyphoscoliosis and lymphocytic thyroiditis.

Thus, non-Ebstein left-sided tricuspid regurgitation was present, but was regarded as a relatively minor hemodynamic problem. The main cause of death was thought to be electrophysiologic: the development of complete heart block with ventricular premature contractions, leading to fatal ventricular fibrillation.

Case 14 was a $25\frac{4}{12}$-year-old man with TGA {S,L,L}, a ventricular septal defect of the atrioventricular canal type, and pulmonary outflow tract atresia (infundibular and valvar). He had a secundum atrial septal defect. Subacute bacterial endocarditis led to calcified vegetations of his right-sided mitral valve leaflets. Angiocardiography revealed moderate left-sided tricuspid regurgitation.

Surgical interventions included a left-sided Blalock-Taussig anastomosis at 5½ years of age and a right-sided Blalock-Taussig anastomosis at $13\frac{7}{12}$ years of age. In 1978 at $23\frac{5}{12}$ years of age, a complete surgical repair was undertaken. His ventricular septal defect and atrial septal defect were closed. Both Blalock Taussig anastomoses were taken down, and a valved conduit was placed from the right-sided left ventricle to the main pulmonary artery. Complete heart block appeared postoperatively, treated by pacemaker implantation 1 week postoperatively. Sepsis then developed, with blood cultures positive for *Enterobacter*. Left-sided tricuspid regurgitation was then described as "free," that is, severe, and was associated with pulmonary hypertension.

At $23\frac{9}{12}$ years of age, left-sided tricuspid valve replacement was done using a 31 mm porcine Hancock valve. The postoperative course was characterized by ventricular ectopy and the appearance of serum hepatitis. Progressive biventricular congestive heart failure developed leading to death at $25\frac{4}{12}$ years of age.

In this patient, left-sided tricuspid regurgitation was a very important factor leading to death. Moderate non-Ebstein tricuspid regurgitation progressed to severe regurgitation, forcing tricuspid valve replacement. (Was the left-sided tricuspid valve involved by bacterial endocarditis when *Enterobacter* septicemia occurred? We don't know. We have no history that this was the case, but we did not have the privilege of examining the native tricuspid valve ourselves. The information that we have leads to the conclusion that bacterial endocarditis of the left-sided tricuspid valve was *not* present prior to its surgical removal.)

Hence, our conclusion is that non-Ebstein tricuspid regurgitation in the setting of TGA {S,L,L} can be moderate in severity, and that over time it can become very severe, necessitating tricuspid valve replacement.

Case 16 was a $14\frac{9}{12}$-year-old boy with TGA {S,L,L} with intact ventricular septum, probe patent foramen ovale, severe left-sided non-Ebstein tricuspid regurgitation, and marked cardiomegaly. Pulmonary congestion and edema with Kerley B lines were noted radiologically at 10½ years of age.

Left-sided tricuspid valve replacement was performed in 1980 using a 31 mm porcine Hancock prosthesis. Sydenham's chorea appeared 1 month postoperatively.

Four years postoperatively, stenosis of the left-sided tricuspid valve prosthesis was identified, with a 20 mm Hg end-diastolic gradient across the prosthesis and a left atrial mean pressure of 25 mm Hg.

Consequently, in 1980 at the age of $14\frac{8}{12}$ years, the stenotic Hancock tricuspid prosthesis was surgically replaced with a 29 mm St. Jude prosthesis, and a pacemaker was implanted into the epicardial surface of the right-sided left ventricle.

Sudden unexpected death occurred 1 month postoperatively, presumably from ventricular fibrillation. At autopsy, the left-sided tricuspid St. Jude prosthesis appeared unremarkable.

This case illustrates that left-sided non-Ebstein tricuspid regurgitation with TGA {S,L,L} can be extremely important. In this patient, non-Ebstein tricuspid regurgitation dominated the clinical picture, necessitating two tricuspid valve replacements.

Just in case you may have been wondering, how can we be sure that this is *non-Ebstein* tricuspid regurgitation when the tricuspid valve has been surgically removed? There are many clues that permit this differential diagnosis: What did the preoperative echocardiograms and angiocardiograms show? Was there a deep curtain-like anterior leaflet? Was the septal leaflet downwardly displaced? What did the surgeon think? Were the septal and posterior leaflets downwardly displaced or not?

Can the pathologic anatomy permit an accurate diagnosis, even when the left-sided tricuspid valve has been surgically removed? Yes. One can see whether or not the septal (and posterior) leaflets were downwardly displaced. Does the morphologically right ventricular septal surface myocardium extend up to the atrioventricular junction? If the answer is yes, then Ebstein's anomaly was not present. If the answer is no, then Ebstein's was present. Remember that in Ebstein's anomaly, not only is the septal leaflet downwardly displaced, but so too is the right ventricular septal surface myocardium. In Ebstein's malformation, *above* the downwardly displaced septal leaflet of the tricuspid valve, the septal surface of the atrialized right ventricle is "smooth as a baby's bottom"—because there is no right ventricular septal surface myocardium above the downwardly displaced septal leaflet. In Ebstein's, the failure of delamination and the failure of ascent of the septal and posterior tricuspid leaflets involves not only failure of these *leaflets* to ascend normally to the atrioventricular junction, but also involved is failure to lay down right ventricular septal *myocardium*. So, even when the tricuspid leaflets are excised, the right ventricular myocardium of the septal and posterior right ventricular surfaces tells the story, because Ebstein's is a malformation not only of the tricuspid valve leaflets, but also of the right ventricular myocardium.

Case 38 was a 6½-year-old boy with TGA {S,L,L}, intact ventricular septum, valvar aortic stenosis with a bicommissural (bicuspid) aortic valve, severe non-Ebstein left-sided tricuspid regurgitation, left atrial hypertrophy and enlargement, and a patent ductus arteriosus (6 mm in internal diameter). In

1965, he underwent tricuspid valve replacement, the valve being placed within the left atrium 1 cm above the atrioventricular junction. Left-sided tricuspid regurgitation was this patient's dominant hemodynamic problem.

Case 47 was a 3½-month-old boy with TGA {S,L,L} with ventricular septal defect and severe left-sided non-Ebstein tricuspid regurgitation. The tricuspid valve had abnormally short chordae tendineae and impaired leaflet mobility. The left-sided right ventricle was markedly enlarged. This patient also had a bicommissural (bicuspid) pulmonary valve with subpulmonary stenosis produced by redundant right-sided mitral valve tissue. This pulmonary outflow tract stenosis may well have contributed to the severe anoxic (blue) spell that led to death. The non-Ebstein severe tricuspid regurgitation was thought to be of major clinical importance.

Case 61 was an 8⁸⁄₁₂-year-old girl with TGA {S,L,L}, intact ventricular and atrial septa, and severe left-sided non-Ebstein tricuspid regurgitation. Left-sided right ventricular hypertrophy and enlargement were severe, and left atrial hypertrophy and enlargement were massive. In 1968 the left-sided tricuspid valve was replaced with a #7 Shiley prosthesis. Right-sided mitral regurgitation was observed at surgery, but at autopsy the right-side mitral valve appeared morphologically unremarkable. In this patient, non-Ebstein left-sided tricuspid regurgitation was the major hemodynamic problem.

Case 67 was a 3-year-old girl with TGA {S,L,L}, a ventricular septal defect, and severe left-sided non-Ebstein tricuspid regurgitation that we saw in consultation in 1985. The ventricular septal defect was of the conoventricular type and it had been surgically closed with a patch. The left-sided tricuspid valve had been replaced with a Bjork-Shiley prosthesis. The congenital tricuspid regurgitation was a major part of this patient's hemodynamic handicap.

Case 78 was a 14¹¹⁄₁₂-year-old boy with TGA {S,L,L}, a small conoventricular type of ventricular septal defect, complete heart block with a heart rate of 60 beats/minute, and marked left-sided non-Ebstein tricuspid regurgitation. In 1993 he was treated surgically with left-sided tricuspid valve replacement using a #33 St. Jude prosthesis, and permanent epicardial pacemaking leads were placed. Again, the congenital left-sided non-Ebstein tricuspid regurgitation was regarded as a very important part of this patient's cardiac disability.

Conclusions. Patients with discordant L-loop ventricles in visceroatrial situs solitus, as in TGA {S,L,L} and DORV {S,L,L}, can have significant congenital left-sided tricuspid regurgitation either because of left-sided Ebstein's malformation (Tables 13.2 and 13.6), or because of left-sided non-Ebstein congenital tricuspid regurgitation (Table 13.10).

Does congenital tricuspid regurgitation occur with discordant D-loop ventricles in visceroatrial situs inversus, as in TGA {I,D,D} and DORV {I,D,D}, either because of right-sided Ebstein's malformation or because of right-sided non-Ebstein tricuspid regurgitation? At present, we do not know the answers to these questions. It is noteworthy that none of these mirror-image possibilities was found in our data. We speculate that these anomalies may well exist, and that our failure to document them may be related to the rarity of visceroatrial situs inversus.

Congenital Non-Ebstein Tricuspid Regurgitation Associated With Trisomies

Tricuspid regurgitation associated with trisomies and having nothing to do with Ebstein's anomaly was found in 5 of these 80 patients (6.25%, Table 13.10): trisomy 18 in 3 patients (Fig. 13.28), and trisomy 13 in 2.

Trisomy 18. Case 39 was a 1-day-old boy with trisomy 18, karyotype proved. His problems included prematurity (33 weeks of gestation, birth weight 1300 grams) and multiple congenital anomalies: bilaterally small palpebral fissures, down-slanting eyes, micrognathia, retrognathia, absence of the left half of the vertebral body of the seventh thoracic vertebra, camptodactyly (bent or flexed fingers, irreducible), absence of distal flexion creases of the hands, nail hypoplasia of fingers and toes, low-arched dermal ridges in 8 of 10 fingers, syndactyly of toes 2 to 4 bilaterally, equinovarus deformity of the right foot, and absence of the right adrenal gland.

His congenital heart disease consisted of a ventricular septal defect of the conoventricular or membranous type and polyvalvar disease: multiple blood cysts of the atrial surface of the tricuspid valve leaflets, myxomatous thickening and redundancy of tricuspid valve leaflets, elongation and redundancy of tricuspid valve chordae tendineae and of the anterior papillary muscle of the right ventricle, mild to moderate tricuspid regurgitation with tricuspid valve prolapse (echocardiography), redundant pulmonary valve leaflets, redundant mitral valve leaflets, with an underdeveloped intercoronary commissure of the aortic valve ("pseudo-bicuspid" aortic valve, that is, only two well formed aortic valve commissures), a common brachiocephalic trunk (an aortic arch artery that gives rise to the right subclavian, the right common carotid, and the left common carotid arteries,

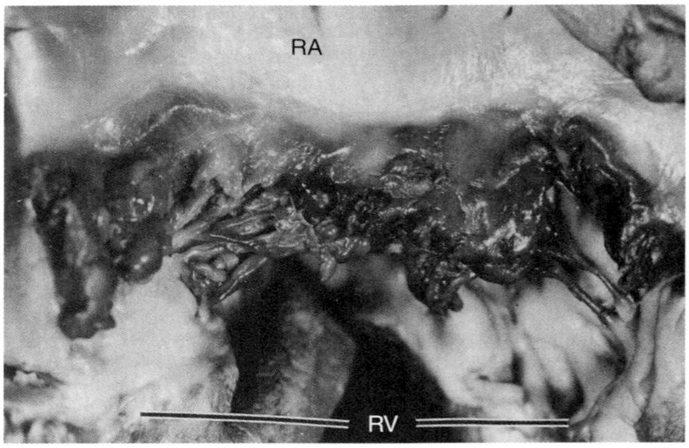

Fig. 13.28 Dysplastic tricuspid valve in trisomy 18 syndrome. The valve leaflets are thickened with gelatinous nodular formations. The chordae tendineae are thickened and shortened, and they also display focal nodules. Many of the interchordal spaces are obliterated with dysplastic fibrous tissue, and the right ventricular papillary muscles are dysplastic. Similar abnormalities are present in almost all cardiac valves in both full and partial trisomy 18 patients. *RA,* Right atrium; *RV,* right ventricle. (Reproduced with permission from Matsuoka R, Yamamoto Y, Kuroki Y, Matsui I: Phenotypic expression of the trisomic segments in partial trisomy 18. In: Van Praagh R, Takao A (eds), *Etiology and Morphogenesis of Congenital Heart Disease.* Futura Publishing Co, Mt Kisco, NY, 1980, p. 41.)

there being only two branches from the aortic arch—the common brachiocephalic trunk and the left subclavian artery), and a patent ductus arteriosus with bidirectional blood flow (echocardiography) indicating elevated pulmonary artery resistance (not unusual during the first day of postnatal life).

Case 40 was a stillborn black male fetus, who died spontaneously in utero at 37½ weeks of gestation (not a medically induced abortion). Trisomy 18 was karyotype proved. His congenital heart disease consisted of a large conoventricular type of ventricular septal defect (10 × 6 mm) and polyvalvar disease. He had congenital mitral stenosis with hypoplasia of the anterolateral papillary muscle of the left ventricle and absence of the posteromedial papillary muscle. All of the mitral chordae tendineae inserted into the small anterolateral papillary muscle, and there was absence of the mitral interchordal spaces. Hence, this fetus with a divided atrioventricular canal (not a common atrioventricular canal) had a **rare form of parachute mitral valve.** Usually with parachute mitral valve and a divided atrioventricular canal, it is the anterolateral papillary muscle group that is absent, and typically all of the mitral chordae tendineae insert into the posteromedial papillary muscle. This patient had the reverse, as above. When the atrioventricular canal is in common, usually all of the mitral chordae tendineae insert into the anterolateral papillary muscle group, resulting in potentially parachute mitral valve (after the atrioventricular canal has been divided surgically). Hence, this patient had the kind of potentially parachute mitral valve that occurs with common atrioventricular canal—except that this fetus did not have common atrioventricular canal.

The tricuspid valve was abnormal with redundant elongated chordae tendineae and hypoplastic papillary muscles of the right ventricle. Congenital tricuspid regurgitation was thought to have been present in utero.

The pulmonary valve was bicuspid (bicommissural) and redundant. The aortic valve was also bicuspid (absence of the right coronary-noncoronary commissure) and redundant. Septum primum (the flap valve of the foramen ovale) was also redundant, but the patent foramen ovale nonetheless appeared to have been valve competent (it would have prevented left-to-right shunting at the atrial level).

Thus, all five of this fetus's cardiac valves were abnormal: mitral, aortic, tricuspid, pulmonary, and atrial septum. One should not forget that the atrial septum (septum primum and the superior limbic band of septum secundum) constitute a unidirectional flap valve in utero, permitting right-to-left atrial blood flow (the *via sinistra*), but normally preventing left atrial-to-right atrial regurgitation. Embryologically, septum primum is thought to be the major component of the left sinoatrial venous valve mechanism, which is bifid consisting of a small left venous valve to the right and a large septum primum to the left. In visceroatrial situs solitus, the interoseptovalvular space lies between septum primum (to the left) and the left venous valve (to the right), and both the left venous valve and septum primum are directly continuous with the left wall of the inferior vena cava (see Chapter 2 for more information and embryonic photomicrographs). *Normally, septum primum is the largest and one of the most hemodynamically important venous valves in the human body.*

The presence of polyvalvar disease should immediately raise the diagnostic question: Is a trisomy present? Once one realizes that septum primum really is a venous valve, the presence of a redundant septum primum along with redundancy of the other four cardiac valves becomes easier to understand. Indeed, one should expect redundancy of septum primum along with redundancy of the other four cardiac valves in trisomy 18.

There are really five cardiac valves: septum primum, plus the other four.

Why not six? Aren't we forgetting the thebesian valve of the coronary sinus? Yes, we are, intentionally. We are "forgetting" the thebesian valve because it is so often incompetent (i.e., small or absent) and thus is not known to matter hemodynamically. (We could be wrong about this. Regurgitation of the thebesian valve may be of hemodynamic importance; but this has not been discovered as yet, to the best of my knowledge.)

So, suffice it to say that regurgitation of at least five of the cardiac valves are now definitely known to be of hemodynamic significance: aortic regurgitation, mitral regurgitation, pulmonary regurgitation, tricuspid regurgitation, and *atrial septal regurgitation,* that is, *ostium secundum atrial septal defect* caused by deficiency of the major left sinoatrial valve leaflet component—septum primum. It is not generally understood that a secundum ASD is really a cardiac valvar regurgitation. This clearly is the situation in utero. Regurgitation of blood from the left atrium into the right atrium decreases left-heart block flow (the *via sinistra*) and increases the right heart blood flow (the *via dextra*).

Case 56 was a 42-week-old stillborn female fetus with karyotype-proved trisomy 18. This fetus had multiple congenital anomalies including lobster claw feet, short thumbs, syndactyly involving fingers 2 to 4, left diaphragmatic hernia with abdominal organs in the left chest, severely hypoplastic lungs, large conoventricular type of ventricular septal defect, high origins of the coronary ostia above the aortic sinuses of Valsalva, a small persistent left superior vena cava to the coronary sinus, and polyvalvar disease involving the tricuspid, mitral, pulmonary and aortic valves. The tricuspid valve leaflets were redundant and myxomatous, with blood cysts involving the leaflets, and the right ventricular papillary muscles were hypoplastic. Tricuspid regurgitation was thought to have been present in utero. The posteromedial left ventricular papillary muscle of the mitral valve was very hypoplastic, and there were blood cysts of the mitral leaflets. The aortic and pulmonary valve leaflets were redundant. Thus, this fetus displayed a very severe trisomy 18 phenotype with multiple congenital anomalies (noncardiovascular and cardiovascular), again with a large ventricular septal defect, and polyvalvar disease involving all four of the postnatally functional cardiac valves.

In a review of 16 cases of full trisomy 18, and of 21 patients with partial trisomy 18, Matsuoka and colleagues[224] found no differences in cardiac pathology between partial and full trisomy 18. The salient congenital heart disease findings in patients with trisomy 18 were as follows:[224]

- dysplastic tricuspid valve, 100% (Fig. 13.28);
- polyvalvar disease, 100%;
- ventricular septal defect, 87%;

- high takeoff of right coronary ostium, 80%;
- patent ductus arteriosus, 73%;
- common brachiocephalic trunk, 47%;
- coarctation of the aorta, 20%; and
- mitral atresia with hypoplastic left ventricle, 7%.

Thus, our three patients with trisomy 18 and non-Ebstein congenital tricuspid regurgitation were characteristic of trisomy 18. Ebstein's anomaly and trisomy 18 are *not* associated, to our knowledge.

Trisomy 13. **Case 35** was a 16-day-old girl with trisomy 13 (caused by a 13/13 translocation, karyotype proved). She had multiple congenital anomalies including a cleft palate, double phalanges of the great toe bilaterally, malformed external ears (pinnae), down-slanting eyes, small forehead, large occiput, extra digit of the right hand, café-au-lait spot above the labia, prominent nasal bones, and agenesis of the corpus callosum.

Congenital heart disease consisted of secundum atrial septum defects (four small fenestrations of septum primum), tricuspid regurgitation with myxomatous and redundant tricuspid valve leaflets, a small and poorly formed anterior papillary muscle of the right ventricle, and the other right ventricular papillary muscles also being abnormally small. The immediate cause of death at 16 days of age was necrotizing enterocolitis.

Case 79 was a female fetus with a gestational age of 26 weeks who had karyotype proved trisomy 13. This fetus had a bicommissural (bicuspid) aortic valve because of marked underdevelopment of the left coronary-noncoronary commissure. (This is a rare form of bicuspid [bicommissural] aortic valve. Even in unicuspid [unicommissural] aortic valves, the left coronary-noncoronary commissure is almost always preserved and relatively well formed.)

Tricuspid regurgitation was thought to have been present in utero because of the abnormal attachments of the chordae tendineae to the underside (ventricular surface) of the anterior tricuspid leaflet, rather than to the free margin of this leaflet. Right ventricular enlargement was associated with marked right atrial hypertrophy and enlargement. Hence, in this fetus, non-Ebstein congenital tricuspid regurgitation was thought to be related to the above-described abnormality of the tensor apparatus (the chordae tendineae) of the anterior tricuspid leaflet.

Comment. The above-described cases of trisomy 18 and trisomy 13, all karyotype proved, illustrate an interesting generalization. Individuals with a trisomy (18, 13, or 21) seem always to have normal segmental anatomy, that is, {S,D,S}. To our knowledge, trisomic individual always have situs solitus of the viscera and atria—never visceroatrial situs inversus, or visceroatrial heterotaxy with or without congenital asplenia or polysplenia. Similarly, trisomic patients seem always to have D-loop (noninverted) ventricles, never L-loop (inverted) ventricles. Trisomic individuals always have essentially solitus normally related great arteries (including tetralogy of Fallot), never typical transposition of the great arteries with a subaortic conus, or double-outlet right ventricle with a bilateral (subaortic and subpulmonary) conus, and so on.

Exceptions to these generalizations should be sought and, if found, well documented.

Trisomies may be regarded as genetic "overdoses." Despite their many deleterious effects, trisomies appear to guarantee cardiac segmental situs normalcy, that is, {S,D,S}.

We speculate that abnormalities of visceral and cardiac segmental situs (situs inversus, and heterotaxy) may represent genetic "underdosage," that is, a lack of the normal controlling genetic information, permitting segmental situs discordance (as opposed to the normal segmental situs concordance). Our hypothesis is that when the normal controlling genetic information (genes, or gene regulators) is missing, then the four independent cardiac segments (atria, ventricular sinuses, conus, and truncus) may develop their patterns of anatomic organization (or situs) in an unregulated, uncoordinated way, resulting in a segmental situs "salad" or mixture that we call complex congenital heart disease. If unregulated, segmental situs may develop at random, by chance. The phenotypic segmental result may appear either normal, or abnormal, when segmental situs develops at random or by chance. It is hoped that it soon may be possible to test this stochastic hypothesis by molecular genetic techniques.

It should be added that the fifth diagnostically and surgically important cardiac segment, the atrioventricular canal or junction, appears *not* to be an independent variable. The pattern of anatomic organization (the situs) of the atrioventricular valves appears to correspond to that of the ventricular loop. Hence, we regard the atrioventricular canal as a dependent variable, not as an independent variable.

The five trisomic cases presented above all had normal cardiac segmental anatomy, that is, {S,D,S}, despite their many cardiac anomalies, and hence they conform to the foregoing hypothesis that trisomies "guarantee" segmental situs concordance (all solitus, that is, usual or normal in their pattern of anatomic organization, not inverted, and not indecipherable).

Non-Ebstein Congenital Tricuspid Regurgitation in Marfan Syndrome

The sixth most common cause of non-Ebstein congenital tricuspid regurgitation in this series of 80 postmortem cases was Marfan syndrome: $n = 4$ (5%, Table 13.10), Cases 2, 31, 55, and 66 (Figs. 13.29 and 13.30).

Case 2 was an 11-month-old girl with infantile Marfan syndrome.[225] The right atrium was huge. Both the tricuspid valve and the mitral valve were redundant and regurgitant (Fig. 13.29). Dilation of the aortic and pulmonary valves was characterized by aneurysmal dilatation of the sinuses of Valsalva of both semilunar valves (Fig. 13.29B). Congestive heart failure was present with dilation of all cardiac chambers. Cardiomegaly was marked; the heart weighed 80 grams (normal = 40 grams), 100% greater than normal. Marfan lung disease was also observed, with marked lobular emphysema. High origins of the coronary ostia were noted.

This patient with infantile Marfan syndrome also had numerous additional congenital anomalies: small cranium, right coronal synostosis, loose skin, poor muscle development, bilateral wrist drop, bilateral dislocation of the hips, high-arched palate, arachnodactyly, lenticular densities (but without ectopia), esphoria, delayed dentition, arthrogryposis, and osteochrondrodystrophy.

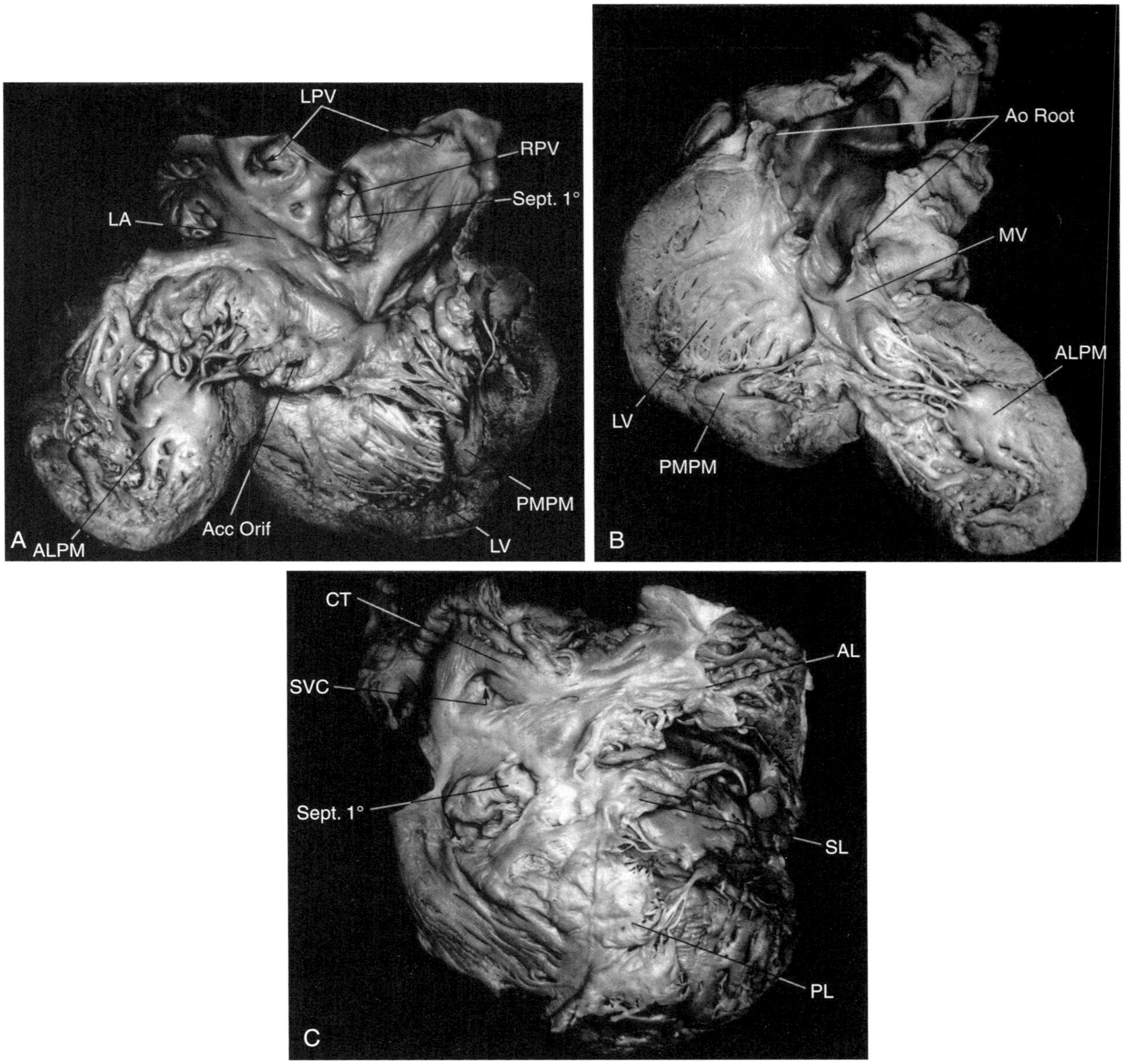

Fig. 13.29 Infantile Marfan syndrome in a girl who died at 11 months of age from congestive heart failure in 1958. (A) Opened left atrium *(LA),* mitral valve, and left ventricular outflow tract *(LV).* (B) Opened LV outflow tract, aortic root *(Ao root),* and ascending aorta. (C) Opened right atrium, tricuspid valve, and right ventricular inflow tract. In (A), the thickened and redundant mitral valve leaflets herniate upward, toward the LA, creating a "hemorrhoidal" appearance when the mitral valve is viewed from above. The mitral chordae are thickened, elongated, and redundant. There is a small accessory orifice *(Acc Orif)* in the anterior mitral leaflet. The LA is markedly hypertrophied and enlarged, reflecting the severity of the mitral regurgitation. Even the ostia of the left pulmonary veins *(LPV)* and the right pulmonary veins *(RPV)* are enlarged. Septum primum *(Sept. 1°)* is redundant; all cardiac valves are redundant, and septum primum—the flap valve of the foramen ovale—is a cardiac valve antenatally. Left ventricular hypertrophy and enlargement are generalized, also involving the anterolateral and the posteromedial papillary muscles (*ALPM* and *PMPM*), but greater of the ALPM than of the PMPM. In (B), note the elongation and redundancy of the chordae tendineae of the mitral valve *(MV).* The Ao root is markedly dilated at the sinuses of Valsalva. The aortic leaflets are dilated and redundant; but note that their leaflet margins are thin and delicate (not thick and rolled), indicating that little or no aortic regurgitation had occurred. Thus, this patient died of massive congestive heart failure at 11 months of age because of marked mitral and tricuspid regurgitation, *before* significant aortic and pulmonary regurgitation had appeared. *Mitral and tricuspid regurgitation is prominent in infantile Marfan syndrome, but is much less so in the adolescent-adult form of Marfan syndrome.* In (C), the anterior leaflet *(AL),* the septal leaflet *(SL),* and the posterior leaflet *(PL)* of the tricuspid valve are thickened, redundant, and protrude upward into the right atrium that is markedly hypertrophied and enlarged. *CT,* Crista terminalis (terminal crest); *SVC,* superior vena cava. This patient was diagnosed as having the Marfan syndrome at birth. Her family history was negative. Weight was less than the 3rd percentile. Height was at the 50th percentile. Arachnodactyly, contractures, kyphoscoliosis, joint hyperelasticity, high-arched palate, and myopia were present. Additional associated anomalies were also found (see text, regarding Case 2). (Reproduced from Geva T, Sanders SP, Diogenes M, Rockenmacher S, Van Praagh R: Two-dimensional and Doppler echocardiographic and pathologic characteristics of the infantile Marfan syndrome. *Am J Cardiol* 1990;65:1230.)

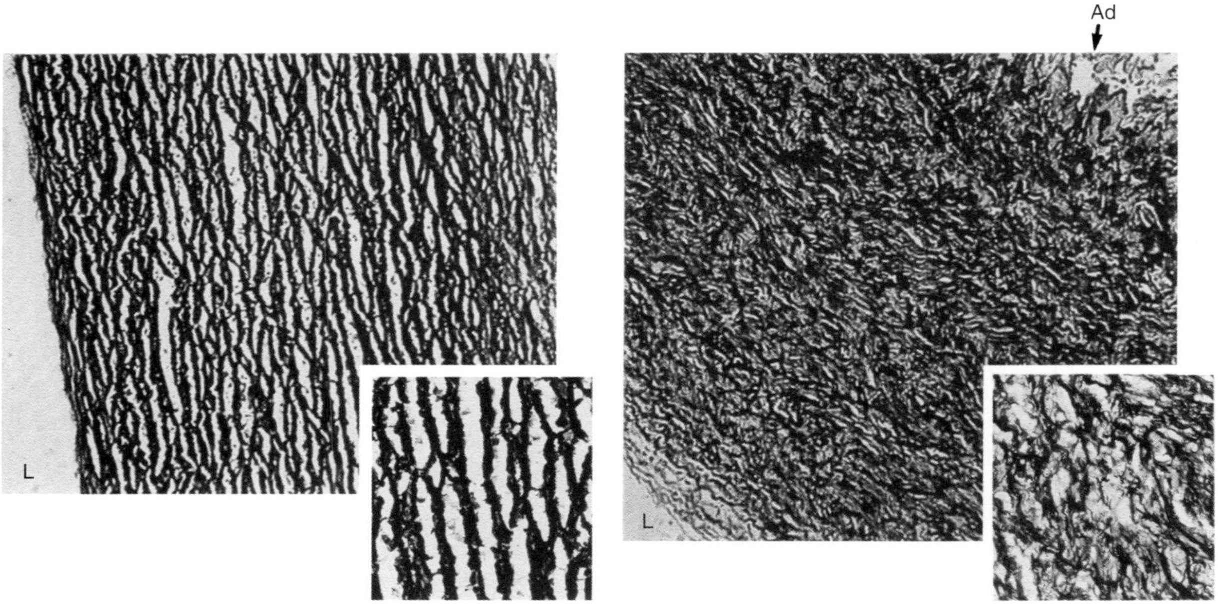

Fig. 13.30 Histologic characteristics of infantile Marfan syndrome. (A) Sections from the ascending aorta at the level of the sinuses of Valsalva: *Left,* normal control; *Right,* from a 10-month-old girl with infantile Marfan syndrome (Case 55). Note the fragmentation and disarray of the elastic fibers, and the increased interfiber ground substance in the patient (×100). *Inset,* high-power magnification (×400) showing details of elastic fibers in infantile Marfan syndrome *(right)* compared with the elastic laminae in the normal control *(left).* Verhoeff-Van Gieson stain for elastic fibers. *Ad,* Adventitia; *L,* lumen. (Reproduced with permission from Geva T, Sanders SP, Diogenes M, Rockenmacher S, Van Praagh R: Two-dimensional and Doppler echocardiographic and pathologic characteristics of the infantile Marfan syndrome. *Am J Cardiol* 1990;65:1230.)

Case 31 was a 13-year-and-21-day old girl with a familial connective tissue disorder (present in one other sibling) that was considered to be Marfanoid. She had arachnodactyly, an increased lower body segment, hyperextensible joints, contractures of the toes, kyphosis, osteoporosis, and wedged dorsal vertebrae. Chronic congestive heart failure was present. Echocardiography revealed moderate tricuspid regurgitation and severe mitral regurgitation with a flail mitral valve. This cachectic young girl underwent mitral valve replacement in 1988 with a #29 St. Jude prosthesis. Postoperatively, acute aortic dissection and a massive right hemothorax resulted in death.

Case 55 was a 10-month-old boy with infantile Marfan syndrome[225] that was characterized by marked hyperextensibility of the joints; bilateral inguinal hernias treated with herniorrphaphies; hypertrophic pyloric stenosis treated with pyloromyotomy (Ramstedt operation) at 7 weeks of age; progressive congestive heart failure that appeared at 5 months of age; severe mitral regurgitation with marked mitral valve prolapse; marked left atrial enlargement; clinical and angiocardiographic evidence of tricuspid regurgitation, with hemorrhoidal anatomic appearance of the atrial surfaces of the tricuspid valve leaflets, tricuspid valve prolapse with thickened leaflets, and elongated redundant tricuspid chordae tendineae; secundum atrial septal defect; moderate left ventricular enlargement; severe failure to thrive; pectus excavatum; arachodactyly; high-arched palate; ventricular arrhythmias at 10 months of age consisting of ventricular premature beats with bigeminy and trigeminy; contractures of the elbows, knees, and ankles; and upward eventration of the right-sided portion of the central fibrous tendon of the diaphragm.

At 10 months of age in 1978, the patient underwent mitral valve replacement with a #19 Hancock prosthesis. Cardiac arrest and death occurred on the second postoperative day.

Autopsy revealed infarction of the posterior papillary muscles of the right ventricle. Severe bilateral pulmonary emphysema with blebs was found. The aortic and pulmonary valve leaflets and sinuses of Valsalva were redundant and enlarged, but without evidence of aortic regurgitation or pulmonary regurgitation. Dilation and thinning of the walls of the ascending aorta and main pulmonary artery were also observed.

Case 66 was a 1-day-old boy with infantile Marfan syndrome.[225] Salient features included arachnodactyly, contractures, and massive cardiomegaly. Marked regurgitation of all four cardiac valves (tricuspid, mitral, pulmonary, and aortic) led to fatal congestive heart failure. There was tricuspid valve prolapse with focal absence of tricuspid leaflet tissue in the region of the anterosuperior commissure. A large secundum atrial septal defect was caused by deficiency and fenestration of septum primum.

Comment. Three of these four patients had the more severe *infantile* form of the Marfan syndrome (Cases 2, 55, and 66) that was described by Geva and his colleagues[225] in 1990, while one patient (Case 31) had the somewhat milder *adolescent-adult* form of the Marfan syndrome. None of these four patients had isolated tricuspid regurgitation; on the contrary, all had multiple other important congenital anomalies, which makes sense when one considers what is now known about Marfan syndrome.[226,227]

Marfan syndrome is caused by mutations in the gene that encodes **fibrillin-1** *(FBN1)*.[226,227] Fibrillin-1 is the major constituent of microfibrils that are one of the main components of the extracellular matrix. Elastic fibers are composed of microfibrils and tropoelastin. Fragmentation and disorganization of elastic fibers, for example, in the aortic media (so-called cystic medial necrosis), are characteristic of Marfan syndrome (Fig. 13.30). However, similar microscopic pathology also occurs in other conditions, such as in familial aortic aneurysms and the aging process. All of the many different manifestations of Marfan syndrome are now believed to be due to a **defect in microfibrils.**[227] More than 100 different mutations have been identified in *FBN1,* the gene that encodes fibrillin-1. *FBN1* is a large gene with approximately 9000 nucleotides in its mRNA. Unfortunately, molecular genetic diagnosis of Marfan syndrome is complicated by the fact that mutations in *FBN1* also cause other (different) clinical syndromes: autosomal dominant ectopic lentis, familial tall stature, the MASS phenotype (*m*itral valve, *a*orta, *s*kin, *s*keletal), and familial aortic aneurysm.[227]

Thus, Marfan syndrome is one of the fibrillinopathies, that is, a widespread abnormality of fibrillin-1, caused by mutations of the gene *FBN1*[226,227] that result in a distinctive clinicopathologic phenotype. Hence, at least at the present time, Marfan syndrome remains a clinicopathologic diagnosis. But our understanding of its genetic etiology is rapidly improving.

Historical question. As noted by Geva and colleagues,[225] the question arises: Did Marfan really report the first case of Marfan syndrome in 1896? In the original case report of Gabrielle P, a 5½-year-old girl, Marfan described in detail the characteristic musculoskeletal anomalies that he called dolichostenomelia (*dolichos* = long, *stenosis* = narrow, *melos* = limb, all Greek), not arachnodactyly (*arachne* = spider, *daktylos* = finger, Greek). Marfan did not mention cardiovascular or ocular abnormalities in his patient. Later investigators have therefore suggested that Marfan's patient may really have had what is now called *congenital contractural arachnodactyly.* In 1912, **Salle**—a German pediatrician—described the first case with cardiac involvement, an infant who died at 2½ months of age with failure to thrive and progressive dyspnea. Autopsy revealed massive cardiomegaly with redundant and thickened mitral and tricuspid leaflets, similar to our Case 2 (Fig. 13.29). Thus, Salle's report appears to be not only the first documented case of what is now known as Marfan syndrome with cardiac involvement, but also the first known case of infantile Marfan syndrome (as opposed to the better known adolescent-adult form of Marfan syndrome).

In our 9 cases of infantile Marfan syndrome reported by Geva et al,[225] tricuspid valve prolapse was present in 8 (89%), with tricuspid regurgitation in 6 (67%). Mitral valve prolapse was present in all (100%), with mitral regurgitation in 8 (89%).

Congenital Non-Ebstein Tricuspid Regurgitation With Uhl's Disease

Congenital tricuspid regurgitation with Uhl's disease was found in 3 of these 80 postmortem-proved cases (3.75%, Table 13.10, Cases 59, 74, and 80) (Figs. 13.31 and 13.32).

Case 59 was a 40-year-old woman with Uhl's disease.[10] Autopsy revealed marked thinning of the right ventricular free wall that measured approximately 1 mm in thickness. The right ventricular free wall transilluminated brilliantly, particularly the diaphragmatic surface of the right ventricular free wall. The right ventricular free wall consisted mostly of subepicardial fat. Although the tricuspid valve was structurally normal, tricuspid regurgitation had developed because of gradual right ventricular dilation secondary to Uhl's disease. The presence of tricuspid regurgitation was confirmed anatomically by right atrial jet lesions above the septal and posterior leaflets of the tricuspid valve.

In 1967, this patient was treated surgically with tricuspid annuloplasty (plication) in an attempt to reduce her tricuspid regurgitation. She had a history of peripheral thromboembolism to the first and fifth toes of the right foot. She also had a history of severe cardiac arrhythmias, with an episode of cardiac standstill, which she survived. The clinical picture of congestive heart failure developed and she died suddenly because of ventricular fibrillation that was documented electrocardiographically.

Comment. In 1952, Uhl[10] published a previously undescribed congenital malformation of the heart, namely, almost total absence of the right ventricular myocardium. Consequently, in 1967 when this patient (Case 59) was studied, we made the diagnosis of Uhl's disease, as above.

However, looking back from the vantage point of 2007 (present time of writing), our question now is: Why shouldn't this case be diagnosed as an example of **arrhythmogenic right ventricular dysplasia,**[228-230] of which we were not aware in 1967? We think it probably should be diagnosed as arrhythmogenic right ventricular cardiomyopathy/dysplasia. However, our diagnosis confusion/uncertainty is instructive, which is why we are publishing *both* diagnoses.

Our present conclusion is: When an infant or young child presents with little or no right ventricular free wall myocardium, the correct pathologic anatomic and clinical diagnosis is Uhl's disease.[10] However, when an adolescent or adult presents with marked right ventricular free wall thinning, with fatty or fibrofatty infiltration, and prominent ventricular arrhythmias, then the appropriate pathologic and clinical diagnosis is right ventricular arrhythmogenic cardiomyopathy/dysplasia.[228-230] One should be aware both of the similarities and of the differences concerning these two similar but somewhat different phenotypes.

From the etiologic perspective, it is now known that arrhythmogenic right ventricular dysplasia can be sporadic (nonfamilial) or familial. When familial, genetic abnormalities have been mapped to chromosomes 1 and 14q23-q24,[230,231] and also to chromosome 10.[232]

When the genetic etiologies of Uhl's disease and arrhythmogenic right ventricular dysplasia are fully known, then the similarities and the differences of these two phenotypes will be more reliably understood.

Case 74 was a female fetus of 20 weeks gestational age. The right ventricle was markedly dilated, with a very thin and wrinkled free wall. The septal leaflet of the tricuspid valve was absent, congenital tricuspid regurgitation was massive, and right atrial hypertrophy and enlargement were marked. The anterior leaflet

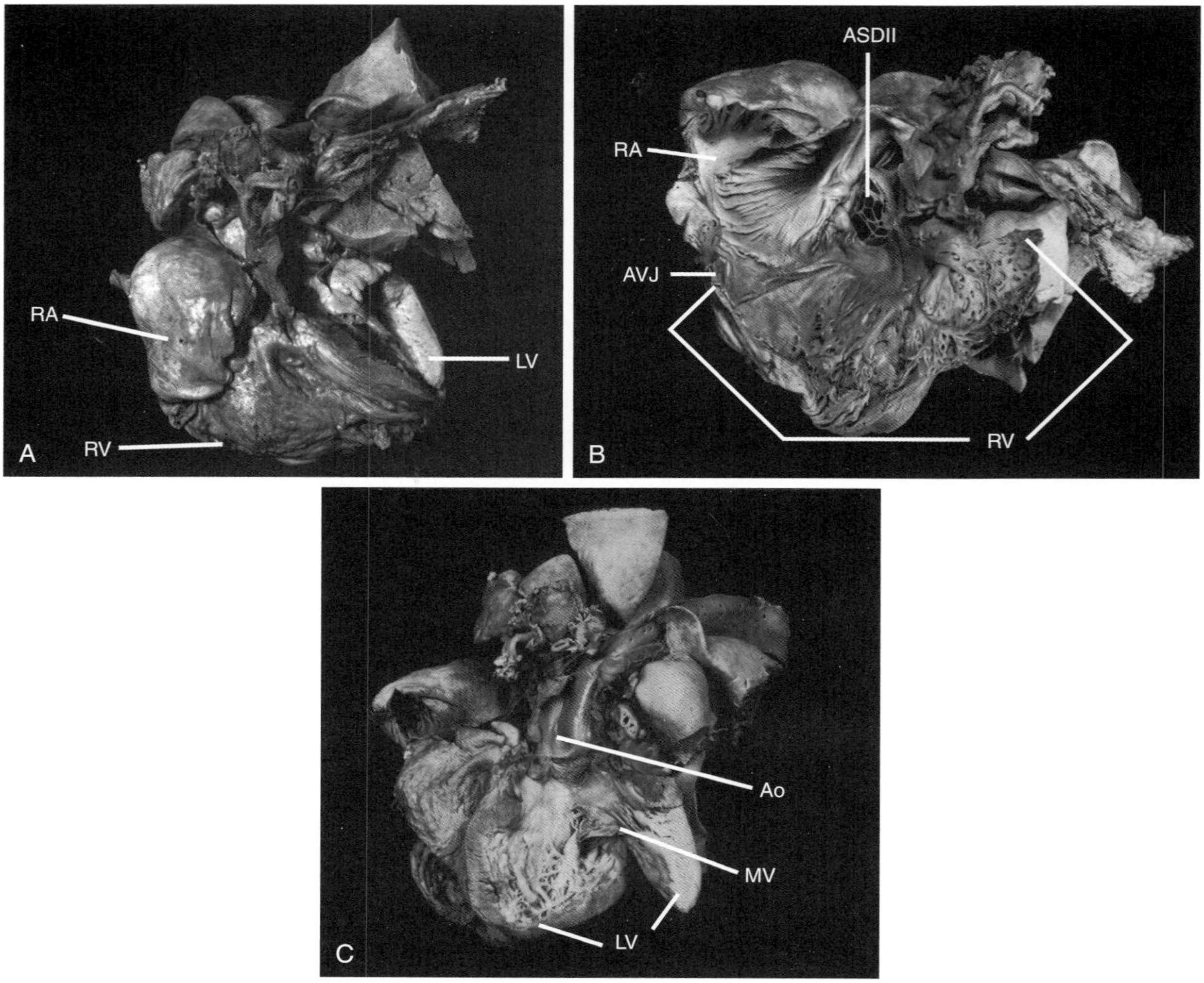

Fig. 13.31 Congenital tricuspid regurgitation because of congenitally unguarded tricuspid orifice, with Uhl's disease (parchment right ventricle). This 2-week-old black boy had pulmonary atresia (valvar), intact ventricular septum, Uhl's disease, and congenitally unguarded tricuspid orifice. (A) External frontal view of the heart. (B) Opened right atrium *(RA)* and right ventricle *(RV)*. (C) Opened left ventricle *(LV)* and ascending aorta *(Ao)*. In (A), the right ventricular free wall looks very thin and wrinkled; it has a "scrotal" appearance. By contrast, the right atrium appears hypertrophied and enlarged. The main pulmonary artery is small, consistent with pulmonary valvar atresia. The segmental anatomy is normal, i.e., {S,D,S}. (B) This image confirmed that the right atrium is markedly hypertrophied and enlarged. A large secundum type of atrial septal defect *(ASDII)* is seen because septum primum (the flap valve of the foramen ovale) is very deficient: a cobweb appearance, with multiple large fenestrations in septum primum. The tricuspid leaflets, chordae tendineae, and papillary muscles are totally absent. Thus, the right atrioventricular orifice is wide open, but totally unguarded, because all elements of the tricuspid valve (leaflets, chordae, and papillary muscles) are absent; only the orifice is present. The right ventricular septal surface below the right atrioventricular junction *(AVJ)* is smooth, or non-trabeculated (reminiscent of the right ventricular septal surface above the downwardly displaced septal leaflet in Ebstein's anomaly—except here, there is no downwardly displaced septal leaflet of the tricuspid valve). The right ventricular free wall is almost paper thin, and its trabecular architecture is abnormally fine (not normally coarse); i.e., the right ventricular free wall's trabecular architecture is dysplastic. The ventricular septal surface is intact (no ventricular septal defect), and the pulmonary outflow tract is atretic. In (C), the architecture of the mitral valve *(MV)*, left ventricle, aortic valve, and ascending aorta is unremarkable.

of the tricuspid valve was deep, with a thickened and rolled free margin confirming tricuspid regurgitation. The tricuspid annulus was not downwardly displaced; hence we did not make the diagnosis of Ebstein's malformation. Our diagnoses were as follows: **Uhl's disease** (virtual absence of right ventricular free wall myocardium), with **partially unguarded tricuspid orifice** (congenital absence of the septal leaflet of the tricuspid valve), and severe **congenital tricuspid regurgitation** without downward displacement of the tricuspid ring.

Comment. Are we happy with this diagnosis? No, not entirely. Why not? Well, in Uhl's original case, the tricuspid valve was structurally normal; not so in this patient (as above). The problem is that many clinicopathologic diagnoses have

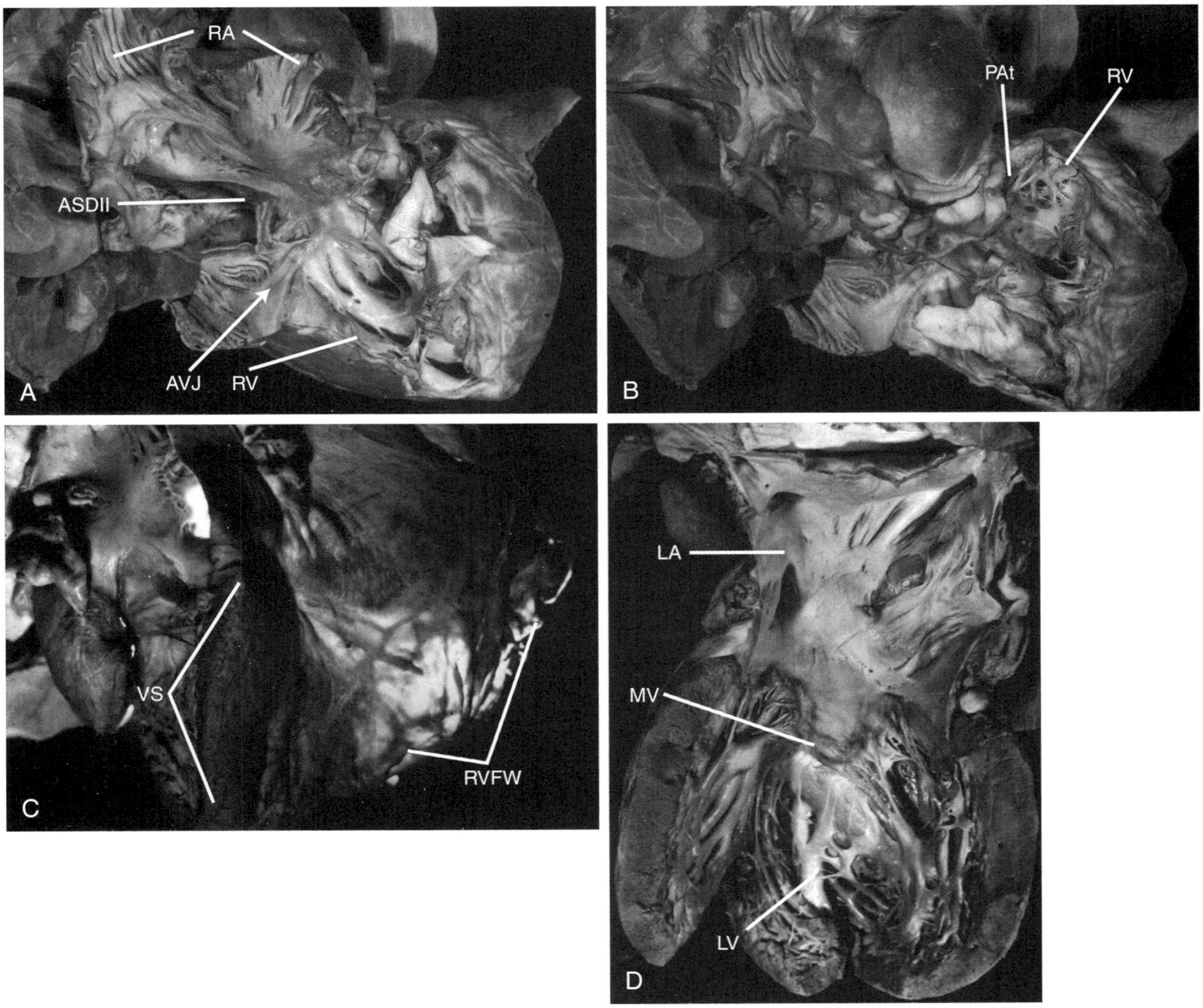

Fig. 13.32 Another patient, an 18-month-old white boy, with congenital tricuspid regurgitation because of congenitally unguarded tricuspid orifice and associated with Uhl's disease, valvar pulmonary atresia, and an intact ventricular septum. In (A), the opened right atrium *(RA)* and right ventricle *(RV)* reveal almost total absence of tricuspid leaflet tissue—just a few thread-like strands are present—at or below the right atrioventricular junction *(AVJ)*. The right atrium is markedly hypertrophied and enlarged. A secundum type of atrial septal defect *(ASDII)* is seen. The right ventricular free wall *(RV)* is extremely thin. The ventricular septum is intact, and there is no patent pulmonary outflow tract. (B) The paper-thin right ventricular free wall *(RV)* and the blind pulmonary outflow tract *(PAt)*. (C) Posterior viewing showing that the very thin right ventricular free wall *(RVFW)* transilluminates brilliantly. *VS*, Ventricular septum. (D) The opened left atrium *(LA)*, mitral valve *(MV)*, and left ventricle *(LV)* are all morphologically unremarkable.

uncomfortable partial forms, such as Uhl's disease with an anomalous tricuspid valve, and congenitally unguarded tricuspid orifice that is only partial, not complete (with functional absence of all three leaflets). This is why we present the conventional diagnoses (such as Uhl's disease, or congenitally unguarded tricuspid orifice) and also describe the pathologic anatomy—particularly when partial forms, so-called *formes frustes*, are present. (*Forme fruste* literally means a worn form. *Fruste* denotes worn by rubbing, and hence literally defaced—as with an old coin. French.)

Case 80 was sent to us as a consultation in 1992; unfortunately we do not know the patient's age or sex. The heart specimen has pulmonary atresia (valvar and infundibular) with intact ventricular septum and a dysplastic tricuspid valve. The anterior tricuspid leaflet was deep and curtain-like. The septal leaflet of the tricuspid valve was muscular (not membranous) and was normally attached at the atrioventricular junction. The posterior leaflet of the tricuspid valve was muscular and was also normally attached at the atrioventricular junction. Congenital tricuspid regurgitation was thought to have been present because of the immobility of the muscular septal and posterior leaflets of the tricuspid valve. **Muscular tricuspid valve** is a rare and little known congenital malformation.

The anterior right ventricular free wall was thin and parchment-like, characteristic of Uhl's disease.[10]

Comment. Again, this was not a typical case of Uhl's disease[10] because pulmonary infundibular and valvar atresia coexisted, as did muscular tricuspid valve involving the septal and posterior leaflets (which were not downwardly displaced beneath the right atrioventricular junction).

Looked at in another way, it is helpful to know that **pulmonary atresia with an intact ventricular septum** occasionally can have much more than these two features. A parchment right ventricular free wall (Uhl's disease),[10] a muscular tricuspid valve (failure of demuscularization), and congenital non-Ebstein tricuspid regurgitation can all coexist.

Thus, parchment right ventricular free wall (Uhl's disease) can occur in isolation, as in Uhl's original case,[10] or with other associated anomalies (such as pulmonary outflow tract atresia and muscular tricuspid valve with congenital tricuspid regurgitation, as in this patient).

Congenital Polyvalvar Disease With Congenital Non-Ebstein Tricuspid Regurgitation

This group of anomalies also occurred in 3 of these 80 patients (3.75%, Table 13.10, Cases 12, 30, and 41).

Case 12 was an 11-month-old girl with a redundant tricuspid valve and mild tricuspid regurgitation (documented by two-dimensional echocardiography), a redundant mitral valve without mitral regurgitation, and a mildly redundant aortic valve with mild aortic regurgitation; thus, congenital polyvalvar disease was present. But, as will soon be seen, mild congenital tricuspid regurgitation with congenital polyvalvar disease was not the patient's main hemodynamic problem. She had multiple congenital anomalies (karyotype unfortunately unknown) with a conoventricular paramembranous ventricular septal defect, a secundum atrial septal defect, and a moderate-sized patent ductus arteriosus. A posterior fossa subdural hematoma was diagnosed at 8 days of age in 1991. Ligation of the patent ductus arteriosus and banding of the main pulmonary artery were performed at 17 days of age. Microcephaly with developmental delay gradually became apparent.

At 5 months of age, stenosis of the left pulmonary veins was diagnosed, followed by diagnosis of stenosis of the right pulmonary veins. Thus, the clinical diagnosis was made of **idiopathic stenosis of individual pulmonary veins,** which at the present time remains a dreaded diagnosis with an exceedingly poor prognosis (virtually 100% fatal, despite all therapeutic efforts). Hydrocephalus appeared and increased, and was associated with premature closure of the cranial sutures.

At 6 months of age, a gastrostomy was performed. At 7 months of age, patch closure of the ventricular septal defect was performed. The main pulmonary artery band was removed, following which the band site was resected, with end-to-end anastomosis of the main pulmonary artery. Fibrous tissue was resected from the orifices of the left pulmonary veins, and the secundum atrial septal defect was closed primarily (without a patch).

At 10 months of age, pulmonary venous dilation and stenting were undertaken: A 7 mm stent was placed into the right upper lobe pulmonary vein; and dilation and stenting were also performed of the left lower lobe pulmonary vein. At 11 months of age, inexorable pulmonary distress led to death. Autopsy confirmed all of the above-mentioned findings and established that the tricuspid leaflets were redundant and thickened.

Comment. This patient illustrates that congenital non-Ebstein tricuspid regurgitation can indeed be associated with congenital polyvalvar disease. But perhaps more important, this case shows that congenital tricuspid regurgitation, although present, was of minor clinical importance in a clinical picture dominated by other more important associated anomalies, most notably by severe and ultimately fatal idiopathic stenosis of individual pulmonary veins.

In a well-formulated diagnosis, not only should all findings be listed, but the relative importance of each should also be indicated or understood. This little girl illustrates that congenital non-Ebstein tricuspid regurgitation can be present, but of little clinical importance.

Case 30 was a 5⁶⁄₇-week-old boy with significant congenital tricuspid regurgitation (documented by two-dimensional echocardiography, cardiac catheterization, and angiocardiography), mild thickening of the pulmonary valve leaflets (with an 8 mm Hg gradient), and with obliteration of some of the interchordal spaces of the mitral valve. Hence, this patient did have polyvalvar disease, unrelated to Ebstein's anomaly. Unfortunately, the karyotype of this patient is not known. (We say "unfortunately" because polyvalvar disease suggests the possibility of a trisomy, as in item 5 of Table 13.10.)

Other associated findings included a secundum atrial septal defect, a conoventricular type of ventricular septal defect, marked right ventricular hypertrophy and enlargement, right ventricular endocardial sclerosis, unusual and abnormal right ventricular myocardial architecture, and a **left ventricular moderator band** (an abnormal band of left ventricular myocardium running from the left ventricular septal surface anteroseptally and then proceeding to, or toward the anterolateral papillary muscle of the left ventricle). This patient also had a positive family history of congenital malformations. The previous pregnancy ended with a spontaneous abortion at 6 months' gestation, the fetus having hydrocephalus.

Comment. The congenital tricuspid regurgitation in this patient was clinically important, but the polyvalvar disease was far from isolated, similar to the previous case.

Case 41 was a 15½-year-old girl with congenital polyvalvar disease (unrelated to Ebstein's anomaly) with intellectual disability and a seizure disorder. There was marked thickening and myxomatous change of the tricuspid valve (congenital tricuspid regurgitation was thought to have been present); the right atrium was hypertrophied and enlarged. The pulmonary valve leaflets were thick and myxomatous (but we thought the pulmonary valve was probably normal functionally). The mitral leaflets were thick and myxomatous. (We were not sure whether some degree of mitral stenosis and regurgitation had been present in life.) The aortic valve was quadricuspid, with thick and myxomatous leaflets. (We thought that aortic stenosis and regurgitation probably had been present in life.)

The ventricular septum was intact. Left ventricular hypertrophy and enlargement were present, as was marked left ventricular endocardial sclerosis. Again, the karyotype was not known.

Comment. As far as the patient's heart is concerned, congenital myxomatous polyvalvar disease was isolated. However, this patient also had an intellectual disability and seizures.

Thus, in these three cases, congenital myxomatous polyvalvar disease with tricuspid regurgitation was never isolated; instead, it was always associated with other cardiovascular or noncardiovascular abnormalities. It always appeared to be part of something bigger.

Congenital Tricuspid Regurgitation Associated With Transposition of the Great Arteries {S,D,D} and (Usually) Dysplastic Tricuspid Valve

This defect occurred in 3 of these 80 patients (3.75%, Table 13.10, Cases 5, 11, and 21).

Case 5 was a 7-day-old girl with transposition of the great arteries {S,D,D}, that is, with situs solitus of the viscera and atria ({S,-,-}), D-loop ventricles ({S,*D*,-}), and D-transposition ({S,D,*D*}). There was atrioventricular AV concordance, with the right-sided morphologically right atrium (RA) opening appropriately or concordantly into the right-sided morphologically right ventricle (RV), and the left-sided morphologically left atrium (LA) opening concordantly or appropriately into the left-sided morphologically left ventricle (LV). But there was ventriculoarterial (VA) discordance with the right-sided RV ejecting inappropriately or discordantly into the right-sided transposed aorta (Ao) and the left-sided LV ejecting discordantly or inappropriately into the left-sided transposed pulmonary artery (PA). All of the foregoing is to be expected in TGA {S,D,D}, unless specifically stated to the contrary. For example, if there is straddling of the tricuspid valve or double-inlet LV with TGA {S,D,D}, this is stated so that one immediately understands that the usual AV concordance is not present. Hence, saying that Case 5 has TGA {S,D,D}, without further qualification of the atrioventricular alignment, means that the usual segmental anatomy ({S,D,D}) and segmental alignments (AV discordance with VA discordance, and hence physiologic uncorrection of the systemic venous and the pulmonary venous circulations) are present. All of this should be immediately understood, unless qualified to the contrary.

But now here comes the interesting part. This newborn girl with TGA {S,D,D} had a hypoplastic RV. Consequently, the tricuspid annulus was also hypoplastic. Hence, the patient had one type of congenital tricuspid stenosis—because of the hypoplastic tricuspid valve and right ventricular sinus. In addition, there was a small membranous ventricular septal defect, a hypoplastic transposed aortic valve, a hypoplastic aortic arch, coarctation of the aorta, and a patent ductus arteriosus.

Surprisingly, cardiac catheterization and angiocardiography (in 1988) revealed moderately severe tricuspid regurgitation. Mystified, we reexamined this heart specimen and found that the tricuspid valve was small (i.e., hypoplastic). But otherwise it was a well-formed, undeformed tricuspid valve: a beautiful, normal miniature.

This cardiac catheterization was performed when the patient was moribund (dying). Our conclusion is that marked tricuspid regurgitation can occur through an intrinsically normal (although small) tricuspid valve, if the patient is moribund at the time of the study, and if TGA is present, that is, if the tricuspid valve is functioning as the systemic atrioventricular valve. Suffice it to say that we were surprised to learn that moderately severe tricuspid regurgitation can occur through a normal (if miniature) tricuspid valve, under the aforementioned conditions. We expected to find some anatomic anomaly of the tricuspid valve (apart from hypoplasia), but we did not. We think that this is a lesson to be remembered.

Case 11 was an 8-month-old boy with TGA {S,D,D}, intact ventricular septum, and pulmonary valvar stenosis (bicuspid, myxomatous, with a 40 to 50 mm Hg gradient). This patient had mild tricuspid regurgitation, but without right atrial jet lesions. The tricuspid valve was abnormally formed, the anterolateral papillary muscle of the right ventricle inserting directly into the tricuspid leaflet tissue, without intervening free chordae tendineae or interchordal spaces. There was mild thickening and rolling of the free margin of the anterior tricuspid leaflet. This little boy's mild tricuspid regurgitation was thought *not* to be one of his main clinical problems.

He also had stenosis of the left upper lobe pulmonary vein. A balloon atrial septostomy was attempted on the first day of life (in 1974), but it failed. Consequently, a Blalock-Hanlon surgical atrial septectomy was performed on the first day of postnatal life. Postoperatively, a wound infection of the median sternotomy developed. Subsequently, a Mustard procedure was performed in this patient with TGA {S,D,D} and unrelieved valvar pulmonary stenosis (40 to 50 mm Hg gradient). Following this atrial switch operation, low cardiac output developed, leading to death 13 hours postoperatively.

Our conclusion was that this patient's mild congenital tricuspid regurgitation related to tricuspid valvar dysplasia did not help hemodynamically, but this little boy had other more major problems. In other words, mild congenital tricuspid regurgitation was present, but was not the major problem. We now know that an atrial switch operation such as the Mustard procedure is contraindicated in a patient with TGA {S,D,D} if significant pulmonary outflow tract stenosis coexists and cannot be relieved.

Case 21 was a $9^{1.5}/_{12}$-year-old boy with TGA {S,D,D}, a small to moderate-sized conoventricular type of ventricular septal defect, a bilateral conus (subaortic and subpulmonary), pulmonary stenosis (infundibular and valvar, with a bicuspid pulmonary valve), and congenital tricuspid regurgitation because of a dysplastic tricuspid valve. The tricuspid valve had an accessory right ventricular papillary muscle arising from the right ventricular free wall, with multiple fenestrations in the anterior tricuspid leaflet. Moderately marked congenital tricuspid regurgitation occurred through these multiple fenestrations, and multiple jet lesions were present of the right atrial endocardium.

This patient, who died in 1979, had additional problems. The left coronary artery originated from the right coronary ostium. The left coronary artery then ran posteriorly to the transposed main pulmonary artery and then appeared anteriorly and to the left as a preventricular branch. There was a small communication between this preventricular termination of the left coronary artery and the LV cavity. This left coronary artery–to–left ventricular communication was 2 mm in diameter and was probe patent. This **left coronary artery–to–left ventricular fistula** created the unusual angiocardiographic picture of "aortic" regurgitation between the right-sided D-transposed aorta and the left-sided left ventricular cavity.

A balloon atrial septostomy was performed when the patient was 2 months of age. At 3³⁄₁₂ years of age, a right Blalock-Taussig anastomosis was done to the upper lobe branch of the right pulmonary artery. When the patient was 8⁹⁄₁₂ years old, an anatomic repair was performed (in 1979). Intraventricular rerouting was done between the left ventricle and the D-transposed aorta via a tunnel-like patch. The ventricular septal defect was enlarged by excision of the conal septum superiorly. The pulmonary valve was closed. A 20 mm valved Hancock conduit was placed externally from the right ventricle to the distal end of the main pulmonary artery. Hence, this anatomic repair involved both intraventricular (LV-to-Ao) and extraventricular (RV-to-PA) rerouting. Left ventricular pump failure appeared 4 months postoperatively. A surgical attempt to close a residual ventricular septal defect was associated with intraoperative death.

Our conclusion was that moderately marked congenital tricuspid regurgitation was present because of a dysplastic tricuspid valve, but that this was only one part of a complex clinical and surgical management problem. Again, it is essential to understand the presence of significant congenital tricuspid regurgitation *in context* with everything else that was a hemodynamic problem for the patient.

Tricuspid Valve Prolapse Causing Congenital Non-Ebstein Tricuspid Regurgitation

This defect was found in 2 of these 80 patients (2.5%, Table 13.10, Cases 22 and 25).

Case 22 was a 9¾-month-old black girl with Down syndrome. Echocardiography revealed mild to moderate tricuspid regurgitation with tricuspid valve prolapse. The anterior leaflet of the tricuspid valve had a hooded and redundant appearance. The anterior tricuspid leaflet was also deep and curtain-like, but the septal leaflet was not downwardly displaced (and hence Ebstein's anomaly was not diagnosed). The atrioventricular canal was normally divided into mitral and tricuspid valves. The ventricular septum was intact, but the patient had a large secundum atrial septal defect (14 × 7 mm) because of deficiency of septum primum; and a patent ductus arteriosus (3 mm in internal diameter) was also present. Heart block with bradycardia appeared 4 days prior to death. Thrombus with almost completely luminal occlusion of the superior vena cava was found at the superior vena caval–right atrial junction. She had diffuse pulmonary alveolar disease that was thought probably to be caused by respiratory syncytial virus pneumonia (not virologically proved).

To summarize, diffuse syncytial pneumonia was the principal cause of death. Tricuspid valve prolapse with congenital mild to moderate tricuspid regurgitation was present, but was thought *not* to be a major cause of disability or death.

Case 25 was a 12-year-old boy with tetralogy of Fallot {S,D,S}, a bicuspid pulmonary valve, and tricuspid valve prolapse with mild to moderate tricuspid regurgitation. In 1962, he developed a right frontal brain abscess caused by *Staphylococcus aureus* that led to cerebral edema, hemorrhage, and death.

Thus, tricuspid valve prolapse and tricuspid regurgitation were present. But these problems were overshadowed clinically by the congenital heart disease (tetralogy of Fallot) and its complication (brain abscess).

Comment. In both of these patients, tricuspid valve prolapse and tricuspid regurgitation were present; but in neither were these problems the main causes of disability and death.

Dysplastic Right Ventricle and Tricuspid Valve

These defects were present in 2 of these 80 patients (2.5%, Table 13.10, Cases 19 and 64).

Case 19 was a 10-month-old girl with a ventricular septal defect of the atrioventricular canal type, without mitral or tricuspid valve clefts. There was dysplasia of the right ventricular sinus (body or inflow tract) with anomalous muscle bands, abnormal papillary muscles, and abnormal tricuspid chordae tendineae. All of the foregoing was associated with congenital tricuspid regurgitation. The papillary muscles of the right ventricle were short and very hypertrophied. The tricuspid chordae tendineae were also very short and thick. The leaflets of the tricuspid valve were extremely thickened with rolled edges (consistent with tricuspid regurgitation). An enlarged right ventricular cavity was associated with marked right ventricular hypertrophy. Right atrial hypertrophy and enlargement coexisted. An abnormal muscle band of the right ventricle ran from the septum to the right ventricular free wall. This anomalous right ventricular band did not resemble the moderator band; it appeared to be truly anomalous. This patient died in 1976. Ebstein's anomaly was not present.

Our assessment was that in this case, congenital tricuspid regurgitation was exceedingly important—the most important anomaly in this patient. Note that *all* levels of this tricuspid valve were anomalous: the leaflets, the chordae tendineae, the papillary muscles, and the underlying right ventricular myocardium. It should be recalled that there is an important right ventricular myocardial component in the development of the tricuspid valve, as is indicated by Ebstein's anomaly and by muscular tricuspid valve.

Case 64 was a 3-day-old boy with severe congenital tricuspid regurgitation. The tricuspid leaflets were nodular and myxomatous. There was also dysplasia of the right ventricular sinus. The septal surface of the right ventricular sinus (inflow tract) was smooth (nontrabeculated). A small muscular ventricular septal defect was present anterosuperiorly, half way between the ventricular apex and the base, at the junction of the ventricular septum and the anterior free walls of the right and left ventricles. There was also a large secundum atrial septal defect because of a deficient septum primum; and a patent ductus arteriosus was also present.

Thus, severe non-Ebstein congenital tricuspid regurgitation was considered to be this newborn's main hemodynamic problem.

Comment. In both of these patients, severe congenital tricuspid regurgitation was considered to be the main cause of death.

Double-Inlet and Double-Outlet Right Ventricle (DIDO RV) With Congenital Non-Ebstein Tricuspid Regurgitation

This defect occurred in 2 patients (2.5%, Table 13.10, Cases 24 and 69).

Case 24 was a 1-year-old boy with DORV {S,L,L}, that is, double-outlet right ventricle with situs solitus of the viscera and atria, L-loop ventricles, and L-malposition of the great arteries. The morphologically left ventricle (LV) was absent; that is, following a very careful search, no vestige of the LV was identified. Consequently, single right ventricle was present. There was a double-inlet right ventricle (DIRV) with congenital tricuspid regurgitation of the left-sided tricuspid valve and congenital mitral stenosis of the right-sided mitral valve. Thickening and rolling was present of the tricuspid leaflet margins and there were jet lesions of the left atrial endocardium, both confirming the presence of left-sided tricuspid regurgitation. Dextrocardia was present (usual for a ventricular L-loop). This patient also had pulmonary outflow tract atresia.

To summarize, this patient with complex congenital heart disease had DIDO RV {S,L,L} with single RV (L), absent LV (R), congenital TR (L) and congenital MS (R), with PAt and dextrocardia.

Therapeutic interventions in 1983 included a right-sided Blalock-Taussig anastomosis at 2 days of age, a central shunt at 9 months of age using a 4 mm Gore-Tex conduit between the ascending aorta and the left pulmonary artery, plus a Gore-Tex patch plasty of a stenosis between the left and right pulmonary artery branches and of the right Blalock-Taussig anastomotic site. Failure of the single right ventricle occurred, with right ventricular end-diastolic pressures of 23 to 30 mm Hg, leading to death at 1 year of age.

Thus, congenital non-Ebstein tricuspid regurgitation was considered to be one important hemodynamic handicap that led to the death of this patient with DIDO RV {S,L,L} and pulmonary atresia.

Case 69 was a 15-year-old girl with congenital heart disease that was similar to that of the previous patient. This teenager had a single RV (absent LV), DIRV, DORV {S,L,L}, bilateral conus (subaortic and subpulmonary), mild pulmonary stenosis with a bicuspid pulmonary valve, severe TR (L), left atrial hypertrophy and enlargement with jet lesions, and two coronary ostia originating from the left septal sinus of Valsalva of the aortic valve. The left-sided tricuspid valve had thickened and rolled margins, confirming the presence of severe left-sided TR.

Comment. It is noteworthy that both of these patients with double-inlet right ventricle and double-outlet right ventricle had single right ventricle (absent left ventricle) with {S,L,L} segmental anatomy (without visceral heterotaxy or splenic anomaly), and with significant congenital left-sided tricuspid regurgitation without Ebstein's anomaly.

Congenitally Unguarded Tricuspid Orifice

Absence or very marked underdevelopment of the tricuspid valve leaflets, but with a widely patent tricuspid orifice, was the cause of very severe congenital non-Ebstein tricuspid regurgitation in 1 case (1.25%, Table 13.10, Case 18). This was a male fetus, 29 weeks gestational age, who was a stillborn macerated abortus weighing 2.75 lb (1247 grams). Intrauterine death was spontaneous (natural), not medically induced. Fetal echocardiography had revealed free tricuspid regurgitation, with intrauterine congestive heart failure (hydrops fetalis). Thus, congenital tricuspid regurgitation was very important as a cause of intrauterine death. The anterior leaflet of the tricuspid valve was very hypoplastic. The posterior leaflet was slightly better developed, but it too was also very hypoplastic. The septal leaflet of the tricuspid valve was virtually absent, just a minimal vestige being present. Right atrial hypertrophy and enlargement were marked. The segmental anatomy was normal, that is, {S,D,S}, and apart from the marked hypoplasia of the tricuspid leaflets, the heart was otherwise structurally normal. (Note that pulmonary valvar atresia with intact ventricular septum was *not* present, as it was in the previously presented cases of congenitally unguarded tricuspid orifice (Figs. 13.31 and 13.32).

Multiple congenital anomalies were present: hypertelorism, microphthalmia, micrognathia, bilateral epicanthal folds, widely spaced nipples, low hairline posteriorly, posterior displacement of the anus, and talipes equinovarus (typical club foot).

This was also a case of familial congenital heart disease. An older brother had tetralogy of Fallot with pulmonary outflow tract atresia and severe tricuspid regurgitation (but with a well-formed tricuspid valve). We could find no evidence that a karyotype had been done.

Comment. Thus, congenitally unguarded tricuspid orifice in the setting of multiple congenital anomalies was yet another cause of very severe congenital non-Ebstein tricuspid regurgitation—so severe that it led to fatal intrauterine congestive heart failure and death.

Downward Displacement of the Anterior Tricuspid Leaflet With Blood Cysts of the Tricuspid Valve Leaflets

These anomalies were associated with massive tricuspid regurgitation in 1 patient (1.25%, Table 13.10, Case 3). This patient was a 3-year-old boy who died in 1961. There was marked dilation of the right atrium that almost filled the entire thorax. The right atrium measured 12 × 9 × 9 cm (i.e., 4.7 × 3.5 × 3.5 inches). There was a pronounced bulge of the anterior chest wall because of the enormous right atrial enlargement. The heart weighed 95 grams. The tricuspid annulus was enlarged with a circumference of 14 cm (5.5 inches). The right ventricle was hypertrophied and enlarged with a thickness of 6 mm. Histology showed myocardium in all sections of the right atrium.

The conclusion following postmortem examination was that this patient had massive congenital tricuspid regurgitation because of dysplasia of the tricuspid leaflets, not idiopathic dilation of the right atrium (as had been thought clinically). In other words, the basic anomaly was thought to be at the level of the tricuspid valve leaflets, resulting in massive tricuspid regurgitation, the very marked right atrial enlargement being regarded as secondary to tricuspid regurgitation. Following autopsy, the right atrial enlargement was no longer considered to be idiopathic.

Congenital Mitral Regurgitation With Pulmonary Hypertension, Pulmonary Vascular Obstructive Disease, and Tricuspid Regurgitation

This combination of abnormalities was associated with tricuspid regurgitation in 1 of these 80 patients (1.25%, Table 13.10, Case 4).

Case 4 was a $15\,^{8}/_{12}$-year-old girl with congenital mitral regurgitation, ventricular septal defect, secundum atrial septal defect, pulmonary hypertension, mild valvar pulmonary stenosis, and aberrant right subclavian artery. At 10 years of age in 1960, she underwent mitral valvuloplasty for congenital mitral regurgitation ("reefing" of the annulus) and atrial septal defect closure. Pulmonary artery hypertension and severe pulmonary vascular obstructive disease (Heath and Edwards grades III and IV) were also found to be present. Left ventricular hypertrophy, right ventricular hypertrophy, tricuspid regurgitation, and right atrial enlargement were also found.

At 12 years of age, atrial fibrillation appeared that was quinidine resistant. Congestive heart failure appeared. The patient was cyanotic, dyspneic, and had a pulsatile hepatic margin 3 cm below the right atrial margin.

Cardiac catheterization at $15\,^{5}/_{12}$ years showed a ventricular septal defect with bidirectional shunt, pulmonary artery hypertension (106/24 mm Hg), pulmonary vascular obstructive disease, marked dilation of the pulmonary arteries, and tricuspid regurgitation.

At $15\,^{8}/_{12}$ years of age (in 1965), she underwent surgical ventricular septal defect closure, mitral valve replacement with a Starr-Edwards ball-valve prosthesis, and tricuspid annuloplasty. Postoperatively, she received a tracheostomy and her clinical condition deteriorated, leading to death 2 days postoperatively. Autopsy confirmed all of the foregoing findings and also revealed 6 accessory splenuli and a common mesentery, but without visceral heterotaxy. She also had talipes cavus—an abnormally high arch of the foot. Mild cardiac cirrhosis and widespread phlebosclerosis were also noted.

Thus, this patient illustrated that tricuspid regurgitation can be associated with congenital mitral regurgitation, ventricular septal defect, and secundum atrial septal defect when pulmonary hypertension progresses to pulmonary vascular obstructive disease and congestive heart failure.

Was this patient's tricuspid regurgitation truly congenital, that is, was it present at birth? The answer to this question is not known to us. All that we can say with confidence is that this patient's tricuspid regurgitation was based on the deleterious hemodynamic effects of her other forms of congenital heart disease (congenital mitral regurgitation, ventricular septal defect, atrial septal defect) and her acquisition of pulmonary vascular obstructive disease. Thus, her tricuspid regurgitation may have been acquired—appearing postnatally—but based on her other congenital heart disease. We simply do not know the answer to this question with certainty. So the reader may prefer to delete this case from our list of *congenital* non-Ebstein tricuspid regurgitation (Table 13.10). However, this tricuspid regurgitation has a congenital basis in the sense that it is based on her *other* congenital heart disease, as above. Congenital heart disease can predispose to other abnormalities with variable times of clinical appearance.

Hypoplastic Pulmonary Arteries With Pulmonary Artery Hypertension and Congenital Tricuspid Regurgitation

This rare combination of abnormalities occurred in 1 of these 80 patients (1.25%, Table 13.10, Case 54). This patient was a 29-day-old girl with severe pulmonary artery hypertension that was unresponsive to vasodilators. Two-dimensional echocardiography revealed tricuspid regurgitation.

Differential diagnoses included persistent pulmonary hypertension of the newborn, and primary pulmonary hypertension.

However, postmortem examination in 1984 revealed that the pulmonary intraparenchymal arteries all were markedly hypoplastic, more so than were the extraparenchymal pulmonary artery branches that accompanied the bronchi. Postmortem pulmonary arteriography showed that the branching pattern was normal, but that the arterial luminal diameters were much smaller than normal relative to the lung volume. There was also minimal background haze because the intraparenchymal arteries seen histologically were markedly hypoplastic.

Although anatomically normal, the tricuspid valve permitted significant tricuspid regurgitation (documented echocardiographically) in association with severe pulmonary artery hypertension. In turn, the pulmonary artery hypertension was caused by the marked hypoplasia of the pulmonary artery branches that was most marked within the pulmonary parenchyma. Goldstein, Rabinovitch, Van Praagh, and Reid[233] published another very similar case in 1979. This is a rare cause of significant congenital tricuspid regurgitation associated with an anatomically normal tricuspid valve.

SUMMARY

Apart from Ebstein's anomaly, there are many other situations in which congenital tricuspid regurgitation can occur (Table 13.10). To our knowledge, these other settings in which congenital tricuspid regurgitation can take place have never been presented in detail, and consequently are not widely recognized.

To summarize, our database revealed that congenital non-Ebstein tricuspid regurgitation (n = 80) occurred in the following settings (Table 13.10):

1. pulmonary atresia with intact ventricular septum (22.5%);
2. double-inlet left ventricle (16.25%);
3. hypoplastic left heart syndrome (15%);
4. transposition of the great arteries (11.25%);
5. trisomies 18 and 13 (6.25%);
6. Marfan syndrome (5%);
7. Uhl's disease (3.75%);
8. myxomatous tricuspid valve with polyvalvar disease (3.75%);
9. transposition of the great arteries with dysplastic tricuspid valve (3.75%);
10. tricuspid valve prolapse (2.5%);

11. dysplastic right ventricle and tricuspid valve (2.5%);
12. double-inlet and double-outlet right ventricle (2.5%);
13. congenitally unguarded tricuspid orifice (1.25%);
14. downward displacement of anterior tricuspid leaflet and blood cysts (1.25%);
15. with congenital mitral regurgitation, ventricular and atrial septal defects, and pulmonary vascular obstructive disease (1.25%); and
16. with hypoplastic pulmonary artery branches and pulmonary hypertension (1.25%).

There may, of course, be other anatomic types of congenital non-Ebstein tricuspid regurgitation that are not represented in our database.

TRICUSPID ATRESIA

Although we have described tricuspid atresia in association with Ebstein's anomaly (imperforate Ebstein's malformation), now we must consider the more common forms of tricuspid atresia.

History. The earliest known definite description of tricuspid atresia was by F. L. Kreysig[234] in Berlin in 1817. This reference was kindly sent to me by Dr. William J. Rashkind, whose translation from German is as follows:

> *"Opening of the right atrium showed much more solid construction than usual; the trabeculae of the auricle were hypertrophied and in the place where the opening into the right ventricle should have been, but was absent, instead there was convergence to a dimple."*

(Dr. Bill Rashkind, as he was known to all of his many friends, was not only the father of interventional cardiology because of his invention of balloon atrial septostomy to improve mixing in patients with transposition of the great arteries. He was also an expert in medical history and in medical art.)

There is an even earlier publication, also sent to me by Dr. Bill Rashkind, that dates to 1812, which reports a newborn infant who died at 7 days of age. This neonate definitely had pulmonary atresia and *probably* had tricuspid atresia. Published by the editors of the *London Medical Review,*[235] these authors stated (in part): "Upon dissection the pulmonary artery was found to be deficient, and instead of it there was a slender impervious ligament, extending from the situation of the right ventricle to the ductus arteriosus. The right ventricle was nearly obliterated. There was a mere depression in its situation. The right auricle was large, and communicated by an extensive foramen ovale of which the valve was very imperfect, with the left auricle. The left ventricle and the aorta were natural. The ductus arteriosus was very large and divided into two branches, which entirely supplied the lungs, without receiving any blood from the pulmonary artery."

So, what do you think? My interpretation is: atresia of the pulmonary valve and main pulmonary artery; and an ostium secundum type of atrial septal defect because of deficiency of septum primum. I think the right ventricle was present, but very small ("nearly obliterated").[235] If there had been any communication between the right atrium and the right ventricle, the authors would have described it; but they did not. In a good pathologic anatomic description, one can safely assume that if something is not mentioned, it is not present; one describes what is there, not what is not there. Nonetheless, I agree that brevity can be overdone. That may have been the case here. The problem with this report is that the evidence is *negative*. A failure to describe something is less persuasive than is a *positive* description of the abnormal findings. This is why I have some hesitation in asserting with certainty that what these authors in 1812 called "a singular malformation of the heart"[235] is the earliest known description of tricuspid atresia. But I think it *probably* is, and so did Dr. Bill Rashkind. I think that this is what Dr. Jesse Edwards and his colleagues about 140 years later would call tricuspid atresia type Ia.[236,237]

After these initial case reports from London[235] and Berlin,[234] other definite early reports of tricuspid atresia followed.[238-240]

Classification

Edwards and colleagues[236,237] introduced in 1949, and later, an influential classification of tricuspid atresia (Fig. 13.33). Although used less now than formerly, this classification should be understood as an aid to the comprehension of the literature on tricuspid atresia. **Type I** means that the great arteries are normally related, and **type II** indicates that transposition of the great arteries coexists. **Type a** means that pulmonary atresia is present, typically with no ventricular septal defect (VSD). **Type b** denotes that a small VSD is present, while **type c** denotes that a larger unrestrictive VSD coexists. See the legend to Fig. 13.33: the meanings of subtypes *a* and *b* are different, depending on whether the great arteries are normally related or transposed.[236,237]

The advantages of this classification are that it allows one to express three important anatomic features with brevity and accuracy. For example, **tricuspid atresia type Ib** (Fig. 13.33) is the most common anatomic type. This designation indicates: (1) that tricuspid atresia is present; (2) that the great arteries are normally related (type I); and that a small VSD is present (type b), constituting subpulmonary stenosis with reduced pulmonary blood flow.

What are the disadvantages of this early classification (Fig. 13.33) of tricuspid atresia? Briefly, congenital heart disease with tricuspid atresia is much more complicated than can be classified using only these two variables (type of relationship between the great arteries, and the presence and size of the VSD—which helps to determine the size of the pulmonary blood flow). For example, subaortic stenosis (not just subpulmonary stenosis or atresia) can be present. The atria are not always in situs solitus. A ventricular D-loop is not always present. Other types of infundibuloarterial anatomy can be present—such as truncus arteriosus, double-outlet right ventricle, doublet-outlet left ventricle, and anatomically corrected malposition of the great arteries. This is one of the reasons why the segmental approach to diagnosis and classification is now used: (1) The segmental approach always applies accurately, no matter how complex the anatomy. (2), Also, the segmental approach is a general classification that applies to all forms of congenital heart disease, not just to a special classification that pertains to tricuspid atresia only. (See Chapters 3 and 4 for more details concerning the

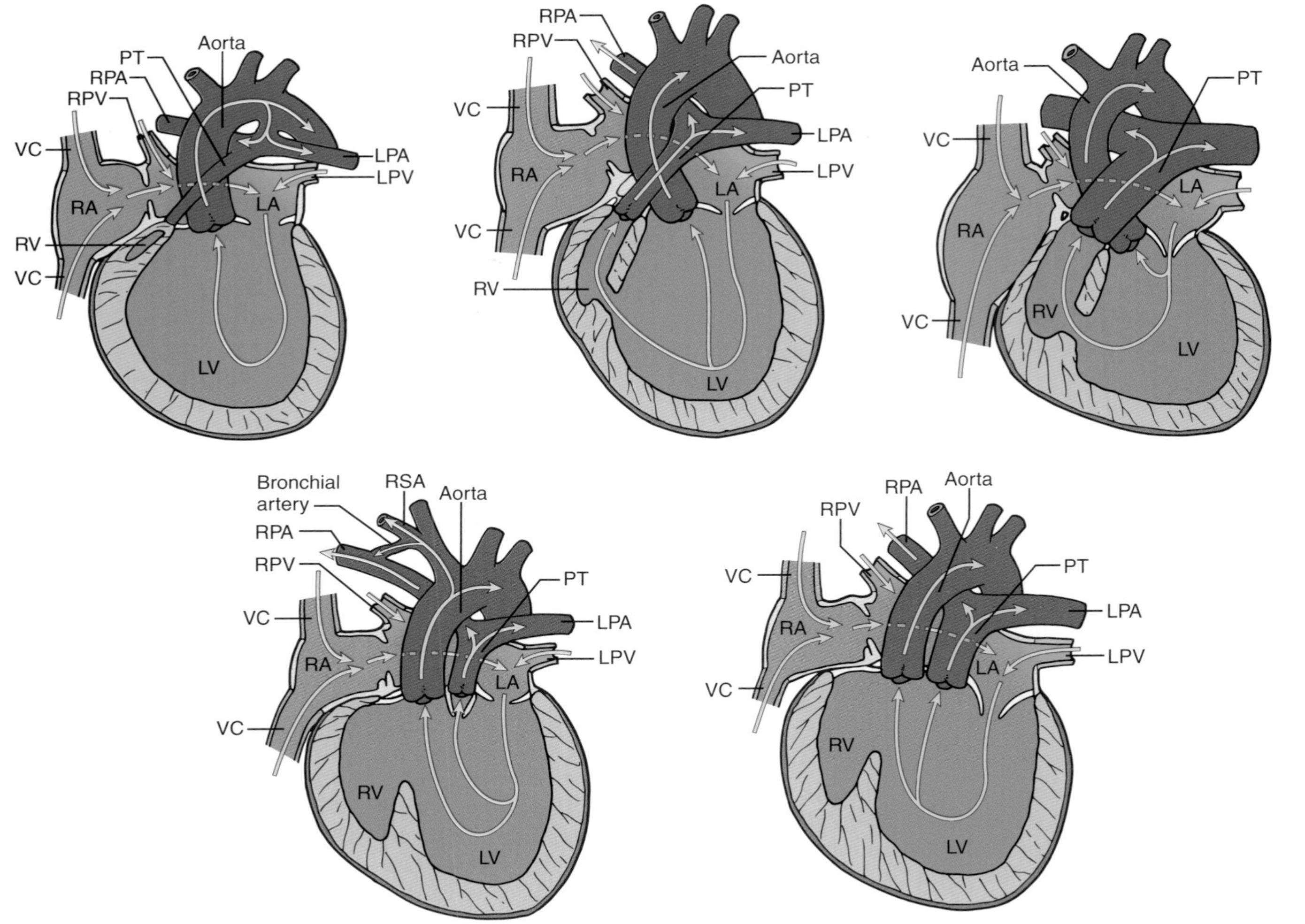

Fig. 13.33 Classification of tricuspid atresia by Edwards and colleagues.[236,237] *Upper,* Tricuspid atresia with normally related great arteries, type I. *Lower,* Tricuspid atresia with transposition of the great arteries, type II. *Upper Left,* **Tricuspid atresia type Ia.** Tricuspid atresia is present, meaning that there is no direct communication between the right atrium *(RA)* and the ventricular part of the heart. All of the systemic venous blood passes from the superior and inferior venae cavae *(VC)* into the RA and thence across the atrial septum into the left atrium *(LA)* and from there across the mitral valve into the left ventricle *(LV)*. In type Ia, because there is no ventricular septal defect (the ventricular septum is intact) and because there is pulmonary valvar atresia, all of the systemic venous blood (from the RA) and all of the pulmonary venous blood (from the LA) is ejected from the LV into the ascending aorta. Then some blood shunts from left to right through the patent ductus arteriosus into the left pulmonary artery *(LPA)* and the right pulmonary artery *(RPA)* to the lungs where it is oxygenated. Thus, in tricuspid atresia type Ia, there is no antegrade blood flow from the small right ventricle *(RV)* into the small pulmonary trunk *(PT)*. Pulmonary blood flow is ductus dependent or collateral artery dependent. *Upper Center,* **Tricuspid atresia type Ib.** The great arteries are normally related (type I). But now there is a small ventricular septal defect *(VSD)* between the LV and the RV (type b). Because it is small, the VSD constitutes subpulmonary stenosis. A relatively small amount of blood shunts left to right across this small VSD from the LV into the RV and thence to the lungs. Hence, pulmonary blood flow is reduced. No patent ductus arteriosus is shown. *Upper Right,* **Tricuspid atresia type Ic.** The great arteries are normally related (type I). But now, a relatively large VSD is present, which does not constitute subpulmonary stenosis (type c). Consequently, pulmonary blood flow is normal, or it can be increased; whereas in tricuspid atresia types Ia and Ib, the pulmonary blood flow typically is reduced. *Lower Left,* **Tricuspid atresia type IIa.** Transposition of the great arteries is present (type II). Subpulmonary stenosis (type a) coexists; hence pulmonary blood flow is reduced. *Lower Right,* **Tricuspid atresia type IIb.** No pulmonary stenosis is present (type b). *Note:* The meanings of subtypes *a, b, and c* change, depending on whether the great arteries are normally related (type I) or transposed (type II). This may be why Edwards and his colleagues deemphasized the use of these subtypes in their later work.[237] Some of us just misremembered. For me, tricuspid atresia type II*a* meant with pulmonary outflow tract atresia (Edwards et al[236,237] did not classify this type). For me, tricuspid atresia type II*b* had pulmonary outflow tract stenosis (instead of *no* pulmonary stenosis, as Edwards and colleagues did it, as in the lower right diagram).[237] For me, tricuspid atresia type II*c* meant no pulmonary outflow tract stenosis (which should have been type II*b*, as above).[236,237] In other words, I made the mental error of assuming that subtypes *a, b, and c* meant the same things, no matter whether their great arteries were normally related or transposed. My error was easier to remember; but it was an error nonetheless. To minimize confusion, I would suggest that the meanings of symbols used in classification should be constants (not variables). Such meanings should not change; as in arithmetic, *2* must always mean *two.* (From Edwards JE, Burchell HB: Congenital tricuspid atresia: classification. *Med Clin North Am* 1949;33:1177–1196, with permission.)

segment-by-segment approach to the diagnosis and classification of congenital heart disease.)

Nonetheless, Edwards and Burchell's classification of tricuspid atresia (Fig. 13.33)[236,237] was very helpful and influential when it was introduced, because of what it *could* do. Its deficiencies only became apparent over time, as our knowledge and understanding increased.

Personal Note. In 1956 to 1957 (July 1 to June 30), I was an Assistant Resident in Pathology at the Children's Medical Center (as it was then known) in Boston, in the Department of Dr. Sidney Farber, the world-famous father of chemotherapy for leukemia and lymphoma, with Dr. John M. Craig as my immediate and greatly admired supervisor. I was a 26-year-old resident in Pediatrics, doing my year of basic science. One of my autopsies was a patient with tricuspid atresia. The fascinating thing was that this patient's anatomic type of tricuspid atresia did not fit into the then extant and widely accepted classification of tricuspid atresia (Fig. 13.33).[236,237] If memory serves, I think my patient had tricuspid atresia with transposition of the great arteries, but with *subaortic stenosis*. I realized that I was looking at a previously undescribed anatomic type of tricuspid atresia.

This chance occurrence stimulated me to do a study of the pathologic anatomy of tricuspid atresia, which in turn led me in the directions of pediatric cardiology and pediatric cardiac pathology and embryology. Briefly, I became fascinated by these interrelated fields and decided to devote my professional life to them.

Perhaps I should add that I never published my study of tricuspid atresia because, when Keith, Rowe, and Vlad's first edition of *Heart Disease in Infancy and Childhood* appeared in 1958,[241] I discovered that the chapter on tricuspid atresia (that I would later learn had been written by my old friend and teacher Dr. Peter Vlad) said almost everything I wanted to say about tricuspid atresia. As Dr. John Craig told all of his pathology residents at that time, "To merit publication, a paper has to be only two things. It has to be true. And it has to be new." I knew that my prospective paper on tricuspid atresia was true. But I also knew that it was no longer new. So this is why I did not publish my first tricuspid atresia study.

However, I owe a great debt of gratitude to my old friend and teacher, Dr. Jesse Edwards, and his classification of tricuspid atresia (Fig. 13.33).[236,237] Trying to amplify his classification led me into my life's work.

Is Tricuspid Atresia a Form of Single Left Ventricle? In 1960–1961, when I was a fellow in the Cardiac Catheterization Laboratory at the Mayo Clinic in Rochester, Minnesota, under the direction of Dr. Jeremy Swan, I was given the project of figuring out single ventricle (see Chapter 17). Largely because of Dr. Jesse Edwards' classification of tricuspid atresia (cited above), we thought we understood tricuspid atresia and we excluded it from single ventricle.

In retrospect, we now realize that this was not a very good reason for excluding tricuspid atresia from the diagnostic category of single left ventricle. We now think that some cases of tricuspid atresia can have a single left ventricle in the sense that the morphologically right ventricle sinus (body, or inflow tract) can be absent, the small right ventricle consisting of the infundibulum or conus arteriosus only. Other cases of tricuspid atresia can have a small amount of right ventricular sinus. When the morphologically right ventricular sinus is absent, it is accurate to state that the morphologically left ventricle is single, that is, that only one ventricular sinus is present; hence, tricuspid atresia can have an *anatomically* single left ventricle.

Tricuspid atresia typically has a *physiologically* single left ventricle because even if a small right ventricular sinus remnant is present, it usually is clinically and surgically useless as a ventricle.

Anatomically and developmentally it should also be understood that the infundibulum or conus is really not a ventricle. Instead, the infundibulum is a connecting segment, not a main segment. The infundibulum is how the great arteries connect with the underlying ventricular sinuses—or sinus, if anatomically single ventricle is present. This is why the embryologists speak about the *conotruncus;* the conus (infundibulum) is part of the conotruncal segment (i.e., the subsemilunar part of the infundibulum is not an integral, inseparable part of either ventricle). This is why the subsemilunar part (the parietal band part) of the conus can straddle the ventricular septum to virtually any degree, demonstrating that the subsemilunar or parietal band part of the conus arteriosus is clearly not an integral, inseparable part of the morphologically right ventricle.

Consequently, the infundibular outlet chamber is really *not* a small right ventricle. The infundibulum "belongs" to the great arteries (the conotruncus), not to either ventricular sinus. Again, this appears to be why the distal (or subsemilunar) part of the conus can connect with the underlying ventricles (meaning ventricular sinuses) in so many different ways: The distal or subsemilunar part of the conus can be entirely above the right ventricle (in double-outlet right ventricle); entirely above the left ventricle (in double-outlet left ventricle); or overriding the ventricular septum to any degree—mostly above the right ventricle, or mostly above the left ventricle, or about equally above both ventricles.

But the important point in the interests of understanding is that in 1960, tricuspid atresia and/or mitral atresia were not what physicians *meant* when they talked about single (or common) ventricle. They thought they understood, at least anatomically, what tricuspid atresia is and what mitral atresia is. What they did not understand was: What is the anatomy of the ventricular part of the heart in *cor triloculare biatriatum* and in *cor biloculare*? When a heart has three chambers with two atria *(cor triloculare biatriatum),* or two chambers with one atrium and one ventricle *(cor biloculare),* in both situations there is (or appears to be) only one ventricle. What is this single ventricle? That was my project.

So, this is what was meant by single ventricle. Tricuspid atresia and mitral atresia were excluded from consideration only in an effort to define what was meant by single ventricle. Hence, the exclusion of tricuspid and mitral atresia was *arbitrary*—not because anyone thought that atresia of either atrioventricular valve and single ventricle did not, or could not, coexist. Dr. Edwards has solved the pathologic anatomic problem of tricuspid atresia. I was assigned the project of trying to understand the pathologic anatomy of single ventricle *without* atrioventricular valvar atresia.

To summarize, Dr. Jesse Edwards' classification of tricuspid atresia (Fig. 13.33)[236,237] was very influential not only in the understanding of tricuspid atresia, but also in the definition of single ventricle. This is why the premorphologic definition of single ventricle in the early 1960s was *the anomaly or anomalies in which both atrioventricular valves or a common atrioventricular valve open entirely or predominantly into one ventricular chamber;* that is, double-inlet or common-inlet ventricle (see Chapter 17). Tricuspid and mitral atresia were thus arbitrarily (not morphologically) excluded from the diagnostic category of single ventricle.

Note that one variable (the status of the atrioventricular valves) was being used to define another variable (the myocardial morphology of the ventricular part of the heart). Using one variable to define another variable is a fundamental error in logic. Each variable should be defined primarily in terms of itself.

So this, then, is the relevant background information.

FINDINGS

The following is a study of **non-Ebstein tricuspid atresia** (Fig. 13.34). The original records of each case were restudied. Flow sheets were made. Then the data were carefully analyzed, just as we have always done for all of our scientific papers. (This is our modus operandi for all chapters in this book. This chapter is an original, data-based study.)

Number of cases: 97.

Gender: male = 55; females = 41; not known =1. Males/females = 55/41 = 1.34/1.

Age at death or cardiac transplantation: $n = 95$ (not known = 2).

Mean: $4\frac{11}{12} \pm 9\frac{8}{12}$ years.

Range: 4.5 hours to 55 years.

Median: 7.5 months.

We regard the median age at death (there were only 2 cardiac transplants) as more accurately reflective of the true situation in this series: the median equals only 7.5 months. The mean age at death ($4\frac{11}{12}$ years) is misleadingly "old" because of the longevity of some of our patients: 16 of these 95 patients (17%) were more than 10 years of age.

Classifications

Now we must endeavor to answer the question: How many anatomic types of tricuspid atresia are there? We are intentionally excluding Ebstein's anomaly with tricuspid atresia, that is, imperforate Ebstein's anomaly, only because we have already considered this malformation. Thus, the question should be rephrased as follows: **In addition to imperforate Ebstein's**

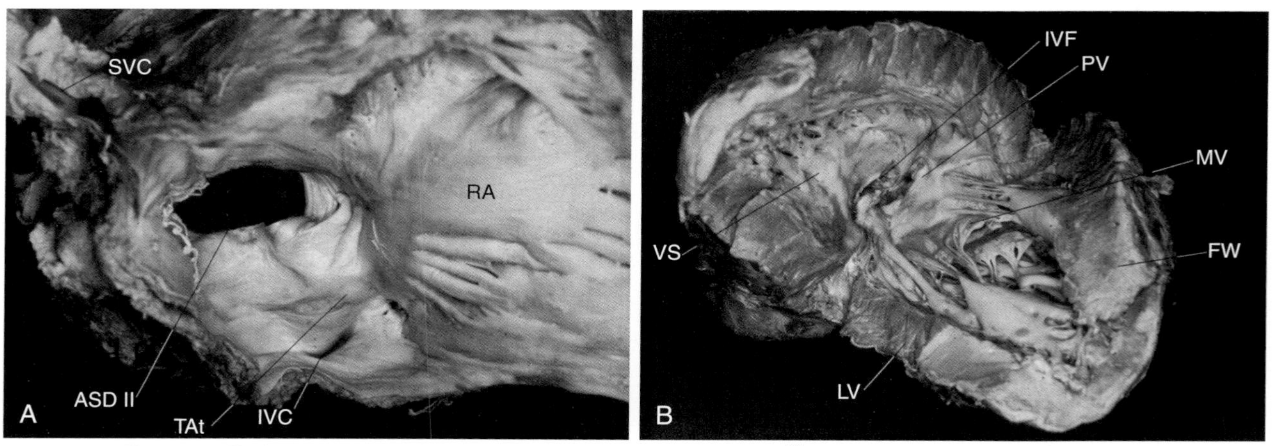

Fig. 13.34 Typical muscular tricuspid atresia *(TAt)* (non-Ebstein) in a $4\frac{11}{12}$-year-old boy with transposition of the great arteries {S,D,D} a small interventricular foramen causing subaortic stenosis, a large secundum type of atrial septal defect (deficient septum primum) *(ASD II),* marked hypoplasia of right ventricular sinus, and no pulmonary stenosis (Case 32). (A) Opened right atrium *(RA).* (B) Opened left ventricle *(LV).* In (A), note the flat muscular floor of the right atrium in the expected site of the tricuspid valve, with no suggestion of the tricuspid valve, typical of tricuspid atresia *(TAt).* The large ostium secundum type of atrial septal defect *(ASD II leader),* the deficient septum primum (below the ASD II), and the normal return of the inferior vena cava *(IVC)* and of the superior vena cava *(SVC)* are well seen. The RA is hypertrophied and enlarged. In (B), note the hypertrophy and enlargement of the left ventricle *(LV),* the transposed pulmonary valve *(PV),* the unremarkable appearing mitral valve *(MV),* and the small interventricular foramen *(IVF)* (or ventricular septal defect) that resulted in subaortic stenosis. At 7 weeks of age, the main pulmonary artery was banded. At $4\frac{11}{12}$ years of age, transinfundibular enlargement of the stenotic IVF was attempted surgically, leading to surgically induced complete heart block and intraoperative death (in 1977). Pulmonary histology was unremarkable, indicating that the pulmonary vascular bed had been effectively protected by the main pulmonary artery band. This patient illustrates that aortic outflow tract stenosis (not just pulmonary outflow tract stenosis) can be very important in patients with typical TAt. *FW,* Left ventricular free wall; *VS,* left ventricular septal surface. (From Edwards JE, Burchell HB: Congenital tricuspid atresia: a classification, *Med Clin North Am,* July 1949, p 1177; and Edwards JE, Carey LS, Neufeld HN, Lester RG: *Congenital Heart Disease, Correlation of Pathologic Anatomy and Angiocardiography.* Philadelphia, 1965, WB Saunders Co, p 347; with permission.)

anomaly, how many other anatomic types of tricuspid atresia are there?

Table 13.11 represents our attempt to answer this question, based on an analysis of our database (*n* = 94). (Cases were excluded when the data were considered not adequate for accurate analysis, as, for example, when the records were illegible.) It should be understood that other anatomic types of tricuspid atresia may well exist that we have not encountered in our database.

We are initially going to attempt to answer this question by following as closely as possible the approach of Dr. Jesse Edwards and his original classification of tricuspid atresia,[236,237] because it is useful and widely understood. However, it should also be appreciated that Edwards' initial classification of tricuspid atresia[236,237] was not really a classification of tricuspid atresia *per se*. Instead, it was a classification of some of the situations in which tricuspid atresia occurs. Edwards' classification[236,237] considers two questions: What is the relationship between the great arteries? And what is the status of the pulmonary outflow tract? These are clinically and surgically important variables, but they have nothing to do with the pathologic anatomy of tricuspid atresia itself.

Later, we will attempt to answer the question, **How many anatomic types of tricuspid atresia *per se* are there?** But first, let us begin with Dr. Jesse Edwards' clinically and surgically useful approach (Table 13.11).

TABLE 13.11 Classification of Non-Ebstein Tricuspid Atresia (*n* = 94)

Anatomy	No. of Cases	% of Series*
1. With normally related great arteries and pulmonary outflow tract atresia†	5	5
2. With normally related great arteries and pulmonary outflow tract stenosis†	44	47
3. With normally related great arteries and unobstructed pulmonary outflow tract†	6	6
4. With truncus arteriosus†	3	3
5. With D-loop transposition of the great arteries	18	19
6. With double-outlet right ventricle†	2	2
7. With double-outlet left ventricle†	1	1
8. With anatomically corrected malposition of the great arteries†	2	2
9. With L-transposition of the great arteries†	11	11
10. With isolated noninversion of the great arteries†	1	1
11. With conjoined twins	1	1

*All percentages are rounded off to the nearest whole number.
†Segmental anatomy:
All cases with normally related great arteries: {S,D,S}.
D-loop transposition of the great arteries: TGA {S,D,D} = 15; TGA {S,D,A} = 2; TGA {S,D,L} = 1.
Double-outlet right ventricle: DORV {S,D,D} = 2.
Double-outlet left ventricle: DOLV {S,D,L} = 1.
Anatomically corrected malposition of the great arteries: ACM {S,D,L} = 2.
L-transposition of the great arteries: TGA {S,L,L} =11.
Isolated noninversion of the great arteries with visceroatrial heterotaxy and polysplenia: {A,(I),L,S} = 1.

Using the now classical Edwardian approach,[236,237] there are at least 11 different anatomic types of tricuspid atresia (Table 13.11). A few words of explanation concerning the table may be helpful: Our anatomic types 1, 2, and 3 correspond to Edwards' types Ia, Ib, and Ic. Our type 5 corresponds to Edwards' type II. Most of our other anatomic types of tricuspid atresia are more recently discovered and described anomalies (Table 13.11) that were not envisioned by, and not included in, earlier classifications. As mentioned earlier, there may well be other anatomic types of tricuspid atresia that we have not been privileged to see and study. So Table 13.11 should be regarded as provisional—the best we can do at the present time (September 2007), based on the data available to us.

Why did we talk about *D-loop* transposition of the great arteries (type 5, Table 13.11), rather than simply D-transposition of the great arteries? Because there were two patients with TGA {S,D,A} and one with TGA {S,D,L} (see table footnote). Thus, although D-loop ventricles were present in all, the semilunar interrelationships were those of A-TGA in two and L-TGA in one (not D-TGA) (Table 13.11).

What does *isolated noninversion of the great arteries* mean? This anomaly (type 10, Table 13.11) is so rare that the meaning of the aforementioned designation may not be immediately obvious. Again, the segmental anatomy spells out the anatomy clearly (footnote): {A(I),L,S} with polysplenia, meaning situs ambiguus (A) of the viscera and atria, with basically situs inversus of the atria (I), with concordant L-loop ventricles (L), and with solitus normally related great arteries (S). Hence, only the great arteries are not inverted, whereas both the atrial and the ventricular segments are inverted; thus isolated noninversion of the great arteries is present. However, for rarities like this, we prefer the spelled-out segmental anatomic designation rather than an unfamiliar verbal term. {A(I),L,S} with polysplenia is clear—as long as one understands segmental anatomy. The segmental anatomy also indicates that there is atrioventricular concordance (between inverted atria and L-loop ventricles) and ventriculoarterial concordance (between L-loop ventricles and solitus normally related great arteries). If either concordance (AV or VA) is altered by additional anomalies, such additional malformations must also be described. In a well formulated diagnosis, when additional anomalies are not mentioned, their absence may be assumed.

Specifically what does *conjoined twins* mean (type 11, Table 13.11)? Patient 30 was a 4.5-hour-old female (the youngest in this series), conjoined twin B of thoracopagus twins, with multiple congenital anomalies. She had **atresia of all four cardiac valves,** a unique finding to our knowledge.

Relative frequencies: What is the most common anatomic type of tricuspid atresia, and which is the rarest? Based on our 94 postmortem cases, the relative frequencies of the anatomic types of tricuspid atresia were found to be as follows (Table 13.11):

1. The most common was tricuspid atresia {S,D,S} with pulmonary outflow tract stenosis (47%). (As expected.)
2. Second in frequency (and this was a surprise to us) was tricuspid atresia with D-loop transposition of the great arteries (19%) (Fig. 13.34).
3. Third in frequency (and also a surprise) was left-sided tricuspid atresia with TGA {S,L,L} (11%) (Fig. 13.35).

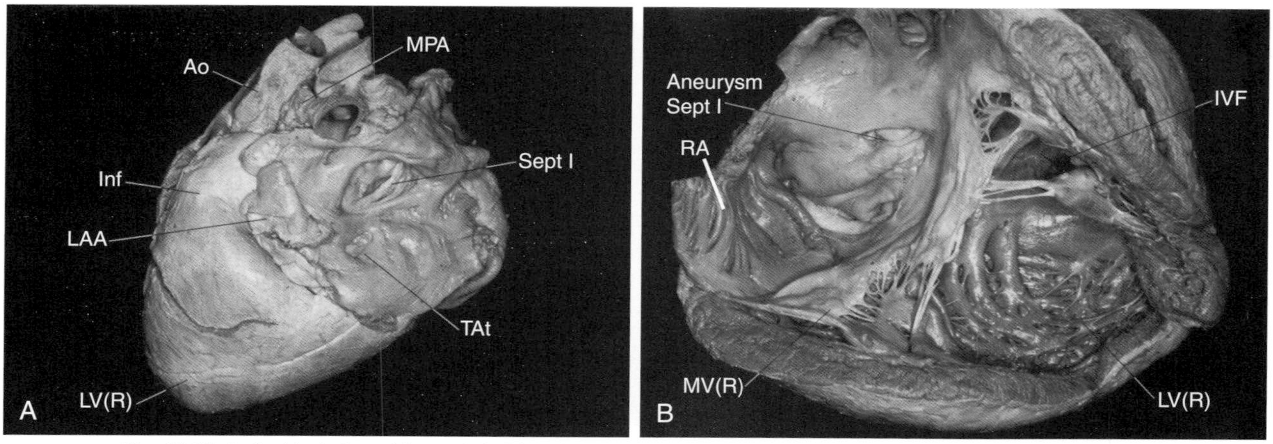

Fig. 13.35 Left-sided tricuspid atresia in TGA {S,L,L} is illustrated by Case 71, a 14-year-old boy who died from ventricular fibrillation in 1957. He also had atrial fibrillation. The atrial septum was normally formed and hence obstructive, with an aneurysm of septum primum bulging into the right atrium. (A) Opened left atrium. (B) Opened right atrium *(RA),* mitral valve, and morphologically left ventricle. In (A), note the left-sided tricuspid atresia *(TAt),* the hypertrophied and enlarged left atrial appendage *(LAA),* and the well-formed and redundant septum primum *(Sept I).* Also seen are the exteriors of the right-sided morphologically left ventricle, *LV(R);* the left-sided and superior infundibulum *(Inf),* from which the L-transposed aorta *(Ao)* originates; and the transposed main pulmonary artery *(MPA),* which arises posteriorly and to the right of the Ao from the LV(R). In (B), note the obstructive and aneurysmal *Sept I* bulging into the hypertrophied and enlarged right atrium *(RA).* The right-sided morphologically mitral valve, *MV(R),* opens into the hypertrophied and enlarged morphologically left ventricle that is positionally right-sided, *LV(R). IVF,* Interventricular foramen (or ventricular septal defect). *Thus, the morphology of the atrioventricular (AV) valves corresponds to that of the ventricles of entry, not to that of the atria of exit.* Here we see a morphologically mitral valve (right-sided) exiting a right-sided RA and entering a right-sided LV. More generally, *the morphology of the AV valves corresponds to that of the ventricular loop with which they are associated, rather than to that of the atria.* This rule applies whether or not an AV valve opens into a ventricle: for example, this rule applies in tricuspid atresia (as in this case) and in mitral atresia. This rule also applies in double-inlet ventricle. For example, in double-inlet LV, when a ventricular D-loop is present, the tricuspid valve is right-sided relative to the mitral valve; but when a ventricular L-loop is present, the tricuspid valve is left-sided relative to the mitral valve. (See Chapter 17 for more data.) Thus, the morphology of the AV valves in this case illustrates an important general principle.

4. Fourth was tricuspid atresia {S,D,S} with an unobstructed pulmonary outflow tract (6%).
5. Fifth was tricuspid atresia with pulmonary outflow tract atresia (5%).
6. Sixth in frequency was tricuspid atresia with truncus arteriosus (3%) (Figs. 13.36 to 13.38). This anatomic association tends to raise the eyebrows of even the cognoscente because truncus arteriosus does not appear in any of the well-known classifications of tricuspid atresia, and conversely tricuspid atresia is not part of the classifications of truncus arteriosus. So this combination—tricuspid atresia with truncus arteriosus—often still comes as a surprise.
7. The other rare associations are similarly surprising to many well-informed observers, such as tricuspid atresia with double-outlet right ventricle {S,D,D} (2%), or with anatomically corrected malposition of the great arteries {S,D,L} (2%) (Fig. 13.39).
8. The rarest association of tricuspid atresia in our experience were with double-outlet left ventricle {S,D,L}, {A(I),L,S} with polysplenia, and with thoracopagus conjoined twins (1% each).

ANATOMIC DETAILS

Although we have listed the 11 main anatomic types of tricuspid atresia (Table 13.11), we have not as yet considered any of the anatomic features of each type. Let us do so in order of descending frequency, beginning with the numerically most common anatomic type.

Tricuspid Atresia {S,D,S} with Pulmonary Outflow Tract Stenosis

This is Dr. Jesse Edwards' type Ib (n = 44 patients, 47% of this series, Table 13.11).

Gender: males = 28; females = 16; males/females = 1.75/1. In other words, a male predominance was found, with males being 75% more frequent than females.

Age at death or cardiac transplantation: mean = $3\frac{7}{12} \pm 6\frac{10}{12}$ years; range = 1 day to $29\frac{4}{12}$ years; and median = 5¼ months. There was only 1 cardiac transplant in this series of 44 patients (2%).

Again it is noteworthy that the median age at death (5¼ months) is much younger than the mean age at death ($3\frac{7}{12}$ years). We think that the younger median age at death more accurately reflects the gravity of tricuspid atresia {S,D,S} with pulmonary outflow tract stenosis than does the older mean age at death. The standard deviation ($\pm 6\frac{10}{12}$ years) is relatively large because this series of 44 postmortem cases contained 5 teenagers (11%), skewing the mean in an older direction ($16\frac{2}{12}$, 17½, 19, $22\frac{9}{12}$, and $29\frac{4}{12}$ years).

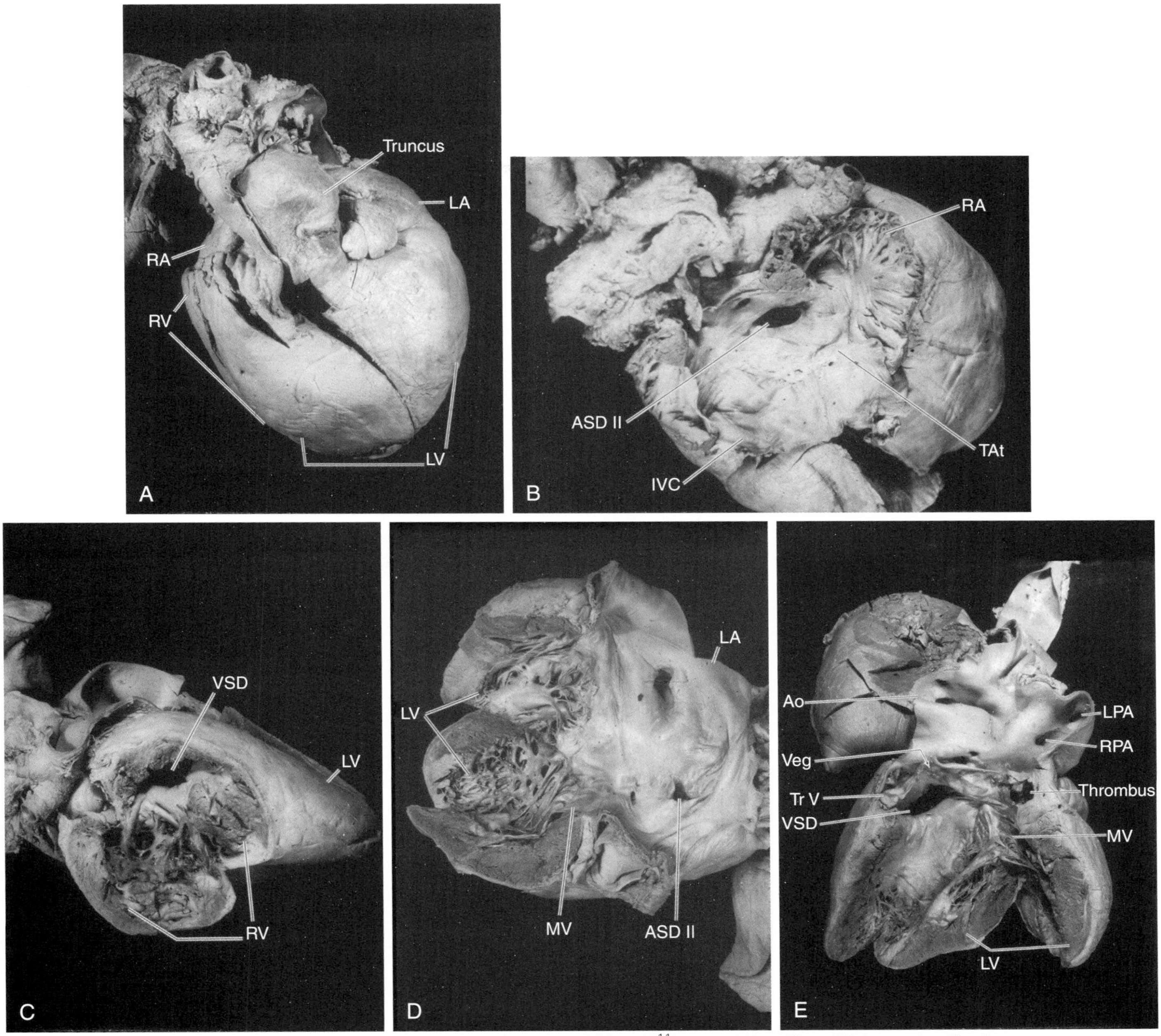

Fig. 13.36 Tricuspid atresia with truncus arteriosus type A2 in a 12 11/12-year-old boy (Case 49). In our classification of truncus arteriosus, type *A* means that a ventricular septal defect (VSD) is present, and type *2* means that there is no aortopulmonary septal remnant. The truncal valve was bicuspid (bicommissural) because of a rudimentary right coronary-noncoronary commissure. A large secundum type of atrial septal defect was present. The VSD was high, large, and subtruncal in location. There was truncal valve–mitral valve direct fibrous continuity (as in normally related great arteries and as in tetralogy of Fallot). Although the coronary ostia were abnormally located (e.g., the right coronary ostium was located above the rudimentary right coronary-noncoronary commissure), this anomaly was thought to be of little or no hemodynamic importance. There was subacute bacterial endocarditis, with vegetations of the truncal valve. The truncal valve was mildly calcified. There was a minimal cleft of the anterior leaflet of the mitral valve with mild fusion of the chordae tendineae. (A) External frontal view of the heart. (B) Interior of the opened right atrium. (C) Interior of the small right ventricle. (D) Opened left atrium, mitral valve, and left ventricular inflow tract. (E) Opened left ventricular outflow tract and truncus arteriosus. In (A), the external view of the right atrium *(RA)*, the small right ventricle *(RV)*, the left atrium *(LA)*, the large left ventricle *(LV)*, and the truncus arteriosus *(Truncus)* are seen. In (B), the opened RA reveals typical muscular tricuspid atresia *(TAt)*, a secundum atrial septal defect *(ASD II)*, and a normally connected inferior vena cava *(IVC)*. In (C), the interior of the small RV, a right-sided view of the ventricular septal defect *(VSD)*, and the exterior of the large LV that forms the ventricular apex are seen. In (D), the interior of the LA, a left atrial view of the ASD II, the opened mitral valve *(MV)*, and the interior of the LV inflow tract are shown. In (E), note the LV outflow tract; the large conoventricular type of subtruncal VSD; the bicuspid truncal valve *(TrV)*; the presence of TrV-MV fibrous continuity; the vegetation *(Veg)* of subacute bacterial endocarditis on the TrV; an old organized thrombus on the TrV; the prominent high coronary arterial ostium above the rudimentary right coronary-noncoronary commissure; the ostia of the right pulmonary artery *(RPA)* and the left pulmonary artery *(LPA)* arising from the truncus arteriosus, which we think is really the ascending aorta *(Ao)*; and the absence of any aortopulmonary septal remnant. Hence, this is what is known as truncus arteriosus type A2. Tricuspid atresia with truncus arteriosus type A2 typically has increased pulmonary blood flow.

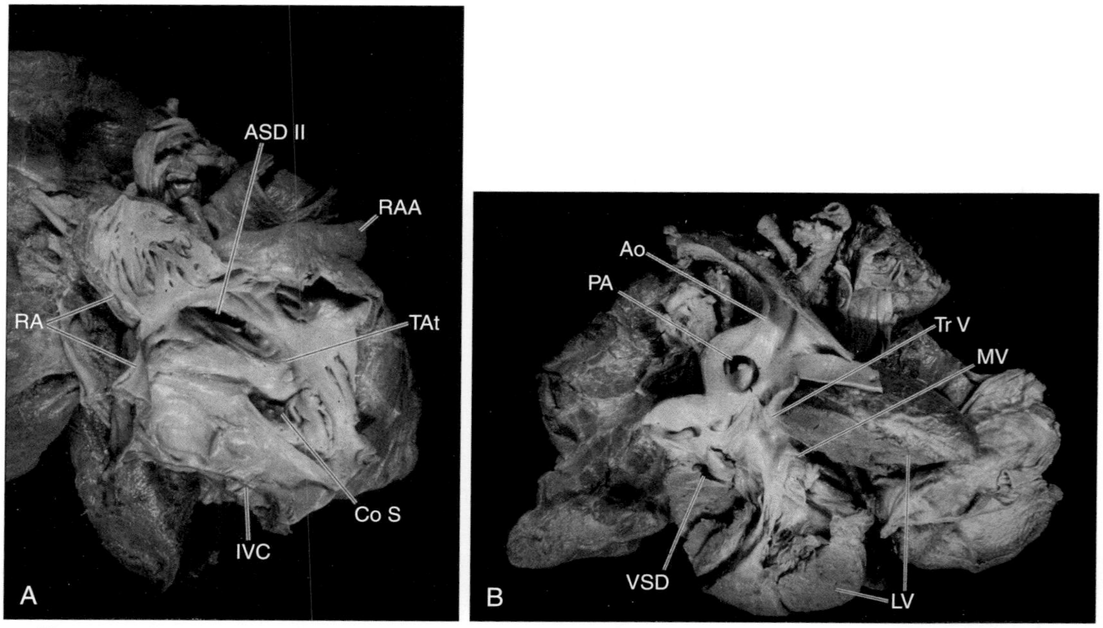

Fig. 13.37 Case 80 was a 6-month-old girl with tricuspid atresia and truncus arteriosus type A2. The ductus arteriosus was absent. She experienced pulmonary flooding with very increased Qp and developed congestive heart failure. She was treated with banding of the left pulmonary artery (in 1964). Subsequently, she developed purulent meningitis due to *Staphylococcus aureus,* leading to death. Autopsy confirmed the aforementioned findings and revealed pulmonary vascular obstructive disease in the unbanded right lung. (A) The opened right atrium *(RA)* revealed tricuspid atresia *(TAt)* and an ostium secundum type of atrial septal defect *(ASD II)*. *Co S,* Coronary sinus; *IVC,* inferior vena cava; *RAA,* right atrial appendage. (B) The opened left ventricular outflow tract *(LV)* shows the mitral valve *(MV)*, the truncal valve *(Tr V)*, TrV-MV fibrous continuity, the subtruncal ventricular septal defect *(VSD)*, and the origin of the pulmonary artery branches *(PA)* from the posterior aspect of the ascending aorta. There is no aortopulmonary septal remnant; hence this is truncus arteriosus type A2.

Anatomic features: In this type of tricuspid atresia, pulmonary outflow tract stenosis is not always due to the presence of a small ventricular septal defect, contrary to what is often said and thought. In fact, the ventricular septal defect can be relatively quite large; but if this large ventricular sepal defect is associated with pulmonary infundibular and/or pulmonary valvar stenosis, then one has pulmonary outflow tract stenosis with a large ventricular septal defect.

Tetralogy of Fallot–like pulmonary infundibular stenosis—with anterosuperior deviation of the conal septum (parietal band), resulting in a relatively large ventricular septal defect, with or without pulmonary valvar stenosis—was found in 6 of these 44 cases (14%). When a tetralogy of Fallot type of infundibuloarterial malformation coexists with tricuspid atresia, we customarily do *not* make the diagnosis of tetralogy with tricuspid atresia—even though that is really what is present. Why do we not make this diagnosis? Perhaps because the addition of tricuspid atresia is more than the four anomalies of the classical tetrad. This conventional diagnostic inhibition really makes no sense. Similarly, tetralogy of Fallot can occur with common atrioventricular canal, or with congenital mitral stenosis, and so on. We now make these diagnoses, even though the total number of malformations is greater than four. So, why not tetralogy with tricuspid atresia, or vice versa? We understand that diagnostic conventions change slowly, and we are not suggesting a change in diagnostic terminology. Instead, our real point is this: One should *understand* that tricuspid atresia and a tetralogy of Fallot type of infundibuloarterial malformation can indeed coexist, explaining the apparent paradox of a large ventricular septal defect in association with pulmonary outflow tract stenosis.

A bicuspid (bicommissural) pulmonary valve was found in 11 of these 44 cases (25%).

An ostium secundum type of atrial septal defect was present in 17 of these 44 patients (39%). Conversely, a prominent **aneurysm of septum primum,** bulging into the left atrium and indicating an obstructive atrial septum, was observed in only 2 (5%). In one patient, the aneurysm of septum primum was described as *giant;* it bulged into the mitral orifice from above and appeared capable of obstructing not only the systemic venous return from the venae cavae, but also the pulmonary venous return from the normally connected pulmonary veins.

A persistent left superior vena cava drained into the coronary sinus and thence to the right atrium in 7 patients (16%).

A prominent **right venous valve** (Eustachian valve of the inferior vena cava) or Chiari's network (filamentous remnants of the right venous valve within the right atrium) were found in 5 (11%).

Multiple congenital anomalies were present in 12 of these patients (27%). No pattern of extracardiovascular anomalies was found to predominate. Many different systems were involved:

1. **Oro-facial.** Case 5 had a left-sided cleft lip and a cleft palate. This 6-month-old girl also had a *brachiocephalic artery,* that

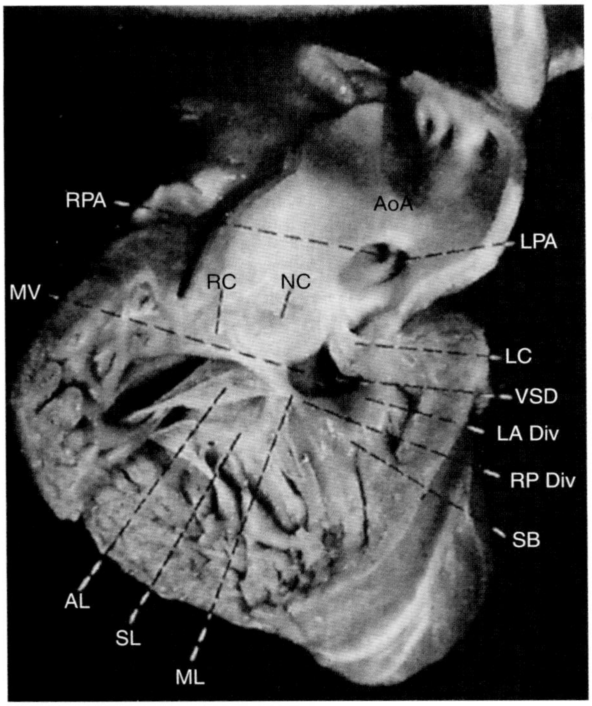

Fig. 13.38 Absence of the pulmonary outflow tract that we used to call truncus arteriosus communis, type A2. The whole pulmonary outflow tract is absent, including the subpulmonary infundibulum, the pulmonary valve, and main pulmonary artery, but not the right and left pulmonary artery branches. Absence of the main pulmonary artery excludes the diagnosis of truncus (common aortopulmonary trunk). The above anomaly has a solitary aortic trunk, not a common aortopulmonary trunk. This anomaly, absence of the whole pulmonary outflow tract, is closely related to tetralogy of Fallot, which has variable underdevelopment of the pulmonary outflow tract but not complete absence of the pulmonary outflow tract. This is a fascinating new insight into what tetralogy of Fallot really is, namely, underdevelopment of the normal adaptation that permits land-living and air-breathing. In tetralogy of Fallot, underdevelopment of the subpulmonary infundibulum and pulmonary valve can be very severe, but never absent, as in this patient. Finally, we understand that tetralogy of Fallot is one of the most common forms of underdevelopment of a basic mechanism that permits land-living and air-breathing in mammals, as opposed to water-living and water-breathing by fish that do not have lungs or a pulmonary outflow tract. This patient had no pulmonary outflow tract but did have lungs. The pulmonary artery branches in this patient arise from the aortic sac, which is where the pulmonary artery branches normally begin but then migrate on the sixth aortic arches to join the main pulmonary artery (MPA). However, in this patient, pulmonary artery branches did not migrate from the aorta to the MPA because the MPA was absent. Background to this discovery is found in the publication by Vizcaino and colleagues in 2002 (see source data below). *AL,* Anterior leaflet of the tricuspid valve; *LA Div,* left anterior division of the septal band; *LC,* left coronary leaflet of the aortic valve; *LPA,* left pulmonary artery; *ML,* muscle of Lancisi/Lushka; *MV,* mitral valve; *RPA,* right pulmonary artery; *RP Div,* right posterior division of the septal band; *SB,* septal band; *SL,* septal leaflet of the tricuspid valve; *VSD,* ventricular septal defect. (From Vizcaino A, Campbell J, Litovsky S, Van Praagh R: Single origin of right and left pulmonary artery branches from ascending aorta with nonbranching main pulmonary artery: relevance to a new understanding of truncus arteriosus. *Pediatr Cardiol* 2002;23:230-234; with permission.)

is, one aortic arch artery giving rise to both the right common carotid and the left common carotid arteries. In addition, she had an aberrant right subclavian artery that arose from the descending thoracic aorta.

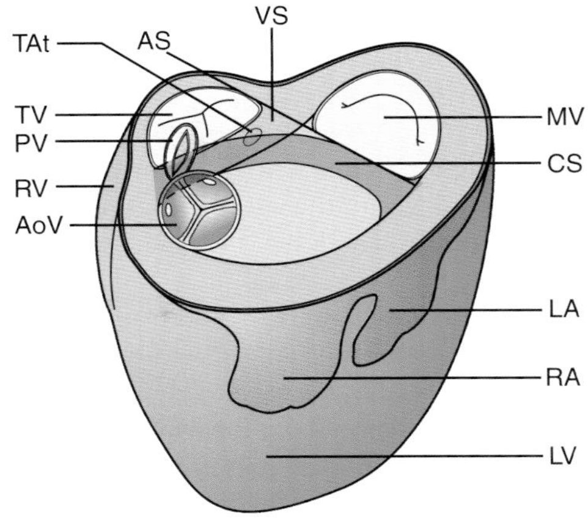

Fig. 13.39 Tricuspid atresia with anatomically corrected malposition of the great arteries {S,D,L} and dextrocardia, in a 2-year-and-20-day-old girl, geometric diagram, view from above. Tricuspid atresia, *TAt.* The expected site of the tricuspid valve is located immediately above the ventricular septum *(VS);* this case illustrates the ventriculoatrial malalignment of typical (non-Ebstein) tricuspid atresia. The mitral valve *(MV)* was unremarkable. There is left-sided juxtaposition of the atrial appendages, the appendage of the right atrium *(RA)* lying immediately beside the appendage of the left atrium *(LA)*—both to the left of both great arteries, because of levomalposition of the right atrial appendage that normally lies to the right of both great arteries. The **cardiac geometry** is very abnormal when measured relative to the anteroposterior plane (the Z axis) and projected onto the horizontal plane: The angle of the atrial septum *(AS)* = 60° left; normal is 30° left. The angle of the ventricular septum *(VS)* = 60° right; normal = 35° to 40° left. The ventriculoatrial (or atrioventricular) septal angle = 120°; normal = 5° to 10°. The conal septal angle = 65° right; normal = 65° right. The conoventricular septal angle = 5°; normal = 100°. Rotation of the semilunar valves (measuring the normal, nonstenotic aortic valve, *AoV*) = 20° left; normal = 150° right. The pulmonary valve *(PV)* is bicuspid (bicommissural) and stenotic. The segmental anatomy is ACM {S,D,L}. *ACM,* Anatomically corrected malposition, meaning that the great arteries are very malpositioned, but that despite this fact, each great artery nonetheless arises above the anatomically (morphologically) correct ventricle: AoV above the LV, and PV above the RV. The viscera and atria are in situs solitus: {*S*,-,-}. However, the AS is further to the left than is normal in situs solitus. D-loop ventricles are present, i.e., {S,*D*,-}, despite the fact that the VS is angulated much further to the right than normal. L-malposition of the great arteries is present, i.e., {S,D,*L*}, the aortic valve having rotated far enough to the left to be located above the LV, and the pulmonary artery having rotated far enough posteriorly and to the right to arise above the RV. Hence, the ventriculoarterial alignments are those of ACM. Consequently, the segmental anatomy is *ACM* {S,D,L}. In ACM, the ventricles and the great arteries loop or twist in opposite directions. In this case, which illustrates the most common form of ACM, the ventricles have looped to the *right* and the great arteries have rotated to the *left.* The contralaterality of these morphogenetic movements appears to explain why ACM is so rare. Usually, the ventricles loop and the conotruncus twists in the same direction—both to the right, or both to the left. ACM used to be called anatomically corrected *transposition* of the great arteries,[633] before it was agreed that *transposition* should be defined literally: as ventriculoarterial discordance. (Reproduced with permission from Van Praagh R, Van Praagh S: Anatomically corrected transposition of the great arteries. *Br Heart J* 1967;29:112.)

2. **Facial-hand-foot.** Patient 12, a 7-day-old boy, had facial dysmorphism with hypertelorism, low-set ears, bilateral simian creases, and syndactyly of the second and third toes bilaterally.
3. **Nasal.** Patient 33, a 1-day-old girl, had choanal atresia.

4. **Eye-neck-chest-genital-central nervous system.** Patient 38, a 6 9/12-year-old boy, had facial dysmorphism with anisocoria (unequal pupil sizes), webbed neck, broadly spaced nipples, one testis, slow motor development, and an intellectual disability. This patient also had a rare cardiovascular anomaly: a **supramitral band** within the left atrium, that appeared to be composed of mitral valve tissue, and that had no physiologic importance.
5. **Brain-lung-hand.** Patient 41, a 2-month-old girl, had hydrocephalus, bilaterally trilobed lungs (without visceral heterotaxy or splenic anomaly), and a left-sided simian crease. She also had small follicular cysts of the ovaries.
6. **Genitourinary-osseous.** Patient 47, a 4-week-old boy, had agenesis of the right kidney, hydronephrosis of the upper pole of the left kidney, a double right renal artery, an undescended right testis, radial deviation of the right hand, thoracic scoliosis, and anomalous ribs (7 on the right side).
7. **Tracheoesophageal.** Patient 56, a 22-year-old girl, had a trachea-esophageal fistula. Esophageal atresia was associated with a fistula between the distal end of the trachea posteriorly and the distal esophagus.
8. **Gastrointestinal.** Three patients had gastrointestinal malformations. Patient 78, an 8-month-old boy, had a Meckel's diverticulum and malrotation of the colon. This little boy also had a perforated peptic ulcer of the first portion of the duodenum and peritonitis. Noteworthy cardiovascular anomalies included **absence of the ductus arteriosus and absence of the bronchial arteries.** (I studied this patient as a Pathology resident in 1956.) Patient 83, a 2 8/12-year-old girl, had ectopic gastric mucosa at the upper end of the esophagus. Patient 94, a 6-week-old boy, had duodenal atresia and an annular pancreas.
9. **Gastrointestinal-renal.** Patient 82, a 5½-month-old boy, had a horseshoe kidney and an imperforate anus.

Unfortunately, no genetic information is available concerning any of the foregoing patients (karyotypes, etc.). No recognized syndromes or other etiologic diagnostic clues are known to us.

To conclude this point, patients with tricuspid atresia {S,D,S} and pulmonary outflow tract stenosis had *isolated* congenital heart disease in 73% of these cases. But *nonisolated* congenital heart disease was found in more than one-quarter of these patients (27%) because of the coexistence of a wide variety of noncardiovascular anomalies.

Anatomic types of tricuspid atresia per se: The great majority of these patients with tricuspid atresia {S,D,S} and pulmonary outflow tract stenosis had the usual **muscular type of tricuspid atresia** (Fig. 13.14). When one looks at the floor of the right atrium where the tricuspid valve should be, one sees no suggestion of a tricuspid valve—just muscle. This is why we call it the muscular type of tricuspid atresia. There is often a little "dimple," a small downward depression in the middle of the floor of the right atrium. This little dimple is widely regarded as part of the membranous septum, that is, the atrioventricular portion of the pars membranacea septi.

Occasionally, the tricuspid atresia can be membranous, as in Case 39. The infrequent **membranous type of tricuspid atresia** was characterized by a fibrous remnant of tricuspid leaflet tissue and chordae tendineae. It is noteworthy that left-sided juxtaposition of the atrial appendages was *not* present; that is, the right atrial appendage was not malposed posteriorly and to the left of the great arteries. Why is this fact noteworthy? Because, as will be seen subsequently, the membranous type of tricuspid atresia (that transilluminates brilliantly) occurs quite often with left-sided juxtaposition of the atrial appendages.

Case 39 was a 29 4/12-year-old woman with a tetralogy of Fallot type of infundibuloarterial anomaly, plus tricuspid atresia, who died in 1989. When she was 7½ months of age, a Potts anastomosis was done (between the left pulmonary artery and the descending thoracic aorta). The anastomosis was judged to be 5 mm in diameter (too big; 3 mm is thought to be optimal). Subsequently, she developed congestive heart failure with pneumonia, which was successfully treated with digoxin and antibiotics. She was maintained thereafter on digoxin.

A Fontan procedure was considered, but not done, when the patient was 21 years of age because cardiac catheterization revealed (not surprisingly) that she had pulmonary artery hypertension, with 70% of the pulmonary blood flow going to the left lung and 30% to the right lung.

It was also noted that her pulmonary infundibular stenosis had progressed to pulmonary infundibular atresia. Thus, in Edwardian terms, her tricuspid atresia type Ib had progressed to tricuspid atresia Ia,[236,237] this progression being possible because she was living on the Potts anastomosis. **Acquired infundibular atresia** is a phenomenon with which those caring for adult patients with congenital heart disease are, no doubt, familiar.

She also had significant periodontal disease. At 24 years of age she developed **bacterial endocarditis** caused by streptococcus viridians. This, too, was well treated.

Very much wanting to have a baby despite her congenital heart disease, at 27 7/12 years of age **she successfully delivered a normal baby girl** at 33 weeks gestation with a birth weight of 1400 grams (3 lb 1 oz). The baby daughter subsequently did well.

The mother, our patient, then developed **nephrotic syndrome** with peripheral edema, and an episode of **gout,** at 28 years of age; both were satisfactorily managed.

At 29 years of age, this courageous young mother died suddenly and unexpectedly because of **occluded Potts anastomosis.** Autopsy revealed the surprising finding that her initially 6 × 4 mm Potts anastomosis had undergone gradual, aseptic, fibrous tissue occlusion. A recent thrombus was identified histologically that was judged to be of less than 2 days' duration. There was a small, residual luminal patency, less than 1 mm in diameter. Her left lung had grade 4 Heath-Edwards changes and grade B Reid-Rabinovitch changes. Her right lung had grade 3 Heath-Edwards changes and grade 0 Reid-Rabinovitch changes. Thus, pulmonary vascular obstructive disease was present, as above, but was not the cause of her sudden, unexpected death.

The history of this 29 4/12-year-old woman is recounted in some detail to illustrate that congenital heart disease is not just about embryos, fetuses, neonates, and children. Congenital heart disease is also very much about adolescents and adults. Indeed, **congenital heart disease in the adult** is regarded as one of the fastest growing specialties in adult cardiology and cardiac surgery. It is also a scary area because as of 2021 (and we hope this will change), relatively few adult cardiologists and cardiac surgeons have an in-depth understanding of congenital heart disease. This study and this book are intended to help the diagnostic and therapeutic understanding of patients with congenital heart disease *of all ages*.

Now, to return to the topic of the anatomic types of tricuspid atresia, we have mentioned two anatomic types thus far:

1. The common **muscular type**; and
2. The infrequent **membranous type.**

There is a third anatomic type that occurs with **partial or incomplete forms of common atrioventricular canal** (Fig. 13.40). This unfamiliar form was illustrated by 3 of these 44 patients (7%).

Patient 33 was a 1-day-old girl with tricuspid atresia {S,D,S} type Ib of Edwards and Burchell[236] (Fig. 13.41). There was a common AV canal with an ostium primum atrial septal defect, a restrictive ventricular septal defect of the atrioventricular canal type (4 × 5 mm), and with no cleft in the anterior mitral leaflet. There was no opening from the right atrium into the small right ventricle. The only inlet into the small right ventricle was via the restrictive ventricular septal defect of the atrioventricular canal type. The anterior mitral leaflet had a raphé-like attachment to the left ventricular septal surface. The pulmonary valve was bicuspid (bicommissural) because the nonseptal–left septal commissure was rudimentary. This patient had multiple congenital anomalies (choanal atresia).

At 11 hours of age during cardiac catheterization, a Berman catheter balloon ruptured with the release of gas. Marked ischemic changes appeared in the electrocardiogram. A Waterston anastomosis (between the ascending aorta and the right pulmonary artery) was performed at 15 hours of age (in 1975) and was revised at 33 hour of age, leading to intraoperative death.

Autopsy revealed that the Waterston anastomosis had been well done (3 × 2 mm). Histology of the left ventricular myocardium showed recent hemorrhage, but the findings of left ventricular myocardial infarction were not present. Our interpretation was that this patient had suffered gas embolism to the coronary arteries, and that it may have been too soon (22 hours) for the histologic signs of left ventricular myocardial infarction to have developed in this neonate.

Differential diagnosis. There is at least one other way that Case 33 could be viewed. One might perhaps contend that this patient had an extremely left-sided form of common atrioventricular canal, opening only from the left atrium and emptying only into the left ventricle, with absence of the tricuspid component of the common atrioventricular valve. The common atrioventricular valve had fused, obliterating the mitral cleft. This interpretation was in fact favored by a highly respected colleague, Dr. Stella Van Praagh.

Perhaps we were saying the same thing with different words. I favor the diagnoses as first presented, namely, tricuspid atresia with complete atrioventricular septal defect (i.e., ostium primum atrial septal defect with ventricular septal defect of the atrioventricular canal type) because (a) there was no opening from the right atrium into the right ventricle (tricuspid atresia), and (b) because the atrioventricular valve opened only from the left atrium (like a mitral valve), not from both atria (like a common atrioventricular valve).

I agree that no identifiable tricuspid valve tissue was present. But remember that "atresia" just means "no hole" or "no opening." Tricuspid atresia does not mean that tricuspid valve tissue must be present and that there is no tricuspid orifice. In the common muscular form of tricuspid atresia, the anatomic findings strongly support the view that the tricuspid valve tissue is not present (or, at least, is not anatomically identifiable as such) and that the right ventricular sinus (body or inflow tract) also often appears not to be present.

So I agree that identifiable tricuspid valve tissue is not present in this case. So that's why I think we were saying the same things with slightly different words.

I also agree that this anomaly may be regarded as a **markedly left-sided type of common atrioventricular canal (or atrioventricular septal defect).**

All observers agreed that the anterior mitral leaflet was not cleft.

To summarize this case, a complete atrioventricular septal defect, without a cleft anterior mitral leaflet, and with tricuspid atresia is a very rare form of common atrioventricular canal. We regard this as a *partial* or *incomplete* form of common atrioventricular canal, despite the presence of a *complete* atrioventricular septal defect because the cleft in the anterior mitral leaflet had fused (closed) and because tricuspid atresia was present. This case illustrates that a complete atrioventricular septal defect can be present in an incomplete or partial form of common atrioventricular canal. Atrioventricular septal defect and common atrioventricular canal are not synonymous. Atrioventricular septal defect is one important part of common atrioventricular canal. The mitral and tricuspid valve anomalies are the other important parts of common atrioventricular canal, as Case 33 demonstrates. (For further information on common atrioventricular canal, see Chapter 11.)

Case 42 was our second rare case of tricuspid atresia {S,D,S} with pulmonary outflow tract stenosis in which tricuspid atresia occurred in the setting of partially common atrioventricular canal. This 19-year-old young man had an ostium primum type of atrial septal defect (i.e., a partial atrioventricular septal defect). The left-sided atrioventricular valve was cleft. Tricuspid atresia was associated with atresia of the right ventricular sinus; that is, there was nothing posteroinferior to the septal band. There was no ventricular septal defect of the atrioventricular canal type; hence, a partial atrioventricular was present. We regard this patient as having a *partial* form of common atrioventricular canal because:

1. there was no ventricular septal defect of the atrioventricular canal type, just an ostium primum type of atrial septal defect (the most common partial form of atrioventricular septal defect); and
2. tricuspid atresia was present (i.e., the common atrioventricular valve had no anatomically identifiable tricuspid valve component).

Is this diagnosis of a partial form of common atrioventricular canal really correct? Well, it sounds right until one starts to think

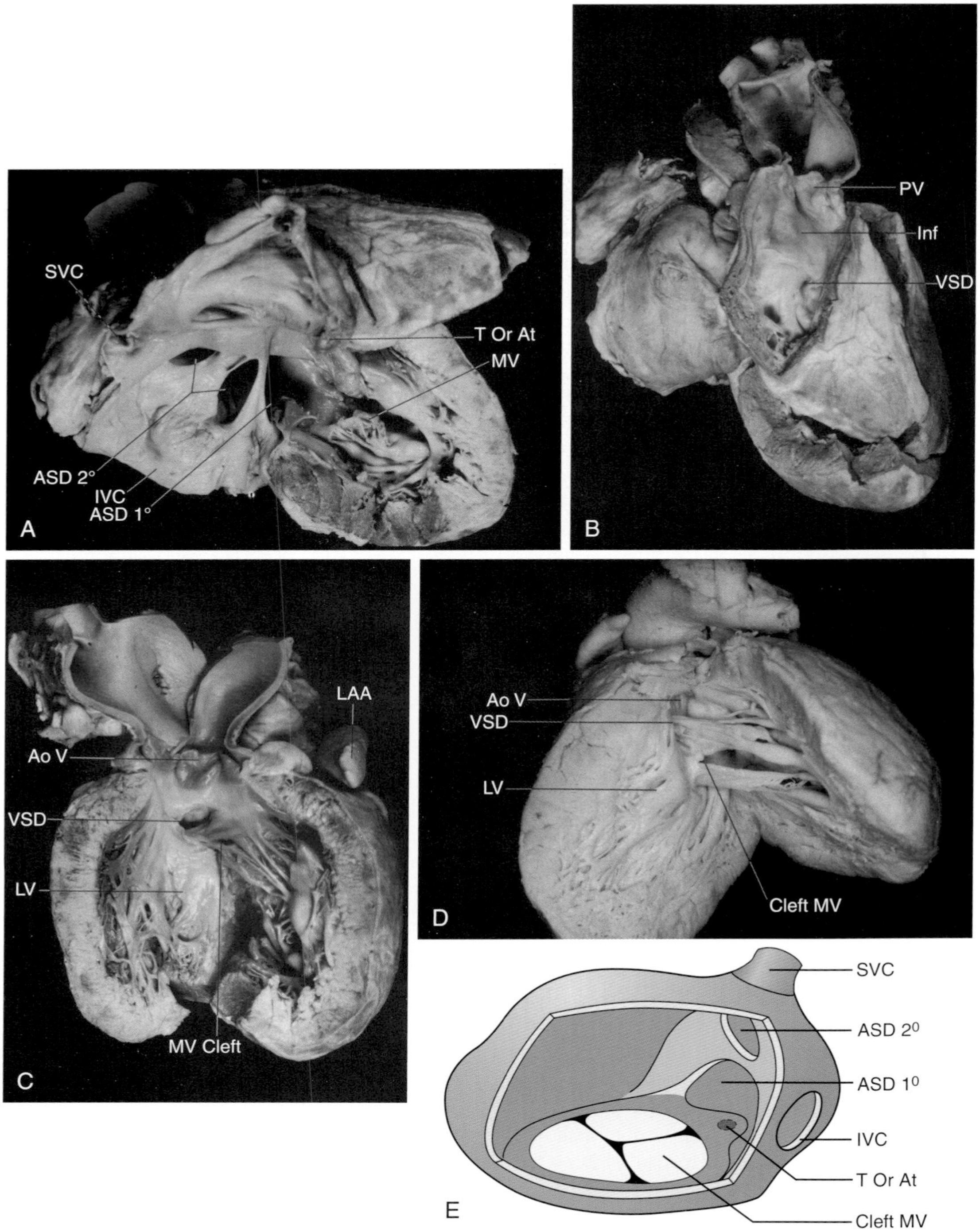

Fig. 13.40 Case 27 was a girl (age not known by us) who had tricuspid atresia with incompletely common atrioventricular canal. (A) The opened right atrium with two secundum atrial septal defects *(ASD 2°)*, a large ostium primum type of defect *(ASD 1°)*, atresia of the tricuspid orifice *(T Or At)* that potentially would have opened into the right ventricle (reflected upward), the mitral valve *(MV)* opening into the large left ventricle, and normal connections of the inferior vena cava *(IVC)* and superior vena cava *(SVC)*. (B) The opened small right ventricle, which really is the subpulmonary infundibulum *(Inf)*, no entering tricuspid valve, a small ventricular septal defect *(VSD)*, and the leaflets of the pulmonary valve *(PV)*. (C) The opened left ventricle *(LV)*, the small conoventricular type of VSD between the conal septum above and the ventricular septum below, and the cleft anterior leaflet of the mitral valve *(Cleft MV)*. Note that this VSD is *above* the superior endocardial cushion component of the anterior mitral leaflet (*not below* the inferior endocardial cushion component of the anterior mitral leaflet). Hence, this is a VSD (or bulboventricular foramen) of the conoventricular (outflow) type, not a VSD of the AV canal (or inlet) type. Consequently, this is an *incomplete* type of common AV canal—because the VSD is not of the AV canal or inlet type. This is tricuspid atresia {S,D,S} type Ib with an ASD I and a cleft anterior mitral leaflet. (D) Another case of the same type in which the cleft of the anterior leaflet of the mitral valve is better seen than in (C). (E) Diagrammatic posterior view of the incomplete form of common AV canal with an ASD 1°, a cleft anterior leaflet of the MV, atresia of the tricuspid orifice *(T Or At)*, an ostium secundum type of ASD (unlabeled), and normally connected IVC and SVC. (This was a consultation sent to us by Dr. Milton H. Paul, Children's Memorial Hospital, Chicago.)

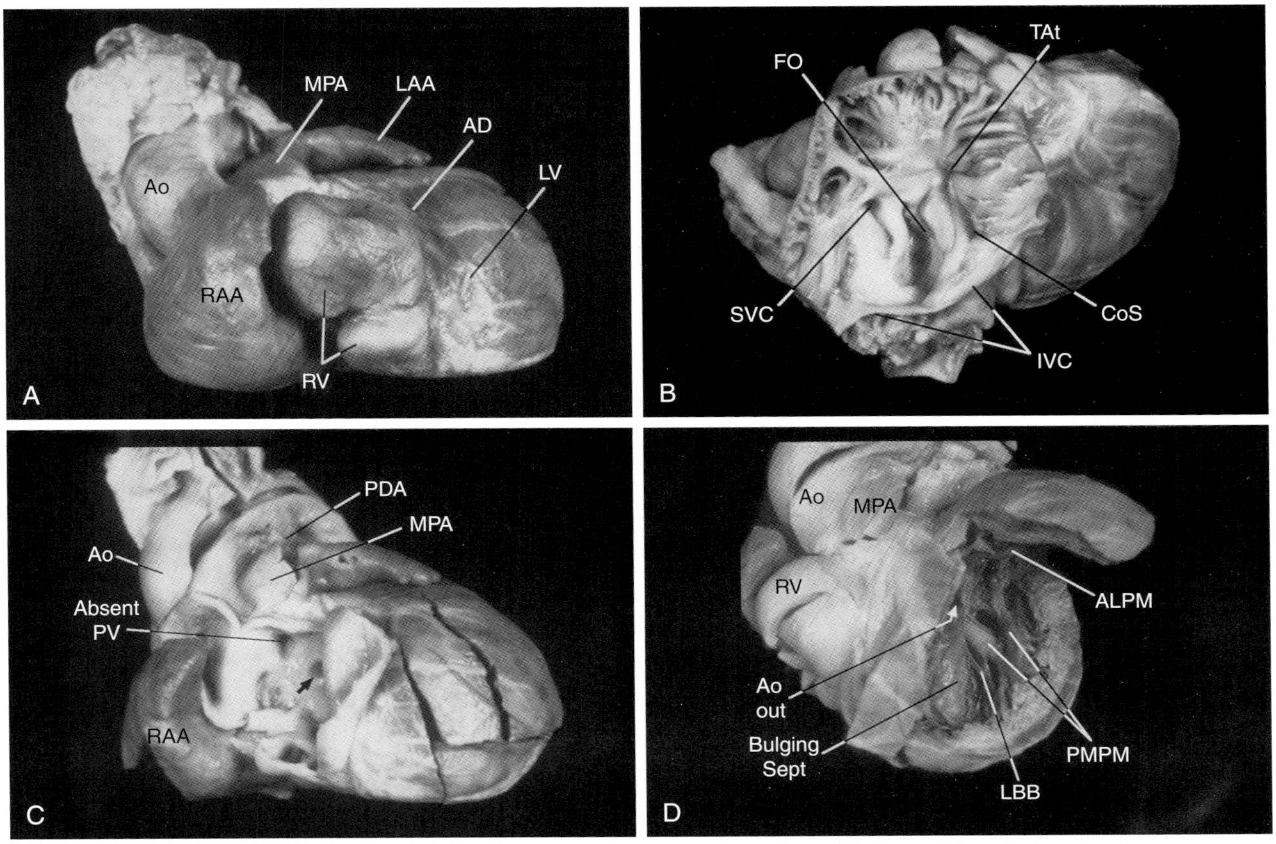

Fig. 13.41 Tricuspid atresia {S,D,S} with absent pulmonary valve leaflets. (A) External frontal view showing a markedly hypertrophied and enlarged right atrial appendage *(RAA)*. Note the deep incisura between the RAA and the lobulated right ventricle *(RV)*. This deep depression has been called the "tricuspid window" by Dr. Helen Taussig upon fluoroscopic examination; i.e., in patients with tricuspid atresia, the right ventricular inflow tract is very deficient, creating an abnormally deep external depression between the large RAA and the abnormally small RV. The lower right ventricular bulge represents the markedly hypoplastic right ventricular sinus. The upper larger right ventricular bulge is the subpulmonary infundibulum. The composite nature of the RV is evident on external inspection, with a sulcus between the lower hypoplastic RV sinus or inflow tract and the upper RV infundibulum or outflow tract. The hypoplasia of the RV is also clearly indicated by the location of the left anterior descending coronary artery *(AD)*. The AD bisects the anterior surface of the ventricles. Far too much of the left ventricle *(LV)* is visible in this anterior view because the RV is so hypoplastic. This abnormally rightward location of the AD coronary artery is typical of tricuspid atresia. *Ao,* Ascending aorta; *LAA,* left atrial appendage; *MPA,* main pulmonary artery. (B) The opened right atrium shows typical muscular tricuspid atresia *(TAt)*. Right atrial hypertrophy and enlargement are confirmed. The other findings are unremarkable. *CoS,* Coronary sinus; *FO,* foramen ovale; *IVC,* inferior vena cava; *SVC,* superior vena cava. (C) The opened right ventricle shows the site of the absent pulmonary valve leaflets *(Absent PV)*. The *black arrow* points at the small ventricular septal defect. *PDA,* Patent ductus arteriosus. (D) The opened left ventricle showing the anterolateral papillary muscle group *(ALPM)*, the posteromedial papillary muscle group *(PMPM)*, the nearby posterior radiation of the left bundle branch of the conduction system *(LBB)*, the convexly bulging left ventricular septal surface *(Bulging Sept)* that is wrapping around the abnormally small RV, and the aortic outflow tract *(Ao out)*. *Note:* We received this consultation in 1997 after the database had been closed (in 1996) to permit data analysis to begin. Hence, this rare case was not included in this series. However, these photographs are included here to document this rarity: TAt {S,D,S} with absence of the pulmonary valve leaflets.

about it. You see, one might very well object, as follows. Because the right ventricular sinus was atretic, or absent—with nothing posteroinferior to the septal band remnant, this means that there could not be a ventricular septal defect of the atrioventricular canal type (which typically lies medially to the septal leaflet of the tricuspid valve) and which opens into the right ventricular sinus (inflow tract). Since there could not be a ventricular septal defect of the atrioventricular canal type, the differential diagnosis between *complete* versus *partial* atrioventricular septal defect is moot (unresolved). This is a good example of the breakdown of the classification of common atrioventricular canal. The basic problem of this classification (and of many others) is that we are trying to classify one variable (whether the atrioventricular canal is undivided or unfused, as opposed to divided or fused) in terms of other variables (the ventricular septum and the atrial septum). Defining one variable in terms of other different variables is an error in logic (and mathematics). Logically, each variable should be defined primarily in terms of itself. We are often tempted, however, to use these other different variables as defining criteria because of their clinical and surgical importance. And when these other variables are relatively normally developed, our definitions and classifications usually work quite well. But when another important defining variable, such as the ventricular sinuses and the ventricular septum, are themselves very abnormally developed, then conventional classification breaks down, as in Case 43.

We are *not* trying to change customary classifications and definitions. Instead, the point is that the weaknesses and breakdowns of conventional definitions and classifications should be *understood*. We classified this patient has having a *partial* form of common atrioventricular canal for the purposes of quick and clear communication: people will readily understand what this means. But we do this with something of a blush and a wink, in view of our deeper understanding (as above).

This young man had a tetralogy of Fallot type of infundibuloarterial anomaly that was associated with a conoventricular type of ventricular septal defect (not a VSD of the AV canal type), measuring 13 mm in horizontal length and 16 mm in vertical height.

At 13 years of age, his regurgitant common atrioventricular valve was replaced with a 33 mm bileaflet St. Jude prosthesis. The ostium primum type of atrial septal defect was patch occluded, and a modified Fontan procedure was performed, placing a conduit from the right atrium to the pulmonary artery. Postoperatively, the patient had atrial flutter with attempted electrophysiologic ablation. In 1995, at 19 years of age, cardiac transplantation was successfully performed.

To summarize, this 19-year-old man had the rare combination of tetralogy of Fallot, a "partial" form of common AV canal with an ostium primum type of atrial septal defect but without a ventricular septal defect of the atrioventricular canal type, with tricuspid atresia—that is, with no communication between the right atrium and the right ventricle, with single left ventricle—that is, absence of the right ventricular sinus or inflow tract, with an infundibular outlet chamber leading to the stenotic pulmonary outflow tract (the os infundibuli pulmonalis measuring 5 × 5 mm), with a conoventricular type of ventricular septal defect (13 × 16 mm), with common-inlet single left ventricle (common AV valve opening only into the left ventricle), and with regurgitation of the common AV valve with atrial flutter.

Problem of interpretation: Was this cleft atrioventricular valve the whole common AV valve? Or was it just the mitral component of the common AV valve? The right atrium did not communicate with the rudimentary right ventricle. This fact is customarily diagnosed as tricuspid atresia. We made this conventional diagnosis. But we could identify no atretic tricuspid valve tissue. Does that support the view that this common AV valve is really the *whole* common AV valve? We think that is certainly possible.

But, in typical muscular tricuspid atresia, we usually cannot identify any atretic tricuspid valve tissue. Does this mean that what we call the mitral valve in typical muscular tricuspid atresia is really the whole common AV valve that has fused its superior and inferior endocardial cushion components—and hence morphologically becomes the mitral valve? Yes, we think that that, too, is a plausible interpretation.

If the latter interpretation is true, does this mean that there really is no such thing as typical muscular tricuspid atresia? We think that the answer is yes. **In typical so-called tricuspid atresia, the tricuspid valve is not atretic; instead, it is absent.** I think it is helpful to lift the curtain on our uncertainties. These words are written in the interests of understanding. I am not trying to change conventional terminology or classification.

Case 63 was a 3-month-old girl with tricuspid atresia {S,D,S} and severe pulmonary outflow tract stenosis. She had a common atrium with fenestrations in the remnant of septum primum. But she did not have a ventricular septal defect of the atrioventricular type. Instead, she had a very small muscular ventricular septal defect, 1 mm in diameter, that constituted marked subpulmonary stenosis. Right ventricular hypoplasia was severe. The common atrioventricular valve opened only into the left ventricle. Blood could enter the small right ventricle only via the highly restrictive muscular ventricular septal defect. In 1966, this patient received no surgical therapy.

In conclusion, tricuspid atresia {S,D,S} with common AV canal characterized by an ostium primum type of atrioventricular septal defect, but without a ventricular septal defect of the atrioventricular canal type, and associated with pulmonary outflow tract stenosis remains an infrequent and little known anatomic type of tricuspid atresia. (Conversely, it also constitutes an infrequent anatomic type of common AV canal.)

Other rare but noteworthy findings in these 44 postmortem cases of tricuspid atresia {S,D,S} with pulmonary outflow tract stenosis (Table 13.11, item 2, type Ib of Edwards and Burchell[236]) include the following:

1. right aortic arch with mirror-image branching of the brachiocephalic arteries in 1 of 44 patients (2%);
2. aberrant right subclavian artery in 2 patients (5%);
3. sinus venosus aneurysm, underlying the left ventricle, and communicating with the coronary sinus, in 1 patient (2%);
4. anterior descending coronary artery arising from the right coronary and supplying the anterior descending coronary artery via a prominent conus coronary artery, in 1 patient (2%);
5. restrictive atrial septum, but without an aneurysm of septum primum, in 1 patient (2%);
6. muscular ventricular septal defect, in 4 patients (9%);
7. two ventricular septal defects, in 1 patient (2%);
8. marked hypoplastic of the main pulmonary artery and both branches, in 1 patient (2%);
9. bicuspid aortic valve, in 1patient (2%); and
10. membranous tricuspid atresia, without juxtaposition of the atrial appendages, in 1 patient (2%).

Tricuspid Atresia With D-Loop Transposition of the Great Arteries

The second most common anatomic type of tricuspid atresia was with D-loop transposition of the great arteries: 18 patients, 19% of 94 cases of tricuspid atresia (Table 13.11, item 5). There were three anatomic subtypes:

1. TGA {S,D,D} in 15 of these 18 patients (83%) (Fig. 13.34);
2. TGA {S,D,A} in 2 (11%); and

3. TGA {S,D,L} in 1 (6%).*

Tricuspid atresia with D-loop TGA corresponds to Edwards, Burchell, and colleagues[236,237] tricuspid atresia type II. Type II tricuspid atresia was subclassified in terms of the status of the pulmonary outflow tract: type IIa, with D-TGA and pulmonary outflow tract atresia; type IIb, with D-TGA and pulmonary outflow tract stenosis; and type IIc, with D-TGA and no pulmonary outflow tract obstruction.

Gender: In patients with tricuspid atresia and TGA {S,D,D}, males = 9; females = 5. (Not known = 1.) Males/females = 9/5 (1.8/1.0). Thus, a strong male predominance was found, males being 80% more frequent than females.

Ages at death (no cardiac transplants):
Mean = $6\frac{7}{12} \pm 9\frac{2}{12}$ years.
Range = 3 days to 28 years.
Median = $2\frac{4}{12}$ years.

In our 2 patients with **tricuspid atresia and TGA {S,D,A}** the gender was male = 1 and female = 1. The ages at death were 19 days and 7.5 months.

In our patient with **tricuspid atresia and TGA {S,D,L}**, the gender was female and the age at death was $5\frac{10}{12}$ years.

The salient anatomic findings in these 18 patients with tricuspid atresia and D-loop transposition of the great arteries (TGA {S,D,D} = 15, TGA {S,D,A} =2, and TGA {S,D,L} = 1) are presented in Table 13.12.

Comparison of Tricuspid Atresia With Normally Related Great Arteries Versus Tricuspid Atresia With Transposition of the Great Arteries. There are important differences between these two groups—in addition to the ventriculoarterial alignments and connections. One of the most significant differences has to do with the status of the great arterial outflow tracts (compare Tables 13.11 and 13.12).

Pulmonary outflow tract obstruction (stenosis or atresia) was much more frequent with normally related great arteries (49 of 55 patients, 89%) than with D-loop transposition of the great arteries (6 of 18 patients, 33%). This difference is statistically highly significant ($p = 0.00000978$, Fisher's exact test).

The converse is equally important clinically. An unobstructed pulmonary outflow tract was much more common in patients with tricuspid atresia and D-loop transposition of the great arteries (12 of 18, 67%) than in patients with tricuspid atresia and solitus normally related great arteries (6 of 55 patients, 11%) ($p = 0.00000978$, Fisher's exact test). (There are no patients in this series with inverted normally related great arteries.)

Aortic outflow tract obstruction (stenosis) was much more common in patients with tricuspid atresia and D-loop transposition of the great arteries (10 of 18, 56%) than in patients with tricuspid atresia and solitus normally related great arteries, that is, {S,D,S} (0 of 55, 0%). This difference is statistically highly significant ($p = 0.00000007043$, Fisher's exact test). (We are talking about *congenital,* not acquired, pulmonary and aortic outflow tract obstruction.)

The above-noted highly significant differences make hemodynamic sense. One would expect in patients with tricuspid atresia that the great artery arising from the infundibular chamber (the "small right ventricle") would be prone to obstruction because the blood flow has to pass through the bulboventricular foramen (which is so-called when the right ventricular sinus is absent), or the ventricular septal defect (when the right

TABLE 13.12 Salient Anatomic Findings in Tricuspid Atresia With D-loop TGA (*n* = 18)

Anatomic Findings	No. of Cases	% of Series*
No pulmonary outflow tract obstruction	12	67
Pulmonary outflow tract stenosis	3	17
Pulmonary outflow tract atresia	3	17
Aortic outflow tract stenosis	10	56
Aortic coarctation or atresia	7	39
Ventricular septal defect, conoventricular, large	3	17
Ventricular septal defect, conoventricular, small	6	33
Ventricular septal defect, muscular, very small	5	28
Secundum atrial septal defect	8	44
Obstructive aneurysm of septum primum (supramitral stenosis)	1	6
Obstructive atrial septum without aneurysm of septum primum	1	6
Left-sided JAA	8	44
Membranous tricuspid atresia with left-sided JAA	3	17
Tricuspid valve tissue remnant	1	6
Muscular tricuspid atresia	15	83
Right aortic arch	4	22
Dextrocardia	2	11
Multiple congenital anomalies	2	11
Bicuspid pulmonary valve	1	6
Bicuspid aortic valve	1	6
Absence of pericardium, left-sided	1	6
Atresia of the main pulmonary artery with discontinuous pulmonary artery branches	1	6
Stenosis of the coronary sinus ostium	1	6
Absent right coronary artery ostium resulting in "single" left coronary artery	1	6
Partially anomalous pulmonary venous connection	1	6

JAA, Juxtaposition of the atrial appendages.
*All percentages are rounded off to the nearest whole number.

**TGA {S,D,D}* denotes transposition of the great arteries with the segmental anatomic set of situs solitus of the viscera and atria, D-loop ventricles, and D-transposition of the great arteries. *TGA {S,D,A}* indicates TGA with the set of solitus viscera and atria, D-loop ventricles, and A-TGA (aortic valve directly anterior to the pulmonary valve). *TGA {S,D,L}* designates TGA with the segmental anatomic set of solitus viscera and atria, D-loop ventricles and L-TGA (transposed aortic valve to the left of the transposed pulmonary valve). All three anatomic subtypes have physiologically uncorrected complete TGA with atrioventricular concordance, but with ventriculoarterial discordance. AV concordance and VA discordance may be modified by additional anomalies, which are specified when present. For additional information regarding TGA, see Chapter 22.

ventricular sinus is small, but present). This outlet foramen leading to the right ventricular great artery is often restrictively small, resulting in pulmonary outflow tract obstruction when the great arteries are normally related, that is, {S,D,S}, or in aortic outflow tract obstruction when D-loop transposition is present (TGA {S,D,D}, or TGA {S,D,A}, or TGA {S,D,L}). In addition to the size of the ventricular septal defect, it should be remembered that with normally related great arteries, pulmonary infundibular and valvar stenosis are also frequent, that is, a tetralogy of Fallot type of conotruncus. So, there are two good reasons why pulmonary outflow tract obstruction so often complicates tricuspid atresia {S,D,S} (Table 13.11): (1) an obstructively small bulboventricular foramen/ventricular septal defect; and (2) a tetralogy of Fallot type of infundibular obstruction (stenosis or atresia) with or without pulmonary valvar obstruction (stenosis or atresia).

Coarctation of the aorta or aortic arch atresia coexisted in 7 of the 10 patients with tricuspid atresia and D-loop TGA (70%), but occurred in none of our 55 patients with tricuspid atresia and normally related great arteries, that is, {S,D,S} (0%).

The early classification of tricuspid atresia by Edwards and Burchell[236] was very helpful and was widely used. But it focused on the presence or absence of *pulmonary* outflow tract obstruction and on the relationship between the great arteries (normal or transposed). But it omitted the problem of *aortic outflow tract obstruction* that is a frequent and important problem in patients with tricuspid atresia and D-loop transposition. (As a Pathology resident in 1956–1957, the importance of the aortic outflow tract was one of the things that I hoped to draw attention to in my unpublished tricuspid atresia study. Better late than never.)

The left juxtaposition of the atrial appendages syndrome is yet another pearl to be found in Table 13.12 (Fig. 13.39). Even though this syndrome is not widely recognized, it is well worth knowing about. Left-sided juxtaposition of the atrial appendages (left-sided JAA) means that both atrial appendages are buying side-by-side (juxtaposed) to the left of the great arteries, instead of being separated normally by the vascular pedicle. Since all of these patients with tricuspid atresia and D-loop transposition (TGA {**S**,D,D} in 15, TGA {**S**,D,A} in 2 and TGA {**S**,D,L} in 1) had situs solitus of the viscera and atria, consequently left-sided JAA means that it is the morphologically *right* atrial appendage that is malposed to the left of the great arteries (Fig. 13.39). (In visceroatrial situs solitus, it is normal for the left atrial appendage to lie to the left of the great arteries.)

In this series of 18 patients with tricuspid atresia and D-loop transposition of the great arteries, left-sided juxtaposition of the atrial appendages with leftward malposition of the morphologically right atrial appendage occurred in 8 cases (44%, Table 13.12). Left-sided JAA occurred in none of the 55 patients with tricuspid atresia and normally related great arteries ({S,D,S}, Table 13.11). This difference is statistically highly significant ($p = 0.000003255$, Fisher's exact test).

We first realized that left-sided juxtaposition of the atrial appendages is a **syndrome** in 1968.[242] Left-sided JAA was associated with **abnormally related great arteries** such as transposition or anatomically corrected malposition (Fig. 13.39), not with normally related great arteries. **Dextrocardia** was more frequent with left-sided JAA (22%) than in transpositions without left-sided JAA (12%).[242] In the present study, dextrocardia was found in 2 of 18 patients (11%); both had left-sided JAA. An **abnormally small right ventricle** was present in 71% (compared with 20% in 100 control transpositions without left JAA), and **tricuspid atresia** or **very severe stenosis** was found in 40% (versus in 4% of transpositions without left-sided JAA).[242]

Thus, left-sided JAA occurs with infundibuloarterial alignment anomalies such as TGA, with dextrocardia, and with tricuspid atresia or severe stenosis. Developmentally, left-sided JAA is normally present at the early D-loop stage. Between embryonic days 23 and 27 in the normal human embryo, left-sided JAA is gradually "cured" as the ventricles swing horizontally from right to left. The great arteries atop the developing ventricles are carried from right to left during this time, bringing the vascular pedicle sufficiently leftward so that the great arteries come to lie between the atrial appendages, rather than to the right of both—which is normal prior to embryonic day 23.[242] (For more information, see Chapter 10.)

Thus, left-sided JAA is a syndrome because leftward malposition of the right atrial appendage, dextrocardia, tricuspid atresia, small right ventricle, and transposition or other infundibuloarterial anomaly of the great arteries all appear to be developmentally interrelated. All of these findings may be regarded as indicative of an idiopathic development arrest at the normal pre–embryonic-day-23 stage. These findings are "anomalies" or "malformations" if viewed with "postnatal" eyes; but if viewed with "embryologic" eyes, many of these findings represent a normal early stage of development, prior to embryonic day 23. This also is why these findings of the left JAA syndrome are a syndrome: they are nonrandom; they all fit together.

Later we would learn that not only left-sided juxtaposition of the atrial appendages with levomalposition of the morphologically right atrial appendage was part of a syndrome associated with *tricuspid atresia*,[242,243] but also that right-sided juxtaposition of the atrial appendages (with dextromalposition of the morphologically left atrial appendage) was part of a syndrome associated with *mitral atresia*.[244] This discovery was primarily due to the work of Dr. Stella Van Praagh.[243,244] We realized that there are *two* "mirror-image" syndromes of JAA:

1. JAA involving malposition of the morphologically right atrial appendage, associated with tricuspid atresia or severe stenosis;[242,243] and
2. JAA involving malposition of the morphologically left atrial appendage, associated with mitral atresia or severe stenosis.[244]

When we speak about *left JAA*, or *left-sided JAA*, we are assuming that situs solitus of the viscera and atria is present. Similarly, when we talk about *right JAA* or *right-sided JAA*, we are assuming visceroatrial situs solitus. Usually, of course, visceroatrial situs solitus *is* present. But not always.

I think Dr. Stella Van Praagh was the first to understand that the conventional "sidedness" approach to JAA (left-sided vs. right-sided) did not always work. Only the *morphologic approach* always applies accurately: malposition of the morphologically right atrial appendage (RAA), or malposition of the morphologically left atrial appendage (LAA), bearing in mind the type of visceroatrial situs that is present (solitus or inversus).[243,244]

It is **malposition of the morphologically right atrial appendage** that is associated with tricuspid atresia and TGA. In visceroatrial situs solitus, this results in *left-sided* JAA, but in visceroatrial situs inversus, malposition of the morphologically right atrial appendage results in *right-sided* JAA;[243] in visceroatrial situs inversus, the morphologically right atrial appendage usually lies to the left of the great arteries.

Similarly, it is **malposition of the morphologically left atrial appendage** that is associated with mitral atresia;[244] this results in *right-sided* JAA in visceroatrial situs solitus, and in *left-sided* JAA in visceroatrial situs inversus.

Thus, the key to understanding JAA is to know *morphologically* which atrial appendage is malpositioned. Morphology is the constant. Relative positions (left-sided and right-sided JAA) are variables. So, morphologic anatomy remains the open-sesame to positional anatomic understanding.[243,244]

Membranous tricuspid atresia that transilluminates brilliantly was found in 3 of the 8 cases of left-sided juxtaposition of the atrial appendages (37.5%) (Table 13.12). In 1 of these 3 patients, a *tricuspid valve tissue remnant* or tag was present, that may have produced an insignificant degree of pulmonary outflow tract stenosis. Otherwise, membranous tricuspid atresia has no functional or surgical significance, to our knowledge.

Rarely, membranous or fibrous tricuspid atresia can occur without left-sided juxtaposition of the atrial appendages, as in Case 39. The patient was a 29 4/12-year-old woman with tricuspid atresia {S,D,S} and a tetralogy of Fallot type of infundibuloarterial anomaly. Living on a Potts anastomosis that had been performed when she was 7½ months of age, she developed acquired infundibular atresia, progressing from Edwards and Burchell's tricuspid atresia type Ib to their type Ia.[236] Mentioned earlier, this was the 27 7/12-year-old mother who delivered a normal baby daughter, and who died suddenly and unexpectedly in 1989 at 29 years of age because her Potts anastomosis underwent occlusion. Autopsy revealed membranous tricuspid atresia, with a fibrous remnant of tricuspid tissue and chordae tendineae.

Almost always, the tricuspid atresia was of the **muscular type** (in 90 of these 94 cases, 96%, Table 13.11). When one looks at the floor of the right atrium where the tricuspid valve should be, in typical muscular tricuspid atresia, what does one see? "Nothing," that is, no suggestion of a tricuspid valve. Just muscle, often with a dimple—which is generally regarded as the atrioventricular portion of the membranous septum. Typically, one sees no vestige of the tricuspid valve. The tricuspid valve appears to be absent. The right ventricular sinus, body, or inflow tract (proximal or upstream relative to the septal band and moderator band remnants) also is either absent or diminutive.

Consequently, so-called typical muscular tricuspid atresia appears to be characterized by absence of the tricuspid valve leaflets and tensor apparatus (chordae tendineae and most or all of the papillary muscles), absence of the tricuspid orifice, and absence or marked hypoplasia of the right ventricular sinus, body, or inflow tract.

The "small right ventricle" is the infundibular outlet chamber, beginning at the septal, moderator, and parietal bands and extending up to the semilunar valve(s). As noted earlier, a small remnant of the right ventricular sinus may or may not be present.

Thus, in a literally accurate sense, the designation *tricuspid atresia* (atresia meaning "no hole," Greek) is not entirely satisfactory. The problem is not that the tricuspid valve has no hole or opening. That is what one does find in imperforate Ebstein's anomaly, or Ebstein's with tricuspid atresia. In "typical" so-called tricuspid atresia (both muscular and membranous), the problem is that the tricuspid valve and orifice are both absent, and the right ventricular sinus is also absent or diminutive. Membranous tricuspid atresia, so-called, may well just have an unusually large atrioventricular portion of the membranous septum.

What really is typical tricuspid atresia? As indicated above, our conclusion is that typical tricuspid atresia, including both the muscular and the membranous forms (Tables 13.11 and 13.12), but excluding imperforate Ebstein's anomaly, usually consists of:

1. absence of the tricuspid valve leaflets and tensor apparatus;
2. absence of the tricuspid orifice; and
3. absence or marked hypoplasia of the right ventricular sinus (inflow tract).

Ironically, the only real form of tricuspid atresia is imperforate Ebstein's anomaly. In the other forms of so-called tricuspid atresia—the "typical" forms (Tables 13.11 and 13.12)—the tricuspid valve and orifice are really absent. In typical tricuspid atresia, the problem is not that the tricuspid valve is present, but lacks an orifice. The problem really is agenesis of the tricuspid valve and its orifice. Briefly, typical tricuspid atresia is really **tricuspid agenesis, plus agenesis or marked hypoplasia of the right ventricular sinus.**

Again, these words are written not in an attempt to change our diagnostic terminology, but in the hope of deepening anatomic, developmental, and etiologic understanding.

The "price" of each advance in understanding must not be a change in diagnostic terminology. Otherwise, in the name of clarity, we will create a tower of Babel that will only increase confusion. Instead, let us wisely pour the "wine" of new understanding into the old "bottles" of our shared diagnostic terminology. Changes in terminology will continue to occur, but they should occur as slowly as possible, to minimize confusion.

So, we plan to continue to use the term *tricuspid atresia,* like almost everyone else does, but with the understanding that it is really tricuspid agenesis. Tricuspid *atresia* is not entirely wrong; there is no hole. But the reason there is no hole is that the tricuspid valve, its orifice, and the underlying right ventricular sinus typically have failed to form.

Left-Sided Tricuspid Atresia With Transposition of the Great Arteries {S,L,L}. The third most common anatomic type of tricuspid atresia was also a surprise. It was not one of the more familiar and hence expected anatomic types of Edwards and Burchell[236] (types Ia, Ib, Ic or IIa, IIb, or IIc). Instead, it was left-sided tricuspid atresia associated with transposition of the great arteries {S,L,L} (Fig. 13.35). In other words, these 11 patients (11% of the whole series of 94 cases, Table 13.11) had the classical form of congenital physiologically corrected transposition of the great arteries, complicated by left-sided tricuspid atresia. It is associated anomalies such as tricuspid atresia that often make the designation of *congenital physiologically corrected* transposition such a cruel joke—because left-sided tricuspid atresia vitiates the potential physiologic correction of the systemic venous and the pulmonary venous circulations.

The segmental anatomy quickly conveys the "floor plan" of such hearts. There is situs solitus (the usual anatomic pattern) of the viscera and the atria, the morphologically right atrium (RA) being right-sided as usual, and the morphologically left atrium (LA) being left-sided, also as usual: {S,-,-}.

But L-loop ventricles are present: {S,L,-}. This means that the morphologically right ventricle (RV) is typically left-sided and left-handed, while the morphologically left ventricle (LV) is usually right-sided and right-handed. Thus, atrioventricular (AV) discordance is typically present, barring associated anomalies. Consequently, in the absence of additional malformations, the RA should open into the right-sided LV, and the LA should open into the left-sided RV; that is, AV discordance should be present.

But tricuspid atresia is also present. It is important to know that the atrioventricular valves correspond to the ventricles of entry, not to the atria of exit. This is why the tricuspid valve usually is left-sided with segmental anatomy of {S,L,-}. The tricuspid valve typically is left-sided because the RV usually is left-sided with L-loop ventricles.

A more general way of stating this principle concerning the morphological identity of the tricuspid valve (TV) and the mitral valve (MV) is as follows: *The morphologic identity of the AV valves corresponds to the anatomic type of ventricular loop into which the AV valves open*. This principle applies both when the AV vales open into two different ventricles (TV into RV, left-sided, and MV into LV, right-sided) and when both AV valves open into the same ventricle (TV and MV both opening into the LV, right-sided, as in double-inlet LV, right-sided).

Thus, both with single-inlet ventricle and with double-inlet ventricle, the morphologic anatomic identity of the AV valves is indicated by and is the same as the morphologic anatomic identity of the ventricle loop (D- or L-). Both with single-inlet ventricle and with double-inlet ventricle, when a ventricular D-loop is present the TV is right-sided and the MV is left-sided. Conversely, when a ventricular L-loop is present, the TV is left-sided and the MV is right-sided. Because left-sided tricuspid atresia is present in these 11 patients, AV discordance cannot be present. The right-sided RA ejects into the right-sided LV. But because of the left-sided tricuspid atresia, the left-sided LA cannot open into the left-sided RV or its remnant.

To complete the segmental anatomy of these patients, they all had L-TGA. So their segmental anatomy was TGA {S,L,L}. There was ventriculoarterial (VA) discordance, in the following sense. The right-sided LV ejected into the transposed main pulmonary artery (MPA). And the left-sided "small RV" ejected into the ascending aorta (Ao). If you accept the foregoing, then VA discordance is present.

However, in terms of anatomic accuracy, one could object as follows. If the left-sided RV sinus is absent, then there is no RV sinus to eject into the Ao. There is really only the subaortic infundibulum or conus. The conus arteriosus is really part of the great arteries (the conotruncus). The true RV, that is, the RV sinus, is absent. So, VA discordance is only half present (LV to MPA), just as AV discordance is also only half present (RA to LV). However, in some cases of tricuspid atresia, a small amount of RV sinus can be present. As a practical matter, we have adopted the view—as have almost all other students of this subject—that in TGA {S,L,L} with left-sided tricuspid atresia, *TGA* is indeed present, as follows.

There is ventriculoarterial discordance in the sense that the LV ejects into the MPA (definitely correct) and the RV, *or its remnant,* ejects into the aorta. The aorta definitely is placed across the plane of the ventricular septal remnant and so arises above the malformed RV. This is what *transposition* means etymologically: *trans* = across, *ponere* = to place (Latin). In TGA {S,L,L} with tricuspid atresia (left-sided), the aorta is placed across the plane of the ventricular septal remnant and hence originates above the malformed RV. So we think that the term *transposition* is not anatomically wrong when applied to single LV or to tricuspid atresia, even when one cannot identify the remnant of the RV sinus.

The foregoing are the reasons why we support the terms and concepts of tricuspid *atresia* and *transposition*, as in TGA {S,L,L} with tricuspid atresia, left-sided, as currently used. Neither term is beyond reproach, we agree. But neither is totally wrong, either, and hence does not have to be changed. In situations like this we think it is the better part of wisdom to accept our common usage, in the interests of clarity of understanding and communication.

Other terminologic concerns. Now that we are considering problems associated with terminology, we'll briefly mention some other important issues of nomenclature that are relevant to this chapter, and indeed to this whole book.

Reasons for coining new terms. We think that there are only two good reasons for coining new anatomic terms:

1. if there is no term for the entity described; and/or
2. if the extant term(s) is (are) factually very inaccurate.

In the interests of clarity of communication and so one generation will be able to understanding the next, we think it is very important to be *conservative* in terminology. Anatomic nomenclature should be *morphologic* and as *unchanging* as possible.

Why do we not describe the ventricles and the great arteries in terms of concordance and discordance? We are fond of the terms and concepts of *concordance* and *discordance*; indeed, we introduced them in 1964.[244a] However, they, too, have limitations. Let us consider atrioventricular (AV) discordance. AV discordance means one thing in visceroatrial situs solitus (ventricular L-loop), the opposite thing in visceroatrial situs inversus (ventricular D-loop), and nothing in visceroatrial situs ambiguus—because the anatomic situs of the atria is itself uncertain or unknown.

In order to analyze diagnostically large series of complex cases of congenital heart disease, it is essential to use anatomic descriptions that have specific and unchanging meanings, such as ventricular D-loop and L-loop. Each of the major cardiac segments (atria, ventricles, great arteries) must be diagnosed specifically; for example, the ventricular situs must be diagnosed *per se,* and its designation must not be dependent on the diagnosis of the atrial situs. If the ventricular situs is atrial-situs-dependent, then AV discordance at the ventricular level means one thing in visceroatrial situs solitus (L-loop), the opposite in visceroatrial situs inversus (D-loop), and nothing in visceroatrial situs ambiguus—as above.

Chirality or handedness, which we introduced at the World Congress of Pediatric Cardiology in London in 1980,[244b] has provided anatomic definitions for *D-loop* ventricles and *L-loop* ventricles. These definitions in terms of chirality provide *anatomic* definitions of ventricular D- and L-loops, in addition to their *embryologic* meanings.

These anatomically defined concepts were subsequently widely accepted. Our British colleagues call D-loop ventricles *right-hand topology* because the D-loop right ventricle (RV) is right-handed; and they call L-loop ventricles *left-hand topology* because the L-loop RV is left-handed.

We call this handedness *chirality* because this is what these patterns are called scientifically, as in elementary particle physics. The designation *chirality* was suggested to us by Dr. David Gordon—one of our coauthors who left elementary particle physics to become a pediatric cardiologist. During this study, we learned that chirality or handedness is a fundamental property of matter. For example, neutrinos are left-handed and antineutrinos are right-handed.

We also think that the concept of topology, as applied to ventricular D- and L-loops, is wrong. In topology, consider a Möbius strip. The straight heart tube is like a Möbius strip before it is twisted. Draw a right-handed RV on it. Then twist the strip so it folds to the right, forming a D-loop. The RV diagram looks normal, as it should in D-loop ventricles.

Then untwist the Möbius strip, so it returns to the straight tube, unlooped condition.

Now twist the Möbius strip in the opposite direction so that it folds to the left, forming an L-loop. Look at your drawing of the RV. It does *not* look like one sees in mirror-image dextrocardia {I,L,I}. The RV diagram is upside down—not right side up as it is in mirror-image dextrocardia.

Whether the RV is right-handed (as in a D-loop) or left-handed (as in an L-loop) does not depend on ventricular looping—or on how one twists the Möbius strip (topology). This is why one can diagnose whether a D-loop is present (as in situs solitus totalis) or an L-loop is present (as in situs inversus totalis) *before* ventricular looping has occurred—at the straight tube stage, as in superoinferior ventricles with the RV superior, the LV inferior, and with the ventricular septum approximately horizontal.

Right-handed (D-loop) chirality and left-handed (L-loop) chirality are present at—and long before—the straight tube (unlooped) stage and are not determined by looping. Thus, right-handed and left-hand RV patterns are not determined by topology or twisting, as the Möbius strip illustrates. In mathematics, topology is defined as the study of the properties of geometric configurations that are *invariant* under transformation, as shown by continuous mappings.

At the straight tube (preloop) stage, the right-handed (D-loop) and left- handed (L-loop) RV configurations are opposites (stereoisomers); they are not invariant (one and the same) and determined by twisting or the direction of loop, as in topology. We are dealing with **isomers or situs** (not topology), as in situs solitus (normal) and situs inversus (its mirror-image, in which everything is right-left reversed, but without superoinferior or anteroposterior change).

However, looping (topology) is important. Looping determines ventricular spatial relations, for example, whether the ventricles are superoinferior or side-by-side. But looping does not determine ventricular chirality or situs (D-loop versus L-loop anatomic patterns, such as whether the RV is right-handed or left-handed).

The foregoing is concerned with background understanding. Now let us consider the data found in the present study of 11 postmortem cases of left-sided tricuspid atresia with TGA {S,L,L}.

Gender: males = 8; females = 3; and males/females = 2.67/1.
Thus, a strong male preponderance was found in this small series.

Age at death (no cardiac transplants): The mean age was $9^{11}/_{12} \pm 16^{3}/_{12}$ years. The range was from 26 hours to 55 years. The median was 5 years (1459 days).

It is of interest that the median age of death of these patients with left-sided tricuspid atresia and TGA {S,L,L} (4 years) was much older than the median age at death in this series as a whole (7.5 months), and was distinctly older than in the most common anatomic type of tricuspid atresia {S,D,S} with pulmonary outflow tract stenosis (5.25 months). This is new information for us, and we don't really understand why this difference was present. Speculative possibilities include the following: Tricuspid atresia {S,D,S} with pulmonary outflow tract stenosis may be more ductus arteriosus dependent; that is, normal ductal closure may be more devastating for patients with tricuspid atresia {S,D,S} with pulmonary outflow tract stenosis than for those with TGA {S,L,L} without pulmonary outflow tract obstruction. However, the foregoing is just one hypothesis concerning this apparent difference in natural history. More data are needed.

Salient findings in left-sided tricuspid atresia with TGA {S,L,L} are summarized in Table 13.13.

Pulmonary Outflow Tract Obstruction

Tricuspid atresia (left-sided) with TGA {S,L,L} had a low incidence of pulmonary outflow tract obstruction (2 patients, 18%, Table 13.13) when compared with tricuspid atresia (right-sided) with normal segmental anatomy ({S,D,S}) (49 patients, 89%, Table 13.11), a statistically highly significant difference (p = 0.000005941, Fisher's exact test).

Pulmonary outflow tract obstruction in tricuspid atresia with TGA {S,L,L} was only about half as frequent (18%) as it was with tricuspid atresia and (D-loop) TGA (33%, Table 13.12), but this difference was not statistically significant (p = 0.24, Fisher's exact test).

Aortic outflow tract obstruction in patients with left-sided tricuspid atresia and TGA {S,L,L} (3 of 11 cases, 27%, Table 13.13) was more common than in patients with right-sided tricuspid atresia and normally related great arteries, that is, {S,D,S} (0 of 55 cases, Table 13.11), a statistically significant difference (p = 0.0036, Fisher's exact test).

Aortic outflow tract obstruction in patients with left-sided tricuspid atresia and TGA {S,L,L} (3 of 11 cases, 27%, Table 13.13) was only about half the frequency of that in patients with right-sided tricuspid atresia and D-loop TGA (10 of 18 cases, 56%, Table 13.12), but this difference was not statistically significant ($p = 0.11$, Fisher's exact test).

It is noteworthy that one of these patients with tricuspid atresia and TGA {S,L,L} had interruption of the aortic arch type A, and another had preductal coarctation of the aorta (Table 13.13).

In view of the increased frequency of subaortic stenosis and the decreased frequency of pulmonary outflow tract stenosis in patients with TGA (D-loop and L-loop), it is important *not* to perform main pulmonary artery banding in such patients. Not surprisingly the combination of aortic outflow tract stenosis and pulmonary artery banding is not well tolerated hemodynamically, as was illustrated by a 4-year-old girl (in 1974).

These findings and statistical analyses confirm that pulmonary outflow tract obstruction was significantly more frequent in patients with tricuspid atresia and normal segmental anatomy ({S,D,S}) than it was in patients with D-loop or L-loop TGA. In addition, these findings show that there was no significant difference in the frequency of pulmonary or aortic outflow tract obstruction in our patients with tricuspid atresia and D-loop or L-loop transposition of the great arteries.

Obstructive atrial septum. The atrial septum was obstructive or restrictive in more than half of our patients with left-sided tricuspid atresia and TGA {S,L,L} (6 of 11 cases, 55%, Table 13.13). This is not surprising when one reflects that in visceroatrial situs solitus, the atrial septum is a unidirectional flap valve that normally opens prenatally from right to left, but not from left to right. Hence, if normally formed, the atrial septum "should" be obstructive in a left-to-right direction in patients with left-sided tricuspid atresia with TGA {S,L,L}.

However, two ways of naturally decompressing the otherwise obstructed left atrium and pulmonary veins in such cases were also observed: *A secundum type of atrial septal defect* was present in 2 (18%, Table 13.13). *A coronary sinus septal defect* coexisted in 1 patient (9%, Table 13.13). In other words, there was a defect in the partition that normally separates the cavity of left atrium from the lumen of the coronary sinus (in the so-called coronary sinus septum), making it possible for the pulmonary venous blood to escape from the obstructed left atrium into the coronary sinus and thence to the right atrium.

Was the atrial septum more frequently obstructive in left-sided tricuspid atresia with TGA {S,L,L} than in right-sided tricuspid atresia with TGA {S,D,D/A/L}?

The answer is yes: 6 of 11 (55%) in left-sided tricuspid atresia versus 2 of 18 (11%) in right-sided tricuspid atresia, and this difference is statistically significant ($p = 0.02$, Fisher's exact test). So, what one would think intuitively was supported by the data.

Table 13.13 contains other noteworthy findings:

Arrhythmias were prominent in almost half of these patients with tricuspid atresia (left-sided) and TGA {S,L,L} (5 of 11 cases, 45%). One of these patients, a 4-year-old girl, died from ventricular fibrillation in the catheterization laboratory in 1974. Another patient, a 13³⁄₁₂-year-old boy, died suddenly and unexpectedly while sitting in class at school.

A prominent interseptovalvular space was found in a 55-year-old man. A prominent space between septum primum to the left and an abnormally well developed left venous valve to the right constitutes a rare form of **cor triatriatum.** This space sits between the right and left atrial cavities, but does not obstruct any veins. The pulmonary veins open normally to the left of septum primum, and the venae cavae and coronary sinus open normally to the right of the unusually prominent left venous valve. The interseptovalvular space is well seen in normal human embryos at about 33 days follow ovulation (see Fig. 8.9). Postnatally, as in our Case 15, this is an asymptomatic form of cor triatriatum because it is not associated with any venous obstruction. It is helpful to know about this anomaly in order to avoid unnecessary interventional or surgical procedures.

A prominent right venous valve (Eustachian valve of the inferior vena cava) was present in 2 patients (18%, Table 13.13). There were no associated adverse hemodynamic sequelae.

Extreme leftward deviation of septum primum was present in a 26-hour-old boy. The left atrium consequently appeared to be very small. Balloon atrial septostomy was attempted in the cardiac catheterization laboratory. Because of the marked leftward deviation of septum primum, this septum was not crossed by the balloon-tipped catheter and the left atrial free wall was ruptured, resulting in cardiac tamponade. Surgical rescue was attempted, with suture closure of an 8 mm long tear in the left atrial free wall and appendage. Septum primum was resected, the main pulmonary artery was banded, and the patent ductus

TABLE 13.13 Salient Findings in Left-Sided Tricuspid Atresia With TGA {S,L,L} ($n = 11$)

Findings	No. of Cases	% of Series*
Obstructive atrial septum	6	55
Aneurysm of septum primum bulging into RA	1	9
Arrhythmias Catheter laboratory death (1) Sudden death in class (1)	5	45
Congestive heart failure	3	27
Subaortic stenosis	3	27
Secundum atrial septal defect	2	18
Pulmonary vascular obstructive disease	2	18
Pulmonary outflow tract stenosis	2	18
Multiple congenital anomalies	2	18
Prominent right venous (Eustachian) valve	2	18
Preductal coarctation of aorta	1	9
Interrupted aortic arch, type A	1	9
Absent left-sided coronary arterial ostium	1	9
Mitral regurgitation, right-sided	1	9
Brain abscess	1	9
Sepsis	1	9
Septum primum, markedly deviated leftward	1	9
Prominent interseptovalvular space	1	9

RA, Morphologically right atrium; *TGA*, transposition of the great arteries.
*All percentages are rounded off to the nearest whole number.

arteriosus was ligated. The patient could not be weaned from cardiopulmonary bypass, leading to intraoperative death (in 1990). We hope that the other findings presented in Table 13.13 will be self-explanatory.

In order of descending frequency (Table 13.11), the next anatomic type is:

Tricuspid Atresia {S,D,S} Without Pulmonary Outflow Tract Obstruction

Tricuspid atresia with normal segmental anatomy {S,D,S} and without pulmonary outflow tract obstruction—Edwards and Burchell's[236] type Ic—occurred in 6 of these 94 patients (6%, Table 13.11).

Gender: males = 2; and females = 4. Males/females = 0.5/1.0. In view of the small number of cases ($n = 6$), no conclusions are drawn concerning gender predominance or the lack of it. More data are needed.

Age at death (no cardiac transplants): mean =10.36 ± 8.44 months; range = 5 days to 1 10/12 years; and median = 10 months.

It is of interest that the median age of death of patients with tricuspid atresia {S,D,S} *without* pulmonary outflow tract stenosis (10 months of age) was almost twice that of patients with tricuspid atresia {S,D,S} *with* pulmonary outflow tract stenosis (5.25 months). Is this difference representative and statistically significant? We do not know. In view of the small size of the no-pulmonary-outflow-tract obstruction group ($n = 6$), no conclusions are drawn. Salient anatomic findings in this anatomic type of tricuspid atresia are summarized in Table 13.14.

Note that in this anatomic type of tricuspid atresia, there were no cases of aortic outflow tract obstruction, which is not surprising because the aorta arises from the large left ventricle, but very different from tricuspid atresia with TGA in which the aorta originates from the small RV: aortic outflow tract obstruction with D-loop TGA = 56% (Table 13.12) and with L-loop TGA = 27% (Table 13.13).

TABLE 13.14 Tricuspid Atresia {S,D,S} Without Pulmonary Outflow Tract Obstruction ($n = 6$)

Findings	No. of Cases	% of Series
Large ventricular septal defect	3	50
Large secundum atrial septal defect	2	33
Congestive heart failure	2	33
Multiple congenital anomalies	2	33
Left superior vena cava to coronary sinus to right atrium	2	33
Right ventricular sinus not confluent with infundibular outlet chamber	1	17
Restrictive probe patent foramen ovale	1	17
Common atrium	1	17
Polyvalvular disease	1	17
Totally anomalous pulmonary venous connection	1	17
Bicuspid pulmonary valve and bicuspid aortic valve	1	17
Anomalous muscle bundles of the left ventricle	1	17

One of these patients, a 22-month-old girl (Case 3), had a somewhat underdeveloped right ventricular sinus beneath the absent right atrioventricular connection. The right ventricular sinus was larger than one usually sees with typical tricuspid atresia. But the fascinating finding was that *the smallish right ventricular sinus (inflow tract) did not connect with the infundibular outflow tract chamber.* The infundibulum communicated only with the morphologically left ventricle via an unobstructive bulboventricular foramen. This patient displayed a *natural experiment* showing that the right ventricular sinus and the subpulmonary infundibulum really are two different chambers—that in this rare case did not communicate at all. **Noncommunication (total separation) of the right ventricular sinus and subpulmonary infundibulum,** as in this patient, appears clearly to illustrate that the "small right ventricle" of typical tricuspid atresia is really the subpulmonary infundibulum—not the right ventricular sinus. The right ventricular sinus typically makes little or no contribution to what is often called "the small RV" of typical tricuspid atresia, as this patient's heart shows with unusual clarity. This is why Becker and Anderson[245] have long called typical tricuspid atresia **univentricular heart of left ventricular type with absent right atrioventricular connection.** We prefer the briefer conventional diagnosis of *tricuspid atresia.* But we want to indicate that we agree with Becker and Anderson[245] concerning the morphologic anatomy of typical tricuspid atresia: the right ventricular sinus is *anatomically* absent or diminutive, and is *functionally* useless.

It should be added that in *mitral atresia,* as will be seen, the morphologically left ventricle is often present anatomically but diminutive and usually is functionally of little or no use.

So we do not want to paint with too broad a brush. Anatomically, in *tricuspid atresia* the right ventricle (i.e., the RV sinus) often is absent; thus, a single morphologically left ventricle is present anatomically—often, but not always.

By contrast, in *mitral atresia* the morphologically left ventricular usually is present, but small. So, mitral atresia typically is a biventricular heart, not a univentricular one, in terms of accurate morphologic anatomy. Physiologically, however, mitral atresia typically has only one effective ventricle (the morphologically right ventricle) and hence functionally, if not anatomically, it too is univentricular.

The foregoing is written in support of the following proposition: **The cure for confusion is accuracy (both anatomic and physiologic).** Oversimplification does not help, because it is not accurate, as most observers will ultimately discover for themselves.

Anomalous muscle bundles of the left ventricle were also present in this patient (Case 3) (Table 13.14). Conal musculature extended on the left ventricular septal surface and into the left ventricular cavity. These anomalous left ventricular muscle bundles had no obvious deleterious sequelae.

Congestive heart failure was prominent in 2 of these 6 patients (33%, Table 13.14). This finding is not surprising given that both great arterial outflow tracts were unobstructed and both great arteries had systemic pressure.

Multiple congenital anomalies coexisted in 2 of these 6 patients (33%, Table 13.14). Case 19 was a 17-month-old girl with the cat-eye syndrome (coloboma of iris and anal atresia syndrome).[246] She had bilateral colobomata at 6 o'clock, imperforate anus with rectovaginal fistula, malformed right pinna with atretic right external auditory canal, cleft palate, hirsutism (particularly of the face), extrahepatic biliary atresia, marked hypoplasia of the gallbladder, severe biliary cirrhosis, 5 accessory spleens, and incomplete lobation of the lungs (incomplete right major fissure, rudimentary right minor fissure, and incomplete left major fissure). Her karyotype (performed in 1971) was described as female, with a small extra acrocentric fragment.

Case 69 was a 7-month-old black girl with a Meckel's diverticulum (unobliterated yolk sac remnant, confluent with the ileum) and a suppurating pilomidal sinus in the coccygeal region containing a tuft of hair.

Case 19 also had **polyvalvular disease** consisting of prominent noduli Albinii of the mitral valve, aortic valve, and pulmonary valve—in addition to tricuspid atresia. (Giuseppe *Albini,* 1827–1911, was professor of physiology at Naples who described the minute nodules at the margins of the tricuspid and mitral valves in 1856.) Strictly speaking, only nodules involving the tricuspid and mitral valves, but not the pulmonary and aortic valves, should be described as Albini's nodules (or *nodule Albinii,* in Latin).

This same patient (Case 19) also had **multiple venous anomalies.** The inferior vena cava was hypoplastic, only half the normal size. The azygos vein was enlarged to 2 to 3 times the normal size.

Totally anomalous pulmonary venous connection (Table 13.14) was also present in 1 patient. The common pulmonary vein was *observed* to be atretic. An anomalous vein connected all of the pulmonary veins to the right superior vena cava, inferior and medial to the entry of the enlarged azygos vein. We thought that pulmonary venous obstruction was *not* present. Although totally anomalous pulmonary venous connection is thought to result from agenesis or atresia of the common pulmonary vein, resulting in the persistence of earlier pulmonary venous-to-systemic venous connections, it is rare to *find* an atretic common pulmonary vein in a patient with totally anomalous pulmonary venous connection, as in this case.

We hope that the other findings in Table 13.14, which we have not commented on, will be self-explanatory.

Tricuspid Atresia {S,D,S} With Pulmonary Outflow Tract Atresia

In order of decreasing frequency, tricuspid atresia {S,D,S} with pulmonary outflow tract atresia occurred in 5 of these 94 cases (5%, Table 13.11).

Gender: males = 2; females = 3; and males/females = 0.67/1.0.

Age at death (no heart transplants): mean = $5^{10}/_{12} \pm 11^{4}/_{12}$ years, ranging from 1 day to 26 years. The median was 6 months.

Salient findings: summarized in Table 13.15.

These 5 patients showed that there are at least two different anatomic types of pulmonary outflow tract atresia associated with tricuspid atresia {S,D,S}:

1. **A tetralogy of Fallot type of infundibuloarterial anomaly** can result in pulmonary outflow tract atresia, as in 2 of these 5 patients (40%, Table 13.15).
2. **Pulmonary valvar atresia with intact ventricular septum** can also coexist with tricuspid atresia, resulting in pulmonary outflow tract atresia, as in 1 of these 5 patients (20%, Table 13.15).

A rare type of partially common atrioventricular canal was found in 1 of these 5 patients (20%, Table 13.15), a 26-year-old woman (the oldest case with this anatomic type of tricuspid atresia). There was a common atrioventricular canal type of cleft in the anterior leaflet of the mitral valve, no ostium primum type of atrial septal defect, a small ventricular septal defect of the atrioventricular canal type, and tricuspid atresia. There was marked mitral regurgitation through the mitral valve cleft with thickening and rolling of the leaflet margins. Autopsy also revealed that a classical right Blalock-Taussig (subclavian-pulmonary) anastomosis had enlarged to 13 mm internal diameter in the fixed state. Blalock-Taussig anastomoses usually do not enlarge over time, although they can—as this case illustrates; whereas Waterston and Potts anastomoses often do enlarge over time—with very deleterious hemodynamic sequelae (such as congestive heart failure) and pulmonary sequelae (hypertensive pulmonary vascular obstructive disease).

This rare partial form of common atrioventricular canal could be very confusing diagnostically, even at open heart surgery—emphasizing the great importance of accurate preoperative diagnosis. From the right atrial perspective, without accurate preoperative diagnosis, the surgeon might never guess that there was a complete cleft of the anterior mitral leaflet—because there was no associated ostium primum type of atrial septal defect and because the ventricular septal defect of the atrioventricular canal type was misleadingly small. Needless to say, a complete mitral cleft typically is associated with a large ostium primum type of atrial septal defect, with or without a ventricular septal defect of the atrioventricular canal type: but not in this rare and hence potentially diagnostically confusing case.

TABLE 13.15 Salient Findings in Tricuspid Atresia {S,D,S} With Pulmonary Outflow Tract Atresia (n = 5)

Findings	No. of Cases	% of Series
Pulmonary valvar atresia	4	80
Pulmonary infundibular atresia (? acquired)	1	20
Tetralogy of Fallot type of infundibuloarterial anomaly	2	40
Pulmonary atresia with intact ventricular septum	1	20
Pulmonary valvar atresia with ventricular septal defect of atrioventricular canal type and partial form of common atrioventricular canal	1	20
Pulmonary valvar atresia with absence of the main pulmonary artery	1	20
Tetralogy of Fallot with infundibular and valvar pulmonary atresia and an aortopulmonary window	1	20
Secundum atrial septal defect	2	40
Multiple congenital anomalies	1	20
Cyanotic spells	1	20

What really is truncus arteriosus with a ventricular septal defect and without an aortopulmonary septal remnant (truncus arteriosus type A2)? One of these patients, a 2½-year-old boy (Case 51), appeared to display a "natural experiment" that answers this question (Fig. 13.38). In addition to tricuspid atresia, he also had a tetralogy of Fallot type of infundibuloarterial anomaly with pulmonary infundibular and valvar atresia, plus an aortopulmonary window (a "congenital Waterston anastomosis") that opened into the right pulmonary artery, which was confluent with a good-sized left pulmonary artery (Table 13.15). By contrast, the main pulmonary artery was very hypoplastic. This looked to us like an *interface case* between tetralogy of Fallot and truncus arteriosus (type A2).[247] If the extremely hypoplastic main pulmonary artery had undergone complete involution, this would have been our anatomic diagnosis: truncus arteriosus with ventricular septal defect (type A) and with no aortopulmonary septal remnant (type 2)—hence type A2.[247] Both pulmonary artery branches would appear to arise from the posterior surface of the ascending aorta.

This case illustrates why we think that truncus arteriosus type A2 really is the following:

1. tetralogy of Fallot with pulmonary infundibular and valvar atresia;
2. involution of the main pulmonary artery; and
3. an anteroposterior (AP) window between the ascending aorta and the right pulmonary artery.

Developmentally, it should be recalled that the pulmonary artery branches originate from the aortic sac and later become confluent with the main pulmonary artery. The aorticopulmonary window or communication is a normal early developmental stage.

Our hypothesis also appears highly relevant to several other questions:

1. In truncus arteriosus type A2, why is there no aorticopulmonary septal remnant? Because the truncus arteriosus is the ascending aorta only. This is why we omit *communis:* truncus arteriosus (not truncus arteriosus *communis*). The main pulmonary artery, diminutive in this patient, typically undergoes involution. We think that truncus arteriosus type A2 is a truncus aorticus solitarius—a solitary aortic trunk, not a truncus arteriosus communis—a common aorticopulmonary trunk.
2. The apparent left pulmonary artery in truncus arteriosus type A2 consist of the normally definitive left pulmonary artery (to the left of the involuted main pulmonary artery) and the normally definitive proximal right pulmonary artery (to the right of the involuted main pulmonary artery and to the left of the "congenital Waterston anastomosis"—the AP window).

Thus, tetralogy of Fallot, truncus arteriosus, and aorticopulmonary septal defect (window) all appear to be closely interrelated anomalies that are illuminated by this rare "interface" patient.

Multiple congenital anomalies, that is, significant extracardiovascular malformation, was found in one patient, Case 72, a 1-day-old boy (Table 13.15). He had an esophageal erosion because of ectopic gastric mucosa at the upper end of the esophagus.

Tricuspid Atresia With Truncus Arteriosus

Truncus arteriosus coexisted with tricuspid atresia in 3 of these 94 patients (3%, Table 13.11) (Figs. 13.36 and 13.37).

Gender: males = 2; female = 1; and male/female = 2/1.

Age at death (no cardiac transplants): mean = $4\frac{6}{12} \pm 7\frac{4}{12}$ years; range from 11 days to $12\frac{11}{12}$ years; and median = 6 months. The ages at death were 11, 180, and 4710 days.

When tricuspid atresia and truncus arteriosus type A2 coexisted, as in all three patients, **the pulmonary outflow tract was unobstructed in all** (hemodynamically similar to Edwards and Burchell's type Ic).[236] Pulmonary flooding (excessive Qp) with congestive heart failure was prominent in 1 (Case 80, a 6-month-old girl).

All patients had **truncal valve-to-mitral valve direct fibrous continuity,** as in typical truncus arteriosus (and as in typical tetralogy of Fallot).

All of the entries in Table 13.16 should be self-explanatory, except for **multiple congenital anomalies** that were found in 1 patient, the 11-day-old boy (Case 42). In addition to tricuspid atresia {S,D,S} with truncus arteriosus type A2 and without pulmonary outflow tract obstruction, he also had the following: accessory splenuli in the left upper quadrant, 3; right cleft lip with bilateral cleft palate; multiple contractions; intestinal malrotation with the cecum beneath the liver in the right upper quadrant; extrahepatic biliary atresia with absence of the gallbladder; and extreme hypoplasia of the pancreas that was identified histologically, but not with certainty grossly. Pregnancy had been characterized by first trimester bleeding. Delivery at 36 weeks gestation in 1983 was by cesarean section because of breech presentation and fetal distress.

Tricuspid Atresia With Double-Outlet Right Ventricle {S,D,D}

Tricuspid atresia with DORV {S,D,D} occurred in 2 of these 94 patients (2%, Table 13.11). DORV {S,D,D} means that both great arteries arise above the morphologically right ventricle (or its

TABLE 13.16 Findings in Tricuspid Atresia With Truncus Arteriosus ($n = 3$)

Findings	No. of Cases	% of Series
Truncus arteriosus type A2	3	100
Absent ductus arteriosus	2	67
Bicuspid (bicommisural) truncal valve	2	67
Secundum atrial septal defect	2	67
Dextrocardia	1	33
Right aortic arch	1	33
Collateral artery from ascending aorta to right lung	1	33
Poorly incorporated common pulmonary vein	1	33
Abnormal locations of both coronary ostia	1	33
Accessory splenuli, 3, left upper quadrant	1	33
Multiple congenital anomalies	1	33
Old subacute bacterial endocarditis	1	33
Acute purulent meningitis, *Staphylococcus aureus*	1	33

remnant, given that tricuspid atresia coexists) and that the segmental anatomy is situs solitus of the viscera and atria (DORV {*S*, -,-}), with D-loop ventricles (DORV {S,*D*,-}), and D-malposition of the great arteries (DORV {S,D,*D*}); that is, D-malposition indicates that the malposed aortic valve lies to the right (Dextro or D) relative to the malposed pulmonary valve.

Gender: males = 0; and females = 2.

Ages at death (no cardiac transplants): 14 months and $5\frac{4}{12}$ years. The mean = $3\frac{3}{12} \pm 2\frac{11}{12}$ years, and the median = $3\frac{3}{12}$ years.

Findings

The 14-month-old girl (Case 45) with tricuspid atresia and DORV {S,D,D} had left-sided juxtaposition of the atrial appendages (Lt JAA), with a secundum atrial septal defect because of a deficient septum primum.

Thus, one of the lessons that this case teaches is that Lt JAA occurs not only with tricuspid atresia and transposition of the great arteries (as we have already seen in patients with tricuspid atresia and D-loop TGA, Table 13.11), but also with tricuspid atresia and DORV.

This patient had pulmonary outflow tract stenosis produced in part by a remnant of tricuspid valve tissue.

Again, it is noteworthy that in a patient with tricuspid atresia, rarely one can have a physiologically significant tricuspid leaflet remnant.

There were additional factors contributing to this patient's pulmonary outflow tract stenosis. There was conal septal posterior malalignment; hence the conal septum encroached on the posteriorly located pulmonary outflow tract. And there was pulmonary valvar stenosis with a bicuspid (bicommissural) pulmonary valve.

The posterior conal septal malalignment was associated with a large ventricular septal defect that was of the confluent conoventricular and atrioventricular canal types.

Thus, this was tricuspid atresia with pulmonary outflow tract stenosis and DORV {S,D,D}, which is not classifiable using the Edwards and Burchell classification.[236] It is close to tricuspid atresia type IIb,[236] except that DORV—not TGA—was present.

In this patient, the infundibulum was large, and the right ventricular sinus was almost absent. Consequently one could say that this patient really had **double-outlet infundibular outlet chamber,** not double-outlet right ventricle (because the right ventricular sinus—the real RV) was virtually absent. We agree with this view in terms of accurate morphologic anatomy; however, many observers continue to call such cases DORV {S,D,D}, rather than the less familiar **DOIOC {S,D,D}.**

A bilateral conus (subaortic and subpulmonary) was present. The large ventricular septal defect was closer to the pulmonary valve than to the aortic valve; but because of the coexistence of fibrous (tricuspid leaflet remnant) and muscular (posteriorly malaligned conal septum) pulmonary outflow tract stenosis, the VSD was functionally subaortic, not subpulmonary, even though the aortic valve was further from the VSD than was the pulmonary valve.

Thus, in DORV and DOIOC, whether a VSD is subaortic or subpulmonary is a question not only of semilunar valve–VSD proximity, but also of outflow tract accessibility (presence or absence of obstruction).

Following a classical right Blalock-Taussig anastomosis in 1962, the patient died because of a massive mucous plug in the lower tracheobronchial tree.

The other patient, a $5\frac{4}{12}$-year-old girl with tricuspid atresia and DORV {S,D,D} or DOIOC {S,D,D}, had subaortic stenosis with aortic hypoplasia, and no pulmonary outflow tract stenosis. Not surprisingly, she also had histologic evidence of pulmonary vascular obstructive disease. No form of surgical treatment was undertaken and she died in 1954.

Tricuspid Atresia With Anatomically Corrected Malposition of the Great Arteries {S,D,L}. Tricuspid atresia with anatomically corrected malposition of the great arteries {S,D,L} was found in 2 of these 94 patients (2%, Table 13.11) (Fig. 13.39). *Anatomically corrected malposition* of the great arteries means that despite the fact that the great arteries are very malposed, they nonetheless arise above the anatomically correct ventricles—the aorta above the anatomically left ventricle and the pulmonary artery above the anatomically right ventricle.

How is that possible? The answer appears to be: The ventricles loop in one direction, let us say to the right, and the conotruncus (the infundibulum and the great arteries) twist in the opposite direction, let us say to the left. That is exactly what ACM {S,D,L} means (Fig. 13.39). The viscera and atria are in situs solitus, that is, ACM {*S*, -,-}; D-loop ventricles are present, that is, ACM {S,*D*,-}; and the infundibulum and great arteries have twisted to the left, that is, ACM {S,D,*L*}.

In ACM {S,D,L}—the most common form of ACM—the L-malposed aorta (Ao) is anterior and to the left, above the morphologically or anatomically left ventricle (LV); and the malposed main pulmonary artery (MPA) is posterior and to the right of the Ao, and the MPA is located above the morphologically or anatomically right ventricle (RV).

Typically, in ACM {S,D,L}, there is *atrioventricular (AV) concordance* with the morphologically right atrium (RA) opening into the RV and the morphologically left atrium (LA) opening into the LV. There is also *ventriculoarterial (VA) concordance,* with the RV ejecting into the MPA and the LV ejecting into the Ao.

It is noteworthy that *VA concordance and normally related great arteries* are not synonyms.

Indeed, there are **two anatomic types of VA concordance**:

1. normally related great arteries, that is, solitus normally related great arteries, that is, {-,-,*S*} and inversus normally related great arteries, that is, {-,-,I}; and
2. anatomically corrected malposition of the great arteries, that is, ACM {S,D,L}; ACM {S,L,D}; ACM {I,L,D}; and ACM {I,D,L}.

In the these two patients with ACM {S,D,L}, the data are as follows:

Gender: male = 1; and female = 1.

Age at death (no cardiac transplants): $16\frac{8}{12}$ years (6080 days) and 4 months (120 days). The mean age at death was $8\frac{6}{12} \pm 11\frac{7}{12}$ years, and the median was $8\frac{6}{12}$ years.

Findings. The $16\frac{8}{12}$-year-old boy displayed the **syndrome of left-sided juxtaposition of the atrial appendages:**[242] dextrocardia, anatomically corrected malposition {S,D,L}, membranous tricuspid atresia, large secundum atrial septal defect

(40 × 23 mm), relatively small conoventricular type of ventricular septal defect (9 × 4 mm), small-chambered and thick-walled right ventricle, bilateral (subaortic and subpulmonary) conus, severe ring-like subpulmonary stenosis (7 mm internal diameter), and bicuspid pulmonary valve with underdeveloped septal commissure. There was also a mild degree of fibrous subaortic stenosis produced by accessory subaortic mitral valve fibrous tissue. The aortic valve was anterior and to the left of the pulmonary valve, with the aortic valve above the left ventricle and the ventricular septum, and the pulmonary valve above the right ventricle. Both semilunar valves were at approximately the same height, with 7 mm of conal muscle beneath each. Left ventricular hypertrophy was marked and left ventricular enlargement was moderate.

At 15 months of age in 1956, this patient had a classical right Blalock-Taussig anastomosis. At 16⁸⁄₁₂ years of age in 1971, an attempt was made to resect the subaortic stenosis and to perform a Waterston anastomosis (between the ascending aorta and the right pulmonary artery). The postoperative period was characterized by atrial flutter–fibrillation with reduction in cardiac output, leading to congestive heart failure and death.

The 4-month-old black girl also had **left-sided juxtaposition of the atrial appendages syndrome**[242] that was characterized by mesocardia with rightward pointing ventricular apex, anatomically corrected malposition of the great arteries {S,D,L}, tricuspid atresia, restrictive patent foramen ovale, conoventricular type of ventricular septal defect, bilateral conus, pulmonary stenosis (infundibular and valvar, marked), anomalous origin of both coronary arteries (both arising from the aortic nonseptal sinus of Valsalva—that usually is noncoronary), and right aortic arch. The malposed aorta arose anteriorly and to the left, above the morphologically left ventricle. The malposed pulmonary artery originated posteriorly and to the right, above the infundibular outlet chamber. The right ventricular sinus was slit-like—almost totally atretic or absent.

What are the anatomic features of the left-sided JAA syndrome, and why do we think it is a syndrome?

The juxtaposition of the atrial appendages syndrome were referred to earlier in this chapter.[243,244] What follows is further information concerning our first study of JAA.[242]

In 1968, Dr. Barbara Melhuish and I published a study of juxtaposition of the atrial appendages in which we compared 42 cases of JAA with 100 cases with conotruncal malformations (such as transposition of the great arteries or double-outlet right ventricle), but without JAA.[242] The control series was randomly selected, except that JAA was excluded.

Why did the control series consist of conotruncal malformations (TGA and DORV)? Because JAA occurs almost always with such conotruncal anomalies. Indeed, only 3 of these 42 patients (7%) with JAA had a normal subpulmonary type of conus and no infundibuloarterial alignment anomaly such as TGA or DORV.

Patients with left-sided JAA had a whole constellation of anomalies that were seen significantly more frequently than did similar patients without left-sided JAA.[242] These characteristic malformations constitute the *left-sided JAA syndrome* (in which

TABLE 13.17 Features of Left-Sided Juxtaposition of the Atrial Appendages Syndrome (JAA)

Anatomic Features	With JAA* No. (%)	Without JAA* No. (%)	χ^2	*p* Value
1. Secundum atrial septal defect	30 (71)	23 (23)	29.46	<0.001
2. Tricuspid atresia or severe tricuspid stenosis	17 (40)	4 (4)	30.47	<0.001
3. Small or absent right ventricular sinus	30 (71)	20 (20)	34.05	<0.001
4. Ventricular septal defect	37 (88)	57 (57)	13.01	<0.001
5. Bilateral conus	30 (71)	25 (25)	26.71	<0.001
6. Pulmonary outflow tract stenosis or atresia	22 (52)	19 (19)	15.80	<0.001
7. Aortic outflow tract stenosis	16 (38)	8 (8)	18.55	<0.001
8. Anatomically corrected malposition of the great arteries	4 (10)	0 (0)	—	0.0069

*In the total series with JAA, *n* = 42, and in control series without JAA, *n* = 100.[242] χ^2 = chi square. All percentages in parentheses (%) are rounded off to the nearest whole number. In item 8, there is no χ^2 number because Fisher's exact test was required.

From Melhuish BPP, Van Praagh R: Juxtaposition of the atrial appendages, a sign of severe cyanotic congenital heart disease, *Br Heart J* 1968;30:269, with permission.

the morphologically right atrial appendage of solitus atria is malposed to the left of both great arteries (Table 13.17).

So, what does the left-sided juxtaposition of the atrial appendages syndrome[242,243] **really mean?** It means that when levomalposition of the right atrial appendage is present, a whole group of anomalies are significantly more likely to be present than when left-sided JAA is absent (Table 13.17).[242] These malformations are all clinically important:[242]

1. **secundum atrial septal defect** in 71% (versus 23% in controls);
2. **tricuspid atresia or severe tricuspid stenosis** in 40% (versus in 4% of controls);
3. **small or absent right ventricular sinus or inflow tract** in 71% (versus 20% in controls);
4. **ventricular septal defect** in 88% (versus 57% in the control series);
5. **bilateral conus**, that is, a muscular subaortic and a muscular subpulmonary infundibulum in 71% (versus in 25% of controls);
6. **pulmonary outflow tract stenosis or atresia** in 52% (versus in 19% of controls);
7. **aortic outflow tract stenosis** in 38% (versus 8% of controls); and
8. **anatomically corrected malposition of the great arteries** in 10% (versus 0 in the control series).

All eight of these differences are statistically highly significant (Table 13.17).

It should also be remembered that there is a second syndrome concerning juxtaposition of the atrial appendages, namely, **the right-sided juxtaposition of the atrial appendages syndrome.**[244] More accurately, this is the **malposition of the morphologically left atrial appendages**—to the *right* of the great arteries in visceroatrial situs solitus, and to the *left* of the great arteries in visceroatrial situs inversus, as was shown by Dr. Stella Van Praagh and her colleagues.[244] Just as malposition of the morphologically right atrial appendage resulting in JAA is a syndrome of tricuspid and right ventricular aplasia or hypoplasia,[242,243] conversely—malposition of the morphologically left atrial appendage resulting in JAA is a syndrome of mitral and left ventricular aplasia or hypoplasia[244]—as we shall see when we study congenital mitral atresia and severe stenosis (see Chapter 10). Thus, the morphology of the atrial appendages is the key to understanding JAA, whether it is left-sided or right-sided.[243,244]

It should be added that we previously thought that **dextrocardia** was part of the (usually left-sided) JAA syndrome (caused by levomalposition of the morphologically right atrial appendage in situs solitus, or caused by dextromalposition of the morphologically right atrial appendage in visceroatrial situs inversus). In our 1968 study,[242] dextrocardia was present in 9 of 42 cases with JAA (21%), and was found in 12 of 100 controls without JAA (12%). However, this difference is *not* statistically significant: $\chi^2 = 1.94$ and $p < 0.25$ but > 0.10.

Similarly, **right aortic arch** was present in 8 of 42 patients with JAA (19%), compared with 10 of 100 controls (10%).[242] This difference also is not statistically significant ($\chi^2 = 2.02$, and $p < 0.25$ but > 0.10). This is the first time that statistical analysis has been published concerning these JAA data (Table 13.17).

Now returning to Table 13.11, it will be noted that the usual type of tricuspid atresia (excluding imperforate Ebstein's anomaly) occurred in one patient each in three different anatomic settings that have not as yet been mentioned.

Tricuspid Atresia With Double-Outlet Left Ventricle {S,D,L}. Case 58 was a 29-year-old woman with tricuspid atresia and double-outlet left ventricle {S,D,L}, whose heart specimen we had the privilege of studying in 1985 thanks to a consultation from Professor E. Rainer de Vivie of Köln (Cologne), Germany. Dr. Stella Van Praagh did this fascinating consultation.

As the segmental anatomy indicates, the patient with DOLV {S,D,L} had situs solitus of the viscera and atria, a ventricular D-loop, and right-sided tricuspid atresia, She had a patent foramen ovale and a conoventricular type of ventricular septal defect.

The truly fascinating aspect was that the infundibuloarterial part of the heart was abnormal and inverted; the segmental anatomy was DOLV {S,D,**L**}. This patient had what may be called "the inverted tetralogy of Fallot type" of DOLV.

One needs to understand that the most common type of DOLV (in our experience) is what may be called the tetralogy type of DOLV {S,D,D}. There is aortic-mitral fibrous continuity, with aortic overriding of the ventricular septal defect. The pulmonary artery also originates above the left ventricle, with a very short muscular subpulmonary infundibulum that is also stenotic. But the conotruncus usually is not inverted; it is of the D-malposition type with the aortic valve to the right and somewhat posteroinferior relative to the left-sided stenotic subpulmonary infundibulum and pulmonary valve. (If necessary, see Chapter 24 for more information.)

But in this rare patient, the infundibuloarterial part of the heart was inverted or of the L-malposition type, that is, DOLV {S,D,L}. The aortic valve arose predominantly above the left ventricle, and also to a small degree above the infundibular outlet chamber (the small "right ventricle"); in other words, the aortic valve was overriding, as in tetralogy of Fallot. The aortic-mitral fibrous continuity was between the right coronary leaflet of the aortic valve and the anterior leaflet of the mitral valve.

The pulmonary valve lay to the *right* of the aortic valve and there was pulmonary valve—mitral valve direct fibrous continuity. There was pulmonary stenosis, subvalvar and valvar. There was no subpulmonary conal musculature, facilitating pulmonary valve—mitral valve direct fibrous continuity.

The coronary arterial origins were inverted, as is appropriate for an inverted type of conus—but as is not appropriate for a D-loop (or noninverted) ventricular segment. The right coronary arterial ostium supplied the anterior descending coronary artery; that is, its distribution was inverted.

Hence, the infundibulum resembled an inverted or mirror-image tetralogy of Fallot, with absence of subpulmonary conal musculature. The pulmonary valve was tricommissural (tricuspid). However, the pulmonary artery was entirely above the left ventricle, with pulmonary valve—mitral valve fibrous continuity. Hence this was DOLV of the inverted tetralogy of Fallot type, with ventricular noninversion and right-sided tricuspid atresia, in visceroatrial situs solitus; or briefly, tricuspid atresia with DOLV {S,D,L} with marked pulmonary outflow tract stenosis.

Although the noninverted tetralogy of Fallot type is the most common anatomic type of DOLV, that is, DOLV {S,D,**D**}, the inverted tetralogy of Fallot type of DOLV is rare, as in this 29-year-old woman with tricuspid atresia and DOLV (S,D,**L**} with aortic-mitral and pulmonary-mitral fibrous continuity and with pulmonary stenosis.

Tricuspid Atresia, Left-Sided {A(I),L,S} With Polysplenia and Multiple Congenital Anomalies. Case 48 was a 1-day-old boy who was born prematurely in 1975 with congenital complete heart block, severe congestive heart failure, ascites (800 mL), generalized edema, anemia, and multiple congenital anomalies. He had a polycystic and hypoplastic right kidney, polysplenia, and dextrocardia.

He had a left-sided inferior vena cava, a left-sided superior vena cava, a common atrium, ipsilateral pulmonary veins, and one atrioventricular valve. My interpretation was: tricuspid atresia, left-sided; mitral valve, right-sided, opening only from the left atrium, right-sided, into the left ventricle, right-sided, with solitus normally related great arteries.

Hence, the segmental anatomy was {A(I),L,S}. In other words, there was viscera heterotaxy with polysplenia and situs ambiguus {**A**-,-,-}, but the atria were in situs inversus {A(**I**),-,-}. A ventricular L-loop was present {A(I),**L**,-}. And the infundibulum and great arteries were of the solitus normal type {A(I),L,**S**}. Thus, the segmental set or combination—that is what the braces {} mean—was that of infundibuloarterial noninversion, with the atria and the ventricles being inverted. At the time (1975–1976), we thought that this was a newly discovered form of congenital heart disease; that is, a newly recognized segmental set. Basically, the segmental combination was {I,L,S}. We did not call this *isolated* infundibuloarterial noninversion (although we were tempted), because there were so many other associated cardiovascular and noncardiovascular anomalies. (But the situs or pattern of organization of the infundibulum and great arteries was of the noninverted type—and hence was "isolated"—in the sense that the situs of the atrial and ventricular segments were both inverted.) {I,L,S} says it clearly and briefly.

There was severe subaortic stenosis because the conal septum was posteriorly malaligned and hence too close to the right-sided mitral valve. The aortic valve was tricuspid (tricommissural), but hypoplastic. There was marked hypoplasia of the ascending aorta and aortic arch, with an aberrant right subclavian artery.

The pulmonary outflow tract was unobstructed. A large main pulmonary artery continued into a large patent ductus arteriosus that arched over the right main stem bronchus and into the descending thoracic aorta.

Tricuspid Atresia in Conjoined Twins

Case 30 was conjoined twin B in a pair of thoracopagus twins. She was a female with multiple congenital anomalies who died at 4½ hours of age. Her heart had **atresia of all four cardiac valves,** a unique finding in our experience. Blood flow in twin B was described as nonpulsatile. The hypothetical circulation in twin B was speculated to be as follows: from twin A via an intercostal arteriovenous fistula to the right atrium of twin B; then to the left atrium; then via a left superior vena cava–like vessel to perfuse twin B. Then blood from twin B returned to twin A via the hepatic arteries of twin B and then via the hepatic veins of twin A.

Pulmonary hypoplasia was bilateral and marked. The pulmonary lobation was abnormal: right bilobed and left unilobed. Twin B, who was smaller than twin A, had microcephaly, a sloping forehead, a prominent nasal bridge, low-set ears, two vaginae, and two uteri. One ovary was long and slender; the other was normal.

A long, looping internal mammary–like artery passes from twin A to the right atrium of twin B. This was regarded as **an arteriovenous fistula** from twin A to twin B—beginning as an artery in twin A and ending as a vein in twin B.

There was **microcardia** with an intact pericardial sac. An **incomplete form of common atrioventricular canal** was found with a large ostium primum type of atrial septal defect (an incomplete atrioventricular septal defect). No atrioventricular valve exited from the morphologically right atrium; hence in this sense, **tricuspid atresia** was present.

Two diminutive atrioventricular valves were observed in the floor of the left atrium, aligned with the underlying left ventricle, and both atrioventricular valves were atretic. Hence, another interpretation is that double-inlet left ventricle was potentially present, but both potential atrioventricular valves were atretic. The right-sided atretic atrioventricular valve could also be interpreted as tricuspid atresia.

There were no papillary muscles in the left ventricle. The left ventricle was diminutive. The right ventricular sinus (inflow tract) was absent. An infundibular outlet chamber was identified. The pulmonary valve was atretic. A tiny bulboventricular foramen was found, less than 1 mm in diameter. Valvar aortic atresia was found. The segmental anatomy was normal, that is, {S,D,S}. Marked hypoplasia of the ascending aorta was observed. A small, low aortopulmonary window (0.5 mm in diameter) was present. Coronary ostia were not found. The aortic isthmus was hypoplastic (1 mm in diameter). The patent ductus arteriosus also had a small opening (1 mm in diameter). The foramen ovale was well formed and the pulmonary veins connected normally with the left atrium.

The left superior vena cava opened into the left atrium to the left of the left pulmonary veins. The coronary sinus was not identified.

Echocardiography failed to show a heart in twin B (our patient) and, as mentioned heretofore, the blood flow in twin B appeared to be nonpulsatile.

There was one liver in common between twins A and B.

The twins were separated surgically, sacrificing twin B. Twin A died in the operating room after 7 hours of surgery.

In summary, twin B had much more than tricuspid atresia. Nonetheless, we think that this patient, unique in our experience, merits description and hence is included here. Atresia of all cardiac valves can reach postnatal life only in conjoined twins, in which one twin supports **the functionally acardiac twin** (as in our twin B).

Discussion of Typical Tricuspid Atresia

By "typical" tricuspid atresia, we mean tricuspid atresia that is not associated with Ebstein's disease, that is, non-Ebstein tricuspid atresia.

At the time of writing (2007), it is now clear that typical tricuspid atresia is much more complex than was known when my friends Dr. Jesse Edwards and Dr. Howard Burchell[236] made their first excellent attempt to describe and classify tricuspid atresia in 1949 at the Mayo Clinic in Rochester, Minnesota. In the present series of 94 postmortem cases, 11 different anatomic types of tricuspid atresia were found (Table 13.11):

1. with normally related great arteries and pulmonary outflow tract atresia (5%);
2. with normally related great arteries and pulmonary outflow tract stenosis (47%);
3. with normally related great arteries and no pulmonary outflow tract obstruction (6%);
4. with truncus arteriosus (3%);
5. with D-loop transposition of the great arteries (19%);
6. with double-outlet right ventricle (2%);
7. with double-outlet left ventricle (1%);
8. with anatomically corrected malposition of the great arteries (2%);
9. with L-loop transposition of the great arteries (11%);
10. with inverted atria, L-loop ventricles, and solitus normally related great arteries (1%); and
11. with conjoined twins (1%).

The salient features of each of these 11 anatomic types of tricuspid atresia are presented in some detail (Tables 13.12 to 13.16). The clinical and surgical importance not only of pulmonary outflow tract obstruction, but also of aortic inflow tract obstruction is emphasized. The anatomic type of ventricular loop (D-loop or L-loop) determines whether the tricuspid atresia is right-sided (with D-loop), or left-sided (with L-loop). Left-sided juxtaposition of the atrial appendages (because of levomalposition of the morphologically right atrial appendage in visceroatrial situs solitus) is recognized as a syndrome that is associated with D-loop tricuspid atresia (Table 13.17).[242,243] Now let us consider the literature in somewhat greater detail than we did previously.

Earliest descriptions. As mentioned heretofore, the earliest probable description of tricuspid atresia known to us was by the editors of the *London Medical Review* in 1812;[235] this reference was kindly sent to me by Dr. Bill Rashkind. Here is what the editors wrote (reported here for the reader's convenience): "The child died on the seventh day. Upon dissection the pulmonary artery was found to be deficient, and instead of it there was a slender impervious ligament, extending from the situation of the right ventricle to the ductus arteriosus. The right ventricle was nearly obliterated. There was a mere depression in its situation. The right auricle was large, and communicated by an extensive foramen ovale of which the valve was very imperfect, with the left auricle. The left ventricle and the aorta were natural. The ductus arteriosus was very large and divided into two branches, which entirely supplied the lungs, without receiving any blood from the pulmonary artery."

The first definite description of tricuspid atresia came 5 years later in 1817 from Kreysig in Berlin.[234] Dr. Rashkind's translation was as follows: "The opening of the right atrium showed a much more solid construction than usual; the trabeculae of the auricle were hypertrophied and in the place where the opening into the right ventricle should have been, but was absent, instead there was convergence to a dimple." Exactly (Fig. 13.10).

Another early definite description of what we now call tricuspid atresia was that of Brown in 1824,[238] also courtesy of Dr. Bill Rashkind.

By 1858, in his first edition, Peacock calls this malformation *"absence of the right auriculo-ventricular aperture."* Note that by this time, the designation is becoming specific (no longer *malformation of the heart*). *Absence of the right auriculo-ventricular aperture* is an excellent, accurate designation—although perhaps a bit too long for current clipped tastes. But I like it because it is accurate and specific. So, too, do Dr. Robert H. Anderson, Dr. Robert M. Freedom, and other contemporary authorities. For example, Freedom et al[248] calls the classic (or typical) form of tricuspid atresia *absent right atrioventricular connection*.

Where does tricuspid *atresia* come from? *Atresia* is derived from Greek: *a*, absence of, *tresis*, hole.

The literature is full of fascination and surprises. Consider this publication from 1955: Hurwitt, Young, and Escher[249] published a paper titled "The rationale of anastomosis of the right auricular appendage to the pulmonary artery in the treatment of tricuspid atresia. Application of this procedure to a case of cor triloculare." This paper was published in the *Journal of Thoracic Surgery*. Dr. Ursula Sauer of München (Munich) pointed this out to me in November 1980.

I was not aware of this pre-Fontan publication. And I think that this work by Hurwitt and his colleagues[249] has been largely forgotten by pediatric cardiologists and cardiac surgeons. For example, this reference is not cited in Freedom et al[248]—who usually are an excellent source for references to the literature; however, the Hurwitt reference[249] is cited by Kirklin and Barratt-Boyes.[250] These authors also make reference to earlier experimental work in dogs by Isaac Starr and colleagues in 1943 showing that right ventricular destruction did not result in systemic venous hypertension; by Rodbard and Wagner in 1949 showing that the right ventricle could be bypassed; and by Warden, DeWall, and Varco showing in 1954 the feasibility of bypassing the right ventricle by a right atrial to pulmonary artery anastomosis. Kirklin and Barratt-Boyes[250] then state that based on the aforementioned studies, Hurwitt and colleagues[249] reported an unsuccessful attempt in 1955 to correct tricuspid atresia by a right atrial to pulmonary artery anastomosis.

Examination of the publication by Hurwitt and colleagues[249] reveals several interesting things:

1. This patient did not have tricuspid atresia; this was the preoperative misdiagnosis. Instead, autopsy revealed double-inlet common ventricle (as the authors called it) with a stenotic pulmonary outflow tract with a subpulmonary infundibulum, and a bicuspid pulmonary valve, and a moderately hypoplastic main pulmonary artery. The mitral valve was large, and the tricuspid valve was described as "rudimentary." My guess is that this patient had a Holmes heart {S,D,S} with double-inlet left ventricle and with tricuspid stenosis. There was an interatrial communication and the ductus arteriosus was closed. Physiologically, therefore, this patient's anomaly resembled classical tricuspid atresia, or even more closely—congenital tricuspid stenosis.
2. Hurwitt's patient[249] really died intraoperatively, before the surgical procedure was completed. Moribund preoperatively, this little boy did not die because the operation failed. Instead, he died intraoperatively from his untreated cyanotic congenital heart disease.
3. Hurwitt,[249] in this brave pioneering attempt, anastomosed the tip of the right atrial appendage to the side of the hypoplastic main pulmonary artery. We now know from experience that this particular technique is almost always obstructive (stenotic). It usually does not work. One needs a much larger right atrial-to-pulmonary artery communication to avoid iatrogenic obstruction, or the use of another technique altogether—such as a lateral tunnel, or a cavopulmonary anastomosis. We only know this now—in 2007—because hindsight is 20/20.

Thus, **right ventricular bypass** has an important—one might say essential—pre-Fontan history involving Isaac Starr, Rodbard and Wagner, Warden, DeWall, and Varco,[250] and Hurwitt and colleagues.[249] The glory has gone to Francis Fontan and his colleagues[17,18] of Bordeaux, not because of the originality of the concept of right ventricular bypass, but because they were the first to achieve success in human patients.

Now an attempt will be made to record many of the scientific publications concerning tricuspid atresia that we have found helpful, in approximately chronological order, from 1965 to the present time.[251-522] These publications document the growth and development of diagnostic and therapeutic understanding over the latter third of the twentieth century and into the twenty-first, a period of more than 40 years.

As always, I apologize to those authors whose work I may have inadvertently omitted. This literature review should be regarded as a useful sample of the literature, but certainly not as all of the literature. Careful perusal of this literature[251-522] reveals a fascinating tale. In the interests of brevity and focus, I am going to have to let most of these references speak for themselves.

From the anatomic standpoint, what did we learn in this study of 94 postmortem cases of classical tricuspid atresia (Tables 13.11 to 13.16)?

Salient novel findings included the following: Typical tricuspid atresia can occur with truncus arteriosus (3%), double-outlet right ventricle (2%), double-outlet left ventricle (1%), anatomically corrected malposition of the great arteries (2%), with visceral heterotaxy and polysplenia (1%), and in conjoined twins (1%).

This study confirmed that tricuspid atresia with normally related great arteries and pulmonary outflow tract stenosis (type Ib of Edwards and Burchell)[236,237] is by far the most common anatomic type (47%) . Tricuspid atresia {S,D,S} with no pulmonary outflow tract obstruction (type Ic)[236] (6%) and tricuspid atresia {S,D,S} with pulmonary outflow tract atresia (type Ia)[236] (5%) are much less frequent. Tricuspid atresia with D-loop transposition of the great arteries accounted for almost one-fifth of our cases (19%),[264,275] while left-sided tricuspid atresia with L-loop transposition of the great arteries made up 11%.

Abrams and colleagues[283] reported in 1975 a patient with tricuspid and pulmonary valvar atresia (type Ia) who survived to 21 years of age apparently because of the coexistence of a circle of Vieussens-like aortopulmonary fistula between a conal branch of the right coronary artery and the proximal main pulmonary artery.

In 1974, Tandon and Edwards[279] updated the anatomic classification of Edwards and Burchell of 1949.[236] Based on a study of 45 postmortem cases, they included the following:[279] tricuspid atresia with normally related great arteries (their type I, 56% of their series, with pulmonary outflow tract obstruction in 84%); tricuspid atresia with transposition of the great arteries (their type II, 42% of the series, with pulmonary outflow tract obstruction in 32%); and tricuspid atresia with truncus arteriosus (1 case, 2%).

In patients with tricuspid atresia, when the great arteries are *transposed* (by which Tandon and Edwards[279] meant abnormally related—a very broad definition of transposition similar to that of Maude Abbott), these authors[279] recognized that the conus can be subaortic (only), which they called type IIA, or subaortic and subpulmonary which they called a double conus and classified as type IIb. Tandon and Edwards' double conus[279] is what we call a bilateral conus, meaning both subaortic and subpulmonary.

This updated classification of tricuspid atresia as much more inclusive than the initial version of 1949,[236] which was a good thing. But the updated version *per force* was more complicated and difficult to remember. Consequently, what most pediatric cardiologists and cardiac surgeons did was simply to describe the anatomy (rather than classifying it)—such as tricuspid atresia with D-transposition of the great arteries, bilateral conus, and pulmonary outflow tract stenosis. Nonetheless, the Tandon and Edwards reclassification[279] of tricuspid atresia served a useful purpose: It summarized many of the newly discovered anatomic complexities that can be associated with tricuspid atresia, which constituted diagnostically and surgically important information.

The authors[279] also pointed out that pulmonary outflow tract obstruction is much more common with normally related great arteries (84%) than with transposition (only 32%). As noted previously, this finding makes sense as follows: Pulmonary outflow tract obstruction is to be expected when the pulmonary artery arises from the "small right ventricle," as it does with normally related great arteries, because the bulboventricular foramen or the subpulmonary conus or the pulmonary valve can be obstructive. But pulmonary outflow tract obstruction is anticipated to be much less frequent when the pulmonary artery originates from the large left ventricle, as it does in transposition of the great arteries, because there usually is no subpulmonary conal musculature that can be obstructive.

Also in 1974, Tandon, Marín-García, Moller, and Edwards published a paper titled "Tricuspid atresia with L-transposition."[284] On rereading, this paper turns out to be much more interesting than its title suggests. Of their five postmortem cases of tricuspid atresia, only one (Case 1) had what we would now call L-transposition of the great arteries. This patient had left-sided tricuspid atresia with **TGA {S,L,L}**.

Case 2[284] had right-sided tricuspid atresia with anatomically corrected malposition of the great arteries {S,D,L}. The aorta (Ao) arose anteriorly and to the left above the morphologically left ventricle (LV). A muscular subaortic conus separated the aortic valve above from the mitral valve below. The atretic pulmonary outflow tract was posterior and to the right of the L-malposed aorta. The pulmonary artery (PA) was located above the morphologically right ventricle (RV). A rightward pointing ventricular apex and a right aortic arch were also present. So, their Case 2[284] had what we would now diagnose as **ACM {S,D,L}**. Anatomically corrected malposition is characterized by ventriculo-arterial concordance: Ao above LV and PA above RV. Hence, this is now known as L-*malposition* of the great arteries of the anatomically corrected malposition type, not as L-*transposition,* which now means ventriculoarterial discordance (RV aligned with the Ao, and LV with the PA). As Tandon and colleagues[284] correctly pointed out, their Case 2 had isolated bulbar inversion, that is, *isolated infundibuloarterial inversion*, the atria and the ventricles being noninverted—as the segmental anatomic diagnosis indicates: ACM {S,D,L} with right-sided tricuspid atresia, and so on.

Malposition of the great arteries includes *all* ventriculoarterial malposition. Hence, the anatomic type of VA malposition must be diagnosed specifically. VA malposition includes transposition of the great arteries (TGA), double-outlet right ventricle (DORV), double-outlet left ventricle (DOLV), and the anatomically corrected malalignment (ACM). So, ACM, as in their Case 2,[284] is just one of several possible VA malpositions. Naming the various anatomic types of ventriculoarterial malalignment *specifically* (e.g., TGA, DORV, DOLV, and ACM), instead of calling them all transpositions, as used to be the custom, greatly aids clarity.

Case 3 of Tandon et al[284] also has tricuspid atresia with **ACM {S,D,L}**, a ventricular septal defect, a subaortic conus separating the L-malposed aortic valve above from the normally located mitral valve below, no pulmonary outflow tract obstruction, and left-sided juxtaposition of the atrial appendages (because of levomalposition of the right atrial appendage to the left of the great arteries).

Absence of pulmonary outflow tract obstruction makes it possible to establish with certainty that PA arises above the small RV. When there is pulmonary outflow tract atresia, as in the authors' Case 2[284] mentioned above, it is more difficult to be certain that the PA originates above the RV. From a hemodynamic standpoint, the "small RV" in their Case 2 (consisting of the infundibulum + a remnant of the RV sinus) in fact did not eject into the PA—because of the coexistence of pulmonary outflow tract atresia. However, this logical and diagnostic difficulty did not exist in Tandon's Case 3[284]—because there was no pulmonary outflow tract obstruction.

Cases 4 and 5 of Tandon and colleagues[284] had tricuspid atresia with **DOLV {S,D,L}**. Both had a subaortic conus (preventing aortic-mitral fibrous continuity) and no subpulmonary conus (permitting pulmonary-mitral fibrous continuity). Case 4 had pulmonary outflow tract stenosis. Case 5 had dextrocardia (or at least a rightward pointing ventricular apex).

To summarize, Tandon et al[284] presented in 1974 several of the rarer anatomic types of tricuspid atresia: left-sided tricuspid atresia with TGA {S,L,L}, and right-sided tricuspid atresia with ACM {S,D,L} and DOLV {S,D,L}.

Freedom and Rowe[302] in 1976 described tricuspid atresia with **aneurysm of the atrial septum.** Echocardiographically, it resembled a ping pong ball going from the right atrium into the left atrium. Such an aneurysm of the atrial septum can occur when the interatrial communication is restrictive, reflecting right atrial outlet stenosis. Aneurysm of septum primum in tricuspid atresia can also result in pulmonary venous obstruction and in supravalvar mitral stenosis.

Attempts to rename tricuspid atresia[306,310,319,325,329,330,360,379] (e.g., univentricular heart of left ventricular type with absent right atrioventricular connection[330]) were ultimately not adopted, even by their proponents.[355,382,415,436,507,509,514] Our thought, mentioned earlier, has long been that the "wine" of new understanding should be poured into the old "bottles" (the established terminology), insofar as possible, in order to avoid confusion. The price of each advance in basic understanding must not be a change in diagnostic terminology; otherwise, in the name of clarification, we will create a tower of Babel.

The arterial blood supply of the right atrium and sinus node in classical tricuspid atresia was studied by Battistessa, Ho, Anderson, Smith, and Deverall[436] in 1988, who found that the artery to the sinoatrial node—the pacemaker of the heart—originated from in right coronary artery in 38% of their cases, from the left coronary artery in 59%, and form both the right and left coronary arteries in 3%.

The significance of a **coronary sinus septal defect** (typically a communication between the coronary sinus and the left atrium) in patients undergoing the Fontan procedure was highlighted by Kurosawa and colleagues[389] in 1985.

Perusal of this sample of the world literature on tricuspid atresia[251-522] makes it clear that many attempts have been made, and are still being made, to improve the **right ventricular bypass procedure** that is necessitated by tricuspid atresia. In 1990, Fontan, Kirklin, Fernandez, Costa, Naftel, Tritto, and Blackstone[457] pronounced the Fontan operation, even when "perfect," to be a palliative, not a curative, procedure. We and many others have been trying to figure out how to improve the right ventricular bypass operation.[510,513]

Causes of Death Following the Modified Fontan Procedure. As the cardiac pathologist of Children's Hospital Boston, I thought that the first thing we had to do was to establish what the causes of death following the Fontan operation really were (Table 13.18).[513] Our hope was that by understanding and whenever possible avoiding the causes of postoperative death, it may be possible to improve the results of right ventricular bypass procedures.

Why was congestive heart failure by far the leading cause of post-Fontan death (82%, Table 13.18)? We did not know. So we decided to do some morphometry in the hope that it might be illuminating.

The basic assumption of the Fontan-Kreutzer procedure[17,18,277] was that it is satisfactory to have a normal-sized main pulmonary artery–like vessel or conduit arising from the right atrium.

Dr. George Falkowksi, at a postgraduate course that he was directing at the Bakoulev Institute of Cardiovascular Surgery in Moscow to which I had been invited, mentioned to me that the cross-sectional area of the normal tricuspid valve is twice that of the normal pulmonary valve. I said "Wow!" and we both agreed

TABLE 13.18 Main Causes of Death Following the Modified Fontan Procedure (n = 33 Postmortem Cases)*

Main Cause of Death	No. of Patients	Percent of Series
1. Congestive heart failure	27	82
2. Arrhythmias	4	12
3. Central nervous system dysfunction†	2	6

*16 of these 32 patients (48%) had a hypoplastic atretic, or absent right ventricular sinus, while 17 had a hypoplastic left ventricular sinus.
†2 patients had severe central nervous system dysfunction, thought probably to be related to air embolism, a technically avoidable cause of death that will not be considered further.
From Kiaffas MG, Van Praagh R, Hanioti C, Green DW: The modified Fontan procedure: morphometry and surgical implications, *Ann Thorac Surg* 1999;67:1746, with permission.

that this bit of normal morphometry could be highly relevant to the Fontan procedure. My job was to investigate and find out because in Boston we had the requisite pathologic anatomic data (Fontan heart specimens and normal controls).

Drs. Maria Kiaffas, Chrysoula Hanioti, Douglas Green, and I[513] found that normally, the pulmonary valve area (PVA) averages only 0.42 compared with the tricuspid valve area (TVA) (Table 13.19).

In somewhat greater detail, the PVA/TVA averaged 0.42 ± 0.22, and ranged from a low of 0.19 to a high of 0.60 (Table 13.19).[513] Thus, on average, the cross-sectional area of the normal pulmonary valve was only 42% of that of the normal tricuspid valve. In other words, the normal pulmonary valve cross-sectional area was 58% less than that of the normal tricuspid valve.

We thought that these observations might well explain why the free wall of the morphologically right atrium (RA) is normally so much thinner than that of the morphologically right ventricle (RV): 1 mm versus 3 to 4 mm, respectively. These observations in turn suggest that the original design and concept of the Fontan procedure may be obstructive.

When the tricuspid valve area (TVA) is indexed to the normal systemic vein area (SVA), that is, to the cross-sectional area of the inferior vena cava (IVC) + the cross-sectional area of the superior vena cava (SVC), the TVA/SVA ratio averaged 1.98 ± 0.68, ranging from 0.73 to 5.0 (Table 13.19). The PVA/SVA ratio averaged 0.77 ± 0.27, ranging from 0.31 to 2.07 (Table 13.19). Thus, the normal PVA averaged 61% less than the normal TVA, when both were indexed to the SVA. And it should be remembered that all of the data in Table 13.19 concern *normal* cardiac morphometry.

The next point is that the *morphometry in our Fontan patients* (Table 13.20) usually was very different from normal, that is, much less favorable. With the atriopulmonary anastomosis type of Fontan procedure, the Fontan area (FA) to systemic vein area (SVA) ratio is shown diagrammatically in Fig. 13.42A: FA/SVA = c/a + b. With the lateral tunnel type of Fontan (Fig. 13.42B), FA/SVA = d + b ± c/a + b ± c.

The FA/SVA averaged only 0.54 ± 0.22, ranging from a low of 0.13 to a high of 0.98. The average FA/SVA ratio of 0.54 was 73% less than the normal TVA/SVA of 1.98.

When the tricuspid and the pulmonary valve areas were indexed to the body surface area (BSA), instead of to the systemic vein area (SVA), very similar results were found (Table 13.21).

The FA/BSA averaged 143.52 compared with TVA/BSA average of 471.25 (Table 13.21).[513] Thus, the Fontan area averaged 70% less than normal when indexed to BSA, compared with 73% less than normal when the Fontan area was indexed to the SVA.

The SVA in our Fontan patients (average = 240.41 mm^2, Table 13.20) was 21% greater than in normal controls (average = 198.44 mm^2, Table 13.19). This was a statistically significant difference ($p < 0.01$). The greater SVA in our Fontan patients was thought to be consistent with obstruction of the Fontan pathway, or systemic ventricular myocardial dysfunction, or both. The significant abnormal enlargement of the systemic vein area (IVC + SVC) in our Fontan patients suggests that indexing the TVA and the PVA to the BSA (Table 13.21)[513] may well be preferable to indexing to the SVA.

However, when we indexed the TVA and the FA to the SVA (Fig. 13.43A) or to the BSA (Fig. 13.43B), there was no appreciable difference. Either method of indexing showed that there was no overlap between the much smaller FAs and the normal TVAs.

Of the 27 Fontan patients who died from congestive heart failure, 6 (22%) died early. Morphometry revealed that the FA/SVA ratio averaged only 0.36 ± 0.08, 82% less than normal, well below the average FA/SVA ratio (0.54 ± 0.22, Table 13.20).

Regarding the lateral tunnel type of Fontan (Fig. 13.42B), we found that the normal SVCA (the cross-sectional area of the

TABLE 13.19 Normal Morphometry (n = 66)

Areas and Ratios	Mean (mm^2)	SD (mm^2)	Range (mm^2)
SVCA + IVCA (SVA)	198.44	103.01	64.11–511.49
TV area (TVA)	365.93	163.87	136.7–854.86
PV area (PVA)	140.13	60.01	45.34–301.56
TVA/SVA	1.98	0.68	0.73–5
PVA/SVA	0.77	0.27	0.31–2.07
PVA/TVA	0.42	0.22	0.19–0.6
TVA/PVA	2.68	0.73	1.65–5.2
SVCA/IVCA	0.31	0.15	0.06–0.81

IVCA, Inferior vena caval area; *PV,* pulmonary valve; *PVA,* pulmonary valve area; *SD,* standard deviation; *SVA,* systemic venous area; *SVCA,* superior vena caval area; *TV,* tricuspid valve; *TVA,* tricuspid valve area. The mean ratios were calculated from each individual ratio.
From Kiaffas MG, Van Praagh R, Hanioti C, Green DW: The modified Fontan procedure: morphometry and surgical implications, *Ann Thorac Surg* 1999;67:1746, with permission.

TABLE 13.20 Fontan Morphometry

Areas and Ratios	Mean (mm^2)	SD (mm^2)	Range (mm^2)
SVCA + IVCA (SVA)	240.41	192.24	57.86–979
Fontan area (FA)	106.95	55.37	31.4–336.62
FA/SVA	0.54*	0.22	0.13–0.98
TPA/SVA	0.79*	0.67	0.24–2.6
TPA/FA	1.37*	1.1	0.41–4.79

IVCA, Cross-sectional area of the inferior vena cava where it enters the right atrium; *SVA,* systemic vein area; *SVCA,* cross-sectional area of the superior vena cava where it enters the right atrium; *TPA,* total pulmonary area, i.e., cross-sectional area of right pulmonary artery + cross-sectional area of left pulmonary artery; in first three-rows, n = 33 cases; in last two rows, n = 14 cases.
From Kiaffas MG, Van Praagh R, Hanioti C, Green DW: The modified Fontan procedure: morphometry and surgical implications, *Ann Thorac Surg* 1999;67:1746, with permission.
*Mean ratios calculated from each individual ratio, not from overall averages.

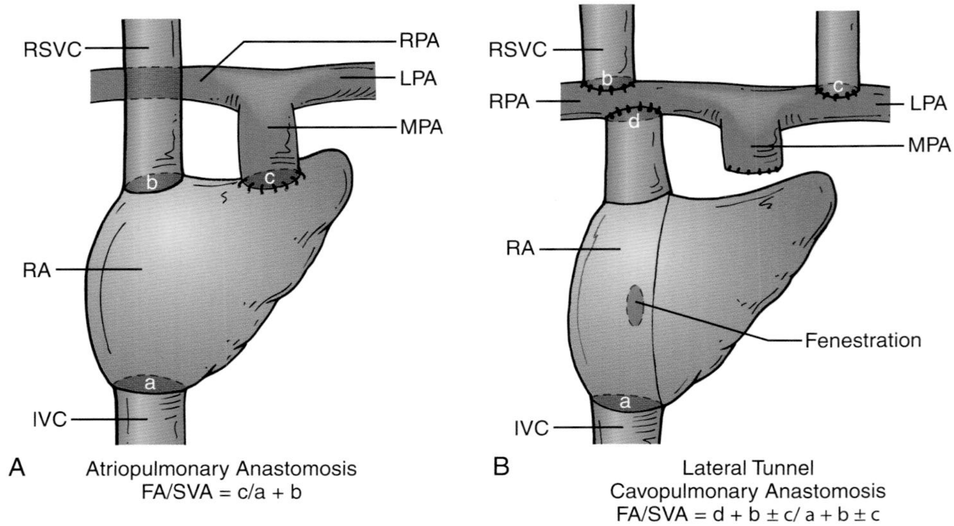

Fig. 13.42 Fontan Morphometry. What is the Fontan anastomosis? Briefly, any and all of the anastomoses to the pulmonary artery and its branches. For example, in the original Fontan-Kreutzer procedure shown in (A), the Fontan area *(FA)* divided by the systemic vein area *(SVC)* equals *c,* the cross-sectional area of the anastomosis between the main pulmonary artery *(MPA)* and the appendage of the right atrium *(RA),* divided by *a,* the cross-sectional area of the opening of the inferior vena cava *(IVC)* into the RA plus *b,* minus the cross-sectional area of the right superior vena cava *(RSVC)* into the RA. Briefly, FA/SVA = c/a + b. In (B), the later lateral tunnel modification of the Fontan procedure, the Fontan area–to–systemic vein area index is as follows: FA/SVA = d + b + c/a + b + c. A persistent left superior vena cava *(LSVC)* may or may not be present. If present, the LSVC is anastomosed to the left pulmonary artery *(LPA); ±,* with or without. The RSVC is anastomosed to the right pulmonary artery *(RPA).* A decompressing fenestration may or may not be present between the lateral tunnel to the right and the rest of the RA to the left (± fenestration). In both Fontan modifications (A and B), the ratio of the FA to the SVA was called the FA/SVA index, and its components varied depending on which surgical modification was performed, as shown. (Reproduced with permission from Kiaffas MG, Van Praagh R, Hanioti C, Green DW: The modified Fontan procedure: morphometry and surgical implications. *Ann Thorac Surg* 1999;67:1746.)

TABLE 13.21 Morphometry Indexed to Body Surface Area

Areas	Mean (mm^2/M^2)	SD (mm^2/M^2)	Range (mm^2/M^2)
Normal Hearts (n = 57)			
TVA/BSA	471.25	123.61	279.95–955.15
PVA/BSA	179.42	43.44	94.39–293.56
SVA/BSA	260.16	106.36	78.18–698.77
Fontan Hearts (*n* = 28)			
FA/BSA	143.52	50.01	55.09–261.67
SVA/BSA	312.79	182.80	101.51–866.37

BSA, Body surface area; *FA,* Fontan area; *PVA,* pulmonary valve area; *SVA,* systemic venous area; *TVA,* tricuspid valve area.
From Kiaffas MG, Van Praagh R, Hanioti C, Green DW: The modified Fontan procedure: morphometry and surgical implications, *Ann Thorac Surg* 1999;67:1746, with permission.

superior vena cava where it enters the RA) divided by the normal IVCA (the cross-sectional area of the inferior vena cava where it enters the RA) averaged only 0.31 ± 0.15, ranging from 0.06 to 0.81 (Table 13.19). In other words, obstruction may occur at the SVC-RA junction because the IVC is often quite a bit larger than the SVC. Stenosis at the level of the SVC may explain, at least in part, why *fenestration* can be hemodynamically and clinically advantageous in lateral-tunnel Fontan patients. The fenestration may well help to decompress the subtly obstructed lateral tunnel pathway, resulting in less congestive heart failure, fewer pleural effusions, less ascites, and less protein-losing enteropathy. I say *subtly* obstructed because there may be little or no pressure gradient to signal that significant obstruction in fact is present.

Wiesman and colleagues[522] made this important point in a paper titled "Energy-depleting fluid-flow distributions associated with small pressure change: relevance to obstructed total cavopulmonary connections." Using a computer-based model of nonpulsatile fluid flow to simulate anatomic obstructions in systemic venous–to–pulmonary venous pathways, they showed that significant anatomic obstruction can coexist with very small pressure changes (<1 mm Hg). Wedge-like or circumferential narrowing, with 40% reduction in conduit cross-sectional area, led to an average gradient of 0.2 mm Hg. Despite these tiny pressure gradients, prominent regions of flow stagnation and flow reversal were found in their model distal to these obstructions.

These authors[522] concluded that "the treatment strategy in post-Fontan patients should be to anatomically streamline cavopulmonary passages, either by surgery or interventional catheterization procedures, in order to achieve the most gradual alterations of flow characteristic possible, and thereby

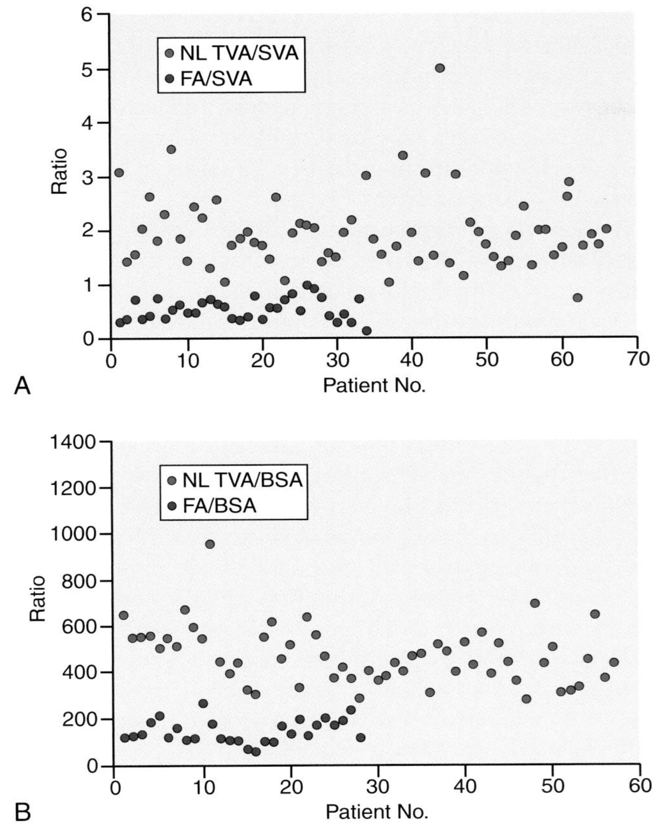

Fig. 13.43 **Was the Fontan Obstructive?** In (A), the areas of the Fontan anastomoses are indexed to the systemic vein area, i.e., FA/SVA. These ratios are shown as *blue circles*. The normal tricuspid valve areas, which are the normal right atrial outlet areas, are also indexed to the systemic vein areas, i.e., TVA/SVA. These normal control ratios are shown as *red circles*. There is almost no overlap between the much smaller Fontan indices *(black circles)* and the normal control indices *(white circles)*. In (B), the Fontan areas are indexed to the body surface areas, i.e., FA/BSA *(black circles)*. The normal control tricuspid valve areas are also indexed to the body surface area, i.e., TVA/BSA *(white circles)*. Comparison of the Fontan indices *(black circles)* with the normal tricuspid valve indices *(white circles)* reveals that there is no overlap between the much smaller Fontan ratios and the much larger normal tricuspid valve ratios. (Reproduced with permission from Kiaffas MG, Van Praagh R, Hanioti C, Green DW: The modified Fontan procedure: morphometry and surgical implications. *Ann Thorac Surg* 1999;67:1746.)

materially reduce energy wastage. We believe that maintaining an energy-efficient cavopulmonary circulation will undoubtedly improve the long-term clinical outcome of modified Fontan patients."

Exactly. And this is also why such "no-gradient" obstructions must be detected, not hemodynamically, but with echocardiography (including Doppler) and/or magnetic resonance imaging or with other methodologies that will not be deceived by very small or absent pressure gradients. Our study[513] persuaded us that clinical morphometry, searching for obstruction sites in the Fontan pathways, could be very helpful both diagnostically and therapeutically in postoperative Fontan patients.

We were assuming that the normal tricuspid valve area, bearing in mind the age and body surface area of the patient, is the optimal right atrial exit dimension; this we regarded as the normal value.[513] However, the blood flow characteristics may also be important, as was pointed out to me in a conference by an experienced cardiac surgeon, Dr. Douglas M. Behrendt. Normally, the tricuspid valve is faced with *pulsatile* blood flow, and most of the transtricuspid blood flow occurs during right atrial systole. However, following the Fontan procedure (atriopulmonary anastomosis, or cavopulmonary anastomosis, or both), the blood flow is *nonpulsatile* and occurs throughout the cardiac cycle (systole and diastole), rather than mostly during right atrial systole. Consequently, the normal tricuspid valve area may be larger than is necessary for a nonpulsatile continuous-flow Fontan pathway. On the other hand, a nonpulsatile continuous-flow Fontan pathway typically lacks the assistance of the right atrial "kick." In view of the foregoing reservations, the assumption that the tricuspid valve area is the normal right atrial exit dimension applicable to the Fontan pathway(s) may be too generous (larger than necessary). The tricuspid valve area may need to be multiplied by a correction factor, the value of which is unknown at present.

Nonetheless, if the narrowest point in the Fontan pathway equals or closely approximates the normal tricuspid valve area for the patient, then prepulmonary stenosis has been avoided. This would be an important surgical achievement, not found in any of our Fontan fatalities (Fig. 13.43A and B).

The Fontan anastomosis or anastomoses (Fig. 13.42A and B) often were not the only sites of obstruction in Fontan pathways. The pulmonary artery branches frequently were also sites of obstruction. To quantitate the degree of pulmonary artery branch obstruction, the narrowest cross-sectional area of the right pulmonary artery (RPA) and the narrowest cross-sectional area of the left pulmonary artery (LPA) were summed in 14 Fontan heart specimens; the RPA area plus the LPA area was termed the total pulmonary artery (TPA) (Table 13.20). The TPA/SVA averaged 0.79 ± 0.67, and ranged from a low of 0.24 to a high of 2.60.

In our Fontan patients, the pulmonary artery branches usually were not as obstructive as the Fontan anastomoses: TPA/SVA averaged 0.79 ± 0.67, range 0.24 ± 0.22, versus FA/SVA, which averaged 0.54 ± 0.22 and ranged from 0.13 to 0.98 (Table 13.20). However, as the standard deviation and the lower end of the range of the TPA/SVA indicate, the total pulmonary area was occasionally much smaller than the average Fontan anastomosis area. Thus, small pulmonary artery branches can be a very important problem in the management of Fontan patients, and this unfortunately cannot be fixed by surgical redesign or improved surgical technique.

Our therapeutic thoughts regarding the problem of very small pulmonary artery branches include (1) the possibility of a pre-Fontan aortopulmonary shunt, which may have the advantage of making the pulmonary artery branches grow, but which may also have the disadvantage of leading to systemic ventricular hypertrophy with associated diastolic dysfunction; and (2) heart and lung transplant, also a suboptimal therapeutic option for an infant or young child at the present time (because of accelerated coronary atherosclerosis leading to the need for multiple cardiac transplants).

Systemic ventricular hypertrophy and enlargement is another factor that is important concerning the leading cause of death in our Fontan patients, congestive heart failure (82% of fatalities, Table 13.18). Systemic ventricular hypertrophy and enlargement—*left* ventricular hypertrophy and enlargement in our patients with tricuspid atresia—were often marked in these Fontan hearts, compared with normal controls (Table 13.22).[513]

After the modified Fontan procedure, systemic left ventricular hypertrophy is disadvantageous not only because it leads to left ventricular diastolic dysfunction,[523] which in turn is associated with reduced cardiac output, but also because systemic ventricular hypertrophy is an independent risk factor for sudden arrhythmic death.[524]

ARRHYTHMIAS

The second main cause of death following the Fontan procedure in our experience was arrhythmias (12%, Table 13.18).[513] In the lateral tunnel Fontan, the baffle was often sutured to the crista terminalis, just lateral to the entry of the superior vena cava into the right atrium. The crista terminalis (terminal crest) internally corresponds to the sulcus terminalis externally, where the sinoatrial node—the pacemaker of the heart—is located. Deep sutures into the crista terminalis can traumatize the SA node and can lead to thrombosis of the sinoatrial nodal artery, resulting in sick sinus syndrome. The problem is that sick sinus syndrome is associated with sudden arrhythmic death.

This is also what happened following an otherwise successful Mustard atrial switch procedure for transposition of the great arteries: downtown, shopping with Mommy, and suddenly the child dropped dead (sudden arrhythmic death). This was a tragically frequent post-Mustard story, that helped to discredit this atrial switch operation for transposition. Similarly, the lateral tunnel modification of the Fontan procedure, despite its energy-conserving advantages, looks as though it were designed to produce sick sinus syndrome and other atrial arrhythmias. The total cavopulmonary anastomosis with an extracardiac conduit from the inferior vena cava to the right pulmonary artery promises to be a significant improvement in terms of arrhythmias. But as always, time will tell.

Please do not misunderstand. I am not casting aspersions. The Mustard procedure was an epochal improvement in the management of patients with transposition of the great arteries when it was introduced. I began my training in pediatrics and pediatric cardiology at the Hospital for Sick Children in Toronto, and Dr. Bill Mustard was a good personal friend. Similarly, the lateral-tunnel Fontan was considered by almost all observers to be an important and favorable modification when it was introduced. But over time, we all gradually learned what its advantages and its disadvantages were. My task is to try to tell the truth—to the degree to which we currently understand it, without offending anyone. It should also be emphasized that some of what we currently think may well prove to be wrong, or only part of the truth. I am reminded of a lecture that I was privileged to hear by Dr. Paul Wood, the legendary cardiologist from London, England (a native Australian). His concluding words were: "Half of what I have told you today is wrong. Unfortunately, I don't know which half. It will be up to you to find out."

TABLE 13.22 Ventricular Wall Thickness

Ventricular Free Wall Thickness (mm)	No. of Cases	Mean	SD	Range
Normal Hearts				
RV inlet	66	3.1	0.96	2–6
RV outlet	66	2.4	0.66	1–4
LV posterior wall	66	6.9	1.79	4–14
LV anterior wall	66	6.3	0.96	3–12
Fontan Hearts, Systemic Ventricles				
RV inlet	15	10.6	1.21	9–13
RV outlet	15	9.7	2.09	7–14
LV posterior wall	14	10.5	2.9	6–16
LV anterior wall	14	9.7	2.09	7–14

The normal left ventricular free-wall thickness averaged 6.6 mm, compared with 10.1 mm in these Fontan hearts (Table 13.22), 53% greater than normal.
LV, Left ventricle; *RV*, right ventricle.

Surgical Implications

Since the two main causes of death following the modified Fontan procedure were congestive heart failure (82%) and arrhythmias (12%) (Table 13.18),[513] the guiding principles in surgical management should be (1) to eliminate or minimize all forms of prepulmonary stenosis that obstruct the Fontan pathways to the lungs and (2) to eliminate or minimize all causes of atrial and ventricular arrhythmias. A vital dye (such as tricarbocyanine dye II and Evans blue) may be instilled into the aortic root with the cardioplegia solution, making the sinoatrial nodal artery more readily visible, thereby helping to avoid inadvertent surgical injury of this important artery. This suggestion of visualizing the SA nodal artery was made to me by Dr. "Billy" Kreutzer of Buenos Aires, the independent co-inventor of the **Fontan-Kreutzer procedure.**

1. It is important that the lungs be perfused with hepatic blood so as to avoid the development of pulmonary arteriovenous malformations.
2. The pulmonary artery branches should be relatively well developed and nonobstructive.
3. Pulmonary vascular obstructive disease should be absent or minimal.
4. Mitral regurgitation or stenosis should be absent or minimal.
5. Left ventricular hypertrophy and enlargement should be absent or minimal.
6. To detect significant obstruction of the Fontan pathways postoperatively, patients should be studied morphometrically, because important stenosis can be present with little or no gradient. The cross-sectional area of the Fontan anastomosis or anastomoses (FA) can be indexed to the

cross-sectional area of the inferior vena cava plus the cross-sectional area of the superior vena cava (called the systemic vein area [SVA]), that is, the FA/SVA ratio; or the FA can be indexed to the body surface area (BSA), that is, the FA/BSA ratio. Either of these ratios can then be compared with normal, the tricuspid valve cross-sectional area (TVA), which can be indexed to the SVA or the BSA, that is, the TVA/SVA or the TVA/BSA ratio. Then the Fontan ratio (FA/SVA or FA/BSA) can be compared with what is anatomically normal (TVA/SVA or TVA/BSA). This comparison indicates quantitatively whether the Fontan anastomosis/anastomoses is/are obstructive or not, and if obstructive, by what percentage compared with normal.

7. Similarly, morphometry can be used to assess whether or not the pulmonary artery branches are obstructive. The cross-sectional area of the RPA plus the cross-sectional area of the LPA (called the total pulmonary area [TPA]) can be indexed to the venae cavae (TPA/SVA) or to the body surface area (TPA/BSA). These ratios may then be compared with the anatomically normal: TVA/SVA or TVA/BSA.
8. If the SVA (IVC area + SVC area) is found to be enlarging post-Fontan, this observation suggests either that obstruction is present in the Fontan pathway, or that some degree of heart failure is present.

We hope that imaging morphometry will prove to be helpful in the diagnosis and management of these patients.

The Evolution of the Right Ventricle and Tricuspid Valve and Its Relation to the Diagnosis and Surgical Management of Congenital Heart Disease. Can an understanding of the evolution (phylogeny) and of the embryology (ontogeny) of the morphologically right ventricle (RV) and tricuspid valve (TV) help in the understanding of tricuspid atresia? I think so and consequently I am going briefly to tell you this tale.[525]

Dr. Billy Kreutzer asked me to investigate these questions. He organized an international symposium on right ventricular bypass in Buenos Aires (October 23–26, 1994), and this is one of the things he asked me to talk about.[525] The questions were many:

How, why, and when did the RV evolve?

Does ontogeny (embryology) really recapitulate phylogeny (evolution), as Ernst Haeckel (1834–1919) of Jena famously said?

Does an understanding of the evolution and the embryology of the human heart—with a focus on the RV—help to make congenital heart disease, including tricuspid atresia, more comprehensible? The answer is more than yes. This is a fascinating story for virtually all serious students of biology.

First, who discovered evolution? Was it Darwin[526] and Wallace, as is usually said? The answer is no. As far as we have been able to discover, evolution was in fact discovered by (or before) **Empedocles,** the brilliant pre-Socratic physicist who lived from 495 to 435 BC in Acragas (now Agrigento) in Sicily, which at the time was part of Magna Graecia (Great Greece).

Empedocles realized not only the existence of evolution, but how it works: the occurrence by *chance* of favorable changes that favor survival and reproduction.[527,528]

Anaximander (ca. 611–547 BC) of Miletus, a student of Thales, also is thought to have been convinced of evolution a century before Empedocles. Anaximander credits the **Syrians** with this understanding before him. The Syrians thought that man had evolved from fish and consequently the Syrians revered fish as their ancestor. But it was **Empedocles,** a pre-Socratic materialist or physicist who first clearly described the theory of evolution, by natural selection, leading to survival of the fittest.[527,528]

Professional historians, such as Will Durant,[529] have long known about Empedocles and have attributed the discovery of evolution to him. But this understanding has seldom filtered down to the level of modern physicians and other modern biological scientists. Consequently, what I am writing here may come as quite a surprise, even a shock, to modern medical readers.

Empedocles deserves the credit for having understood evolution and for having persuaded the scientifically minded of the ancient world. For example, Empedocles' concept of evolution was incorporated by the ancient Roman writer Lucretius (99 or 95 to 55 or 51 BC) into his famous work *De Rerum Natura (On the Nature of Things).*[529]

Darwin[526] deserves the credit for having *rediscovered* evolution and for having persuaded the scientific modern world. The historian Will Durant ironically refers to the nineteenth century as that echo chamber of ancient science.[529]

PHYLOGENY

Homo sapiens sapiens—our modest name for ourselves (meaning "man wise wise," or "wise wise man") belongs to the *phylum chordata,* which includes all animals with a notochord (meaning a back cord, Greek). The notochord marks the long axis of the embryo, indicating where the vertebrae and the brain will develop. (So, the notochord really is the back cord.) The chordates are essentially synonymous with the vertebrates.

From the phylogenetic (evolutionary) standpoint, our remote ancestors were the **ancient fish** of the Ordovician period and the upper Devonian period, 500 million to 345 million years ago.[520]

So, as we now know, Empedocles, Anaximander, and the Syrians were essentially right. Man did evolve from an aquatic vertebrate ancestor; and this understanding is more than 2500 years old.

In craniate vertebrates such as fish (Fig. 13.44),[530] the heart is a specialized pulsatile part of the primary longitudinal ventral blood vessel that pumps venous blood from the ducts of Cuvier and the hepatic veins forward and upward through the gills, where oxygenation takes place.[530]

As long as our vertebrate ancestors "breathed" water, there was a single circulation and no need for an RV.

But in the early Carboniferous period about 325 million years ago, **amphibians** evolved. These animals developed lungs and so could breathe air, but they still had to breed in the water, like modern frogs.

From these primitive amphibians evolved not only modern amphibians, but also fully terrestrial animals that did not need to breed in the water. These were the **Amniota**—all animals with

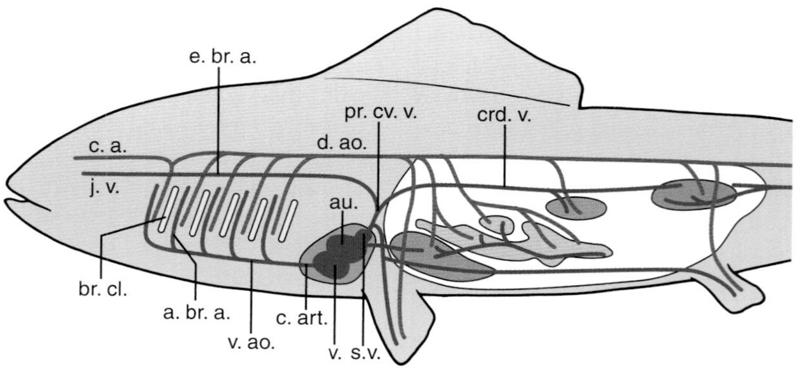

Fig. 13.44 In craniate vertebrates such as fish, the cardiovascular system is specialized for "breathing" water. There is a single cardiovascular system, the systemic (not a double cardiovascular system—systemic and pulmonary—as in air-breathing animals: Reptilia, Aves, and Mammalia). The vertebrate heart began as a specialized pulsatile part of the primary longitudinal ventral blood vessel. The heart of the fish has four chambers, but these four chambers are different from those of an air-breathing mammal. Systemic venous unoxygenated blood *(stippled)* returns to the common cardinal vein or duct of Cuvier (*pr. cv. v.* = precaval vein) and then passes into the sinus venosus *(s.v.)*, which is the first of the four cardiac chambers of the piscine heart. The sinus venosus is the small chamber to which all of the systemic venous blood returns—from the cranial part of the body (*j. v.* = jugular vein) and from the caudal part of the body (*crd. v.* = cardinal vein). From the sinus venosus, the blood passes into the atrium (*au.* = auricle), which is the second cardiac chamber or compartment. Then, the systemic venous unoxygenated blood passes into the ventricle *(v.)*, the third cardiac compartment. Last, the blood is pumped into the conus arteriosus *(c. art.)*, the fourth cardiac compartment. All of the arterial blood is ejected from the conus arteriosus into the ventral aorta *(v. ao.)*, all still unoxygenated. Another way of viewing the fish heart is to say that it has only two chambers, an atrium and ventricle, with one systemic venous connection and one systemic arterial connection. (*Sinus, ūs* = a bending, a curve, a fold, Latin, fourth declension masculine noun. *Conus,-i*, a cone, Latin, second declension masculine noun.) Blood is pumped from the conus arteriosus into the v. ao. and thence via the afferent branchial arteries *(a. br. a.)* up to the gills, where oxygenation occurs (oxygenated blood is shown as *black*; *br. cl.* = brachial cleft). Then the oxygenated blood passes to the head via the carotid artery *(c. a.)* and to the lower body via the dorsal aorta *(d. ao.)*. Many details are omitted from this diagram, such as the sinoatrial valve, the atrioventricular valve, the semilunar valves in the conus arteriosus, and the coronary arteries (that arise from the efferent branchial arteries and bring oxygenated blood down to the heart). (Reproduced with permission from Robb JS: *Comparative Basic Cardiology*. New York, Grune & Stratton, 1965.)

an amniotic sac. (If you would like to review what the amniotic sac is, or the ducts of Cuvier, etc., see Chapter 2.)

The amniotic sac surrounds a "mare internum" (internal sea) of amniotic fluid in which the embryo and later the fetus floats, like our aquatic vertebrate ancestors. The terrestrial Amniota then evolved into reptiles, birds (feathered reptiles), and mammals (furry or hairy reptiles).

The amniotic sac was one of the most important developments that made possible the colonization of the land. Amniotes did not need to return to the water to breed. Land-living and air-breathing had become possible.

Internal fertilization by copulation was another very important evolutionary development in the vertebrate conquest of the land, or flight from the water. (Which was it? We may never know.) Aquatic vertebrates (fish and amphibian) spread their sperm over the eggs in the water (external fertilization); but this was no longer an option for the fully terrestrial amniotes (hence internal fertilization).

Mammals evolved during the Jurassic period some 180 million years ago when reptiles—including giant dinosaurs (meaning fearful or monstrous lizards, Greek)—were lords of the earth.

Although fish and amphibian have no right ventricle, higher reptiles, birds, and mammals do.

The evolution of the right ventricle from the conus arteriosus was one of the most important cardiovascular adaptations of the Amniote vertebrates to air-breathing and land-living. In higher reptiles, birds, and mammals, the RV is the lung pump. The ancient ventricle of our phylum, now the morphologically left ventricle (LV), remains the body or systemic pump.

The evolution of the RV was a critically important part of the development of a **double circulation**—pulmonary and systemic—in fully terrestrial vertebrates. By contrast, in fully aquatic and partially aquatic vertebrates, there is only a single circulation—the systemic, which also supplies the organs of respiration (gills, lungs, and skin).

Why is the RV the **right** ventricle? Because D-loop formation places the conus arteriosus, from which the RV sinus develops, to the right of the ventricle of the bulboventricular loop. D-loop formation also makes the ventricle of the bulboventricular loop the **left** ventricle (LV).

D-loop formation is normal for our phylum chordata and it occurred before the double circulation evolved. For example, sharks are ancient cartilaginous fish (Chondrichthyes), and shark hearts display D-bulboventricular loops.[525] D-loop formation is part of visceral **situs solitus**—the usual anatomic pattern of the viscera (*solitus* = customary, habitual, usual; Latin).

Occasionally in vertebrates, **situs inversus totalis** occurs in which all of the viscera are mirror-images of those in situs solitus. Mirror-imagery is characterized by right-left reversal, but without anterior-posterior or superior-inferior change.

In situs inversus totalis, **bulboventricular L-loop formation** occurs, placing the morphologically right ventricle to the left of the morphologically left ventricle. Hence, with L-looping, the RV is left-sided relative to the LV, which is right-sided. Briefly, L-loop formation results in RV (L) and LV (R).

Because of the variations in bulboventricular loop formation that can occur, in complex congenital heart disease it is essential to identify the ventricles both *morphologically* (RV or LV) and *positionally* (right-sided, left-sided, superior, inferior, anterior, posterior).

Chirality or handedness can be very helpful in figuring out which type of ventricular situs is present, particularly when bulboventricular loop formation is very abnormal, as in superoinferior ventricles. With **solitus ventricles,** in which D-loop formation has—or "should have"—occurred, the RV is right-handed and the LV is left-handed.[525] Conversely, with **inversus ventricles,** in which L-loop formation has—or "should have"—occurred, the RV is left-handed and the LV is right-handed. D-loop ventricles in situs solitus and L-loop ventricles in situs inversus totalis are stereoisomers.

Why are visceroatrial situs solitus and bulboventricular D-loops vastly more frequent than visceroatrial situs inversus and bulboventricular L-loops in both aquatic and terrestrial vertebrates? The answers to these questions are unknown at present, but they may well prove to be genetic.[531] However, even when the genetic cascades controlling the development of visceroatrial situs solitus and bulboventricular D-loop formation are fully identified, the question may well still remain, Why were these genetic systems selected and not others? Did vertebrate life evolve only once, and is what we call situs solitus what our original ancestors (male and female) had?

Ontogeny*

From the ontogenetic or embryologic standpoint in human embryos, the **cardiogenic crescent** of precardiac mesoderm appears between 16 and 20 days following ovulation (Streeter's horizons 8 and 9), when the first pair of somites is appearing and when the human embryo is 1.5 mm in length (as in Davis's Carnegie embryo #5080).[525]

The **straight tube or pre-loop stage** is reached in humans by 20 to 22 days of age in utero (horizon 10, as in Davis's Carnegie embryo #4216, which has seven pairs of somites and is now 2.2 mm long). D-loop formation begins at this stage. The human heartbeat also probably begins at this time (estimate based on our chick embryo studies).

D-loop formation normally is completed in the human embryo between 22 and 24 days (horizon 11, as in Davis's Carnegie embryo #470, which has 16 pairs of somites and is 3.3 mm long). No outpouchings or evaginations of the future LV and RV sinuses have as yet occurred. There is a **single in-series circulation** beginning in the human embryo, reminiscent of the circulation of a fish: right atrium (RA), to left atrium (LA), to future LV, to future RV, and to future great arteries.

At this stage (normally 22 to 24 days of age at the completion of D-loop formation, horizon 11), the bulbus cordis or conus arteriosus lies to the right of and mildly posterior to the ventricle of the bulboventricular D-loop.

For a pediatric cardiologist, radiologist, or cardiac surgeon, this is a fascinating stage in normal human cardiac development because so many different forms of congenital heart disease are potentially present:[525]

1. The conotruncus lies to the right of the right atrial appendage; that is, **left-sided juxtaposition of the atrial appendages** is present (levomalposition of the right atrial appendage, which lies to the left of the great arteries).
2. The developing ventricular apex points to the right; that is, **dextrocardia** is present.
3. The single in-series circulation resembles that of **tricuspid atresia,** and that of **double-inlet or common-inlet left ventricle.** The blood goes from the RA into the LA, and then from the LA into the future LV.
4. Both developing great arteries are located above the future RV sinus; that is, **double-outlet right ventricle** is potentially present. ("Potentially" means that unless normal development continues, DORV would be present.)

Thus, if normal cardiovascular development is arrested at horizon 11 or 22 to 24 days of age in utero, the foregoing is a list of those forms of congenital heart disease that one may expect.

By **26 to 28 days of age** in utero (horizon 13, as in Carnegie embryo #836, which has 30 pairs of somites and is 4 mm long), both the LV sinus and the RV sinus are beginning to outpouch or evaginate from the greater curvature of the bulboventricular D-loop. The LV sinus is developing faster and is larger than the RV sinus. The RV sinus is still somewhat posterior to the LV sinus. The developing ventricular apex is still pointing to the right; that is, dextrocardia is still present. The right atrial appendage is starting to bulge to the right of the great arteries, so the earlier left-sided juxtaposition of the atrial appendages is starting to be "cured" during horizon 13 (26 to 28 days of age).

By **30 to 32 days of age** in utero (horizon 15, as in Carnegie embryo #3385, which is 8.3 mm in length), considerably more outpouching of the ventricular sinuses has normally occurred. Although the RV sinus is still smaller than the LV sinus, the growth of the RV sinus is catching up with that of the LV. The ventricles have swung horizontally leftward so that the developing ventricular septum occupies an approximately sagittal plane. Mesocardia is now present. Dextrocardia has been "cured." Left-sided juxtaposition of the atrial appendages has by now normally completely disappeared because the right atrium lies entirely to the right of the great arteries.

By **32 to 34 days of age** (horizon 16), ostium primum has been almost completely closed by the growth of the endocardial cushions of the atrioventricular canal (as in Carnegie embryo #6510, which is 10.1 mm in length).

By **34 to 36 days of age** (horizon 17), ostium primum normally is completely closed. The tricuspid valve now opens into the RV, and the RV is almost as large as the LV. Mesocardia is still present.

*See Chapter 2 for appropriate figures, as needed.

By **38 to 40 days of age,** the ventricular apex normally points leftward; levocardia has been achieved (as in Carnegie embryo #6520, which is 14.2 mm in length). The RV sinus is now as large as the LV sinus; normally a fully biventricular heart has now developed. Cardiac morphogenesis is now largely complete, except that the interventricular foramen (the ventricular septal defect) is still open.

By **38 to 45 days of age** in utero, the interventricular foramen normally is closed, at its rightmost end, adjacent to the tricuspid valve. As all pediatric cardiologists know, the interventricular foramen can take much longer to close; it can remain patent until after birth, accounting for "spontaneous closure" of ventricular septal defects. Spontaneous closure is late or delayed VSD closure, "spontaneous" meaning surgically or interventionally unassisted VSD closure.

What is the membranous septum (pars membranacea septi)? It is superior endocardial cushion tissue that is intimately related to the tricuspid valve. The membranous septum lies between the anterior and the septal leaflets of the tricuspid valve. A membranous septal defect here can result in a **left ventricular-to-right atrial shunt,** often called a Gerbode shunt, that goes through the tricuspid valve. A defect below this superior commissure of the tricuspid valve results is a defect in the interventricular portion of the membranous septum, this being a **typical membranous VSD.** A defect above the superior commissure of the tricuspid valve (between the anterior and septal leaflets) results in an **LV-to-RA shunt**. Thus, where the shunt goes on the right side of the heart depends on what part of the membranous septum is involved in the defect.

(Perhaps I should add parenthetically that I have had the privilege of studying the above-mentioned Carnegie embryos in person, both the histologic slides and the reconstructions. Many of these embryos are presented pictorially in Chapter 2 and hence are not repeated here. All of the embryos are presented photographically in the 1995 paper.[525])

So, does ontogeny (embryology) recapitulate phylogenic (evolution), as Ernst Haeckel said in his famous biogenic law? Yes. As we have seen, the human heart beings at 20 days of age as a single in-series circulation similar to that of a fish, and ends 25 days later at 45 days of age as the double in-parallel circulations of an air-breathing and land-living mammal. These approximately 25 days of human cardiac development—from the straight heart tube at day 20 to the closure of the interventricular foramen at day 45—do indeed recapitulate the 500-million-year history of the cardiovascular system of our phylum Chordata. The genes, with their many favorable mutations, have an amazingly long and accurate memory. But it is also the occasional copying errors—the mutations—that have made it all possible: no mutations, no evolution.

While some mutations are favorable to survival and reproduction, many are not. Those responsible for much of congenital heart disease exemplify unfavorable mutations, as our molecular geneticists are now discovering.

We should remember **Ernst Haeckel** (1834–1919) not only for his biogenic law or recapitulation theory. He was also **the founder of modern morphology.** Born in Potsdam, he studied medicine at Wurzberg, Berlin, and Vienna. He quit medicine to become professor of zoology at Jena in 1862. In 1866, he published *General Morphology*. His other publications included *Natural History of Creation* in 1868 and *Anthropogeny or the Evolution of Man* in 1874, the latter being a study of human embryology. He coined the terms **"ontogeny," "phylogeny,"** and **"ecology."**

What Is Tricuspid Atresia From the Phylogenetic and Ontogenetic Viewpoints?

In our phylum Chordata, the LV is the ancient "professional" systemic pump. It is at least 500 million years old and is seldom involved in primary malformation. By contrast, the RV is a "Johnny Come Lately," a relative newcomer. It is only about 180 million years old, only 36% as old as the LV. The RV is very much more prone to malformation than is the LV, apparently because the RV is a much more complex, more recently evolved, and much more composite structure than is the LV.

Viewed segmentally (Fig. 13.5a), the normal definitive RV is composed as follows:

1. There is a proximal connecting segment, the atrioventricular (AV) canal or junction (component 1, Fig. 13.5a);
2. A distal connecting segment, the conus arteriosus or infundibulum (components 3 and 4, Fig. 13.5a); and
3. A relatively small main segment, the RV sinus or pumping portion (component 2, Fig. 13.5a).

Each of the four components of the definitive normal RV has an important function:

1. The atrioventricular canal or junction (component 1, Fig. 13.5a) forms the tricuspid valve, which prevents right ventriculoatrial regurgitation. It also plays an important role in septation, forming the atrioventricular septum.
2. The relatively small RV sinus is the pumping portion. It is located below and behind the ring of conal musculature formed by the conal septum and parietal band, the septal band, and the moderator band (component 2, Fig. 13.5a). The definitive normal RV is approximately half RV sinus (inflow tract) and half outflow tract (conus arteriosus); whereas the definitive normal LV is almost all sinus (or pumping portion), very little conus normally being fused with the LV sinus.
3. The septal band (component 3, Fig. 13.5A) is the proximal or apical part of the conus. The septal band appears to be the "mother" of the RV sinus. The septal band and the RV sinus never dissociate (whereas the parietal band and the RV sinus frequently do). Whenever an RV sinus is present, it is always located right beneath the septal band. So it is from, or just beneath, this part of the conus that the RV sinus evolved and normally develops in humans.
4. The conal septum, parietal band, and contiguous subsemilunar free wall (component 4, Fig. 13.5a) is the distal or subsemilunar part of the conus arteriosus or infundibulum that can be involved in conotruncal malformations such as transposition of the great arteries.

What is the subsemilunar conus doing there in the normal heart? It is not a good pump. Comparative anatomy and physiology[11] have revealed that in some animals, the conus squeezes in order to help prevent arterioventricular regurgitation, and in other animals it moves little or not at all.

The distal or subsemilunar part of the conus arteriosus normally performs nature's arterial switch operation. The starting position following D-loop formation is DORV {S,D,D} with a bilateral conus, reminiscent of the Taussig-Bing malformation. Normally, the subaortic conal free wall undergoes resorption (apoptosis), while the subpulmonary conal free wall grows and expands. Involution of the subaortic conal free wall permits aortic-mitral approximation and direct fibrous continuity via the intervalvular fibrosa. Expansile growth and development of the subpulmonary part of the conus elevates the pulmonary valve superiorly and carries it anteriorly, away from the VSD. Then the interventricular foramen closes at its rightmost or tricuspid end, separating the ventricles and making the aorta draining the LV only, and the pulmonary artery the RV only.

This process is called the crossing of the circulations because this is how it looks in a lateral view (angiocardiographically, for example). Normally, the *posterior* LV ejects into the *anterior* aortic arches 4, while the *anterior* RV ejects into the *posterior* pulmonary arches 6. The normal unilateral resorption of the subaortic conal free wall and growth of the subpulmonary conal free wall switches the developing aortic valve posteriorly toward the mitral valve, and switches the developing pulmonary valve anteriorly—away from both AV valves. So, normal conal development (resorption and growth) literally does switch the semilunar valves, like a railway switch changing the direction of train tracks.

This arterial switch maneuver is not performed if the wrong half of the conus undergoes resorption (of the subpulmonary conal free wall, permitting pulmonary-mitral approximation and fibrous continuity) and if the wrong half of the conus undergoes growth (the subaortic conal free wall, preventing aortic-AV valve fibrous continuity, as in transposition of the great arteries). In the lateral view, transposed great arteries then appear parallel, not crossed. The *anterior* RV ejects into the *anterior* aortic arches 4, and the *posterior* LV ejects into the *posterior* pulmonary arches 6.

Phylogenetically and ontogenetically, what is tricuspid atresia? Approximately 180 million years of vertebrate cardiac evolution have been partially erased. The tricuspid valve is totally or partially absent, and the right ventricular sinus is totally or partially absent: components 1 and 2 of the normal definitive RV are missing (Fig. 13.5A). This is the situation when tricuspid atresia is associated with normally related great arteries, as it was in 59% of our cases (Table 13.11, 55 of 94 = 58.51%, or 59%). However, tricuspid atresia was associated with infundibuloarterial (conotruncal) malformations (we think basically *conal* malformations) in the remaining 41% of our patients (Table 13.11).

Transposition of the great arteries, double-outlet right ventricle, double-outlet left ventricle, anatomically corrected malposition of the great arteries, and "corrected" transposition of the great arteries all have infundibular malformations. (For more information, see the appropriate chapters.) "Corrected" transposition has a ventricular anomaly in addition to an infundibular malformation. Truncus arteriosus has both infundibular and great arterial malformations.

Thus, more than 40% of these patients had more than tricuspid atresia (Table 13.11).

From both a phylogenetic and an ontogenetic perspective, we have long thought that **"tricuspid atresia" is really absence of the RV sinus and absence of the tricuspid valve.** In other words, the emphasis really should go on absence (or extreme hypoplasia) of the RV sinus. Absence of the tricuspid valve is really secondary to absence of the RV sinus. In our first study of juxtaposition of the atrial appendages,[242] absence or marked hypoplasia of the RV sinus (71%) was almost twice as common as was tricuspid atresia or extreme stenosis (40%), suggesting that absence or marked hypoplasia of the RV sinus was the more basic anomaly, with tricuspid atresia or severe congenital tricuspid stenosis also often being present, but not always. In the anomaly known as tricuspid atresia, up until that time (1968),[242] we had thought that the small or absent right ventricular sinus was secondary to the presence of tricuspid atresia. But the above-mentioned data (absent or very hypoplastic RV sinus = 71% and tricuspid atresia or severe stenosis = "only" 40%)[242] made us realize that the basic anomaly probably was absence or extreme hypoplasia of the right ventricular sinus, not so-called tricuspid atresia, in which this valve also typically appeared to be absent (not present but imperforate).

As mentioned earlier, this also suggests that "tricuspid atresia" and single LV with double-inlet or common-inlet LV are very closely related anomalies. We think that the "tricuspid valve" of double-inlet LV is not the normal tricuspid valve. Instead, it appears that in double-inlet LV, the essentially mitral valve has undergone subdivision relative to the overlying atrial septum; that is, we think that what is known as double-inlet LV may well really be double-orifice mitral valve with both ostia opening into the single LV.

Both tricuspid atresia and double-inlet LV typically have absence of the RV sinus: This is the real common denominator, we think, despite the differing anatomy of the mitral valve: undivided in tricuspid atresia; and subdivided in double-inlet LV. The latter is presented as a hypothesis. The "real" or "true" tricuspid valve must have a right ventricular component, as Ebstein's anomaly indicates. Normally, the septal leaflet of the tricuspid valve delaminates from the right ventricular septal surface and then ascends to or toward the right atrioventricular junction, this being what fails to happen in typical Ebstein's malformation.

One may say that the tricuspid valve in double-inlet LV is the "real" or "true" tricuspid valve, except that it lacks a right ventricular component to its septal leaflet. This may prove to be correct.

Again, we are not suggesting any change in diagnostic terminology. The foregoing is written only in the interests of better understanding.

What Is the Significance of Right Ventricular Evolution to Human Congenital Heart Disease?

Malformation of the LV is uncommon. By contrast, much of what we call congenital heart disease consists of anomalies of that evolutionary "newcomer," the RV. The RV evolved as one of our major adaptations to air-breathing and land-living:

1. The RV sinus serves as a lung pump, but normally has never served as the systemic pump. This point is relevant to the atrial switch procedures (Mustard and Senning) for transposition of the great arteries, and to the modified Fontan procedures with a systemic RV.
2. The tricuspid valve plays an important role in septation, being intimately related to the membranous septum.

3. The subsemilunar part of the conus arteriosus crosses the circulations, which is essential to avoid physiologic uncorrection of the circulations (as in transposition and in double-outlet RV).
4. The small RV sinus is essential to achieving a double circulation, pulmonary as well as systemic: no RV sinus, no double circulation. The other components of the RV can be normal, but to no avail physiologically. The proximal connecting segment, the tricuspid valve, can be (or appear to be) normal. But when the small RV sinus is absent, the result is double-inlet LV *per force* (because there is no RV sinus to open into). The distal connecting segment, the conus, can be normal, but to no avail. The result is a Holmes heart: single LV with double-inlet (or common-inlet) LV, with normally related great arteries. Thus, the RV sinus is the *sine qua non* of a double circulation.

What are some of the anomalies of the RV? They include the following:

1. tricuspid atresia;
2. single LV with double-inlet or common-inlet LV;
3. Ebstein's anomaly of the tricuspid valve and RV sinus;
4. congenitally unguarded tricuspid orifice, with partial or complete absence of the tricuspid leaflets, but with a patent "tricuspid" orifice;
5. Uhl's disease, that is, parchment right ventricle with small or large areas of the right ventricular free wall having little or no right ventricular free wall myocardium;
6. hypoplasia of the RV sinus with congenital tricuspid stenosis, or straddling tricuspid valve, or superoinferior ventricles, or crisscross AV relations;
7. double-chambered RV, with an abnormally prominent wall of muscle in the mid-RV, separating the RV sinus or inflow tract proximally from the infundibulum or conus arteriosus or outflow tract distally, that may or may not be associated with a hemodynamically demonstrable obstruction (stenosis, or rarely atresia) at the level of the mid-RV;
8. tetralogy of Fallot, that is, obstruction (stenosis or atresia) of the subpulmonary conus and the sequelae thereof (the classical tetrad);
9. truncus arteriosus, typically atresia of the subpulmonary infundibulum and pulmonary valve with an aortopulmonary septal defect;
10. transposition of the great arteries, that is, ventriculoarterial discordance (as Dr. John W. Kirklin was the first to call it), which results from several anomalies of the subsemilunar conus arteriosus;
11. double-outlet right ventricle, in which both great arteries arise entirely or predominantly above the RV, typically caused by anomalies of the subsemilunar conus arteriosus;
12. double-outlet left ventricle, in which both great arteries arise entirely or predominantly above the LV, again typically related to anomalies of the conus arteriosus; and
13. anatomically corrected malposition of the great arteries, characterized by malformations of the subsemilunar conus arteriosus and by rotational anomalies of the infundibulum and great arteries relative to the ventricles.

This list is not complete. For further information on any of these anomalies, see the appropriate chapter.

Thus, it is difficult to overstate the importance of malformation of the right ventricle in the causation of human congenital heart disease. Anomalies of the tricuspid valve (this chapter) are only part of the story.

Congenital heart disease, the most common malformation that occurs in humans, represents our continuing difficulties with our cardiovascular adaptations to air-breathing and land-living. These adaptations, which began about 180 million years ago in our prehuman vertebrate ancestors, are successful in about 99% of live-born humans. But evolution is still ongoing, which comes as no surprise when one realizes that fully modern man, a category that includes all living humans, is only about 60,000 years old.[532-534] Thus, we are a very recent life form, but with a long and fascinating evolutionary history.[532-534]

CONGENITAL TRICUSPID STENOSIS

What really is congenital tricuspid stenosis? Based on 70 postmortem cases, the answer to this question is summarized in Table 13.23.

Small-Volume Right Ventricular Sinus Cavity

A small-volume right ventricular sinus cavity, that is, a small-volume RV inflow tract, was by far the most common setting in which congenital tricuspid stenosis (TS) occurred in this series of 70 postmortem cases (48 patients, 69%, Table 13.23).

Pulmonary atresia (valvar) with intact ventricular septum was much the most frequent subset within this group (23 of 48 patients, 65%). With pulmonary valvar atresia and intact ventricular septum, typically the right ventricular cavity is small-chambered and thick-walled. Traditionally this is regarded as congenital tricuspid stenosis because the tricuspid orifice is much smaller than normal. The tricuspid valve may be a normally formed miniature, or it may be malformed, for example, with obliteration of interchordal spaces. However, there is little or no antegrade blood flow across the tricuspid valve (preoperatively), and hence from a hemodynamic standpoint, the typical tricuspid valvar and annular hypoplasia is not really a stenosis hemodynamically because of the absence of antegrade trans-tricuspid blood flow caused by the coexistence of pulmonary valvar atresia and intact ventricular septum. So this so-called congenital tricuspid "stenosis" is, in the natural (preoperative) state, potential (not actual).

TABLE 13.23 Anatomic Types of Congenital Tricuspid Stenosis ($n = 70$)

Anatomic Type	No. of Cases	% of Series
With small RV sinus	48	69
Pulmonary atresia or severe stenosis + intact ventricular septum {S,D,S} (31)		
Other (17)		
With absent RV sinus + double-inlet single LV	11	16
Ebstein's anomaly with tricuspid stenosis	10	14
Rhabdomyoma of ventricular septum	1	1

LV, Morphologically left ventricle; *RV*, morphologically right ventricle.

However, if an attempt is made to open up the right ventricular outflow tract surgically (with myocardial resection, pulmonary valvotomy or partial valvectomy, and right ventricular outflow tract patching), then the hypoplastic and sometimes dysplastic tricuspid valve and the small tricuspid annulus can become a very real and hemodynamically important tricuspid stenosis. This fact can lead to low cardiac output and death postoperatively, as we and many others have learned.

The hypoplastic and potentially stenotic tricuspid valve can permit tricuspid regurgitation. When there is little or no tricuspid regurgitation, the RV can do pressure work, but little or no flow work. The result is the typical small-chambered and thick-walled RV. But when tricuspid regurgitation occurs, the RV can do both pressure work and retrograde flow work, resulting in a larger right ventricular cavity. Thus, although pulmonary valvar atresia with an intact ventricular septum typically is small-chambered and thick-walled when little or no tricuspid regurgitation coexists, the RV cavity can be much larger when tricuspid regurgitation is present (Fig. 13.25), as was appreciated by Davignon, Edwards, and their colleagues in 1961.[218]

It should also be mentioned at this point that **pulmonary valvar atresia with intact ventricular septum is really a syndrome** that also includes tricuspid valve anomalies (hypoplasia, stenotic dysplasia, or Ebstein's anomaly), right ventricular endocardial sclerosis or fibroelastosis, right ventricular–to–coronary arterial sinusoids, coronary mural thickening with luminal narrowing or interruption where the sinusoids connect with the coronary arteries (Fig. 13.45), and a prominent right venous valve (right sinoatrial valve) that may result in a right atrial rete Chiari (Chiari's network) or an obstructive supratricuspid membrane, as was pointed out by Kauffman and Andersen[535] in 1963.

Congenital Tricuspid Stenosis With Pulmonary Atresia or Severe Pulmonary Valvar Stenosis and Intact Ventricular Septum. The salient findings in our 31 postmortem cases of congenital tricuspid stenosis with pulmonary valvar atresia or severe pulmonary valvar stenosis and intact ventricular septum—by far the largest anatomic subtype—are summarized in Table 13.24.

Looking over Table 13.24, perhaps a few words of explanation may be helpful.

How could the gender be unknown in one case? It was a fetal consultation from another hospital. We were only shown the heart specimen, and we forgot to inquire about the patient's gender.

Regarding the ages at death or cardiac transplantation, note the huge difference between the mean (average) age (1 8/12 years) and the median age (29.5 days). The mean age at death is misleadingly old, because of the long survival of a few of our patients, the oldest of whom had a successful transplant at 14 3/12 years of age (see the footnote, Table 13.24). The young median age of death gives a much more accurate picture of what a lethal anomaly pulmonary atresia or very severe stenosis with intact ventricular septum and congenital tricuspid stenosis has in fact been in our experience.

Regarding the anatomy of the tricuspid valve (Table 13.24), all 31 cases were *hypoplastic* because the right ventricle was thick-walled and small-chambered. In 10 of these cases (32%), the tricuspid valve was also *dysplastic* or malformed, with obliteration of interchordal spaces and with some degree of leaflet fusion. In 6 of these patients (19%), there was also pathologic anatomic evidence of tricuspid *regurgitation*—with thickening and rolling of the tricuspid leaflet margins and with right atrial jet lesions (areas of endocardial thickening related to the impact of tricuspid regurgitant jets).

Two of these 31 patients (6%) had *Ebstein's anomaly* with severe congenital tricuspid stenosis. Case 28 was a 17-week-old girl, the only openings through her tricuspid valve being interchordal spaces related to the anterior and posterior leaflets. A right ventricular outflow tract reconstructive repair was attempted in 1986, but without tricuspid valvuloplasty, leading to intraoperative death. Case 48 was the aforementioned 14 3/12-year-old girl who underwent successful orthotopic heart transplantation in 1993. Her explanted heart specimen revealed infantile Ebstein's malformation with severe congenital tricuspid stenosis, a 5 × 2 mm opening into the subpulmonary infundibulum, just beneath the atretic pulmonary valve. The tricuspid valve appeared to have rotated inferiorly, then anteriorly and superiorly—the anterosuperior tricuspid commissure being the apparently fixed point beneath which tricuspid valve "rotation" occurred. The tricuspid valve was located in the right ventricular outflow tract and opened into the subpulmonary infundibulum beneath the atretic pulmonary valve. There was a major component of tricuspid leaflet absence, below the very displaced tricuspid valve reminiscent of congenitally unguarded tricuspid orifice. There was also a prominent aneurysm of the diaphragmatic surface of the right ventricular free wall, with marked thinning of the right ventricular free wall myocardium, reminiscent of Uhl's disease or parchment right ventricle. Hence, this patient demonstrated the tricuspid leaflet and right ventricular myocardial features of the most severe (infantile form) of Ebstein's malformation of the tricuspid valve and right ventricle. The tricuspid valve was almost imperforate (atretic).

Quotation marks are used around "rotation" above. We think that, in fact, the tricuspid valve failed to grow, develop, delaminate, and move in the *opposite* direction: inferiorly, posteriorly, and then superiorly to reach the right atrioventricular junction. The conventional description of the tricuspid valve in Ebstein's anomaly is based on a comparison with the normal location of the tricuspid valve (downward displacement of the tricuspid valve, into the right ventricle). However, bearing in mind normal tricuspid and right ventricular sinus (inflow tract) morphogenesis, one understands *why* the tricuspid valve appears so downwardly and even anterosuperiorly displaced in Ebstein's malformation: because the tricuspid valve has *failed to ascend* to, or toward, the right atrioventricular junction in the normal way.

The therapeutic odyssey of this 14-year-old young woman is instructive. She appears to have survived because her pulmonary valvar atresia and severe tricuspid stenosis were not addressed directly. Instead, they were bypassed. At 10 days of age, a right Blalock-Taussig anastomosis and ligation of her patent ductus arteriosus were performed. Then an unsuccessful Fontan anastomosis (right atrial appendage to the pulmonary artery) led to a takedown and a Waterston anastomosis (ascending aorta to right pulmonary artery). At 3 9/12 years of age, the Waterston was replaced with a central shunt, a 5 mm Gore-Tex conduit from the ascending aorta to the right pulmonary artery.

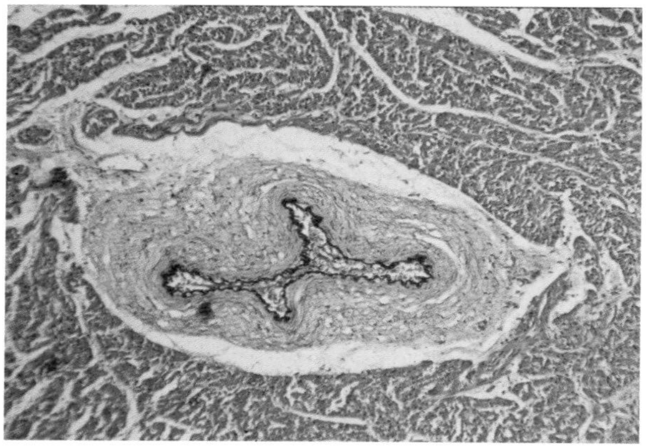

Fig. 13.45 Sinusoid from the infundibular apical recess (anterior to septal and moderator bands) to the left anterior descending coronary artery. This large collapsed sinusoid is seen traversing the left ventricular myocardium; original magnification ×10; elastic tissue stain. This 5½-month-old girl displayed most of the features of the *syndrome of pulmonary valvar atresia or extreme stenosis with intact ventricular septum:* extreme pulmonary valvar stenosis with intact ventricular septum; small-chambered and thick-walled right ventricle; moderate endocardial sclerosis of the right ventricle; hypoplasia (stenosis) of the tricuspid valve consistent with the hypoplasia of the RV inflow tract; anomalous muscle bundles of the right ventricle; high takeoff of a moderator band–like structure from the septal band; as above—sinusoid from the infundibular apical recess to the left anterior descending coronary artery, with nonobstructive coronary mural thickening and luminal narrowing close to junction with sinusoid; and prominent right venous valve (Eustachian valve) of the inferior vena cava, nonobstructive. This syndrome was identified in 1963 by Kauffman and Andersen[535] and was called the *persistent venous valve syndrome.* We think that this syndrome is better understood as *the pulmonary valvar atresia or severe stenosis with intact ventricular septum syndrome.* The larger point is that this type of congenital tricuspid stenosis, with or without sinusoids, are parts of this syndrome. This patient did *not* have Uhl's disease, also a potential part of this syndrome. The diagnosis of pulmonary valvar atresia or severe stenosis with intact ventricular septum should trigger a careful search for all of the other aforementioned associated anomalies.

Following a failed repeat Fontan attempt at $7\frac{1}{12}$ years of age, a right Glenn anastomosis (right superior vena cava–to–right pulmonary artery) was done. By $12\frac{10}{12}$ years of age, because her right Glenn anastomosis had thrombosed, the central shunt was taken down, a shunt was placed from the right superior vena cava to the right pulmonary artery, and a modified left Blalock-Taussig anastomosis was also done. So, this was the background to her successful heart transplant at $14\frac{3}{12}$ years. (*Per ardua ad astra.* Through adversity to the stars.)

The prominent right venous valve (right sinoatrial valve or Eustachian valve of the inferior vena cava) was never clinically important, as far as we could tell: that is, never truly a supratricuspid stenosing membrane (5 cases, 16%, Table 13.24).

Sinusoids (Fig. 13.45) were observed in 5 of these 31 patients (16%, Table 13.24)—small but macroscopic communications (1 to 2 mm in internal diameter) between the right ventricular cavity and the coronary arteries. The sinusoids connected the hypertensive right ventricular cavity with the left anterior descending coronary artery in 4 of these 5 patients (80%). One patient had three sinusoids between the hypertensive right ventricular cavity and the left anterior descending coronary artery, plus an additional sinusoid between the right ventricular cavity and the right coronary artery (20%). The right ventricular–to–right coronary artery sinusoid lay between the RV and the right coronary artery in the inferior (posterior, or diaphragmatic) portion of its course. This part of the right coronary artery displayed a thick wall and a small (but not interrupted) lumen; that is, the characteristic **coronary arteriopathy** associated with sinusoidal communications was found in 1 of these 5 patients (20%), in the only patient with multiple sinusoids.

TABLE 13.24 Salient Findings in Congenital Tricuspid Stenosis With Pulmonary Valvar Atresia or Severe Pulmonary Valvar Stenosis and Intact Ventricular Septum (n = 31)

Finding	No. of Cases	% of Series*
Pulmonary valvar atresia	27	87
Extreme pulmonary valvar stenosis	4	13
Gender:		
Male	16	53
Female	14	47
Male/Female = 1.14/1		
Age at death or transplant†		
Mean = $1\frac{8}{12} \pm 3\frac{10}{12}$ years		
Range = 0 to $14\frac{3}{12}$ years		
Median = 29.5 days		
Tricuspid valve:		
Hypoplastic	31	100
Dysplastic	10	32
Regurgitant	6	19
Ebstein's	2	6
Prominent right venous valve	5	16
Sinusoids	5	16
Coronary anomalies	4	13
Anomalous muscle bundles of the right ventricle	2	6
Multiple congenital anomalies	7	23
Coronary sinus septal defect	1	3
Twin, monozygotic	1	3
Complete heart block	1	3
Hydrops fetalis	1	3
Mitral valve anomaly	1	3

*All percentages are rounded off to the nearest whole number.
†There were 3 fetuses in this series; their postnatal ages were regarded as 0 (zero) for these calculations. There was one orthotopic cardiac transplantation, performed successfully in 1993, in a girl of $14\frac{3}{12}$ years who had Ebstein's anomaly with severe congenital tricuspid stenosis (5 × 2 mm); she was the oldest patient in this subset. Thus, 30 of these 31 patients were fatalities (97%).

Of the 4 patients with a single sinusoid, there were 2 males and 2 females (no gender predilection). The ages at which these sinusoids were found also varied widely: 2 days, 4½ days, 11 days, and $9\frac{8}{12}$ years. Thus, no age predilection was apparent. The one patient with four sinusoids was a 17-week-old female.

Why did some patients with pulmonary atresia, intact ventricular septum, and tricuspid stenosis have sinusoids (16%), whereas the majority (84%) did not? We cannot answer this question. However, a word of caution is in order here. We found that the best way of detecting sinusoids was by means of selective right ventricular premortem angiocardiography. Another good way is by postmortem coronary arterial dissection. Upon opening up the coronary arteries by longitudinal incision, one should look carefully for abnormally large communications opening into the coronary arteries. This may well be how the presence of a sinusoid is recognized. And one should also look for areas of coronary mural thickening and luminal narrowing (a coronary "jet lesion") adjacent to the entry of a sinusoid. Thus, at postmortem examination, the presence of sinusoids may be subtle—not immediately obvious, and hence may be underdiagnosed. We always did our best, but this word of caution is still in order.

Coronary anomalies, 4 cases (13%, Table 13.24): specifically, what does that mean? These patients are in addition to those mentioned above who were known to have sinusoids.

Case 9 was a female fetus, 30 weeks gestational age, with multiple coronary arterial anomalies: a short sinoatrial nodal artery, terminating at the beginning of the right atrial appendage, not reaching the sinoatrial junction; and absence of the left anterior descending coronary artery, after the origin of the left circumflex coronary artery (distal territory of the left anterior descending coronary artery supplied by an elongated posterior descending coronary artery). This fetus had complete heart block and severe hydrops fetalis.

Case 11 was an 8-week-old boy who experienced sudden unexpected death during a heel stick to draw blood. Autopsy (in 1966) revealed that the left anterior descending coronary artery was focally very thick-walled, with an almost nonexistent lumen. Histology showed ischemic changes of the left ventricular myocardium. Sinusoids were not described.

Case 57 was an 8-day-old boy. Autopsy in 1955 showed that the left anterior descending coronary artery had a markedly thickened wall and a very reduced lumen. Again, no sinusoid or coronary-cameral communication was described.

Case 65 was a 7-month-old girl with absence of the ostium of the right coronary artery. The right coronary artery was supplied by anastomoses with the left coronary artery.

Parenthetically, cases like this are often reported inaccurately as having a single left coronary artery. In fact, the right coronary artery was present and normal, except that the right coronary arterial ostium was atretic.

The total number of coronary abnormalities in these 32 cases of pulmonary atresia or severe stenosis with intact ventricular septum and tricuspid stenosis + tricuspid regurgitation was 9 patients (28%, Table 13.24: sinusoids, 5, plus coronary anomalies without proved sinusoids, 4).

Anomalous muscle bundle of the right ventricle was documented in 2 of these 31 patients (6%, Table 13.24). This is mentioned because this, too, is a subtle diagnosis. When a moderator band–like muscle takes off abnormally high from the septal band, it may or may not result in stenosis in the middle of the right ventricle—between the right ventricular sinus proximally (upstream) and the infundibulum or conus (downstream). When so-called anomalous muscle bundle of the right ventricle (also known as double-chambered right ventricle) is associated with pulmonary valvar atresia with intact ventricular septum, the stenosis at mid–right ventricle is hemodynamically potential, but not real—because of the absence of antegrade right heart blood flow.

However, if and when the right ventricular outflow tract and the pulmonary valve are opened up surgically (or perhaps interventionally), then the stenosis at the mid–right ventricular level can become hemodynamically real.

The point is as follows. Before the right ventricular outflow tract is opened up, the presence of anomalous muscle bundles is often *not* apparent. But after right ventricular outflow tract reconstruction, the space just distal to the anomalous muscle bundle can open up. A virtual space becomes a real and demonstrable space.

Then the question becomes: has the right ventricle really grown postoperatively, and if so, by how much?

That is when it may become important for all concerned to understand that the right ventricular cavity has not really grown all that much. Instead, the virtual (collapsed or unexpanded) space distal to the anomalous infundibular muscle bundle often undergoes postoperative expansion, becoming a real space. What may look like remarkable right ventricular *growth* is often the becoming manifest of a previously collapsed and therefore inapparent virtual space downstream from the anomalous infundibular muscle bundle. Consequently, we strongly suspect that our statement that there were 2 of 32 patients (6%, Table 13.24) with anomalous right ventricular muscle bundles is a considerable underestimate. This point is mentioned here in the interests of understanding.

Supramitral stenosis. Rarely, pulmonary atresia or very severe stenosis with intact ventricular septum can also have significant supramitral stenosis:

1. **A large aneurysm of septum primum** (the flap valve of the foramen ovale) can obstruct the inflow through the mitral valve from above (Fig. 13.46).

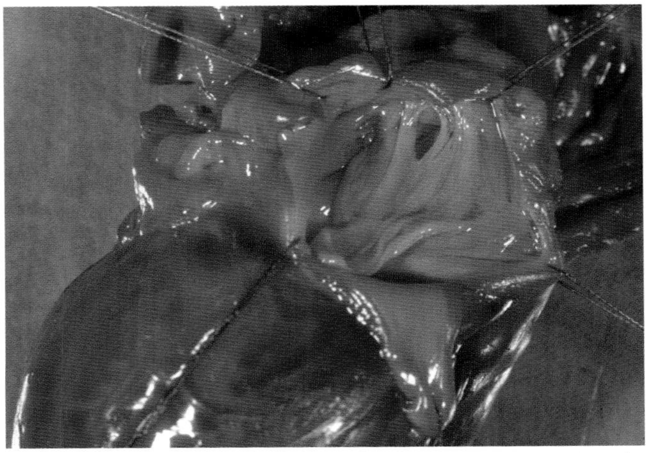

Fig. 13.46 Aneurysm of septum primum that prolapses into the mitral orifice. Large aneurysm capable of obstructing mitral orifice completely. The immediate cause of death at 25 hours of age was thought to be obstruction of the mitral orifice by this large and redundant aneurysm of septum primum. This is the opened left atrial view of a newborn boy with pulmonary valvar atresia {S,D,S}, intact ventricular septum, small right ventricular sinus, hypoplasia and dysplasia of the tricuspid valve with some tricuspid incompetence, small secundum type of atrial septal defect, restrictive atrial septum with large aneurysm of septum primum (as above), and patent ductus arteriosus. In the first day of life (in 1976), the patient received prostaglandin E1 intravenously to maintain ductal patency, followed by surgical pulmonary valvotomy and right ventricular outflow tract augmentation and formalin infiltration of the ductus arteriosus. Shortly postoperatively, the patient became acutely hypotensive, cyanotic, and with electromechanical dissociation leading to death. Only at autopsy was the patient's "functional mitral atresia" understood.

2. **The left atrial appendage can undergo intussusception**, literally folding inside-out (like what can happen to your shirt sleeve in the washing machine). The inside-out left atrial appendage now protrudes into the left atrial cavity. Then the intussuscepted left atrial appendage can prolapse down into the mitral orifice, producing significant mitral stenosis (Fig. 13.47). To my knowledge, this is a previously unknown form of intussusception. (*Intus* = within + *suscipere* = to receive. Latin.)

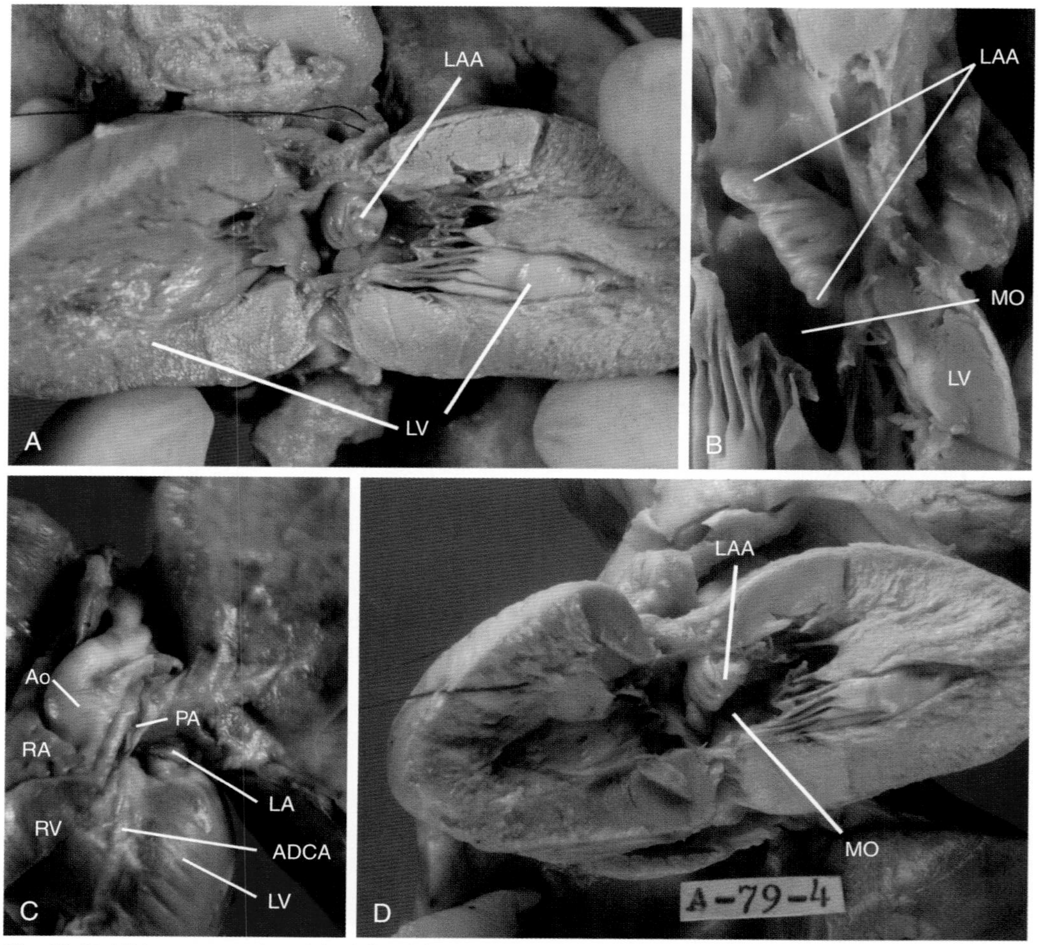

Fig. 13.47 (A) Intussusception of the left atrial appendage *(LAA)* that has prolapsed down and into the mitral orifice, producing significant mitral stenosis. Opened left ventricle, the ventricular septum to the viewer's left, the left ventricular free wall to the viewer's right, the mitral valve leaflets and orifice between these two structures. The mitral orifice, between the mitral leaflets, is filled by the inside-out (intussuscepted) and downwardly prolapsed left atrial appendage. This patent also had valvar pulmonary atresia, intact ventricular septum, thick-walled and small-chambered right ventricle, tricuspid hypoplasia (appropriate to the small cavity of the right ventricle), tricuspid stenosis with thickening and semicartilaginous change of portions of the tricuspid leaflets (not a normal but miniature tricuspid valve), right atrial hypertrophy and enlargement, prominent right venous valve (Eustachian valve) but not obstructive, large unrestrictive patent foramen ovale, several tiny fenestrations of septum primum inferiorly (small secundum atrial septal defects), brachiocephalic artery (innominate and left common carotid arteries, both arising from a common brachiocephalic trunk), and closing patent ductus arteriosus. (B) Opened left atrium, mitral valve, and left ventricle *(LV)* showing the inside-out left atrial appendage *(LAA)* protruding into the left atrial cavity and down into the mitral orifice *(MO)*. (C) External frontal view showing very hypertrophied and enlarged right atrium *(RA)*. Note that the left atrial appendage *(LA)* appears remarkably small, with an atypical rounded external appearance; it looks as though the left atrial appendage may have been amputated. Note the small main pulmonary artery *(PA)*, the much larger ascending aorta *(Ao)*, and the left anterior descending coronary artery *(ADCA)* bisecting the anterior ventricular surface, with a characteristically small right ventricle to the right, and a hypertrophied and enlarged left atrium to the left. The external appearance is also consistent with normal segmental anatomy {S,D,S}, and pulmonary atresia with intact ventricular septum. (D) Another view of the obstructive inside-out left atrial appendage *(LAA)* prolapsing down into the mitral orifice *(MO)*. Photograph A was taken in Boston. Photographs B, C, and D were taken at the Hospital Infantil de Mexico. This is a patient of Dr. Alfredo Vizcaino-Alarcon of Mexico City, presented here with his kind permission. Dr. Vizcaino presented this case at the World Congress of Paediatric Cardiology in London, England, in 1980. Dr. Vizcaino presented this very rare case as an example of previously unknown form of intussusception of the left atrial appendage, with protrusion into the left atrial cavity, and

Continued

Fig. 13.47 cont'd with downward prolapse of this inside-out left atrial appendage into the mitral orifice, resulting in a very rare form of supramitral stenosis. Having examined and photographed this heart specimen, I wish to confirm Dr. Vizcaino's findings and interpretation. *Note:* Could this be a hoax (a "Piltdown" heart)? Dr. Vizcaino and I do not think so. Dr. Vizcaino dissected this heart specimen himself; there was no prior pathologic examination of this heart specimen. We decided against calling this an *inverted* left atrial appendage for two reasons: (1) *Invert* literally means upside down or inside out: *invertere, in* = in, or inward + *vertere* = to turn. (2) But in cardiology, *inversion* now has the well established connotation of mirror-imagery, as in situs inversus totalis, meaning right-left reversal, but without superoinferior or anteroposterior change—as in an image in a mirror. We thought it would not be wise to use the same term (inverted, or inversion) but with a different meaning from that which is generally accepted. First-hand examination showed that this left atrial appendage really is *intussuscepted* and downwardly *prolapsed*. Is it possible to reduce the intussusception of the left atrial appendage? Yes. Dr. John Papagiannis, who was one of our fellows at this time (1981), did it. This is why we can be sure that it is readily possible to reduce this rare intussusception, and this is also one of the reasons that we can be sure that this is a solitus (noninverted) left atrial appendage. Any therapeutic implications? Yes. If correctly diagnosed, this intussuscepted left atrial appendage could be reduced (*un*intussuscepted) at open heart surgery. We think that it might be wise then to amputate the left atrial appendage—so that this rare form of mitral obstruction, which is potentially fatal, could not recur.

Multiple congenital anomalies were present in one-quarter of these patients (7 cases, 23%, Table 13.24). Specifically, what are we talking about?

The diagnosis of *multiple congenital anomalies* does not refer to their number. Instead, it means that malformations *not* involving the cardiovascular system were also present; that is, other organ systems were also malformed. Clinically and surgically, this can be a very important fact.

Gender: males, 4; females, 3; and males/females = 1.33/1.

Age at death: mean = 3.2 ± 4.3 months (95.25 ± 129.30 days), ranging from 1 day to 1 year. The median age at death was 45.5 days (1.52 months).

Other Organ Systems Involved

Three patients with multiple congenital anomalies had **anomalies of the gastrointestinal tract** only (37.5%). Two patients (a 2-week-old girl and a 7-week-old girl) had a Meckel's diverticulum (a sacculation or appendage of the ileum, derived from an unobliterated stalk of the yolk sac). The third was a 7-month-old girl with a pancreatic choristoma of the first part of the duodenum, that is, pancreatic heterotropic tissue (*choristos* = separated, Greek).

Two patients had additional anomalies of the **genitourinary system** only: a 3-day-old boy with absence of the right kidney, right renal artery, right renal vein, and right ureter, with left hydronephrosis, cryptorchidism, and hypospadias; and a 3-month-old boy with left hydronephrosis and ureteropelvic stenosis.

A **mitral valve anomaly** was found in one of these patients (Table 13.24). A 9⁸⁄₁₂-year-old black boy with pulmonary atresia and intact ventricular septum {S,D,S} had a very small-chambered and thick-walled right ventricle. At autopsy, we described the right ventricle as tiny. The tricuspid valve had a markedly hypoplastic annulus with thickened and myxomatous tricuspid leaflets. Many of the potential interchordal spaces were filled and obliterated with unresorbed leaflet-like tissue. Angiocardiography demonstrated a sinusoid between the diminutive right ventricle and the left anterior descending coronary artery. There was a large secundum atrial septal defect, a prominent right venous valve (of no apparent functional significance), and no thickening of the right ventricular endocardium (i.e., no endocardial fibroelastosis or endocardial sclerosis).

But the really unusual finding was that the mitral valve was also very abnormal. The mitral leaflets were thickened and myxomatous, with rolling of the mitral leaflet's margins and documented mitral regurgitation. Typically, the mitral valve is essentially normal; but not in this patient.

Multisystem involvement was present in 2 of these 7 patients (29%) with multiple congenital anomalies (Table 13.24): Case 49 was a 6-week-old boy who had multiple congenital anomalies with multisystem malformations: facial dysmorphism with a small left palpebral fissure, webbed neck, sternal skin tag, and hypospadias with chordee.

Case 53, a 1-year-old boy, was the other patient with multisystem anomalies consisting of bilateral cleft lip, bilateral cleft palate, partial DiGeorge syndrome, mild hypothyroidism, difficulty swallowing with aspiration and vomiting, left hydronephrosis and hydroureter and a small left kidney, arthrogryposis of both wrists, small penis, and undescended left testis (in the inguinal canal).

Congenital Tricuspid Stenosis With Small Right Ventricle but Without Pulmonary Valvar Atresia/Severe Stenosis and Without Intact Ventricular Septum. There were 17 such patients with congenital tricuspid stenosis but *without* pulmonary atresia/severe stenosis with intact ventricular septum, summarized as *Other (17)* in Table 13.23. These 17 patients constituted 24% of all of these cases of congenital tricuspid stenosis, and 35% of all cases of congenital tricuspid stenosis with a small right ventricle (Table 13.23). These 17 cases of congenital tricuspid stenosis with small right ventricles that were *not* associated with pulmonary atresia or severe stenosis and intact ventricular septum {S,D,S} are presented in greater detail in Table 13.25.

Segmental anatomy: Braces {} mean the set or combination of. Transposition of the great arteries (TGA) means VA alignment discordance. TGA occurred with three different segmental sets: {S,D,D} = solitus atria, D-loop ventricles, D-TGA (aorta valve to the right of the pulmonary valve). There was AV alignment concordance with VA alignment discordance. TGA {S,D,L} = TGA with solitus atria, D-loop ventricles, and L-TGA (aortic valve to the left of the pulmonary valve). There were AV concordance and VA discordance. TGA {S,L,L} = TGA with the

TABLE 13.25 Congenital Tricuspid Stenosis With Small Right Ventricle Not Associated With Pulmonary Atresia and Intact Ventricular Septum ($n = 17$)

Anatomy	No. of Cases	% of Series* ($n = 17$)
Transposition of the great arteries {S,D,D} = 2 {S,D,L} = 1 {S,L,L} = 1	5	29
Tricuspid stenosis without severe PS	4	24
Tetralogy of Fallot	3	18
AV discordance with VA concordance {S,L,S} = 1 {S,L,I} = 1	2	12
Completely common AV canal	2	12
Double-outlet right ventricle {S,D,L} = 1	1	6

AV, Atrioventricular; *PS*, pulmonary stenosis; *VA*, ventriculoarterial.
*All percentages are rounded off to the nearest number.

segmental anatomic combination of solitus atria, L-loop ventricles, and L-TGA. There were AV alignment discordance and VA alignment discordance. Thus, 3 patients had physiologically uncorrected complete TGA, and 1 patient had congenitally physiologically corrected TGA.

There were two different anatomic types of AV discordance with VA concordance: {S,L,S} = solitus atria, L-loop ventricles, and solitus normally related great arteries; and {S,L,I} = solitus atria, L-loop ventricles, and inverted normally related great arteries. {S,L,S} is called *isolated ventricular inversion;* only the ventricles are inverted, whereas the atria and the great arteries are not.

Double-outlet right ventricle (DORV) occurred with the segment situs set of {S,D,L}, which means solitus atria, D-loop ventricles and L-malposition of the great arteries (aortic valve to the left of the pulmonary valve). The segmental alignments were AV discordance, with the VA alignments of DORV.

Transposition of the Great Arteries

When TGA was associated with congenital tricuspid stenosis and a hypoplastic right ventricle, was there anything special, interesting, different about these 5 patients (Table 13.25)? We think the answer is yes, in several respects. The ages at death of these 3 boys and 2 girls were very young: mean = 13.4 ± 16.56 days; range = 2 to 42 days; and median = 7 days.

Of the two patients with TGA {S,D,D}, one was a 7-day-old girl with a secundum type of atrial septal defect, a hypoplastic right ventricle, a hypoplastic tricuspid valve that functionally was both stenotic and regurgitant, a small membranous ventricular septal defect, a hypoplastic ascending aorta and aortic arch with preductal coarctation of the aorta, and a closing patent ductus arteriosus. The combination of a small right ventricle and tricuspid valve with a secundum atrial septal defect facilitated right-to-left shunting at the atrial level, away from the transposed aorta and aortic isthmus which were hypoplastic and obstructive (coarcted). Functional closure of the ductus arteriosus and severe preductal coarctation of the aorta is a fatal combination. This patient did not undergo any form of surgical or interventional therapy. Congestive heart failure led to anasarca and death.

The other patient with TGA {S,D,D} was a 13-day-old boy with a small right ventricular sinus (inflow tract), a hypoplastic tricuspid valve that was functionally stenotic, a small conoventricular type of ventricular septal defect (4 × 2 mm), a left circumflex coronary artery arising from the right coronary artery and passing behind the pulmonary valve, and preductal coarctation of the aorta. At 1 day of age, a balloon atrial septostomy was done, in the hope of increasing mixing of the systemic and pulmonary venous blood streams at the atrial level. At 5 days of age he underwent an arterial switch procedure, patch closure of the ventricular septal defect, ligation and division of the patent ductus arteriosus, and augmentation of the neopulmonary artery (native aortic arch and preductal coarctation) with glutaraldehyde-fixed pericardium. The postoperative course was characterized by transient complete heart block, low cardiac output, hypotension, disseminated intravascular coagulation, and marked edema. At 13 days of age on the 8th postoperative day, repeat balloon atrial septostomy and balloon dilation were performed, resulting in death in the cardiac catheterization laboratory. The tricuspid stenosis was associated with a transtricuspid gradient of 3 to 6 mm Hg. At autopsy, the effective tricuspid orifice measured 4 × 5 mm, compared with a normal mitral orifice of 9 × 7 mm. Treating both the tricuspid orifice and the mitral orifice as an ellipse, and recalling that the area of an ellipse = $\pi \times r_1 \times r_2$, where r_1 = one-half of the major axis and r_2 = one-half of the minor axis, the area of the tricuspid orifice = 15.708 mm^2, and the area of the mitral orifice = 49.480 mm^2. These approximations suggest that the cross-sectional area of the tricuspid orifice is approximately 68% less than the cross-sectional area of the mitral orifice. (The % change between 49.480 and 15.708 = −68.25%.)

At autopsy, we thought that the major lessons of this case were as follows:

1. The hypoplastic type of preductal coarctation of the aorta should be regarded as a sign of upstream obstruction with shunting away from the aorta.
2. A hypoplastic right ventricle (the sinus or inflow tract) and a consequently stenotic (hypoplastic) tricuspid valve constitute a serious problem for the arterial switch procedure in patients with TGA because the tricuspid hypoplasia and the RV hypoplasia cannot be enlarged surgically ("at the present time" should be understood). It does not help hemodynamically to relieve the aortic coarctation if the causal obstruction is upstream at the level of the right ventricle and tricuspid valve and cannot be treated (enlarged) surgically.
3. A balloon atrial septostomy cannot help hemodynamically if the causal obstructions at the tricuspid valve and right ventricular inflow tract levels cannot be relieved surgically. Indeed, successful balloon atrial septostomy may make hemodynamic matters worse by facilitating atrial shunting away from the right ventricle and the neopulmonary artery.

4. We thought that the following principles merit serious consideration in this type of difficult case:
   a. Switch the aorta to the good-sized left ventricle.
   b. Repair the aortic hypoplasia and coarctation.
   c. Ligate and divide the ductus arteriosus.
   d. Bypass the hypoplastic right ventricle and tricuspid valve by a cavopulmonary or Fontan type of procedure.

(These are our best present thoughts. We expect that our cardiologic and surgical colleagues in the future may well be able to develop better ways of handling this difficult therapeutic problem than are presently evident to us. Heart transplantation and mechanical hearts suggest themselves as hopeful possibilities.)

The point of the foregoing is to say an emphatic yes: a small right ventricle and tricuspid valve leading to functional tricuspid and subtricuspid stenosis are serious and important problems in patients with TGA.

One patient, a 6-week-old boy, had TGA {S,D,L} (Table 13.25). This is a D-loop transposition in which the aortic valve lay to the *left* of the pulmonary valve, correctly suggesting that the bulboventricular D-loop had undergone some sort of malrotation (unusual rotation for a D-loop). This patient had superoinferior ventricles with a superior right ventricle, an inferior left ventricle, and an approximately horizontal ventricular septum. As is usual with superoinferior ventricles, the right ventricular sinus was small, resulting in tricuspid hypoplasia (stenosis hemodynamically). Although small, the tricuspid valve was otherwise normally formed (not dysplastic). This patient may have had unrecognized subaortic stenosis produced by the hypoplastic tricuspid valve and right ventricular sinus. However, the patient also had a conoventricular type of ventricular septal defect and did not have preductal coarctation of the transposed aorta. This patient underwent atrial septal defect creation and banding of the main pulmonary artery, which led to postoperative death. Obstruction of *both* the aortic outflow tract (tricuspid and right ventricular sinus hypoplasia) and of the pulmonary outflow tract (banding of the main pulmonary artery) was not well tolerated. The human heart can tolerate obstruction of one great arterial outflow tract, but not both. (The patient was Case 4 in the publication by Dr. Stella Van Praagh and her colleagues concerning superoinferior ventricles in 1980.[536])

Case 52 was a 2-day-old boy with TGA {S,L,L}, dextrocardia, a large conoventricular type of ventricular septal defect, marked pulmonary outflow tract stenosis, and a closing patent ductus arteriosus. The left-sided morphologically right ventricle was thick-walled and small-chambered, and the left-sided tricuspid valve was consequently hypoplastic (stenotic). The patient died in 1975 during an attempted Waterston procedure. Although this one case may not prove that right ventricular and tricuspid hypoplasia are important management problems in patients with discordant L-loop TGA, consider the difficulty of trying to do a double-switch procedure (arterial switch and atrial switch) in such a patient. This is why we suspect that congenital tricuspid stenosis (left-sided) and right ventricular hypoplasia (left-sided) in patients with TGA {S,L,L} will prove to be important management problems.

Case 14 was a 3-day-old girl with TGA {S,L,L}, moderately marked hypoplasia of the left-sided morphologically right ventricle, and with moderately severe hypoplasia of the left-sided tricuspid valve that resulted in left-sided congenital tricuspid stenosis. A conoventricular type of ventricular septal was slit-like (very small). The L-transposed aortic valve was hypoplastic and bicuspid because the right coronary—left coronary commissure was rudimentary. Preductal coarctation of the aorta was associated with a large but closing patent ductus arteriosus.

In 1976, management involved surgical resection of the preductal coarctation of the aorta and of the patent ductus arteriosus, anastomosis of the aortic arch to the descending thoracic aorta, banding of the main pulmonary artery, and atrial septectomy, which led to intraoperative death.

Our assessment postmortem was that surgical repair of downstream sequelae such as preductal coarctation of the aorta is futile, unless its intracardiac cause (congenital tricuspid and right ventricular sinus hypoplasia) can be addressed in some effective way, either by enlargement, or by bypass. Since enlargement of the hypoplasia of the right ventricular cavity and of the tricuspid valve is impossible at present, we thought that some sort of surgical right ventricular bypassing procedure might facilitate successful management of this very difficult therapeutic problem.

Congenital Tricuspid Stenosis Without Severe Pulmonary Stenosis

What does this heading mean (Table 13.25)? It means that either there was no pulmonary stenosis, or, if pulmonary stenosis was present, it was much less severe than the tricuspid stenosis. (This is the opposite of what one sees with pulmonary atresia or severe stenosis, with intact ventricular septum and tricuspid stenosis; in the latter anomaly, obstruction at the pulmonary valve level is typically much more severe than at the tricuspid valve level.) These 4 cases constituted 25% of the present group (Table 13.25).

There were 2 boys and 2 girls. Their ages at death had a mean of 2 4/12 years, with a standard deviation of 2 3/12 years, a range from 3 days to 4½ years, and median of 2 4/12 years (850 days).

Case 34 was a 4½ year old girl who died in 1962. She had severe congenital tricuspid stenosis {S,D,S}, right ventricular hypoplasia, and left ventricular hypertrophy. The tricuspid valve measured only 10 mm in diameter, compared with a mitral valve diameter of 22 mm; the tricuspid valve's diameter was approximately 45% of the mitral valve's diameter (% change from 22 to 10 = −55%). Autopsy revealed evidence of old bacterial endocarditis with vegetations covering the tricuspid valve and the ventricular septal defect. The patient had a history of cyanotic congenital heart disease with clubbing of fingers and toes, and polycythemia. Autopsy revealed multiple thrombi in the brain, spleen, heart, submaxillary glands, pancreas, and tonsils.

This patient also had multiple congenital anomalies consisting of left hydronephrosis, double left renal pelves and ureters, double vaginae, and bicornuate uterus. She had recurrent urinary tract infections. She died in 1962 of hemorrhage postoperatively following a Potts procedure.

Thus, this patient with congenital tricuspid stenosis probably also had an important component of acquired tricuspid stenosis produced by the vegetations covering her abnormally small tricuspid valve.

Case 58, a 4-year-old boy who died at 4 years of age in 1954, had a common atrium, congenital tricuspid stenosis (7 mm in diameter), and a very small-chambered right ventricle that was also thick-walled (13 to 14 mm thick) with a slit-like restrictive ventricular septal defect (9 × 4 mm). The subpulmonary infundibulum, pulmonary valve, and main pulmonary artery were dilated. The patient was thought to have an anomalous pulmonary venous connection. The lower left pulmonary vein was anastomosed to the left atrium just behind the left atrial appendage. The patient died 35 hours postoperatively. The impression at autopsy was that an anomalous pulmonary venous connection was not present. The congenital tricuspid stenosis and common atrium were regarded as important, resulting in right-to-left shunting at the atrial level. Left-to-right shunting through the relatively small ventricular septal defect may well have accounted for the good-sized pulmonary infundibulum and pulmonary artery.

Case 63 was a 3-day-old girl with a small tricuspid valve, a small-chambered and thick-walled right ventricle, and a normal sized pulmonary valve and main pulmonary artery. This patient also had mild postductal coarctation of the aorta, valvar aortic stenosis, subaortic stenosis, and endocardial sclerosis of the left ventricle. Her ductus arteriosus was patent. So, this patient had the difficult hemodynamic dilemma of obstruction of both the right and left sides of the heart. In addition, she had multiple congenital anomalies with hypoplasia of the abdominal wall musculature, double pelvis and double ureter of the left kidney, and megacolon.

Case 66 was an 8-month-old boy with a very hypoplastic tricuspid valve (1.5 mm in diameter) and a tiny saccular right ventricle with a 2 mm thick wall and a cavity that measured 15 × 15 × 15 mm. The tiny right ventricle was yellowish and fibrotic, with white endocardium. There was a muscular ventricular septal defect. The subpulmonary infundibulum and pulmonary valve were also smallish but not nearly as hypoplastic as the tricuspid valve; the pulmonary valve measured 12 mm in diameter.

The left heart was normally developed: the mitral valve measured 48 mm in diameter, the aortic valve 22 mm in diameter and the left ventricular wall 8 to 10 mm in thickness. There was a large secundum atrial septal defect (12 mm in diameter). Coarctation (marked narrowing) of the proximal left pulmonary artery was present opposite the left ligamentum arteriosum (closed ductus arteriosus). The musculature of the ductus arteriosus can lasso the descending thoracic aorta, and when this encircling musculature contracts it can produce an adult type of coarctation of the aorta (not present in this patient). The musculature of the ductus arteriosus can also lasso the proximal left pulmonary artery, and when this encircling musculature contracts it can produce coarctation (marked focal stenosis) of the proximal left pulmonary artery (present in this patient). **Hence, the musculature of the ductus arteriosus is a "double threat" to its neighbors—the descending thoracic aorta ("adult" coarctation of the aorta) and the proximal left pulmonary artery (coarctation or focal stenosis of the proximal left pulmonary artery).** (Etymologically, coarctation is derived from *coarctare,* to press together, Latin.)

This patient also had multiple congenital anomies: There was a partial inclusion of the right adrenal gland within the liver. This patient also had scoliosis and brachycephaly.

Stenosis and hypoplasia of the right coronary artery were found. Sinusoids were not observed.

This patient had large collateral arteries, 2 mm in diameter, one to the hilum of each lung. This patient died in 1962 because of a kinked and thrombosed left Blalock-Taussig anastomosis.

Multiple congenital anomalies were present in 3 of these 4 patients (75%). It is striking that non-Ebstein congenital tricuspid stenosis seems never to occur in isolation.

Congenital Tricuspid Stenosis With Tetralogy of Fallot

Three patients had congenital tricuspid stenosis that was associated with tetralogy of Fallot (19% of this group, Table 13.25). There were 2 boys and 1 girl and their ages at death were very young (1 day, 4 days, and 7 days): mean = 4 ± 3 days, ranging from 1 to 7 days, median = 4 days. All had pulmonary outflow tract atresia, with a right ventricle that was thick-walled and small-chambered—resulting in a hypoplastic tricuspid valve that was hemodynamically stenotic.

In **Case 56,** the 4-day-old boy, the tricuspid valve had abnormal attachments to the inferior surface of the anterosuperiorly deviated conal septum and to the ventricular septum. The ventricular septal defect was largely obstructed by tricuspid valve tissue. Sinusoids communicated with the right coronary artery, which displayed mural thickening and marked luminal narrowing. There was absence of the ostium of the right coronary artery, resulting in what is often erroneously called single left coronary artery; so multiple sinusoids communicated with an abnormally low pressure right coronary artery. No sinusoids connected with the anterior descending branch of the left coronary artery. There was a prominent right venous valve and the secundum atrial septal defect was small (fenestrations within septum primum).

Thus, the cardiac malformations in this patient closely simulated those of pulmonary atresia with intact ventricular septum from a hemodynamic standpoint, even though Case 56 had tetralogy of Fallot, not pulmonary atresia with intact ventricular septum. Case 56 had **tetralogy of Fallot with suprasystemic right ventricle**—because the ventricular septal defect was largely obstructed by abnormally attached tricuspid valve tissue. This hemodynamic insight appears to explain not only why the right ventricle was small-chambered and thick-walled, and why there was tricuspid hypoplasia resulting in hemodynamic stenosis, but also why there were right ventricular sinusoids, right coronary arteriopathy with luminal narrowing, and a prominent right venous valve. Thus, tetralogy of Fallot with suprasystemic right ventricle can display most of the features of the pulmonary atresia with intact ventricular septum syndrome.

As was pointed out by Flanagan and colleagues[537] in 1980, **tetralogy of Fallot with obstruction of the ventricular septal defect**—also known as tetralogy of Fallot with suprasystemic right ventricular pressure—can have a distressingly high surgical mortality rate, perhaps because of the greater than usual right ventricular myocardial hypertrophy (possibly a risk factor for sudden arrhythmic death), and perhaps also because of undetected sinusoids and coronary arteriopathy with luminal narrowing. (More work is needed on this problem.)

Whatever the cause or causes of this elevated surgical mortality may prove to be, these facts are stark and should be remembered: in 1988, the surgical mortality in our patients with tetralogy of Fallot and suprasystemic right ventricular pressure because of a restrictively small ventricular septal defect was 75%, compared with our overall experience in tetralogy in which the surgical mortality rate was 6%.[537] So this is a small but deadly subset.

In **Case 64,** a 7-day-old girl, autopsy revealed tetralogy of Fallot with valvar pulmonary atresia, a small ventricular septal defect (3 mm in internal diameter), a small-chambered and thick-walled (9 mm) right ventricle, a hypoplastic tricuspid valve (7 mm in diameter), a secundum atrial septal defect (fenestrated septum primum), and an aberrant right subclavian artery. A Blalock-Taussig anastomosis was performed in 1963 by end-to-end anastomosis of the aberrant right subclavian and left pulmonary arteries, with ligation of the ductus arteriosus.

Case 32, a 1-day-old boy, had tetralogy of Fallot {S,D,S} with infundibular and valvar pulmonary atresia, a thick-walled and small-chambered right ventricle, and consequently a hypoplastic (stenotic) tricuspid valve. The anterior papillary muscle of the right ventricle was absent and the ductus arteriosus was closing.

This patient also had multiple congenital anomalies. Those in Cardiology and the Cardiac Registry favored the diagnosis of the Cornelia de Lange syndrome, whereas those in General Pathology preferred the diagnosis of the Rubenstein-Taybi syndrome. (To my knowledge, this differential diagnostic question was never resolved to the satisfaction of all.) He had marked generalized hirsutism, syndactyly of the second and third toes bilaterally, thin lips, micrognathia, micromelia, a high-arched palate, microcephaly (280/335 grams, 84% of normal, or −16%), abnormal dermatoglyphics (a crease of the thenar eminence bilaterally), low birth weight for dates (5 lb 6 oz or 2438 grams at full term), and short stature (45/50 cm, 90% of normal). He did not have synophrys or long curly eyelashes (both typical of the de Lange syndrome).

Summary. So what are we really talking about in this section concerning congenital tricuspid stenosis with tetralogy of Fallot? Are we really talking about congenital tricuspid stenosis? Basically, not really. The important thing to understand is that tetralogy of Fallot can hemodynamically resemble pulmonary atresia with intact ventricular septum when the VSD in TOF is restrictive, resulting in TOF with suprasystemic RV. TOF with pulmonary outflow tract atresia and an obstructed VSD also develops a thick-walled and small-chambered RV, similar to pulmonary atresia with intact ventricular septum. In TOF with a thick-walled and small-chambered RV, the tricuspid valve had to be hypoplastic to open in the small-chambered RV. So then we make the diagnosis, correctly enough, of congenital tricuspid stenosis. But this is a *secondary* type of congenital tricuspid stenosis—secondary to TOF with pulmonary outflow tract atresia, an obstructed VSD, and little or no tricuspid stenosis. The point is: It is important to understand *why* congenital tricuspid stenosis is present. These cases are about much more than just a small tricuspid valve. Often it is essential to understand the *whole* case in order to comprehend any one part of it (such as the status of the tricuspid valve). This is why we are using a *case* presentation approach, rather than just a *lesion* presentation approach.

AV DISCORDANCE WITH VA CONCORDANCE

Two of the patients in this group (congenital tricuspid stenosis, but without pulmonary atresia and intact ventricular septum) had atrioventricular (AV) discordance with ventriculoarterial (VA) concordance (12.5% of this group, Table 13.25) (Fig. 13.48).

The segmental anatomy was {S,L,S} in an 8¾-month-old (263 days) boy and was {S,L,I} in a 2-day-old boy (Case 25 and Case 13, respectively).

Since AV discordance with VA concordance is rare and therefore unfamiliar, a few introductory words may be helpful. The segmental anatomic set of {S,L,S} means that there is situs solitus of the viscera and atria {S,-,-}, with L-loop ventricles {S,*L*,-}, and with solitus normally related great arteries {S,L,*S*}. As this segmental combination suggests, there is AV discordance: right-sided morphologically right atrium (RA) opens into the right-sided morphologically left ventricle (LV), and left-sided morphologically left atrium (LA) opens into left-sided morphologically right ventricle (RV). As the segmental anatomy also indicates, there is VA concordance: the right-sided LV ejects through the right-sided aortic valve (AoV) into the aorta (Ao), and the left-sided RV ejects through the left-sided pulmonary valve (PV) into the main pulmonary artery (MPA).

Since there is only one segmental discordance (at the AV junction), the systemic and pulmonary venous circulations are physiologically uncorrected (as in physiologically uncorrected or complete transposition of the great arteries). The blue systemic venous blood in the right side of the heart goes from the RA to the LV to the Ao. The bright red pulmonary venous blood in the left side of the heart goes from the LA to the RV to the MPA. Therapeutically, {S,L,S} needs an atrial switch operation (Mustard or Senning). One would not want to do an arterial switch operation, because the great arteries are solitus normally related.

Why are the great arteries *solitus* normally related? Because the aortic valve lies to the right of the pulmonary valve; there is aortic valve–to–mitral valve direct fibrous continuity, typical of normally related great arteries; there is a muscular subpulmonary conus (infundibulum) also typical of normally related greater arteries and the main pulmonary artery passed to the *left* of the ascending aorta—as in situs solitus totalis.

When visceroatrial situs solitus is associated with discordant L-loop ventricles, almost always the great arteries are transposed, as in TGA {S,L,L}, or malposed, as in DORV {S,L,L}. But rarely, the infundibuloarterial segment can be solitus normally related to the underlying ventricular sinuses and the atrioventricular canal and valves, resulting in the rare segmental combination of {S,L,S}. We described the {S,L,S} heart in 1966[538] and called this segmental anatomic set **isolated ventricular inversion,** meaning that only the ventricles were inverted, but the atria and the great arteries were not inverted.

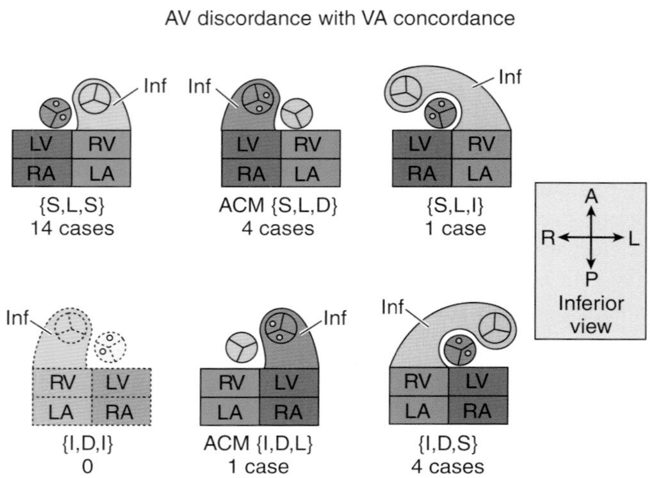

Fig. 13.48 The anatomic types of atrioventricular *(AV)* discordance with ventriculoatrial *(VA)* concordance. The diagrams are drawn as though these hearts were seen from below, as in a subxiphoid two-dimensional echocardiogram. There were five known anatomic types of AV discordance with VA concordance as of 1988:[539] (1) **{S,L,S}**, also known as **isolated ventricular inversion**,[538] in 14 of these 24 cases (58%, the most common anatomic type). The circulations are physiologically uncorrected, as expected, with one segmental discordance (at the AV level); hence an atrial switch procedure, if feasible, is indicated.[540] Note that the infundibulum *(Inf)* is subpulmonary. There is direct fibrous continuity between the aortic valve (indicated by the coronary ostia) and the right-sided mitral valve that opens into the right-sided morphologically left ventricle *(LV)*. A subpulmonary infundibulum and aortic-mitral fibrous continuity are characteristic of normally related great arteries. {S,L,S} means the set of solitus viscera and atria {*S*,-,-}, discordant L-loop ventricles {S,*L*,-}, and solitus (as opposed to inversus) normally related great arteries {S,L,*S*}. (2) ***ACM* {S,L,D}** indicates anatomically corrected malposition (ACM) consisting of the set or combination of solitus viscera and atrial {*S*,-,-}, discordant L-loop ventricles {S,*L*,-}, and D-malposition of the great arteries {S,L,*D*}. Note that the infundibulum is subaortic, typical of malpositions of the great arteries (as opposed to the subpulmonary infundibulum of normally related great arteries). This malposition of the great arteries is regarded as anatomically corrected because, despite the great arterial malposition, each great artery nonetheless arises above the anatomically correct ventricle: malposed aortic valve above the right-sided LV, and malposed pulmonary valve (no coronary ostia) above the left-sided RV. Thus, ventriculo-arterial concordance can be present not only with normally related great arteries, but also with ACM. ACM is thought to be rare because the ventricles loop in one direction, but the great arteries twist in the opposite direction, as the segmental anatomy indicates: ACM {S,*L*,*D*}. Although ACM {S,L,D} is corrected anatomically or morphologically, it is uncorrected *physiologically* because there is one segmental discordance at the AV level: {S,L,-}. There is VA concordance, by definition, in ACM. Surgically, therefore, an atrial switch procedure is indicated, if feasible. ACM {S,L,D} was tied for second place in frequency with {I,D,S}: 4 of 24 (17%). (3) **{S,L,I}** means the set of solitus viscera and atrial {*S*,-,-}, with L-loop ventricles {S,*L*,-} and therefore AV discordance, with inverted normally related great arteries {S,L,*I*}. One cannot call {S,L,I} isolated ventricular inversion because the infundibuloarterial part of the heart (the conotruncus) is also inverted. In addition to the inverted normal semilunar relationship, the main pulmonary artery passes to the *right* of the ascending aorta (instead of to the *left* as in solitus or noninverted great arteries). Surgically, because of physiologic uncorrection of the circulations, if feasible one would want to do an atrial switch procedure. {S,L,I}—which can also be spelled out in words (as above)—was one of the rarest anatomic types of AV discordance with VA concordance: 1 of 24 cases (4%). (4) **{I,D,I}**, the mirror-image of {S,L,S}, to our knowledge had not been documented in 1988 when we did this study.[539] (5) **ACM {I,D,L}** denotes ACM with the segmental anatomic set of situs inversus of the viscera and atria {*I*,-,-}, with discordant D-loop ventricles {I,*D*,-} and with anatomically corrected L-malposition of the great arteries {I,D,*L*}, also one of the rarest anatomic types of ACM in our study: 1 of 24 cases (4%). Segmentally, ACM {I,D,L} is a mirror-image of ACM {S,L,D}. Physiologically the systemic and pulmonary circulations are uncorrected (only one intersegmental discordance, at the AV level). Surgically, an atrial switch operation would merit consideration. (Since VA concordance is present, presumably one would want *not* to do an arterial switch operation.) (6) {I,D,S} means the set of visceroatrial situs inversus, with D-loop ventricles (therefore AV discordance), with solitus normally related great arteries (therefore VA concordance). Since the circulations are physiologically uncorrected, and because the great arteries are normally related to the underlying ventricles and AV valves, if feasible one surgically would consider an atrial switch (not a ventricular switch) operation. {I,D,S} was tied with ACM {S,L,D} as the second most common anatomic type of AVD with VAC in our study.[539] (Reproduced with permission from Pasquini L, Sanders SP, Parness I, Colan S, Keane JF, Mayer JE, Kratz C, Foran RB, Marino B, Van Praagh S, Van Praagh R: Echocardiographic and anatomic findings in atrioventricular discordance with ventriculoarterial concordance. *Am J Cardiol* 1988;62:1256.)

{S,L,I} means the segmental anatomic combination of visceroatrial situs solitus, with L-loop ventricles (and AV discordance), and with inverted normally related great arteries (with VA concordance). In {S,L,S} and {S,L,I}, the segmental alignments are the same. Both have AV discordance and VA concordance and consequent physiologic uncorrection of the systemic and pulmonary venous circulations.

The anatomic difference between {S,L,*S*} and {S,L,*I*} is that the infundibuloarterial segments are mirror-images. In {S,L,*I*}, the infundibulum and great arteries are as in situs inversus totalis. The aortic valve typically is to the left of the pulmonary valve. There is aortic-mitral direct fibrous continuity, typical of normally related great arteries. There is a subpulmonary muscular infundibulum or conus—preventing pulmonary-to-AV valve fibrous continuity, also typical of normally related great arteries. No matter what the spatial relationship between the semilunar valves may be (it can be artifactually altered), the main pulmonary artery passes to the *right* of the ascending aorta—reliably indicating that inverted normally related great arteries are present. (With solitus normally related great arteries, the main pulmonary artery passes to the *left* of the ascending aorta.)

Just as there are two anatomic types of TGA (D-TGA or solitus TGA, and L-TGA or inverted TGA), so too there are two anatomic types of normally related great arteries (NRGA) (solitus NRGA and inverted NRGA) that are symbolized in the third element of the cardiac segmental set as S, that is, {-,-,S} and I, that is, {-,-,I}.

{S,L,S} and {S,L,I} are only two of the six anatomic types of AV discordance with VA concordance.[539] The other four anatomic types of AV discordance with VA concordance (Fig. 13.48) include anatomically corrected malposition of the great arteries (ACM): ACM {S,L,D}, {I,D,I}, {I,D,S}, and ACM {I,D,L}.

When considering AV discordance with VA concordance, it is easy to forget about ACM, in which there is VA concordance (LV ejecting into the aorta and RV into the pulmonary artery), but in which the VA connections (the conus arteriosus) and the AV valve—great arterial relations are very abnormal. VA concordance is not synonymous with NRGA, because ACM also exists. When we reported the anatomic types of AV discordance with VA concordance,[539] we were not aware of a definitely well documented example of {I,D,I}, which is why it is depicted with broken lines (Fig. 13.48). I still am uncertain about this; hence only five (of the potentially six) anatomic types of AV discordance with VA concordance have been proved to exist.

Only the {S,L,S} heart can be called **isolated ventricular inversion.** In the {S,L,I} heart, not only are the ventricles inverted, but so too are the inverted normally related great arteries.

AV discordance cannot be diagnosed in the heterotaxy syndromes with asplenia and polysplenia when the atrial situs cannot be diagnosed with confidence. In the heterotaxy syndrome with *polysplenia,* the atrial situs usually can be diagnosed with confidence. In the heterotaxy syndrome with *asplenia,* diagnosis of the atrial situs (solitus or inversus) is more difficult than with polysplenia. But quite often, the diagnosis of the atrial situs in asplenia patients is possible. However, when the atrial situs defies confident diagnosis, which is not rare with asplenia, we make the diagnosis of *atrial situs ambiguus,* which just means that we do not know for sure. Atrial situs ambiguus does *not* imply that *atrial "isomerism,"* right isomerism or left isomerism, is present. Accurately speaking, we think that the concept of atrial isomerism is an error.[21] For further data, see Chapter 29.

As was pointed out by Konstantinov and colleagues in 2004,[540] AV discordance with VA concordance constitutes a remaining indication for the atrial switch operation because, as mentioned above, one does not want to do an arterial switch operation in these rare anomalies because the great arteries are normally related, or at least VA concordance is present with ACM. (Much of this essential background information is repeated, for the reader's convenience, in the legend of Fig. 13.48. The foregoing words are much easier to understand when one is also looking at a diagram.)

Case 25, the 8¾-month-old boy, had the segmental set of **{S,L,S}**. There were superoinferior ventricles, with an underdeveloped RV sinus superiorly, a well-developed LV inferiorly, and an approximately horizontal ventricular septum in between. The tricuspid annulus was not hypoplastic, measuring 4.1 cm in circumference (compared with a normal control heart specimen of 3.3 cm). However, congenital tricuspid stenosis was present in the sense that the tricuspid valve opened into the right ventricular septal surface and into the hypoplastic right ventricle; that is, immediately subvalvar tricuspid stenosis was present. There was a ventricular septal defect of the atrioventricular canal type, but without a common atrioventricular valve. There was aortic outflow tract stenosis. The aortic outflow tract ran between the medial leaflets of the right-sided and inferior mitral valve and the left-sided and superior tricuspid valve. The aortic valve was hypoplastic and bicuspid (lack of development of the right coronary-noncoronary commissure). The aortic arch and isthmus were hypoplastic; clinically, the patient was considered to have a pseudocoarctation, plus a patent ductus arteriosus.

At 23 days of age in 1975, a 10 mm Dacron conduit was placed from the ascending to the descending thoracic aorta, the patent ductus arteriosus was ligated, and the main pulmonary artery was banded. At 28 days of age, the band of the main pulmonary artery was tightened. At 33 days of age, the banding of the main pulmonary artery was loosened and a surgical atrial septal defect was created under inflow occlusion.

The postoperative course was characterized by recurrent pneumonia, chronic congestive heart failure, and failure to thrive.

At 8 months of age, a Blalock-Hanlon atrial septectomy was performed. Postoperatively the patient had ectopic atrial rhythms, intermittent 2/1 atrioventricular block, episodes of bradycardia and hypotension, and oliguria appeared. Sepsis developed related to genitourinary tract infection with *Escherichia coli* and gram-negative septicemia (multiple species of flavobacterium) associated with hypothermia and thrombocytopenia, leading to death at 8¾ months of age.

Was this patient's congenital subtricuspid stenosis clinically important? At autopsy, we thought that obstruction of the tricuspid inflow tract had been of relatively little clinical importance because of the coexistence of a large ventricular septal defect of the AV canal type that facilitated increased pulmonary blood flow, despite the smallness of the right ventricle. The subaortic stenosis produced by the approximation of the medial leaflets of the AV valves, and the aortic valvar stenosis related to the hypoplasia of this bicommissural aortic valve could not be relieved surgically. Consequently, the aortic outflow tract obstruction could not be significantly improved by the placement of a conduit distally to bypass the aortic isthmic hypoplasia. Banding of the main pulmonary artery added pulmonary outflow tract obstruction to unrelieved aortic outflow tract obstruction, leading to failure to thrive, congestive heart failure, and death. (Needless to say, none of these comments is meant critically. Instead, these thoughts represent our best attempts to learn, in order to improve both diagnosis and management. It is our duty to do our very best to learn, which is the main purpose and the highest hope of the book.)

Case 13 was the 2-day-old boy with **{S,L,I}.** He was the infant of a diabetic mother. At 36 weeks gestation, echocardiography revealed severe congestive heart failure (hydrops fetalis), with complete heart block and severe bradycardia (35 to 50 beats/minute).

Death occurred on the second postnatal day. Autopsy revealed dextrocardia, which is appropriate for inverted or L-loop ventricles. A large left superior vena cava returned to the coronary sinus and thence to the right atrium. The right superior vena cava was small and returned to the right atrium. The left-sided tricuspid valve was markedly hypoplastic (diameter = 3 mm) compared with the right-sided mitral valve (15 mm in diameter). The left-sided right ventricle was thick-walled (11 mm thick) and small-chambered with areas of endocardial fibroelastosis. The right-sided left ventricle appeared normal in size and its wall was 10 mm thick. There as a moderate sized subaortic conoventricular type of ventricular septal defect, 6 mm in diameter. The inverted normally related main pulmonary artery had an internal diameter of 8 mm. The internal diameter of the inverted normally related aorta was 12 mm. The patent ductus arteriosus had an internal diameter of 3 mm.

Thus, the hypoplasia of the left-sided tricuspid valve corresponded to the small size of the left-sided right ventricular cavity. In non-Ebstein congenital tricuspid stenosis, the hypoplasia of the tricuspid valve usually corresponds to that of the right ventricular inflow tract into which the tricuspid valve opens, as in this patient.

Complete Form of Common AV Canal With Congenital Tricuspid Stenosis

Congenital tricuspid stenosis associated with completely common atrioventricular canal occurred in 2 of these 16 patients (12.5%, Table 13.25) (Fig. 13.49).

Case 1 was a 19 11/12-year-old woman with visceral heterotaxy and the polysplenia syndrome. She had seven splenuli in the left upper quadrant and malrotation of the gut, with the small bowel right-sided, the large bowel left-sided, and a common gastrointestinal mesentery. The segmental anatomy was {S,D,S}. The inferior vena cava was interrupted. A prominent left azygos vein returned to the left superior vena cava. There were bilateral superior venae cavae with absence of the left innominate vein. The larger left superior vena cava drained into the left side of a common atrium and a smaller right superior vena cava opened into the right side of the common atrium.

The liver was in situs solitus. The hepatic segment of the inferior vena cava and the hepatic veins drained into the right side of the common atrium close to the midline. The lungs were bilaterally bilobed and the pulmonary veins returned to the left side of the common atrium, also close to the midline.

Earlier in her life, she was thought to have mesocardia with sagittal orientation to the ventricular septum. Later, she was felt to have dextrocardia because of progressive right ventricular hypertrophy.

A complete form of common atrioventricular canal was present, with a few small ventricular septal defects anterior to the superior leaflet of the common atrioventricular valve. It resembled an ostium primum atrial septal defect, with a few small ventricular septal defects. The mitral valve component of this common atrioventricular valve was cleft, with mild to moderate mitral regurgitation, with thickening and rolling of the margins of the cleft.

The tricuspid component of the common atrioventricular valve was abnormally formed, with abnormal insertions into the right ventricular septal surface, resulting in subtricupsid stenosis.

Surgical repair involved septation of the common atrium and common atrioventricular valve. The postoperative course was characterized by low cardiac output and pulmonary edema, that was thought to be secondary to a redundant atrial baffle that led to pulmonary venous obstruction.

This patient's mild tricuspid stenosis was not thought to be important preoperatively. The important preoperative clinical problems were the common atrium, the completely common atrioventricular canal with mitral regurgitation, and congestive heart failure. The important postoperative hemodynamic problem was pulmonary venous obstruction with pulmonary edema and low cardiac output.

Case 43 was a 32-day-old black boy with normal segmental anatomy, that is, {S,D,S}, but with completely common atrioventricular canal and extremely severe stenosis of the tricuspid component of the common AV valve and a very small right ventricular sinus.

The patient was born prematurely at 37 weeks gestation with a birth weight of 2300 grams. Karyotype revealed a chromosomal anomaly of chromosome 11p. He had intrauterine growth retardation, gram negative sepsis, congestive heart failure, and necrotizing enterocolitis. Autopsy revealed *E. coli* meningitis and ventriculitis that was judged to be subacute. Cardiorespiratory failure was regarded as the cause of death.

Autopsy confirmed the presence of severe congenital tricuspid stenosis in the setting of completely common AV canal. A left superior vena cava opened into the coronary sinus and thence into the right atrium. There was an ostium primum type of atrial septal defect, with a ventricular septal defect of the atrioventricular canal type that was restrictive. There was a wide cleft of the mitral component of the common atrioventricular valve with mitral regurgitation.

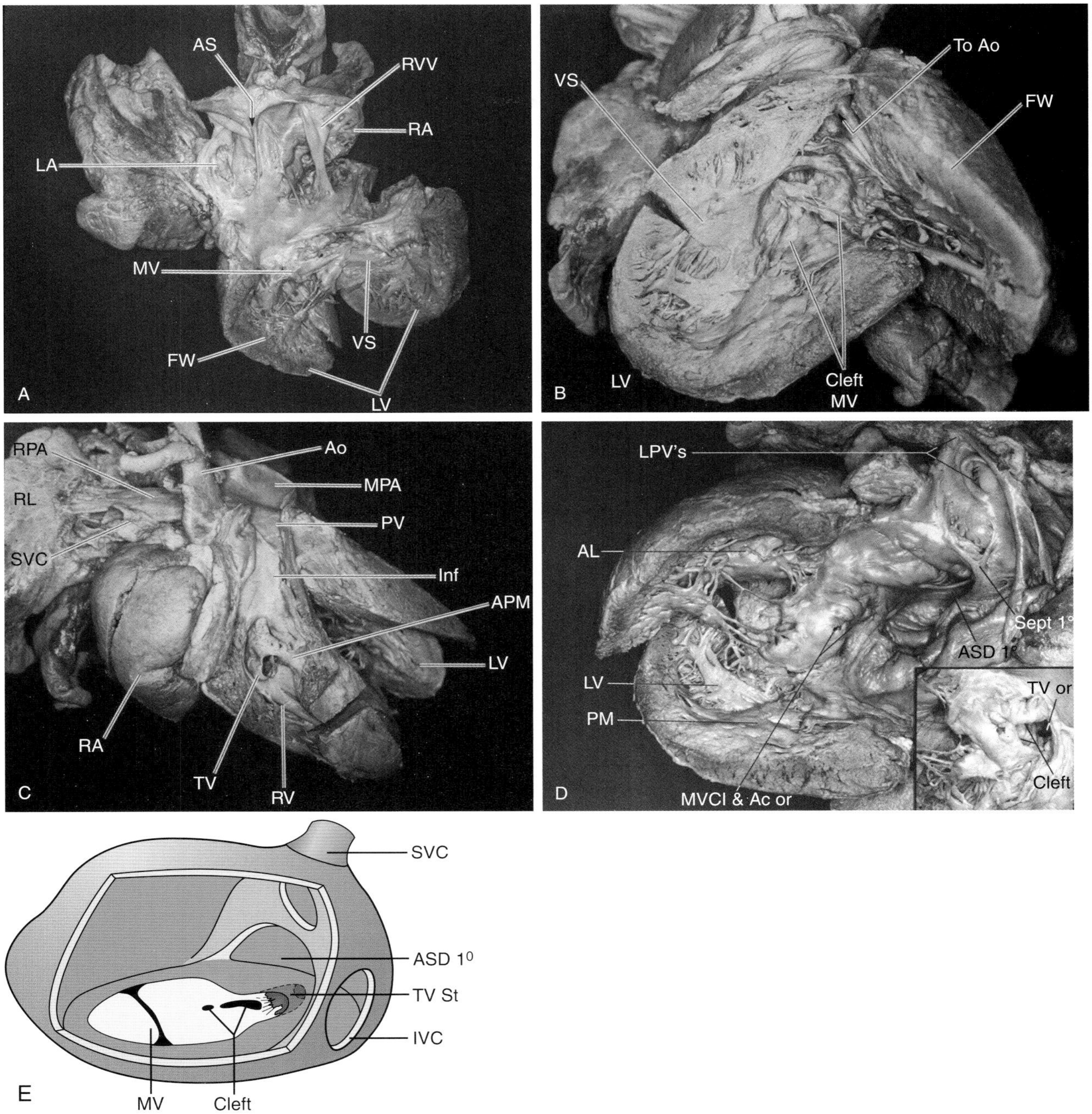

Fig. 13.49 Complete form of common atrioventricular canal (CCAVC) with congenital tricuspid stenosis and small right ventricle. (A) The opened common atrium with a vestigial atrial septum *(AS)* demarcating the morphologically right atrium *(RA)* to the viewer's right *(posterior view)* and the morphologically left atrium *(LA)* to the viewer's left. A right venous valve *(RVV)* remnant is seen to the right of the vestigial AS. The morphologically left ventricle *(LV)* is hypertrophied and enlarged, with the LV's free wall *(FW)* to the left and the LV's ventricular septal surface to the right. The mitral valve component *(MV)* of the common atrioventricular valve is seen. (B) The outflow tract of the LV leading toward the aortic valve. The cleft in the anterior leaflet component of the mitral valve is seen. (C) The very small morphologically right ventricle *(RV)*, which permits the entry of only a small tricuspid valve *(TV)* component of the common AV valve. The tricuspid orifice measured only 7 mm in greatest dimension: marked stenosis of the tricuspid component of this common AV valve. The ventricular septal defect of the AV canal type was restrictive and slit-like (9 × 4 mm). What is conventionally known as congenital tricuspid stenosis is often, as seen here, **a very hypoplastic RV** into which the TV component of the common AV valve can open only minimally. This situation is also known as the **left ventricular type of common AV canal** in which the common AV valve opens almost exclusively into the LV—because the RV is so small. *Ao,* Ascending aorta; *APM,* anterior papillary muscle of the RV; *Inf,* infundibulum; *MPA,* main pulmonary artery; *PV,* pulmonary valve; *RL,* right lung; *RPA,* right pulmonary artery; *SVC,* superior vena cava.

Fig. 13.49 cont'd (D) The opened left atrium, common AV canal, and large LV. The *inset* shows the extremely small orifice of the TV as seen from above *(TV or)*. *AL,* Anterolateral papillary muscle of the left ventricle; *ASD 1°,* atrial septal defect of the ostium primum type (more accurately, atrioventricular septal defect); *LPV's,* left pulmonary veins; *MVCl + Ac or,* mitral valve cleft and accessory orifice; *PM,* posteromedial papillary muscle of the left ventricle; *Sept 1°,* septum primum. (This is Case 58, a 4-year-old boy.) (E) Diagram of another patient with very similar anatomy. The windowed left atrium is viewed from behind. The tricuspid valve stenosis *(TVSt)* is marked. The common AV valve has an incomplete cleft. The ASD 1° is large. An unlabeled ostium secundum type of atrial septal defect is located above ASD 1°. *IVC,* Inferior vena cava. (From Van Praagh R, Litovsky S: Pathology and embryology of common atrioventricular canal. *Progress in Pediatric Cardiology* 1999;10:115–127; with permission.)

Our assessment was that congenital tricuspid stenosis with marked hypoplasia of the right ventricle was only one part of this complex problem. Other more clinically prominent problems included the cleft mitral valve with severe mitral regurgitation, congestive heart failure, necrotizing enterocolitis, gram-negative sepsis, and neonatal meningitis.

Double-Outlet Right Ventricle

Congenital tricuspid stenosis occurred in one patient, a 2-month-old boy, with double-outlet right ventricle {S,D,L} (6%, Table 13.25). The malposed aortic valve was anterior and to the left of the atretic pulmonary outflow tract. Left-sided juxtaposition of the atrial appendages coexisted, the neck of the levomalpositioned right atrial appendage being compressed by the hypoplastic main pulmonary artery. A moderately large secundum atrial septal defect was present. The right ventricle was thick-walled and small-chambered, with moderate hypoplasia of the tricuspid valve, resulting in hemodynamic tricuspid stenosis. A ventricular septal defect of the AV canal type was present (without other evidence of common AV canal). A left aortic arch and a left-sided patent ductus arteriosus (2 mm internal diameter) were present. This patient had a brachiocephalic artery—the first branch of the aortic arch giving origin to the right subclavian, right common carotid, and left common carotid arteries. In 1978, this patient underwent unsuccessful formalinization of the ductus arteriosus (injection of formalin into the wall of the ductus arteriosus to denature its constricting musculature and prevent ductal closure). This surgical procedure was soon abandoned at our hospital because of lack of success, as in this patient. The most clinically important features of this case were pulmonary outflow tract atresia and a closing ductus arteriosus.

To summarize, by far the most common anatomic type of congenital tricuspid stenosis was associated with a small right ventricular sinus (inflow tract) cavity (48 of 70 cases, 69%, Table 13.23). Of these 48 patients, 31 had pulmonary atresia or severe stenosis with intact ventricular septum (31/70 = 44% of the whole series).

There were 17 other patients with congenital tricuspid stenosis and a small-chambered right ventricular sinus, but who did not have pulmonary atresia or severe stenosis with intact ventricular septum (17/70 = 24% of the whole series). These 17 patients had the following (Table 13.25):

1. congenital tricuspid stenosis {S,D,S}, but without severe pulmonary stenosis, 4;
2. transposition of the great arteries (5), with TGA {S,D,D} 2, TGA {S,D,L} 1, and TGA {S,L,L} 2;
3. tetralogy of Fallot {S,D,S} 3;
4. AV discordance with VA concordance 2, with {S,L,S} 1 and {S,L,I} 1;
5. completely common AV canal 2; and
6. double-outlet right ventricle {S,D,L} 1.

Congenital Tricuspid Stenosis With Absence of the Right Ventricular Sinus (Inflow Tract) and Double-Inlet Single Left Ventricle. Is it really possible to have congenital tricuspid stenosis when the right ventricular sinus (inflow tract) is absent? Indeed it is; as Table 13.23 shows, this was the second most common type of congenital tricuspid stenosis, being found in 11 of these 70 patients (16%).

One must quickly add, however, that some degree of skepticism seems well merited. The question is as follows: In double-inlet left ventricle with single left ventricle (meaning absence of the right ventricular sinus), is what we call the tricuspid valve really the tricuspid valve? Remembering the lessons that we learned from Ebstein's anomaly, we know that the normal tricuspid valve has an important right ventricular component. Failure of the normal delamination and ascent of the septal and posterior leaflets of the tricuspid valve results, in Ebstein's anomaly, in the marked downward displacement of the septal and posterior leaflets into the right ventricular cavity, far below the right atrioventricular junction. This means that the tricuspid valve, which is right-sided with ventricular D-loop and left-sided with a ventricular L-loop, cannot be a *normal* tricuspid valve. At "best," it can be a tricuspid valve without its right ventricular component. At "worst," it may not be the tricuspid valve at all. Perhaps this "tricuspid valve" may be a subdivided portion of the atrioventricular valve that in the early embryo opens from the left atrium into the left ventricle. Later in development, this AV valve comes to underlie both atria, not just the left atrium, but also the right atrium. Then this atrioventricular valve undergoes division relative to the overlying atrial septum, resulting in a ventricular D-loop in what we call the mitral valve between the left-sided left atrium and the left part of the underlying single left ventricle, and resulting in what we call the tricuspid valve between the right-sided right atrium and the right part of the underlying single left ventricle.

If the latter concept is correct, and this is the view that we favor, the tricuspid valve consists of its normal atrioventricular canal components, but lacks *per force* its normal right ventricular components.

Thus, in double-inlet left ventricle, we think that what we have been calling the tricuspid valve is the tricuspid valve, but it is not an entirely normal tricuspid valve because this valve lacks its normal right ventricular components.

Gender: males = 8, females = 3, males/females = 8/3 (2.67/1).

In this small series, there was a strong male preponderance.

Age at death: mean = $1^{2}/_{12} \pm 2^{2}/_{12}$ years, ranging from 12 hours to $6^{11}/_{12}$ years, with a median of 23.5 days.

Segmental anatomy: Three different segmental combinations were found in this series of 11 cases with double-inlet left ventricle and congenital tricuspid stenosis:

1. TGA {S,L,L} in 6 (55%);
2. {S,D,S} in 3 (27%); and
3. TGA {S,D,D} in 2 (18%)

Ventriculoatrial malalignment appeared to be the basic mechanism causing congenital tricuspid stenosis (Fig. 13.50). If there was not enough space immediately beneath the tricuspid valve, then the result was congenital tricuspid stenosis. For example, the tricuspid valve might open directly into the underlying left ventricular free wall, or directly into the ventricular septal remnant—instead of opening into the unobstructed left ventricular cavity.

Case 12, a $2^{5}/_{12}$-year-old boy, exemplifies **ventriculoatrial malalignment** and its sequelae of congenital tricuspid stenosis (with or without congenital tricuspid regurgitation). He had single left ventricle with an infundibular outlet chamber and TGA {S,L,L} with double-inlet left ventricle. The left-sided tricuspid valve opened onto the left ventricular free wall, without subjacent chordae tendineae or papillary muscles. The hemodynamic result was left-sided congenital tricuspid stenosis and regurgitation, both moderately severe. Pulmonary outflow tract stenosis was present and the atrial septum was well formed. Congestive heart failure appeared at 3 months of age.

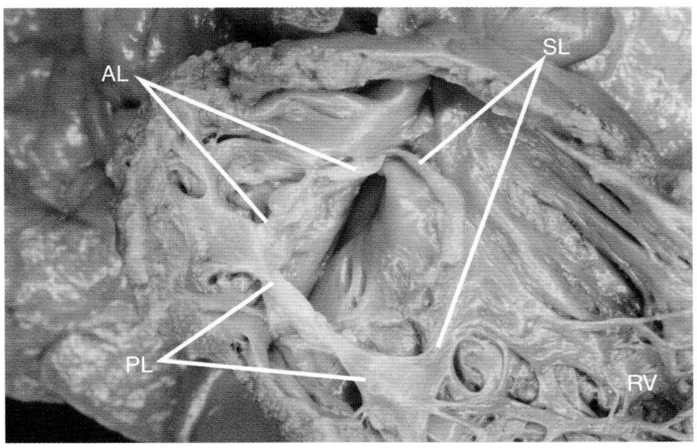

Fig. 13.50 Marked hypoplasia of tricuspid valve leaflets, associated with severe congenital tricuspid regurgitation leading to hydrops fetalis and intrauterine death at 29 weeks gestation. The anterior tricuspid leaflet *(AL)* was present but very hypoplastic. The posterior leaflet *(PL)* was somewhat better developed, but still markedly hypoplastic. The septal leaflet *(SL)* was vestigial (partially absent). The heart was structurally otherwise unremarkable with normal segmental anatomy {S,D,S}. If congenitally unguarded tricuspid orifice is defined strictly as absence of all tricuspid valve leaflets and their tensor apparatus (chordae tendineae and papillary muscles), then anatomically, the patient does not have congenitally unguarded tricuspid orifice; physiologically, however, that is precisely what this patient had and that is the diagnosis that was made. Anatomically and physiologically, this case could certainly be regarded as having a variant of congenitally unguarded tricuspid orifice.

At 22 months of age in 1986, atrial septectomy was performed. Postoperatively, congestive heart failure increased and the postpericardiotomy syndrome occurred. At 29 months of age, a modified Fontan procedure was performed. The right atrial appendage was anastomosed to the main pulmonary artery and the right pulmonary artery, the pulmonary valve was sutured closed, and an intraatrial Gore-Tex baffle was placed creating right AV valve "atresia" so that all the systemic venous blood was directed to the pulmonary artery. Neither atrioventricular valve was touched surgically. The postoperative course was characterized by low cardiac output, leading to a Fontan takedown 2 days postoperatively with placement of a 5 mm central shunt, resulting in intraoperative death.

Case 21 also exemplifies **ventriculoatrial malalignment** leading to subtricuspid obstruction. This $3^{2}/_{12}$-year-old boy with single left ventricle and an infundibular outlet chamber with normally related great arteries {S,D,S} had severe tricuspid stenosis because the tricuspid valve straddled the ventricular septal remnant. This was a Holmes heart with severe congenital tricuspid stenosis, the bulboventricular foramen being obliterated by the adherent tricuspid leaflet tissue. The occluded bulboventricular foramen resembled a potential ventricular septal defect of the AV canal type that was totally occluded by the straddling and adherent tricuspid leaflet tissue. This patient also had pulmonary infundibular and valvar atresia. The mitral valve was thickened and redundant with mitral regurgitation. This patient had multiple congenital anomalies with microcephaly and partial deletion of chromosome 8. The cause of death was an obstructed modified Fontan pathway.

Case 45, a 23-day-old boy, had single left ventricle with an infundibular outlet chamber and **truncus arteriosus type 2** and with normal segmental anatomy, that is, {S,D,S} and double-inlet left ventricle with very severe congenital tricuspid stenosis (1 mm in diameter opening) compared with the mitral valve (14 mm in diameter).

Truncus arteriosus with single LV is a very rare combination. Type 2 indicates that there was no aorticopulmonary septal remnant. This patient also had left-sided juxtaposition of the atrial appendages because of levopmalposition of the right atrial appendage, with a large secundum atrial septal defect (18 × 9 mm). It is worthy of being remembered that **the left-sided juxtaposition of the atrial appendage syndrome** includes severe tricuspid obstruction (stenosis or atresia), marked underdevelopment of the right ventricle, and a secundum atrial septal defect.[242,243] This patient also had **congenital absence of the ductus arteriosus.**

If our understanding of what **truncus arteriosus** really is proves to be correct, then truncus type 2 {S,D,S} has pulmonary infundibular and valvar atresia, with absence of the main pulmonary artery component and hence absence of an aortopulmonary septal remnant. Absence of the pulmonary infundibulum, pulmonary valve, and main pulmonary artery would also help to explain why the ductus arteriosus is absent in this case. Ductal development is thought to depend on right-to-left blood flow in utero from the main pulmonary artery through the ductus arteriosus and into the descending thoracic aorta. But in what is known as truncus arteriosus type 2, atresia or functional absence of the pulmonary infundibulum, valve, and main pulmonary artery would explain why there is no ductus arteriosus: no right-to-left blood flow from the main pulmonary artery through the ductus to the descending thoracic aorta.

One final rare detail: This patient died at 23 days of age of a ventricular arrhythmia (it was thought at the New England Medical Center, Boston, by Dr. Jonathan Rhodes and his colleagues, to whom we are deeply indebted for this fascinating consultation).

Thus, we think type 2 truncus arteriosus is not really a truncus arteriosus *communis* (a common aortopulmonary trunk), because the main pulmonary artery component is absent. Hence, our hypothesis is that trunucs arteriosus type 2 is really a **solitary aortic trunk,** or if one prefers Latin, **truncus aorticus solitarius,** not a truncus arteriosus *communis.*

Congenital Tricuspid Stenosis With Ebstein's Anomaly

Congenital tricuspid stenosis caused by Ebstein's anomaly was the third most frequent type of congenital tricuspid stenosis, occurring in 10 of these 70 postmortem cases (14%, Table 13.23). This should probably come as no surprise because it is now widely understood that Ebstein's malformation can have many different hemodynamic sequelae, varying from congenital tricuspid regurgitation to tricuspid atresia (imperforate Ebstein's anomaly). Ebstein's with congenital tricuspid stenosis may be viewed as representing the stage moving towards imperforate Ebstein's malformation, but not quite so extreme.

Gender: males = 7, females = 3, and males/females = 2.3/1.

Age at death or cardiac transplantation: mean = 5.1 ± 8.0 months, ranging from 2.5 days to 2$^{1}/_{12}$ years, with a median of 24 days.

Of these 10 patients, 9 died, but 1 (**Case 37,** a 2$^{1}/_{12}$-year-old boy) underwent successful heart transplantation. He was the oldest patient in this series. His explanted heart specimen confirmed that he had Ebstein's anomaly {S,D,S} with congenital tricuspid stenosis. He had extremely reduction of interchordal spaces, these potential spaces being filled with valve-like tissue. The interchordal spaces are an important component of the normal tricuspid orifice; hence the obliteration of these spaces leads to congenital tricuspid stenosis. This patient had only two openings through his tricuspid valve: a 3 mm long slit that faced upwards toward the right ventricular outflow tract; and a 16 × 5 mm opening that faced inferiorly and opened into the right ventricular free wall (not into the right ventricular cavity).

He had two ventricular septal defects: a high large muscular ventricular septal defect (20 mm internal diameter); and a moderate sized membranous ventricular septal defect that opened into the atrialized right ventricle and permitted a left ventricular-to-right atrial shunt.

This patient also had **bizarre left ventricular architecture** with myocardial bridges joining the anterolateral and the posteromedial papillary muscles of the left ventricle.

The superior endocardial cushion component of the anterior mitral leaflet inserted directly into the left ventricular septal surface, resulting in a noncanal type of cleft of the mitral valve, but without significant associated mitral regurgitation.

There was striking thinning of the ventricular septum below the muscular ventricular septal defect. The muscular ventricular septum deviated in a rightward direction and wrapped around the small right ventricular sinus. The left ventricular conduction system ran freely within the left ventricular cavity, there being a space between the conduction system to the left and the rightwardly deviated ventricular septum to the right. Thus, this patient with Ebstein's anomaly of the tricuspid valve and the right ventricular sinus also had the rare associated finding of mitral and left ventricular dysplasia. **Ebstein's malformation with biventricular atrioventricular valvar and biventricular myocardial dysplasia** is both rare and noteworthy.

His pulmonary valve was bicuspid (because of a rudimentary nonseptal–right septal commissure). He had valvar pulmonary stenosis with thickened myxomatous leaflets, a small annulus, and a 40 to 60 mm Hg gradient. He had moderate endocardial fibroelastosis of the right ventricle.

Cyanosis had been noted at 3 hours of age. Echocardiography revealed Ebstein's anomaly with severe left ventricular dysfunction. Left ventricular contraction were seen only at the base and at the apex of the left ventricle. Cardiac output was very low. Bifrontal cerebral infarctions were noted, associated with seizures.

Successful cardiac transplantation at 2½ years of age in this boy with **Ebstein's anomaly and biventricular pathology** is noteworthy.

Segmental anatomy: In these 10 patients with congenital tricuspid stenosis and Ebstein's anomaly, the segmental anatomy was normal, that is {S,D,S} in 8 (80%), but was TGA {S,L,L} in 1 (10%), and was DORV {A(S),D,D} in 1 asplenic patient. (DORV {A(S),D,D} means double-outlet right ventricle with situs ambiguus of viscera and atria, but with the atria thought to be in situs solitus, with D-loop ventricles, DORV and with D-malposition of the great arteries.)

These 10 patients with Ebstein's anomaly and congenital tricuspid stenosis had many noteworthy anatomic findings, some of which are as follows:

Case 2, a 6-month-old boy with asplenia syndrome and DORV {A(S),D,D}, had an incomplete form of common AV canal: an ostium primum type of atrial septal defect, but no ventricular septal defect of the AV canal type. He had a double-orifice mitral valve, and an almost imperforate Ebstein's anomaly of the tricuspid valve, there being only one probe patent interchordal space where the anterior tricuspid leaflet inserted into the anterior papillary muscle group of the right ventricle. All other interchordal spaces of the anterior tricuspid leaflet were filled with leaflet-like tissue. The posterior leaflet of the tricuspid valve was downwardly displaced, its medial portion being absent. The septal leaflet of the tricuspid valve was absent. This case of Ebstein's anomaly displayed **a partial form of**

congenitally unguarded tricuspid orifice (congenital absence of tricuspid valve leaflets), which is typical of Ebstein's anomaly.

There was an obstructive muscle bundle of the right ventricle, with only a small opening above the obstructing anomalous muscle bundle.

There was a bilateral conus (subaortic and subpulmonary), with pulmonary outflow tract atresia (infundibular, valvar and also of the main pulmonary artery). The right and left pulmonary artery branches were discontinuous. A conoventricular type of ventricular septal defect measured 9 × 3 mm.

In this case of the heterotaxy syndrome with asplenia, the liver was symmetrical (often erroneously described as "midline"), the stomach was in the left upper quadrant, and the noninterrupted (intact) inferior vena cava connected with the right-sided right atrium. No coronary sinus ostium was found, presumably due to unroofing of the left sinus horn (or failure of formation of the coronary sinus septum that normally separates the coronary sinus posteriorly from the left atrium anteriorly).

This case illustrates that Ebstein's anomaly can be associated with the incomplete form of common atrioventricular canal in the heterotaxy syndrome with asplenia.

I had the privilege of studying this case in 1982 with Dr. Rumiko Matsuoka, now a leading investigator at Tokyo Women's Medical University, Tokyo, Japan. We are greatly indebted to Dr. Kathy Heidelberger of the University of Michigan Medical School in Ann Arbor for the privilege of studying this rare case in consultation.

It should be understood that much of what we have learned at the Cardiac Registry of Children's Hospital Boston has never been published previously. This chapter is an excellent example of that.

Case 15, a 21-day-old boy, illustrates that Ebstein's anomaly with congenital tricuspid stenosis can occur in a discordant ventricular L-loop. The segmental anatomy was TGA {S,L,L}—the classical form of congenitally physiologically "corrected" transposition of the great arteries. Unfortunately, as so often happens, associated anomalies conspired to spoil the potential physiologic correction of the circulations. In the severely stenotic left-sided tricuspid valve, only the anterior leaflet was present. The septal and the posterior leaflets of the tricuspid valve were absent. There was **double-orifice of the tricuspid valve (DOTV)** with straddling of the left-sided tricuspid valve that was located above the ventricular septum. The result was **double-outlet left atrium (DOLA).** The left-sided orifice of the tricuspid valve opened into the left-sided right ventricle; and the right-sided orifice of the tricuspid valve opened into the right-sided left ventricle. Both tricuspid orifices were markedly stenotic.

The right atrial ostium of the coronary sinus was atretic. There was a small and restrictive secundum atrial septal defect (3 × 2 mm); septum primum bulged into the right atrium, reflecting the obstruction of the stenotic left-sided Ebstein tricuspid valve. A conoventricular type of ventricular septal defect was slit-like (exceedingly small). Hypoplasia of the aortic isthmus and preductal coarctation of the aorta were thought to reflect reduced anterograde aortic blood flow, caused by the combination of severe congenital tricuspid stenosis (left-sided) plus a very small ventricular septal defect.

This case is significant not only because it illustrates **stenotic Ebstein's anomaly in TGA {S,L,L}**, but also because it exemplifies **double-orifice tricuspid valve** resulting in **double-outlet left atrium** (opening into RV and LV, both ostia stenotic) in the setting of **straddling tricuspid valve.**

In 1970, I had the pleasure of studying the foregoing rare case with the late Dr. Masahiko Ando, founder of the Cardiac Registry of Tokyo Women's Medical University, Tokyo, Japan, and with the late Dr. Stella Van Praagh, my incomparable wife. We are indebted to Dr. William T. Dungan of the University of Arkansas Medical Center in Little Rock for the privilege of studying this rare case in consultation.

Case 24, an 11-month-old girl, had Ebstein's anomaly {S,D,S} with congenital tricuspid stenosis and marked thinning of the right ventricular free wall (a Uhl's disease component, common in Ebstein's anomaly). The septal and posterior tricuspid leaflets were absent (a congenitally unguarded tricuspid valve component, common in Ebstein's anomaly). Right-to-left shunting occurred at the atrial level, leading to marked systemic desaturation (72% to 74% oxygen saturation) and polycythemia (hemoglobin 20 gm%, hematocrit 60% at cardiac catheterization). At 4½ months of age, a right Blalock-Taussig shunt was done (in 1983). The systemic oxygen saturation increased to 80%. But congestive heart failure developed, which later improved with decongestive therapy. Acute meningitis caused by *Haemophilus influenzae* claimed her life at 11 months of age.

This patient illustrates stenotic Ebstein's anomaly that led to marked right-to-left shunting at the atrial level, requiring a Blalock-Taussig anastomosis at 4½ months of age, and with fatal acute meningitis at 11 months of age.

This patient illustrates that **stenotic Ebstein's anomaly can be a form of cyanotic congenital heart disease.** By right-to-left atrial shunting that permits much of the systemic venous return not to pass through the "filter" of the pulmonary circulation, congenital tricuspid stenosis may have facilitated the development of this patient's fatal meningitis. We do not usually think of Ebstein's anomaly as a form of cyanotic congenital heart disease; but if complicated by tricuspid stenosis or atresia, Ebstein's malformation becomes a form of cyanotic congenital heart disease, with all of the increased associated risks.

Case 27, a boy who died at only 2½ days of age, reinforces the importance of Ebstein's anomaly with congenital tricuspid stenosis (7 × 5 mm) as a form of **rapidly lethal cyanotic congenital heart disease.** The segmental anatomy was normal, that is, {S,D,S}. The patient also had thickened and myxomatous pulmonary valve leaflets, that were not otherwise stenotic (no leaflet fusion, etc.). Cyanosis was present at birth; systemic oxygen saturation was 74%, pO_2 = 45 mm Hg, and arterial pH = 7.28. Cardiomegaly was considered to be massive. His clinical course was characterized by cyanotic spells with hypoxemia, cyanosis, acidosis, and oliguria, leading to death.

Case 29, an 11-day-old girl, had Ebstein's anomaly with severe congenital tricuspid stenosis. The solitary anterosuperior opening measured only 4 mm in length. The septal tricuspid leaflet was absent; so too was the medial component of the posterior leaflet. The right ventricular free wall was very deficient anteroinferiorly (Uhl's disease component). The pulmonary valve was only mildly hypoplastic.

At 3 days of age, while surgical therapy was being initiated in the operating room, intraoperative **ventricular fibrillation** occurred. Despite immediately and intensive therapy, her course was downhill. Her chest was left open, covered with silastic. Her postoperative course was characterized by episodes of sinus tachycardia, junctional rhythm, ascites, anasarca, oligura, anuria, and death on the 8th postoperative day.

Lethal arrhythmias, well known to be associated with Ebstein's anomaly, were thought to be much more important than the congenital tricuspid stenosis in this particular patient.

Case 42, a boy who died at 2 weeks of age, had Ebstein's anomaly with marked congenital tricuspid stenosis, a prominent Uhl's disease component (the right ventricular free wall was very thin and was described as "scrotal"), mild valvar pulmonary stenosis (thickened and dysplastic leaflets), patent foramen ovale, a moderator band of the left ventricle, and **abnormal left ventricular myocardial architecture** with origin of the posteromedial papillary muscle partly from the left ventricular septal surface. This is the second patient in this small group of 10 patients with Ebstein's anomaly and congenital tricuspid stenosis to have **associated left ventricular myocardial dysplasia.** The other patient was Case 37 (above) who underwent cardiac transplantation.

When the present patient (Case 42) was 2 weeks of age (in 1980), the stenotic Ebstein tricuspid valve was replaced with a #21 St. Jude prosthesis, the patent foramen ovale was closed with a Gore-Tex patch, and the patent ductus arteriosus was ligated. The postoperative course was characterized by complete heart block, low cardiac output, and death 4 hours postoperatively.

Autopsy confirmed all of the pathologic anatomic findings presented heretofore, and also revealed iatrogenic right coronary arterial stenosis. A suture used to place the tricuspid valve prosthesis was found to have compressed the right coronary artery in the right atrioventricular groove approximately 2 cm from the ostium of the right coronary artery.

To summarize, this was the second case with biventricular myocardial dysplasia in association with Ebstein's anomaly and congenital tricuspid stenosis (Cases 37 and 42) (2/10, 20%).

Case 46, a 6-month-old boy, had Ebstein's anomaly {S,D,S} with exceedingly severe congenital tricuspid stenosis. The small and obstructive tricuspid valve was located just beneath the normally located pulmonary valve. This is what we call the **"infantile form" of Ebstein's anomaly.** The degree of displacement of the tricuspid valve is spectacular. At first glance, it looks as though there are two pulmonary valves, one on top of the other. The more distal pulmonary valve is the real pulmonary valve, in the normal location. The valve just beneath the pulmonary valve is the small, obstructive, and extremely displaced tricuspid valve. It looks as though the tricuspid valve has hung from its anterosuperior commissure, and has then rotated inferiorly, then anteriorly, and then superiorly—like an accomplished gymnast—to end up only slightly beneath the normally located pulmonary valve.

This description of the apparent morphogenetic movement of this exceedingly displaced Ebstein's tricuspid valve is made by comparing this subpulmonary tricuspid valve with a normally located tricuspid valve. We do this only for the purposes of first attempted description.

What we think has really happened—or, in fact, what has failed to happen—is that this very displaced subpulmonary tricuspid valve has failed to delaminate and to move in the *opposite* direction: inferiorly, posteriorly, and superiorly up to the right atrioventricular junction—all of this normal morphogenetic movement and rotation occurring around the anterosuperior commissure of the tricuspid valve between the most anterior aspects of the anterior and septal tricuspid leaflets. The papillary muscle of the conus (also known as the medial papillary muscle, or the muscle of Lushka, or the muscle of Lancisi)—this is approximately the hub around and beneath which this normal rotatory morphogenetic movement of the tricuspid valve normally occurs, but fails to occur in this—the most severe form of Ebstein's anomaly.

This patient also had a huge apical muscular ventricular septal defect (12 × 10 mm). As seen from the left ventricular perspective, one realizes that the entire finely trabeculated apical portion of the muscular ventricular septum is missing. The part that is missing is the ventricular sinus septum, the part that is formed by the outpouching of the neighboring or adjacent left and right ventricular sinuses.

It should be recalled that when we talk about the delamination and migration and ascent of the septal leaflet of the tricuspid valve, we are also talking about the laying down of right ventricular septal myocardium just beneath this migrating septal tricuspid leaflet. If the tricuspid valve failed to delaminate and migrate, then not only would that explain the bizarre subpulmonary location of the tricuspid valve, but it might perhaps also help to explain the presence of a large muscular apical ventricular septal defect—because not only did the tricuspid valve fail to migrate; the ventricular septal myocardium also did not get laid down. This hypothesis may help to make this large muscular VSD more comprehensible; but it does not explain why the *left* ventricular component of the ventricular septal myocardium must also have failed to form. If Ebstein's should be viewed as really a *biventricular* myocardial dysplasia, then absence of both RV and LV septal myocardial components could perhaps become more understandable.

I do *not* want to suggest that Ebstein's anomaly typically is a biventricular myocardial dysplasia: this is *not* what one usually sees. But we now know that occasionally biventricular myocardial dysplasia can be associated with Ebstein's anomaly (Cases 37 and 42 above).

This heart displayed another rare anomaly: a large (39 × 25 mm) **aneurysm of the right horn of the sinus venosus** underlying the right ventricle. The large orifice (22 × 13 mm in internal diameter) leading into this aneurysm did not have any valve between the right atrium and the aneurysm. The wall of the aneurysm was 2 mm thick. (For further information on sinus venosus aneurysms, see Chapter 6.)

The patent foramen ovale was valve competent. A Chiari's network (right venous valve remnants) were present within the right atrium.

This patient had a history of WPW syndrome and of supraventricular tachycardia. The appearance of congestive heart failure had responded appropriately to banding of the main pulmonary artery.

Case 54, a boy who died at 9 days of age, also had Ebstein's anomaly with severe congenital tricuspid stenosis caused by the **infantile or primitive form of Ebstein's malformation**. The tricuspid valve consisted of cauliflower-like excrescences in an immediately subpulmonary location, the internal diameter of the tricuspid valve measuring 3 to 4 mm. There was also a small slit-like orifice (a patent interchordal space) just lateral to the anterior papillary muscle of the right ventricle (1 mm in width).

The atrialized right ventricle displayed diffuse thickening and whitening of the right ventricular endocardium. Septum primum bulged aneurysmally into the left atrium. There was marked deficiency of tricuspid leaflet tissue septally, posteriorly, and inferiorly. The anterior tricuspid leaflet was deep and curtain-like. The small remnant of the septal leaflet of the tricuspid valve had a blood cyst on it, 2 mm in diameter. There was also a very small blood cyst on the inflow surface of the mitral valve (<1 mm in diameter).

Other findings of interest included a small membranous ventricular septal defect, a diminutive right coronary arterial ostium (functionally a single left coronary artery), a bicuspid aortic valve (diminutive right coronary-left coronary commissure); and a closing patent ductus arteriosus (1 mm in internal diameter).

Ebstein's Anomaly: Additional Thoughts

Before leaving Ebstein's anomaly, at least one other thing needs to be said.

A confession: our **classification** of the anatomic types of congenital tricuspid stenosis based on 70 postmortem cases (Table 13.23) is not perfect. (Perhaps no classification can be?) We have one patient, **Case 28,** that had congenital tricuspid stenosis with a small right ventricle and with pulmonary atresia and an intact ventricular septum {S,D,S}. Our problem is that this 17-week-old girl also had Ebstein's anomaly; none of the other 30 patients in this group did (Table 13.23).

Why did we not put case 28 in the group with all of the other Ebstein's patients with tricuspid stenosis (n = 10, Table 13.23)? Our answer is: Because none of these 10 patients resembled pulmonary atresia with an intact ventricular septum and tricuspid stenosis {S,D,S}. These 10 cases had a ventricular septal defect and often many other anomalies in addition, as we have just seen. So, from a hemodynamic standpoint, we thought that Case 28 belonged where we put it (with pulmonary atresia and intact ventricular septum, which this patient also had). But if anyone wishes to reduce the pulmonary atresia or severe stenosis and intact ventricular septum group from 31 to 30 patients, and to add one patient to the Ebstein's group (from 10 to 11 cases), this would be more correct if one considers Ebstein's anomaly only. Thus, there were 11 of 70 patients with Ebstein's malformation (16%, not 14%, Table 13.23).

Congenital Tricuspid Stenosis Produced by Rhabdomyoma of the Ventricular Septum. Case 69 was an 11-day-old girl with a relatively huge rhabdomyoma of the ventricular septum (Fig. 13.51) that greatly widened her ventricular septum and compressed both atrioventricular valves, resulting in secondary tricuspid stenosis and mitral stenosis (Table 13.23). This secondary, extrinsic, compression of both the tricuspid and the mitral orifices was thought to be an important cause of death.

The tricuspid valve was normally formed, but about three quarters of the tricuspid orifice was filled by large gray-pink fleshy rounded masses of protruding tumor tissue, resulting in marked stenosis of the tricuspid orifice. The tricuspid leaflets themselves were involved by two tumor masses, larger mass being 5 mm (about 1/5th of an inch) in diameter. The greatly thickened ventricular septum bulged convexly into the right ventricular cavity, and combined with the tumor masses in the tricuspid leaflets appeared to result in a marked degree of tricuspid stenosis, as viewed from below. The moderator band was somewhat flattened, and showed a couple of blood-filled cysts that measured 3 × 1 and 2 × 1 mm, respectively.

The right ventricular outflow tract was not obstructed and the pulmonary valve appeared normal. The pulmonary veins were moderately dilated and the mitral valve was also involved by tumor tissue. The segmental anatomy was {S,D,S} and examination was otherwise unremarkable.

DISCUSSION

So what really is congenital tricuspid stenosis? What do the data teach us (Tables 13.23 to 13.25)? Have any mechanisms become apparent? I think the answer is yes (Table 13.26).

Mechanisms Resulting in Congenital Tricuspid Stenosis

As is summarized in Table 13.26, there appear to be four main anatomic mechanisms that result in congenital tricuspid stenosis:

1. **Small tricuspid valve and right ventricular inflow tract.** When the right ventricular sinus (inflow tract) is small-chambered, the tricuspid valve has a small annulus resulting in hemodynamic stenosis. The tricuspid leaflets and tensor apparatus (chordae tendineae and papillary muscles) may be hypoplastic, but otherwise normal, or dysplastic (malformed). Congenital tricuspid stenosis resulting from a small tricuspid valve and a small-chambered right ventricular inflow tract was by far the most common anatomic type of congenital tricuspid stenosis encountered in this study (48 of 70 cases, 69%, Table 13.26) and occurred in seven different settings:
    a. with pulmonary atresia and intact ventricular septum {S,D,S} (31/70 cases, 44%);
    b. with TGA (5/70 cases, 7%) of three different segmental anatomic types:
        a. TGA {S,D,D} = 2,
        b. TGA {S,D,L} = 1, and
        c. TGA {S,L,L} = 2;
    c. with normal segmental anatomy, that is, {S,D,S}, but without severe pulmonary outflow tract obstruction and usually with a ventricular septal defect (4/70 cases, 6%);

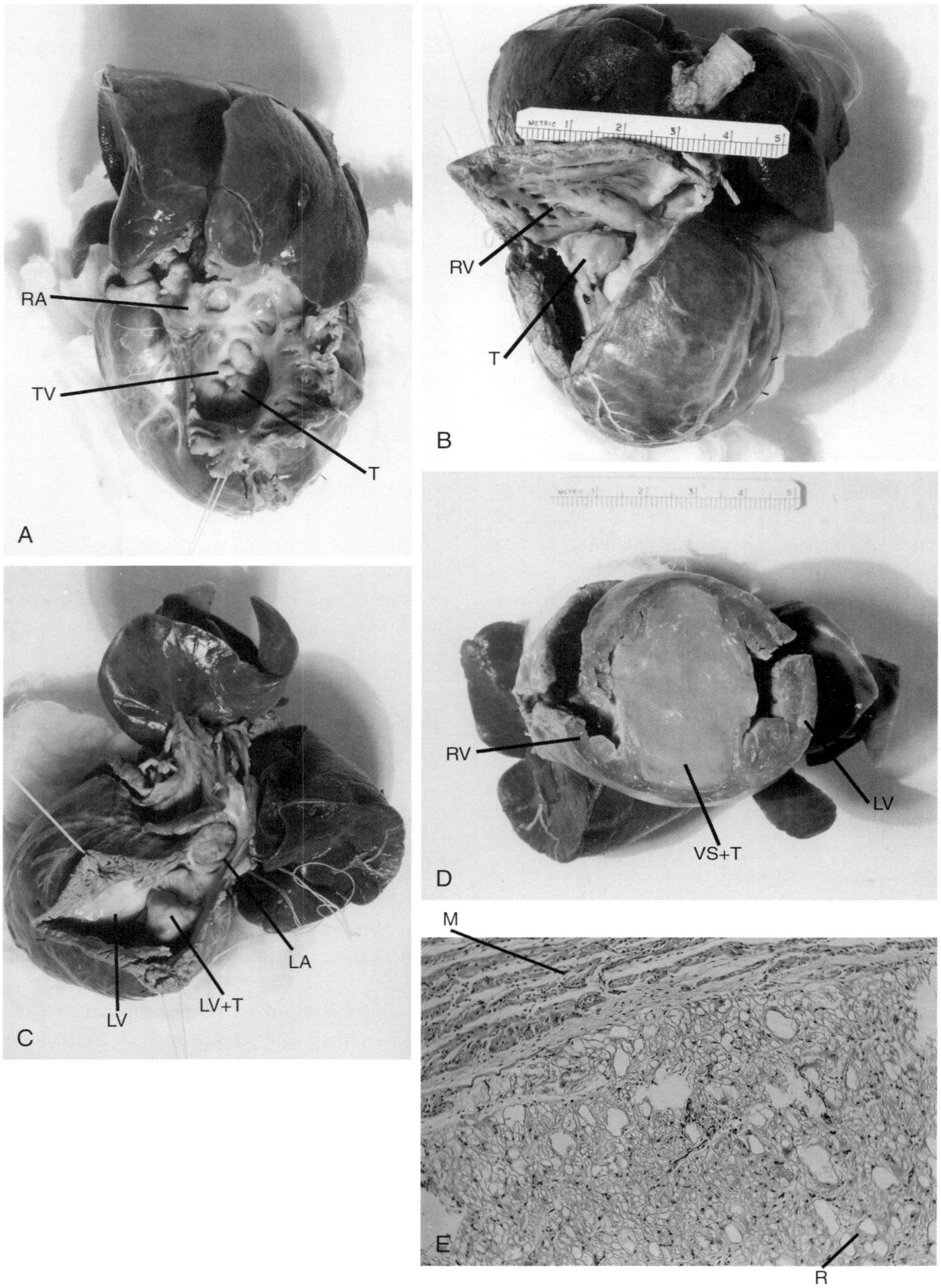

Fig. 13.51 Huge rhabdomyoma of the ventricular septum in an 11-day-old girl. (A) View of the right atrium *(RA)* and the tricuspid valve *(TV)* from above. The tumor *(T)* narrowed the tricuspid orifice, a rare form of congenital tricuspid stenosis. (B) Opened right ventricle *(RV)* and main pulmonary artery (PA). The tumor (T) filled about three quarters of the tricuspid orifice with gray-pink fleshy rounded masses of tumor, producing severe tricuspid stenosis. The tricuspid leaflets were normally formed, but the leaflets were engulfed by two tumor masses, the larger being 5 mm in diameter. The greatly thickened ventricular septum bulged convexly into the right ventricular cavity, contributing to stenosis of the tricuspid valve and right ventricular inflow tract. The right ventricular outflow tract was not obstructed. (C) Opening of the left atrium *(LA)* and left ventricle *(LV)* revealed that the tumor had also involved the mitral valve (MV), producing congenital mitral stenosis. The left ventricular septal surface bulged convexly into the left ventricular cavity. (D) A cross section of the ventricles near the base of the heart revealed a very large rhabdomyoma of the interventricular septum (VS). The left ventricle (LV) is to the viewer's right and the right ventricle (RV) is to the viewer's left, as though one were standing at the foot of the bed and looking cranially (short-axis view). (E) Histologic section showing normal ventricular myocardium and rhabdomyoma *(R)*. (H&E ×185). (All photographs were taken at the time of autopsy in 1957. As an Assistant Resident in Pathology, I was the photographer in D.)

TABLE 13.26 Mechanisms Causing Congenital Tricuspid Stenosis ($n = 70$)

Mechanisms	Examples	No. of Cases	% of Series
1. Small tricuspid valve	Small RV with PAt + IVS	48 31*	69
	Small RV:		
	• with TGA	5	
	• without severe PS	4	
	• with TOF	3	
	• with AVD		
	• with VAC	2	
	• with CCAVC	2	
	• with DORV	1	
2. Ventriculoatrial malalignment	Absent RV with DILV	11	16
	• TGA {S,L,L}	6	
	• {S,D,S}	3	
	• TGA {S,D,D}	2	
3. Arrested or abnormal development of TV + RV sinus	Ebstein's anomaly*	10	14
4. Tumor of ventricular septum	Rhabdomyoma	1	1

AVD, Atrioventricular discordance; *CCAVC*, completely common atrioventricular canal; *DILV*, double-inlet left ventricle; *DORV*, double-outlet right ventricle; *IVS*, intact ventricular septum; *PAt*, pulmonary atresia; *PS*, pulmonary stenosis; *RV*, morphologically right ventricle; *{S,D,D}*, the set of solitus atria, ventricular D-loop, and D-transposition/malposition of the great arteries; *{S,D,S}*, the set of solitus atria, ventricular D-loop, and solitus normally related great arteries; *{S,L,L}*, the set of solitus atria, ventricular L-loop, and L-transposition/malposition of the great arteries; *TGA*, transposition of the great arteries; *TOF*, tetralogy of Fallot; *TV*, tricuspid valve; *VAC*, ventriculoarterial concordance.
*One of our patients, a 17-week-old girl (Case 28), had *both* pulmonary atresia with intact ventricular septum *and* Ebstein's anomaly. We classified her in the pulmonary atresia intact ventricular septum group ($n = 31$); but she could also be classified in the Ebstein group ($n = 10$), which we did not do. So, if one wishes to focus on Ebstein's anomaly, Case 28 could be included with the Ebstein's group (revised $n = 11$, revised % = 15%). (We did not classify her in both groups, which would have made our total number of cases wrong: total $n = 70$, not 71.)

d. with tetralogy of Fallot {S,D,S} (3/70 cases, 4%)
e. with atrioventricular discordance and ventriculoarterial concordance (2/70 cases, 3%) of two different anatomic types:
   i. {S,L,S}, that is, isolated ventricular inversion, in 1, and
   ii. {S,L,I} in 1:
f. with completely common atrioventricular canal (2/70 cases; 3%); and
g. with double-outlet right ventricle {S,D,L} (1/70 cases, 1%).

2. **Ventriculoatrial malalignment with double-inlet left ventricle.** The second most common mechanism resulting in congenital tricuspid stenosis involved double-inlet left ventricle (11/70 cases, 16%, Table 13.26) (Fig. 13.52). When the right ventricular sinus or inflow tract is absent, resulting in single left ventricle, the tricuspid valve can be malaligned relative to the underlying single (unpaired) left ventricle. The tricuspid valve can "open" into the left ventricular free wall, or into the interventricular septal remnant, resulting in congenital obstruction of the tricuspid valve and orifice. The cause of this ventriculoatrial and ventriculo-atrioventricular valvar malalignment almost always appears to be the underlying ventricular part of the heart. The atria typically are not malpositioned, but the ventricular segment (which is a "professional contortionist") often is malpositioned. Malposition of the ventricular segment of the heart relative to the atrial and atrioventricular valvar segments (which we call ventriculoatrial malalignment for convenient brevity) occurred in three different settings:
   a. with TGA {S,L,L} in 6/70 cases (9%);
   b. with {S,D,S} in 3/70 cases (4%); and
   c. with TGA {S,D,D} in 2/70 cases (3%).
3. **Arrested or abnormal development of the tricuspid valve and of the right ventricular sinus: Ebstein's anomaly.** Ebstein's anomaly was present in 11 of 70 postmortem cases of congenital tricuspid stenosis (16%). As the footnote to Table 13.26 indicates (see asterisk), Ebstein's anomaly also occurred in one of the 31 patients with pulmonary atresia and intact ventricular septum.

In an ideal classification, each characteristic (in our case, anomaly) should occur in one group only. Each group should be mutually exclusive of all other groups. The problem is that reality is not always like that. Different characteristics occasionally can and do coexist, defying our hopes for mutual exclusivity.

Ebstein's anomaly illustrates that the tricuspid valve is the "child" of the right ventricular sinus. Their mutually interdependent and interrelated development and anatomy have been presented and illustrated above: The typical failure of formation of the interchordal spaces of the anterior leaflet, which is hemodynamically stenotic; the failure of the septal leaflet to ascending from the conus (septal band) below to the right atrioventricular junction above—and the associated failure to lay down right ventricular septal surface myocardium above the unascending septal tricuspid leaflet; and the thin diaphragmatic surface aneurysm of the right ventricular free wall—another indication of a failure to lay down right ventricular myocardium—not only of the septum, but also of the inferior right ventricular free wall; the Uhl's disease component with marked thinning of the right ventricular free wall anteriorly; and the frequent absence of the septal leaflet and of the septal portion of the posterior leaflet—the congenitally unguarded tricuspid valvar component of severe Ebstein's cases. All of the foregoing can be understood as an arrest or failure of development of both the tricuspid valve and of the right ventricular sinus.

4. **Rhabdomyoma.** I remember this case well from 1957; as a resident I was the photographer (Fig. 13.52). The medial compression of the tricuspid orifice and the valvar invasion by the tumor were unforgettable, and fortunately rare.

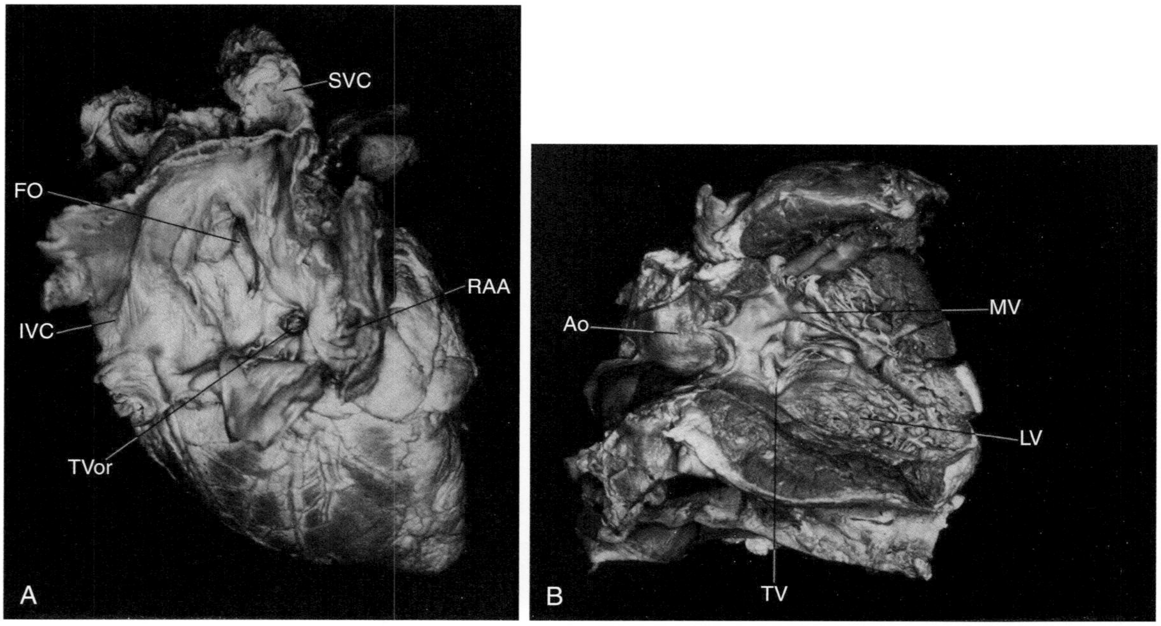

Fig. 13.52 Double-inlet left ventricle {S,D,S} with severe congenital tricuspid stenosis. (A) Opened right atrium showing diminutive tricuspid valve orifice *(TVor). FO,* Foramen ovale; *IVC,* inferior vena cava; *RAA,* right atrial appendage; *SVC,* superior vena cava. (B) Opened left ventricle *(LV)* and ascending aorta *(Ao)* showing normal mitral valve *(MV),* and very stenotic tricuspid valve *(TV)* that barely opens into the LV immediately above the interventricular septum. This is a good example of **ventriculoatrial septal malalignment** causing congenital tricuspid stenosis. If the ventricular septum had been displaced further to the right, then the TV would have opened unimpeded into the LV. If the ventricular septum had been displaced slightly further to the left, then the result would have been tricuspid atresia, i.e., the tricuspid orifice would have been totally blocked by the ventricular septum. An understanding of **ventriculoatrial septal geometry** aids the comprehension of many anomalies of the atrioventricular valves, including atresia, stenosis, straddling, and double-inlet of the AV valves. Cardiac geometry is an underexploited approach to understanding.

SUMMARY

Thus, four mechanisms greatly simplify congenital tricuspid stenosis, helping to make it understandable and memorable (Table 13.25):

1. a small tricuspid valve and right ventricular inflow tract (69%);
2. ventriculoatrial malalignment with double-inlet left ventricle (16%);
3. arrested or abnormal development of the tricuspid valve and of the right ventricular inflow tract: Ebstein's anomaly (14%); and
4. rhabdomyoma (1%).

Congenitally Unguarded Tricuspid Orifice, Also Known as Congenital Absence of Tricuspid Leaflets and Tensor Apparatus

In this very rare anomaly,[541-551] the tricuspid leaflets, chordae tendineae, and papillary muscles are absent. Consequently, the tricuspid orifice is unguarded, resulting in free tricuspid regurgitation. For photographs of congenitally unguarded tricuspid orifice, see Figs. 13.32 and 13.33.

The first case known to us was published by Kugel[541] in 1932. His patient, a 6-month-old girl, was found at autopsy to have total absence of tricuspid valve leaflets and tensor apparatus, associated with pulmonary atresia and intact ventricular septum.

The second case, reported by Klein[542] in 1938, occurred in a 4-year-old girl, who also had absence of tricuspid leaflets and tensor apparatus associated with pulmonary atresia and intact ventricular septum.

In reporting the third known case of congenital absence of the tricuspid leaflets and tensor apparatus associated with pulmonary atresia and intact ventricular septum in 1964, Kanjuh, Stevenson, Amplatz, and Edwards[543] proposed the term *congenitally unguarded tricuspid orifice*. The authors[543] realized that the potential diagnostic term "absence of the tricuspid valve" invites confusion with tricuspid atresia; whereas their proposed designation—*unguarded tricuspid orifice*—avoids this confusion. The point to be understood is that typical tricuspid atresia has absence of all three valvar components: (1) leaflets, (2) tensor apparatus, and (3) orifice. By contrast, congenitally unguarded tricuspid orifice has absence of only two of the three valvar components: (1) leaflets and (2) tensor apparatus. But the tricuspid orifice is present, permitting free tricuspid regurgitation, which functionally is the opposite of tricuspid atresia.

In 1969, Abella, Van Praagh, Novak, Miller, and Hastreiter[544] published two patients with congenital absence of the tricuspid valve leaflets, again with pulmonary atresia and intact ventricular septum. (Note that we were careful to call this anomaly congenital absence of the tricuspid valve *leaflets,* which we thought was another good way of ensuring clarity of meaning, and of avoiding confusion.) Both patients were boys who died at 19 months and 14 days of age, respectively. Noteworthy clinical features included cyanosis since birth, a single S2 (second heart sound), and no murmurs.

Autopsy[544] also revealed that the right ventricular free wall was very thin, with areas of marked right ventricular free wall hypoplasia alternating with areas of right ventricular free wall absence; that is, Uhl's disease was also present. The Uhl's disease component explained why the right ventricle had been so poorly contractile at cardiac catheterization and angiography, and why the *v* wave was so much less prominent than the *a* wave. A giant right atrium with marked hypertrophy and enlargement was found at autopsy, and the tricuspid leaflets were totally absent.

In 1970, Edalgi Kumar, Gilbert, Aerichidé, and Van Praagh[545] proposed that Ebstein's anomaly, Uhl's disease, and congenital absence of tricuspid valve leaflets are all really different features of the **tricuspid and right ventricular dysplasia syndrome.** Why is there so much anatomic overlap between these three supposedly distinct and different "entities"? Because these three anomalies are interrelated, because they are all really parts of something bigger—the tricuspid and right ventricular dysplasia syndrome. We are not trying to displace or get rid of the names of these three anomalies as they are generally defined and understood. Instead, we seek to point out the *anatomic interrelationships* among these three malformations, as a way of deepening understanding.

These interrelationships are very evident in the data.[545] Of 14 postmortem cases with the phenotype of Ebstein's anomaly, absence of demonstrable right ventricular sinus septal myocardium was observed in 11 (79%). Dysplastic right ventricular sinus septal myocardium was found in 3 (21%). Uhl's disease involved the posteroinferior right ventricular free wall in 4 (29%), and involved the entire right ventricular free wall in 1 (7%). Thus, a significant Uhl's disease component was present in 36% of these patients with Ebstein's anomaly.[545] The septal and posterior tricuspid leaflets were partially absent in 4 of these 14 patients with Ebstein's malformation (29%); and the septal and posterior tricuspid leaflets were totally absent in 1 (7%). Hence an important component of tricuspid leaflet absence was observed in 36% of this sample of Ebstein's anomaly.

Imperforate Ebstein's' anomaly (with membranous or valvar tricuspid atresia) was found in 2 patients (14%); imperforate Ebstein's was a newly recognized anomaly at that time (in 1970).[545] Ebstein's was also found with transposition of the great arteries {S,D,D} in 1 patient (7%); this was the first reported such case, to our knowledge.

Left-sided Ebstein's anomaly in transposition of the great arteries {S,L,L} was present in 2 patients (14%);[545] these were the first two described such patients, to our knowledge. Other important anomalies associated with Ebstein's anomaly[545] included ventricular septal defect in 5 (36%); pulmonary atresia in 2 (14%); pulmonary stenosis in 2 (14%); and aortic atresia (valvar) in 1 (7%).

The developmental basis of this newly recognized **tricuspid and right ventricular dysplasia syndrome** was hypothesized to be the intimate relation that is known to exist between the embryonic development of the tricuspid valve and of the right ventricular sinus[545] (presented above).

In 1975, Haworth, Shinebourne, and Miller[546] presented an intriguing hemodynamic paradox: right-to-left shunting at the atrial level, but with normal right ventricular pressure. How could this happen? Their Case 1 had pulmonary atresia, intact ventricular septum, Uhl's disease, and tricuspid valvar dysplasia with tricuspid regurgitation. Consequently, right-to-left atrial shunting had to be 100%, and right ventricular hypertension could not develop because of Uhl's disease plus tricuspid dysplasia with regurgitation.

Their Case 2,[546] a boy who died at 7½ years of age, had absence of the tricuspid valve leaflets—again precluding the development of right ventricular hypertension.

Three other patients[546] (Cases 3, 4, and 5) had isolated right ventricular hypoplasia.

In 1978, Brenner, Bharati, Winn, and Lev[547] presented the first known case of left-sided congenitally unguarded tricuspid orifice in a 36-hour-old boy with transposition of the great arteries {S,L,L}. We had been privileged to study in consultation the heart of a similar patient of Dr. Peter Vlad from the Buffalo Children's Hospital.

In 1986, Gussenhoven, Essed, and Bos[548] presented the case of a 32-day-old boy with congenitally unguarded tricuspid orifice who also had two-chambered right ventricle (also known as anomalous muscle bundles of the right ventricle).

In 1990, Anderson, Silverman, and Zuberbuhler[549] presented the differential diagnoses between Ebstein's malformation and congenitally unguarded tricuspid orifice when each is also associated with pulmonary atresia and intact ventricular septum. Their diagnostic pearl: Echocardiographically, look at the mural (i.e., the anterior) tricuspid leaflet. In Ebstein's anomaly, it is very much present (deep, curtain-like, it waves at you). But in congenitally unguarded tricuspid orifice, the anterior (or mural) tricuspid leaflet is absent.

We agree. You can't trust the septal or the posterior tricuspid leaflets, because—as we've already seen—they can be absent or very dysplastic in Ebstein's anomaly and in congenitally unguarded tricuspid orifice.

Also in this paper, Anderson and his colleagues[549] studied 46 postmortem cases of **pulmonary atresia with intact ventricular septum** (from the Pittsburgh collection). How common is Ebstein's anomaly in this setting? Their finding: 17 of 46 cases (37%). How common is congenitally unguarded tricuspid orifice in this setting? Their answer: 3 of 46 patients (7%).

Is it possible to treat patients effectively with congenitally unguarded tricuspid orifice? Yes, it is possible, as was described (in a letter to the editor) by Magotra, Agrawal, Mall, and Parikh[550] (from Bombay) in 1990. Their patient, a 7-year-old girl, had tricuspid valve replacement with a 31 mm bileaflet mechanical valve (Cardiomedics, Inc.). This is the first known surgical repair of isolated congenitally unguarded tricuspid orifice. The patient did well postoperatively.

In 1996, Agarwala, Waldman, and Carbone[551] confirmed that congenitally unguarded tricuspid orifice can coexist with Uhl's malformation.

OUR SERIES

In our series of 3216 autopsied cases of congenital heart disease, only 2 patients were classified as having congenitally unguarded tricuspid orifice (0.062%). This suggests that in our experience, congenitally unguarded tricuspid orifice is one of the rarest forms of congenital heart disease.

I should state that initially, I thought we had 3 such cases. But on reexamination of our original records (which I have done in all of our cases), I discovered that we had misclassified one patient as having congenitally unguarded tricuspid orifice because the septal leaflet of the tricuspid valve was totally absent, and the posterior leaflet was almost totally absent. However, a deep curtain-like anterior tricuspid leaflet was present, resulting in an imperforate Ebstein's anomaly. We now know that absence of the septal and posterior leaflets of the tricuspid valve—**a partial form of congenitally unguarded tricuspid orifice**—occurs frequently with Ebstein's anomaly.

We have only made the diagnosis of congenitally unguarded tricuspid orifice when *all three leaflets* (including the anterior or parietal or free-wall leaflet) are virtually absent.

The potential difficulties in making the differential diagnosis between Ebstein's anomaly with a partial form of congenitally unguarded tricuspid orifice (absence of the septal and posterior tricuspid leaflets) and the complete form of congenitally unguarded tricuspid orifice (in which the anterior tricuspid leaflet is also absent) illustrate the **tricuspid and right ventricular dysplasia syndrome** in which Ebstein's anomaly, Uhl's disease, and absence of tricuspid valve leaflets often occur together, rather than as separate entities.[545] Each of the "entities" can merge into one another.

Case 1, a 4-week-old girl, was a patient of Dr. James Reynolds of Southern Baptist Hospital in New Orleans. I had the privilege of studying this heart in consultation in 1973 with Dr. Stella Van Praagh. The pathologic anatomic findings may be summarized as follows:

Congenital absence of all tricuspid valve leaflets and tensor apparatus
Marked hypoplasia of the right ventricular sinus
Extreme paucity of right ventricular free-wall myocardium (Uhl's disease)
Double-chambered right ventricle (also known as anomalous muscle bundles of the right ventricle)
No communication between the right ventricular sinus (inflow tract) and the infundibulum (outflow tract), that is, atresia of the proximal os infundibuli with total separation of right ventricular sinus and right ventricular infundibulum
Normal segmental anatomy {S,D,S} with subpulmonary conus and aortic-mitral fibrous continuity
Ventricular septal defect between left ventricle and infundibulum (no communication with right ventricular sinus)
Functionally double-outlet left ventricle with the aorta arising normally from left ventricle, and a widely patent pulmonary artery originating from subpulmonary infundibulum that communicates via a nonrestrictive VSD with the left ventricle only, that is, functionally DOLV {S,D,S} (rare form of DOLV)

PATENT FORAMEN OVALE

Status Post–Waterston Anastomosis

In addition to congenitally unguarded tricuspid orifice and a rare form of functionally DOLV with normal segmental anatomy, that is, without a conotruncal malformation [DOLV {S,D,S}], this case also had a very dramatic **separation or noncommunication between the RV sinus (inflow tract) and the RV infundibulum (outflow tract),** illustrating that the RV sinus and the RV infundibulum really are different cardiac chambers. Normally, the RV sinus and the RV infundibulum look like different parts of the right ventricle, as this ventricle is conventionally understood. But this case is a rare natural experiment demonstrating that the RV sinus and the infundibulum (conus) are really two different chambers. The conus (infundibulum) belongs to the great arteries (the conotruncal segment). The conus is how the great arteries connect with the underlying ventricular sinuses (inflow tracts) and the atrioventricular valves. The sinuses are the real pumps, systemic and pulmonary. The conal connector is not a good pump. The conus is there for structural reasons—to cross the circulations, when the conotruncus develops normally (see Chapter 2). This case demonstrates the *separateness* of the RV sinus (that normally is the lung pump) and the subpulmonary conus or infundibulum (that normally is the connecting segment between the ventricular sinuses and the great arteries).

Case 2 was a male fetus, the estimated age at the time of abortion being 29 weeks, that I studied as a consultation from the Beth Israel Hospital in 1986 with Dr. Maurice Kakou and Dr. Ronald Foran. Our diagnoses were as follows (Fig. 13.50):

Congenitally unguarded tricuspid orifice, forme fruste, with very marked underdevelopment of the tricuspid leaflets (but not absence)
Anterior tricuspid leaflet present, but very hypoplastic
Posterior leaflet of the tricuspid valve somewhat better developed, but still markedly hypoplastic
Septal leaflet of the tricuspid valve minimally present (virtually absent)
Tricuspid regurgitation, severe (fetal echocardiography)
Right atrial hypertrophy and enlargement, marked
Patent ductus arteriosus
No other cardiovascular pathology
Multiple congenital anomalies
Probably intrauterine growth retardation (weight at 29 weeks, 2¾ pounds)
Microphthalmia
Hypertelorism
Micrognathia
Bilateral epicanthal folds
Midfacial hypoplasia
Hydrops fetalis, that is, intrauterine congestive heart failure, with ascites (6 mL), pericardial effusion (5 mL), pericardial sac not tense
Widespread maceration, consistent with intrauterine death
Talipes equinovarus
Widely spaced nipples
Posterior displacement of anus

Flat posterior aspect of head
Low hairline posteriorly

As our diagnoses indicates, small nubbins of anterior, posterior, and septal leaflets of the tricuspid valve were present. But they were so small that the patient had no functionally effective tricuspid leaflet tissue. Noteworthy were the absence of the right ventricular outflow tract obstruction, and the presence of a mildly small patent ductus arteriosus. The ductus was the same size as the left pulmonary artery, rather than being the same size as the descending thoracic aorta (which would be normal). Interestingly, this patient's older brother had tetralogy of Fallot with pulmonary outflow tract obstruction, with a normally formed tricuspid valve (autopsy confirmed), but with severe tricuspid regurgitation (premortem echocardiography). We were never clear why the older brother had severe tricuspid regurgitation with an anatomically normal tricuspid valve. (He may have been moribund when studied. [?])

Did our patient with congenitally unguarded tricuspid orifice have a known syndrome? Our geneticists though he might have a variant of the cerebro-oculo-facio-skeletal syndrome; however, they were not sure. But multiple congenital anomalies definitely were present (as above).

Hypoplastic Tricuspid Valve

We made the diagnosis of hypoplastic tricuspid valve in 6 cases (6 of 3216 cases of congenital heart disease = 0.19%).

Gender: boys = 2, girls = 3, unknown = 1; males/females = 2/3 (0.67).

Ages at death: mean = 51 ± 89 days, ranging from 4¼ hours to 7 months, median = 13 days.

What did we mean by hypoplastic tricuspid valve? The right ventricle was always small-chambered. The tricuspid annulus was always small, appropriate to the size of the right ventricular cavity that it opened into. Typically, the tricuspid leaflets were thin and delicate, with well-formed interchordal spaces—a normal but miniature tricuspid valve. In this anatomic sense, congenital tricuspid stenosis was not present. In a hemodynamic sense, a miniature but otherwise normal tricuspid valve can certainly be stenotic or restrictive, as can the underlying small-chambered right ventricular sinus.

However, congenital hypoplasia of the tricuspid valve was never a primary diagnosis; it was always secondary to something else. The important associated diagnoses in these 6 cases were as follows:

1. tetralogy of Fallot with pulmonary outflow tract atresia, small-chambered right ventricular sinus, and hypoplastic tricuspid valve;
2. pulmonary atresia with intact ventricular septum, bicuspid aortic valve, diminutive right ventricle; and very small tricuspid valve;
3. very severe pulmonary valvar stenosis (unicommissural pulmonary valve), intact ventricular septum, thick-walled and small-chambered right ventricle and hypoplastic tricuspid valve;
4. transposition of the great arteries {S,D,D} with moderately severe right ventricular hypoplasia, hypoplastic tricuspid valve, conoventricular type of ventricular septal defect, hypoplastic ascending aorta, aortic arch, and isthmus;
5. DORV {S,D,D} with left-sided juxtaposition of the atrial appendages, pulmonary atresia, conoventricular ventricular septal defect, moderate right ventricular hypoplasia, and moderate tricuspid hypoplasia; and
6. DORV {S,D,D}, conoventricular ventricular septal defect, mitral valve straddling through the ventricular septal defect, superoinferior ventricles with hypoplastic right ventricle and tricuspid valve superior, well developed left ventricle and large mitral valve inferior, and ventricular septum approximately horizontal.

There is no sharp and valid distinction between tricuspid hypoplasia and tricuspid stenosis. Indeed, the anatomist's tricuspid hypoplasia often is the hemodynamicist's and the surgeon's tricuspid stenosis. For example, the patient with TGA {S,D,D}, RV hypoplasia, and tricuspid hypoplasia died following an arterial switch operation in low cardiac output, we thought because of the hemodynamic restriction (stenosis) imposed by the small right ventricle with hypoplastic tricuspid and aortic valves with aortic hypoplasia.

The purpose of this brief entry on tricuspid hypoplasia is to promote deeper understanding. As Ebstein's anomaly teaches us, remember that the tricuspid valve is the "child" of the right ventricle. When the right ventricular sinus (inflow tract) is small-chambered, the tricuspid valve also is very likeably to be hypoplastic. Even if the tricuspid valve looks like an otherwise normal miniature, it may very well be significantly stenotic from a hemodynamic standpoint. Finally, it should be understood that **the basic diagnosis is a small-chambered right ventricular sinus,** not tricuspid hypoplasia. In other words, when the right ventricular inflow tract has a hypoplastic chamber, tricuspid hypoplasia (small orifice) should be expected as a corollary.

Thus, the most common type of tricuspid hypoplasia is **tricuspid orifice hypoplasia,** often resulting hemodynamically in congenital tricuspid *stenosis*.

A second far rarer form of tricuspid hypoplasia is **tricuspid leaflet hypoplasia,** resulting in massive congenital tricuspid *regurgitation*. We presented this case above as a forme fruste of congenitally unguarded tricuspid orifice (Fig. 13.50). The tricuspid leaflets, chordae, and papillary muscles were very hypoplastic, but not absent.

A third anomaly in which the tricuspid valve may, at first glance from the right atrium appear hypoplastic—but in fact is not—has to do with **tethering anomalies of the tricuspid tensor apparatus** (Fig. 13.53). Viewed from the right atrium (A), the tricuspid leaflet may look too small, preventing leaflet coaptation and resulting in congenital tricuspid regurgitation. However, inspection of the interior of the right ventricle (B) reveals that the problem really is malformation of the tensor apparatus. The anterior tricuspid leaflet really is of good size, but it is bound down or tethered by abnormally short chordae tendineae and small papillary muscles just to the right of the anterior leaflet. This anomaly of the tensor apparatus means that it is not possible for the anterior leaflet to move far enough medially to achieve coaptation and close the tricuspid orifice.

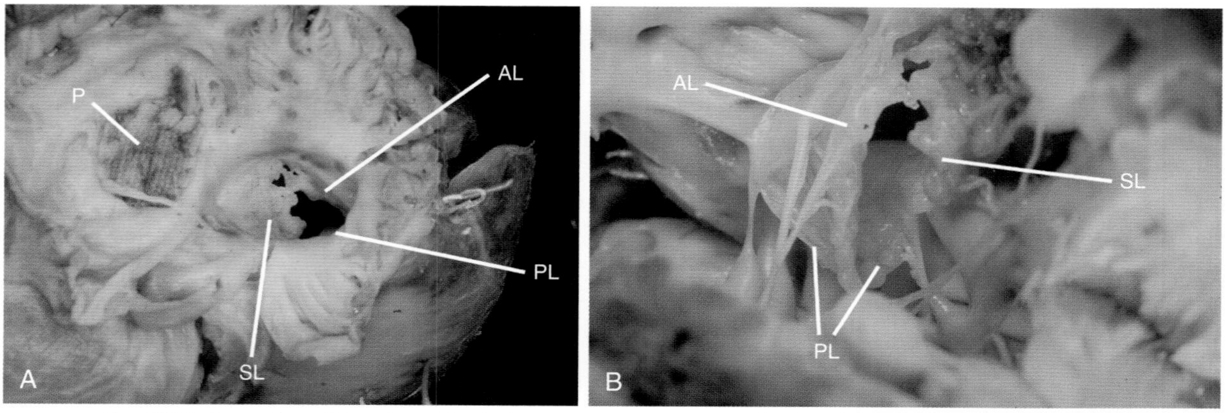

Fig. 13.53 Anomalies of the tricuspid valve's tensor apparatus can make the tricuspid valve look hypoplastic, as seen from above (A). The anterior leaflet *(AL)* looks small and the posterior leaflet *(PL)* seems to be absent. The septal leaflet *(SL)* looks well developed. An atrial septal defect was closed surgically with a patch *(P)*. Malformed chordae tendineae and papillary muscles (B) can bind down tricuspid leaflets, making leaflet coaptation impossible, resulting in tricuspid regurgitation. This is the heart of a 6-week-old boy.

Myxomatous Tricuspid Valve

Eight patients were classified as having a myxomatous tricuspid valve (Table 13.1), giving a frequency of 8 of 3216 autopsied cases of congenital heart disease (0.25%).

Gender: males = 4, females = 3, unknown = 1 (a macerated fetus). The male/female ratio was 4/3 (1.3/1).

Age at death: mean = 9.18 years (3349.4 days) ± 15.4 years (5619.55 days), ranging from 0 postnasal days (a 17 to 18 week gestation fetus) to 41 years. The median age at death was 1½ months (45 days).

Pathology: What is *myxomatous* tricuspid valve? By myxomatous valve leaflets we mean that the leaflets are thickened and flipper-like. Histologically, such leaflets have primitive-appearing connective tissue cells separated by a mesenchymal, gelatinous appearing stroma. The Greek word *myxa* means mucus. The English *myxo* (as in myxomatous) means that histologically the cells are separated by an abnormal amount of mucus-like substance. As a practical matter, we use the term myxomatous valve to mean a thickened, flipper-like immature appearing and abnormal appearing valve leaflets. The term does not mean that we have necessarily examined the valve microscopically; usually we have not. Thus, myxomatous tricuspid valve denotes the aforementioned gross appearance.

What kinds of patients have myxomatous tricuspid valve? Cases that we and the other pathologists at Children's Hospital Boston diagnosed and classified as having myxomatous tricuspid valve always have had other anomalies: myxomatous tricuspid valve never occurred in isolation. Often myxomatous tricuspid valve was just one small part of a total body metabolic or chromosomal syndrome:

1. **mucopolysaccharidosis,** 2 of 8 patients (25%);
2. **chromosomal trisomy,** 2 of 8 patients 925%); and
3. **polyvalvar disease,** 4 of 8 patients (50%).

Each of these apparently three different groups will be described in somewhat greater detail:

1. **Mucopolysaccharidosis.** Our first patient with a mucopolysaccharidosis, an 8-year-old boy who died in 1966, had the severe form of **Hurler's disease** with involvement of the heart, brain, bones and cartilage, liver, spleen, intestinal tract, skin, and tongue. There was cardiomegaly, the heart weight 36% more than normal (150 grams/110 grams). Epicardial thickening and atrial endocardial thickening were noted.

Thickening of the tricuspid, mitral, pulmonary, and aortic leaflets were found. The coronary arterial walls were thickened, most markedly of the left main coronary artery, but without luminal obstruction. The ascending aorta was moderately dilated. Aortic and pulmonary regurgitation were thought probably to have been present; but no hemodynamic data were available. Histology showed a widespread atherosclerosis-like pattern. In all organs, the histiocytes were markedly swollen. The nuclei of the neurons of the brain were swollen and eccentric.

Chemical tests were not done because the diagnosis of Hurler's syndrome was thought to be evident clinically and pathologically.

The Hurler syndrome (mucopolysaccharidosis 1H) is inherited as an autosomal recessive. The primary defect is absence of lysosomal α-L-iduronidase in all tissues, which results in the accumulation of mucopolysaccharides in parenchymal and mesenchymal tissues.[552]

The immediate causes of death were head trauma following a fall and aspiration of food while eating lunch.

Our second patient was a 24 3/12-year-old man with **Hunter's syndrome** (mucopolysaccharidosis II) who died in 1985. His brother also had this syndrome; that is, this was a case of familial Hunter syndrome.

Autopsy revealed an unusual prominent infundibular leaflet between the anterior and septal leaflets of the tricuspid valve. Thus, the tricuspid valve appeared somewhat redundant, displaying this infundibular leaflet at its superior commissure, but was otherwise structurally unremarkable.

The mitral valve also was redundant, displaying unusually prominent leaflets at both the anterolateral and posteromedial commissures. Distinct thickening of the mitral valve leaflets and chordae tendineae were also present. Both the pulmonary and the aortic valves were unremarkable.

To summarize, the abnormality of the tricuspid valve was minimal, and of the mitral valve was mild.

Echocardiography at another institution was interpreted as showing thickening of the aortic and mitral valve leaflets, with mitral insufficiency and mitral stenosis. The patient was thought to have a left expectancy of only a few months because of cardiac disease.

Autopsy findings (described above) did not support these clinical impressions. The coronary arteries were also unremarkable at autopsy. The immediate causes of death were associated with multiple dental extractions (15, for dental caries). Inability to intubate the patient for the induction of anesthesia led to tracheostomy. Postoperatively, bleeding occurred around the tracheostomy. A coagulopathy was diagnosed with a circulating antibody (a lupus-like anticoagulant). Postoperatively the patient could not be weaned from the trachesotomy. A gastrostomy was performed. A wound infection developed around the gastrostomy site *(Staphylococcus aureus)*. This was followed by massive arterial bleeding from the tracheostomy site, leading to death despite resuscitative measures.

The Hunter syndrome has an X-linked inheritance, the primary defect being a deficiency in iduronate sulfatase. Excess dermatan sulfate and heparin sulfate are found in the urine.[553]

Our impression is that these mild tricuspid valve abnormalities found in our patients with mucopolysaccharidosis, while definitely present, were of little or no clinical importance.

2. **Chromosomal trisomies.** One patient had trisomy D **(chromosomes 13, 14, and 15),** the Patau syndrome, and the other had **trisomy 18** (Fig. 13.28).

The patient with trisomy D (involving a trisomy of the chromosome 13.15 group) was a 3-day-old girl who died in 1981. Our pediatric cardiologists thought that the tricuspid valve was huge and that it prolapsed into the right atrium. Autopsy confirmed that she had a dysplastic, myxomatous, and redundant tricuspid valve, with abnormal septal attachments. The segmental anatomy was normal, that is, {S,D,S}. Additional findings included dextrocardia, a membranous (conoventricular) type of ventricular septal defect, two small apical muscular ventricular septal defects, severe preductal coarctation of the aorta (isthmic hypoplasia 5 mm long and 3 mm wide), a large but closing patent ductus arteriosus, a bicuspid aortic valve (absence of the right coronary-noncoronary commissure) that did not appear stenotic, persistent left superior vena cava to the coronary sinus, a large secundum type of atrial septal defect, and multiple other associated congenital anomalies typical of trisomy 13.15.

How clinically important was the tricuspid valve anomaly? **Polyvalvar disease** is typical of trisomies. But the immediate cause of death in this patient was thought to be the combination of severe preductal coarctation of the aorta and a closing ductus arteriosus.

The second case was a fetus of 17 to 18 weeks gestational age, severely macerated and of undetermined sex, who had karyotype-proved trisomy 18. The salient cardiac anomalies consisted of myxomatous, thick septal and anterior tricuspid leaflet, large ventricular septal defect, and reduced interchordal spaces of the posteromedial commissure of the mitral valve—characteristic of trisomy 18.[554]

3. **Polyvalvar disease.** Four of these 8 patients (50%) with myxomatous tricuspid valve had polyvalvar disease:

(a) A 41-year-old man died in 1991 with focal myxomatous thickening of the tricuspid valve that was thought to be of little or no functional significance. All tricuspid leaflets had areas of nodular thickening, up to 3 mm in thickness; these nodular thickenings were prominent where the chordae tendinae attached. There was slight rolling of the leaflet margins. The chordae tendineae were thin and delicate.

The pulmonary valve leaflets showed marked myxomatous change, with elongation of the leaflets. The pulmonary leaflets were up to 1 mm in thickness, with rolled free margins. The pulmonary leaflet were 3 cm in length from the free margin to the deepest aspect of the pulmonary sinuses of Valsalva. The pulmonary annulus was 3 cm in diameter. We thought that pulmonary valve stenosis was probably present in life; but we were aware of no hemodynamic data with which to check the accuracy of our anatomic impression. The pulmonary valve was tricommissural and tricuspid.

The mitral valve was markedly myxomatous with probable mitral valve prolapse, and with evidence of marked mitral regurgitation. The mitral leaflet displayed nodular myxomatous thickening, similar to the tricuspid valve, up to 5 mm in thickness and prominent where the chordae tendineae attached. The mitral leaflets showed hooding between chordal attachments, with billowing toward the left atrial cavity, and with rolling of the free margins. The gross appearance of the mitral valve was "hemorrhoidal"—Dr. Jesse Edwards' unforgettable description of mitral valve prolapse (Barlow syndrome). The left atrium was markedly enlarged with diffuse endocardial thickening and with septum primum bulging into the right atrial cavity. The aortic valve was tricommissural (and therefore tricuspid), with mild diffuse leaflet thickening. The aortic annulus was 2.4 cm in diameter.

The coronary orifices and arteries were unremarkable. This patient's karyotype was not known to us. (We studied this fixed and dissected heart specimen as a consultation from another institution.)

In addition to polyvalvar disease, this patient also had other diagnoses of importance including status epilepticus, low-grade oligodendroglioma of the corpus callosum, neurofibromatosis, pneumonia, alcoholism, and an intellectual disability.

We hypothesized that this patient may have had an unrecognized heritable disorder of connective tissue, which might explain the coexistence of myxomatous polyvalvar disease, neurofibromatosis, intellectual disability, and the thickened corpus callosum with a low-grade oligodendroglioma. We are far from sure that this hypothesis is correct.

But at least one thing is clear: Myxomatous tricuspid valve does not occur alone (in our experience to date). Indeed, this diagnosis should initiate a search for other abnormalities: metabolic (such as mucopolysaccharidosis), or chromosomal (trisomies), or currently idiopathic (not really understood etiologically, as in this patient).

(b) A stillborn male fetus had double-outlet right ventricle {S,D,D} with hypoplastic left heart. As often occurs with DORV when hypoplastic left heart coexists, a unilateral conus (not a bilateral conus) was present. So it was in this case who had the paradox of DORV, but with a normal subpulmonary type of conus, and with absence of the subaortic conal free wall permitting aortic-mitral and aortic-tricuspid direct fibrous continuity.

What kind of hypoplastic left heart was present? Severe congenital mitral stenosis was found with absence of recognizable left ventricular papillary muscles. There was a single focus of insertion of mitral chordae tendineae into the junction between the left ventricular septal surface and the left ventricular free wall posteromedially. Interchordal spaces were absent, the chordae tendineae were shortened, and the only orifice of the mitral valve was at the posteromedial commissure. This severe form of congenital mitral stenosis was regarded as a variant of parachute mitral valve. The left ventricle was small-chambered and thick-walled.

There was a large conoventricular type of ventricular septal defect between the conal septum superiorly and the ventricular septum inferiorly, with posterior extension of the ventricular septal defect into the septum of the atrioventricular canal.

The aorta arose predominantly above the large right ventricle, and there was subaortic stenosis between the conal septum anterosuperiorly and the atrioventricular valves (mainly the tricuspid valve) posteroinferiorly. The aortic annulus was moderately hypoplastic, but the aortic valve was tricommissural and tricuspid. Aortic isthmic hypoplastic was severe, with discrete preductal coarctation of the aorta. The coronary arteries were basically normal, except for the hypoplasia of the left anterior descending coronary artery and the left circumflex-reflecting the hypoplasia of the left ventricle.

The tricuspid valve has absence of the commissure between the anterior and the septal leaflets which are continuous, apparently because of absence of the papillary muscle of the conus (into which both the anterior and the septal leaflets normally insert, thereby forming the antero-superior commissure of the tricuspid valve). The free edges of the tricuspid leaflets showed myxomatous thickening. Some tricuspid chordae tendineae inserted directly into the crest of the muscular ventricular septum in the region of the ventricular septal defect.

This stillborn fetus also had multiple congenital anomalies that are unknown to us; this was a cardiac consult from another hospital.

To summarize this case, as you can see, this patient *did* have a myxomatous tricuspid valve; but this was one of this individual's least important problems. This case is really a clinic on DORV with hypoplastic left heart, illustrating a very severe form of parachute mitral valve, and demonstrating the tendency of DORV with hypoplastic left heart to have stenosis of the posterior great arterial outflow tract (in this case, subaortic and aortic annular stenosis) and the sequelae of this posterior great artery outflow tract stenosis (in this case, severe isthmic hypoplasia with preductal coarctation of the aorta). DORV with hypoplastic left heart often has an unilateral conus, that may be subpulmonary as in this case) or subaortic. When the conus is subaortic, the posterior great arterial outflow tract is the pulmonary; and often there is pulmonary outflow tract stenosis, with its sequelae.

(c) This patient was a 12-day-old girl with double-outlet right ventricle {S,D,A} with a well-expanded subaortic conus, pulmonary valve–to–tricuspid valve fibrous continuity, severe subpulmonary stenosis, bicommissural and bicuspid stenotic pulmonary valve, and ventricular septal defect of conoventricular type with posterior extension medial to septal leaflet of the tricuspid valve.

The tricuspid and mitral valves both appear immature, with large myxomatous nodules at the free edges of these leaflets. Other findings include left-sided juxtaposition of the atrial appendages; a secundum type of atrial septal defect; left superior vena cava to coronary sinus to right atrium; and a dominant right coronary artery giving origin to a large conus coronary that extends into the lower half of the anterior descending coronary artery territory; the right coronary artery also supplies the posterior descending coronary artery; and the left coronary artery supplies the superior or proximal portion of the anterior descending coronary artery territory and the left circumflex coronary artery. The semilunar interrelationship is anterior-posterior, with the aortic valve directly anterior to the pulmonary valve, as is indicated by DORV {S,D,**A**}.

The left ventricle was morphologically normal, the free wall measuring 4.5 mm in thickness in the fresh state. The right ventricle displayed marked hypertrophy (wall 8 mm thick in the fresh state), but with only mild enlargement.

There was a left aortic arch with a right-sided ductus arteriosus. The ductus extended from the innominate artery to the proximal right pulmonary artery, the ductus being long (2.1 cm), narrow, and still patent at 12 days of age. A vascular ring was not present.

At 3 days of age, a modified left Blalock-Taussig shunt was performed using a 4 mm Gore-Tex conduit. Episodes of desaturation postoperatively led at 11 days of age to a central shunt from the ascending aorta to the right pulmonary artery, using a 3.5 mm Gore-Tex conduit. Postoperatively, increased pulmonary blood flow, generalized edema, and cardiac arrest occurred. Intensive efforts to rescue this patient in 1991, including partial clip obliteration of the central shunt, were unsuccessful.

Summary of this case. This patient illustrates that one can have DORV with a *unilateral* conus (subaortic, with pulmonary-tricuspid fibrous continuity) *without* hypoplastic left heart. This case again demonstrates that in DORV with a unilateral (as opposed to a bilateral) conus, the posterior great arterial outflow tract (in this case, the pulmonary outflow tract) is prone to significant obstruction. This patient also illustrates the difficulties that can be associated with palliative surgery.

Once again, the myxomatous tricuspid valve appears to have been of no clinical importance.

(d) This 1½-month-old girl had the following diagnoses: prematurity, with estimated gestational age of 35 weeks, but with birth weight of 3.8 kg (8 lb 6 oz), that is, macrosomia; spastic quadriparesis with multiple seizures; history of meconium aspiration; persistent fetal circulation; supraventricular tachycardia with onset at 3½ weeks of age, characterized by episodes of persistent tachycardia (260/min, associated with hypotension) due to atrial flutter with 1:1 conduction or with variable block (2:1 and 3:1); and episodes of hypoglycemia, acidosis, and hypocalcaemia; prolonged apnea associated with seizures.

Following a period of normal sinus rhythm, the patient suddenly went into ventricular fibrillation, from which she could not be converted, leading to death.

Her presentation at birth with macrosomia, hypoglycemia, and visceromegaly (enlarged liver and prominent adrenals on abdominal ultrasound examination) suggested the Beckwith-Wiedemann syndrome.[555] But this diagnosis was questioned because of the absence of certain features (omphalocele and ear creases), and because of the presence of other findings not associated with the Beckwirth-Wiedemann syndrome (neurological abnormalities and a cutis laxa-like hyperextensibility of the skin).

Autopsy revealed massive cardiomegaly: the heart weighed 50 grams, normal being 18. Hence, the heart weight was 177% greater than normal. Or, the heart weight/normal = 2.77/1. Myocardial hypertrophy was generalized and marked: left ventricular free wall = 12 mm in thickness; right ventricular free wall = 8 to 9.5 mm; ventricular septum = 13 to 15.5 mm in thickness; left atrial free wall = 1.5 to 2.5 mm thick; and right atrial free wall = 1 to 3 mm in thickness. Both ventricles were strikingly thick-walled and small-chambered.

The leaflets of the tricuspid valve and of the mitral valve were thick and myxomatous—so much so that at autopsy we wondered whether or not tricuspid and mitral stenosis might perhaps have been present in life. However, no hemodynamic data were available to establish or disprove this speculative possibility.

To summarize this rare care, although the tricuspid valve was myxomatous, we thought that this was one of this patient's least important problems. I have a strong feeling that we do not understand what the basic diagnosis is in this patient. Are we dealing with a poorly understood metabolic abnormality, perhaps of carbohydrate metabolism—as is suggested by the hypoglycemia? Left ventricular hypertrophy is known to be an independent risk factor for sudden arrhythmic death. Is this why this patient died suddenly from ventricular fibrillation?

What does myxomatous tricuspid valve mean? From a diagnostic and surgical viewpoint, it means: *Keep looking.* Although seldom clinically important *per se,* myxomatous tricuspid valve can be associated with other major problems that include mucopolysaccharidoses, chromosomal trisomies, and polyvalvar disease.

It should be understood that in our definition of myxomatous tricuspid valve, we have excluded cases in which the tricuspid valve was clearly dysfunctional and therefore clinically important, such as congenital tricuspid stenosis or regurgitation. In such cases, the tricuspid valve also may well be thickened and myxomatous. But in such patients, we (and virtually everyone else) make the diagnosis of congenital tricuspid stenosis or regurgitation (not myxomatous tricuspid valve). Thus, the fact that the diagnosis of myxomatous tricuspid valve, as presented in this section, is not clinically or surgically important is true because of our definition and usage of *myxomatous tricuspid valve* in our database. Nonetheless, the diagnosis of myxomatous tricuspid valve is significant because it strongly suggests that the heart is abnormal. Even though nonspecific, this finding should heighten one's diagnostic suspicions and should invite the investigator to look further. The question should be: What else is wrong?

Tricuspid Valve Prolapse

We made the diagnosis of tricuspid valve prolapse in 4 of these 3400 postmortem cases of heart disease in infants and children (Table 13.1) (0.12%). The question, of course, is: What kind of cases were these?

Gender: males = 3; females = 1; male/female ratio = 3.1.

Age at death: mean = 6.24 years (2277.5 days) ± 10.91 years (3981.81 days). The range was from 0 (a 21-week-gestation fetal abortus) to 22 7/12 years (8240 days). The median age at death was 1.19 years (435 days).

PATHOLOGY

Case 1 was a 22 7/12-year-old man who died in 1991. His main diagnoses were as follows: double-outlet right ventricle {S,D,D} with subaortic conus and wide aortic-tricuspid separation and no subpulmonary conus with pulmonary-tricuspid fibrous continuity; superoinferior ventricles with abnormally horizontal ventricular septum and marked underdevelopment of the superior right ventricle and a well developed inferior left ventricle; multiple ventricular septal defects with a large conoventricular (outlet) ventricular septal defect (20 × 12 mm) and a large muscular inlet ventricular septal defect (35 × 25 mm) that did not extend up to the insertion of the septal leaflet of the tricuspid valve and hence was not classified as a VSD of the AV canal type; and pulmonary outflow tract stenosis.

The tricuspid valve did not straddle the abnormally horizontal ventricular septum, connecting only with the small superior right ventricle. Multiple fenestrations were present within the tricuspid valve leaflets, varying from less than 1 mm to 4 or 5 mm in diameter. This **"filigree" tricuspid valve** permitted severe tricuspid regurgitation. The tricuspid valve leaflets were markedly redundant, with severe prolapse of the tricuspid leaflets into the right atrial cavity.

The mitral valve displayed a "hemorrhoidal" appearance, with marked upward hooding of the interchordal mitral leaflet tissue, mitral valve prolapse, and mitral regurgitation. The free margins of the mitral leaflets were thickened and rolled, confirming the presence of mitral regurgitation.

Right atrial hypertrophy and enlargement were marked, reflecting, in part, the severity of the tricuspid regurgitation.

Thus, this patient had the devastating combination of double-outlet right ventricle with a small right ventricle, two large ventricular septal defects, and prolapse and regurgitation of both the tricuspid and the mitral valves.

He also had duplication of the right ureter—of no known functional significance. But he therefore did have **multiple**

congenital anomalies, ***that is,*** malformations not only of the cardiovascular system, but also of an additional system—in this case the genitourinary.

At 6½ months of age, he had a right Blalock Taussig anastomosis and surgical trial septal defect creation. Subsequently he did well until 9$^{1}/_{12}$ years of age when he developed subacute bacterial endocarditis with blood cultures positive for *Streptococcus viridans*. Appropriate antibiotic treatment led to full recovery.

Cardiac catheterization at 13½ years of age revealed mild kinking of the right pulmonary artery at the insertion of the right Blalock-Taussig anastomosis. Repeat cardiac catheterization at 16$^{5}/_{12}$ years of age showed reduced left and right ventricular function, leading to a modified Fontan procedure at 16$^{10}/_{12}$ years of age: The right Blalock-Taussig shunt was ligated. The pulmonary valve was closed. The tricuspid orifice was closed with a patch. The interatrial communication was also closed with a patch. The right atrium was connected with the right pulmonary artery by a right atrial flap and a Tascon graft.

Postoperatively, dehiscence of the tricuspid valve patch superiorly was repaired with pledgetted sutures and a cloth patch. One month later, atrial flutter with 2:1 atrioventricular block appeared; cardioversion was successful.

By 21½ years of age, chronic edema and protein-losing enteropathy had appeared. Despite intensive therapeutic efforts, heart failure worsened, leading to death.

Autopsy revealed massive cardiomegaly (1440 grams in the fresh state), with marked right ventricular hypertrophy (wall thickness 13 to 15 mm), marked left ventricular hypertrophy and enlargement (wall thickness 14 to 16 mm), large tricuspid annulus (43 mm in diameter), large mitral annulus (43 mm in diameter), an opening in the atrial septum immediately posterior to the patch (3 mm in diameter), and a long linear opening in the tricuspid patch measuring 15 mm (0.6 inch) that permitted tricuspid regurgitation. The anastomosis between the amplified right atrial appendage and the right pulmonary artery measured 21 × 11 mm (0.8 × 0.4 inch).

Note that both the tricuspid and the mitral annulus measured 43 mm (1.7 inch) in diameter. Thus, the Fontan anastomosis was 51% less in diameter than were the orifices of the tricuspid and mitral valves, suggesting that the Fontan anastomosis may have been stenotic. Tricuspid regurgitation (through the defect in the patch) and untreated mitral regurgitation were thought also to be significant factors leading to this patient's death.

Summary of this case. Tricuspid valve prolapse with many small leaflet fenestrations ("filigree" tricuspid valve)—a rare anomaly—resulted in severe tricuspid regurgitation, which was one important component of this patient's complex hemodynamic handicap. In this patient, tricuspid and mitral prolapse occurred together in the setting of double-outlet right ventricle with small right ventricle, two large ventricular septal defects, superoinferior ventricles, and pulmonary outflow tract stenosis.

Case 2 was a 19-month-old boy with polyvalvar disease: severe congenital mitral stenosis with marked thickening of mitral leaflet tissue, small anterolateral papillary muscle group and large posteromedial papillary muscle group of the left ventricle, but with chordal insertions into both papillary muscle groups; hypoplastic and bicuspid aortic valve with absence of the intercoronary commissure; marked tricuspid regurgitation, with noncoaptation or large redundant and thickened anterior tricuspid defect (4 mm gap between anterior and septal leaflets of the tricuspid valve) and with tricuspid valve prolapse observed angiocardiograpically. The patient's chromosomal status (a trisomy?) was unknown to us.

Thus, this patient had the combination of severe congenital mitral stenosis and severe congenital tricuspid regurgitation with prolapse of the tricuspid valve.

Other important findings included the following: a small left ventricle, preductal coarctation of the aorta, massive right ventricular hypertrophy and enlargement (right ventricular free wall thickness = 7 to 10 mm), marked right atrial hypertrophy and enlargement (wall thickness = 2 to 5 mm) with moderate right atrial endocardial fibroelastosis (jet lesion, related to marked tricuspid regurgitation); ostium of left coronary artery abnormally close to the left coronary–noncoronary commissure of aortic valve (of no known functional significant); and absence of left circumflex coronary artery.

Therapeutic efforts included the following: resection of aortic coarctation with end-to-end anastomosis (at 2 weeks of age); balloon angioplasty of coarctation site, reducing gradient to 2 mm Hg (at 9 months of age); and mitral valve replacement surgically using a 16 mm Carbomedics prosthesis (at 19 months of age). Left ventricular outflow tract obstruction by the prosthesis led to intraoperative death.

Thus, tricuspid valve prolapse was just one important part of complex congenital heart disease with polyvalvar disease (severe congenital mitral stenosis with small left ventricle and aortic valvar hypoplasia with preductal coarctation of the aorta). Tricuspid valve regurgitation and prolapse should be understood in context: an important part of a larger picture.

Case 3 was a 10-month-old boy with infantile Marfan syndrome (Figs. 13.29, 13.30, and 13.54).[225] Salient features included the following: facial dysmorphism with large ears, and high-arched, narrow palate; marked arachondactyly of upper and lower extremities; pectus excavatum; severe mitral regurgitation with marked mitral valve prolapse; left atrial enlargement, marked; tricuspid regurgitation with tricuspid valve prolapse; mild to moderate dilation of the aortic root, without aortic regurgitation; secundum atrial septal defect, 6 × 5 mm; moderate left ventricular enlargement; contractures of elbow joints, knee joints, and ankle joints; eventration of the central tendon portion of the diaphragm, right-sided; and absence of a family history of Marfan syndrome, that is, no autosomal dominant genetic family history.

Other clinically important details include the following: bilateral inguinal hernia repair, at 3 weeks of age; pyloromyotomy (Ramstedt operation) for hypertrophic pyloric stenosis; body cast (spica) for bilateral congenital dislocation of the hips, done at 4 months of age, for a duration of 4 months; progressive congestive heart failure, appearing at 5 months of age, with subsequent failure to thrive; ventricular arrhythmias including ventricular premature beats, bigeminy, and trigeminy, at 10 months of age; and mitral valve replacement using a #19 Hancock prosthesis at 10 months and 25 days of age.

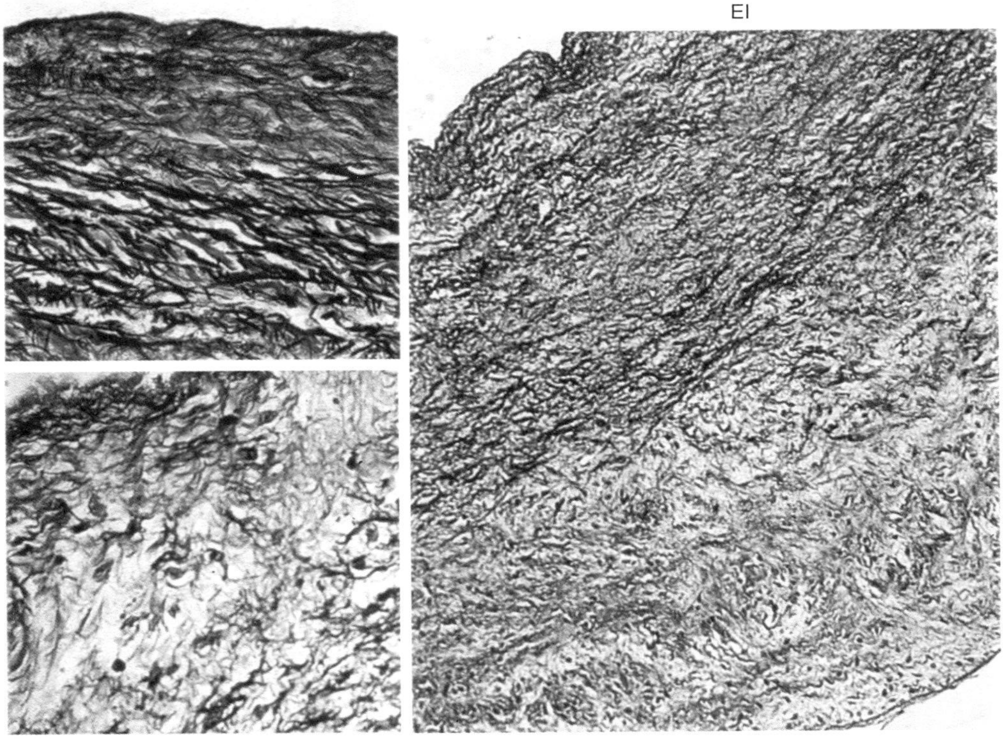

Fig. 13.54 Histology of the **mitral valve** in infantile Marfan syndrome, Case 2 (same patient as in Fig. 13.29). *Right,* Low-power magnification (×40) showing thickening of the elastica *(El)* with disruption, fragmentation, and disarray of the elastic fibers. In the fibrosa *(Fib)*, the collagen fibers are numerous and fragmented, with increased interstitial ground substance. *Bottom Left,* High-power magnification (×400) of the elastica showing details of the fragmented elastic fibers, compared with an age-matched normal control with its unfragmented, longitudinally arranged elastic fibers *(Top Left)*. (Verhoeff-Van Gieson stain for elastic fibers.) (Reproduced with permission from Geva T, Sanders SP, Diogenes M, Rockenmacher S, Van Praagh R: Two-dimensional and Doppler echocardiographic and pathologic characteristics of the infantile Marfan syndrome. *Am J Cardiol* 1990;65:1230.)

The postoperative course was characterized by low cardiac output and hypoxemia. A left-sided pneumothorax was treated with a chest tube. Cardiac arrest leading to death occurred on the second postoperative day (in 1978).

Autopsy revealed severe bilateral pulmonary emphysema with many small blebs in the subpleural region of both lungs, which helped to explain the postoperative pneumothorax. The tricuspid leaflets were thickened and redundant, with elongation (but without rupture) of the chordae tendineae; these findings were consistent with the clinical and angiocardiographically observed tricuspid valvar regurgitation and prolapse. The pulmonary valve leaflets were redundant, but without anatomic evidence of pulmonary regurgitation. The walls of the ascending aorta and main pulmonary artery appeared dilated and thinned.

Genetic history: Although there was no family history of Marfan syndrome *per se,* as above, a grandfather apparently had a Marfanoid appearance. The mother, an 18-year-old white woman, is said to have had an elastin abnormality of her collagen, but this abnormality was not regarded as diagnostic of any specific syndrome. This is all the genetically related information that is known to us.

Case 3 exemplifies why Geva and his colleages[225] in 1990 reported the ***infantile* Marfan syndrome** (Fig. 13.54). It is clinically more devastating and rapidly progressive than the more familiar adolescent-adult form of this disease, apparently because of major involvement of the atrioventricular valves—with severe mitral and tricuspid regurgitation and prolapse. When this boy died at 10 months of age, aortic (and pulmonary) regurgitation had not as yet appeared. The clinically fatal features were the massive bilateral atrioventricular valvar regurgitation, leading to irreversible left and right congestive heart failure, that was not rescued by mitral valve replacement.

In general, Marfan syndrome (or Marfan's syndrome, the latter being the older usage) is the most common and best characterized of the connective tissue disorders with serious cardiovascular manifestations.[556] Marfan's is an autosomal dominant, multisystem disorder. Phenotypic expression involves the cardiovascular, skeletal, ocular, and other systems. Mutations involve the gene *FBN1* that is important in the formation of connection tissue protein fibrillin-1.[556]

In our experience, tricuspid valve prolapse has been associated with tricuspid regurgitation, and tricuspid valve prolapse has never occurred in isolated in our experience to date. (We are not suggesting that tricuspid valve prolapse *cannot* occur without tricuspid regurgitation, or that tricuspid prolapse *cannot* occur alone. But as a factual matter, we have not as yet found either of these possibilities.)

Case 4 was a female fetus, estimated gestational age 17.5 weeks. The mother was 34 years old, gravida 3, para 2. The fetus had hydrops fetalis, massive cystic hygromas (lymphagiectasia) of the nuchal skin, pleural effusions, and ascites.

Examination of the fetal heart revealed polyvalvar disease: The tricuspid valve was redundant, and the anterior papillary muscle of the right ventricle was hypoplastic. We thought that the tricuspid valve would have prolapsed into the right atrium; but this is a hypothesis because tricuspid valve prolapse was not documented echocardiographically.

The mitral valve was also redundant. The excessive valve tissue created an upward bulging aneurysm, again creating the appearance of prolapse of the mitral valve into the left atrium (hypothesis based on anatomic appearance).

The pulmonary and aortic valves were both bicuspid (bicommissural) and redundant.

The fetal karyotype (trisomy?) is not known by us. Hence, we must regard this case of polyvalvar disease as etiologically idiopathic, in a patient with lymphangiectasis (including large cystic hygromas of the nuchal skin) and hydrops fetalis.

Summary. In this small series ($n = 4$), tricuspid valve prolapse did not occur in isolation. Indeed it always occurred with polyvalvar disease (4 of 4). Tricuspid valve prolapse was associated with congenital heart disease in half of these patients: double-outlet right ventricle (Case 1), and congenital mitral stenosis with preductal coarctation (Case 2). Tricuspid valve prolapse occurred once in a patient with infantile Marfan syndrome (Case 3), and once in a hydropic fetus with lymphagiectasia (cystic hygromas) and polyvalvar disease (Case 4).

Muscular Tricuspid Valve

Muscular tricuspid valve, also known as **incompletely demuscularized tricuspid valve,** was found in 1 of the 3216 autopsied cases of congenital heart disease (0.03%, Table 13.1) (Fig. 13.6). The patient was a 1-year-old white girl with transposition of the great arteries {S,D,D}, ventricular septal defect (subpulmonary, conoventricular type), single right coronary artery arising from the anterior (nonseptal) sinus of Valsalva, and also giving off a separate conal branch and the left main coronary artery. The transposed aortic valve was quadricuspid because an underdeveloped commissure subdivided the right septal aortic leaflet. The presence of this unusual, undeveloped aortic commissure was of no known functional significance.

The tricuspid valve had incomplete demuscularization of the anterior and posterior leaflets, adjacent to the tricuspid annulus.

There was mild valvar pulmonary stenosis, the pulmonary valve being tricuspid and tricommissural, but with thickened leaflets (observed echocardiographically before banding of the main pulmonary artery, and confirmed at autopsy). The patient also had a right aortic arch, which is unusual with TGA {S,D,D}.

Therapy included ligation of a patent ductus arteriosus and banding of the main pulmonary artery via a left thoacotomy at 6 weeks of age because of intractable heart failure.

At 1 year of age (in 1986), an atrial switch operation was attempted (a modified Senning operation): Gore-Tex patch closure of the ventricular septal defect, pericardial augmentation of the left atrial–to–tricuspid pulmonary venous pathway, and debanding of the main pulmonary artery. The operation was complicated by bleeding associated with a coagulopathy. The postoperative course was associated with low cardiac output leading to death 12 days postoperatively.

Autopsy also revealed severe *Klebsiella* pneumonia, and *congenital diabetes mellitus with agenesis of the pancreatic islets of Langerhans and of pancreatic exocrine tissue.* There was also a Meckel's diverticulum.

Our impression was that the abnormal tricuspid valve morphology (incomplete demuscularization of the anterior and posterior leaflets) was just one anatomic abnormality, suggesting a developmental arrest, but without identified functional importance, in a patient with multiple other congenital anomalies. Absence of pancreatic function, both exocrine and endocrine, with *congenital diabetes mellitus,* we thought was a rare and lethal metabolic anomaly. The incompletely demuscularized tricuspid valve appeared to be a lesser clinical problem.

Multiple-Orifice Tricuspid Valve: Double-Orifice, Triple-Orifice, and "Filigree" Tricuspid Valve. The tricuspid valve can have more than one orifice. When there is one accessory orifice, the result is **double-orifice tricuspid valve.** When there are two accessory orifices, the result is **triple-orifice tricuspid valve.** Rarely, there can be multiple orifices within the tricuspid valve leaflets, resulting in **"filigree" tricuspid valve**, as above.

Number: In this series of 3216 cases of congenital heart disease, we recorded 16 cases as having more than one tricuspid orifice (0.5%): double-orifice tricuspid valve in 12, triple-orifice tricuspid valve in 3; and "filigree" tricuspid valve in 1 rare patient who also had tricuspid valve prolapse and severe congenital tricuspid regurgitation (presented above). The sex and age data for the multiple-tricuspid-orifice patients as a whole are as follows:

Sex: males = 8, females = 8, males/females = 1.

Age at death: mean = 3.05 ± 5.82 years (1114.57 ± 2125.68 days); range from 9 hours to 22 7/12 years; and median = 4 months (120 days).

Double-Orifice Tricuspid Valve

Of these 16 patients with multiple-orifice tricuspid valve, 12 (75%) had double-orifice tricuspid valve (DOTV). There were 6 males and 6 females, the male/female ratio being 1/1.

Age at death: mean = 1.21 ± 2.48 years (441.098 ± 903.44 days); range = 9 hours to 7 4/12 years; and median = 24 days.

Settings: What were the settings or situations in which DOTV occurred? In other words, what were the salient associated anomalies that occurred with DOTV? My best attempt to answer this question is summarized in Table 13.27.

A brief word of explanation is probably indicated at the outset. *Double-orifice tricuspid valve* (DOTV) is largely *terra incognita* at the present time. Most books don't even mention it, and those that do have little or no detailed information about this anomaly. But it is present in our database; so we must attempt to understand it. Consequently, these cases with DOTV will be presented in detail so that we will be able to see the various

TABLE 13.27 Settings in Which Double-Orifice Tricuspid Valve Occurred ($n = 12$)

Associated Anomalies	No. of Cases	% of Series*
1. Ebstein's anomaly	5	42
2. Common AV canal	3	25
3. Aortic atresia, valvar, with IVS	3	25
4. Double-inlet left ventricle	1	8

AV, Atrioventricular; *IVS*, intact ventricular septum.
*Percentages are rounded off to the nearest whole number.

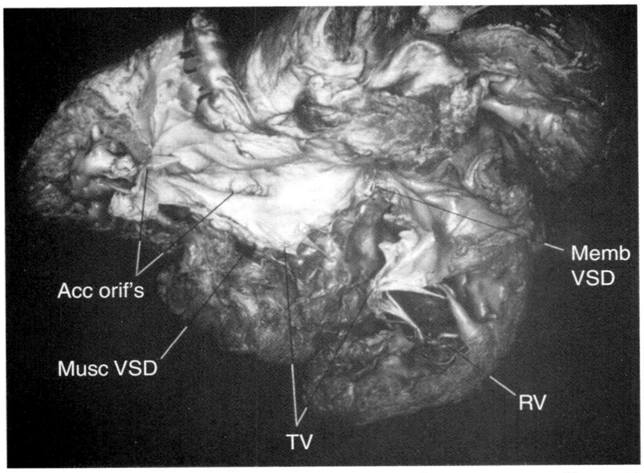

Fig. 13.55 Ebstein's anomaly with two small accessory orifices *(Acc orif's)* in the septal leaflet of the tricuspid valve *(TV)*: opened right atrium, TV, and right ventricle *(RV)*. A 10 mm in diameter membranous ventricular septal defect *(Memb VSD)* and a 30 mm in diameter muscular ventricular septal defect *(Musc VSD)* are also seen. The small accessory orifices in the septal leaflet of the tricuspid valve were thought to be of little or no hemodynamic importance. This 4 9/12-year-old girl died shortly following an attempt to close her VSDs surgically in 1960.

settings in which DOTV occurs, and we shall also try to assess how important DOTV is clinically, hemodynamically, and surgically.

Ebstein's anomaly was most often associated with DOTV (5 of 12 cases, 42%, Table 13.27): Cases 2, 6, 9, 12, and 14. A patient with Ebstein's anomaly and two small accessory orifices in the septal leaflet is presented in Fig. 13.55. This could be called **triple-orifice tricuspid valve.**

Case 2 was a 6-month-old boy with DORV {S,L,L}, pulmonary atresia, patent foramen ovale, superoinferior ventricles with the small right ventricular sinus superiorly and the well-developed left ventricle inferiorly, Ebstein's anomaly of the superior and left-sided tricuspid valve, severe tricuspid regurgitation, a large conoventricular type of ventricular septal defect, straddling of the right-sided and inferior mitral valve through the aforementioned large ventricular septal defect, and a small apical muscular ventricular septal defect (2 × 3 mm).

The left-sided DOTV in this Ebstein's tricuspid valve consisted of a small probe-patent orifice within the tricuspid leaflet substance that was thought at autopsy to be of little or no hemodynamic significance. This small accessory orifice was not associated with thickening or rolling of its leaflet margins.

In 1992, this boy was given a modified right Blalock-Taussig shunt with a Gore-Tex conduit from the right subclavian artery to the right pulmonary artery at 2 days of age, because of his pulmonary outflow tract atresia.

At 6 months of age, a cavopulmonary anastomosis was attempted consisting of patch closure of the left-sided regurgitant tricuspid valve, atrial septectomy, patch closure of the right superior vena cavo–right atrial junction, transection of the proximal right pulmonary artery, anastomosis of the right-sided portion of the right pulmonary artery to the right side of the right superior vena cava (end-to-side), and anastomosis of the left-sided portion of the right pulmonary artery to the left side of the right superior vena cava (end-to-side). Thus, a bidirectional Glenn procedure was performed, plus occlusion of the regurgitant left-sided Ebstein's tricuspid valve and the surgical creation of a common atrium.

The postoperative course was characterized by atrial fibrillation, followed by junctional rhythm and low cardiac output, leading to death 7 hours postoperatively.

Autopsy revealed infarction of the right-sided and inferior left ventricle, with suture stenosis of the inverted left coronary artery.

Thus, the small double-orifice of the left-sided Ebstein tricuspid valve was thought to be of little or no clinical or surgical importance.

Case 6 was a 32-hour-old boy with extremely severe pulmonary valvar stenosis (a pinhole opening), an intact ventricular septum, and an Ebstein-like anomaly of the tricuspid valve. The anterior tricuspid leaflet was deep and curtain-like, with no interchordal spaces. The septal leaflet was bound down, but without downward displacement. The accessory tricuspid orifice was located in the posterior leaflet. But this accessory orifice did not have thickened and rolled margins and was thought *not* to be significantly malfunctional. However, the anterior and septal leaflets of the tricuspid valve were myxomatous, and tricuspid regurgitation was marked. The right ventricle was enlarged and the wall was thin.

From the therapeutic standpoint, in 1985 the patient was delivered by cesarean section at 37 weeks gestation because of fetal tachycardia. The prenatal echocardiographic diagnosis was pulmonary valvar atresia, intact ventricular septum, and Ebstein's anomaly.

At 1 day of age utilizing deep hypothermic circulatory arrest, the interatrial communication was enlarged, and the superior and inferior venae cavae and coronary sinus were patched into the left atrium. The patent ductus arteriosus was ligated, and a 3 mm central Gore-Tex shunt was constructed from the ascending aorta to the main pulmonary artery.

The postoperative course was complicated by cardiac arrest, followed by idioventricular rhythm, systemic hypotension, and low cardiac output leading to death 6 hours postoperatively.

Autopsy revealed postoperative hematoma and sutures at the inferior margin of the atrial baffle, within the triangle of Koch (the expected location of the atrioventricular node).

Thus, the small accessory orifice in the posterior tricuspid leaflet was thought *not* to be important clinically or surgically. Instead, the important anatomic features were considered to be virtual pulmonary valve atresia with intact ventricular septum, and an Ebstein-like anomaly of the tricuspid valve with myxomatous anterior and septal leaflets, and with a bound-down and largely immobilized nonfunctional septal leaflet—this combination resulting in severe tricuspid regurgitation.

Case 9 was a 27-day-old girl with multiple congenital anomalies that included a left diaphragmatic hernia (foramen of Bochdalek) that was repaired at 1 day of age. The patient was placed on extracorporeal membrane oxygenation (ECMO) at 1 day of age. Cardiac catheterization at 1 day of age (in 1985) revealed a patent ductus arteriosus with right-to-left shunt and systemic pressures in the pulmonary artery.

By 3 days of age, right heart failure with anasarca appeared. Bilateral pneumothoraces occurred that were treated with chest tubes. Fever appeared at 27 days of age, leading to death.

Autopsy confirmed the presence of dysmorphic facial features: hypertelorism, large ears, and short neck. As expected, the left lung was hypoplastic. The pancreas was globular, with underdevelopment of the tail of the pancreas.

A very large secundum type of atrial septal defect was present because septum primum was almost totally absent, resulting in a common atrium.

Ebstein's anomaly of the tricuspid valve was found, with marked downward displacement of the septal and posterior leaflets. Congenital tricuspid stenosis was spent, with a small orifice opening superiorly into the right ventricular outflow tract, and with a very small slit-like orifice opening into the right ventricular inflow tract.

Hence, double-orifice tricuspid valve was present in this patient with Ebstein's anomaly and multiple congenital anomalies. But the hemodynamically interesting feature was that double-orifice tricuspid valve was associated with congenitally tricuspid *stenosis*—not congenital tricuspid regurgitation as one might expect.

Another anatomically interesting feature is that both tricuspid orifices were reduced portions of what "should" have been the tricuspid orifice. Neither was an *accessory* orifice in the sense of an abnormal opening within a tricuspid leaflet. Instead, this was a subdivided tricuspid orifice, resulting in congenital tricuspid stenosis in a patient with Ebstein's anomaly and with multiple other congenital malformations (karyotype unfortunately unknown).

A large conoventricular type of ventricular septal defect was present.

This patient also has *triple-orifice mitral valve.* A prominent pillar-like muscle that was confluent with the anterolateral papillary muscle group of the left ventricle extended cephalad, almost to the level of the aortic annuls, subdividing the mitral orifice into a relatively small anterolateral compartment and a relatively large posteromedial compartment. The comparatively large posteromedial mitral orifice was again subdivided by a bridge of fibrous tissue, thereby creating triple-orifice mitral valve—a rare anomaly. We thought that congenital mitral stenosis may have been present based on the anatomic appearance; but relevant hemodynamic data were not available.

This patient had polyvalvar disease: Ebstein's anomaly with congenital tricuspid stenosis and DOTV; triple-orifice mitral valve (with possible congenital mitral stenosis?); mild myxomatous thickening of pulmonary valve leaflets (tricuspid and tricommisural) and mild myxomatous thickening of aortic valve leaflets, with left coronary leaflet much smaller than the other two leaflets.

This patient also had preductal coarctation of the aorta (2 mm internal diameter) and a closed ductus arteriosus; but the patient had been maintained on ECMO.

Case 12 was a 3-week-old boy with transposition of the great arteries {S,L,L}, a straddling left-sided tricuspid valve with Ebstein's anomaly, and severe congenital tricuspid stenosis with DOTV. Both tricuspid orifices were obstructive. The superior tricuspid orifice (at a 12 o'clock position) measured 1.25 × 1.6 cm and opened into the left-sided morphologically right ventricle. The inferior tricuspid orifice (at a 6 o'clock position) measured only 2 mm in internal diameter and opened into the right-sided morphologically left ventricle. Hence, the left atrium, which was normally left-sided, opened through separate orifices into two different ventricles.

This is a rare anomaly known as **double-outlet left atrium.** When both tricuspid orifices open into the *same* ventricle, this is known as double-orifice tricuspid valve. But when double-orifice tricuspid valve occurs in a straddling tricuspid valve, and each tricuspid orifice opens into a different ventricle, the diagnosis of *double-outlet left atrium* indicates that the left atrium opens into both ventricles through separate atrioventricular valvar orifices.

When the left atrium (or the right atrium) opens into both ventricles through *one* typically straddling atrioventricular valvar orifice, we do not make the diagnosis of double-outlet (left or right) atrium. This we simply call this situation straddling atrioventricular valve (tricuspid, mitral, or common). But when one atrium opens into both ventricles through *two* separate atrioventricular valve orifices, this much rarer situation we call double-outlet atrium—double-outlet right atrium or double-outlet left atrium—as in this rare patient whose heart specimen was kindly sent to us as a consultation in 1970 by Dr. W. T. Dungan, Department of Pediatrics, University of Arkansas Medical Center, Little Rock. In the interests of accuracy and clarity, we always use the term *double-outlet* literally: only when there really are two outlets.

It is noteworthy that there was no ventricular septal defect of the atrioventricular canal (inlet) type. The straddling tricuspid valve adhered to the ventricular septum, obliterating this type of ventricular septal defect that is often associated with straddling tricuspid valve.

But there was a slit-like conoventricular (outlet) type of ventricular septal defect. Other findings included atresia of the coronary sinus ostium, preductal coarctation of the aorta, and a patent ductus arteriosus.

To summarize this case of TGA {S,L,L} from the standpoint of left-sided double-orifice tricuspid valve: DOTV was associated with Ebstein's anomaly, straddling tricuspid valve, severe tricuspid stenosis, and double-outlet left atrium. Again, DOTV was associated with severe congenital tricuspid *stenosis*—not the congenital tricuspid regurgitation that one might expect *a priori* to be associated with DOTV.

Clinically, how important was the DOTV? This is, we think, a difficult question to answer because there were so many other anomalies. DOTV was far from "isolated." In the complex of TGA {S,L,L} with left-sided Ebstein's malformation and congenital tricuspid stenosis, the fact that the tricuspid valve had two orifices could readily be regarded as an interesting detail, but hardly the main problem, even if one focuses only on the left-sided AV valve. So our conclusion is that DOTV was one small part of a much larger problem.

Case 14 was a 9-hour-old female infant who was born by cesarean section at 33½ weeks estimated gestational age in 1986 with a birth weight of 7 lb 4 oz (3288 grams) with massive hydrops fetalis, indicating severe intrauterine congestive heart failure. Vigorous resuscitation was complicated by a right tension pneumothorax that led to death.

Autopsy revealed completely common atrioventricular canal, type A of Rastelli, with a large ostium primum type of atrial septal defect component and a small ventricular septal defect beneath the anterosuperior leaflet only of the common AV valve. There was a wide cleft (or gap) in the potentially anterior leaflet of the mitral valve component, that was associated with moderate to severe "mitral" regurgitation.

The tricuspid component of the common atrioventricular valve was associated with Ebstein's anomaly. The anterior and posterior leaflets of the potentially tricuspid valve were deep and curtain-like, with incomplete demuscularization. The septal leaflet of the tricuspid valve component was markedly displaced inferiorly, and was so severely hypoplastic as to be judged functionally absent. Double-orifice tricuspid valve was present. Severe congenital tricuspid regurgitation was observed echocardiographically and confirmed pathologically.

Double-orifice of the tricuspid valve component of this common atrioventricular valve with Ebstein's anomaly and severe congenital "tricuspid" and "mitral" regurgitation with terminal intrauterine heart failure appeared to be but one small part of a much larger problem: DO "TV" was, at most, a minor part of this patient's clinical problem.

Summary. Ebstein's anomaly was the most common setting in which double-orifice tricuspid valve occurred (5 of 12 cases, 42%, Table 13.27). But the presence of double-orifice tricuspid valve never appeared to be clinically important.

Common atrioventricular canal was the second most common setting in which double-orifice "tricuspid valve" was found (3 of 12 patients, 25%, Table 13.27).

Case 1 was a 10-month-old boy with completely common atrioventricular canal, type A, with normal segmental anatomy {S,D,S}, and a patent foramen ovale. The left ventricle was small, and there was right ventricular hypertrophy and enlargement. This was the *right-sided* type of completely common atrioventricular canal also known as the *dominant right ventricular type*. Some have interpreted this anomaly as being due to excessive right-shift of the atrioventricular canal or junction. Our hypothesis is that the left ventricle is relatively hypoplastic (compared with the right ventricle), and consequently the ventricular septum is shifted abnormally leftward relative to the atrioventricular canal and the atrial septum. The common atrioventricular valve underlying both atria opens predominantly into the large right ventricle, and opens much less into the small left ventricle.

The *ventriculoatrial malalignment* becomes very important surgically when one tries to patch closed the atrioventricular septal defect. It looks as though the ventricular loop (which developmentally is highly mobile—a "professional contortionist") has shifted abnormally far to the left, carrying the ventricular septum and left ventricle too far to the left relative to the AV junction and the atrial septum. The result is that the potential mitral orifice is much smaller than the potential tricuspid orifice; consequently, most of the atrial blood flows into the right ventricle, resulting in right ventricular hypertrophy and enlargement, with relative left ventricular hypoplasia and potential mitral stenosis following surgical septation.

Thus, our hypothesis is that the right ventricular dominant type of common atrioventricular canal is related to ventriculoatrial malalignment with abnormal left-shift of the ventricular loop relative to the atrioventriuclar canal and the atria. This understanding appears important in this patient's management.

At 10 months of age at another institution (we studied this case as a consultation in 1989), the atrioventricular septal defect was closed with a glutaraldehyde treated pericardial patch. The mitral cleft was suture-closed completely. The postoperative course was characterized by mitral stenosis, subaortic stenosis, and complete heart block, leading to death.

Autopsy revealed severe iatrogenic mitral stenosis (the mitral orifice = 3 × 4 mm). A prominent anterolateral muscle of the left ventricle (muscle of Moulaert) largely filled and obstructed the subaortic outflow tract of the small-chambered left ventricle postoperatively. The aortic isthmus was moderately hypoplastic (4.8 mm, calculated diameter), but not coarcted. The double-orifice of the tricuspid component of the common atrioventricular valve was thought to be of no hemodynamic significance.

Case 3 was a 5½-year-old girl with a complete form of common atrioventricular canal and pulmonary valvar stenosis. In 1958, repair of the atrioventricular septal defect was performed using an Ivalon patch, with suture closure of the mitral cleft and of the gap between the anterior and septal leaflets of the tricuspid valve. The pulmonary valve was thickened and myxomatous and a commissurotomy was performed between the nonseptal and left septal pulmonary leaflets. The postoperative course was characterized by heart failure and low cardiac output leading to death 9 days postoperatively.

Autopsy revealed that the ventricular septal defect component of the atrioventricular septal defect was patent. The right coronary artery originated, as did the left coronary artery, from the left coronary sinus of Valsalva of the aortic valve. The left coronary artery gave rise normally to the left anterior descending and left circumflex coronary artery branches. The right coronary artery passed to the right, between the aortic root posteriorly and the pulmonary root anteriorly and thence to the right atrioventricular sulcus.

The septal leaflet of the tricuspid valve displayed a double orifice that was 10 mm in length and 8 mm in maximal width.

The orifice of the repaired mitral valve admitted only a finger tip, before the mitral valve was opened by dissection of autopsy. No measurement of the examiner's finger tip was made in 1958; but this observation suggests the probability of iatrogenic mitral stenosis in this 5½-year-old girl.

The double-orifice of the tricuspid valve was thought to be an interesting incidental finding of no obvious clinical importance; but there are no hemodynamic data with which to assess this impression.

Case 14 was described above: the last patient with Ebstein's anomaly who also had common AV canal and double-orifice tricuspid valve. DOTV appeared to be of little or no clinical importance.

Summary. In none of these 3 patients with common AV canal did DOTV appear to be a significant clinical and hemodynamic problem (Table 13.27).

Valvar Aortic Atresia With Intact Ventricular Septum and Double-Orifice Tricuspid Valve

This group was also the second most common setting in which DOTV occurred, being tied with common AV canal, occurring in 3 of 12 patients (25%, Table 13.27).

Case 4 was a 2-month-old boy with aortic atresia, intact ventricular septum, and extremely severe congenital mitral stenosis (2 pinhole openings). This patient with the hypoplastic left heart syndrome had marked hypoplasia of the left ventricle without endocardial fibroelastosis, and with marked hypertrophy and enlargement of the left atrium, right atrium, and right ventricle.

In 1980, this boy had an early Norwood procedure consisting of surgical atrial septal defect creation; augmentation of the ascending aorta and aortic arch and proximal main pulmonary artery with Gore-Tex; placement of a conduit from the infundibular part of the right ventricle to the transected distal main pulmonary artery just proximal to the origins of the right and left pulmonary artery branches; clipping of the conduit in order to introduce a degree of pulmonary stenosis; and occlusion of the patent ductus arteriosus. (Note how similar this operation is to what we now call the **Sano modification of the Norwood procedure.**) Unfortunately, the patient died intraoperatively.

Autopsy confirmed the foregoing and revealed a DOTV. Both the main and the accessory tricuspid orifices appeared functionally normal (neither regurgitant, nor stenotic). Hence, we thought that the presence of DOTV was of no clinical or hemodynamic or surgical significance, insofar as we were able to determine.

Case 7, a 12-day-old girl, had mitral atresia, aortic valvar atresia, intact ventricular septum, a tiny left ventricle, patent foramen ovale, juxtaductal coarctation of the aorta, marked right ventricular hypertrophy and enlargement, and tricuspid regurgitation (documented by two-dimensional echocardiography and by cineangiocardiography).

At 9 days of age in 1983, she underwent a Norwood procedure consisting of atrial septectomy, ligation and division of the patent ductus arteriosus, anastomosis of the small ascending aorta (2 mm in diameter) to the main pulmonary artery, closure of the distal main pulmonary artery with a Gore-Tex patch, and placement of a 4 mm Gore-Tex conduit from the innominate artery to the right pulmonary artery (modified right Blalock-Taussig anastomosis). The postoperative course was complicated by difficulty weaning from cardiopulmonary bypass, low cardiac output, and metabolic acidosis, leading to death 3 days postoperatively.

Autopsy confirmed the above-mentioned anatomic findings and revealed infarction of the anterior right ventricular free wall. Other noteworthy findings included generalized petechiae, infarction of the lower pole of the left kidney, and a thrombus in the aorta from the origin of the inferior mesenteric artery to the origin of the umbilical arteries.

Autopsy also revealed DOTV with an accessory orifice in the anterior tricuspid leaflet, associated with small chordae tendineae and an abnormally small papillary muscle attached to the anterior right ventricular free wall. This accessory tricuspid orifice was not associated with thickening or rolling of its margins—nothing to suggest regurgitation or other malfunction of this small accessory tricuspid orifice.

Case 10 (Fig. 13.56) was a 2-day-old girl with membranous mitral atresia, aortic valvar and subvalvar atresia, intact ventricular septum, and extreme left ventricular hypoplasia. This patient had a small secundum type of atrial septal defect (6 mm in diameter), a prominent Eustachian valve of the inferior vena cava, and a large but functionally closing ductus arteriosus at 2 days of age.

No surgical therapy was undertaken. We had the privilege of studying this patient's heart at autopsy in 1974, which was before the advent of the Norwood procedure for the hypoplastic left heart syndrome.

Autopsy also revealed the presence of DOTV. The anterolateral tricuspid orifice was 8 mm in diameter and was interpreted as the main tricuspid orifice. A very small accessory tricuspid orifice was located posteromedially (1.0 mm in diameter). Malfunction of the tricuspid valve was not thought to be present clinically, hemodynamically, or at autopsy. Hence, DOTV was considered to have been of no functional importance in this patient.

Discussion. In these 3 patients with hypoplastic left heart syndrome and DOTV (Cases 4, 7, and 10), tricuspid valve malfunction—that is, tricuspid regurgitation—was thought to be present in only 1 (Case 7). Even in this patient, the small accessory tricuspid orifice did not display thickening and rolling of its margins consistent with tricuspid regurgitation. How should these findings be interpreted?

First, we agree that these findings are somewhat confusing and that interpretation may be perilous (i.e., wrong). Nonetheless we are tempted to try:

1. DOTV may not be malfunctional; it is not necessarily associated with tricuspid regurgitation.
2. Even when tricuspid regurgitation is present, the regurgitation is not necessarily because of the presence of an accessory tricuspid orifice (see below).
3. As has been noted previously, it should be understood that the anatomy of the tricuspid valve is not optimal to occlude an approximately circular systemic atrioventricular orifice, whereas that of the mitral valve is. The tricuspid valve normally is "cleft," between the anterior and the septal leaflets;

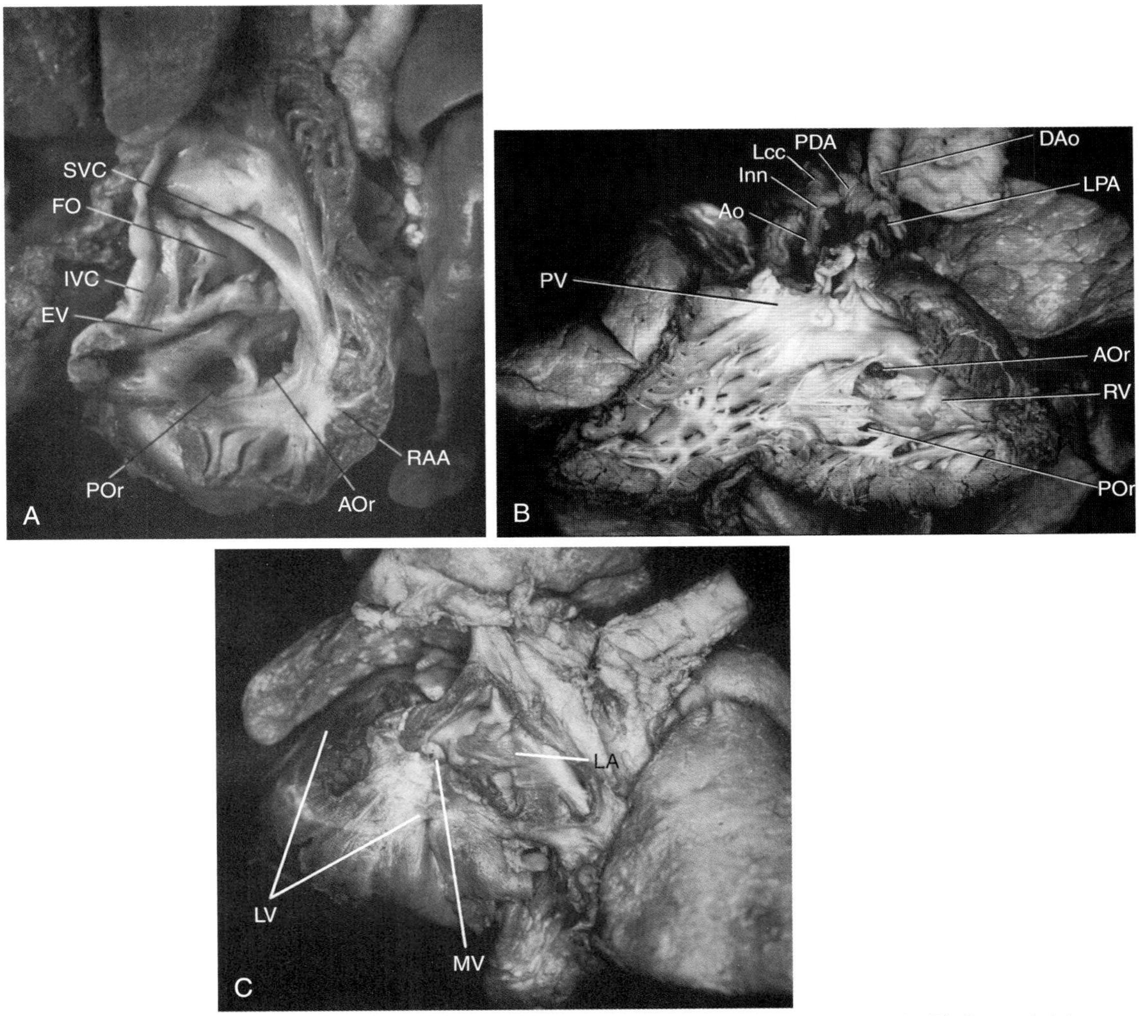

Fig. 13.56 Double-orifice tricuspid valve with hypoplastic left heart syndrome (Case 10). (A) Opened right atrium looking down on the tricuspid valve from above. The anterolateral orifice *(AOr)* of the tricuspid valve measured 8 mm in maximum dimension and was the main tricuspid orifice. The posteromedial orifice *(POr)* measured only 1 mm in diameter. The presence of double-orifice tricuspid valve was thought to be of little or no functional importance. *EV,* Eustachian valve; *FO,* foramen ovale (a small secundum atrial septal defect, 6 mm in diameter, was present); *IVC,* inferior vena cava; *RAA,* right atrial appendage; *SVC,* superior vena cava. (B) The opened right ventricle *(RV)* is markedly hypertrophied, and the large anterolateral orifice (AOr) is superior to the diminutive posteromedial orifice (POr). The POr is seen to a small interchordal space. What should be other interchordal spaces are filled with valve-like fibrous tissue. This is why the anterior tricuspid leaflet appears to insert directly into the prominent anterior papillary muscle of the RV—except where the POr is. Hence, the POr is really the only approximately normally formed interchordal space. *Ao,* Small ascending aorta (this 2-day-old girl had aortic valvar and immediately subvalvar atresia, plus membranous mitral atresia, and an intact ventricular septum); *DAo,* descending aorta; *Inn,* innominate artery; *Lcc,* left common carotid artery; *LPA,* left pulmonary artery; *PDA,* patent ductus arteriosus (that was functionally closing); *PV,* pulmonary valve. (C) Opened left atrium *(LA)* revealing membranous mitral atresia. *MV,* Mitral valve remnant; *LV,* left ventricle (the leaders show how small the LV is).

whereas the mitral valve normally is not cleft, this being one of the main hemodynamic problems associated with common AV canal—because the mitral cleft permits regurgitation.

The papillary muscles of the tricuspid valve are numerous, relatively small, and attached to both the septal and free wall surfaces of the right ventricle. If the right ventricle is subjected to volume and pressure overload, the septal and free-wall insertions of the tricuspid valve make it possible to pull the tricuspid valve apart, resulting in tricuspid regurgitation. By contrast, the papillary muscles of the mitral valve normally are few (two large groups, the anterolateral and the posteromedial) and both groups are attached only to the left ventricular free wall. Hence, pressure and volume overload, by distending the left ventricle, does not tend to pull the mitral valve apart, resulting in mitral regurgitation.

The coronary artery blood supply of the left ventricle (two arteries, the left anterior descending and the circumflex) is better than that of the right ventricle (one artery, the right coronary).

The conduction system of the mitral valve and left ventricle is better (two main radiations, the anterior that runs to the anterolateral papillary muscles and the posterior that runs to the posteromedial papillary muscle) than that of the right ventricle which has only an anterior (or superior) radiation—the right bundle branch, the posterior (or inferior) radiation being absent in the right ventricle.

Thus, *multiple anatomic features* make the mitral valve a better systemic atrioventricular valve than the tricuspid valve, that is, less likely to regurgitate: leaflet anatomy, papillary muscles, coronary arterial blood supply, and conduction system.

In view of the foregoing considerations, it is not surprising that tricuspid regurgitation can be a problem in postoperative patients with the hypoplastic left heart syndrome that often have a large and more circular than normal tricuspid orifice. Indeed, the status of the tricuspid valve and its function should be carefully monitored longterm in postoperative patients with the hypoplastic left heart syndrome. What proportion of these patients will ultimately require tricuspid valvuloplasty or replacement is unclear at present.

So, when we say that patients with hypoplastic left heart syndrome and DOTV may have tricuspid regurgitation that is not necessarily related to the coexistence of DOTV, what we mean, and why, should now be clear.

On the other hand, in some of these patients, tricuspid regurgitation may indeed be present because of DOTV. If so, it may be possible to avoid tricuspid valve replacement in such patients by patch occlusion of the accessory regurgitant tricuspid orifice.

Double-Inlet Left Ventricle With Double-Orifice Tricuspid Valve

Case 13, a 7 4/12-year-old girl, had transposition of the great arteries {S,L,D} with single left ventricle and an infundibular outlet chamber, and double-inlet left ventricle. This was the least frequent setting in which DOTV occurred: 1 patient, 8% (Table 13.27).

As the segmental anatomy indicates, there was situs solitus of the viscera and atria {S,-,-}, a discordant L-loop at the ventricular level {S,*L*,-}, and D-TGA at the great arterial level {S,L,*D*}—indicating that the transposed aortic valve lay to the right (dextro or D) relative to the transposed pulmonary valve. There was double-inlet left ventricle, the tricuspid valve lying to the left of the mitral valve (as is usual with a ventricular L-loop).

Because there was double-orifice of the left-sided tricuspid valve, one may regard this patient as having **triple-inlet left ventricle.** The accessory orifice of this left-sided tricuspid valve had short aberrant chordae tendineae that inserted directly into the abnormally located left ventricular septal surface, which was situated anteriorly and to the left in the ventricular part of the heart; hence, the left ventricular septal surface faced posteriorly and to the right. The accessory tricuspid orifice was closely adjacent to this abnormally located left ventricular septal surface.

The bulboventricular foramen leading from the single left ventricle into the infundibular outlet chamber was obstructively small, resulting in subaortic stenosis. The left ventricle was *single* in the sense that the right ventricular sinus (body, or inflow tract) was absent, which is why there was double-inlet left ventricle, there being no right ventricle for the tricuspid valve to open into.

There was a vascular ring formed by a right aortic arch that gave rise to an aberrant left subclavian artery that originated from a diverticulum of Kommerell. The ring was closed by a left-sided patent ductus arteriosus that ran from the aberrant left subclavian artery to the left pulmonary artery.

At 5 months of age (in 1966), the left ductus arteriosus was surgically divided. The aberrant left subclavian artery was "tacked" to the left chest wall posteriorly, and the main pulmonary artery was banded.

When the patient was 7 5/12 years of age (in 1973), surgical correction of her single left ventricle was undertaken. The single left ventricle was divided into right-sided and left-sided chambers with a Dacron septum. The conal septum (above the bulboventricular foramen) and the ventricular septal crest (below this foramen) were excised to remove subaortic stenosis, and the main pulmonary artery was debanded and repaired with a Dacron gusset to correct the iatrogenic pulmonary arterial stenosis produced by the main pulmonary artery band.

The postoperative course was characterized by complete heart block and low cardiac output, leading to death 2 days postoperatively.

Autopsy confirmed the above-mentioned anatomic findings and suggested that the prosthetic ventricular septum had buckled and produced subpulmonary stenosis.

The double-orifice of the left-sided tricuspid valve (described above) was thought not to have been of any hemodynamic importance. However, it was illuminating concerning the pathogenetic mechanism of double-orifice tricuspid valve.

Pathogenic Mechanism of DOTV

DOTV is an anomaly of tricuspid leaflet tissue and of the subjacent tensor apparatus.[557] Our hypothesis is that at least one mechanism for developing DOTV is an abnormal ring of chordae tendineae that insert into the ventricular surface of a tricuspid (or mitral) leaflet (Fig. 13.55). This abnormal ring of chordae does not insert into the leaflet free margins, as chordae normally do.

Both leaflets and chordae tendineae are formed from the same embryonic leaflet substance (the endocardial cushions). Apparently because the endocardial cushion tissue is limited in amount (there is only so much of it), and because leaflets and chordae are both made out of the same endocardial cushion tissue, the endocardial cushion tissue can form either leaflet, or chordae, but not both at the same location. *There is an inverse relationship anatomically between leaflet tissue and chordae tendineae.* Where leaflet tissue is maximal, chordae are minimal (as at the deepest part of the anterior mitral leaflet). Conversely, where chordae tendineae are maximal, leaflet tissue is minimal (as at the anterolateral and posteromedial mitral commissures).

So, what happens when an abnormal ring of chordae tendineae forms and attaches to the ventricular surface of a tricuspid leaflet, as in this patient with double-inlet left ventricle? Apparently because of the inverse relationship between the formation of chordae tendineae and leaflet tissue (either one, or the other, but not both at the same location), when an abnormal ring of chordae forms, there is no leaflet tissue within the abnormal chordal ring. This is what we call an accessory orifice, and it results in a double-orifice tricuspid valve[557] (or a double-orifice mitral valve[558]).

This inverse relationship between leaflet substance and chordae tendineae of atrioventricular valves[557,558] reminds me of the law of conservation of mass and energy in physics: it is either one, or the other, and essentially nothing is lost in the transitions between one form and the other. This hypothesis[557,558] is presented in an attempt to make accessory orifices comprehensible developmentally and anatomically.

How important an accessory orifice (or orifices) is (are) depends on its (their) location, size, number, and the associated tensor apparatus.

This patient appears to illustrate the aforementioned hypothesis:[557,558] an abnormal chordal ring, and nothing within the chordal ring—resulting in an accessory tricuspid orifice, and hence triple-inlet single left ventricle.

Does this hypothesis always work? In other words, is an abnormal chordal ring inserting into the ventricular surface of a tricuspid leaflet always associated with an accessory tricuspid orifice, resulting in DOTV?

The answer is no. In 1986 we studied a 17-month-old girl whose heart had a deep dimple in the posterior tricuspid leaflet—within a ring of chordae tendineae. However, there was no opening into the tricuspid leaflet (no accessory orifice). But it looked like a potential DOTV, or an imperforate form. We wondered whether or not embryonic or fetal hemodynamics might also be important. For example, does leaflet movement pull a hole in the tricuspid leaflet substance because of tethering by the abnormal chordal ring? Most anomalies have *formes frustes*. Accessory tricuspid orifice may be no exception.

DISCUSSION

How important clinically, hemodynamically, and surgically was the presence of an accessory tricuspid orifice resulting in double-orifice tricuspid valve in this series of 12 postmortem cases (Table 13.27)? To summarize, we were not able to prove that an accessory tricuspid ostium resulting in double-orifice tricuspid valve was important clinically, hemodynamically, or surgically. We are aware, of course, that more sophisticated studies in the future may indicate that our conclusion is not necessarily correct. However, the conclusion that we are presenting here must be based on the data that are available to us at the present time.

DOTV occurred in four different settings, always with complex congenital heart disease—never as an isolated malformation (Table 13.27): with Ebstein's anomaly (42%), with common atrioventricular canal (25%), with hypoplastic left heart syndrome (25%), and with single left ventricle and double-inlet left ventricle (8%). Thus, DOTV appeared to be a "fellow traveler"—associated with complex congenital heart disease, but (in our experience) not the cause *per se* of significant hemodynamic disability.

Specifically, in the 5 patients with DOTV and **Ebstein's anomaly** (Table 13.27), 3 had severe congenital tricuspid regurgitation (Cases 2, 6, and 14) and 2 had significant congenital tricuspid stenosis (Cases 9 and 12). In all 5 patients, the hemodynamic tricuspid disability appeared to be related to the Ebstein's anomaly or other associated cardiac malformations, not to the presence of an accessory tricuspid orifice.

Similarly, in the 3 patients with DOTV and **common atrioventricular canal** (Table 13.27), 1 (Case 14) had severe tricuspid regurgitation related to Ebstein's anomaly of the tricuspid valve component of the common AV valve, the septal leaflet being functionally absent, the DOTV not being the hemodynamic problem. The other 2 patients (Cases 1 and 3) did not have identified tricuspid valve malfunction.

In the 3 patients with DOTV and **hypoplastic left heart syndrome** (Table 13.27), 2 (Cases 4 and 10) did not have identified tricuspid valve malfunction, whereas the one who did (Case 7) had severe tricuspid regurgitation that was thought to be related to post-Norwood right ventricular infarction, not to DOTV.

In the 1 patient (Case 13) with DOTV and **double-inlet left ventricle** (Table 13.27), neither atrioventricular valve was thought to be malfunctional. Instead, the postoperative problem following attempted septation of the single left ventricle was thought to be iatrogenic subpulmonary stenosis related to buckling of the Dacron prosthetic ventricular septum, leading to low cardiac output.

Triple-Orifice Tricuspid Valve

Triple-orifice tricuspid valve means that there are three tricuspid orifices. Typically, in addition to the usual tricuspid orifice there are two accessory tricuspid orifices (Fig. 13.55).

Triple-orifice tricuspid valve was found in 3 patients (Case 8, 15, and 16), constituting 19% of the 16 patients with more than one tricuspid orifice, and making up 0.09% of the 3216 cases of congenital heart disease on which this book is based (Table 13.1).

Sex: males 1, females 2, and male/female ratio = ½ (0.5).

Age at death: mean = 3.93 ± 2.93 years (1433.33 ± 1067.81 days), ranging from 7½ months to 6$^2/_{12}$ years. The median age at death was 5 years (1825 days).

Case 8 was a 6$^2/_{12}$-year-old girl with multiple congenital anomalies and a chromosomal abnormality, that is, a chromosome 17 translocation. Her birth weight was 4 lb 10 oz (2098 grams), with an estimated gestational age of 34 to 38 weeks. Her mother was 16 years of age. The patient had micrognathia, a single umbilical artery, a high-arched palate, broad nose, low-set ears, clinodactyly, pectus excavatum, an accessory midline nipple, deafness, severe intellectual disability, and marked delay in physical and psychomotor development. Her brain was malformed with anomalies that included partial absence of the corpus callosum, olfactory aplasia, abnormal gyral pattern of the cerebral hemispheres (broad simple gyri in frontal and parietal regions), and underdevelopment of the hypothalamus.

Her congenital heart disease consisted of tetralogy of Fallot {S,D,S} with severe infundibular and valvar pulmonary stenosis. The main pulmonary artery was hypoplastic, with further areas of hypoplasia (functional stenosis) at the branch points of the right and left pulmonary artery branches. A persistent left superior vena drained into the coronary sinus. An associated coronary sinus septal defect permitted drainage of this bloodstream into both the left and right atria (demonstrated angiocardiographically). The electrocardiogram showed WPW syndrome (ventricular preexcitation). Echocardiography revealed holosystolic prolapse of both the mitral and the tricuspid valves.

Surgical repair of her tetralogy of Fallot was undertaken (in 1977), which included resection of the infundibular stenosis; ventricular septal defect closure (which was difficult because the VSD extended behind the septal leaflet of the tricuspid valve); direct suture closure of the coronary sinus septal defect (3 to 4 mm in diameter); direct suture closure of the patent foramen ovale; and a large pericardial patch of the right ventricular outflow tract, main pulmonary artery and proximal right pulmonary artery, with excision of the pulmonary valve. During the first postoperative night, she developed electromechanical dissociation, could not be resuscitated, and died.

Autopsy confirmed the aforementioned anatomic findings and also revealed a triple-orifice tricuspid valve. At the superior commissure of the tricuspid valve there were two accessory orifices. The most medial was the smallest. Just lateral to this lay a somewhat larger accessory orifice. Then, further laterally lay the main tricuspid orifice, the margins of which were thickened and rolled, consistent with mild to moderate tricuspid regurgitation. This interpretation was also consistent with the echocardiographically observed tricuspid valve prolapse. The morphology of the mitral valve—also observed to prolapse—was unremarkable.

It is interesting that neither of the small superior accessory tricuspid orifices appeared to be the site of tricuspid regurgitation. Instead, the thickening and rolling of the leaflet margins suggested that the main tricuspid orifice was the site of tricuspid regurgitation.

Assessment. Clinically and surgically, how important was the presence of triple-orifice tricuspid valve? We thought that triple-orifice tricuspid valve was only one small part of this patient's much larger problem. Much more important, we thought, were the chromosomal 17 translocation and the multiple congenital anomalies, including severe tetralogy of Fallot.

Case 15, a 7½-month-old boy, had **isolated dextrocardia {S,D,S}**. In other words, the cardiac position in the chest was right-sided (inverted), but nothing else was—all of the cardiac segments being in situs solitus (noninverted). This is an infrequent anatomic type of dextrocardia, varying from 7% to 18% in various series.[559] A persistent left superior vena cava drained into the coronary sinus and thence into the right atrium.

There was a large left-to-right shunt at the atrial level, the Qp/Qs being 4/1. An incomplete form of common atrioventricular canal was present, that is, with an ostium primum and an ostium secundum types of atrial septal defect.

The mitral cleft was atypical, running anterosuperiorly (rather than horizontally, at right angles to the left ventricular septal surface, as is usual with incomplete common AV canal). There was congenital mitral stenosis with a parachute mitral valve, with all of the chordae tendineae inserting into the *anterolateral* papillary muscle group of the left ventricle. A small posteromedial papillary muscle group was present, but received no chordal insertions. (Note that when parachute mitral valve is associated with common atrioventricular canal, all of the chordae tendineae often insert into the *anterolateral* papillary muscle group, as in this case, rather than into the *posteromedial* papillary muscle group which is the rule when parachute mitral valve is associated with a normally divided AV canal, not a common AV canal.[560])

Thickening and rolling of the margins of the cleft mitral valve suggested that congenital mitral regurgitation was also present—in addition to congenital mitral stenosis. However, there were no left atrial jet lesions, suggesting that the congenital mitral regurgitation was only mild to moderate in degree (not severe).

So, this patient displayed the unusual finding of a cleft parachute mitral valve that was both stenotic and regurgitant.

Thickened and fibrotic mitral valve leaflet tissue attached to the left ventricular outflow tract, perhaps contributing to some degree of left ventricular outflow tract stenosis (but no hemodynamic data were available on this point). The aortic valve was mildly hypoplastic, with mild underdevelopment of the left coronary-noncoronary commissure. Mild narrowing of the aortic isthmus (3.5 mm internal diameter) was noted, but coarctation was thought not to be present.

The left ventricular dimensions were normal (compared with normal controls), but hypertrophy and enlargement of the right atrium and right ventricle were marked, reflecting the 4/1 Qp/Qs shunt at the atrial level, in turn related to the mitral valve dysfunction (stenosis and regurgitation).

Triple-orifice tricuspid valve was present because there were two small accessory ostia involving the posteroinferior portion of the septal leaflet. These accessory orifices were thought to be of no functional significance, without thickening or rolling of the leaflet margins about the accessory ostia. However, there was mild myxomatous change of the anterior tricuspid leaflet with mild thickening and rolling of the anterior leaflet margin, suggesting that mild tricuspid regurgitation may have been present through the main tricuspid orifice; however, we were uncertain about this possibility. If present, tricuspid regurgitation appeared to have been mild. In this patient, the major hemodynamic problems involved the mitral (not the tricuspid) valve.

Surgical repair of this patient's congenital heart disease was undertaken (in 1986) at 7½ months of age. The primum and secundum atrial septal defects were closed with a large pericardial patch. The muscular inferior limbic band of septum secundum was excised, making the secundum atrial septal defect above confluent with the primum atrial septal defect below. A single suture was placed in the mitral cleft paraseptally (adjacent to the left ventricular septal surface).

The postoperative course was characterized by elevation of left atrial pressure with prominent "a" waves (18 mm Hg). Also prominent were tachypnea, an apical diastolic murmur, and the appearance of an electrocardiographic pattern of left atrial hypertrophy. Sudden clinical deterioration occurred 7 days postoperatively, leading to death.

Assessment. We thought that the triple-orifice tricuspid valve was of little or no hemodynamic or surgical importance. This patient's major hemodynamic problem was predominantly congenital mitral stenosis with parachute mitral valve in the setting of the incomplete form of common atrioventricular canal.

Case 16, a 5-year-old girl (whose heart we were privileged to study as a consultation from Argentina in 1994), had transposition of the great arteries {S,D,D} with single left ventricle, absence of the right ventricular sinus, and a well-developed infundibular outlet chamber. The left-sided mitral valve displayed normal morphology and opened into the single left ventricle.

The right-sided tricuspid straddled the ventricular septal remnant, opening partly into the left ventricle, and partly into the infundibular outlet chamber. The straddling tricuspid valve had three orifices, but the tricuspid valve was not thought to be significantly malfunctional—neither stenotic, nor regurgitant. Because of the straddling tricuspid valve, the right atrium opened both into the left ventricle and into the infundibular outlet chamber.

She had had an arterial switch operation for transposition of the great arteries and division of a patent ductus arteriosus. (Other details are not known to us.)

Her final admission was for brain abscess, and cyanosis on exercise. She was treated with antibiotics and neurosurgery, but finally died.

Autopsy revealed not only the findings recorded above, but also polysplenia (more than one spleen) in the right upper quadrant. There were two well-formed spleens weighing 67 grams, and 4 or 5 smaller splenuli, 0.5 cm each, in the presplenic fat. The liver was predominantly left-sided, and so too was the duodenum. However, the cecum was located normally in the right lower quadrant.

These abdominal findings, reported to us by a respected and knowledgeable colleague, suggest that visceral heterotaxy with polysplenia were present. Some of the abdominal viscera appear to have been arranged in a fashion similar to situs inversus (the liver and the duodenum), but the atria were definitely in situs solitus.

Consequently, we suspect that this patient had **visceroatrial situs discordance with visceral heterotaxy and polysplenia:** situs inversus of some of the abdominal viscera (liver and duodenum), with situs solitus of the atria. This type of visceroatrial situs discordance we have seen before in visceral heterotaxy with *polysplenia.*

Assessment. How important was this patient's triple-orifice tricuspid valve? We thought that triple-orifice tricuspid valve in this case was of little or no clinical importance. Instead, the important aspects were thought to be (1) the presence of single ventricle, making the occurrence of brain abscess more likely (all of the blood did not have to go through the "filter" of the pulmonary circulation); and (2) the development of brain abscess, which was judged to be the immediate cause of death.

Summary. Based on this very small sample of triple-orifice tricuspid valve, the following conclusions appear to be justified:

1. Triple-orifice tricuspid valve always occurred with other forms of complex congenital heart disease, not in isolation.
2. Triple-orifice tricuspid valve never appeared to be the patient's main cardiovascular disability. In 1 of these 3 cases, it was associated with mild to moderate tricuspid regurgitation.

MULTIPLE FENESTRATIONS ("FILIGREE") TRICUSPID VALVE

One patient (Case 5), a 22 7/12-year-old man, was the oldest patient in this series of 16 cases of multiple-orifice tricuspid valve. This patient was also described above in relation to tricuspid valve prolapse. For the reader's convenience, this rare case is represented here.

Multiple fenestrations of the tricuspid valve leaflets, or more briefly—*"filigree" tricuspid valve*—is a rare anomaly: 1/16 = 6.25% of our cases with more than one tricuspid orifice; and 1/3216—0.03% of cases of congenital heart disease on which this study is based.

His complex congenital heart disease consisted of the following: double-outlet right ventricle {S,D,D}; subaortic conus with aortic-tricuspid wide separation, and with pulmonary-tricuspid direct fibrous continuity; superoinferior ventricles with abnormally horizontal ventricular septum, superior morphologically right ventricle and inferior morphologically left ventricle; marked underdevelopment of the right ventricle, and left ventricle well developed; high large conoventricular type of ventricular septal defect between conal septum and ventricular septum (20 × 12 mm); large muscular ventricular septal defect involving inlet portion of ventricular sinus septum (35 × 25 mm); pulmonary outflow tract stenosis (100 mm Hg gradient); tricuspid valve connecting only with small right ventricle (not straddling); multiple fenestrations of tricuspid valve leaflets, resulting in "filigree" tricuspid valve with many small openings within the tricuspid leaflets, varying from less than 1 mm in diameter to 4 to 5 mm, and associated with severe tricuspid regurgitation; marked redundancy of tricuspid leaflets with severe tricuspid valve prolapse; "hemorrhoidal" appearing mitral valve with marked upward hooding of interchordal mitral leaflet tissue, with mitral valve prolapse and mitral regurgitation indicated by thickening and rolling of mitral leaflet margins; and very marked right atrial hypertrophy and enlargement. He also had duplication of the right ureter (not known to have been of any functional importance). Nonetheless, this patient had multiple congenital anomalies, that is, malformations of more than one system (cardiovascular and genitourinary).

Therapeutically at 6½ months of age (in 1969) this patient had surgical atrial septal defect creation and a right Blalock-Taussig shunt.

At 9½ years of age (in 1978), he had an episode of subacute bacterial endocarditis, with blood cultures positive for *S. viridans.* Antibiotic therapy with penicillin for 28 days led to full recovery.

In 1982 at 13½ years of age, cardiac catheterization revealed mild kinking of the right pulmonary artery at the insertion of the right Blalock-Taussig anastomosis. In 1985 at 16 5/12 years of age, reduced left and right ventricular function were documented by cardiac catheterization.

In 1986 at 16 10/12 years of age, a modified Fontan procedure was performed consisting of ligation of the right Blalock-Taussig shunt, closure of the pulmonary valve, patch closure of the tricuspid orifice, patch closure of the interatrial communication, and anastomosis of the right atrium to the right pulmonary artery utilizing a right atrial flap and a Tascon graft.

Six months postoperatively, cardiac catheterization revealed dehiscence of the tricuspid valve patch with moderate tricuspid regurgitation into the right atrium, with a 4 to 6 mm Hg gradient between the right atrium and the pulmonary artery.

1½ months later (in 1986), this now 17 5/12-year-old young man had surgical closure of the dehiscence of the superior aspect of the tricuspid valve patch utilizing pledgetted sutures and a clot patch.

One month postoperatively, atrial flutter was documented with 2/1 atrioventricular block, that was successfully treated with cardioversion.

About 3½ years later, when the patient was 21½ years of age (in 1990), chronic edema and protein-losing enteropathy appeared. His subsequent course was characterized by worsening pitting edema, pleural effusions, ascites, low serum albumin, and low serum protein level with reduction of immunoglobulins.

Severe biventricular failure was documented. Stenosis of the right lower lobe pulmonary artery was treated with balloon dilation, but without a change in the gradient. The atrial septal defect patch was fenestrated interventionally (Brockenbrough technique followed by balloon dilations). Worsening pump failure led to death in 1991 at 22 7/12 years of age.

Autopsy confirmed the above-mentioned anatomic findings and revealed massive cardiomegaly (1440 grams), marked right ventricular hypertrophy (13 to 15 mm wall thickness), marked left ventricular hypertrophy and enlargement (14 to 16 mm wall thickness), large mitral annulus (43 mm in diameter), and large tricuspid annulus (43 mm in diameter). There was an opening in the posterior part of the tricuspid patch that measured 15 mm in length and that permitted tricuspid regurgitation that had been observed echocardiographically and at cardiac catheterization. The margins of this linear opening were coated with neopseudointima, consistent with the interpretation that this discontinuity in the tricuspid patch was old.

There was a 3 mm opening in the atrial septum immediately posterior to the atrial septal defect patch. The anastomosis of the amplified right atrial patch with the right pulmonary artery measured 21 × 11 mm.

In the fresh state, the tricuspid valve was described by Dr. John Papagiannis as "extremely dysplastic with redundant leaflets having multiple fenestrations (like a venous valve) with no central orifice, but with multiple eccentric orifices."

Assessment. Multiply fenestrated ("filigree") tricuspid valve was unquestionably important, both hemodynamically and surgically. Indeed, attempts to patch closed the tricuspid orifice, to prevent tricuspid regurgitation and tricuspid valve prolapse, failed, as autopsy revealed, despite one reoperation undertaken specifically to repair the dehiscence of the tricuspid valve patch.

Nonetheless, significant tricuspid regurgitation was just one of this patient's cardiovascular handicaps. Other important problems included mitral valve prolapse and regurgitation; small-chambered right ventricle with superoinferior ventricles—necessitating a right ventricular bypass type of surgical palliation (the modified Fontan operation); and the post-Fontan appearance of protein-losing enteropathy syndrome with hypoproteinemia and anasarca. Double-outlet right ventricle {S,D,D} with significant pulmonary outflow tract stenosis was treated with a Blalock-Taussig anastomosis but gradually led to reduced biventricular function (incipient heart failure), leading to the Fontan. Mitral regurgitation (untreated) and tricuspid regurgitation (not successfully treated because of repeated dehiscence of the tricuspid valve patch) led to post-Fontan heart failure—with protein-losing enteropathy and anasarca.

So, the tricuspid regurgitation associated with "filigree" tricuspid valve was definitely *one* important factor leading to fatal heart failure that began pre-Fontan and became progressively worse post-Fontan.

Was the Fontan pathway itself stenotic,[513] and did this go unrecognized despite our autopsy examination? We did this autopsy examination in 1991, which is before we had studied the modified Fontan pathways by morphometry. By 1999, we had come to understand that Fontan pathways can be stenotic, and that this fact may well not be evident without morphometry.[513] In this case, for example, the atriopulmonary anastomosis (between the right atrium and the right pulmonary artery) is analogous to the patient's tricuspid valve (diameter = 43 mm). But the maximal diameter of this atriopulmonary anastomosis was only 21 mm, which is 51% less than the patient's tricuspid (and mitral) diameters. Or, to say it another way, the Fontan (cardiopulmonary) anastomosis was only 49% as big as it "should" have been (21/43 = 0.488).

Was the fact that the atriopulmonary anastomosis was slightly less than half as big as it normally should have been important in the post-Fontan course of this patient? Was this too-small atriopulmonary anastomosis at least one of the reasons why this patient developed protein-losing enteropathy and fatal pump failure? We now think so. There were other factors too, noted above (regurgitation of both atrioventricular valves).

This patient also had polyvalvar disease (tricuspid, mitral and the pulmonary valves were thickened and myxomatous). One wonders—trisomy? Unfortunately, we cannot answer this question (karyotype unknown).

Multiple fenestrations of the tricuspid valve leaflets (filigree tricuspid valve) may be a *forme fruste* of congenitally unguarded tricuspid orifice (absence of tricuspid valve leaflets). Filigree tricuspid valve was definitely important both clinically and surgically.

LITERATURE

Straddling Tricuspid Valve

In 1999, Pessotto and colleagues[219] published a morphometric study of 19 postmortem cases of straddling tricuspid valve (Fig. 13.57). These results were compared with 32 normal control heart specimens. In hearts with a straddling

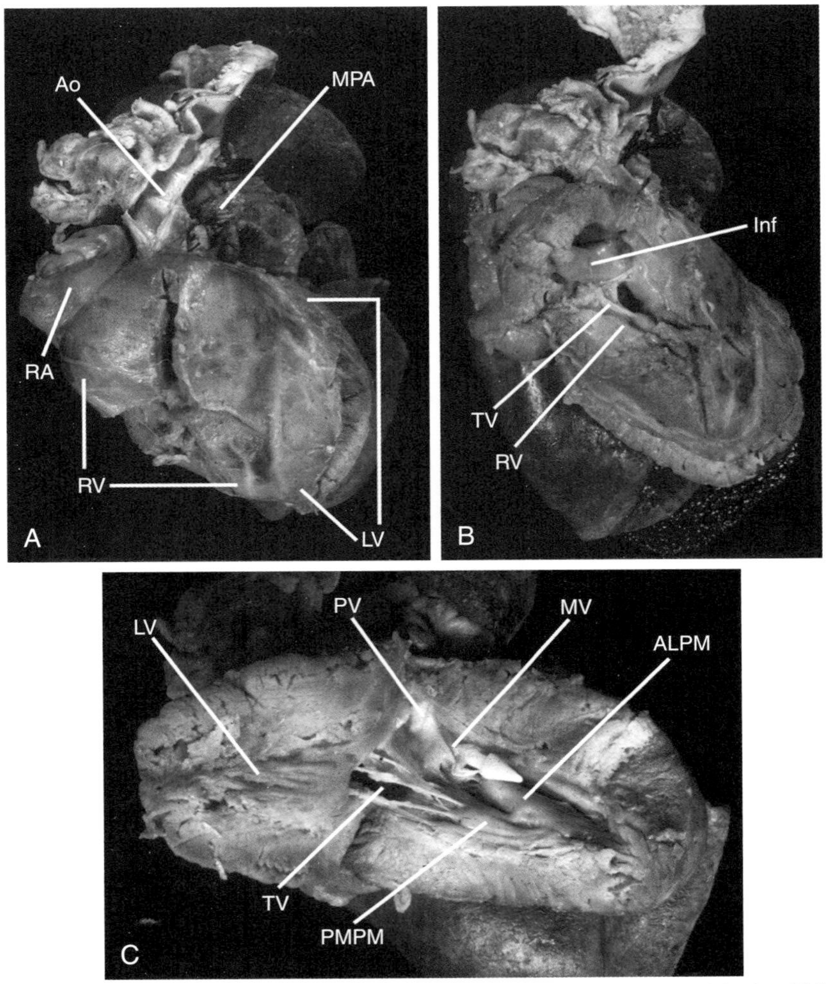

Fig. 13.57 Straddling tricuspid valve. *Straddling* tricuspid valve means that the tricuspid valve *(TV)* has bicameral tensor apparatus. *Overriding* tricuspid valve means that the tricuspid annulus overlooks the plane of the ventricular septum and is located above the right ventricle and also above the left ventricle, but the tensor apparatus of the TV inserts only into the right ventricle: the tensor apparatus of the TV is unicameral, not bicameral. (A) External frontal view of the heart of a 19-day-old white boy correctly suggests TGA {S,D,D}. A large transposed aorta *(Ao)* arises above the right ventricle and a banded main pulmonary artery *(MPA)* originates above the left ventricle *(LV)*; hence transposition of the great arteries (TGA) seems likely. Internal inspection is necessary for certainty. The broad triangular shape of the right-sided atrial appendage looks like the morphologically right atrium *(RA)*, suggesting visceroatrial situs solitus, i.e., TGA {*S*,-,-}. The ventricular configuration suggests D-loop ventricles, i.e., TGA {S,*D*,-}. Note that the right-sided morphologically right ventricle *(RV)* appears small compared with the much larger morphologically left ventricle *(LV)*. The LV forms the ventricular apex. Much too much LV is visible from the front. The transposed main pulmonary artery (MPA) is posterior and to the left of the transposed aorta; hence the segmental anatomy appears to be TGA {S,D,D}. Concerning the atrioventricular valves, the smallness of the RV should raise the diagnostic question: straddling tricuspid valve (TV)? (B) The opened RV showed that the TV does indeed open into this small RV chamber. *Inf*, Subaortic infundibulum. (C) The opened LV shows that the TV straddles through a ventricular septal defect of the atrioventricular canal type and inserts into the posteromedial papillary muscle group of the LV. The mitral valve *(MV)*, with a *white arrowhead* through the orifice, also opens into the LV and its chordae tendineae insert only into the anterolateral papillary muscle *(ALPM)* of the LV, similar to a parachute mitral valve *(MV)*. The LV is hypertrophied and enlarged. There is direct fibrous continuity between the MV and the straddling TV and the transposed pulmonary valve *(PV)*. Hence, this TGA has a muscular subaortic conus (only), well seen in B (above the straddling TV), with no subpulmonary muscular conus, permitting PV-MV and PV-straddling TV direct fibrous continuity.

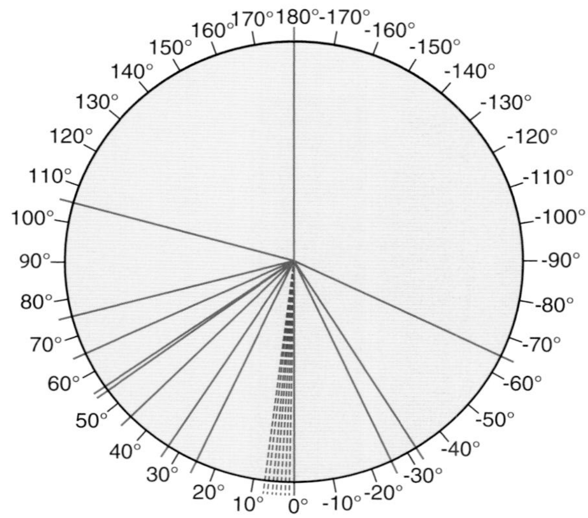

Fig. 13.58 Ventriculoatrial septal angles in straddling tricuspid valve *(solid lines)* compared with normal controls *(broken lines),* viewed in short-axis projection, seen from the front. *Vertical lines* from 0° to 180° represents the plane of the atrial septum, which is the frame of reference. *All other lines* represent the planes of the ventricular septum. There was no overlap between the abnormally large ventriculoatrial septal angles in straddling TV (mean = 61° ± 24°, and mean = 60°) and the normally small ventriculoatrial septal angles (mean = 5° ± 2°, and median = 6°) (p <0.001). The ventriculoatrial septal angle is a quantitative method of expressing the malalignment of the ventricles as a whole (not just the ventricular septum) relative to the atria as a whole (not just the atrial septum). With straddling tricuspid valve, the ventricular septum is *laterally displaced* and *angulated* relative to the atrial septum. The inflow tract or ventricular sinus septum is displaced toward the side of the underdeveloped morphologically right ventricular sinus—reminiscent of the displacement of the mediastinum in the direction of a small or absent lung. Thus, with D-loop ventricles, the ventricular septum is displaced toward the small right ventricular sinus (RV), i.e., to the *right,* and it is also angulated relative to the atrial septum. These ventriculoatrial septal angles are expressed in *positive degrees.* Similarly with L-loop ventricles, the ventricular septum is displaced toward the small RV sinus, i.e., to the *left,* and it is also angulated relative to the atrial septum. These ventriculoatrial septal angles are expressed in *negative degrees.* For statistical analysis, *absolute numbers* (without sign) were used; for example, |60°|, not +60° or −60°. (Reproduced with permission from Pessotto R, Padalino M, Rubino M, Kadoba K, Büchler JR, Van Praagh R: Straddling tricuspid valve as a sign of ventriculoatrial malalignment: a morphometric study of 19 postmortem cases. *Am Heart J* 1999;138:1184.)

tricuspid valve, marked malalignment of the ventricles was always found relative to the atria. In order to express this ventriculoatrial malalignment quantitatively, the angle between the plane of the ventricular septum and the plane of the atrial septum was measured in short-axis projection (from the ventricular apex ventrally to the atrial septum dorsally). In hearts with straddling tricuspid valve, the ventriculoatrial septal angle averaged 61° ± 24°, whereas the normal ventriculoatrial septal angle measured 5° ± 2° (p <0.001) (Fig. 13.58).[219]

A heart specimen with **double-outlet right atrium** is presented in Fig. 13.59.[219] Double-outlet right atrium can result when a straddling tricuspid valve becomes adherent to the malpositioned ventricular septal crest, obliterating the ventricular septal defect of the atrioventricular canal type, resulting in an intact ventricular septum. The result is a heart with *three atrioventricular valves:* an RA-to-small RV valve, that is, the nonstraddling TV; an RA-to-large LV valve, that is, the straddling part of the tricuspid valve; and the LA-to-LV valve, that is, the mitral valve, which may or may not be stenotic—depending on the septal geometry. As will be seen, this patient (Fig. 13.59) also had the polysplenia syndrome, accessory orifices in both the nonstraddling and straddling components of the TV, and congenital mitral stenosis.

When the tricuspid valve had two or more ostia that opened into the same ventricular chamber, this is known as double- or triple-orifice TV (as above). But when the TV opens into two different chambers, then this situation is called double-outlet right atrium. Double-outlet right atrium occurred in 4 of 19 patients with straddling TV (21%).[219]

With straddling tricuspid valve, the right ventricular sinus (inflow tract) was significantly smaller than the left (p <0.01) (Table 13.28).

The degree of straddling of the TV was estimated by the ratio of the portion of the tricuspid annulus connected with the LV to the total tricuspid annulus, expressed as a percentage. The mean was 47.09 ± 14.84%, ranging from 17% to 74%. The median was 46.5%.

The RV inflow index (RV inflow length/LV inflow length × 100): mean = .71 ± .17; range from .38 to 1.0; median = .67.

Ventriculoatrial septal angle was expressed in positive degrees when the ventricular septum was angulated to the right of the atrial septum, as was usual with D-loop ventricles. The ventriculoatrial septal angle was expressed in negative degrees when the ventricular septum lay to the left of the atrial septum, as was usual with L-loop ventricles. Mean = 61.21 ± 24.14°, ranging from 25° to 110°; median = 60°. For these calculations, absolute values (without sign) were used; for example, |60°|, not +60° or −60°. When the straddling tricuspid valve adhered to the ventricular septal crest, obliterating the ventricular septal defect of the AV canal type and resulting in double-outlet right atrium, the degree of tricuspid straddling was recorded as – (inapplicable) because the nonstraddling RA-to-RV valve always straddled by 0%, whereas the straddling RA-to-LV valve always straddled by 100%, by definition, hence no tricuspid straddling.

A ventricular septal defect was present in 79%: atrioventricular canal type in 42%, atrioventricular canal type confluent with a conoventricular type in 26%, and a conoventricular type only in 11%.

In the 21% of cases (n = 4) without a ventricular septal defect (VSD), the straddling tricuspid valve had adhered to the muscular crest of the ventricular septum, obliterating the VSD. In addition to an intact ventricular septum, the other result of adherence of the tricuspid valve leaflet tissue was **double-outlet right atrium** (Figs. 13.59 and 13.60). The nonstraddling part of the tricuspid valve opened into the small right ventricle, and the straddling part of the tricuspid valve opened into the larger left ventricle. The mitral valve also opened into the left ventricle.

Thus, hearts with straddling tricuspid valve and double-outlet right atrium had **three atrioventricular valves:** (1)

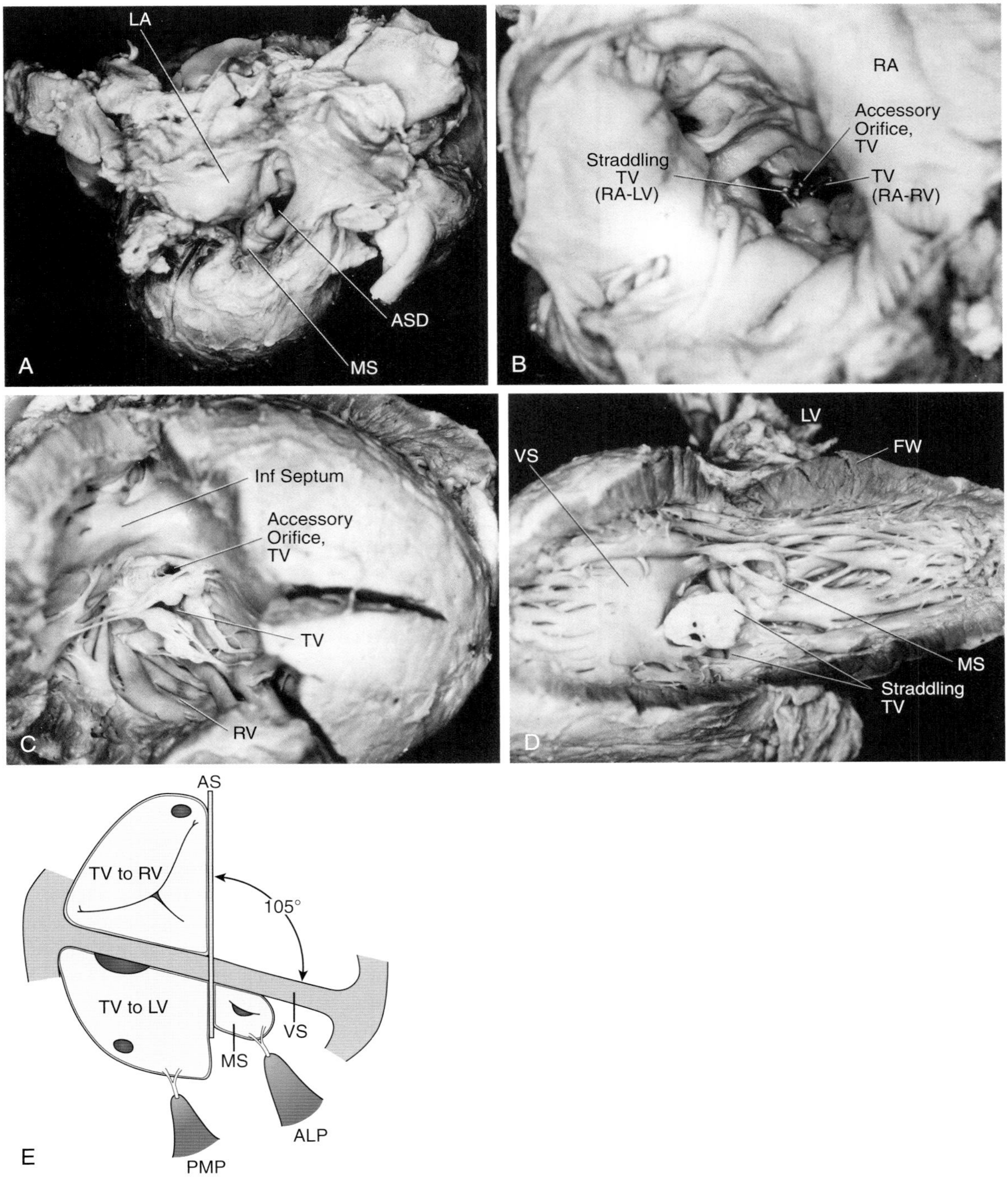

Fig. 13.59 Double-outlet right atrium. (A) Opening the left-sided left atrium *(LA)* reveals severe congenital mitral stenosis *(MS)* and a secundum type of atrial septal defect *(ASD)*. (B) Opening the right-sided right atrium *(RA)* shows double-outlet right atrium. The nonstraddling tricuspid valve *(TV)* opens from the RA into the right ventricle *(RV)*, i.e., the RA-to-RV valve *(RA-RV)*. The straddling TV opens from the RA into the left ventricle *(LV)*, i.e., the RA-to-LV valve *(RA-LV)*. Superiorly, the nonstraddling TV (RA-RV valve) has an accessory orifice. Hence, in this patient with double-outlet right atrium, the nonstraddling TV has double-orifice tricuspid valve. (C) The nonstraddling TV is seen opening into the RV. The accessory orifice of the TV is seen within the anterior tricuspid leaflet. The RV was somewhat small. The RV inflow index was 0.84 (i.e., RV inflow length/LV inflow length divided by the normal control RV inflow length/normal LV inflow length). *Inf Septum,* infundibular septum. (D) Opening the LV reveals the straddling TV with two small accessory orifices, i.e., triple-orifice straddling tricuspid valve, and severe congenital MS. The straddling RV inserts into the posteromedial papillary muscle of the LV, whereas the mitral valve (MV) inserts only into the anterolateral papillary muscle group of the LV. Hence, this stenotic mitral valve resembles parachute mitral valve, except that both papillary muscle groups are present. The tensor apparatus (chordae tendineae and papillary muscles) of the straddling TV and of the MV were always separate; they did not crisscross or interdigitate. Surgically, this could be important because it would be anatomically possible to separate these two valves with a prosthetic ventricular septum. In this patient, for example, the MV and the straddling TV did not share papillary muscles: MV into the anterolateral papillary muscle group only; and straddling TV into the posteromedial

Continued

Fig. 13.59 cont'd papillary muscle group only. Both the MV and the straddling TV were stenotic. *Parachute MV* and *parachute straddling TV* coexist in this patient. Parachute TV is not a widely recognized entity. Parachute MV and TV means that there is only one "man" (papillary muscle) beneath the shroud or leaflets of an atrioventricular valve, rather than the normal two papillary muscles (or more in the case of the tricuspid valve). This is one of Dr. Jesse Edwards' graphic and unforgettable coinages: When an AV valve attaches to only one papillary muscle, it resembles a parachutist. Why is this concept important? Because, as in this patient, when an AV valve attaches to only one papillary muscle group, it is likely to be stenotic. Why? Because the interpapillary muscle distance is a major component of the orifice of an AV valve; and the interchordal spaces are the other. When there is no inter-papillary muscle distance (e.g., between the anterolateral and the posteromedial papillary muscles of the MV), then the valvar orifice is likely to be significantly reduced, leading to stenosis. Note the absence of a ventricular septal defect of the AV canal type in both (D) and (C). Hence, this case of straddling TV has double-outlet right atrium. The billowing leaflets of the straddling TV caused fibrous left ventricular outflow tract stenosis. *FW,* Free wall; *VS,* ventricular septum. (E) Septal geometry, in short-axis projection. The plane of the atrial septum (AS) is normal, i.e., vertical or straight up and down. But the plane of the ventricular septum (VS) is very abnormal. The ventriculoatrial septal angle is huge: 105°. Why? Because the ventricular part of the heart is very malaligned relative to the normally positioned atria. The VS is approximately horizontal, i.e., 15° more than horizontal; a ventriculoatrial septal angle of 90° would have a perfectly horizontal VS, with RV above and LV below. So this heart has superoinferior ventricles. In this case, the effect of this ventriculoatrial malalignment has been to place the ventricular septum under the straddling TV, with the nonstraddling TV *(TV-to-RV)* lying above the VS, and the straddling TV *(TV-to-LV)* lying below the VS. Another effect of this ventriculoatrial malalignment was that the VS compressed the MV from above, reducing the size of the LA-to-LV inflow tract and contributing to the congenital MS. The opened LV (D) photograph is positioned for comprehensibility. How was it positioned really? Rotate the photo of the LV (D) 90° clockwise. That is how it really was positioned; (D) shows how it "should" have been positioned. **The basic diagnosis** in this case is revealed by the cardiac geometry (E). Ventriculoatrial malalignment, as expressed quantitatively by the ventriculoatrial septal angle (105°), resulted in several important sequelae: straddling TV with double-outlet right atrium and congenital MS. Straddling TV is not a primary diagnosis; it is a secondary diagnosis. The TV is not the "sinner"; it is the "sinned against." The TV (and the MV) are the innocent victims; ventriculoatrial malalignment is the real "villain," the primary anatomic diagnosis. Cardiac geometry is an underused but very helpful approach to the understanding of complex congenital heart disease. *ALP,* Anterolateral papillary muscle; *PMP,* posteromedial papillary muscle. (Reproduced with permission from Pessotto R, Padalino M, Rubino M, Kadoba K, Büchler JR, Van Praagh R: Straddling tricuspid valve as a sign of ventriculoatrial malalignment: a morphometric study of 19 postmortem cases. *Am Heart J* 1999;138:1184.)

TABLE 13.28 Morphometry in Straddling Tricuspid Valve (n = 19)

No.	Degree of Straddling (%)	Right Ventricular Inflow Index	Ventriculoatrial Septal Angle (°)
1	60	0.88	+55
2	47	0.93	+54
3	32	0.57	+75
4	17	0.88	+33
5	30	1.00	+70
6	35	0.38	+65
7	40	0.84	+105
8	—	0.62	+25
9	55.5	0.515	+55
10	—	0.61	+45
11	—	0.84	+60
12	58	0.69	+55
13	43	0.85	+90
14	40	—	+80
15	50	0.64	+110
16	74	0.71	65
17	66	0.545	−32
18	60	0.625	−25
19	46	0.65	−64

Reproduced with permission from Pessotto R, Padalino M, Rubino M, Kadoba K, Büchler JR, Van Praagh R: Straddling tricuspid valve as a sign of ventriculoatrial malalignment: a morphometric study of 19 postmortem cases, *Am Heart J* 1999;138:1184.

nonstraddling tricuspid valve (RA to RV), (2) straddling tricuspid valve (RA to LV), and (3) mitral valve (LA to LV). Congenital mitral stenosis was present in 26% of this series.[219]

In the anomaly known as straddling tricuspid valve, we realized that the tricuspid valve is the "victim," not the "villain." The real "villain" is the malalignment of the ventricular part of the heart relative to the atria and the atrioventricular canal (the atrioventricular valves) (Fig. 13.59). Indeed, straddling tricuspid valve (and straddling mitral valve) both are signs of ventriculoatrial malalignment. In both, the atrioventricular valves are the "sinned against," not the "sinners." In imaging studies (two- and three-dimensional echocardiography, and magnetic resonance imaging), cardiac geometry of the ventricles relative to the atria could be very illuminating (Table 13.29).

Attachments of the Straddling Tricuspid Valve[219]

The straddling tricuspid valve showed four different patterns of left ventricular attachment:

1. to the posteromedial papillary muscle group, shared with the mitral valve in 9 of 19 patients (47%) (Fig. 13.60);
2. to the posteromedial papillary muscle group, not shared with the mitral valve, in 8 of 19 cases (42%) (Fig. 13.59);
3. to the posteromedial and anterolateral papillary muscle groups of the left ventricle, the latter shared with the mitral valve, in 1 of 19 patients (5%); and
4. to the anterolateral papillary muscle group of the left ventricle, shared with the mitral valve, in 1 of 19 cases (5%) (Fig. 13.61).

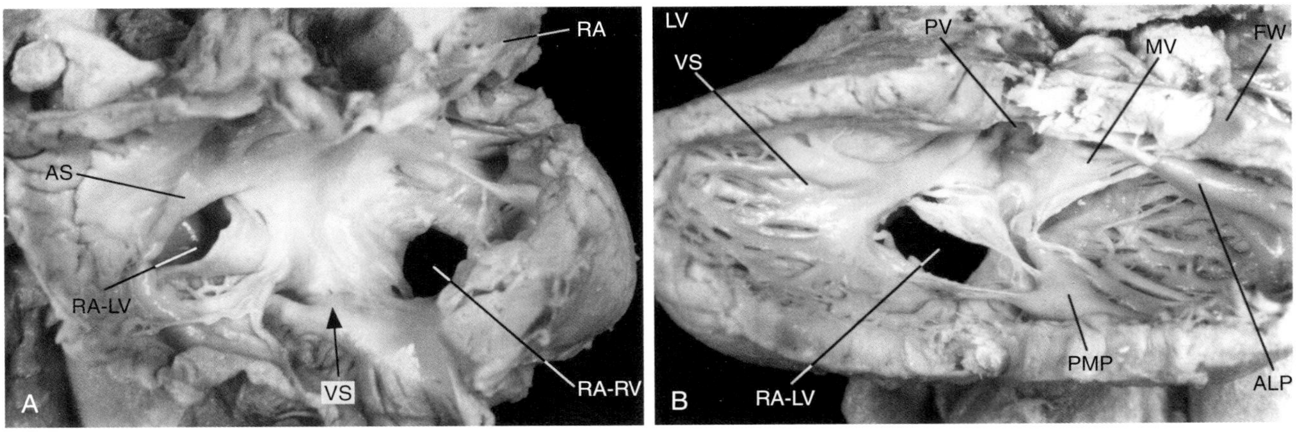

Fig. 13.60 Double-outlet right atrium. (A) Opened right atrium *(RA)* showing double-outlet right atrium. The right-sided valve opens from the RA into the small right ventricle (RV): *RA-RV*. The left-sided valve opens from the RA into the large left ventricle *(LV)*: *RA-LV*. The plane of the ventricular septum *(VS)* lies far to the right of the atrial septum *(AS)*, and the VS is angulated relative to the AS (ventriculoatrial septal angle = 55°). (B) Opened LV shows that there is no ventricular septal defect because the straddling tricuspid valve is firmly attached to the crest of the muscular VS. The nonstraddling TV is right-sided and opens only into the moderately hypoplastic RV (RV inflow index = 0.69). The straddling TV (RA-LV) seen here opens only into the LV and inserts into the posteromedial papillary muscle *(PMP)* of the LV that the straddling TV shares with the mitral valve *(MV)*. Transposition of the great arteries {S,D,D} is present. The transposed pulmonary valve is in direct fibrous continuity with the MV and the straddling TV. The anterolateral papillary muscle *(ALP)* and the PMP are well separated and there is no congenital mitral stenosis. Hence, this heart with straddling TV and double-outlet RA has three atrioventricular valve: a nonstraddling TV, a straddling TV, and an MV. (This is Case 12 of Pessotto R, Padalino M, Rubino M, Kadoba K, Büchler JR, Van Praagh R: Straddling tricuspid valve as a sign of ventriculoatrial malalignment: a morphometric study of 19 postmortem cases. *Am Heart J* 1999;138:1184, reproduced with permission.)

TABLE 13.29 What Kinds of Heart Had Straddling Tricuspid Valve?

Types of Heart	*N*	% (*n* = 19)
1. Tetralogy of Fallot {S,D,S}*	5	26
2. Transposition of the great arteries {S,D,D}†	4	21
3. Transposition of the great arteries {S,L,L}	3	16
4. Transposition of the great arteries {S,D,A}†	2	11
5. Normal type of heart {S,D,S}	2	11
6. Tetralogy of Fallot {S,D,I}*	1	5
7. Double-outlet right ventricle {S,D,D}	1	5
8. Double-outlet left ventricle {S,D,L}	1	5

*If one combines TOF {S,D,S} and TOF {S,D,I} as TOF in visceroatrial situs solitus, then there are 6 cases (32%).

†If one combines TGA {S,D,D} and TGA {S,D,A} as D-loop TGA, there are 6 cases (32%). Then physiologically uncorrected complete TGA and TOF are tied for first place in the frequency of the settings in which straddling TV occurred.

From Pessotto R, Padalino M, Rubino M, Kadoba K, Büchler JR, Van Praagh R: Straddling tricuspid valve as a sign of ventriculoatrial malalignment: a morphometric study of 19 postmortem cases, *Am Heart J* 1999;138:1184, with permission.

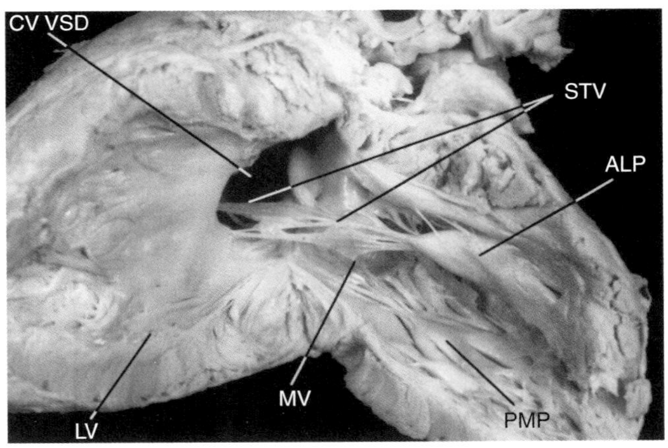

Fig. 13.61 Straddling tricuspid valve *(STV)* inserting into the anterolateral papillary muscle *(ALP)* of the left ventricle *(LV)* through a conoventricular (outlet) type of ventricular septal defect *(CV VSD)*. Both the STV and the mitral valve share the ALP. Only the *MV* inserts into the posteromedial papillary muscle *(PMP)* of the LV. Insertion of the STV into the ALP muscle group is unusual. Typically, the STV inserts into the PMP muscle group, as in Fig. 13.60. (Reproduced with permission from Pessotto and colleagues.[219])

Attachments of the Mitral Valve When Straddling Tricuspid Valve Coexists.[219] Five different patterns of mitral valve (MV) attachment were found:

1. Normal attachments of the MV were found in 10 of 19 patients (53%), with insertions of mitral chordae tendineae into both the anterolateral and the posteromedial papillary muscle groups of the left ventricle.
2. Mitral chordal attachments were to the anterolateral papillary muscle group only in 6 of 19 cases (32%) (Fig. 13.59). Congenital mitral stenosis occurred in 4 of these 6 patients (67%) in whom all mitral chordae inserted only into the

anterolateral papillary muscle group. The 4 cases with congenital mitral stenosis had only one focus of chordal insertion into the anterolateral papillary muscle group whereas the 2 patients without congenital mitral stenosis had two separate foci of chordal insertion into the anterolateral papillary muscle group.
3. Mitral chordae attached to the anterolateral papillary muscle group and to the subaortic left ventricular septal surface in 1 of 19 patients (5%).
4. Mitral chordae inserted into the posteromedial papillary muscle group and into the left ventricular free wall, the anteropapillary muscle group being absent, in 1 of 19 cases (5%).
5. The tricuspid and mitral valves both straddled the ventricular septum in one rare case of transposition of the great arteries {S,L,L} (5%) (Fig. 13.62). The tricuspid valve straddled above the inlet part of the ventricular septum, and the mitral valve straddled above the outlet part of the ventricular septum. The mitral chordae tendineae inserted into the anterolateral papillary muscle of the left ventricle and into an anterosuperior papillary muscle of the right ventricle located above the anterior papillary muscle of the right ventricle.

The literature on straddling tricuspid valve is noteworthy.[561-579] Who was it who coined the term "straddling" tricuspid (and mitral) valve? I think it may have been Dr. Maurice Lev of Chicago.[561] I remember that he used to call them "straddlers." Others spoke of "overriding" tricuspid valve.[562,565]

In 1979, Milo and colleagues[571] proposed that *straddling* be used to denote biventricular chordal insertions and the *overriding* be used to mean annular overlooking (relative to the plane of the ventricular septum). In a study of 57 heart specimens, these authors found that there could be straddling without overriding, and overriding without straddling. This was a helpful distinction between AV valve *straddling* and *overriding* that has been generally adopted.

In 1989, Isomatsu and colleagues[566] reported straddling tricuspid valve without a ventricular septal defect of the atrioventricular canal type that resulted in *double-outlet right atrium.*

In 1982, Wenink and Gittenberger-de Groot[572] pointed out that straddling tricuspid valve typically has a ventricular septal defect of the atrioventricular canal type (that they called an inlet septal defect), whereas, as we shall see (in Chapter 14), straddling mitral valve typically has a conoventricular type of ventricular septal defect (that they called an infundibular septal defect).

These authors[572] also clarified several other terms:

- The *parietal band* (of Lev and other American workers) they called the *infundibular septum.*
- The *septal band* (of American workers) they called the *bulboventricular septum.*
- The *moderator band* (of American workers) they called the *trabecula septomarginalis;* the latter is Tandler's term.
- The *ventricular sinus septum* they called the *inlet septum.*[572]

This glossary is included here to aid mutual understanding.

The surgical management of straddling tricuspid valve has been the focus of several publications.[567,569,574,575,580] For example, in 1998 van Son and coworkers[580] reported suspension of the straddling tricuspid valve chordae into the morphologically right ventricle. In two patients, straddling tricuspid chordae and the papillary muscle head were successfully anchored to the right ventricular septal surface.[580] This, in turn, facilities surgical closure of the ventricular septal defect of the atrioventricular canal type.

Why do we prefer the term *ventricular septal defect of the AV canal type* to *inlet ventricular septal defect?* Because *two* anatomically different types of VSD occur in this area: (1) a VSD of the AV canal type that is confluent with the tricuspid valve leaflet tissue, as in straddling tricuspid valve; and (2) a muscular VSD in the ventricular sinus septum that does not extend up to the level of the tricuspid valve tissue and hence is not confluent with the tricuspid valve. *Inlet VSD* does not make this distinction. Or, one may accurately say that there are two anatomic types of inlet VSD: (1) a VSD of the AV canal type (a complete or partial form of AV septal defect); and (2) a muscular VSD in the inlet (sinus) septum.

Why do we prefer *conoventricular* (or *infundibuloventricular*) type of VSD to *infundibular VSD,* which some favor (as noted above)? Again, anatomic specificity and accuracy are our reasons. Such VSDs can occur between the conal septum above and the septal band and the ventricular septum below, without displacement of one septum relative to the other, or with displacement of one septum relative to the other (as in tetralogy of Fallot, or the Taussig-Bing malformation, etc.). But VSDs also can occur of (or within) the conal (infundibulum) septum, resulting in a typical subpulmonary (or subsemilunar) VSD. The latter really is an infundibular septal defect, that is, a defect of or within the infundibular septum. Whereas in a conoventricular type of VSD—as in the Taussig-Bing malformation—is a conal septal defect present? We are not sure. The conal septum is clearly very malaligned relative to the ventricular septum and the septal band; but the conal septum *per se* often looks well developed—not as though a defect is present within the conal septum itself. By contrast, in a typical subpulmonary VSD in a segmentally normal heart, that is, {S,D,S}, a conal septal defect definitely is present, as all agree.

Thus, we distinguish between a *conoventricular type of VSD,* that is, a defect between the conal septum and the ventricular septum, in which either the conal or the ventricular septum may or may not be deficient, and a *conal septal defect* in which the conal septum definitely is deficient. For further information and illustrations, see Chapter 16.

Again, these distinctions are recorded here to facilitate mutual understanding.

Other Topics

What else merits mention in the literature concerning the tricuspid valve? Looking over my notes that I have been making on 5 × 8 inch cards since the late 1950s, the following papers merit specific mention:

the morphology of the normal human tricuspid valve, by Silver et al;[581]

the membranous ventricular septum and the tricuspid valve in Down syndrome without common atrioventricular canal, by Rosenquist and colleagues;[582]

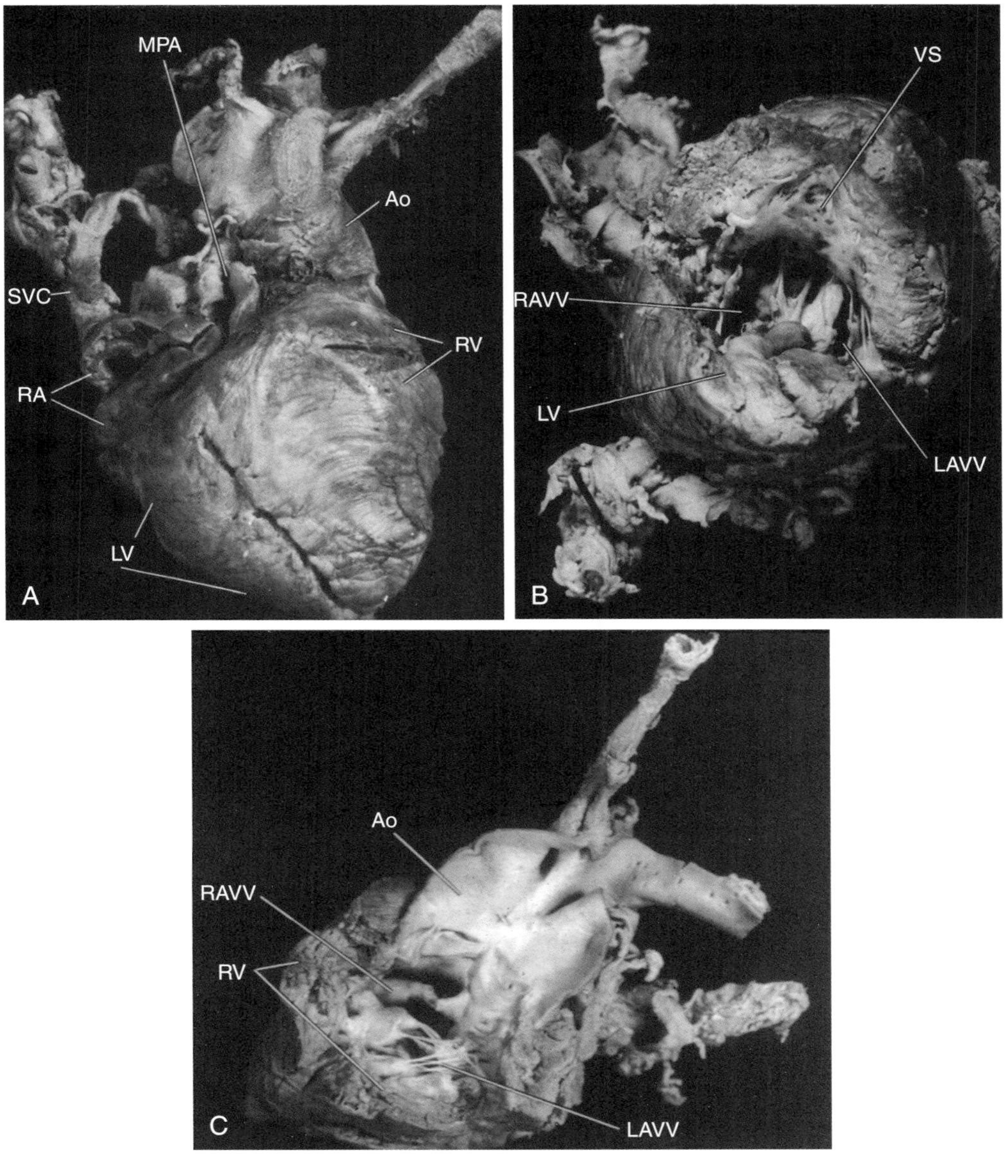

Fig. 13.62 Straddling of *both* the tricuspid valve and the mitral valve in a 13-day-old white girl with transposition of the great arteries {S,L,L}, large ventricular septal defect (confluent conoventricular and atrioventricular canal type), and hypoplasia of the morphologically right ventricle (left-sided). (A) External frontal view of transposition of the great arteries {S,L,L}. Note the right-sided right atrium *(RA)* and superior vena cava *(SVC)*. Most of the ventricular part of the heart consists of a large right-sided morphologically left ventricle *(LV)*. The apex of the heart is formed by the *LV*. The morphologically right ventricle *(RV)* is small and sits on the left anterosuperior portion of the ventricular mass. The L-transposed aorta *(Ao)* is large, indicating that the aortic outflow tract is not obstructed; whereas the main pulmonary artery *(MPA)* is smaller than expected, consistent with pulmonary outflow tract obstruction; pulmonary valve stenosis (bicuspid) and subvalvar stenosis (a fibrous ring) were found. (B) View of the opened LV from the apex, showing that the left-sided atrioventricular valve *(LAVV)*, which is the left-sided tricuspid valve (with L-loop ventricles), and the right-sided atrioventricular valve *(RAVV)*, which is the right-sided mitral valve (with L-loop ventricles), both straddle the ventricular septum *(VS)*. Note that the left ventricular septal surface *(VS)* faces posteriorly and to the right, typical of L-loop ventricles. The right-sided LV is markedly hypertrophied and enlarged. (C) The opened RV, sitting on the left "shoulder" of the ventricular mass, is very small-chambered. This RV is left-handed, typical of L-loop ventricles. The small RV receives the left-sided tricuspid valve *(LAVV)*, which straddles across the inlet portion of the right ventricular septal crest. The right-sided mitral valve *(RAVV)* straddles across the outlet portion of the right ventricular septal crest. The L-transposed ascending aorta (Ao) is large and unobstructed despite the subaortic straddling of both AV valves. **Straddling of both AV valves is rare.**

normal attachments of the tricuspid valve to the membranous system, and relevance to left ventricle-to-right atrial shunts, by Rosenquist and Sweeney;[583]
accessory tricuspid leaflet tissue producing right ventricular outflow tract stenosis, by Pate et al[584] and by Cosio et al;[585]
double-orifice tricuspid valve by Cascos et al,[586] by Pisenti,[587] and by Sierra-Quiroga et al;[588]
prominent and potentially obstructive right venous valve, that is, Eustachian valve of the inferior vena cava by Folger,[589] Paloheimo,[590] and Weinberg and colleagues;[591]
obstructive giant blood cyst of tricuspid valve in an infant, by Gallucci and colleagues;[592]
congenital papillary tumor of the tricuspid valve obstructing the right ventricular outflow in a neonate with trisomy E, by Anderson and colleagues;[593]
congenital tricuspid regurgitation caused by absence of papillary muscles and chordae tendineae to the posterior leaflet;[594]
severe congenital tricuspid stenosis with right ventricular hypoplasia and intact ventricular septum;[595]
calcific tricuspid incompetence in childhood;[596]
first case of successful porcine valve replacement of congenital tricuspid stenosis in a 21-year-old man, reported in 1973;[597]
severe congenital tricuspid regurgitation in the neonate;[598]
19-year-old male heroin addict who did well following total tricuspid valvectomy, without prosthetic valve replacement, in the treatment of *Pseudomonas* endocarditis;[599]
the hemodynamic consequences of total tricuspid valvulectomy, without tricuspid valve replacement, in 10 heroin addicts with *Psuedomonas* tricuspid endocarditis[600] (their answer: no congestive heart failure in 7; congestive heart failure in 3; and inability to differentiate between these two outcome groups preoperatively);[600]
prolapse of the tricuspid leaflets in the systolic murmur-click syndrome[601] (findings in 61 patients: mitral valve prolapse in 85%; prolapse of the tricuspid valve leaflets in 52%; prolapse of the tricuspid valve leaflets only in 15%);[601]
precordial honk due to tricuspid regurgitation in a 49-year-old woman;[602]
review of congenital tricuspid regurgitation;[603]
spontaneous resolution of massive congenital tricuspid regurgitation;[604]
severe congenital pulmonary stenosis and congenital tricuspid stenosis in a 30-year-old man, with impressive clinical improvement following surgical pulmonary valvotomy, infundibulectomy, and tricuspid valve replacement with a #29 porcine xenograft;[605]
transient tricuspid insufficiency in neonates, with elevation of serum creatine phosphokinase MB fraction within 6 hours of myocardial infarction (necrosis of anterolateral papillary muscle of the right ventricle), with peak at 24 hours, and return to normal by 36 hours;[606]
congenital tricuspid incompetence simulating pulmonary atresia with intact ventricular septum;[607]
tricuspid valve excision without replacement in a patient with endocarditis associated with drug abuse;[608]
detection of tricuspid valve prolapse with two-dimensional echocardiography by using a subxiphoid approach;[609]
parachute tricuspid valve;[610]
surgical correction of congenital tricuspid stenosis;[611]
severe tricuspid regurgitation in a 9-year-old girl with myxomatous tricuspid leaflets and elongated tricuspid chordae, in a patient with systemic lupus erythematosus, mistakenly thought to have Liebman-Sacks endocarditis (no tricuspid vegetation found), successfully treated with tricuspid valve replacement using a #27 Bjork-Shiley prosthesis;[612]
non-Ebstein tricuspid and mitral dysplasia in newborns;[613]
transient neonatal tricuspid regurgitation, possibly related to premature closure of ductus arteriosus in utero, leading to massive tricuspid regurgitation that recovers when the pulmonary arteriolar resistance falls postnatally;[614]
congenital isolated tricuspid regurgitation in a 46-year-old-woman caused by absence of the anterior tricuspid leaflet and its chordae and papillary muscles, successfully treated with tricuspid valve replacement;[615]
tricuspid regurgitation caused by annular dilation and failure of leaflet coaptation;[616]
traumatic rupture of the tricuspid valve in a 10-year-old girl involved in an automobile accident, repaired by chordal replacements using pericardial strips of autogenous pericardium and annuloplasty;[617]
rupture of tricuspid valve papillary muscle during pulmonary balloon valvuloplasty;[618]
the normal, dilated and markedly dilated tricuspid annulus in adults;[619,620] findings: annulus <12 cm is normal, 12 to 14 cm is dilated; >14 cm is markedly dilated; language note: *annulus*, pleural *annuli; annulus* = a ring (Latin), diminutive of *annus* = a year, originally a circuit; *anulus,* pleural *anuli; anulus* is diminutive of *anus,* Latin, said originally to have been derived from an Anglo-Saxon word meaning to sit; *anus* in medicine means the terminal orifice of the alimentary canal; *anulus* means little anus; thus *annulus* and *anulus* are both correct, are both derived from different Latin roots, and have different etymologies; we prefer *annulus* to mean a valve ring, because *anulus* literally means little anus (source of the foregoing etymologies: *Dorland's Illustrated Medical Dictionary,* 24th edition, W.B. Saunders Co., Philadelphia and London, 1965);
transient neonatal tricuspid regurgitation, and the importance of Doppler echocardiography to distinguish between severe functional neonatal tricuspid regurgitation and a structural anomaly of the tricuspid valve;[620]
thrombotic lesions of the tricuspid valve in a premature male newborn, their surgical management, and the etiology of the tricuspid thrombi not clear;[621]
a 46-year-old woman with isolated probably congenital tricuspid stenosis, treated with percutaneous tricuspid balloon valvotomy;[622]
pacemaker-lead puncture of the posterior tricuspid leaflet, accurate diagnosis and successful surgical repair;[623]
the first report in the tricuspid valve position of strut fracture of a Björk-Shiley valve with embolization of the occluder disc in a 39-year-old woman;[624]
diagnosis and surgical management of tricuspid annular stenosis in complex cardiac anomalies; recommendation: if the

tricuspid annulus is less than 70% of normal, do a Glenn or a bidirectional cavopulmonary shunt;[625]
windsock diverticulum of the tricuspid valve producing right ventricular outflow tract obstruction;[626]
deficient anterior leaflet of the tricuspid valve, resembling a cleft, resulting in severe tricuspid regurgitation in adults;[627]
surgical repair of dilated congenital tricuspid regurgitation that does not have downward displacement of the septal leaflet; technique:
1. gathering suture of anterior leaflet;
2. artificial chordal implantation; and
3. ring annuloplasty;[628]

repair of congenital tricuspid valve abnormalities with artificial chordae tendineae;[629]
the de Vega tricuspid annuloplasty for tricuspid regurgitation in children—provides excellent, safe relief;[630] and
tethered tricuspid valve, a cause of severe tricuspid regurgitation.[631]

Can Pectus Excavatum Cause Tricuspid Compression?

The answer is: usually it does not,[632-634] but occasionally it can.[635,636] Womble and colleagues[635] report the case of a 15-year-old girl with pectus excavatum. At age 9 years she was found to have supraventricular tachycardia and a mild pectus excavatum deformity. Echocardiography showed mild mitral valve prolapse with mild mitral valve insufficiency, patent foramen ovale, and moderate tricuspid valve stenosis. By age 15 years, she had a more pronounced pectus excavatum deformity. During her competitive dance activities, she noted shortness of breath with long routines. Repeat echocardiography revealed right atrial and left atrial enlargement consistent with restrictive cardiac physiology. Right ventricular pressures were estimated to be 70% to 80% of systemic pressure, consistent with moderate to severe pulmonary hypertension. Significant compression of the tricuspid annulus was observed. Moderate tricuspid stenosis was found, the peak tricuspid inflow pressure gradient being 8 mm Hg, with a right ventricular–to–right atrial pressure gradient of 71 mm Hg. Mitral valve prolapse was also present.

The patient underwent an open modified Ravich pectus excavatum repair without complication. Three months postoperatively, her mild symptoms had resolved. Echocardiography showed that the tricuspid annulus size had increased, now with only mild tricuspid stenosis: the peak tricuspid inflow pressure gradient postoperatively was 3.5 mm Hg (compared with 8 mm Hg preoperatively, a 56% reduction). The right ventricular–to–right atrial pressure gradient postoperatively was 29 mm Hg (compared with 71 mm Hg preoperatively, a 59% reduction). The estimated right ventricular pressure postoperatively was 35% of systemic (compared with 70% to 80% systemic preoperatively, a 53% reduction). Thus, right ventricular and pulmonary artery pressures fell to within the normal range. Right and left atrial enlargement was reduced postoperatively (from moderate preoperatively to mild postoperatively). Mitral valve prolapse was also reduced (from mild to moderate preoperatively to mild postoperatively).

Although most patients with pectus excavatum are asymptomatic, cardiovascular compression[635,636] by the dorsally malpositioned sternum and rib cage have been associated with early fatiguability and with a restrictive pulmonary pattern in exercise pulmonary function tests. A well-known association with mitral valve prolapse, namely right heart compression, can include tricuspid stenosis and the compressed innominate vein syndrome. Postoperative studies in pectus excavatum patients have shown improvement in maximum voluntary ventilation, maximum oxygen utilization, total lung capacity, and total exercise time.[635,636]

Thus, in addition to its psychosocial benefits—particularly during adolescence—open pectus excavatum repair can also have beneficial results by reducing cardiopulmonary compression.

CHAPTER SUMMARY

Because this has been a lengthy exploration, frequently of unfamiliar territory, and because an attempt has been made to present the various tricuspid anomalies in clinical and surgical context, an attempt will now be made to summarize the main anatomic and physiologic points very briefly. Table numbers will be included to help the reader find relevant details.

1. Twelve different anatomic types of TV malformation, Table 13.1, n = 359 of 3216 cases of congenital heart disease (11.16%).
2. Ebstein's anomaly, in 4 different anatomic settings, Table 13.2, n = 78 (2.43%).
3. Ebstein's anomaly with tricuspid regurgitation: associated findings, Table 13.3, n = 25 (0.78%).
4. Ebstein's anomaly with tricuspid stenosis: associated findings, Table 13.4, n = 11 (0.34%).
5. Ebstein's anomaly with tricuspid atresia (imperforate TV), n = 2 (0.06%).
6. Ebstein's anomaly with tricuspid regurgitation, associated with pulmonary atresia or severe stenosis and intact ventricular septum, Table 13.5, n = 12 (0.37%).
7. Ebstein's anomaly with tricuspid stenosis, associated with pulmonary atresia and intact ventricular septum, n = 2 (0.06%).
8. Left-sided Ebstein's anomaly: associated findings, Table 13.6, n = 14 (0.44%).
9. Ebstein's anomaly with incomplete form of common atrioventricular canal and tricuspid atresia or severe stenosis: associated findings, Table 13.7, n = 6 (0.19%).
10. Ebstein's anomaly with incomplete form of common atrioventricular canal and tricuspid regurgitation: associated findings, Table 13.8, n = 3 (0.09%).
11. Tricuspid valve function in 78 cases of Ebstein's anomaly: Table 13.9.
12. Ebstein's anomaly: literature review.[1-216]
13. Congenital tricuspid regurgitation (non-Ebstein's): associated findings, Table 13.10, n = 80 (2.49%), 16 different anatomic subsets.
14. Tricuspid atresia (non-Ebstein): associated findings, Table 13.11, n = 94 (2.92%), 11 different anatomic types.

15. Tricuspid atresia with D-loop transposition of the great arteries: associated findings, Table 13.12, $n = 18$ (0.56%).
16. Left-sided tricuspid atresia with TGA {S,L,L}: associated findings, Table 13.13, $n = 11$ (0.34%).
17. Tricuspid atresia {S,D,S} without pulmonary outflow tract obstruction: associated findings, Table 13.14, $n = 6$ (0.19%).
18. Tricuspid atresia {S,D,S} with pulmonary outflow tract atresia: associated findings, Table 13.15, $n = 5$ (0.16%).
19. Tricuspid atresia with truncus arteriosus {S,D,S}: associated findings, Table 13.16, $n = 3$ (0.09%).
20. Tricuspid atresia with double-outlet right ventricle {S,D,D}: $n = 2$ (0.06% of 3216 cases of congenital heart disease).
21. Tricuspid atresia with anatomically corrected malposition of the great arteries {S,D,L}: $n = 2$ (0.06%).
22. Features of the left-sided juxtaposition of the atrial appendages syndrome that is associated with tricuspid atresia: findings in 42 cases and statistical comparison with 100 cases that did not have juxtaposition of the atrial appendages, Table 13.17.[242]
23. Tricuspid atresia with double-outlet left ventricle {S,D,L}: $n = 1$ (0.03%).
24. Left-sided tricuspid atresia in a patient with visceral heterotaxy and polysplenia {A(I),L,S}: $n = 1$ (0.03%).
25. Tricuspid atresia in a functionally acardiac thoracopagus conjoined twin, segmental anatomy {S,D,S}, all cardiac valves atretic: $n = 1$ (0.03%).
26. Tricuspid atresia literature review.[234-243,245,248-525]
27. Main causes of death following the modified Fontan procedure: Table 13.18, $n = 33$.[513]
28. Normal morphometry: Table 13.19, $n = 66$.[513]
29. Fontan morphometry: Table 13.20.[513]
30. Normal and Fontan morphometry indexed to body surface area; Table 13.21.[513]
31. Ventricular free wall thickness, normal hearts and Fontan hearts (systemic ventricle): Table 13.22.[513]
32. The evolution (phylogeny) and embryology (ontogeny) of the morphologically right ventricle and tricuspid valve.[525]
33. The discoverers of evolution were the Syrians, followed by Anaximander (611–547 BC), and Empedocles (495–435 BC). Darwin[526] and Wallace rediscovered evolution by natural selection (joint presentation, 1858).
34. Haeckel (1834–1919) discovered that phylogeny (evolution) recapitulates ontogeny (embryology). Haeckel founded modern morphology and coined the terms "phylogeny," "ontogeny," and "ecology."
35. From the phylogenetic standpoint, in tricuspid atresia approximately 180 million years of vertebrate evolution have been partially erased.
36. From the ontogenetic viewpoint, tricuspid atresia closely resembles Streeter's horizon 11 (22–24 days of age in utero).
37. The development of the right ventricle, tricuspid valve, and infundibulum (conus) are of great importance in congenital heart disease. Examples include tricuspid atresia; single left ventricle (absence of the right ventricular sinus) with double-inlet or common-inlet left ventricle; Ebstein's anomaly; congenitally unguarded tricuspid orifice; Uhl's disease; hypoplasia of the right ventricular sinus with congenital tricuspid stenosis, or straddling tricuspid valve, or superoinferior ventricles, or crisscross atrioventricular relations; double-chambered right ventricle (anomalous muscle bundles of the right ventricle); tetralogy of Fallot; truncus arteriosus, transposition of the great arteries; double-outlet right ventricle; double-outlet left ventricle; and anatomically corrected malposition of the great arteries.
38. Congenital tricuspid stenosis: Table 13.23, anatomic types, $n = 70$ (2.18%).
39. Congenital tricuspid stenosis with pulmonary valvar atresia or severe stenosis and intact ventricular septum: associated findings, Table 13.24, $n = 31$ (0.96%).
40. Congenital tricuspid stenosis with small right ventricle, but without pulmonary valvar atresia or severe stenosis, and without intact ventricular septum: associated findings, Table 13.25, $n = 17$ (0.53% of total series of congenital heart disease, $n = 3216$).
41. Congenital tricuspid stenosis with absent right ventricular sinus, single left ventricle, and double-inlet left ventricle: Table 13.23, n = 11 (0.34%). Segmental anatomy: TGA {S,L,L} in 6, {S,D,S} in 3, and TGA {S,D,D} in 2.
42. Congenital tricuspid stenosis with Ebstein's anomaly: Table 13.23, $n = 10$ (0.31%).
43. Congenital tricuspid stenosis caused by rhabdomyoma of the ventricular septum: Table 13.23, $n = 1$ (0.03%).
44. Congenital tricuspid stenosis: four causative mechanisms, Table 13.26.
45. Congenitally unguarded tricuspid orifice: $n = 2$ (0.06%).
46. The tricuspid and right ventricular dysplasia syndrome:[545] the findings of Ebstein's anomaly, Uhl's disease, and congenitally unguarded tricuspid orifice often merge into one another because these three entities are parts of the larger tricuspid and right ventricular dysplasia syndrome; hence the observed overlap of anatomic findings.
47. Hypoplastic tricuspid valve: $n = 6$ (0.19%).
48. Myxomatous tricuspid valve: $n = 8$ (0.25%).
49. Tricuspid valve prolapse: $n = 4$ (0.12% of the wide series of congenital and acquired heart disease, $n = 3400$, because TV prolapse can have an important acquired component to its pathogenesis, that is, not definitely only congenital).
50. Muscular tricuspid valve, that is, incompletely demuscularized tricuspid valve: $n = 1$ (0.03% of 3216 cases of congenital heart disease).
51. Multiple-orifice tricuspid valve: double-orifice tricuspid valve, Table 13.27, $n = 12$ (0.37%); triple-orifice tricuspid valve, $n = 3$ (0.09%); and multiply fenestrated (filigree) tricuspid valve, $n = 1$ (0.03%).
52. Straddling tricuspid valve: the morphometry of ventriculoatrial malalignment (Tables 13.28 and 13.29).[219]
53. Additional literature concerning the normal and abnormal tricuspid valve.[581-631]
54. The importance of ventriculoatrial septal geometry to diagnostic understanding of complex anomalies of the tricuspid and mitral valves has been illustrated in Fig. 13.58, Fig. 13.59E, and Fig. 13.63.

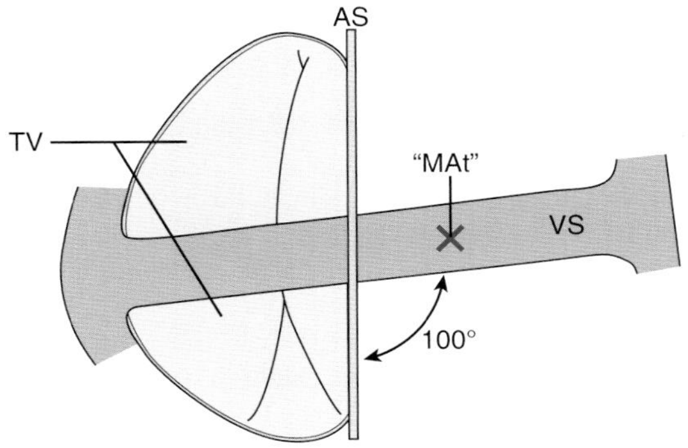

{S,D,S}. "MAt", Large LV, Small RV
(C72-147)

Fig. 13.63 The importance of ventriculoatrial septal geometry to the understanding of anomalies of the atrioventricular valves. Short-axis view from the ventricular apex of the atrial septum *(AS)*, which is normally located, and the ventricular septum *(VS)*, which is very abnormally located. This patient, a 2½-month-old boy, had normal segmental anatomy, i.e., {S,D,S}, with mitral atresia *("MAt")*, a normally formed and hence obstructive atrial septum with a patent foramen ovale bulging into the right atrium, a large left ventricle, and an infundibular outlet chamber with a small right ventricular sinus. The VS, instead of being normally vertical (as the atrial septum is), is approximately horizontal. The ventriculoatrial septal angle, measured inferiorly, is 100° (normal = 5° to 7°). The ventricular septum is located directly beneath the expected site of the mitral orifice. The malposition of the VS appears to be responsible for the presence of mitral atresia. We put quotation marks around "MAt" in an effort to suggest that this case of MAt appears to have had little or nothing to do with the mitral valve itself. This MAt (or left atrial outlet atresia) appears to be secondary to the malposition of the VS that blocks the mitral orifice from below. This secondary MAt may also help to explain why the left ventricle (below the plane of the VS) was large. Malposition of the VS also appears to explain why the tricuspid valve *(TV)* straddles the VS through a ventricular septal defect of the AV canal type. The malpositioned VS runs directly beneath the large TV; hence the TV straddles the VS, opening both into the small right ventricle above the plane of the VS and into the large left ventricle *(LV)* below the plane of the VS. Thus the ventriculoatrial septal geometry anatomically explains both the "MAt" and the straddling TV. This case was very nearly a Holmes heart,[221] i.e., single left ventricle with infundibular outlet chamber and normally related great arteries {S,D,S}. However, all observers thought that a very small right ventricular sinus was also present. Thus, *anatomically* this was not quite a single LV, but *physiologically* it was. This is the anomaly that Dr. Manuel Quero of Madrid reported[220] in 1972: single left ventricle with mitral atresia, i.e., mitral atresia but with a *large* LV and an infundibular outlet chamber. In Quero's anomaly,[220] many questions of interpretation remain incompletely understood: Is this really mitral atresia? Can one really have mitral atresia with a *large* left ventricle? Should we be making the diagnosis of left atrial outlet atresia (rather than mitral atresia)? Or absent left atrioventricular connection? Is what we are calling the straddling tricuspid valve really the TV? Or is it a common AV canal (without an ostium primum defect)? Here, we have used conventional terminology for comprehensibility, as Quero did.[220] No matter what interpretation (and hence terminology) are ultimately shown to be correct, the abnormal cardiac geometry appears to be the primary anatomic diagnosis—with "mitral atresia" and straddling "tricuspid valve" being secondary diagnoses, i.e., sequelae of ventricular malalignment relative to the atria and the atrioventricular valves. Thus **cardiac geometry** is diagnostically important. (This consultation was sent to us in 1972 by Dr. Marian E Molthan, Phoenix, Arizona.)

REFERENCES

1. Freedom RM, Mawson JB, Yoo S-J, Benson LN. *Congenital Heart Disease, Textbook of Angiocardiography*. Armonk, NY: Futura Publishing Company, Inc; 1997:349.
2. Ebstein W. Ueber einen sehr seltenen fall von insufficienz der valvula tricuspidalis, bedingt durch eine angeborene hochgradige Missbildung derselben. *Arch Anat Physiol Wiss Med.* 1866;238.
3. Sebastian A. *A Dictionary of the History of Medicine*. New York: The Parthenon Publishing Group; 1999:270.
4. Schiebler GL, Gravenstein JS, Van Mierop LHS. Ebstein's anomaly of the tricuspid valve. Translation of original description with comments. *Am J Cardiol.* 1968;22:867.
5. Mann RJ, Lie JT. The life story of Wilhelm Ebstein (1836-1912) and his almost overlooked description of a congenital heart disease. *Mayo Clin Proc.* 1979;54:197.
6. Shampo MA. Wilhelm Ebstein, internist, pathologist, and medical historian. *Prog Pediatr Cardiol.* 1993;2:1.
7. Feldt RH. Ebstein's anomaly, a historical overview. *Prog Pediatric Cardiol.* 1993;2:2.
8. Edwards WD. Embryology and pathologic features of Ebstein's anomaly. *Prog Pediatr Cardiol.* 1993;2:5.
9. Van Mierop LHS, Kutsche LM, Victorica BE. Ebstein anomaly. In: Adams FH, Emmanouilides GC, Riemenschneider TA, eds. *Moss' Heart Disease in Infants, Children, and Adolescents.* 4th ed. Baltimore: Williams and Wilkins; 1989:361.
10. Uhl HSM. A previously undescribed congenital malformation of the heart: almost total absence of the myocardium of the right ventricle. *Bull Johns Hopkins Hosp.* 1952;91:197.
11. Robb JS. *Comparative Basic Cardiology*. New York: Grune & Stratton; 1965.
12. Keane JF, Fyler DC. Tricuspid valve problems. In: Keane JF, Lock JE, FylerDC, eds. *Nadas' Pediatric Cardiology*. 2nd ed. Philadelphia; 2006:761.
13. Kumar AE, Fyler DC, Miettinen OS, Nadas AS. Ebstein's anomaly: clinical profile and natural history. *Am J Cardiol.* 1971;28:84.
14. Jaiswal PK, Balakrishan KG, Saha A, Venkitachalam CG, Tharakan J, Titus T. Clinical profile and natural history of Ebstein's anomaly of tricuspid valve. *Internat J Cardiol.* 1994;46:113.
15. Reich JD, Auld D, Hulse E, Sullivan K, Campbell R. The pediatric radiofrequency ablation registry's experience with Ebstein's anomaly. Pediatric Electrophysiology Society. *J Cardiovasc Electrophysiol.* 1998;9:1370.
16. Baño-Rodrigo A, Van Praagh S, Trowitzsch E, Van Praagh R. Double-orifice mitral valve: a study of 27 postmortem cases with developmental, diagnostic, and surgical considerations. *Am J Cardiol.* 1988;61:152.
17. Fontan F, Mounicot F-B, Baudet E, Simonneau J, Gordo J, Gouffrant J-M. "Correction" de l'atresie tricuspidienne. Rapport de deux cas "corrigés" par l'utilisation d'une technique chirurgicale nouvelle. *Ann Chir Thorac Cardio-Vasc.* 1971;10:39.
18. Fontan F, Baudet E. Surgical repair of tricuspid atresia. *Thorax.* 1971;26:240.
19. Kauffman SL, Andersen DH. Persistent venous valves, maldevelopment of the right heart, and coronary artery-ventricular communications. *Am Heart J.* 1963;66:664.
20. Kumar AE, Gilbert C, Aerichidé N, Van Praagh R. Ebstein's anomaly, Uhl's disease, and absence of tricuspid leaflets: a new spectrum. *Am J Cardiol.* 1970;25:111.

21. Van Praagh R, Van Praagh S. Atrial isomerism in the heterotaxy syndromes with asplenia, or polysplenia, or normally formed spleen: an erroneous concept. *Am J Cardiol.* 1990;66:1504.
22. Van Praagh S. Cardiac malpositions and the heterotaxy syndromes. In: Keane JF, Lock JE, Fyler DC, eds. *Nadas' Pediatric Cardiology.* Philadelphia; 2006:675.
23. Ticho BS, Goldstein AM, Van Praagh R. Extracardiac anomalies in the heterotaxy syndromes with focus on anomalies of midline-associated structures. *Am J Cardiol.* 2000;85:729.
24. Kilby RA, DuShane JW, Wood EH, Burchell HB. Ebstein's malformation: a clinical and laboratory study. *Medicine.* 1956;35:161.
25. Becu LM, Swan HJC, DuShane JW, Edwards JE. Ebstein malformation of the left atrioventricular valve in corrected transposition of the great vessels with ventricular septal defect. *Proc Staff Meet Mayo Clin.* 1955;30:483.
26. Hunter SW, Lillehei CW. Ebstein's malformation of the tricuspid valve: study of a case, together with suggestion of a new form of surgical therapy. *Dis Chest.* 1958;33:297.
27. Hardy KL, May IA, Webster CA, Kimball KG. Ebstein's anomaly: a functional concept and successful definitive repair. *J Thorac Cardiovasc Surg.* 1964;48:927.
28. De Leon AC, Perloff JK, Blanco P. Congenital pulmonic stenosis complicating Ebstein's anomaly of the tricuspid valve. *Am J Cardiol.* 1964;14:695.
29. Kalke BR, Carlson RG, Lillehei CW. Evolution of surgery for complete correction of Ebstein's anomaly. *Circulation.* 1966;34:suppl 3–138.
30. Makous N, Vander Veer JB. Ebstein's anomaly and life expectancy, report of a survival to over age 79. *Am J Cardiol.* 1966;18:100.
31. Gueron M, Hirsch M, Stern J, Cohen W, Levy MJ. Familial Ebstein's anomaly with emphasis on the surgical treatment. *Am J Cardiol.* 1966;18:105.
32. Watson H. Electrode catheters and the diagnosis of Ebstein's anomaly of the tricuspid valve. *Br Heart J.* 1966;28:161.
33. Moller JH, Lynch RP, Edwards JE. Fetal cardiac failure resulting from congenital anomalies of the heart. *J Pediatr.* 1966;68:699.
34. Lillehei CW, Kalke BR, Carlson RG. Evolution of corrective surgery for Ebstein's anomaly. *Circulation.* 1967;35(suppl 1):111.
35. Genton E, Blount SG. The spectrum of Ebstein's anomaly. *Am Heart J.* 1967;73:395.
36. Watson H, Emslie-Smith D, Lowe KG. The intracardiac electrocardiogram of human atrioventricular conducting tissue. *Am Heart J.* 1967;74:66.
37. Rebolledo JR. Ebstein's anomaly with right aortic arch. Review of the cardiovascular defects associated with Ebstein's malformation of the tricuspid valve. *J Pediat.* 1967;71:66.
38. Elliott LP, Hartmann AF. The right ventricular infundibulum in Ebstein's anomaly of the tricuspid valve. *Radiology.* 1967;89:694.
39. Pérez-Alvarez JJ, Pérez-Treviño C, Gaxiola A, Reta-Villalobos A. Ebstein's anomaly with pulmonic stenosis. Implantation of a tricuspid valvular prosthesis. *Am J Cardiol.* 1967;20:411.
40. Newfeld EA, Cole RB, Paul MH. Ebstein's malformation of the tricuspid valve in the neonate. Functional and anatomic pulmonary outflow tract obstruction. *Am J Cardiol.* 1967;19:727.
41. Donegan CC, Moore M, Wiley TM, Hernandez FA, Green JR, Schiebler GL. Familial Ebstein's anomaly of the tricuspid valve. *Am Heart J.* 1968;75:375.
42. Macruz R, Tranchesi J, Ebaid M, Pileggi F, Romero A, Décourt LV. Ebstein's disease, electrovectorcardiographic and radiologic correlations. *Am J Cardiol.* 1968;21:653.
43. Lowe KG, Emslie-Smith D, Robertson PGC, Watson H. Scalar, vector, and intracardiac electrocardiograms in Ebstein's anomaly. *Br Heart J.* 1968;30:617.
44. Pocock WA, Tucker RBK, Barlow JB. Mild Ebstein's anomaly. *Br Heart J.* 1969;31:327.
45. Hardy KL, Roe BB. Ebstein's anomaly, further experience with definitive repair. *J Thorac Cardiovasc Surg.* 1969;58:553.
46. Littler WA. Successful pregnancy in a patient with Ebstein's anomaly. *Br Heart J.* 1970;32:711.
47. Lev M, Liberthson RR, Joseph RH, et al. The pathologic anatomy of Ebstein's disease. *Arch Patch.* 1970;90:334.
48. Saigusa M, Mizuno A, Ukishima H, Hasegawa T, Kobayashi H. Tricuspid valve replacement with a preserved aortic valve homograft for Ebstein's malformation, a case report. *J Thorac Cardiovasc Surg.* 1971;62:55.
49. Lev M, Gibson S, Miller RA. Ebstein's disease with Wolff-Parkinson-White syndrome: report of a case with a histopathologic study of possible conduction pathways. *Am Heart J.* 1955;49:724.
50. Watson H. Natural history of Ebstein's anomaly of the tricuspid valve in childhood and adolescence. *Br Heart J.* 1971;33:143.
51. Simcha A, Bonham-Carter RE. Ebstein's anomaly, clinical study of 32 patients in childhood. *Br Heart J.* 1971;33:46.
52. Fontana ME, Wooley CF. Sail sound in Ebstein's anomaly of the tricuspid valve. *Circulation.* 1972;46:155.
53. Follath F, Hallidie-Smith KA. Unusual electrocardiographic changes in Ebstein's anomaly. *Br Heart J.* 1972;34:513.
54. Bialostozsky D, Horowitz S, Espino-Vela J. Ebstein's malformation of the tricuspid valve, a review of 65 cases. *Am J Cardiol.* 1972;29:826.
55. Bialostozsky D, Medrano GA, Munoz L, Contreras R. Vectorcardiographic study and anatomic observations in 21 cases of Ebstein's malformation of the tricuspid valve. *Am J Cardiol.* 1972;30:354.
56. Crews TL, Pridie RB, Benham R, Leatham A. Auscultatory and phonocardiogrpahic findings in Ebstein's anomaly. Correlation of first heart sound with ultrasonic records of tricuspid valve movement. *Br Heart J.* 1973;34:681.
57. Balkoura-Christopoulos MH, Kittle CF. Post superior vena cava—right pulmonary artery shunt, total surgical correction of Ebstein's anomaly with Starr-Edwards prosthesis. *Chest.* 1973;63:120.
58. Tajik AJ, Gau GT, Guiliani ER, Ritter DG, Schattenberg TT. Echocardiogram in Ebstein's anomaly with Wolff-Parkinson-White preexcitation syndrome, type B. *Circulation.* 1973;47:813.
59. From AHL, Mazzitello WF, Judd AS, Edwards JE. Ebstein's malformation of the tricuspid valve associated with valvular stenosis and cor triatriatum. *Chest.* 1973;64:248.
60. Lundström N-R. Echocardiography in the diagnosis of Ebstein's anomaly of the tricuspid valve. *Circulation.* 1973;47:597.
61. Rao PS, Jue KL, Isabel-Jones J, Ruttenberg HD. Ebstein's malformation of the tricuspid valve with atresia. Differentiation from isolated tricuspid atresia. *Am J Cardiol.* 1973;32:1004.
62. Watson H. Natural history of Ebstein's anomaly of tricuspid valve in childhood and adolescence. An international cooperative study of 505 cases. *Br Heart J.* 1974;36:417.
63. Sekelj P, Beufey BG. Historical landmarks: Ebstein's anomaly of the tricuspid valve. *Am Heart J.* 1974;88:108.
64. Yuste P, Minguez I, Aza V, Señor J, Asin E, Martinez-Bordiu C. Echocardiography in the diagnosis of Ebstein's anomaly. *Chest.* 1974;66:273.

65. Nora JJ, Nora AH, Toews WH. Lithium, Ebstein's anomaly, and other congenital heart defects. *Lancet*. 1974;2:594.
66. Kerber RE, Marcus M, Wolfson PM. Demonstration of Ebstein's anomaly by simultaneous catheter-tip localization of the tricuspid valve and right coronary artery visualization: a new method. *Chest*. 1975;68:99.
67. Soloff LA. Ebstein's anomaly. *Am Heart J*. 1975;89:129.
68. Kastor JA, Goldreyer BN, Josephson ME, et al. Electrophysiologic characteristics of Ebstein's anomaly of the tricuspid valve. *Circulation*. 1975;52:987.
69. McFaul RC, Davis Z, Guiliani ER, Ritter DG, Danielson GK. Ebstein's malformation, surgical experience at the Mayo Clinic. *J Thorac Cardiovasc Surg*. 1976;72:910.
70. Gerlis LM, Anderson RH. Cor triatriatum dexter with imperforate Ebstein's anomaly. *Br Heart J*. 1976;38:108.
71. Emanuel R, O'Brien K, Ng R. Ebstein's anomaly, genetic study of 26 families. *Br Heart J*. 1976;38:5.
72. Senoo Y, Ohishi K, Nawa S, Teramoto S, Sumada T. Total correction of Ebstein's anomaly by replacement with a biological aortic valve without plication of the atrialized ventricle. *J Thorac Cardiovasc Surg*. 1976;72:243.
73. Jugdutt BI, Brooks CH, Sterns LP, Callaghan JC, Rossal RE. Surgical treatment of Ebstein's anomaly. *J Thorac Cardiovasc Surg*. 1977;73:114.
74. Hirschklau MJ, Sahn DJ, Hagan AD, Williams DE, Friedman WF. Cross-sectional echocardiographic features of Ebstein's anomaly of the tricuspid valve. *Am J Cardiol*. 1977;40:400.
75. Monibi AA, Neches WH, Lenox CC, Park SC, Mathews RA, Zuberbuhler JR. Left ventricular anomalies associated with Ebstein's malformation of the tricuspid valve. *Circulation*. 1978;57:303.
76. Takayasu S, Obunai Y, Konno S. Clinical classification of Ebstein's anomaly. *Am Heart J*. 1978;95:154.
77. Ports TA, Silverman NH, Schiller NB. Two-dimensional echocardiographic assessment of Ebstein's anomaly. *Circulation*. 1978;58:336.
78. Anderson KR, Danielson GK, McGoon DC, Lie JT. Ebstein's anomaly of the left-sided tricuspid valve. Pathologic anatomy of the valvular malformation. *Circulation*. 1978;58(suppl I):87.
79. Anderson KR, Lie JT. Pathologic anatomy of Ebstein's anomaly of the heart revisited. *Am J Cardiol*. 1978;41:739.
80. Price JE, Amsterdam EA, Vera Z, Swenson R, Mason DT. Ebstein's disease associated with complete atrioventricular block. *Chest*. 1978;73:542.
81. Bove EL, Kirsh MM. Valve replacement for Ebstein's anomaly of the tricuspid valve. *J Thorac Cardiovasc Surg*. 1979;78:229.
82. Melo J, Saylam A, Knight R, Starr A. Long-term results after surgical correction of Ebstein's anomaly, report of two cases. *J Thorac Cardiovasc Surg*. 1979;78:233.
83. Seward JW, Tajik AJ, Feist DJ, Smith HC. Ebstein's anomaly in an 85-year-old man. *May Clin Proc*. 1979;54:193.
84. Danielson GK, Maloney JD, Devloo RAE. Surgical repair of Ebstein's anomaly. *Mayo Clin Proc*. 1979;54:185.
85. Anderson KR, Lie JT. The right ventricular myocardium in Ebstein's anomaly, a morphometric histopathologic study. *Mayo Clin Proc*. 1979;54:181.
86. Anderson KR, Zuberbuhler JR, Anderson RH, Becker AE, Lie JT. Morphologic spectrum of Ebstein's anomaly of the heart, a review. *Mayo Clin Proc*. 1979;54:174.
87. Giuliani ER, Fuster V, Brandenberg RO, Mair DD. Ebstein's anomaly, the clinical features and natural history of Ebstein's anomaly of the tricuspid valve. *Mayo Clin Proc*. 1979;54:163.
88. Zuberbuhler JR, Allwork SP, Anderson RH. The spectrum of Ebstein's anomaly of the tricuspid valve. *J Thorac Cardiovasc Surg*. 1979;77:202.
89. Barbero-Marcial M, Verginelli G, Awad M, Ferreira S, Ebaid M, Zerbini EJ. Surgical treatment of Ebstein's anomaly. Early and late results in twenty patients subjected to valve replacement. *J Thorac Cardiovasc Surg*. 1979;78:416.
90. Otero Coto E, Quero Jimenez M, Deveral PB, Camanas A. Morphological findings in Ebstein's anomaly. *Jap Heart J*. 1979;20:43.
91. Koiwaya Y, Narabayashi H, Koyanagi S, et al. Early closure of the tricuspid valve in a case of Ebstein's anomaly with type B Wolff-Parkinson-White syndrome. *Circulation*. 1979;60:446.
92. Marcelletti C, Düren DR, Schuilenburg RM, Becker AE. Fontan's operation for Ebstein's anomaly. *J Thorac Cardiovasc Surg*. 1980;79:63.
93. Gussenhoven WJ, Spitaels SEC, Bom N, Becker AE. Echocardiographic criteria for Ebstein's anomaly of tricuspid valve. *Br Heart J*. 1980;43:31.
94. Otero-Coto E, Perez-Martinez V, Palacios V, Caffarena JM. Ebstein's anomaly of the left-sided atrioventricular (AV) valve in AV discordance. *Thorac Cardiovasc Surgeon*. 1980;28:364.
95. Shigenobu M, Mendez MA, Zubiate P, Kay J. Thirteen years' experience with the Kay-Shiley disc valve for tricuspid replacement in Ebstein's anomaly. *Ann Thorac Surg*. 1980;29:423.
96. Daniel W, Rathsack P, Walpurger G, et al. Value of M-mode echocardiography for non-invasive diagnosis of Ebstein's anomaly. *Br Heart J*. 1980;43:38.
97. Schmidt-Habelmann P, Meisner H, Struck E, Sebening F. Results of valvuloplasty for Ebstein's anomaly. *Thorac Cardiovasc Surgeon*. 1981;29:155.
98. Caralps JM, Aris A, Bonnin JO, Solanes H, Torner M. Ebstein's anomaly: surgical treatment with tricuspid replacement without right ventricular plication. *Ann Thorac Surg*. 1981;31:277.
99. Charles RG, Barnard CN, Beck W. Tricuspid valve replacement for Ebstein's anomaly, a 19 year review of the first case. *Br Heart J*. 1981;46:578.
100. Cabin HS, Wood TP, Smith JO, Roberts WC. Ebstein's anomaly in the elderly. *Chest*. 1981;80:212.
101. Cabin HS, Roberts WC. Ebstein's anomaly of the tricuspid valve and prolapse of the mitral valve. *Am Hear J*. 1981;101:177.
102. Castaneda-Zuniga W, Nath HP, Moller JH, Edwards JW. Left-sided anomalies in Ebstein's malformation of the tricuspid valve. *Pediatr Cardiol*. 1982;3:181.
103. Smith WM, Gallagher JJ, Kerr CR, et al. The electrophysiologic basis and management of symptomatic recurrent tachycardia in patients with Ebstein's anomaly of the tricuspid valve. *Am J Cardiol*. 1982;49:1223.
104. Westaby S, Karp RB, Kirklin JW, Waldo AL, Blackstone EH. Surgical treatment in Ebstein's malformation. *Ann Thorac Surg*. 1982;34:388.
105. Danielson GK. Ebstein's anomaly: editorial comments and personal observations. *Ann Thorac Surg*. 1982;34:396.
106. Danielson GK, Fuster V. Surgical repair of Ebstein's anomaly. *Ann Surg*. 1982;196:499.
107. Willis PW, Craige E. First heart sound in Ebstein's anomaly: observations on the cause of wide splitting by echophonocardiographic studies before and after operative repair. *J Am Coll Cardiol*. 1983;2:1165.
108. Sugrue D, Dickie S, McKenna WJ, et al. The sequence of right heart contraction in Ebstein's anomaly: non invasive assessment by phase analysis of krypton-81M radionuclide angiography. *Circulation*. 1983;68:suppl III–13.

109. Abe T, Komatsu S. Valve replacement for Ebstein's anomaly of the tricuspid valve, early and long-term results of eight cases. *Chest.* 1983;84:414.
110. Silver MA, Cohen SR, McIntosh CL, Cannon RO, Roberts WC. Late (5 to 132 months) clinical and hemodynamic results after either tricuspid valve replacement or annuloplasty for Ebstein's anomaly of the tricuspid valve. *Am J Cardiol.* 1984;54:627.
111. Zuberbuhler JR, Becker AE, Anderson RH, Lenox CC. Ebstein's malformation and the embryological development of the tricuspid valve, with a note on the nature of "clefts" in the atrioventricular valves. *Pediatr Cardiol.* 1984;5:289.
112. Shiina A, Seward JB, Edwards WD, Hagler DJ, Tajik AJ. Two-dimensional echocardiographic spectrum of Ebstein's anomaly: detailed anatomic assessment. *J Am Coll Cardiol.* 1984;3:356.
113. Crupi G, Villani M, Di Benedetto G, et al. Tricuspid atresia with imperforate valve: angiographic findings and surgical implications in two cases with AV concordance and normally related great arteries. *Pediatr Cardiol.* 1984;5:49.
114. Rossi L, Thiene G. Mild Ebstein's anomaly associated with supraventricular tachycardia and sudden death. Clinicomorphologic features in 3 patients. *Am J Cardiol.* 1984;53:332.
115. Gussenhoven EJ, Stewart PA, Becker AE, Essed CE, Ligtvoet KM, De Villeneuve VH. "Offsetting" of the septal tricuspid leaflet in normal hearts and in hearts with Ebstein's anomaly. Anatomic and echocardiographic correlation. *Am J Cardiol.* 1984;53:172.
116. Gussenhoven EJ, Essed CE, Bos E, de Villeneuve VH. Echocardiographic diagnosis of overriding tricuspid valve in a child with Ebstein's anomaly. *Pediatr Cardiol.* 1984;5:209.
117. Raj Behl P, Blesovsky A. Ebstein's anomaly: sixteen year's experience with valve replacement without plication of the right ventricle. *Thorax.* 1984;39:8.
118. Otero Coto E, Quero Jimenez M, Deverall PB. Rare anomalies of atrioventricular connection: hidden or supernumerary valves with imperforate right atrioventricular connection. *Internat J Cardiol.* 1984;6:149.
119. Davido A, Maarek M, Jullien JL, Corone P. Maladie d'Ebstein associée à une tétralogie de Fallot. À propos d'une observation familiale, revue de la littérature, implication embryologique et génétique. *Arch Mal Coeur.* 1985;78:752.
120. Piéard LA, Henrard L, Demouiln J-C. Persistent atrial standstill in familial Ebstein's anomaly. *Br Heart J.* 1985;53:594.
121. Barber G, Danielson GK, Heise CT, Driscoll DJ. Cardiorespiratory response to exercise in Ebstein's anomaly. *Am J Cardiol.* 1985;56:509.
122. Radford DJ, Graff RF, Neilson GH. Diagnosis and natural history of Ebstein's anomaly. *Br Heart J.* 1985;54:517.
123. Oh JK, Holmes DR, Hayes DL, Porter C-BJ, Danielson GK. Cardiac arrhythmias in patients with surgical repair of Ebstein's anomaly. *J Am Coll Cardiol.* 1985;6:1351.
124. Nihoyannopoulos P, McKenna WJ, Smith G, Foale R. Echocardiographic assessment of the right ventricle in Ebstein's anomaly: relation to clinical outcome. *J Am Coll Cardiol.* 1986;8:627.
125. Driscoll DJ, Mottram CD, Danielson GK. Spectrum of exercise intolerance in 45 patients with Ebstein's anomaly and observations on exercise tolerance in 11 patients after surgical repair. *J Am Coll Cardiol.* 1988;11:831.
126. Leung MP, Baker EJ, Anderson RH, Zuberbuhler JR. Cineangiographic spectrum of Ebstein's malformation: its relevance to clinical presentation and outcome. *J Am Coll Cardiol.* 1988;11:154.
127. Knight WB, Shinebourne EA. Imperforate tricuspid valve with single cardiac outlet from right ventricle. *Br Heart J.* 1988;60:259.
128. DiLello F, Flemma RJ, Mullen DC, Kleinman LH, Werner PH. Tricuspid valve replacement for Ebstein's anomaly in childhood with a Starr-Edwards caged-ball prosthesis, 21-year follow-up. *Chest.* 1988;94:1096.
129. Carpentier A, Chauvaud S, Macé L, et al. A new reconstructive operation for Ebstein's anomaly of the tricuspid valve. *J Thorac Cardiovasc Surg.* 1988;96:92.
130. Lott M, Lin F-Y, Jong Y-S, Tseng Y-Z, Wu T-L. Ebstein's anomaly with ventricular tachycardia: evidence for the arrhythmogenic role of the atrialized ventricle. *Am Heart J.* 1989;117:959.
131. Marino JP, Mihaileanu S, El Asmar B, et al. Echocardiography and color-flow mapping evaluation of a new reconstructive surgical technique for Ebstein's anomaly. *Circulation.* 1989;80(suppl I-197).
132. Roberson DA, Silverman NH. Ebstein's anomaly: echocardiographic and clinical features in the fetus and neonate. *J Am Coll Cardiol.* 1989;14:1300.
133. Kirklin JK. Christian Barnard's contribution to the surgical treatment of Ebstein's malformation. *Ann Thorac Surg.* 1991;51:147.
134. Saxena A, Fong LV, Tristam M, Ackery DM, Keeton BR. Late noninvasive evaluation of cardiac performance in mildly symptomatic older patients with Ebstein's anomaly of tricuspid valve: role of radionuclide imaging. *J Am Coll Cardiol.* 1991;17:182.
135. Hornberger LK, Sahn DJ, Kleinman CS, Copel JA, Reed KL. Tricuspid valve disease with significant tricuspid insufficiency in the fetus: diagnosis and outcome. *J Am Coll Cardiol.* 1991;17:167.
136. Plowden JS, Kimball TR, Bensky A, et al. The use of extracorporeal membrane oxygenation in critically ill neonates with Ebstein's anomaly. *Am Heart J.* 1991;121:619.
137. Sharlan GK, Chita SK, Allan LD. Tricuspid valve dysplasia or displacement in intrauterine life. *J Am Coll Cardiol.* 1991;17:944.
138. Rheuban KS, Carpenter MA, Everett AD, Gutgesell HP. Successful balloon pulmonary valvuloplasty in a neonate with Ebstein's anomaly and critical pulmonic stenosis. *Am Heart J.* 1991;121:1565.
139. Bennett MR, Shiu MF. Ebstein's anomaly associated with splenomegaly and reversible hypersplenism. *Br Heart J.* 1991;65:223.
140. Lang D, Oberhoffer R, Cook A, et al. Pathologic spectrum of malformations of the tricuspid valve in prenatal and neonatal life. *J Am Coll Cardiol.* 1991;17:1161.
141. Balaji S, Dennis NR, Keeton BR. Familial Ebstein's anomaly: a report of six cases in two generations associated with mild skeletal abnormalities. *Br Heart J.* 1991;66:26.
142. Starnes VA, Pitlick PT, Bernstein D, Griffin ML, Choy M, Shumway NE. Ebstein's anomaly appearing in the neonate, a new surgical approach. *J Thorac Cardiovasc Surg.* 1991;101:1082.
143. Donnelly JE, Brown JM, Radford DJ. Pregnancy outcome and Ebstein's anomaly. *Br Heart J.* 1991;66:368.
144. Quaegebeur JM, Sreeram N, Fraser AG, et al. Surgery for Ebstein's anomaly: the clinical and echocardiography evaluation of a new technique. *J Am Coll Cardiol.* 1991;17:722.
145. Pressley JC, Wharton JM, Tang ASL, Lowe JE, Gallager JJ, Prystowsky EN. Effect of Ebstein's anomaly on short- and long-term outcome of surgically treated patients with Wolff-Parkinson-White syndrome. *Circulation.* 1992;86:1147.
146. Mori K, Ando M, Satomi G, Nakazawa M, Momma K, Takao A. Imperforate tricuspid valve with dysplasia of the right ventricular myocardium, pulmonary valve, and coronary artery: a clinicopathologic study of nine cases. *Pediatr Cardiol.* 1992;13:24.

147. Gentles TL, Calder AL, Clarkson PM, Neutze JM. Predictors of long-term survival with Ebstein's anomaly of the tricuspid valve. *Am J Cardiol*. 1992;69:377.
148. Leung MP, Lee J, Lo RNS, Mok CK. Modified Fontan procedure for severe Ebstein's malformation with predominant tricuspid stenosis. *Ann Thorac Surg*. 1992;54:523.
149. Celermajer DS, Cullen S, Sullivan ID, Spiegelhalter DJ, Wyse RKH, Deanfield JE. Outcome in neonates with Ebstein's anomaly. *J Am Coll Cardiol*. 1992;19:1041.
150. Danielson GK, Driscoll DJ, Mair DD, Warnes CA, Oliver WC. Operative treatment of Ebstein's anomaly. *J Thorac Cardiovasc Surg*. 1992;104:1195.
151. Ivy D, Loehr J, Schaffer M. Prolonged prostaglandin infusion in neonates with severe Ebstein's anomaly. *Cardiol Young*. 1993;3:I–92 (abstract 300).
152. Connolly HM, Warnes CA. Ebstein's anomaly—outcome of pregnancy. *Cardiol Young*. 1993;3:I–45. abstract 133.
153. Hagler DJ, O'Leary PW, Seward JB, Tajik AJ, Danielson GK. Intraoperative transesophageal echocardiography assessment of Ebstein's anomaly. *Cardiol Young*. 1993;3:I–32. abstract 95.
154. Zabal C Attie F, Buendia A, et al. Natural history of 144 cases with Ebstein's anomaly. *Cardiol Young*. 1993;3:I–32.
155. Wenink ACG, Wisse LJ, Poelmann R, Gittenberger-de Groot A. Developmental pathology of the right ventricular inlet portion. *Cardiol Young*. 1993;3:I–31. abstract 91.
156. Lamberti A, Mihaileanu S, Chauvaud S, et al. Correlation of echocardiography (transthoracic and esophageal) with surgical anatomy in Ebstein's anomaly. *Cardiol Young*. 1993;3:I–132. abstract 459.
157. Blumenthal-Barby CC, Bartel J, Sandring KH, Luning M, Streichan F. Ebstein's anomaly—magnetic resonance imaging for noninvasive assessment with regard to surgical approach. *Cardiol Young*. 1993;3:I–131. abstract 456.
158. Hong YM, Moller JH. Ebstein's anomaly: a long-term study of survival. *Am Heart J*. 1993;125:1419.
159. Seward JB. Ebstein's anomaly: ultrasound imaging and hemodynamic evaluation. *Echocardiography*. 1993;10:641.
160. Chauvaud S, Carpentier A, Mihaileanu S, Marino J-P, Lamberti A. Conservation surgery of Ebstein's anomaly—results of valvuloplasty associated with ventriculoplasty. *Cardiol Young*. 1993;3:I–32. abstract 96.
161. Celermajer DS, Bull C, Till JA, et al. Ebstein's anomaly: presentation and outcome form fetus to adult. *J Am Coll Cardiol*. 1994;23:170.
162. Kumar N, Gallo R, Al-Halees Z, Al-Fadley F, Duran CMG. Unstented semilunar homograft replacement of tricuspid valve in Ebstein's malformation. *Ann Thorac Surg*. 1995;59:320.
163. Misaki T, Watanabe G, Iwa T, et al. Surgical treatment of patients with Wolff-Parkinson-White syndrome and associated Ebstein's anomaly. *J Thorac Cardiovasc Surg*. 1995;110:1702.
164. Chandar JS, Tamer DF, Young M-L, Moller JH. Surgical outcome in Ebstein's anomaly: (multicenter study). *Pediatrics*. 1996;98(suppl 525):s526.
165. MacClellan-Tobert SG, Driscoll DJ, Mottram CD, Mahoney DW, Wallan PC, Danielson GK. Exercise tolerance in patients with Ebstein's anomaly. *J Am Coll Cardiol*. 1997;29:1615.
166. Augustin N, Schmidt-Habelmann P, Wottke M, Meisner H, Sebening F. Results after surgical repair of Ebstein's anomaly. *Ann Thorac Surg*. 1997;63:1650.
167. Ammash NM, Warnes CA, Connolly HM, Danielson GK, Seward JB. Mimics of Ebstein's anomaly. *Am Heart J*. 1997;134:508.
168. Daliento L, Angelini A, Ho SY, et al. Angiographic and morphologic features of the left ventricle in Ebstein's malformation. *Am J Cardiol*. 1997;80:1051.
169. Marianeschi SM, McElhinney DB, Reddy VM, Silverman NH, Hanley FL. Alternative approach to the repair of Ebstein's malformation: intracardiac repair with ventricular unloading. *Ann Thorac Surg*. 1998;66:1546.
170. Augustin N, Schreiber C, Wottke M, Meisner H. Ebstein's anomaly: when should a patient have operative treatment? *Herz*. 1998;23:287.
171. Kiziltan HT, Theodoro DA, Warnes CA, O'Leary PW, Anderson BJ, Danielson GK. Late results of bioprosthetic tricuspid valve replacement in Ebstein's anomaly. *Ann Thorac Surg*. 1998;66:1539.
172. Pavlova M, Fouron J-C, Drblik SP, et al. Factors affecting the prognosis of Ebstein's anomaly during fetal life. *Am Heart J*. 1998;135:1081.
173. Vargas FJ, Mengo G, Granja MA, Gentile JA, Rannzini ME, Vazquez JC. Tricuspid annuoloplasty and ventricular plication for Ebstein's malformation. *Ann Thorac Surg*. 1998;65:1755.
174. Hetzer R, Nagdyman N, Ewert P, et al. A modified repair technique for tricuspid incompetence in Ebstein's anomaly. *J Thorac Cardiovasc Surg*. 1998;115:857.
175. Yetman AT, Freedom RM, McCrindle BW. Outcome in cyanotic neonates with Ebstein's anomaly. *Am J Cardiol*. 1998;81:749.
176. Schreiber C, Cook A, Ho SY, Augustin N, Anderson RH. Morphologic spectrum of Ebstein's malformation: revisitation relative to surgical repair. *J Thorac Cardiovasc Surg*. 1999;117:148.
177. Ho SY, Goltz D, McCarthy K, et al. The atrioventricular junctions in Ebstein malformation. *Heart*. 2000;83:444.
178. Knott-Craig CJ, Overholt ED, Ward KE, Razook JD. Neonatal repair of Ebstein's anomaly: indications, surgical technique, and medium-term follow-up. *Ann Thorac Surg*. 2000;69:1505.
179. Tanaka M, Ohata T, Fukuda K, Kigawa I, Yamashita Y, Wanibuchi Y. Tricuspid valve supra-annular implantation in adult patients with Ebstein's anomaly. *Ann Thorac Surg*. 2001;71:582.
180. Chauvaud SM, Brancaccio G, Carpentier AF. Cardiac arrhythmia in patients undergoing surgical repair of Ebstein's anomaly. *Ann Thorac Surg*. 2001;71:1547.
181. Wu Q, Huang Z. Anatomic correction of Ebstein's anomaly. *J Thorac Cardiovasc Surg*. 2001;122:1237.
182. Ahel V, Kilvain S, Rožmanić V, Taylor JFN, Vukas D. Right atrial reduction for tachyarrhythmias in Ebstein's anomaly in infancy. *Texas Heart Inst J*. 2001;28:297.
183. Sano S, Ishino K, Kawada M, et al. Total right ventricular exclusion procedure: an operation for isolated congestive right ventricular failure. *J Thorac Cardiovasc Surg*. 2002;123:640.
184. Knott-Craig CJ, Overholt ED, Ward KE, Ringewald JM, Baker SS, Razook JD. Repair of Ebstein's anomaly in the symptomatic neonate: an evolution of technique with 7-year follow-up. *Ann Thorac Surg*. 2002;73:1786.
185. Chauvaud S, Berrebi A, d'Attellis N, Mousseaux E, Hernigou A, Carpentier A. Ebstein's anomaly: repair based on functional analysis. *Eur J Cardio Thorac Surg*. 2003;23:525.
186. Wu Q, Huang Z. A new procedure for Ebstein's anomaly. *Ann Thorac Cardiovasc Surg*. 2004;77:470.

187. Inai K, Naskanish T, Mori Y, Tominatsu H, Nakazawa M. Left ventricular diastolic dysfunction in Ebstein's anomaly. *Am J Cardiol.* 2004;93:255.
188. Ullmann MV, Born S, Sebening C, Gorenflo M, Ulmer HE, Hagl S. Ventricularization of the atrialized chamber: a concept of Ebstein's anomaly repair. *Ann Thorac Surg.* 2004;78:918.
189. Hajar Albinali HA. Ebstein's anomaly in an adult. *Heart Views.* 2004;5:64.
190. Khositseth A, Danielson GK, Dearani JA, Munger TM, Porter CJ. Supraventricular tachyarrhythmias in Ebstein anomaly: management and outcome. *J Thorac Cardiovasc Surg.* 2004;128:826.
191. Tede NH, Shivkumar K, Perloff JK, et al. Signal-averaged electrocardiogram in Ebstein's anomaly. *Am J Cardiol.* 2004;93:432.
192. Chen JM, Mosca RS, Altmann K, et al. Early and medium-term results for repair of Ebstein anomaly. *J Thorac Cardiovasc Surg.* 2004;127:990.
193. Hancock Friesen CL, Chen R, Howlett JG, Ross DB. Posterior annular plication: tricuspid valve repair in Ebstein's anomaly. *Ann Thorac Surg.* 2004;77:2167.
194. Sharland G, Tingay R, Jones A, Simpson J. Atrioventricular and ventriculoarterial discordance (congenitally corrected transposition of the great arteries): echocardiographic features, associations, and outcome in 34 fetuses. *Heart.* 2005;91:1453.
195. McElhinney DB, Salvin JW, Colan SD, et al. Improving outcomes in fetuses and neonates with congenital displacement (Ebstein's malformation) or dysplasia of the tricuspid valve. *Am J Cardiol.* 2005;96:582.
196. Wald RM, Adatia I, Van Arsdell GS, Hornberger LK. Relation of limiting ductal patency to survival in neonatal Ebstein's anomaly. *Am J Cardiol.* 2005;96:851.
197. Koh M, Yagihara T, Uemura H, et al. Intermediate results of the double-switch operations for atrioventricular discordance. *Ann Thorac Surg.* 2006;81:671.
198. Boston US, Dearani JA, O'Leary PW, Driscoll DJ, Danielson GK. Tricuspid valve repair for Ebstein's anomaly in young children: a 30-year experience. *Ann Thorac Surg.* 2006;81:690.
199. Sarris GE, Giannopoulos NM, Tsoutsinos AJ, on behalf of the European Congenital Heart Surgeons Association, et al. Results of surgery for Ebstein anomaly: a multicenter study from the European congenital heart surgeons association. *J Thorac Cardiovasc Surg.* 2006;132:50.
200. Chauvaud SM, Hernigou AC, Mousseaux ER, Sidi D, Hébert J-L. Ventricular volumes in Ebstein's anomaly: x-ray multislice computed tomography before and after repair. *Ann Thorac Surg.* 2006;81:1443.
201. Reemtsen BL, Fagan BT, Wells WJ, Starnes VA. Current surgical therapy for Ebstein anomaly in neonates. *J Thorac Cardiovasc Surg.* 2006;132:1285.
202. Iturralde P, Nava S, Salica G, et al. Electrocardiographic characteristics of patients with Ebstein's anomaly before and after ablation of an accessory atrioventricular pathway. *J Cardiovasc Electrophysiol.* 2006;17:1332.
203. Ortigado Matamala A, Garcia Garcia A, Jimenez Bustos JM. Ebstein's anomaly and lithium exposure during pregnancy. *An Pediatr.* 2006;65:626.
204. Kothari S, Gupta AK, Lokhandwala YY, Vora AM, Kerkar PG, Thakur RK. Atriofascicular pathways: where to ablate? *Pacing Clin Electrophysiol.* 2006;29:1226.
205. Kanter RJ. Ebstein's anomaly of the tricuspid valve: a Wolf(f) in sheep's clothing. *J Cardiovasc Electrophysiol.* 2006;17:1337.
206. Betrian Blasco P, Galladro Agromayor E. Ebstein's anomaly and left ventricular noncompaction association. *Int J Cardiol.* 2006;23.
207. Parranon S, Abadir S, Acar P. New insight into the tricuspid valve in Ebstein anomaly using three-dimensional echocardiography. *Heart.* 2006;92:1627.
208. da Silva JP, Baumgratz JF, da Fonseca L, et al. The cone reconstruction of the tricuspid valve in Ebstein's anomaly. The operation: early and midterm results. *J Thorac Cardiovasc Surg.* 2007;133:215.
209. Cyrus C, Cyril E, Cherian KM, Kulkarni S, Nallathambi C. Down syndrome with tandem 21;21 rearrangement and Ebstein's anomaly—a case report. *Int J Cardiol.* 2007;115.
210. Lopez JA, Leachman DR. Successful use of transvenous atrial and bifocal left ventricular pacing in Ebstein's anomaly after tricuspid prosthetic valve surgery. *Ann Thorac Surg.* 2007;83:1183.
211. Macfarlane AJ, Moise S, Smith D. Caesarean section using total intravenous anesthesia in a patient with Ebstein's anomaly complicated by supraventricular tachycardia. *Int J Obstet Anesth.* 2007.
212. Bichell DP, Mora BN, Mathewson JW, Kirkpatrick SK, Tyner JJ, McLees-Palinkas T: Modified technique for the surgical treatment of severe tricuspid valve deformity in Ebstein's anomaly, *Ann Thorac Surg* , 207; 83:678.
213. Ogus NT, Indelen C, Yildirim T, Selimoglu O, Basaran M. Pericardial patch augmentation of both anterior and septal leaflets in Ebstein's anomaly. *Ann Thorac Surg.* 2007;83:676.
214. Attenhofer Jost CH, Connolly HM, Dearani JA, Edwards WD, Danielson GK. Ebstein's anomaly. *Circulation.* 2007;115:277.
215. Lai CH, Wu JM, Yang YJ. Ebstein's anomaly of the tricuspid valve in combination of tetralogy of Fallot: total correction in infancy. *Ann Thorac Surg.* 2007;83:304.
216. Kiernan TJ, Fahy G. Multiple accessory pathways, dual AV nodal physiology, non-compacted myocardium and patent foramen ovale in patient with Ebstein's anomaly: report of a case. *Int J Cardiol.* 2007;114:412.
217. Perls TT, Silver MH, Lauerman JF. *Living to 100, Lessons in Living to Your Maximum Potential at Any Age.* Basic Books; 1999.
218. Davignon AL, Greenwold WE, DuShane JW, Edwards JE. Congenital pulmonary atresia with intact ventricular septum. Clinicopathologic correlation of two anatomic types. *Am Heart J.* 1961;62:591.
219. Pessotto R, Padalino M, Rubino M, Kadoba K, Büchler JR, Van Praagh R. Straddling tricuspid valve as a sign of ventriculoatrial malalignment: a morphometric study of 19 postmortem cases. *Am Heart J.* 1999;138:1184.
220. Quero M. Coexistence of single ventricle with atresia of one atrioventricular orifice. *Circulation.* 1972;46:794.
221. Holmes WF. Case of malformation of the heart. *Trans Med-Chir Soc Edinburgh.* 1824;1:252.
222. Sano S, Kawada M, Yoshida H, et al. Norwood procedure to hypoplastic left heart syndrome. *Jpn J Thorac Cardiovasc Surg.* 1998;46:1311.
223. Norwood WI, Lang P, Hansen DD. Physiologic repair of aortic atresia—hypoplastic left heart syndrome. *N Engl J Med.* 1983;308:23.
224. Matsuoka R, Yamamoto Y, Kuroki Y, Matsui I. Phenotypic expression of the trisomic segments in partial trisomy 18. In: Van Praagh R, Takao A, eds. *Etiology and Morphogenesis of Congenital Heart Disease.* Mt Kisco, NY: Futura Publishing Co; 1980:41.

225. Geva T, Sanders SP, Diogenes M, Rockenmacher S, Van Praagh R. Two-dimensional and Doppler echocardiographic and pathologic characteristics of the infantile Marfan syndrome. *Am J Cardiol.* 1990;65:1230.
226. Pyeritz RE. The Marfan syndrome. *Ann Rev Med.* 2000;51:481.
227. Pyeritz RE. Genetics and cardiovascular disease. In: Braunwald E, Zipes DP, Libby P, eds. *Heart Disease, A Textbook of Cardiovascular Medicine.* Philadelphia: W.B. Saunders Co; 2001:1997.
228. Lee AH, Morgan JM, Callagher PJ. Arrhythmogenic right ventricular cardiomyopathy. *J Pathol.* 1993;171:157.
229. Yamabe H, Okumura K, Tsuchiya T, Yasue H. Demonstration of entrainment and presence of slow conduction during ventricular tachycardia in arrhythmogenic right ventricular dysplasia. *Pacing Clin Electrophysiol.* 1994;17:172.
230. Corrado D, Basso C, Thiene G, et al. Spectrum of clinicopathologic manifestations of arrhythmogenic right ventricular cardiomyopathy/dysplasia: a multicenter study. *J Am Coll Cardiol.* 1997;30:1512.
231. Corrado D, Basso C, Schiavon M, Thiene G. Screening for hypertrophic cardiomyopathy in young athletes. *N Engl J Med.* 1998;339:364.
232. Li D, Ahmad F, Gardner MJ, et al. The locus of a novel gene responsible for arrhythmogeneic right ventricular dysplasia characterized by early onset and high penetrance maps to chromosome 10p12-p14. *Am J Hum Genet.* 2000;66:148.
233. Goldstein JD, Rabinovitch M, Van Praagh R, Reid L. Unusual vascular anomalies causing persistent pulmonary hypertension in a newborn. *Am J Cardiol.* 1979;43:962.
234. Kreysig FL. Berlin. *Die Krankheiten des Herzens.* Vol 3. 1817:104. Case 19.
235. The Editors. Case of a singular malformation of the heart. *London Med Rev.* 1812;5:263.
236. Edwards JE, Burchell HB. Congenital tricuspid atresia: a classification. *Med Clin N Amer.* 1949:1177.
237. Edwards JE, Carey LS, Neufeld HN, Lester RG. *Congenital Heart Disease, Correlation of Pathologic Anatomy and Angiocardiography.* Philadelphia: WB Saunders Co; 1965:347.
238. Brown B. Case of singular malformation of the heart. *London Med Repository.* 1824;1:127.
239. Favell. Malformation of heart. *Prov Med & Surg J.* 1842;13:440.
240. Peacock TB. *On Malformations, Etc of the Human Heart with Original Cases.* London: John Churchill; 1858:20–100.
241. Keith JD, Rowe RD, Vlad P. *Heart Disease in Infancy and Childhood.* New York: Tricuspid Atresia, Macmillan Publishing Co; 1958:434.
242. Melhuish BPP, Van Praagh R. Juxtaposition of the atrial appendages, a sign of severe cyanotic congenital heart disease. *Br Heart J.* 1968;30:269.
243. Van Praagh S, O'Sullivan J, Brili S, Van Praagh R. Juxtaposition of the morphologically right atrial appendage in solitus and inversus atria: a study of 35 postmortem cases. *Am Heart J.* 1996;132:382.
244. Van Praagh S, O'Sullivan J, Brili S, Van Praagh R. Juxtaposition of the morphologically left atrial appendage in solitus and inversus atria: a study of 18 postmortem cases. *Am Heart J.* 1996;132:391.
244a. Van Praagh R, Van Praagh S, Vlad P, Keith JD. Anatomic types of congenital dextrocardia: diagnostic and embryologic implications. *Am J Cardiol.* 1964;13:510–531.
244b. Van Praagh R, David I, Gordon D, Wright GB, Van Praagh S. Ventricular diagnosis and designation. In: Godman M, ed. *Paediatric Cardiology 1980.* Edinburgh and London: Churchill Livingston; 1981:163.
245. Becker AE, Anderson RH. Absence of an atrioventricular connection (AV valve atresia). In: *Pathology of Congenital Heart Disease.* London: Butterworths; 1981:257.
246. Jones KL. *Smith's Recognizable Patterns of Human Malformation.* 4th ed. Philadelphia: W.B. Saunders Co; 1988:62.
247. Van Praagh R, Van Praagh S: The anatomy of common aorticopulmonary trunk (truncus arteriosus communis) and its embryologic implications, a study of 57 necropsied cases,. *Am J Cardiol* 16:4061965.
248. Freedom RM, Mawson JB, Yoo S-J, Benson LN. *Congenital Heart Disease, Textbook of Angiocardiography.* Vol II. Armonk, NY: Futura Publishing Co Inc; 1997:1171.
249. Hurwitt ES, Young D, Escher DJW: The rationale of anastomosis of the right auricular appendage to the pulmonary artery in the treatment of tricuspid atresia. Application of this procedure to a case of cor triloculare, *J Thorac Surg* 30:5031955.
250. Kirklin JW, Barratt-Boyes BG. *Cardiac Surgery. Morphology, Diagnostic Criteria, Natural History, Techniques, Results and Indications.* 2nd ed. New York, Edinburgh: Churchill Livingstone; 1993:1055.
251. Subramanian S, Carr I, Waterston DJ, Bonham-Carter RE. Palliative surgery in tricuspid atresia, forty-two casers. *Circulation.* 1965;32:977.
252. Gamboa R, Gersony WM, Nadas AS. The electrocardiogram in tricuspid atresia and pulmonary atresia with intact ventricular septum. *Circulation.* 1966;34:24.
253. Jordan JC, Sanders CA. Tricuspid atresia with prolonged survival, a report of two cases with a review of the world literature. *Am J Cardiol.* 1966;18:112.
254. Gallaher ME, Fyler DC. Observations on changing hemodynamics in tricuspid atresia without associated transposition of the great vessels. *Circulation.* 1967;35:381.
255. Guller B, Titus JL. Morphological studies in tricuspid atresia. *Circulation.* 1968;38:977.
256. Edwards WS, Bargeron LM. The superiority of the Glenn operation for tricuspid atresia in infancy and childhood. *J Thorac Cardiovasc Surg.* 1968;55:60.
257. Marcano BA, Riemenschneider TA, Ruttenberg HD, Goldberg SJ, Gyepes M. Tricuspid atresia with increased pulmonary blood flow, an analysis of 13 cases. *Circulation.* 1969;40:399.
258. Guller B, DuShane JW, Titus JL. The atrioventricular conduction system in two cases of tricuspid atresia. *Circulation.* 1969;40:217.
259. Guller B, Titus JL, DuShane JW. Electrocardiographic diagnosis of malformations associated with tricuspid atresia: correlation with morphologic features. *Am Heart J.* 1969;78:180.
260. Levin AR, Spach MS, Canent RV, Boineau JP. Dynamics of interatrial shunting in children with obstruction of the tricuspid and pulmonic valves. *Circulation.* 1970;41:503.
261. Davachi F, Lucas RV, Moller JH. The electrocardiogram and vectocardiogram in tricuspid atresia. Correlation with pathologic anatomy. *Am J Cardiol.* 1970;25:18.
262. Gabriele OF. Progressive obstruction of pulmonary blood flow in tricuspid atresia. *J Thorac Cardiovasc Surg.* 1970;59:447.
263. Leatham A, Scully RE. Cyanotic congenital heart disease with death at the age of fifty-eight years. *New Engl J Med.* 1969;280:317.
264. Folger GM, Witham AC, Ellison RG. Tricuspid atresia with transposition of the great vessels. *J Pediat.* 1969;74:946.
265. Rashkind W, Waldhausen J, Miller W, Friedman S. Palliative treatment in tricuspid atresia. Combined balloon atrioseptos-

tomy and surgical alteration of pulmonary blood flow. *J Thorac Cardiovasc Surg.* 1969;57:812.
266. Lenox CC, Zuberbuhler JR. Balloon septostomy in tricuspid atresia after infancy. *Am J Cardiol.* 1970;25:723.
267. Rosenquist GC, Levy RJ, Rowe RD. Right atrial—left ventricular relationships in tricuspid atresia: position of the presumed site of the atretic valve as determined by transillumination. *Am Heart J.* 1970;80:493.
268. Levy RJ, Rosenquist GC. Anatomical variations in tricuspid atresia: report of two cases with previously undescribed lesions. *Hopkins Med J.* 1970;126:177.
269. Becker MJ, Amplatz K, Burchell HB, Becker AE, Edwards JE. Clinical pathologic conference. *Am Heart J.* 1971;81:264.
270. Baron MG. Hypoplasia of the inflow portion of the right ventricle: an angiocardiographic sign of tricuspid atresia. *Circulation.* 1971;44:746.
271. Karp RB, Soto B, Bargeron LM, Barcia A. The collateral venous circulation after Glenn anastomosis. *Am J Cardiol.* 1972;29:272.
272. Oparil S, Goldblatt A, Hendren WH. Left-superior-vena-cava steal syndrome. *New Engl J Med.* 1972;286:303.
273. Glenn WWL, Fenn JE. Axillary arteriovenous fistula, a means of supplementing blood flow through a cava-pulmonary shunt. *Circulation.* 1972;46:1013.
274. Taussig HB, Keinonen R, Momberger N, Kirk H. Long-time observations on the Blalock-Taussig operation. IV: tricuspid atresia. *Hopkins Med J.* 1973;132:135.
275. Neches WH, Park SC, Lenox CC, Zuberbuhler JR, Bahnson HT. Tricuspid atresia with transposition of the great arteries and closing ventricular septal defect. Successful palliation by banding of the pulmonary artery and creation of an aorticopulmonary window. *J Thorac Cardiovasc Surg.* 1973;65:538.
276. Stanford W, Armstrong RG, Cline RE, King TD. Right atrium-pulmonary artery allograft for correction of tricuspid atresia. *J Thorac Cardiovasc Surg.* 1973;66:105.
277. Kreutzer G, Galíndez E, Bono H, de Palma C, Laura JP. An operation for the correction of tricuspid atresia. *J Thorac Cardiovasc Surg.* 1973;66:613.
278. Miller RA, Pahlajani D, Serratto M, Tatooles C. Clinical studies after Fontan's operation for tricuspid atresia. *Am J Cardiol.* 1974;33:157.
279. Tandon R, Edwards JE. Tricuspid atresia, a re-evaluation and classification. *J Thorac Cardiovasc Surg.* 1974;67:530.
280. Karp RB, Bargeron LM. Late results of superior vena cava—right pulmonary artery anastomosis for tricuspid atresia. In: Kirklin JW, ed. *Advances in Cardiovascular Surgery.* New York: Grune & Stratton; 1973:37.
281. Cokkinos DV, Plessas ST, Tolis G, Voridis EM. Tricuspid atresia with dextroversion, a not very rare combination. *J Thorac Cardiovasc Surg.* 1974;68:268.
282. Walker DR, Sbokos CG, Lennox SC. Correction of tricuspid atresia. *Br Heart J.* 1975;37:282.
283. Abrams R, Saldana M, Kastor JA, Shelburne JC. Tricuspid and pulmonary valve atresia with aortopulmonary fistula: survival of a patient to 21 years of age. *Chest.* 1975;68:263.
284. Tandon R, Marín-Garciá J, Moller JH, Edwards JE. Tricuspid atresia with l-transposition. *Am Heart J.* 1974;88:417.
285. Roe BB. Aorto-pulmonary shunt in premature infant. Technical considerations. *J Thorac Cardiovasc Surg.* 1975;69:437.
286. Somerville J, Ross DN. Tricuspid atresia—new hope with radical palliative surgery. *Br Heart J.* 1975;37:782.
287. Henry JN, Danielson GK. Tricuspid atresia: successful surgical "correction" in two patients using porcine xenograft valves: results of a detailed anatomical study. *Ann Royal College of Physicians and Surgeons of Canada.* 1975;8:18.
288. Henry JN, Devloo RAE, Ritter DG, Mair DD, Davis GD, Danielson GK. Tricuspid atresia, successful surgical "correction" in two patients using porcine xenograft valves. *Mayo Clin Proc.* 1974;49:803.
289. Dick M, Fyler DC, Nadas AS. Tricuspid atresia: clinical course in 101 patients. *Am J Cardiol.* 1975;36:327.
290. Kyger ER, Reul GT, Sandiford FM, Wukasch DC, Hallman GL, Cooley DA. Surgical palliation of tricuspid atresia. *Circulation.* 1975;52:685.
291. Bailey LL, Freedom RM, Fowler RJ, Trusler GA. Nonoperative management of late failure of a Glenn anastomosis. Transvenous wafer occlusion of patent superior vena cava—right atrial junction. *J Thorac Cardiovasc Surg.* 1976;71:371.
292. Anderson RH, Shinebourne EA, Becker AE, et al. Tricuspid atresia. *J Thorac Cardiovasc Surg.* 1977;74:325.
293. Bharati S, Lev M. Reply. *J Thorac Cardiovasc Surg.* 1977;74:328.
294. Laks H, Mudd JG, Standeven JW, Fagan L, Willman VL. Long-term effect of the superior vena cava—pulmonary artery anastomosis on pulmonary blood flow. *J Thorac Cardiovasc Surg.* 1977;74:253.
295. Rao PS. Natural history of the ventricular septal defect in tricuspid atresia and its surgical implications. *Br Heart J.* 1977;39:276.
296. Bharati S, Lev M. The conduction system in tricuspid atresia with and without regular (d-) transposition. *Circulation.* 1977;56:423.
297. LaCorte MA, Dick M, Scheer G, La Farge CG, Fyler DC. Left ventricular function in tricuspid atresia. Angiographic analysis in 28 patients. *Circulation.* 1975;52:996.
298. Quero Jiménez M, Maître Azcárate MJ, Alvarez Bejarano H, Vázquez Martul E. Tricuspid atresia, an anatomical study of 17 cases. *Europ J Cardiol.* 1975;3:337.
299. Gago O, Salles CA, Stern AM, Spooner E, Brandt RL, Morris JD. A different approach for the total correction of tricuspid atresia. *J Thorac Cardiovasc Surg.* 1976;72:209.
300. Schatz J, Krongrad E, Malm JR. Left anterior and left posterior hemiblock in tricuspid atresia and transposition of the great vessels. Observations and electrocardiographic nomenclature and electrophysiologic mechanisms. *Circulation.* 1976;54:1010.
301. Serratto M, Miller RA, Tatooles C, Ardekani R. Hemodynamic evaluation of Fontan operation in tricuspid atresia. *Circulation.* 1976;54:III–99.
302. Freedom RM, Rowe RD. Aneurysm of the atrial septum in tricuspid atresia. Diagnosis during life and therapy. *Am J Cardiol.* 1976;38:265.
303. Williams WG, Rubis L, Fowler RS, Rao MK, Trusler GA, Mustard WT. Tricuspid atresia; results of treatment in 160 children. *Am J Cardiol.* 1976;38:235.
304. Bini R, Thiene G. Associazioni malformative che accompagnano l'atresia della tricuspside: quadric comuni e variant rare. *Boll Soc Ital Cardiol.* 1975;20:725.
305. Bharati S, McAllister HA, Tatooles CJ, et al. Anatomic variations in underdeveloped right ventricle related to tricuspid atresia and stenosis. *J Thorac Cardiovasc Surg.* 1976;72:383.
306. Anderson RH, Wilkinson JL, Gerlis LM, Smith A, Becker AE. Atresia of the right atrioventricular orifice. *Br Heart J.* 1977;39:414.
307. Shariatzadeh AN, King H, Girod D, Shumacker HB. Tricuspid atresia, a review of 68 cases. *Chest.* 1977;71:538.
308. Treistman B, Cooley DA. Total physiologic correction of tricuspid atresia with atrial septal defect. Ventricular septal defect

closure and a right atrium – right ventricle non-valved conduit: case report. *Cardiovasc Dis Bull Texas Heart Inst.* 1978;5:406.
309. Quero Jimenez M, Maitre Azcarate MJ, Moreno Granado F, Perera C, LopezVarea F. Tricuspid atresia. Morphology in 19 cases. *Magyar Pediat.* 1978;12(suppl 4):3.
310. Becker AE, Meyboom EJ, Wilkinson JL, Smith A, Anderson RH. "Tricuspid atresia" is a form of univentricular heart: a concept supported by the anatomy of the atrioventricular conduction tissue. *Magyar Pediat.* 1978;12(suppl 4):3.
311. Rashkind WJ. Tricuspid atresia; certain historical aspects. *Magyar Pediat.* 1978;12(suppl 4):3.
312. Beppu S, Nimura Y, Tamai M, et al. Two-dimensional echocardiography in diagnosing tricuspid atresia. Differentiation from other hypoplastic right heart syndromes and common atrioventricular canal. *Br Heart J.* 1978;40:1174.
313. Bowman FO, Malm JR, Hayes CJ, Gersony WM. Physiological approach to surgery for tricuspid atresia. *Circulation.* 1978;58:I–83.
314. Patel R, Fox K, Taylor JFN, Graham GR. Tricuspid atresia, clinical course in 62 cases (1967–1974). *Br Heart J.* 1978;40:1408.
315. Seward JB, Tajik AJ, Hagler DJ, Ritter DG. Echocardiographic spectrum of tricuspid atresia. *Mayo Clin Proc.* 1978;53:100.
316. Serratto M, Pahlajani DB. Electrophysiologic studies in tricuspid atresia. *Am J Cardiol.* 1979;42:983.
317. Björk VO, Olin CL, Bjarke BB, Thorén CA. Right atrial—right ventricular anastomosis for correction of tricuspid atresia. *J Thorac Cardiovasc Surg.* 1979;77:452.
318. Bharati S, Lev M. The concept of tricuspid atresia complex as distinct from that of the single ventricle complex. *Pediatr Cardiol.* 1979;1:57.
319. Anderson RH, Becker AE, Macartney FJ, Shinebourne EA, Wilkinson JL, Tynan MJ. Is "tricuspid atresia" a univentricular heart? *Pediatr Cardiol.* 1979;1:51.
320. Sauer U, Mocellin R. Angiocardiographic left ventricular volume determination in tricuspid atresia. Comparison of patients with and without palliative surgery. *Herz.* 1979;4:248.
321. Gravinghoff LM, Keck EW. Changing aspects in the treatment of tricuspid atresia. *Magyar Pediat.* 1978;12(suppl 4):4.
322. Choussat A, Fontan F, Besse P, et al: Cardiac performance in tricuspid atresia, *Magyar Pediat* 1978;12(suppl 4):5.
323. Yacoub M, Radley-Smith R. Right atrial function after the Fontan operation. *Magyar Pediat.* 1978;12(suppl 4):6.
324. Sauer U. Angiographic left ventricular volume determination in patients with tricuspid atresia before and after palliative surgery. *Magyar Pediat.* 1978;12(suppl 4):8.
325. Shinebourne EA, Zuberbuhler JR, Miller GH, Anderson RH. Tricuspid atresia type III equals absent left atrioventricular connexion with univentricular heart. *Magyar Pediat.* 1978;12(suppl 4):8.
326. Karczenski K, Karczenski J. Development and pathology of tricuspid atresia based on postmortem study of 41 cases. *Magyar Pediatr.* 1978;12(suppl 4):9.
327. Takahashi O, Eshaghpour E, Kotler MN. Tricuspid and pulmonary valve echoes in tricuspid and pulmonary atresia. *Chest.* 1979;76:437.
328. Sharratt GP, Johnson AM, Monro JL. Persistence and effects of sinus rhythm after Fontan procedure for tricuspid atresia. *Br Heart J.* 1979;42:74.
329. Dickinson DF, Wilkinson JL, Smith A, Anderson RH. Atresia of the right atrioventricular orifice with atrioventricular concordance. *Br Heart J.* 1979;42:9.
330. Dickinson DF, Wilkinson JL, Smith A, Becker AE, Anderson RH. Atrioventricular conduction tissues in univentricular hearts of left ventricular type with absent right atrioventricular connection ("tricuspid atresia"). *Br Heart J.* 1979;42:1.
331. Sauer U, Hall D. Spontaneous closure or critical decreased in size of the ventricular septal defect in tricuspid atresia with normally connected great arteries: surgical implications. *Herz.* 1980;5:369.
332. Freedom RM, Williams WG, Fowler RS, Trusler GA, Rowe RD. Tricuspid atresia, transposition of the great arteries, and banded pulmonary artery. Repair by arterial switch, coronary artery reimplantation, and right atrioventricular valve conduit. *J Thorac Cardiovasc Surg.* 1980;80:621.
333. Anderson RH, Shinebourne EA, Becker AE, Macartney FJ, Wilkinson JL, Tynan MJ. Tricuspid atresia and univentricular heart. *Pediatr Cardiol.* 1980;1:165.
334. Bharati S, Lev M. Reply. *Pediatr Cardiol.* 1980;1:165.
335. Weinberg PM. Anatomy of tricuspid atresia and its relevance to current forms of surgical therapy. *Ann Thorac Surg.* 1980;29:306.
336. Trusler GA, Williams WG. Long-term results of shunt procedures for tricuspid atresia. *Ann Thorac Surg.* 1980;29:312.
337. Annecchino FP, Fontan F, Chauve A, Quaegebeur J. Palliative reconstruction of the right ventricular outflow tract in tricuspid atresia: a report of 5 patients. *Ann Thorac Surg.* 1980;29:317.
338. Behrendt DM, Rosenthal A. Cardiovascular status after repair by Fontan procedure. *Ann Thorac Surg.* 1980;29:322.
339. Jennings RB, Crisler C, Johnson DH, Brickman RD. Tricuspid atresia with dextrotransposition, dextrocardia, and mitral insufficiency: successful circulatory correction. *Ann Thorac Surg.* 1980;29:369.
340. Rosenthal A. Current status of treatment for tricuspid atresia: introduction to symposium. *J Thorac Surg.* 1980;29:304.
341. Baum VC, Tarnoff H, Hoffman JIE. Pulsus paradoxus in a patient with tricuspid atresia and hypoplastic right heart. *Circulation.* 1980;62:651.
342. Rao PS. A unified classification for tricuspid atresia. *Am Heart J.* 1980;99:799.
343. Gale AW, Danielson GK, McGoon DC, Wallace RB, Mair DD. Fontan procedure for tricuspid atresia. *Circulation.* 1980;62:91.
344. Otero Coto E, Calabro R, Marsico F, Lopez Arranz JS. Right atrial outlet atresia with straddling left atrioventricular valve, a form of double outlet atrium. *Br Heart J.* 1981;45:317.
345. Nishioka K, Kamiya T, Ueda T, et al. Left ventricular volume characteristics in children with tricuspid atresia before and after surgery. *Am J Cardiol.* 1981;47:1105.
346. Doty DB, Marvin WJ, Lauer RM. Modified Fontan procedure. Methods to achieve direct anastomosis of right atrium to pulmonary artery. *J Thorac Cardiovasc Surg.* 1981;81:470.
347. Dick M, Behrendt DM, Byrum CJ, et al. Tricuspid atresia and the Wolff-Parkinson-White syndrome: evaluation methodology and successful surgical treatment of the combined disorders. *Am Heart J.* 1981;101:496.
348. Ben-Shachar G, Nicoloff DM, Edwards JE. Separation of neointima from Dacron graft causing obstruction. Case following Fontan procedure for tricuspid atresia. *J Thorac Cardiovasc Surg.* 1981;82:268.
349. Stanton RE, Lurie PR, Lindesmith GG, Meyer BW. The Fontan procedure for tricuspid atresia. *Circulation.* 1981;64:II–140.
350. Reder RF, Yeh H-C, Steinfeld L. Aneurysm of the interatrial septum causing pulmonary venous obstruction in an infant with tricuspid atresia. *Am Heart J.* 1981;102:786.
351. Santalla A, Quero M, Yen-Ho S, Fernández Espino R, Brito JM, Arteaga M. New surgical approach to palliate tricuspid atresia in infants. *Ann Thorac Surg.* 1982;33:297.

352. Kreutzer GO, Vargas FJ, Schlichter AJ, et al. Atriopulmonary anastomosis. *J Thorac Cardiovasc Surg*. 1982;83:427.
353. Williams DB, Kiernan PD, Schaff HV, Marsh HM, Danielson GK. The hemodynamic response to dopamine and nitroprusside following right atrium—pulmonary artery bypass (Fontan procedure). *Ann Thorac Surg*. 1982;34:51.
354. Rashkind WJ. Tricuspid atresia. A historical review. *Ped Cardiol*. 1982;2:85.
355. Deanfield JE, Tommasini G, Anderson RH, Macartney FJ. Tricuspid atresia: analysis of coronary artery distribution and ventricular morphology. *Br Heart J*. 1982;48:485.
356. Lins RFA, Lins MFA, Cavalcanti C, Miranda RP, Mota JH. Orthoterminal correction of congenital heart disease: double cava-pulmonary anastomosis. *J Thorac Cardiovasc Surg*. 1982;84:633.
357. Shachar GB, Fuhrman BF, Wang Y, Lucas RV, Lock JE. Rest and exercise hemodynamic after the Fontan procedure. *Circulation*. 1982;65:1043.
358. Sanders SP, Wright GB, Keane JF, Norwood WI, Castaneda AR. Clinical and hemodynamic results of the Fontan operation for tricuspid atresia. *Am J Cardiol*. 1982;49:1733.
359. Weinberg PM. Pathologic anatomy of tricuspid atresia. In: Rao S, ed. *Tricuspid Atresia*. Mt Kisco, NY: Futura Publishing Co; 1982:49.
360. Ho SY, Milo S, Anderson RH, et al. Straddling atrioventricular valve with absent atrioventricular connection, report of 10 cases. *Br Heart J*. 1982;47:344.
361. Rigby ML, Gibson DG, Joseph MC, et al. Recognition of imperforate atrioventricular valves by two dimensional echocardiography. *Br Heart J*. 1982;47:329.
362. Patterson W, Baxley WA, Karp RB, Soto B, Bargeron LL. Tricuspid atresia in adults. *Am J Cardiol*. 1982;49:141.
363. Sabbagh AH, Riveros M, Fritz JM, Fernandez J. Fontan operation: modification of the valve position in conduit with brief review of the literature. *Texas Heart Inst J*. 1983;10:183.
364. Rao PS. Further observations on the spontaneous closure of physiologically advantageous ventricular septal defects in tricuspid atresia: surgical implications. *Ann Thorac Surg*. 1983;35:121.
365. Bull C, deLeval MR, Stark J, Taylor JFN, Macartney FJ. Use of a subpulmonary ventricular chamber in the Fontan circulation. *J Thorac Cardiovasc Surg*. 1983;85:21.
366. de Brux J-L, Zannini L, Binet J-P, et al. Tricuspid atresia, results of treatment in 115 children. *J Thorac Cardiovasc Surg*. 1983;85:440.
367. Uretzky G, Puga FJ, Danielson GK. Modified Fontan procedure in patients with previous ascending aorta-pulmonary artery anastomosis. *J Thorac Cardiovasc Surg*. 1983;85:447.
368. Fontan F, Deville C, Quaegebeur J, et al. Repair of tricuspid atresia in 100 patients. *J Thorac Cardiovasc Surg*. 1983;85:647.
369. De Leon SY, Idriss FS, Ilbawi MN, et al. The role of the Glenn shunt in patients undergoing the Fontan operation. *J Thorac Cardiovasc Surg*. 1983;85:669.
370. Breisch EA, Wilson DB, Laurenson RD, Mazur JH, Bloor CM. Tricuspid atresia (type Ia): survival to 21 years of age. *Am Heart J*. 1983;106:149.
371. Sanchez GR, Mehta AV, Black IFS: Cardiac rhythm following Fontan–type procedures in children. *Northeast Ped Cardiol Soc Program for Scientific Sessions*. 1983:25–27.
372. Lemmer JH, Coran AG, Behrendt DM, Heidlelberger KP, Stern AM. Liver fibrosis (cardiac cirrhosis) five years after modified Fontan operation for tricuspid atresia. *J Thorac Cardiovasc Surg*. 1983;86:757.
373. Cloutier A, Ash J, Smallhorn J, et al. Pulmonary blood flow distribution (PBF) after Fontan procedure. *Circulation*. 1983;68:III–276.
374. Hellenbrand W, Glenn W, Laks H, et al. Cava-pulmonary artery anastomosis, a 25 year follow-up. *Circulation*. 1983;68:III–212.
375. Nouri S, Pennington DG, Ho J. Hemodynamic assessment of Fontan's operation. *Circulation*. 1983;68:III–212.
376. Nakazawa M, Nakanishi T, Okuda H, et al. Dynamics of right heart flow in patients after Fontan procedure. *Circulation*. 1984;69:306.
377. Kreutzer GO. Atrioventricular connections versus atriopulmonary anastomosis. *J Thorac Cardiovasc Surg*. 1984;87:147.
378. deLeval MR. Reply. *J Thorac Cardiovasc Surg*. 1984;87:147.
379. Scalia D, Russo P, Anderson RH, et al. The surgical anatomy of hearts with no direct communication between the right atrium and the ventricular mass—so-called tricuspid atresia. *J Thorac Cardiovasc Surg*. 1984;87:743.
380. Ishikawa T, Neutze JM, Brandt PWT, Barratt-Boyes BG. Hemodynamics following the Kreutzer procedure for tricuspid atresia in patients under two years of age. *J Thorac Cardiovasc Surg*. 1984;88:373.
381. Gomes AS, Benson L, George B, Laks H. Management of pulmonary arteriovenous fistulas after superior vena cava – right pulmonary artery (Glenn) anastomosis. *J Thorac Cardiovasc Surg*. 1984;87:636.
382. Gerlis LM, Anderson RH, Scott O. Interventricular and subarterial obstruction in tricuspid atresia resulting from an endocardial tissue tag. *Am J Cardiol*. 1984;54:236.
383. Alboliras ET, Porter CJ, Danielson GK, et al. Results of the modified Fontan operation for congenital lesions in patients without preoperative sinus rhythm. *J Am Coll Cardiol*. 1985;6:228.
384. Laks H, Milliken JC, Perloff JK, et al. Experience with the fontan procedure. *J Thorac Cardiovasc Surg*. 1984;88:939.
385. Nakae S, Imai Y, Harada Y, et al. Assessment of left ventricular function before and after Fontan's operation for the correction of tricuspid atresia. Changes in left ventricular function determined by left ventricular volume change. *Heart Ves*. 1985;1:83.
386. Ottenkamp J, Wenink ACG, Quaegebeur JM, et al. Tricuspid atresia. Morphology of the outlet chamber with special emphasis on surgical implications. *J Thorac Cardiovasc Surg*. 1985;89:597.
387. Del Torso S, Kelly MJ, Kalff V, Venables AW. Radionuclide assessment of ventricular contraction at rest and during exercise following the Fontan procedure for either tricuspid atresia or single ventricle. *Am J Cardiol*. 1985;55:1127.
388. DiSessa TG, Yeatman LA, Williams RG, Lois JF, Friedman WF, Laks H. Thrombosis complicating balloon angioplasty of left pulmonary artery stenosis after Fontan's procedure: successful treatment with intravenous streptokinase. *Am J Cardiol*. 1985;55:610.
389. Kurosawa H, Yagi Y, Imamura E, et al. A problem in Fontan's operation: sinus septal defect complicating tricuspid atresia. *Heart Ves*. 1985;1:48.
390. Mair DD, Rice MJ, Hagler DJ, Puga FJ, McGoon DC, Danielson GK. Outcome of the Fontan procedure in patients with tricuspid atresia. *Circulation*. 1985;72:II–88.
391. Jacobstein MD, Fletcher BD, Goldstein S, Riemenschneider TA. Magnetic resonance imaging in patients with hypoplastic right heart syndrome. *Am Heart J*. 1985;110:154.
392. Cleveland DC, Kirklin JK, Naftel DC, et al. Surgical treatment of tricuspid atresia. *Ann Thorac Surg*. 1984;38:447.

393. Juaneda E, Haworth SG. Pulmonary vascular structure in patients dying after a Fontan procedure. The lung as a risk factor. *Br Heart J*. 1984;52:575.
394. Hess J, Kruizinga K, Bijleveld CMA, Hardjowijono R, Eygelaar A. Protein-losing enteropathy after Fontan operation. *J Thorac Cardiovasc Surg*. 1984;88:606.
395. Gidding SS, Rosenthal A, Rocchini AP, Dick M. Response to Valsalva maneuver after the Fontan procedure for tricuspid atresia, single ventricle, or pulmonic valve atresia. *Am J Cardiol*. 1985;56:905.
396. De Leon SY, Ilbawi MN, Idriss FS, et al. Persistent low cardiac output after the Fontan operation. Should takedown be considered? *J Thorac Cardiovasc Surg*. 1986;92:402.
397. Dobell ARC, Trusler GA, Smallhorn JF, Williams WG. Atrial thrombi after the Fontan operation. *Ann Thorac Surg*. 1986;42:664.
398. Vargas FJ, Mayer JE, Jonas RA, Castaneda AR. Atrioventricular valve repair or replacement in atriopulmonary anastomosis: surgical considerations. *Ann Thorac Surg*. 1987;43:403.
399. Humes RA, Mair DD, Porter C-BJ, Puga FJ, Schaff HV, Danielson GK. Results of the modified Fontan operation in adults. *Am J Cardiol*. 1988;61:602.
400. Mayer JE, Helgason H, Jonas RA, et al. Extending the limits for modified Fontan procedures. *J Thorac Cardiovasc Surg*. 1986;92:1021.
401. Tazelaar HD, Moore GW, Hutchins GM. Ventricular Inversion and Tricuspid Atresia (VITA complex): long survival without surgical treatment. *Pediatr Cardiol*. 1986;6:187.
402. Warnes CA, Somerville J. Tricuspid atresia in adolescents and adults: current state and complications. *Br Heart J*. 1986;56:535.
403. Mathews K, Bale JF, Clark EB, Marvin WJ, Doty DB. Cerebral infarction complicating Fontan surgery for cyanotic congenital heart disease. *Pediatr Cardiol*. 1986;7:161.
404. Ilbawi MN, Idriss FS, Muster AJ, et al. Effects of elevated coronary sinus pressure on left ventricular function after the Fontan operation, an experimental and clinical correlation. *J Thorac Cardiovasc Surg*. 1986;92:231.
405. Girod DA, Fontan F, Deville C, Ottenkamp J, Choussat A. Long-term results after the Fontan operation for tricuspid atresia. *Circulation*. 1987;75:605.
406. Vargas FJ, Mayer JE, Jonas RA, Castañeda AR. Anomalous systemic and pulmonary venous connections in conjunction with atriopulmonary anastomosis (Fontan-Kreutzer). Technical considerations. *J Thorac Cardiovasc Surg*. 1987;93:523.
407. Lamberti JJ, Grehl T, Waldman J, Kirkpatrick S. The cavopulmonary shunt. *Bergamo International Cardiac Surgical Symposium*. 1988:132. Abstracts.
408. Squarcia U, Agnetti A, Zavota L, Carano N, Cavalli C. Percutaneous balloon angioplasty in postoperative Fontan patients with pulmonary artery stenosis. *Bergamo International Cardiac Surgical Symposium*. 1988;125. Abstracts.
409. Faidutti B, Freidli B, Oberhänsli I, Rouge JC. Palliation of complex non-correctable heart defects with bidirectional cavopulmonary anastomosis (Haller operation). *Bergamo International Cardiac Surgical Symposium*. 1988:92. Abstracts.
410. Sano S, Brawn WJ, Mee RBB. Experience with the modified Fontan operation. *Bergamo International Cardiac Surgical Symposium*. 1988:83. Abstracts.
411. Aru GM, Chin AJ, Murphy JD, et al. Norwood WI: modified Fontan operation: correctable anastomotic causes of low cardiac output, persistent pleural effusions, late onset effusions, and protein losing enteropathy. *Bergamo International Cardiac Surgical Symposium*. 1988:79. Abstracts.
412. Leung MP, Benson LN, Smallhorn JF, Williams WG, Trusler GA, Freedom RM. Abnormal cardiac signs after Fontan operation—a clue to hemodynamic disturbances. *Bergamo International Cardiac Surgical Symposium*. 1988:79. Abstracts.
413. Rigby ML, Knight WB, Oldershaw PJ, Shinebourne EA. Comparison of left ventricular function in tricuspid atresia and double inlet left ventricle. *Bergamo International Cardiac Surgical Symposium*. 1988:80. Abstracts.
414. Del Torso S, Milanesi O, Bui F, et al. Lung perfusion after the Fontan procedure. *Bergamo International Cardiac Surgical Symposium*. 1988:81. Abstracts.
415. Yen Ho S, Battistessa SA, Anderson RH, Smith A, Deverall PB. The arterial supply to the right atrium and sinus node in classical tricuspid atresia. *Bergamo International Cardiac Surgical Symposium*. 1988:81. Abstracts.
416. Sawatari K, Imai Y, Kurosawa H, Fukuchi S, Aoki M, Ohta J. New selection criteria for Fontan procedure: pulmonary artery clamping test and the pulmonary vascular resistance in increased pulmonary blood flow. *Bergamo International Cardiac Surgical Symposium*. 1988:82. Abstracts.
417. de Vivie ER, Horst M, Kottof S. Hemodynamic follow-up and protein losing enteropathy after the Fontan operation. *Bergamo International Cardiac Surgical Symposium*. 1988:69. Abstracts.
418. Kreutzer G. Tricuspid atresia: long term follow-up of anterior and posterior approaches in the bypassing of the right ventricle. *Bergamo International Cardiac Surgical Symposium*. 1988:69. Abstracts.
419. Laks H, Wu A, Pearl K, Haas G, George B. UCLA experience with the Fontan procedure including use of an adjustable intra-atrial communication. *Bergamo International Cardiac Surgical Symposium*. 1988. Abstracts.
420. Graham TP, Moreau G. Postoperative ventricular function and exercise capability after the Fontan procedure. *Bergamo International Cardiac Surgical Symposium*. 1988:70. Abstracts.
421. Paul MH, Seliem MA, Muster AJ, Benson DW. Relationship of left ventricular muscle mass to the outcome of Fontan procedure in patients with tricuspid atresia. *Bergamo International Cardiac Surgical Symposium*. 1988:71. Abstracts.
422. Anderson RH. The surgical anatomy of the Fontan procedure. *Bergamo International Cardiac Surgical Symposium*. 1988:67. Abstracts.
423. Virmani R. The tricuspid valve. *Mayo Clin Proc*. 1988;63:943.
424. Hauck AJ, Freeman DP, Ackermann DM, Danielson GK, Edwards WD. Surgical pathology of the tricuspid valve: a study of 363 cases spanning 25 years. *Mayo Clin Proc*. 1988;63:851.
425. Hurwitz RA, Caldwell RL, Girod DA, Wellman H. Left ventricular function in tricuspid atresia: a radionuclide study. *J Am Coll Cardiol*. 1986;8:916.
426. Driscoll DJ, Danielson GK, Puga FJ, Schaff HV, Heise CT, Staats BA. Exercise tolerance and cardiorespiratory response to exercise often the Fontan operation for tricuspid atresia or functional single ventricle. *J Am Coll Cardiol*. 1986;7:1087.
427. Nakazwa M, Nojima K, Okuda H, et al. Flow dynamics in the main pulmonary artery after the Fontan procedure in patients with tricuspid atresia or single ventricle. *Circulation*. 1987;75:1117.
428. von Scheidt W, von Arnim T, Schneider B, Erdmann E. Balloon embolization of a pulmonary arteriovenous fistula after cavopulmonary anastomosis in tricuspid atresia. *Am Heart J*. 1988;116:182.

429. Patel MM, Overy DC, Konzonis MC, Hadley-Fowlkes LL. Long-term survival in tricuspid atresia. *J Am Coll Cardiol.* 1987;9:338.
430. Tam CKH, Lightfoot NE, Finlay CD, et al. Course of tricuspid atresia in the Fontan era. *Am J Cardiol.* 1989;63:589.
431. Stellin G, Mazzucco A, Bortolotti U, et al. Tricuspid atresia versus other complex lesions. Comparison of results with a modified Fontan procedure. *J Thorac Cardiovasc Surg.* 1988;96:204.
432. Annecchino FP, Brunelli F, Borghi A, Abbruzzese P, Melo M, Parenzan L. Fontan repair for tricuspid atresia: experience with 50 consecutive patients. *Ann Thorac Surg.* 1988;45:430.
433. Coles JG, Leung M, Kielmanowicz S, et al. Repair of tricuspid atresia: utility of right ventricular incorporation. *Ann Thorac Surg.* 1988;45:384.
434. Voci G, Diego JN, Shafia H, Alavi M, Ghusson M, Banka VS. Type Ia tricuspid atresia with extensive coronary artery abnormalities in a living 22 year old woman. *J Am Coll Cardiol.* 1987;10:1100.
435. Kondoh C, Hiroe M, Nakanishi T, et al. Left ventricular characteristics during exercise in patients after Fontan's operation for tricuspid atresia. *Heart Ves.* 1988;4:34.
436. Battistessa SA, Ho SY, Anderson RH, Smith A, Deverall PB. The arterial supply to the right atrium and the sinus node in classic tricuspid atresia. *J Thorac Cardiovasc Surg.* 1988;96:816.
437. de Leval MR, Kilner P, Gewillig M, Bull C. Total cavopulmonary connection: a logical alternative to atriopulmonary connection for complex Fontan operations. Experimental studies and early clinical experience. *J Thorac Cardiovasc Surg.* 1988;96:682.
438. Mitchell IM, Goh DW, Abrams LD. Creation of brachial artery-basilic vein fistula, a supplement to the cavopulmonary shunt. *J Thorac Cardiovasc Surg.* 1989;98:214.
439. Fyfe DA, Gillette PC, Jones JS, Danielson GK. Successful pregnancy following modified Fontan procedure in a patient with tricuspid atresia and recurrent atrial flutter. *Am Heart J.* 1989;117:1387.
440. Sade RM, Gillette PC. Fontan operation in a case of single functional pulmonary artery. *J Thorac Cardiovasc Surg.* 1989;98:153.
441. Puga FJ. The modified Fontan operation. *J Thorac Cardiovasc Surg.* 1989;98:150.
442. de Leval MR. Reply to the editor. *J Thorac Cardiovasc Surg.* 1989;98:150.
443. Glenn WWL. Superior vena cava—pulmonary artery shunt. *Ann Thorac Surg.* 1989;47:62.
444. Leung MP, Benson LN, Smallhorn JF, Williams WG, Trusler GA, Freedom RM. Abnormal cardiac signs after Fontan type of operation: indicators of residua and sequelae. *Br Heart J.* 1989;61:52.
445. Ottenkamp J, Wenink ACG. Anomalies of the mitral valve and of the left ventricular architecture in tricuspid valve atresia. *Am J Cardiol.* 1989;63:880.
446. Mazzera E, Corno A, Picardo S, et al. Bidirectional cavopulmonary shunts: clinical applications as staged or definitive palliation. *Ann Thorac Surg.* 1989;47:415.
447. De Leon SY, Ilbawi MN, Idriss FS, et al. Direct tricuspid closure versus atrial partitioning in Fontan operation for complex lesions. *Ann Thorac Surg.* 1989;47:761.
448. Seliem M, Muster AJ, Paul MH, Benson DW. Relation between preoperative left ventricular muscle mass and outcome of the Fontan procedure in patients with tricuspid atresia. *J Am Coll Cardiol.* 1989;14:750.
449. Weber HS, Hellenbrand WE, Kleinman CS, Perlmutter RA, Rosenfeld LE. Predictors of rhythm disturbances and subsequent morbidity after the Fontan operation. *Am J Cardiol.* 1989;64:762.
450. Fontan F, Fernandez G, Costa F, et al. The size of the pulmonary arteries and the results of the Fontan operation. *J Thorac Cardiovasc Surg.* 1989;98:711.
451. Fernandez G, Costa F, Fontan F, Naftel DC, Blackstone EH, Kirklin JW. Prevalence of reoperation for pathway obstruction after Fontan operation. *Ann Thorac Surg.* 1989;48:654.
452. Gewillig MH, Lundström UR, Deanfield JE, et al. Impact of Fontan operation on left ventricular size and contractility in tricuspid atresia. *Circulation.* 1990;81:118.
453. Moore JW, Kirby WC, Madden WA, Gaither NS. Development of pulmonary arteriovenous malformations after modified Fontan operations. *J Thorac Cardiovasc Surg.* 1989;98:1045.
454. Geggel RL, Mayer JE, Fried R, Helgason H, Cook EF, Reid LM. Role of lung biopsy in patients undergoing a modified Fontan procedure. *J Thorac Cardiovasc Surg.* 1990;99:451.
455. Marcelletti C, Corno A, Giannico S, Marino B. Inferior vena cava—pulmonary artery extracardiac conduit. A new form of right heart bypass. *J Thorac Cardiovasc Surg.* 1990;100:228.
456. Julsrud PR, Danielson GK. A modification of the Fontan procedure incorporating anomalies of systemic and pulmonary venous return. *J Thorac Cardiovasc Surg.* 1990;100:233.
457. Fontan F, Kirklin JW, Fernandez G, et al. Outcome after a "perfect" Fontan operation. *Circulation.* 1990;81:1520.
458. Gewillig MH, Lundström UR, Bull C, Wyse RKH, Deanfield JE. Exercise responses in patients with congenital heart disease after Fontan repair: patterns and determinants of performance. *J Am Coll Cardiol.* 1990;15:1424.
459. Bartmus DA, Driscoll DJ, Offord KP, et al. The modified Fontan operation for children less than 4 years old. *J Am Coll Cardiol.* 1990;15:429.
460. Rhodes J, Garafano RP, Bowman FO, Grant GP, Bierman FZ, Gersony WM. Effect of right ventricular anatomy on the cardiopulmonary response to exercise. Implications for the Fontan procedure. *Circulation.* 1990;81:1811.
461. Lamberti JJ, Spicer RL, Waldman JD, et al. The bidirectional cavopulmonary shunt. *J Thorac Cardiovasc Surg.* 1990;100:22.
462. Qureshi SA, Richheimer R, McKay R, Arnold R. Doppler echocardiographic evaluation of pulmonary artery flow after modified Fontan operation: importance of atrial contraction. *Br Heart J.* 1990;64:272.
463. Tchervenkov CI, Béland MJ, Latter DA, Dobell ARC. Norwood operation for univentricular heart with subaortic stenosis in the neonate. *Ann Thorac Surg.* 1990;50:822.
464. Kürer CC, Tanner CS, Norwood WI, Vetter VL. Perioperative arrhythmias after Fontan repair. *Circulation.* 1990;82:IV–190.
465. Caspi J, Coles JG, Rabinovitch M, et al. Morphological findings contributing to a failed Fontan procedure, twelve-year experience. *Circulation.* 1990;82:IV–177.
466. Bridges ND, Jonas RA, Mayer JE, Flanagan MF, Keane JF, Castaneda AR. Bidirectional cavopulmonary anastomosis as interim palliation for high-risk Fontan candidates. Early results. *Circulation.* 1990;82:IV–170.
467. Mair DD, Hagler DJ, Puga FJ, Schaff HV, Danielson GK. Fontan operation in 176 patients with tricuspid atresia. Results and a proposed new index for patient selection. *Circulation.* 1990;82:IV–164.
468. Trusler GA, Williams WG, Cohen AJ, et al. The cavopulmonary shunt. Evolution of a concept. *Circulation.* 1990;82:IV–131.

469. Bridges ND, Lock JE, Castaneda AR. Baffle fenestration with subsequent transcatheter closure. Modification of the Fontan operation for patients at increased risk. *Circulation*. 1990;82:1681.
470. Kopf GS, Laks H, Stansel HC, Hellenbrand WE, Kleinman CS, Talner NS. Thirty-year follow-up of superior vena cava-pulmonary artery (Glenn) shunts. *J Thorac Cardiovasc Surg*. 1990;100:662.
471. Sade RM, Wiles HB. Pleuroperitoneal shunt for persistent pleural drainage after Fontan procedure. *J Thorac Cardiovasc Surg*. 1990;100:621.
472. Nakazawa M, Katayama H, Imai Y, et al. A quantitative analysis of hemodynamic effects of the right ventricle included in the circulation of the Fontan procedure. *Circulation*. 1991;83:822.
473. Holmes G, Wagman AJ, Epstein ML. Anomalous systemic venous to left atrial connection in tricuspid atresia with severely restrictive interatrial communication. *Pediatr Cardiol*. 1991;12:241.
474. Rychik J, Piccoli DA, Barber G. Usefulness of corticosteroid therapy for protein-losing enteropathy after the Fontan procedure. *Am J Cardiol*. 1991;68:819.
475. Park I-S, Yoo S-J, Kim KS, Hong CY. Tricuspid atresia associated with double-orifice mitral valve and coronary sinus septal defect. *Texas Heart Inst J*. 1991;18:202.
476. Rothman A, Snyder J. Protein-losing enteropathy following the Fontan operation: resolution with prednisone therapy. *Am Heart J*. 1991;121:618.
477. Akagi T, Benson LN, Green M, et al. Ventricular function during supine bicycle exercise in univentricular connection with absent right atrioventricular connection. *Am J Cardiol*. 1991;67:1273.
478. Danilowicz D, Langsner A, Colvin SB. Successful modified Fontan procedure in an adolescent after left pneumonectomy. *Pediatr Cardiol*. 1991;12:186.
479. Zellers TM, Porter CJ, Driscoll DJ. Pseudo-preexcitation in tricuspid atresia. *Texas Heart Inst J*. 1991;18:124.
480. Pearl JM, Laks H, Stein DG, Drinkwater DC, George BL, Williams RG. Total cavopulmonary anastomosis versus conventional modified Fontan procedure. *Ann Thorac Surg*. 1991;52:189.
481. Rao P, Levy JM, Nickicicz E, Gilbert-Barness EF. Tricuspid atresia: association with persistent truncus arteriosus. *Am Heart J*. 1991;122:829.
482. Frommelt PC, Snider R, Meliones JN, Vermilion RP. Doppler assessment of pulmonary artery flow patterns and ventricular function after the Fontan operation. *Am J Cardiol*. 1991;68:1211.
483. Weil J, Horowitz E, Cullen S, Shinebourne E, Redington A, Rigby M. Does transesophageal echocardiography improve diagnostic accuracy in congenital atrioventricular valve abnormalities? *Cardiol Young*. 1993;3:I–27.
484. Penny DJ, Redington AN. Doppler echocardiographic evaluation of pulmonary blood flow after the Fontan operation: the role of the lungs. *Br Heart J*. 1991;66:372.
485. Serraf A, Lacourt-Gayet F, Nicolas F, Bruniaux J, Houyel L, Planché C. Cavopulmonary bypass for surgical decision making in total cavopulmonary connections. *Cardiol Young*. 1993;3:I–98 (abstract).
486. Muster AJ, Zales VR, Backer CL, Ilbawi MN, Mavroudis C. Bilateral pulsatile pulmonary blood flow in correction of "one and one half" ventricular hearts. *Cardiol Young*. 1993;3:I–12.
487. Bridges ND, Lock JE, Castaneda AR. Results of test occlusion after the fenestrated Fontan operation. *Cardiol Young*. 1993;3:I–12.
488. Julsrud P, Van Son J, Weigel T, et al. Relationship of ventricular morphology to outcome in Fontan patients. *Cardiol Young*. 1993;3:I–11.
489. Matsuda H, Shimazaki Y, Arisawa J, et al: Hemodynamic comparison of total cavopulmonary connection in modified Fontan operation, *Cardiol Young* 3:I-11.
490. Reybrouck RR, Dumoulin M, Daenen W, Van Hove M, Van der Hauwaert L, Gewilling M. Cardiorespiratory response to exercise after the Fontan operation. *Cardiol Young*. 1993;3:I–4.
491. Connelly M, Redington A, Somerville J. Cardiopulmonary function in adult patients late after the Fontan operation. *Cardiol Young*. 1993;3:I–4.
492. Jahangiri M, Ross D, Redington A, Lincoln C, Shinebourne E. Thromboembolism following Fontan procedure and its modifications. *Cardiol Young*. 1993;3:I–4.
493. Javidi D, de Leval M, Elliott M, Stark J, Bull C, Cooper M. Early and medium-term experience with total cavopulmonary connection. *Cardiol Young*. 1993;3:I–3.
494. Penny DJ, Rigby ML, Redington AN. Abnormal patterns of intraventricular flow and diastolic filling after the Fontan operation: evidence for incoordinate ventricular wall motion. *Br Heart J*. 1991;66:375.
495. Sánchez JA, Doyle T, Dewar M, et al. Thrombotic and thromboembolic complications following the Fontan procedure—a role for routine anticoagulation. *Cardiol Young*. 1993;3:I–150 (abstract 534).
496. Lundstrom U, Nisula L, Pesonen E, Sairanen H, Louhimo I, Wallgren EI. Pulmonary artery growth failure after Fontan operations—cause and consequence. *Cardiol Young*. 1993;3:I–148 (abstract 526).
497. Miura T, Shimazaki Y, Kadoba K, et al. Comparisons of ventricular pump function, myocardial contractility and stiffness before and after modified Fontan operation. *Cardiol Young*. 1993;3:I–149.
498. Rubio MD, Merino JL, Castro C, et al. Doppler assessment of diastolic function after the Fontan operation. *Cardiol Young*. 1993;3:I–150. abstract 532.
499. Sett SS, Williams WG, Trusler GA, Coles JG, Rebeyka IM, Freedom RM. Long-term results of palliation using the Glenn shunt. *Cardiol Young*. 1993;3:I–3.
500. Mitani Y, Tamura T, Higa T, et al. Evaluation of pulmonary vascular lesion associated with tricuspid atresia and single ventricle after the Glenn procedure in the long-term follow-up period. *Cardiol Young*. 1993;3:I–149.
501. Chang AC, Hanley FL, Wernovsky G, et al. Early bidirectional cavopulmonary shunt in young infants. Postoperative course and early results. *Circulation*. 1993;88(part 2):149.
502. Michielon G, Gharagozloo F, Julsrud PR, Danielson GK, Puga FJ. Modified Fontan operation in the presence of anomalies of systemic and pulmonary venous connection. *Circulation*. 1993;88(part 2):141.
503. Malcic I, Sauer U, Stern H, et al. The influence of pulmonary artery banding on outcome after the Fontan operation. *J Thorac Cardiovasc Surg*. 1992;104:743.
504. Akagi T, Benson LN, Williams WG, Freedom RM. Regional ventricular wall motion abnormalities in tricuspid atresia after the Fontan procedure. *J Am Coll Cardiol*. 1993;22:1182.
505. Day RW, Orsmond GS, Sturtevant JE, Hawkins JA, Doty DB, McGough EC. Early and intermediate results of the Fontan procedure at moderately high altitude. *Ann Thorac Surg*. 1994;57:170.
506. Harake B, Kuhn MA, Jarmakani JM, et al. Acute hemodynamic effects of adjustable atrial septal defect closure in the lateral tunnel Fontan procedure. *J Am Coll Cardiol*. 1994;23:1671.
507. Thoele DG, Ursell PC, So SY, et al. Atrial morphologic features in tricuspid atresia. *J Thorac Cardiovasc Surg*. 1991;102:606.

508. Geva T, Ott DA, Ludomirsky A, Argyle SJ, O'Laughlin MP. Tricuspid atresia associated with aortopulmonary window: controlling pulmonary blood flow with a fenestrated patch. *Am Heart J.* 1992;123:260.
509. Orie JD, Anderson C, Ettedgui JA, Zuberbuhler JR, Anderson RH. Echocardiographic-morphologic correlations in tricuspid atresia. *J Am Coll Cardiol.* 1995;26:750.
510. Van Praagh R, Kiaffas MG, Hanioti C. Causes of death following the modified Fontan-Kreutzer procedure: a study of 14 postmortem cases. *Rev Argentina Cardiol.* 1996;64:265.
511. Ho SY, Jackson M, Kilpatrick L, Smith A, Gerlis LM. Fibrous matrix of ventricular myocardium in tricuspid atresia compared with normal heart, a quantitative analysis. *Circulation.* 1996;94:1642.
512. Pinto RJ, Deshpande J, Dalvi BV. Mitral valve anomalies in tricuspid atresia: an autopsy study of 54 hears. *Cardiol Young.* 1997;7:163.
513. Kiaffas MG, Van Praagh R, Hanioti C, Green DW. The modified Fontan procedure: morphometry and surgical implications. *Ann Thorac Surg.* 1999;67:1746.
514. Sanchez-Quintana D, Climent V, Ho SY, Anderson RH. Myoarchitecture and connective tissue in hearts with tricuspid atresia. *Heart.* 1999;81:182.
515. Mair DD, Puga FJ, Danielson GK. The Fontan procedure for tricuspid atresia: early and late results of a 25-year experience with 216 patients. *J Am Coll Cardiol.* 2001;37:933.
516. Binotto MA, de Lourdes, Higuchi M, Demarchi AV. Left ventricular remodeling in hearts with tricuspid atresia. Morphologic observations and possible basis for ventricular dysfunction after surgery. *J Thorac Cardiovasc Surg.* 2003;126:1026.
517. Sittiwangkul R, Azakie A, Van Arsdell GS, Williams WG, McCrindle BW. Outcomes of tricuspid atresia in the Fontan era. *Ann Thorac Surg.* 2004;77:889.
518. Nürnbeg JH, Ovroutski S, Alexi-Meskishvili V, Ewert P, Hetzer R, Lange PE. New onset arrhythmias after the extracardiac conduit Fontan operation compared with the intraatrial lateral tunnel procedure: early and midterm results. *Ann Thorac Surg.* 2004;78:1979.
519. Fogel MA, Durning S, Wernovsky G, Pollock AN, Gaynor JW, Nicolson S. Brain versus lung: hierarchy of feedback loops in single-ventricle patients with superior cavopulmonary connection. *Circulation.* 2004;110(suppl II):II-147.
520. Dodge-Khatami A, Rahn M, Prêtre BU. Dual chamber epicardial pacing for the failing atriopulmonary Fontan patient. *Ann Thorac Surg.* 2005;80:1440.
521. Morales DLS, Dibardino DJ, Braud BE, et al. Salvaging the failing Fontan: lateral tunnel versus extracardiac conduit. *Ann Thorac Surg.* 2005;80:1445.
522. Wiesman JP, Gaver DP, Ross-Ascuitto NT, Ascuitto RJ. Energy-depleting fluid-flow disturbances associated with small pressure change: relevance to obstructed total cavopulmonary connections. *Congenital Cardiol Today.* 2006;4:1.
523. Grossman W, Bain DS, eds. *Cardiac Catheterization, Angiography, and Intervention.* 4th ed. Philadelphia: Lea and Febiger; 1990:333.
524. Myerburg RJ, Castellanos A. Cardiac arrest and sudden cardiac death. In: Braunwald E, ed. *Heart Disease: A Textbook of Cardiovascular Medicine.* 4th ed. Philadelphia: WB Saunders Co; 1992:756.
525. Van Praagh R. The evolution of the right ventricle and its relation to the surgical management of congenital heart disease. La evolución del ventrículo derecho y su relación con el manejo quirúrgico de las cardiopatiás congénitas. *Rev Arg Cardiol.* 1995;63:417.
526. Darwin C. *The Origin of Species.* New York: Mentor Books, The New American Library, (originally published in 1859); 1958.
527. Van Praagh R. *Survival, A New Approach from the Life Sciences to the Major Problem of Our Time.* Phoenix: Falcon Press; 1985:96.
528. Aristotle. *The Physics (Vol IV, Books 1-4) with English Translation by PW Wicksteed and FM Cornfornford, London and Cambridge.* W Heinemann Ltd, Harvard University Press, the Loeb Classical Library; 1970:168.
529. Durant W. *The Story of Civlization. II, The Life of Greece.* New York: Simon and Schuster; 1939:342. 345, 355-357, 530.
530. Robb JS. *Comparative Basic Cardiology.* New York and London: Grune and Stratton; 1965:43.
531. Van Praagh R, Layton WM, Van Praagh S. Morphogenesis of normal and abnormal relationships between the great arteries and the ventricles: pathologic and experimental data. In: Van Praagh R, Takao A, eds. *Etiology and Morphogenesis of Congenital Heart Disease.* Mt Kisco, NY: Futura Publishing Co Inc; 1980:271.
532. Wells S. *The Journey of Man, A Genetic Odyssey.* New York: Random House Trade Paperbacks; 2003:70–72.
533. Wade N. *Before the Dawn, Recovering the Lost History of Our Ancestors.* New York: The Penguin Press; 2006:1,2,5, 265.
534. Dawkins R. *The Ancestor's Tale. A Pilgrimage to the Dawn of Evolution.* Boston: Houghton Mifflin Co; 2004:35.
535. Kauffman SL, Andersen DH. Persistent venous valves, maldevelopment of the right heart, and coronary artery—ventricular communications. *Am Heart J.* 1963;66:664.
536. Van Praagh S, LaCorte M, Fellows KE, et al. Supero-inferior ventricles: anatomic and angiocardiographic findings in ten postmortem cases. In: Van Praagh R, Takao A, eds. *Etiology and Morphogenesis of Congenital Heart Disease.* New York: Futura Publishing Co, Mt Kisco; 1980:317.
537. Flanagan MF, Foran RB, Sanders SP, Jonas R, Van Praagh R. Tetralogy of Fallot with obstruction of the ventricular septal defect: spectrum of echocardiographic findings. *J Am Coll Cardiol.* 1980;11:386.
538. Van Praagh R, Van Praagh S. Isolated ventricular inversion. A consideration of the morphogenesis, definition, and diagnosis of nontransposed and transposed great arteries. *Am J Cardiol.* 1966;17:395.
539. Pasquini L, Sanders SP, Parness I, et al. Echocardiographic and anatomic findings in atrioventricular discordance with ventriculoarterial concordance. *Am J Cardiol.* 1988;62:1256.
540. Konstantinov IE, Lai L, Colan SD, et al. Atrioventricular discordance with ventriculoarterial concordance: a remaining indication for the atrial switch operation. *J Thorac Cardiovasc Surg.* 2004;128:944.
541. Kugel MA. Congenital heart disease. A clinical and pathological study of two cases of truncus solitarius aorticus (pulmonary atresia). *Am Heart J.* 1932;7:262.
542. Klein H. Über einen seltenen Fall von Herz missbildung mit rudimentärer Entwicklung des rechten Ventrickels und Defekt der Ticuspidalklappen. *Virchows Arch path Anat.* 1938;301(1).
543. Kanjuh VI, Stevenson JE, Amplatz K, Edwards JE. Congenitally unguarded tricuspid orifice with co-existent pulmonary atresia. *Circulation.* 1964;30:911.
544. Abella JB, Van Praagh R, Novak G, Miller RA, Hastreiter AR. Congenital absence of tricuspid valve leaflets. *Am J Cardiol.* 1969;23:104.

545. Edalgi Kumar A, Gilbert G, Aerichidé N, Van Praagh R. Ebstein's anomaly, Uhl's disease, and absence of tricuspid leaflets: a new spectrum. *Am J Cardiol.* 1970;25:111.
546. Haworth SG, Shinebourne EA, Miller GAH. Right-to-left interatrial shunting with normal right ventricular pressure. A puzzling hemodynamic picture associated with some rare congenital malformations of the right ventricle and tricuspid valve. *Br Heart J.* 1975;37:386.
547. Brenner JI, Bharati S, Winn WC, Lev M. Absent tricuspid valve with aortic atresia in mixed levocardia (atrial situs solitus, L-loop), a hitherto undescribed entity. *Circulation.* 1978;57:836.
548. Gussenhoven EJ, Essed CE, Bos E. Unguarded tricuspid orifice with two-chambered right ventricle. *Pediatric Cardiol.* 1986;7:175.
549. Anderson RH, Silverman NH, Zuberbuhler JR. Congenitally unguarded tricuspid orifice: its differentiation from Ebstein's malformation in association with pulmonary atresia and intact ventricular septum. *Pediatr Cardiol.* 1990;11:86.
550. Magotra RA, Agrawal NB, Mall SP, Parikh SJ. Severe dysplasia of the tricuspid valve (unguarded tricuspid anulus): clinical presentation and surgical treatment. *J Thorac Cardiovasc Surg.* 1990;99:174.
551. Agarwala B, Waldman JD, Carbone M. Unguarded tricuspid orifice with Uhl's malformation. *Cardiol Young.* 1996;6:177.
552. Jones KL. Hurler syndrome (mucopolysaccharidosis 1H): coarse facies, stiff joints, mental deficiency, cloudy corneas by one to two years. In: *Smith's Recognizable Patterns of Human Malformation.* 4th ed. Philadelphia: WB Saunders Co; 1988:406.
553. Jones KL. Hunter syndrome (mucopolysaccharidosis II): coarse facies, growth deficiency, stiff joints by two to four years, clear corneas. In: *Smith's Recognizable Patterns of Human Malformation.* 4th ed. Philadelphia: WB Saunders Co; 1988:412.
554. Matsuoka R, Yamamoto Y, Kuroki Y, Matsui I. Phenotypic expression of the trisomic segments in partial trisomy 18. In: Van Praagh R, Takao A, eds. *Etiology and Morphogenesis of Congenital Heart Disease.* Mt Kisco, NY: Futura Publishing Co; 1980:41.
555. Jones KL. Beckwith-Wiedemann syndrome (exophthalmos-macroglossia-gigantism syndrome: macroglossia, omphalocele, macrosomia, ear creases). In: *Smith's Recognizable Patterns of Human Malformation.* 4th ed. Philadelphia: WB Saunders Co; 1988:136.
556. Lacro RV. Dysmorphology and genetics. Single gene disorders. Marfan syndrome. In: Keane JF, Lock JE, Fyler DC, eds. *Nadas' Pediatric Cardiology.* 2nd ed. Saunders Elsevier; 2006:65.
557. Bano-Rodrigo A, Van Praagh S, Trowitzsch E, Hernandez-Latuff P, Van Praagh R: Double-Orifice Atrioventricular Valves: Pathologic Anatomy in 28 Postmortem Cases, with Diagnostic and Surgical Implications. *Pediatric Cardiology,* New York, 1986, Springer-Verlag Inc, p 915.
558. Bano-Rodrigo A, Van Praagh S, Trowitzsch E, Van Praagh R. Double-orifice mitral valve: a study of 27 postmortem cases with developmental, diagnostic, and surgical considerations. *Am J Cardiol.* 1988;61:152.
559. Van Praagh R, Vlad P. Dextrocardia, mesocardia, and levocardia: the segmental approach to diagnosis in congenital heart disease. In: Keith JD, Rowe RD, Vlad P, eds. *Heart Disease in Infancy and Childhood.* 3rd ed. New York: MacMillan Publishing Co, Inc; 1978:638.
560. David I, Castaneda AR, Van Praagh R. Potentially parachute mitral valve in common atrioventricular canal: pathologic anatomy and surgical importance. *J Thorac Cardiovasc Surg.* 1982;84:178.
561. Liberthson RR, Paul MH, Muster AJ, Arcilla RA, Eckner FAO, Lev M. Straddling and displaced atrioventricular orifices and valves with primitive ventricles. *Circulation.* 1971;43:213.
562. Scheff D, Christianson SD, Rosenquist GC. Overriding right atrioventricular valve with ventricular septal defect. *Johns Hopkins Med J.* 1972;130:259.
563. Tandon R, Becker AE, Moller JH, Edwards JE. Double inlet left ventricle. Straddling tricuspid valve. *Br Heart J.* 1974;36:747.
564. Seward JB, Tajik AJ, Ritter DG. Echocardiographic features of straddling tricuspid valve. *Mayo Clin Proc.* 1975;50:427.
565. LaCorte MA, Fellows KE, Williams RG. Overriding tricuspid valve: echocardiographic and angiocardiographic features. Eight cases of ventricular septal defect of atrioventricular canal type. *Am J Cardiol.* 1976;37:911.
566. Isomatsu Y, Kurosawa H, Imai Y. Straddling tricuspid valve without a ventricular septal defect. *Br Heart J.* 1989;62:222.
567. Tabry IF, McGoon DC, Danielson GK, Wallace RB, Tajik AJ, Seward JB. Surgical management of straddling atrioventricular valve. *J Thorac Cardiovasc Surg.* 1979;77:191.
568. Bharati S, McAllister HA, Lev M. Straddling and displaced atrioventricular orifices and valves. *Circulation.* 1979;60:673.
569. Pacifico AD, Soto B, Bargeron LM. Surgical treatment of straddling tricuspid valves. *Circulation.* 1979;60:655.
570. Aziz KU, Paul MH, Muster AJ, Idriss FS. Positional abnormalities of atrioventricular valves in transposition of the great arteries including double outlet right ventricle. Atrioventricular valve straddling and malattachment. *Am J Cardiol.* 1979;44:1135.
571. Milo S, Ho SY, Macartney FJ, et al. Straddling and overriding atrioventricular valves: morphology and classification. *Am J Cardiol.* 1979;44:1122.
572. Wenink ACG, Gittenberger-de Groot A. Straddling mitral and tricuspid valves: morphologic differences and developmental backgrounds. *Am J Cardiol.* 1982;49:1959.
573. Barron JV, Sahn DJ, Valdes-Cruz LM, et al. Two-dimensional echocardiographic evaluation of overriding and straddling atrioventricular valves associated with complex congenital heart disease. *Am Heart J.* 1984;107:1006.
574. Rice MJ, Seward JB, Edwards WD, et al. Straddling atrioventricular valve: two-dimensional echocardiographic diagnosis, classification, and surgical implications. *Am J Cardiol.* 1985;55:505.
575. deVivie R, Van Praagh S, Bein G, Eigster G, Vogt J, Van Praagh R. Transposition of the great arteries with straddling tricuspid valve. Report of two rare cases with acquired subaortic stenosis after main pulmonary artery banding. *J Thorac Cardiovasc Surg.* 1989;98:205.
576. Anderson RH. Straddling tricuspid valve. To the editor. *J Thorac Cardiovasc Surg.* 1990;100:631.
577. deVivie R, Van Praagh S, Van Praagh R. Reply to the editor. *J Thorac Cardiovasc Surg.* 1990;100:632.
578. Reddy VM, Liddicoat JR, McElhinney DB, Brook MM, van Son JAM, Hanley FL. Biventricular repair of lesions with straddling tricuspid valves using techniques of chordal translocation and realignment. *Cardiol Young.* 1997;7:147.
579. Anderson RH. Surgical repair of straddling and overriding tricuspid valve. *Cardiol Young.* 1997;7:122.
580. van Son JAM, Hambsch J, Mohr FW. Suspension of straddling tricuspid valve chordae into the appropriate ventricle. *Ann Thorac Surg.* 1998;65:850.
581. Silver MD, Lam JHC, Ranganathan N, Wigle ED. Morphology of the human tricuspid valve. *Circulation.* 1971;43:333.
582. Rosenquist GC, Sweeney LJ, McAllister HA. Relationships of the tricuspid valve to the membranous ventricular septum in

Down's syndrome without endocardial cushion defect: study of 28 specimens, 14 with a ventricular septal defect. *Am Heart J.* 1975;90:458.
583. Rosenquist GC, Sweeney LJ. Normal variations in tricuspid valve attachments to the membranous ventricular septum; a clue to the etiology of left ventricle-to-right atrial communication. *Am Heart J.* 1975;89:186.
584. Pate JW, Richardson RL, Giles HH. Accessory tricuspid leaflet producing right ventricular outflow obstruction. *New Engl J Med.* 1968;279:867.
585. Cosio FG, Wang y, Nicoloff DM. Membranous right ventricular outflow obstruction. *Am J Cardiol.* 1973;32:1000.
586. Cascos AS, Rábago P, Sokolowski M. Duplication of the tricuspid valve. *Br Heart J.* 1967;29:943.
587. Pisenti G: Di una rarissma anomalia della tricuspide, *Annali Perugia, Facoltà di Medicinae Chirugia* 3:107, 1887/1888.
588. Sierra-Quiroga JL, Rubio-Alvarez J, Fuster Siebert M, Iglesias Carreño C, Durán D, Garcia-Bengochea JB. Duplication of the right atrioventricular orifice in a patent with common atrium and mitral cleft. *Texas Heart Inst J.* 1988;15:68.
589. Folger GM. Supravalvular tricuspid stenosis. Association with developmental abnormalities of the right heart and derivatives of the sixth aortic arch. *Am J Cardiol.* 1968;21:81.
590. Paloheimo JA. Thread-like strand from right atrium into the right ventricle as leader of freely moving ball thrombus. *Br Heart J.* 1973;35:223.
591. Weinberg PM, Peyser K, Hackney JR. Fetal hydrops in a newborn with hypoplastic left heart syndrome: tricuspid valve "stopper". *J Am Coll Cardiol.* 1985;6:1365.
592. Gallucci V, Stritoni P, Fasoli G, Thiene G. Giant blood cyst of tricuspid valve. Successful excision in an infant. *Br Heart J.* 1976;38:990.
593. Anderson KR, Fiddler GI, Lie JT. Congenital papillary tumor of the tricuspid valve. An unusual cause of right ventricular outflow obstruction in a neonate with trisomy. *E. Mayo Clin Proc.* 1977;52:665.
594. Antia AU, Osunkoya BO. Congenital tricuspid incompetence. *Br Heart J.* 1969;31:664.
595. Horne MK, Rowlands DT. Hypoplastic right heart complex in a 46-year-old woman. *Br Heart J.* 1971;33:167.
596. Clarke M. Calcific tricuspid incompetence in childhood. *Br Heart J.* 1972;34:859.
597. Dimich I, Goldfinger P, Steinfeld L, Lukban SB. Congenital tricuspid stenosis. Case treated by heterograft replacement of the tricuspid valve. *Am J Cardiol.* 1973;31:89.
598. Barr PA, Celermajer JM, Bowdler JD, Cartmill TB. Severe congenital tricuspid incompetence in the neonate. *Circulation.* 1974;49:962.
599. Robin E, Belmaric J, Thoms NW, Arbulu A, Ganguly SN. Consequences of total tricuspid valvulectomy without prosthetic replacement in treatment of Pseudomonas endocarditis. *J Thorac Cardiovasc Surg.* 1974;68:461.
600. Robin E, Thoms NW, Arbulu A, Ganguly SN, Magnisalis K. Hemodynamic consequences of total removal of the tricuspid valve without prosthetic replacement. *Am J Cardiol.* 1975;35:481.
601. Maranhão V, Gooch AS, Yang SS, Sumathisena DR, Goldberg HH. Prolapse of the tricuspid leaflets in the systolic murmur-click syndrome. *Cath Cardiovasc Diagnosis.* 1975;1:81.
602. Upshaw CB. Precordial honk due to tricuspid regurgitation. *Am J Cardiol.* 1975;35:85.
603. Aaron BL, Mills M. Congenital tricuspid insufficiency, definition and review. *Chest.* 1976;69:637.
604. Boucek RJ, Graham TP, Morgan JP, Atwood GF, Boerth RC. Spontaneous resolution of massive congenital tricuspid insufficiency. *Circulation.* 1976;54:795.
605. Mehl SJ, Kaltman AJ, Krouzon I, Dworkin L, Adams P, Spencer FC. Combined tricuspid and pulmonic stenosis. Clinical, echocardiographic, hemodynamic, surgical, and pathologic features. *J Thorac Cardiovasc Surg.* 1977;74:55.
606. Nelson RM, Bucciarelli RL, Eitzman DV, Egan EA, Gessner IH. Serum creatine phosphokinase MB fraction in newborns with transient tricuspid insufficiency. *New Engl J Med.* 1978;298:146.
607. Berman W, Whitman V, Stanger P, Rudolph AM. Congenital tricuspid incompetence simulating pulmonary atresia with intact ventricular septum: a report of two cases. *Am Heart J.* 1978;96:655.
608. Sethia B, Williams BT. Tricuspid valve excision without replacement in a case of endocarditis secondary to drug abuse. *Br Heart J.* 1978;40:579.
609. Inoue D, Furukawa K, Matsukubo H, Watanabe T, Katsume H. Subxiphoid two-dimensional echocardiographic detection of tricuspid valve prolapse. *Chest.* 1979;76:693.
610. Milo S, Stark J, Maccartney FJ, Anderson RH. Parachute deformity of the tricuspid valve. *Thorax.* 1979;34:543.
611. Smith MD, Sagar KB, Mauck HP, Crowley MJ, Lower RR. Surgical correction of congenital tricuspid stenosis. *Ann Thorac Surg.* 1982;34:329.
612. Laufer J, Frand M, Milo S. Valve replacement for severe tricuspid regurgitation caused by Libman-Sacks endocarditis. *Br Heart J.* 1982;48:294.
613. Gallo P, Bastianon V, Colloridi V, Grillo LR. Non-Ebstein concomitant dysplasia of tricuspid and mitral valves in newborns. *Appl Pathol.* 1983;1:283.
614. Berry TE, Muster AJ, Paul MH. Transient neonatal tricuspid regurgitation: possible relation with premature closure of the ductus arteriosus. *J Am Coll Cardiol.* 1983;2:1178.
615. Sakai K, Inoue Y, Osawa M. Congenital isolated tricuspid regurgitation in an adult. *Am Heart J.* 1985;110:680.
616. Come PC, Riley MF. Tricuspid annular dilatation and failure of tricuspid leaflet coaptation in tricuspid regurgitation. *Am J Cardiol.* 1985;55:599.
617. Katz NM, Pallas RS. Traumatic rupture of the tricuspid valve. Repair by chordal replacement and annuoloplasty. *J Thorac Cardiovasc Surg.* 1986;91:310.
618. Ittia I, Weinhaus L, Walls JT, Lababidi Z. Rupture of tricuspid valve papillary muscle during balloon pulmonary valvuloplasty. *Am Heart J.* 1987;114:1233.
619. Waller BF, Moriarty AT, Eble JN, Davey DM, Hawley DA, Pless JE. Etiology of pure tricuspid regurgitation based on annular circumference and leaflet area: analysis of 45 necropsy patients with clinical and morphologic evidence of pure tricuspid regurgitation. *J Am Coll Cardiol.* 1986;7:1063.
620. Gewillig M, Dumoulin M, Van der Hauwaert LG. Transient neonatal tricuspid regurgitation: a Doppler echocardiographic study of three cases. *Br Heart J.* 1988;60:446.
621. Hartyánszky IL, Kádár K, Huttl T, Sapi E, Losádi K. Thrombotic lesions of the tricuspid valve in a newborn: surgical management. *Pediatr Cardiol.* 1989;10:109.
622. Robalino BB, Whitlow PL, Marwick T, Casale PN. Percutaneous balloon valvotomy for the treatment of isolated tricuspid stenosis. *Chest.* 1991;100:867.
623. Rubio PA, Al-Bassam MS. Pacemaker-lead puncture of tricuspid valve, successful diagnosis and treatment. *Chest.* 1991;99:1519.

624. Silver MA. Strut fracture and embolization of a Björk-Shiley valve from the tricuspid valve position. *Am J Cardiol.* 1991;68:1253.
625. Fukuda T, Suzuki T, Nakamichi T. Diagnosis and surgical management of tricuspid annular stenosis in complex cardiac anomalies. *Cardiol Young.* 1993;3:I–58.
626. Gerlis LM, Ho SY, Rigby ML. Right ventricular outflow obstruction by anomalies of the tricuspid valve: report of a windsock diverticulum. *Pediatr Cardiol.* 1992;13:59.
627. Eichhorn P, Ritter M, Suetsch G, von Segesser LK, Turina M, Jenni R. Congenital cleft of the anterior tricuspid leaflet with severe tricuspid regurgitation in adults. *J Am Coll Cardiol.* 1992;20:1175.
628. Katogi T, Aeba R, Ito T, et al. Surgical management of isolated congenital tricuspid regurgitation. *Ann Thorac Surg.* 1998;66:1571.
629. Reddy VM, McElhinney DB, Brook MM, Silverman NH, Stanger P, Hanley FL. Repair of congenital tricuspid valve abnormalities with artificial chordae tendineae. *Ann Thorac Surg.* 1998;66:172.
630. Kanter KR, Doelling NR, Fyfe DA, Sharma S, Tam VKH. De Vega tricuspid annuloplasty for tricuspid regurgitation in children. *Ann Thorac Surg.* 2001;72:1344.
631. Kobza R, Kurz DJ, Oechslin EN, et al. Aberrant tendinous chordas with tethering of the tricuspid leaflets: a congenital anomaly causing severe tricuspid regurgitation. *Heart.* 2004;90:319.
632. Van Praagh R, Ongley PA, Swan HJC. Anatomic types of single or common ventricle in man. Morphologic and geometric aspects of 60 necropsied cases. *Am J Cardiol.* 1964;13:367.
633. Van Praagh R, Plett JA, Van Praagh S. Single ventricle: pathology, embryology, terminology, and classification. *Herz.* 1979;4:113.
634. Van Praagh R, Van Praagh S. Anatomically corrected transposition of the great arteries. *Br Heart J.* 1967;29:112.
635. Womble J, Fountain-Dommer R, Downing MT, Leinwand MJ. An example of pectus excavatum causing tricuspid valve compression. *Congenit Cardiol Today.* 2008;6:1.
636. Fonkalsrud EW. Current management of pectus excavatum. *World J Surg.* 2003;27:502.

14

Mitral Valve Anomalies

What anomalies involve the mitral valve? Our database of cardiac pathologic conditions provides an answer that is summarized in Table 14.1.

It seems likely that the adjective *mitral* was applied to the valve that normally resides between the left atrium (LA) and the left ventricle (LV) because this valve is bicuspid—with two "peaks" reminiscent of the hat worn by popes, bishops, and abbotts.[1a,b]

Let us begin a detailed consideration of the pathologic anatomy of the mitral valve with **mitral atresia,** which from the hemodynamic and surgical standpoints is perhaps the worst malformation that befalls the mitral valve.

MITRAL ATRESIA

In the pathologic anatomic database of the Cardiac registry of Boston Children's Hospital and Harvard Medical School, mitral atresia was found to be third in frequency of mitral valve anomalies (177 cases), or 5.50% of 3216 cases of all patients with congenital heart disease on which this book is based, right behind congenital mitral stenosis (224 cases, or 6.97% of all congenital heart disease) and congenital mitral regurgitation (216 cases, or 6.72%) (see Table 14.1).

Some of the questions for consideration are:

1. How many anatomic types of mitral atresia are there?
2. Specifically, what are they?
3. What are the relative frequencies of each?

Why does an understanding of the anatomic types of mitral atresia matter? Because this understanding is the basis of accurate and complete diagnosis and of successful cardiologic intervention and successful cardiovascular surgery.

The salient anatomic findings in these 177 postmortem cases of mitral atresia are summarized in Table 14.2 and in Fig. 14.1. These cases of mitral atresia constitute 5.50% of all 3216 cases of congenital heart disease that form the basis of this study.

Mitral atresia may be classified into six different groups (see Table 14.2 and Fig. 14.1):

1. mitral atresia with normal segmental anatomy, that is, {S,D,S}, in 118 patients (66.67%);
2. mitral atresia with double-outlet right ventricle (DORV) or transposition of the great arteries (TGA) in visceroatrial situs solitus with concordant D-loop ventricles, in 40 cases (22.60%);
3. mitral atresia with DORV or TGA in visceroatrial situs solitus with discordant L-loop ventricles, in 5 patients (2.82%);
4. mitral atresia with DORV in visceroatrial situs inversus with concordant L-loop ventricles, in 1 case (0.56%);
5. mitral atresia with DORV or TGA in visceroatrial situs inversus with discordant D-loop ventricles, in 5 patients (2.82%); and
6. mitral atresia with DORV in the heterotaxy syndromes of polysplenia or asplenia with visceroatrial situs ambiguus, and with D-loop or L-loop ventricles, in 3 cases (1.69%).

Within these six different groups, *18 different anatomic types of mitral atresia* were found (see Table 14.2 and Fig. 14.1). It is understood that these 18 different anatomic types of mitral atresia may be reorganized or consolidated into fewer *hemodynamics,* or *surgical,* or *etiologic* types of mitral atresia. The purpose of this study is to present the anatomic findings with sufficient

TABLE 14.1 Mitral Valve Anomalies

Mitral Valve Anomalies	No. of Cases	% of Series (n = 3216)[a]
1. Mitral atresia	177	5.50
2. Congenital mitral stenosis	201	6.25
3. Congenital mitral regurgitation	216	6.72
4. Congenital absence of mitral valve leaflets[b]	1	0.03
5. Adherent mitral valve	1	0.03
6. Cleft mitral valve	43	1.34
7. Mitral valve dysplasia	2	0.06
8. Hypoplasia of the mitral valve	26	0.81
9. Mitral valve anomaly causing left ventricular outflow obstruction	1	0.03
10. Myxomatous mitral valve	6	0.19
11. Mitral valve prolapse	11	0.34

Language Note: What does *mitral* mean? One might reply that it is an adjective meaning *like a miter*. So the question becomes, what is a miter? The dictionary[1a] defines *miter* as "a headdress; specifically *a)* a tall, ornamented cap with peaks in front and back, worn by the Pope, bishops, and abbots as a mark of office."

Miter has descended to us in modern English through middle English and the old French *mitre,* from Latin and Greek *mitra* where it meant a belt or a headband (a fillet), or a turban.

[a]Of the 3400 autopsied cases of heart disease, mostly in infants and children, on which this book is based, 3216 patients had congenital heart disease, that is, developmental structural heart disease that one is born with, and 184 patients had acquired heart disease.

[b]Also known as *congenitally unguarded mitral orifice.*

TABLE 14.2 Anatomic Classification of Mitral Atresia (n = 177 Postmortem Cases)

	No.	%
1. Mitral Atresia With Normal Segmental Anatomy (n = 118/177 [66.67%])		
1. MAt, {S,D,S}, IVS, AoVAt	80	45.20
2. MAt, {S,D,S}, IVS, AoV patent	2	1.13
3. MAt, {S,D,S}, VSD, AoV patent	27	15.25
4. MAt, {S,D,S}, VSD, AoVAt	5	2.82
5. MAt, {S,D,S}, VSD, Truncus arteriosus	1	0.56
6. MAt, {S,D,S} or other,[a] VSD or BVF, large LV and small RV, or single LV and absent RV	2 (of 7)[a]	1.13 (of 3.95)
7. MAt, {S,D,S}, IVS, TAt, PAt, AoVAt, conjoined thoracopagus twin	1	0.56
2. Mitral Atresia With Double-Outlet Right Ventricle or Transposition of the Great Arteries in Visceroatrial Situs Solitus With Concordant D-Loop Ventricles (n = 40/177 [22.60%])		
8. MAt, VSD, DORV {S,D,D/"S"}[b]	28	16.38
9. MAt, no VSD, DORV {S,D,D}	7	3.95
10. MAt, ± VSD, TGA {S,D,D}	5	2.82
3. Mitral Atresia With Double-Outlet Right Ventricle or Transposition of the Great Arteries in Visceroatrial Situs Solitus With Discordant L-Loop Ventricles (n = 5/177 [2.82%])		
11. MAt (R), VSD, DORV {S,L,L}	4	2.26
12. MAt (R), IVS, TGA {S,L,L}	1	0.56
4. Mitral Atresia With Double-Outlet Right Ventricle in Visceroatrial Situs Inversus With Concordant L-Loop Ventricles (n = 1/177 [0.56%])		
13. MAt (R), IVS, DORV {I,L,L}	1	0.56
5. Mitral Atresia With Double-Outlet Right Ventricle or Transposition of the Great Arteries in Visceroatrial Situs Inversus With Discordant D-Loop Ventricles (n = 5/177 [2.82%])		
14. MAt (L), ± VSD, DORV {I,D,D}	3	1.69
15. MAt (L), IVS, TGA {I,D,D/A}	2	1.13
6. Mitral Atresia With Double-Outlet Right Ventricle in the Heterotaxy Syndromes of Polysplenia and Asplenia (n = 3/177 [1.69%])		
16. MAt, No VSD, DORV {A (S),D,D}, + polysplenia	1	0.56
17. MAt, VSD, DORV {AS,D,L} + asplenia	1	0.56
18. MAt, VSD, DORV {A,L,L} + asplenia	1	0.56

AoVAt, Aortic valvular atresia; *AoV,* aortic valve; *BVF,* bulboventricular foramen; *DORV {A,D,D/L},* double-outlet right ventricle with the segmental anatomic set of situs ambiguus (A) of the viscera and atria, D-loop ventricles (D), and D-malposition (D) or L-malposition (L) of the great arteries; *DORV {AS,D,L},* DORV with situs ambiguus (A) of the viscera and situs solitus (S) of the atria, D-loop ventricles (D), and L-malposition of the great arteries (L); *DORV {I,D,D},* DORV with situs inversus of the viscera and atria (I), D-loop ventricles (D), and D-malposition of the great arteries (D); *DORV {I,L,L},* DORV with situs inversus of the viscera and atria, (I), L-loop ventricles (L), and L-malposition of the great arteries (L); *DORV {S,D,D/"S"},* DORV with situs solitus of the viscera and atria (S), D-loop ventricles (D), and D-malposition of the great arteries (D) or a solitus-normal-like malposition of the great arteries ("S") with a subpulmonary conus and AoV-TV (tricuspid valve) direct fibrous continuity; *DORV {S,L,L},* DORV with situs solitus of the viscera and atria (S), L-loop ventricles (L), and L-malposition of the great arteries (L); *IVS,* intact ventricular septum; *LV,* morphologically left ventricle; *MAt,* mitral atresia; *MAt (L),* mitral atresia, left-sided; *MAt (R),* mitral atresia, right-sided; *n* and *No.,* number; *PAt,* pulmonary atresia (valvar); *RV,* right ventricle; *{S,D,S},* the segmental anatomic set of situs solitus (S) of the viscera and atria, D-loop ventricles (D), and solitus normally related great arteries (S); *TAt,* tricuspid atresia; *TGA {I,D,D/A},* transposition of the great arteries with the segmental anatomic set of situs inversus (I) of the viscera and atria, D-loop ventricles (D), and D-TGA (D) or A-TGA (A) of the great arteries; *TGA {S,D,D},* TGA with solitus (S) viscera and atria, D-loop (D) ventricles, and D-TGA (D); *TGA {S,L,L},* TGA with solitus viscera and atria (S), L-loop ventricles (L), and L-TGA (L); *VSD,* ventricular septal defect.

[a] In mitral atresia with a large LV or a single LV (no right ventricular sinus, body, or inflow tract), the segmental anatomy was: {S,D,S} in 2; TGA {S,D,D} in 1; TGA {S,D,A} in 1; TGA {S,L,D} in 1; DORV {S,D,A} in 1; and DOIOC {S,L,L} in 1. *DOIOC,* Double-outlet infundibular outlet chamber, the right ventricular sinus being absent.

[b] *DORV {S,D,"S"}* occurred in 18 of these 34 cases of DORV with MAt (53%). Thus, DORV with a subpulmonary conus only and AoV-TV fibrous continuity was quite common with MAt. The relationship of the great arteries to each other was like solitus normally related great arteries. However, the relationship of the aortic valve to the atrioventricular valves (AoV-TV fibrous continuity), and the relationship between the aortic valve to the left ventricle (DORV) were both different from that with solitus normally related great arteries; hence, the quotation marks: DORV {S,D, *"S"*}.

clarity so as to facilitate any kind of reorganization of the data, for whatever purpose one may have in mind.

For example, one way of trying to simplify the anatomic classification of mitral atresia is to do it in terms of the types of relationship between the great arteries (Table 14.3). Classifying the pathologic anatomy of hearts with mitral atresia in terms of the type of relationship between the great arteries apparently reduces the anatomic types of mitral atresia from 18 to 5 (see Table 14.3). Although perhaps helpful, this approach is not really an improvement, either diagnostically or surgically because, for patient management, one really *has* to know the anatomic status of all three major cardiac segments, not just that of the infundibuloarterial segment. This is why we prefer the approach shown in Table 14.2 and in Fig. 14.1.

Table 14.2 and Fig. 14.1 should be understood, not memorized. One of the advantages of *the segmental approach to the diagnosis of congenital heart disease*[2-14] is that it replaces memorization with understanding.

Now each of these 18 anatomic types of mitral atresia will be presented in greater detail.

Anatomic Types of Mitral Atresia
n = 177

1. With normal segmental anatomy: {S,D,S}, n = 118 (66.7%)

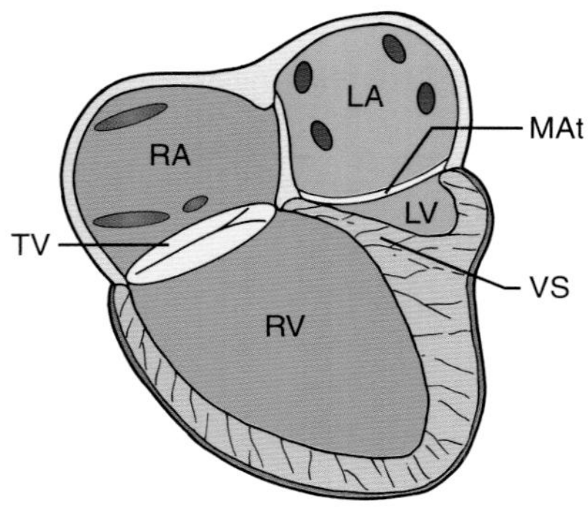

	No.	%
(1) IVS, AoV At	80	45.20
(2) IVS, AoV patent	2	1.13
(3) VSD, AoV patent	27	15.25
(4) VSD, AoV At	5	2.82
(5) VSD, truncus Art	1	0.56
(6) VSD or BVF, large LV or single LV	2 (of 7)	1.13 (of 3.95)
(7) IVS, atresia of all valves, conjoined twin	1	0.56

2. With DORV or TGA and concordant D-loop ventricles, n = 40 (22.60%)

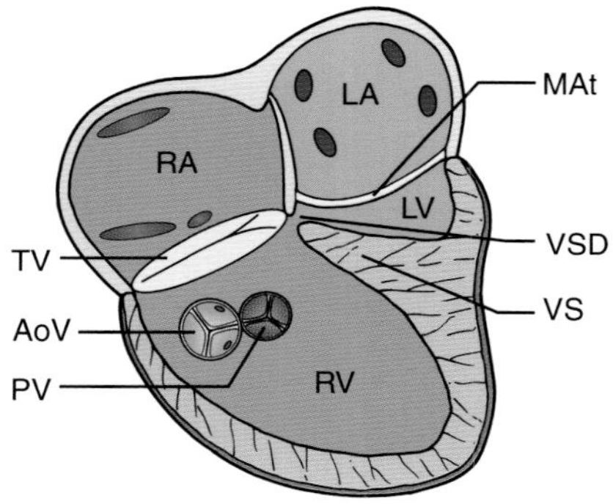

	No.	%
(8) VSD, DORV {S,D,D/"S"}	28	15.82
(9) No VSD, DORV, {S,D,D}	7	3.95
(10) ±VSD, TGA {S.D.D}	5	2.82

3. With DORV or TGA and discordant L-loop ventricles, n = 5 (2.82%)

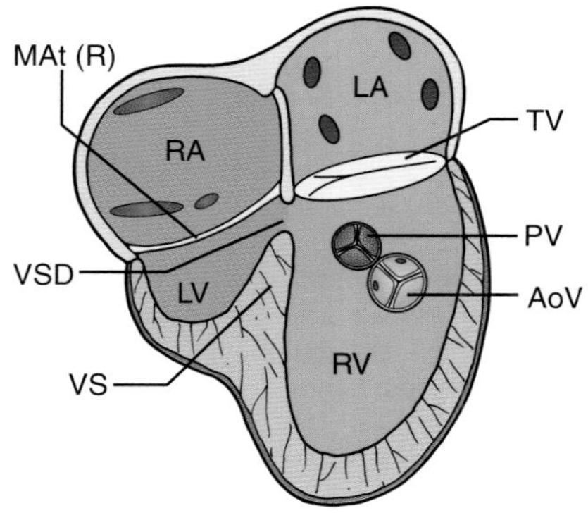

	No.	%
(11) VSD, DORV {S,L,L}	4	2.26
(12) IVS, TGA, {S,L,L}	1	0.56

Fig. 14.1 cont'd

Anatomic Types of Mitral Atresia (cont.)

4. With DORV In situs inversus and concordant L-loop ventricles,
n = 1 (0.56%)

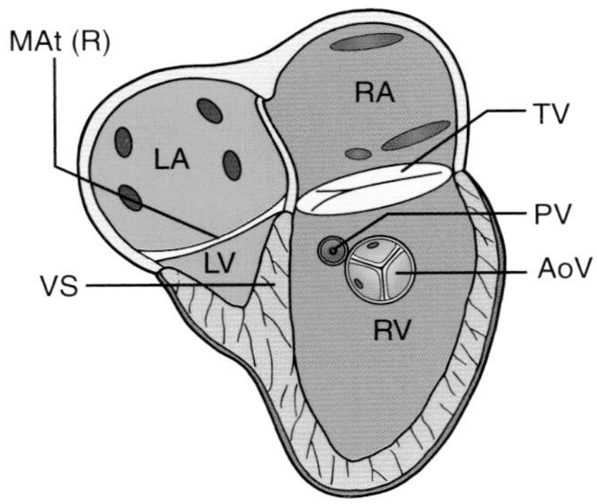

	No.	%
(13) IVS, DORV {I,L,L}	1	0.56

5. With DORV or TGA In situs inversus and discordant D-loop ventricles,
n = 5 (2.82%)

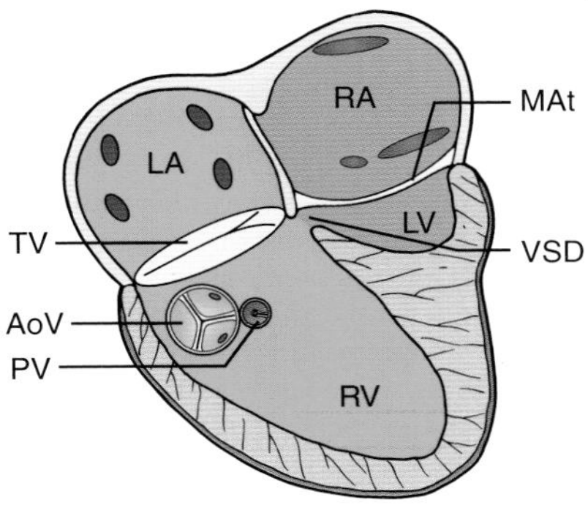

	No.	%
(14) ±VSD, DORV {I,D,D}	3	1.69
(15) IVS, TGA {I,D,D/A}	2	1.13

6. With DORV In the heterotaxy syndromes with polysplenia or asplenia and D-loop or L-loop ventricles,
n = 3 (1.69%)

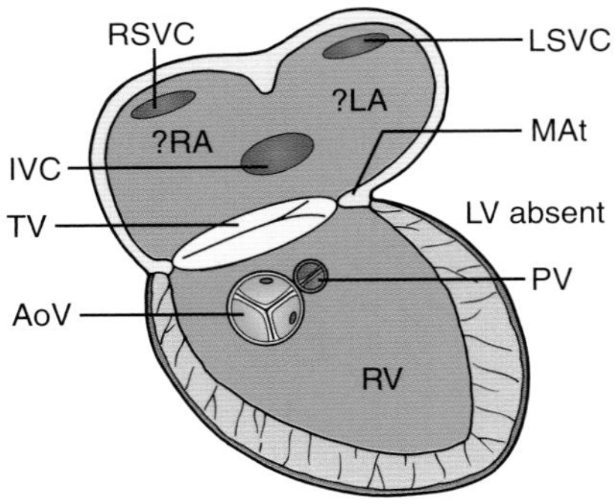

	No.	%
(16) No VSD, DORV {A(S),D,D} and polysplenia	1	0.56
(17) DORV {AS,D,L} and asplenia	1	0.56
(18) DORV {A,L,L} and asplenia	1	0.56

Fig. 14.1 cont'd

TABLE 14.3 Types of Relationship Between the Great Arteries Associated With Mitral Atresia (n = 177)

	No.	%
1. Normally related great arteries	118	66.67
2. Double-outlet right ventricle	46	25.99
3. Transposition of the great arteries	11	6.21
4. Truncus arteriosus	1	0.56
5. Double-outlet infundibular outlet chamber (right ventricular sinus absent)	1	0.56

Mitral Atresia With Normal Segmental Anatomy {S,D,S}

This was by far the largest group of anatomic types in this study of mitral atresia: anatomic types 1 to 7 (see Table 14.2 and Fig. 14.1), which accounted for 118 of these 177 cases (66.67%).

Mitral Atresia With Normal Segmental Anatomy {S,D,S}, Intact Ventricular Septum, and Aortic Valvular Atresia

This was by far the most frequent anatomic type of mitral atresia (Fig. 14.2), occurring in 80 of 177 patients (45.20%; see Table 14.2 and Fig. 14.1).

Fig. 14.1 cont'd The Anatomic Types of Mitral Atresia Found in 177 Postmortem Cases. *{A(S),D,D}*, the set of situs ambiguus of the viscera, probably with situs solitus of the atria, parentheses (S) indicating some uncertainty that the atria are definitely in situs solitus, D-loop ventricles, and D-malposition of the great arteries with the aortic valve *(AoV)* to the right of (dextro- or D-) relative to the pulmonary valve *(PV)*; *{AS,D,L}*, the set of situs ambiguus of the viscera with situs solitus of the atria, D-loop ventricles, and L-malposition of the great arteries with the AoV to the left (levo- or L-) of the PV; *{A,L,L}*, the set of situs ambiguus of the viscera and the atria, L-loop ventricles, and L-malposition of the great arteries; bulboventricular foramen *(BVF)*; *D-loop*, ventricular loop that has looped to the right (dextro- or D-) with a right-handed right ventricle *(RV)* and/or a left-handed left ventricle *(LV)* in terms of ventricular chirality; double-outlet right ventricle *(DORV)*; *{I,D,D}*, the set of visceroatrial situs inversus, D-loop ventricles, and D-malposition of the great arteries; *{I,D,D/A}*, the set of visceroatrial situs inversus, D-loop ventricles, and D- or A-malposition of the great arteries, A-malposition denoting that the AoV is directly anterior (antero- or A-) relative to the PV; *{I,L,L}*, the set of visceroatrial situs inversus, L-loop ventricles, the ventricles having looped to the left (levo- or L-) with left-handed RV and right-handed left ventricular chirality. *{S,D,D}*, the set of visceroatrial situs solitus, ventricular D-loop, and D-malposition of the great arteries; *{S,D,D/"S"}*, the set of visceroatrial situs solitus, ventricular D-loop, and D-malposition of the great arteries or a solitus-normal–like malposition of the great arteries (the quotation marks around *"S"* indicating that the relationship between the great arteries resembles solitus normally related great arteries as in DORV {S,D,"S"} with aortic-tricuspid fibrous continuity and a subpulmonary conus). In DORV {S,D,"S"}, the great arteries are *not really* solitus normal in type because DORV coexists; that is, the conotruncus strongly *resembles* solitus normally related great arteries: *{S,D,S}*, the set of visceroatrial situs solitus, D-loop ventricles, and solitus normally related great arteries; *{S,L,L}*, the set of visceroatrial situs solitus, L-loop ventricles, and L malposition of the great arteries. *±*, With or without; *?*, questionable or uncertain; *At*, atresia; *AoV*, aortic valve; *IVC*, inferior vena cava; *Truncus Art*, truncus arteriosus; *IVS*, intact ventricular septum; *LA*, morphologically left atrium; *LSVC*, left-sided superior vena cava; *LV*, morphologically left ventricle; *MAt*, mitral atresia; *(R)*, right-sided; *RA*, morphologically right atrium; *RSVC*, right-sided superior vena cava; *RV*, morphologically right ventricle; *TGA*, transposition of the great arteries; *TV*, tricuspid valve; *VS*, ventricular septum; *VSD*, ventricular septal defect. The anatomic types of mitral atresia found in 177 postmortem cases. *{A(S),D,D}*, the set of situs ambiguus of the viscera, probably with situs solitus of the atria, parentheses (S) indicating some uncertainty that the atria are definitely in situs solitus, D-loop ventricles, and D-malposition of the great arteries with the aortic valve *(AoV)* to the right of (dextro- or D-) relative to the pulmonary valve *(PV)*; *{AS,D,L}*, the set of situs ambiguus of the viscera with situs solitus of the atria, D-loop ventricles, and L-malposition of the great arteries with the AoV to the left (levo- or L-) of the PV; *{A,L,L}*, the set of situs ambiguus of the viscera and the atria, L-loop ventricles, and L-malposition of the great arteries; bulboventricular foramen *(BVF)*; *D-loop*, ventricular loop that has looped to the right (dextro- or D-) with a right-handed right ventricle *(RV)* and/or a left-handed left ventricle *(LV)* in terms of ventricular chirality; double-outlet right ventricle *(DORV)*; *{I,D,D}*, the set of visceroatrial situs inversus, D-loop ventricles, and D-malposition of the great arteries; *{I,D,D/A}*, the set of visceroatrial situs inversus, D-loop ventricles, and D- or A-malposition of the great arteries, A-malposition denoting that the AoV is directly anterior (antero- or A-) relative to the PV; *{I,L,L}*, the set of visceroatrial situs inversus, L-loop ventricles, the ventricles having looped to the left (levo- or L-) with left-handed RV and right-handed left ventricular chirality. *{S,D,D}*, the set of visceroatrial situs solitus, ventricular D-loop, and D-malposition of the great arteries; *{S,D,D/"S"}*, the set of visceroatrial situs solitus, ventricular D-loop, and D-malposition of the great arteries or a solitus-normal–like malposition of the great arteries (the quotation marks around *"S"* indicating that the relationship between the great arteries resembles solitus normally related great arteries as in DORV {S,D,"S"} with aortic-tricuspid fibrous continuity and a subpulmonary conus). In DORV {S,D,"S"}, the great arteries are *not really* solitus normal in type because DORV coexists; that is, the conotruncus strongly *resembles* solitus normally related great arteries: *{S,D,S}*, the set of visceroatrial situs solitus, D-loop ventricles, and solitus normally related great arteries; *{S,L,L}*, the set of visceroatrial situs solitus, L-loop ventricles, and L malposition of the great arteries. *±*, With or without; *?*, questionable or uncertain; *At*, atresia; *AoV*, aortic valve; *IVC*, inferior vena cava; *Truncus Art*, truncus arteriosus; *IVS*, intact ventricular septum; *LA*, morphologically left atrium; *LSVC*, left-sided superior vena cava; *LV*, morphologically left ventricle; *MAt*, mitral atresia; *(R)*, right-sided; *RA*, morphologically right atrium; *RSVC*, right-sided superior vena cava; *RV*, morphologically right ventricle; *TGA*, transposition of the great arteries; *TV*, tricuspid valve; *VS*, ventricular septum; *VSD*, ventricular septal defect. (From Van Praagh R. Cardiac anatomy: Morphologic and segmental analyses. 1st Annual Aspen Conference on Pediatric Cardiovascular Disease, online syllabus: Delmo Walter EM, Komoda T, Siniawski H, Miera O, Van Praagh R, Hetzer R. Long-term surgical outcome of mitral valve repair in infants and children with Shone's anomaly. *Eur J Cardiothorac Surg.* 2013;43:473-482; and Van Praagh R: The Farber-Landing lecture: Pediatric pathology—the clinician's "open sesame" and its importance in pediatric cardiology and cardiovascular surgery. *Pediatr Dev Pathol.* 2012:15;431-449; with permission.)

Sex: Males, 48 of 80 (60%); females, 31 of 80 (38.75%); and not known, 1 of 80 (1.25%)—a consult from elsewhere, gender not stated. The sex ratio was males to females = 48/31 (1.55:1). Thus a male preponderance was found in this anatomic type of mitral atresia (mitral atresia, aortic atresia, intact ventricular septum), which is one of the forms of the **hypoplastic left heart syndrome (HLHS).**

Age at Death: In these 80 patients, the mean age at death and the standard deviation were 57.39 ± 125.06 days; or expressed in months, the mean was 1.91 ± 4.17 months. The range in the

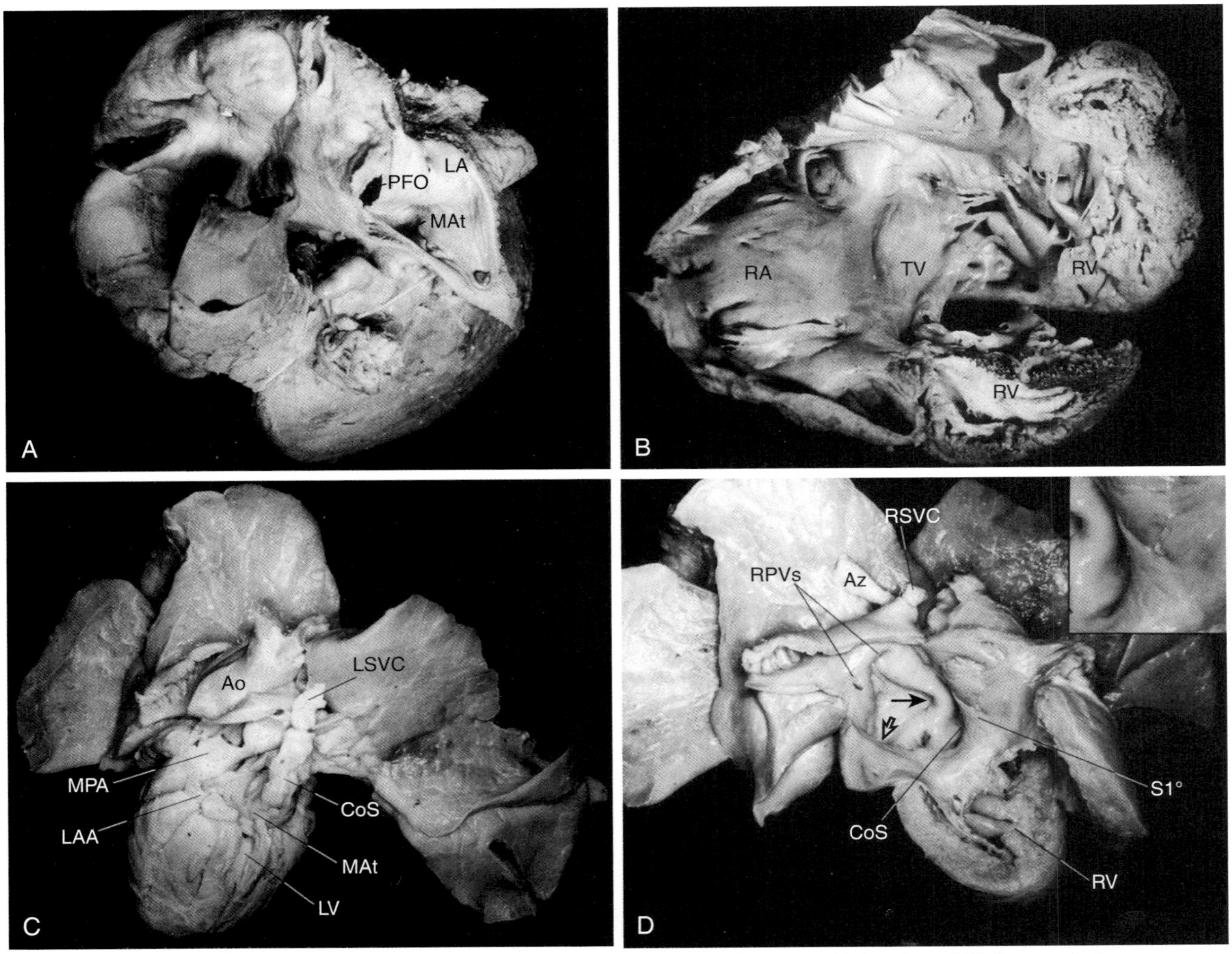

Fig. 14.2 (A) Mitral atresia {S,D,S} with intact ventricular septum. The opened left atrium *(LA)* shows mitral atresia *(MAt)* and patent foramen ovale *(PFO)*. (B) Opened right atrium *(RA)*, tricuspid valve *(TV)*, and right ventricular inflow tract *(RV)*. Right atrial hypertrophy and enlargement and right ventricular hypertrophy and enlargement are marked. The septal leaflet of the TV is thickened and rolled, consistent with tricuspid regurgitation. (C) Another patient with MAt and double-outlet right ventricle (DORV) {S,D,D}, bilateral conus, no pulmonary or aortic outflow tract obstruction, a persistent left superior vena cava *(LSVC)* draining into the coronary sinus *(CoS)* and then into the right atrium, a tiny left ventricle *(LV)* and an intact ventricular septum. The main pulmonary artery *(MPA)* and ascending aorta *(Ao)* were both of good size. (D) The opened right atrium, tricuspid valve, and right ventricular inflow tract (sinus) revealed that septum primum *(S1°)* was very malpositioned with attachments to the posterior left atrial wall, enlarged in the *inset*. Although not fused with the posterior atrial wall, the malpositioned septum primum prevented normal right atrial–to–left atrial blood flow in embryonic and fetal life (the via sinistra), and may have played a role in the development of mitral atresia. The marked malpositioning of the septum primum made it readily possible, from the right atrial side, to see all of the entering venous ostia: the right pulmonary veins *(RPVs)*, the left pulmonary veins *(solid arrow)*, the suprahepatic segment of the inferior vena cava *(open arrow)*, the coronary sinus *(CoS)*, and the right superior vena cava *(RSVC)*. An enlarged azygos vein *(Az)* drained into the RSVC. The right and left pulmonary veins were normally connected with the LA, but they drained totally anomalously into the RA and RV because of the anomalous leftward malposition of the septum primum and the coexistence of mitral atresia. Leftward malposition of the septum primum is a newly recognized cause of totally anomalous pulmonary venous drainage into the right atrium, with normally connected pulmonary veins. Functionally, the leftwardly malpositioned septum primum acted like a supramitral stenosing membrane, which anatomically it was not. A common atrium really was *not* present, despite the fact that the systemic and pulmonary venous blood streams were not separated. These are two tempting *misdiagnoses* (supramitral stenosing membrane, and common atrium) that are mentioned here preemptively, in the hope that these misdiagnoses will *not* be made. The correct, but unfamiliar, diagnosis is *malposition of the septum primum into the left atrium*. This 2½-month-old boy probably had visceral heterotaxy with polysplenia and interruption of the IVC; we thought so, but because the autopsy was limited to heart and lungs, we do not know for sure. Bilaterally hyperarterial bronchi and bilaterally bilobed lungs were present.

Continued

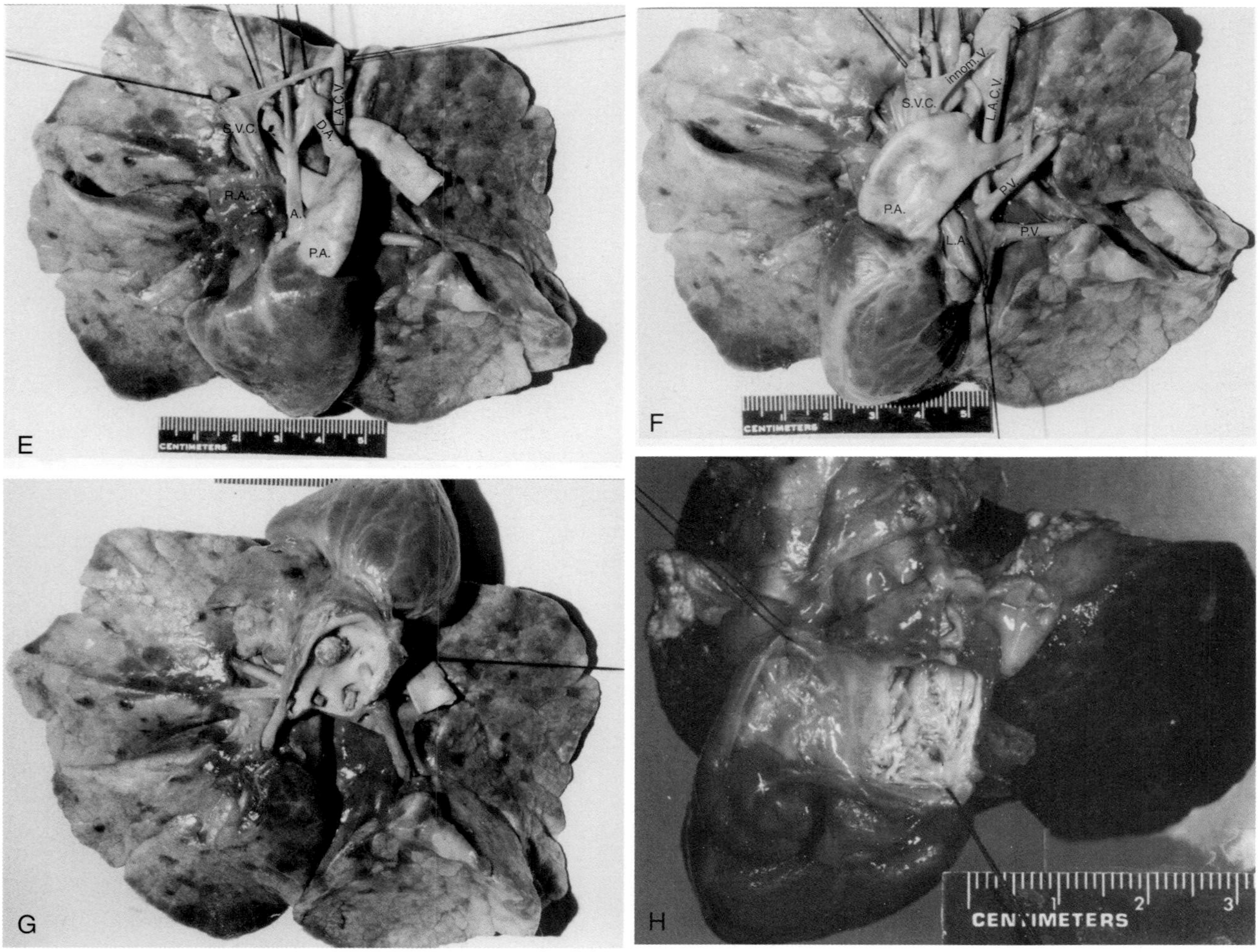

Fig. 14.2 cont'd (E) The exterior view of the heart and lungs of a 4-month-old boy with mitral atresia, aortic atresia, intact atrial septum, intact ventricular septum {S,D,S} segmental anatomy, closing patent ductus arteriosus (PDA), and a persistent LSVC draining into the CoS. The RA and RV (unlabeled) are hypertrophied and enlarged. The closing ductus arteriosus *(D.A.)* is small. The ascending aorta (A) is very hypoplastic, as expected with aortic valvar atresia. The branches of the aortic arch are normal. The diagnosis of levoatrial cardinal vein *(L.A.C.V.)* is incorrect but instructive. This is really a persistent LSVC that communicates with the left innominate vein (unlabeled) that opens into the RSVC and then to the RA. There was a CoS septal defect between the LA anteriorly and the CoS immediately posteriorly. The LA opened into the CoS and then into the persistent LSVC, which is why the prosector who labeled this photo thought that a levoatrial cardinal vein was present. However, a LACV connects with the LA and with pulmonary veins, but not with the CoS, whereas a persistent LSVC typically does connect with the CoS. (F) Left anterior oblique view of this heart specimen showing how large the PA is and revealing the LA. Note how relatively small the LV (unlabeled) is; the course of the anterior descending coronary artery can be seen. Photographs taken at the time of autopsy. (Courtesy of the Department of Pathology, Boston Children's Hospital, Boston, MA) (G) Posterior view of the opened LA. The absence of a mitral valve and orifice is apparent. There is a round antemortem thrombus situated over the PFO, occluding it, and rendering the atrial septum intact. There are probes in the left and right pulmonary veins that connect normally with the LA *(left lung to the viewer's left hand, and right lung to the viewer's right hand)*. The probe second from the *left,* between the left and right pulmonary veins, marks the CoS septal defect, a defect between the LA and the CoS, that in turn communicates both with the RA via the CoS's right atrial orifice and with the persistent LSVC and the left innominate vein. Thus, the CoS septal defect helped to decompress the obstructed LA. (Photographs taken at the time of autopsy in 1955.) (H) The opened LA of a 15-hour-old boy with mitral atresia, aortic valvar atresia, intact ventricular septum, normal {S,D,S} segmental anatomy, and a completely intact atrial septum. The LA is markedly hypertrophied and enlarged, with endocardial fibroelastosis (EFE) of the left atrial endocardium, especially marked in the region of septum primum that is thickened.

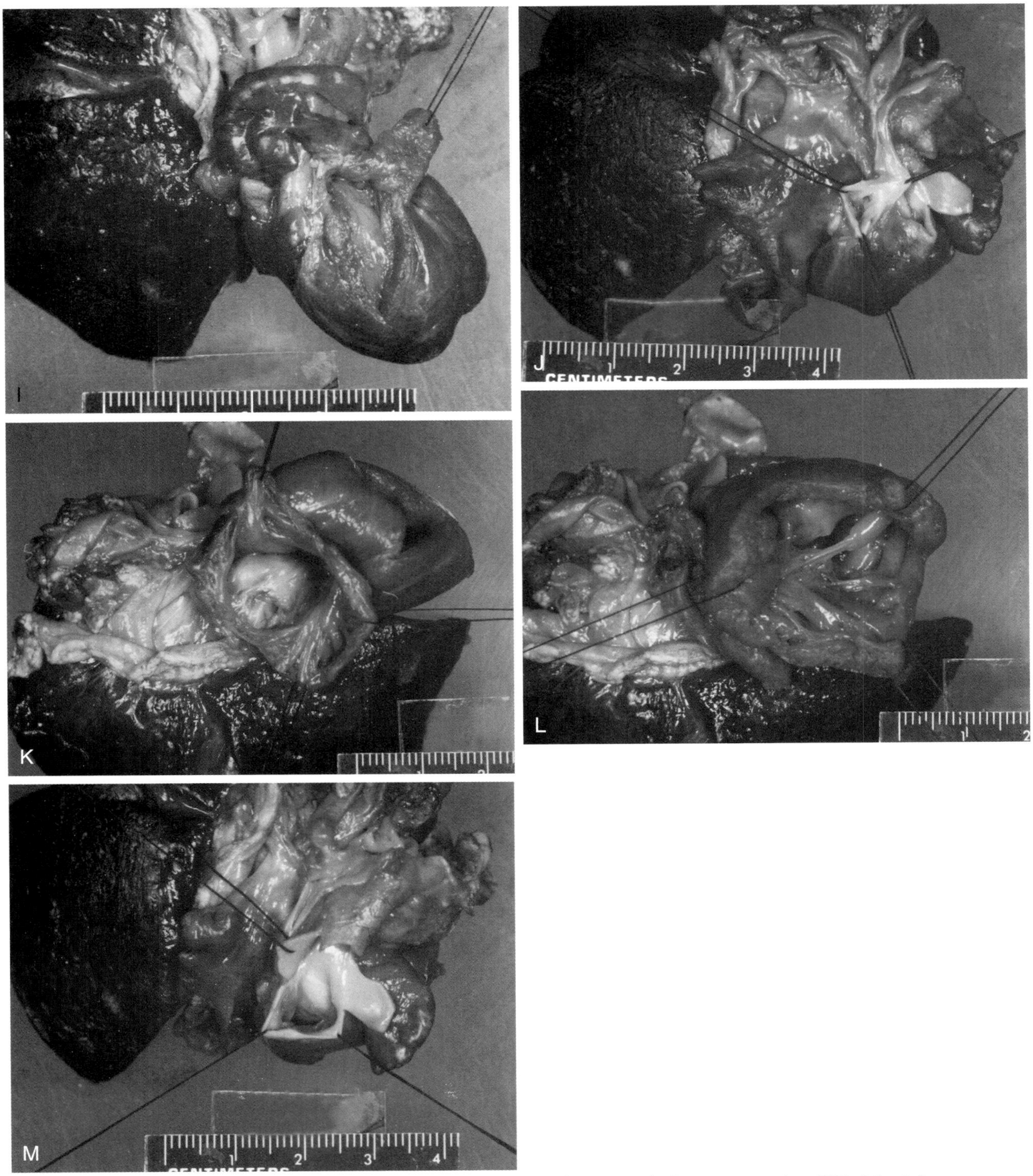

Fig. 14.2 cont'd (I) The opened LV is hypoplastic, with an intact ventricular septum and no EFE of the left ventricular endocardium. Membranous mitral atresia is present, with a myxomatous lumpy appearance of the mitral leaflet tissue and with two hypoplastic left ventricular papillary muscles. The aortic valve is atretic; all three commissures are present but rudimentary. (J) The opened and hypoplastic ascending aorta, with an attempt to show the atretic aortic valve. The brachiocephalic arteries originate normally. (K) The opened RA, showing the atrial septum bulging into the right atrial cavity. The normal atrial septal "landmarks" formed by the superior limbic band of septum secundum and septum primum are not apparent in this intact atrial septum. (L) The opened RV, showing marked hypertrophy and enlargement. (M) The opened MPA showing the large and normally tricommissural pulmonary valve from above. Note how relatively small the opened ascending aorta is, immediately to the right of the very enlarged main pulmonary artery. Photographs taken at the time of autopsy. (Courtesy of the Department of Pathology, Boston Children's Hospital, Boston, MA) *Innom V,* innominate vein; *LAA,* left atrial appendage; *PV,* pulmonary vein. (Reproduced with permission from Van Praagh S, Carrera ME, Sanders SP, Mayer JE, Van Praagh R. Partial or total direct pulmonary venous drainage to right atrium due to malposition of septum primum: Anatomic and echocardiographic findings and surgical treatment—a study based on 36 cases. *Chest.* 1995;107:1488.)

ages at death was from 0 (prenatal death) to 20.92 months. The median age at death was only 10 days.

The median age at death (10 days) is considered to be a more accurate reflection of the history of this—the most common anatomic type of mitral atresia—than is the mean (average) age at death (57 days) because the latter is skewed in an older direction by a few unusually long-lived patients. The median age at death of only 10 days indicates how highly lethal the combination (or complex) of mitral atresia with normal segmental anatomy, intact ventricular septum, and aortic valvular atresia was in this study.

Salient Anatomic Features

For clarity and brevity, the salient anatomic features of this type of mitral atresia are summarized in Table 14.4.

Why Did This Anatomic Type of Mitral Atresia Have Such an Unfavorable History With a Median Age at Death of Only 10 Days?

It is not easy for us to answer this important question because our data reflect not only the *natural* history but also the *iatrogenic* history of the foregoing combination of anomalies. Of these 80 patients (see Table 14.4), 43 died after a modified Norwood procedure (53.75%) and 3 died as the result of a medically induced abortion (3.75%). Consequently the age at death of these patients does not reflect the natural history of this anatomic type of mitral atresia in 46 of these 80 patients (57.5%).

However, the age at death does reflect the natural history in 31 of these 80 patients (38.75%) who had no surgical procedure of any kind and whose ages at death are known to us: mean age at death, 9.65 ± 22.53 days; range, from 0 (spontaneously occurring stillbirth) to 120 days; and median, 2.5 days. Thus, the median age at death of our unoperated patients with this anatomic type of mitral atresia was even worse (younger) than that found in the total series of all patients (operated and unoperated), that is., 2.5 days versus 10 days of age, respectively.

Some of the anatomic features presented in Table 14.4 appear highly relevant to the early lethality of this anatomic type of mitral atresia (type 1; see Table 14.2 and Fig. 14.1). *The atrial septum was observed to be well formed and restrictive or obstructive* to 100% left-to-right atrial shunting in 26 of these 80 cases (32.5%; see Table 14.4). An aneurysm of the septum primum—the flap valve of the foramen ovale—was observed to be bulging

TABLE 14.4 Salient Anatomic Features of Mitral Atresia, {S,D,S}, Intact Ventricular Septum, and Aortic Valvular Atresia (n = 80)

	No.	%		No.	%
Mitral atresia, membranous	14	17.5	Anterior leaflet of tricuspid valve incompletely demuscularized	1	1.25
Blood cyst at site of MV	1	1.25	Supraventricular tachycardia	1	1.25
Atretic parachute MV	1	1.25	Right-sided juxtaposition of the atrial appendages, that is, dextromalposition of the left atrial appendage	1	1.25
Rudimentary LV	39	48.75	Patent ductus arteriosus, restrictive or closing	16	20.0
Absent LV	16	20.0	Coarctation of the aorta, preductal or juxtaductal	10	12.5
LV thick-walled + small-chambered with EFE	1	1.25	Coronary arteriopathy, thick-walled with narrowed lumen	1	1.25
Aortic atresia, valvar + subvalvar	9	11.25	Tiny third coronary artery from aortic root	1	1.25
Cor triatriatum, that is, stenotic common pulmonary vein	1	1.25	Aberrant third coronary artery from proximal LPA	1	1.25
Levoatrial cardinal vein	1	1.25	Aberrant left circumflex coronary artery from proximal RPA	1	1.25
Sinus venosus defect with unroofing of right pulmonary veins	1	1.25	High origin of right coronary artery, above sinus of Valsalva	1	1.25
Partially anomalous pulmonary venous connection	3	3.75	Dextrocardia	1	1.25
Coronary sinus septal defect between LA + CoS to LSVC	4	5.0	Crisscross ventricles	1	1.25
Incompletely common AV canal with MAt and ASD I	1	1.25	Aberrant right subclavian artery	4	5.0
LSVC to CoS to RA	9	11.25	Multiple congenital anomalies	9	11.25
CoS ostial stenosis or atresia	3	3.75	Aspiration pneumonia	1	1.25
Obstructive patent foramen ovale	26	32.5	Acute bacterial endocarditis	1	1.25
Aneurysm of septum I bulging into RA	9	11.25	Two-vessel umbilical cord, that is, single umbilical artery	1	1.25
Intact atrial septum	6	7.5	Prematurity	2	2.50
Leftward displacement of superior portion of septum I	8	10.0	Twin	1	1.25
Atrial septal defect, ostium II type	15	18.75	Fetal abortus	4	1.25
Prominent eustachian valve of IVC	1	1.25	Familial congenital anomalies	1	1.25
Tricuspid regurgitation	9	11.25	Familial congenital heart disease	1	1.25
Double-orifice tricuspid valve	1	1.25			

ASD I, Atrial septal defect of the ostium primum type, that is, incomplete atrioventricular septal defect; *AV*, atrioventricular; *CoS*, coronary sinus; *EFE*, endocardial fibroelastosis; *IVC*, inferior vena cava; *LA*, morphologically left atrium; *LPA*, left pulmonary artery; *LSVC*, left superior vena cava; *LV*, morphologically left ventricle; *MAt*, mitral atresia; *MV*, mitral valve; *ostium II*, ostium secundum; *RA*, morphologically right atrium; *RPA*, right pulmonary artery; *septum I*, septum primum.

into the right atrium (RA), confirming that the atrial septum was obstructive to left-to-right shunting at the atrial level, in 9 of these 80 patients (11.25%; see Table 14.4).

In an additional 6 patients, the atrial septum was found to be *intact* at postmortem examination and hence totally obstructive (7.5%; see Table 14.4). Thus, the atrial septum was significantly obstructive to left-to-right atrial shunting in at least 32 of these 80 patients (40%). A restrictive atrial septum results in pulmonary venous congestion and hypertension, typically leading in turn to the clinical picture of congestive heart failure early in the neonatal period.

However, a **secundum type of atrial septal defect (ASD)** coexisted with mitral atresia in 15 of these 80 patients (18.75%), tending to reduce or eliminate left atrial and pulmonary venous hypertension. The size of the secundum ASD typically determined how much left atrial and pulmonary venous hypertension resulted.

One of these patients with mitral atresia also had **cor triatriatum sinistrum,**[15] that is, stenosis of the common pulmonary vein (see Table 14.4). Consequently, in this patient the presence of pulmonary venous hypertension was unrelated to the anatomic state of the atrial septum.

Other anomalies in addition to a secundum type of ASD can reduce or eliminate left atrial and pulmonary venous hypertension in association with mitral atresia.

A levoatrial cardinal vein[16,17] was present in 1 patient (1.25%; see Table 14.4). As its name suggests, this anomalous vein ran between the LA inferiorly and the left innominate vein superiorly. *A levoatrial cardinal vein is different from a persistent left superior vena cava (LSVC).* A levoatrial cardinal vein does not connect with the coronary sinus, and the course of a levoatrial cardinal vein is more posterior than that of a persistent LSVC. In this patient, the levoatrial cardinal vein was thought to help to decompress the LA.

This patient, a 20-day-old boy, came from a *family with congenital anomalies.* Both parents and the patient's brother had congenital deafness. The patient's father represented a fourth-generation Waardenburg syndrome; the cause of the mother's deafness was not known. The *Waardenburg syndrome*[18,19] is characterized by lateral displacement of the medial canthi, partial albinism, and deafness because of atrophic changes in the spiral ganglion and nerve of the organ of Corti.

This patient also had *familial congenital heart disease:* a cousin with congenital heart disease (type not known by us). This patient had *multiple congenital anomalies* (MCAs) in addition to congenital heart disease: a prominent helix of the right ear; dysplastic toe nails; and a sacral dimple. This patient also had a **partially anomalous pulmonary venous connection:** the left upper lobe pulmonary veins communicated with the levoatrial cardinal vein, and this pulmonary venous blood returned to the RA via the left innominate vein and the right superior vena cava (RSVC). Both the levoatrial cardinal vein and the partially anomalous pulmonary venous connection tended to decompress the LA and reduce the pulmonary venous hypertension.

Partially anomalous pulmonary venous connection was found in 3 of these 80 patients with this type of mitral atresia (3.75%; see Table 14.4). One patient (1.25%; see Table 14.4) had a **sinus venosus defect**[20] **with unroofing of the right pulmonary veins.** Both the posterosuperior interatrial communication and the unroofing of the right pulmonary veins would tend to reduce left atrial hypertension. The interatrial communication would permit left-to-right shunting at the atrial level, and the unroofing of the right pulmonary veins functions as partially anomalous drainage of the right pulmonary veins into the RA.

A coronary sinus septal defect is another way of decompressing the LA and the pulmonary veins when mitral atresia is present. Four patients (5.0%; see Table 14.4) had a so-called coronary sinus septal defect between the coronary sinus posteriorly and the LA anteriorly. Such a defect permits pulmonary venous blood in the LA to flow posteriorly into the coronary sinus and then to the RA, or retrogradely via the LSVC and the left innominate vein to the RSVC and RA.

Three of our patients with the latter type of anomalous pulmonary venous drainage (i.e., decompressing coronary sinus septal defect, permitting pulmonary venous blood to return to the RA via the coronary sinus, or via the LSVC, left innominate vein, and RSVC) also had stenosis or atresia of the right atrial ostium of the coronary sinus (3.75%; see Table 14.4).

An incomplete form of common atrioventricular (AV) canal was found in 1 patient (1.25%; see Table 14.4). The mitral component of the common AV valve was atretic, and a large ostium primum type of defect (i.e., the most common form of incomplete AV septal defect) permitted left-to-right shunting at the atrial level, decompressing the LA. The ventricular septum was intact.

Leftward displacement of the superior portion of the septum primum (see Fig. 14.2) was documented in 8 of these patients (10%; see Table 14.4). We speculate that this curious leftward malposition of the superior portion of the septum primum may have reduced the embryonic and fetal via sinistra (blood flow into the left heart), thereby perhaps contributing to the morphogenesis of mitral atresia. I think that Dr. Paul Weinberg (circa 1976, when Dr. Weinberg was our Cardiac Registry fellow in cardiac pathology) was the first to point out the leftward malposition of the septum primum in patients with mitral atresia, and to draw attention to the potential morphogenetic importance of this atrial septal malposition.

To summarize thus far, the status of the atrial septum, which can be significantly or totally obstructive, and the presence or absence of other anomalies that may influence left atrial and pulmonary venous hypertension, appear important concerning the very unfavorable natural history of this anatomic type of mitral atresia.

The functional status of the ductus arteriosus is another important variable. At autopsy, the ductus arteriosus usually appears to be widely patent, but not always. In the present study, the ductus arteriosus was observed to be restrictive or functionally closing in 16 patients (20%; see Table 14.4). We suspect that this may well be a significant underestimate.

Functional narrowing or near closure of the patent ductus arteriosus (PDA) is thought to be an important factor contributing to the massive right ventricular and right atrial hypertrophy and enlargement that was found in all cases, plus tricuspid regurgitation that was found in 9 patients (11.25%; see Table 14.4) (probably another important underestimate). Functional narrowing of the PDA leads to excessive pulmonary blood flow, increasing pulmonary venous and left atrial hypertension, increasing tricuspid regurgitation, and leading to a clinical picture of increasing left-sided and right-sided congestive heart failure.

Functional narrowing of the large PDA also can contribute to discrete coarctation of the aorta (preductal or juxtaductal), that was observed in 10 of these patients (12.5%; Table 14.4). The ductal medial musculature can encircle the small aortic isthmus, or the aorta opposite the ductal opening, creating a juxtaductal shelf. When the ductus constricts, the coarctation (juxtaductal shelf) becomes more marked; and when the ductal constriction relaxes, the coarctation lessens or disappears.

Functional narrowing of the large PDA acts like an acute "coarctation" of the arterial blood flow in an anterograde direction to the lower body, and in a retrograde direction to the brachiocephalic arteries, very small ascending aorta, and the coronary arteries.

One may wonder why the ascending aorta is so small in the anatomic complex of mitral atresia, intact ventricular septum, and aortic valvar atresia {S,D,S}, as is shown in Fig. 14.2E. Our understanding is that to the degree to which form is determined by function, in this anatomic complex, the ascending aorta typically functions as a *common coronary artery*. This may explain why the ascending aorta in this type of mitral atresia is usually only about two coronary arteries wide (Fig. 14.2E).

To return to the question concerning why the natural history of this anatomic type of mitral atresia is so lethal (median age at death in unoperated patients, 2.5 days of age), we have seen thus far that the inflow into the heart can be significantly obstructed (typically by a restrictive atrial septum) and that the outflow from the heart also can be importantly obstructed (often by a functionally closing PDA). But what happens *between* the inflow tract and the outflow tract is also hemodynamically relevant.

The morphologically LV was specifically described as rudimentary or tiny in 39 of these 80 patients (48.75%; see Table 14.4) and as absent in 16 of these 80 cases (20%; see Table 14.4). *Absence* of the LV means that after making careful serial sections in the expected site of the LV, no vestige of the LV could be found and identified by careful gross examination using loupes.

This means that this anatomic type of mitral atresia (see Table 14.4) can be associated with **anatomically single right RV** (absence of the LV), and with **functionally single RV** (marked hypoplasia of the LV). In turn, this also means that the classic definition of single ventricle is inadequate; that is, that single ventricle is present when *both* AV valves or a *common* AV valve open into one ventricular chamber (univentricular AV connection).[21] This old definition of single ventricle arbitrarily excludes tricuspid atresia and mitral atresia, which we now understand is unsatisfactory.[22-24]

Thus, in 55 of these 80 cases, the LV was specifically described as markedly hypoplastic or absent (68.75%; see Table 14.4). Again, this statistic is regarded as conservative (i.e., as an underestimate).

In only 1 patient (1.25%; see Table 14.4) was the LV described as thick-walled and small-chambered, with endocardial fibroelastosis (EFE) of the LV. A careful search for evidence of a ventricular septal defect (VSD) was negative. This patient, a 22-day-old boy (Case 12), had a modified Norwood procedure at 4 days of age. Autopsy revealed precoronary stenosis: the opening into the coronary compartment at the aortic root was slit-like, nonpatulous, but probe patent (1- × 2-mm internal diameter). Multiple antemortem thrombi were also found in the modified Blalock-Taussig anastomosis. Right-sided juxtaposition of the atrial appendages, with dextromalposition of the left atrial appendage (LAA) that is known to be associated with HLHS, was also found (Fig. 14.3).

However, when the LV is thick-walled and small-chambered, this raises the question: *Is the LV really hypoplastic?* The answer to this question has proved elusive because it is difficult to know precisely how much of the ventricular septum should be included with the left ventricular free wall—if one wishes to weigh such an LV and compare it with normal control LVs. However, this was the only patient with a thick-walled and small-chambered LV that we encountered in these 80 cases of this anatomic type of mitral atresia (see Table 14.4). The overwhelming majority of these patients had LVs that were definitely hypoplastic or absent, as is shown diagrammatically in Fig. 14.1.

In Case 12, the mitral atresia was described as "membranous." A membranous form of mitral atresia was found in 14 of these 80 patients (17.5%; see Table 14.4). More often, the mitral atresia was described as "muscular," that is, looking at the floor of the LA, in the expected site of the mitral valve, one sees a muscular floor, with perhaps a small dimple, where the mitral valve "should" be.

Our speculation concerning the thick-walled and small-chambered LV with EFE of Case 12 is that perhaps the mitral atresia occurred later in intrauterine development than it usually does. If the membranous mitral valve were patent for some time in utero, this might perhaps explain why the free wall of the LV was thick and why there was EFE of the small-chambered LV's endocardium. Or perhaps a VSD had been present but closed premortem. These are hypotheses that we can neither prove nor disprove.

But to return to the main point—a consideration of the hemodynamics in this anatomic type of mitral atresia (see Table 14.4), these patients all had a **functionally single RV.** The tricuspid valve is not optimally designed to occlude an approximately circular systemic AV orifice, whereas the mitral valve is. For further consideration of this important point, please see Chapter 11.

Tricuspid regurgitation was documented in 9 of these patients (11.25%; see Table 14.4); again we suspect that this statistic is probably a significant underestimate. (Autopsy is a good way of establishing structural anomalies, but not of all functional abnormalities.)

Thus, in patients with mitral atresia, intact ventricular septum, aortic valvar atresia, and normal {S,D,S} segmental anatomy, there are multiple hemodynamic handicaps: inflow obstruction, outflow obstruction, and a functionally single pulmonary ventricle (morphologically RV), with a suboptimal AV (tricuspid) valve that is prone to regurgitation when called upon to function as a systemic AV valve.

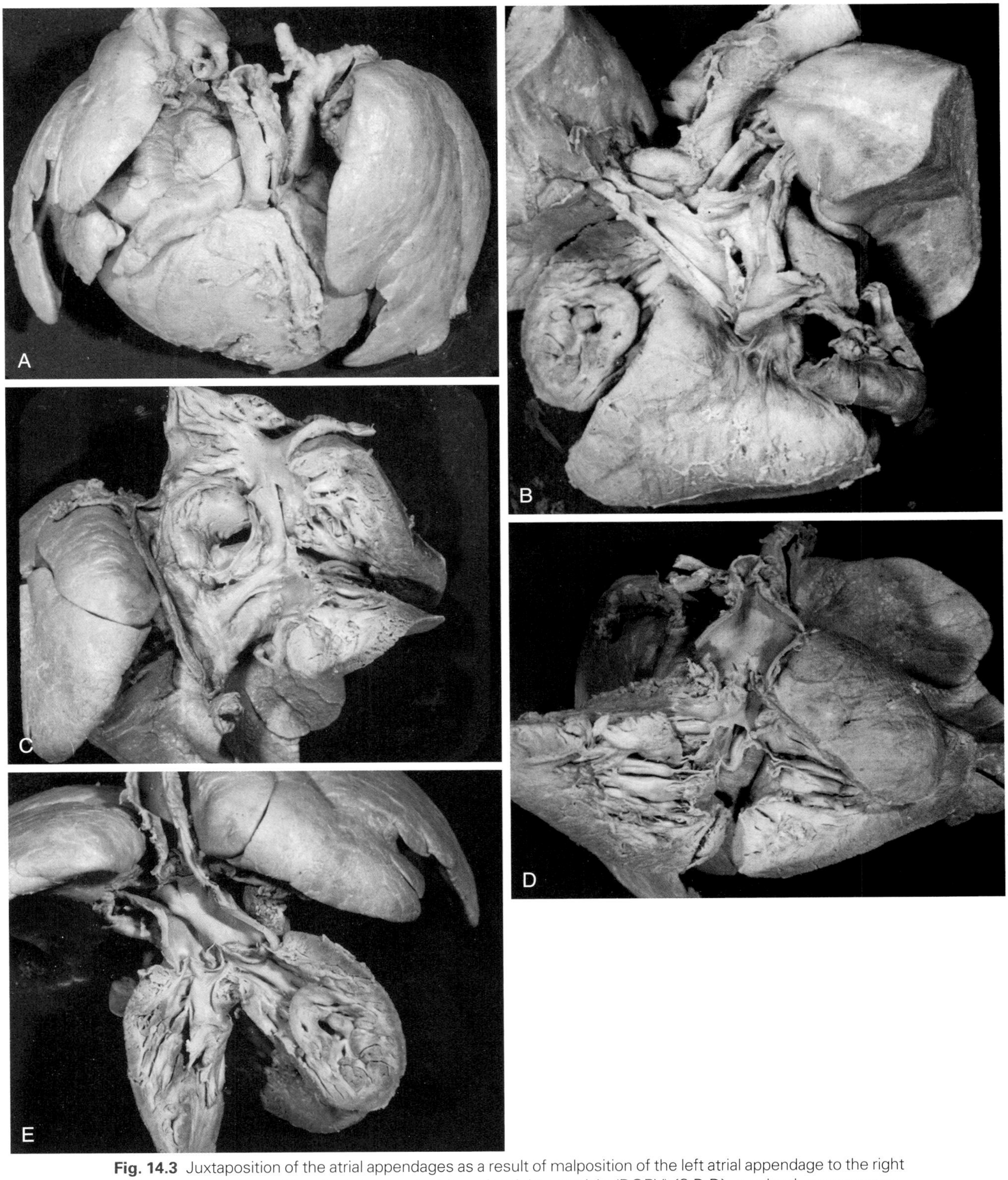

Fig. 14.3 Juxtaposition of the atrial appendages as a result of malposition of the left atrial appendage to the right of the great arteries, with mitral atresia, double-outlet right ventricle (DORV) {S,D,D}, a subpulmonary conus, marked hypoplasia of the aortic isthmus (coarctation of the aorta), PDA, and left subclavian artery arising from the top of the descending thoracic aorta. In A, note the long, thin left atrial appendage lying to the right of both great arteries. The hypoplasia of the distal aortic arch and the origin of the left subclavian artery are also seen. (B) The opened left atrium reveals mitral atresia, an interatrial communication, and normally connecting pulmonary veins. (C) The opened right heart reveals hypertrophy and enlargement of the right atrium and right ventricle. A relatively large ostium secundum type of ASD is due to marked deficiency of the septum primum, the flap valve of the foramen ovale. The tricuspid valve appears unremarkable. (D) The opened right ventricle showing aortic valve–to–tricuspid valve direct fibrous continuity. Subaortic stenosis was thought to be present. (E) The

Continued

Fig. 14.3 cont'd opened right ventricle showing a well-developed nonobstructive subpulmonary muscular conus (partially torn by artifact postmortem), pulmonary valve, and main pulmonary artery. A ductus arteriosus opens into the descending thoracic aorta. Note that there are two syndromes of juxtaposition of the atrial appendages (JAA).[30-32] When JAA involves malposition of the *morphologically left atrial appendage* (LAA) in visceroatrial situs solitus, as in this patient (A), the LAA lies to the *right* of both great arteries. But when JAA involves malposition of the LAA in visceroatrial situs inversus, the LAA lies to the *left* of both great arteries. JAA involving malposition of the LAA, both in visceroatrial situs solitus and in visceroatrial situs inversus, is associated with obstructive lesions of the *left* heart, such as mitral atresia, as in this patient.[31] However, when JAA involves malposition of the *morphologically right atrial appendage* (RAA) in visceroatrial situs solitus, the RAA lies to the *left* of both great arteries.[30,32] But when JAA involves malposition of the RAA in visceroatrial situs inversus, the RAA lies to the *right* of both great arteries. JAA involving malposition of the RAA, both in visceroatrial situs solitus and in visceroatrial situs inversus, is associated with obstructive lesions of the *right* heart, such as tricuspid atresia.[30,32] Thus, there are two keys to the understanding of JAA: (1) Morphologically, which atrial appendage is malpositioned, the RAA or the LAA? (2) What type of visceroatrial situs is present, situs solitus or situs inversus?[30-32] The sidedness of JAA (left-sided or right-sided) is independent of the type of ventricular loop that coexists. With JAA involving malposition of the LAA, the LAA is always superior to the RAA.[30-32]

From a therapeutic standpoint, several other points merit mention:

Because of the importance of narrowing or functional closure of the PDA in the disastrous natural history of this form of HLHS, it is important to know that *prostaglandin E1* can prevent the ductus arteriosus from closing. It is also important to know *not* to give oxygen to a neonate who may have HLHS, because "everything good" (e.g., oxygen) tends to close a PDA, whereas "everything bad" (e.g., hypoxemia) tends to open the neonatal ductus arteriosus. And therapeutically in this situation, one wants to keep the ductus arteriosus open, to avoid *functional "coarctation"* of the aorta.

Regarding the **coronary arteries** in this anatomic type of mitral atresia, the surgeon should know that the coronary arteries are usually normal, but not always. In the present series, an aberrant third coronary artery originated from the inferior surface of the proximal left pulmonary artery in 1 patient (1.25%; see Table 14.4), and an aberrant left circumflex coronary artery arose from the inferior surface of the proximal right pulmonary artery in 1 patient (1.25%; see Table 14.4). This aberrant left circumflex coronary artery was oversewn surgically, an important error.

Thus, the surgeon should resist the urge to "tidy things up" by interrupting such mysterious, small, unidentified arteries that course down to the heart from the proximal left or right pulmonary artery. It may be helpful to know that in sharks the coronary arteries arise from the branchial or gill arches[25] that correspond to the aortic arches in humans: the sixth aortic arches contribute to the pulmonary artery branches and the ductus arteriosi bilaterally. Thus, comparative anatomy[25] helps make coronary arteries arising from the proximal pulmonary artery branches comprehensible.

Aortic atresia can be valvar and subvalvar in this complex of anomalies, as was found in 9 patients (11.25%; see Table 14.4). What does this mean developmentally? We know that mitral valve tissue can become adherent to the left ventricular septal surface, resulting in severe fibrous subaortic stenosis.[26-28]

Indeed, we now think that **discrete fibrous subaortic stenosis** is really a mitral valve malformation, in the sense that this fibrous subaortic tissue appears to be "*un*tidied up" AV endocardial cushion tissue, intimately related to the mitral valve. This subaortic fibrous tissue may also help explain why there was no high (subaortic, conoventricular) type of VSD in this complex of anomalies. In our experience, typical fibrous subaortic stenosis always extends over onto the anterior mitral leaflet. This obstructive tissue always remains fibrous and never becomes muscular. If this subaortic tissue were conal (infundibular), it would become muscular. But it never does. Instead, fibrous subaortic stenosis appears to be fibroelastic AV endocardial cushion tissue, closely related to the mitral valve.

In this type of mitral atresia (see Table 14.4), the fibrous subaortic tissue can extend 2 or 3 mm below the atretic aortic valve. This important detail merits further study. We speculate that perhaps this totally obstructive subaortic fibrous tissue may be responsible for the atresia of the overlying aortic valve.

Does the combination of mitral atresia, intact ventricular septum, aortic valvar atresia, with normal {S,D,S} segmental anatomy usually occur in isolation, or is it often found with other multisystem congenital anomalies?

MCAs—meaning malformations of *other* organ systems in addition to the cardiovascular system—were present in 9 of those 80 patients (11.25%; see Table 14.4). The salient data may be summarized as follows:

Sex: Males, 4; females, 5; males to females = 4/5 (0.8:1.0).

Age at Death: Mean, 5.08 ± 6.57 days; range, 0 (spontaneous stillbirth) to 20 days of age; and median, 2.67 days.

Findings: The salient findings in these 9 patients with mitral atresia, intact ventricular septum, aortic valvar atresia, normal segmental anatomy {S,D,S}, and MCAs (polysystem malformations) are summarized in Table 14.5.

MORPHOGENESIS

What are the morphogenesis and etiology of the anomaly that we now call "mitral atresia"? I wish we knew, but at the present time we do not. However, the following thoughts and observations are recorded here in the hope that they may be of some assistance in solving this basic problem of causation.

Accurately speaking, I think that there is no such thing as "Ebstein anomaly" of the mitral valve, with downward

TABLE 14.5 Multiple Congenital Anomalies in Patients With Mitral Atresia, Intact Ventricular Septum, Aortic Valvar Atresia, and Normal Segmental Anatomy {S,D,S} (n = 9 of 80 [11.25%])

Case No.	Sex	Age at Death	Multiple Congenital Anomalies
1. Case 49	Male	2 days	Incompletely bilobed lungs bilaterally Normal karyotype, 46XY Abnormally formed left ear with absent antihelix and hypoplasia of tragus Webbed neck Clinodactyly Hyperextensible thumbs Sacral pit with hair Generalized hypotonia Small penis Microcephaly
2. Case 55	Female	6 days	Hydronephrosis, left-sided
3. Case 56	Male	Stillborn fetus	Asymmetrical face with frontal (not induced bossing abortion) Abnormal ears and toes Camptodactyly of hands, bilateral Hydronephrosis, bilateral Very small thymus (1/7 ± 3 g)
4. Case 69	Female	11 days	Pectus excavatum
5. Case 84	Female	1½ hours (0.0625 day)	Holoprosencephaly with agenesis of optic nerves Agenesis of olfactory tracts Hypotelorism with single orbit Microphthalmia Single naris Choanal atresia Microstomia Narrow palate Low-set ears Short neck Polydactyly of hands and feet Camptodactyly Abnormal vertebral ossification Duodenal stenosis Double vagina, cervix, and uterus Presacral teratoma Right simian crease
6. Case 138	Female	1 day	Right cleft lip + palate Normal karyotype, 46XX (Paternal cleft lip and palate)
7. Case 150	Female	2.67 days	Supernumerary fissure, right upper lobe of lung Double left renal artery Bifid uvula
8. Case 162	Male	3 days	Male pseudohermaphrodite with relatively large phallus Undescended testes Vagina-like structure Uterus-like structure
9. Case 178	Male	20 days	Prominent helix, right ear Dysplastic toe nails Sacral dimple History of both parents with congenital deafness, patient's father with fourth-generation Waardenburg syndrome

displacement of the septal (anterior) leaflet, without downward displacement of the free wall (or posterior) leaflet, and with an associated left ventricular myocardial deficiency or absence.

Atretic Ebstein anomaly, often called "imperforate" Ebstein malformation, is the only *real* form of tricuspid atresia, as explained in Chapter 13. What I mean is that typical so-called **tricuspid atresia,** of the "muscular" sort, appears to represent a failure of the right ventricular sinus (inflow tract) to develop; that is, typical tricuspid atresia does not appear to be primarily a tricuspid valve problem. Instead, it looks like a right ventricular inflow tract (right ventricular sinus) abnormality, in which both the right ventricular sinus and the tricuspid valve have failed to develop.

In typical tricuspid atresia, the expected site of the tricuspid valve and orifice often is located directly above the posterior portion of the muscular ventricular septum. In other words, *ventriculoatrial malalignment* appears to be very important in the morphogenesis of tricuspid atresia. Why is the posterior part of the ventricular septum right beneath the expected site of the tricuspid valve? We think that the answer is because the right ventricular sinus (inflow tract) is very underdeveloped. When the right ventricular sinus develops and expands normally, the ventricular septum moves further leftward, making it possible for the tricuspid valve to open into the right ventricular sinus. This is our best present hypothesis concerning the morphogenesis of tricuspid atresia, which is based on the pathologic anatomic findings of a very small or absent right ventricular sinus and ventricular septum underlying and blocking the tricuspid orifice.

Mitral atresia, so-called, appears to be similar. Underdevelopment or even absence of the morphologically LV may well be the main problem, with failure of the mitral valve to develop normally and with ventriculoatrial malalignment.

In so-called mitral atresia, what one does *not* see is very impressive. We have never seen an essentially normal looking mitral valve, but with its leaflet margins fused together and, hence, no mitral orifice. Only in a minority of cases (14/80, 17.5%; see Table 14.4) did we find some membranous tissue in the expected site of the mitral valve. Typically, the floor of the LA was muscular (not membranous) where the mitral valve "should" have been. In only 2 of 80 patients did we find an atretic parachute mitral valve—with all chordae tendineae inserting into one small papillary muscle (2.5%). Why was the LV very hypoplastic or absent in the typical case? Two hypotheses suggest themselves:

1. Perhaps the problem is **"primary" underdevelopment of the LV** from the ventricle of the bulboventricular loop, probably for genetic reasons.
2. Or possibly **the ventricular loop is malaligned relative to the atria and the AV canal.** Bearing in mind that the ventricular loop is "a professional contortionist"—undergoing complex morphogenetic movements in the process of D-loop (or L-loop) formation (see Chapter 2)—**VA malalignment** could narrow or occlude what normally would be the mitral orifice. For example, in visceroatrial situs solitus, if the ventricular D-loop becomes *right-shifted* relative to the atria and the AV canal, this might place the developing left ventricular free wall directly beneath the expected site of the mitral orifice, thereby narrowing or occluding what normally would be the mitral orifice. *Rightward malalignment* of the ventricular loop relative to the AV canal and the atria during the complex process of ventricular loop formation may explain both the hypoplasia or the apparent absence of the LV and the absence of a mitral orifice in the anomaly known as mitral atresia. If mitral atresia were primarily a problem of the mitral valve, one would expect that there would be an anomaly known as "imperforate mitral valve," but that is not what one typically finds in so-called mitral atresia.

It should be understood that I am not trying to change our conventional diagnostic terminology; instead, I hope to deepen anatomic and developmental understanding. In attempting to solve the important problems of morphogenesis and etiology, it is helpful to understand where the basic anomaly is located. In mitral atresia, I suspect that the mitral valve may be the victim, not the perpetrator. This possibility will become even more persuasive when we consider mitral atresia with a large or single LV (see later).

MITRAL ATRESIA {S,D,S}, INTACT VENTRICULAR SEPTUM, AND PATENT AORTIC VALVE

This anatomic type of mitral atresia is the same as the previous one, except that the aortic valve is patent, rather than atretic (see Table 14.2, anatomic type 2, and Fig. 14.1, anatomic type 2). The hypoplastic aortic valve is often called *congenital aortic stenosis,* even though no anterograde aortic blood flow goes through the typically small aortic valve because of the coexistence of mitral atresia and an intact ventricular septum. This anatomic type of mitral atresia was found in only 2 of 177 postmortem cases (1.13%; see Table 14.2).

Thus, when mitral atresia is associated with an intact ventricular septum and normal segmental anatomy (n = 82; see Table 14.2), the aortic valve is almost always atretic (80/82 cases, 97.5%; see Table 14.2 and Fig. 14.1). Only in a very small minority of patients is the aortic valve patent but hypoplastic, as in this anatomic type of mitral atresia (2/177 patients, 1.13%; see Table 14.2 and Fig. 14.1).

Because there is no obvious hemodynamic difference between mitral atresia {S,D,S} with intact ventricular septum, and aortic valvar *atresia* (n = 80 patients; see Table 14.2) and mitral atresia {S,D,S} with intact ventricular septum, and aortic valvar *hypoplasia* (n = 2 patients; see Table 14.2), both of these anatomic types of mitral atresia could be lumped together as mitral atresia {S,D,S}, intact ventricular septum, and aortic valvar atresia or hypoplasia (see Table 14.2 and Fig. 14.1). In our experience, this was by far the largest anatomic type of mitral atresia (82/177 cases, 46.33%; see Table 14.2 and Fig. 14.1).

Anatomic Findings

The salient anatomic findings in these 2 rare cases of mitral atresia with normal {S,D,S} segmental anatomy, intact ventricular septum, and aortic valvar patency and hypoplasia may be summarized as follows:

Sex: Male, 1; female, 1; and male to female = 1/1 = 1.

Age at Death: Mean, 302.5 ± 427.80 days, ranging from 0 days (a 22-week abortus) to 605 days (1 8/12 years), and median,

302.5 days (10.08 months, or 10 months and 2 days). These statistics are included only as data. They are thought to have no statistical significance because of the very small size of this group (n = 2).

Because this rare anatomic subset of mitral atresia consists of only 2 cases, each will be summarized individually.

Case 45 was a 1 8/12-year-old boy who died in 1986. Mitral atresia occurred with normal {S,D,S} segmental anatomy. At autopsy, the ventricular septum was intact; however, a jet lesion involving the left ventricular apex suggested that an old apical muscular VSD had been present at some time before death but had undergone spontaneous closure. Hence, at autopsy, the ventricular septum was found to be intact. The left ventricular papillary muscles were absent. The aortic valve was bicuspid (more accurately, bicommissural), because the intercoronary commissure was absent. Although bicommissural, valvar aortic stenosis was thought not to be present. Left atrial hypertrophy was present, without enlargement. A patent foramen ovale was thought to be restrictive. The RA was both hypertrophied and enlarged. A rete Chiari was present in the RA because of the presence of a prominent right venous valve remnant. Although morphologically unremarkable, tricuspid regurgitation had been documented both angiocardiographically and echocardiographically (two-dimensional echo). Right ventricular hypertrophy and enlargement were massive. A discrete juxtaductal coarctation of the aorta was found, associated with hypoplasia of the aortic arch between the innominate and the left common carotid arteries, the internal diameter of this portion of the aortic arch measuring 3 mm. A restrictive PDA was also present. Hydronephrosis of the right kidney was an associated anomaly.

From a therapeutic standpoint, this boy underwent a modified Norwood procedure (i.e., a stage 1 palliation of HLHS) at 21 days of age. A 10-mm Gore-Tex tube was placed between the proximal main pulmonary artery (MPA) and the distal aortic arch where it merges into the descending thoracic aorta. Pulmonary arterial blood flow was supplied by a modified Blalock-Taussig anastomosis using a 4-mm Gore-Tex conduit.

The unreconstructed transverse aortic arch, with an internal diameter of only 3 mm, became important after spontaneous closure of the apical muscular VSD. After VSD closure, all of the blood flow to the innominate artery, the pulmonary arteries, and the coronary arteries had to pass through the hypoplastic (3-mm internal diameter) transverse aortic arch. The patient died suddenly at home at 1 8/12 years of age.

Case 127 was a female fetus, aborted at 22 weeks gestational age. Again, the salient anatomic findings were mitral atresia, normal segmental anatomy {S,D,S}, and an intact ventricular septum. There was premature closure of the foramen ovale. Left ventricular hypoplasia was moderate, and the left ventricular papillary muscles were absent. The aortic valve was hypoplastic but patent, with severe congenital aortic hypoplasia, the orifice being only 1 mm in diameter. Right atrial hypertrophy and enlargement, with very marked right ventricular hypertrophy and enlargement, and a moderate-sized PDA were also found.

This fetus had MCAs. The right lung displayed abnormal lobation with partially anomalous pulmonary venous connection of the scimitar syndrome type. The right pulmonary veins did not connect with the LA. Instead, the right pulmonary veins left an abnormal and large lateral lobe of the right lung and coursed downward, passing through the right leaf of the diaphragm and into the abdomen. The precise connection of this anomalous right pulmonary vein within the abdomen was not described (because the autopsy was limited to the thorax). Nonetheless, this fetus was thought to have the scimitar syndrome with the characteristically anomalous right pulmonary venous connection and drainage.

The right lung had a very small upper lobe, a large lower lateral lobe, and a smaller medial lobe. No anomalous pulmonary arterial supply to the right lung was described. So this fetus had **MCAs** with normal cardiac segmental anatomy, mitral atresia, intact ventricular septum, severe congenital aortic valvar "stenosis" (hypoplasia), the scimitar syndrome, and a dysmorphic spleen with a downward dangling "tail."

Familial HLHS was also found in this patient's family. Two previous female infants had autopsy-proved diagnoses of HLHS. Our present patient, this 22-week-old aborted fetus, was the third female infant with a definite diagnosis of HLHS. The first sibling died at 4 days of age in 1978. The second died at 3½ weeks of age in 1981. Our patient died in 1984. It is noteworthy that a normal *male* infant was born to this family in 1979. Some of the father's siblings have or had congenital heart disease; no other details are known to us. The history suggests that familial HLHS may have been inherited from the father. Be that as it may, this case history appears definitely to document that **familial HLHS can and does occur.**

MITRAL ATRESIA {S,D,S}, VENTRICULAR SEPTAL DEFECT(S), AND PATENT AORTIC VALVE

Mitral atresia occurred with normal segmental anatomy, that is, {S,D,S}, VSD(s), and a patent aortic valve in 27 of these 177 postmortem cases, 15.25%, anatomic type 3; see Table 14.2 and Fig. 14.1. Thus, when the aortic valve is patent in association with mitral atresia, it is much more usual for one or more VSDs to be present than for the ventricular septum to be intact (15.25% versus 1.13%, respectively; see Table 14.2). This anatomic type of mitral atresia makes up 22.88% of patients with mitral atresia and normal segmental anatomy (27/118) (see Fig. 14.1).

Sex: Males, 11; females, 16, male to females = 0.6875.

Age: The age at autopsy in these 27 patients was: Mean, 127.023 ± 383.420 days, or 4.23 ± 12.78 months; range, 0 to 1825 days, or 0 days (stillborn) to 5 years; and median, 9 days.

Again, the *median* age at death (9 days) is thought to reflect the highly lethal nature of this subset of mitral atresia better than does the mean age ± the standard deviation (4.23 ± 12.87 months).

Salient Anatomic Features

What were these 27 cases of mitral atresia with normal segmental anatomy, one or more VSDs, and a patent aortic valve really like? First of all, it will be appreciated that this group is hemodynamically the opposite of the previous much larger group (n = 80 patients, 45% of all of our cases of mitral atresia; see Table 14.2, item 1, and Fig. 14.1, item 1) in the sense that when the aortic valve is patent, blood can flow in an anterograde (normal) direction in the ascending aorta, whereas when the aortic valve is atretic, the blood must flow in a retrograde ("backward") direction to perfuse the coronary arteries and the brachiocephalic arteries. In this hemodynamic sense, the present group is very different from the previous one.

Atrial Septum. The typical finding was a well-formed atrial septum that was obstructive to left-to-right atrial shunting necessitated by mitral atresia. The worst case was *premature closure of the foramen ovale,* resulting in an intact or impervious atrial septum, that we found in 3 of these 27 patients (11.1%; Cases 71, 92, and 118). However, in a few patients, the atrial septum was not at all obstructive to left-to-right shunting at the atrial level.

Common atrium was found in 1 patient (1/27 = 3.7%; Case 66) who also had MCAs that included Meckel diverticulum, tracheo-esophageal fistula with esophageal atresia, duodenal atresia, a web at the ampulla of Vater, a two-vessel umbilical cord, low-set ears, and a vertebral anomaly (T8 was bifid because of an incompletely fused vertebral body).

The incomplete form of common AV canal with mitral atresia occurred in 1 patient (3.7%; Case 66), who also had MCAs that included Meckel diverticulum, tracheo-esophageal fistula with esophageal atresia, duodenal atresia, a web at the ampulla of Vater, a two-vessel umbilical cord, low-set ears, and a vertebral anomaly: T8 was bifid because of an incompletely fused vertebral body.

The incomplete form of common AV canal with mitral atresia occurred in 1 patient (3.7%; Case 154). The ostium primum type of AV septal defect (also known as an incomplete AV septal defect) was huge and almost constituted a common atrium.

A septum primum malposition ASD[29] was found in 2 of these 27 patients (7.4%; Cases 169 and 170; see Fig. 14.3). The septum primum (the flap valve of the foramen ovale) was normally attached inferiorly. But the superior rim of the septum primum was displaced far to the left, into the LA. Consequently, the septum primum had an abnormally horizontal lie and leftward displacement into the LA. Because the superior limbic band of septum secundum was normally located between the "roof" of the right and left atria, and because the superior edge of the septum primum was displaced abnormally far to the left, the superior edge of the septum primum could not close against the superior limbic band of septum secundum in the normal way. This inability of the septum primum to occlude the interatrial communication and to prevent left-to-right atrial shunting we have called a *septum primum malposition type of ASD*[29] (see Fig. 14.3).

It should be understood that a septum primum malposition ASD is different from the much more common secundum type of ASD. The usual type of ostium secundum ASD is caused by deficiencies of septum primum (the atrial septal "door"), deficiency of the superior limbic band of septum secundum (the "door jamb"), or both. However, in a secundum ASD, the septum primum, or its remnant, is normally located. Not so in a septum primum malposition ASD, in which septum primum is approximately horizontal, not approximately vertical (which, of course, is normal) (see Fig. 14.3). Septum primum malposition defect is often associated with HLHS,[29] as in these two patients, whereas the typical secundum ASD can be associated with "anything."

Case 169, an 11-day-old girl with a septum primum malposition ASD, had a large dysmorphic mass involving the inferior limbic band that measured 9 mm in length, 7 mm in width, and 11 mm in height. The tricuspid valve was dysmorphic and displayed tricuspid regurgitation. The tricuspid leaflets were myxomatous, and there were multiple blood cysts involving the tricuspid leaflets.

The other patient with septum primum malposition ASD, Case 170 (a 22½-month-old boy), did *not* have an additional anomaly of the inferior limbic band of septum secundum—from which the septum primum develops and normally grows upward[15]—and no additional anomaly of the tricuspid valve. Consequently, we think that this abnormally leftward and horizontal lie of the septum primum (see Fig. 14.3), resulting in an uncloseable interatrial communication, is not necessarily associated with additional demonstrable malformations of the inferior limbic band and/or of the tricuspid valve.

Malposition of the septum primum into the LA[29] is often better seen echocardiographically (see Fig. 14.3) than anatomically (see Fig. 14.2D) because echocardiographically there is no spatial distortion that may be associated with organ removal and positioning for photography. In this apical four-chamber view (see Fig. 14.3), note that the inferior origin of the septum primum is normally located. But what is normally the more superior portion of the septum primum is instead displaced far to the left into the LA. The septum primum is almost horizontally oriented. It is malpositioned to the left of both the right and left pulmonary veins, resulting in totally anomalous pulmonary venous *drainage* into the RA and then into the right ventricle (see Fig. 14.3). The pulmonary veins are normally *connected* to the LA.

This patient did *not* have mitral atresia. The diagnosis in this 2½-year-old boy was tetralogy of Fallot (TOF) {S,D,S} with totally anomalous pulmonary venous drainage to the RA. The malpositioned and approximately horizontally oriented septum primum can simulate and be mistaken for a supramitral stenosing membrane with common atrium (see Fig. 14.3).

Right-sided juxtaposition of the atrial appendages[30-32] has recently been described as juxtaposition of the atrial appendages to the right of both great arteries because of rightward malposition of the LAA[31] (Fig. 14.4), that occurred in only 1 of these 23 patients with mitral atresia (3.7%; Case 104). The latter designation specifies that it was malposition of the morphologically LAA to the right of the great arteries that resulted in juxtaposition of the atrial appendages. In this study we encountered no patients with the more common form of juxtaposition of the atrial appendages caused by malposition of the morphologically right atrial appendage (RAA) to the left of the great arteries.[32]

I have very recently realized that the aforementioned descriptions[31,32] of the atrial appendages as *malpositions* relative to the great arteries in juxtaposition of the atrial appendages (JAA) is, in fact, wrong. The morphologically RAA or the morphologically LAA are not malpositioned, of necessity, in JAA. The appendages *can be* malpositioned, but that is not the essence of JAA. Instead, the atrial appendages in JAA are more like "innocent bystanders," that is, essentially normal. *The appearance of*

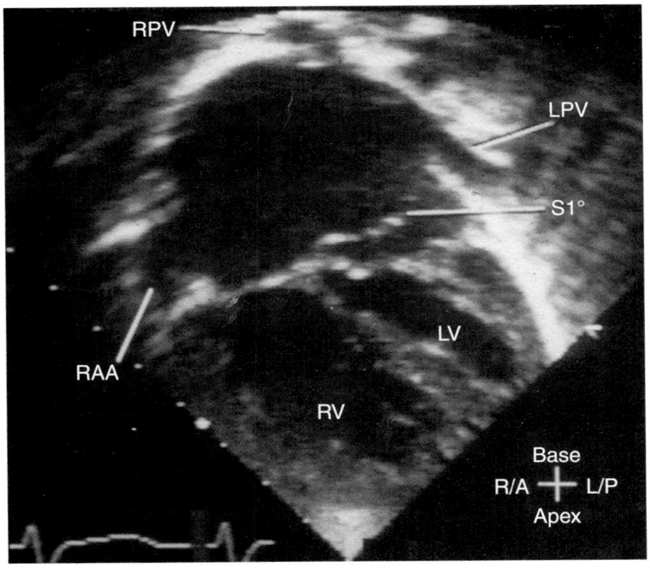

Fig. 14.4 Marked leftward malposition of septum *(S1°)* resulting in supramitral stenosis and in totally anomalous pulmonary venous drainage into the right atrium (RA). Both the left pulmonary vein *(LPV)* and the right pulmonary vein *(RPV)* are normally connected to the left atrium (LA), but both drain anomalously into the RA because of the marked leftward malposition of S1°. This is an apical four-chamber view of the heart of a 2-year-old infant with an interrupted inferior vena cava with atrial situs solitus, D-loop ventricles, and solitus normally related great arteries with tetralogy of Fallot. The segmental anatomy was normal, that is, {S,D,S}. Note that the superior limbic band appears to be absent. Hence, the septum primum had nothing to attach to superiorly, which may explain why the septum primum was so markedly levopositioned. There were multiple fenestrations in the septum primum. This echocardiographic picture may suggest the erroneous diagnosis of common atrium with a supramitral membrane. Marked leftward malposition of septum occurs predominantly in patients with the heterotaxy syndrome, usually with polysplenia. *LV,* left ventricle; *RAA,* right atrial appendage; *RV,* right ventricle. (Reproduced with permission from Van Praagh S, Carrera ME, Sanders SP, Mayer JE, Van Praagh R. Partial or total direct pulmonary venous drainage to right atrium due to malposition of septum primum: Anatomic and echocardiographic findings and surgical treatment—a study based on 36 cases. *Chest.* 107:1488, 1995.)

JAA is produced by abnormal ventricular morphogenetic movement. With solitus atria and D-loop ventricles, that is {S,D,-}, normal D-loop formation is "a two-step dance." *Step one:* the straight heart tube loops to the right, forming a ventricular D-loop. *Step two:* the ventricles swing horizontally from right to left, passing from dextrocardia, through mesocardia, to normal definitive levocardia.

In the normal human embryo at 23 days of age in utero, the conotruncus lies to the right of both atrial appendages; that is, left-sided JAA is normally present.[30] By 27 days of age, the ventricles have swung far enough leftward so that the conotruncus, mounted atop the ventricles, now runs between the RAA and the LAA, thereby "curing" the left-sided JAA.[30] Thus, a subnormal step 2—a deficient right-to-left swing of the ventricles—results in left-sided JAA. A supernormal or excessive step 2 appears to result in right-sided JAA. *Left-sided JAA typically has a hypoplastic right heart syndrome.*[30,31] *Right-sided JAA* often has HLHS.[32]

In the conventional description of JAA, the "malpositioned" atrial appendage is the atrial appendage that is adjacent to (closer to) the great arteries. In the conventional description of JAA, the *adjacent* atrial appendage is considered to be malpositioned *relative to* the great arteries, and *relative malposition* of the adjacent atrial appendage is indeed present.

However, as suggested earlier, a more basic understanding of JAA is now considered to be that the atrial appendages are essentially normal and can serve as markers of deficient or excessive ventricular movement during development.

Is *HLHS,* often with a hypertrophied and enlarged LV, responsible for subnormal ventricular right-to-left movement, resulting in left-sided JAA? Is *HLHS,* with a hypertrophied and enlarged RV, responsible for excessive ventricular right-to-left movement, resulting in right-sided JAA? *These findings suggest that right ventricular development may be very important in ventricular right-to-left movement:*

1. When there is a hypoplastic right heart syndrome with a normal or hypertrophied LV, right-to-left movement is deficient, indicated by left-sided JAA in which both great arteries remain to the right of both atrial appendages.
2. When HLHS is present, with a normal or hypertrophied RV, ventricular right-to-left movement is excessive, as is indicated by right-side JAA, in which both great arteries have been carried to the left of both atrial appendages.

These observations suggest that right ventricular development may be very important in normal right-to-left movement of the ventricles, that is, in step 2 of the normal ventricular D-loop "dance."

In addition, both left-sided JAA and right-sided JAA are syndromes, because of their characteristic and opposite associations[30-32]:

1. left-sided JAA and the hypoplastic right heart syndrome; and
2. right-sided JAA and HLHS.

Case 104 was a 19-day-old girl, a nonidentical twin, with MCAs, including epicanthal folds, hypertelorism, a cervical rib, and a bifid spleen. The other twin had a cleft palate and hare lip. As will become increasingly apparent, *MCAs* are an important reality in patients with this type of mitral atresia (see later).

Totally anomalous pulmonary venous connection (TAPVC) is potentially another way of avoiding the deleterious hemodynamic consequences of a normally formed and, hence, obstructive atrial septum leading to pulmonary venous congestion and low cardiac output postnatally. There were only 2 such cases in these 27 patients (7.4%; see Table 14.2, anatomic type 3):

Case 144 was a 1-day-old boy with a TAPVC to the left innominate vein and then to the RSVC and RA. This, the classic "snowman" type of supracardiac TAPVC, did not have anatomic evidence of obstruction. This newborn boy also had a secundum type of ASD because of a deficient septum primum. The PDA was large. Why, then, did this patient die at only 1 day (30 hours) of age? He also had severe unicuspid aortic valvar stenosis with an aortic valvar orifice of only 1 to 1.5 mm in diameter.

Case 76, the second patient, had TAPVC to the coronary sinus, also without anatomically evident pulmonary venous stenosis. This 15-day-old boy had **absence of the morphologically LA. To my knowledge, absence of the LA is a previously unknown and undescribed form of congenital heart disease.**

Using loupes, we searched unsuccessfully for any evidence of the LA. No patent foramen ovale or fossa ovalis was found.

In view of the rarity of this anomaly—**absence of the LA**—this heart merits detailed, individual description: mitral atresia; {S,D,S}; moderate left ventricular hypoplasia; two VSDs, a small membranous VSD and a large apical muscular VSD; a hypoplastic bicuspid aortic valve with a rudimentary right coronary–noncoronary (RC/NC) commissure; preductal coarctation of the aorta; right atrial hypertrophy and enlargement; a morphologically normally formed tricuspid valve, but with cardiac catheterization evidence of tricuspid regurgitation and with anatomic confirmation of regurgitation in the form of thickening and rolling of the free margins of the anterior and septal tricuspid leaflets; right ventricular hypertrophy and enlargement; and a PDA. (It should be understood that virtually all patients with mitral atresia and {S,D,S} have right atrial and right ventricular hypertrophy and enlargement.)

Therapeutically, in 1987, this patient (Case 76) at 4 days of age had a subclavian flap angioplasty for coarctation of the aorta, ligation of the PDA, and banding of the MPA. Because of a persisting coarctation gradient, at 15 days of age the patient underwent a modified Damus-Kaye-Stansel procedure in which a 6-mm Gore-Tex tube graft was placed between the proximal MPA and the descending thoracic aorta. Death occurred 6½ hours postoperatively.

Based on our experience with fetal and postnatal congenital heart disease, we now think that **all cardiac chambers can be absent, except the morphologically RA.** We have never seen or heard of a case in which the RA was absent. Because the RA is in part the systemic venous confluence forming the first cardiac chamber, we think that an RA is essential to the existence of a heart with a systemic circulation.

Partially anomalous pulmonary venous connection was found in 4 of these 27 patients (see Table 14.2, anatomic type 3; Cases 18, 64, 121, and 122).

In **Case 18,** a 6-day-old girl, all of the left upper lobe drained anomalously to the RA via a "snowman" pathway (left vertical vein to left innominate vein to RSVC). The right lung drained normally to the LA and anomalously to the RSVC. There was incomplete incorporation of the common pulmonary vein into the LA, but without stenosis of the common pulmonary vein.

This patient also had *MCAs* with a mongoloid slant of the eyes, an increased carrying angle of the arms, a shield-shaped chest, widely spaced nipples, and pectus excavatum.

In addition, this family exemplified *familial congenital heart disease.* This patient's older brother died at 4 9/12 years of age in 1970, and autopsy revealed an incomplete form of common AV canal with a large ostium primum type of ASD (the most common type of incomplete AV septal defect), no VSD of the AV canal type, congenital mitral stenosis with a rudimentary mitral valve with a diminutive cleft of the anterior mitral leaflet, thickening and rolling of the free margins of the anterior and septal leaflets of the tricuspid valve consistent with tricuspid regurgitation, right atrial hypertrophy and enlargement (marked), right ventricular hypertrophy and enlargement, and dilatation of the MPA. Thus, not only did this family display familial congenital heart disease but also the anatomic types of congenital heart disease were similar: mitral atresia in our 6-day-old female patient (Case 18) and a very severe congenital mitral stenosis in her 4 9/12-year-old brother.

Case 64 was a 9-day-old girl with *scimitar syndrome.* All of the right pulmonary venous blood coursed through and below the diaphragm in a vein that connected with the ductus venosus. An anomalous systemic artery passed upward through the diaphragm and supplied the lower right lung. And there was sequestration of the right lung. Once again there were *MCAs,* in addition to the right pulmonary sequestration, including accessory spleens or polysplenia (one large spleen and seven splenuli), bilaterally unilobed lungs, and a bicornuate uterus with a continuous vaginal septum.

Case 121 was a 2-day-old boy with a partially anomalous pulmonary venous connection: a very small pulmonary vein (internal diameter = 1 mm) ran from the hilum of the right lung to the RSVC, slightly above the connection of the azygos vein. This patient was premature (36 weeks estimated gestational age, birth weight 1870 g or 4.12 lb), and an "identical" twin. The co-twin was a normal boy. This family was also afflicted with *familial congenital heart disease.* An older brother, 2 years old, had a VSD with mild pulmonary valvar stenosis. This older brother was also a twin, the co-twin being stillborn.

Case 122 was a stillborn female fetus who underwent a spontaneous intrauterine death at an estimated gestational age of 32 to 34 weeks, with a weight of 1900 g (4.19 lb). This patient was also considered to have a partially anomalous pulmonary venous connection. The right pulmonary veins connected normally with the LA. The left lung was markedly hypoplastic, and *no* left pulmonary veins were found at autopsy. In other words, no left pulmonary veins connected with the LA or with any other site. *The left pulmonary veins were considered to be absent.* Note that *absence* of the left pulmonary veins is different from a partially anomalous pulmonary venous connection. Here we are dealing with *a partially anomalous pulmonary venous nonconnection.* The problem is that the finding of **partial absence of the pulmonary veins** is very rare and does not fit into the widely used classification of totally[33] and partially anomalous pulmonary venous connections. I cannot remember ever having seen another such case. This finding is exceedingly rare and perhaps unique. However, this case of absence of the left pulmonary veins did *not* occur in isolation. Absence of the left pulmonary veins was associated with marked hypoplasia of the left lung, probably a very important additional fact.

This patient also had *MCAs* (marked hypoplasia of the left lung, as earlier). *Left ventricular hypoplasia* was the rule in association with mitral atresia and VSD (see Table 14.2, anatomic type 3). *Absence of tensor apparatus* (no mitral chordae tendineae and no left ventricular papillary muscles) was specifically described in 8 of these 27 patients (29.63%). Hypoplastic left ventricular papillary muscles were described in 3 patients (11.11%). Therefore, the status of the mitral tensor apparatus was variable.

One or more *VSDs* were present in all 27 patients. A single VSD was present in 16 of 27 cases (59.26%), and multiple VSDs were found in 11 (40.74%). The anatomic types of VSD were as follows:

1. conoventricular, 15 of 27 (55.56%);
2. muscular, 11 of 27 (40.74%); and
3. AV canal type, 2 of 27 (7.41%).

The aortic valve, although patent, was frequently hypoplastic and *bicuspid* (15/27 patients, 55.56%); more accurately, it was often *bicommissural* because of the deficiency or absence of one commissure. Typically with bicommissural aortic valves, all three leaflets were present anatomically, but functionally such aortic valves have only two functioning leaflets.

The number of well-developed commissures equals the number of functional leaflets[28]:

1. A bicommissural aortic valve is a functionally bicuspid aortic valve.
2. A unicommissural aortic valve is a functionally unicuspid aortic valve.
3. When no well-developed commissure is present, such an aortic valve typically is atretic, with no functional aortic valve leaflet(s). Rarely, however, it is possible to have an acommissural aortic valve with hypoplastic ("stenotic") aortic leaflets and a patent aortic valvar orifice. In such a rare patient, as was presented previously, attempted balloon dilation of the aortic valve led to tearing of the unsupported aortic leaflets, followed by aortic valvar regurgitation.

Which aortic valve commissure was deficient or absent was recorded in 12 of these 15 cases of bicommissural aortic valve:

1. The RC/LC commissure was deficient or absent in 6 of 12 patients (50%).
2. The RC/NC commissure was deficient or absent in 3 of 12 cases (25%).
3. The LC/NC commissure was deficient or absent in 3 of 12 patients (25%).

A unicuspid aortic valve with only one well-developed commissure was described in only 2 of these 27 patients (7.41%; see Table 14.2, anatomic type 3). The commissures were described in only one of these two patients (Case 10): The RC/LC commissure was well formed, whereas the LC/NC and the RC/NC commissures were rudimentary.

Note that surgical and pathology reports of abnormal aortic valves should always describe the status of the commissures specifically, as earlier, making it possible for others to understand the precise anatomic abnormality. Statements such as "the aortic valve is bicuspid," or "the aortic valve is unicuspid" leave one wondering, What exactly is wrong with the aortic valve? Which commissure(s) is (are) absent? For clarity, anatomic descriptions must be specific. Specific description of the commissural anatomy revealed that deficiency or absence of the intercoronary commissure (RC/LC) was twice as common a cause of bicuspid aortic valve as were the other two possible types of commissural deficiency (RC/NC and LC/NC) in this subset of mitral atresia (see Table 14.2, anatomic type 3).

In the area of improving diagnostic and surgical reports concerning congenital heart disease department, **the anatomic type of conus (infundibulum)** also always should be described specifically. Was it **subpulmonary,** with aortic–AV valvar fibrous continuity? Was it **subaortic,** with pulmonary–AV valvar fibrous continuity? Was it **bilateral,** that is, subaortic and subpulmonary, with no semilunar–AV valvar fibrous continuity? Or was it bilaterally **absent or very deficient** with bilateral semilunar–AV valvar fibrous continuity? The conus is the often "forgotten," but very important connecting segment between the great arteries and the ventricles.[34] The conus is part of the great arteries (not part of either ventricle), which is why it is known developmentally as the **conotruncal segment.** The conus plays a key role in determining the definitive ventriculoarterial (VA) alignments and connections, both normally and abnormally. This is why the conus merits careful study and specific description.[34]

Subaortic stenosis was diagnosed in 5 of these 27 patients (18.52%). Further description in 2 of these patients indicated that *posterior malalignment* of the conal septum compressed or "squeezed" the immediately subaortic outflow tract. Not included in this estimate of subaortic stenosis (5 patients, 18.52%) is the probable role of a restrictively small VSD(s). Suffice it to say that we regard this statistic (18.52%) to be a significant underestimate of the true incidence of subaortic stenosis from all causes. This impression is heightened by the much higher prevalence of preductal coarctation.

Preductal coarctation of the aorta[35] was found in 12 of these 27 patients (44.44%) with this variety of mitral atresia; see Table 14.2, anatomic type 3). Preductal coarctation of the aorta (isthmic hypoplasia) is considered to result from a reduction in anterograde aortic blood flow, which in turn points to the hemodynamic importance of mitral atresia, restrictively small VSD(s), subaortic stenosis, and aortic valvar stenosis. There was also 1 patient with *interruption of the aortic arch type B*[36] (between the left common carotid and the left subclavian arteries). If one includes this case, the incidence of preductal coarctation of the aorta and interruption of the aortic arch becomes 13 of those 27 patients (48.15%).

Hence, these data suggest that at least half of these patients with mitral atresia (see Table 14.2, item 3) suffered from significantly reduced anterograde aortic blood flow. None had pulmonary outflow tract obstruction (stenosis or atresia). However, two patients (Cases 77 and 98) did have a bicuspid (bicommissural) pulmonary valve.

Case 77 was a 4-day-old boy with trisomy 18 (karyotype proved). He had typical polyvalvar disease with redundant pulmonary leaflets. **Case 98,** a 2-day-old boy, had MCAs, including a tracheo-esophageal fistula, bilateral cryptorchidism, malrotation of the intestines, Meckel diverticulum, dilatation of the ureters and hypertrophy of the bladder (posterior urethral valves or other obstruction not described), kernicterus (without jaundice), and intrauterine growth failure (birth weight at term = 4 lb 6 oz). *Both semilunar valves were bicuspid.* The aortic valve had a rudimentary LC/NC commissure. The pulmonary valve's commissural anatomy was not described.

Although there was typically a large PDA, it was described as functionally closing in 7 of these 27 patients (25.93%). This, too, may be a significant underestimate. Narrowing or closure of a PDA in a patient with mitral atresia can be the immediate cause of death. This is true if the ductus arteriosus is the main, or the only, pathway for anterograde blood flow to the lower body or to the entire systemic arterial circulation. In this hemodynamic situation, narrowing or closure of the ductus arteriosus is equivalent to an acute coarctation of the aorta, or to complete interruption of the descending thoracic aorta. Normal ductal narrowing or closure in this situation is a hemodynamic disaster.

A persistent LSVC opened into the coronary sinus and then into the RA in 5 of these 27 patients (18.52%).

Absence of the right atrial ostium of the coronary sinus was found in **Case 13,** a 22¾-month-old boy. The coronary sinus blood flow passed into a left vertical vein and then into the left innominate (brachiocephalic) vein, the RSVC, and RA. This anomaly may be regarded as *anomalous cardiac venous drainage* of the supracardiac type via a snowman pathway, caused by atresia of the right atrial ostium of the coronary sinus. We do not know if this anomalous cardiac venous drainage was *total* or *partial* because we do not know if some of the cardiac venous blood returned to the heart via thebesian venous pathways, which, however, is thought to have been probable.

It is also noteworthy that we are talking about *cardiac* veins, not *coronary* veins. Anatomists prefer to reserve the term *coronary* for the arteries of the heart, not for the veins of the heart, because only the arteries form a crown (*corona,* Latin) for the ventricles of the heart, whereas the cardiac veins do not. However, many widely used medical dictionaries do not follow this convention.

Anomalous cardiac venous drainage is not a widely recognized anomaly. Textbooks devoted to congenital heart disease often do not even mention anomalous cardiac venous drainage.

An aberrant subclavian artery (or arteries) was (were) found in 3 of these 27 patients (11.11%).

MCAs were prominent in patients with this type of mitral atresia (13/27 patients, 48.15%), and they were highly variable. The term *MCAs* means that not only was the cardiovascular system involved, but also that *other systems* of the body were malformed as well. These additional associated anomalies include a tracheo-esophageal fistula with esophageal atresia (5/27 patients, 18.52%); Meckel diverticulum (2/27, 7.41%); anomalous vertebral bodies with failure of normal fusion (2/27, 7.41%); duodenal atresia (1/27, 3.70%); cleft palate, low-set ears, midline skin tag of the neck anteriorly; bilateral simian transverse palmar creases, hypoplastic finger nails, absent thymus (DiGeorge syndrome?), horseshoe kidney, and hydroureter associated with a balanced translocation involving chromosomes 9 and 22, the mother being the carrier of this chromosomal anomaly (1/27, 3.7%); polycystic kidneys (1/27, 3.7%); shield-shaped chest, widely spaced nipples, pectus excavatum, increased carrying angle of the arms, and mongoloid slant of the eyes, associated with familial congenital heart disease. An older brother had incompletely common AV canal with a large ostium primum defect, severe congenital mitral stenosis, and tricuspid regurgitation (1/27, 3.7%); duodenal atresia (1/27, 3.7%); trisomy 18 (1/27, 3.7%); malrotation of the intestines (1/27, 3.7%); dilatation of the bladder and ureters (no obstruction such as posterior urethral valves being identified); kernicterus without jaundice in a patient with intrauterine growth restriction, birth weight at term being 4 lb 6 oz (1/27; 3.7%); epicanthal folds, hypertelorism, cervical rib, and bifed spleen in a nonidentical twin (1/27, 3.7%); marked hypoplasia of the left lung with absence of the left pulmonary veins in a stillborn 32- to 34-week fetus who weighed 1900 g (1/27, 3.7%); syndactyly of the left foot (1/27, 3.7%); and left diaphragmatic hernia of the foramen of Bochdalek type with stomach, spleen, pancreas, left lobe of liver, and a portion of small bowel, cecum, and appendix in the left hemithorax, with marked hypoplasia of a unilobed left lung (1/27, 3.7%).

Familial congenital heart disease was found in the families of 2 (Cases 18 and 121) of these 27 patients with this variety of mitral atresia (7.41%; see Table 14.2, anatomic type 3). Both of these families have already been mentioned.

Case 18 was the 6-day-old girl with MCAs (mongoloid slant of the eyes, increased carrying angle of the arms, shield-shaped chest, widely spaced nipples, and pectus excavatum) whose 4 9/12-year-old brother had the incomplete form of common AV canal with severe congenital mitral stenosis and tricuspid regurgitation.

Case 121 was the 2-day-old boy—a twin—whose "identical" twin brother was normal. Their older brother, who was 2 years old, had a VSD with mild pulmonary stenosis. This older brother was also a twin, but his twin was a stillborn fetus.

Coronary Anomalies. Two noteworthy coronary anomalies were found in these 27 patients. **Case 64** was a 9-day-old white girl with an *anomalous left coronary artery arising from the bifurcation of the MPA.* The right coronary artery originated normally from the aortic root. This patient also had scimitar syndrome and MCAs.

As has been mentioned previously, it is important, particularly for surgeons, to know that it is possible for coronary arteries to arise from the pulmonary artery, from its bifurcation or from the proximal portion of either pulmonary artery branch. One should resist the urge to "tidy up the field" by interrupting this mysterious strand that should not be arising from the pulmonary arterial tree. From the standpoint of understanding, it may well help to know that in sharks, the coronary arteries normally arise from the branchial arches, from their efferent sides, immediately after the branchial arch blood has been oxygenated in the gills.[25] The human pulmonary artery branches are homologous with the shark's branchial arches in the sense that the pulmonary artery branches (like the afferent branchial arteries) are leading the blood to be oxygenated.[25] Coronary arteries arising from the pulmonary arterial tree certainly appear to be atavistic. Consequently, *a vessel-like structure arising from the pulmonary artery tree and running to the heart should be regarded as an anomalous coronary artery until proved otherwise.* Such a structure should be left alone, not ligated and divided.

Case 154, a 5-year-old girl, had an anomalous origin of the left circumflex coronary artery from the right aortic sinus of Valsalva. The anomalously originating left circumflex coronary artery ran posteriorly and to the left, behind the aortic root, and emerged to the left of it. Then, proceeding anteriorly to the left of the great arteries, it reached the AV junction, from where it ran leftward in the normal course of the left circumflex coronary artery. The left coronary ostium was normally located and gave rise only to the left anterior descending coronary artery.

MITRAL ATRESIA {S,D,S}, VENTRICULAR SEPTAL DEFECT, AND AORTIC VALVAR ATRESIA

There were 5 patients with mitral atresia {S,D,S}, VSD, and aortic valvar atresia among the 118 cases with mitral atresia and normal, {S,D,S}, segmental anatomy (see Table 14.2, anatomic type 4, and Fig. 14.1), constituting 4.24% of patients with normal segmental anatomy (5/118) and 2.82% of all patients with mitral atresia and any kind of segmental anatomy (5/177).

Sex: Males, 2; females, 3; males to females = 0.67.

Age at Death: Mean, 4.4 ± 3.29 days; range, 0 (17-week fetal abortion) to 9 days; and median, 5 days.

Salient Anatomic Features: *Secundum* ASD, 2 of 5 patients (40%); *leftward malalignment of the septum primum,* 1 of 5 (20%); *LSVC to coronary sinus to RA,* 2 of 5 (40%); *atresia of the proximal coronary sinus* (adjacent to the RA), 1 of 5 (20%); *VSD,* present in all patients (100%) by definition in this group, always small; conoventricular type of VSD, 3 (60%); muscular VSD, 3 (60%); and multiple VSDs, 2 (40%); *aberrant subclavian artery,* 2 (40%), aberrant right, 1, and aberrant left, 1; PDA, 5 (100%), closing PDA, 1, and bilateral ductus arteriosi, 1; and *MCAs,* 1 (20%), with hypoplastic kidneys bilaterally, unilobed lungs bilaterally, and nonobstructive vascular ring.

Perhaps the lesson of this group (see Table 14.2, anatomic type 4), is that occasionally it is possible for patients with mitral atresia, normal segmental anatomy, and a VSD(s) to have aortic valvar atresia, particularly when the VSD (or VSDs) is (are) *small.* From a functional standpoint, these 5 patients were very similar to the much larger group of patients with mitral atresia {S,D,S} and an intact ventricular septum (80 cases, 45.20%; see Table 14.2; anatomic type 1). When the VSD is sizeable, the aortic valve can be patent, if often hypoplastic (see Table 14.2, anatomic type 3, 27 patients, 15.17%). Thus, the status of the ventricular septum (i.e., the size of the VSD, if present) and the status of the aortic valve (atretic or patent) appear to vary directly:

1. When the ventricular septum is intact (no VSD), the aortic valve typically is atretic (no aortic valvar orifice), as in Table 14.2, anatomic type 1.
2. When the VSD is sizeable, the aortic valve can be patent, if hypoplastic, as in Table 14.2, anatomic type 3, 15.17%.
3. When a VSD is present, but small, the aortic valve seldom is patent, as in Table 14.2, anatomic type 2, accounting for only 1.69% of this series of patients with mitral atresia.

MITRAL ATRESIA {S,D,S}, VENTRAL SEPTAL DEFECT, AND TRUNCUS ARTERIOSUS

In 1994 we studied a 9-day-old girl with mitral atresia, normal {S,D,S} segmental anatomy, and a high conoventricular type of VSD **(Case 171).** The rare finding was the coexistence of *truncus arteriosus* (Fig. 14.5).[37-40] Anatomically, she had truncus arteriosus type A3[37]; type A means that a VSD of the usual conoventricular type is present, and type 3 means that only one pulmonary artery branch is present. In her case, the proximal left pulmonary artery was absent, the distal left pulmonary artery being supplied by the left-sided PDA. Bilateral SVCs were present, the persistent LSVC flowing into the coronary sinus and then into the RA. The left innominate (brachiocephalic) vein was present. The atrial septum was restrictive, and this was treated at 9 days of age by a surgical atrial septectomy. There was partially anomalous pulmonary venous connection, the right pulmonary veins connecting with the RSVC. The LV was hypoplastic, without papillary muscles.

The truncal valve (which we thought was the aortic valve) was bicuspid and the leaflets were redundant. The truncal valve originated almost entirely above the RV, but it also overrode the hypoplastic LV to a small degree above a conoventricular type of VSD. Both coronary ostia, were abnormally located: the right coronary ostium was abnormally high, above the RC/NC commissure. The left coronary artery arose within a sinus of Valsalva, but was abnormally close to a commissure.

A complete muscular subtruncal conus arteriosus (infundibulum) was present that was shown well angiocardiographically (see Fig. 14.5 A–B). Anatomically, the conal musculature prevented truncal valve-to-tricuspid valve fibrous continuity (see Fig. 14.5 C–D). This very rare example of *the right ventricular type of truncus arteriosus* with a complete subtruncal conus was kindly sent to us as a consult by Dr. Jami Shakibi of Teheran, Iran.

The right subclavian artery was aberrant, arising as the last brachiocephalic artery from the top of the descending thoracic aorta and then coursing rightward to supply the right arm.

Surgery at 9 days of age consisted (as mentioned previously) of atrial septectomy, and removal of the right pulmonary artery branch from the truncus arteriosus, occlusion of the left PDA, end-to-end anastomosis of the right and left pulmonary artery branches, and placement of a modified Blalock-Taussig anastomosis. The patient died intraoperatively. Autopsy revealed marked hypoplasia of both the right and left pulmonary artery branches.

To the best of our present knowledge, mitral atresia is not included in any extant classification of truncus arteriosus, and, conversely, truncus arteriosus is not included in any classification of mitral atresia of which we are aware. Consequently, this is a rare and noteworthy case (see Table 14.2, anatomic type 5).

MITRAL ATRESIA {S,D,S} WITH A VENTRICULAR SEPTAL DEFECT OR A BULBOVENTRICULAR FORAMEN, WITH A LARGE LEFT VENTRICLE AND A SMALL RIGHT VENTRICLE, OR A SINGLE LEFT VENTRICLE AND AN ABSENT RIGHT VENTRICLE

The anomaly of mitral atresia {S,D,S}, VSD or bulboventricular foramen, large LV and small RV or single LV and absent RV (see Table 14.2, mitral atresia type 6, and Fig. 14.1, type 6) sounds like a developmental impossibility: mitral atresia with a large LV? And with a small or absent RV? The ventricular anatomy is counterintuitive—exactly the opposite of what we have been considering thus far (see Fig. 14.1 and Table 14.2, anatomic types of mitral atresia types 1 to 5, inclusive).

This developmental "impossibility" is what we are now going to present; mitral atresia anatomic type 6 (see Fig. 14.1 and Table 14.2) consists of 7 cases, 3.95% of all of these patients with mitral atresia. However, as will soon be seen, only 2 of these 7 patients had normal segmental anatomy, hence, "2 (of 7)" in

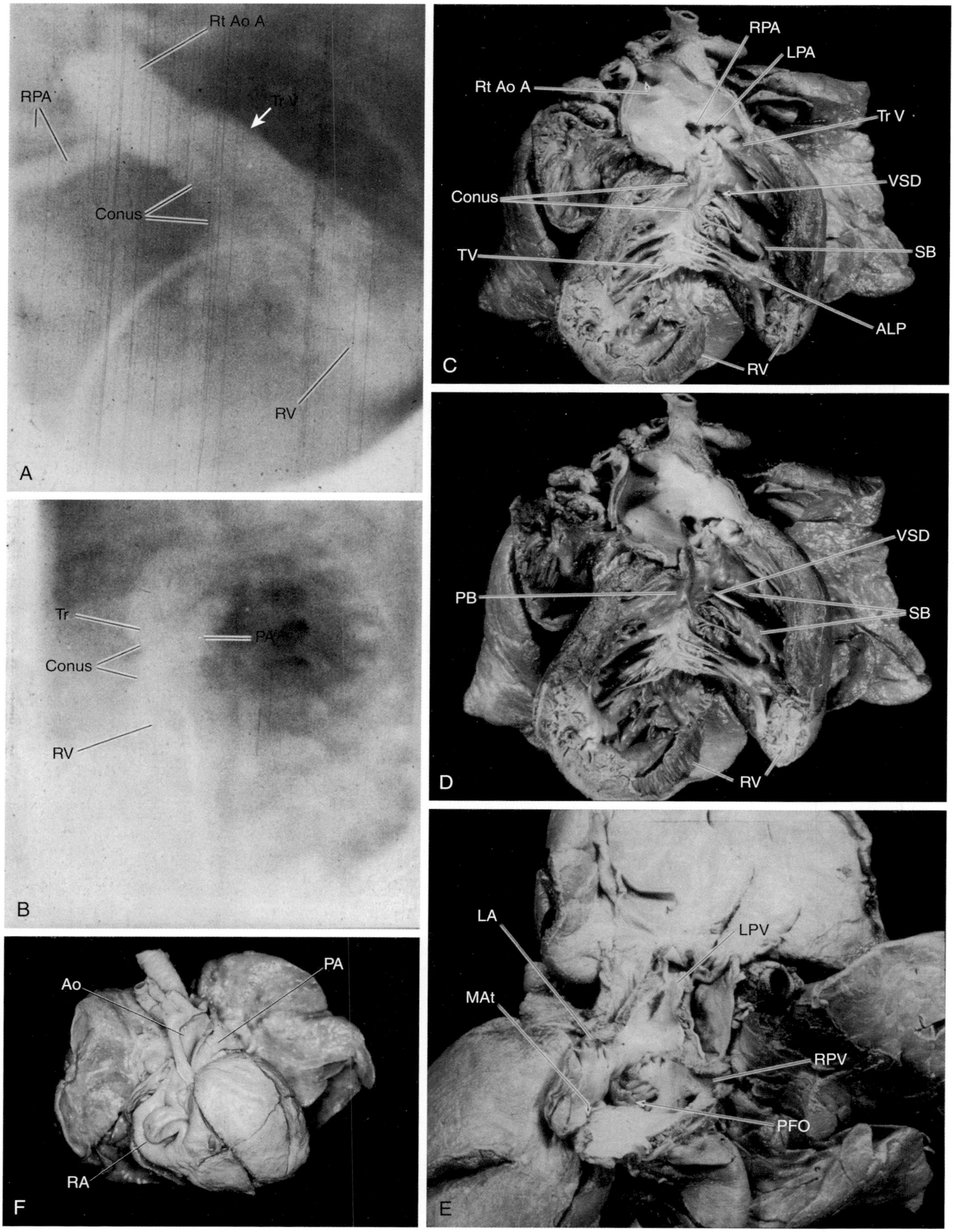

Fig. 14.5

Continued

Fig. 14.5 Mitral atresia with a right ventricular truncus arteriosus and complete subtruncal muscular conus. (A) Selective right ventricular angiocardiogram, posteroanterior projection, showing a morphologically right ventricle *(RV)* giving rise to a truncus arteriosus with a right aortic arch *(Rt Ao A)*. The truncal valve *(TrV)* sits high above a well-developed subtruncal muscular conus. The right pulmonary artery *(RPA)* can be seen arising from the truncus. The more posterior origin and course of the left pulmonary artery *(LPA)* is not visible in this projection. (B) In this simultaneous left lateral projection, the posterior origin of the pulmonary artery (PA) from the truncus (Tr) can be seen. (C) Opened RV showing tricuspid valve *(TV)*, septal band *(SB)*, anterolateral papillary muscle *(ALP)*, muscular subtruncal conus separating type of TrV above from TV below, small conoventricular type of ventricular septal defect *(VSD)* between conal musculature above and ventricular septal crest below, origins of the RPA and the LPA from the posterior and leftward portion of the truncus arteriosus, no aorticopulmonary septal remnant, no main pulmonary artery component, and right aortic arch. Thus, this is a rare case of right ventricular truncus arteriosus {S,D,D} type A2 with a muscular subtruncal conus and mitral atresia. (Truncus type A means that a VSD is present. Truncus type 2 means that both pulmonary artery branches arise from the truncus, with no aortopulmonary septal remnant and no main pulmonary artery component.)[37,38] The rare features of this case are the presence of truncus arteriosus arising entirely above the RV, the presence of a complete subtruncal muscular conus preventing truncal valve–to–atrioventricular valve fibrous continuity, and the coexistence of mitral atresia. (D) A probe through the small VSD indicates the location of this defect more clearly than in C. The parietal band *(PB)*, indicating that the subtruncal conal musculature runs out onto the right ventricular free (or parietal) wall. (E) Opened morphologically left atrium (LA), showing the marked hypertrophy of the left atrial walls, the presence of mitral atresia, the normal connections of the left pulmonary veins *(LPV)* and the right pulmonary veins *(RPV)*, and the patent (but obstructive) foramen ovale *(PFO)*. (F) The opened morphologically left ventricle is markedly hypoplastic compared with the RV, and the very small VSD is indicated by a *white arrow*. *Ao,* Aorta; *RA,* right atrium. (This very rare case was kindly sent to us as a consult in 1976 by Dr. Jami Shakibi, pediatric cardiologist of Teheran, Iran.)

mitral atresia type 6 (see Fig. 14.1). For convenience, all 7 cases of this rare form of mitral atresia will be considered here.

Sex: Males, 3; females, 4; males to females = 0.75.

Age at Death: Mean, 848 ± 1417.16 days (2.3 ± 3.9 years); range, from 0 postnatal days (fetus aborted at 18 weeks gestational age) to 3405 days (9.3 years); and median, 75 days (2.5 months).

Salient Anatomic Features

Segmental anatomy:

1. {S,D,S} in 2 of 7 (28.6%);
2. TGA in 3 to 7 (42.9%):
   TGA {S,D,D}, 1;
   TGA {S,D,A}, 1; and
   TGA {S,L,D}, 1 in which the mitral atresia (or atrial outlet atresia) was *right-sided;*
3. DORV in 1 of 7 (14.3%):
   DORV {S,D,A}, 1; and
4. double-outlet infundibular outlet chamber (DOIOC):
   DOIOC {S,L,L} in 1 of 7 (14.3%), in which the mitral atresia (or atrial outlet atresia) was *right-sided.* The identity of the AV valves corresponds to that of the ventricular loop of entry, not to that of the atria of exit. In a *ventricular L-loop,* the *tricuspid valve is left-sided* and the *mitral valve is right-sided.*

What does double-outlet from the infundibulum outlet chamber (DOIOC) mean? Both great arteries arise from the infundibular outlet chamber or conus arteriosus. This designation also means that neither great artery originates above a right or a left ventricular sinus or inflow tract. A description of the associated ventricular anatomy is necessary for full comprehension.

Ventricular Anatomy

A *single LV* was present in 4 of these 7 patients (57.1%) (Cases 46, 57, 72, and 93) because the RV (the right ventricular sinus, body, or inflow tract) was absent. *A large LV and a small RV (sinus)* were found in 3 of these 7 patients (42.9%) (Cases 23, 111, and 148). The presence of a small or hypoplastic RV in a few of these cases made it possible to have DORV, as mentioned earlier.

Other important anatomic findings in this rare form of mitral atresia with a single LV and no right ventricular sinus or with a large LV and a small right ventricular sinus were as follows:

- obstructive atrial septum in 2 of 7 patients;
- coronary sinus ostial atresia with an associated persistent LSVC in 1;
- cor triatriatum in 1;
- straddling tricuspid valve in the 3 patients with a hypoplastic right ventricular sinus; preductal coarctation of the aorta in 3 patients, and interrupted aortic arch (type B, distal to the left common carotid artery) in 1, associated with aortic outflow tract obstruction caused by a restrictive bulboventricular foramen;
- pulmonary infundibular outflow tract stenosis in 1;
- an aberrant right subclavian artery in 1;
- a single left coronary artery (absence of the right coronary arterial ostium) in 1; high ostium of the left coronary artery in 1; and hypoplasia of the left coronary arterial ostium in 1 patient, with enlargement of the right coronary arterial ostium; and closing PDA in 2 of these 7 patients.

Now it is time to present this infrequent form of mitral atresia with a large morphologically LV and a small or absent morphologically right ventricular sinus photographically (Fig. 14.6 to Fig. 14.14, inclusive). These figures and their legends merit careful consideration.

Developmental Hypothesis

Saying that mitral atresia with a large morphologically LV is a "developmental impossibility," as I did by way of introduction to this rare form of mitral atresia is, of course, itself an

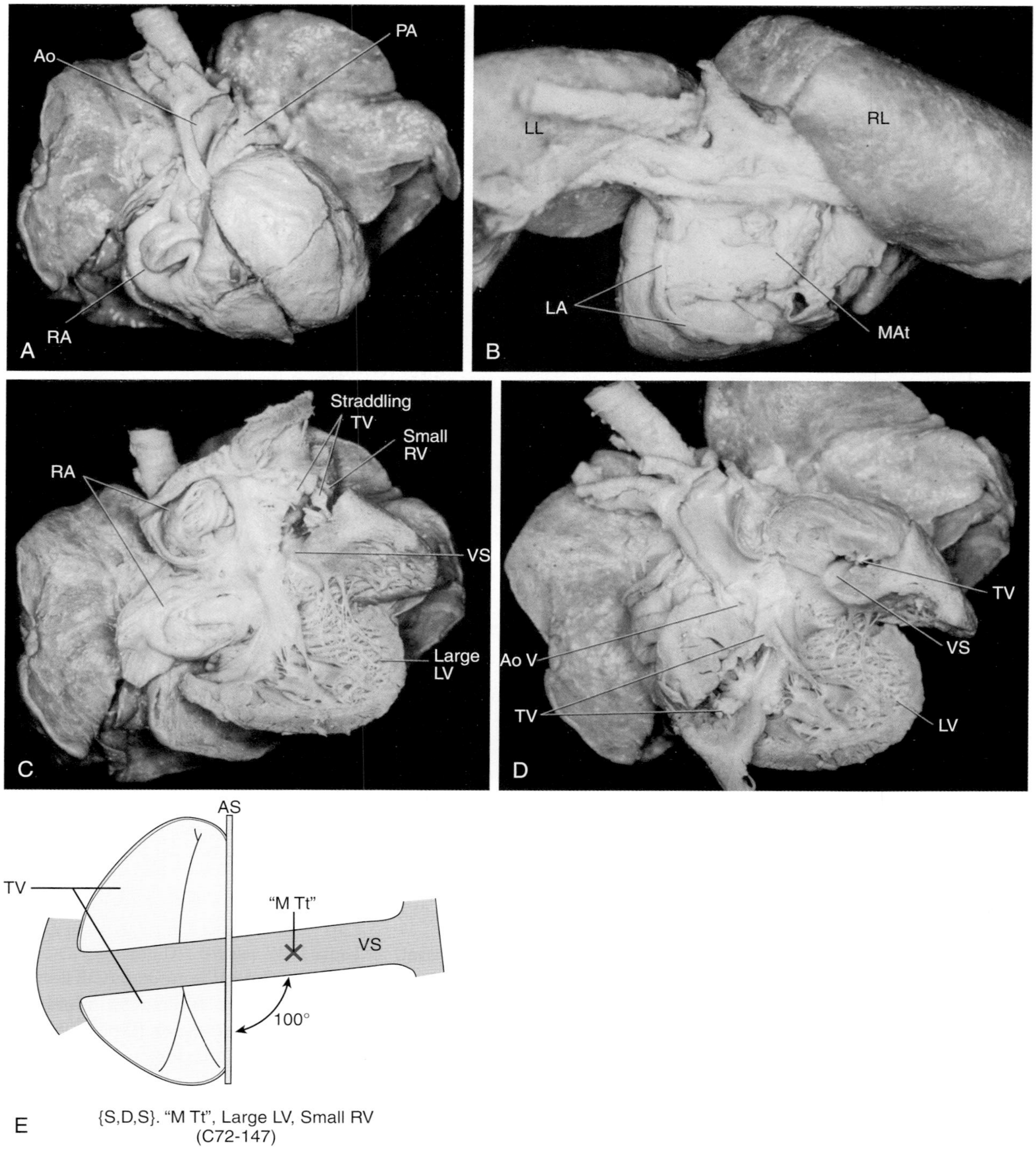

Fig. 14.6 Mitral atresia *(MAt)* {S,D,S} with large left ventricle *(LV)*, small right ventricle *(RV)*, and straddling tricuspid valve *(TV)*. The patient was a 2½-month-old white boy. (A) External frontal view showing the right atrium *(RA)*, the ventricular segment (unlabeled), and normally related great arteries. The right and left lungs and trachea are unlabeled. (B) Posterosuperior view of the opened left atrium *(LA)* showing MAt, that is, no mitral orifice or leaflets. (C) Opened RA, TV, large LV, and small RV. The RA is markedly hypertrophied and enlarged. The TV opens predominantly into the large LV but also straddles above the ventricular septum *(VS)* into a small RV. C is a view of the ventricular outflow tract. Note that the straddling TV attaches to the crest of the muscular VS. (D) Part of the ventricular outflow tract from the large LV into the normally related aorta. The aortic valve *(AoV)* is in direct fibrous continuity with the underlying atrioventricular valve, indicating that the subaortic infundibular free wall has undergone resorption, typical of normally related great arteries. A subpulmonary conus was present (not seen in this view), also typical of normally related great arteries. (E) Cardiac septal geometry, as seen from an apical four-chamber perspective. The atrial septum is normally vertical. The ventricular septum is very abnormally located, being almost horizontal. The ventriculoatrial septal angle measured 100°. The normal ventriculoatrial septal angle is 5° to 7°, median = 6°. The marked malalignment of the ventricular segment relative to the atrial segment appears to have resulted in mitral atresia and in straddling tricuspid valve. The VS immediately underlay where the mitral orifice "should" have been located, and the VS also underlay the TV, apparently predisposing to straddling of the tricuspid valve. *Ao,* Ascending aorta. *LL,* left lung; *PA,* main pulmonary artery; *RL,* right lung. This case was kindly sent to us as a consult in 1972 by Dr. Marian Molthan of the Good Samaritan Hospital in Phoenix Arizona. (This case was presented by R. Van Praagh[89] in 1985 at the Second World Congress of Pediatric Cardiology in New York City, but this figure is published here for the first time.)

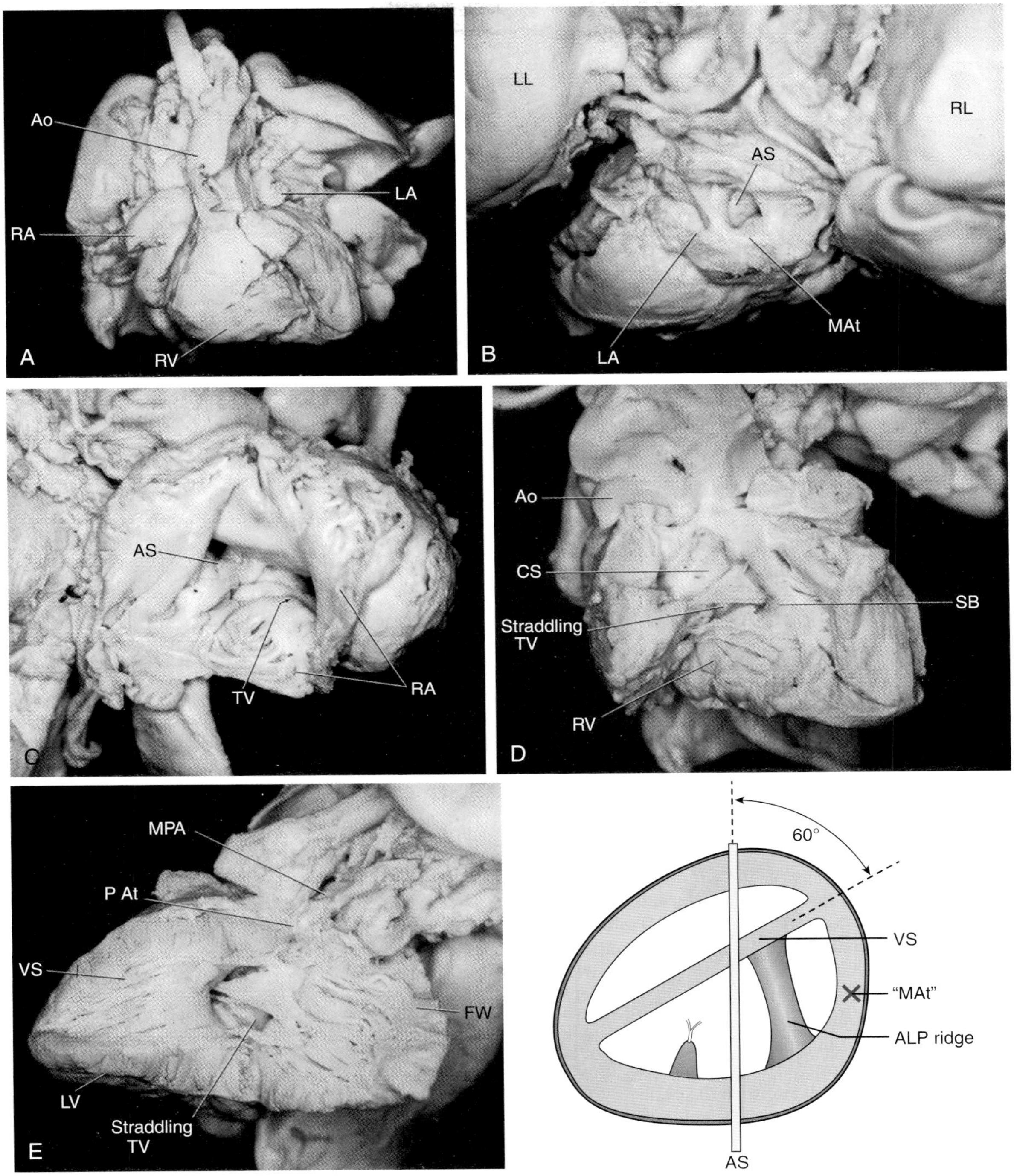

F TGA {S,D,D}, "MAt", absent ALP muscle (A71-111)

Fig. 14.7 This is the heart and lung specimen of a 24-day-old boy who died in 1971. Autopsy revealed transposition of the great arteries {S,D,D} with pulmonary atresia (infundibular and valvar), a ventricular septal defect (VSD) of the atrioventricular (AV) canal type, straddling tricuspid valve *(TV)*, and mitral atresia *(MAt)*. The left ventricle *(LV)* was of normal size. There was right atrial hypertrophy and enlargement, and right ventricular hypertrophy and enlargement. (Note that in this patient the right ventricle *[RV]* was *not* significantly small-chambered [hypoplastic].) On day 1 of postnatal life, a surgical atrial septal defect was created and a Waterston anastomosis (between the ascending aorta and the right pulmonary artery, side-to-side, 2 × 3 mm) was performed. Aspiration of gastric contents led to death. (A) External frontal view of the heart and lungs showing the morphologically right atrium *(RA)*, the morphologically left atrium (LA), and the morphologically right ventricle (RV) from which the D-transposed aorta *(Ao)* arises. (B) Posterosuperior view of the opened LA showing MAt, that is, absence of a left AV valve and orifice. The surgically created defect in the atria septum *(AS)*, and the posterior aspects of the left lung *(LL)* and right lung *(RL)* are also seen. (C) A right lateral view of the opened RA reveals marked right atrial hypertrophy and enlargement, a right atrial view of the AS and the

Continued

Fig. 14.7 cont'd surgically created atrial septal defect, and the approaches to the TV. (D) The opened RV shows the straddling TV, the septal band *(SB)*, the conal septum *(CS)*, and the opened aortic valve (unlabeled) and ascending Ao of the D-transposed Ao. The Waterston anastomosis (unlabeled) is seen in the middle of the posterior surface of the ascending Ao. (E) The opened LV, the straddling TV, the VSD of the AV canal type (unlabeled), the infundibular and valvar pulmonary atresia *(P At)*, and the small main pulmonary artery *(MPA)* are seen. The left ventricular septal surface (VSD) and free wall *(FW)* are labeled for orientation. (F) The cardiac geometry, shown in an apical four-chamber perspective, shows the ventriculoatrial malalignment. When we drove a needle through the expected site of the mitral valve as viewed from within the LA (as in B), the needle emerged within the FW of the LV (× marks the spot of the "MAt"). The atrial septum (AS) occupied a normally vertical orientation. But the ventricular septum *(VS)* was markedly abnormally angulated relative to the AS. The ventriculoatrial septal angle measured 60° (the normal ventriculoatrial septal angle = 5° ± 2°, median = 6°).[41] The LV (unlabeled) is inferior and to the left of the VS, and the RV (unlabeled) is superior and to the right of the VS. The anterolateral papillary (ALP) muscle of the LV is absent, replaced by an abnormal ALP ridge. The posteromedial papillary muscle of the LV (unlabeled) was well developed and received the chordae tendineae of the straddling TV. Quotation marks are placed around the MAt label ("MAt") to indicate that in this case, we think that the absence of a left AV valve and orifice is not primarily because of a malformation of the mitral valve (MV). The MV appears to have been the "sinned against," not the "sinner," that is, the "victim," not the "perpetrator." In this patient the left atrial outlet atresia appears to be due to ventriculoatrial malalignment. The left ventricular free wall is immediately beneath the site of the expected MV and orifice, apparently causing the left atrial outflow tract atresia. If the MV had little or nothing to do with causing this case of so-called "mitral" atresia, what is the straddling TV really? Is it the TV only? Or is it a combination of tricuspid and mitral valve tissue? We do not know the answer to this question. Our use of conventional terminology (mitral atresia with straddling tricuspid valve)[41] should not obscure this unsolved underlying mystery. Cardiac geometry reveals the more basic diagnosis: this entity is a particular type of ventriculoatrial malalignment, as photographed and diagrammed earlier. (Reproduced with permission from Van Praagh R, Visner MS. The postoperative pathology of congenital heart disease. *Am J Cardiol.* 1976;38:225, 1976.)

impossibility. Anything that in fact occurs cannot be developmentally impossible. (But it can be mind boggling.)

How is it possible to have a large LV, or even a single LV, in association with mitral atresia? Almost always with mitral atresia, the LV is diminutive. But occasionally, the LV can be large. Why? *Our hypothesis is that the small or absent right ventricular sinus is the key.* When the RV inflow tract is hypoplastic or absent, the ventricular septum, or its remnant, is displaced toward the side of the hypoplastic or absent RV—to the right with a ventricular D-loop or to the left with a ventricular L-loop. This *ventricular septal displacement* is one type of **ventriculoatrial malalignment.** The geometry of ventriculoatrial malalignment in this type of mitral atresia is presented in Fig. 14.15.

With D-loop ventricles, for example, rightward displacement of the ventricular septum places the LV abnormally to the right of the atrial septum, beneath the right-sided RA and the tricuspid valve. Consequently, the blood from the left and right atria flows through the tricuspid valve and into the abnormally right-sided LV, permitting the LV to grow and become large.

Usually with typical mitral atresia, when the right ventricular sinus or inflow tract develops well and the LV is diminutive, the ventricular septum comes to underlie the atrial septum. Because of typical mitral atresia, blood cannot flow from the embryonic and fetal LA into the LV; hence, the LV, deprived of pressure work and flow work, remains diminutive. The RV grows and develops and becomes functionally the systemic ventricle of the embryo and fetus in *typical* cases of mitral atresia, such as those considered previously.

Ventricular septal displacement toward the side of the absent ventricle is what one sees in hearts with single LV,[21,22] which 4 of these 7 patients with mitral atresia, large LV, and absent right ventricular sinus had. Displacement of the ventricular septum toward the side of the hypoplastic RV is what one sees anatomically in straddling tricuspid valve,[41] which is what 3 of these 7 patients had. When a lung is hypoplastic or absent, a very similar phenomenon occurs: the mediastinum is displaced toward the side of the hypoplastic or absent lung.

Summary

Mitral atresia with a large LV and a small or absent right ventricular sinus and with the resulting **ventriculoatrial malalignment** occurred with normally related great arteries and normal {S,D,S} segmental anatomy (2/7, 28.6%), with TGA and D-loop TGA {S,D,D} and TGA {S,D,A} (2/7, 28.6%), with L-loop TGA (S,L,D} (1/7, 14.3%), with D-loop DORV {S,D,A} (1/7, 14.3%), and with L-loop DOIOC {S,L,L} (1/7, 14.3%). Absence of the right ventricular sinus occurred in 4 of 7 patients (57.1%), resulting in single LV, and hypoplasia of the right ventricular sinus was found in 3 of 7 (42.9%), resulting in a large LV and a small RV.

To the best of our knowledge, this anomaly was first reported by Dr. Manuel Quero[23] of Madrid, Spain in 1970. Dr. Quero, a good friend, was trying to show us that a single ventricle could occur with AV valvar atresia, that is, that the then accepted definition of single ventricle was wrong. The classic premorphologic definition was single ventricle is present if both AV valves or a common AV valve open entirely or predominantly into one ventricular chamber.[21] Quero's point, to quote Cole Porter, was "It ain't necessarily so." Look at this case of mine,[23] he was saying. It has a single LV with absence of the right ventricular sinus and normally related great arteries. The segmental anatomy is normal {S,D,S}, but it also has mitral atresia. In fact, this is a **Holmes heart with mitral atresia.**[23]

Our Case 93 is Dr. Manuel Quero's case,[23] which he very kindly sent to us, just in case we had any lingering doubts. We did not. We fully agreed that Quero was right. We also knew

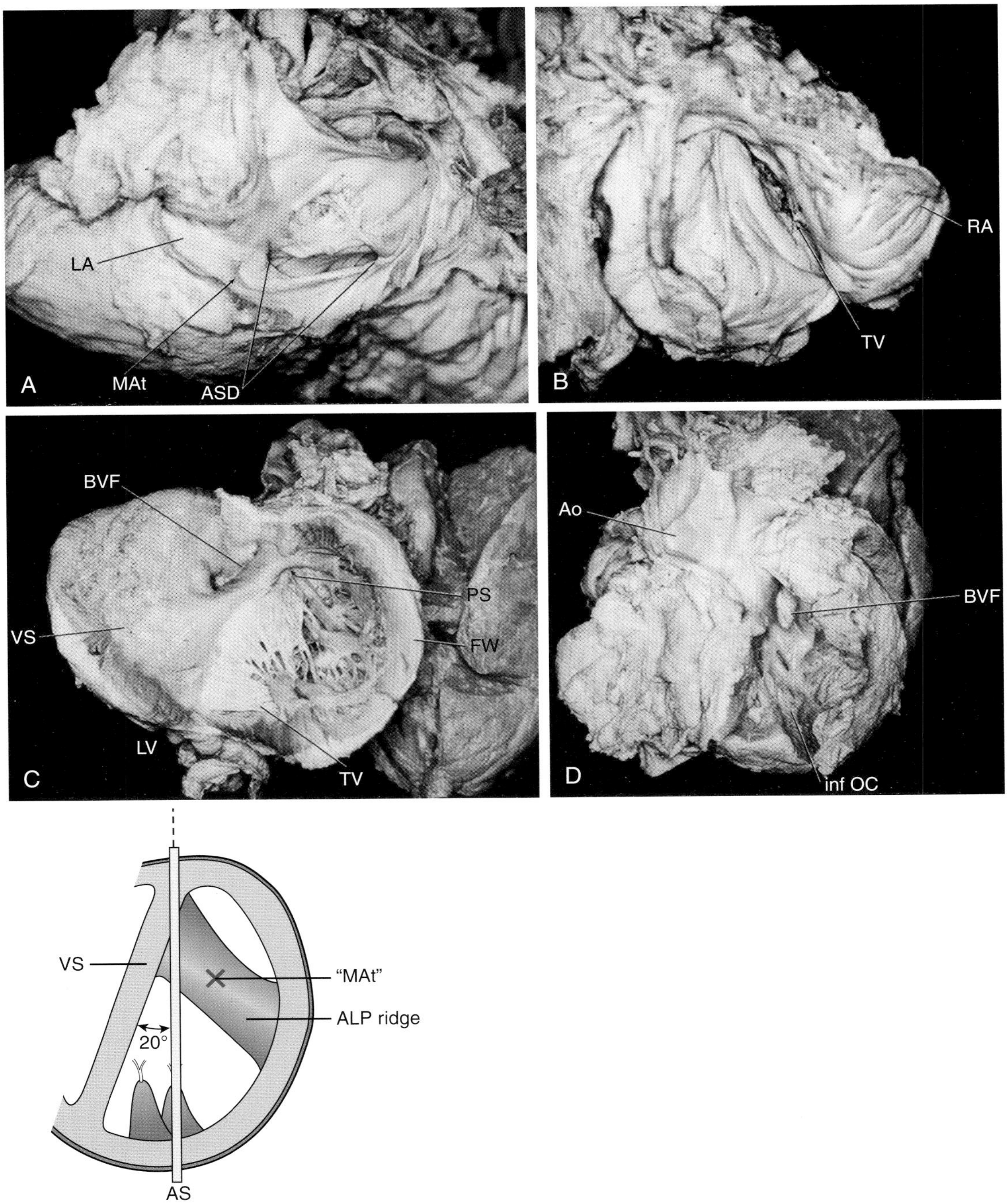

Fig. 14.8 The heart of a 12 7/12-year-old boy with transposition of the great arteries (TGA) {S,D,D} with mitral atresia *(MAt)*, single left ventricle *(LV)* (absence of the right ventricular sinus), infundibular outlet chamber (inf OC), and subpulmonary stenosis. (A) Posterosuperior view of opened left atrium *(LA)* showing MAt and surgically created atrial septal defect *(ASD)*. (B) Right lateral view of opened right atrium *(RA)*, which shows hypertrophy and enlargement, and the large unopened tricuspid valve *(TV)* seen from above. (C) The opened single LV, left posterolateral view. The TV opens only into the LV, which is not surprising when one remembers that the right ventricular sinus is absent. Note that the TV attaches mostly to the posteromedial papillary muscle group of the LV. The anterolateral papillary muscle is abnormally small and posteriorly located. The thickened and rolled edges of the TV at its anterior commissure reflect tricuspid regurgitation, which clinically was severe. The left ventricular septal surface *(VS)* and the left ventricular free wall *(FW)* are labeled for orientation. The bulboventricular foramen *(BVF)* leads from the LV into the infundibular outlet chamber from which the D-transposed aorta arises. The transposed pulmonary artery originates from the single LV. The conal

Continued

Fig. 14.8 cont'd septum is malaligned posteriorly, causing subpulmonary stenosis *(PS)*. (D) The opened infundibular outlet chamber *(inf OC)*, right anterior view, showing the BVF and the opened D-transposed aorta *(Ao)*. Through the BVF one can see the TV leaflet tissue opening into the single LV. (E) Cardiac geometry, as seen from the apical four-chamber perspective. The atrial septum *(AS)* is vertical and normally located. The single LV is abnormally displaced to the right and is angulated relative to the AS. The angle between the ventricular septum (VSD) and the AS equals 20 degrees, which is abnormally large (normal median = 6 degrees). Beneath the expected site of the mitral orifice is a prominent anterolateral papillary *(ALP)* muscular ridge (× marks the spot). MAt is placed between quotation marks ("MAt") to suggest that the absence of a mitral valve (MV) and orifice appears not to be due to a malformation of the MV per se, but instead appears to reflect the presence of ventriculoatrial malalignment. A prominent muscular ridge, interpreted as an ALP muscle ridge, is located immediately beneath the expected site of the MV and orifice. Again, these anatomic findings strongly suggest that the MV is not the "sinner," but the "sinned against" (the "victim," not the "perpetrator"). In other words, these data suggest that the real diagnosis is not MAt, meaning an anomaly of the MV itself; instead, it appears to be left atrial outlet atresia caused by ventriculoatrial malalignment, resulting in the mitral orifice being blocked by immediately subjacent left ventricular musculature. Is the "TV," shown in C, really the TV? It cannot be a normal TV, remembering the contribution of the right ventricular septal surface in the normal morphogenesis of the TV, as illustrated by Ebstein anomaly because the RV (sinus) is absent in the present case. If this "TV" is not developmentally and anatomically the normal TV, is it really the MV, or a combination of the TV and the MV? The developmental and anatomic identity of this large valve entering the LV is uncertain at the present time. Because there is left atrial outlet atresia, it is conventional to make the diagnosis of MAt; the right-sided valve therefore "must" be the TV. It is important to realize that this conventional way of thinking may in fact be wrong, as the cardiac geometry strongly suggests. (Reproduced with permission from Van Praagh R, Visner MS. The postoperative pathology of congenital heart disease. *Am J Cardiol.* 1976;38:225.)

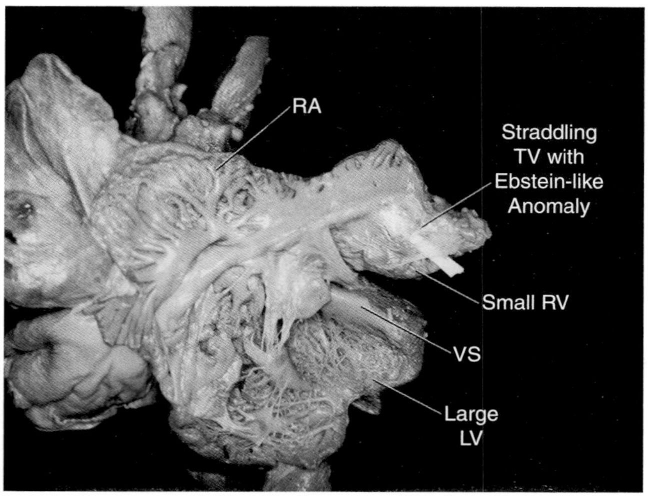

Fig. 14.9 The heart has normal {S,D,S} segmental anatomy, mitral atresia, large left ventricle *(LV)*, small right ventricle *(RV)*, straddling tricuspid valve *(TV)*, ventricular septal defect of the atrioventricular canal type (unlabeled) and an Ebstein-like anomaly of the TV. The rightward and anterior malalignment and angulation of the ventricular septum *(VS)* relative to the atrial septum (not labeled) is also evident. The right atrium *(RA)* is hypertrophied and enlarged. The deep, curtain-like anterior leaflet of the TV adjacent to the right ventricular free wall is very Ebstein-like (indicated by a *white probe*).

that the classic premorphologic definition of single ventricle cited earlier was wrong for several additional reasons:

1. **Double-inlet or common-inlet RV** typically has a small LV. An anatomically single RV usually is *not* present; instead, one finds morphologically that there is a large RV and a diminutive LV[42] (not a single RV).
2. **The Lambert heart**[43,44] also violates the classic definition of single ventricle because double-inlet LV (DILV) is *not* present. Instead, the tricuspid valve opens predominantly or entirely into the infundibular outlet chamber.

We refer to mitral atresia with a single LV, an absent right ventricular sinus, an infundibular outlet chamber, and normally related great arteries with normal {S,D,S} segmental anatomy as **the Quero heart,** in his honor.[23]

One may ask why we put all 7 of these cases of mitral atresia with a large LV and a small or absent right ventricular sinus together into anatomic type 6 (see Table 14.2 and Fig. 14.1), despite the fact that there are several very different segmental combinations in these 7 patients. The answer is that we think of mitral atresia with a large LV and a small or absent right ventricular sinus as one anatomic type of mitral atresia, which occurred in five different segmental anatomic sets: (1) {S,D,S} in 2; TGA {S,D,D/A} in 2; TGA {S,L,D} in 1; DORV {S,D,A} in 1; and DOIOC {S,L,L} in 1 patient.

An alternative way of classifying mitral atresia with a large LV and a small or absent right ventricular sinus would be to regard each of the five foregoing segmental sets as an anatomic type of mitral atresia. The disadvantage of the latter approach is that it would increase the anatomic types of mitral atresia from 18 (see Table 14.2 and Fig. 14.1) to 23. As a practice matter, our preference has been to keep the number of anatomic types of mitral atresia (and of all other anomalies) as low as possible, without oversimplifying the data.

In geometric Fig. 14.15 and in those preceding this figure, note that in this infrequent type of so-called mitral atresia with a large LV and with a small or absent right ventricular sinus, ventriculoatrial malalignment often resulted in *blocking from below* what should have been the mitral orifice. This occurred both with D-loop ventricles (see Fig. 14.15 A–F, inclusive) and L-loop ventricles (see Fig. 14.15G–H). Often, ventriculoatrial malalignment placed the left ventricular free wall beneath what should have been the mitral orifice (see Fig. 14.15A–E, H). Occasionally, a prominent muscular ridge in the LV underlay appeared to block what should have been the mitral orifice (see Fig. 14.15 F–G).

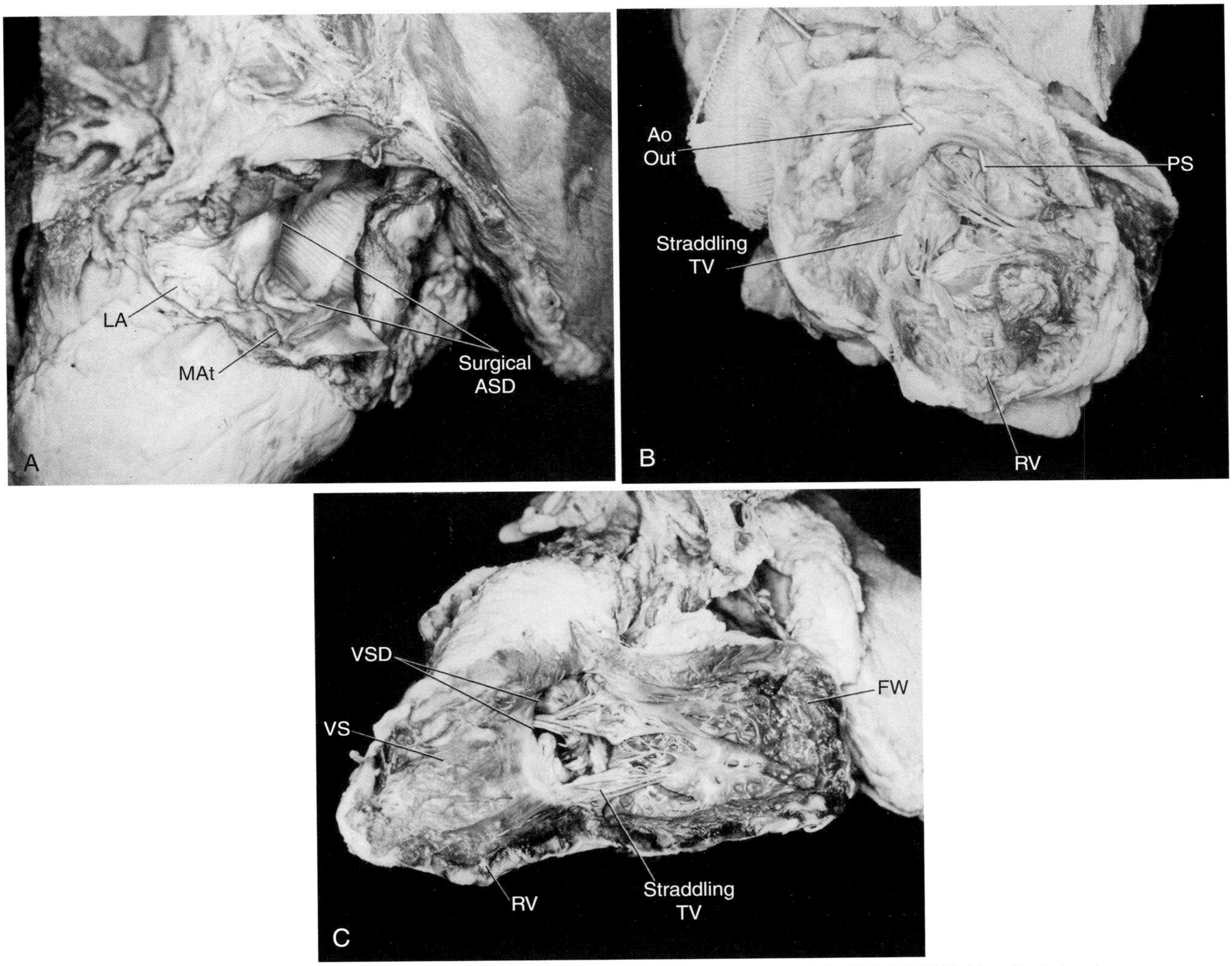

Fig. 14.10 The heart of a 9 4/12-year-old boy with double-outlet right ventricle (DORV) {S,D,A}, mitral atresia *(MAt)*, restrictive patent foramen ovale, small right ventricular sinus, large left ventricle, straddling tricuspid valve *(TV)*, ventricular septal defect *(VSD)* of the atrioventricular (AV) canal type, bilateral conus (subaortic and subpulmonary) with leftward malalignment of conal septum and subpulmonary stenosis, hypoplasia of ostium of left coronary artery, and enlargement of two right coronary arteries. In DORV {S,D,A}, *A* means that the aortic valve was directly anterior to the pulmonary valve, that is, that *antero*malposition of the great arteries was present. (A) Opened left atrium *(LA)* showing MAt and a surgically created atrial septal defect *(Surgical ASD)*. A surgically placed atrial septum is also seen. (B) The opened small right ventricle *(RV)* showing the straddling TV, the stenotic pulmonary outflow tract *(PS)* and the unobstructed aortic outflow tract *(Ao Out)*. (C) The opened left ventricle, the straddling TV, and the VSD of the AV canal type. The straddling TV inserts into one papillary muscle group of the LV. The ventricular septum *(VS)* and the left ventricular free wall *(FW)* are labeled for orientation.

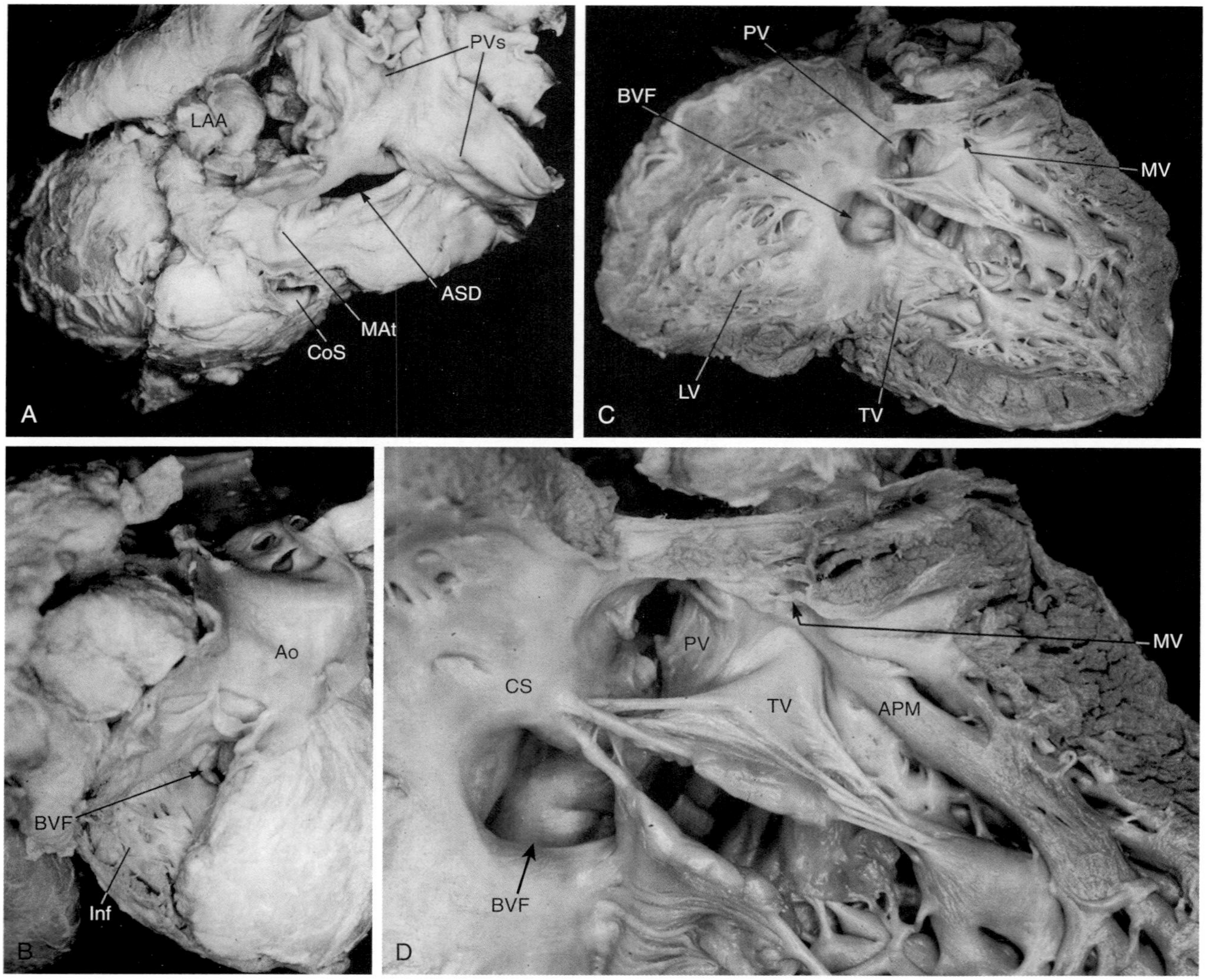

Fig. 14.11 The heart of a 1 3/12-year-old boy with transposition of the great arteries {S,D,D}, mitral atresia *(MAt),* left atrial hypertrophy, a surgically enlarged atrial septal defect *(ASD)* and pulmonary artery banding at 6 weeks of age, right atrial hypertrophy and enlargement, absence of the right ventricular sinus resulting in single left ventricle *(LV),* left ventricular hypertrophy and enlargement, left superior vena cava to coronary sinus *(CoS),* atresia of the right atrial ostium of the CoS, and tiny coronary sinus septal defect. (A) Opened left atrium showing MAt, the normally connected pulmonary veins *(PVs)* with markedly hypertrophied walls, the surgically enlarged atrial septal defect *(ASD),* the unopened left atrial appendage *(LAA),* and the dilated CoS reflecting atresia of the right atrial ostium. (B) The opened infundibular outlet chamber *(Inf),* D-transposed aorta *(Ao),* and bulboventricular foramen (*BVF)* are seen. (C) The opened single LV. The tricuspid valve *(TV)* opens only into the LV. The location of the atretic mitral valve *(MV)* is shown. The left ventricular outflow tracts through the transposed PV and through the BVF into the infundibular outlet chamber and the D-transposed aorta are both unobstructed. (D) A close-up of the LV shows that the TV is tricuspid and tricommissural. The anterosuperior tricuspid leaflet inserts into the left ventricular anterolateral papillary muscle; the posteroinferior tricuspid leaflet attaches into the posteromedial papillary muscle of the LV. Both the superior and inferior tricuspid leaflets insert into the left ventricular surface of the conal septum *(CS)* above the BVF. The mural or free wall leaflet of the TV runs between the anterolateral and the posteromedial papillary muscle groups of the LV. The free margins of the superior and inferior tricuspid leaflets are thickened and rolled, consistent with tricuspid regurgitation. The MV leader points to a very small membranous pouch that is close to the left ventricular free wall, immediately beneath the atretic mitral orifice, and somewhat to the left of the transposed PV. These details indicate how malaligned the ventricular part of the heart is relative to the atria and the AV valves. More usually, with typical double-inlet into a single LV, the AV valves are side-by-side. The MV is not superior to the TV, as in this patient. The MV usually is inferior to the PV, not to the left of the PV as in this patient. For the TV and the MV of this patient to be side-by-side, one has to rotate this photograph (D) through almost 90° in a clockwise direction: this indicates how malaligned the ventricular segment of this patient's heart is compared with a more usual double-inlet single LV without MAt in which the AV valves are side-by-side, not superoinferior as in this case. (Reproduced with permission from Van Praagh R, Visner MS. The postoperative pathology of congenital heart disease. *Am J Cardiol.* 1976;38:225.)

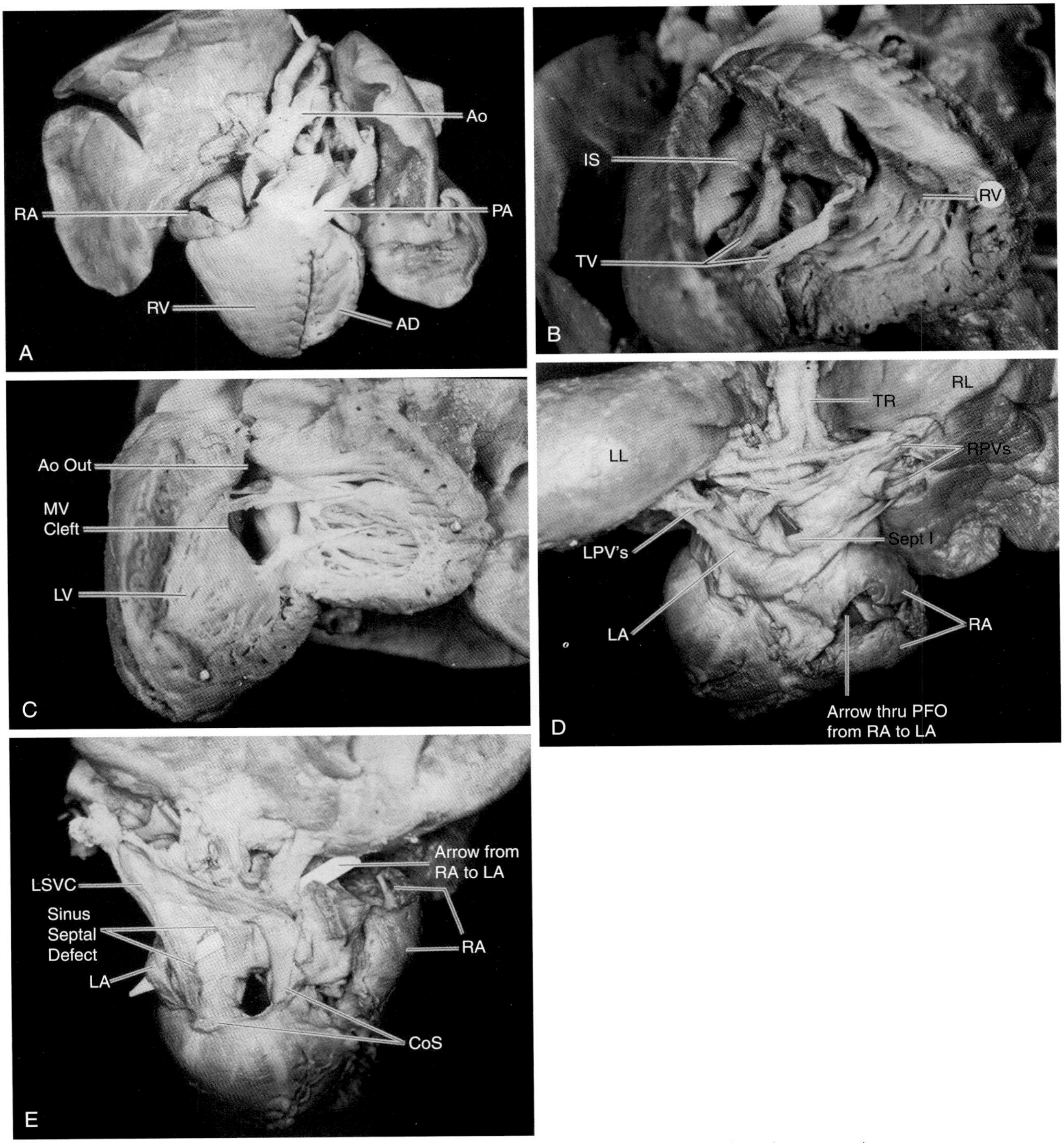

Fig. 14.12 The heart and lungs of a 4-month-old boy with left atrial outlet atresia, a decompressing coronary sinus *(CoS)* septal defect, a persistent left superior vena cava *(LSVC)* to the coronary sinus to the right atrium *(RA)*, atresia of the right superior vena cava, normal segmental anatomy {S,D,S}, a patent but competent foramen ovale, an intact atrial septum, ventriculoatrial malalignment such that the expected site of the mitral orifice as seen from the atrial aspect is located directly above the left ventricular free wall, common atrioventricular (AV) canal with a common AV valve (Rastelli type A) and a ventricular septal defect of the AV canal and with the common AV valve opening into both ventricles, right ventricular hypertrophy and enlargement, left ventricular hypertrophy and enlargement, subaortic stenosis produced by superior leaflet of common AV valve, bicuspid aortic valve with rudimentary intercoronary commissure, moderate hypoplasia of aortic arch and isthmus (coarctation not diagnosed), high ostium of right coronary artery, and ligamentum arteriosum. (A) External frontal view of the heart and lungs. The segmental anatomy is normal, that is, {S,D,S}. The morphologically RA is right-sided, hypertrophied, and enlarged. The morphologically right ventricle *(RV)* is

Continued

Fig. 14.12 cont'd right-sided and anterior, as well as hypertrophied and enlarged. The anterior descending *(AD)* coronary artery indicates the location of the ventricular septum that separates the RV from the morphologically left ventricle (unlabeled) that is left-sided and posterior as well as hypertrophied and enlarged. The great arteries are solitus normally related, the main pulmonary artery *(PA)* arising anteriorly and to the left relative to the aorta *(Ao)* that originates posteriorly and to the right. The PA is enlarged, reflecting the huge Qp/Qs of 5/1 (cardiac catheterization); and the Ao is somewhat small, reflecting the subaortic stenosis and the left-to-right shunt through the ventricular septal defect of the AV canal type. (B) The opened RV, showing the tricuspid valve *(TV)* component of the common AV valve, the hypertrophy and enlargement of the RV, and the infundibular septum *(IS)*—also hypertrophied—that extends out into the right ventricular parietal (or free) wall as the parietal band. The pulmonary outflow tract (unlabeled) lies above the IS. (C) The opened morphologically left ventricle *(LV)* showing the cleft mitral valve *(MV Cleft)* component of the common AV valve. The "scooped out" crest of the left ventricular septal surface, typical of common AV canal, forms the "floor" of the ventricular septal defect (VSD) of the AV canal type. The "roof" of such a VSD is formed by the superior and inferior bridging leaflets of the common AV valve. Note the narrowed subaortic outflow tract *(Ao Out)*. The floor of the aortic outflow tract is formed by the superior bridging leaflet of the common AV valve. During atrial systole, the superior bridging leaflet became relatively horizontal, forming a striking "goose-neck" pattern angiocardiographically, again typical of a common AV valve. During ventricular systole, a typical "scallops" pattern was seen angiocardiographically. (D) The opened left atrium *(LA)* reveals no AV valve or orifice. This was interpreted as left atrial outlet atresia, not as mitral atresia, for the reasons presented later. Note that an *arrow* passes from the RA through the patent foramen ovale *(PFO)*, above the septum primum (Sept I) into the LA. The left pulmonary veins *(LPVs)* and the right pulmonary veins *(RPVs)* open into the LA. Also seen are the posterior aspects of the left lung *(LL)*, the right lung *(RL)*, and the trachea *(TR)*. (E) The opened LSVC showing the CoS septal defect *(Sinus Septal Defect)* between the LSVC and the CoS posteriorly and the LA anteriorly (highlighted by a *large white arrow*) that passes from RA to LA via the PFO. The CoS is very enlarged as it opens into the RA because the CoS blood flow is greatly increased from the LSVC, and from the pulmonary veins through the CoS septal defect. Note that this case is regarded as a very important "natural experiment." As mentioned earlier, marked ventriculoatrial malalignment was present, with the expected site of the mitral valve (MV) and orifice being above the left ventricular free wall. Both ventricles were well developed (rather than having hypoplasia, atresia, or absence of one ventricle—RV or LV—as in the other cases presented in this study). Remembering that the AV endocardial cushion tissue is located about the atrial outlets and the ventricular inlets, the question is what is the anatomic and developmental identity of the AV valve that opens from the RA into both ventricles? Is it a common AV valve that straddles the ventricular septum and has some chordal attachments to the ventricular septal crest, as in a Rastelli type A common AV valve? Or is this really mitral atresia with a straddling TV that also is associated with a VSD of the AV canal type and that also can attach to the underlying scooped out ventricular septal crest? Or is it impossible to make this differential diagnosis with confidence, one way or the other? I favored the diagnosis of left atrial outlet atresia with a common AV canal and valve because of the striking ventriculoatrial malalignment. I think that all, or almost all, of this patient's AV endocardial cushion tissue surrounding the inlets to the well-developed RV and LV is probably to be found in this large AV valve that exits the RA only and that opens into both well-developed ventricles approximately equally. A small amount of potentially MV tissue may have been used to close this patient's ostium primum, resulting in an intact atrial septum with only a PFO between the RA and the LA. Dr. Stella Van Praagh, whose opinion and judgment I valued very highly, favored the opposite view, that is, that this really *is* mitral atresia with a straddling TV.[88] Why did she favor the latter interpretation? I think because she had studied similar cases with congenital mitral *stenosis* (not atresia) with straddling TV,[88] that looked very similar to the present case. She was extrapolating. She was less impressed with the ventriculoatrial malalignment than I was. I record her interpretation here, not only out of fairness, but because she may have been right and I may be wrong. But from a developmental standpoint, remembering the AV endocardial cushion tissue surrounding the inlet into the malaligned LV is potential MV tissue, I cannot believe that this large AV valve is composed *only* of TV tissue. I think it is very probably made up of *both* potential TV and MV tissue, and therefore that this really is a common AV valve, not a TV only. I present this as an unsolved anatomic and developmental problem, with the pros and cons of two different interpretations. This patient was not included by Dr. Stella Van Praagh in the study of Shinpo et al[87] because this patient's RV was well developed (not small or absent). We would *not* call this kind of case *double-outlet right atrium*, as some of our friends and colleagues have done, because one AV valve opens into two different ventricles. Accurately speaking from an anatomic standpoint, this anomaly has single-outlet RA because only *one* AV valve also exits the RA. This one AV valve straddles the ventricular septum and opens into both ventricles. In what we call *double-outlet right atrium (DORA)*,[41] two AV valves exit the RA, one opening into the RV and the other opening into the LV. A MV also exits the LA and opens in the LV. Thus, there are three AV valves. DORA occurs with *double-inlet left ventricle (DILV)*.[41] *RL*, Right lung.

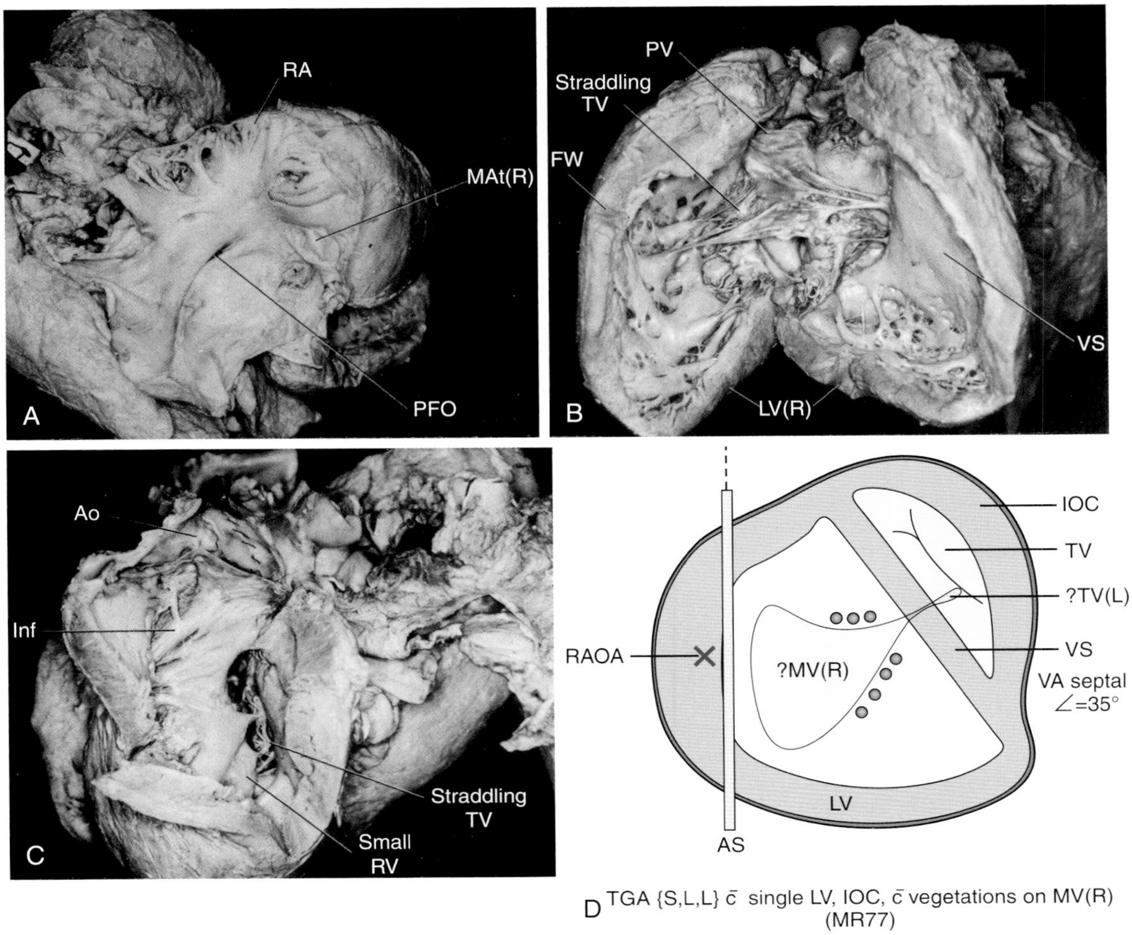

Fig. 14.13 The heart of a 27-year-old man with transposition of the great arteries *(TGA)* {S,L,L} and right atrial outlet atresia. The conventional diagnosis would be mitral atresia (right-sided) *(MAt[R])* because a discordant ventricular L-loop is present. Similarly, the large left-sided atrioventricular (AV) valve would conventionally be regarded as a tricuspid valve (TV) (left-sided), again because a ventricular L-loop is present. In the interests of intellectual honesty, I am not going to disguise the fact that Dr. Stella Van Praagh et al[88] had one interpretation of the anatomy of this heart (they labeled the heart photographs, Fig. 14.13A–C, inclusive), whereas I had a somewhat different view (I made the short-axis geometric drawing, Fig. 14.13D). (A) The opened right atrium (RA) shows that the right-sided atrioventricular (AV) valve is atretic, that is, that there is no right-sided AV valve and/or orifice exiting the RA and opening into the ventricular segment; these data were interpreted as mitral atresia, right-sided, that is, *MAt(R)* by Shinpo et al.[87] A small patent foramen ovale *(PFO)*, and right atrial hypertrophy and enlargement are also seen. (B) The opened morphologically left ventricle *(LV)* is right-sided, that is, *LV(R)*, and inverted (i.e., right-handed; the LV in D-loops is left-handed). The left ventricular septal surface *(VS)* is right-sided, with a smooth nontrabeculated surface superiorly and with numerous fine trabeculae carneae inferiorly and apically. The left ventricular free wall *(FW)* is to the viewer's left hand. Left ventricular hypertrophy and enlargement are present. A large AV valve, interpreted as a left-sided straddling tricuspid valve (straddling TV),[88] receives mixed venous blood from the left atrium. (Note the unusual AV alignments that are *concordant* between the solitus atrial segments and the inverted or L-loop ventricular segment.) There is AV *alignment* concordance, but with AV *situs* discordance.) This large AV valve inserts into a broad multihead papillary muscle on the left ventricular FW and inserts into the muscular crest of the "scooped-out" VS. There is a ventricular septal defect (VSD) of the AV canal type. The transposed pulmonary valve *(PV)* is in direct fibrous continuity with the large left-sided AV valve, and there is no left ventricular outflow tract obstruction. (C) The opened left-sided and anterior subaortic ventricular chamber and the L-transposed aorta *(Ao)*. The subaortic chamber consists of an hypertrophied and enlarged infundibulum *(Inf)*. Dr. Stella Van Praagh et al[88] thought that a very small right ventricular sinus (small RV) was also present because the large AV valve that was almost entirely left ventricular inserted minimally into this chamber. Dr. Stella et al[88] may be right about this (their Figure 2C, reproduced here). I think that the septal band, moderator band, and the anterior papillary muscle of the RV are all infundibular structures, that mark the proximal or upstream boundary of the infundibulum. The true right ventricular sinus lies upstream to this conal (infundibular) ring that in its entirety consists of the conal septum, parietal band, septal band, moderator band, and the anterior papillary muscle of the RV. My interpretation comes from studies of single ventricle and anomalous muscle bundles

Continued

Fig. 14.13 cont'd of the RV (i.e., double-chambered RV). I thought there was no definite right ventricular sinus upstream to the septal band and moderator band remnants in this heart. This is why I thought that this heart had single LV with an infundibular outlet chamber. Note that this infundibular outlet chamber is left-handed (inverted). The straddling of the TV is minimal into the infundibular outlet chamber, typical of single LV (i.e., absence of the right ventricular sinus). The rare feature of this heart is the presence of right-sided AV valve atresia (so-called), that is, the absence of double-inlet LV (DILV). (D) Geometric diagram of the AV portion of this heart in an apical four-chamber projection. This diagram clarifies what has happened developmentally to this heart. The atrial septum (AS) is vertical and normally oriented. But notice that the expected location of the right-sided AV valve and orifice (that usually would be a right-sided mitral valve [MV]) is located above the left ventricular FW. The × marks the spot when one pushes a needle through the expected AV valve location as seen from the RA (as in A) into the ventricular portion of the heart. Thus, right atrial outlet atresia *(RAOA)* appears to have been caused by the FW of the left ventricle being immediately below the expected site of the right-sided AV valve. Why did that happen? We do not know, but happen it did. Notice how far to the left of the AS the VS is. Relative to the atria and the atrial septum, the ventricular part of this heart had undergone marked displacement to the patient's left *(toward the viewer's right hand).* Not only is the ventricular L-loop displaced markedly to the left relative to the atria and the AS, but the ventriculoatrial septal angle of 35° is much greater than normal (5 ° to 7 °).[41] Thus, the ventriculoatrial malalignment involves both left lateral displacement and angulation of the ventricular L-loop relative to the solitus (normally located) atria. These findings suggest that the RAOA was not caused by an anomaly of the MV itself; that is, *mitral atresia* thus appears to be a misnomer. Remembering that the AV endocardial cushion tissue that forms the MV is located around the inlet into the ventricle of the bulboventricular loop that forms the LV, I wonder whether this large AV valve that opens into the LV is not a malformed MV component of a common AV valve that is right-sided, that is, ? *MV(R),* relative to a small left-sided TV valve component, that is, ? TV (L). There is a ventricular septal defect of the AV canal type that is consistent with common AV canal. The absence of an ostium primum type of interatrial communication suggests that the right lateral component of the AV endocardial cushion tissue entering the LV may have fused the atrial septum above with the left ventricular FW below, creating a highly obstructed RA, with the only outlet being a relatively small PFO (as seen in A). This 27-year-old man had thickened and rolled free margins of the regurgitant large AV valve opening principally into the LV, with evidence of vegetations indicating old healed bacterial endocarditis. Hence, my hypothesis (indicated by the question marks) is that this anomaly may be regarded as an incomplete form of common AV canal opening almost entirely into a single LV (i.e., a left ventricular type of incompletely common AV canal). I present this interpretation as a *hypothesis* for future consideration. I am relatively certain that this anomaly really is *not* right-sided MAt with a straddling left-side TV, even though this might remain the conventional diagnosis until it becomes widely understood that these findings result from a particular type of ventriculoatrial malalignment, as the cardiac geometry indicates. (Figs. 14.13A–C, inclusive are reproduced with permission from Shinpo H, Van Praagh S, Parness I, Sanders S, Motthan M, Castañeda A. Mitral atresia with a large left ventricle and an underdeveloped or absent right ventricular sinus: Clinical profile, anatomic data, and surgical considerations. *J Am Coll Cardiol.* 1992;19:1561. Fig. 14.13D was presented by R. Van Praagh at the Second World Congress of Pediatric Cardiology held in New York City in 1985, but was not published in this paper[89] because of lack of space.)

Thus, in this infrequent anatomic type of mitral atresia (see Fig. 14.1 type 6), the primary problem appears to be ventriculoatrial malalignment, not atresia of the mitral valve.

Mitral atresia, that is, **atrial outlet atresia** with a large LV and a small or absent RV, can be diagnosed angiocardiographically (Fig. 14.16) and echocardiographically (Fig. 14.17).

MITRAL ATRESIA {S,D,S}, AORTIC VALVAR ATRESIA, TRICUSPID ATRESIA, AND PULMONARY VALVAR ARESIA IN A CONJOINED TWIN

Case 80 was a female thoracopagus conjoined twin who died at 4½ hours of age. Autopsy revealed what may well be a unique case with microcardia and atresia of all four cardiac valves, as indicated earlier. This rare case was included in Chapter 13 concerning tricuspid valve anomalies; but for the reader's convenience, the salient findings are repeated here.

Both atretic AV valves were aligned as in DILV, with a single morphologically LV, absence of the right ventricular sinus (body or inflow tract), absence of a bulboventricular foramen, an infundibular outlet chamber, and normally related great arteries. Hence, this patient had a Holmes heart[45] with atresia of both AV valves and atresia of both semilunar valves. Our patient was designated as twin B.

From an intercostal artery of twin A, a vessel connected with the RA of our patient (twin B) and then to the LA of our patient via an ostium primum defect (the most common but not the only form of incomplete AV septal defect). From the LA, the blood then flowed into persistent LSVC of twin B via a coronary sinus septal defect. Our hypothesis is that the blood then flowed retrogradely to perfuse twin B with nonpulsatile blood flow.

How did the blood return to twin A in this rare and *naturally occurring cross-circulation system*? Our hypothesis is that the blood flowed into the liver of twin B via the hepatic veins, which then anastomosed with the hepatic veins of twin A, permitting the blood to return to twin A. It should be emphasized that only the anatomic findings of this rare case can be regarded as evidence-based (definite); our physiologic interpretation should be regarded as hypothetical.

However, it may be stated with confidence that twin B had a *biatrial but an aventricular circulation.* From the surgical standpoint, twin B was sacrificed in the operating room in an attempt to separate the thoracopagus conjoined twins, at 1 hour into

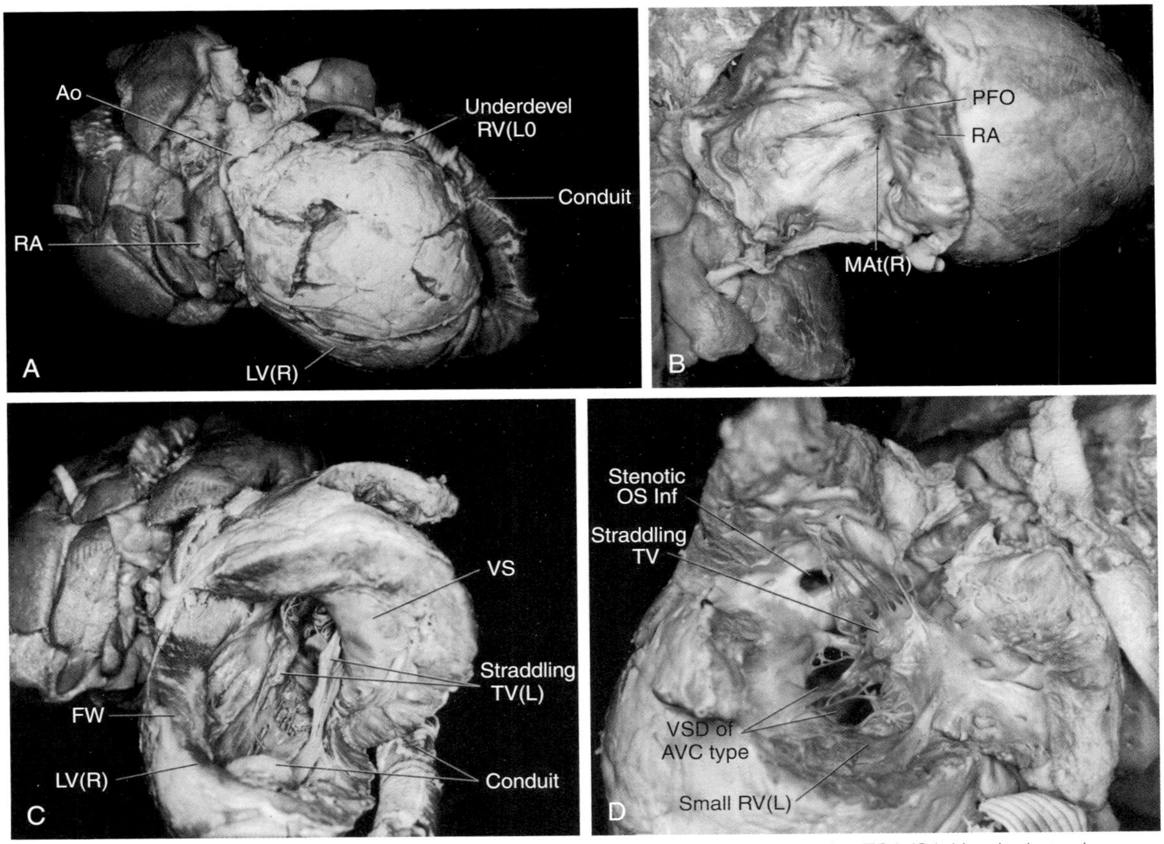

Fig. 14.14 The heart of a 2 10/12-year-old boy with transposition of the great arteries TGA {S,L,L}, mitral atresia (right-sided) *(MAt[R])*, restrictive atrial septum with patent foramen ovale *(PFO)*, a large left ventricle (right-sided) *(LV[R])*, small right ventricle (left-sided) *(RV[L])*, straddling tricuspid valve (left-sided) *(TV[L])*, ventricular septal defect *(VSD)* of atrioventricular [AV] canal type, double-chambered right ventricle (left-sided) with restrictive os infundibuli resulting in subaortic stenosis, subaortic conus with pulmonary-tricuspid valvar fibrous continuity, hypoplastic aortic isthmus (moderate), unobstructed pulmonary outflow tract, and large patent ductus arteriosus (PDA). Because the right atrium *(RA)* was highly obstructive, the patient had the clinical picture of right heart failure (in this case right atrial failure) with hepatomegaly, ascites, and prominent right atrial pulsations in the venae cavae ("a" wave = 26 mm Hg at cardiac catheterization). Thus, right-sided MAt can produce severe *systemic* venous obstruction. At 4 months of age, the patient underwent banding of the main pulmonary artery and ligation of the PDA. (Inadvertently, this produced obstruction of both great arterial outflow tracts—the pulmonary [by banding] and the aortic because of unrecognized and obstructive double-chambered right ventricles.) At 2 10/12 years of age, severe heart failure and suprasystemic left ventricular pressure were found; there as a gradient of 48 mm Hg between the left ventricle (LV) and the aortic root. Misdiagnosed as a restrictive bulboventricular foramen, the patient was treated with a conduit from the left ventricular apex to the descending thoracic aorta; he died 20 hours postoperatively. (A) External frontal view showing the right-sided RA; the large morphologically LV that is right sided, that is, LV(R); the underdeveloped morphologically right ventricle (RV) that is left-sided and superior, that is, *Underdevel RV(L);* the anterior transposed aorta *(Ao);* and a conduit from the left ventricular apex (seen) to the descending thoracic aorta (not seen in this photo). (B) The opened RA showing the presence of MAt, right-sided, that is, *MAt(R)*, and the obstructive PFO. (C) The opened LV(R), which is markedly hypertrophied and enlarged; the straddling TV(L) with thickened and rolled leaflet margins consistent with tricuspid regurgitation; the TV straddling through the ventricular septal defect *(VSD)* of the AV canal type *(VSD of the AVC type);* the left ventricular septal surface: the left ventricular free wall *(FW);* and the conduit originating from the left ventricular apex and passing posteriorly on the left (to the descending thoracic aorta, which is not shown). (D) The small RV(L) has been opened showing the straddling TV, the VSD of the AVC type; and the stenotic os infundibuli *(Os Inf)* associated with double-chambered RV (i.e., anomalous muscle bundles of the RV). Here, the stenotic os infundibuli is seen from the right ventricular sinus or upstream perspective. Note that the right ventricular sinus, although small-chambered, is nonetheless very hypertrophied, reflecting the stenosis of the subaortic outflow tract caused by the small os infundibuli. (E) The stenotic os infundibuli as seen from within the opened subaortic infundibular compartment. The L-transposed Ao sits atop a well-developed subaortic infundibulum (SubAo Inf). The aortic valve has not been opened and hence cannot be seen in this view. Although we have used conventional terminology in describing this heart (e.g., right-sided *MAt* and left-sided *straddling TV,* we nonetheless do so with the mental reservations expressed previously. We strongly suspect that *right atrial outlet atresia* is more accurate than "right-sided mitral atresia." Similarly, we think that a *common atrioventricular valve* as part of an *incomplete form of common AV canal* is more accurate than "left-sided straddling tricuspid valve." The AV canal is *incomplete* in the sense that there is no ostium primum type of defect at the atrial septal level. Because the interpretation of the anatomy is controversial at the present time, I have presented both views here. My colleagues Shinpo et al[87] presented this patient, their Case 18, but these figures are published here for the first time.

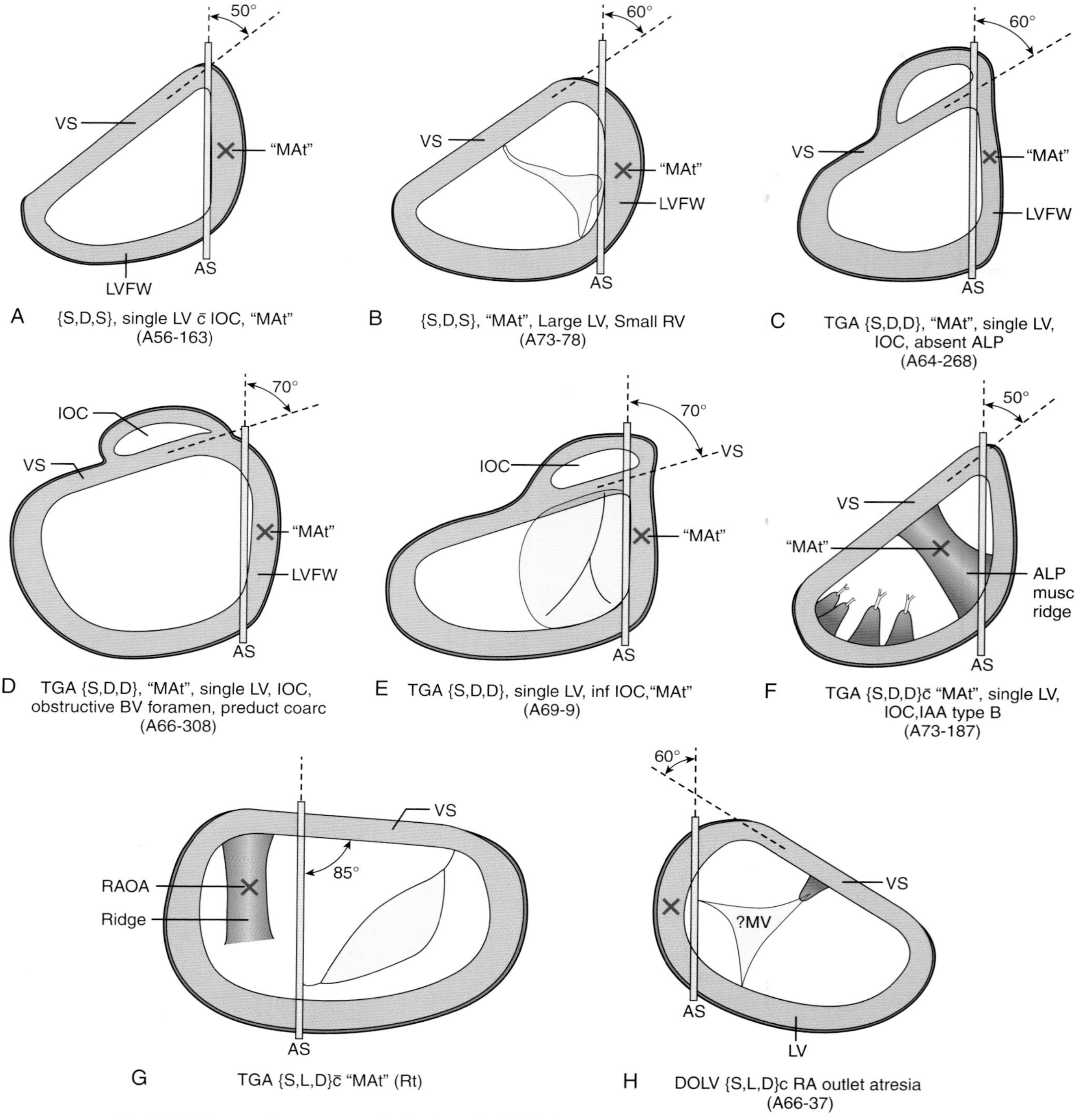

Fig. 14.15 The cardiac geometry of mitral atresia *(MAt)* with large morphologically left ventricle *(LV)*, as seen from the apical four-chamber perspective. In these representative cases, the expected site of the mitral valve (MV), as seen from the atrial perspective, is established at the ventricular level by passing a long straight needle through the expected mitral location at the atrial level directly into the ventricular segment. The × marks the spot where the needle emerged at the ventricular level. Immediately beneath the expected site of the MV and orifice there was always ventricular myocardium. In A, the geometry of the heart of a 2-day-old boy is presented (Case 1 of Shinpo et al[87]). He had normal segmental anatomy, that is, {S,D,S} a single morphologically LV, that is, an absent right ventricular sinus, with an infundibular outlet chamber *(IOC)* and "mitral atresia," that is, left atrial outlet atresia. {S,D,S} means the set of solitus viscera and atria, ventricular D-loop, and solitus normally related great arteries. He also had subpulmonary stenosis. Thus, this patient had a Holmes heart,[45] with "mitral atresia." The atrial septum (AS) was normally located and vertical. But the ventricular segment was malaligned markedly in a rightward direction. Consequently, the expected site of the MV was located immediately above the left ventricular free wall *(LVFW)*, resulting in "mitral atresia" (or left atrial

Continued

Fig. 14.15 cont'd outlet atresia). The ventricular septum (VSD) was displayed far to the right of the AS, and the VSD was markedly abnormally angulated relative to the plane of the AS. The ventriculoatrial septal angle was 50° (the normal ventriculoatrial septal angle = 6°, median).[41] The IOC is not shown. Thus, the ventriculoatrial malalignment that appears to be responsible for this patient's left atrial outlet atria and for the presence of a large LV involves an idiopathic right shift and angulation of the ventricular segment relative to the atrial segment, placing the free wall immediately beneath the expected site of the MV, making it impossible for the MV to open into the LV. In B, the geometry of a 6.5-year-old girl is presented (Case 3 of Shinpo et al[87]). Again, this patient had normal {S,D,S} segmental anatomy. But in addition to a large LV, a small right ventricle *(RV)* is also present; hence, single LV is not present because the heart has two ventricular sinuses. The small RV is not diagrammed. The important geometric features are very similar to the heart shown in A; again, the ventricular part of the heart is markedly malaligned to the right relative to the atria and the normally situated AS. The ventricular septum *(VS)* again is markedly abnormally angulated relative to the plane of the AS, the ventriculoatrial septal angle measuring 60° (normal median = 6°). The rightward malalignment of the ventricles relative to the atria appears responsible for placing the LVFW immediately beneath the expected site of the MV, resulting in left atrial outlet atresia, now called "mitral atresia" (MAt). (C) Geometry of a heart of a 10-day-old boy with transportation of the great arteries (TGA) {S,D,D}, with "mitral atresia," a large and single LV because of absence of the right ventricular sinus, IOC diagrammed but not labeled, located anteriorly and to the right of the VS remnant. *TGA* {S,D,D} is a convenient abbreviation for transposition of the great arteries with the set (or combination) of situs solitus of the viscera and atria, ventricular D-loop, and D-transposition of the great arteries. The anterolateral papillary *(ALP)* muscle of the LV is absent. The ventricular segment is markedly right-shifted and angulated relative to the atria and the AS. The ventriculoatrial septal angle measures 60° (much greater than normal, which is 5° to 7°).[41] The × marks the expected location of the MV, which is immediately above the LVFW. (This is Case 6 of Shinpo et al.[87]). (D) Cardiac geometry of a 7-week-old girl with TGA {S,D,D}, "mitral atresia" ("MAt"), single LV because of absence of the right ventricular sinus, IOC, obstructive bulboventricular *(BV)* foramen, and preductal coarctation of the aorta *(preduct coarc)*. Again, the expected site of the mitral orifice (×) is directly above the LVFW. The ventricular part of this heart is markedly right-shifted and angulated relative to the atria and the AS. The ventriculoatrial septal angle is huge (70°) (normal = 5° to 7°).[41] (This is Case 11 of Shinpo et al.[87]) (E) Cardiac geometry of a 2-month-old girl with TGA {S,D,D}, "mitral atresia" ("MAt"), single LV (absence of the right ventricular sinus) with an IOC, expected site of the mitral orifice (×) above the LVFW, marked right shift of the ventricular part of the heart relative to the atria and the AS, with marked angulation of the VS plane relative to the atrial septal plane (AS) (the ventriculoatrial septal angle = 70°, the normal ventriculoatrial septal angle = 5° to 7°).[41] The AV valve opens from the RA into the LV only, without straddling into the IOC, and inserts into the anterolateral and posteromedial papillary muscles of the LV and into the conal septum. This valve was tricommisural. The BV foreman is restrictive (2 × 6 mm), the aortic valve is bicommissural (bicuspid), and preductal coarctation of the aorta is also present. The pulmonary outflow tract from the single LV is unobstructed. A persistent left superior vena cava drains into the coronary sinus, but the coronary sinus has luminal atresia. The cardiac veins drain individually into the right atrium. A small PDA is also present. (This patient is Case 12 of Shinpo et al.[87]). (F) Cardiac geometry of a 5-day-old boy is presented with TGA {S,D,D}, "mitral atresia," ("MAt"), single LV (absence of the right ventricular sinus) with an IOC (not diagrammed), and type B interrupted aortic arch without aortic outflow tract stenosis. (Type B interruption is distal to the left common carotid artery.) The AS was obstructive. There was a large but functionally closing patent ductus arteriosus (PDA) between the main pulmonary artery (MPA) and the descending thoracic aorta (Ao). This is a fatal combination: an interrupted aortic arch involving the aortic isthmus, plus a closing PDA between the MPA and the descending thoracic aorta, that is, little or no blood flow to the lower body. In this patient, the muscular obstruction of the MV (×) did not involve the LVFW. Instead, it was produced by an anomalous anterolateral papillary muscular ridge *(ALP Musc Ridge)*. The ventricular segment again was markedly right-shifted and angulated relative to the atria and the AS (ventriculoatrial septal angle = 50°). Thus, when there is a large LV, the left atrial outlet atresia is not always produced by an immediately subjacent obstructing LVFW. Other muscular structures within the LV can obstruct the left atrial outlet, as in this patient. (This was Case 15 of Shinpo et al.[87]) (G) The cardiac geometry of a 5 4/12-year-old girl with TGA {S,L,D} with right-sided "mitral atresia" ("MAt") (R) and a large LV (right-sided), absence of the right ventricular sinus (left-sided) and therefore a single left ventricular IOC (not diagrammed). TGA {S,L,D} is a conveniently brief way of indicating that transposition of the great arteries is present with the segmental anatomic set of situs solitus of the viscera and atria, with a ventricular L-loop (right-handed LV and left-handed IOC), and D-transposition of the great arteries (the transposed aortic valve to the right [dextro- or D-] relative to the transposed pulmonary valve. This is the first case in Fig. 14.15 in which a discordant ventricular L-loop has been present with right-sided "mitral atresia" resulting in right atrial outlet atresia *(RAOA)*. The × marks the spot where the expected site of the right-sided mitral orifice "should" have been, as judged from the atrial aspect. However, immediately beneath the expected location of the right-sided MV, there was a prominent left ventricular muscle ridge, that appeared to block the opening of the right-sided atrioventricular valve and orifice. There was a secundum type of atrial septal defect (8 × 14 mm). The left-sided "tricuspid valve (TV)" did not straddle into the IOC, opening only into the single LV; the valve was tricommissural, attaching to the posteromedial papillary muscle of the LV and inserting on to the left ventricular septal surface. The valve leaflets were thick and redundant, with evidence of valvar regurgitation. The BV foramen measured 15 × 12 cm, and there was posterior malalignment of the conal septum causing mild subpulmonary stenosis. Note how marked the ventriculoatrial malalignment is. The AS is normally located (vertical), but the ventricular septum (VS) is approximately horizontal, the ventriculoatrial septal angle measuring 85°. (This is Case 20 of Shinpo et al.[87]). (H) Geometry of the heart of a 3-week-old boy with double-outlet left ventricle *(DOLV)* {S,L,D}

Continued

Fig. 14.15 cont'd with right atrial outlet atresia: × marks the expected site of the right-sided MV, directly above the LVFW. The left-sided right ventricular sinus is absent. Consequently this patient has a single LV with an IOC; the IOC is not diagrammed. DOLV {S,L,D} is an abbreviation of double-outlet left ventricle with segmental anatomic set of situs solitus of the viscera and atria, ventricular L-loop, and D-malposition of the great arteries (with the aortic valve to the right [dextro- or D-] relative to the pulmonary valve). There is a secundum atrial septal defect (12 × 10 mm). The left-sided AV valve opens only into the LV, is tricommissural, and attaches on to the left ventricular septal surface and inserts into the posteromedial papillary muscle of the LV. We speculate that this left-sided AV valve, instead of being the left-sided TV, may in fact be a cleft mitral valve *(?MV)*. Why do we think that? Because there is very marked ventriculoatrial malalignment with considerable left shift and angulation of the ventricular segment relative to the atria and the AS (the ventriculoatrial septal angle = 60°) (normal median ventriculoatrial septal angle = 6°).[41] The RAOA appears to have been caused by ventriculoatrial malalignment (right-sided AV valve and orifice blocked by the LVFW, ×), not by an anomaly of the right-sided MV itself. If so, then what happened to the AV valve tissue that is located around the inlet into the developing LV and the developing RV? The right ventricular sinus failed to develop. Consequently, we speculate that most, if not all, of this patient's AV endocardial cushion tissue must have gone into the formation of this AV valve that enters the LV. If this inference is correct, this AV valve may well be a common (undivided) AV valve or perhaps mostly the MV because the right ventricular sinus failed to develop and hence the RV's contribution to the development of the TV may not have occurred (?MV). If this AV valve is essentially the undivided (common) AV valve, why is it undivided? The answer may be that the AS lies too far to the right to have played a role in septating or dividing the AV valve, although septation at the rightmost side of the AV valve may have closed the AS, creating the appearance of right-sided MAt. Similarly, the angulated VS is too far to the left to have played its role in the division of the AV valve. Thus, this AV endocardial cushion tissue could not "find" an AS or a VS to partner with, that is, to anchor the upper and lower extremities of the atrioventricular septum, which is necessary for the AV valve to undergo septation or division into mitral and tricuspid components. Briefly, this AV valve is very likely to remain a common (undivided) AV valve because of the ventriculoatrial malalignment, which places the AS too far to the right, and which places the VS too far to the left for septation of the AV valve to occur. This is why I strongly suspect that the AV valve that opens into the large LV, and which looks like a common AV valve, really is just that—a common (undivided) AV valve in a previously unrecognized rare, incomplete form of common AV canal (incomplete because the ostium primum has been closed). But there typically is a VSD of the AV canal type. Closure of the ostium primum creates the appearance of "mitral atresia." **But the cardiac geometry indicates that the problem does not primarily involve the MV; instead, the basic diagnosis is ventriculoatrial malalignment.** Because this is not primarily a MV anomaly, this observation also explains how and why it is possible to have "mitral atresia" with a *large* LV. This sounds like a contradiction in terms, that is, like an oxymoron, and it is. That is our hypothesis. We thought that this patient had DOLV because our observation was that the malposed aorta arose mostly above the large LV, not mostly above the IOC. Shinpo et al[87] thought that the aorta originated mostly above the IOC; hence, they made the diagnosis of TGA, not DOLV. This was Case 21 of Shinpo et al.[87] (The diagrams shown in Figs. 14.15B, E, and H are reproduced with permission from Shinpo H, Van Praagh S, Parness I, Sanders S, Motthan M, Castañeda A. Mitral atresia with a large left ventricle and an underdeveloped or absent right ventricular sinus: Clinical profile, anatomic data, and surgical considerations. *J Am Coll Cardiol.* 19:1561, 1992.)

surgery. The heart of twin B was left in the body of twin A. At 7½ hours into surgery, twin A died. Accurate anatomic description of the heart of twin B was possible because twin A also underwent autopsy.

Twin B also had MCAs, including microcephaly, sloping forehead, micrognathia, high-arched palate, low-set ears, marked bilateral pulmonary hypoplasia, duplicate vaginae, two uteri, and one normal ovary, with the other being long and slender (but not a streak ovary).

MITRAL ATRESIA WITH DOUBLE-OUTLET RIGHT VENTRICLE OR TRANSPOSITION OF THE GREAT ARTERIES IN VISCEROATRIAL SITUS SOLITUS WITH CONCORDANT D-LOOP VENTRICLES

We are now leaving the largest group of mitral atresia, that is, those patients with normally related great arteries and normal segmental anatomy (118/177 patients, 66.67%; see Table 14.2) and are about to consider in detail the second largest group of patients with mitral atresia—those with DORV or with TGA in visceroatrial situs solitus with concordant D-loop ventricles (40/177 patients, 22.60% of the series; see Table 14.2 and Fig. 14.1).

MITRAL ATRESIA WITH VENTRICULAR SEPTAL DEFECT AND DOUBLE-OUTLET RIGHT VENTRICLE {S,D,D/"S"}

Mitral atresia with a VSD and DORV was by far the largest anatomic type of mitral atresia with abnormal segmental anatomy (see Table 14.2, anatomic type 8): n = 28, or 15.82% of the entire series of 177 patients and 51.85% of the 54 cases of mitral atresia with abnormal segmental anatomy; see Fig. 14.1).

Sex: Males, 10; females, 18; males to females = 10/18 (0.56). There appears to be a female preponderance in this anatomic type of mitral atresia; however, it should be remembered that this is a small series (n = 28).

Age at Death: Mean, 682.89 ± 1527.38 days, or 1.87 ± 4.18 years; range, 0 (fetal death) to 6205 days, or 0 to 17 years; and median, 97.5 days or 3.25 months.

It is noteworthy that the median age at death of this mitral atresia subset (3¼ months) is the "best," that is, the oldest, of any

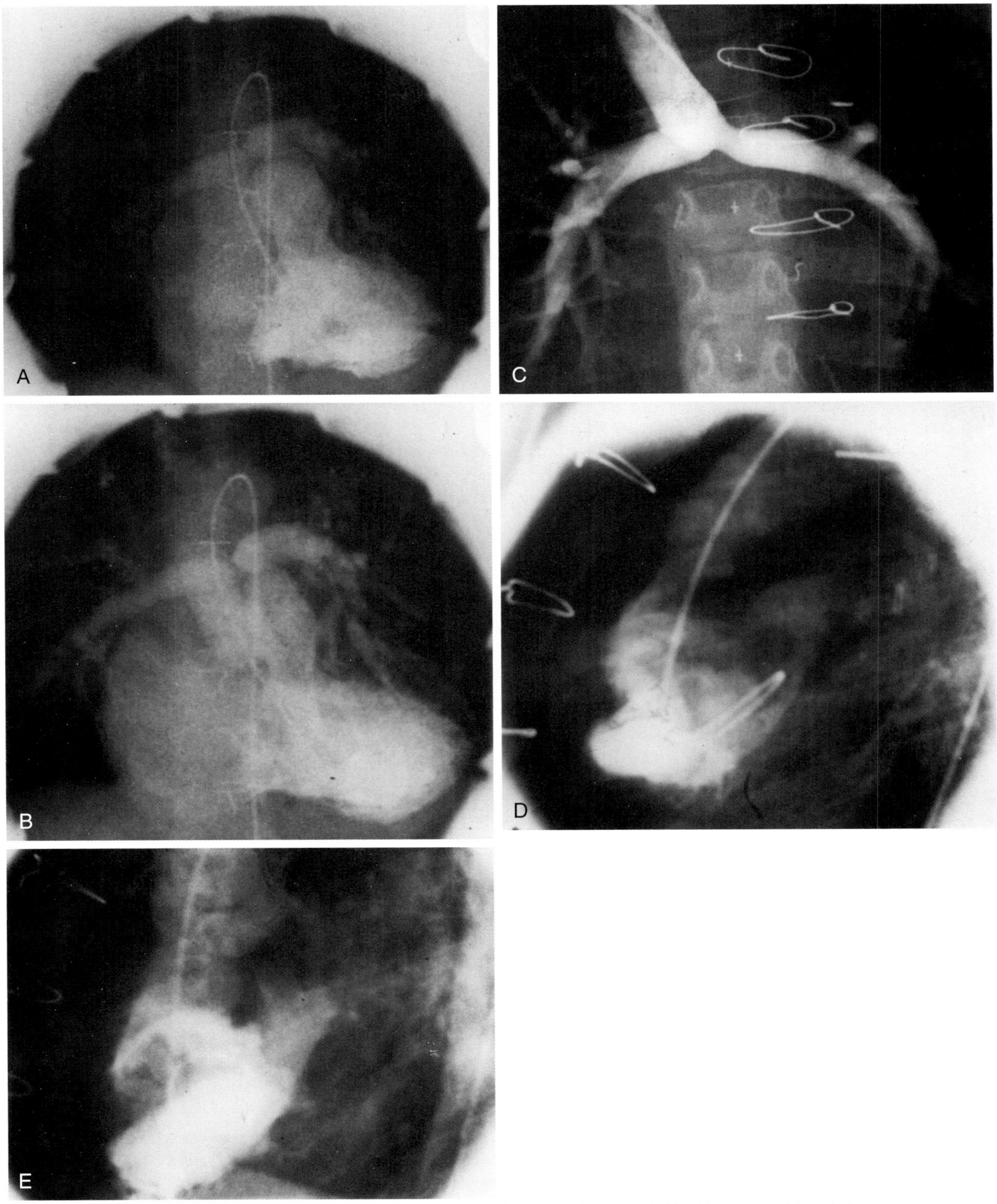

Fig. 14.16 Angiocardiographic findings are presented in a 7 11/12-year-old girl with transposition of the great arteries (TGA) {S,D,D}, left-sided mitral atresia, large left ventricle (LV), small right ventricle (RV), straddling right-sided atrioventricular (AV) valve, large surgically created atrial septal defect, a large ventricular septal defect of the AV canal type, left superior vena cava (LSVC) to the coronary sinus, right superior vena cava occluded or atretic, superoinferior ventricles, subaortic muscular stenosis, and mild regurgitation of the straddling right-sided AV valve. This is patient 9 of Shinpo et al[87] who was alive at the time of this report in 1992. Diagnosis is based on cardiac catheterization, angiocardiography, and surgical observation. At 2.5 months of age, she had atrial septal resection and banding of the main pulmonary artery (MPA). At 5 years of age, mild cyanosis and mildly decreased exercise tolerance were noted. At 5 4/12 years of age, the MPA

Continued

Fig. 14.16 cont'd was transected and oversewn, and the LSVC was anastomosed to the left pulmonary artery (which was in continuity with the right pulmonary artery); that is, a bidirectional Glenn procedure was performed. At 6 4/12 years of age, a subaortic muscular stenosis was diagnosed with a pressure gradient of 70 to 80 mm Hg. Consequently, at 6 5/12 years of age, subaortic stenosis resection and an AV valvuloplasty for regurgitation were performed. Postoperatively, the subaortic pressure gradient was reduced to 5 mm Hg and the AV valvar regurgitation was considered to be mild. Clubbing and cyanosis persisted. A and B show selective left ventricular angiocardiograms in the posteroanterior projection. In both A and B, the banded MPA can be seen. In B, the D-transposed aorta and left aortic arch are seen. AV valve regurgitation from the large LV into the large right atrium is also visualized. C shows the bidirectional Glenn anastomosis (slightly right anterior oblique projection). Contrast has been injected into the LSVC, with good filling of both the right and left pulmonary artery branches. D and E show a selective left ventricular injection, in left lateral projection, following subaortic stenosis resection and MPA transection. The inferior large LV, and the superior small RV and the lack of subaortic stenosis are seen. Although this case was published by Shinpo et al[87] (as earlier), these angiocardiograms are published here for the first time.

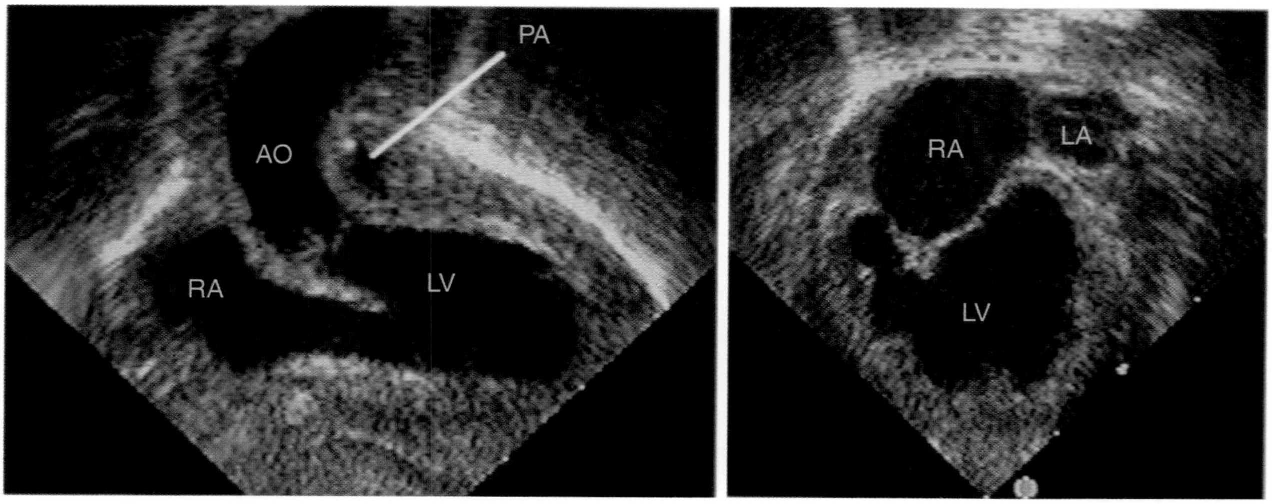

Fig. 14.17 Magnetic resonance images kindly given to us of "mitral atresia" and large left ventricle *(LV)* by Dr. Tal Geva. The *left panel* in posteroanterior projection shows normal {S,D,S} segmental anatomy: the right atrium *(RA)* is right-sided; the LV is left-sided; and the great arteries look solitus normally related, the pulmonary artery *(PA)* being superior and to the left, the aortic valve *(Ao)* being inferior and to the right and in direct continuity with the atrioventricular (AV) valve that opens into the LV. The *right panel* shows the heart in a left anterior oblique–like projection. The left atrium *(LA)* is located directly above the posterior free wall of the LV. No AV valve opens from the LA into a ventricular cavity; hence, left atrial outlet atresia is present. A large AV valve opens from the RA into the LV.

group that we have considered thus far (see Table 14.2, anatomic types 1 to 8, inclusive). Although mitral atresia is a highly lethal form of congenital heart disease with a very unfavorable natural history, some anatomic types have better natural histories than others, as judged by their median ages at death (Table 14.6). What do the varying median ages at death in these 8 anatomic types of mitral atresia suggest concerning the natural history of these anatomic types? The worst was that of the thoracopagus conjoined twin with atresia of all four cardiac valves at 4½ hours of age. This death was also importantly related to a surgical attempt to separate these twins, our patient being intentionally sacrificed in the hope that the other twin might survive, which, alas, she did not.

Turning to the common anatomic types of mitral atresia (see Table 14.6), our impression is that when the aorta "escapes" from the diminutive LV, the natural history (reflected by median age at death) improves sharply. Compare types 1 to 5, inclusive (average median age at death of 11.53 days) with types 6 and 7 (average median age at death of 86.25 days). When the aorta is not confined to a very small LV, but instead arises above a RV or above an infundibular outlet chamber, the antegrade aortic blood flow often is much better than when the aorta is "imprisoned" within a diminutive LV. Thus, the apparent differences in the natural history of these 8 anatomic types of mitral atresia (see Table 14.6) appear to be comprehensible in terms of their variable and very different pathophysiologies.

Anatomic Features

The salient anatomic features of these 28 patients with mitral atresia, DORV{S,D,D/"S"}, and VSD (see Table 14.2, anatomic type 8) are summarized in Table 14.7.

In the interests of attempted brevity, I must let Table 14.7 largely speak for itself. However, there are several noteworthy aspects that do require some explanation.

When DORV occurs in association with HLHS—of which mitral atresia is an excellent example, *the conus (infundibulum) is often unilateral—subpulmonary (only), or subaortic (only)—* rather than bilateral, as is typical of DORV with two well-developed ventricles.

TABLE 14.6 Median Ages at Death in Eight Anatomic Types of Mitral Atresia

Anatomic Type of Mitral Atresia	Median Age at Death
1. MAt {S,D,S}, thoracopagus conjoined twin with atresia of all fourth cardiac valves	4.5 hours
2. MAt {S,D,S}, VSD, Ao At	5 days
3. MAt {S,D,S}, VSD, patent AoV	9 days
4. MAt {S,D,S}, VSD, truncus arteriosus	9 days
5. MAt {S,D,S}, IVS, Ao At	10 days
6. MAt {S,D,S}, IVS, patent AoV	36 days
7. MAt {S,D,S}, VSD/BVF, large or single LV and small or absent RV	75 days
8. MAt, DORV {S,D,D/ "S"}, VSD	97.5 days

Ao At, Aortic atresia, valvar; *AoV,* aortic valve; *BVF,* bulboventricular foramen; *DORV {S,D,D/"S"},* double-outlet right ventricle with the segmental anatomic set of situs solitus of the viscera and atria, D-loop ventricles, and D-malposition of the great arteries with the aortic valve to the right of the pulmonary valve, that is, DORV {S,D,D}, or a normal solitus type of relationship between the great arteries in which a subpulmonary conus is present, the pulmonary valve being anterior, superior, and to the left of the aortic valve, and the aortic valve being rightward, posterior, inferior and in direct fibrous continuity with the tricuspid valve, closely similar to solitus normally related great arteries, except that DORV is in fact present—the latter may be represented as DORV {S,D,"S"}: the quotation marks around "S" indicate that the relationship between the great arteries resembles solitus normally related great arteries (S), but this really is *not* present because DORV coexists—hence, quotes are like a wink—a "not really" sign; *IVS,* intact ventricular septum; *MAt,* mitral atresia; *{S,D,S},* the normal anatomic segmental set of solitus atria, D-loop ventricles, and solitus normally related great arteries; *VSD,* ventricular septal defect.

TABLE 14.7 Mitral Atresia, DORV {S,D,D/"S"}, and Ventricular Septal Defect (n = 28)

Anatomy	No. Cases	% of Group
Subpulmonary conus, with aortic-tricuspid fibrous continuity	18	64.29
Tetralogy of Fallot–like infundibulum and great arteries	4	14.29
Subaortic conus, with pulmonary-tricuspid fibrous continuity	2	7.14
Bilateral (subaortic and subpulmonary) conus with no semilunar-tricuspid fibrous continuity	3	10.71
Restrictive atrial septum	12	42.86
Persistent left superior vena cava to coronary sinus to right atrium	8	28.57
Absence of left atrium	1	3.57
Absence of left atrial appendage	2	7.14
Partially anomalous pulmonary venous connection	2	7.14
Totally anomalous pulmonary venous connection	1	3.57
Agenesis of left pulmonary veins	1	3.57
Membranous mitral atresia	4	14.29
Parachute mitral valve with mitral atresia	2	7.14
Absence of left ventricular chordae tendineae and papillary muscles	5	17.86
Leftward malalignment of septum primum	2	7.14
Right-sided juxtaposition of the atrial appendages	1	3.57
Sinus venosus aneurysm	2	7.14
Polysplenia syndrome	2	7.14
Visceroatrial situs discordance with polysplenia and DORV{ IS,D,D}	1	3.57
Coronary sinus septal defect	1	3.57
Tricuspid valve anomaly with low insertion of anterior and posterior leaflets with underdevelopment of right ventricular sinus and diverticulum at RA-RV junction communicating with RA via circular hole in posterior tricuspid leaflet	1	3.57
Tricuspid regurgitation	2	7.14
Multiple VSDs	8	28.57
Absent LV resulting in single RV	1	3.57
Subaortic stenosis	13	46.43
Bicuspid aortic valve	5	17.86
Aortic valvar stenosis	4	14.29
Preductal coarctation of aorta	8	28.57
Interrupted aortic arch, type B	1	3.57
Atresia of aortic arch, type B	1	3.57
Bicuspid AoV and PV	2	7.14
Right aortic arch	2	7.14
MAPCAs	1	3.57
Double-chambered RV	1	3.57
Aberrant left coronary artery from MPA	1	3.57
Congenital stenosis of ostium of right coronary artery	1	3.57
Single right coronary artery, that is, absence of ostium left coronary artery	1	3.57
High origins of both coronary arteries	1	3.57
Crossed origins of pulmonary artery branches	1	3.57
Pulmonary atresia valvar and infundibulum	1	3.57
Absent ductus arteriosus	1	3.57
Congenital isolation of both subclavian arteries, both ostia surrounded and occluded by ductus arteriosus tissue	1	3.57
Aberrant right subclavian artery	2	7.14
Aberrant left subclavian artery	1	3.57
Wolff-Parkinson-White syndrome	1	3.57

DORV with the segmental anatomic set of situs inversus of the abdominal viscera situs solitus of the atria, D-loop of the ventricle.
AoV, Aortic valve; *DORV {IS,D,D},* double-outlet right ventricle with the segmental anatomic set of situs inversus of the abdominal viscera with situs solitus of the atria, D-loop ventricles, and D-malposition of the great arteries; *MAPCAs,* major aortopulmonary collateral arteries; *MPA,* main pulmonary artery; *PV,* pulmonary valve; *RA,* morphologically right atrium; *RV,* morphologically right ventricle.

Note that a **subpulmonary conus with aortic-to-tricuspid direct fibrous continuity** occurred in 18 of these 28 cases (64%; see Table 14.7 and Figs. 14.3D–E and 14.18B–C). Of these 18 patients, 4 had a TOF-like infundibulum and great arteries, with pulmonary outflow tract stenosis. Because the conotruncus was basically of the normal type, on external and internal inspection, the great arteries looked *almost* solitus normally related. But DORV was present, so the great arteries were not entirely normally related; hence, the designation DORV {S,D,D/"S"}. "S" indicates that the great arteries were *almost* solitus normally related, as mentioned earlier. So, in this sense, these cases displayed *the almost normally related great arteries type of DORV*. And when the subpulmonary infundibulum and the pulmonary valve were obstructive, such cases exemplified what may be called *the TOF type of DORV*.

When the pulmonary outflow tract was widely patent with a subpulmonary infundibulum, this situation was often associated with aortic outflow tract obstruction. Because the subaortic infundibular free wall was resorbed, permitting aortic-tricuspid fibrous continuity, the subaortic outflow tract was often "squeezed" between the conal septum anteriorly and the tricuspid valve posteriorly, resulting in subaortic stenosis. Note the high incidence of subaortic stenosis (13 patients, 46%; see Table 14.7). This was not the only mechanism of subaortic stenosis but also was a frequent and important one.

When the subpulmonary infundibulum was underdeveloped, resulting in a TOF-like conotruncus, the infundibular septum was deviated anteriorly, superiorly, and leftward—away from the tricuspid valve, which opened up the aortic outflow tract.

Note also the prevalences of bicuspid aortic valve (5 patients, 18%), aortic valvar stenosis (4 patients, 14%), preductal coarctation of the aorta (8 patients, 29%), and interrupted or atretic aortic arch (type B) (2 patients, 7%), all indicating aortic outflow tract obstruction.

The other type of unilateral conus, subaortic only, with pulmonary-tricuspid fibrous continuity, resulted in **the transposition type of DORV** associated with mitral atresia. On external and internal inspection, the great arteries looked very much like TGA, except that DORV was in fact present. The transposition-like type of DORV occurred in only 2 patients (7%; see Table 14.7).

A bilateral conus (subaortic and subpulmonary) was found in only 3 of these cases of DORV with mitral atresia (11%; see Table 14.7 and Fig. 14.18). Although a bilateral conus is the rule in association with DORV and two well-developed ventricles, it was the exception in those patients with *HLHS*.

Although all 28 of these patients with mitral atresia had a VSD, **multiple VSDs** were found in 8 patients (29%; see Table 14.7). When VSDs were multiple (typically two), there was always a high conoventricular type of VSD and a lower muscular type of VSD.

Other noteworthy findings in Table 14.7 include:

- absence of the LA (in 1, 4%);
- absence of the LAA (in 2, 7%);
- leftward malalignment of the septum primum[29] (in 2, 7%) and right-sided juxtaposition of the atrial appendages (in 1, 4%).

MITRAL ATRESIA WITH NO VENTRICULAR SEPTAL DEFECT AND DOUBLE-OULET RIGHT VENTRICLE {S,D,D}

How is it possible to have DORV with the segmental anatomic set of solitus atria, D-loop ventricles, and D-malposition of the great arteries, *but with no VSD* (see Table 14.2, type 9)? In the widely used classifications of DORV,[46-56] there is almost always a VSD, which may be subpulmonary (as in the Taussig-Bing, malformation),[46-50] subaortic, beneath both great arteries, or remote from both great arteries (uncommitted). *But absent?* Perhaps one should not be too surprised that cases with no VSD are rarely included in conventional classifications of DORV. Neither is mitral atresia, nor is the unilateral conus (subpulmonary or subaortic). The advantage of studying the primary data (as we are doing in this chapter) is that the data contain many important surprises.

Once again we are exploring *terra incognita*—the domain of the unknown, or at least of the very rare malformations. *The heart specimens are the real professors. All of the rest of us are merely students of various ages.* So, we must discover how it is possible for DORV not to have a VSD. Megarity et al[53] published one such case in 1972. The only outlet from the LV was via a LV-RA shunt. There was no interventricular septal defect (IVSD).[53]

Sex: Males, 4; females, 3; males to females = 1.33/1.0.

Age at Death: Mean, 152.00 ± 336.60 days, or 5.07 months ± 0.92 year; range, from 0 (stillborn) to 913 days, or from 0 to 2.5 years; and median, 36 days

Anatomic Features

First, let's answer the question posed by the very existence of this anatomic type of mitral atresia: how is it possible to have DORV {S,D,D} without a VSD? There are two logical possibilities, and both were found to occur.

First, *the ventricular septum can indeed be intact,* as in 4 of these 7 rare cases (57%): **Cases 157, 158, 167,** and **173** (Fig. 14.19). In 3 of these 4 patients, the LV was diminutive or tiny (Cases 157, 167, and 173). However, in 1 patient with *membranous mitral atresia* (not the more common *muscular mitral atresia* in which there may be a dimple in the floor of the LA but no sign of membranous mitral valve tissue), the ventricular septum was intact (no VSD), but the *LV was small-chambered and thick-walled,* that is, not definitely hypoplastic (Case 158).

Thus, it is interesting to realize that in HLHS, not only is the LA often hypertrophied (not at all hypoplastic), but also the LV may not be definitely hypoplastic. When the LV is thick-walled but small-chambered (because it is doing pressure work, but no flow work), whether the LV is truly hypoplastic is uncertain.

Hypoplastic (adjective) and *hypoplasia* (noun) in pathology mean weighing significantly less than is normal for the age, often qualified as meaning more than 2 standard deviations below the mean that is normal for the age. The reason this has been a difficult problem to solve in HLHS when a thick-walled but small-chambered LV is present is as follows. It is easy to weigh the left ventricular free wall. But what about the left ventricular component of the interventricular septum? How much

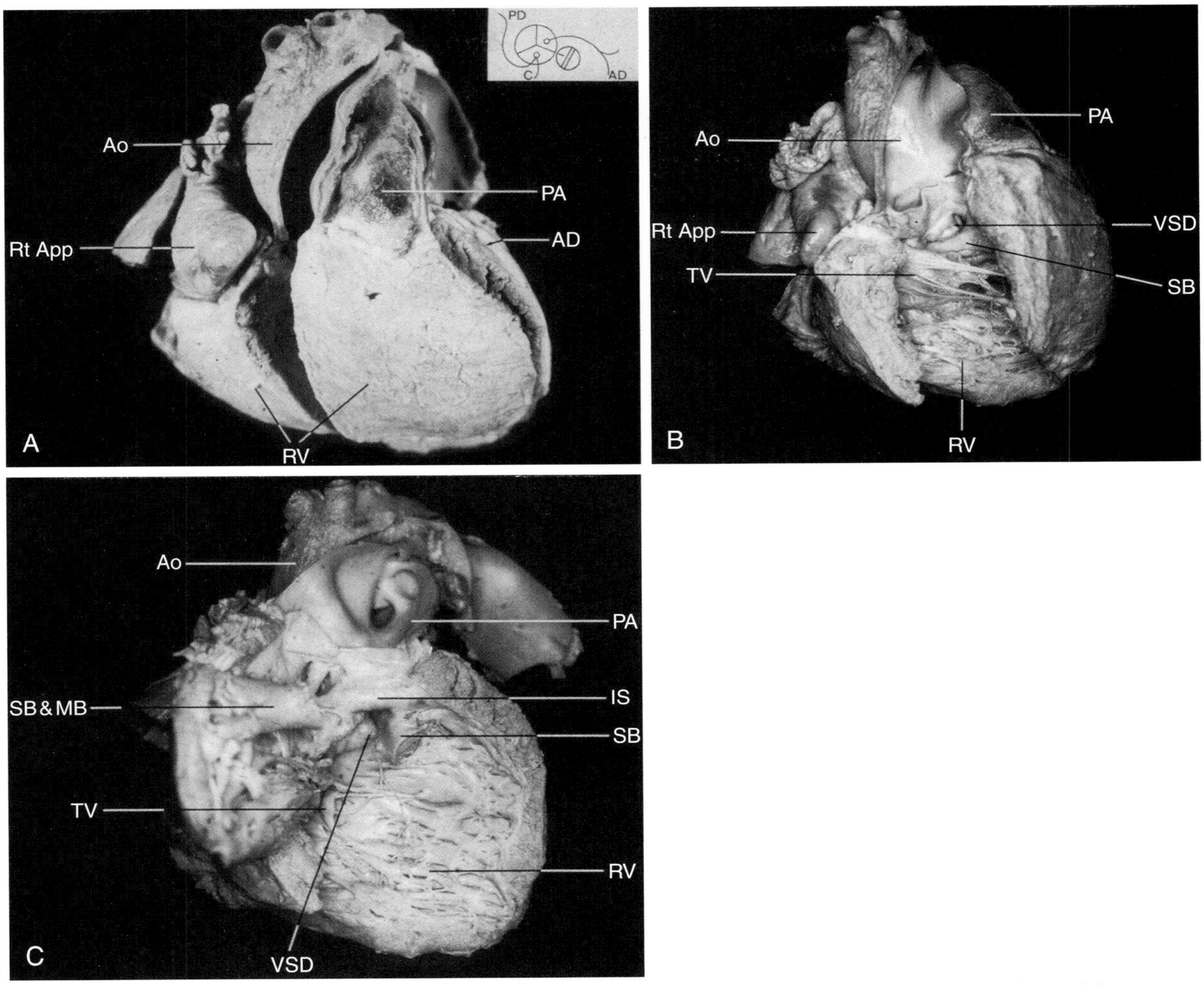

Fig. 14.18 This is the heart of an 11-month-old girl with mitral atresia, a small left ventricle (LV), a large right ventricle *(RV),* a good-sized main pulmonary artery *(PA),* and a large aorta *(Ao).* Why was the ascending aorta large instead of being "typically" small? Because this patient had double-outlet right ventricle (DORV) {S,D,D} with a large conoventricular type of ventricular septal defect *(VSD)* (8 × 3 mm) without subaortic stenosis, not normally related great arteries {S,D,S}. DORV {S,D,D} is an abbreviation meaning DORV with the segmental anatomic contribution (set) of situs solitus of the viscera and atria, D-loop ventricles, and D-malposition of the great arteries in which the aortic valve is to the right (dextro- or D-) relative to the pulmonary valve. {S,D,S} is the normal anatomic set of solitus viscera and atria, D-loop ventricles, and solitus normally related great arteries. (A) External frontal view of the heart showing that the right atrial appendage *(Rt App)* is right-sided, the RV is large and right-sided, the PA is left-sided and of good size, and the aorta is right-sided and also of good size (not hypoplastic). The anterior descending *(AD)* coronary artery is seen, but almost nothing of the small LV is visible form the front. The *inset* shows that the pulmonary valve is bicommissural (bicuspid) and that the aortic valve is large and tricommissural (tricuspid). The origin and courses of the coronary arteries are normal (*C,* conal branch; and *PD,* posterior descending branch). (B) The opened RV shows the tricuspid valve *(TV),* the subaortic VSD with a probe in the defect, the septal band *(SB),* and the pulmonary artery (PA). There is marked right ventricular hypertrophy and enlargement. (C) The opened RV showing the pulmonary outflow tract. Although the pulmonary valve is bicommissural, it is not stenotic. The pulmonary outflow tract and the PA and branches are all of good size. (The SB runs through the moderator band to reach the right ventricular free wall.) Thus, in this case, the aorta "escaped" from the small LV associated with typical mitral atresia because DORV was present. This patient had a very restrictive atrial septum, the patent foramen ovale measuring only 1 to 2 mm in maximal patent dimension. In 1965, a surgical atrial septectomy was planned, but not accomplished, because the patient died intraoperatively. *IS,* Infundibular septum; *SB&MB,* septal band and moderator band.

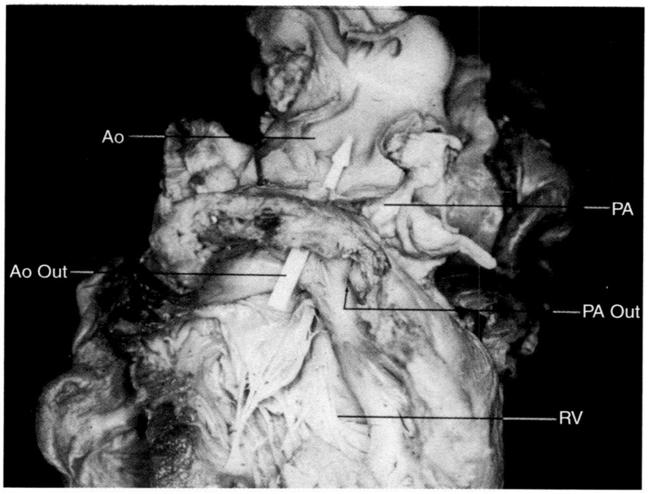

Fig. 14.19 The heart of a 2½-year-old boy with membranous mitral atresia, a small-chambered and thick-walled left ventricle (LV) (not definitely hypoplastic), with an intact ventricular septum, an obstructive atrial septum with a small secundum atrial septal defect (3 mm in maximal dimension) and diffuse left atrial endocardial sclerosis, and double-outlet right ventricle (DORV) {S,D,D} with a bilateral conus (subaortic and subpulmonary) with no semilunar valvar–to–tricuspid fibrous continuity, pulmonary outflow tract stenosis both infundibular (moderate) and valvar (a 3- to 4-mm in diameter dome stenosis). DORV {S,D,D} denotes DORV with the segmental anatomic set of solitus viscera and atria, D-loop ventricles, and D-malposition of the great arteries with the malposed aortic valve to the right (dextro- or D-) relative to the malposed pulmonary valve. The photograph shows the markedly hypertrophied and enlarged right ventricle *(RV)*, the entering tricuspid valve (unlabeled), the widely patent aortic outflow tract *(Ao Out)* shown by a *large white arrow*, and the stenotic pulmonary outflow tract *(PA Out)* indicated by a *small black arrow*. This case is noteworthy for several reasons. It is possible to have membranous mitral atresia with a thick-walled but small-chambered LV with an intact ventricular septum (no ventricular septal defect). When a bilateral conus is present, neither great artery arises from the LV; that is, the aorta *(Ao)* "escapes" from the small-chambered LV and the aortic outflow tract, valve, and ascending aorta can be of good size. This patient was successfully treated with a Blalock-Hanlon surgical atrial septal defect creation at 16 months of age, creating a 21 × 11 mm atrial septal defect. At 2 5/12 years of age, a modified right Blalock-Taussig anastomosis was performed to palliate the pulmonary outflow tract stenosis using a 4-mm Gore-Tex conduit, which unfortunately kinked, leading to conduit thrombosis and death in 1979.

of the muscular interventricular septum belongs to the LV (as opposed to the RV), and how much septal myocardium should be weighed to give an accurate weight of the LV as a whole, meaning the left ventricular free wall and the LV component of the muscular ventricular septum? It is because of uncertainty concerning how much of the ventricular septal myocardium to include in the weight of the whole LV that this question has thus far eluded a definite answer. However, it is suspected that such a thick-walled and small-chambered LV, as in Case 158, my well *not* be significantly hypoplastic.

Another perhaps more important problem associated with the diagnosis of *HLHS* is its nonspecificity. What are we talking about—mitral atresia, aortic atresia, both, or neither? In individual cases, we prefer specific diagnoses, such as mitral atresia. However, we agree that HLHS may be a useful general heading covering the many different anomalies that can be associated with hypoplasia of the LV.

Now, to return to the question, *How can DORV {S, D, D} have no VSD?* The first mechanism, as earlier, is yes, indeed, *the ventricular septum can be intact with DORV,* both when the LV is tiny and when the LV is thick-walled and small-chambered (and only questionably hypoplastic). These are anatomic facts. The real question is How is it possible for such a patient to survive prenatal life? We speculate that the via sinistra is minimal to nonexistent, with little or no inferior vena cava (IVC) blood flow going into the LA because of the presence of mitral atresia. In addition, the pulmonary venous return to the LA late in pregnancy must be able to shunt left-to-right from the LA into the RA.

The second mechanism is when the LV is absent, resulting in an anatomically single RV. When the LV is absent, there can be no VSD. It should be understood that VSD is a short form for IVSD. There can be no IVSD between the RV and the LV unless both ventricles are present.

With single RV, there is no bulboventricular foramen. Again, it should be understood that *bulboventricular foramen* is a short form for infundibulo-left ventricular foramen, when the right ventricular sinus is absent, as in single LV with an infundibular outlet chamber. In single LV, one cannot talk accurately about a VSD, because the RV (meaning the right ventricular sinus, body, or inflow tract) is missing. There can be no IVSD (or VSD) when the RV is absent and only the LV is present; hence, the term *bulboventricular foramen* is used, not VSD, in the interests of anatomic accuracy.

This is one reason why it is important to understand that *the infundibulum or conus arteriosus is not a ventricle.*[57] The conal or infundibular outlet chamber is often mistakenly regarded as a small, deformed, or hypoplastic RV. In fact, the conus arteriosus and the ventricles belong to different cardiac segments. The conus is the crucial *connecting segment* between the great arteries and *both* ventricles (not just the RV). The RV is part of a *main cardiac segment* (the ventricular loop) that normally provides the systemic pump (the left ventricular sinus) and the pulmonary pump (the right ventricular sinus). The infundibulum or conus is not a good pump; its function normally is to perform an aortic switch from above the RV to above the LV during cardiogenesis to achieve concordant VA alignments. The conus is an embryonic "architect" but not a good pump.

The LV was absent, resulting in single RV, in 3 of these 7 patients (43%): ***Cases 39, 153,*** *and* ***164.*** The anatomic type of mitral atresia (9) (see Table 14.2 and Fig. 14.1) is called mitral atresia with *no VSD* and DORV {S,D,D}, *not* mitral atresia with *intact ventricular septum* and DORV {S,D,D}, because when the LV is *absent*, there can be no VSD. With single RV and absent LV, it is difficult to identify the ventricular septum with certainty when there is no left ventricular septal surface. The designation "intact ventricular septum" suggests that there could be a VSD, but the ventricular septum has been identified, examined, and found to be intact. However, when the LV is absent, none of the foregoing connotations is correct. There cannot be a VSD, and the ventricular septum has not been identified precisely and examined. Hence, "no VSD" is preferred to "intact ventricular septum" in Fig. 14.1, mitral atresia type 9.

It is also noteworthy that single RV is not included in conventional classifications of DORV. **Other important findings** in these 7 cases of mitral atresia with DORV {S,D,D}, single RV (absent LV), and no VSD are summarized in Table 14.8. In Table 14.8, the atrial septum was highly obstructive in 3 of these 7 patients, totally obstructive in 1, and not obstructive in 3.

The patient with a large ostium primum type of defect had common AV canal with atresia of the mitral component of the common AV valve. Because this patient also had absence of the LV, resulting in a single RV, the patient had no ventricular septum. Consequently, it was impossible to say whether a VSD of the AV canal type was present or would have been present had a ventricular septum been present anatomically. This is why our diagnosis was common AV canal, *not otherwise qualified*. Was this a *complete* form of common AV canal or a *partial* form? We do not know.

This is an instructive problem. Conventionally, we classify common AV canal (AV septal defect) not in terms of itself, but

TABLE 14.8 Mitral Atresia With Single RV (Absent LV), DORV {S, D, D}, and No Ventricular Septal Defect (n = 7)

Anatomy	No. of Cases	% of Group
Restrictive atrial septum	3	42.86
Premature closure of foramen ovale	1	14.29
Common atrium	1	14.29
Ostium primum defect, large	1	14.29
Common atrioventricular canal with mitral atresia	1	14.29
Left superior vena cava to coronary sinus to right atrium	2	28.57
Rightward malposition of septum primum, on RA side	1	14.29
Totally anomalous pulmonary venous connection to RA	1	14.29
Tricuspid valve redundant and myxomatous	1	14.29
Subpulmonary conus with AoV-TV continuity	2	28.57
Subaortic stenosis with subpulmonary conus	1	14.29
Unicuspid aortic valve, RC/NC commissure well formed	1	14.29
Bilateral conus	3	42.86
Pulmonary stenosis, infundibular and valvar, with bilateral conus	2	28.57
Bilateral hyparterial bronchi, bilaterally trilobed lungs (state of spleen NK: ? polysplenia)	1	14.29
Multiple congenital anomalies, both with foramen of Bochdalek diaphragmatic hernias	2	28.57

AoV-TV, Aortic valve–to–tricuspid valve; *NK*, not known; *RC/NC*, right coronary/noncoronary.

in terms of another variable, the ventricular septum, to decide whether the common AV canal is complete or partial. This approach works well, except when the other variable is abnormal, or nonexistent as in Case 164. Then one understands the weakness of classifying one variable (such as the anatomic status of the AV junction) in terms of another variable (such as the ventricular septum).

Classifying one variable primarily in terms of a different variable is a fundamental error in logic and mathematics. Then why do we physicians do this so often? Because these other variables are clinically and surgically so important. Despite being illogical, this method of classification works well as long as the other variable (or variables) is (are) relatively normal. But when the other variable—such as the ventricular septum in the classification of common AV canal—is very abnormal, this practical, if illogical, approach to classification breaks down, as in Case 164 (earlier). The point is that when such breakdowns in classification occur, we should not be too surprised because classifying one variable in terms of another variable, instead of in terms of itself, is fundamentally flawed, an error in logic.

Rightward malposition of the septum primum, that is, when the septum primum is on the right atrial side (instead of being on the left atrial side, which is normal) is a noteworthy finding (see Table 14.8). Heretofore, we have considered *leftward* malposition of the septum primum in association with various types of HLHS. In *rightward* malposition of the septum primum, this septum (the flap valve of the foramen ovale) lies to the right of the superior limbic band of septum secundum, thereby placing the septum primum on the right atrial side. Rightward malalignment of the septum primum is often associated with the heterotaxy syndrome and polysplenia with interruption of the IVC. Was the polysplenia syndrome present in our patient (Case 167)? Unfortunately we do not know; this autopsy was limited to the heart and lungs and did not include the abdomen. However, because Case 167 had bilaterally hyparterial bronchi, bilaterally bilobed lungs, and rightward malposition of the septum primum, we strongly suspect that the heterotaxy syndrome with polysplenia was indeed present, but we shall never know for sure.

Rightward malposition of the septum primum may well be related to the abnormal hemodynamics associated with interruption of the IVC, which is common with visceral heterotaxy and polysplenia. When the IVC is interrupted, the via sinistra of the IVC's normal blood flow into the RA and through the patent foramen ovale into the LA and then to the left heart and up to the brain is greatly reduced because the venous blood flow from the lower body is conveyed to the SVC (right, left, or both) by a necessarily enlarged azygos vein(s), which is often called an "azygos extension."

Normally, the via sinistra "pushes" the septum primum into the LA, to the left of the superior limbic band of the septum secundum. But when the IVC is interrupted, as is frequent with the polysplenia syndrome, there is much less blood flowing into the RA via the hepatic and suprahepatic portions of the IVC, and, hence, the hemodynamic forces "pushing" the septum primum into the LA are considerably reduced. Consequently, with interruption of the IVC in the polysplenia syndrome, the septum primum can be startlingly right-sided—on the right atrial side, instead of on the LA side, which is normal. This is our best *hypothesis* to explain rightward malposition of septum primum, which we have repeatedly found in association with the heterotaxy syndrome and polysplenia.

It also should be understood that it is almost always possible to diagnose the atrial situs (solitus, or inversus) in the heterotaxy syndrome with polysplenia[58,59] because the concept of atrial isomerism in the heterotaxy syndromes with asplenia, polysplenia, or occasionally with a normally formed but right-sided spleen, is anatomically erroneous[58-60] (see Chapter 29 for further discussion).

MITRAL ATRESIA WITH OR WITHOUT A VENTRICULAR SEPTAL DEFECT AND TRANSPOSITION OF THE GREAT ARTERIES {S,D,D} (N = 5, TABLE 14.2, TYPE 10)

Sex: Males, 2; females, 3; males to females = 0.67

Age at Death: n = 5; mean, 163.2 ± 135.53 days, or 5.44 ± 4.52 months; range, from 24 to 330 days, or from 24 days to 11 months; and median, 150 days, or 5 months.

It is noteworthy that this median age at death of 150 days is the "best" (i.e., the oldest) of any of the 10 anatomic types of mitral atresia that we have studied thus far (Table 14.9).

When we say that mitral atresia with or without a VSD and with TGA {S,D,D} had a better (older) median age at death than did any other anatomic type of mitral atresia studied thus far, that is, 150 days (see Table 14.9), we should quickly add that everything is relative: 150 days, or only 5 months of age, is still a very early median age at death, emphasizing what a highly lethal anomaly mitral atresia has been in our experience (see Table 14.9).

TABLE 14.9 Median Ages at Death in the 10 Anatomic Types of Mitral Atresia Considered Thus Far

Anatomic Type of MAt	N	Median Age (days)
1. MAt {S,D,S}, IVS, AoVAt	80	10
2. MAt {S,D,S}, IVS, patent AoV	3	36
3. MAt {S,D,S}, VSD, patent AoV	27	9
4. MAt {S,D,S}, VSD, AoVAt	5	5
5. MAt {S,D,S}, VSD, truncus arteriosus	1	9
6. MAt {S,D,S}, VSD/BVF, large/single LV	7	75
7. MAt {S,D,S}, mo VSD, TAt, PVAt, AoV At, thoracopagus conjoined twin	1	0.19
8. MAt, VSD, DORV {S,D,D/"S"}	28	97.5
9. MAt, No VSD, DORV {S,D,D}	6	20
10. MAt, ± VSD, TGA {S,D,D}	5	150

Ao, Aorta; *AoV*, aortic valve; *AoVAt*, aortic valvar atresia; *BVF*, bulboventricular foramen; *DORV {S,D,D/"S"}*, double-outlet right ventricle with the segmental anatomic set of solitus atria, D-loop ventricles, D-malposition of the great arteries, or similar to solitus normally related great arteries; *IVS*, intact ventricular septum; *LA*, morphologically left atrium; *LV*, morphologically left ventricle; *MAt {S,D,S}*, mitral atresia with the segmental anatomic set of solitus atria, D-loop ventricles, and solitus normally related great arteries (in MAt {S, D, S}, atrioventricular concordance is only half present because of MAt: RA opens into RV, but LA does not open into LV; in MAt {S,D,S}, ventriculoarterial concordance may be fully present or only half present, depending on the status of the AoV: when the AoV is patent, ventriculoarterial concordance is (fully) present, RV to PA and LV to Ao, but when the AoV is atretic, ventriculoarterial concordance is only half present: RV to PA, but LV *not* to Ao; PA, main pulmonary artery); *PV At*, pulmonary valvar atresia; *RA*, morphologically right atrium; *RV*, morphologically right ventricle; *TAt*, tricuspid atresia; *TGA {S,D,D}*, transposition of the great arteries with the segmental anatomic set of solitus atria, D-loop ventricles, and D-transposition of the great arteries; *VSD*, ventricular septal defect; *± VSD*, with or without a VSD.

Anatomic Features

The atrial septum was highly restrictive in 2 of these 5 patients (Cases 16 and 41) (40%). TAPVC of the supracardiac type occurred in 1 of these 5 cases (20%) (Case 60). The anomalous venous pathway included a stenotic vertical vein to the RSVC. A persistent LSVC that drained into the coronary sinus was not part of the anomalous pulmonary venous pathway. A persistent LSVC connected with the coronary sinus and then to the RA in 2 patients (Cases 60 and 91) (40%). Rightward displacement of the septum primum that lay to the right of the superior limbic band of the septum secundum was present in 1 patient (Case 60) (20%); that is, the septum primum was on the right atrial side, instead of being on the left atrial side, which is normal. A straddling tricuspid valve, through a VSD of the AV canal type, was associated with a small right ventricular sinus (body, or inflow tract) in 1 patient (Case 14) (20%). Absence of the RV (the right ventricular sinus) resulted in single LV with an infundibular outlet chamber and D-TGA in 1 patient (Case 16) (20%). An intact ventricular septum was found in 1 of these 5 patients (Case 91) (20%). This patient also had stenosis of the proximal left pulmonary artery at the ductal insertion site (20%). It is well to remember that *a closing ductus arteriosus can cause important obstruction at both of its ends:* superiorly, ductal medial musculature can encircle and constrict the aorta, causing discrete coarctation of the aorta; and inferiorly, ductal medial musculature can encircle and constrict a proximal pulmonary artery branch, as in this patient.

The transposed great arterial outflow tracts were obstructed in all cases, which was a striking finding; pulmonary outflow tract atresia was present in 4 of these 5 patients (Cases 14, 41, 60, and 91) (80%). This is what one would expect in association with mitral atresia and D-TGA in which the pulmonary artery arises from a typically diminutive LV. However, in the infrequent form of mitral atresia with a single LV (Case 16) (20%), the transposed pulmonary artery arises from a large LV, and in this situation the pulmonary outflow tract typically is widely patent, and so it was in this patient. When a D-transposed aorta arises from an infundibular outlet chamber, the patient is vulnerable to subaortic stenosis from a restrictively small bulboventricular foramen, if the conal septum above the bulboventricular foramen is aligned too well with the ventricular septal remnant below the bulboventricular foramen. Then the foramen can be restrictively small, as was the case in Case 16.

Proof of the significant reduction in anterograde aortic blood flow was provided by hypoplasia of the ascending aorta and aortic arch and preductal coarctation of the aorta (internal diameter 1 mm). The *coup de grâce* in this 7-week-old girl was that the PDA was also closing, depriving her lower body of adequate systemic arterial blood flow.

The ductus arteriosus was found to be closing in 3 of these 5 patients (Cases 16, 41, and 60) (60%). In view of the very high prevalence of great arterial outflow tract obstruction in this anatomic type of mitral atresia (100%)—pulmonary outflow tract atresia in 80% and aortic outflow tract obstruction in 20%—normal or even delayed closure of the ductus arteriosus, although a normal phenomenon, is in these patients a hemodynamic catastrophe, as noted earlier.

Mitral Atresia With DORV {S,L,L} or TGA {S,L,L}. Now we are leaving left-sided mitral atresia with concordant D-loop ventricles (see Table 14.2, anatomic types 1 to 10, inclusive) that accounts for 163 of these 177 patients with mitral atresia (92.09%). In group 3 mitral atresia, we are about to consider patients with *right-sided* mitral atresia and discordant L-loop ventricles (n = 5/177 cases, 2.82%) that have either DORV {S,L,L} or TGA {S,L,L,} (see Table 14.2 and Fig. 14.1).

It will be recalled that the AV valves (tricuspid and mitral) correspond to the ventricles of entry, not to the atria of exit. It would be even more accurate to say that the AV valves correspond to the *ventricular loop of entry,* not to the atria of exit.

L-loop ventricles are often referred to as *inverted ventricles,* meaning mirror-image ventricles. In a mirror image, there is right-left reversal (hence, the tricuspid valve is left-sided and the mitral valve is right-sided), without anteroposterior or superoinferior change. Front and back are unchanged, as are top and bottom.

With - {S,L,-} segmental anatomy, not only is the atretic mitral valve right-sided but also the obstructed atrium is the morphoplogically RA, not the morphologically LA. Because the atrial septum normally opens from the RA to the LA in utero, one might expect that an obstructive atrial septum would not be a problem in patients with right-sided mitral atresia and discordant L-loop ventricles in visceroatrial situs solitus. Surprisingly, this was *not* what was found, as we will soon see.

MITRAL ATRESIA (RIGHT-SIDED) WITH VENTRICUAL SEPTAL DEFECT AND DOUBLE-OUTLET RIGHT VENTRICLE {S, L, L} (N = 4, 2.26% OF THE SERIES)

Sex: Males, 3; females, 1; males to females = 3/1.

Age at Death or Cardiac Transplantation: Mean, 1600.00 ± 1905.38 days, or 4.38 ± 5.22 years; range, 50 to 4380 days, or 7 1/7 weeks to 12 years; and median, 985 days, or 2.70 years.

This median age at death or cardiac transplantation is the "best" (i.e., the oldest) that we have encountered thus far (compare with Table 14.9). Case 166, a boy, underwent successful cardiac transplantation at 12 years of age; in 1978 we examined the explanted heart specimen in consultation.

Anatomic Features

The atrial septum was obstructive in all 4 of these patients (Cases 7, 59, 125, and 166). In one patient (Case 7), a finely fenestrated but obstructive septum primum bulged far into the LA; this aneurysm of septum primum constituted supratricuspid stenosis above the left-sided tricuspid valve (Fig. 14.20). All four patients had visceroatrial situs discordance.

Why is the atrial septum often restrictive with right-sided mitral atresia? When the atrial septum is normally formed, with a well-formed septum primum (the "door" that normally opens into the LA prenatally) and a well-formed superior limbic band of septum secundum (the "door jamb" against which the septum primum normally closes postnatally) and when the pulmonary veins are normally connected with the LA, after birth and expansion of the lungs, the bright red pulmonary venous blood comes flooding into the LA, tending to close the septum primum against the septum secundum in the normal way.

However, this normal narrowing of the interatrial communication makes the atrial septum obstructive when all of the right atrial systemic venous return must shunt right-to-left because of right-sided mitral atresia. *Consequently, if the atrial septum is well formed, it usually is obstructive regardless of whether the mitral atresia is left-sided or right-sided.*

Dextrocardia was present in 2 of these 4 patients (Cases 7 and 125) (50%) (see Fig. 14.20). Why? Because L-loop ventricles "belong" in the right hemithorax, just as D-loop ventricles "belong" in the left hemithorax. Ventricular loop formation may be regarded as a two-step "dance." Normally, the straight heart tube first loops to the right (forming a D-loop); and then later the ventricular apex swings from right to left, ending up predominantly in the left hemithorax, resulting in levocardia. Abnormally, the straight heart tube first loops to the left (L-loop formation), and later the ventricular apex may then swing in the opposite direction, to the right, resulting in dextrocardia, as in situs inversus totalis. When L-loop ventricles are present in a *left-sided* heart, levocardia is an additional (often unrecognized) abnormality.

The anatomic type of conus was recorded in 2 of these 4 patients: it was bilateral in 1 (Case 7) and subaortic (only) in 1 (Case 59). Thus, a *unilateral conus, subaortic only,* with pulmonary-to-AV valve direct fibrous continuity, also occurs with discordant L-loop ventricles with right-sided HLHS.

Case 59, a 2 10/12-year-old boy, has several other lessons to teach us. He had an infrequent form of incompletely common AV canal with no ostium primum type of ASD, a common AV valve with right-sided mitral atresia, and an undivided and unattached anterior leaflet of the common AV valve (type C–like), and a large VSD of the AV canal type. This patient had a mildly small right ventricular sinus (left-sided), a double-chambered RV (left-sided), and a stenotic subaortic os infundibuli that was associated with moderate hypoplasia of the aortic isthmus (but the hypoplasia was not severe enough to warrant the diagnosis of preductal coarctation of the aorta). But the remarkable finding was that this patient with right-sided mitral atresia had *hypertrophy and enlargement of the*

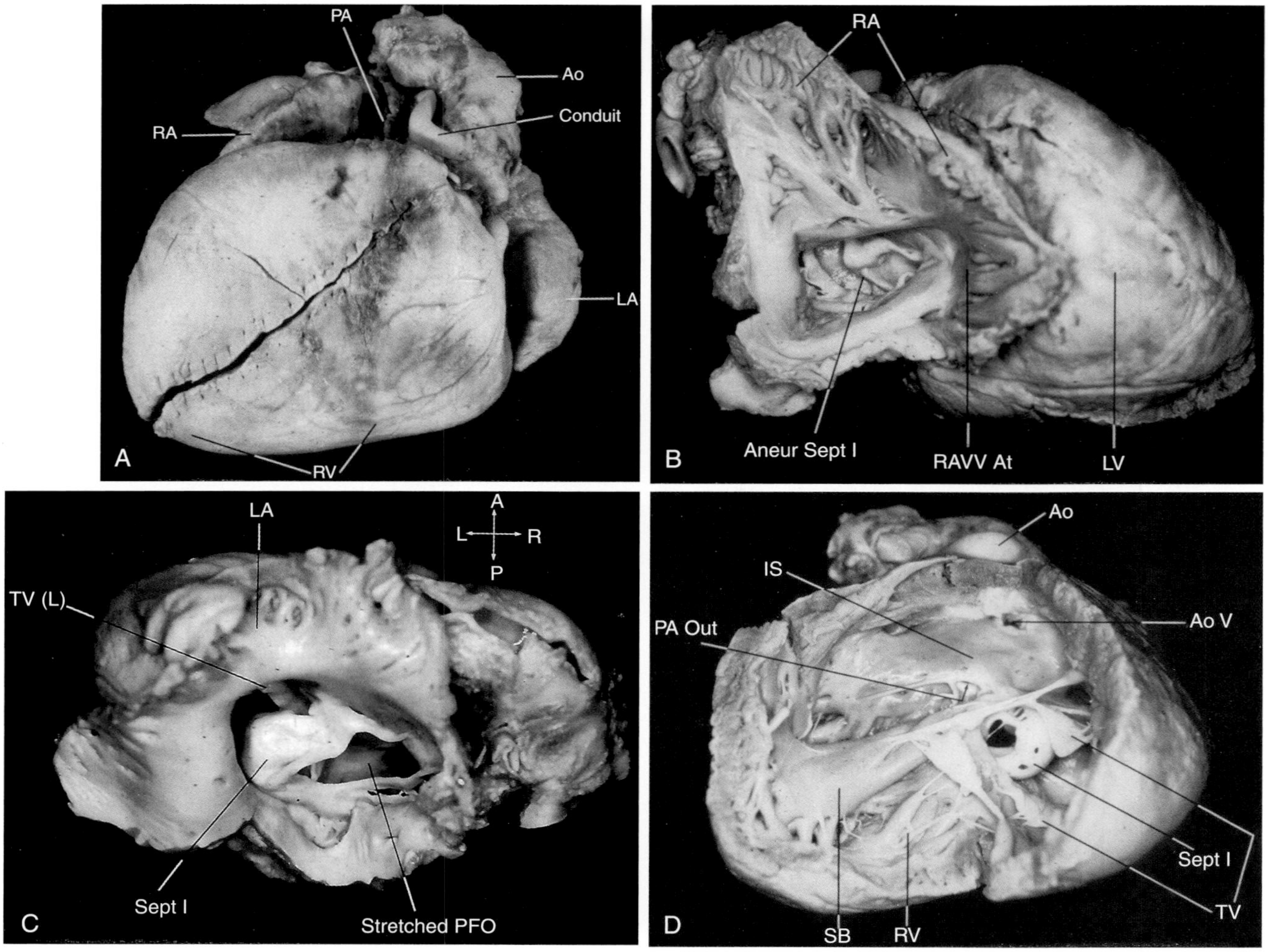

Fig. 14.20 The heart of a 2 7/12-year-old boy with mitral atresia (right-sided) and double-outlet right ventricle (DORV) {S,L,L}, a bilateral conus (subaortic and subpulmonary), pulmonary outflow tract stenosis (infundibular and valvar) with a bicuspid pulmonary valve, a secundum type of atrial septal defect consisting of multiple fenestrations of the septum primum, an aneurysm of septum primum bulging into the left atrium and down into the left-sided tricuspid orifice and constituting supratricuspid stenosis, and dextrocardia. DORV {S,L,L} briefly denotes DORV with a segmental anatomic set of solitus viscera and atria, L-loop ventricles, and L-malposition of the great arteries with the malposed aortic valve lying to the left (levo- or L-) relative to the malposed pulmonary valve. (A) An external frontal view of the heart, note that the atria are in situs solitus, with the morphologically right atrium *(RA)* lying to the patient's right and the morphologically left atrium *(LA)* lying to the patient's left. Dextrocardia is present, with the ventricular apex pointing to the patient's right. The ascending aorta *(Ao)* is left-sided and large (unobstructed) relative to the main pulmonary artery *(PA)*, which is smaller (obstructed) and relatively right-sided. A Gore-Tex Conduit runs from the ascending aorta to the PA. The entire anterior surface of the ventricular part of the heart is formed by an inverted or L-loop morphologically right ventricle *(RV)*, which is markedly hypertrophied and enlarged. (B) Right lateral view of the opened RA and the small and unopened morphologically left ventricle *(LV)* that is positionally to the right of the hypertrophied and enlarged RV (seen externally in A). The hypoplastic LV is demarcated by the anterior and posterior descending coronary arteries (unlabeled). The right-sided atrioventricular valve, that is, the mitral valve, is atretic *(RAVV At)*. The aneurysmal, obstructive, and fenestrated septum primum *(Aneur Sept I)* is seen from the right atrial perspective. (C) The opened LA, the stretched foramen ovale *(PFO)*, the left-sided tricuspid valve *(TV [L])* as glimpsed from above, and the aneurysmal septum primum *(Sept I)* herniating down into the left-side TV orifice. (D) The opened, left-sided RV. Note that the RV is left-handed (inverted in its anatomic pattern), typical of L-loop ventricles. The TV is left-sided. A septum primum aneurysm is seen bulging down into the TV orifice, constituting a supratricuspid stenosis. The septal band *(SB)* is inverted. The infundibular septum *(IS)* is well developed. The unopened aortic valve *(Ao V)* is seen from below and is widely patent. However, the pulmonary outflow tract *(PA Out)* is "squeezed" or compressed by the large posteriorly malaligned IS, resulting in PA Out stenosis. A right Blalock-Taussig anastomosis was performed at 2 4/12 years of age and was revised 2 months later. One month later, the Blalock-Taussig anastomosis was ligated and was replaced by a central Gore-Tex shunt from the ascending aorta into the main pulmonary artery (MPA). Then, thinking that his pulmonary blood flow had become excessive and was causing congestive heart failure, his physicians attempted to reduce the pulmonary blood flow to that delivered by the conduit by ligating the proximal MPA below the conduit anastomosis. However, as soon as the MPA was crossclamped, cardiac arrest occurred. Resuscitation was unsuccessful, resulting in intraoperative death. The important anatomic features of this patient are considered to be right-sided mitral atresia, a hypoplastic right-sided LV, a single small ventricular septal defect, L-loop ventricles, DORV {S,L,L} with a bilateral conus, significant pulmonary outflow tract obstruction, no aortic outflow tract obstruction, and a restrictive septum primum aneurysm that resulted in left-sided supratricuspid stenosis. Orientation symbols: *A*, Anterior; *P*, posterior; *L*, left; and *R*, right.

right-sided LV. So this patient with mitral atresia did *not* have HLHS (meaning the hypoplastic morphologically LV syndrome). How is this possible? We thought that the presence of a large VSD beneath the anterior and posterior leaflets of the common AV valve may have made it possible for the LV to perform enough pressure and flow work, in combination with the mild hypoplasia of the RV, for the LV to become hypertrophied and enlarged, despite the coexistence of mitral atresia. We interpreted the VSD as a confluent conoventricular plus AV canal type of VSD. One may also conclude that this patient demonstrates that it is possible for right-sided mitral atresia to be associated with a *large LV* (right-sided) and a *mildly small RV* (left-sided). At the AV valvar and ventricular levels, these findings are a mirror-image of the findings presented earlier in mitral atresia type 6 with left-sided mitral atresia and a ventricular D-loop (see Fig. 14.1). This same patient also had an obstructive atrial septum that resulted in *right atrial congestive heart failure* with hepatomegaly, ascites, and prominent right atrial pulsations in the venae cavae. At cardiac catherization, the "a" wave measured 26 mm Hg. It will be recalled that this patient's incomplete form of common AV canal had no ostium primum type of ASD.

This patient illustrates yet another important point, namely, *that mitral atresia can occur in association with common AV canal*. In other words, mitral atresia with common AV canal is one of the anatomic types of mitral atresia; conversely, common AV canal with mitral atresia is one of the anatomic types of common AV canal. Although they are two different diagnoses, mitral atresia and common AV canal are not mutually exclusive malformations and can occur together.[61] The same is true of tricuspid atresia and common AV canal; they too can coexist.[62]

The great arterial outflow tracts in these 4 patients with right-sided mitral atresia and DORV {S,L,L} were very suboptimal. There was pulmonary outflow tract obstruction in 3 of these 4 patients (75%): pulmonary outflow tract stenosis in 2 (Cases 7 and 166), and pulmonary outflow tract atresia in 1 (Case 125).

Case 166 had *congenital absence of pulmonary valve leaflets* in association with severe subvalvar pulmonary outflow tract stenosis (3 to 4 mm in internal diameter). Congenital absence of the pulmonary valve (leaflets) is usually associated with TOF, and is seen only rarely in other settings,[63] such as in Case 166. Case 166 also had marked left-sided *tricuspid regurgitation,* with thickening and rolling of the tricuspid leaflet free margins.

Finally, Case 166 had one other noteworthy finding: *membranous* mitral atresia. Typically, when one examines the atrial "floor" where the mitral valve is expected to be, one often sees nothing, that is, no fibrous mitral valve–like tissue but rather only muscle. This we call the *muscular* type of mitral (or tricuspid) atresia. But in this patient, there was membranous tissue where the mitral valve was expected to be. Perhaps in cases of membranous mitral atresia, the *concept of mitral atresia* may be accurately valid. Perhaps a mitral valve was present but failed to develop an orifice. The etymology of *atresia* is: *a,* without, and *tresis,* hole, Greek. By contrast, in the so-called muscular form of mitral atresia, the mitral valve may well be absent; hence, the concept of mitral atresia may not be accurate in *muscular mitral atresia*. The alternative concept of *absent AV connection* has the advantage of, at the least, not being developmentally and/or anatomically wrong. We clearly have much to learn about the cause and morphogenesis of what is generally known as mitral atresia.

Absence of the right-sided morphologic LV resulted in a *single morphologically RV* in a 50-day-old girl with right-sided mitral atresia, DORV {S,L,L}, and pulmonary outflow tract atresia. Accurately speaking, this would be a case of *the aplastic LV syndrome* (not HLHS).

Again it should be remembered that I am not trying to change conventional diagnostic terminology. Instead, my hope is to deepen anatomic and developmental understanding. We continue to use the conventional designations *mitral atresia* (and *tricuspid atresia*), even though we fully agree that we have much to learn concerning their etiology, morphogenesis, and anatomy.

MITRAL ATRESIA (RIGHT-SIDED) WITH INTACT VENTRICULAR SEPTUM AND TRANSPOSITION OF THE GREAT ARTERIES {S,L,L}

Case 47, a 2-month-old girl, had right-sided mitral atresia, a minute and slit-like right-sided LV, pulmonary outflow tract atresia, TGA {S,L,L}, dextrocardia, and a closing ductus arteriosus (1 mm internal diameter) (see Table 14.2 and Fig. 14.1, type 12, 0.56% of this series of 177 postmortem cases of mitral atresia.)

TGA{S,L,L} is the classic form of congenitally physiologically corrected TGA. Unfortunately, however, the potential physiologic correction of the systemic and pulmonary venous circulations is often spoiled by additional associated malformations, for example, by HLHS (right-sided): mitral atresia, minute LV, pulmonary outflow tract atresia, and a closing ductus arteriosus.

As is appropriate for L-loop ventricles, dextrocardia was present. This kind of right-sided heart is sometimes referred to as *isolated* dextrocardia, meaning dextrocardia *without* situs inversus viscerum.

Group 4 is characterized by mitral atresia (right-sided) with DORV (left-sided) in visceroatrial situs inversus with concordant L-loop ventricles (see Table 14.2 and Fig. 14.1, type 13). There was only 1 such patient (Case 152) in this series of mitral atresia (1/177 = 0.56%).

ANATOMIC TYPE 13 WITH MITRAL ATRESIA (RIGHT-SIDED), INTACT VENTRICULAR SEPTUM, AND DOUBLE-OUTLET RIGHT VENTRICLE {I,L,L}

One may ask why anatomic type 13 of mitral atresia is so rare. The answer appears to be, at least in part, because visceroatrial situs inversus is between 1/5000 and 1/15,000 times *less* frequent than visceroatrial situs solitus (see Table 14.2 and Fig. 14.1).

Case 152 was a 1-day-old boy whose segmental anatomic set indicates that visceroatrial situs inversus (I) is present: DORV {*I*, L, L}. As the segmental anatomy also indicates, there was *situs concordance* between the visceroatrial segment (DORV {*I*,-,-})

and the ventricular segment (DORV {I,*L*,-}). The atrial situs and the ventricular situs are concordant, or appropriate to each other, that is, the same: both are inverted (mirror-images of normal).

Alignment concordance between the atria and the ventricles is only half present because of the coexistence of mitral atresia (right-sided). On the left side, the morphologically RA is aligned with and opens into the left-sided morphologically RV. But on the right side, the morphologically LA may not be normally aligned with, and certainly does not open into, the right-sided morphologically LV. So in this patient, alignment concordance is only half present: the RA opens into the RV on the left side, but the LA does not open into the LV on the right side. Hence, it is important to be aware that **there are two different kinds of AV concordance and discordance:** *situs* concordance or discordance and *alignment* concordance or discordance.

We think that the concept of *connections* concordance and discordance is erroneous because, accurately speaking, the atria do not normally connect with the ventricles muscle-to-muscle, except at the bundle of His, because of the interposition of fibroelastic AV canal or junction. Similarly, the ventricles do not normally connect tissue-to-tissue with the great arteries because of the interposition of the conus arteriosus. What some of our colleagues call AV and VA *connections* we prefer to call *AV and VA alignments,* in the interests of anatomic accuracy. Thus, in DORV {I,L,L} with right-sided mitral atresia, there is AV *situs* concordance; but the concept of AV *alignment* concordance does not apply well because of the presence of mitral atresia. It also should be understood that the concepts of AV and VA concordance/discordance can apply well to the *alignments* of the *main* cardiac segments—atria, ventricles, and great arteries—in blood flow (anterograde) order, but not to the *connecting* cardiac segments themselves, the AV canal or junction, and the conus or infundibulum. These connecting segments are like Janus, the Roman god of doorways: they "look" in opposite directions simultaneously. The AV canal connects both with the ventricles and with the atria. Similarly, the conus connects both with the ventricles and with the great arteries.

In DORV {S,L,L}, for example, consider the tricuspid portion of the AV canal. The left-sided tricuspid valve connects with the left-sided RV, that is, a concordant connection. But this same left-sided tricuspid valve connects with the left-sided LA, which is a discordant connection. So, in DORV {S,L,L}, the left-sided tricuspid valvar connection is both concordant and discordant, depending on in which direction one looks, anterogradely or retrogradely. This is an example of why the concept of concordance/discordance can apply well to the alignments of the main segments but does not apply well to the connecting segments per se. When people speak of AV and VA *connections* they mean AV and VA *alignments.*

Case 152, the newborn boy with DORV {I,L,L} and mitral atresia (right-sided), had an incomplete form of common AV canal with an ostium primum defect but without a VSD of the AV canal type. The right-sided LV was extremely hypoplastic, with no mitral tensor apparatus (no chordae tendineae and no papillary muscles). The ventricular septum was intact. Although the patent foramen ovale was valve competent, this did not prevent right-to-left shunting from the LA (right-sided) to the RA (left-sided) via the incomplete AV septal defect (i.e., the ostium primum defect).

Pulmonary outflow tract stenosis was very severe (nearly atretic). A left aortic arch was present, inconsistent with visceroatrial situs inversus. A *brachiocephalic artery* was present; the first branch from the aortic arch gave origin to the right subclavian artery, the right common carotid artery, and the left common carotid artery. The left subclavian artery arose as the second branch from the aortic arch. This 1-day-old boy had a ductus arteriosus that was tortuous and minimally patent. This type of tortuous and small PDA is characteristic of severe pulmonary outflow tract stenosis or atresia because ductal development depends on right-to-left blood flow in utero from the MPA through the ductus arteriosus into the descending thoracic aorta. This right-to-left blood flow prenatally is greatly reduced or eliminated by severe pulmonary outflow tract obstruction—hence, the tortuous and small-caliber ductus arteriosus of this patient.

This patient had a bilateral conus—subaortic (to the left) and subpulmonary (to the right). Consequently, there was no fibrous continuity between either semilunar valve (aortic or pulmonary) and the left-sided tricuspid valve. The right-sided subpulmonary part of the conus was very poorly expanded, that is, tightly stenotic, and the pulmonary valve was also very small (as earlier). The left-sided subaortic part of the conus was only several millimeters in height; consequently, the unobstructed aortic valve was almost in direct fibrous continuity with the left-sided tricuspid valve. Hence, the infundibuloarterial part of this heart closely approximated that of inverted or mirror-image TOF. This was almost a unilateral (subpulmonary only) conus, except for 2 or 3 mm of subaortic conal free wall myocardium that separated the aortic valve above from the tricuspid valve below. It will be recalled that we encountered DORV with a unilateral conus (subpulmonary only, or subaortic only) in association with HLHS in other cardiotypes (presented earlier). Case 152 was nearly the same thing: DORV with an almost unilateral conus in association with HLHS, now in the rare cardiotype (segmental anatomic combination) of DORV {I,L,L}.

Case 152 also exemplified **familial congenital heart disease:** an older sibling had the heterotaxy syndrome and was stillborn. It also had *MCAs:* the *Meckel-Gruber syndrome* or a variant thereof. This syndrome is characterized by *dysencephalia splanchnocystica.* In greater detail, the Meckel-Gruber syndrome typically has an encephalocele, polydactyly, and cystic kidneys. It is inherited as an autosomal recessive condition. This case had an occipital defect with only partial skin covering, brittle skull bones, a large and open anterior fontanelle, hypertelorism, a small chest, scoliosis, bilaterally undescended testes, six digits on all extremities, clubbing of both feet, omphalocele, abnormal facies, hypoplastic lungs, cystic kidneys, and a normal male karyotype (46XY).

Anatomic group 5 of mitral atresia had DORV or TGA in visceroatrial situs inversus, but with D-loop ventricles (see Table 14.2 and Fig. 14.1). Consequently the mitral atresia was *left-sided.* Group 5 contained two anatomic types of mitral atresia, types 14 and 15 (see Fig. 14.1).

MITRAL ATRESIA (LEFT-SIDED) WITH OR WITHOUT A VENTRAL SEPTAL DEFECT AND DOUBLE-OUTLET RIGHT VENTRICLE {I,D,D}

Three of these 177 cases (1.69%; see Table 14.2) had left-sided mitral atresia in association with DORV that had a segmental anatomic set of situs inversus of the viscera and atria, discordant D-loop ventricles, and D-malposition of the great arteries, or briefly DORV {I, D, D} (see Fig. 14.1, type 14, and Fig. 14.2). Because D-loop (noninverted) ventricles were present, the mitral atresia was left-sided. As the segmental anatomy indicates—DORV {I,D,D}—there was AV *situs* discordance (inverted atria with noninverted ventricles). AV *alignment* discordance was only half present because of left-sided mitral atresia. On the right side, the LA opened into the RV. But on the left side, the RA did *not* open into the LV because of mitral atresia.

Sex: In this small series of 3 rare cases (see Fig. 14.1, anatomic type 14), there were 2 boys, no girls, and in 1 case (a consult from Brooklyn, New York) the gender of the patient was unknown to us. Hence, males to females = 2/0, with unknown = 1.

Age at Death: $n = 2$ (not known = 1); mean, 1358.5 ± 1861.81 days, or 3.72 ± 5.10 years; range, from 42 to 2675 days, or from 6 weeks to 7.33 years; and median, 1358.5 days or 3.72 years.

Anatomic Features

The cardiac position in the thorax was noteworthy in two patients. **Case 62** had *dextrocardia,* which is normal for visceroatrial situs inversus but abnormal for D-loop ventricles. Case 25 had *mesocardia,* which is always abnormal. Mesocardia may be regarded as incomplete cardiac morphogenetic movement in the following sense. Ventricular looping to the right (D-loop formation) has occurred, but the subsequent swing of the ventricular apex from right to left was incomplete. In this patient, mesocardia is regarded as *half way to levocardia* (which is normal for D-loop ventricles, but abnormal for viscerotrial situs inversus). Perhaps mesocardia in DORV {I,D,D} may be regarded as a "compromise" between what is normal for visceroatrial situs inversus (i.e., dextrocardia) and what is normal for D-loop ventricles (i.e., levocardia); however, this is speculation.

The atrial septum was restrictive in 2 of these 3 patients (Cases 25 and 160). In the third patient (Case 62), an incompletely common AV canal with mitral atresia had a large typical ostium primum defect that did not restrict left-to-right shunting at the atrial level necessitated by left-sided mitral atresia. This same patient (Case 62, a 7 4/12-year-old boy) had visceral heterotaxy but with a normal spleen. In other words, this rare patient had the asplenia syndrome, but with a normally formed left-sided spleen, and with atrial situs inversus (not atrial situs ambiguus, and not "right atrial isomerism"). The right-sided IVC veered to the left at the level of the liver, received the hepatic veins, and then drained into the left-sided RA. A right-sided SVC drained into the coronary sinus and then to the left-sided RA. A LSVC connected with the left-sided RA; hence, there were bilateral SVCs. There was TAPVC to the junction of the LSVC with the left-sided RA, without obstruction of the pulmonary venous return. This relatively "old" patient (7 4/12 years) had significant and hemodynamically disadvantageous *tricuspid regurgitation.*

Case 62's segmental anatomy was DORV {*AI*,D,D}; *A* indicates situs ambiguus of the viscera; and *I* means situs inversus of the atria. Note that *A* and *I* are not separated by a comma because the viscera and the atria are regarded as different parts of the same cardiac segment, that is, the visceroatrial segment.

This kind of case has taught us that it is definitely possible to have visceral heterotaxy, very similar if not identical to that of the asplenia syndrome, but with a normally formed spleen. This is why we prefer **the heterotaxy syndrome** as the main diagnosis (rather than the asplenia syndrome); but we always describe the anatomic state of the spleen with care (in view of its importance in the body's defenses against infectious diseases). *Also, the spleen can be present, but hypoplastic* in mitral atresia with DORV {I,D,D}, as in Case 25, in which the spleen weighed only 60% of the normal weight. The LV was hypoplastic in all 3 patients. In 2, absence of the mitral tensor apparatus—absence of chordae tendineae and papillary muscles—was documented. The ventricular septum was intact in 2 of these 3 patients: in Case 160,[a] and in Case 62 with an incomplete form of common AV canal. Case 25 had a high, small conoventricular type of VSD.

The anatomic type of conus was recorded in 2 of these 3 patients: bilateral in 1 (Case 25), and subaortic (only) in 1 (Case 160). Pulmonary outflow tract obstruction was found in 2 of these 3 patients: pulmonary infundibular and valvular stenosis in Case 25, who had a bilateral conus, and pulmonary outflow tract atresia in Case 160, who had a subaortic conus. Case 25 had a right aortic arch, a closing right-sided ductus arteriosus, stenosis ("coarctation") of the proximal right pulmonary artery at the ductal insertion site, and a vascular ring that compressed the morphologically left mainstem bronchus that was positionally right-sided. The vascular ring about the right-sided bronchus was formed by the right aortic arch superiorly and posteriorly, the right pulmonary artery branch anteriorly, and the closing right ductus arteriosus superiorly and anteriorly where it inserted into the proximal right pulmonary artery. The proximal left pulmonary artery also played a role because it lay immediately to the left of the right-sided bronchus that was compressed by its neighboring structures (Fig. 14.21). When **Dr. Louise Calder** and I studied this 42-day-old boy in 1970, we thought that ligation and division of the right-sided ductus arteriosus would have decompressed the entrapped right-sided left mainstem bronchus.

---

[a]Although it is impossible to thank all of our many friends and colleagues from all over the world, I would like to acknowledge **Dr. Walter Silver** and **Dr. Nakul Chandra** from Maimonides Medical Center in Brooklyn, NY, who kindly sent Case 160 to Dr. Stella Van Praagh and me for consultation in 1987. Because of the kindness and generosity of so many friends, we have learned much that we have never previously been able to publish. This work is an attempt to say thank you and to make amends.

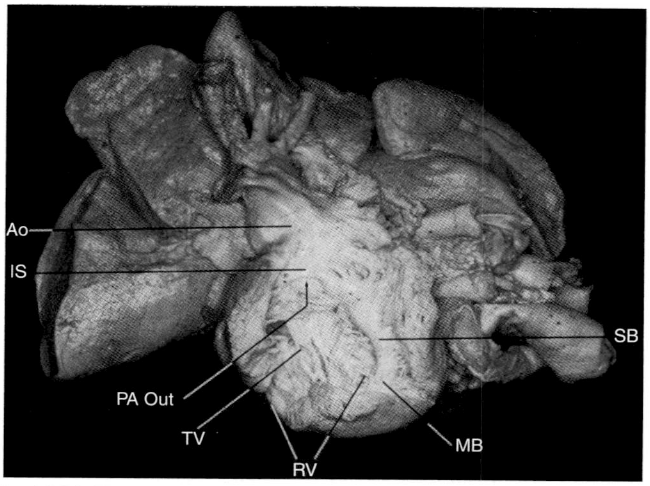

Fig. 14.21 This is the opened right-sided morphologically right ventricle *(RV)* of a 42-day-old boy with mesocardia, left-sided mitral atresia, and double-outlet right ventricle (DORV) {I,D,D} and a high small conoventricular type of ventricular septal defect. The morphologically left ventricle is hypoplastic with absence of left ventricular papillary muscles. DORV {I,D,D} briefly denotes DORV with the segmental anatomic set of situs inversus of the viscera and atria, D-loop ventricles, and D-malposition of the great arteries with the malposed aortic valve lying to the right (dextro- or D-) relative to the malposed pulmonary valve. Thus, this was one of those rare patients with situs inversus "totalis," except for the heart. This segmental anatomy suggests that he "should" have had the rare form of congenitally physiologically corrected transposition of the great arteries in visceroatrial situs inversus, except for a few additional anomalies that vitiated the potential physiologic correction of the circulations, such as mitral atresia, bilateral conus, DORV, and pulmonary outflow tract stenosis (infundibular and valvar). The pulmonary valve was unicuspid (i.e., unicomissural). In the photograph, one can see that the opened RV is markedly hypertrophied and enlarged. The situs (pattern of anatomic organization) of the RV is right-handed, that is, that of D-loop ventricles. The entering tricuspid valve *(TV)* is right-sided. The hypertrophied septal band *(SB)* and moderator band *(MB)* are quite left-sided, all appropriate for a D-loop RV, and the opposite of the anatomic pattern of an L-loop RV (compare with Fig. 14.20D). A bilateral conus (subaortic and subpulmonary) is present. The outflow tract to the D-malposed aorta *(Ao)* is wide open (unobstructed). But the pulmonary outflow tract *(PA Out)* is very stenotic. The infundibular septum *(IS)* is posteriorly malaligned, compressing or "squeezing" the pulmonary outflow tract. The aortic arch was right-sided (appropriate for visceroatrial situs inversus). The patent ductus arteriosus (PDA) was also right-sided (again, appropriate for visceroatrial situs inversus); but the right-sided PDA was also closing functionally, an important problem in view of the severe pulmonary outflow tract stenosis, but to be expected at (or before) 6 weeks of age. This patient had a vascular ring with compression of the right-sided left mainstem bronchus. The vascular ring was formed by the left pulmonary artery, the right pulmonary artery, the right patent ductus arteriosus, and the right aortic arch. There was hypoplasia of the proximal right pulmonary artery (3 mm internal diameter). The right-sided spleen was hypoplastic (60% of expected weight). This was identified as mitral atresia (left-sided) in the rare setting of DORV {I,D,D}.

MITRAL ATRESIA (LEFT-SIDED) WITH INTACT VENTRICULAR SEPTUM AND TRANSPOSITION OF THE GREAT ARTERIES {I,D,D/A}

Mitral atresia is left-sided in this type because D-loop ventricles are present. TGA {I,D,D/A} is potentially congenitally physiologically corrected TGA in visceroatrial situs inversus. Please forgive all the adverbs, but each is important: *potentially,* because additional congenital malformations frequently vitiate the potential physiologic correction of the systemic and pulmonary venous circulations, as this type of mitral atresia exemplifies; *congenitally,* because we are not talking about *surgically* corrected TGA; and *physiologically,* because we are not talking about an anomaly now known as anatomically corrected malposition (ACM) of the great arteries that used to be regarded as a type of TGA. Suffice it to say that we fully agree that *potentially congenitally physiologically corrected TGA* is far too much of a mouthful to be clinically practical; we essentially never use this designation. At most, we may talk about *congenitally corrected* TGA, or simply *corrected* TGA, with all of the foregoing being understood. Frequently, we do not talk about *corrected TGA* at all, because the concept of physiologic correction is often such a cruel joke in hearts with AV and VA discordance (double discordance). Instead, we prefer to use segmental anatomy, which is accurate and brief.

For example, in these two rare patients (see Fig. 14.1, type 15) **Case 17,** a 6-year-old girl, had *TGA {I,D,D}* with left-sided mitral atresia, and **Case 65,** a 16-day-old boy, had *TGA {I,D,A}* with left-sided mitral atresia. As the segmental anatomy indicates, Case 17 had D-TGA (meaning that the transposed aortic valve was to the right [*dextro-* or D-] relative to the transposed pulmonary valve), whereas Case 65 had A-TGA (meaning that the transposed aortic valve was directly anterior [*antero-* or A-] relative to the transposed pulmonary valve). Although we prefer to make our diagnoses in terms of brief, accurate segmental anatomy, we also think that the older physiologic concepts such as congenitally physiologically corrected TGA should be understood, despite their frequent physiologic inaccuracies.

Sex: Male, 1; female, 1; and male to female = 1.

Age at Death: Mean, 1103 ± 1537.25 days, or 3.02 ± 4.21 years; range, from 16 to 2190 days, or from 16 days to 6 years; and median, 1103 days or 3.02 years.

This type of mitral atresia (left-sided) with congenitally "physiologically corrected" TGA in situs inversus with segmental anatomy of TGA {I,D,D} or TGA {I,D,A} occurred in the previously mentioned 2 patients, composing 1.13% of this series of 177 postmortem cases of mitral atresia (see Table 14.2 and Fig. 14.1, anatomic type 15).

Anatomic Features

The **atrial septum** was obstructive in both cases, despite the fact that the atrial septum in visceroatrial situs inversus is designed to open from left to right, that is, from the left-sided RA into the right-sided LA.

An interesting mechanism for decompressing the left-sided RA was found in **Case 17**. There was a large *coronary sinus septal defect* between the coronary sinus and the right-sided LA. Thus, in addition to shunting left-to-right through the restrictive atrial septum, systemic venous blood from the left-sided RA could flow retrogradely through the coronary sinus ostium and then through the large coronary sinus septal defect into the right-sided LA and then into the right-sided RV.

The other patient, Case 65, had an *aneurysm of septum primum* that bulged into the right-sided LA and down into the right-sided tricuspid orifice, producing *supratricuspid stenosis.*

- *The left-sided LV* was markedly hypoplastic in both patients.
- *Pulmonary outflow tract atresia* was present in both cases.
- *A closing ductus arteriosus* was found in both patients.
- *Isolated levocardia* was considered to be present in both patients; that is, the heart was left-sided but the viscera and atria were in situs inversus.
- *A right aortic arch* was present in both patients, which is usual for visceroatrial situs inversus.

The mother of Case 65 with TGA {I,D,A} and mitral atresia (left-sided) was addicted to cocaine. Her son, who died at 16 days of age (Case 65), had signs of methadone withdrawal. The presence of *maternal cocaine addiction* is recorded here, in case cocaine may prove relevant to the cause and/or morphogenesis of mitral atresia with TGA {I,D,A} or a similar anomaly.

Mitral Atresia With the Heterotaxy Syndromes of Polysplenia or Asplenia. Does mitral atresia occur in the heterotaxy syndromes with polysplenia or asplenia? Judging from our database, the answer is yes, but very infrequently. We have only one patient with mitral atresia and visceral heterotaxy and polysplenia (0.56% of our series of mitral atresia; see Table 14.2 and Fig. 14.1, anatomic type 16) and only two of 177 patients with mitral atresia had visceral heterotaxy and asplenia (1.13%; see Table 14.2 and Fig. 14.1 anatomic types 17 and 18).

All 3 patients had DORV. These 3 patients with mitral atresia in the heterotaxy syndromes constitute mitral atresia group 6, which contains 3 different anatomic types: types 16, 17, and 18 (see Table 14.2 and Fig. 14.1).

MITRAL ATRESIA WITH DOUBLE-OUTLET RIGHT VENTRICLE {A(S),D,D} AND VISCERAL HETEROTAXY

Heterotaxy With Polysplenia

Case 82 was a 7½-month-old boy who died in 1951. He had DORV {A(S),D,D} with mitral atresia and polysplenia. The A (S) part of his segmental anatomy means he had situs ambiguus (A) of the viscera and we thought the atrial situs very probably was solitus (S). DORV {A(S),D,D} indicates that he definitely had visceral situs ambiguus and that we thought that he *probably* had atrial situs solitus. The S symbol is placed in parentheses to indicate some doubt: we thought the atria very probably were in situs solitus, but we could not be entirely certain.

The patient had two spleens; in that sense polysplenia was present. The liver was bilaterally symmetrical. The lungs were bilaterally trilobed (more like the asplenia syndrome than the polysplenia syndrome). There was TAPVC to the RSVC-atrial junction. A LSVC also connected with the poorly septated atrial segment. The left innominate vein was absent. The IVC was midline, not interrupted, and connected with the atrial segment. There was an ostium primum defect. To the left of the atrial septal remnant, there was no patent AV valve or valvar component. Mitral atresia was considered to be present. No vestige of the morphologically LV was found. The patient had a *single morphologically RV.* The RV was of the right-handed or solitus type in terms of its chirality. A ventricular D-loop with a single RV and an absent LV was our diagnosis. The tricuspid valve lay to the right of the atrial septal remnant and opened into the RV. The segmental anatomy, as earlier, was DORV {A(S),D,D}. A common AV canal was thought to be present because of the ostium primum defect (the most common incomplete form of AV septal defect).

As is usual with single RV, because of absence of the LV, no ventricular septum or ventricular septal remnant could be identified. Consequently, we could not say whether this was a complete form or a partial form of common AV canal. In other words, was a VSD of the AV canal type present or not? When a ventricular septal remnant cannot be identified, and the morphologically LV is absent, this question cannot be answered (to the best of our present understanding).

A bilateral conus was present (subaortic and subpulmonary). Pulmonary outflow tract stenosis (infundibular and valvar) was present, with no aortic outflow tract obstruction. The pulmonary valve was bicuspid (bicommissural). The ductus arteriosus was absent. There was a right aortic arch. The small and large bowel had a common mesentery.

In summary, the mitral valve and the morphologically LV were both absent; in this sense, mitral atresia was diagnosed. It is noteworthy that we still do not know how to distinguish between *mitral atresia* (mitral valve present, but with no orifice) and *mitral valve absence.* At present, the diagnosis of mitral atresia appears to include both potential anomalies. The same applies to the tricuspid valve: our uncertain ability to distinguish between tricuspid valvar atresia (which definitely occurs with the Ebstein anomaly, that is, with imperforate Ebstein malformation) and tricuspid valvar absence. Typical tricuspid and mitral atresia, that is, so-called muscular tricuspid atresia and muscular mitral atresia, may well represent tricuspid valvar *absence* and mitral valvar *absence,* not a lack of an opening in either valve. Imperforate Ebstein anomaly may be the only real form of tricuspid valvar atresia because the tricuspid leaflets are definitely present, but with no valvar opening (imperforate). In other words, "typical" tricuspid atresia and typical mitral atresia (the "muscular" forms) may well be *erroneous concepts,* accurately speaking. Perhaps *membranous* atresia and *muscular* atresia (both mitral and tricuspid) may distinguish between AV valvar atresia, as opposed to AV valvar absence, respectively. Much remains to be learned.

MITRAL ATRESIA WITH DOUBLE-OUTLET RIGHT VENTRICLE AND D-LOOP VENTRICLES IN THE HETEROTAXY SYNDROME WITH ASPLENIA

Case 83 was a newborn female infant who died at 1 hour of age with not only the previously listed anomalies, but also with the Meckel-Gruber syndrome (see later). This is the 17th anatomic type of mitral atresia present in our database. This case constitutes 0.56% of all of our postmortem cases of mitral atresia (see Table 14.1 and Fig. 14.1).

This patient had visceral heterotaxy with asplenia. The segmental anatomy of DORV {AS,D,L} means DORV *with situs ambiguus of the viscera and with situs solitus of the atria,* D-loop ventricles, and L-malposition of the great arteries (with the aortic valve lying to the left [*levo-* or L-] relative to the pulmonary valve). There was *right-sided juxtaposition of the atrial appendages* because of dextromalposition of a small LAA. This type of juxtaposition of the atrial appendages has a strong tendency to be associated with HLHS with D-loop ventricles.[31] A common atrium was present, separated by only a thin atrial septal remnant. A large ostium primum defect was present. Bilateral SVCs were found. The RSVC opened into what was interpreted as a right-sided RA, and a persistent LSVC opened into the left-sided LA. The septum primum was largely absent, contributing to the previously mentioned common atrium. A VSD of the AV canal type was present. Mitral atresia was of the "muscular" type. The LV was diminutive, with no papillary muscles. The VSD of the AV canal type was subdivided by what we interpreted as a conduction tissue band. A bilateral conus (with subaortic and subpulmonary conal musculature) was present. Subvalvar pulmonary stenosis was present, without aortic outflow tract obstruction. There was a single right coronary artery; that is, the left coronary ostium was absent. There was a left aortic arch, and the ductus arteriosus was absent. This patient was a twin; her co-twin was a normal girl.

Why did this patient die at only 1 hour of age? In addition to visceral heterotaxy with asplenia and the previously mentioned congenital heart disease, she also had the Meckel-Gruber syndrome, that is, dysencephalia splanchnocystica (which we have considered heretofore). Case 83 had an encephalocele, microcephaly, mircophthalmia, sloping forehead, short and webbed neck, polydactyly, polycystic kidneys, hydrocephalus, lobulated tongue, and hypoplastic lungs.

MITRAL ATRESIA WITH DOUBLE-OUTLET RIGHT VENTRICLE AND L-LOOP VENTRICLES IN THE HETEROTAXY SYNDROME WITH ASPLENIA

Case 19 was a boy who died at 18 days of age with the heterotaxy syndrome and asplenia. He had dextrocardia, meaning only that the heart was predominantly in the right hemithorax (with no implications concerning the segmental anatomy). The heart had DORV {A,L,L} segmental anatomy, meaning DORV with the segmental anatomic set of situs ambiguus of the viscera and atria, L-loop ventricles, and L-malposition of the great arteries (see Table 14.2 and Fig. 14.1, type 18). The ventricles could not be described as concordant or discordant because the atrial situs (solitus or inversus) was itself unknown (and hence was called situs ambiguus). The SVCs were bilateral. The IVC was right-sided. The stomach was left-sided, and the liver was bilaterally symmetrical. This finding is often called a "midline" liver, meaning that the liver was neither predominantly right-sided nor predominantly left-sided, that is, approximately bilaterally symmetrical. Accurately speaking, however, there is no such thing as a *midline* liver—*if* one means a liver confined to the midline. All of the pulmonary veins connected with the right side of a common atrium. (Was this TAPVC, or were the pulmonary veins normally connected? Not knowing the atrial situs, we could not answer this question.)

There was a completely common AV canal, in the following sense. As noted earlier, there was a common atrium. (Dr. Jesse Edwards used to say that common atrium is the forgotten form of common AV canal.) And there was a very small VSD of the AV canal type between the tiny right-sided morphologically LV and the hypertrophied, enlarged, and left-sided morphologically RV. Hence, a complete AV septal defect was present. However, in another sense, this AV canal was *not* completely in common because right-sided mitral atresia coexisted. Nonetheless, it is customary to classify this kind of anatomy as *completely* common AV canal because an AV septal defect is present both at the interatrial level and at the interventricular level, if not at the level of the AV valve itself because of the presence of mitral atresia (right-sided).

In the interests of anatomic accuracy, I think that the aforementioned anatomy may accurately be regarded as an *intermediate form* of common AV canal. *Intermediate* common AV canal means intermediate between the typical complete and the typical partial forms of common AV canal. In this patient, an ostium primum defect and a VSD of the AV canal type are present. Hence, a complete AV and septal defect is present. *However, the AV valve itself is not completely in common* in this case because of mitral atresia. Another way of saying this is that this patient has *almost completely* common AV canal defect, except for the presence of mitral atresia (right-sided). Only the *tricuspid component* of the common AV valve opens into the large left-sided RV.

In this diagnostic analysis, I am tacitly accepting the conventional interpretation that the mitral valve is present, but imperforate (i.e., atretic), even though the floor of the common atrium above the tiny right-sided LV is muscular, with no visible suggestion of fibrous mitral leaflet tissue. What if we consider the alternative hypothesis mentioned earlier, namely, that the mitral component of the common AV valve is really absent (not just imperforate)? Even in this interpretation, the AV canal is not completely in common, because the mitral valvar component is missing. Thus, my interpretation is that the AV canal is almost completely in common. However, it is not completely in common because of the right-sided mitral atresia. Could my interpretations be wrong? Yes. How? If the AV valve that we are calling the tricuspid valve is really the common AV valve, *all of it,* this really is a complete form of common AV canal. My bad joke about this situation is that even at the level of gross anatomy, sometimes diagnostic certainty is not possible, at least at the present time. *Werner Heisenberg's uncertainty principle* seems not to be confined to the subatomic world of the very small, as in quantum theory. Situs ambiguus in the heterotaxy syndromes, as in mitral atresia (see Fig. 14.1, types 16, 17, and 18) is another example of diagnostic uncertainty at the level of gross anatomy.

A bilateral conus (with subaortic and subpulmonary conal musculature) was present in this patient. The left-sided aortic outflow tract was widely patent, but the right-sided and posterior pulmonary outflow tract was atretic. There was pulmonary infundibular and valvular atresia, with marked hypoplasia of the pulmonary arteries. The internal diameter of the MPA was 1.5 mm, of the left pulmonary artery was 1.0 mm, and of the right pulmonary artery was 3.0 mm. Multiple aortopulmonary collateral arteries **(MAPCAs)** were found, but no ductus arteriosus was identified. The aortic arch was left-sided. MAPCAs usually are associated with TOF that has pulmonary outflow tract atresia; but not always, as this rare case illustrates.

Common AV canal with mitral atresia, as in this patient, is an extreme example of what Dr. Maurice Lev called the *right ventricular type of common AV canal (or orifice)* because the AV valve opens predominantly or entirely into the RV (entirely, in this patient). Thus, the common AV canal can be *balanced,* the common AV valve opening approximately equally into the RV and LV; the common AV canal can be of the *left ventricular type,* the common AV valve opening predominantly or entirely into the LV; or the common AV canal can be of the *right ventricular type,* the common AV valve opening predominantly or entirely into the RV as in Case 19. **Thus, common AV canal is classified in terms of several different anatomic considerations:**

1. the AV septal defect (complete or partial);
2. the leaflets of the AV valve (unfused, partly fused, completely fused); and
3. the ventricles or ventricle of entry (balanced, left ventricular type, or right ventricular type).

We do not classify common AV canal only in terms of the status of the AV septal defect, because of the clinical and surgical importance of the other two considerations mentioned previously:

1. the status of the AV valve or valves; and
2. the atrial and ventricular alignment(s) of the AV valve(s).

Mitral atresia and **tricuspid atresia** seldom are included in **classifications of common AV canal.** They should be, in view of their clinical importance in patients, such as Case 19.

Summary and Discussion: Pathologic Anatomy of Mitral Atresia

Table 14.2 and diagrammatic **Figs. 14.1 to 14.21** summarize the salient features of the pathologic anatomy of mitral atresia that were found in 177 postmortem cases. The findings were classified into six anatomic groups, and into 18 anatomic types of mitral atresia. The median ages at death (or cardiac transplantation) in the 18 anatomic types of mitral atresia are summarized in Table 14.10. Table 14.10 is also a convenient summary of the salient features of the 18 different anatomic types of mitral atresia.

The mean age at death or cardiac transplantation (only 1 patient had a transplant) for the series as a whole (all 18 anatomic types) was 231 • 24 ± 431 • 42 days, or 7.7 months ± 1.18 years, **ranging** from 1 hour to 3.72 years, with a **mean** of 28 days.

The classic forms of mitral atresia had normal segmental anatomy {S,D,S} in 118 of these 177 cases (66.67%, types 1 to 7 inclusive). In type 6 with a single LV and absence of the right ventricular sinus, that is, the right ventricular inflow tract, or a large LV and a very small RV, only 2 of these 7 cases had

TABLE 14.10 Median Ages At Death or Cardiac Transplantation in the 18 Anatomic Types of Mitral Atresia (n = 177)

Anatomic Type	N	Median Age (days)
1. MAt {S,D,S}, IVS, AoV At	80	10
2. MAt {S,D,S}, IVS, patent AoV	3	36
3. MAt {S,D,S}, VSD, patent AoV	27	9
4. MAt {S,D,S}, VSD, AoV At	5	5
5. MAt {S,D,S}, VSD, truncus arteriosus	1	9
6. MAt {S,D,S}, VSD/BVF, large/single LV	7	75
7. MAt {S,D,S}, No VSD, thoracopagus conjoined twin	1	0.19
8. MAt, VSD, DORV {S,D,D/"S"}	28	97.5
9. MAt, No VSD, DORV {S,D,D}	6	20
10. MAt, ± VSD, TGA{S,D,D}	5	150
11. MAt, VSD, DORV {S,L,L}	4	985
12. MAt, IVS, TGA {S,L,L}	1	60
13. MAt, IVS, DORV {I,L,L}	1	1
14. MAt, ± VSD, DORV {I,D,D}	3	1358.5
15. MAt, IVS, TGA {I,D,D/A}	2	1103
16. MAt, No VSD, DORV {A(S),D,D}, and polysplenia	1	225
17. MAt, DORV {AS,D,L} and asplenia	1	0.04
18. MAt, DORV {A,L,L} and asplenia	1	18

normal {S,D,S} segmental anatomy (see Table 14.2 and Fig. 14.1). Patients with an intact ventricular septum and aortic valvar atresia predominated (45%). Infrequently, patients with mitral atresia and an intact ventricular septum had a patent but hypoplastic aortic valve (1%). But when the aortic valve was patent, it was more usual for a VSD to coexist (15%). Nonetheless, despite the presence of a VSD, aortic valvar atresia was found in 3% of these patients with mitral atresia and normal segmental anatomy (see Table 14.2 and Fig. 14.1).

Rare and noteworthy cases were encountered in group 1 with mitral atresia and normal {S,D,S} segmental anatomy:

1. **A large morphologically LV and a small or absent morphologically right ventricular sinus** were found in 2 of these 118 patients with mitral atresia {S,D,S} (1 • 69%); these 2 cases constitute 1 • 13% of all patients with mitral atresia in this study (see Table 14.2 and Fig. 14.1). Single LV with absence of the right ventricular sinus and an infundibular outflow chamber with mitral atresia {S,D,S} is the **Quero heart.**[23]
2. **Truncus arteriosus** occurred in a rare patient with mitral atresia {S,D,S} (0.56%; see Table 14.2 and Fig. 14.1).
3. One patient was a **functionally acardiac thoracopagus conjoined twin** with atresia of all four cardiac valves.
4. Mitral atresia occurred in hearts with *normal segmental anatomy,* {S,D,S}, in 118 of 177 patients (66.67%) (see Table 14.2 and Fig. 14.1), as earlier. Mitral atresia also occurred in hearts with *abnormal segmental anatomy* in 59 of 177 patients (33.33%). To simplify and make this easier to remember, in

mitral atresia the segmental anatomy was *normal in two-thirds of cases* and was *abnormal in one-third of cases.*

In the one-third of patients with mitral atresia and abnormal segmental anatomy (n = 59), the infundibuloarterial (conotruncal) anomalies were DORV in 47 of 177 patients (26.55%), TGA in 11 of 177 patients (6.21%), and DOIOC with absence of the right ventricular sinus in 1 of 177 patients (0.56%).

When examining the statistics in Table 14.2 and Fig. 14.1, remember that type 6 mitral atresia contains only 2 patients with normal {S,D,S} segmental anatomy. Type 6 also contains TGA {S,D,D/A} in 2, TGA {S,L,D} in 1, DORV {S,D,A} in 1, and DOIOC {S,L,L} in 1. It is necessary to remember this for all the members to add up correctly.

Most textbook accounts of mitral atresia assume that the segmental anatomy is normal. This assumption does not apply accurately to about one-third of patients with mitral atresia (see Table 14.2 and Fig. 14.1).

Absence of the morphologically LA was another exceedingly rare finding. To my knowledge, absence of the LA is a previously unknown anomaly. This patient was **Case 135,** autopsy number A76-8, a 10-day-old boy with mitral atresia, anatomic type 8, that is, mitral atresia with VSD and DORV {S,D,D/"S"} (see Table 14.2 and Fig. 14.1).

DORV in association with mitral atresia often had a unilateral conus, that is, *a subpulmonary conus* with aortic-tricuspid fibrous continuity (made possible by resorption of the subaortic conal free wall) or *a subaortic conus* with pulmonary valve-tricuspid valve direct fibrous continuity (made possible by resorption of the subpulmonary conal free wall). DORV with a unilateral conus—subpulmonary only or subaortic only—is very different from the *bilateral conus* (with subaortic and subpulmonary infundibular musculature) that is usual when DORV is associated with two well-developed ventricles.

Although not widely recognized, DORV with a unilateral conus (subpulmonary or subaortic) occurring in association with HLHS is a specific anatomic type of DORV. DORV with a unilateral conus (subpulmonary only or subaortic only) is as specific an anatomic type of DORV as is the Taussig-Bing malformation with two well-developed ventricles and[46,50] a bilateral (subpulmonary and subaortic) conus. DORV with a unilateral conus merits wider recognition because of its importance in the understanding of mitral atresia with DORV.

What the Literature Teaches Concerning the Pathologic Anatomy of Mitral Atresia

If one consults many of the excellent contemporary textbooks that deal with pediatric cardiology and/or congenital heart surgery, there is a remarkable dearth of detailed anatomic information concerning mitral atresia, absent left AV connection, imperforate left AV connection, or atresia of the left AV connection, these being synonyms that some of our colleagues currently favor. However, the journal literature remains a rich source of information. Pioneering studies include those of Edwards and Rodgers[64] in 1947 and of Edwards and DuShane[65] in 1950 in which these authors also describe premature closure of the foramen ovale and a decompressing levo-atrio-cardinal vein between the LA and the left innominate vein. In 1955, Friedman, Murphy, and Ash[66] emphasized the hypoplastic nonfunctioning left heart associated with mitral atresia. Three years later, in 1958, Noonan and Nadas[67] focused on the same aspect and named it HLHS. In 1960, Watson, Rowe, Conen, and Duckworth[68] reported 11 cases of mitral atresia in which the aortic valve was of normal size, not hypoplastic. In 1962, Lucas, Lester, Lillehei, and Edwards[17] again described the combination of mitral atresia with a levoatrial cardinal vein; note the updated spelling of levoatrial.

Classification

In 1965, Dr. Jesse Edwards and colleagues attempted to classify mitral atresia, based on a study of 32 postmortem cases. Eliot, Shone, Kanjuh, Ruttenberg, Carey, and Edwards[69] proposed the following anatomic classification of mitral atresia, using three variables to classify mitral atresia:

1. the presence or absence of TGA;
2. the presence or absence of hypoplasia of left-sided cardiac structures; and
3. the presence or absence of a VSD.

How did they do? As well as was possible at that time, I thought. Their group I was clear: 24 of 32 cases (75%) had normally related great arteries; 14 of these patients (43.75%) had aortic valvular atresia with marked left ventricular hypoplasia. Of these 14 with aortic valvular atresia, 13 (92.86%) had an intact ventricular septum and only 1 had a VSD. The aortic valve was patent but hypoplastic in 10 patients (31.25%). In group II,[69] with "transposition" of the great arteries (TGA in 8 of 32 patients [25%] and with "common" ventricle in 7 of these 8 patients [87.5%]), the diagnostic analysis becomes much less clear, for now very understandable reasons.

In 1965, TGA was still being used—by "everybody"—in Abbott's[70] sense, meaning any abnormal relationship between the great arteries themselves, and/or between the great arteries and the underlying ventricles, ventricular septum, and AV valves. It was not until the latter half of the 1960s and the early 1970s that it was appreciated that for diagnostic clarity, it is essential that the various VA alignments—normal and abnormal—*must* be defined with literal accuracy. For example, *transposition* of the great arteries must mean that both great arteries are "placed across" (*trans* = across, and *ponere* = to place, Latin) the ventricular septum; hence, each arises above the morphologically inappropriate ventricle: aorta above the RV and pulmonary artery above the LV.[71,72] In other words, *transposition* must be used with literal anatomic accuracy. It does not matter if the aortic valve is anterior to the pulmonary valve, beside the pulmonary valve, or posterior to the pulmonary valve.[71,72] What matters clinically, hemodynamically, and surgically is which ventricle each great artery arises above, not the anteroposterior relationship between the great arteries. We had introduced the concepts of *concordance* and *discordance* of the AV alignments in 1964.[73] Dr. John Kirklin extended the concept of *concordance and discordance* to the VA alignments in 1973 concerning ACM of the great arteries.[74] In many subsequent publications, Dr. Robert H. Anderson of London, England and his colleagues did much to popularize the use of AV and VA concordance or discordance in the description and classification of congenital heart disease. Hence, by the late 1960s and early 1970's,[71-74] TGA was redefined, with literal anatomic accuracy, as VA discordance, meaning that the RV ejected (inappropriately or discordantly) into the ascending aorta, and the LV ejected inappropriately into the MPA. Similarly, DORV, double-outlet LV, and ACM of the great arteries quickly came to be used with literal anatomic accuracy. Before this time, any and all VA malalignments were regarded as some type of TGA,[70] with this term then being used in a very broad and imprecise way. So, what did Edwards and his colleagues[64] mean by "transposition" of the great arteries in 1965? Because of the broad general usage of *transposition*[70] then current, it is now difficult to be certain what the precise VA alignments were in this pioneering paper.[69] For example, almost certainly some of these "transpositions"[69] would today be called DORV. But as I said at the outset, these authors did as well as could be done in 1965. Whether we realize it or not, we are all "prisoners" of our time.

In 1965, *nonmorphologic terminology* was still being used to designate the various cardiac chambers: "venous" atrium and arterial "atrium" and "venous" ventricle and "arterial" ventricles. These hemodynamic terms ("venous" and "arterial") lead to the questions of, anatomically, which is the "arterial" ventricle? Is it the morphologically LV, or is it the morphologically RV? The answers to these questions can be very unclear, particularly when "transposition" of the great arteries—used in the old way[70]—coexisted. In other words, one of Dr. Maurice Lev's most important papers,[75] published in 1954, was concerned with how to diagnose the morphologic anatomic identity of the various cardiac chambers, no matter what the spatial location of the cardiac chambers may be, by examining the morphologic anatomic features of the septal surfaces of the atria and ventricles. *This was an essential key to the understanding and accurate anatomic diagnosis of complex congenital heart disease.*[75]

Ten years later, in 1964, Van Praagh, Ongley, and Swan[21] used a modification of Lev's morphologic method[75] to understand the pathologic anatomy of what was then called "single" or "common" ventricles. Van Praagh et al[21] used not only the morphologic anatomic features of the ventricular septal surfaces, as Lev[75] had done, but also extended the morphologic anatomic analysis to include *the ventricular free walls.* Anatomic and embryologic study in humans had convinced Van Praagh et al[21,22] that the morphologic features of the ventricular free walls were every bit as specific, different, and diagnostically informative as the morphologic features of the ventricular septal surfaces. Because the morphologic anatomy of the ventricular septal surfaces can be altered or absent in single ventricle, the additional use of the morphologic anatomic features of the ventricular *free walls* made it possible to understand the pathologic anatomy of the single ventricle.[21,22]

What did Eliot et al[69] mean in 1965 by *common ventricle*? The premorphologic meaning of *single* or *common* ventricle was that both AV valves or a common AV valve open entirely or predominantly into one ventricular chamber.[21] The designation *common* ventricle, that was used by Edwards et al[64] in this first attempted classification of mitral atresia (Table 14.11), suggests that the ventricles may be in common, or undivided by a ventricular septum. The systemic and pulmonary venous blood streams certainly appeared to be in common, or undivided. Hence, the question became morphologically or anatomically, what is a single or common ventricle? This is the question that Van Praagh et al[21] had tried to solve in 1964, presumably when the study of Eliot et al[69] was being written.

TABLE 14.11 Classification of Mitral Atresia—1965

Group I	Normally related great arteries and hypoplasia of the left-sided cardiac structures
Type A	Aortic valvular atresia with markedly hypoplastic left ventricle 1. With intact ventricular septum 2. With ventricular septal defect
Type B	Aortic valvular and left ventricular hypoplasia 1. With intact ventricular septum 2. With ventricular septal defect
Group II	Transposed great arteries
Type A	Common ventricle 1. With inverted infundibulum 2. With noninverted infundibulum
Type B	Two ventricles present

From Eliot RS, Shone JD, Kanjuh VI, et al. Mitral atresia: A study of 32 cases. *Am Heart J.* 1965;70:6; with permission.

So, 1965[69] was the very early days. To summarize, the problems that Eliot et al[69] faced unknowingly in 1965 were:

1. *TGA* was still being used in a very broad and anatomically imprecise way[70]; hence, the meaning of "transposition" of the great arteries in their classification[69] (see Table 14.11) is imprecise.
2. *The initial morphologic method* of cardiac chamber identification, pioneered by Dr. Maurice Lev[75] in 1954, still was not widely understood. It should be added that Dr. Lev himself thought his morphologic method could not be used in single or common ventricle anomalies because he thought that the ventricular septal surface morphologies were either abnormal or absent in these malformations.
3. *The extended or full morphologic method* using both the septal surface and the free-wall morphologies, pioneered by Van Praagh et al,[21,22] had revealed that there are two anatomic types of single ventricle: (1) single (unpaired) morphologically LV caused by absence of the morphologically right ventricular sinus in about 75% of cases and (2) single (unpaired) RV, caused by absence of the LV, in about 25% of cases. However, in 1965, Eliot et al[69] could not be expected to understand this, because it was still in the early days—hence, the *common* ventricle of their classification (see Table 14.11).[69]
4. The year 1965[69] was also too early for the adoption of *the segmental approach* to the diagnostic understanding of congenital heart disease pioneered by Van Praagh et al.[2-14]

This diagnostic method, based on both morphologic anatomy and embryology, was used by Van Praagh et al since 1964, but was not formally named and presented until 1972.[2] The segmental approach was developed and tested repeatedly both clinically and pathologically from 1960 to 1972. We were trying to develop a diagnostic method that always worked, no matter how complex the congenital heart disease. No "exceptions" or other excuses were accepted. Only when we could not find anything wrong with it did we present it.[2]

Thus, by 1965, the necessary understanding and methods for the accurate anatomic diagnosis of large series of complex cases of congenital heart disease had not been completely worked out. This is why I said at the outset that these outstanding investigators[69] did the best that they could do in 1965 (see Table 14.11).

In 1968, Summerell et al[76] expanded the classification of Eliot et al[69] by reporting that it is possible for mitral atresia with normally related great arteries and left ventricular hypoplasia to have a normal-sized aortic valve, thereby confirming the findings of Watson et al[68] in 1960.

In 1969, Navarro-Lopez et al[77] described a patient with mitral atresia who had an occlusive left atrial thrombus and who survived for 11 years. We have not seen a patient with a left atrial thrombus. The oldest patient found in their literature review was 22 years of age. Of the approximately 160 cases of mitral atresia studied at autopsy, they also found that 10 had lived for more than 1 year (6.25%). Their literature review found that only 25% of patients had normally related great arteries, whereas 75% had "transposition" of the great arteries; these findings are the opposite of ours (see Table 14.2 and Fig. 14.1) and the opposite of those of Eliot[69] and Edwards et al,[64] perhaps explaining the relative longevity of the patients in the literature review of Navarro-Lopez et al.[77]

In 1970, Dr. Manuel Quero[23] from Madrid, Spain reported a patient with a Holmes heart {S,D,S} with single LV and an infundibular outlet chamber who had mitral atresia, that is, mitral atresia with a large LV, an absent right ventricular sinus, and normally related great arteries. This type of mitral atresia was thought at the time to be unique; hence, we called this anomaly[23] **the Quero heart,** in his honor. In 1972, Quero[24] did it again. He published the case of a 3-month-old girl with TGA {S,L,D} with right-sided mitral atresia, a large right-sided morphologically LV, and a left-sided infundibular outlet chamber. In other words, a single LV with an infundibular outlet chamber, but this time with right-sided mitral atresia, a ventricular L-loop, and D-TGA. Quero demonstrated that mitral atresia could occur with a single LV both in a ventricular D-loop (1970)[23] and a ventricular L-loop (1972).[24] It should be recalled that the old premorphologic definition of single (or common) ventricle was as follows: Single or common ventricle is present if both AV valves or a common AV valve open entirely or predominantly into one ventricular chamber. In other words, the old definition of single ventricle excluded mitral or tricuspid atresia. Dr. Manuel Quero was proving that single LV and mitral atresia could indeed coexist, suggesting that tricuspid atresia and mitral atresia should not be excluded from the category of single LV.

Edwards et al had described and classified both tricuspid and mitral atresia, but nobody yet understood double-inlet single ventricle. In 1974, Dr. Glen Rosenquist[78] published 3 cases of mitral atresia with a normal-sized LV, a straddling tricuspid valve, and a small RV; 2 of these patients had TGA. Also in 1974, Cabrera et al[79] published the case of a 14-day-old boy with TGA {S,D,D} with left-sided mitral atresia, single LV with infundibular outlet chamber, and coarctation of the aorta. This case was similar to Quero's 1972 report,[24] except that the patient of Cabrera et al[79] had a ventricular D-loop (not a ventricular L-loop). The case of Cabrera et al[79] was thought to be the first published case of its type. In 1974, Bjørnstad and Michalsen[80] published a case of mitral atresia with aortic atresia and intact ventricular septum in siblings, suggesting the possibility of a heritable genetic etiology in this anatomic type of mitral atresia with HLHS. In 1976, Moreno, Quero, and Perez Diaz[81] reported 18 cases of mitral atresia with a normal aortic valve, confirming earlier reports.[68,76] Also in 1976, Friedman et al[82] reported a rare hemodynamic cause for failure of a Blalock-Taussig anastomosis to relieve inadequate pulmonary blood flow: mitral atresia with premature closure of the foramen ovale, resulting in pulmonary venous and pulmonary arterial hypertension. Creation of an ASD helped.[82] In 1979, Ostermeyer et al[83] reported the case of a 6 8/12-year-old girl with mitral atresia, VSD, *normal-sized ventricles,* and D-TGA. Rarely, mitral atresia can be associated with *two well-developed ventricles*—not with hypoplastic LV syndrome—if a good-sized VSD coexists. In 1980, Mickell, Mathews, Park, Lenox, Fricker, Neches, and Zuberbuhler[84] reported 40 cases of left AV valvar atresia. They understood that 31 of these patients had mitral atresia (77.5%) and 9 had left-sided tricuspid atresia (22.5%). In other words, they were aware that the identity of the *left-sided* AV valve is ventricular-loop dependent: mitral, when a ventricular D-loop is present and tricuspid, when a ventricular L-loop coexists. The study of Mickell et al[84] was focused primarily on clinical management. In 1981, Thiene, Daliento, Frescura, DeTommasi, Macartney, and Anderson[85] reported an anatomic study and **classification** of 62 postmortem cases of mitral atresia, that they preferred to call *atresia of the left AV orifice.* When Thiene et al[85] used the conventional term *mitral atresia,* they put mitral between quotation marks: "mitral" atresia. However, they used the conventional diagnosis tricuspid atresia, unadorned with quotation marks. This study merits careful consideration because the first author and the senior author are both world-class congenital heart pathologists. By 1981, Dr. Gaetano Thiene and Dr. Robert H. Anderson and their colleagues[85] had learned many significant lessons, including the importance of morphologic anatomy for cardiac chamber identification, and the utility of the segmental approach for diagnostic data analysis. Consequently their study and classification represent an advance over earlier pioneering investigations.

Classification of Thiene, Anderson, and Colleagues. As we will see, Thiene, Anderson et al[85] adopted Dr. Jesse Edwards' approach,[64] at least in part.

I. Left AV atresia with aortic valvular atresia (n = 32)
   a. Imperforate left AV valve with AV concordance and a biventricular heart (n = 5)
   b. Absent left AV connection with univentricular heart of right ventricular type (n = 27), rudimentary chamber of left ventricular type posteriorly and left-sided in all
II. Left AV atresia with patent aortic valve (n = 30)
   a. Imperforate left AV valve, AV concordance, and biventricular heart (n = 5)
   b. Absent left AV connection with univentricular heart of right ventricular type (n = 15), with rudimentary LV always posteriorly on the left

c. Absent left AV connection with univentricular heart of left ventricular type (n = 9), with the rudimentary chamber of right ventricular type situated anteriorly to the right in 2, and anteriorly and to the left in 7
d. Imperforate left AV valve with univentricular heart of left ventricular type and double inlet (n = 1)

Comment. **Alphanumeric classification,** that is, classification based on arbitrary and intrinsically meaningless letters and numbers, is difficult if not impossible to remember and hence is little used clinically. For example, what is left AV atresia type IIc?[86] Most readers have to go back and look up this type in order to understand what it means.

By contrast, one of the advantages of the segmental approach is that no memorization is necessary because all of the designations are abbreviation of anatomic terms, and hence are not arbitrary and intrinsically meaningless. For example, what does TGA {S,D,D} mean? These designations literally spell out the answer to this question: TGA with the segmental anatomic set of solitus atria, D-loop ventricles, and D-TGA. Anatomic understanding, without memorization, is all that is required.

In single variable analysis versus multivariable analysis, the authors[86] use single variable analysis, not set analysis, which considers multiple variables simultaneously. Complex congenital heart disease, like mitral atresia, requires multivariable analysis because usually there is more than one abnormal variable. This is why set analysis, which is a form of multivariable analysis, is so helpful diagnostically.

1. The visceroatrial situs is one variable.
2. The type of ventricular loop is a second variable.
3. The great arterial anatomy is a third variable.

The foregoing are the three main cardiac segments. The two connecting cardiac segments are:

4. the AV canal or junction; and
5. the conus arteriosus or infundibulum.

Thus, the segment-by-segment approach to diagnosis routinely considers *five variables:* the three main cardiac segments (atria, ventricles, great arteries) and the two connecting cardiac segments (the AV canal or junction, and the conus arteriosus or infundibulum).

In the segmental approach, *associated malformations*—such as ASDs, VSDs, and pulmonary outflow tract obstruction—are always included.

In the 62 cases of Thiene et al,[85] how many different kinds of heart are there? And exactly what are they? Because their univariate analysis is not fully integrated, the reader is unable to answer these questions.

The Infundibulum or Conus. These distinguished authors (Thiene et al[85]) do not regard the infundibulum or conus arteriosus as a connecting segment between the ventricles and the great arteries, as we do. Instead, they regard the infundibulum as part of the RV.[85] The difficulty with this view is that the infundibulum can override the ventricular septum to any degree. Indeed, the conus can be located entirely, or almost entirely, above the morphologically LV, indicating that the infundibulum or conus arteriosus cannot be regarded as an exclusively right ventricular structure. Instead, the anatomic data demonstrate that the infundibulum forms part of the outflow tract of *both* ventricles. The conus arteriosus is how the great arteries connect with the underlying ventricles, ventricular septum, and AV valves. This problem is resolved by the realization that the conus arteriosus belongs neither to the RV nor the LV. Instead, the conus "belongs to," or "is part of" the great arteries, as its developmental name indicates. *Conus arteriosus* means "arterial cone" (Latin). The conoarterial segment connects with the underlying ventricles, ventricular septum, and AV canal in various ways. This insight makes both the normal and the abnormal conotruncal anatomic findings understandable. The authors[85] do not describe the infundibulum specifically as subpulmonary, subaortic, or bilateral (subaortic and subpulmonary), or as bilaterally absent or very deficient. Similarly, they do not describe semilunar-AV fibrous continuity or discontinuity.

Mitral Valve Between Right Atrium and Large Left Ventricle. Thiene et al[85] state that in their cases with left AV atresia in which the RA opens into a large morphologically LV, the AV valve is a *morphologically mitral valve.* However, they do not further describe or otherwise justify this potentially very important conclusion. I agree with Thiene et al.[85] However, some later authors[87] (including Dr. Stella Van Praagh) did not agree, maintaining that this patent AV valve opening from the RA into a large LV is a *morphologically tricuspid valve.*

Why is this AV valvar identification important? If, as Thiene et al[85] state, this valve is a large mitral valve, the left AV atresia cannot be due to *mitral* atresia; logically one cannot have mitral atresia and a large patent mitral valve in the same patient. Thus, Aristotle's *law of contradiction* appears to apply: *A cannot be both A and not A.* Hence, a heart cannot have mitral atresia and a patent mitral valve. In logic, Aristotle's law of the excluded middle also seems relevant: A must be either A or not A. Thus, left AV atresia is either mitral atresia or it is not mitral atresia. To continue the use of logic, one can combine both of these Aristotelian laws of logic as follows. The left AV atresia is either mitral atresia or it is not mitral atresia (law of the excluded middle). This proposition seems reasonable, even inescapable.

One cannot have mitral atresia and a patent mitral valve in the same heart (the law of contradiction). This proposition also seems reasonable. But we are assuming that a heart can have only one mitral valve. Although this assumption appears to be correct, can we exclude the possibility of an exception?

Turning from logic to morphology, the most reasonable interpretation of the findings of Thiene et al[85] may be that left AV atresia is not mitral atresia and that the mitral valve opens from the RA into the LV. Are Thiene et al[85] right about this? Briefly, I think that they were right about this.[86] *The morphology of the AV valve corresponds to that of the ventricle of entry, not to that of the atrium of exit.* This is true when one AV valve enters one ventricular sinus, that is, in single inlet in each ventricle. *When two AV valves enter one ventricular sinus, the morphology of the AV valves corresponds to that of the type of ventricular loop that is present:* right-sided tricuspid valve and left-sided mitral valve with a ventricular D-loop (solitus ventricular loop) and left-sided tricuspid valve and right-sided mitral valve with a ventricular L-loop (inverted ventricular loop).

AV and VA "Connections"

Thiene et al[85] write about AV and VA connections because they do not regard the AV junction or canal and the infundibulum or conus arteriosus as separate connecting cardiac segments between the atria and the ventricles and between the ventricles and the great arteries, respectively, as we do.

In the interests of anatomic accuracy, as noted earlier, we prefer the concepts of AV *alignments* and VA *alignments* (not connections). Why, exactly? Because the atria and the ventricles normally do not connect tissue-to-tissue, because of the interposition of the AV canal and valves. Similarly, the ventricles and the great arteries normally do not connect tissue-to-tissue, because of the interposition of the conus arteriosus or infundibulum.

Their *nonconnection* explains why the main cardiac segments can be aligned in so many different ways, accounting for much of the complexity of congenital heart disease. For example, if the morphologically RA really were connected with the morphologically RV muscle-to-muscle, and if the morphologically LA really were connected with the morphologically LV muscle-to-muscle, then discordant L-loop ventricles would be developmentally impossible. It is because the atria are not connected muscle-to-muscle with the ventricles that the AV alignments can be so variable: concordant, discordant, double-inlet, right atrial outlet atresia, left atrial outlet atresia, etc. Similarly, if the RV really were connected to the MPA, and if the LV really were connected with the aorta, conotruncal anomalies such as TGA, DORV, double-outlet left ventricle (DOLV), and ACM would be developmentally impossible. It is because the ventricles and the great arteries are *not* connected tissue-to-tissue that virtually any conceivable VA alignment can and does exist. Note that our concern has nothing to do with terminologic preference; rather, it has everything to do with anatomic and embryologic accuracy.

Because so many of our friends and colleagues like to talk about AV and VA *connections*, one may well wonder why we cannot somehow make *connections* anatomically correct. I would say that of course we can. All it takes is a little grammatical "subterfuge," as follows: It is anatomically accurate to say that the atria *are connected* to the ventricles by the AV canal or junction. Similarly, the ventricles and the great arteries *are connected* by the infundibulum or conus arteriosus. In these two sentences, the verb *are connected* is in the **passive voice,** the meaning of which is anatomically correct. By contrast, in the sentence the atria *connect* with the ventricles, the verb connect is in the **active voice,** the meaning of which is anatomically incorrect. So, use of the passive voice solves the problem; only the active voice is anatomically wrong. But if grammar was never your strong suite, don't worry. What really matters is *meaning*. Grammar is the slave of meaning. When some of our colleagues say "the atria connect with the ventricles" what they mean is "the atria *are connected* with the ventricles" in this or that way.

Preselection of Data. All of the authors'[85] cases had visceroatrial situs solitus (a term that they use). Apparently excluded were patients with visceroatrial situs inversus and cases with visceroatrial heterotaxy and asplenia or polysplenia that may or may not have had atrial situs ambiguus (atrial situs uncertain or indeterminate).

In the present study (see Fig. 14.1 and Table 14.2), no case has been excluded for any "reason." **The avoidance of preselection of data**[88] is a basic principle, essential to full anatomic understanding.

If one wonders, why these authors apparently exclude all patients who did *not* have visceroatrial situs solitus, the following considerations may be illuminating. Their title could no longer be "atresia of the left AV orifice" if one means *left* in a positional, not in a morphologic, sense. In visceroatrial situs inversus, the morphologically LA is *right-sided*. In visceroatrial heterotaxy with *asplenia*, if one thinks that the RA is bilateral, as in right atrial "isomerism," there is *no morphologically LA. Hence, atresia of the left* AV *orifice cannot occur*. In visceral heterotaxy with *polysplenia*, if one thinks that left atrial "isomerism" is present, that is, that the morphologically LA is bilateral, perhaps there are two mitral orifices, that is, a bilateral mitral orifice. *Mitral atresia, or atresia of the left AV orifice, might then be bilateral, involving both left-sided and right-sided AV valves.*

I hasten to add that we have long understood that the concept of atrial "isomerism" or mirror imagery is anatomically erroneous.[58-60,89] This applies to isomerism of the atria as a whole, to isomerism of just the atrial appendages, or to isomerism of only the musculi pectinati (pectinate muscles) of the atrial appendages. This oversimplification is not supported by the anatomic data.

In a study of 104 autopsied cases with visceral heterotaxy, we found that the atrial situs (solitus or inversus) often can be determined anatomically.[89] When the atrial situs was morphologically uncertain or indeterminate, we made the diagnosis of atrial situs ambiguus, meaning that the atrial situs was uncertain or unknown, without the implication that either right or left atrial isomerism was present, because isomerism was not supported by the morphologic data.[58-60,89]

Once one realizes that atrial level "isomerism" is an error, this realization opens the door to diagnosing the anatomic type of atrial situs in the visceral heterotaxy syndromes, be it solitus, inversus, or unknown. If, for the sake of argument, one assumes that the concepts of right and left atrial isomerism are correct, this assumption leads to some very strange conclusions concerning left AV atresia, as outlined earlier. We think that all of the conclusions mentioned previously, based on the erroneous concept of atrial level "isomerism," are themselves erroneous and therefore should not be taken seriously. By excluding visceroatrial situs inversus and visceral heterotaxy, the authors[85] avoided coming to terms with the previously mentioned problems.

I wish to emphasize that there is nothing personal in the previously mentioned scientific disagreements. Drs. Gaetano Thiene and Robert Henry Anderson are personal friends and distinguished colleagues. Differences in scientific opinion and interpretation are to be encouraged and discussed. If everyone thinks the same thing, then no one is thinking. Some of our friends dismiss these discussions as "terminology wars." That is an understandable, but superficial, read, a view from the "outside." What is really going on is a very serious attempt to get a better understanding of the pathologic anatomy, embryology, and genetics. Ironically, words have very little to do with what is occurring. *It is about accuracy of meaning, not about terminology preferences.*

Single Ventricle and Ventricular Situs. Let me build bridges—a glossary—between our terminology and that of Thiene, Anderson, et al[85] so that everyone will be able to understand. Their *univentricular heart of right ventricular type*[85] means single-inlet into a large morphologically RV, but with a small or diminutive morphologically LV also present. This is what we regard as a *functionally single RV*, but not an *anatomically* single RV, because a small or tiny LV was also always present.

The hypoplastic LV was always located posteriorly and to the left relative to the large RV. This means that *D-loop* (or noninverted) ventricles probably were present in all of these cases. Hence, the title of their paper[85] was accurate: it was about left-sided mitral atresia. Although the authors did not comment on the ventricular situs, I think they understood the foregoing.

Ventricular chirality, as an aid to diagnosing ventricular situs, had been introduced only 1 year previously, in 1980.[90,91]

Univentricular heart of left ventricular type[85] means single-inlet into a single LV, with absence of the right ventricular sinus (inflow tract) and with an infundibular outlet chamber. Thiene et al[85] call this infundibular outlet chamber a *rudimentary chamber of right ventricular type.* Our interpretation is that there is nothing rudimentary about the infundibular outlet chamber (i.e., the conus is not rudimentary). The problem is that the right ventricular *sinus* is absent. Thiene et al[85] did not distinguish between the right ventricular sinus (the inflow tract) and the conus (the outflow tract); they[85] lump the right ventricular sinus and the infundibulum together, regarding them both as parts of the RV, which of course they normally are. Hence, this is the conventional view. Viewed in this way, the infundibular outlet chamber may be regarded as a rudimentary RV because the right ventricular sinus is absent. We prefer a more analytic interpretation that recognizes that the right ventricular sinus and the infundibulum in fact belong to different cardiac segments. The right ventricular sinus is part of the ventricular loop. The conus is part of the conotruncus. The more analytic approach identifies and pinpoints the anomaly—absence of the right ventricular sinus.

Did none of the authors' patients have a *hypoplastic* right ventricular sinus (which we found), as opposed to an *absent* right ventricular sinus? The reader cannot tell because everything was lumped together under the diagnosis of *rudimentary chamber of right ventricular type,* which is morphologically imprecise.

The authors[85] indicated whether the infundibular outlet chamber was anterior and to the right relative to the large LV, indicating that probably a ventricular *D-loop* was present, or anterior and to the left, indicating that a ventricular *L-loop* probably was present.

They call the bulboventricular foramen the *outlet foramen,*[85] which we regard as a nonmorphologic anatomic synonym. Normally related great arteries they call *ventriculoarterial concordance.*[85] *Transposition of the great arteries* they preferred to call *ventricularterial discordance.*[85] These were the contributions of Dr. John W. Kirklin et al.[74]

However, linguists and philologists frown on replacing terms with their definitions, which is what the authors[85] are doing. Why do students of language discourage this practice? Because the definitions tend to be longer than the terms, leading to unnecessary and undesirable wordiness. For example, single LV becomes "univentricular heart of left ventricular type," single RV becomes "univentricular heart of right ventricular type," and so forth. By definition, one synonym cannot be better than another, because both are (approximately) equal, by definition. In the English language and in scientific terminology, clarity and brevity are highly prized. Prolixity is not regarded as an asset. Nonetheless, others may regard such synonymizing as an enrichment of our cardiologic lexicon. In language, the only constant we know is change. This is why we must continue to strive for clarity, brevity, and the use of morphologic anatomic terminology in our diagnoses.

In conclusion, the study and classification of Thiene et al[85] represents the work of expert morphologists and cardiologists whose views have been and continue to be both important and influential. Their study[85] represents a considerable improvement on the work that preceded it. The present study (see Table 14.2 and Fig. 14.1) and the foregoing suggestions are intended in an entirely constructive spirit to improve the understanding of the anomaly that we still call mitral atresia.

In 1982, Restivo, Ho, Anderson, Cameron, and Wilkinson[92] published a paper entitled "Absent Left AV Connection With RA Connected to the Morphologically Left Ventricular Chamber, Rudimentary Right Ventricular Chamber, and Ventriculoarterial (VA) Discordance. Problem of Mitral Versus Tricuspid Atresia." Based on 4 autopsied cases, the authors concluded: "The observations from these cases have been used to emphasize problems concerning the use of the confusing terms 'tricuspid' and 'mitral' atresia to describe such hearts."

My analysis of their cases is as follows:

Case 1 is TGA {S,D,D} with *left atrial outlet atresia,* a large and single LV, and an infundibular outlet chamber. The bulboventricular foramen is partly occluded by the right-sided AV valve.

Case 2 is TGA {S,L,D} with *tricuspid atresia (left-sided)* and large LV (right-sided) with small RV (left-sided).

Case 3 is TGA {S,L,D} with *tricuspid atresia (left-sided),* large LV (right-sided), and rudimentary RV (left-sided).

Case 4 is TGA {S,L,L} with *tricuspid atresia (left-sided),* LV (right-sided), hypoplastic RV (left-sided), with hypoplastic aortic arch and isthmus.

So, I did not find these interesting cases "confusing," as the authors said.[92] Case 1 was (so-called) mitral atresia (left-sided) with a ventricular D-loop; whereas Cases 2, 3, and 4 all had tricuspid atresia (left-sided) with a ventricular L-loop. In other words, the type of ventricular loop (D- or L-) determines the expected anatomic identity of the apparently atretic left-sided AV valve.

The authors[92] used *positional* anatomy, "absent *left* AV connection," meaning absent *left-sided* AV connection, not *morphologic* anatomy. The authors augmented the confusion against which they inveighed by combining a ventricular D-loop (Case 1) with ventricular L-loops (Cases 2 to 4). The cure for this type of confusion is to use both positional and morphologic anatomy. Restivo's[92] Case 1 has left-sided mitral atresia. Cases 2, 3, and 4 have left-sided tricuspid atresia. The morphologic identity of the missing (so-called atretic) AV valve is indicated by:

1. the morphologic anatomic identity of the ventricle or ventricles, leading to the diagnosis of the anatomic type of ventricular loop that is present, either D-loop or L-loop; and by
2. the morphologic anatomic identity of the AV valve that is present.

Once one knows these two things, then the morphologic anatomic identity of the missing (atretic) AV valve can readily be deduced.

In 1984, Gittenberger-de Groot and Wenink[93] of Leiden replied to Anderson's critique, that is, the communication of Restivo et al,[92] in a paper entitled "Mitral Atresia, Morphological Details."[93] In a careful study of 30 heart specimens, all {S,D,-}, they found that dense fibrous tissue connected the floor of the LA to the LV in all cases. They proposed that when a fibrous membrane is detectable macroscopically, the diagnosis should be *"imperforate membrane."* But when the fibrous strand is detectable only microscopically, then the diagnosis should be *"absent* AV *connection."* These authors[93] also understood that this distinction could not be made clinically or by current imaging techniques. This may be why they used the conventional term *mitral atresia* in the title of this paper.[93] These authors[93] also stated that diagnostically, it is important to know if one is dealing with atresia of the mitral valve or with atresia of the tricuspid valve, which depends on the type of ventricular loop that is present. This is the same point that I was making earlier concerning the study by Restivo et al.[92]

In 1986, Starc and Gersony[94] pointed out that progressive obstruction of the foramen ovale can occur in patients with left AV valve atresia. Consequently, these authors proposed that balloon atrial septostomy be done in the neonatal period, even if there is no demonstrable gradient between the atria. Our anatomic observations (noted earlier) would strongly support their proposal.[94]

In 1986, at the Second World Congress of Pediatric Cardiology in New York City, I presented[86] a paper entitled "The Importance of Ventriculoatrial Malalignment in Anomalies of the AV Valves, Illustrated by 'Mitral Atresia' and Congenital Mitral Stenosis With Large LV."

From our studies of single ventricle,[21,22] we knew that when the right ventricular sinus (inflow tract) fails to develop, the result typically is single LV, with double-inlet or common-inlet LV, and with an infundibular outlet chamber. With a ventricular D-loop, the ventricular septal remnant lies to the *right* of and somewhat anterior to the right-sided tricuspid valve. With a ventricular L-loop, the ventricular septal remnant lies to the *left* of and somewhat anterior to the left-sided tricuspid valve. Both with a D-loop and with an L-loop, there is DILV (if two AV valves are present) or common-inlet LV (if a common AV canal with a common AV valve is present).

When the LV sinus (body or inflow tract) fails to develop, the opposite happens.[21,22] With a ventricular D-loop, the ventricular septal remnant lies to the *left* of the left-sided mitral valve, typically resulting in double-inlet RV (DIRV) (right-sided). When a ventricular L-loop is present, the ventricular septal remnant lies to the *right* of the right-sided mitral valve, again typically resulting in DIRV (left-sided).

Consequently, **the ventricular septum moves toward the side of the small or absent ventricular inflow tract,** just as the mediastinum moves toward the side of a small or absent lung. The same principle applies in straddling tricuspid valve[41] and in double-outlet RA.[41] However, more than lateral (right or left) movement of the ventricular septal remnant occurs. The ventricular septal remnant also rotates[86]: it becomes more coronal—more right-to-left oriented—than normal. The abnormal position of the ventricular septal remnant was measured relative to the normal location of the atrial septum using long (lumbar puncture) needles, projected on the coronal plane.[86] The abnormally rightward or leftward displacement of the ventricular septum was noted. To measure the rotation of the ventricular septum relative to the atrial septum, the ventriculoatrial septal angle was measured using long needles and a circular (360 degree) protractor.

The normal mean ventriculoatrial septal angle was found to be only 5 degrees, the normal ventricular septum lying only 5 degrees to the left of the normal atrial septum, as viewed from the ventricular apex (as in an apical four-chamber view). In 19 postmortem cases (12 with mitral atresia and large LV, and 7 with mitral stenosis and large LV), the ventriculoatrial septal angle averaged 60 degrees, ranging from a minimum of 20 degrees to a maximum of 100 degrees.[86] Because of limitation of space, I was not allowed to publish any figures (photographs) with this paper; fortunately, however, Dr. Stella Van Praagh and her colleagues[89] published three of these geometric drawings and measurements in 1992. All of these geometric diagrams are included here: Figs. 14.6E, 14.7F, 14.8E, 14.13D, 14.15A–H. To summarize, the ventriculoatrial septal angle in these 19 cases was much greater than normal.[86] The atrial septum was vertical (normal), but the ventricular septum was much more horizontal than normal (when the heart position was horizontal, as in newborns and infants), or was much more coronal than normal (when the heart position was vertical or semivertical, as in older children and adults). The ventricular part of the heart was found to have very abnormal *lateral displacement*[86]:

1. *rightward displacement* in 8 of the 9 patients with D-loop ventricles (89%), so that the expected site of the mitral orifice was directly above the left ventricular free wall (see Figs. 14.7F, 14.15A–E); or
2. *leftward displacement* of the ventricular part of the heart in all 3 cases with a ventricular L-loop (see Fig. 14.13D).

In these 12 cases of mitral atresia with a large LV, 10 (83%) had an absent mitral orifice that was located directly above the left ventricular free wall (as shown by the cardiac geometry mentioned previously),[86] apparently because of strikingly abnormal ventriculoatrial malalignment. In 2 of these 12 patients (17%) with "mitral atresia" and a large LV, another muscular structure (not the left ventricular free wall) blocked the expected site of the mitral orifice from below. In 1 patient, the very malpositioned *ventricular septum* (ventriculoatrial septal angle = 100 degrees) underlaid the expected site of the mitral orifice (see Fig. 14.6E). This patient had left atrial outlet atresia ("mitral atresia") with normal segmental anatomy {S,D,S}, a large LV, a small RV, and a straddling tricuspid valve. In the other patient (see Fig. 14.8E), an abnormal prominent muscular ridge in the location of the *anterolateral papillary muscle group that was absent* blocked the expected site of the mitral orifice from below. This patient had TGA {S,D,D} with a single LV (absent RV inflow tract), infundibular outlet chamber, and rightward malposition of the ventricular segment relative to the atria and the atrial septum, with an abnormally large ventriculoatrial septal angle of 20 degrees.

Although the atria are relatively immobile, being held in place by the venae cavae, the pulmonary veins, the diaphragm, and the lungs, from a developmental perspective the ventricular part of the heart is a "professional contortionist." The ventricles have much more opportunity to undergo abnormal morphogenetic movement than do the atria.

Normally, the human straight heart tube begins to loop to the right during Streeter's horizon 10 (20 to 22 days of age). D-loop formation normally is completed during horizon 11 (22 to 24 days of age). The LV develops faster than the RV, and the ventricular apex swings from right to left. Levocardia is normally achieved by horizon 18 (36 to 38 days of age in utero). Thus, the real questions from an anatomic and embryologic standpoint seem to be:

1. Why is there such striking ventriculoatrial malalignment in this anatomic type of "mitral atresia" with a large LV and a small or absent RV inflow tract?
2. There is no doubt that **left atrial outlet atresia** is present with ventricular D-loops and that **right atrial outlet atresia** is present with ventricular L-loops. But are these mitral valves (left-sided with D-loop ventricles and right-sided with L-loop ventricles) really atretic, or do these mitral valves really open into the large LV in these rare cases?
3. Has it been *assumed* that mitral atresia is present, and therefore that logically the valve opening into the large LV must be the morphologically tricuspid valve?

It will be recalled that Thiene and Anderson et al[85] thought that the AV valve opening from the RA into the large LV was the *mitral valve morphologically*. Were they wrong? This is the "heart" of Restivo's mystery.[92] If Thiene et al[85] are right, one would think that their left-sided AV orificial atresia cannot be mitral atresia, just as they are suggesting. Similarly, if Thiene et al[85] are right, the confusion that Restivo et al[92] are highlighting is very real.

The problem of ventriculoatrial malalignment[86] deserves much serious consideration. In tricuspid atresia, an exploratory needle through the expected site of the tricuspid orifice often runs into the immediately subjacent posterior part of a rightwardly displaced ventricular septal remnant: again, this looks like ventriculoatrial malalignment.

The AV valves—mitral and tricuspid—often seem to be the "sinned against," not the "sinners"—the "victims" of ventriculoatrial malalignment, not the "villains."[86]

I would like to emphasize that I agree with most of what Shinpo et al,[87] including Dr. Stella Van Praagh, wrote concerning this subject, that is, so-called mitral atresia with a large morphologically LV and an underdeveloped or absent right ventricular sinus. There is also an addition I would like to add to their contribution.[87] But first, the points of agreement. The study published in 1992 by Dr. Stella Van Praagh and colleagues (i.e., by Shinpo et al)[87] was the largest investigation published up to that time of mitral atresia with a large LV and an underdeveloped or absent right ventricular sinus. This investigation was based on 15 postmortem cases and on the echocardiograms and angiocardiograms in 10 living patients. Companion studies were also done of 55 postmortem cases with DILV and 72 heart specimens with tricuspid atresia.[87] So this was a very large study, based on 142 postmortem cases, with the companion investigations being done in the interests of balance and perspective.[87] Shinpo and colleagues[87] reached the following conclusions:

1. The identity of the AV valves (tricuspid or mitral) is reflected more accurately by the attachments of their chordae tendineae, than by their leaflet morphology.
2. The identity of the AV valves depends on the type of ventricular loop that is present; typically, the tricuspid valve is right-sided with a ventricular D-loop and is left-sided with a ventricular L-loop.
3. The identity of an AV valve (tricuspid or mitral) is expressed by the number and position of its papillary muscle attachments, which are usually recognizable echocardiographically and also can be used to diagnose the type of ventricular loop (D- or L-) present. The tricuspid valve is "septophilic," with numerous small papillary muscle attachments into the ventricular sinus septum; whereas the mitral valve is "septophobic," with few large papillary muscles that typically do not insert into the ventricular septum.
4. Tricuspid regurgitation is a significant hemodynamic and surgical problem in patients with mitral atresia and a large LV.
5. Shinpo et al[87] also presented the concept of ventriculoatrial malalignment in their Fig. 14.10.

The anatomic details presented by Shinpo et al[87] are noteworthy. In their main study of mitral atresia with a large LV, the right ventricular sinus was underdeveloped, but not absent, in 11 of 25 patients (44%). In these cases, the single AV valve straddled the ventricular septum through a VSD of the AV canal type just as in straddling tricuspid valve. When the right ventricular sinus was absent (in 14/25 patients, 56%) the single AV valve did not straddle the ventricular septum and opened only into the large single LV, just as the tricuspid valve does with DILV into a single LV with absent right ventricular sinus. Thus, in both situations (small right ventricular sinus, and no right ventricular sinus), the single AV valve behaved like a tricuspid valve. If it were a mitral valve, one would expect the single AV valve to straddle through a conoventricular (outlet) type of VSD, not through a VSD of the AV canal (or inlet) type.

No matter whether the tricuspid valve was biventricular or exclusively left ventricular, it was tricommissural in 22 of 25 patients (88%). The attachments of the chordae tendineae of this single AV valve were paraseptal, or into the ventricular septal crest, or into the conal septum like a tricuspid valve and not like a mitral valve. The tricuspid valve is "septophilic," as these chordal attachments were, not "septophobic" as is characteristic of a mitral valve. Thiene et al[85] stated that this single AV valve opening from the RA into the LV was mitral in morphology, but with no further morphologic anatomic details or discussion of this critical question.

The addition I would like to add to the study and conclusions of Shinpo et al[87] in 1992 is as follows. **Ventriculoatrial malalignment** appears to be a fundamental morphogenetic and anatomic problem in the anomaly currently known as mitral atresia with large LV and small or absent right ventricular sinus.[86] In other words, "mitral atresia" (or left atrial outlet atresia) and malalignment of the morphologically LV to a position beneath the morphologically RA both appear to be sequelae of ventriculoatrial malalignment. In this developmental and anatomic sense, mitral atresia appears to be a hemodynamically important sequel, but not the primary embryologic and anatomic problem. Shinpo et al[87] agreed that striking ventriculoatrial malalignment is present in this anomaly.

Underdevelopment or absence of the right ventricular sinus may well explain the movement of the ventricular septum or its remnant abnormally to the right (in ventricular D-loops), in turn accounting for the LV underlying the RA, and the left ventricular free wall underlying the expected site of the mitral orifice.

The AV endocardial cushion tissue may perhaps have remained partly beneath the LA, helping to seal the left atrial floor and resulting in "mitral atresia" and closing the ostium primum type of partial AV septal defect. Some AV endocardial cushion tissue also may have remained adherent to the left ventricular inlet and may have made an important developmental contribution to the single AV valve opening from the RA into the LV.

So, with all due respect to Aristotle's laws of logic mentioned earlier, I am not sure that it is *im*possible to have left-sided mitral atresia (with an important contribution by the underlying left ventricular free wall), with a right-sided mitral valve or common AV valve opening from the RA into the large LV and straddling through a VSD of the AV canal type when a hypoplastic right ventricular sinus is present.

The problem with the identification of the AV valves is that they are a *dependent variable;* their morphology is ventricular-loop dependent. This is why we have never seen a heart with two well-developed ventricles and two separate AV valves in which a morphologically tricuspid valve opens into a morphologically LV and a morphologically mitral valve opens into a morphologically RV. This seems to be why the morphologies of the tricuspid valve and the mitral valve correspond to the morphologies of the ventricles of entry, or at least to the morphology of the ventricular loop (D- or L-) of entry in DILV or in DIRV anomalies. Thus, the morphology of the AV valves does *not* correspond to that of the atrium of exit, but to that of the ventricle of entry or the ventricular loop of entry. The problem of the identification of the AV valves (mitral versus tricuspid) is further complicated by their very different embryologic origins: the mitral valve arises from the endocardial cushions of the AV canal and hence is "fibrogenic," whereas the tricuspid valve originates importantly from the right ventricular myocardium and hence is, at least in part, "myogenic" in particular from the right ventricular septal surface, as the Ebstein anomaly indicates. Hence, the morphology of the tricuspid valve and the mitral valve may be, at least in part, primary or intrinsic, not entirely secondary or extrinsic.

Thus, the question arises in complex situations, such as the anomaly under consideration, how far can one "trust" AV valve morphology for their identification realizing that the morphology seems mostly to be *not* intrinsic or primary, but appears largely to be secondary, impressed on the AV valves by the tensor apparatus (chordae tendineae and papillary muscles),[87] which in turn is determined by the ventricular myocardial morphology and perhaps also by the very different hemodynamics of each AV valve. The tricuspid valve normally is a ventricular inflow valve only, whereas the mitral valve normally is both a ventricular inflow valve and a ventricular outflow valve.

All of the other four diagnostically important cardiac segments are *independent variables,* not dependent variables: the viscera and atria, the ventricles, the conus arteriosus, and the great arteries.

Because the morphology of the tricuspid valve and the mitral valve are ventricular-dependent or ventricular-loop dependent, the question concerning how far one can "trust" AV morphology for AV valve identification in complex anomalies such as the one under consideration becomes a matter of real concern. I think that caution is indicated. AV valve morphology appears to be a dependent variable, largely secondary to ventricular and ventricular loop anatomy and development. Diagnostically, it is important to understand how complex this problem of AV valve identification really is.

However, there is one matter concerning which there is no doubt or uncertainty: striking ventriculoatrial malalignment is an anatomic fact in mitral atresia with large LV. But why that occurs remains to be discovered.

ALIGNMENT CONCORDANCE AND DISCORDANCE VERSUS SITUS CONCORDANCE AND DISCORDANCE

As Shinpo et al[87] correctly pointed out, there are the previously mentioned two different kinds of concordance and discordance: alignment and situs. For example, in visceroatrial situs solitus with left atrial AV outlet atresia, with rightward malalignment of a D-loop ventricular segment and with single inlet from the RA into the right-shifted LV, there is AV *alignment discordance* because the RA opens into the LV. But there is AV *situs concordance* because of the presence of visceroatrial situs solitus and a D-loop (solitus, or noninverted) ventricular segment. More precisely, there is *one-half AV alignment discordance:* the RA opens into the LV, but the LA opens into nothing.

When a small right ventricular sinus coexists with a large LV, the AV alignments get even more complex: the AV alignments are both discordant (RA to LV) and concordant (RA to RV). This is why we always describe the ventricular situs (as D-loop or L-loop, or in terms of chirality) and do not rely on AV alignment ("connection") concordance or discordance (which we introduced in 1964)[73] because we have long understood that these useful concepts do not always apply. The same is also true of VA alignment concordance or discordance. Difficulties also occur with DORV and DOLV (VA alignments are both concordant and discordant) and with ACM. In ACM, the VA alignments are concordant, by definition, but these VA alignments are very abnormal.

Thus, there are *two very different types of VA concordance:* (1) with normally related great arteries, that is, solitus normally related (S) and inversus normally related (I), and (2) with ACM. With ACM, the VA alignments are concordant (by definition) and also are very abnormal (also by definition).

In 1993, Schulze-Neick et al[95] published a new method of producing an atrial septal perforation in mitral atresia by using radiofrequency energy, followed by blade atrial septostomy, followed by balloon atrial septostomy. These authors found that they could not do a conventional balloon atrial septostomy in a patient with mitral atresia because the LA was small and the atrial septum was leftwardly displaced and touched the left atrial free wall. They found that no force is needed when using radiofrequency energy. The left atrial pressure dropped from 32 mm Hg to 8 mm Hg.[95]

OCCLUSION OF THE MITRAL ORIFICE BY A LARGE, BALL-LIKE RHABDOMYOMA RESULTING IN STILLBIRTH

Just in case you may be wondering if there any other anatomic types of mitral atresia in addition to those that are diagrammed in Fig. 14.1, I strongly suspect that the answer will prove to be yes. In 1975, we had the privilege of studying the heart of a 3250-g (7 lb 3 oz) male stillborn fetus in which the mitral orifice was functionally occluded by a relatively large, ball-like rhabdomyoma (Fig. 14.22).[96] This patient had **functional mitral atresia,** but no *anatomic* mitral atresia because the mitral valve and orifice per se were widely patent, but filled with a downwardly prolapsing tumor (see Fig. 14.22D–F).

Usage

As pediatric cardiology increasingly becomes *fetal* cardiology, it is noteworthy that our customary distinction between *congenital* heart disease and *acquired* heart disease can break down. *Congenital* literally means born together (*congenitus,* Latin). It refers to conditions that are present at and before birth. One cannot say, with a straight face, that this rhabdomyoma (see Fig. 14.22) was a form of *acquired* heart disease (meaning acquired postnatally), not *congenital* heart disease, because this tumor was certainly present at and before birth: literally, this tumor was *congenital;* it was also *acquired prenatally.* However, *congenital*—as in *congenital* heart disease—is used to mean **structural heart disease** or **cardiac malformative heart disease,** typically as opposed to *degenerative* or *neoplastic* heart disease.

Designating diseases by the time when their clinical presentation used to occur (e.g., pediatric cardiology versus adult cardiology, congenital heart disease as opposed to acquired heart disease) now may break down, as this patient (see Fig. 14.22) illustrates. What we used to call *congenital* heart disease, and often still do, is really *heart disease caused by malformation during cardiac development,* that is, *malformative, developmental, or structural heart disease.* As we become increasingly more familiar with heart disease in utero, the foregoing more accurate designation of "congenital" heart disease may become increasingly important. This book is really mostly about malformative, developmental, or structural heart disease that can be clinically important at any age—prenatally, during infancy, childhood, adolescence, adulthood, or even during old age (e.g., bicuspid aortic valve, with premature aortic valvar calcification).

One final question is raised by the patient presented in Fig. 14.22. **Is this rhabdomyoma really a form of congenital malformative, developmental, or structural heart disease?** This tumor appears to have originated from the AV septum, that is, from the intera or "ostium primum" part of the AV septum that is formed by the AV endocardial cushion tissue. Histologically, rhabdomyomas strongly resemble *embryonic* AV endocardial cushion tissue. *Is so-called rhabdomyoma really an AV endocardial cushion tissue tumor?* I do not know the answer to this question, but it may well merit further consideration. Thus, the fascinating possibility exists that rhabdomyoma may be a form of congenital heart disease in the appropriate sense of a developmental malformation of cardiac tissue in utero and therefore present at birth.

CONGENITAL MITRAL STENOSIS

In 1978, Dr. Roger Ruckman and I[97] published a study of congenital mitral stenosis based on 49 autopsied cases that will serve as an introduction to the present much larger study of 201 necropsied patients.

First, however, it is essential to be familiar with several salient morphologic features of the **normal mitral valve** (Fig. 14.23). The relatively deep anterior or aortic leaflet and the much shallower posterior or mural leaflet of the mitral valve normally are thin, delicate, and pliable. The chordae tendineae (tendinous cords) are relatively long and thin, and they insert into the anterolateral and posteromedial papillary muscle groups. The interchordal spaces normally are well formed. The interpapillary muscle distance between the anterolateral and posteromedial papillary muscle groups is relatively wide. The mitral orifice consists of the interpapillary muscle space plus the interchordal spaces. There are no bands of fibrous tissue running from the anterior mitral leaflet to the left ventricular septal surface. Both papillary muscle groups are approximately equal in size, the posteromedial being inferior, medial, and paraseptal relative to the anterolateral, which is superior and more lateral, just as its name indicates.

When the great arteries are normally related, there is aortic-mitral direct fibrous continuity because normally there is no subaortic conal (infundibular) free wall myocardium to separate the aortic valve above from the mitral valve below (see Fig. 14.23).

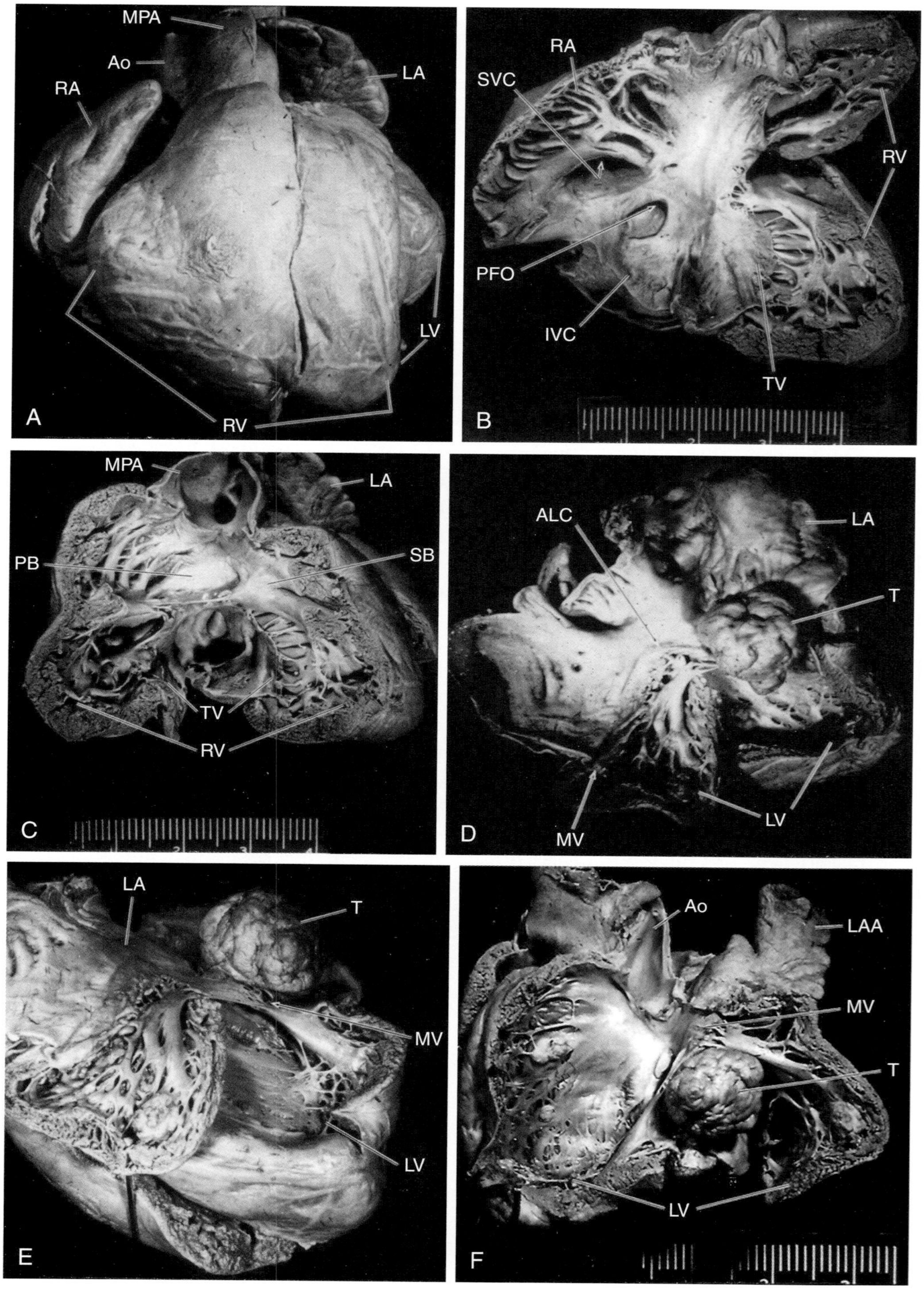

Fig. 14.22 Rhabdomyoma occluding the mitral orifice of a stillborn child. (A) External frontal view of the heart. The heart is normally formed with normal {S,D,S} segmental anatomy. {S,D,S} denotes the anatomic set or combination of solitus viscera and atria, with D-loop ventricles, and solitus normally related great arteries. A spectacular degree of right heart and left atrial hypertrophy and enlargement are apparent. The right atrial appendage *(RA)* is extremely hypertrophied and enlarged. So too is the right ventricle *(RV)*; indeed the RV is the only ventricle that forms the ventricular apex. The main pulmonary artery *(MPA)* is enlarged. The left atrial appendage *(LA)* is enormous. The left ventricle *(LV)* is so relatively small that it looks like a curious "side pocket" on the ventricular mass. The anterior interventricular sulcus is greatly exaggerated; instead of being a slight indentation, in this heart it has become a deep ravine because of the extraordinary right ventricular

Continued

Fig. 14.22 cont'd hypertrophy and enlargement that is juxtaposed with relatively left ventricular smallness. The aorta *(Ao)* is glimpsed posteriorly on the right, in its normal location, but is not well enough seen to merit further description. (B) The opened RA, tricuspid valve *(TV)*, and right ventricular inflow tract as viewed form a right lateral projection. This is a picture of normal anatomy, greatly exaggerated by hypertrophy and enlargement. The inferior vena cava *(IVC)* connects normally with the RA. Note that the IVC extends upward and its left wall is continuous with the septum primum, above which is the patent foramen ovale *(PFO)*. The septum primum (unlabeled) is the largest venous valve in the body, responsible for preventing regurgitation from the LA into the RA, both prenatally and postnatally. The septum primum is the flap valve of the foramen ovale (oval foramen), the "door" that normally opens from the RA into the LA prenatally, the via sinistra (left road) of the embryonic and fetal circulation. The eustachian valve of the IVC lies to the right of its orifice. This right venous valve component is usually thought of as the valve of the IVC. What is seldom recognized is that the IVC has two venous valves (or leaflets)—a right venous valve (eustachian) and a left venous valve (septum primum). (See Chapters 2 and 3 for more on this.) Of the IVC's two venous valves, the left one, the septum primum, is much more important. The "roof" of the PFO is the superior limbic band of septum secundum, which functions as the "door jamb" for the normally unidirectional (RA to LA only) flap valve of the prenatal circulation. The ostium of the coronary sinus and the triangle of Koch can be seen between the right venous valve remnant of the IVC and the origin of the septal leaflet of the TV. The superior vena cava *(SVC)* can be seen entering the RA. To the right of the SVC's entry is the crista terminalis (terminal crest), which marks the termination medially of the musculi pectinati (pectinate muscle) component derived from the primitive atrium. Medial to the terminal crest is the smooth venous component of the RA derived from the right horn of the sinus venosus. External to the crista terminalis is the sinoatrial node, making the crista terminalis an important landmark. Medial to the entry of the SVC is the superior limbic band of septum secundum (normally the "roof" of the PFO). "Pectinate" means like the teeth of a comb, well seen here. Despite the mitral occlusion, the septum primum has not herniated into the RA. The right ventricular inflow tract or sinus is well seen. This is the true RV, the pumping portion. The infundibulum, conus, or outflow tract, begins with the conal ring formed by the septal band (well seen here), by its extension the moderator band, by the inferior rim of the conal septum, and by its parietal or free wall extension, the parietal band. The right ventricular sinus (the "real" RV) is smaller than most realize, and the infundibulum or conus is larger than is often understood. (The ruler is marked off in cm and mm.) (C) The right ventricular inflow tract and the right ventricular outflow tract are opened widely, showing the conal septum and parietal band *(PB)*, the septal band *(SB)*, the intact ventricular septum, the opened pulmonary valve and large main pulmonary artery (MPA). The extreme right ventricular hypertrophy and enlargement are again noted. (D) The opened LA, viewed from above, showing the relatively large rhabdomyoma tumor *(T)*, located just above the opened mitral valve *(MV)*. One can also see the interior of the left atrial appendage *(LAA)* and its musculi pectinati. The anterolateral commissure *(ALC)* of the MV is labeled for orientation. One can also see down into the relatively small and finely trabeculated LV. (E) In this apical view of the opened LV, MV, and LA, one can see that the large rhabdomyoma (T) is originating from the left atrial septal surface just above the MV. (F) In this view of the opened LV, one can see that the large left atrial tumor herniates down into the orifice of the MV, thereby essentially totally occluding it. This is very rare case of **prenatally acquired mitral atresia** that caused stillbirth. Note that normal aortic-mitral fibrous continuity, the relatively small-chambered and thin-walled LV, the relatively small ascending Ao, and the very fine left ventricular trabeculations, and one can even see the left bundle branches of the atrioventricular conduction system coursing down the left ventricular septal surface in a normal way. The LAA is hugely hypertrophied and enlarged. This heart displays the most extreme example of hypertrophy and enlargement of the right heart (RA, RV, MPA) and LA that I think I have ever seen. *The question is: How was it possible for this extreme degree of hypertrophy and enlargement of the RA, RV, MPA and LA to occur, in contrast to the relative hypoplasia of the LV and the Ao?* My hypothetical answer is that the patient was a fetus. Because he did not have to breathe air on this own, but could rely on his mother's placenta for his respiration and oxygenation, this patient achieved a degree of differential hypertrophy and enlargement of the right heart and left atrium, compared with the relative hypoplasia of the left ventricle and aorta that I have never seen equaled by a postnatal patient. Have another look at Fig. 14.22A: it is amazing. (This patient was published as Case 2 of Geva et al,[96] but the photographs shown in Fig. 14.22 are published here for the first time.)

Normally, the LC/NC commissure of the aortic valve is located directly above the middle of the anterior mitral leaflet. The RC/NC commissure normally is located directly above the pars membranacea septi (the membranous septum). The RC/LC commissure of the aortic valve normally is located immediately above the conal (infundibular) septum. There normally is no supramitral ring.

ANATOMIC TYPES OF CONGENITAL MITRAL STENOSIS

Some of the important anatomic types of congenital mitral stenosis will now be presented pictorially, to help the reader visualize what the following text will describe.

Congenital mitral stenosis associated with HLHS, that is, with aortic valvar atresia or with severe congenital aortic valvar stenosis and an intact ventricular septum is shown in Fig. 14.24. Typically, the LV is thick-walled and small-chambered with severe EFE of the LV. The anterolateral and posteromedial papillary muscles are abnormally small and are involved by EFE. The chordae tendineae are short and the interchordal spaces are absent. The free margin of the anterior mitral leaflet is thickened and rolled, consistent with some degree of congenital mitral regurgitation, in addition to congenital mitral stenosis. The arched inferior margin of the anterior mitral leaflet has been called a congenital mitral arcade. The LA is hypertrophied and enlarged. The septum primum (the flap valve of the foramen

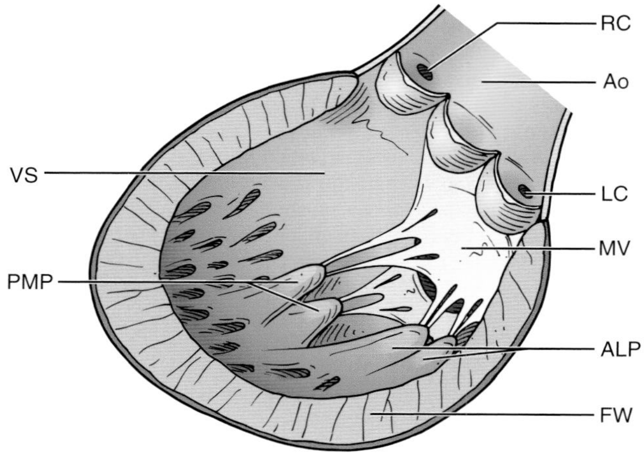

Fig. 14.23 The normal mitral valve *(MV)*. The morphologically left ventricle has been opened, the left ventricular septal *(VS)* surface being right and superior, and the left ventricular free wall *(FW)* being inferior. The valve of the aorta *(Ao)* has also been opened. The ostium of the right coronary *(RC)* artery and the ostium of the left coronary *(LC)* artery are visible within their respective sinuses of Valsalva. The MV has not been opened. The deep anterior leaflet of the MV, also known in normally formed hearts as the deep aortic leaflet of the MV is well seen. The shallow posterior or mural leaflet of the MV can be glimpsed between the papillary muscles. The anterolateral papillary muscle *(ALP)* and the posteromedial papillary muscle *(PMP)* are both relatively large. Both normally arise from the left ventricular FW. The PMP muscle is posterior (or inferior), medially, and paraseptal, that is, adjacent to the inferior left VS surface. In the intact, unopened LV, the ALP muscle is anterior (superior) and lateral relative to the PMP muscle. Note that the spaces between the MV's chordae tendineae (tendinous cords) are well formed, and that the space between the ALP muscle group and the PMP muscle group is relatively large. The mitral orifice normally consists of the space between the anterior and posterior mitral leaflets, plus the interchordal spaces, plus the interpapillary muscle space. A supramitral ring, not seen in this drawing, can abnormally narrow the inlet into the MV. The MV orifice is really the MV canal, with an inlet (stenosing supramitral ring), a middle portion (mitral valve leaflets), and an outlet (interchordal spaces and the interpapillary muscle space). Normally related great arteries typically have direct fibrous continuity between the aortic valve and the anterior leaflet of the MV via the intervalvar fibrosa. The three leaflets of the normal opened aortic valve are well seen: the right coronary (RC) leaflet, the left coronary (LC) leaflet, and the unlabeled noncoronary leaflet between the RC and LC leaflets. Note the following surgically important relationships in normally formed hearts: (1) the NC/LC commissure of the aortic valve normally is located directly above the middle of the anterior mitral leaflet and (2) the NC/RC commissure of the aortic valve normally is located directly above the membranous ventricular septum, which in turn normally is directly above the atrioventricular conduction system. These normal anatomic relationships are important for a surgeon doing transaortic surgery through the aortic valve from above. This heart specimen is from autopsy number A65-12, precisely drawn by Janis Cirulis. (Reproduced with permission from Ruckman RN, Van Praagh R. Anatomic types of congenital mitral stenosis: Report of 49 autopsy cases with consideration of diagnosis and surgical implications. *Am J Cardiol.* 1978;42:592.)

ovale) is redundant, suggesting that the atrial septum may well have been restrictive to left-to-right atrial shunting, with herniation of the septum primum into the right atrial cavity. This portrait (see Fig. 14.24) is a highly accurate representation[97] by Janis Cirulis, a gifted artist.

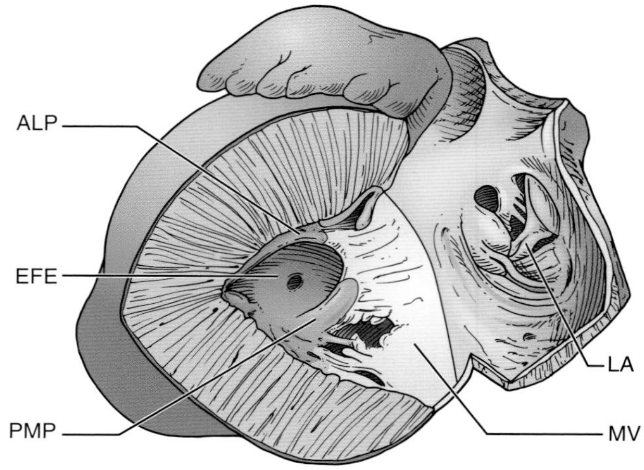

Fig. 14.24 Congenital mitral stenosis in a 12-day-old patient with the hypoplastic left heart syndrome. This patient had severe congenital aortic stenosis with an intact ventricular septum. The left ventricle was small-chambered and thick-walled, with severe endocardial fibroelastosis *(EFE)*. The anterolateral papillary *(ALP)* muscles and the posteromedial papillary *(PMP)* muscles were atrophied, and the interchordal spaces were absent. The free margin of the anterior mitral leaflet was thickened and rolled, forming what Dr. Jesse Edwards called a congenital mitral arcade. The hypertrophy and enlargement of the left atrium *(LA)* are well shown. The mitral orifice was only 20% of normal size and the left ventricular cavity was only 43% the size of normal control heart specimens. We called this **the hypoplastic type of congenital mitral stenosis** because it was part of the hypoplastic left heart syndrome. *MV,* Mitral valve. (Reproduced with permission from Ruckman RN, Van Praagh R. Anatomic types of congenital mitral stenosis: Report of 49 autopsy cases with consideration of diagnosis and surgical implications. *Am J Cardiol.* 1978;42:592.)

Congenital mitral stenosis not associated with aortic valvar atresia or severe aortic valvar stenosis is presented in Figs. 14.25 through 14.28.[97] These four anatomic types of congenital mitral stenosis are also summarized diagrammatically in Fig. 14.29.[97]

In Fig. 14.25, the anterior leaflet of the mitral valve is thickened and bulges into the left ventricular cavity. The chordae tendineae appear shortened, and the interchordal spaces are occluded by fibrous tissue. The space between the anterolateral and the posteromedial papillary muscles is mildly reduced (compared with age-matched normal controls). Thus, congenital mitral stenosis resulted from reduction of the interleaflet space, absence of the interchordal spaces, and reduction of the interpapillary muscle space below the mitral orifice (Case 9).[97]

In Fig. 14.26 the anterolateral and the posteromedial papillary muscles are fused; hence, the interpapillary muscle distance has been reduced to zero. Both papillary muscles receive chordae tendineae. However, the space between these two foci of chordal insertion is greatly reduced. The only other mitral orifice is a small interchordal space at the anterolateral commissure of the mitral valve (see Fig. 14.26). The other interchordal spaces are occluded by fibrous tissue.

A subaortic fibrous ridge extends from the anterior leaflet of the mitral valve onto the left ventricular septal surface, immediately beneath the aortic valve leaflets. Although physiologically insignificant, this subaortic fibrous ridge suggests that fibrous subaortic stenosis (not present in this patient) results from

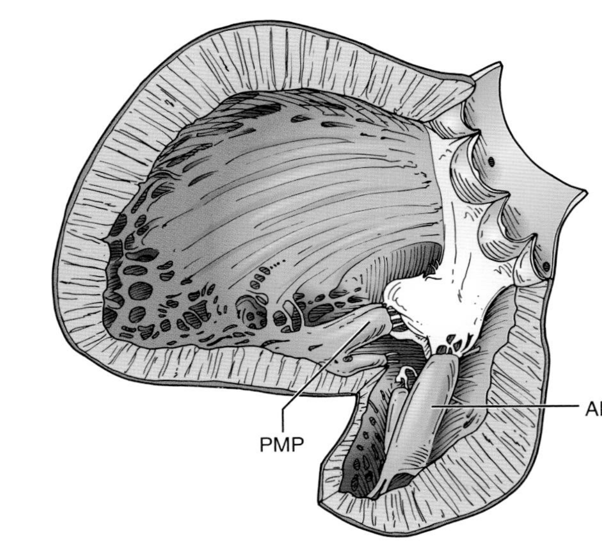

Fig. 14.25 A 4-month-old patient with **typical congenital mitral stenosis.** A thickened anterior mitral leaflet bulges into the left ventricular cavity. The mitral chordae tendineae are shortened, and the interchordal spaces are obliterated by fibrous tissue. The interpapillary muscle distance between the anterolateral papillary muscle *(ALP)* and the posteromedial papillary muscle *(PMP)* is mildly reduced. The mitral orifice size was only 69% of normal, but the left ventricular cavity size was 100% of normal. In typical congenital mitral stenosis, transmitral obstruction typically is produced by a combination of reduced interleaflet space, reduction or absence of interchordal spaces, and reduction of interpapillary muscle space. (Reproduced with permission from Ruckman RN, Van Praagh R. Anatomic types of congenital mitral stenosis: Report of 49 autopsy cases with consideration of diagnosis and surgical implications. *Am J Cardiol.* 1978;42:592.)

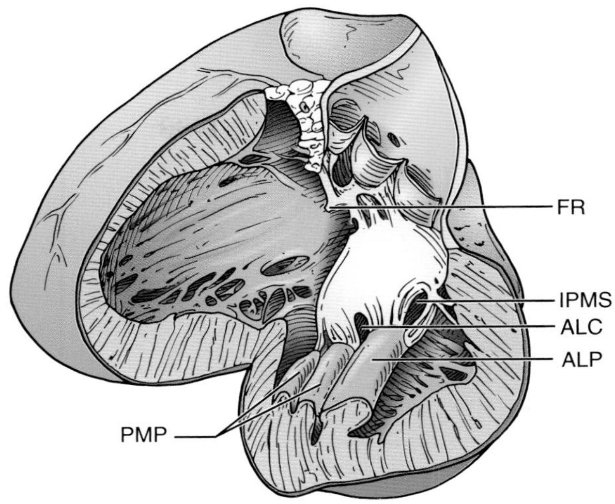

Fig. 14.26 Congenital mitral stenosis with fusion of the anterolateral papillary muscle *(ALP)* and the posteromedial papillary muscle *(PMP).* The upward extension of what normally is the interpapillary muscle space *(IPMS),* that normally is the main portion of the mitral orifice, is greatly narrowed. All of what normally are the interchordal spaces are obliterated by fibrous tissue, except for one interchordal space at the anterolateral commissure *(ALC).* The result is severe congenital mitral stenosis with double-orifice mitral valve. This case also may be viewed as a forme fruste of parachute mitral valve. Although two papillary muscle groups are present (ALP and PMP), they are fused, essentially forming one large papillary muscle group. A physiologically insignificant subaortic fibrous ring *(FR)* extends from the anterior mitral leaflet to the left ventricular septal surface. (Reproduced with permission from Ruckman RN, Van Praagh R. Anatomic types of congenital mitral stenosis: Report of 49 autopsy cases with consideration of diagnosis and surgical implications. *Am J Cardiol.* 1978;42:592.)

"untidied up" fibroelastic tissue of the AV endocardial cushions that form the anterior mitral leaflet. (This is a portrait of Case 18.)

Fig. 14.27 illustrates typical parachute mitral valve in a patient with a divided AV canal, that is, having separate mitral and tricuspid valves, and with normally related great arteries. There is a large solitary posteromedial papillary muscle into which all of the chordae tendineae insert. The anterolateral papillary muscle is absent. The interchordal spaces are obliterated by fibrous tissue. The small mitral orifice opens into the left ventricular free wall. The mitral valve is both stenotic and eccentric.

Dr. Jesse Edwards et al[98] with Dr. John Shone as first author coined the term "parachute mitral valve": the single papillary muscle is likened to a person hanging from a parachute. When the AV canal is in common (undivided), often the single papillary muscle receiving all of the chordae tendineae is the anterolateral papillary muscle (not the posteromedial). This is known as a *potentially parachute mitral valve,*[99] meaning that following surgical repair of the common AV canal, one is left with a parachute mitral valve, in which it is usually wise not to suture closed the cleft in the anterior mitral leaflet because this would worsen the congenital mitral stenosis.

Finally, it is possible for two papillary muscle groups to be present, but for all of the chordae tendineae to insert into only one papillary muscle group. Thus, the bottom-line surgical consideration is not how many papillary muscle groups are present, but rather, *how many foci of chordal insertion there are.* (Fig. 14.27 is a portrait of the heart of Case 49.[97])

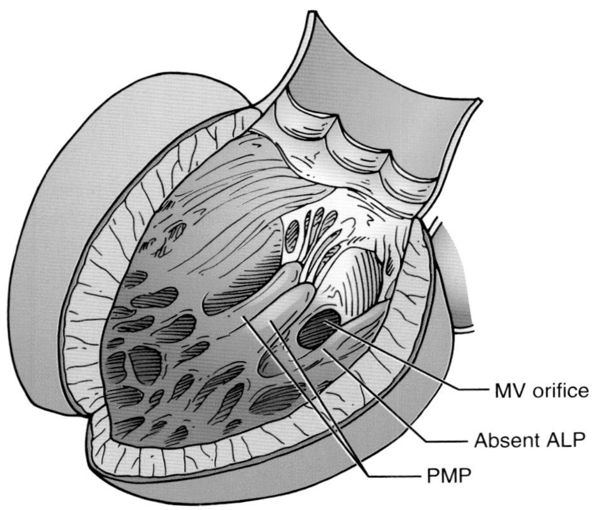

Fig. 14.27 Congenital mitral stenosis with parachute mitral valve. In this 20-year-old patient, the anterolateral papillary muscle group was absent *(Absent ALP).* The posteromedial papillary muscle group *(PMP)* was present and enlarged. All of the thickened chordae tendineae inserted into the PMP muscle group. The orifice of the mitral valve *(MV)* opened laterally and inferiorly into the left ventricular free wall. The orifice of the MV was eccentric and stenotic. The mitral orifice measured 84% of normal size, and the left ventricular cavity size was 136% of normal size. (Reproduced with permission from Ruckman RN, Van Praagh R. Anatomic types of congenital mitral stenosis: Report of 49 autopsy cases with consideration of diagnosis and surgical implications. *Am J Cardiol.* 1978;42:592.)

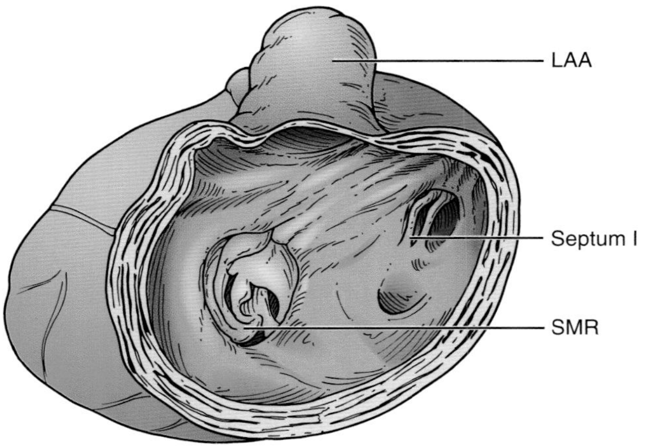

Fig. 14.28 Congenital mitral stenosis with supramitral ring *(SMR)*. This 5½-year-old patient had a mild form of typical congenital mitral stenosis, similar to that shown in Fig. 14.25. This patient did not have parachute mitral valve (MV), as in Fig. 14.27. Hence, this patient did not have Shone syndrome,[98] that is, supramitral stenosing ring of the left atrium, parachute MV, subaortic stenosis, and coarctation of the aorta. However, this patient did have tetralogy of Fallot. Note the marked hypertrophy and enlargement of this patient's left atrium, including the left atrial appendage *(LAA)*. The septum primum *(Septum I)* sealed the foramen ovale, as is typical with left atrial hypertension. The SMR was severely stenotic. Note that one does not see the mitral valve beneath the SMR. (Reproduced with permission from Ruckman RN, Van Praagh R. Anatomic types of congenital mitral stenosis: Report of 49 autopsy cases with consideration of diagnosis and surgical implications. *Am J Cardiol*. 1978;42:592.)

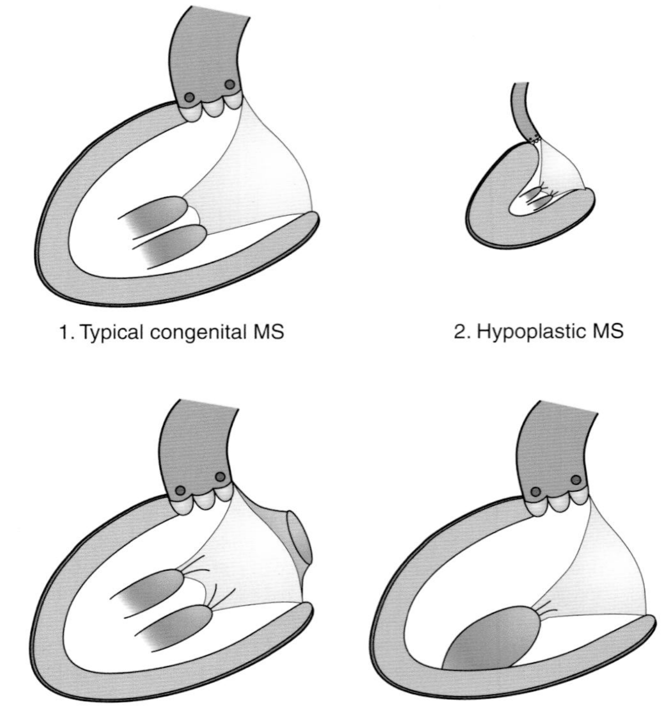

Fig. 14.29 Diagrammatic summary of the four main anatomic types of congenital mitral stenosis *(MS)*, found in 49 autopsied cases: typical, 49%; hypoplastic, 41%; supramitral ring, 12%; and parachute, 8%. Two anatomic types of congenital MS were found in 6 of 49 patients (12.24%). (Reproduced with permission from Ruckman RN, Van Praagh R. Anatomic types of congenital mitral stenosis: Report of 49 autopsy cases with consideration of diagnosis and surgical implications. *Am J Cardiol*. 1978;42:592.)

Fig. 14.28[97] illustrates a supramitral stenosing ring. This is stenosis of the inlet into the mitral canal. The supramitral ring is continuous with the subjacent mitral valve leaflets. This patient (Case 2)[97] had mild stenosis of the underlying mitral valve and TOF. The septum primum sealed the foramen ovale, making it a fossa ovalis, which explains the severe hypertrophy and enlargement of the LA (see Fig. 14.28).[97] The supramitral stenosing ring is part of **Shone syndrome,**[98] another of Dr. Jesse Edwards' outstanding contributions. Shone syndrome—named in honor of my friend Dr. John Shone—consists of a supramitral ring, parachute mitral valve, subaortic stenosis, and preductal coarctation of the aorta.[98]

The foregoing (Figs. 14.24 to 14.29) are not all of the anatomic types of congenital mitral stenosis that are now known to exist; but this is a good beginning, which will help make the following findings comprehensible.

Many modern textbooks of pediatric cardiology and cardiac surgery contain no illustrations of the various anatomic types of congenital mitral stenosis, and little or no detailed description of the various anatomic types. Consequently, the following presentation, based on 201 autopsied cases, will endeavor to answer the following questions:

How many anatomic types of congenital mitral stenosis are now known to exist? What are they? What are the relative prevalences of each? What are the diagnostic and therapeutic implications of these anatomic findings?

In the present series of 201 autopsied cases, congenital mitral stenosis occurred in 7 subsets (anatomic and developmental groups or complexes) that are summarized in Table 14.12.

Excluded cases of mitral stenosis were 1 patient with rheumatic mitral stenosis, this section being devoted to the analysis of congenital (not acquired) mitral stenosis; 3 patients who, on careful reassessment, were thought not to have definite congenital mitral stenosis; and 5 patients who had the complete form of common AV canal with a common AV valve, that is, without separate mitral and tricuspid valves. These 5 patients had *potential* congenital mitral stenosis following surgical repair of the completely common AV canal; but because congenital mitral stenosis was not present preoperatively, these 5 cases were excluded.

CONGENITAL MITRAL STENOSIS WITH HYPOPLASTIC LEFT HEART SYNDROME, THAT IS, WITH AORTIC VALVAR ATRESIA OR SEVERE CONGENITAL AORTIC VALVAR STENOSIS

Congenital mitral stenosis with HLHS (i.e., aortic valvar atresia or congenital aortic valvar stenosis) was by far the most common anatomic type of congenital mitral stenosis (see Fig. 14.24) found in this study of 201 autopsied cases, occurring in 130 patients (64.7% of this series) (see Table 14.12). The prevalence of this anatomic type of congenital mitral stenosis was much higher in the present large study than it was in our

TABLE 14.12 Anatomic Types of Congenital Mitral Stenosis in 201 Postmortem Cases

	No	%
1. Congenital MS with HLHS, that is, AoVAt or severe AS	130	64.7
2. Congenital MS without HLHS and without other major mitral anomalies	48	23.9
3. Congenital MS with ICAVC	13	6.5
4. Congenital MS with straddling TV or with DILV, ± single LV	6	3.5
5. Congenital MS with DIRV, ± single RV	2	1.0
6. Congenital MS caused by rhabdomyoma	1	0.5
7. Congenital MS in a conjoined twin	1	0.5
Totals	201	100.1[a]

AS, Aortic stenosis, valvar; *AoVAt*, aortic valvar atresia; *DILV*, double-inlet left ventricle; *DIRV*, double-inlet right ventricle; *HLHS*, hypoplastic left heart syndrome; *ICAVC*, incompletely common atrioventricular canal; *LV*, morphologically left ventricle; *MS*, mitral stenosis; *No.*, *number; RV*, morphologically right ventricle; *TV*, tricuspid valve.
[a]Percentages are rounded off.

earlier study based on 49 necropsied cases (65% versus 41%, respectively). This difference is highly significant statistically: $x^2 = 9.25$, the probability that this is a random event occurring by chance being less than 0.005; that is, $p < .005$. This unexpected finding raises the question: What is the difference between the present larger study of congenital mitral stenosis based on 201 autopsied cases (see Table 14.6) and our earlier smaller study based on 49 autopsied cases?[99] The difference may be that in the present larger series an attempt has been made to include *all* autopsied patients with congenital mitral stenosis seen at Boston Children's Hospital with retained necropsy specimens since World War II, as opposed to a less all-inclusive sample.[99] (Sex: males, 87 [66.9%] and females, 43 [33.1%].) Thus, a strong male preponderance (males to females = 2.02/1) was found in this subset of congenital mitral stenosis.

Aortic Valvar Atresia Versus Aortic Valvar Stenosis

Of these 130 cases with HLHS, 74 (56.9%) had aortic valvar atresia and 56 (43.1%) had severe aortic valvar stenosis. This distinction may not matter much clinically or surgically, but it is of some interest hemodynamically. Congenital mitral stenosis is present in the *anatomic* and *pathologic* sense that the mitral orifice is abnormally small (see Fig. 14.24). *Stenosis* is new Latin from Greek *stenosis,* from *stenoun,* to constrict, from *stenos,* narrow. ("New Latin" means that you are unlikely to find *stenosis* in your Latin dictionary, because it was a learned borrowing from Greek by physicians who initially wrote in Latin.)

However, when stenosis is construed *hemodynamically,* it is noteworthy that the usual meaning (difficulty passing through an abnormally small orifice, resulting in a pressure gradient) may well not apply to the mitral valve when aortic valvar *atresia* is associated with an intact ventricular septum (see Fig. 14.24). In this situation, which pertained in the majority of these patients with HLHS (57%), little or no blood may have flowed through the mitral valve from the LA into the LV because, barring a significant sinusoidal connection between the left ventricular cavity and the coronary arterial system, there was no pathway for anterograde blood flow out of the left ventricular cavity. Hence, in this hemodynamic sense, we are confronted with *functional* congenital mitral "atresia," that is, with little or no anterograde blood flow across the mitral valve, with or without some degree of congenital mitral regurgitation. It is interesting to understand that one can have *functional* mitral atresia with a patent mitral orifice.

I am not suggesting any change in diagnostic terminology. We continue to make the diagnosis of congenital mitral stenosis in this situation (aortic valvar atresia with intact ventricular septum) because it makes sense anatomically, if not hemodynamically.

Why is the LV typically thick-walled and small-chambered in HLHS with aortic valvar atresia or severe aortic valvar stenosis and an intact ventricular septum (see Fig. 14.24)? We think that the answer is that because in this situation, the LV can do only pressure work but little or no flow work, barring significant sinusoidal communication(s) between the left ventricular cavity and the coronary arteries and/or significant mitral regurgitation.

Why is left ventricular EFE so characteristic of this anatomic type of HLHS (see Fig. 14.24)? We think that left ventricular EFE results from global endocardial and subendocardial myocardial ischemic necrosis or infarction. When left ventricular intracavitary pressure remains high throughout the cardiac cycle (systole and diastole), because of aortic valvar atresia or severe aortic valvar stenosis with an intact ventricular septum and a relatively competent mitral valve, the subendocardial left ventricular myocardium, including the left ventricular papillary muscles of the mitral valve, do not receive adequate oxygenation and nutrition in diastole, resulting in subendocardial ischemic necrosis. The endocardial and subendocardial fibrosis and elastosis consist of the fibroelastic "houses" (the perimysium and endomysium) within which the now vanished cardiac myocytes used to live.

This interpretation of the typical left ventricular EFE of HLHS (see Fig. 14.24), that is, that it results from endocardial and subendocardial myocardial ischemic necrosis, is supported by other observations. When the congenital mitral stenosis is very severe, with only a tiny orifice, left ventricular EFE tends *not* to occur, or to be only focal, not global. Or, if a sizeable VSD coexists, EFE typically is *not* present. Why not? When the LV is able to do anterograde flow work and to decompress itself through the VSD, left ventricular intracavitary pressure does not remain high during the entire cardiac cycle. At the end of systole, left ventricular intracavitary pressure can fall in diastole, permitting left ventricular myocardial oxygenation and nutrition during diastole in the normal way. Hence, subendocardial ischemic necrosis of the myocardium does not occur. The fibroelastic endomysium and perimysium remain inhabited by viable cardiac myocytes.

Why does aortic valvar atresia or severe stenosis occur, resulting in HLHS with congenital mitral stenosis? We think that at least part of the answer to this question has to do with the development of the commissures of the aortic valve. Normally, the three aortic commissures elevate and separate the leaflets between which they develop. When one commissure is underdeveloped or absent, the aortic valve is bicommissural and functionally bicuspid (instead of being normally tricommissural and tricuspid). Usually, it is the intercoronary (or RC/LC) commissure, or the right coronary-noncoronary commissure that is poorly formed or absent, resulting in a bicommissural, functionally bicuspid aortic valve. It should be understood that typically, all three leaflets are present. But the valve superficially looks and acts as though only two leaflets are present, because *the number of well-developed commissures determines the number of functional leaflets that are present.*[28] When two commissures are absent or poorly developed, and only one commissure is well developed (typically *the LC/NC commissure* is the only well-developed commissure), the result is a unicommissural and hence a functionally unicuspid aortic valve.[28]

What happens when all three aortic commissures are absent or very poorly developed? We hypothesize that typically, the result is aortic valvar atresia. Why? Apparently because no commissure developed well enough *to elevate and separate* the adjacent aortic valve leaflets. Our hypothesis is that adjacent aortic valve leaflets that are not separated and elevated by a well-developed commissure can adhere to each other, forming a large double leaflet, rather than forming two normally separated and supported aortic leaflets.

When congenital mitral stenosis is associated with aortic valvar atresia or severe aortic valvar stenosis resulting in HLHS, the congenital mitral stenosis appears to be *secondary* to the aortic valvar atresia or severe stenosis. All of the other characteristic features of HLHS also appear to be *secondary* to aortic valvar atresia or severe stenosis (see Fig. 14.24): the thick-walled and small-chambered LV, the left ventricular EFE, and the occurrence of sinusoids between the left ventricular cavity and the coronary arteries.

The segmental anatomy of HLHS with congenital mitral stenosis (see Fig. 14.24) typically is normal, that is {S,D,S}. There is situs solitus of the viscera and atria {*S*,-,-}, D-loop or noninverted ventricles {S,*D*,-}, and solitus normally related great arteries {S,D,*S*}. The AV and VA alignments typically are both concordant (appropriate).

Because HLHS is highly lethal, it inspired the development of the **Norwood procedure**[100] and **infantile cardiac transplantation.**[101] **The ages at death** of these 130 patients with HLHS and congenital mitral stenosis were as follows: mean, 165.81 ± 760.47 days, and range, 0 to 7665 days. In other words, the mean or average age at death was 5.53 months, and the standard deviation was huge, ± 2.08 years. Are these numbers really representative of the ages at death of patients with HLHS? I do not think so. Why? Because these numbers were skewed toward older ages by several unusually old patients in this series. The **median** age at death was only 9 days, accurately reflecting the high, early lethality that is characteristic of the natural history of HLHS.

Other Features of Interest

Let us now reexamine these 130 cases of congenital mitral stenosis with aortic valvar atresia or severe stenosis and intact ventricular septum, looking for interesting or unusual features that we have not mentioned as yet. But first, two "typical" cases:

Case 2, described by Dr. Ben Landing in 1951 (A51-294), is typical of this anatomic type of congenital mitral stenosis. The patient was a 3-week-old girl with severe congenital mitral stenosis. The papillary muscles of the LV were small and indistinct. The interchordal spaces were obliterated by fibrous tissue. EFE of the LV was present. Aortic valvar stenosis was severe, and the commissures of the aortic valve were poorly formed.

Case 4 was a consult that I did in 1987 (C87-281) concerning a boy who was 6 months and 21 days old. Congenital mitral stenosis was severe, with failure of formation of most of the interchordal spaces and reduction of the interpapillary muscle distance to 2 mm. EFE of the LV was mild and focal, we thought because the congenital mitral stenosis was so severe, limiting the entry of blood into the left ventricular cavity. Aortic valvar stenosis was also extremely severe, the aortic valve being unicommissural and unicuspid. The only well-developed commissure was the LC/NC; the other two commissures were absent. The aortic orifice, situated beneath the LC/NC commissure, was only 1 mm in internal dimension. The segmental anatomy was normal, that is, {S,D,S}, and the ventricular septum was intact. The LV was thick-walled and small-chambered. Right ventricular hypertrophy and enlargement were massive. A Norwood procedure[100] had been performed at 6 days of age. Autopsy revealed a moderate "coarctation" (narrowing) of the aorta at the distal end of the aortic arch reconstruction leading into the descending thoracic aorta, the "coarctation" measuring 3 mm in internal dimension.

These first 2 cases had fairly typical congenital cardiac pathology. But because we are looking for the *unusual,* we will now say farewell to the routine type of pathologic anatomy in HLHS.

Case 6 was a 17-day-old boy whom I studied in 1991 with Drs. John Papagiannis and Walter Jung (A91-52). The patient had severe congenital mitral stenosis *associated with abnormal left ventricular myocardial architecture.* A prominent *muscle of Moulaert, that is, the anterolateral muscle of the LV,* was found (Fig. 14.30).[102] This muscle was confluent with the anterolateral papillary muscle group and then extended upward as a prominent muscular pillar toward the semilunar valve (the aortic valve) at the left ventricular outlet. This patient had normal segmental anatomy {S,D,S}. *The prominent anterolateral muscle of the LV (muscle of Moulaert)* crowded the mitral valve, which was diminutive, with thin and delicate leaflets. A narrow aortic valve–to–mitral valve intervalvar fibrosa, typically of normally related great arteries, was present.

An abnormal accessory posteromedial papillary muscle group originated from the left ventricular septal surface inferiorly and inserted into the anterior leaflet of the mitral valve.

The previously mentioned muscle of Moulaert largely filled the left ventricular outflow tract, creating left ventricular subaortic obstruction (stenosis). Congenital aortic valvar stenosis was also present. The aortic valve was hypoplastic, bicuspid, and bicommissural, with the RC/LC commissure being absent. The internal dimension of the aortic valvar orifice was 4 mm. The ascending aorta and aortic arch were hypoplastic, and a preductal coarctation of the aorta was present.

A small muscular VSD was present posteroinferiorly (1.5 to 2.0 mm internal dimension). Left atrial hypertrophy, right atrial

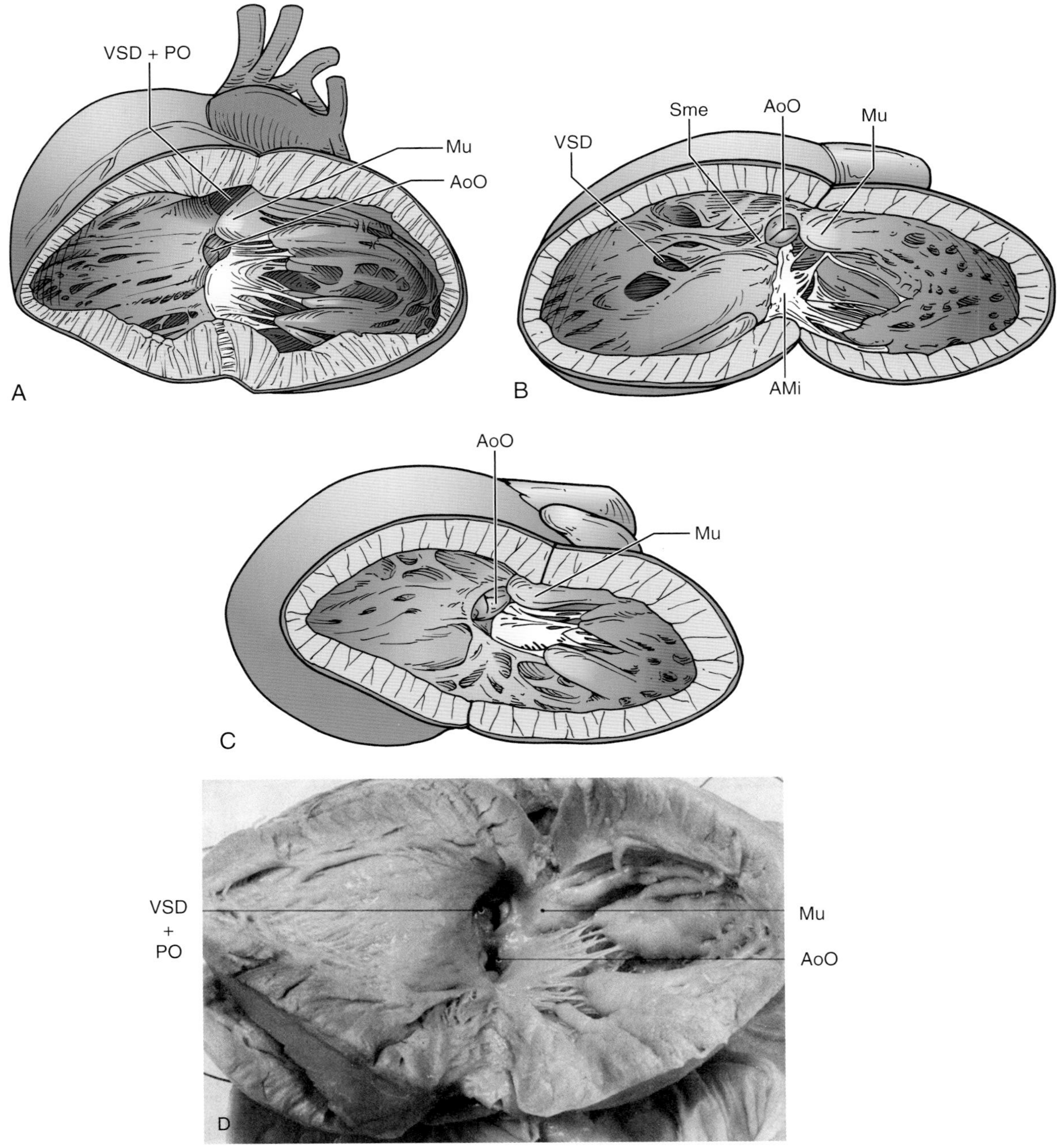

Fig. 14.30 The anterolateral muscle of the left ventricle (LV), also known as the **muscle of Moulaert.** To my knowledge, the anterolateral muscle of the LV was first described and diagrammed by Dr. André J. M. G. Moulaert in his medical thesis from the University of Leiden in 1974. These drawings are from his book entitled, *Ventricular Septal Defects and Anomalies of the Aortic Arch:* A, his figure 15b; B, figure 32B; C, figure, 21B; and D, figure 16a. All of these figures depict an opened morphologically LV. (A) The anterolateral muscle of the LV, abbreviated as *Mu,* lies above the anterolateral papillary muscle of the LV and extends distally to lie between the pulmonary valve superiorly, that overrides the LV minimally, and a bicuspid stenotic aortic valve inferiorly. There is an infundibular subpulmonary ventricular septal defect *(VSD).* (B) The Mu bulges into the left ventricular outflow tract and may narrow the mitral inflow tract. Thus, the muscle of Moulaert can be hemodynamically important. (C) This patient had the Eisenmenger complex. The aortic valve orifice *(AoO)* was displaced to the right (aortic overriding), a subaortic VSD was present, and no right ventricular outflow tract obstruction was present. So the Eisenmenger complex has been described as tetralogy of Fallot *without* pulmonary outflow tract obstruction. Mu was not obstructive to left ventricular inflow or outflow. (D) Dr. Moulaert thought that the anterolateral muscle of the LV (Mu) displaced the anterior leaflet of the mitral valve (MV) toward the anterolateral wall of the LV. But no hemodynamic data were presented to support this hypothesis. *AMi,* Anterior leaflet of mitral valve; *AoO,* aortic orifice; *Sme,* septum membranaceum; *VSD + PO,* ventricular septal defect and pulmonary orifice. (From Vizcaino A, Campbell J, Litovsky S, Van Praagh R. Single origin of right and left pulmonary artery branches from ascending aorta with nonbranching main pulmonary artery: Relevance to a new understanding of truncus arteriosus. *Pediatr Cardiol.* 2002;23:230-234; with permission.)

hypertrophy and enlargement, marked right ventricular hypertrophy and enlargement, and left ventricular hypoplasia were found. The left lung was unilobed (i.e., absence of lobation).

A Norwood procedure[100] had been performed at 2 days of age. Autopsy revealed a residual coarctation of the aorta, a nonpatulous (stenotic appearing) left coronary ostium, thrombotic occlusion of the modified right Blalock-Taussig shunt (thought to be the cause of death), and multiple other antemortem thromboses. Postmortem blood cultures grew *Escherichia coli*, suggesting that *gram-negative sepsis* may well have been the cause of the multiple thromboses.

Returning to the pathologic anatomy, we thought that this patient had **a newly recognized anatomic type of congenital mitral stenosis** characterized by a squeezed or compressed and hence diminutive but otherwise normal mitral valve and abnormal left ventricular myocardial architecture (anomalous anterolateral muscle of the LV, also known as the muscle of Moulaert) that was the agent of the mitral crowding and apparent compression.

Careful review of this entire anatomic subset of congenital mitral stenosis, with a prominent anterolateral muscle of the LV (muscle of Moulaert) contributing to muscular subaortic stenosis, revealed one other such patient: Case 103 (2/130 such patients = 1.54% of this anatomic subset).

In somewhat greater detail, **Case 103** (A89-89) was an 11½-month-old boy with premature closure of the foramen ovale. Congenital mitral stenosis was present, the mitral valve being hypoplastic. The papillary muscles were abnormally close together, but distinct and not fused. Chordae tendineae went to both the anterolateral and the posteromedial papillary muscle groups. Subaortic muscular stenosis was produced by a localized protrusion of the ventricular septum into the left ventricular outflow tract medially and a prominent anterolateral muscle of the LV (muscle of Moulaert) laterally. Congenital aortic valvar stenosis was present, the aortic valve being bicuspid and bicommissural, because of absence of the *LC/NC commissure*. It is rare for *this* aortic valve commissure to be absent. Typically, this is the one well-developed commissure when severe, unicuspid, and unicommissural aortic valvar stenosis is present. In this anatomic subset of 130 autopsied patients with congenital mitral stenosis and HLHS, there were only 3 patients (2.31%) in whom the LC/NC commissure was absent (**Cases 103, 107,** and **195**).

Case 103 also had coarctation of the aorta. Although this patient had *multilevel left ventricular outflow tract obstruction* (congenital mitral stenosis, subaortic muscular stenosis of the left ventricular outflow tract, aortic valvar stenosis, and coarctation of the aorta), it differed from Shone syndrome[98] in *not* having a supramitral stenosing ring and in not having a parachute mitral valve.

The other findings of interest associated with congenital mitral stenosis and HLHS are summarized in Table 14.13. Although these features are statistically infrequent in this study, it would be a mistake to dismiss them as "rare birds" of no consequence. Some are important causes of death, such as a *closing PDA,* which was observed in 11 of these 130 patients (8.46%) (see Table 14.13) (in how many more patients did this occur, but was not detectable at autopsy?). An *intact atrial septum* was observed in 9 of these 130 patients (6.92%) (but in how many more was the atrial septum significantly restrictive to left-to-right shunting at the atrial level, thereby contributing to early mortality?). Other associated findings (see Table 14.13) may well prove to be of etiologic (molecular genetic) importance, such as the occurrence of *MCAs* (in 15/130 patients, 11.54%) and the occurrence of *familial congenital heart disease* (in 6/130 patients, 4.62%) (see Table 14.13).

MCAs were the most common associated finding in this series of 130 postmortem cases of congenital mitral stenosis with HLHS occurring in 15 of these patients (11.5%; see Table 14.13).

MCAs means that malformations were present not only of the cardiovascular system but of other systems as well, such as the gastrointestinal system and/or the urogenital system, etc. Thus, MCAs means that *multiple-system malformations* coexisted; that is, more than one organ system was involved. However, the trouble is that "multiple congenital anomalies" has no *specific* anatomic meaning. What does this category (see Table 14.13) *really* mean? Without further explanation, this category would remain a mystery. Table 14.8 presents the specific anatomic findings in these 15 patients. There was a marked female preponderance in this small series: males, 4 of 15 (26.7%), and females, 11 of 15 (73.3%); females to males = 11/4 = 2.75/1. All 4 male patients had congenital aortic valve stenosis (100%), and none had aortic valvar atresia. But 8 of 11 female patients had aortic valvar atresia (72.7%), and only 3 had congenital aortic valvar stenosis (27.3%) (Table 14.14). MCAs may involve only one other system, as in Case 9, who had a polycystic left kidney, or may include malformations of many other systems in addition to the cardiovascular system.

The cause of the MCAs may be at least partially understood, as in patients with a *chromosomal anomaly:* an anomaly involving the short arm of chromosome 5 (5p), as in **Case 42** (see Table 14.8), or the long arm of chromosome 6 (6 q+), as in **Case 105** (see Table 14.8).

MCAs can be associated with *known syndromes* such as Williams syndrome **(Case 166),** Turner syndrome **(Case 186),** or Albright syndrome **(Case 193)** (see Table 14.8). MCAs also can be associated with *familial congenital heart disease,* as in **Cases 178, 185,** and **192** (see Table 14.8). MCAs also may be associated with *familial MCAs,* as in **Case 193** (see Table 14.8). The cause of other cases of multiple anomalies remains largely unknown at the present time. Phenotypic similarities suggest that we are dealing with currently recognized syndromes: several recurrent themes are thought to be developmentally significant (see Table 14.14):

Urogenital dysgenesis (Cases 9, 105, 178, 185, 193, and 196);
Dysmorphic facies (Cases 14, 17, 42, 105, 116, 166, 185, 189, 192, and 193);
Cerebral malformation (Cases 42, 105, 185, 189); and
Congenitally dislocated hips (Cases 124 and 196).

These findings strongly suggest that *molecular genetic anomalies,* many of which remain to be elucidated, will prove to be of etiologic significance.

TABLE 14.13 **Findings Associated With Congenital Mitral Stenosis and the Hypoplastic**

Finding	No.	%
LEFT HEART SYNDROME (N = 130)		
1. Multiple congenital anomalies	15	11.5
2. Patent ductus arteriosus, closing	11	8.5
3. Intact atrial septum	9	6.9
3. Sinusoid(s) from LV cavity to coronary artery (arteries)	9	6.9
4. Familial congenital heart disease	6	4.6
5. Fusion of anterolateral and posteromedial papillary muscles	5	3.9
6. Parachute mitral valve with absent ALPM	4	3.1
7. Aortic atresia, valvar and subvalvar	3	2.3
7. Absence of left coronary-noncoronary commissure of AoV	3	2.3
8. Double-orifice mitral valve	2	1.5
8. LV myocardial dysplasia with diverticulum (or diverticula)	2	1.5
8. Prominent anterolateral muscle of the LV (muscle of Moulaert) contributing to muscular subaortic stenosis	2	1.5
8. No endocardial fibroelastosis of LV	2	1.5
8. Subaortic fibrous stenosis related to anterior leaflet of MV	2	1.5
8. Congenital MS with HLHS and VSD(s)	2	1.5
8. MV = normal miniature, that is, hypoplasia only	2	1.5
8. Shone syndrome variant	2	1.5
8. With incomplete form of CAVC	2	1.5
9. Double-inlet right ventricle	1	0.8
9. Brachiocephalic artery (bovine trunk)	1	0.8
9. Septum primum with leftward displacement superiorly	1	0.8
9. Abnormal pulmonary arterial histology (considered to be under estimate)	1	0.8
9. Left superior vena cava opening into LA, that is, unroofing of CoS (coronary sinus septal defect)	1	0.8
9. {AIS,L,I} and asplenia syndrome	1	0.8
9. With stenosis of individual pulmonary veins	1	0.8
9. Downward displacement of anterior leaflet of MV, resembling Ebstein-like anomaly of MV	1	0.8
9. Double-orifice tricuspid valve	1	0.8
9. Congenital unicuspid aortic valvar stenosis, the only well-formed commissure being the right coronary-noncoronary	1	0.8
9. Muscular bridge 1 mm above hypoplastic MV	1	0.8
9. Right-sided juxtaposition of the atrial appendages, with dextromalposition of the left atrial appendage	1	0.8
9. Left atrial appendage posterior to great arteries and pointing superiorly, ? forme fruste of right-sided JAA	1	0.8
9. Right aortic arch, without vascular ring	1	0.8
9. Right aortic arch, without vascular ring	1	0.8
9. Right aortic arch, with vascular ring	1	0.8
9. Insertion of mitral chordae tendineae into LV endocardium, with no papillary muscles	1	0.8
9. With severe valvar pulmonary stenosis, aortic valvar atresia, and severe MS	1	0.8

{AIS,L,I}, The segmental anatomic set of visceroatrial situs ambiguus (A) with predominantly situs inversus (I) of the abdominal viscera with a left-sided inferior vena cava, that switched from left to right at the level of the liver and drained into the right-sided right atrium in atrial situs solitus (S), with discordant L-loop (inverted) ventricles (L), and with inverted normally related great arteries (I); *ALPM,* anterolateral papillary muscle; *AoV,* aortic valve; *CAVC,* common atrioventricular canal; *CoS,* coronary sinus; *HLHS,* hypoplastic left heart syndrome; *JAA,* juxtaposition of the atrial appendages; *LA,* morphologically left atrium; *LV,* morphologically left ventricle; *mm,* millimeter; *MS,* mitral stenosis; *MV,* mitral valve; *No.,* number; *VSD(s),* ventricular septal defect(s).

In addition to MCAs, the other important findings associated with congenital mitral stenosis and HLHS that are presented in Table 14.13 are much more self-explanatory:

A closing PDA (observed in 11/130 autopsied cases, or 8.5%) is a very important and probably underobserved finding. A large but functionally closing PDA is thought to be one of the major immediate causes of death in HLHS. When aortic valvar atresia or severe aortic valvar stenosis coexists, a large and widely patent ductus arteriosus is essentially the only pathway from the heart to the systemic circulation, including the coronary arteries. Significant constriction of the ductus arteriosus not only reduces the flow of blood to the body (Qs), it also deleteriously increases the blood flow to the lungs (Qp) via the left and right pulmonary artery

TABLE 14.14 Multiple Congenital Anomalies in Patients With Congenital Mitral Stenosis and the Hypoplastic Left Heart Syndrome (n = 15)

Case No. (Autopsy No.)	Gender (AoVAt or St)	Findings
Case 9 (A83-142)	F AoVAt	Lt polycystic kidney.
Case 14 (A79-41)	F AoVSt	Single palmar crease (rt-sided), hypertelorism, micrognathia, low-set ears, Meckel diverticulum.
Case 17 (A78-2)	F AoVAt	Low-set ears, short neck, flection contractures (upper and lower extremities), overriding third toes bilateral, bicornuate uterus, accessory lobation of lungs, kidneys, and liver.
Case 42 (A86-116)	F AoVAt	None recorded.
Case 105 (A90-60)	M AoV St	Chromosomal anomaly: extra chromosomal material on long arm of chromosome 6 (6 q+) (?duplication, or unbalanced translocation); dysmorphic features: flat head; hypertelorism; absent eyelashes, upper and lower; ears small and low-set; broad nose; small chin; contractures of hips and knees; deep sacral dimple; partial absence of corpus callosum; pelvic horseshoe kidney; maternal grandmother exposed to diethylstilbestrol (DES).
Case 116 (A85-197)	F AoVAt	Dysmorphic facies.
Case 124 (C83-248)	M AoVSt	Bilateral hip dislocations; pulmonary hypoplasia, bilateral, both unilobed (no fissures).
Case 166 (A93-4)	M AoVSt	Williams syndrome with diffuse thickening of the ascending aorta (2.5–3.0 mm thick) and brachiocephalic arteries; diffuse thickening of pulmonary arterial tree (MPA = 3–5 mm thick); bilaterally trilobed lungs.
Case 178 (A89-117)	F AoVAt	Familial congenital heart disease: mother and maternal aunt with situs inversus and dextrocardia. This patient: imperforate anus with cloaca.
Case 185 (A94-28)	F AoVAt	Familial congenital heart disease; older sister (A92-80) with normal karyotype, renal dysgenesis, anophthalmia, absence of left lung, and tetralogy of Fallot. {S,D,S} with pulmonary outflow tract atresia. This patient: bilateral anophthalmia, bilateral unilobed lungs, left superior vena cava to coronary sinus to right atrium with absence of left innominate vein, crossed pulmonary artery branches with RPA ostium (2–3 mm) beneath and somewhat to the left of the LPA ostium (1.5–2 mm) and with LPA ostium above and somewhat to the right of the RPA ostium.
Case 186 (A94-19)	F AoVAt	Turner syndrome 45X0; prematurity, 35 weeks gestation, birthweight 2.2 kg (4.85 lb).
Case 189 (A93-88)	F AoVAt	Dysmorphic facies with micrognathia, microcephaly, small ears (left smaller than right) and hyperfolded helix, mild midface hypoplasia, flat nasal bridge, small anterior fontanelle (1.5 × 3.0 cm), para-anal dimple, hairy patch at base of spine.
Case 192 (A93-53)	F AoVSt	Familial congenital heart disease: brother with bicuspid aortic valve and unusual facies. This patient: macroglossia, similar facies, small height and weight, abnormal lobation of the lungs bilaterally (right and left lingual middle lobes consist of several small lobules).
Case 193 (A93-42)	M AoVSt	Familial multiple congenital anomalies: mother with Albright-McCune-Sternburg syndrome, that is; asymmetrical disease of the bones (osteitis fibrosa cystica) with melanotic pigmentation of the skin and sexual precocity in females. This patient: dysmorphic facial features with low-set ears, epicanthal folds, flat nasal bridge, hypothyroidism, and renal dysfunction (elevated BUN + creatinine).
Case 196 (A96-11)	F AoVSt	Renal dysplasia, bilateral, severe; bilaterally dislocated hips; severe stenosis of origins of left anterior and left middle cerebral arteries.

AoVAt, Aortic valve atresia; *AoVSt,* aortic valve stenosis; *BUN,* blood urea nitrogen; *F,* female; *Lt,* left; *LPA,* left pulmonary artery; *M,* male; *MPA,* main pulmonary artery; *RPA,* right pulmonary artery; *{S,D,S},* the set of visceroatrial situs solitus (S), concordant D-loop ventricles (D), and solitus normally related great arteries (S), that is, normal segmental anatomy; *Rt,* right.

branches. Instead of being normally approximately equal per unit of time, the Qs and the Qp become reciprocals of each other because of ductal constriction. As the Qs decreases, the Qp tends to increase. The femoral pulses disappear, the lungs become more congested, and the liver edge descends into the right upper quadrant of the abdomen. When the ductus arteriosus relaxes and opens, these changes reverse. The femoral pulses return, the lungs become less congested, and the liver edge ascends out of the right upper abdominal quadrant. With constriction of the ductus arteriosus, the increased Qp becomes deleterious because the blood has difficulty exiting the left heart because of the coexistence of congenital mitral stenosis; a typically intact ventricular septum; aortic valvar atresia or severe congenital aortic valvar stenosis; a thick-walled, small-chambered, and uncompliant LV typically with left ventricular EFE; and an atrial septum that is often restrictive to left-to-right atrial shunting, or that can be intact. Hence, ductal narrowing can lead to pulmonary congestion, edema, and hemorrhage. Thus, normal closure or marked narrowing of the PDA in HLHS is a hemodynamic catastrophe, leading typically to early postnatal death.

An intact atrial septum, observed in 9 of 130 patients (6.9%; see Table 14.7) also contributes to early death in HLHS by preventing the physiologically essential left-to-right shunting at the atrial level, as mentioned earlier.

One or more sinusoids were found between the left ventricular cavity and the coronary arterial system in 8 of these 130 patients (6.2%; see Table 14.13).

First, what is a *sinusoid*? A sinusoid is defined as resembling a sinus. More specifically, a *sinusoid* is a form of terminal blood channel consisting of a large, irregular anastomosing vessel with a reticuloendothelial lining, but with little or no adventitia. Sinusoids are found in the liver, adrenal glands, heart, parathyroid, carotid gland, spleen, and pancreas. *Sinus* (Latin) means a bending, curve, fold, or hollow. *Eidos* (Greek) means "form."[103] In medical usage, *sinus* usually denotes a hollow space. A *sinusoid* typically denotes a fistula-like communication that is not interrupted by capillaries.

In **Case 25** (A90-59), a boy who died at 1 day of age with aortic valvar atresia, sinusoids were found at the left ventricular apex that communicated with the left anterior descending coronary artery. Angiocardiography revealed *retrograde* blood flow from the left anterior descending coronary artery into the aortic root. The proximal coronary sinus and the coronary sinus ostium both were enlarged, indicating increased blood flow that was made possible by the sinusoidal communication between the left ventricular cavity and the left anterior descending coronary artery.

Case 69 (A89-80), a 19-day-old boy with aortic valvar atresia, also was found to have a fistula between the left ventricular cavity and the left anterior descending coronary artery.

Case 98 (A89-98), a 17-day-old boy with aortic valvar atresia and a parachute mitral valve, had *multiple sinusoids* connecting the left ventricular cavity with epicardial coronary arteries demonstrated best by angiocardiography and two-dimensional echocardiography.

Case 132 (A89-76) was a 26-hour-old girl with congenital aortic valvar stenosis and congenital mitral stenosis who had a sinusoid between the left ventricular cavity and the posterior descending coronary artery. The left anterior descending coronary artery was tortuous and rope-like, with a relatively thick wall and narrowed lumen. As this case suggests, sinusoids can be associated with *significant congenital coronary arteriopathy*. The hypothesis is that suprasystemic left ventricular intracavitary pressure can be conveyed to the coronary arterial system via one or more sinusoids, resulting in "jet lesions" of the walls of the coronary arterial system, leading to coronary arterial mural thickening and luminal narrowing or occlusion.

Case 167 (A92-102), a 23-day-old girl, had aortic valvar atresia and congenital mitral stenosis with severe left ventricular EFE and diminutive anterolateral and posteromedial papillary muscles. She also had two sinusoids between the left ventricular cavity and the left circumflex coronary artery. Thus, sinusoids can connect between the left ventricular cavity and any nearby coronary artery: the anterior descending, the posterior descending, the left circumflex, or the obtuse marginal epicardial branches.

Case 184 (A94-39), a 3-day-old girl, had aortic valvar atresia, severe congenital mitral stenosis (2 mm opening), and a sinusoid between the left ventricular cavity with severe EFE and the left circumflex coronary artery.

Case 185 (A94-28), a 2-hour-old girl with aortic valvar atresia, extreme congenital mitral stenosis (opening less than 1 mm), and MCAs (bilateral anophthalmia), had a large sinusoid (1.3 mm in diameter) between the left ventricular cavity and a diagonal branch (or obtuse marginal branch) of the left coronary artery. Case 185 also exemplified familial congenital heart disease (TOF {S,D,S} with pulmonary outflow tract atresia).

Case 189 (A93-88), a 12-day-old girl with aortic valvar atresia, congenital mitral stenosis with double-orifice mitral valve (DOMV), and MCAs was found to have a left anterior descending coronary artery that was unusually prominent and thick-walled. A sinusoid connected the left ventricular cavity at the apex with this thick-walled and narrow-lumened coronary artery.

Case 202 (S95-4007A) consisted of an explanted heart specimen after orthotopic cardiac transplantation in a 17-day-old girl. The native heart specimen had aortic valvar atresia and marked congenital mitral stenosis (1.5 mm opening). A large sinusoid between the left ventricular cavity and the proximal left anterior descending coronary artery resulted in retrograde coronary arterial blood flow and in antegrade aortic blood flow. The ascending aorta was larger than is usually seen with aortic valvar atresia.

Familial congenital heart disease was found in 6 of these 130 patients with congenital mitral stenosis and HLHS (4.6%; see Table 14.13).

Case 15 (C89-247) was a boy whose gestation was terminated at 22 weeks by an elective abortion. This patient had aortic valvar atresia, extreme congenital mitral stenosis, and EFE of the LV. His older brother also had HLHS with hypoplasia of the mitral valve, LV, aortic valve, and aortic arch. He also had multiple VSDs and a secundum ASD. His older brother died at 5 months of age from sepsis after multiple operations. Our patient also had a living half-sister (the same mother but a different father) who was born with gastroschisis, that is, a congenital fissure of the anterior abdominal wall, not involving insertion of the umbilical cord, through which small bowel and a portion of large bowel protruded. The half-sister's heart was normal. Thus, Case 15 exemplifies familial congenital heart disease (familial HLHS) and familial malformation involving a different organ system—the anterior abdominal wall. It has been said, only partly in jest, that the genes are not good pathologists, meaning that the same pathologic type of congenital heart disease seldom recurs in identical twins and in familial congenital heart disease. But Case 15 is an exception to that generalization: When both parents were the same, both children had HLHS.

Case 80 (A88-15), a 3-day-old boy, seems to emphasize the aforementioned point. Our patient had aortic valvar atresia and severe congenital mitral stenosis. The mother had congenital aortic stenosis with a bicuspid aortic valve. From a developmental and etiologic perspective, this mother's congenital heart disease may be related to that of her son, Case 80.

Case 178 (A89117) a 3-day-old girl, again illustrates the adage that the genes are not necessarily good pathologists. Case 178 had MCAs (an imperforate anus and cloaca) with aortic valvar atresia and severe congenital mitral stenosis (3-mm opening). But our patient's mother and her maternal aunt both had situs inversus and dextrocardia, which are anatomically very different anomalies.

Case 185 (A94-28) was a 2-hour-old girl with aortic valvar atresia, extreme congenital mitral stenosis (<1 mm opening), no tensor apparatus (no papillary muscles and no chordae tendineae), a large sinusoid (1.3 mm in diameter) between the left ventricular cavity and a diagonal branch of the left coronary artery, a thick-walled and small-chambered LV *without* EFE, and preductal coarctation of the aorta (2.5 mm in internal diameter). She also had MCAs: bilateral anophthalmia. Our patient (Case 185) had an older sister who died at 7 hours of age. An autopsy performed at Boston Children's Hospital (A92-80) revealed that she too had MCAs consisting of bilateral anophthalmia, renal dysgenesis, and absence of the left lung, with a normal karyotype. This older sister also had congenital heart disease: TOF {S,D,S} with pulmonary outflow tract atresia. Consequently, the family of Case 185 displayed *familial MCAs and familial congenital heart disease.* These two patients are thought to constitute **a newly recognized syndrome** characterized by familial MCAs, including anophthalmia and familial congenital heart disease.

Case 192 was an 8 5/12-year-old girl with aortic annular stenosis and fibrous subaortic stenosis (2 to 4 mm in internal diameter in the fresh state). The aortic valve leaflets were normal. Congenital mitral stenosis with thickened and myxomatous leaflets were present, with failure of formation of the interchordal spaces. The papillary muscles were very small. Tricuspid regurgitation was also present, with thickening and rolling of the free margins of the anterior and septal leaflets. This patient also had MCAs: macroglossia, unusual facies, and small height and weight. Case 192 also had a brother with similar dysmorphic facies and with congenital heart disease consisting of a bicuspid aortic valve. Thus, Case 192 is another example of *familial MC and familial congenital heart disease.*

Case 207 (S94-4270) was the explanted native heart specimen after orthotopic cardiac transplantation of a 1-year-old boy with congenital aortic valve stenosis that was severe, unicuspid, and unicommisural. The LC/NC commissure was the only commissure present. The aortic leaflet tissue was very thickened and domed. Severe congenital mitral stenosis was present with thick myxomatous leaflets, two hypoplastic papillary muscles, and EFE of the LV. This boy's father had a VSD. Hence, *familial congenital heart disease* was present.

Other Categories Presented in Table 14.13

In the interests of brevity, it is hoped that the other entries in Table 14.13 will be clear with little or no additional explanation.

Fusion of the anterolateral and posteromedial papillary muscles of the LV may be regarded as a forme fruste of Shone syndrome[98] (5/130 cases, 3.9%; see Table 14.7). With a divided AV canal (as opposed to a common AV canal), when a parachute mitral valve is present, typically it is the anterolateral papillary muscle group that is absent, with only the posteromedial papillary muscle group being present, as in 4 of these 130 patients (3.1%; see Table 14.7).

When the AV canal is in common (undivided), often the reverse situation pertains: The posteromedial papillary muscle group is absent, and only the anterolateral group is present.[99] This is important because surgical division of the common AV canal results in a potentially parachute mitral valve,[99] in which it is often wise not to suture closed the cleft, so as not to increase the mitral stenosis postoperatively. *Potentially* parachute mitral valve means that parachute mitral valve is present only postoperatively because no mitral valve is present preoperatively when the AV valve is in common (undivided).

In HLHS with aortic valvar atresia, is it the aortic valve only that is atretic? Occasionally, there also can be fibrous *subaortic atresia,* as in 3 of these patients (2.3%; see Table 14.7). Why is this noteworthy? Because fibrous subaortic obstruction, typically *stenosis,* appears to be produced by fibrous tissue of the AV canal that also forms the anterior leaflet of the mitral valve.[28] These 3 cases also suggest that fibrous tissue of the endocardial cushions of the AV canal can also contribute to or cause *fibrous subaortic atresia.*

Absence of the LC/NC commissure of the aortic valve is also noteworthy. Why? Because, as noted previously, this is the only commissure that almost always is present in unicuspid and unicommissural aortic valves with congenital aortic valvar stenosis.[28] Why is the LC/NC commissure almost always present in unicommissural aortic valvar stenosis—the worst form of congenital aortic valvar stenosis? The answer is unknown at the present time. But finding the LC/NC commissure to be absent is a rare anomaly (3/130 cases, 2.3%; see Table 14.13). When the LC/NC commissure of the aortic valve was absent, which commissure(s) was (were) present? In two patients (Cases 103 and 195), the congenitally stenotic aortic valve was bicuspid and bicommissural: the RC/LC and the RC/NC commissures were both present. In one patient (Case 107), only the RC/NC commissure was present, the congenitally stenotic aortic valve being unicommisural and hence unicuspid.

DOMV[104] can be associated with congenital mitral stenosis, as in 2 of these patients (1.5%; see Table 14.13). Case 107 (A82-124), a 21-day-old girl, had congenital mitral stenosis with hypoplasia of the mitral valve and DOMV. There was a thin tongue of mitral valvar tissue between the anterior and posterior leaflets holding the anterior leaflet in approximately the closed position and dividing the mitral opening into a somewhat larger anterolateral orifice (6 mm in internal dimension) and a somewhat smaller posteromedial orifice (3.5 mm in internal dimension). There were also multiple small blood cysts of the mitral valve. The congenital aortic valvar stenosis was unicuspid and unicommissural, the only well-formed commissure being the *RC/NC,* which is a rare finding, as mentioned earlier. The LV was moderately hypoplastic, a large nonrestrictive secundum ASD was present, and a large PDA was closing. Thus, this patient had a rare form of congenital mitral stenosis with DOMV and an uncommon form of unicommissural congenital aortic valvar stenosis, with only the RC/NC commissure being well formed.

The other patient with DOMV,[104] Case 189 (A93-88), was a 12-day-old girl with aortic valvar atresia and very severe congenital mitral stenosis. The anterolateral orifice was smaller than the posteromedial. This infant had MCAs consisting of dysmorphic facies with micrognathia, microcephaly, small ears (left smaller than right) with hyperfolded helix, mild midfacial hypoplasia, flat nasal bridge, small anterior fontanelle (1.5 × 3.0 cm), para-anal dimple, and hairy patch at the base of the spine.

Congenital mitral stenosis with DOMV[104] is an anatomic type of congenital mitral stenosis that we had not encountered in our earlier study (1978) of 49 autopsied cases.[97] However, in a later study (1988) of 27 autopsied cases of DOMV,[104] we found that 26% (7 cases) had congenital mitral stenosis. To complete the picture, another 26% (7 cases) of DOMV had *congenital mitral regurgitation,* and in the remaining 48% (13 cases), the mitral valve was functionally normal, despite the presence of DOMV.

Left Ventricular Myocardial Dysplasia With Diverticulum or Diverticula

Left ventricular myocardial dysplasia with a diverticulum or diverticula was found in 2 of these patients (1.5%; see Table 14.13) with congenital mitral stenosis and HLHS. **Case 105** (A90-60) was a 3-month-and-24-day old male infant with severe congenital mitral stenosis with thickened leaflets and multiple hypertrophied papillary muscles. The left ventricular free wall was dysmorphic: a diverticulum-like structure was present. There was left ventricular endocardial sclerosis, and left atrial hypertrophy and enlargement were massive. Congenital aortic valvar stenosis was severe with a small annulus, thickened aortic leaflets, and a bicuspid bicommissural aortic valve with a rudimentary RC/LC commissure. This patient had a chromosomal anomaly with extra chromosomal material on the long arm of chromosome 6 (6q+). Whether this finding represented a duplication or an unbalanced translocation remained uncertain. This patient also had MCAs: flat head, hypertelorism, absent eyelashes (upper and lower), small and low-set ears, broad nose, small chin, contractures of hips and knees, deep sacral dimple, partial absence of corpus callosum, and a pelvic horseshoe kidney.

The other patient with left ventricular dysplasia was **Case 151** (A67-6), a 2-day-old boy with severe congenital aortic valvar stenosis (1 mm opening) and congenital mitral stenosis with marked hypoplasia. The ascending aorta, aortic arch, and aortic isthmus were also markedly hypoplastic. There was focal failure of muscularization of the left ventricular free wall, and two large muscular VSDs were also present. Thus, myocardial dysplasia involving deficiency and absence involved both the left ventricular free wall and the left ventricular component of the interventricular septum.

Left ventricular dysplasia was another anomaly that we did not encounter in our 1978 study of congenital mitral stenosis.[97] It was not until 2001 that we did a detailed study of congenital left ventricular aneurysm with Dr John Papagiannis et al[105] (Fig. 14.31).

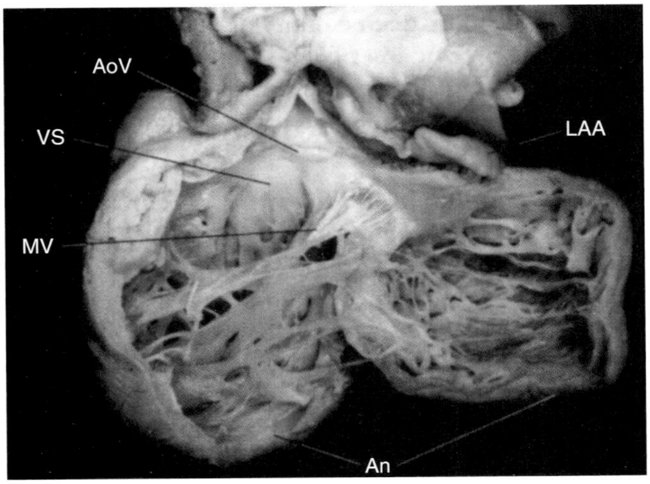

Fig. 14.31 This is the opened left ventricle of a 23-week-old male fetus with trisomy 13. Pregnancy was interrupted. Note **the large congenital aneurysm *(An)* of the left ventricular free wall,** which is thin and lined with dysplastic fibromuscular trabeculations. There are no well-formed papillary muscles of the mitral valve *(MV).* Fibromuscular strands run from the mitral leaflets into the aneurysm. The ventricular septum *(VS)* shows endocardial fibroelastosis. The aortic valve *(AoV)* is normally formed. *LAA,* Left atrial appendage. (Reproduced with permission from Papagiannis J, Van Praagh R, Schwint O, et al. Congenital left ventricular aneurysm: Clinical, imaging, pathologic, and surgical findings in severe new cases. *Am Heart J.* 2001;141:491.)

Prominent Anterolateral Muscle of the Left Ventricle (Muscle of Moulaert)

Also mentioned above concerning Case 6 (A91-52), a prominent anterolateral muscle of the LV is an abnormality of left ventricular myocardial architecture. Confluent with or close to the anterolateral papillary muscle, the abnormal anterolateral muscle extends upward toward the exiting semilunar valve, normally toward the aortic valve. It is as though the aortic valve needs a subjacent papillary muscle, just as the mitral valve does.

This abnormality of left ventricular myocardial free wall architecture can have two deleterious effects. It can crowd the nearby mitral valve, resulting in a diminutive mitral valve that may have thin and delicate leaflets (as in Case 6, mentioned previously, a 17-day-old boy).

A muscle of Moulaert also can contribute to muscular left ventricular free wall obstruction (as in both Case 6 and Case 103). The latter was an 11 1/2-month-old boy. These 2 cases constituted 1.5% of our patients with congenital mitral stenosis and HLHS (see Table 14.13). In Case 103, the mitral valve was hypoplastic and the interpapillary muscle distance between the anterolateral and the posteromedial papillary muscles was reduced.

In Case 103, the muscular subaortic stenosis resulted from a localized protrusion of the ventricular septum into the left ventricular outflow tract medially, plus a prominent muscle of Moulaert that narrowed the left ventricular outflow tract laterally.

When Is There No Left Ventricular EFE in HLHS? When the congenital mitral stenosis is extreme (nearly atresia), there may be no left ventricular EFE. This is one answer, as in **Case 111** (A80-88), a 2-month-old boy with aortic valve atresia with extremely severe congenital mitral stenosis: the mitral orifice consisted of only two pin-hole openings.

Another possibility is when the congenital aortic valve stenosis is only moderately severe, as in **Case 168** (A89-103), a 10-day-old boy. The moderately severe congenital aortic valvar stenosis consisted of a bicuspid and bicommissural aortic valve: the septal (RC/LC) commissure was very underdeveloped. Moderate congenital aortic valvar stenosis was associated with quite severe congenital mitral stenosis; the papillary muscles were fused at their bases (a forme fruste of parachute mitral valve), and the interchordal spaces were not formed.

We think that if, for whatever reason, the left ventricular intracavitary pressure does not remain above the coronary arterial perfusion pressure in diastole, subendocardial myocardial oxygenation can occur, preventing so-called **EFE, which we think is an extensive subendocardial myocardial ischemic necrosis.** The fibroelastic endomysium and perimysium persist, after their more oxygen-dependent "residents"—the cardiac myocytes—have died, creating the gross and histologic picture of EFE. However, the *absence* of EFE in HLHS is rare (2 of 130 Cases, or 1.5%; see Table 14.7); the *presence* of EFE with aortic valvar atresia or severe stenosis and congenital mitral stenosis is certainly the rule (128 or 130 patients, 98.5%).

What is the morphogenetic cause of fibrous subaortic stenosis? We think that the answer is fibroelastic tissue of the endocardial cushions of the AV canal. Why? Because one can see fibrous tissue extending from the anterior leaflet of the mitral valve over onto the ventricular septum beneath the aortic valve, as in 2 of these 130 patients (1.5%; see Table 14.13).

More specifically, **Case 65** (A93-28), a 22-day-old boy, had congenital mitral stenosis and congenital mitral regurgitation with marked myxomatous thickening of both the anterior and the posterior mitral leaflets. Almost all of the interchordal spaces were obliterated by fibrous tissue, and there was moderate reduction of the interpapillary muscle distance. *The thick myxomatous anterior mitral leaflet filled up much of the subaortic space, causing fibrous left ventricular outflow tract stenosis.* Congenital aortic valvar stenosis was caused by a unicuspid, unicommissural valve, the LC/NC commissure being the only well-developed commissure.

Case 188 (C94-32), a 21-week-gestation female fetus, had congenital mitral stenosis with absence of interchordal spaces and papillary muscles that were very close together. There was fibrous subaortic stenosis, and congenital aortic valvar stenosis with a bicommissural aortic valve.

CONGENITAL MITRAL STENOSIS WITH HYPOPLASTIC LEFT HEART SYNDROME AND VENTRICULAR SEPTAL DEFECT(S)

Congenital mitral stenosis with HLHS almost always has an intact ventricular septum. But 2 of these 130 patients (1.5%) had one or more VSDs, with normal segmental anatomy, that is, {S,D,S}.

Case 164 (A93-36), a 4-day-old boy, had congenital mitral stenosis with moderate valvar hypoplasia, and aortic valvar atresia. A small membranous (or conoventricular) type of VSD was found. The LV was larger than that usually seen with aortic valve atresia, and EFE of the LV was *not* present. We thought that both of these features may well have been related to the presence of a VSD, which permitted the LV to do some antegrade flow work (hence, the larger-than-usual left ventricular cavity size) and to decompress itself during diastole (hence, no EFE).

Case 208 (A94-68 and S94-4549) was a 3-month-old boy with aortic valvar atresia {S,D,S}, HLHS, and **double-inlet right ventricle (DIRV).** The mitral valve opened only into the RV and did not straddle into the LV. The tricuspid valve was thickened and enlarged (22 by 15 mm, internal dimension), with congenital tricuspid regurgitation (echocardiography). There was congenital mitral stenosis (5 mm in diameter) with crowding of the submitral area.

Multiple VSDs were present: a high, small, conoventricular (membranous) VSD, 2 mm (2-mm internal dimension), and a VSD of the AV canal type (4 mm in internal dimension). A LSVC drained into the coronary sinus and hence into the RA; the left innominate vein was absent. An aberrant right subclavian artery, with a left aortic arch, was also present. The LV was small-chambered, but *not* thick-walled (5 to 7 mm in thickness). Right ventricular hypertrophy and enlargement were marked (9 to 11 mm in thickness). At 3 months of age, an orthotopic cardiac transplantation was performed; death occurred 5 days postoperatively.

What Is Congenital Mitral Stenosis?

As we have already seen, congenital mitral stenosis may involve an anomaly of the inlet to the mitral canal, that is, a supramitral stenosing ring (see Fig. 14.28), thickened and myxomatous mitral valve leaflets with failure of formation of the interchordal spaces (see Figs. 4.25 and 14.26), reduction of the interpapillary muscle distance (see Fig. 14.26), and absence of a papillary muscle group, typically absence of the anterolateral papillary muscle group (see Fig. 14.27). These four anatomic types of congenital mitral stenosis are shown diagrammatically in Fig. 14.29.

But is it possible for congenital mitral stenosis to have an intrinsically **normally formed, but miniature mitral valve** with thin, delicate leaflets, well-formed interchordal spaces, and two papillary muscle groups? Yes, but infrequently: 2 of 130 patients (1.5%; see Table 14.13).

Case 82 (A69-168), a 42-hour-old boy, had aortic valvar atresia, intact ventricular septum, a small-chambered and thick-walled LV with severe EFE. The mitral valve was markedly hypoplastic, but otherwise normal—a normal miniature. This patient had a right aortic arch (without a vascular ring) and a large left-sided PDA that was closing—the latter being the immediate cause of death.

Case 92 (A58-262) was a 5-day-old girl with valvar aortic atresia, intact ventricular septum, EFE of the LV, and hypoplasia of the mitral valve. Conventionally, such mitral valvar hypoplasia is regarded as *functional mitral stenosis.* But as noted previously, from a hemodynamic standpoint, this situation is more like *functional mitral atresia,* with a patent but hypoplastic mitral valve. Why? Because with aortic valvar atresia, an intact ventricular septum, and no sinusoidal communication between the left ventricular cavity and the coronary arteries, there can be little or no anterograde flow of blood across the mitral valve. So, this is congenital mitral "stenosis" with a wink. More accurately, this is *congenital mitral hypoplasia.*

The larger point is that mitral *stenosis* and mitral *regurgitation* are both basically *hemodynamic,* not anatomic, concepts. This is why there are various "anatomic types" of congenital mitral stenosis (see Figs 14.24 to 14.29), that is, anatomically different anomalies that can obstruct blood flow across the *mitral canal—at the inlet, and/or middle, and/or outlet.*

Shone Syndrome Variants

Shone syndrome[98] consists of supramitral stenosing ring, parachute mitral valve, fibrous subaortic stenosis, and preductal coarctation of the aorta. Neither of our 2 patients had all features of Shone syndrome; hence, we refer to them as Shone syndrome variants. However, both had *multilevel* left ventricular obstruction.

Case 190 (S93-3855 and A93-80) was a 3½-year-old boy with congenital mitral stenosis (but without supramitral stenosing ring and without parachute mitral valve). Severe, discrete, fibrous subaortic stenosis was present. So too was congenital aortic valve stenosis with a small annulus, myxomatous leaflets, and a unicuspid valve—the only well-formed commissure being the LC/NC. (Aortic valvar stenosis was not part of Shone syndrome[98] as originally described.) The LV was thick-walled and small-chambered, with severe EFE. No preductal coarctation of the aorta was present in this patient. (However, preductal coarctation is part of Shone syndrome.[98])

Shone syndrome[98] had *four* levels of left ventricular inflow and outflow tract obstruction: supramitral ring, parachute mitral valve, fibrous subaortic stenosis, and preductal coarctation of the aorta. Case 190 had *three* sites of left ventricular obstruction: congenital mitral stenosis, subaortic fibrous stenosis, and congenital unicuspid aortic valvar stenosis. From a pathophysiologic point of view, the uncompliant, thick-walled, small-chambered LV with EFE also may be viewed as a fourth level of systemic ventricular obstruction. So, Case 190 certainly had multilevel left ventricular obstruction, even if the sites of obstruction were not identical to those originally reported by Shone et al.[98]

Case 195 (C93-60) was a 10-month-old female patient with supramitral stenosing ring, congenital mitral stenosis with two partly fused papillary muscles, a tunnel type of fibrous left ventricular outflow tract stenosis, and congenital bicuspid aortic valvar stenosis. *The LC/NC commissure was absent, a rare finding.* Coarctation of the aorta was not present. Other findings included a persistent LSVC to coronary sinus to RA, a secundum type of ASD, a PDA , and a left aortic arch with an aberrant right subclavian artery. Thus, Case 195 had four levels of left ventricular obstruction, two at the left ventricular inlet (the supramitral stenosing ring and the congenital mitral stenosis) and two at the left ventricular outlet (fibrous subaortic stenosis and congenital aortic valvar stenosis).

In summary, Shone syndrome variants with multilevel left ventricular obstruction were found in 2 of these 130 patients (1.5%; see Table 14.13) with congenital mitral stenosis and HLHS.

The incomplete form of common AV canal occurred in 2 of these patients (1.5%; see Table 14.7). **Case 134** (A65-276) was a 60-hour-old girl with an ostium primum type of AV septal defect, no VSD of the AV canal type, no cleft in the anterior mitral leaflet, and extreme congenital mitral stenosis with a very marked congenital aortic valve stenosis. Left ventricular hypoplasia was marked. There were hypertrophy and enlargement of the LA, RA, and RV. The PDA was large, but closing.

The other patient with congenital mitral stenosis with incompletely common AV canal, **Case 138**, had the asplenia syndrome and is presented in detail here.

A number of findings occurred in only 1 patient in this series (0.8%; see Table 14.7):

DIRV. Case 208 (S94-4549 and A94-68) was a 3-month-old boy with DIRV. The segmental anatomy was normal {S,D,S}. The LV was not absent; that is, single RV was not present. Instead, the LV was very small-chambered and posterior. But it was not thick-walled (5 to 7 mm thick) and EFE was not present. The mitral valve did not straddle into the LV, even though a small VSD of the AV canal type coexisted. A high small (2 mm in internal dimension) conoventricular type of VSD was also present. Congenital mitral stenosis was present, the internal maximal dimension being only 5 mm, and there was crowding of the submitral area. The tricuspid valve was thickened and enlarged (22- × 15-mm internal dimensions). Echocardiography revealed that congenital tricuspid regurgitation was present. Aortic valvar atresia was found. So here we have *a rare anatomic type of HLHS* with {S,D,S} segmental anatomy, aortic valve atresia, DIRV with congenital mitral stenosis (hypoplasia and submitral crowding), and congenital tricuspid regurgitation, multiple VSDs, and no left ventricular EFE. Right ventricular hypertrophy and enlargement were marked, the right ventricular free wall (right ventricular free wall) being 9 to 11 mm thick.

A brachiocephalic artery, also known as a bovine trunk was found in 1 patient (0.8%; see Table 14.7). **Case 204** (A95-10) was a 4-day-old girl with severe congenital mitral stenosis and aortic valve atresia. Only two arteries originated from the aortic arch, the brachiocephalic artery (bovine trunk) and the left vertebral artery. The brachiocephalic artery gave origin to all of the major aortic arch branches: right subclavian, right common carotid, left common carotid, and left subclavian arteries.

Leftward deviation of septum primum. To my knowledge, Dr. Paul Weinberg was the first (ca 1976) to focus on this finding that can be associated with HLHS. The septum primum arises normally and caudally is confluent with the left wall of the IVC. But then as it extends superiorly or cephalad, the septum primum deviates leftward, into the left atrial cavity. Then, as Drs. Stella Van Praagh, Stephen Sanders et al[29] showed in 1995, the superior margin of the septum primum can lie to the left of the right pulmonary veins, resulting in partially anomalous pulmonary venous *drainage,* even though all of the pulmonary veins are normally *connected* with the LA. And the superior portion of septum primum can even lie to the left of the left pulmonary veins (in visceroarterial situs solitus), resulting in totally anomalous pulmonary venous drainage, even though all of the pulmonary veins are connected normally with the LA.[29]

If associated with HLHS, as in Case 189 (A93-88)—a 12-day-old girl with congenital mitral stenosis with DOMV, aortic valvar atresia, and MCAs—leftward deviation of the septum primum superiorly would help prevent the atrial septum from becoming restrictive or highly obstructive to left-to-right atrial shunting. Hence, leftward deviation of the septum primum may be hemodynamically beneficial in HLHS. When the septum primum is deviated to the left, it is surprisingly *firm* and *difficult to move.* When leftwardly deviated superiorly, the septum primum tends to stay in this "open" position: open to the right atrial–to–left atrial blood flow of the normal prenatal *via sinistra* and also open to shunting in the opposite direction from LA to RA.

When leftward deviation of the septum primum is extreme, it can lie approximately horizontally, above but close to the mitral orifice. In this situation, the markedly leftward deviated septum primum constitutes *a rare form of congenital supramitral stenosis.*

Abnormal pulmonary arterial histology was described by Dr. Marlene Rabinovitch in one of our patients with congenital mitral stenosis, congenital aortic stenosis, and a thick-walled and small-chambered LV with severe EFE. **Case 172** (A77-10) was a 25-hour-old boy. Dr. Marlene Rabinovitch became an expert in pulmonary histologic morphometry under the guidance of Professor Lynne M. Reid. Dr. Rabinovitch's conclusion was that abnormal extension of muscle with increased wall thickness of small peripheral pulmonary arteries is seen with severe congenital mitral stenosis or mitral atresia, and with severe congenital aortic stenosis or aortic valvar atresia within the first few days of postnatal life. These pulmonary histologic changes that were found with HLHS in this patient who died after only 1 day of postnatal life, seem clearly to have been congenital, that is, present at, and before, the time of birth, unroofing of the coronary sinus.[20]

When a persistent LSVC connects with the coronary sinus, this systemic venous blood stream does not always flow into the RA, not if the coronary sinus is unroofed. In this case, the blood may flow, as least in part, into the LA. Unroofing of the coronary sinus is also known as a **coronary sinus septal defect.** When such a defect is present, there is absence not only of the anterior (ventral) wall of the coronary sinus, but also of the posterior (dorsal) wall of the adjacent LA. Thus, the so-called coronary sinus septum consists of two different walls, not just one.[20]

Case 145 (A83-33) was a 6-day-old boy with congenital mitral stenosis, aortic valvar atresia, an intact ventricular septum, and a LV that was thick-walled and small-chambered with severe EFE, a typical case of HLHS except that the LSVC drained into the LA.

At that time (1983), everyone was very impressed by the patient's clinical improvement after the administration of prostaglandin E1, which dilated the patient's PDA. It was becoming clear that functional closure of the ductus arteriosus was the immediate cause of death in HLHS. This patient died after a modified Norwood procedure.

The Segmental Anatomy in HLHS. In our experience, the segmental anatomy and the AV and VA alignments are almost always normal. We must say *almost* always, because exceptions do exist.

In our experience, the segmental anatomy of congenital mitral stenosis with HLHS is always normal, that is {S,D,S}, unless **the heterotaxy syndrome with congenital asplenia** is also present. Then one should expect a "segmental situs salad," as in Case 138 (A89-68), a 2-day-old boy.

But first, **what does {S,D,S} mean?** It denotes *the set of* (that is, what braces { } signify: situs solitus [S] of the viscera and atria, i.e., {*S*, -,-}; with D-loop ventricles, i.e., {S, *D*, -}; and with solitus normally related great arteries, i.e., {S,D,*S*}). The situs (anatomic pattern) of each of the *three main cardiac segments*—the atria, ventricles, and great arteries—constitutes the elements of the *segmental situs set.* The segmental anatomy largely determines what the AV and the VA *alignments* are, that is, what opens into what. In {S,D,S}, one expects that both the AV and the VA alignments are concordant (appropriate, i.e., normal). When this is not the case, the AV and/or VA alignments are described specifically.

In Case 138, with asplenia, the segmental anatomy was {AIS,L,I}. The segmental anatomic situs set consisted of situs ambiguus (A) of the viscera and atria, that is {*A*, -,-}; there was situs inversus (I) of the abdominal viscera, that is, {A*I*,-,-}. The IVC was left-sided within the abdomen. Then, at the level of the liver, the IVC switched from left to right and drained into a right-sided RA, the atria being in situs solitus (S). So visceroatrial situs was {AIS,-,-}. There was visceroatrial situs discordance (IS) in this asplenic patient with visceroatrial situs ambiguus (also known as visceroatrial heterotaxy). L-loop ventricles (L) were present, that is, {AIS,*L*,-}. The great arteries were inverted normally related (I) {AIS,L,*I*}. Thus, this patient's segmental anatomy was more complex than usual but not rare in the heterotaxy syndrome with apslenia. It is noteworthy that this asplenia patient has inverted normally related great arteries with aortic valvar atresia, all three aortic valvar commissures being very underdeveloped. It is rare for the asplenia syndrome to have *normally related great arteries (solitus or inversus).* It is also rare for an asplenic patient to have aortic outflow tract obstruction (aortic valvar atresia). With asplenia, typically there is no aortic outflow tract obstruction, with pulmonary outflow tract stenosis or atresia, in the setting of DORV or TGA. Consequently, this patient's segmental anatomy {AIS,L,I} is decidedly unusual and noteworthy.

In this patient with the asplenia syndrome there was a common atrium. The incomplete form of common AV canal was present, with no VSD of the AV canal type; the ventricular septum was intact.

The incompletely common AV canal opened mostly into the left-sided morphologically RV and only a small amount into the diminutive right-sided morphologically LV. Congenital right-sided mitral stenosis was marked, with failure of formation of the interchordal spaces. A subpulmonary conus was well developed, typical of inverted normally related great arteries, and the pulmonary outflow tract was widely patent. A severe juxtaductal coarctation of the aorta was found, the PDA was large, the coronary sinus was unroofed, and a right aortic arch was present.

The liver was right-left symmetrical, and the gallbladder was left-sided. The stomach was in the right upper quadrant of the abdomen, and the colon was inverted. The lungs were bilaterally trilobated. The heart was left-sided (levocardia). Bilateral SVCs drained into ipsilateral atria. The IVC was not interrupted. There was TAPVC below the diaphragm, connecting with the ductus venous and draining into the IVC and the portal venous system. The pulmonary venous return was obstructed.

In this series of patients with HLHS, when the aortic valve was atretic, it was always with normally related great arteries: Almost always, the great arteries were *solitus* normally related, when the segmental anatomy was normal, that is {S,D,S}. This patient (Case 138) was the only one in this study with aortic valvar atresia and *inverted* normally related great arteries. We think that this rare finding was related to the coexistence of visceral heterotaxy with asplenia, in which a segmental situs "salad" (i.e., an unusual and often discordant combination of segmental situs) is the rule.

Stenosis of individual pulmonary veins occurred in Case 132 (A89-76), a 26-hour-old girl with moderately severe congenital mitral stenosis (myxomatous leaflets, failure of formation of interchordal spaces, reduction of the interpapillary muscle distance, marked atrophy of the papillary muscle), very severe congenital aortic valvar stenosis (myxomatous leaflets, small annulus, unicommissural, with only the LC/NC commissure being well formed; orifice equals 1 mm), small-chambered and thick-walled LV with moderate EFE. The surprise finding in this patient was *stenosis of individual pulmonary veins*. The right upper pulmonary venous orifice measured 2 mm (internal dimension), and the left upper pulmonary venous orifice also measured 2 mm (internal dimension) in the fresh state. There was premature closure of the foramen ovale in this 1-day-old girl with the septum primum fused with the superior limbic band of septum secundum.

Left atrial endocardial sclerosis was severe, the left atrial endocardium measuring 1.5 mm in thickness. Left atrial hypertrophy was marked—3 mm thick in the fresh state. Coarctation of the aorta, tubular hypoplasia of the aortic arch and isthmus, and a sinusoid between the left ventricular cavity and the posterior descending coronary artery were also found. The left anterior descending coronary artery was rope-like, tortuous, and with a reduced lumen.

An Ebstein-like anomaly of the mitral valve was also observed in **Case 114** (A77-179), a 5-week-old boy. There was downward displacement of the anterior mitral leaflet. No interchordal spaces were formed and the papillary muscles were absent. The mitral orifice was very small and stenotic. Because the mitral valve leaflets had no mobility (they could not move), we thought there was also some degree of mitral regurgitation. The mitral valve formed a skirt-like shelf of fibrous tissue, thought to represent endocardial cushion tissue of the AV canal, that was attached very tightly to the left ventricular free wall. Congenital aortic valvar atresia was also present. To the best of my knowledge, there is no such thing as Ebstein anomaly of the mitral valve, *accurately speaking*. This anomaly was only somewhat reminiscent of Ebstein's because of the *downward displacement of the anterior mitral leaflet*, very rare malformation that was associated with congenital mitral stenosis and regurgitation.

Double-orifice tricuspid valve[106] was found in **Case 111** (A80-88), a 2-month-old boy with extremely severe congenital mitral stenosis (two pinhole openings) and aortic valvar atresia. The markedly hypoplastic LV had no EFE. The double-orifice tricuspid valve was thought to have been of little or no functional importance. Death occurred intraoperatively, during a Norwood procedure.

Autopsy revealed *precoronary stenosis*. What does that mean? The opening leading into the aortic root and the coronary arteries was probe patent but was nonpatulous. One could not see the coronary ostia from within the arterial repair. The opening into the atretic aortic valve and the coronary ostia should look like a soprano singing a high C—wide open.

Congenital unicuspid aortic valvar stenosis, the only well-formed commissure being the RC/NC. This is a rare anomaly. Almost always when the aortic valve is unicommissural, it is the *LC/NC commissure* that is the only well-formed commissure.[28] This rare commissural malformation, a solitary RC/NC commissure, was found in Case 107 (A82-124), a 21-day-old girl with congenital mitral stenosis and DOMV, and the previously mentioned congenital aortic valvar stenosis (0.8%; see Table 14.7).

The rare finding of a **muscular bridge 1 mm above a hypoplastic mitral valve** was the rare finding observed in **Case 99** (A65-139), a 5¼-hour-old boy with congenital mitral stenosis, marked left ventricular hypoplasia, and aortic valvar atresia (0.8%; see Table 14.13).

Right-sided juxtaposition of the atrial appendages with dextromalposition of the LAA[31] was found in **Case 90** (A80-146), a 6½-week-old boy with severe congenital mitral stenosis and aortic valvar atresia (0.8%; see Table 14.13). I was surprised that we did not find more such cases.[31,32] There was 1 other patient, **Case 67** (A83-49), a 19-day-old boy with very severe congenital mitral stenosis (1-mm opening at the posteromedial commissure) and aortic valvar atresia in whom the LAA was found to be posterior to the normally related great arteries—the segmental anatomy being normal, that is, {S,D,S}—with the malpositioned LAA pointing superiorly (cephalad). We thought that this malpositioned LAA probably represented a forme fruste of right-sided juxtaposition of the atrial appendages (0.8%; see Table 14.13).

Juxtapositions of the atrial appendages I will always think of as Dr. Stella Van Praagh's syndromes.[31,32] It was she who first pointed out that juxtaposition of the atrial appendages should be analyzed morphologically, not positionally.[31,32]

In visceroatrial situs solitus, the malpositioned RAA is *left-sided*, that is, to the left of both great arteries, as in Case 90. But in visceroatrial situs inversus, the malpositioned RAA is *right-sided*, that is, to the right of both great arteries. Both in visceroarterial situs solitus and in visceroatrial situs inversus, when juxtaposition of the atrial appendages with *malposition of the LAA* is present, there is a high probability that HLHS coexists.[31] Dr. Stella Van Praagh found that juxtaposition involving malposition of the LAA had left atrial outlet obstruction in 69%, left ventricular hypoplasia in 67%, and aortic outflow tract obstruction in 39%.[31] The findings in *juxtaposition with malposition of the RAA* are typically the opposite.[32] Juxtaposition with malposition of the LAA typically has a hypoplastic LV and a normal conus with normally related great arteries,[31] whereas juxtaposition with malposition of the RAA typically has a hypoplastic RV and an abnormal conus with abnormally related great arteries.[32,30]

The *sidedness* of a malpositioned atrial appendage with juxtaposition of the atrial appendages depends on the type of visceroatrial situs that is present. *In visceroarterial situs solitus*, juxtaposition of the atrial appendages (JAAs) with malposition of the RAA, the RAA is *left-sided*.[30,32] *In visceroarterial situs solitus*, JAA with malposition of the LAA, the LAA is *right-sided*, as in Case 90.[31] *In visceroatrial situs inversus,* JAA with malposition of the RAA, the RAA is *right-sided.*[32]

In visceroatrial situs inversus, JAA with malposition of the LAA, the LAA is *left-sided.*[31]

Thus, the sidedness of the malpositioned atrial appendage in JAA depends on the type of visceroatrial situs that is present (not on the type of ventricular loop that coexists, as used to be thought). This is why JAA is best understood morphologically, that is, in terms of morphology of the malposed atrial appendage and of the visceroatrial situs, not positionally because each malpositioned atrial appendage in JAA can be either right-sided or left-sided, depending on the visceroatrial situs.[31,32]

This type of left-sided JAA also has been called **left-sided JAA with levomalposition of the RAA.** It is abnormal for the RAA to lie to the left of the conotruncus. But it is normal for the LAA to lie to the left of the conotruncus.

JAA should be understood both positionally and morphologically. It occurs in association with both types of ventricular situs (D-loop and L-loop) and with both types of visceroatrial situs. The foregoing is how Dr. Stella Van Praagh liked to think about JAA. My addition would be as follows. **JAA** appears to have nothing primarily to do with the atrial appendages. Instead, it really reflects subnormal ventricular loop formation. Ventricular looping is really a "two-step cardiovascular dance." Normally, the straight heart tube loops in a rightward or dextral direction, forming a bulboventricular D-loop *(step one).* Then, the D-loop normally swings horizontally to the left. Thus, normally, dextrocardia becomes mesocardia and finally levocardia *(step two).* If the leftward swing of the D-loop (step two) is performed subnormally, the infundibulum and great arteries remain to the right of the morphologically RA, instead of being carried leftward and so coming to lie normally between the appendages of the RA and the morphologically LA. This creates the appearance of left-sided JAA: both atrial appendages are lying to the left of the infundibuloarterial segment with nothing between the atrial appendages.

In HLHS, **vascular rings** are rare. Why? One reason is that there is usually a left aortic arch. But even if a right aortic arch is present with a left-sided PDA, a vascular ring may not result, as in **Case 82** (A69-168), a 42-hour-old boy who died after a Norwood procedure from suture line dehiscence and massive hemothorax.

A vascular ring was present in **Case 25** (A90-59), a 1-day-old boy who had a right aortic arch and a large left-sided PDA. Why did Case 82 not have a vascular ring, whereas Case 25 did, despite the fact that they had similar vascular anatomy? I think the answer may lie in the details of Case 25, who did have that rare finding—a vascular ring in HLHS. The aortic arch passed over the right mainstem bronchus (this being the definition of a right aortic arch). The branching pattern of the brachiocephalic arteries, from left to right, was as follows. The left common carotid artery originated farthest to the left. Then to the right arose the right common carotid artery. Then farther to the right, the right subclavian artery originated. Finally, farthest to the right and inferiorly, an aberrant left subclavian artery arose and passed from right to left behind the esophagus to reach the left arm. At the time of this autopsy in 1990, we thought that the vascular ring with indentations of the right and left sides of the trachea immediately above the carina had been produced by the combination of a right aortic arch and a large left-sided PDA. Although these two vessels clearly played an important role in producing this compressing vascular ring, I now think that the aberrant left subclavian artery also played an important role. The pressure of an aberrant left subclavian artery running behind the esophagus prevented the trachea and esophagus from moving somewhat more posteriorly (dorsally) to escape from the pincers of the right aortic arch and the left PDA. The difference between Case 25 (with a compressing vascular ring) and Case 82 (with no compressing vascular ring) was that Case 25 had an aberrant left subclavian artery that closed the ring posteriorly, whereas Case 82 did not have an aberrant left subclavian artery and hence the ring was open posteriorly.

Is it possible for the mitral chordae tendineae to insert directly into the left ventricular endocardium, without intervening papillary muscles? We were surprised to learn that the answer is yes, as in Case **62** (A67-200), a 2-week-old boy with extreme congenital mitral stenosis and hypoplasia, aortic valvar atresia, marked hypoplasia of the LV with severe EFE, and a closing PDA. Marked hypoplasia of the mitral valve's papillary musculature is characteristic of HLHS with aortic valvar atresia or severe congenital stenosis, congenital mitral stenosis, and severe left ventricular EFE. We thought that this uncommon patient displayed extreme papillary muscle hypoplasia or aplasia. I did this case in 1967 with Dr. Robert M. Freedom, when he was one of our fellows in Cardiology at Children's Hospital Medical Center in Boston, as our hospital was then known.

Severe pulmonary valvar stenosis in HLHS sounds like a hemodynamic impossibility. But this is what **Case 39** (C86-439) had. She was a stillborn macerated fetus with an estimated gestational age of 26 weeks. There was a maternal history of three abortions, two spontaneous and one elective. Severe congenital mitral stenosis was present with marked hypoplasia of the mitral valve. The LV was thick-walled (6 mm) and small-chambered. The ventricular septum was intact, the aortic valve was atretic, and the segmental anatomy was normal, that is {S,D,S}. The surprise finding was extreme pulmonary valvar stenosis with a unicommissural pulmonary valve (which commissure was present and which were absent is not stated in our report).

This patient certainly had polyvalvar disease, suggesting the possibility that perhaps a trisomy or other chromosomal anomaly was present. However, viable tissue was not available to investigate this hypothesis in this macerated fetus. Severe pulmonary valvar stenosis was considered to be the cause of spontaneous fetal death in this case.

Summary

A. Of the seven different anatomic types of congenital mitral stenosis that were found in 201 postmortem cases, congenital mitral stenosis with HLHS aortic valvar atresia, or severe aortic valvar stenosis, was by far the most common anatomic type (130 cases, 64.7% of the total series; see Table 14.12 and Fig. 14.24).

B. Clinically and surgically important findings associated with congenital mitral stenosis and HLHS are summarized in Table 14.13 and are considered in the text:
1. MCAs (11.5%),
2. closing PDA (8.5%),
3. intact atrial septum (6.9%),
4. sinusoids from the left ventricular cavity to the coronary arteries (6.9%),
5. familial congenital heart disease (4.6%),
6. fusion of the anterolateral and posteromedial papillary muscles of the LV (3.9%),
7. parachute mitral valve with absence of the anterolateral papillary muscle of the LV (3.1%),
8. valvar and subvalvar aortic atresia (2.3%),
9. absence of the LC/NC commissure of the aortic valve (2.3%),
10. DOMV (1.5%),
11 left ventricular myocardial dysplasia with diverticulum or diverticula (1.5%),
12. prominent anterolateral muscle of the LV (muscle of Moulaert) contributing to muscular subaortic stenosis (1.5%),
13. absence of EFE of the LV (1.5%),
14. fibrous subaortic stenosis related to the anterior leaflet of the mitral valve (1.5%),
15. VSD(s) with congenital mitral stenosis and HLHS (1.5%),
16. normal miniature mitral valve, with mitral hypoplasia only (1.5%),
17 Shone syndrome variant (1.5%),
18. congenital mitral stenosis with the incomplete form of common AV canal (1.5%),
19. congenital mitral stenosis with DIRV and HLHS (0.8%),
20. brachiocephalic artery (bovine trunk) giving origin to all of the major brachiocephalic arteries (0.8%),
21. leftward displacement of the septum primum superiorly into the left atrial cavity (0.8%),
22. unroofing of the coronary sinus (coronary sinus septal defect) with persistent LSVC opening into the LA (0.8%),
23. heterotaxy syndrome with asplenia and discordant segmental anatomy {AIS,L,I} (0.8%);
24. stenosis of individual pulmonary veins (0.8%),
25. downward displacement of anterior mitral leaflet (0.8%),
26. double-orifice tricuspid valve (0.8%),
27. unicuspid and unicommissural aortic valve with the only well-developed commissure being the RC/NC (0.8%),
28. supramitral muscular bridge 1 mm above a hypoplastic mitral valve (0.8%),
29. right-sided juxtaposition of the atrial appendages in visceroarterial situs solitus with dextromalposition of the LAA (0.8%),
30. LAA posterior to the great arteries and pointing superiorly (0.8%),
31. right aortic arch with left-sided ductus arteriosus and no vascular ring (0.8%),
32. right aortic arch with left-sided ductus arteriosus and aberrant left subclavian artery, with compressing vascular ring (0.8%),
33. insertion of mitral chordae tendineae into left ventricular endocardium with no papillary muscles (0.8%), and
34. severe pulmonary valvar stenosis with aortic valvar atresia and severe congenital mitral stenosis leading to intrauterine death (0.8%).

C. The MCAs associated with congenital mitral stenosis and HLHS are summarized in Table 14.14.

Congenital Mitral Stenosis Without the Hypoplastic Left Heart Syndrome and Without Other Major Atrioventricular Anomalies

This was the second most frequent anatomic type of congenital mitral stenosis that was found in 48 of these 201 postmortem cases (23.9%; see Table 14.12).

Without HLHS is clear. But what does *without other major AV anomalies* mean, specifically? This disclaimer means: without any of the other major cardiovascular anomalies listed in Table 14.6 (anatomic types 3 to 7). One cannot call this anatomic type of congenital mitral stenosis (type 2; see Table 14.12) *isolated* congenital mitral stenosis because many other problems can coexist, as we shall soon see.

Ages at Death. The ages at death in those 47 patients with congenital mitral stenosis without HLHS were as follows:

The **number** (n) of these patients was 47, not 48, because the age at death was unknown to us in one consult from the Mayo Clinic in 1974 (Case 198).

The **mean** age at death was 1032.38 days, or 2 10/12 years.

The **standard deviation** was 1724.95 days, or 4 9/12 years.

The **range** in the ages at death postnatally (minimum to maximum) varied from 0 (i.e., intrauterine death) to 7300 days or 20 years.

The **median** age at death was 120 days or 4 months of age.

The ages at death in these patients with congenital mitral stenosis, but *without* HLHS were distinctly better (i.e., older) than in our patients with congenital mitral stenosis *with* HLHS (Table 14.15).

The median ages at death are thought to reflect most clearly the severity of congenital mitral stenosis without, and with, HLHS. Although both anatomic types of congenital mitral stenosis are highly lethal, congenital mitral stenosis *with* HLHS is distinctly worse than congenital mitral stenosis *without* HLHS: median ages at death with HLHS are 9 days, versus without HLHS of 4 months (see Table 14.15). This difference in ages at death is attributed to the presence of HLHS in only one of these two relatively common anatomic types of congenital mitral stenosis.

TABLE 14.15 Ages at Death in Congenital Mitral Stenosis: Without Versus With Hypoplastic Left Heart Syndrome

	Without HLHS	With HLHS
Mean	2 10/12 years	5½ months
Range	0–20 years	0–21 years
Median	4 months	9 days

HLHS, Hypoplastic left heart syndrome.

What is congenital mitral stenosis without HLHS? It is many different things, a *spectrum* of anatomic and developmental anomalies of the mitral valve (Table 14.16). This group includes other cardiovascular and noncardiovascular malformations (see Table 14.10). Congenital mitral stenosis without HLHS is *not* one specific anatomic type of congenital mitral stenosis (see Table 14.16). Also, this group does *not* include other significantly different anatomic types of mitral malformation, such as the incomplete form of common AV canal with a cleft anterior leaflet of the mitral valve, DILV, DIRV, or congenital mitral stenosis caused by rhabdomyomata, or congenital mitral stenosis in conjoined twins (items 3 to 7 inclusive; see Table 14.12), which will be presented separately and in detail later. Thus, congenital mitral stenosis without HLHS is a group heading (see Table 14.16), not one specific anatomic type of congenital mitral stenosis.

MULTIPLE CONGENITAL ANOMALIES

Of these 48 postmortem patients with congenital mitral stenosis who did not have HLHS, MCAs (meaning multisystem malformations) were the most common finding: 20 patients, 42% (see Table 14.16).

Sex: Males, 9, females, 11; males to females = 0.82/1.0. No sex predilection was evident in this small series.

Phenotypes

The most common phenotype was characterized by low-set ears, small mouth, webbed neck, and shield chest (with other variations) in 6 of these 20 patients (30%): Cases 41, 49, 85, 110, 142, and 147. The karyotype, when done, was normal.

Case 41, a 6-day-old boy, had low-set and posteriorly rotated ears, a small mouth, micrognathia, a prominent broad nose, a speckled iris, a short neck, hypospadias, bilateral cryptorchidism, short upper arms, clinodactyly of the fifth fingers, a single right transverse palmar crease, a prominent occiput, an imperforate anus, and a right pelvic kidney.

Case 49, a 5½-year-old boy, had slightly low-set ears, an antimongoloid slant to the eyes, a short mildly webbed neck, a protruding lower jaw with malocclusion, and accessory lobation of both lungs.

Case 85, a 27-day-old boy, was described as having dysmorphic facies, a small mandible, and thick nuchal folds.

Case 110, a 1-day-old boy, had low-set ears, a webbed neck, hypertelorism, a shield chest with widely spaced nipples, facial dysmorphism, and horseshoe kidneys.

Case 142, a 6-day-old boy, had dysmorphic facies with microphthalmus, low-set ears, absent right radius, Meckel diverticulum, a bifid fifth thoracic vertebral body, and agenesis of the corpus callosum.

Case 147, a 10 2/12-year-old girl, had a webbed neck and bilateral simian creases.

Although these 6 patients share certain broad similarities, they also have numerous and important individual differences. Consequently, they are not regarded as constituting a single phenotypic group. Nonetheless, when one sees a patient with dysmorphic facies, low-set ears, a webbed neck, and a shield chest, etc., with a normal karyotype, this clinical picture should immediately suggest *MCAs* and trigger a diagnostic search to delineate what all of these malformations are.

TABLE 14.16 Congenital Mitral Stenosis Without The Hypoplastic Left Heart Syndrome: Anatomic Findings in 48 Postmortem Patients

Anatomic Findings	No. of Cases	% of Series
Multiple congenital anomalies	20	42
"Typical" congenital mitral stenosis	16	33
Parachute mitral valve	12	25
Double-outlet right ventricle	5	10
Left ventricular outflow obstruction	5	10
Trisomy, proved by karyotype	4	8
Double-orifice mitral valve	3	6
Tetralogy of Fallot	2	4
Ebstein anomaly of the tricuspid valve	2	4
Transposition of the great arteries {S,D,S}	1	2
Heterotaxy syndrome with polysplenia	1	2
Right-sided juxtaposition of the atrial appendages {S,D,S}	1	2
Familial congenital heart disease	1	2
Common ventricle, that is, very deficient ventricular septum	1	2

Percentages rounded off to the nearest whole number.

Trisomies

Chromosomal trisomies were found in 4 of these 20 patients (20%) with congenital mitral stenosis without HLHS and with MCAs (see Table 14.16): trisomy 8 in 1, and trisomy 18 in 3.

Syndromes

Established syndromes were identified in 4 of these 20 patients (20%): Noonan syndrome in 2, Coffin-Iris syndrome in 1, and Alagille syndrome in 1.

An acquired intrauterine syndrome was found in 1 patient, a 6½-year-old boy: the phenyl hydantoin syndrome in the child of a mother who was taking phenytoin (Dilantin) and mysoline for seizure control.

Other Findings

Additional anomalies were found in only 1 patient each among these 20 cases with MCAs (see Table 14.16): bronchus suis (pig bronchus, Latin) right upper lobe bronchus arising directly from the trachea, rather than from the right bronchus, which is normal, with hemivertebrae and fused ribs, right upper lobe bronchial stenosis, underdeveloped right kidney with multicystic ovaries, familial MCAs and familial congenital heart disease, and congenital hydrocephalus with polysplenia (but without the heterotaxy syndrome).

Typical Congenital Mitral Stenosis Without the Hypoplastic Left Heart Syndrome

This was the most common form of congenital mitral stenosis when HLHS (aortic valvar atresia or severe congenital aortic valvar stenosis) was not present, occurring in 16 of 48 patients (33%; see Table 14.16). In these patients, congenital mitral stenosis was often the patient's main diagnosis. (By contrast, when HLHS coexisted, it typically was the primary cardiac diagnosis, and congenital mitral stenosis was merely a "fellow traveler," virtually a part of HLHS.) So these are the patients in whom the diagnosis of congenital mitral stenosis was of *primary* importance. It is in this sense that these patients may be considered to have *"typical"* congenital mitral stenosis (see Table 14.16).[97]

Sex: Males, 11; females, 5; males to females = 2.2/1.0. Thus, in this small series of 16 patients with congenital mitral stenosis and without HLHS, there was a strong male preponderance.

Ages at Death: n = 16; mean, 1483 ± 2070.70 days, 4.06 ± 5.67 years, or 4 years and 22 days ± 5 8/12 years; *range,* 1 day to 20 years; median, 559 days, or 1 year, 6 months, and 14 days.

Again, a large difference was found between the *median* age at death (1.53 years) and the *mean* age at death (4.06 years). The median age at death is regarded as more accurately reflective of the severity of typical congenital MS without HLHS than is the mean (average) age at death, because the mean is skewed in an older direction by a few relatively old patients.

It will be recalled that the median age at death in our 130 autopsied patients with congenital mitral stenosis and *with* HLHS was only 9 days; whereas the median age at death in our 16 necropsied patients with typical congenital mitral stenosis but *without* HLHS was 559 days (1.53 years), that is, 62 times older. This difference reflects the lethal effect of HLHS as a cause of neonatal death (i.e., within the first month of postnatal life). Still, a median age at death of only 1.53 years represents very serious disease in the toddler age group.

The Morphologic Features of "Typical" Congenital Mitral Stenosis (Without Hypoplastic Left Heart Syndrome)

"Typical" congenital mitral stenosis without HLHS has been presented graphically in Fig. 14.25. However, one may ask what are the relative frequencies of the various morphologic features that together make up so-called typical congenital mitral stenosis. In an effort to answer this question, the descriptions of these 16 postmortem cases were analyzed with care and the findings are summarized in Table 14.17.

Thus, **typical congenital mitral stenosis** (see Fig. 14.25) has a failure of formation of interchordal spaces (in at least 44%; see Table 14.17), a reduced interpapillary muscle distance (in at least 25%; see Table 14.17), hypoplasia of the mitral valve and orifice (in at least 19%), and myxomatous mitral leaflets (in at least 19%). (I say "in at least" because a morphologic feature is not included in Table 14.17 unless it was specifically described in the heart description of our Cardiac Registry Report. Consequently some of the morphologic findings listed in Table 14.11 may be underrepresented.)

The *papillary muscles* in typical congenital mitral stenosis are noteworthy. They can be hypoplastic to virtually absent. In one

TABLE 14.17 Typical Congenital Mitral Stenosis: Findings in 16 Postmortem Patients

Finding		No. of Cases	% of Series[a]
1.	Failure of formation of interchordal spaces	7	44
2.	Preductal coarctation of the aorta	6	37.5
3.	Multiple congenital anomalies	5	31
4.	Reduced interpapillary muscle distance	4	25
1.	Ventricular septal defect	4	25
	Membranous VSD2	2	12.5
	Muscular VSD	2	12.5
2.	Myxomatous mitral leaflets	3	19
5.	Hypoplasia of the mitral valve	3	19
5.	Polyvalvar disease	3	19
5.	Mild congenital aortic valvar stenosis with bicommissural aortic valve	3	19
5.	Hypoplasia of the mitral valve	3	19
6.	Tricuspid regurgitation with thickened and rolled free margins of the anterior leaflet	2	12.5
6.	Intact atrial septum	2	12.5
3.	Persistent left superior vena cava to coronary sinus to right atrium	2	12.5
6.	Muscularized septum primum bulging into the right atrium	2	12.5
6.	Absence of the left circumflex coronary artery	2	12.5
	Left ventricular papillary muscles thin and wide	1	6
7.	Mitral leaflets inserting directly into the papillary muscle	1	6
7.	Chordae tendineae attached to the left ventricular septal surface	1	6
7.	Chordae tendineae attached to the left ventricular free wall surface	1	6
7.	Small anterolateral papillary muscle group	1	6
7.	Submitral network of chordae tendineae	1	6
7.	Prominent muscle of Moulaert (anterolateral muscle of the left ventricle)	1	6

Continued

TABLE 14.17 Typical Congenital Mitral Stenosis: Findings in 16 Postmortem Patients—cont'd

Finding		No. of Cases	% of Series[a]
7.	Abnormal left and right ventricular myocardial architecture	1	6
7.	Duplicate anterior papillary muscle of the right ventricle	1	6
7.	Short moderator band of the right ventricle	1	6
7.	Abnormal lung lobation	1	6
7.	Totally anomalous pulmonary venous drainage below the diaphragm to the ductus venosus, obstructed	1	6
7.	Acute *Staphylococcus aureus* pneumonia (1953), fatal	1	6
7.	Right-sided juxtaposition of the atrial appendages	1	6
7.	Common atrium, that is, absence of septum primum	1	6
7.	Large secundum atrial septal defect	1	6
7.	Congenital mitral stenosis and congenital mitral regurgitation	1	6
7.	Absent right coronary arterial ostium resulting in so-called "single" left coronary artery	1	6
7.	Transection of conus coronary artery supplying right ventricle in patient with so-called single LCA resulting in death	1	6
7.	Prominent right and left venous valve leaflets of sinoatrial valve in right atrium	1	6
7.	Pulmonary hypertensive vascular disease involving pulmonary veins and arteries in oldest patient (20-year-old man) in 1963	1	6
7.	Congenital mitral arcade	1	6
7.	Eisenmenger complex {S,D,S} with intact atrial septum and postpulmonary stenosis—distal to the lungs—at the mitral valve	1	6

LCA, Left coronary artery; *No.*, number; *{S,D,S}*, the set of situs solitus of viscera and atria, D-loop ventricles, and solitus normally related great arteries; *VSD*, ventricular septal defect.
[a]All percentages are rounded off to the nearest whole number.

patient, they were described as thin and wide, that is, hypoplastic (see Table 14.17). In another patient, the chordae tendineae were described as inserting into the left ventricular septal surface. Remembering that the posteromedial papillary muscle of the LV is paraseptal (i.e., very close to the left ventricular septal surface), marked hypoplasia of this papillary muscle may explain the septal insertion of these chordae tendineae. In another patient, the chordae tendineae were described as being attached to the left ventricular free wall surface (see Table 14.17). Remembering that the antero*lateral* papillary muscle is much further away from the left ventricular septal surface than is the previously mentioned postero*medial* papillary muscle, marked hypoplasia of the anterolateral papillary muscle may explain the apparent insertion of the mitral chordae tendineae directly into the left ventricular free wall. In another patient, the mitral leaflets inserted directly into the papillary muscles of the LV, with apparently no intervening chordae tendineae (see Table 14.17). This appearance can be understood as follows. The chordae tendineae of the mitral valve are in fact present, as transillumination of the mitral valve leaflets shows. But the interchordal spaces have failed to form and are still filled by mitral leaflet–like tissue. Consequently, it looks as though the mitral leaflets are inserting directly into the papillary muscles, because the chordae tendineae are effectively disguised by leaflet-like tissue that still fills what normally should be the interchordal spaces. A less severe form of the same process produces the appearance of *short chordae tendineae.*

The finding of a *submitral network or mesh of chordae tendineae* was a startling and rare finding in 1 patient (see Table 14.17).

One patient, a 5½-year-old boy, presented in 1954 with cyanosis and squatting, a TOF-like clinical picture. A young Dr. Alex Nadas, just 5 years after he had founded the Department of Cardiology at Boston Children's Hospital, knew that his patient had *functional pulmonary stenosis*. His clinical impression was correct. But autopsy revealed that the patient had the *Eisenmenger complex*. The segmental anatomy was normal, that is, {S,D,S} (see Table 14.17). The conal septum was deviated anterosuperiorly, similar to that in TOF, but not enough to produce pulmonary infundibular or pulmonary valvar stenosis. Instead, the patient was found to have an undiagnosed congenital mitral stenosis with an intact atrial septum. Thus, this patient had *postpulmonary stenosis*—beyond the pulmonary valve, artery, and lungs—at the mitral valvar level, not *pre*pulmonary stenosis at the pulmonary infundibular and valvar levels proximal to the lungs as in TOF. This patient had pulmonary hypertension because of congenital mitral stenosis with an intact atrial septum, not pulmonary hypotension as in TOF. But this patient's pulmonary hypertension resulted in right-to-left shunting through the large VSD, simulating the clinical picture of TOF with squatting.

Victor Eisenmenger (1864–1932) was a German physician who, in 1897, described the congenital anomaly of a large subaortic VSD, overriding aorta, and right ventricular hypertrophy (i.e., TOF, but *without* pulmonary outflow tract obstruction). This is what Dr. Nadas' patient had, plus congenital mitral stenosis with an intact atrial septum (our Case 160 in this series). It is very unusual for an untreated 5½-year-old patient with the Eisenmenger complex to have a clinical picture simulating TOF with cyanosis and squatting, unless congenital mitral obstruction (stenosis or atresia) and an intact atrial septum also coexist.

Thinking of eponyms, it should be mentioned that many of these patients had **Lutembacher syndrome**. Rene Lutembacher

(1884–1968) of Paris, France first described the combination of ASD and mitral stenosis in 1916.

Both of these eponymous diagnoses, the Eisenmenger complex and/or syndrome and the Lutembacher syndrome, appear to be fading into disuse. They are included here for the sake of completeness and to facilitate understanding of the older medical literature.

Other noteworthy findings in patients with typical congenital mitral stenosis (see Fig. 14.11) include the relatively high frequencies of preductal coarctation of the aorta (37.5%), MCAs (31%), VSD (25%), polyvalvar disease (19%), mild congenital aortic valvar stenosis with bicommissural ("bicuspid") aortic valve (19%), and significant tricuspid regurgitation (at least 12.5%). (I say "at least" because tricuspid regurgitation can occur without thickening and rolling of the tricuspid leaflets' free margins.)

Parachute Mitral Valve in Patients With Congenital Mitral Stenosis and Without Hypoplastic Left Heart Syndrome

Parachute mitral valve, in its complete or partial forms, was found in 12 of 48 patients (25%) with congenital mitral stenosis, but without HLHS (see Table 14.16).

Sex: Males, 5 (33%); females, 8 (67%); and males to females = 4/8 or 0.5. Thus, a strong female preponderance was found in this small series.

Age: Mean, 2.25 ± 4.15 years; range, 7 days to 14 3/12 years; and median, 112.5 days or 3 3/34 months.

ANATOMIC TYPES OF PARACHUTE MITRAL VALVE

Parachute mitral valve may be complete or partial:

In the *complete form,* usually only one papillary muscle is present and it receives all of the mitral chordae tendineae.

In the *partial forms,* both papillary muscle groups (anterolateral and posteromedial) are present, but the papillary muscles are partially fused or they are closely separated (i.e., much too close together). When the papillary muscle groups are close together (≤4 mm), this has been called *parachute mitral valve, forme fruste.*

In the complete form, only one papillary muscle receiving chordae tendineae was present in 8 of these 12 patients (67%). But which papillary muscle was present and which was absent? Or were both really present? Based on location, careful gross examination in these 8 patients with only one papillary muscle indicated that the solitary papillary muscle was *the anterolateral in 3* (37.5%) (Cases 54, 159, and 183); *the posteromedial in 3* (39.5%) (Cases 50, 65, and 86); and was composed of the *visibly fused anterolateral and posteromedial papillary muscles in 2 (25%)* (Cases 35 and 85).

The foregoing findings were a surprise. I had previously thought that when the AV canal is divided with separate mitral and tricuspid valves (as opposed to a common AV canal with a common AV valve), the parachute mitral valve typically has a single *posteromedial* papillary muscle with absence of the anterolateral papillary muscle.[99] These findings are somewhat different. In this small series, a single *anterolateral* papillary muscle was just as common as a single posteromedial papillary muscle (3/3). And in two patients, a single papillary muscle was composed of *both* the anterolateral and the posteromedial papillary muscles that had fused.

Let us look more closely at the papillary muscle anatomy and at other aspects of these 8 cases of definite parachute mitral valve.

Single Anterolateral Papillary Muscle Receiving All Chordae Tendineae

Case 54, a 3-month-old girl, had moderately severe congenital mitral stenosis with two high, small papillary muscles in the position of the anterolateral papillary muscle group. The posteromedial papillary muscle group was absent. There was marked reduction of the interpapillary muscle space because all of the chordae tendineae inserted into the high small anterolateral papillary muscle group. This patient also had normal {S,D,S} segmental anatomy, right-sided juxtaposition of the atrial appendages, a secundum ASD, a high and large subaortic VSD of the conoventricular type, and bilaterally trilobed lungs with a normally formed spleen.

Case 159, a 48-day-old girl, had severe congenital mitral stenosis, with the internal diameter of the mitral orifice being only 3 mm. She had a parachute mitral valve in which the chordae tendineae attached only to the anterolateral papillary muscle group. *A posteromedial papillary muscle group was present but received no chordae tendineae.* Two anomalous left ventricular muscle bundles were found: from the left ventricular septal surface to the anterolateral papillary muscle group; and from the left ventricular septal surface to the posteromedial papillary muscle group. Hence, this patient had anomalous left ventricular myocardial architecture that was not confined to the papillary muscles. The stenotic mitral orifice was located above the anterolateral papillary muscle group because that is where all of the mitral chordae inserted.

This patient also had MCAs, probably Alagille syndrome. Alagille syndrome is characterized by a paucity of intrahepatic bile ducts; cholestasis without cirrhosis; hypercholesterolemia; neonatal jaundice that clears by 4 years of age; lifelong pruritus; hemivertebrae, "butterfly" vertebrae, spina bifida occulta, rib anomalies; peripheral pulmonary stenosis; mild intellectual disability; retinal degeneration; and strabismus. In addition, peripheral pulmonary stenosis, ASD, VSD, PDA, and coarctation of the aorta have been reported. The kidneys are characterized by decreased creatinine clearance, increased blood urea nitrogen, increased serum uric acid, and horseshoe kidney. Hypogonadism, decreased growth hormone with growth retardation, increased testosterone, and hypothyroidism are typical. Peculiar faces with deep set eyes, broad forehead, bulbous nose, and prominent chin are characteristic. Most have a normal life span. It is autosomal dominant. Called **arteriohepatic dysplasia** by Watson and Miller in 1973,[107] these authors were referring to the familial pulmonary arterial stenosis with neonatal liver disease. In 1975, Alagille et al[108] reported the same entity and their title summarized this syndrome well: *"Hepatic ductular hypoplasia associated with characteristic facies, vertebral malformations,* *retarded physical, mental and sexual development and cardiac murmur.*" The mother had hyperprolactinemia.

REVISED DEFINITION OF PARACHUTE MITRAL VALVE

This patient forced us to reassess parachute mitral valve. This patient and other cases like it have forced us to realize that in parachute mitral valve, what is even more important than the number of papillary muscle groups is **the number of foci of chordal insertion.** If there is only one focus of chordal insertion, parachute mitral valve functionally is present, even if both papillary muscle groups coexist. When there is only one focus of chordal insertion, there is essentially no "interpapillary muscle distance," that is, no distance between the normally two foci of chordal insertion.

The space between the two foci of chordal insertion is one very important component of the normal mitral orifice; and the interchordal spaces are the other (see Fig. 14.23). Both components of the mitral orifice are very reduced in typical parachute mitral valve (see Fig. 14.27), resulting in congenital mitral stenosis.

Case 183, a 2½-year-old boy, had parachute mitral valve, all chordae tendineae inserting into the anterolateral papillary muscle. A small posteromedial papillary muscle was also present that received no chordae tendineae. The interchordal spaces of the chordae tendineae inserting into the anterolateral papillary muscle group had largely failed to form. The mitral orifice consisted of two small patent interchordal spaces. A small (2 mm) apical muscular VSD was also present.

This case, like the previous one (Case 159), illustrates that parachute mitral valve should be defined as one focus of chordal insertion, even when two papillary muscle groups are present. This new definition of parachute mitral valve may constitute a diagnostic challenge, because chordae tendineae may be harder to visualize than papillary muscles. The congenital heart surgeon may well prove to be the most accurate diagnostician because he or she can see the chordae tendineae and the papillary muscle(s) at open heart surgery.

Single Posteromedial Papillary Muscle Receiving All Chordae Tendineae

Case 86 was a 7-day-old girl with parachute mitral valve: the anterolateral papillary muscle group was absent, and all chordae tendineae inserted into a large posteromedial papillary muscle. The mitral leaflets were myxomatous, the interchordal spaces were poorly formed, and left ventricular hypoplasia was marked. She also had a large conoventricular type of VSD and a PDA. In addition, this patient had trisomy 18 (proved by karyotype).

Case 50, a 5 7/12-year-old girl, had a variant of Shone syndrome[98]: a small supramitral fibrous ring (of no physiologic importance, i.e., not causing supramitral stenosis); insertion of all chordae tendineae into the posteromedial papillary muscle; the anterolateral papillary muscle was present but received no chordae tendineae; interchordal spaces were present; a high small subaortic conoventricular type of VSD was found; a bicuspid aortic valve was present, the intercoronary commissure being rudimentary; and a preductal coarctation of the aorta was also present. Thus, the only feature of the classic Shone syndrome[98] that this patient did *not* have was subaortic stenosis. (Instead, she had a hypoplastic bicommissural aortic valve.) So, what his patient had was close to a typical Shone syndrome.

Case 65, a 14 3/12-year-old girl, did have classic Shone syndrome[98]: a supramitral ring that was physiologically insignificant, one large posteromedial papillary muscle group that received all of the mitral chordae tendineae, subaortic fibrous ring with subaortic stenosis, and preductal coarctation of the aorta. This teenager (the oldest parachute mitral valve patient in this series) also had a subaortic conoventricular type of VSD and a PDA, both not parts of Shone syndrome as originally described.[98]

Single Papillary Muscle Resulting From Fusion of Both Papillary Muscle Groups With a Single Focus of Chordal Insertion

In **Case 85,** a 27-day-old boy, a small anterolateral papillary muscle group had fused with a larger posteromedial papillary muscle group, resulting in a single papillary muscle with no interpapillary muscle space and a single focus of chordal insertion. The interchordal spaces also had failed to form. Additional findings included a secundum ASD, a small membranous VSD, left ventricular hypoplasia, a bicuspid pulmonary valve (rudimentary septal commissure), a bicuspid aortic valve (rudimentary RC/NC commissure), polyvalvar disease (abnormal mitral, aortic, and pulmonary valves), {S,D,S}, normal karyotype (46XY), and MCAs with dysmorphic facial features, small mandible, and thick nuchal folds.

Case 35, a girl aged 2 months and 6 days, was similar to the preceding case. Congenital mitral stenosis was severe. There was no interpapillary muscle distance between the fused anterolateral and posteromedial papillary musculature, resulting in one large papillary muscle with a single focus of chordal insertion. The interchordal spaces had largely failed to form. There was a jet lesion on the left ventricular septal surface opposite to a slit-like opening within the tissue of the anterior mitral leaflet.

Parachute Mitral Valve with Two Partially Fused Papillary Muscle Groups

Now we are entering the territory of parachute mitral valve *forme fruste* (partial or "almost" parachute mitral valve).

Case 56, a 7¼-month-old girl, had a hypoplastic mitral valve *with fusion of the anterolateral and posteromedial papillary muscles at their upper tips,* and essentially a single focus of chordal insertion. There were thickening and rolling of the posterior mitral leaflet indicating congenital mitral *regurgitation.* Hence, this patient had both congenital mitral stenosis and congenital mitral regurgitation. This patient also had a relatively large interchordal space anterolaterally and a single moderate-sized conoventricular VSD.

Additional findings included hypoplasia of the LV (abnormally thin left ventricular free wall), with hypoplasia of the aortic annulus, ascending aorta, and aortic arch; an aberrant right subclavian artery (with normal segmental anatomy, {S,D,S}, and a left aortic arch); a persistent LSVC opened into the *coronary* sinus and then to the RA; and MCAs, probably the Coffin-Siris syndrome. *The*

Coffin-Sirus syndrome is characterized by intellectual disability with absence of the fifth fingernail and terminal phalanx.[109]

Case 136, was a 4½-month-old girl with TOF {S,D,S} and severe pulmonary outflow tract stenosis, the os infundibuli measuring only 1 mm in internal diameter, with a bicuspid pulmonary valve measuring 2 mm in internal diameter. She also had congenital mitral stenosis, the orifice measuring 5 mm in internal dimension. *The anterolateral and posteromedial papillary muscles were fused at their bases* with reduction of the interpapillary muscle space, but with two foci of chordal insertion that were abnormally close together. The atrial septum was intact. Hence, this patient was considered to have parachute mitral valve forme fruste. Additional findings included hypoplasia of the LV, a right aortic arch, and a persistent LSVC opening into the coronary sinus and then to the RA.

Case 48, a 3 2/12-year-old boy, had congenital mitral stenosis with a supramitral ring that was more marked above the posterior mitral leaflet than above the anterior mitral leaflet. The diameter of the supramitral ring was 12 mm. The orifice of the stenotic mitral valve measured only 6 mm in diameter dimension. The chordae tendineae were attached mostly to a large posteromedial papillary muscle, with only two chordae attaching to a small anterolateral papillary muscle. The left atrial free wall was twice the normal thickness, and the LA was mildly enlarged (on comparison with normal age-matched control heart specimens, which was done routinely, i.e., on all cases). A small secundum ASD was present (3 mm in maximal dimension). A large conoventricular type of VSD and a small PDA (2 mm in internal dimension) were also present.

Neither subaortic stenosis, nor preductal coarctation of the aorta was present; hence, the diagnosis of Shone syndrome was not made. However, this patient could be considered to have a *partial* form of Shone syndrome.

This patient was thought to have a *parachute-like mitral valve*, not a definite parachute mitral valve because both papillary muscle groups were present and there were two foci of chordal insertion. However, there very nearly was a single focus of chordal insertion because *almost all* of the chordae tendineae did insert into the posteromedial papillary muscle.

Case 94, an 11-day-old girl, had severe congenital mitral stenosis with a parachute mitral valve forme fruste. The anterolateral papillary muscle group was large, the posteromedial papillary muscle group was much smaller, and there was considerable reduction of the interpapillary muscle distance (only 4 mm), with failure of formation of the interchordal spaces.

Additional findings included a secundum ASD with septum primum herniating into the RA; a thick-walled and small-chambered LV without EFE; and a very small membranous VSD (1 to 1.5 mm in internal dimension).

To summarize, in these 12 patients, 8 (67%) had definite parachute mitral valve (the complete form) with only one focus of chordal insertion, that is, with all of the chordae tendineae inserting into only one papillary muscle: the anterolateral in 3, the posteromedial in 3, and into fused anterolateral and posteromedial papillary musculature in 2. The remaining 4 patients (33%) had the partial form or forme fruste of parachute mitral valve. In 2, the papillary muscles were partially fused, and in the other 2, the papillary muscles were abnormally closely spaced, that is, much too close together.

What did we learn?

1. I was surprised to find, in this admittedly small series of parachute mitral valve with a divided AV canal (n = 12), that the single focus of chordal insertion was just as often into the anterolateral papillary muscle (3) as into the posteromedial (3). I previously thought that when the AV canal is divided (with separate mitral and tricuspid valves), the single papillary muscle receiving all of the chordae tendineae is usually the posteromedial; whereas with common AV canal and potentially parachute mitral valve, the single papillary muscle receiving all of the chordae tendineae typically is the anterolateral papillary muscle.[99] With more anatomic data, the nature of the papillary muscle malformation in parachute mitral valve with a divided AV canal and with a common AV canal may become clearer.
2. It was of interest that two papillary muscles could be present, but with only one of them receiving chordae tendineae. This realization indicates that parachute mitral valve should be defined as one focus of chordal insertion, not as the presence of only one papillary muscle group (because the latter criterion is a variable).
3. It was also of interest to find that a solitary papillary muscle could be composed of fused anterolateral and posteromedial papillary muscle groups.
4. Finally, I was surprised that only 1 of the 12 patients (Case 65) has the Shone syndrome in its complete classic form.[98]

Shone syndrome[98] represents four-level left heart obstruction, two levels involving the left ventricular inflow tract, that is, the supramitral stenosing ring and parachute mitral valve, and two levels involving the left ventricular outflow tract, that is, subaortic stenosis that may be fibrous, muscular, or both, and preductal coarctation of the aorta. Congenital mitral stenosis seldom comes alone; unlike acquired mitral stenosis (e.g., rheumatic mitral stenosis), congenital mitral stenosis seldom is an anomaly of the mitral leaflets only, as acquired mitral stenosis often is. To my knowledge, congenital mitral stenosis never results from the fusion of two previously separate mitral leaflet margins, whereas this frequently is the case in acquired mitral stenosis.

Thus, congenital mitral stenosis is entirely different from acquired mitral stenosis in many important respects: age at presentation, cause, morphogenesis, and pathologic anatomy. But congenital and acquired mitral stenosis are similar or identical in some respects: the same valve, the mitral valve, is involved in both, and the hemodynamic and clinical sequelae can be similar or identical in both. However, the anatomic differences between congenital and acquired mitral stenosis suggest that the surgical procedures in congenital mitral stenosis must be individualized. For example, mitral commissurotomy, often appropriate in acquired mitral stenosis, is seldom, if ever, appropriate in congenital mitral stenosis, because a commissural leaflet fusion is not the problem in congenital mitral stenosis, as we have seen.

Congenital Mitral Stenosis With Double-Outlet Right Ventricle

DORV associated with congenital mitral stenosis and without HLHS (5 of these 48 patients or 10%; see Table 14.16) is so interesting that DORV in this setting demands further description.

Gender: Males, 4 (80%); female, 1 (20%); males to females, 4/1 (or 4).

Age at Death: Mean = 475.7 days = 1.30 years; standard deviation = 1060.35 days = 2.91 years; range = 0 to 2372.5 days = 6.5 years; and median = 0 (i.e., intrauterine demise).

There were three intrauterine deaths (Cases 44, 139, and 153). None of these prenatal deaths was caused by an elective abortion; all were spontaneous.

There was a strong male preponderance (80%); but this is a very small series (n = 5), and, hence, the significance of these numbers is unclear. More data are needed. There is a startling divergence between the mean age of death (1.3 ± 2.9 years) and the median age at death (0), meaning no days of postnatal life because of prenatal demise.

THE CONUS (INFUNDIBULUM)

A *subpulmonary conus* with aortic-tricuspid fibrous continuity was present in 4 of these 5 cases (80%): Cases 44, 139, 144, and 153. Three were males and one was a girl (Case 153). A *bilateral conus* (subaortic and subpulmonary) was found in 1 patient (Case 41). How should the *segmental anatomy* be represented in these cases? My tentative suggestions are as follows:

1. When DORV is present with a subpulmonary conus and aortic-tricuspid fibrous continuity: **DORV {S,D,"S"} with subpulmonary conus;** and
2. When DORV is present with a bilateral conus: **DORV {S,D,D} with a bilateral conus.**

DORV {S,D,**"S"**} with a subpulmonary conus indicates that a normal type of infundibulum is present. The quotation marks around "S" indicate that a normal solitus type of infundibulum (conus) and great arteries is present, but that despite that fact, DORV is present.

In other words, the "S" symbol in DORV {S,D,"S"} indicates that the conotruncus is very like the solitus normal conotruncus (with a subpulmonary muscular conus and with no subaortic muscular conus). However, the conotruncus is not entirely like a solitus normal conotruncus, because DORV is present. This means that there is aortic-tricuspid (not aortic-mitral) direct fibrous continuity. Hence, the quotation marks (mean "not entirely," or "almost like") are necessary: DORV {S,D,"S"}. If the foregoing approach is regarded as too subtle, the segmental anatomy can be described as DORV {S,D,D} with subpulmonary conus and aortic-tricuspid fibrous continuity. The latter is accurate.

Nonetheless, some may well prefer DORV {S,D, "S"} because this indicates what the heart looks like. The great arteries look like solitus normally related great arteries, that is, like {-,-,S}. But both great arteries arise above the RV; hence, the great arteries are not solitus normally related as far as the ventricles and AV canal are concerned. The segmental anatomy must reflect that, to be accurate: DORV {S,D,"S"}.

This combination of DORV but with a normal solitus type of conotruncus seems like a contradiction in terms, a logical impossibility. But it is not. That is what we observed, as noted earlier. How can this be? It has to do with our tacit, almost subconscious assumptions. In DORV, most of us assume that because DORV is a "conotruncal malformation" (which it is most of the time, but not always) there *must* be something wrong with the conotruncus or more specifically with the conus.

But *DORV is really a relationships diagnosis:* a specific type of alignment between the conotruncus above, and the ventricles, ventricular septum, and AV canal and valves below. More briefly, DORV is a type of alignment between two major cardiac segments: (1) the conotruncus above and (2) the ventricular loop and the AV canal below. Usually, DORV is caused by a malformation of component (1), the conal part of the conotruncus. Component (2), the ventricular loop and the AV canal usually are essentially normally formed.

However, occasionally, the reverse can happen. Component 1, the conotruncus, can be normally formed, whereas component 2, the ventricular loop and the AV canal, can be malformed, resulting in DORV *because DORV is a VA alignments diagnosis between these two major cardiac segments, either of which can be malformed, causing the VA malalignments of DORV.*

So DORV is not always a conal (or "conotruncal") malformation. Sometimes, DORV can result from an anomaly of the AV canal and valves, and of the ventricular segments of the heart as in DORV {S,D,"S"} with a subpulmonary conus, aortic-tricuspid fibrous continuity, and congenital mitral stenosis.

In a specific type of malalignment between two cardiac segments (as in DORV), malformation of either component can result in DORV. It may seem surprising to say that **DORV is not always a conotruncal malformation, but occasionally it can be an AV canal and ventricular anomaly.** But that is exactly what I am saying because of Cases 44, 139, 144, and 153, all of whom had DORV {S,D,"S"}.

One might argue that the quotation marks are unnecessary, even wrong, and that it should be DORV {S,D,**S**}. Why? Because the conotruncal (infundibuloarterial) part of the heart *really* is normally formed. And DORV *really* is present. Hence, the apologetic quotation marks could easily be viewed as unnecessary or even wrong. The entire diagnosis—**DORV** {S,D,**S**}—is anatomically accurate. DORV really can occur with a normally formed infundibuloarterial segment. However, I have decided to retain the quotation marks, as in DORV {S,D,"S"}, because the anatomy of the great arteries is not entirely of the solitus normal type. True, the infundibuloarterial anatomy is solitus normal, as above. However, the *VA alignments* are not of the solitus normal type. Instead, DORV is present, not solitus normally related great arteries.

Thus, DORV {S,D,**"S"**} is intended to indicate all of the foregoing rare features: DORV is present. But the infundibuloarterial anatomy is of the solitus normal type: a normal subpulmonary conal connection is present; and the semilunar valves and great arteries are of the solitus normal type, with the pulmonary valve anterior, superior, and to the left relative to the aortic valve, which is posterior, inferior, and to the right.

DORV {S,D,"S"} is also relevant to the **definition of DORV.** These cases indicate that DORV cannot be defined as abnormally *connected* great arteries for several reasons. First, in these cases, the conal connector is of the normal anatomic type that is, subpulmonary. Second, the concept of VA connections is anatomically wrong. The ventricles do not connect with the great arteries because of the interposition of the conus and the importance of the AV valves with which the semilunar valves of the great arteries do connect. Because the concept of ventriculoarterial *connections* is anatomically inaccurate, we prefer the concept of **VA alignments,** which is anatomically accurate.

These patients clearly illustrate the important differences between VA connections and VA alignments:

1. The VA connections (or connectors) are normal. The muscular conus is subpulmonary. The absent muscular conal free wall is subaortic, permitting aortic–AV valvar direct fibrous continuity (or connection).
2. The VA alignments are abnormal, DORV being present in all.

These cases prove that it is possible to have abnormal VA alignments (DORV) with normal VA connections (subpulmonary conus and absent subaortic conal free wall).

These distinctions also apply to AV alignments and AV connections. AV alignments may be concordant, discordant, double-inlet, straddling, etc. AV connections (or connectors) are the mitral valve, the tricuspid valve, and the common AV valve.

The confusion between alignments and connections is related to a failure to recognize the connecting segments (AV canal and conus arteriosus) as real. The tricuspid valve is not part of the morphologically RV. DILV proves that. The mitral valve (MV) is not part of the LV. DIRV proves that. The conus arteriosus (or infundibulum) is not part of the RV. Double-outlet LV with the conus mostly or entirely above the LV proves that. The connecting segments are real, separate components of the heart, that should be understood as such.

The fact that the atria do not connect with the ventricles (except at the AV bundle of His), because of the interposition of the AV canal, and the fact that the ventricles do not connect with the great arteries because of the interposition of the conus arteriosus or infundibulum; these two facts are very important developmentally. The AV nonconnection and the VA nonconnection help explain how and why it is possible for so many different AV and VA alignments to occur, creating the fascinating complexity of congenital heart disease.

Each of these five cases of DORV with congenital mitral stenosis, but without severe aortic valvar stenosis or atresia (HLHS), will now be presented briefly.

Case 44, a stillborn male fetus, underwent a spontaneous intrauterine death. Autopsy revealed DORV {S,D,"S"} with a well-developed left-sided subpulmonary conus and absence of the right-sided subaortic conal free wall that permitted aortic-mitral and aortic-tricuspid fibrous continuity. Severe congenital mitral stenosis was found, with absence of identifiable papillary muscles. A single focus of chordal insertion attached to the posteromedial left ventricular free wall, adjacent to the left ventricular septal surface. Thus, **a rare form of parachute mitral valve was found with no papillary muscle,** just a single focus of chordal insertion into the left ventricular free wall.

There were absence of interchordal spaces and shortened chordae tendineae, with the only orifice of the mitral valve being at the posteromedial commissure. The LV was small-chambered and thick-walled. A prominent muscle of Moulaert contributed to muscular subaortic stenosis. A conoventricular type of VSD was present.

The tricuspid valve was also abnormal with no papillary muscle of the conus, absence of the commissure between the anterior and septal tricuspid leaflets, and myxomatous thickening of the leaflet margins consistent with tricuspid regurgitation. Also contributing to the muscular subaortic stenosis was narrowing of the right ventricular outflow tract between the conal septum anterosuperiorly and the tricuspid valve posteroinferiorly. There was hypoplasia of the aortic isthmus, preductal coarctation of the aorta, a PDA (not surprising in a fetus), a patent foramen ovale, and MCAs.

To summarize, perhaps the most unusual features of this rare case of DORV {S,D,"S"} are the presence of a subpulmonary conus with aortic-mitral and aortic-tricuspid stenosis, a parachute mitral valve with no demonstrable papillary muscle but a single posteromedial focus of chordal insertion into the left ventricular free wall, with subaortic stenosis and preductal coarctation of the aorta. This fetus had all the features of Shone syndrome except for a supramitral stenosing ring.

Case 139, a second stillborn male fetus who suffered a spontaneous intrauterine demise, weighed 565 g. Autopsy revealed DORV {S,D,"S"} with a subpulmonary infundibulum and aortic-tricuspid fibrous continuity. The patent foramen ovale of the atrial septum was restrictive, with a redundant septum primum herniating into the right atrial cavity like a spinnaker. The LA was small-chambered.

The annulus and leaflets of the mitral valve were hypoplastic. The mitral tensor apparatus was strikingly abnormal, with the chordae tendineae inserted directly into the left ventricular septal surface posteriorly and directly into the left ventricular free wall anteriorly. The mitral chordae tendineae did not insert into any papillary muscle, even though a small posteromedial papillary muscle was present.

Left ventricular hypoplasia was marked. A high small conoventricular type of VSD was found. The tricuspid valve had a deep curtain-like anterior leaflet that was tethered to the right ventricular free wall; this anterior (or parietal) tricuspid leaflet appeared to be minimally functional, that is, largely nonfunctional. The septal leaflet of the tricuspid valve was not downwardly displaced; hence, a diagnosis of Ebstein anomaly was *not* made. Massive tricuspid regurgitation was thought to have been present in life. Right atrial hypertrophy and enlargement and right ventricular hypertrophy and enlargement were both marked. The pulmonary valve was bicuspid and bicommissural because the nonseptal left septal commissure was absent.

Polyvalvar disease was present, with congenital mitral stenosis, congenital tricuspid regurgitation, and a bicommissural pulmonary valve. The pat karyotype was not known by us. (This heart specimen was sent to us as a consultation in 1988.)

Why did both of these last two patients suffer spontaneous intrauterine death? The answer may be because of polyvalvar disease. Specifically, in this last patient, *the combination of severe congenital mitral stenosis and massive tricuspid regurgitation* may well have constituted an insupportable hemodynamic burden. In addition, this patient had a restrictive atrial septum, aortic outflow tract stenosis, and preductal coarctation of the aorta. This patient's pulmonary valve, although bicommissural, was thought not to be hemodynamically significantly abnormal.

Thus, my impression is that patients with severe congenital mitral stenosis can survive into postnatal life if they have an essentially normal tricuspid valve. But if massive tricuspid regurgitation coexists, spontaneous intrauterine death may well occur, as in this last patient.

Case 144, a 6½-year-old boy, had severe congenital mitral stenosis. The interchordal spaces had largely failed to form. The only opening was a cleft in the mitral valve. Both papillary muscles were present.

DORV {S,D,"S"} was present with a subpulmonary conus, and aortic-tricuspid and aortic-mitral (via conoventricular type of VSD) direct fibrous continuity were present. A persistent LSVC drained into the coronary sinus and then to the RA. Left atrial hypertrophy and enlargement, left ventricular hypoplasia, and right ventricular hypertrophy and enlargement were also documented.

Three accessory spleens were found measuring 5 mm, 2.5 mm, and 2.5 mm in greatest dimension.

This patient also had the *diphenyl hydantoin syndrome* because during his gestation his mother had taken Dilantin and mysoline for seizure control. Also known as the *fetal hydantoin syndrome* or the *fetal Dilantin syndrome,* the findings in this patient included hypertelorism, microcephaly, small finger nails, and congenital heart disease.

This patient also exemplified *familial congenital heart disease:* one sibling had a VSD; another sibling had a PDA; and a maternal aunt died at 11 years of age because of congenital heart disease (other details being unknown to us).

Case 153, a female fetus, was our fourth and final patient with congenital mitral stenosis and DORV {S,D,"S"} with a subpulmonary conus. She suffered a spontaneous intrauterine death at an estimated gestational age of 38 weeks. Our patient was one of triplets; the other two sisters are well.

Our patient with congenital mitral stenosis had a hypoplastic anterolateral papillary muscle and a small and tilted mitral orifice. She also had a conoventricular type of VSD with some anterosuperior malalignment of the conal septum, but without pulmonary outflow tract obstruction. In addition, she had a persistent LSVC connecting with the coronary sinus and draining into the RA.

Case 41, a 6-day-old boy was our only patient with congenital mitral stenosis and DORV {S,D,D} with a bilateral conus (subaortic and subpulmonary) and consequently with no semilunar–AV valve direct fibrous continuity. Congenital mitral stenosis was mild (a 4 mm Hg gradient), with hypoplasia of the mitral annulus, marked underdevelopment of the anterolateral papillary muscle group, but without other mitral valvar deformity.

A conoventricular type of VSD was subpulmonary (as in the Taussig-Bing malformation). The pulmonary outflow tract was widely patent. There was mild subaortic stenosis. The right-sided aortic valve had three leaflets, but was smaller than the left-sided pulmonary valve. There was severe hypoplasia of the aortic isthmus and preductal coarctation of the aorta (<1 mm in internal dimension). A PDA was present. He had a ductus-arteriosus-dependent circulation requiring the administration of PGE (prostaglandin E1) because of the extremely severe coarctation of the aorta associated with a PDA. A persistent LSVC connected with the coronary sinus and then to the RA.

This patient with a normal karyotype (46XY) had MCAs, including low-set and posteriorly rotated ears, a small mouth, micrognathia, a prominent and broad nose, specked irides, a short neck, hypospadias, bilateral cryptorchidism, short upper arms, clinodactyly of the right fifth finger, right transverse palmar crease, prominent occiput, imperforate anus, and right pelvic kidney.

In conclusion, congenital mitral stenosis without HLHS was associated with DORV in 5 of 48 postmortem cases (10%; see Table 14.10). Of these 5 patients with DORV, 4 (80%) had a subpulmonary conus (DORV {S,D,"S"}) and only 1 (20%) had a bilateral (subaortic and subpulmonary) conus (DORV {S,D,D}). In our experience, DORV with a subpulmonary conus was always associated with obstructive congenital heart disease involving the left heart, such as congenital mitral stenosis.

Left Ventricular Outflow Tract Obstruction in Patients With Congenital Mitral Stenosis but Without the Hypoplastic Left Heart Syndrome

There were 5 such patients in these 48 autopsied cases (10%; see Table 14.10). But what kinds of left ventricular outflow tract obstruction did they have?

Case 49, a 5½-year-old boy, had very severe subaortic stenosis that was produced by an obstructive anterior mitral leaflet. This leaflet was thick and redundant, with superiorly protruding blood cysts that caused severe left ventricular outflow tract obstruction.

Additional findings included mild fusion of the anterolateral and posteromedial papillary muscle groups, but with two foci of chordal attachment (and hence not regarded as a parachute mitral valve); failure of formation of the interchordal spaces of the chordae to the anterolateral papillary muscle, but with interchordal spaces present between the chordae to the posteromedial papillary muscle; mild congenital mitral regurgitation with jet lesions on the atrial surface of the anterior mitral leaflet; mild myxomatous thickening of the aortic valve leaflets; failure of formation of the interchordal spaces of the anterior tricuspid leaflet, with a hemodynamically insignificant blood cyst on the atrial surface of the septal leaflet of the tricuspid valve; mild thickening of the pulmonary valvar leaflets with mild pulmonary valvar stenosis; polyvalvar disease, all four valves being abnormal (as earlier), suggesting the possibility of a chromosomal or genetic anomaly (not further investigated in 1969); massive concentric left ventricular hypertrophy with myocardial fibrosis; left atrial hypertrophy and enlargement; intact atrial and ventricular septa with normal segmental anatomy, that is {S,D,S}; and MCAs: mildly low-set ears, antimongoloid slant of the eyes, short and mildly webbed neck, mild shield chest, protruding lower jaw with malocclusion, and accessory lobation of both lungs. This patient died after an anoxic spell.

It is noteworthy that tissue related to the anterior mitral leaflet often causes fibrous subaortic stenosis, particularly when the segmental anatomy is normal with normally related great arteries, and made worse when the ventricular septum is intact (i.e., when there is no "escape" into the RV and pulmonary artery). Indeed, **this is what fibrous subaortic stenosis is: abnormal fibrous tissue related to the anterior mitral leaflet.**

Case 108, a 1-month-and-8-day-old girl, had severe left ventricular outflow tract obstruction caused by small knob-like masses of myxomatous tissue of the anterior leaflet of the mitral valve that largely filled the subaortic left ventricular outflow tract, reducing its patent lumen to 1.5 × 1.5 mm.

This patient's congenital mitral stenosis was severe, characterized by thick myxomatous leaflet tissue attached to the ventricular septal crest. The mitral orifice measured only 4 mm in internal dimension in the fresh state. *The mitral tensor apparatus was absent, with no chordae tendineae and no papillary muscles.*

There was normal segmental anatomy—{S,D,S}. A probe-patent foramen ovale, a conoventricular type of VSD (3 × 4 mm), a closing PDA, and an aberrant right subclavian artery were also found. Moderate left ventricular hypoplasia, right atrial hypertrophy and enlargement, and right ventricular hypertrophy and enlargement were also present.

A rare and unexpected finding was **ventriculoatrial malalignment.** The mitral valve was almost unable to open into the LV because of *rightward malposition of the ventricles relative to the atria.* This ventriculoatrial malalignment may help explain the presence of congenital mitral stenosis *with no tensor apparatus*—a rare form of congenital mitral stenosis. It is worth recalling that the atria are relatively fixed in position by the venae cavae and the pulmonary veins, whereas the ventricular loop is a "professional contortionist" (see Chapter 2), which can result in ventriculoatrial malalignment, as in this patient. During this patient's gestation, her mother had a brain tumor; information concerning the mother's therapy is not known to us. Regarding this patient's severe left ventricular outflow tract obstruction, again the cause was obstructive fibrous tissue related to the anterior mitral leaflet.

Case 142 was a 6-day-old premature boy with a birth weight of 2000 g (4 lb 6.5 oz) and an estimated gestational age of 33 weeks (8¼ months). The nature of this patient's subaortic left ventricular outflow tract obstruction was more challenging because autopsy revealed *no discrete fibrous or muscular narrowing.* Instead, the patient was found to have a *dysmorphic LV* with abnormal left ventricular muscle bundles, and abnormal left ventricular septal architecture with multiple VSDs: a relatively large apical muscular defect (3 mm in internal dimension) and a high small membranous defect.

This patient had a rare form of bicuspid (bicommissural) aortic valve without aortic stenosis. *The LC/NC commissure was absent.* This is the commissure that almost always is well formed both in bicommissural and in unicommissural aortic valves. But rarely, the LC/NC commissure can be absent, as this case illustrates.

The patient also had multiple secundum ASDs caused by fenestrations within the septum primum, a relatively frequent defect. This patient also had MCAs: microphthalmos, low-set ears, absent right radius, Meckel diverticulum, a bifid T5 vertebra, and agenesis of the corpus callosum.

To summarize, this patient's left ventricular outflow tract obstruction was thought *not* to be related to a discrete fibrous or muscular obstruction of the left ventricular outflow tract, but rather to be associated with a dysmorphic LV in the setting of MCAs.

Case 147, a 10 2/12-year-old girl, had congenital mitral stenosis with a small annulus with thickened and fibrotic leaflets that caused left ventricular outflow tract obstruction. The interchordal spaces were obliterated by fibrous tissue. EFE of the LV was associated with fibrosis of the papillary muscles. This patient also had MCAs: a webbed neck and bilateral simian creases. (A simian crease is a single transverse palmar crease.) This patient's left ventricular outflow tract obstruction was produced by her thickened and fibrotic anterior mitral leaflet. The importance of the anterior leaflet of the mitral valve in producing subaortic left ventricular outflow tract obstruction is not surprising when one recalls that the anterior mitral leaflet forms the lateral aspect of the left ventricular outflow tract.

Case 198, a boy (age unknown by us), had ACM of the {S,D,L} type. As the segmental anatomy indicates, he had situs solitus of the viscera and atria, a concordant ventricular D-loop, and L-malposition of the great arteries, that is, {S,D,L}. The L-malposition of the great arteries was anatomically corrected, meaning that despite the malposition of the great arteries, each great artery originated above the anatomically correct ventricle: aorta above the morphologically LV, and pulmonary artery above the morphologically RV.[110] The patient had a subaortic conus with pulmonary-tricuspid and pulmonary-mitral fibrous continuity.

The patient also had congenital mitral stenosis with a functionally insignificant supramitral ring. The mitral ring was squeezed or compressed by a relatively huge anterolateral papillary muscle that inserted into the bottom of the conal septum. This muscle of Moulaert (or anterolateral muscle of the LV) produced severe *muscular* left ventricular outflow tract stenosis.[102]

This patient also had a very deficient ventricular septum, that is, a type C *common ventricle.*[21,22] Thus, this patient's heart exemplifies several rarities:

1. ACM {S,D,L} is rare. This segmental anatomic set is both anatomically corrected (as mentioned earlier) and physiologically corrected (because there is both AV and VA concordance).
2. ACM can indeed occur with a subaortic conus, as in this patient. A bilateral conus (subaortic and subpulmonary) is not essential to the morphogenesis of ACM, contrary to what we used to think.[106] In other words, for the ventricles to loop in one direction (say, to the right), and for conotruncus to twist in the opposite direction (to the left), resulting in ACM {S,**D,L**}, a bilateral conus is *not* necessary to completely disconnect the semilunar valves above from the AV valves below.
3. In congenital mitral stenosis, *muscular* subaortic stenosis can occur, even without aortic-mitral fibrous continuity, if a large muscle of Moulaert coexists.
4. *Common ventricle* does exist! Very rarely it is possible for the left ventricular sinus and the right ventricular sinus to be in common (unseparated), if the muscular interventricular septum is very deficient. It is noteworthy that *common*

ventricle, that is, left ventricular sinus and right ventricular sinus essentially unseparated, is anatomically very different from *single* ventricle.[21,22] In single LV, the right ventricular sinus is absent but the infundibulum is present. In single RV, the left ventricular sinus is absent, but the right ventricular sinus and the infundibulum are present.

Thus, in *common* ventricle, both ventricular sinuses (inflow tracts) are present; whereas in *single* ventricle, one ventricular sinus is absent.[21,22]

To summarize, in these 5 cases of congenital mitral stenosis without HLHS that also had left ventricular outflow tract obstruction, the obstruction was fibrous in 4 (80%, Cases 49, 108, 142, and 147) and muscular in 1 (20%, Case 198). The fibrous obstruction was caused by AV endocardial cushion tissue, that is, by tissue related to the anterior mitral leaflet. The muscular obstruction was caused by an anomalous anterolateral muscle of the LV (also known as the muscle of Moulaert).

TRISOMY

Of these 48 patients with congenital mitral stenosis, but without HLHS, 4 (8%) had a trisomy that was proved by karyotype (see Table 14.16). But what kind of trisomy (or trisomies) was (or were) present?

Case 13, a 34-day-old girl, has **trisomy 8** with translocation to the long arm of chromosome 13 (trisomy 8q13). She had TOF {S,D,S} with extremely severe pulmonary outflow tract stenosis, aortic-tricuspid direct fibrous continuity, and aortic-mitral *indirect* fibrous continuity via the tricuspid valve. The tricuspid and mitral valves were in fibrous continuity with each other. Because the aortic valve was right ventricular, this case could also be diagnosed as DORV {S,D,"S"} with a markedly stenotic subpulmonary conus. (We recorded both diagnoses.) There was a large secundum type of ASD (13 × 6 mm) because the septum primum was markedly deficient. Hence, this could be regarded as a case of **pentalogy of Fallot** with very marked aortic overriding, that is, an essentially right ventricular aorta. In 1990, when we did this case, we favored the diagnosis of tetralogy or pentalogy of Fallot, probably because we were less familiar with the relatively rare **DORV {S,D,"S"}**. Now I would favor the diagnosis of **DORV** because the aortic valve was right ventricular and because the aortic-mitral fibrous continuity was *indirect,* via the tricuspid valve.

There were bilateral SVCs, with a small RSVC to the RA, a larger LSVC connecting with the coronary sinus and draining into the RA, and with absence of the left innominate vein.

The tetralogy type of conoventricular VSD was considerably reduced in functional size because myxomatous mitral valve tissue bulged into the VSD from the left ventricular side.

Severe congenital mitral stenosis was characterized by marked myxomatous change of the leaflets, failure of formation of the interchordal spaces, reduction of the interpapillary muscle space, a large blood cyst of the posterior mitral leaflet, and extreme reduction of the mitral orifice (2 mm in internal dimension in the fresh state).

The MPA (3 mm in external diameter) and the right and left pulmonary artery branches (2.5 mm in external diameter) were markedly hypoplastic. The pulmonary valve was very stenotic, myxomatous, and unicommissural, with the only well-formed commissure being the nonseptal–left septal. The ductus arteriosus was closed, a ligamentum arteriosum being found. The aortic leaflets were thick and myxomatous, and the aortic valve was bicuspid and bicommissural: the LC/NC commissure was very poorly formed. *The latter is a rare finding.* Even in unicuspid and unicommissural aortic valves, the LC/NC commissure is the one that almost always is well formed. The tricuspid valve was also markedly myxomatous.

Polyvalvar disease was present, with all valves being anomalous: mitral, aortic, tricuspid, and pulmonary (as described previously). Polyvalvar disease should suggest that a trisomy may be present, as it definitely was in this patient (trisomy 8). *Small MAPCAs* (major aortopulmonary collateral arteries) were also found in this patient with extremely pulmonary outflow tract stenosis. *An aberrant right subclavian artery* was present.

MCAs were also very prominent in this case of *trisomy 8.* Dysmorphic features included a square head, micrognathia, cleft tip of the tongue, hypoplastic nipples, webbed neck, vaginal tag, digital contractures, plantar clefts, sacral dimple, diffuse cerebral atrophy, mild bilateral hydronephrosis, hypoparathyroidism with marked hypocalcemia, esophageal reflux with feeding difficulties and vomiting, malrotation of the gastrointestinal tract, nasopharyngeal reflux, seizure activity with eye rolling and hypertonicity, and a mobile colon.

The other three patients all had **trisomy 18.**

Case 72, a 4-month-old girl, had trisomy 18 with clenched fists, flexed great toes, a fibrous defect of the clavicles, a short sternum, diastasis recti, pancreatic ectopia in the pylorus and duodenum, Meckel diverticulum, underdeveloped olfactory bulbs and cribriform plate, malformation of the middle ear, partial defect of the diaphragm, incomplete rotation of the kidneys, double renal arteries, urachal cysts, hypoplasia of the iliac arteries, delayed and irregular development of the skeletal muscles, a high-arched palate, and a high thymus.

The cardiovascular findings included congenital mitral stenosis with hypoplasia of the mitral annulus, a small patent foramen ovale, venous hypertrophy within the lungs, pulmonary arterial hypertension with pulmonary arteriosclerosis, a PDA, a conoventricular type of VSD, a persistent LSVC to the coronary sinus, and bilateral azygos veins.

Case 86, a 7-day-old girl, had trisomy 18 with congenital mitral stenosis with typical parachute mitral valve, that is, with absence of the anterolateral papillary muscle. The mitral leaflets were myxomatous, and all of the chordae tendineae inserted into the posteromedial papillary muscle. Additional findings included a large conoventricular type of VSD and a PDA .

Case 95 was a stillborn male fetus with an estimated gestational age of 37½ weeks. Trisomy 18 was associated with congenital mitral stenosis and parachute mitral valve. In this patient, the mitral valve was markedly hypoplastic and the posteromedial papillary muscle group was absent—the opposite of the situation found in the previous case. A very small anterolateral papillary muscle group received all of the mitral chordae tendineae, and the interchordal spaces were absent. A large conoventricular type of VSD (10 × 6 mm) was present.

The tricuspid valve was abnormal with redundant leaflets and hypoplastic papillary muscles. The pulmonary valve was bicuspid and its leaflets were redundant. The aortic valve was also bicuspid because of underdevelopment of the RC/NC commissure, and its leaflets were redundant. The septum primum was also redundant, but the foramen ovale was competent nonetheless. (Recall that the foramen ovale is a unidirectional flap-valve in utero.) The LV was mildly underdeveloped, and was much smaller than the RV, which was hypertrophied and enlarged. The ductus arteriosus was patent, as expected prenatally.

Dr. Rumiko Matsuoka et al[111] described the phenotypic expression of complete and partial trisomy 18. In 12 autopsied cases of full trisomy 18 and in 3 autopsied cases of partial trisomy 18, congenital heart disease was present in all. Polyvalvar disease occurred in 100%, membranous (or conoventricular) VSD in 87%, PDA in 73%, and high take-off of the right coronary ostium in 80%. No differences in cardiac pathology were recognized between patients with partial trisomy 18 (n = 3) and those with full trisomy 18 (n = 12).[111] Redundant and dysplastic valves, as in Case 95, were characteristic.[111]

Double-Orifice Mitral Valve

Of these 48 autopsied patients with congenital mitral stenosis without HLHS, DOMV occurred in 3 (6%; see Table 14.16). Because DOMV with congenital mitral stenosis is infrequent and therefore unfamiliar,[104,112] these 3 patients will be presented in detail.

Sex: Male, 1; female, 2; male to female = 0.5.

Age at Death: Mean, 67.33 ± 34.20 days; range, 28 to 90 days; and median, 84 days.

Case 61, a 3-month-old boy, had DOMV[104] with congenital mitral stenosis. There was a 4- to 5-mm long central fibrous tissue tongue between the anterior and posterior mitral leaflets (surgical description, as seen from the atrial aspect). This patient also had TGA {S,D,D} with a subaortic conus and pulmonary-mitral fibrous continuity. There was no demonstrable subaortic gradient, and the transposed pulmonary artery overrode the ventricular septum. There was a large subpulmonary conoventricular type of VSD, and a large secundum type of ASD.

Additional findings included marked stenosis of the right atrial ostium of the coronary sinus. A small persistent LSVC connected the obstructed coronary sinus to the left innominate vein and then to the RSVC and RA.

A coronary anomaly was also found. The left coronary artery originated via a small ostium from the right coronary sinus of Valsalva of the transposed aortic valve, originating just to the left of the normally arising right coronary artery. The left coronary artery then ran posteriorly, to the right of the large transposed pulmonary valve. Then the left coronary artery turned leftward, behind the pulmonary valve where it gave off the left circumflex coronary. Then proceeding further leftward and anteriorly, this anomalously arising coronary artery then supplied the territory of the left anterior descending coronary artery. This anomalously originating left coronary artery was never intramural.

Because of the impression that subaortic (conal) stenosis was present, despite the absence of a demonstrable gradient (there was a large VSD with a large wide-open overriding pulmonary artery), in 1990 a Damus-Kaye-Stansel procedure was done at 3 months of age, with closure of the VSD by a clamshell device in the operating room, leading to death 2 days postoperatively. So this case illustrates that DOMV[104] did not occur in isolation but was part of complex congenital heart disease.

Let us postpone detailed consideration of the DOMV with congenital MS until all 3 cases have been presented. Remember that this DOMV looked like a central tongue of fibrous tissue connecting the anterior and posterior mitral leaflets, dividing the mitral orifice into approximately equal anterolateral and posteromedial orifices. The question for consideration will be: what is the detailed anatomy of the mitral valve in this type of DOMV?

Case 75, a 4-week-old girl, had congenital mitral stenosis with DOMV. Again, the anterolateral and posteromedial mitral orifices were approximately equal in size, separated by a thin and redundant appearing tongue of mitral valve tissue.

The tensor apparatus was very abnormal. The anterolateral papillary muscle group was small, the posteromedial papillary muscle group was much larger, and both papillary muscle groups were confluent or fused, reducing the interpapillary muscle distance to zero.

We thought that this patient had a forme fruste of parachute mitral valve. The severe congenital mitral stenosis had both a valvar and a subvalvar (papillary muscle) component. There was no stenosing supramitral ring. Left atrial hypertrophy was marked (3 mm in thickness) and there was EFE of the LA. A moderate-sized secundum type of ASD was present. Subaortic stenosis was produced by a prominent muscle of Moulaert (anterolateral muscle of the LV).

Other important findings included a conoventricular type of VSD, a preductal coarctation of the aorta, right atrial hypertrophy and enlargement (wall 2- to 3-mm thick), and marked right ventricular hypertrophy and enlargement (11- to 14-mm thick). Thus, multiple levels of left heart obstruction were present: at the mitral leaflets (DOMV), papillary muscles (confluent, with no interpapillary muscle distance), left ventricular subaortic outflow tractor (muscle of Moulaert), and preductal coarctation of the aorta.

Case 115, an 11-week-old girl, had congenital mitral stenosis with a diastolic gradient of 3 mm Hg between the LA and the LV measured at cardiac catheterization. DOMV was found, the anterolateral mitral orifice being smaller than the posteromedial. Again, the impression was that a bridge of fibrous tissue connected the anterior and posterior mitral leaflets. A secundum ASD coexisted, with a large left-to-right shunt at the atrial level, in part because of the presence of congenital mitral stenosis. In 1977, this combination of congenital mitral stenosis, a large secundum ASD, and a large left-to-right shunt at the atrial level was regarded as an example of the **congenital Lutembacher syndrome.**

In 1916, **Rene Lutembacher** (1884–1968) of Paris, France described the combination of an ASD with mitral stenosis, which is almost always the result of acquired rheumatic valvulitis. The additional adjective, *congenital* Lutembacher syndrome, is intended to indicate that the mitral stenosis is congenital (not acquired). The secundum ASD is, of course, always congenital in both the congenital and the acquired forms of the Lutembacher syndrome.

The LV was moderately hypoplastic. Five muscular VSDs were found, and right ventricular hypertrophy and enlargement were also present. (When not stated, one may assume that the segmental anatomy was normal, i.e., {S,D,S}.)

What Is DOMV Anatomically and Developmentally? I will attempt to answer this question based not only on the aforementioned three cases, but also based on our study by Baño-Rodrigo et al[104] of 27 autopsied cases of DOMV.

An anomaly of the tensor apparatus was always found consisting of:

1. a chordal ring;
2. an accessory papillary muscle or muscles;
3. a subdividing muscular ridge; or
4. a central fibrous subdivision.

More than one of these anomalies often coexisted in a single case.

DOMV almost always consisted of abnormal holes in essentially normal leaflets. In other words, DOMV almost never consisted of abnormal fibrous bridges or adhesions between normal leaflets. Consequently, when viewed from above (from the atrial aspect, the surgeon's view), what often looks like abnormal tongues of fibrous tissue between the two mitral orifices should not be transected to join the two mitral orifices together, thereby "curing" the DOMV. Instead, if one does that, the surgeon will discover that he or she has cut through normal mitral leaflet tissue and supporting chordae tendineae, resulting in iatrogenic mitral regurgitation.

The intraoperative diagnostic problem is that the abnormal tensor apparatus of the mitral valve—the real anomaly—can be well seen and well understood only by viewing the mitral valve from *below,* from the ventricular aspect, a view not normally possible for the naked-eye cardiac surgeon.

What Is a Chordal Ring? A chordal ring is an abnormal ring of chordae tendineae inserting into the ventricular surface of the mitral valve, often close to the anterolateral or the posteromedial commissure (Figs. 14.32 and 14.33). Why is there an opening (an orifice) in the middle of a chordal ring? My best hypothesis is the following. There appears to be *an inverse relationship between leaflet tissue and chordae tendineae.* It reminds me of the law of conservation of mass and energy in physics: It's either mass *or* energy.

Similarly, the mitral valve leaflet tissue and chordae tendineae are composed of AV endocardial cushion tissue. There is only so much endocardial cushion tissue, and it forms either leaflet tissue or chordae tendineae. The AV endocardial cushions can produce *either* mitral leaflet tissue *or* mitral chorea tendineae at one location. The endocardial cushions cannot produce *both* leaflet tissue *and* chordae tendineae at the same site.

What happens when an abnormal ring of chordae inserts into the ventricular surface of the AV endocardial cushions? The cushion tissue forms an abnormal chordal ring. Within the chordal ring there is a hole—no leaflet tissue. Why? Because the cushion tissue has all been used up forming these abnormal chordae. So, there is no endocardial cushion tissue left to form leaflet tissue inside (within) the chordal ring. Why not? Because the amount of AV endocardial cushion tissue is limited, not unlimited. This is the morphogenetic hypothesis concerning the formation of DOMV that the anatomic data strongly suggest.

Consider the normal mitral valve. At the middle of the anterior mitral leaflet, leaflet tissue is maximal and chordae tendineae are minimal. As one progresses toward either commissure, the leaflet tissue decreases and the chordae tendineae increase. At the commissures, the leaflet tissue is minimal and the chordae are maximal.

In other words, there is an inverse relationship between leaflet tissue and chordae tendineae:

1. At the center of abnormal anterior mitral leaflet, leaflet tissue is maximal and chordae tendineae are minimal.
2. At the mitral commissures, normally the leaflet tissue is minimal and the chordae tendineae are maximal.

This inverse relationship between leaflet tissue and chordae tendineae is also exemplified by the anatomy of DOMV, as earlier. This normal inverse relationship between chordae and leaflet tissue also appears to explain why anomalies of the tensor apparatus and particularly of the chordae tendineae can result in DOMV. **Briefly, to understand these leaflet malformations, study the chordae tendineae, because the tensor apparatus, especially the chordae, are the real "villains."**

As noted previously, if one has a relatively small chordal ring, it looks as though all of the endocardial cushion tissue is used to form these abnormal chordae, with nothing left within the ring to form leaflet tissue, resulting in an accessory mitral orifice (see Figs. 14.32 and 14.33). A small chordal ring can insert directly into the subjacent left ventricular free wall, *without any intervening papillary muscles,* as in Fig. 14.32C. Or a chordal ring surrounding a small accessory anterolateral orifice can insert into a *high, small anterolateral papillary muscle,* as in Fig.14.32B. Note that the chordal ring surrounding the small anterolateral mitral orifice all insert into the high, small anterolateral papillary muscle (see Fig. 14.32B), whereas the chordae of the much larger chordal ring that surrounds the large posteromedial mitral office all insert into the large posteromedial papillary muscle (see Fig. 14.32A). Hence, *a double parachute mitral valve* may be said to exist because all of the chordae tendineae surrounding each mitral orifice insert into only one papillary muscle.

Fig. 14.32 presents the type of DOMV that was originally reported in the first known case by Greenfield[113] in 1876: the AV canal was divided into separate mitral and tricuspid valves, and there was small accessory anterolateral mitral orifice and a much larger main posteromedial mitral orifice.

In our patient (see Fig. 14.32), the small accessory anterolateral mitral orifice was thought to be of little or no functional importance. But that is not always the case (see Fig. 14.33). In this patient, there was severe congenital mitral regurgitation via the accessory anterolateral orifice. As seen from the left atrial perspective (see Fig. 14.33A), the accessory anterolateral orifice was much larger than in the previous patient (see Fig. 14.32A). The main posteromedial mitral orifice is even larger.

To comprehend this case of DOMV with a regurgitant accessory anterolateral orifice, one must examine the mitral valve

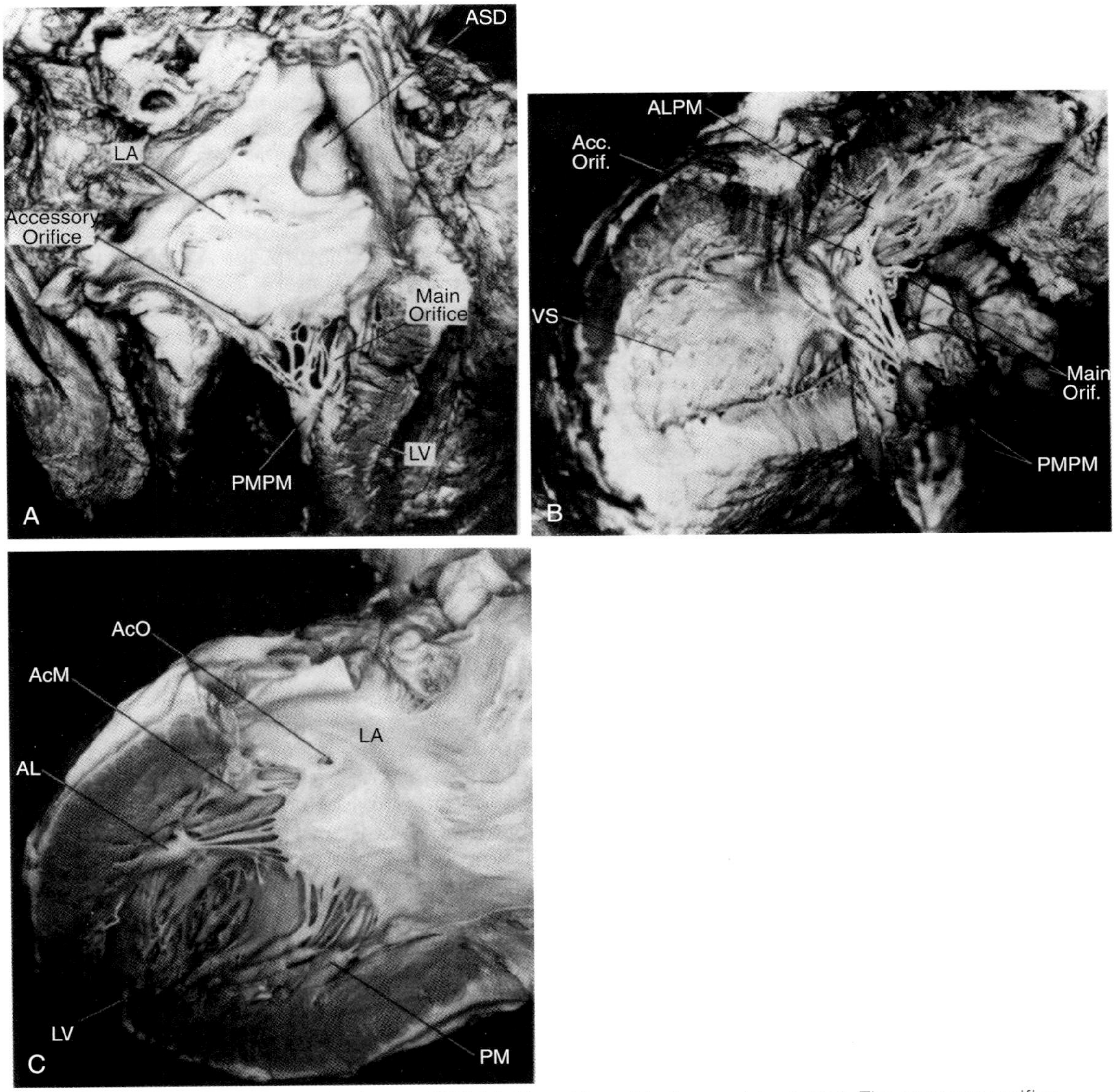

Fig. 14.32 Double-orifice mitral valve (DOMV). The atrioventricular canal is divided. The accessory orifice is at the anterolateral commissure. (A) Left atrial *(LA)* view, Case 1. (B) Left ventricular *(LV)* view, Case 1. (C) Left atrial (LA) and left ventricular view, Case 3. In these two patients, DOMV was of no functional significance. From the left atrial aspect, the accessory mitral orifice resembles a hole in the mitral leaflet tissue at the anterolateral commissure. From the LV aspect, there is a high, small anterolateral papillary muscle *(ALPM)*. In B, note how much smaller the ALPM is compared with the much larger posteromedial papillary muscle *(PMPM)*. Note also that there is a ring of chordae from the small ALPM that inserts into the margin of the small accessory orifice *(Acc Orif)*. The chordae tendineae from the larger PMPM insert only into the margins of the main mitral orifice *(Main Orif)*. This creates DOMV, with a small accessory anterolateral mitral orifice, and a much larger main posteromedial mitral orifice. (C) The accessory mitral orifice *(AcO)* is located at the anterolateral commissure, and the AcO is very small (1 × 3 mm). A ring of small chordae tendineae extends from the circular margins of the small AcO and inserts directly into the left ventricular septal *(VS)* surface, without intervening papillary muscles. *AcM,* Accessory papillary muscle; *ALPM,* antero-lateral papillary muscle. (Reproduced with permission from Baño-Rodrigo A, Van Praagh S, Trowitzsch E, Van Praagh R. Double-orifice mitral valve: A study of 27 postmortem cases with developmental, diagnostic, and surgical considerations. *Am J Cardiol.* 1988;61:152.)

from the ventricular perspective to understand the anomalies of the tensor apparatus—the chordae tendineae and the papillary muscles. The anterolateral papillary muscle of the LV is abnormally large and low. The posteromedial papillary muscle appears normal. The chordae tendineae from the anterior and posterior mitral leaflets insert into both the anterolateral and posteromedial papillary muscle groups, embracing the larger and functionally unremarkable main posteromedial mitral orifice. There is a high, small, accessory anterosuperior papillary muscle above the anterosuperior mitral orifice. The mitral leaflet tissue at the

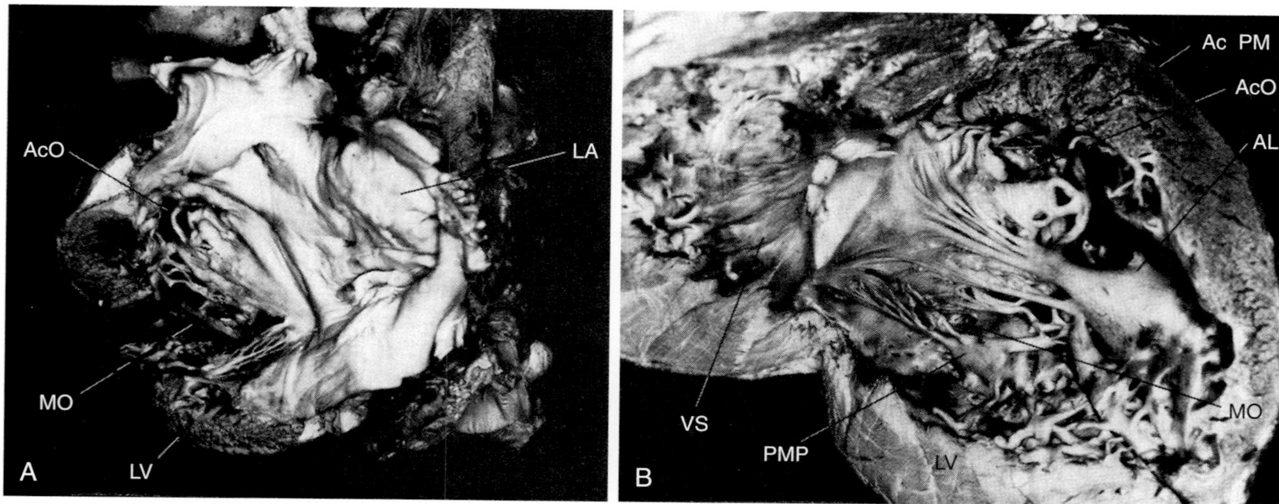

Fig. 14.33 Double-orifice mitral valve with divided atrioventricular canal and accessory anterolateral mitral orifice with severe congenital mitral regurgitation through the accessory anterolateral orifice. (A) View from the left atrium *(LA)* showing the large accessory anterolateral mitral orifice *(AcO)*. The somewhat larger main orifice *(MO)* is posteromedial. (B) View of the opened left ventricle *(LV)* showing an abnormally large and low anterolateral papillary muscle *(ALP)* muscle. A smaller posteromedial papillary *(PMP)* muscle is seen in the expected location. But above the ALPM, there is an abnormal superior accessory papillary muscle *(Ac PM)* and a large poorly supported AcO. Thickened and rolled chordae tendineae from the anterosuperior accessory orifice insert into both the large ALP muscle and abnormal anterosuperior accessory papillary muscle. The MO has chordae tendineae inserting into the ALP muscle and into the PMP muscle. So, this is the three-papillary-muscle type of DOMV, and the accessory mitral orifice was very important because it permitted severe mitral regurgitation. *VS*, Ventricular septum. (Reproduced with permission from Bafio-Rodrigo et A Baño-Rodrigo, S Van Praagh, E Trowitzsch, P Hernandez-Latuff, R Van Praagh. Double-orifice atrioventricular valves: pathologic anatomy in 28 postmortem cases with diagnostic and surgical implications. In: EF Doyle, MA Engle, WM Gersony, WJ Rashkind, NS Talner (Eds.). Pediatric Cardiology, Springer-Verlag, New York (1986), pp. 915-919.)

anterosuperior commissure insert into the high, small accessory papillary muscle superiorly and into the large anterolateral papillary muscle inferiorly. The two papillary muscles of the regurgitant anterosuperior orifice are very poorly matched; the upper is too high and too small, and the lower is too low and too large.

In this patient there are *three papillary muscles:* anterolateral, posteromedial, and accessory anterosuperior. This mitral valve has *three foci of chordal insertion,* not the normal two. The anterolateral commissural portion of the mitral valve is poorly supported. The thickened and rolled chordae tendineae and leaflet tissue bordering the anterolateral orifice of the mitral valve bear silent testimony to the severe mitral regurgitation that occurred through this abnormal opening.

The "law" of the mitral valve is as follows: Whenever there are two foci of chordal insertion, a mitral orifice normally forms between these foci. In this patient (see Fig. 14.33B), there are three papillary muscles, that is, three focus of chordal insertion. Consequently, there are two mitral orifices:

1. between the anterolateral and the posteromedial papillary muscles, this main posteromedial orifice being the normal mitral orifice; and
2. between the small accessory anterosuperior papillary muscle (an abnormal papillary muscle) and the large anterolateral papillary muscle, forming an abnormal and poorly supported accessory anterosuperior orifice.

Thus, the presence of three papillary muscles receiving chordal insertion results in two mitral orifices. This is **the three papillary muscle type of DOMV.**

Another anatomic type of DOMV is **the subdividing muscular ridge type** with congenital mitral stenosis (Fig. 14.34). Viewed from the surgical left atrial perspective, one can see that the mitral orifice is subdivided by a prominent muscular ridge into a larger posteromedial orifice and a smaller anterolateral orifice (see Fig. 14.34A). However, to really understand, one must examine the mitral valve from below, from the ventricular perspective (see Fig. 14.34B). The ventricular view, which can be assessed by modern imaging modalities (two-dimensional echo, three-dimensional echo, magnetic resonance imaging [MRI], etc.), reveals a prominent muscular ridge that runs from the anterolateral papillary muscle group into the mitral orifice, subdividing it. Multiple muscular VSDs are also seen. This patient had a *left ventricular myocardial anomaly* that was confluent with the anterolateral papillary muscle.

DOMV with approximately equal-sized anterolateral and posteromedial orifices, similar to Cases 61 and 75, is presented in Figs. 14.35 and 14.36.[112] In Fig. 14.35A, one can see the appearance from the atrial level (the surgeon's perspective). The anterior leaflet of the mitral valve forms a V-shaped wedge of tissue, subdividing the mitral orifice into approximately equal–sized anterolateral and posteromedial openings. But why? The ventricular view provides the answer (see Fig. 14.35B). Between the anterolateral and the posteromedial papillary muscles, there is a middle papillary muscle arising from the left ventricular free wall that receives chordal insertions from both the anterior and the posterior mitral leaflets.

Another way of getting an abnormally central papillary muscle that receives chordae tendineae from both the anterior and

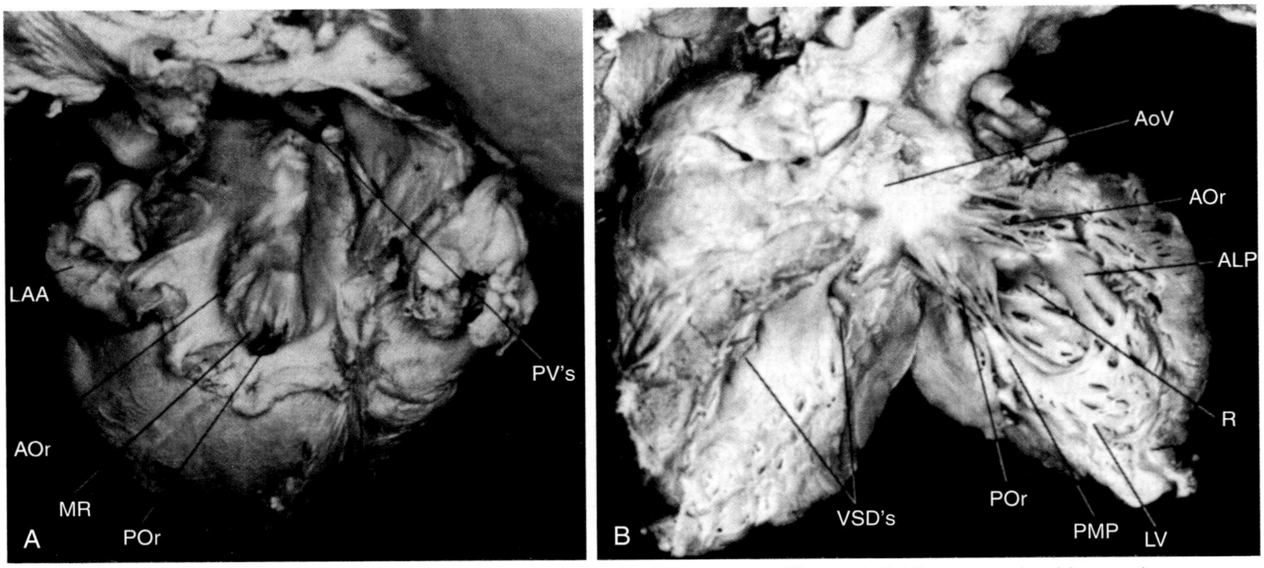

Fig. 14.34 Double-orifice mitral valve with anterolateral accessory orifice, subdividing muscular ridge, and congenital mitral stenosis. (A) View of the left atrium from above showing the posterior mitral orifice *(POr)*, the anterior mitral orifice *(AOr)*, and the subdividing muscular ridge *(MR)*. (B) shows the opened left ventricle *(LV)*. The subdividing muscular ridge *(R)* is confluent with the anterolateral papillary muscle *(ALP)*. R subdivides the mitral valve into an accessory (smaller) anterolateral orifice (AOr), and into the main (larger) posteromedial mitral orifice (POr). The posteromedial papillary muscle *(PMP)* is unremarkable. Multiple muscular ventricular septal defects *(VSDs)* are present. R appears to be an abnormal dorsal and medial extension of the ALP muscle group. *AoV*, Aortic valve; *LAA*, left atrial appendage; *PVs*, pulmonary veins. (Reproduced with permission from Baño-Rodrigo A, Van Praagh S, Trowitzsch E, Van Praagh R. Double-orifice mitral valve: A study of 27 postmortem cases with developmental, diagnostic, and surgical considerations. *Am J Cardiol*. 1988;61:152.)

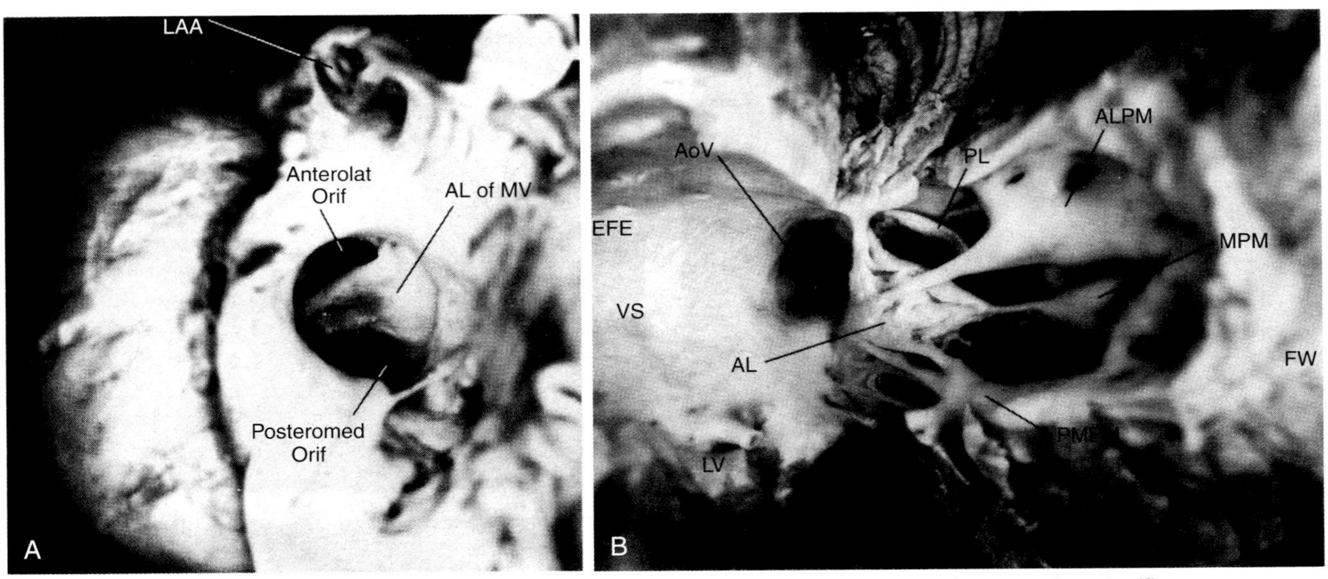

Fig. 14.35 Double-orifice mitral valve (MV) with a divided atrioventricular canal and an anterolateral orifice *(Anterolat Orif)* and a posteromedial orifice *(Posteromed Orif)* that were approximately equal in size. (A) A view of the left atrium and (B) a view of the left ventricle *(LV)*. In B, one sees that the anterior leaflet *(AL)* of the MV *(AL of MV)* is attached by chordae tendineae to a medial papillary muscle *(MPM)*. The AL of the MV forms a V-shaped wedge of MV tissue that subdivides the mitral orifice into approximately equal superior and inferior portions. This MPM arises from the left ventricular free wall (LVFW) below the ALP muscle and above the PMP muscle. *ALPM*, anterolateral papillary muscle; *AoV*, aortic valve; *EFE*, Endocardial fibroelastosis; *LAA*, left atrial appendage; *PL*, posterior leaflet; *VS*, ventricular septum. (Reproduced with permission from Baño-Rodrigo A, Van Praagh S, Trowitzsch E, Van Praagh R. Double-orifice mitral valve: A study of 27 postmortem cases with developmental, diagnostic, and surgical considerations. *Am J Cardiol*. 1988;61:152.)

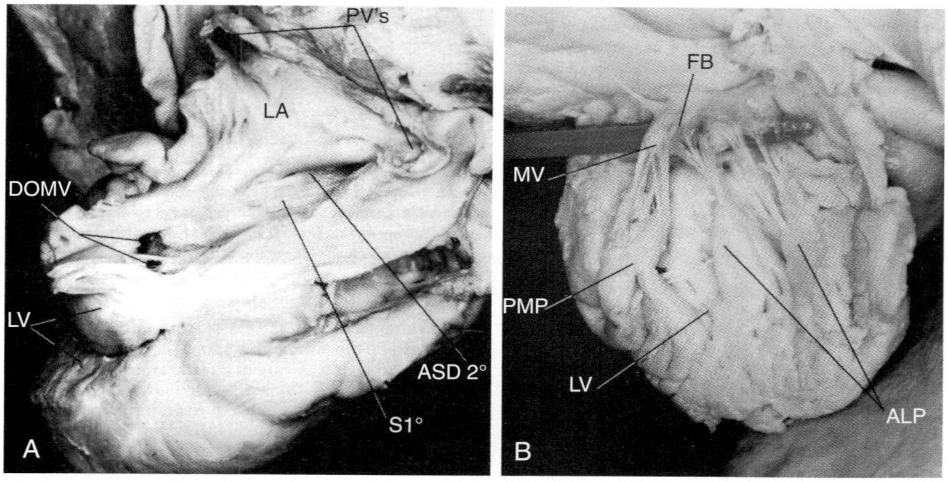

Fig. 14.36 Double-orifice mitral valve *(DOMV)* with a divided atrioventricular canal and with approximately equal-sized superior and inferior orifices, as is seen in the left atrial *(LA)* view in (A). (B) The left ventricular *(LV)* view shows that the anterolateral papillary *(ALP)* muscle and the posteromedial papillary *(PMP)* muscle are too close together, being fused at their bases. There is a fibrous bridge *(FB)* between the anterior and posterior leaflets (A). (B) The ALP muscle and the PMP muscle are artificially separated by largely invisible pins, in order to show the subdividing FB from below. *ASD 2°*, Ostium secundum type of atrial septal defect; *MV*, mitral valve; *S1°*, septum primum. (Reproduced with permission from Baño-Rodrigo A, Van Praagh S, Trowitzsch E, Van Praagh R. Double-orifice mitral valve: a study of 27 postmortem cases with developmental, diagnostic, and surgical considerations. *Am J Cardiol.* 1988;61:152, 1988.)

posterior mitral leaflets is shown in Fig. 14.36. This patient had anterolateral and posteromedial papillary muscles that were abnormally close together, and fused at their bases.

Fig. 14.36A shows the left atrial view. A fibrous bridge between the anterior and posterior mitral leaflets subdivides the mitral orifice into two approximately equal–sized anterolateral and posteromedial mitral orifices. In Fig. 14.36B, the subdividing fibrous bridge is seen from below, that is, from the ventricular viewpoint.

When the chordae tendineae from both the anterior and the posterior mitral leaflets insert into the same central papillary muscle, this produces a commissure in the middle of the mitral orifice. *Commissura* (*commissurae*, plural) means "a joining together" in Latin. This joining together of the anterior and posterior mitral leaflets in the middle of the mitral orifice produces the central fibrous bridge seen from above and below in Fig. 14.25.

Double-orifice of the mitral component of a common AV valve also occurs, as was presented by Baño-Rodrigo et al.[112] This might be called *potentially DOMV; potentially* means "following surgical septation of the common AV canal into mitral and tricuspid canals." A common AV valve can have an accessory mitral orifice at the anterolateral commissure (see Fig. 14.26) or at the posteromedial commissure (Fig. 14.37) of the mitral component of the common AV valve.

In Fig. 14.38, there is an accessory orifice at the anterolateral commissure of the potentially mitral valve. Why? Because of the abnormal tensor apparatus. This patient has an anterolateral papillary muscle. But above that there is an accessory anterosuperior papillary muscle. Thus, the mitral portion of this superior leaflet of this common AV valve has two foci of chordal insertion: the anterolateral papillary muscle below, and the accessory anterosuperior papillary muscle above. Consequently, there is an accessory orifice in the superior leaflet of this common AV valve. Remember the *"law" of the mitral valve:* between two foci of chordal insertion there is a mitral orifice. Why? If the superior leaflet endocardial cushion tissue had not been used to make chordae tendineae to insert into the abnormal accessory anterosuperior papillary muscle, then this endocardial cushion tissue would have formed leaflet tissue, and there would be no accessory orifice in the superior leaflet of this completely common AV valve (type C of Rastelli). This process is what I likened to the law of conservation of mass and energy. As in Einstein's famous equation, $E = mc^2$ (energy = mass multiplied by the speed of light squared), matter exists either as energy or as matter, that is, either as an atomic explosion or as uranium 235, but not as both at the same time.

By analogy, because there is only a certain amount of it, AV endocardial cushion tissue can form a leaflet or chordae, but not both in the same place at the same time. If an abnormal papillary muscle encourages the formation of abnormal chordae tendineae (or vice versa), then there will be an abnormal orifice, because the endocardial tissue has been used to form chordae, not leaflet.

As noted previously, another way to express this same principle is to say that there is *an inverse relationship between leaflet tissue and chordae tendineae in the formation of the mitral valve:* the more chordae tendineae present, the less leaflet tissue and vice versa.

In this same patient (see Fig. 14.38), note that the posteromedial papillary muscle is hypoplastic, poorly formed, and fused with the undersurface of the anterolateral papillary muscle. Note also that the inferior leaflet of the common AV valve inserts only into the anterolateral papillary muscle. The superior leaflet of the common AV valve also inserts, in part, into the anterolateral papillary muscle (see Fig. 14.38). Thus, the main orifice of the mitral component of this common AV valve is

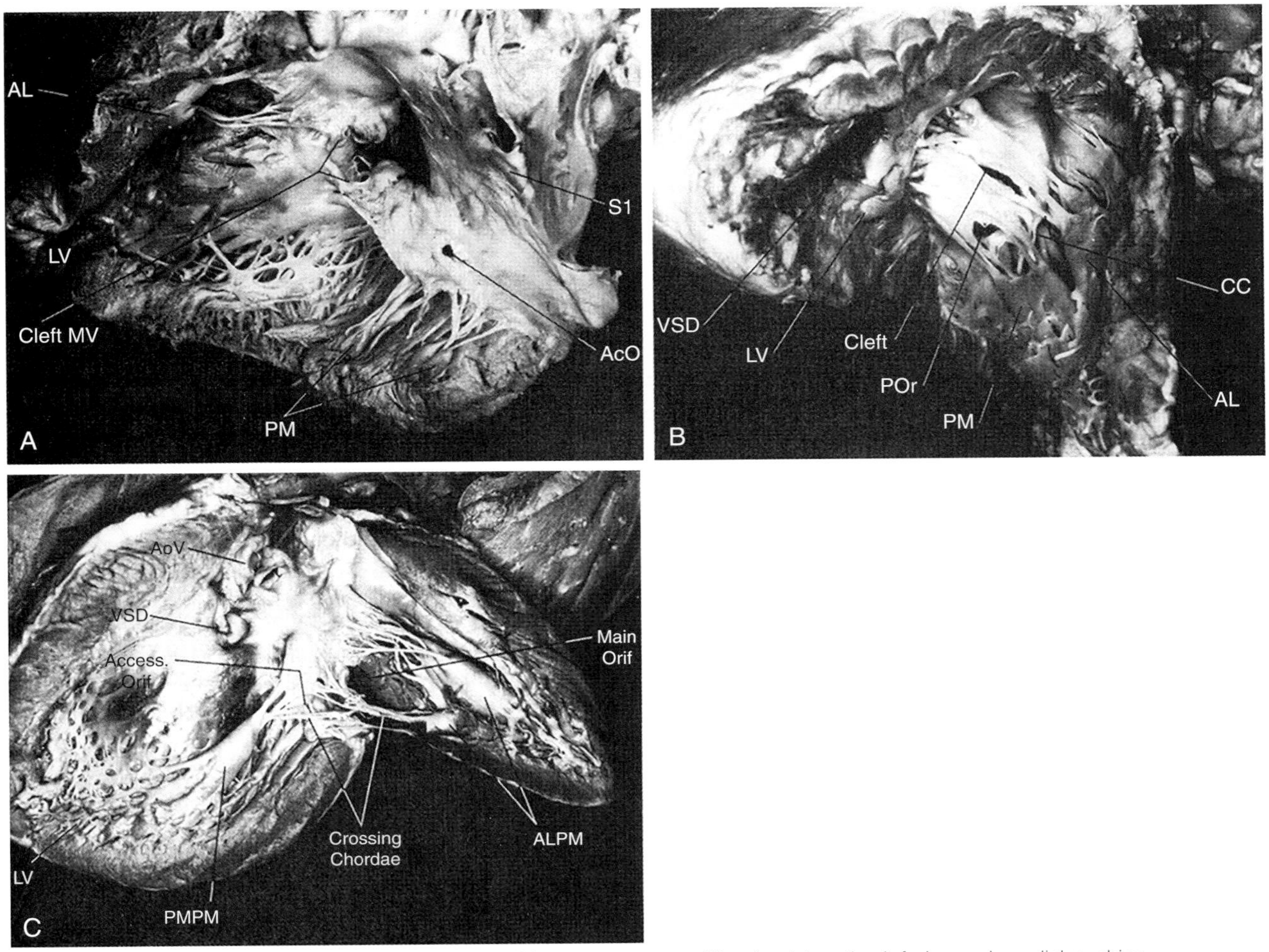

Fig. 14.37 Double-orifice mitral valve with an accessory orifice involving the inferior endocardial cushion component of the mitral valve (MV). (A) This patient has complete common atrioventricular canal (CAVV) type A, showing the opened left atrium, atrioventricular valve, and left ventricle *(LV)*. Note the accessory orifice *(AcO)* of the mitral component of this CAVV at the posteromedial commissure. Beneath this accessory orifice (AcO), there is an abnormal ring of chordae tendineae inserting into the posteromedial papillary musculature *(PM)*. This accessory orifice was thought to be of little or no physiologic significance. Note also septum primum *(S1)*, the cleft in the anterior mitral component of the CAVV, and the anterolateral papillary musculature *(AL)*. (B) Left ventricular view of a patient with CAVV type A. The cleft orifice is the main opening of the mitral component of this CAVV. Above the cleft orifice *(Cleft)* is the superior leaflet component, and below the cleft orifice is the inferior leaflet component. There is a prominent accessory mitral orifice *(POr)* just above the PM. The AL and the PM papillary muscle are abnormally close to each other; they are fused at their bases. The inferior leaflet inserts into the PM papillary muscle group (which is "normal") and into the nearby AL papillary muscle (which is abnormal). The latter is *crossing chordae:* inferior leaflet chordae inserting into the superior (AL) papillary muscle. We think this is why there is an abnormal posteromedial accessory mitral orifice *(Access orif):* the abnormal insertions of the inferior leaflet into the PM papillary muscle group ("normal") and also into the anterolateral (AL) papillary muscle group (abnormal), by means of the abnormal crossing chordae *(CC)*. (C) Left ventricle of a patient with a divided atrioventricular canal. The inferior component of the anterior mitral leaflet inserts into the posteromedial papillary muscle *(PMPM)*, which is normal. But the inferior part of the anterior mitral leaflet also inserts into the anterolateral papillary muscle group *(ALPM)*, which is abnormal, via crossing chordae. The result of these abnormalities of the mitral tensor apparatus is an accessory posteromedial mitral orifice between the normally attached MV to the PMPM and the abnormally attached MV to the ALPM via the inferior-to-superior crossing chordae tendineae. Thus, anomalies of the tensor apparatus—of the chordae tendineae and of the papillary muscles—appear to explain why double-orifices of the MV occur. *AoV,* Aortic valve; *Cleft MV,* cleft mitral valve; *Main Orif,* main orifice; *PM,* papillary muscle; *VSD,* ventricular septal defect. (Reproduced with permission from Baño-Rodrigo A, Van Praagh S, Trowitzsch E, Van Praagh R. Double-orifice mitral valve: A study of 27 postmortem cases with developmental, diagnostic, and surgical considerations. *Am J Cardiol.* 1988;61:152.)

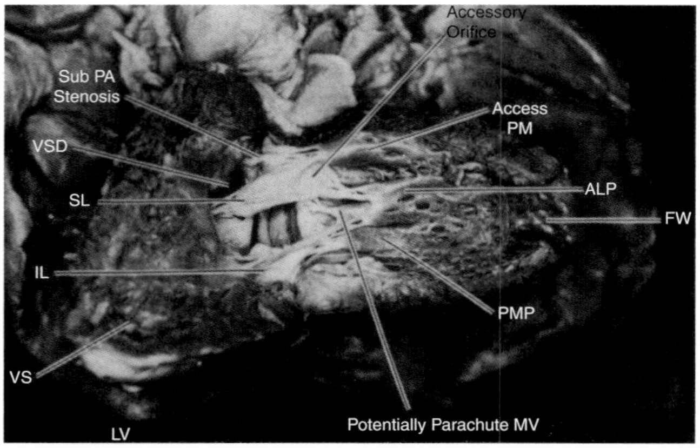

Fig. 14.38 Double-orifice mitral valve (MV) in the setting of completely common atrioventricular (AV) canal type C. Note the malformed papillary muscle architecture. The posteromedial papillary muscle *(PMP)* is hypoplastic and fused with the anterolateral papillary muscle *(ALP)*. There is a very superior accessory papillary muscle *(Access PM)* above the ALP muscle. The superior leaflet *(SL)* of the common atrioventricular valve (CAVV) inserts into the ALP muscle and into the access PM. Between these two separate insertions of the superior leaflet, there is an accessory anterolateral orifice within the superior leaflet of the CAVV. The main orifice of the left ventricular component of the CAVV is formed by the free margins of the superior leaflet (SL) and the inferior leaflet *(IL)*. Both the SL and the IL of the common AV valve insert via chordae tendineae into the ALP muscle, perhaps explaining the hypoplasia of the PMP muscle group. When the IL of a CAVV inserts into the *superior* ALP muscle, instead of into the *inferior* PMP muscle, which is more usual, this is called *crossing chordae*, which is an anomaly of the tensor apparatus of a CAVV. This patient has multiple anomalies of the mitral tensor apparatus. This case exemplifies an accessory orifice in the superior leaflet of a common AV valve, we think caused by the abnormal anterosuperior accessory PM. When chordae tendineae insert into two separate papillary muscles (superior accessory PM and the ALP muscle), the result is an orifice. **The rule of the mitral endocardial cushion tissue** appears to be that it can form leaflet tissue *or* chordae tendineae. But it cannot form both at the same location. If chordae tendineae form in association with normal or abnormal papillary muscles, that is it. There you will find an orifice, not leaflet tissue, because the endocardial cushion tissue has been used to form chordae, not leaflet. The MV displays an inverse (either/or) relationship between leaflet tissue and chordae, apparently because the mitral endocaudial tissue is limited in amount. This patient also exemplifies what may be called *potentially parachute MV*. There is only one well-formed papillary muscle in this LV: the anterolateral. Surgical repair of this kind of common AV canal results in the production of parachute MV because there is only one well-formed papillary muscle (the ALP) receiving all of the main chordae tendineae supporting the main mitral orifice. The accessory orifice in the superior leaflet of this CAVV was thought not to have been physiologically important. *FW*, Free wall; *LV*, left ventricle; *Sub PA*, subpulmonary; *VS*, ventricular septum; *VSD*, ventricular septal defect. (Reproduced with permission from Van Praagh S, Antoniadis S, Otero-Coto E, Leidenfrost RD, Van Praagh R. Common atrioventricular canal with and without conotruncal malformations: An anatomic study of 251 postmortem cases. In: Nora JJ, Takao A, eds. Congenital Heart Disease: Causes and Processes. Mt. Kisco, NY: Futura Publishing, Co.; 1984:599–639.)

a potentially parachute mitral valve, because both the superior and inferior leaflets of the AV valve insert into this one anterolateral papillary muscle.

Another way of expressing this same idea is to say that the inferior leaflet has **crossing chordae.** The chordae tendineae of the inferior leaflet cross from inferiorly to superiorly and therefore insert into the superior papillary muscle (the anterolateral), instead of inserting into the inferior papillary muscle (the posteromedial), which is usual (dare I say "normal"?) for a common AV valve. The understanding of *crossing chordae tendineae*[112] is important. In the usual, "normal" common AV valve, the superior leaflet inserts into the anterolateral papillary muscle (the superior one) and the inferior leaflet inserts into the posteromedial papillary muscle (the inferior one). Any deviation from this usual or "normal" pattern results in *crossing chordae,* which may be associated with DOMV or with parachute mitral valve. There are two anatomic types of crossing chordae:

1. inferior leaflet (or endocardial cushion tissue) with *superiorly crossing chordae* that insert into the anterolateral papillary muscle (see Fig. 14.26); and
2. superior leaflet (or endocardial cushion tissue) with *inferiorly crossing chordae* that insert into the posteromedial papillary muscle.

The understanding of superiorly or inferiorly crossing chordae helps make sense of many otherwise confusion mitral anomalies.

Double-orifice of the mitral component of common AV valves is further exemplified in Fig. 14.37. In the patient shown in Fig. 14.37A, who had completely common AV canal type A, note the accessory orifice at the posteromedial commissure of the mitral valvar component. An abnormal ring of chordae tendineae is inserted into the posteromedial papillary musculature.

In Fig. 14.37B, another patient with completely common AV canal type A, note that the anterolateral and posteromedial papillary muscles are abnormally close together, and are fused at their bases. The cleft orifice is the main orifice of the mitral component of this common AV valve.

However, there is also a prominent posteromedial accessory orifice. Why? Because the inferior leaflet (below the cleft) inserts not only into the posteromedial papillary muscle (which is usual), but also inserts into the superior or anterolateral papillary muscle because of *inferior-to-superior crossing chordae* of the inferior leaflet.

In other words, the inferior leaflet has two foci of chordal insertion: into the lower or posteromedial papillary muscle, and into the upper or anterolateral papillary muscle via the superiorly crossing chordae from the inferior leaflet. These two foci of chordal insertion result in an accessory orifice between these two different foci of chordal attachment (the "law" of the mitral valve).

Do crossing chordae occur only with common AV canal? No, as Fig. 14.37C illustrates. This patient had a divided (not a common) AV canal. But inferior-to-superior crossing chordae from the inferior part of the anterior mitral leaflet insert into the superior (or anterolateral) papillary muscle, and this pattern of chordal insertion was associated with an accessory mitral orifice.

Why? Because the inferior endocardial cushion component of the anterior mitral leaflet inserted not only into the posteromedial papillary muscle of the LV but also into the anterolateral papillary muscle, with an abnormal accessory orifice between these two different foci of chordal insertion (the "law" of the mitral valve, once again).

To the reader scratching his or her head and muttering, "I've never heard of any of this!" I can only say "Courage! These are significant data." I am reminded of a joke that Dr. Jesse Edwards at the Mayo Clinic in Rochester, Minnesota used to tell tired house officers attending his congenital heart pathology teaching sessions. Jesse would say, "The mitral valve is just like a woman. The more you study her, the less you understand her." Having grown up in the sexist 1960s, I realized that this, of course, was not really true. But it was a wonderful way of getting the attention of sleepy house officers who probably had been up for most of the previous night. And as always, there was much truth in what Dr Edwards said. The mitral valve really is fascinating and it does require careful study.

CONGENITAL MITRAL STENOSIS WITH EBSTEIN'S ANOMALY OF THE TRICUSPID VALVE

Of the 48 postmortem patients with congenital mitral stenosis, but without HLHS, 2 had Ebstein's anomaly (4%; see Table 14.10).

Case 37, a 15-year-old boy, had congenital mitral stenosis with a "fish mouth" appearance from the LA. The left ventricular view revealed failure of formation of the interchordal spaces. One year before death, the patient had subacute bacterial endocarditis (SBE). At autopsy, the vegetations of SBE were found on the anterior mitral leaflet and on the right coronary leaflet of the aortic valve. This old vegetation was described as rectangular, granular, and hard. The year was 1965. This 15-year-old boy had normal segmental anatomy, {S,D,S}. Ebstein malformation of the tricuspid valve was found; tricuspid regurgitation had been severe. In addition, this patient had pulmonary valvar stenosis with a hypoplastic pulmonary annulus. Hence, this patient had both congenital and acquired heart disease, with all valves being involved: congenital mitral stenosis, Ebstein anomaly of the tricuspid valve, congenital pulmonary valvar stenosis, and SBE with a vegetation involving both the mitral and the aortic valves.

Case 141 was an 18-hour-old girl with MCAs, including a webbed neck, shield chest, widely spaced nipples, nonpitting edema of the lower extremities, microcephaly, microphthalmia, epicanthal folds, low-set ears, micrognathia, bilateral simian creases, third toe overlapping fourth toe bilaterally, and a normal karyotype: 46XX. She was considered to have **Noonan syndrome**. She also had polyvalvar disease, with all valves having thick myxomatous leaflets. The mitral leaflets were thick and myxomatous, with poorly formed interchordal spaces, resulting in typical congenital mitral stenosis (see Fig. 14.25). The tricuspid valve displayed Ebstein anomaly. Some degree of pulmonary valvar stenosis was also thought to be present because of the myxomatous pulmonary leaflets. Multiple fenestrations of the septum primum resulted in a secundum type of ASD. The ductus arteriosus was closing, and the left innominate vein ran anterior to the thymus in yet another congenital anomaly. In conclusion, the devastating combination of congenital mitral stenosis and Ebstein anomaly of the tricuspid valve with tricuspid regurgitation rarely does occur (4%; see Table 14.10).

I hope that the other entries in Table 14.16 will be self-explanatory. This brings to an end this section on congenital mitral stenosis.

Congenital Mitral Regurgitation

Our unreexamined records indicate that of 3216 autopsied cases of congenital heart disease, congenital mitral regurgitation was present in 216 (6.72% of this entire series; see Table 14.1). Reexamination revealed only half this number of cases (see later). We are now going to take a very careful look at these cases with congenital mitral regurgitation, in an effort to answer many questions:

- **What really is congenital mitral regurgitation anatomically and developmentally?**
- **How many different anatomic types of congenital mitral regurgitation are there?**
- **What does congenital mitral regurgitation occur with, or does it typically occur as an isolated anomaly?**
- **Is there any gender preponderance?**
- **How old were our patients at the time of death or cardiac transplantation?**
- **What are the diagnostic and therapeutic implications of these anatomic findings?**

Material and Methods

After careful reexamination of the records of each case of congenital mitral regurgitation, the salient statistics were as follows:

Sex: n = 108; males, 59, females, 48; gender not known, 1, males to females = 59/48, = 1.2/1.0; males, 59/107 (55%), females, 48/107 (45%).

Age at Death or Cardiac Transplantation: n = 108; age not known, 2; mean, 3313.985 days, or 9.08 years; standard deviation = ± 4490.2015 days, or 12.3 years; minimum = 0 (4 fetuses); maximum, 23,725 days, or 65 years (1 female); median, 2 years.

The median age at death (there was only 1 cardiac transplant) is thought to reflect the severity of congenital mitral regurgitation (i.e., 2 years of age) more accurately than does the mean (average) age at death (i.e., 9.08 years of age, or 9 years and 29 days of age), because the average is skewed to the right (in an older direction) by uncharacteristically old outliers. This is also why the standard deviation is so large (±12.3 years).

This is one of the largest autopsy-proved studies of congenital mitral regurgitation that has been published to date.

Causes of Congenital Mitral Regurgitation

Factors thought to cause or be associated with congenital mitral regurgitation are summarized in Table 14.18. The entries presented in Table 14.18 require explanation. Please note that the data have forced a shift in my approach to the understanding of congenital mitral regurgitation. I am no longer looking just for *anatomic types* of congenital mitral regurgitation, as I expected before doing this study, because, as will be seen, structurally normal mitral valves can and do undergo regurgitation, for *congenital* reasons that may have nothing directly to do with the mitral valve per se. Thus, by **congenital mitral regurgitation** I mean mitral regurgitation that has a congenital (not an acquired) basis in the mitral valve, or elsewhere. The anomalies of the mitral valve in entry 1 of Table 14.18 are summarized in Table 14.19.

TABLE 14.18 Factors Causing or Associated With Congenital Mitral Regurgitation (n = 108)

Causal or Associated Factors		No.	% of Series[a]
1	Abnormal tensor apparatus ± leaflets of the MV	31	29
2	Incomplete form of common AV canal with cleft MV	18	17
3	Multiple congenital anomalies	14	13
4	Severe aortic valvar stenosis or atresia	13	12
5	Dilated cardiomyopathy	12	11
6	Marfan syndrome with or without other congenital anomalies	11	10
7	Transposition of the great arteries	7	6
8	Aberrant left coronary artery from pulmonary artery	5	5
9	Hypertrophic obstructive cardiomyopathy	4	4
9	Tetralogy of Fallot	4	4
10	Single left ventricle	3	3
10	Congenital left ventricular dysplasia/cardiomyopathy	3	3
10	Down syndrome	3	3
11	Double-outlet right ventricle	2	2
11	Left ventricular outflow tract obstruction	2	2
11	Duchenne muscular dystrophy	2	2
12	Large secundum atrial septal defect	1	1
12	Straddling mitral valve	1	1
12	Truncus arteriosus	1	1
12	Pulmonary arterial vascular obstructive disease and pulmonary veno-occlusive disease	1	1
12	Heterotaxy syndrome and polysplenia	1	1
12	Hypoplastic left heart syndrome	1	1
12	Ventricular septal defect	1	1

AV, Atrioventricular; *MV*, mitral valve.
[a]Percentages rounded off to the nearest whole number.

Incomplete Form of Common Atrioventricular Canal With Cleft Mitral Valve

This is entry 2 in Table 14.18: n = 18, constituting 17% of this series of 108 postmortem cases with congenital mitral regurgitation. The meaning of entry 2 (see Table 14.18) is thought to be clear enough to require no further explanation: regurgitation occurring through the cleft in the anterior mitral leaflet in the incomplete form of common AV canal (with an ASD of the ostium primum type and without a VSD of the AV canal type). However, entries 1 and 2 (see Table 14.18) account for less than half of this postmortem-proved series of congenital mitral regurgitation: 46%.

Multiple Congenital Anomalies. Entry 3 in Table 14.18, concerns factors that cause or that are associated with congenital mitral regurgitation (n = 1 4, 13% of this series). In terms of frequency, MCAs were the third most common finding in this study: 13% of these patients had malformations involving systems other than the cardiovascular system. These anomalies did not cause congenital mitral regurgitation but were *associated with* it. What are we talking about? For clarity, entry 3 (see Table 14.18) requires explanation. This entry also means that 87% of these patients with congenital mitral regurgitation did *not* have anomalies involving systems other than the cardiovascular system, detected by careful gross and histologic postmortem examination (Table 14.20)

Severe Aortic Valvar Stenosis or Aortic Valvar Atresia

Severe aortic valvar stenosis or aortic valve atresia was the fourth most common finding in our study of factors causing or associated with congenital mitral regurgitation (n = 13/108 patients or 12% of this series; see Table 14.12). But the question is: how does this work? Why should severe stenosis or atresia of the *aortic* valve cause or be associated with congenital *mitral* regurgitation?

Case 35 (Table 14.21) suggests an important part of the answer. This 3-month-old boy had severe aortic valvar stenosis with a bicuspid aortic valve and marked EFE of the LV. We

TABLE 14.19 Anomalies of the Tensor Apparatus With or Without Leaflets of the Mitral Valve in Congenital Mitral Regurgitation (n = 31)

Case 1, 7 9/12 yr, female	Insertion of the chordae tendineae half way between the leaflet margins and their origins.
Case 4: 30 11/12 yr, male	Paucity of chordae tendineae at the anterolateral commissure, resulting in MR there.
Case 16: 2 days, male	Incomplete form of common AV canal with cleft anterior leaflet of MV, myxomatous thickening and rolling of MV leaflets and obliteration of interchordal spaces. Parachute MV with all primary chordae inserting only into the anterolateral papillary muscle group, with severe MR (echo + angio) though main cleft orifice of MV. Double-orifice MV with small accessory opening posteromedially of no functional significance. *Plus* Uhl disease of the RV, with paper-like thinning of entire right ventricular free wall, and Ebstein anomaly of the tricuspid valve with deep curtain-like anterior leaflet, absence of septal and posterior tricuspid leaflets with diminutive chordae tendineae, marked failure of formation of interchordal spaces, and absence of papillary muscles of the tricuspid valve.
Case 18: 6 3/12 yr, male	Large (9 × 5 mm) congenital perforation in the mid-portion of the posterior MV leaflet.
Case 20: 12 days, female	MV described as "deficient in valve tissue" at MV replacement with no. 16 dura mater valve (surgical assessment).
Case 21: 55 yr male	TGA {S,L,L} with multiple fenestrations of anterior leaflet of right-sided MV
Case 22: 5 7/12 female	Severe congenital MR with thickening and rolling of free margins of MV leaflets, obliteration of some interchordal spaces, short chordae tendineae, and patchy EFE of the LV

TABLE 14.19 **Anomalies of the Tensor Apparatus With or Without Leaflets of the Mitral Valve in Congenital Mitral Regurgitation (n = 31)—cont'd**

Case 23: 4½ mo, female	Cleft anterior leaflet of MV, isolated, without ostium primum interatrial communication and without VSD of AV canal type, but with tetralogy of Fallot.
Case 29: 4 mo, female	Accessory small separate anterolateral papillary muscle of the LV, small jet lesion of left atrium.
Case 42: 5½ mo male	Thickening and rolling of MV free margins, failure of formation of interchordal spaces, leaflets appear to insert directly into papillary muscles.
Case 43: 2 9/12 yr, male	Thickening and rolling of leaflet margins with thickened and shortened chordae tendineae. The posteromedial papillary muscle is large, and the anterolateral papillary muscle is high and small; that is, unbalanced tensor apparatus.
Case 45: Sender and age unknown	Complete MV cleft of the AV canal type, no primum type of interatrial communication, no VSD or the AV canal type.
Case 51: 4 yr female	Holmes heart, single LV {S,D,S} with double-inlet LV, marked thickening of anterior MV leaflet with nodules, marked hypertrophy of papillary muscles with thickened and partly muscularized chordae tendineae. Focal EFE of the LV.
Case 63: 2 yr, female	Anterolateral papillary muscle poorly differentiated—high and small. Thickened margins of both leaflets at anterolateral commissure.
Case 67: 14 9/12 yr male	Rudimentary anterolateral papillary muscle. Jet lesion of left atrial endocardium behind and above anterolateral mitral commissure.
Case 72: 5 weeks, male	Aortic valve atresia, with mitral regurgitation and stenosis, severe. *Ebstein-like anomaly of the left-sided mitral valve,* with marked downward displacement of the anterior mitral leaflet, absence of interchordal spaces, and absence of papillary muscles. The mitral valve has a skirt-like shelf of fibrous tissue that attaches tightly to the left ventricular free wall. The mitral valve has a small, stenotic orifice, and with no leaflet mobility. Consequently, the mitral regurgitation from the blind LV is severe. There is marked EFE of the LV and LA.
Case 76: Stillborn male	Spontaneous fetal death at 31 6/7 weeks gestation from hydrops fetalis. Severe MR observed echocardiographically in utero. Very limited mobility of posterior MV leaflet. A small free wall papillary muscle attached to the ventricular surface of the posterior leaflet, limiting its motion and resulting in severe MR. Posterior leaflet thickened and rolled. Very few interchordal spaces. Unicuspid very stenotic aortic valve. LV markedly dilated, apical portion paper-thin with no trabeculations: left ventricular apical aneurysm and dysplasia. Anterolateral papillary muscular group is very hypoplastic. Left ventricular histologic examination showed "Uhl disease of the LV" with extensive myocardial necrosis and calcification.
Case 81: 1½ yr female	Noonan syndrome with valvar pulmonary stenosis, a large secundum atria septal defect, and congenital mitral regurgitation with myxomatous MV leaflets, obliteration of most interchordal spaces, and reduction of the interpapillary muscle distance, and a jet lesion of the left atrial endocardium. Bilateral pulmonary lymphangiectasia, progressive. Myxomatous tricuspid valve with tricuspid regurgitation. Polyvalvar disease involving mitral, tricuspid and pulmonary valves.
Case 85: 16 day, male	Heterotaxy syndrome with asplenia and double-outlet infundibular outlet chamber {I,D,D}, pulmonary atresia (infundibular and valvar), extreme hypoplasia of the right ventricular sinus, partial form of common AV canal, Ebstein anomaly with tricuspid atresia (imperforate tricuspid valve). Partial form of CAVC because AV valve is not in common because of tricuspid atresia. Double-orifice mitral valve with large central subdividing mass of posteromedial papillary muscle dividing MV orifice into medial and lateral components. This subdividing posteromedial papillary musculature attaches to both anterior and posterior MV leaflets by short, fused chordae tendineae. There are three papillary muscles attached to the left ventricular free wall: the normal anterolateral, the normal posteromedial, and the abnormal subdividing central papillary muscle that attaches to both anterior and posterior MV leaflets, subdividing the mitral orifice, resulting in double orifice MV. This double-orifice MV may have been associated with some degree of congenital mitral stenosis, with well documented congenital mitral regurgitation (angiocardiography).
Case 92: 5 mo, male	*A rare Ebstein-like anomaly of the mitral valve and of the left ventricle* (compare with Case 72 above). The MV is downwardly displaced below the left atrial–left ventricular junction, below the coronary sinus, and below the left circumflex coronary artery. The left ventricular free wall below the left atrioventricular junction and above the downwardly displaced mitral valve is exceedingly thin and aneurysmal. This aneurysm of the left ventricular inflow tract is somewhat similar to the aneurysm of the right ventricular inflow tract with Ebstein anomaly. Hence, this left ventricular inflow tract aneurysm is referred to, with a wink, as "Ebstein anomaly of the left ventricle." This parchment-thin left ventricular inflow tract aneurysm is *not* identical to the right ventricular inflow tract aneurysm with Ebstein. But this left ventricular inflow tract aneurysm is *reminiscent* of Ebstein inflow tract aneurysm. The left ventricular wall is of normal thickness at, and below the level of the downwardly displaced mitral valve. The thinned, parchment-like aneurysmal left ventricular inflow tract above the downwardly displaced MV could be viewed as the atrialized LV. The length of the left AV junction to the left ventricular apex measures 45 mm in length. The very thin left ventricular aneurysm occupies the first 20 mm of this length, that is, 44.4% of the distance from the left AV junction to the left ventricular apex. Only the lower 25 mm (55.6%) of the left ventricular inflow tract is of normal left ventricular free wall thickness. My suggested name for this newly recognized anomaly is **downwardly displaced mitral valve with supramitral aneurysm, an Ebstein-like anomaly of the mitral valve and left ventricle.** Briefly: **downwardly displaced mitral valve with supramitral aneurysm.**
Case 94: 1 day male	Aortic stenosis, unicommissural, very severe (only left coronary–noncoronary commissure is present), with marked global EFE. Congenital MR with high small anterolateral papillary muscle, large low posteromedial papillary muscle, triangular anterior mitral leaflet (like a lateen sail), with thickening and rolling of anterolateral free margin, indicating where MR was occurring.

Continued

TABLE 14.19 Anomalies of the Tensor Apparatus With or Without Leaflets of the Mitral Valve in Congenital Mitral Regurgitation (n = 31)—cont'd

Case 98: 7¼ mo female	Multiple congenital anomalies: intrauterine growth restriction, small anterior fontanelle, depressed neurologic function, prominent breast buds, anteriorly displaced anus, short left fifth finger, short left fifth toe, short right fifth finger, bilateral simian creases (single palmar creases), and congenital heart disease. Hypoplastic mitral valve with fusion of the anterolateral and posteromedial papillary muscle groups at their tops, with thickening and rolling of posterior leaflet, identifying where the congenital MR occurred.
Case 101: 7 yr male	Parachute mitral valve, all chordae inserting into the hypoplastic anterolateral papillary muscle group (ALPMG) and into a fibrous bridge between the ALPMG and the very hypoplastic PMPMG (posteromedial papillary muscle group), with redundant chordae tendineae, double-orifice mitral valve, and moderate EFE of the LV. There is an accessory papillary muscle immediately beneath the anterolateral commissure of the MV that receives chordae from both the MV leaflets, resulting in congenital MR because of inability of MV to close normally. DOMV is present because there are two left ventricular inlets: (1) the normal one between the hypoplastic ALPMG and the PMPMG, and (2) at the AL commissure that cannot close. Thus, congenital MR is due to abnormal tensor apparatus, that is, abnormal papillary musculature (a left ventricular myocardial architectural anomaly).
Case 103: 20 days, female	Multiple congenital anomalies: bilateral cataracts and congenital heart disease. Incomplete form of common AV canal opening mostly into the RV: large ostium primum atrial septal defect, but no VSD of AV canal type, with a 3-mm-wide cleft or gap resulting in congenital MR.
Case 104: Fetus, male	18–19 week fetus, mitral regurgitation seen in fetal echocardiogram, leading to termination of pregnancy. Abnormal mitral valve: absence of interchordal spaces, leaflets attach directly to papillary muscles without intervening free chordae tendineae. Hydrops fetalis (intrauterine heart failure), severe oligohydramnios.
Case 109: 26 yr female	Incomplete type of common AV canal, left-sided type, with right-sided tricuspid atresia, no VSD of AV canal type, cleft of AV canal type with marked congenital MR.
Case 112: 27 yr, female	Thickening of anterior leaflet of MV. Failure of formation of interchordal spaces. Chordae appear shortened. Anterior leaflet of MV inserts directly into ALMP group. Redundancy of MV at AL commissure. Posterior MV leaflet has nodular thickening consistent with MR.
Case 114: Stillborn female	Thickened and rolled edges of anterior leaflet of MV indicating congenital MR, with abnormally small posteromedial papillary muscle, that is, unbalanced tensor apparatus. Multiple congenital anomalies: omphalocele, right hydroureter, right hydronephrosis.
Case 116: 9 3/12 yr, meal	Tetralogy of Fallot {S,D,S} with right aortic arch and congenital MR: thickened anterior leaflet of MV, very short chordae tendineae, two papillary muscle groups are hypertrophied and short. Left atrial hypertrophy and enlargement (twice normal size) with jet lesions in posterior wall of left atrium consistent with mitral regurgitation.
Case 119: 11 9/12 yr, female	Congenital MR, moderate: MV is moderately enlarged. Of the three scallops in the posterior leaflet of the MV, the lateral and middle scallops are large and prolapse into the LA. The edges of the MV leaflets are thickened and rolled. Jet lesions on the walls of the LA immediately above the prolapsing posterior leaflet of the MV. Intact atrial septum. Totally anomalous pulmonary venous connection to the coronary sinus, and to left superior vena cava to coronary sinus to right atrium (with intact atrial septum, the latter being very unusual). Multiple congenital anomalies: hypoplastic left lung, hemivertebrae (lower thoracic spine), congenital double pelvis of the left kidney, hypoplastic right kidney, severe scoliosis.
Case 122: 8½ mo, male	Congenital MR with small, thickened anterior leaflet and with rudimentary chordae tendineae and papillary muscles. The posterior leaflet was described as wide and redundant. The patient suffered from chronic heart failure. An unsuccessful mitral annuloplasty was attempted in 1962.

AL, Anterolateral; *ALPMG,* anterolateral papillary muscle group; *AV,* atrioventricular; *EFE,* endocardial fibroelastosis; *{I,D,D},* the segmental anatomic set of visceroatrial situs inversus (I), ventricular D-loop (D), and D-malposition of the great arteries; *LA,* morphologically left atrium; *LV,* morphologically left ventricle; *MR,* mitral regurgitation; *PMPMG,* posteromedial papillary muscle group; *RV,* morphologically right ventricle; *{S,D,S},* the segmental anatomic set of visceroatrial situs solitus (S), ventricular D-loop (D), and solitus normally related great arteries (S); *TGA* {S,L,L}, transposition of the great arteries (TGA) with the segmental anatomic set of visceroatrial situs solitus (S), ventricular L-loop (L), and L-TGA (L); *VSD,* ventricular septal defect.

thought that this patient's congenital mitral regurgitation was caused by *papillary muscle dysfunction* associated with extreme left ventricular endomyocardial fibrosis.

It should be recalled that EFE associated with severe aortic valvar stenosis or atresia is thought to be caused by left ventricular endocardial sclerosis and subendocardial myocardial ischemic necrosis by global subendocardial myocardial infarction with replacement fibrosis. When left ventricular EFE is severe, it can involve the papillary muscles, resulting in papillary muscle dysfunction, expressed as congenital mitral regurgitation with a structurally normally formed mitral valve.

This is not the whole story, however; it is more complicated than that. The mitral valve also can be malformed. Congenital mitral regurgitation often appears to have a *multifactorial causation.* Mitral regurgitation can also appear to be *partly congenital and also perhaps partly acquired.* Case 55 illustrates these complexities (see Table 14.21).

Case 55 was a 25-year-old man with severe congenital aortic valvar stenosis, a bicuspid aortic valve, and calcification of the right coronary and noncoronary leaflets. The patient also had longstanding moderate aortic valvar regurgitation, moderate supravalvar aortic stenosis, and subaortic stenosis that was

TABLE 14.20 Noncardiovascular Abnormalities Associated With Congenital Mitral Regurgitation (n = 14)

Case No.	Gender	Age	Noncardiovascular Abnormality
1	Female	7 9/12 yr	Familial dwarfism
6	Female	15 8/12 yr	Multiple accessory spleens (7) and common mesentery
7	Male	24 yr	Hypertrophy cardiomyopathy, initially obstructive, later nononbstructive
1	Male	3¾ mo	Heterotaxy syndrome with polysplenia (9 in right upper quadrant adjacent to greater curvature of stomach); interruption of inferior vena cava between renal and hepatic veins; abnormally symmetrical liver—right lobe slightly larger than left; bilaterally bilobed lungs; bilateral superior venae cavae with absence of left innominate vein; solitus normal cardiac segments—{S,D,S}; common atrium with absence of septum primum and poorly formed septum secundum superiorly and anteriorly; hepatic segment of IVC opening mainly into RA, but with larger left hepatic vein opening slightly to the left of the midline into a common atrium; normal pulmonary venous connections; left SVC opening into roof of LA because of absence of coronary sinus septum (i.e., unroofing of coronary sinus); incomplete form of common AV canal with cleft anterior leaflet of MV, with mild thickening and rolling of cleft margins consistent with MR; no VSD.
11	Male	2 days	Hypospadias
19	Male	20 yr	Duchenne progressive muscular dystrophy (also known as pseudo-hypertrophic muscular dystrophy); intellectual disability
36	Male	9 7/12 yr	Hurler syndrome (gargoylism); chronic duodenal ulcer (8 × 8 mm) bleeding with massive gastrointestinal hemorrhage; herpes zoster, right chest, T4 distribution
42	Male	5.5 mo	Ileal atresia
81	Female	1.5 yr	Noonan syndrome
85	Male	16 day	Heterotaxy syndrome with asplenia: bilaterally symmetrical liver; left-sided stomach; IVC right-sided in abdomen, veering leftward at liver and diaphragm; double-outlet infundibular outlet chamber {I,D,D} with pulmonary atresia (infundibular and valvar); partial form of common AV canal with Ebstein anomaly and imperforate tricuspid valve (right-sided tricuspid atresia), and VSD of AV canal type[a]; double-orifice MV produced by prominent muscular subdividing PMPMG; probably some degree of congenital mitral stenosis; well-documented congenital mitral regurgitation (angiocardiography).
95	Male	41 yr	Neurofibromatosis; oligodendroglioma of corpus callosum; status epilepticus; intellectual disability; alcoholism.
98	Female	7¼ mo	Intrauterine growth restriction; small anterior fontanelle; depressed neurologic function; prominent breast buds; anteriorly displaced anus; short left fifth finger, left fifth toe, and right fifth finger; bilateral simian creases
118	Male	20 3/12 yr	William syndrome: idiopathic hypercalcemia (13.2 mgm%); supravalvar aortic stenosis; bilateral peripheral pulmonary stenosis; coarctation of the aorta; left SVC to coronary sinus to RA; intermittent systemic hypertension.
119	Female	11 9/12 yr	Hypoplastic left lung; hemivertebrae, lower thoracic spine; double pelvis, left kidney; hypoplasia, right kidney; severe scoliosis.

AV, Atrioventricular; *{I,D,D},* the anatomic set or combination of visceroatrial situs inversus (I), D-loop ventricles (D), and D-malposition of the great arteries (D); *IVC,* inferior vena cava; *LA,* morphologically left atrium; *mo,* months; *MR,* mitral regurgitation; *MV,* mitral valve; *PMPMG,* posteromedial papillary muscle group; *RA,* morphologically right atrium; *{S,D,S},* the anatomic set (combination) of visceroatrial situs solitus (S), D-loop ventricles (D), and solitus normally related great arteries (S); *SVC,* superior vena cava; *VSD,* ventricular septal defect; *yr,* years.

[a]Note that it is possible for the partial or incomplete form of common AV canal to have a VSD of the AV canal type. This patient (Case 85), has a partial or incomplete form of common AV canal because of the coexistence of tricuspid valvar atresia (Ebstein anomaly with an imperforate tricuspid valve): that is, the AV valve is not completely uncommon (unfused) because the tricuspid component of this valve is fused (not in common). It is true, of course, that the most frequent partial or incomplete form of common AV canal does not have a VSD of the AV canal type. This most frequent type has two AV valves, a cleft anterior leaflet of the mitral valve, an ostium primum type of atrial septal defect, and no VSD of the AV canal type. *There are several other partial (incomplete) forms of common AV canal:* isolated VSD of the AV canal type; isolated cleft of the anterior leaflet of the MV of the AV canal type; and the partial form of common AV canal with mitral atresia. Does isolated ostium primum type of atrial septal defect exist? If so, it must be very rare.

TABLE 14.21 Congenital Mitral Regurgitation Caused by or Associated With Severe Congenital Aortic Stenosis or Atresia (n = 13)

Case 25: 3 mo, female	Severe congenital aortic stenosis with bicuspid aortic valve; EFE of LV, marked; congenital MR caused by *papillary muscle dysfunction* related to severe EFE and extreme LV fibrosis involving papillary muscles.
Case 55: 35 yr, male	Congenital aortic stenosis with bicuspid aortic valve, leaflet thickening, and calcification of right coronary and noncoronary leaflets; aortic valve regurgitation, long-standing; moderate supravalvar aortic stenosis; subaortic stenosis, mainly muscular, with minor fibrous component; left ventricular hypertrophy and enlargement; congenital mitral regurgitation (angiocardiographic documentation); healed vegetations of mitral valve leaflets, consistent with old bacterial endocarditis.
Case 58, 30.5 yr, male	Congenital aortic stenosis (CAS), severe, with bicuspid aortic valve; coarctation of aorta (Coarc), postductal; mitral regurgitation, moderate (clinical and catheterization), thought to be caused by endomyocardial and papillary muscle dysfunction due to severe CAS and Coarc.

Continued

TABLE 14.21 Congenital Mitral Regurgitation Caused by or Associated With Severe Congenital Aortic Stenosis or Atresia (n = 13)—cont'd

Case 74 1 2/12 yr, male	Aortic atresia, valvar and subvalvar; VSD, conoventricular type, moderate in size (angiocardiography); congenital MR, mild, with myxomatous thickening of MV leaflets; jet lesions of left atrial endocardium, two, small, linear, above posterior MV leaflet; mild myxomatous thickening of tricuspid valve; bicuspid pulmonary valve (septal commissure rudimentary) with moderate thickening of pulmonary leaflets; that is, polyvalvar disease: all four leaflets involved; aortic arch interruption, type C, between right common carotid artery (or innominate artery) and left common carotid artery.
Case 79: 5 yr, female	Congenital aortic stenosis, valvar, severe, with bicommissural (hence bicuspid) aortic valve (intercoronary commissure very underdeveloped); and with thick stenotic leaflets; left ventricular hypertrophy, severe, concentric; coarctation of the aorta; congenital MR, with thickening of anterior leaflet of MV and left atrial jet lesion.
Case 90: 5½ wk, female	Congenital aortic stenosis, valvar, severe, unicommisural (only the LC/NC commissure was well developed) and small aortic annulus (4.5-mm internal diameter [ID]), compared with pulmonary annulus ID = 10–11 mm: aortic valvar ID/pulmonary valvar ID = 0.43; endocardial sclerosis of left ventricular septal surface; atrophy of both anterolateral and posteromedial papillary muscle groups; congenital MR, mild to moderate, thought to be the result of papillary muscle dysfunction.
Case 94: 1 day, male	Aortic stenosis, valvar, very severe, unicommissural (LC/NC commissure well developed, other two absent), aortic leaflets thick and myxomatous, with small aortic annulus (ID = 2 mm); EFE of LV marked, global; congenital MR with high small anterolateral papillary muscle and large low posteromedial papillary muscle; triangular anterior mitral leaflet with thickening and rolling of free margin of asymmetrical anterior mitral leaflet; preductal coarctation of aorta; left atrial hypertrophy and enlargement; atrial septum bulging into right atrium, with highly restrictive muscularized septum primum with diminutive patent foramen ovale.
Case 97 13 yr, male	Congenital aortic valvar stenosis, unicommissural (LC/NC commissure incompletely formed, the other two commissures are absent), leaflets markedly thickened; left ventricular hypertrophy, marked; congenital MR, anterior leaflet thickened and nodular adjacent to anterolateral commissure, with left atrial jet lesion; pulmonary valve with only one well-formed commissure (septal), the other two being poorly formed; polyvalvar disease: aortic, mitral, pulmonary; sudden death while riding his bicycle. Marked LVH is an independent risk factor for sudden arrhythmic death.
Case 107: 22 days, male	Congenital aortic stenosis, valvar, unicommissural (LC/NC the only well-developed commissure), small aortic annulus, marked myxomatous thickening of aortic leaflets; severe LVH (thickness = 9–13 mm) and enlargement; congenital MR and MS with marked myxomatous thickening of anterior and posterior mitral leaflets, failure of formation of almost all interchordal spaces; to moderate reduction of the interpapillary muscle distance; apparent narrowing of LVOT: anterior MV leaflet appeared too close to the left ventricular septal surface.
Case 108: fetus, male	This fetus of 26–28 weeks estimated gestational age died an unassisted death in utero (not a planned termination). Congenital aortic stenosis, unicommissural (LC/NC commissure well-formed, others absent), marked hypoplasia of the aortic annulus, aortic leaflets *not* thickened; congenital mitral regurgitation with thickening of the free margin of the anterior mitral leaflet, and marked paucity of interchordal spaces of the MV; LVH and E, with enlargement very marked, LVH and E, enlargement also very marked; premature closure of foramen ovale; intact ventricular septum; normal segmental anatomy, that is, {S,D,S}: the set or combination of visceroatrial situs solitus (S), D-loop ventricles (D), and solitus normally related great arteries (S). *Atrioventricular (AV) concordance and ventriculoarterial (VA) concordance should always be assumed, unless stated to the contrary. If the segmental anatomy is not stated, it should be assumed to be normal.*
Case 111: 5 wk, male	Aortic stenosis, valvar, unicommissural (LC/NC commissure normally formed, the other two absent); LVH + E, marked; congenital MR with marked elongation and fibrosis of both papillary muscle groups of the MV, thickening of MV leaflets, and failure of formation of most interchordal spaces of the MV; and cardiomegaly (2.5 × normal size).
Case 113: 1 day, female	Congenital aortic stenosis, unicommissural (commissures not described), thickened aortic valve leaflets, aortic valve slightly hypoplastic; EFE of LV + LA; congenital MR, severe, and congenital MS, moderate, diminished interchordal spaces with two well-spaced papillary muscles.
Case 118: 20 3/12 yr, male	Williams syndrome with idiopathic hypercalcemia (13.2 mgm%), mild intellectual disability, supravalvar aortic stenosis, bilateral peripheral pulmonary stenosis, coarctation of the aorta, intermittent systemic hypertension; left SVC to CoS to RA; and MR (angiocardiography) with jet lesions of left atrial endocardium; time of appearance of MR unknown, but MR has a congenital basis.

AV, Atrioventricular; *CAS,* congenital aortic valvar stenosis; *Coarc,* coarctation of the aorta; *CoS,* coronary sinus; *EFE,* endocardial fibroelastosis; *ID,* internal diameter; *LA,* morphologically left atrium; *LVH + E,* left atrial hypertrophy and enlargement; LC/NC, left coronary/noncoronary; *LV,* morphologically left ventricle; *LVH,* left ventricular hypertrophy; *LVH + E,* left ventricular hypertrophy and enlargement; *LVOT,* left ventricular outflow tract; *MR,* mitral regurgitation; *MS,* mitral stenosis; *MV,* mitral valve; *RA,* morphologically right atrium; *{S,D,S},* the set of solitus viscera and atria (S), D-loop ventricles (D), and solitus normally related great arteries (S); *SVC,* superior vena cava; *VA,* ventriculoarterial; *VSD,* ventricular septal defect.

mainly muscular, but with a minor fibrous component. The LV was hypertrophied and enlarged. Congenital mitral regurgitation was confirmed angiocardiographically, but autopsy (in 1971) revealed healed vegetations of the mitral valve, consistent with old bacterial endocarditis, raising the possibility that there was an acquired component to this patient's mitral regurgitation.

Another example of the complexity of this group is provided by **Case 94** (see Table 14.21), a 1-day-old boy with severe congenital aortic valvar stenosis. The aortic valve was unicommissural and therefore unicuspid, the only well-developed commissure being the LC/NC. The other two commissures were absent. Left ventricular EFE was marked and global. The anterolateral papillary muscle group was high and small, the posteromedial papillary muscle group was low and large, and the anterior leaflet of the mitral valve was triangular. The thickening and rolling of the asymmetrical anterior mitral leaflet was maximal adjacent to the hypoplastic anterolateral papillary muscle group. Preductal coarctation of the aorta was also present. Thus, in Case 94, although papillary muscle dysfunction of the LV was considered to be present secondary to severe congenital aortic valvar stenosis and marked global EFE, structural anomalies of the mitral papillary muscles and leaflets were also present.

Consequently, it is necessary to present this group in detail, in order to report the data accurately (see Table 14.21).

DILATED CARDIOMYOPATHY

Dilated cardiomyopathy was the fifth factor causing or associated with congenital mitral regurgitation in this series of 108 autopsy-proved cases: 12 patients, 11% of this series. What were these patients really like?

Case 8 was a boy who died at 5 months and 5 days of age. Congestive heart failure appeared at 4 months of age. Echocardiography revealed mild to moderate mitral regurgitation, later confirmed at autopsy by mild thickening and rolling of the free margin of the anterior mitral leaflet. Echocardiography at 4 months of age also revealed mild tricuspid regurgitation and severe left ventricular dysfunction. This patient also had episodes of bradycardia, down to 60/min for approximately 4 minutes, with associated hypotension (40 to 50/– mm Hg). Despite all therapeutic efforts in 1988, a rapidly downhill course led to death at 5 months and 5 days of age. Autopsy revealed marked cardiomegaly, with hypertrophy and enlargement of all chambers. The heart weighed 120 g, the normal being 37 g (120/37 = 3.24/1). Therefore, the heart was 224.3% greater than normal in weight. There was evidence of terminal multisystem failure, including terminal hepatic failure with icterus. Structural congenital heart disease was *not* present. Anasarca was present with marked ascites (400 mL, clear yellow).

In summary, our diagnostic impression was hypertrophic cardiomyopathy, dilated, nonobstructive, and idiopathic, with intractable congestive heart failure, mitral regurgitation, and tricuspid regurgitation. Hypertrophic, dilated, nonobstructive idiopathic cardiomyopathy is also known as dilated cardiomyopathy. Note that these terms are diagnostic fig leaves, currently used to cover our embarrassing diagnostic ignorance. We do not really know what is wrong with the heart muscle in patients like this. This is what Dr. Maurice Lev used to call "a research problem," a problem that needs to be solved to permit deeper understanding.

Case 12 was a boy who died at 10 10/12 years of age. Autopsy in 1988 revealed **primary idiopathic EFE of the LV and LA.** *Primary* EFE means that it is not secondary to severe aortic valvar stenosis or atresia. This condition is also known as *endomyocardial disease* of the LV and LA. Because there was massive cardiomegaly involving all cardiac chambers, this disease is also known as *dilated cardiomyopathy with primary idiopathic EFE*. The heart was structurally normal; that is, no congenital cardiac malformation was found. There was mild thickening of the free margin of the anterior mitral leaflet adjacent to the anterolateral commissure. Massive bilateral pleural effusions were found. Histologically there was no evidence of myocarditis. Left ventricular myocardial fibrosis also was not found. Hence, our diagnostic impression was primary idiopathic EFE of the LV and LA, a process that was thought to be congenital. The mitral valve was normally formed. Mitral regurgitation was *not* this patient's major problem. *Severe primary EFE* was the main problem. Again, it must be clearly stated that because we do not know the cause of this patient's primary EFE, we really do not understand this case. Severe global EFE, primary or secondary (to aortic valvar atresia or severe stenosis), is thought to result in *internal splinting of the LV*, which impairs left ventricular systolic and diastolic function, leading to fatal congestive heart failure.

Case 24, a boy who died at 16 2/12 years of age, had massive cardiomegaly, chronic intractable congestive heart failure, mitral regurgitation with thickening and rolling of the leaflet free margins, and left atrial jet lesions. There was atrophy of the papillary muscles of the LV. Left atrial hypertrophy and enlargement were marked. Endocardial sclerosis of the LV was described as severe of the LV septal surface and mild to moderate of the left ventricular free wall. Mild focal endocardial thickening was also present of the RV.

Endocardial sclerosis is a term used to describe endocardial thickening that is not as marked as EFE (which indicates thickening and whitening, sometimes described as porcelainizing). Mild to moderate pulmonary hypertension was documented at cardiac catheterization (50/25 mm Hg), with only mild intimal thickening being found at autopsy (no lipid streaking or gross atherosclerosis). This patient had idiopathic pericarditis at 10 years of age. The patient had a strong family history of congenital malformations and of left ventricular endomyocardial disease, with eldest sister, normal; second sister, spina bifida with death at 3 weeks of age; third sister, stillborn with encephalocele; fourth sibling, a brother, died at 2½ years of age with autopsy-proved EFE of the LV; fifth sibling, a brother, healthy, death by suicide; and sixth sibling, this patient. To summarize, this devastating family history:

Phenotypically normal, 2 of 6 (33.3%); congenital malformations of the nervous system, 2 of 6 (33.3%); and endomyocardial disease, 2 of 6 (33.3%).

In addition, this patient suffered from cardiac arrhythmias:

- Atrial fibrillation, 12 years of age.
- Stokes-Adams syndrome at 12 10/12 years of age; because of ventricular fibrillation, he was treated with defibrillation, successfully.
- Death occurred in 1980 from intractable congestive heart failure.

Case 26 was a boy who died at 5 2/12 years of age. Cardiomegaly was very marked. Left ventricular hypertrophy and enlargement were extreme, with diffuse endocardial sclerosis. A left ventricular antemortem mural thrombus was attached to the septal-anterolateral free wall junction. Mitral regurgitation and a left atrial jet lesion above the posteromedial commissure were found. Hypertrophy and enlargement of all cardiac chambers were present. Congestive heart failure appeared clinically at 4½ years of age, 13 months before death. The cause was not identified. Acute skeletal rhabdomyolysis also occurred, as did multiple pulmonary emboli. This patient also had pectus carinatum, an anomaly that was thought to have been of no clinical importance. This patient's mitral regurgitation was thought to be secondary to idiopathic, dilated, congestive, nonobstructive cardiomyopathy, also known briefly as dilated cardiomyopathy. It might be objected that this dilated cardiomyopathy did not present clinically until 4½ years of age.

So, how do we know that this cardiomyopathy and the mitral regurgitation associated with it were congenital (not acquired postnatally)? We do not know this for sure. But we think that hypertrophic obstructive and nonobstructive cardiomyopathy that pass through intractable congestive heart failure to death and therefore appear dilated terminally are congenital conditions with a molecular genetic basis. The molecular genetic and other causes of cardiomyopathy are now undergoing intensive investigation.[114] Clinical latent periods and variability of expression are parts of the clinical picture.

Case 27, a boy who died at 17½ years of age, had chronic congestive idiopathic cardiomyopathy, that is, dilated cardiomyopathy with intractable congestive heart failure. At 8½ years of age, cardiac catheterization revealed that his left ventricular end-diastolic pressure was markedly elevated (18 to 27 mm Hg). His cardiac output was very low (1.9 to 2.4 L/min/m^2). At 14 years of age, atrial flutter and atrial fibrillation appeared. By 15 years of age, severe chronic pericardial effusions appeared that were treated by pericardial stripping via median sternotomy. At 14½ years of age, an aortoiliac saddle embolus was removed surgically. Chronic severe diffuse pulmonary calcifications involving the lower lung fields bilaterally appeared during the last 2 years of life (from 15 to 17 years) and were progressive. Autopsy revealed two antemortem right atrial thrombi. Progressive severe osteoporosis occurred with widespread vertebral compression fractures. Two months before death, restrictive cardiomyopathy developed secondary to pericardial stripping and mediastinal fibrosis.

Autopsy revealed early pulmonary atheromata with lipid spots and streaks, moderate right ventricular hypertrophy and enlargement, and right atrial endocardial sclerosis. Mild mitral regurgitation and left atrial jet lesions were also observed. Left ventricular endocardial sclerosis, moderate and generalized, was thought to be typical of dilated cardiomyopathy. Hepatic cirrhosis was thought to be cardiac in origin. Chronic splenic congestion and fibrosis were also found, as was chronic anemia. Varicose veins of the legs were bilateral and severe.

The foregoing history and findings sound like those of an octogenarian, not like those of a 17-year-old young man. Most, if not all, of the foregoing history and findings were caused by chronic severe left-sided and right-sided heart failure, typical of dilated cardiomyopathy.

Case 32, a 12 5/12-year-old girl, had primary EFE of the LV *not* secondary to severe left ventricular outflow tract obstruction. Marked congenital mitral regurgitation was present, with a jet lesion of the left atrial endocardium. Hypertrophy and enlargement were present of all four cardiac chambers. Surgical mitral valve replacement with a Starr-Edwards prosthesis was done in 1966. The patient died 2 days postoperatively. In retrospect, we thought that this was the wrong operation to perform because with dilated cardiomyopathy, the mitral regurgitation typically is secondary to the cardiomyopathy, not a structurally abnormal mitral valve.

Case 46, a 4 7/12-year-old girl, had familial endomyocardial disease, or familial cardiomyopathy, or unknown etiology. The first child, a girl, died at 6 weeks of age with autopsy-proved EFE of the LV. The second pregnancy ended as a spontaneous miscarriage during the first trimester. The third pregnancy ended as a spontaneous miscarriage during the second trimester. The fourth pregnancy, a boy, died at 4 months of age as a crib death (thought to be sudden infant death syndrome). No autopsy was performed. The fifth pregnancy, a girl, is alive and well. The sixth pregnancy was this patient. At 2 months of age, the diagnosis of congestive heart failure was made. Marked cardiomegaly was found on the chest radiograph. The electrocardiogram indicated biventricular hypertrophy and right atrial enlargement. At 4 7/12 years of age, she was admitted to Boston Children's Hospital because of severe congestive heart failure. Although she was thought to respond well to medication (in 1973), she died of inexorable congestive heart failure and right lower lobe pneumonia.

Autopsy confirmed the presence of marked cardiomegaly and revealed severe primary EFE of the LV. The posteromedial papillary muscle of the LV was hypoplastic. Thickening and rolling of the free margin of the anterior mitral leaflet and a mild left atrial jet lesion confirmed the presence of mild mitral regurgitation. The LA displayed hypertrophy, enlargement, and EFE. The RV had hypertrophy, enlargement, and diffuse EFE. There was evidence of chronic congestive heart failure. The right lower lobe bronchus was compressed by the left atrial enlargement, leading to right lower lobe atelectasis and right lower lobe pneumonia. Thus, congenital mitral regurgitation was secondary to familial endomyocardial disease with *primary* EFE of the left heart.

Case 47, a 6 7/12-year-old boy, had dilated cardiomyopathy, also known as idiopathic hypertrophic nonobstructive cardiomyopathy. Cardiomegaly was marked at 263/100 g = 2.63/1, that is, the heart weight was 163% greater than normal. There were hypertrophy and enlargement of the LV, LA, and RV. Congenital mitral regurgitation was moderate, with diffuse left atrial jet lesions. Focal endocardial thickening was found of the LV. There was pneumonia of the right middle lobe. Narrowing of the left mainstem bronchus was caused by left atrial enlargement. Chronic intractable heart failure, both left-sided and right-sided, was reflected by chronic passive congestion of the viscera.

Case 69, a 12 5/12-year-old girl had dilated cardiomyopathy, that is, idiopathic hypertrophic cardiomyopathy without left ventricular outflow tract obstruction and cardiomegaly. Left ventricular hypertrophy was moderately severe, but symmetrical. Ventricular septal and free wall thickness varied from 10 to 20 mm. Left ventricular inflow thickness averaged 13 mm (normal for the age = 10 mm; i.e., 13 mm is 30% above normal). The left ventricular outflow tract averaged 12 mm (normal = 8 mm; i.e., 50% above normal). Chronic mitral regurgitation was present. Left atrial hypertrophy was marked (4 to 5 mm in thickness), with diffuse left atrial jet lesions. Elongation and attenuation of some of the mitral chordae tendineae were observed, but otherwise the mitral valve appeared normal. This was *not* a floppy myxomatous mitral valve. Hypertrophy of the RV and RA was minimal. Cardiomegaly was present; the heart weighed 280 g (normal = 180 g); thus, the heart weight was 56% greater than normal. This 12 5/12-year-old girl also had moderately severe pulmonary vascular obstructive disease (Heath-Edwards grade III changes). Death was sudden and unexpected and was thought probably to be related to ventricular fibrillation (hypothesis, not documented).

Case 86, a 1 10/12-year-old boy, had idiopathic familial cardiomyopathy and skeletal myopathy. The segmental anatomy was normal {S,D,S}, with a patent foramen valve, an intact ventricular septum, and a closed ductus arteriosus (ligamentum arteriosum). Congenital mitral regurgitation was associated with moderate primary EFE of the LV. The anterolateral papillary muscle was displaced superiorly and the interchordal spaces were poorly formed, with many filled with leaflet-like tissue.

Case 89, a 2-day-old boy, had idiopathic primary endomyocardial disease with cardiomegaly. All cardiac chambers were abnormal. The findings included endocardial sclerosis of the RA; patchy diffuse EFE of the RV; patchy EFE of the LA; severe primary EFE of the LV that was widespread but with focal accentuations; a congenital left ventricular aneurysm of a large region of the left ventricular apex[105]; nodular gelatinous thickening of the mitral leaflets; marked congenital mitral regurgitation; patent foramen ovale, with herniation of septum primum into the RA; PDA, not abnormal in a 2-day-old patient; mild congenital aortic regurgitation; and congestive heart failure, with cyanosis, leading to neonatal death (at 2 days of age).

In the area of **congenital left ventricular aneurysm,**[105] the left ventricular wall was greatly thinned. Left ventricular myocardium was markedly reduced, but not absent, and EFE was severe. The inflow half of the LV was severely afflicted with EFE. There was a marked deficiency of the normally numerous, fine, oblique trabeculae carneae of the LV derived from the stratum spongiosum. Thus, a *left ventricular myocardial dysplasia* was present with marked deficiency of both stratum compactum (the compact, coronary supplied myocardium) and of stratum spongiosum (the fine, oblique trabeculae carneae). A poorly contracting LV was observed to be present. The coronary arteries were normal.

Case 117, a 17 9/12-year-old young man, had familial hypertrophic nonobstructive cardiomyopathy. This patient's oldest sibling died at 18 years of age with autopsy-confirmed hypertrophic nonobstructive cardiomyopathy. Left ventricular hypertrophy and enlargement were massive. Diffuse left ventricular myocardial fibrosis was present, with congenital mitral regurgitation and jet lesions of the left atrial endocardium. Right ventricular hypertrophy and enlargement were moderate. Multiple antemortem thrombi were found of the RA, tricuspid valve, and LV. Pulmonary thromboembolism was present, with multiple wedge-shaped pulmonary infarcts. Infarcts were also found of the liver, spleen, and kidneys. Cardiomegaly was massive: 1051 g (normal being 281 to 360 g, with a normal average for this age being 320.5 g). Thus, the weight of this heart was 228% greater than normal.

It should be understood that *dilated cardiomyopathy* is not really an accurate term. It could convey the wrong impression to the uninitiated. *Dilated* should mean enlarged, but without hypertrophy, and therefore having a wall that is thinner than normal. But, as we have seen repeatedly, so-called *dilated cardiomyopathy* typically has mural hypertrophy with, for example, a left ventricular free wall that is much thicker than normal, as well as being *enlarged*. Cardiac chamber *enlargement* is different from cardiac chamber *dilatation*. However, those that coined the term *dilated cardiomyopathy* either did not understand this distinction, or they ignored it. *Dilated cardiomyopathy* really just means: cardiomyopathy with cardiac enlargement. "Enlargement" does not imply anything about the thickness of cardiac chamber walls, whereas dilation (or dilatation) does, as mentioned earlier. This distinction should be understood by those interested in *cardiac morphometry*.

This 17 9/12-year-old young man had a significant arrhythmia—the tachycardia-bradycardia syndrome—that was associated with heart failure, both left-sided and right-sided. He was treated (in 1981) with a permanent transvenous pacemaker, but died 3 hours after this procedure.

Marfan Syndrome With or Without Other Congenital Anomalies

This category also accounted for 10% of the autopsy-proved patients with congenital mitral regurgitation (n = 11; see Table 14.12). Each patient will be presented individually to avoid inaccurate generalizations and convey how important congenital mitral regurgitation was, or was not, in the natural history of each patient.

Case 17, a 20 11/12-year-old young man, had the adolescent-adult form of Marfan syndrome with mild congenital mitral region (or, at least, mitral regurgitation with a congenital basis) and mild aortic regurgitation (again, with a congenital basis). Autopsy revealed thickened mitral leaflets with left atrial jet lesions, confirming the mitral regurgitation. Autopsy also revealed slight thickening of the edges of the aortic valve leaflets and dilated sinuses of Valsalva of the aortic valve, corroborating the presence of aortic regurgitation. However, the immediate cause of death was a dissecting aneurysm of the ascending aorta from the aortic valve above the RC/NC commissure to the descending thoracic aorta, with rupture into the pericardial sac leading to hemopericardium, cardiac tamponade, and death. Other findings included left ventricular hypertrophy and enlargement, cardiomegaly (heart weight = 450 g), cystic medial necrosis of the aorta (typical of Marfan syndrome), arachnodactyly, scoliosis, pectus carinatum, and psoriasis. Thus, mild mitral regurgitation was present; but this was *not* this patient's major clinical problem. Aortic dissection, with rupture into the pericardial sac and cardiac tamponade were the immediate causes of death. The underlying cause of death was Marfan syndrome. This patient had the typical *adolescent-to-adult form of Marfan syndrome.*

Case 31, a 10-month-old girl, had *the infantile form of Marfan syndrome*[112] with severe congestive heart failure, mitral regurgitation (with leaflet thickening, left atrial jet lesions, and elongation of the mitral chordae tendineae), tricuspid regurgitation, thickening of aortic leaflets (with histologically increased mucopolysaccharide), and cardiomegaly (57 g, normal being 37 g; therefore 54% greater than normal). Other findings included acute peripheral bronchitis, chronic viral pneumonitis, bilateral pulmonary atelectasis with areas of overdistention, chronic dysplasia of the left hip, high-arched palate, dolichocephaly, arachnodactyly, pectus excavatum, dorsolumbar kyphosis, and chondromalacia of the ears. Thus, the immediate causes of death were congenital mitral regurgitation, plus congenital tricuspid regurgitation leading to severe heart failure—left-sided with viral pneumonitis, and right-sided. The underlying cause of death was the infantile form of Marfan syndrome, which is more severe than the typical adolescent-adult form of this disease.[115]

Case 38, an 11-month-old girl, had the infantile form of Marfan syndrome.[115] She was dead on arrival at Children's Hospital Boston (in 1958). She had redundant mitral and tricuspid leaflets. It was thought that she had had congenital mitral regurgitation (but this is a hypothesis, because of the absence of clinical or cardiac catheterization data). She had both left ventricular hypertrophy and enlargement and left atrial hypertrophy and enlargement. The aortic valve and pulmonary valve were both dilated, as were the ascending aorta and the MPA. A deficiency of elastic tissue development was noted. Cardiomegaly was marked: 80 g (normal = 40 g). Thus, the heart weight was 100% greater than normal. All of the cardiac chambers were enlarged. The lungs were cystic lungs with marked pulmonary emphysema. Other findings included a small cranium, microcephaly, right coronal synostosis, loose skin, poor muscular development, bilateral talipes equinovarus (club foot), bilateral wrist drop, bilateral dislocation of the hips, arthrogryposis, high-arched palate, arachnodactyly, lenticular densities, myopia, esophoria, delayed dentition, and osteochondrodystrophy. Thus, this patient had **infantile Marfan syndrome**[115] **with major associated malformations.** Another way of stating this is **infantile Marfan syndrome within a syndrome of other congenital anomalies** involving other disorders of connective tissue (such as arthrogryposis) and malformations of additional systems such as the central nervous system (e.g., microcephaly).

Case 54, a 19 6.5/12-year-old young man with Marfan syndrome, had mild, chronic, nonprogressive mitral regurgitation. His major clinical problem was dissection of the ascending aorta, aortic arch, and proximal descending thoracic aorta that occurred in 1970, beginning 2 months before his last hospital admission. Severe aortic regurgitation appeared after the aortic dissection. At 19 6/12 years of age, aortic valve replacement was performed, with partial resection of the aortic wall. An attempt was made to obliterate the proximal ostium of the false channel. A massive hemopericardium occurred postoperatively, leading to death.

Autopsy revealed a perforation of the ascending aorta posteriorly, 1 mm in diameter. Double right renal arteries were found. Mild pectus excavatum was confirmed. Bilateral inguinal herniorrhaphies had been done at 5 months of age. The mitral leaflets were slightly thickened and slightly rolled. A minimal jet lesion of the left atrial endocardium was present above the posterior mitral leaflet. Thus, once again, mild mitral regurgitation, with a congenital basis, was present, but was *not* the main clinical problem. Chronic aortic dissection was this patient's major clinical problem. It occurred in three episodes between 2 months and 3 weeks before his last hospital admission. *The immediate cause of death* was a postoperative small perforation (1 mm in diameter) in the wall of the posterior ascending aorta leading to a massive hemopericardium. *The underlying cause of death* was the adolescent-adult form of Marfan syndrome.

Case 64, an 18-year-old young woman with Marfan syndrome, had severe scoliosis that had been arrested by a spinal fusion from T7 to L1 (the seventh thoracic vertebra to the first lumbar vertebra). She had *severe mitral regurgitation* with dilatation of the mitral valve annulus, and rupture of one primary chorda tendinea to the posterior mitral leaflet that attached to the middle and lateral scallops. There was a jet lesion of the left atrial endocardium. Even more serious, she had a *rupture dissecting aneurysm of the ascending aorta* close to the annulus of the aortic valve. The tear involved the base of the aorta and the right coronary sinus of Valsalva; the rupture was 2 cm in length (i.e., 0.7874 inch, approximately 0.8 inch). This patient had a single left coronary ostium, that is, absence of the right coronary ostium. The single left coronary artery supplied the distributions of both the left and right coronary arteries. She had annuloaortic ectasia with aortic regurgitation. The aortic leaflets were thickened. Hypertrophy and enlargement of all cardiac chambers were found. Cardiomegaly was marked, the heart weighing 510 g, compared with a normal control heart weight of 240 g. Thus, the heart weight was 112.5% greater than normal.

The patient had had recurrent episodes of atrial fibrillation.

At 15 years of age, she had had an appendectomy. Pathology did not confirm a convincing appendicitis. There were large numbers of lymphocytes in the serosa, suggesting a viral lymphadenitis.

On the day of her death, she had a severe pain in her left arm all day long. She suddenly collapsed in an ice cream parlor. On coming to Boston Children's Hospital, she was found to be dead on arrival. Autopsy revealed cardiac tamponade: 800 to 1000 mL of blood were found in the pericardial cavity. Another estimate, at the time (in 1975), was that there was 650 mL of blood in the pericardial cavity, with diffuse hemorrhage into the mediastinum.

Annuloaortic ectasia involving the aortic valvar ring was associated with a dissecting aortic aneurysm of the ascending aorta with rupture. There was an oblique 4 cm (1.6 inch) long tear of the right lateral surface of the ascending aorta. In addition to the thickening of the aortic valve leaflets, there was a 1-mm intimal tear in the left coronary sinus of Valsalva. There was also a 1 mm rent of the intima of the noncoronary sinus of Valsalva that appeared to be the proximal ostium of the aortic dissection. The tricuspid leaflets were thickened and redundant, with fibrin deposits on the occlusal surfaces, and the papillary muscles were thin. Degeneration of the elastic tissue of the aorta was observed histologically, typical of Marfan syndrome.

Case 70, a 1-day-old boy, had *infantile Marfan syndrome*[115] with arachnodactyly, contractures, tricuspid valve prolapse into the RA with a hemorrhoidal tricuspid valve, marked deficiency of the tricuspid valve's anterior leaflet beneath the anterosuperior commissure, incomplete demuscularization of the tricuspid valve with retention of muscle of the tricuspid leaflets close to their origins or annular attachments, prominent muscular pillars adjacent to the tricuspid valve right anteriorly and right posteriorly, small blood cyst of the tricuspid valve laterally on the atrial surface, marked tricuspid regurgitation, severe right ventricular hypertrophy and enlargement, right atrial hypertrophy and enlargement that was very marked, a large secundum type of ASD consisting of multiple fenestrations of the septum primum and a large ostium secundum above a deficient septum primum, marked congenital mitral regurgitation, a relatively large anterolateral papillary muscle of the LV and a relatively small posteromedial papillary muscle of the LV, left ventricular hypertrophy and enlargement, massive cardiomegaly (57 g, normal = 18.5 g; therefore heart weight was 208% greater than normal), severe pulmonary valvar regurgitation, severe aortic valvar regurgitation, failure of coaptation of pulmonary and aortic valve leaflet, tortuous course of left anterior descending coronary artery, very large ostia of both right and left coronary arteries, and an unusual accessory strand of thin left ventricular myocardium running immediately anterior to the anterior mitral leaflet and attaching to the aortic-mitral intervalvular fibrosa (of no obvious clinical significance, but a rare morphologic finding like a thin, fine chorda tendinea), and a moderately large PDA.

To summarize, this patient with *infantile Marfan syndrome*[115] had regurgitation of all four cardiac valves, massive heart failure (left-sided and right-sided), with extreme cardiomegaly. Note that patients with *infantile* Marfan syndrome die of massive bilateral heart failure, secondary to regurgitation of most, it not all cardiac valves, whereas patients with the *adolescent-adult Marfan syndrome* often have relatively mild valvar regurgitation, but they may die of aortic dissection with rupture into the pericardial sac (leading to cardiac tamponade), or rupture elsewhere. This difference in the natural history of infantile versus adolescent-adult Marfan syndrome in our patients is striking.

It should be understood that this is a postmortem series of Marfan syndrome; hence, only the worst cases (i.e., the fatal cases) are being presented. Speaking of severity, Case 70 was one of the worst cases of the infantile Marfan syndrome that I have ever seen, with severe regurgitation of all four cardiac valves, leading to massive cardiomegaly and death at 1 day of age. Although this chapter focuses on congenital mitral regurgitation, it is noteworthy that **congenital mitral regurgitation very often does not occur alone and indeed may not be the most clinically important pathophysiologic condition present. That is why these patients are being presented "whole," as complete cases, so that the reader can understand the setting in which congenital mitral regurgitation occurs.** Otherwise, convenient reductionism can be blinding and unrealistic, divorced from clinical reality.

Case 87, a 13-year-old girl, had an *idiopathic familial connective tissue disorder,* as did one sibling. Our patient had a Marfanoid habitus with arachnodactyly, increased lower body segment, hyperextensible joints, contracture of the toes, osteoporosis, and kyphosis with wedge-shaped vertebrae. She had severe congenital mitral regurgitation, moderate tricuspid regurgitation, and severe congestive heart failure. Mitral valve replacement with a no. 29 St. Jude prosthesis was performed in 1988 when she was 13 years of age. Postoperatively, sudden collapse occurred, followed by death. Autopsy revealed an aortic dissection, 10 mm in length (0.4 inch long), starting at the aortic cannulation site, that was associated with severe bleeding. Although this patient was thought not to have typical Marfan syndrome, she certainly had a Marfan-like idiopathic, familial connective tissue disorder. This case also illustrates the risk associated with surgical cannulation of the ascending aorta in patients with Marfan and Marfan-like connective tissue disorder: such cannulation can initiate a dissection of the ascending aorta that may lead to massive fatal postoperative exsanguination.

Beal syndrome[116,117] is contractural arachnodactyly, without heart disease, as in Marfan's original report.[118] Gabrielle P. (Marfan's patient) had no demonstrated heart disease, and her eyes were unremarkable (no dislocation of the lenses). So today, Marfan's patient[118] would not be considered to have Marfan syndrome,[119] but rather Beal syndrome.[116,117] *Hence, Marfan syndrome, as now understood, consists of a spectrum of connective tissue disorders with a Marfanoid bodily habitus.*

Case 105, a 3½-month-old black boy, had infantile Marfan syndrome[115] with the following features: massive cardiomegaly, 72 g (30 g was normal, therefore 140% greater than normal); hypertrophy and enlargement of all four cardiac chambers; mitral valve prolapse into the LA with a markedly myxomatous appearance of the mitral leaflets, upward hooding of mitral leaflet components between chordal attachments and elongation of chordae tendineae, creating the "hemorrhoidal" appearance typical of mitral valve prolapse; linear jet lesions of the left atrial endocardium confirming congenital mitral regurgitation; and marked mitral valve enlargement, (the mitral circumference or perimeter measuring 73 mm, the normal control being 33 mm, i.e., 121% greater than normal); prominent dilatation of the aortic valve, including the sinuses of Valsalva, with an internal diameter of 15 mm; redundancy of the aortic valve leaflets, with some downward prolapse; tricuspid valve prolapse with myxomatous thickening, upward hooding, and marked annular enlargement (79 mm, normal control of 30 mm, therefore 163% larger than normal); small secundum ASDs: two fenestrations within septum primum (7 × 4 mm and 4 × 2 mm); dilatation of the central veins of the liver (histology), consistent with congestive heart failure, tricuspid regurgitation, and pulmonary regurgitation; reduction of the white pulp of the spleen (histology), consistent with the chronic stress of congestive cardiomyopathy; dilatation of the ascending aorta, with disorientation and disarray of the fibroelastic architecture; and no aortic (or other) dissection.

Case 106, a 6 10/12-year-old girl, had Marfan syndrome with severe mitral regurgitation. Mitral valve prolapse was associated with *a partially flail mitral valve* because chordae tendineae to the posterior leaflet, close to the anterolateral commissure, were ruptured.

Left ventricular hypertrophy and enlargement, left atrial hypertrophy and enlargement, aortic root dilatation, and mild tricuspid regurgitation were also present. Other findings included arachnodactyly, subluxation of the ocular lenses, flexion contractures of the extremities, and severe kyphoscoliosis.

In 1993, at the age of 6 10/12 years, she underwent surgical reattachment of the ruptured chordae tendineae. The postoperative course was characterized by episodes of atrial fibrillation, that were successfully treated by cardioversion. Three-dimensional echocardiography revealed that there was still marked prolapse of the mitral valve, but without a partially flail posterior mitral leaflet. Mitral regurgitation had been reduced from severe to moderate. A pericardial effusion (small to moderate) was present. Left atrial pressure had been reduced to 10 mm Hg, and left ventricular function was regarded as moderately depressed. On the fourth postoperative day, mitral regurgitation had again become severe and left atrial pressure had almost doubled (to 19 mm Hg). Reoperation revealed 400 mL of pericardial fluid under pressure (i.e., cardiac tamponade). After evacuation of the pericardial effusion, the patient's cardiovascular status seemed decidedly improved. But the marked redundancy and prolapse of the mitral leaflets and elongation of the chordae tendineae were again observed. Consequently, mitral valve replacement with a no. 33 St. Jude prosthesis was implanted. After this reoperation, severely low cardiac output was observed, leading to death 4 hours postoperatively. Perhaps the most noteworthy aspects of this case were mitral valve prolapse, chordal elongation, and chordal rupture resulting in a partially flail posterior mitral leaflet with very severe mitral regurgitation.

Case 115, a 10-month-old boy with infantile Marfan syndrome[115] had marked hyperextensibility of some of his joints (e.g., wrists and fingers) and bilateral inguinal hernias, with surgical herniorrhaphies at 3 weeks of age. Pylorotomy (a Ramstedt operation) was done at 7 weeks of age for hypertrophic obstructive pyloric stenosis. Severe congenital mitral regurgitation was characterized by marked prolapse of the mitral valve. Left atrial enlargement was marked. Tricuspid valve prolapse and regurgitation were also found. Moderate dilatation of the aortic valve was present, but without aortic valve regurgitation. The leaflets of the pulmonary valve were redundant but also without evidence of pulmonary valvar regurgitation. The walls of the ascending aorta and MPA were dilated and thinned, but without dissection.

A secundum type of ASD was present. Other important findings were severe failure to thrive; pectus excavatum; arachnodactyly; a high-arched palate; and ventricular arrhythmias, including ventricular premature beats, bigeminy, and trigemini (at 10 months of age). There were contractures of his elbow, knee and ankle joints. He had no familial history of Marfan syndrome.

Eventration of the central fibrous tendon of the diaphragm, somewhat right-sided, was also observed.

Progressive heart failure appeared at 5 months of age. At 10 months and 25 days of age in 1978, mitral valve replacement was performed with a no. 19 Hancock prosthesis. The postoperative course was characterized by hypoxemia, a left-sided pneumothorax (treated with a chest tube), and cardiac arrest leading to death. Examination of the explanted mitral valve confirmed that the mitral leaflets were thickened and redundant, with elongated and tortuous chordae tendineae. Examination of the heart specimen at autopsy indicated that the tricuspid valve had very similar findings. Bilateral pulmonary emphysema was found. Areas of old fibrosis of the left ventricular free wall were consistent with old myocardial infarction, that was predicted by the electrocardiographic findings. There was also an infarct of the posterior papillary muscle of the RV. The subaortic area was narrowed by one of the struts of mitral prosthesis; that is, iatrogenic subaortic stenosis was produced by the mitral valve prosthesis.

Case 126, a 10-month-old girl with infantile Marfan syndrome,[115] had chronic left-sided and right-sided heart failure. Congenital mitral regurgitation with leaflet thickening was present. Mitral regurgitation was documented angiocardiographically. So, too, was a secundum type of ASD with a left-to-right shunt. Tricuspid regurgitation was also present. Thickening of aortic valve leaflets with increased amounts of mucopolysaccharide was found histologically.

The immediate causes of death were chronic left-sided and right-sided heart failure, complicated by acute bronchitis and chronic viral pneumonia, with areas of pulmonary atelectasis and overdistention bilaterally. Deformities consistent with Marfan syndrome included congenital dysplasia of the left hip, a high-arched palate, dolichocephaly, arachnodactyly, pectus excavatum, thoracolumbar kyphosis, and chondromalacia of the ears.

Summary

The salient findings in these 11 postmortem cases of congenital mitral regurgitation with Marfan syndrome, or with a closely related connective tissue disorder, with or without additional associated malformations are summarized in Table 14.22.

Infantile form: Mean age at death, 223 days (7.4 months); standard deviation, ±136 days (4.5 months); minimum, 1 day; maximum, 330 days (11 months); median, 300 days (10 months). Sex: Males = 3, females = 3.

Intermediate form: Mean age at death, 3618 days (9.9 years); standard deviation, ±1595 days (4.4 years); minimum, 2490 days (6.8 years); maximum, 4745 days (13 years); median, 3618 days (9.9 years). Sex: Male, 0; females, 2.

Adult form: Mean age at death, 7110 days (19.5 years); standard deviation, ±530 days (1.5 years); minimum = 6570 days (18 years); maximum, 7630 days (20.9 years); median, 7130 days (19.5 years). Sex: Male, 2, female, 1

TABLE 14.22 Congenital Mitral Regurgitation With Marfan Syndrome (n = 11)

Type of Marfan	No. of Cases	% of Series	Salient Findings
Infantile	6	55	Heart failure (L+R)
Intermediate	2	18	Heart failure Partially flail MV
Adult	3	27	Dissecting aneurysm of ascending aorta

FORMS OF MARFAN SYNDROME

How many forms does the Marfan syndrome have? As Table 14.22 suggests, three forms (or grades of severity) appear to be accurate.

The infantile form is the most severe, with the most unfavorable natural history, with a median age at death of 10 months, ranging from 1 day to 11 months, and dominated by severe left-sided and right-sided heart failure, without spontaneous aortic dissection.

The adult form of Marfan syndrome (often also called the *adolescent-adult form*) is the least severe; it has the best natural history, with a median age at death in this series of 19.5 years, ranging from 18 years to 20.9 years. The clinical picture is dominated by spontaneous dissection of the ascending aorta, with or without rupture of mitral chordae tendineae. Rupture of the dissecting aneurysm into the pericardial sac, resulting in fatal cardiac tamponade preoperatively or postoperatively, occurred in all 3 cases. Intractable heart failure was not a problem, except after mitral chordal rupture.

The intermediate form of Marfan syndrome lay between the infantile and the adult forms both in terms of age at death and severity of disease. The median age at death was 9.9 years (neither an infant, nor an adult or even a teenager), ranging from 6.8 years to 13 years. Case 87 (13 years old) with severe mitral and tricuspid regurgitation and heart failure resembled the severe infantile form, except that she also had aortic dissection postoperatively, resembling the adult form of Marfan syndrome.

Case 106 (6 10/12 years of age) had severe mitral regurgitation (suggesting the infantile form), but only because of a ruptured mitral chorda tendinea (reminiscent of the adult form).

It should be understood that attempts to grade the Marfan syndrome in terms of age and severity, for reasons of diagnostic and therapeutic understanding, are of course somewhat arbitrary, like trying to subclassify a spectrum or demarcate parts of a rainbow. Nonetheless, these parts of the rainbow are distinctive and different, and these clinically important differences should be understood.

It will now also be apparent that mitral regurgitation is only part of the Marfan story, very important in the infantile form, along with severe tricuspid regurgitation, but much less important in the adult form, until a mitral chorda breaks, suddenly causing severe mitral regurgitation.

CONGENITAL MITRAL REGURGITATION WITH TRANSPOSITION OF THE GREAT ARTERIES

Why did congenital mitral regurgitation occur with TGA, as in 7 of these 108 postmortem cases (6%), item 7 in Table 14.18? This is the question that we are going to try to answer now. With TGA {S,D,D} there were 3 such patients. TGA {S,D,D} means transposition of the great arteries with the following segmental anatomy: situs solitus of the viscera and atria (S), D-loop ventricles (D), and D-TGA (D). AV concordance and ventriculoarterial (VA) discordance are understood to be present, unless other AV and/or VA alignments are specified.

Case 2, a 1 11/12-year-old boy with TGA {S,D,D}, had left-sided juxtaposition of the atrial appendages, TGA {S,D,D}, and a VSD of the conoventricular type. There was *posterior malalignment of the conal septum,* resulting in pulmonary valvar stenosis (PS), a bicuspid pulmonary valve because of absence of the left septal–nonseptal commissure, and subpulmonary stenosis. Mild mitral regurgitation was present, with thickening of the free margin of the anterior mitral leaflet and a jet lesion of the left atrial endocardium. But the question is *why* was there mitral regurgitation. We think that the answer is as follows. The conal septum was posteriorly malaligned. The anterior mitral leaflet was normally located. Posterior malalignment of the conal septum narrowed the left ventricular outflow tract. The anterior mitral leaflet was abnormally close to the left ventricular septal surface, similar to what can happen with hypertrophic obstructive cardiomyopathy with asymmetrical hypertrophy of the ventricular septum. In our patient, because of posterior conal septal malalignment, the anterior leaflet of the mitral valve was *in* the left ventricular outflow tract, rather than being to the left of the left ventricular outflow tract, which is normal. Consequently left ventricular systole ejected blood not only into the left ventricular outflow tract (to the right of the anterior mitral leaflet), but also into the LA (to the left of the anterior mitral leaflet), and thus mitral regurgitation occurs.

The hemodynamics of the pulmonary outflow tract also may well have been significantly abnormal because of subpulmonary and pulmonary valvar stenosis. Abnormal turbulence and increased velocity may have been present, resulting in abnormal hemodynamic changes of the anterior mitral leaflet such as thickening and rolling, predisposing to mitral regurgitation. However, the coexistence of a conoventricular type of VSD (associated with posterior malalignment of the conal septum) may have lessened the abnormal pulmonary outflow tract hemodynamics by providing an "escape hatch" for the obstructed pulmonary arterial outflow tract blood stream.

Case 48, a 7-month-old boy with TGA {S,D,D}, an intact ventricular septum, and a small secundum ASD had a balloon atrial septostomy at 22 days of age. This created a large interatrial communication. Why did the patient have thickening and rolling of the free margins of a normally formed mitral valve, indicating mitral regurgitation? I really do not know. There was left ventricular hypertrophy and enlargement. Perhaps the left ventricular enlargement with high pulmonary arterial blood flow may have created sufficient mitral annular enlargement to result in mitral regurgitation. Left ventricular fibrosis and papillary muscle dysfunction in a cyanotic patient with unsaturated coronary blood flow are hypothetical possibilities, but I am not certain.

Case 82, a 6½-month-old boy with TGA {S,D,D}, had a small VSD of the AV canal type. The anterior leaflet of the mitral valve had a cleft of the AV canal variety with moderate to severe congenital mitral regurgitation. This patient had a partial form of common AV canal because there was no ostium primum type of interatrial communication. He had a small secundum type of ASD. A blade atrial septostomy was performed at 5 months of age.

In addition, this patient had valvar and subvalvar pulmonary stenosis. Mitral valve tissue caused the subpulmonary left ventricular outflow tract obstruction. A right upper lobe pulmonary vein connected with the RSVC, just below the entry of the azygos vein; thus, a partially anomalous pulmonary venous connection was present. At 6 months of age, a Senning procedure (atrial switch procedure) was performed. The cleft of the anterior mitral leaflet was sutured closed. The VSD was closed directly with two sutures, resulting in a residual VSD. A small PDA was closed. A conduit from the left ventricular apex to the MPA was placed (because of the left ventricular outflow tract obstruction). However, there was severe stenosis at the anastomosis between the LV apex and the conduit, with a 90–mm Hg gradient, the LV pressure being suprasystemic. Low cardiac output and severe congestive heart failure led to death 10 days postoperatively. Hence, in this patient, the cause of congenital mitral regurgitation was clearly understood: an incomplete form of common AV canal, with a *cleft anterior leaflet of the mitral valve,* a small VSD of the AV canal type, and no ostium primum interatrial communication.

Summary

Three patients with TGA {S,D,D} had congenital mitral regurgitation; Case 2 had *posterior malalignment of the conal septum,* causing mitral regurgitation (similar to idiopathic hypertrophic subaortic stenosis). Case 48 was a *mystery:* exactly why mitral regurgitation occurred was not definitely established. Case 82 had a *cleft of the anterior mitral leaflet of the AV canal type* (approximately at right angles to the plane of the left ventricular septal surface).

CONGENITAL MITRAL REGURGITATION WITH TRANSPOSITION OF THE GREAT ARTERIES {S,D,L}

TGA {S,D,L) means TGA with a segmental anatomic set (or combination) of situs solitus of the viscera and atria (S), D-loop ventricles (D), and L-TGA (L). It is understood that there is AV concordance and VA discordance, unless otherwise specified. The presence of *L*-TGA (instead of the more usual *D*-TGA) correctly suggests that the bulboventricular loop may well be malrotated in a clockwise direction, viewed from the front, carrying the transposed aortic valve to the left of the transposed pulmonary valve.

Case 30 had *crisscross AV relations with mild overriding of the mitral valve* that opened mostly into the LV. There was congenital mitral regurgitation with left atrial jet lesions. Two anatomic types of VSD were found: a VSD of the AV canal type and a conoventricular type (i.e., both an inlet and an outlet type of VSD). The right ventricular sinus (the RV inflow tract) was underdeveloped. There was severe pulmonary outflow tract stenosis, subvalvar and valvar. The subvalvar pulmonary stenosis was produced by the medial (septal) leaflet tissue of both AV valves, and the valvar stenosis was caused by a unicommissural and unicuspid pulmonary valve. The transposed pulmonary artery was related to the LV, but it arose above the ventricular septum and hence the pulmonary artery was overriding. A single coronary artery arose from the right septal sinus of Valsalva of the L-transposed aortic valve. The single right coronary artery supplied the distributions of both the right and left coronary arteries (as is usual with so-called "single" coronary arteries, which is a misnomer. Such patients have a single coronary *ostium,* but not a single coronary artery). This 23 10/12-year-old young man, who died in 1977, had two Blalock-Taussig anastomoses. The left was a classic subclavian-pulmonary end-to-side anastomosis, with an internal diameter of only 1 mm. The right was a modified Blalock-Taussig shunt using a ⅝-inch (15.875 mm) Teflon graft from the right subclavian artery to the right pulmonary artery.

The immediate cause of death was a brain abscess. He developed SBE caused by β-hemolytic streptococci, group B, proved by blood culture. He had a history of headache 2 weeks before death, with transient right hemiparesis and right paresthesia. Autopsy revealed a right cerebellar abscess caused by *Hemophilus paraphrophilus* and *Staphylococcus aureus.* The abscess and an associated hematoma had been drained surgically, but the patient did not survive. Hence, this patient had congenital mitral regurgitation in the setting of complex congenital heart disease, complicated by fatal infectious acquired disease. Congenital mitral regurgitation was only one relatively small part of a much more complex clinical picture.

Case 73, a 28½-year-old woman who died in 1987, also had TGA {S,D,L} with a single LV, that is, absence of the right ventricular sinus and an infundibular outlet chamber. There was a DILV. The mitral valve attached to two different papillary muscle groups, and the tricuspid valve attached to the ventricular septum and to papillary muscles. Despite the attachments of the tricuspid valve to the ventricular septum, the bulboventricular foramen (between the infundibular outlet chamber and the single LV) was large and unrestrictive (23 × 17 mm). Mild mitral regurgitation was present, with thickening of the anterior mitral leaflet. Both great arteries were widely patent, and the pulmonary artery was regurgitant. The patient had cyanosis with severe clubbing of fingers and toes. Cardiac catheterization revealed severe pulmonary vascular obstructive disease. Sudden unexpected death occurred; a fatal arrhythmia was suspected. Histology of the lungs revealed Heath-Edwards grade IV changes, confirming the occlusive severity of her obstruction. Again, mitral regurgitation was found to be one small part of a complex clinical problem.

CONGENITAL MITRAL REGURGITATION WITH TRANSPOSITION OF THE GREAT ARTERIES {S,D,A}

Case 88, a 7.5-month-old girl who died in 1992, was the only patient in this study of congenital mitral regurgitation who had TGA {S,D,A}. In TGA {S,D,A}, the segmental anatomy is solitus atria (S), D-loop ventricles (D), and A-TGA, meaning that the transposed aortic valve is directly anterior (antero- or A-) relative to the transposed pulmonary valve. Left-sided juxtaposition of the atrial appendages (Lt JAA) was present. LtJAA is a syndrome that is frequently associated with TGA and tricuspid atresia,[30,32] as it was in this patient: TGA {S,D,A}, tricuspid atresia, mild mitral regurgitation with thickening and rolling of the free margins of both the anterior and posterior leaflets and with left atrial jet lesions, a large secundum type of ASD (25 × 20 mm), left ventricular hypertrophy and enlargement, and a restrictive mid-muscular VSD (4 × 6 mm). Tubular hypoplasia of the transverse aortic arch was present (3 mm in internal diameter) with a preductal coarctation of the aorta. Why were these abnormalities present? Because the mid-muscular VSD leading to the transposed aorta arising from the rudimentary RV was restrictively small, constituting subaortic muscular stenosis. Consequently, a subnormal volume of blood reached the transposed aorta, resulting in tubular hypoplasia of the transverse aortic arch and preductal coarctation of the aorta. Conversely, an excessively large volume of blood went to the transposed pulmonary artery and the ductus arteriosus, resulting in dilatation of the pulmonary artery and branches, and a large PDA. There was a high origin of the left coronary artery reminiscent of the evolutionary fact that in fish, from which we are descended, the coronary arteries arise from the branchial arches.[25] The high origin of this patient's left coronary artery had no deleterious consequences of which we are aware. Beginning at 4 days of age, this patient had multiple operations, including an arterial switch procedure, an aortic arch repair, and a repair of the left pulmonary artery, with unfortunately a fatal outcome. Mitral regurgitation was a minor player in this drama.

CONGENITAL MITRAL REGURGITATION WITH TRANSPOSITION OF THE GREAT ARTERIES {S,L,L}

Case 21, a 55-year-old man who died in 1982, had TGA {S,L,L} with left-sided tricuspid atresia and right-sided mitral regurgitation through multiple congenital fenestrations in the anterior mitral leaflet. There was also considerable calcification of right-sided mitral valve. TGA {S,L,L} means TGA with solitus atria (S), L-loop ventricles (L), and L-TGA (L). One would expect AV discordance, unless otherwise stated, and VA discordance (because those are the VA alignments of TGA). However, as indicated earlier, typical AV discordance was *not* present because of the coexistence of left-sided tricuspid atresia. A secundum type of ASD was associated with a prominent *interseptovalvular space* between the septum primum to the left and the left venous valve to the right. A prominent interseptovalvular space creates a type of cor triatriatum, but without pulmonary venous obstruction that is typical of the left-sided type of cor triatriatum (cor triatriatum sinistrum), and without systemic venous obstruction that can occur with the right-sided type of cor triatriatum (cor triatriatum dextrum). A prominent interseptovalvular space creates a form of *cor triatriatum (triatrial heart) that is central*—neither left-sided nor right-sided, and without venous obstruction. Right atrial hypertrophy and enlargement were very marked, and were associated with atrial fibrillation. Multiple calcifications of the left atrial endocardium were also found. There was pulmonary-mitral direct fibrous continuity, a subaortic conus, no great arterial outflow tract obstruction, and pulmonary vascular obstruction (grade III of Heath and Edwards), with multiple brain abscesses. Terminally, aspiration led to death. Multiple fenestrations of the anterior leaflet of the mitral valve were thought to be congenital. These fenestrations of the anterior mitral leaflet constitute a rare form of congenital mitral regurgitation, in a right-sided mitral valve, associated with left-sided tricuspid atresia.

Summary

A wide variety of mitral valve anatomy was found in these 7 cases of congenital mitral regurgitation (Table 14.23):

A. posterior conal septal malalignment with an intrinsically normally formed mitral valve (Case 2);
B. a normally formed mitral valve with a secundum ASD (Case 48);
   1. a canal type of mitral valve cleft (Case 82);
   2. overriding mitral valve with crisscross AV relations (Case 30);
   3. with double-inlet single LV (Case 73);
   4. with right-sided tricuspid atresia and left-sided juxtaposition of the atrial appendages (Case 88); and
   5. with multiple fenestrations of the anterior leaflet of a right-sided mitral valve, with left-sided tricuspid atresia (Case 21).

CONGENITAL MITRAL REGURGITATION WITH ABERRANT LEFT CORONARY ARTERY FROM THE PULMONARY ARTERY

This condition was found in 5 of these 108 patients with congenital mitral regurgitation (5%; see Table 14.12).

Age at Death: Mean, 1669.2 days, 4.57 years, or 4 7/12 years; standard deviation, 2846.72 days, or 7.8 years, 7 9.7/12 years; minimum, 120 days, or 4 months; maximum, 6720 days, or 18 5/12 years; and median, 330 days, or 11 months

Features Found With Aberrant Left Coronary Artery Arising From the Pulmonary Artery

The segmental anatomy was normal in all 5 patients, that is {S,D,S}. A VSD of the conoventricular type was present in only 1 of 5 patients (Case 62). Extracardiac anomalies were found in 2 patients: congenital ellipsocytosis (Case 28); and a double collecting system of the left kidney (Case 93). The aberrant left coronary artery typically arose from the left septal sinus of

TABLE 14.23 Congenital Mitral Regurgitation Associated With Transposition of the Great Arteries (n = 7) (6%)

	Type of TGA	No. of Cases	% of Series[a] (n = 108)
1	TGA {S,D,D}	3	2.8
2	TGA {S,D,L}	2	1.9
3	TGA {S,D,A}	1	0.9
4	TGA {S,L,L}	1	0.9

As above; please see text.
TGA, Transposition of the great arteries.
All patients with TGA had visceroatrial situs solitus. D-loop TGA accounted for 6 of these 7 cases (86%). L-loop TGA occurred in only 1 (14%).
[a]Percentages rounded off to the nearest whole number.

Valsalva of the MPA. Cardiomegaly was noted in the fresh state in 2 of these 5 patients (40%) with left ventricular hypertrophy and enlargement in 2 (40%), left atrial hypertrophy and enlargement in 3 (60%), and mitral regurgitation in all 5 (100%).

Mitral regurgitation was mild in 1, moderate in 1, and severe in 3. Left ventricular endocardial sclerosis was found in 2. Atrophy and infarction of the anterolateral papillary muscle of the LV were found in 4 of these 5 patients. Atrophy of the posteromedial papillary muscle of the LV was present in 2 patients. A left ventricular apical aneurysm, left ventricular fibrosis, and left ventricular myocardial infarction were found in 1 case each. The patient with left ventricular myocardial infarction (Case 28) was noted in life to have diffuse (widespread) left ventricular myocardial hypokinesis. The normally arising right coronary artery was noted to be dilated and tortuous in 1 patient. Prominent collateral connections were observed between the right and left coronary arteries in another patient. Right ventricular hypertrophy and enlargement were present in 2 patients. Right atrial hypertrophy and enlargement were observed in 1.

Failure to thrive, with no weight gain over two months, was reported in 1 patient, and another was observed to have had chronic pulmonary congestion.

Incidental findings, thought to be unrelated to aberrant left coronary artery and its sequelae, including the following. A quadricuspid aortic valve was found in Case 62. The noncoronary aortic leaflet was incompletely subdivided by a partially formed commissure. Both portions of the incompletely divided noncoronary leaflet were moderately thickened. The right coronary and left coronary leaflets of the aortic valve were normally formed. No evidence was found of aortic valvar regurgitation, or stenosis in this 11-month-old boy. A brachiocephalic trunk was also found in the same patient (Case 62). Only two arteries arose from the aortic arch. The first was the brachiocephalic trunk that gave rise to the right subclavian, right common carotid, and left common carotid arteries. The second branch was the left subclavian artery. The presence of a brachiocephalic trunk was thought to be of no clinical significance in this patient.

In this small series of 5 postmortem cases of aberrant left coronary artery from the MPA, all had mitral regurgitation. The mitral valve was normally formed in all 5 patients. The cause of the mitral regurgitation is thought to have been perfusion of the left coronary artery and its branches by unsaturated blood from the MPA. This unsaturation of the left ventricular blood supply is thought to have led to the observed myocyte necrosis, infarction, fibrosis, and compensatory hypertrophy and enlargement described above.

Left ventricular papillary muscle and mural dysfunction led to disability and death in these 5 patients.

Is there anything "interesting", unusual, or surprising that is revealed by these cases?

1. I was surprised first by the *sex* of these patients: 4 of 5 were female (80%). However, in view of the small size of this sample, no definite conclusion seems warranted. However, the question is raised: Is there a predominance of females in patients with aberrant left coronary artery? Many more carefully studied cases are needed to answer this question.
2. I was also interested by the *ages at death*. This condition is not as rapidly fatal as one might have supposed. The median age at death was 11 months. The youngest fatality was 4 months of age and the oldest was 18 5/12 years.
3. By far the most interesting finding, I thought, was the high prevalence of *myocardial hypertrophy*, or what grossly looks like myocardial hypertrophy but may in fact be a combination of myocyte necrosis, replacement fibrosis, and hypertrophy of surviving myocytes. The causes of myocardial hypertrophy are usually thought perhaps to be: (1) an increase in flow work per unit of time, (2) an increase in pressure work per unit of time, or (3) both, that is, 1 and 2 together.

What is noteworthy about the "natural experiment" that we are now considering (aberrant left coronary artery and its sequelae) is that the heart typically is normally formed (as in 4 of the 5 present patients). Typically, therefore, there is no increase in flow work or pressure work. But, the gross and very impressive appearance of hypertrophy (and enlargement) of the LV, the LA, the RV, and even the RA is what we found (as described previously).

So what is going on? How can, and should, we understand these findings? First, we should not simply dismiss the findings; they are real. In Case 14 (a 5-month and 6-day old girl, studied in 1987), cardiomegaly was described as "massive." In Case 28 (a 4-month-old girl, studied in 1977), cardiomegaly was found to be "marked," and left ventricular hypertrophy and enlargement were described as "very marked." These are just examples, supporting the surprising finding of left ventricular hypertrophy, in the absence of an increase in flow work or pressure work (the usual causes of hypertrophy).

This neonatal, infantile, pediatric, and occasionally adolescent model of left ventricular hypoxemia and its sequelae differs in at least one important respect from the adult and old-age model of left ventricular hypoxemia and anoxia: *growth,* which is present in our pediatric model, but absent in the more familiar adult model of left ventricular hypoxemia. The presence of the growth factor in the pediatric model of left ventricular hypoxemia, and the absence of the growth factor in the adult and senescent model of left ventricular hypoxemia, may help explain the presence of myocardial hypertrophy in the pediatric model, despite the absence of the familiar causes of hypertrophy (e.g., an increase in flow or pressure work).

What may grossly (with the naked eye) look like hypertrophy may histologically be seen to consist of myocyte necrosis, drop-out, and replacement fibrosis, plus hypertrophy of surviving myocytes. The gross appearance of hypertrophy, apparently supported by gross measurements of wall thickness and/or organ weight, should always be investigated microscopically. Histologic examination may well reveal that the gross impression of "hypertrophy" is really much more complicated, as noted previously.

Because all 5 of these patients had mitral regurgitation, they all did in fact have an abnormal increase in flow work involving the LV, the LA, and perhaps even the RV. Consequently, I suspect that chronic, untreated mitral regurgitation, by increasing flow work, may well have played a role in the chamber hypertrophy, enlargement, and cardiomegaly that we found.

CONGENITAL MITRAL REGURGITATION WITH HYPERTROPHIC OBSTRUCTIVE CARDIOMYOPATHY

The combination of congenital mitral regurgitation and hypertrophic obstructive cardiomyopathy was found in 4 of the 108 postmortem cases (4%; see Table 14.12), that is, Cases 7, 60, 96, and 124. (There are 127 patients in this series as a whole, consisting of 108 patients with *congenital* mitral regurgitation and 19 patients with *acquired* mitral regurgitation. This section is focusing only on patients with congenital mitral regurgitation.)

Sex: Males, 3; female, 1.

Age at Death: Mean, 22.33 ± 3.94 years; range, 18.16 to 27 years; and median, 22.08 years.

All four of these patients were young adults, not children, as the foregoing age data indicate.

Severity of Mitral Regurgitation: Mild in 3 of 4 patients (Cases 7, 60, and 124) and moderate in 1 (Case 96).

When the mitral regurgitation was judged to be *mild* clinically and cineangiocardiographically, the findings at autopsy were as follows.

Case 7, a 24-year-old man, had a normally formed mitral valve, but its circumference was enlarged: 82 mm, compared with a normal control of 70 mm. Thus, the circumference of the mitral valve was 17% greater than normal.

Case 60, an 18 2/12-year-old young woman, had a small jet lesion of the left atrial endocardium that was found adjacent to the posterior mitral leaflet.

Case 124, a 20 2/12-year-old man, had only a mild jet lesion of the left atrial endocardium.

Case 96, a 27-year-old man, had what was considered to be *moderate* mitral regurgitation. The entire anterior leaflet of the mitral valve was found to be thickened, and there were diffuse jet lesions of the left atrial endocardium.

Was the mitral regurgitation really congenital in these 4 young adults with hypertrophic cardiomyopathy? I think this is a very fair question or critique. We do not know when the mitral regurgitation first appeared in these patients. By classifying the mitral regurgitation as *congenital,* I mean that it has a congenital basis. I am assuming that hypertrophic cardiomyopathy is caused by a genetic abnormality, as is now being discovered in many such patients, but perhaps not in all. If some forms of hypertrophic cardiomyopathy prove not to be genetic anomalies, the mitral regurgitation in such patients may not have a congenital basis, and perhaps should be regarded as acquired mitral regurgitation. The answer to this question is unresolved at present.

Clinical Profile

Mitral regurgitation was *not* the main clinical problem in any of these patients. Hypertrophic cardiomyopathy was. These four patients with hypertrophic cardiomyopathy had two immediate causes of death:

1. sudden death in 3 of these 4 patients, with ventricular tachycardia progressing to ventricular fibrillation being documented in 1 (Case 124); and
2. intractable heart failure and terminal shock (Case 7).

Case 7 initially presented with the clinical picture of hypertrophic *obstructive* cardiomyopathy at 14 years of age, when he was found to have left ventricular outflow tract stenosis with a gradient of 30 mm Hg. Subsequently, however, severe congestive heart failure appeared, and at 24 years of age *the left ventricular outflow tract gradient had disappeared.*

Autopsy at 24 years of age revealed the impact lesion on the left ventricular septal surface opposite the anterior leaflet of the mitral valve where the left ventricular outflow tract obstruction had occurred, before its disappearance. Autopsy also showed hypertrophy and enlargement of all cardiac chambers, and asymmetrical hypertrophy of the ventricular septum. At the level of the mitral impact lesion, the ventricular septum was 2.8 cm thick. But above the apex, the septum measured only 1.9 cm in thickness, a 32% reduction.

In Case 7, intractable heart failure presented as terminal shock, low cardiac output, renal failure, pulmonary edema, probable pneumonitis, pulmonary congestion, focal hemorrhages, pleural effusions (left = 50 mL, right = 500 mL), hepatic failure secondary to heart failure, and acute tubular necrosis of the kidneys. This patient also had mild psychomotor retardation with low normal intelligence (IQ = 65). Hence, this man had MCAs: not only anomalies of the cardiovascular system but also of the central nervous system.

Sudden (not entirely unexpected) death caused by a ventricular tachyarrhythmia occurred in patients with mild (Cases 60 and 124) and with moderate (Case 96) mitral regurgitation. **Did the "sudden death" group of patients with hypertrophic cardiomyopathy and mild to moderate mitral regurgitation have any distinguishing features? Any warning symptoms or signs?**

Case 60, an 18 2/12-year-old young man had an arrhythmia, Wolff-Parkinson-White syndrome, that was progressive. When he was 15 years of age, he had multifocal ventricular premature beats, episodes of dizziness, and chest pain. His sudden death in 1975, presumably due to ventricular fibrillation, occurred after prolonged palpitations of up to 10 beats in length. Thus, this young man had multiple arrhythmic premonitory warnings before his fatal episode of (presumed) ventricular fibrillation. Autopsy revealed hypertrophy and enlargement of all cardiac chambers, most marked of the LV. Histologic examination revealed extensive diffuse myocardial replacement fibrosis involving the left ventricular free wall, the right ventricular free wall, the papillary muscles, and the ventricular septum. Asymmetric septal hypertrophy was not found at autopsy; but at 15 8/12 years of age, this patient had undergone a transaortic left ventricular septal myectomy for left ventricular outflow tract obstruction.

Case 96, a 27-year-old man, had hypertrophic obstructive cardiomyopathy with asymmetrical ventricular septal hypertrophy. After sudden death, probably caused by ventricular fibrillation, autopsy revealed that the ventricular septum was 35 mm thick, the left ventricular free wall measured 26 to 33 mm in thickness, and the right ventricular free wall was 9 to 10 mm thick. Cardiomegaly with biventricular hypertrophy was present, as the measurements indicate. In 1982, this patient had been treated with propranolol, without surgery. We were not aware of any premonitory cardiac arrhythmias. So, were there no warning symptoms or signs? None, except the presence of ventricular hypertrophy that in this patient was massive, which is an independent risk factor for sudden arrhythmic death.

Case 124, a 20 2/12-year-old young man who died in 1969, had hypertrophic obstructive cardiomyopathy with asymmetrical septal hypertrophy and massive cardiomegaly: the heart at autopsy weighed 1000 g. Sudden death had been documented electrocardiographically, with ventricular tachycardia progressing to ventricular fibrillation. Biventricular and biatrial hypertrophy were present. The ventricular septum was 31 mm thick, compared with the left ventricular free wall, which measured 17 to 22 mm in thickness. The ventricular septal–to–left ventricular free wall ratio was 31/22 (1.4/1) to 31/17 (1.8/1). The right ventricular free wall thickness was 10 mm. The left atrial free wall measured 2.5 mm in thickness. Interstitial fibrosis of the LV was found histologically. We were not aware of any premonitory cardiac arrhythmias in this young man. But his ventricular myocardial hypertrophy was massive, and this appears to be a silent warning sign or risk factor for sudden arrhythmic death.

CONGENITAL MITRAL REGURGITATION WITH TETRALOGY OF FALLOT

Sex: Males, 3; female, 1.

Age at Death: Mean, 10.20 ± 14.43 years; range, from 3 months and 9 days to 30 11/12 years; and median = 4 10/12 years

Although a male predominance was found (males to females = 3/1), this is, of course, much too small a sample to draw any conclusions (n = 4). The ages at death of these patients illustrate that TOF with congenital mitral regurgitation can present a serious clinical problem in childhood, or in adult life. Our youngest fatality occurred at 3.3 months of age, and the median age at death was 4 10/12 years. However, our oldest fatality was 30 11/12 years of age.

Clinical and Anatomic Features

Case 4, a 30 11/12-year-old man (our oldest patient), died in 1977. His mitral regurgitation was regarded as mild, but it was associated with a left atrial jet lesion. The free margins of the mitral leaflets at the anterolateral commissure were thickened and rolled, indicating chronic mitral regurgitation at this site. Careful examination of the mitral valve revealed a paucity of chordae tendineae at and beneath the anterolateral commissure. This malformation of the tensor apparatus is thought to have caused the mitral regurgitation, which was therefore thought to be congenital. No evidence of acquired pathologic conditions was found at this site. However, relatively mild congenital mitral regurgitation was among the least of this patient's problems. His TOF was characterized by severe infundibular stenosis at the proximal os infundibuli. Stenosis at the pulmonary valve level was mild, with a bicuspid pulmonary valve because of a rudimentary septal commissure.

When he was 10 months of age, on January 13, 1947, a Potts anastomosis was done. (This is a side-to-side anastomosis between the left pulmonary artery anteriorly, and the descending thoracic aorta posteriorly.) As we learned from later clinical experience, one of the major problems with the Potts procedure is that the anastomosis can "grow." It can get bigger and bigger over time. By 22½ years of age, in April 1968, this patient was in congestive heart failure because of excessive pulmonary blood flow through the Potts anastomosis. Consequently, in 1968 an attempt was made to repair the TOF, and a direct suture closure of the Potts shunt was performed. Postoperatively, a residual VSD was found with a left ventricular–to–right atrial shunt and severe tricuspid regurgitation. By April 1971, intermittent first-degree heart block, right bundle branch block with left anterior hemiblock, and ventricular premature beats were observed. By 1976, a diagnosis of sick sinus syndrome was made, and the patient was treated with cardioversion. On February 26, 1976, cardiac catheterization revealed mild mitral regurgitation. On March 3, 1976, surgical closure of the VSD and tricuspid valve replacement with a no. 29 Hancock prosthesis were performed. An epicardial pacemaker was also placed. The postoperative course was characterized by recurrent intractable congestive heart failure, leading to death from ventricular fibrillation. Cardiomegaly was enormous, with a cardiothoracic ratio of 85%. This is where we have come from. May we never forget.

Case 23, a 4½-month-old girl, had mild TOF, that is, mild infundibular pulmonary stenosis with a hypoplastic, but trileaflet pulmonary valve. She also had a relatively large secundum type of ASD; hence, she had *pentalogy of Fallot*. She also had a *horizontal cleft in the anterior mitral leaflet,* without an ostium primum type of ASD and without a VSD of the AV canal type. This cleft in the anterior mitral leaflet of the AV canal type was associated with severe congenital mitral regurgitation. A small PDA was also present at autopsy. Other findings included biventricular hypertrophy and enlargement, biatrial hypertrophy and enlargement, and a normal tricuspid valve. The patient had several "blue spells," that is, episodes of hypercyanosis with loss of consciousness. It is noteworthy that blue spells can occur with relatively mild pulmonary outflow tract stenosis in TOF, as in this patient.

Because she was only 4½ months old in 1969, she was regarded as too young for correction on cardiopulmonary bypass, that correction of her severe congenital mitral regurgitation would have required. In 1969, we were still in the era of palliation, not correction of congenital heart disease in infancy. She could have had a Blalock-Taussig shunt or other aortopulmonary anastomosis without cardiopulmonary bypass, but she did not need that because her pulmonary outflow tract obstruction was relatively mild. So she was discharged home, where she died. Hence, in this patient, the pressure of severe congenital mitral regurgitation through an AV canal type of cleft was of major clinical importance.

In this study of 3400 autopsied cases of heart disease (3216 cases of congenital heart disease, and 184 cases of acquired heart disease) between 1946 and 2000, although the anatomy does not change, patient management certainly does, as the foregoing case reminds us. As far as patient management is concerned we are taking a voyage back and forth through the last half of the 20th century. This is the first half century when accurate diagnosis and successful management of almost all forms of congenital heart disease were achieved, at the hospital where successful surgery for congenital heart disease began (with the closure of a PDA on August 26, 1938 by Dr. Robert E Gross).

Case 110, a 3-month-and-9-day old boy, was born by cesarean section at 36 weeks gestation because of fetal distress with bradycardia; his birth weight was 2.4 kg (5.29 lb, or 5 lb and 4.6 oz). In 1984, bilateral pneumothoraces were successfully treated with chest tubes between 4 and 18 days of postnatal age. TOF {S,D,S} with pulmonary outflow tract atresia was diagnosed. The right pulmonary artery was absent, a large collateral artery supplying the right lung. A smaller tortuous collateral artery supplied the left lung. Congenital absence of the ductus arteriosus was also noted. The patent foramen ovale was valve competent. A small fistula (internal diameter = 2 mm) was found between the proximal MPA and the left anterior descending coronary artery (see Fig. 14.38).

The patient underwent surgery at 3 months and 9 days of age in 1984. The MPA was transected, with oversewing of the proximal stump of the MPA and with direct anastomosis of the distal MPA to the ascending aorta (3-mm internal diameter of the anastomosis). The patient could not be weaned from cardiopulmonary bypass, leading to intraoperative death.

Autopsy revealed marked cardiomegaly. The LV was severely hypertrophied and enlarged, with extensive left ventricular myocardial fibrosis that was both subendocardial and transmural. The left ventricular papillary muscles displayed hypertrophy, fibrosis, and infarction. Mitral regurgitation, documented angiocardiographically was thought to be related to papillary muscle dysfunction. Left atrial hypertrophy and enlargement, with mild generalized endocardial thickening were also found.

The orifice of the left coronary artery was stenotic. It arose from the appropriate left coronary sinus of Valsalva and pursued a normal course to the left ventricular apex; it continued around the cardiac apex, reaching the posteroinferior ventricular surface. The left coronary artery also communicated with the root of the MPA, distal to the pulmonary infundibular and valvar atresia, via a *left coronary artery–to–MPA fistula (see* Fig. 14.38). At cardiac catheterization, a gradient had been measured between the aorta and the left coronary artery of 60 to 65 mm Hg. Thus, our diagnostic impression was that, in addition to the *left coronary ostial stenosis,* there had also been a *steal from the left coronary artery into the MPA* via the fistula between these two structures (see Fig. 14.38). Ostial stenosis leading into the left coronary artery, plus a steal from the left coronary artery into the low-pressure MPA were thought to be the main congenital factors leading to papillary muscle fibrosis and infarction and widespread myocardial fibrosis of this patient's left ventricular free wall.

In addition, the right coronary artery was hypoplastic: it was only 2 cm long and did not reach the posteroinferior surface of the heart. This anomaly of the right coronary artery may also have been clinically important per se. In addition, this right coronary hypoplasia may have denied this patient the possibility of developing collaterals from the right coronary artery to compensate for the anomalies of the left coronary artery. Both lungs were unilobed, because of failure of development of the normal pulmonary fissures.

Our reservations concerning the accuracy of the gradient between the aorta and the left coronary artery mentioned above (60 to 65 mm Hg) probably should be explicit. Can one accurately measure the pressure in a left coronary artery after passing an end-hole catheter through a stenotic left coronary ostium in a 3-year-old child? We suspect that the catheter may have contributed to the gradient that was measured.

Nonetheless, because of the anatomic findings, we were convinced that the following diagnoses are correct: (1) ostial stenosis of the left coronary artery; plus (2) left coronary artery steal via a small fistula leading into the very-low-pressure MPA; (3) resulting in left ventricular papillary muscle and free wall ischemic necrosis and replacement fibrosis; and leading to (4) mitral regurgitation with a congenital basis.

Case 116, a 9 3/12-year-old boy, had TOF {S,D,S} with a right aortic arch and congenital mitral regurgitation. The anterior mitral leaflet was thickened, and the chordae tendineae were very short. Two left ventricular papillary muscle groups were present, and both were hypertrophied and short. Complete repair was undertaken in 1970. His postoperative course was characterized by nodal rhythm (related to surgical injury of the sinoatrial node), atrial flutter (treated with quinidine, with good response), and left anterior hemiblock (related to surgical injury, presumably associated with VSD patch placement). Sudden death occurred at home, thought to be related to an arrhythmia. Autopsy revealed, in addition to the foregoing, marked left atrial hypertrophy and enlargement. The LA was twice the normal size. Jet lesions of the posterior left atrial wall confirmed the presence of mitral regurgitation. Thus, this patient with TOF also had *typical congenital mitral regurgitation.*

Summary

The types of congenital mitral regurgitation found in these 4 patients with TOF may be summarized as follows:

1. Case 4: Chordal paucity at the anterolateral commissure.
2. Case 23: Canal cleft of anterior mitral leaflet.
3. Case 110: Left coronary ostial stenosis, plus steal from left coronary artery into low-pressure MPA via a left coronary artery–to–MPA fistula.
4. Case 116: Typical congenital mitral regurgitation, that is, thick anterior mitral leaflet and very short chordae tendineae.

CONGENITAL MITRAL REGURGITATION WITH SINGLE LEFT VENTRICLE

Case 51, a 4-year-old girl had single LV, an infundibular outlet chamber, and normally related great arteries. The segmental anatomy was {S,D,S}. So, she had a Holmes heart, without pulmonary stenosis. The right ventricular sinus displayed extreme hypoplasia; that is, it was essentially absent, resulting in a single, or unpaired, LV. There was DILV, and both AV valves were regurgitant. The left-sided mitral valve had mitral regurgitation, documented both by angiocardiography and echocardiography. Autopsy revealed marked nodular thickening of the anterior mitral leaflet and mild thickening of the posterior mitral leaflet. The anterolateral and posteromedial papillary muscles of the LV were hypertrophied, and the mitral chordae tendineae were partly muscularized. The single LV was hypertrophied and enlarged, the left ventricular free wall measuring 12 mm in thickness in the fresh state. Mild, focal EFE of the LV was also present. The LA was markedly hypertrophied and enlarged, with jet lesions of the left atrial endocardium posteriorly and anterolaterally, confirming the presence of mitral regurgitation.

The right-sided tricuspid valve straddled the ventricular septal remnant (well developed on the left ventricular side, but almost absent on what normally would have been the right ventricular side). This type of straddling tricuspid valve is typical of D-loop single LV with DILV. Therefore, some degree of tricuspid regurgitation is typical; it was judged to be mild by echocardiography and angiocardiography in this patient. But what is unusual in this situation is mitral regurgitation. Typically, in a Holmes heart the mitral valve inserts normally into the left ventricular papillary muscles with little or no mitral dysfunction. The RA was both hypertrophied and enlarged, the right atrial free wall measuring 4 mm in thickness in the fresh state. The septal leaflet of the tricuspid valve was abnormally thickened, reflecting the presence of tricuspid regurgitation.

Multiple VSDs were present: a large VSD of the AV canal type, through which the tricuspid valve straddled; a posterior mid-muscular VSD; and an apical muscular VSD. A word concerning **terminology** may be helpful here. Strictly speaking, all of these VSDs are *bulboventricular foramina,* because the right ventricular sinus was absent. Ventricular septal defect is short for *interventricular septal defect (IVSD).* Logically, an IVSD cannot be present if there is only one ventricle. It should be understood that an infundibular outlet chamber is not a malformed RV. The infundibulum, or infundibular outlet chamber, is normally formed with single LV and normally related great arteries (a Holmes heart). The infundibulum or conus arteriosus is really part of the great arterial segment, the conotruncus. Thus, the infundibulum is really not part of either ventricle. Instead, the infundibulum or conus arteriosus is how the great arteries connect with the subjacent structures—the ventricles, ventricular septum, and AV canal. This is why the infundibulum can override the ventricular septum to any degree; the infundibulum can be mostly above the LV because the infundibulum is *not* an intrinsic part of the RV.

The use of the term *VSD* to describe the aforementioned defects instead of the more correct *bulboventricular foramen,* is an intentional bow to common usage. My wife, Dr. Stella Zacharioudaki Van Praagh, was a native Greek. I soon came to understand that what matters most is *meaning* or *understanding,* not terminology. The same meaning can be conveyed by many different words (in Greek, Italian, French, German, Japanese, etc.). What I am trying to emphasize is meaning and understanding, not terminology. But I also know how important accurate terminology is; hence, this explanatory note.

Now, returning to Case 51, this patient had a systemic level of pulmonary hypertension, with a Qp/Qs of 4.9/1.0. Thus, at 3½ years of age, the patient underwent banding of the MPA (in 1987). At 4 years of age (in 1988), a modified Fontan procedure was performed. The IVC blood stream was directed to the SVC via an intra–right atrial lateral tunnel constructed with a Gore-Tex patch. The SVC was anastomosed to the right pulmonary artery, which also communicated with the left pulmonary artery. The MPA was divided. The atrial septum was resected, and the mitral orifice was closed with a patch. The postoperative period was characterized by hypotension and low cardiac output. In turn, this led to Fontan takedown. Supraventricular tachycardia occurred subsequently and was associated with hypotension, leading to cardiac arrest and death.

The presence of congenital mitral regurgitation prompted patch closure of the mitral orifice. Consequently, in the surgical management of this patient with single LV {S,D,S} in 1988, the presence of congenital mitral regurgitation was of considerable importance. Patch closure of the mitral orifice meant that this patient's only AV valve was a straddling and regurgitation tricuspid valve.

Case 73, a 28½-year-old woman, had single LV with an infundibular outlet chamber and TGA {S,D,L}. (TGA {S,D,L} means TGA with solitus atria [S], D-loop ventricular segment [D], and L-TGA.) The transposed aortic valve was to the left (levo- or L-) relative to the transposed pulmonary valve. Mitral regurgitation was mild, with thickening of the anterior mitral leaflet. The mitral valve's chordae tendineae inserted into the anterolateral and posteromedial papillary muscle groups.

Why did the mitral valve regurgitate? We did not really know. Dr. Stella Van Praagh thought that pulmonary regurgitation may have caused hemodynamic changes in the subjacent mitral valve, leading to mild mitral regurgitation. In other words, the mitral valve was located in an abnormal pulmonary regurgitant flow stream, which may have caused what Dr. Maurice Lev called "hemodynamic change," such as leaflet thickening, fibrosis, and subsequent retraction, leading to mild mitral regurgitation. We were forced to consider such a hypothesis because the anatomy of the mitral valve per se appeared normal.

The bulboventricular foramen leading from the single LV into the infundibular outflow chamber was large and unrestrictive (23 × 17 m); thus there was no subaortic stenosis. As mentioned earlier, there was pulmonary valvar regurgitation. There was no pulmonary outflow tract obstruction. Hence, it is not surprising that this 28½-year-old woman had pulmonary vascular obstructive disease, suggested by cardiac catheterization data. She displayed cyanosis, with severe clubbing of her fingers and toes. This patient had DILV. The tricuspid valve attached to the ventricular septum and to the left ventricular papillary muscles.

This patient experienced a sudden and unexpected death in 1987. A fatal terminal arrhythmia was suspected, but not documented. At autopsy, pulmonary histology revealed grade IV Heath-Edwards changes. In grade IV, the pulmonary arterioles are dilated. The media is abnormally thin, and the lumina are occluded by fibrous tissue. Thus, pulmonary histology confirmed the presence of pulmonary vascular obstructive disease. Consequently, a modified Fontan procedure could not have been performed successfully in 1987.

What can we learn from this case? The importance of an early modified Fontan procedure, before the development of pulmonary vascular obstructive disease and before the development of severe left ventricular hypertrophy, seems to be the most important (if obvious) lesson of this kind of case. This patient was born in 1959, a little more than a decade before the development of the Fontan-Kreutzer procedure (1970–1972). So, she was born at least 10 years too soon. In other words, this case history emphasizes the importance of a timely, preemptive cavopulmonary type of procedure in patients with a single ventricle, particularly if there is no protective pulmonary outflow tract stenosis. The presence of mild mitral regurgitation appears to have been of little clinical importance.

Case 102, a 19-year-old young woman, had single LV with an infundibular outlet chamber and TGA {S,L,L}. (Recall that TGA {S,L,L} means TGA with the segmental anatomy of solitus atria [S], ventricular L-loop [L], and L-TGA [L]. Single LV means that the right ventricular sinus is absent but the infundibulum is present; hence, the presence of an infundibular outlet chamber.) There was DILV with thickening and rolling of the leaflet margins of the left-sided tricuspid valve and of the right-sided mitral valve. Hence, there was regurgitation of both the left-sided tricuspid valve and of the right-sided mitral valve. Both AV valves had abnormal chordal attachments to the conal septum superiorly. There was mild to moderate subaortic stenosis at the level of the bulboventricular foramen that had a fibrous rim of endocardial sclerosis. There was no subaortic infundibular stenosis and no aortic valvar stenosis. Subpulmonary outflow tract stenosis was present. The pulmonary outflow tract was crowded between the medial leaflets of both AV valves, and the pulmonary valve leaflets were also thickened. A PDA was present, with an internal diameter of 3 to 5 mm. A left aortic arch was present. A *brachiocephalic artery* gave rise to the right subclavian, the right common carotid, and the left common carotid arteries. The second branch was the left subclavian artery. It is noteworthy that single LV with an infundibular outlet chamber and TGA {S,L,L} is the most common anatomic type of single ventricle. This woman died in 1981 because of an acute brain abscess. Her right frontoparietal cerebritis was caused by streptococcus MG-intermedius, normal mouth flora.

Again, right-sided mitral regurgitation was not judged to be a major clinical problem. But brain abscess certainly was. One of the advantages of a modified Fontan type of hemodynamic palliation in patients with only one well-formed ventricle has to do with *the lungs' filter function*. In addition to their respiratory function, the lungs also seem very important because they can filter out or catch various different kinds of abnormalities in the systemic venous blood stream, such as thromboemboli, pus, and bacteria. The result in a normally formed heart and pulmonary filter can be pulmonary emboli or foci of pneumonia; but this is better than a stroke or a brain abscess. This is why a patent foramen ovale can be important in a biventricular heart, because it can permit paradoxical (i.e., right-to-left) embolism. But in hearts with only one ventricle, the risk for paradoxical embolism is ever present, as this patient illustrates.

CONGENITAL MITRAL REGURGITATION WITH CONGENITAL ANEURYSM OR DYSPLASIA OF THE LEFT VENTRICLE

There were 3 such patients in this series of 109 postmortem cases of congenital mitral regurgitation (3%; see Table 14.12).

Case 50 was a boy whose age we did not know. This heart specimen was sent as a consult from Hannover, Germany in 1988, courtesy of Prof. Carlo Kallfelz. The boy had a large congenital aneurysm of the LV (Fig. 14.39). The left ventricular dysplasia involved both the left ventricular free wall and the left ventricular septal surface, from the base of the papillary muscles to the left ventricular apex. The aneurysmal left ventricular free wall was thinner (2 mm thick) than the nonaneurysmal left ventricular free wall (5 to 7 mm thick). The interior of the

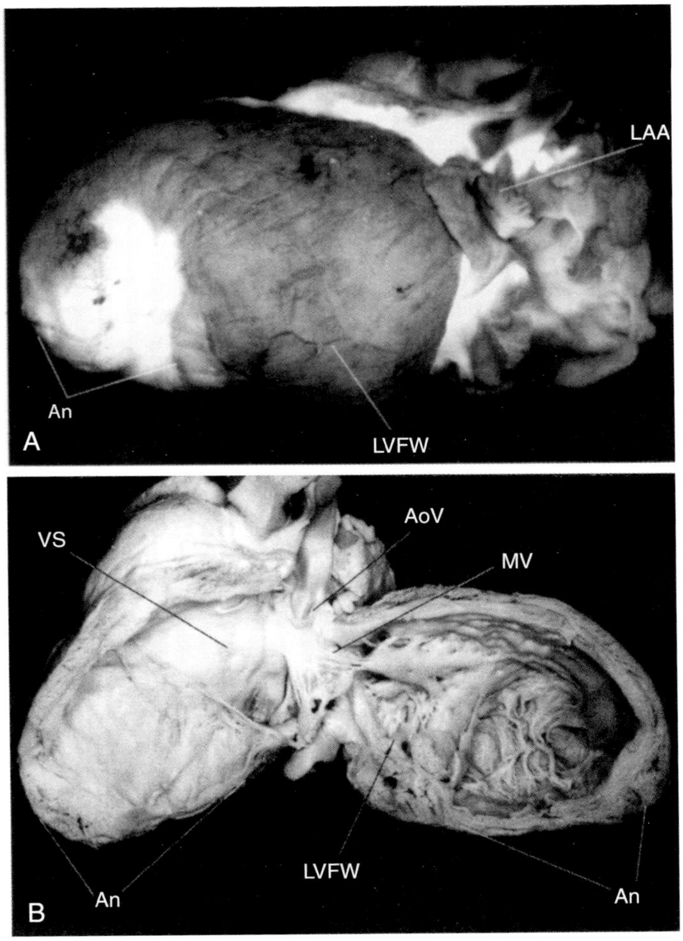

Fig. 14.39 Congenital left ventricular aneurysm with brilliant transillumination of the left ventricular apex *(An)*, whereas the nonaneurysmal left ventricular free wall *(LVFW)* does not transilluminate. (A) External view of the left ventricle. (B) Internal view of the left ventricle (LV). The congenital left ventricular aneurysm is very large, involving the apical half of the LV. There is a prominent circumferential muscular ridge demarcating the proximal nonaneurysmal left ventricular septum and free wall from the apical aneurysm. The aneurysmal left ventricular free wall is dysplastic, displaying rootlet-like structures. The proximal left ventricular septal surface *(VS)* displays endocardial fibroelastosis. This patient was a 2-day-old white male infant who died from congestive heart failure. There was a clinical question of cardiac tamponade. Hence, our study confirmed that congenital left ventricular aneurysm is left ventricular endomyocardial disease. No evidence of viral or other infection was found. *AoV*, Aortic valve; *LAA*, left atrial appendage; *MV*, mitral valve. (Reproduced with permission from Papagiannis J, Van Praagh R, Schwint O, et al. Congenital left ventricular aneurysm: Clinical, imaging, pathologic, and surgical findings in severe new cases. *Am Heart J*. 2001;141:491.)

left ventricular aneurysm was dysplastic, being covered with bizarre membranous trabeculations. The left ventricular septal surface had EFE. The anterolateral papillary muscle of the LV was shortened, and the posteromedial papillary muscle of the LV was hypoplastic (see Fig. 14.39B). Fibrous streamer-like enlargement of the posteromedial papillary muscle extended into the congenital left ventricular aneurysm. The congenital left ventricular aneurysm was relatively large, measuring 4 × 4 cm (length × width). The approximate ratio of the volume of the left ventricular aneurysm to the volume of the nonaneurysmal left ventricular cavity was 3:1. In other words, the volume of left ventricular aneurysm was approximately 3 times as big as that of the nonaneurysmal LV. Thickening and rolling of the free margins of the anterior and posterior mitral leaflets confirmed the presence of congenital mitral regurgitation. The LA was hypertrophied and enlarged. The septum primum bulged into the RA. Right ventricular hypertrophy and a PDA were also found. This was a patient with a large congenital left ventricular aneurysm, with dysplasia of the left ventricular free wall and septal surfaces, involvement of the left ventricular anterolateral and posteromedial papillary muscles, and with congenital mitral regurgitation. Polymerase chain reaction studies revealed no evidence of viral myocarditis.

Case 80, a 14-month-old boy, had a clinical diagnosis of cardiomyopathy. (This heart specimen was sent to us as consultation in 1984 by Dr. James Reynolds of New Orleans, Louisiana). Autopsy revealed left ventricular dysplasia with areas of marked left ventricular thickening, widespread areas of marked left ventricular thinning, bizarre left ventricular architecture, and congenital mitral regurgitation. Massive left ventricular hypertrophy involved both of the papillary muscle groups—anterolateral and posteromedial—and focal areas of the left ventricular free wall posteroinferiorly that were 18 mm thick. Amazingly, there was a *cavity* within the left ventricular free wall posteroinferiorly. There were also widespread areas of left ventricular free wall thinning that measured between 3 and 7 mm in thickness. EFE of the left ventricular was also present. Thickening and rolling of the anterior mitral leaflet were also found, consistent with mitral regurgitation in life. Left atrial hypertrophy and enlargement were found, with marked endocardial sclerosis. Right ventricular hypertrophy was regarded as mild to moderate in degree. But the septal band and the papillary muscle of the conus were described as huge.

Terminal convulsions and unconsciousness led to death. Autopsy revealed thrombosis of the transverse (or coronal) and sagittal sinuses of the dura mater, hydrocephalus, and recent hemorrhage in the posterior fossa. Our hypothesis concerning the immediate cause of death in this 14-year-old boy was as follows: antemortem left ventricular mural thrombosis probably led to fatal cerebral thromboembolism (i.e., a stroke). However, it should be emphasized that the foregoing is a *hypothesis;* no definite evidence of antemortem left ventricular mural thrombus was found.

What should we call this patient's cardiomyopathy? I think this is an unknown anatomic type of cardiomyopathy. Let us call the entity **hypertrophic and hypoplastic cardiomyopathy.** This designation embraces two of its most striking anatomic features: simultaneous focal hypertrophy and hypoplasia of the LV. Other features displayed by this patient (C84-169) include left ventricular EFE (hence, this is an *endomyocardial dysplasia*), a cavity within the focally hypertrophied left ventricular free wall, and mitral regurgitation. The mitral regurgitation was thought to be related to the left ventricular cardiomyopathy. The mitral valve was normally formed per se; but the subjacent left ventricular myocardium, including the papillary muscles, were very dysplastic. Another way of saying this is that the mitral regurgitation appeared to be related to the papillary muscles (very hypertrophied) and the left ventricular myocardium (very dysplastic), not the mitral leaflets and chordae tendineae. What was the cavity within the very hypertrophied left ventricular free wall posteroinferiorly? It should be stated that the cardiac segmental anatomy was normal, that is {S,D,S} and that the ventricular septum was intact.

We entertained the possibility that this perhaps was a *"dissection cavity"* within the markedly hypertrophied left ventricular free wall. But, although aortic mural dissections are well known in connective tissue disorders such as Marfan syndrome, I have never heard of a left ventricular free wall dissection. However, such things may occur before a left ventricular free wall rupture (hypothesis). Suffice it to say that I do not really know what this **left ventricular intramural cavity** is. It may be a previously unrecognized congenital malformation.

HYPERTROPHIC AND HYPOPLASTIC CARDIOMYOPATHY

Case 89, a boy who died at 2 days of postnatal age, had primary (i.e., idiopathic) endomyocardial disease or cardiomyopathy involving all cardiac chambers: endocardial sclerosis of the RA; patchy diffuse EFE of the RV; patchy EFE of the LA; severe EFE of the LV that was focal, but widespread; congenital left ventricular aneurysm involving a large region of the left ventricular apex (see Fig. 14. 38); marked congenital mitral regurgitation with nodular gelatinous thickening of the mitral leaflets; patent foramen ovale with herniation of the septum primum into the RA; and mild aortic regurgitation. To my knowledge this is the first report of hypertrophic and hypoplastic cardiomyopathy. He had a history of severe congestive heart failure with cyanosis, leading to neonatal death (at 2 days of age). In the area of congenital left ventricular aneurysm involving much of the left ventricular apex, the greatly thinned left ventricular free wall transilluminated brilliantly (see Fig. 14.39A). Histologically, the left ventricular myocardium was greatly thinned but not absent and left ventricular EFE was severe. The dysplastic and aneurysmal left ventricular myocardium had a marked deficiency of numerous, fine, oblique trabeculae carneae (see Fig. 14.39B). Thus, the area of the congenital left ventricular aneurysm displayed marked deficiency of stratum compactum (the outer, compact myocardium supplied by the coronary arteries) and of stratum spongiosum (from which the numerous, fine, oblique left ventricular trabeculae carneae normally develop). The coronary arteries were normal.

Thus, the poorly contracting LV, observed by imaging studies during life, were well explained by the postmortem findings.

Regarding cause, polymerase chain reaction studies revealed no evidence of viral myocarditis.

Histologic Findings of Congenital Left Ventricular Aneurysm

The histologic features of congenital left ventricular aneurysm in two autopsied patients are shown in Fig. 14.40. Fig. 14.40A shows extensive transmural fibrosis, with little remaining normal-appearing left ventricular free wall myocardium. However, Fig. 40B shows, apart from left ventricular free wall myocardial thinning, histologically unremarkable myocardium, without fibrosis, necrosis, calcification, or inflammation. Thus, left ventricular histologic examination did not reveal the cause or the morphogenesis of congenital left ventricular aneurysm. Both remain unknown at the present time.

CONGENITAL MITRAL REGURGITATION WITH DOWN SYNDROME

Down syndrome was the 10th situation in which congenital mitral regurgitation was found (3 patients, 3% of the series; see Table 14.12). Case 9, a 5½-year-old girl; Case 65, a 14-month-old girl; and Case 84, a 35-year-old woman all had an incomplete form of common AV canal with an ostium primum type of interatrial communication, no VSD, and a cleft anterior leaflet of the mitral valve that permitted congenital mitral regurgitation. None had undergone surgery. The clinically significant difference among these 3 patients had to do with the severity of the mitral regurgitation, which in turn was reflected by their ages at death.

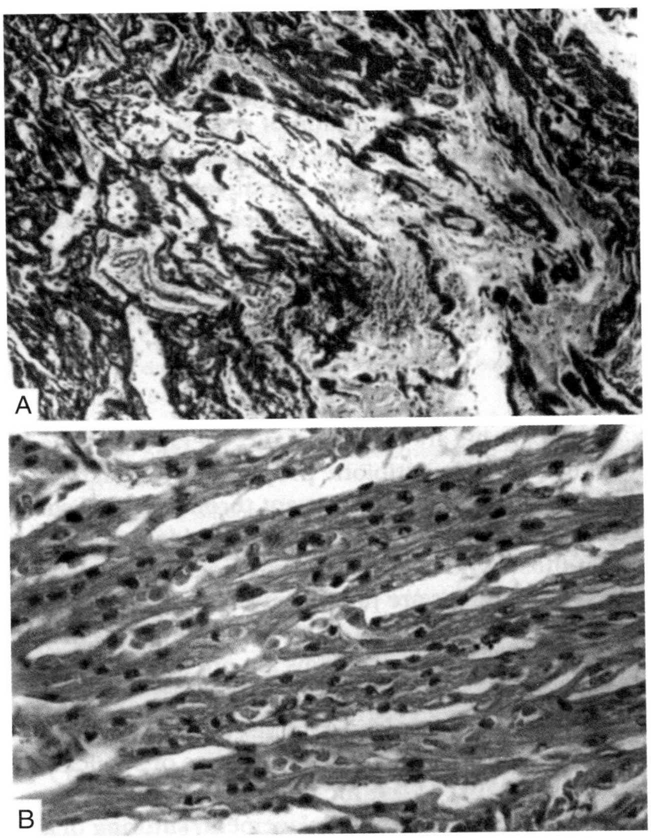

Fig. 14.40 Histology of congenital left ventricular aneurysm, from two autopsied cases. (A) Gomori trichrome, original magnification ×100. Considerable transmural fibrosis, with little normal-appearing myocardium. (B) Hematoxylin and eosin, original magnification ×400. Apart from left ventricular free wall thinning, histologically unremarkable ventricular myocardium without fibrosis, necrosis, calcification, or inflammation. (Reproduced with permission from Papagiannis J, Van Praagh R, Schwint O, et al. Congenital left ventricular aneurysm: Clinical, imaging, pathologic, and surgical findings in severe new cases. *Am Heart J.* 2001;141:491.)

Case 65, a 14-month-old girl, was the youngest, with the most severe mitral regurgitation. She had a very wide cleft in the anterior mitral leaflet: it was a gap measuring 1 cm (or 0.4 inch) in width. She also had a small cleft between the anterior and septal leaflets of the tricuspid valve. In 1971, she had a history of chronic congestive heart failure and recurrent episodes of pneumonia. Autopsy revealed cardiomegaly (71 g, normal being 54 g, i.e., 31% greater than normal), with hypertrophy and enlargement of all cardiac chambers. She also had a very small blood cyst on the left ventricular septal surface, adjacent to the gap in her anterior mitral leaflet. Thus, the salient finding in this case was *marked deficiency of the anterior mitral leaflet,* resulting in a 1-cm-wide gap (much wider than the usual cleft).

Case 9, a 5½-year-old girl, had moderate mitral regurgitation through a cleft in the anterior mitral leaflet. Marked thickening and rolling of the free margins of the regurgitant cleft and widespread left atrial endocardial jet lesions were present. Other findings included a small ostium secundum type of ASD (3 mm in maximal dimension); cardiomegaly with hypertrophy and enlargement of all chambers; an ostium primum type of interatrial communication, with no VSD; a history of Qp/Qs = 3.1/1; an aberrant right subclavian artery; and a history of chronic congestive heart failure that led to death in 1983. Thus, the salient finding of this patient with Down syndrome and a typical incomplete form of common AV canal was *moderate mitral regurgitation through a cleft of the anterior leaflet of the mitral valve.*

Case 84, a 35-year-old woman with Down syndrome, died in 1992. She, too, had *normal cardiac segmental anatomy {S,D,S}, as patients with trisomy 21 always do, in our experience,* and an incomplete or partial form of common AV canal characterized by a large ostium primum type of interatrial communication (20 × 8 mm), a prominent aneurysm of the membranous septum (14 mm long), and an *incomplete cleft of the anterior leaflet of the mitral valve.* There was a short paraseptal fusion of the superior and inferior components of the anterior mitral leaflet. Mitral regurgitation occurred through this incomplete (or partial) cleft of the anterior mitral leaflet. A prominent left atrial jet lesion extended 3 cm (1.2 inches) above the posteromedial commissure of the mitral valve. Mild tricuspid regurgitation was also present.

Other very significant findings at autopsy were acute bronchopneumonia; cerebral edema that was acute, bilateral, diffuse, severe, and associated with tonsillar herniation; lymphocytic thyroiditis (Hashimoto thyroiditis); fecal impaction, most marked in the sigmoid colon; and aspirated material in the airways.

The salient finding as far as congenital mitral regurgitation is concerned was an incomplete cleft in the anterior mitral leaflet associated with mitral regurgitation that was mild enough to permit a relatively "long" life to 35 years of age.

All three cases exemplify the highly variable relatively *natural history* of the incomplete form of common AV canal with mitral regurgitation, in which open heart surgery was *not* performed. Severe congenital mitral regurgitation led to death at 4 months of age; moderate mitral regurgitation led to death at 5½ years of age; and milder mitral regurgitation permitted survival until 35 years of age.

CONGENITAL MITRAL REGURGITATION WITH DOUBLE-OUTLET RIGHT VENTRICLE

Congenital mitral regurgitation occurred in 2 patients with DORV (2% of this series of 108 autopsied patients with congenital mitral regurgitation; see Table 14.2). Both had malformed mitral valves.

Case 101, a 7-year-old boy, had DORV {S,D,D}, a bilateral conus, a subaortic VSD, a bicommissural aortic valve (the intercoronary commissure was underdeveloped, but the aortic valve was not stenotic), and an aberrant right subclavian artery. Congenital mitral regurgitation was related to abnormal left ventricular tensor apparatus and an anomaly of left ventricular architecture. Both papillary muscles of the LV were abnormally small. The posteromedial papillary muscle was very small. The anterolateral papillary muscle group was somewhat larger, but much smaller than normal. An accessory papillary muscle immediately beneath the anterolateral commissure of the mitral valve received chordae tendineae from both mitral leaflets. These abnormal chordal attachments into this accessory papillary muscle resulted in mitral regurgitation because of inability of the mitral valve to close normally. Left ventricular hypertrophy and moderate left ventricular EFE were also found. Right ventricular hypertrophy and enlargement were present. At 1 year of age (in 1961), banding of the MPA had been performed. At 7 years of age (in 1966), complete repair was undertaken. Death occurred because the patch leading from the VSD to the aortic valve was obstructive. Thus, as far as congenital mitral regurgitation is concerned, the salient problem was *a malformation of the tensor apparatus of the mitral valve: an accessory papillary muscle receiving all of the mitral chordae tendineae, with inability of the mitral leaflets to close.*

Case 114, a stillborn girl, had evidence of congenital mitral regurgitation. The anterior mitral leaflet had a thickened and rolled edge. The posteromedial papillary muscle was abnormally small, and its chordal attachments were abnormal (that was how they were described). DORV {S,D,D} with a bilateral conus (subaortic and subpulmonary) was also present. The subaortic conal free wall was only 2 to 3 mm in height, but this prevented aortic-tricuspid and aortic-mitral direct fibrous continuity. The conotruncus was otherwise similar to that in mild TOF. There was a large subaortic VSD with mild anterosuperior malalignment of the conal septum. Although the pulmonary valve was bicuspid, it was neither hypoplastic nor stenotic. There was a single left coronary artery. The ostium of the right coronary artery was absent, and the right coronary artery per se was absent, *a rare finding.* This patient also had MCAs: an omphalocele, a right hydroureter, and right hydronephrosis. To summarize the congenital mitral regurgitation, this stillborn girl had *abnormal tensor apparatus with hypoplastic posteromedial papillary muscle and abnormal chordae tendineae.*

CONGENITAL MITRAL REGURGITATION WITH LEFT VENTRICULAR OUTFLOW TRACT OBSTRUCTION

How is it possible for left ventricular outflow tract obstruction to be responsible for congenital mitral regurgitation? The answer is *the left ventricular outflow tract squeeze.* Posterior malalignment of the conal septum squeezes the left ventricular outflow tract between the abnormally posteriorly located conal septum superiorly and anteriorly and the normally located mitral valve posteriorly and inferiorly. The normally located mitral valve cannot get out of the way. The anterior leaflet of the mitral valve forms part of the posteroinferior surface of the left ventricular outflow tract. When the great arteries are normally related, the posteriorly deviated conal septum results in aortic outflow tract stenosis. But when TGA is present, the result is pulmonary outflow tract obstruction. In either case, posteroinferior malalignment of the conal septum lowers the "roof" of the left ventricular outflow tract creating subarterial stenosis. The accelerated outflow tract velocity and turbulence associated with left ventricular outflow tract obstruction produces thickening and hemodynamic change of the anterior mitral leaflet, predisposing to mitral regurgitation. The mechanism of mitral regurgitation in this situation is somewhat similar to what can happen in hypertrophic obstructive cardiomyopathy, in which the asymmetric septal hypertrophy can bulge into the left ventricular outflow tract, significantly narrowing it. The anterior mitral leaflet is *in* the left ventricular outflow tract, rather than lying to the left of it. Another analogy that may aid understanding is the following. Posteroinferior malalignment of the conal septum is the opposite of TOF. (In tetralogy, the conal septum is malaligned anterosuperiorly.) Hence, the hemodynamic effects of posteroinferior malalignment of the conal septum are the opposite of tetralogy—hence, left ventricular outflow tract obstruction rather than right ventricular outflow tract obstruction.

Case 29, a 4-month-old girl, had normal segmental anatomy {S,D,S}, a conoventricular type of VSD that was more subpulmonary than subaortic, and posteroinferior deviation of the conal septum. The posteroinferior malalignment of the conal septum had multiple effects: subaortic stenosis (by lowering the "roof" of the left ventricular outflow tract); aortic annular hypoplasia (resulting in aortic annular stenosis); mild to moderate hypoplastic of the ascending aorta, aortic arch, and becoming maximal at the aortic isthmus (internal diameter = 3 mm), resulting in a mild to moderate preductal coarctation of the aorta and mild to moderate mitral regurgitation with a small jet lesion of the LA. At 2½ months of age in 1981, the patient was operated on to close the VSD. The postoperative course was characterized by a myocardial infarction. Subsequently, pneumonitis of the right lung caused by respiratory syncytial virus led to death at 4 months of age. This combination of anomalies, which may be thought of as **anti**-TOF, that is, the opposite of TOF, is still not widely understood.

Should one be surprised that this patient died after the surgical closure of her VSD? Would you be surprised if a patient with TOF died after surgical closure of the VSD, if nothing else was done? No. Why not? Because "everyone" knows how important it is to repair the pulmonary outflow tract obstruction in TOF. Exactly. But think about a patient with the opposite of TOF. In anti-TOF, is it not hemodynamically important to repair the subaortic stenosis, aortic valvar (annular) stenosis, hypoplasia of the aorta, and coarctation of the aorta? Just as TOF is much more than just a VSD, so too the opposite of TOF is much more than just a VSD. Many pediatric cardiologists do not know that there is an opposite to TOF. Perhaps that is why the combination of anomalies has no name. I tentatively suggest *anti*-TOF. Whether this suggestion will meet with approval is much too early to say. No matter what one may prefer to call this combination of anomalies, it is important to know that such a combination of malformations does indeed exist, because this understanding may then permit successful surgical repair. Anti-tetralogy has one feature that is not the opposite of tetralogy: mitral regurgitation. Why is this so? Because in tetralogy, the malalignment of the conal septum is *away* from the AV valves, in an anterosuperior direction; whereas in anti-tetralogy, the deviation of the conal septum is *toward* the mitral valve, in a posteromedial direction. So, only in the opposite of tetralogy does the conal septum interfere with mitral valve function.

Case 2, a 1 11/12-year-old boy, had TGA {S,D,D}. (Recall that TGA {S,D,D} means TGA with the segmental anatomic set of situs solitus of the viscera and atria [S], D-loop ventricles [D], and D-transposition of the great arteries [D].) The conus was subaortic, permitting pulmonary-mitral direct fibrous continuity. The VSD was of the conoventricular anatomic type (between the conal septum above and the ventricular septal below). The conal septum was malaligned posteriorly and inferiorly, narrowing the subpulmonary area and the pulmonary valve. There was subpulmonary stenosis and pulmonary valvar stenosis. The pulmonary valve was bicuspid because of absence of the left septal–nonseptal commissure. Mitral regurgitation was mild, with thickening of the middle portion of the free margin of the anterior mitral leaflet. A Rastelli procedure was done, with a conduit between the RV and the MPA to bypass the pulmonary outflow tract stenosis. Autopsy revealed that the left anterior descending coronary artery was narrowed by the RV-to-MPA conduit. Mild mitral regurgitation was thought to be caused by the posteroinferior malalignment of the conal septum that was abnormally close to the normally located anterior leaflet of the mitral valve, resulting in left ventricular outflow tract stenosis. The thickening of the middle third of the anterior mitral leaflet and the left atrial jet lesion prove that mitral regurgitation was indeed present. The RV was hypertrophied and enlarged, an unusual finding with D-TGA and left-sided juxtaposition of the atrial appendages. Right ventricular hypoplasia, often with tricuspid stenosis or atresia, is a usual finding with TGA {S,D,D} and left-sided juxtaposition of the atrial appendages.

CONGENITAL MITRAL REGURGITATION WITH DUCHENNE MUSCULAR DYSTROPHY

Duchenne muscular dystrophy, named after Guillaume Benjamin Armand Duchenne, a French neurologist (1806–1875), was described by him in Paris, France in 1868. Duchenne muscular dystrophy is an X-linked recessive form of progressive muscular dystrophy occurring in early childhood, mostly in boys. The gene marker was discovered by Kay Davies and Robert Williamson in 1983. In 1986, Louis M. Kunkle and Eric P. Hoffmann and colleagues discovered that the protein dystrophin is absent in Duchenne muscular dystrophy.

Duchenne, a neurologist from Boulogne, studied under the direction of Rene Laënnec, Guillaume Dupuytren, and Francois Magendie in Paris. Duchenne was one of the earliest workers on the electrophysiology of muscles, and he published *De Electerisation Locale* in 1825.

Duchenne muscular dystrophy is the most common and severe type of pseudohypertrophic muscular dystrophy. It is chronic and progressive. It begins in early childhood with weakness of the pelvic and shoulder girdles, with pseudohypertrophy of the muscles, followed by atrophy, lordosis, and a swaying gait with the legs kept wide apart. Affected individuals seldom survive to maturity. Death is usually due to respiratory or cardiac failure.

Case 19, a man who died at 20 years of age in 1970, had Duchenne progressive muscular dystrophy, also known as pseudohypertrophic muscular dystrophy. He was markedly cachectic, weighing only 32 kg (70.5 lb). All organs were underweight, except for the heart (350 g, normal being 300 g, 16.7% greater than normal). He also had an intellectual disability, which is not part of Duchenne muscular dystrophy. He had a history of congestive heart failure, with cardiomegaly, and pericardial and pleural effusions.

Autopsy revealed bilateral bronchopneumonia, acute bronchitis, and obstruction of both main bronchi by micropurulent material. Focal pulmonary hemorrhages were found in the right lower lobe. Multiple flexion contractures were present in the arms and legs. He had a history of Wolff-Parkinson-White syndrome, with episodes of tachycardia, followed by brief episodes of cardiac arrest (of approximately 1 minute in duration). Left ventricular hypertrophy was marked, with mild left ventricular enlargement. There was evidence of chronic mitral regurgitation, with fibrosis and calcification of the free margins of the mitral leaflets and left atrial jet lesions. This patient's main clinical problem was Duchenne muscular dystrophy. The chronic mitral regurgitation was thought to be part of the chronic, progressive, and ultimately fatal muscular dystrophy.

Case 57, a boy who died at 15 4/12 years of age, had *Duchenne muscular dystrophy, Becker variant*. Becker muscular dystrophy closely resembles Duchenne muscular dystrophy, but it typically has a later onset and a slowly progressive course. It, too, is transmitted as an X-linked recessive trait. This male adolescent had a history of congestive heart failure with pitting edema of the lower extremities. He also had a history of supraventricular tachycardia and low cardiac output.

Autopsy confirmed the presence of marked cardiomegaly with enlargement of all cardiac chambers. Diffuse left ventricular myocardial fibrosis was found. Mitral regurgitation with thickening of the mitral leaflets and left atrial jet lesions were found. The mitral regurgitation was thought to be caused by left ventricular papillary muscle dysfunction, by left ventricular myocardial failure, and by left ventricular chamber enlargement. The RV was dilated, with marked thinning of the right ventricular free wall.

CONGENITAL MITRAL REGURGITATION WITH LARGE SECUNDUM ATRIAL SEPTAL DEFECTS

Case 10, a 65-year-old woman, was found to have severe mitral regurgitation (1 patient, 1% of this series; see Table 14.12). The mitral leaflets were markedly thinned and calcified. These changes were more marked of the posterior mitral leaflet than of the anterior leaflet. The posterior mitral leaflet ballooned into the LA; that is, **mitral valve prolapse involving the posterior leaflet** was present. We did not think that the mitral valve looked rheumatic; for example, there was no thickening, shortening, and adhesion of the chordae tendineae. Other potentially significant findings included two large ostium secundum type of ASDs consisting of two large fenestrations of the septum primum: 32 × 15 mm, and 18 × 7 mm. She had atrial fibrillation. An embolus to the left middle cerebral artery resulted in a right-sided stroke. How should the mitral regurgitation of this case be understood? First, there is no doubt that mitral regurgitation and mitral valve prolapse of the posterior leaflet were present. But why did these things happen to a normally formed mitral valve? Dr. Stella Van Praagh and I thought that the two large secundum ASDs may have been important. Dr. Maurice Lev has ascribed *hemodynamic change* (leaflet thickening) of the mitral valve leaflets to the abnormal hemodynamics associated with a large secundum ASD. Lev's hypothesis is that when the RA contracts, slightly before the LA, a right-to-left jet of blood streams through the large secundum ASD, striking the left lateral aspect of the atrial surfaces of the mitral leaflets, traumatizing them. Shortly thereafter, left atrial contraction sends a stream of blood from left to right, resulting in a net left-to-right shunt at the atrial level. Left-to-right atrial shunting not only results from left atrial contraction but also may be aided by subsystemic right ventricular pressures, right ventricular compliance greater than left, and pulmonary vascular resistance less than systemic. However, as far as the mitral valve is concerned, the important part of this hypothesis is the *mitral valve jet lesion* on the lateral aspect of the mitral leaflets. Lev called this jet lesion *hemodynamic change* to emphasize that this pathologic process is not infectious, rheumatic, or a congenital malformation of the mitral valve per se. Instead, it is hemodynamic trauma, permitted by a large secundum ASD, when the RA contracts slightly before the LA when the patient is in normal sinus rhythm. The hypothesis is that a lifetime of abnormal hemodynamics, secondary to large secundum ASDs, may have contributed to the thickening and calcification of this patient's mitral valve leaflets and the atrial prolapse of her posterior mitral leaflet, resulting in severe mitral regurgitation. This explanation is presented as an hypothesis because I am not certain that it has been well documented (the early right-to-left jet component). But this type of hemodynamic change of the mitral valve, when searched for carefully, often has been found in association with a large secundum ASD, hence, this hypothesis. Hemodynamic trauma led to leaflet thickening, fibrosis, leaflet retraction, mitral regurgitation, and leaflet calcification. We regard this patient's mitral regurgitation as congenital, in the sense that the large secundum ASDs (congenital anomalies) may well have played an important role in the pathogenesis of this woman's severe mitral regurgitation.

Congenital Mitral Regurgitation With Straddling Mitral Valve

Case 30, a 23 10/12-year-old man, had dextrocardia (a predominantly right-sided heart) with TGA {S,D,L}. (Recall that TGA {S,D,L} means TGA with visceroatrial situs solitus [S], D-loop ventricles [D], and L-TGA, that is, with the transposed aortic valve to the left [L- or levo-] relative to the transposed pulmonary valve.) There were crisscross AV relations. This means that after ventricular D-looping had occurred with the establishment of concordant AV alignments and connections between the solitus atria and the D-loop ventricles, then, for reasons unknown, the ventricular part of the heart rotated in the wrong direction—to the left instead of the right.

Consequently, the morphologically RV starts normally on the right side, where it connects normally with the RA. But then the RV twists to the left, where it leads up to the transposed aorta. The morphologically LV starts on the left side, where it connects with the LA. Then, the LV twists abnormally to the right, where it leads to the transposed pulmonary artery. Thus, each ventricle is bilateral, with the RV starting on the right and then twisting superiorly and to the left, whereas the LV starts on the left and twists inferiorly and to the right.

"Dance" this spatially, with your hands. Your right hand is initially superior, palm facing down. Your left hand is initially inferior, palm facing up. Put both hands together, fingers pointing in front (ventrally). Your hands are modeling the superoinferior ventricles stage, that is, the straight tube or preloop stage. Now twist your hands 90 degrees clockwise, so the RV is right-sided, the LV is left-sided, and the ventricular septum is straight up and down (vertical, not horizontal). This models the normal D-loop stage of ventricular development.

Now, to model what happens in this kind of crisscross AV relations (with a ventricular D-loop, in visceroatrial situs solitus, with AV concordance). The D-loop untwists, in the wrong direction, to the *left*. The hands twist back to the superoinferior ventricles stage, after AV concordance has been achieved. Leftward twisting of the ventricular loop places the RV superiorly, with the right ventricular apex pointing leftward. The LV again becomes inferior, with AV concordance, and the left ventricular apex points to the right. Once you understand it in three-dimensional space, crisscross AV relations become a "piece of cake"—easy to understand. There are two essential steps: (1) normal D-loop formation with the establishment of AV discordance and (2) then twisting in the wrong direction, to the left, making both ventricles bilateral. Both ventricles crisscross each other, like a narrow St. Andrew's cross.

The right ventricular sinus typically is underdeveloped superiorly. The left ventricular sinus usually is well developed inferiorly. That is why *dextrocardia* is present, because the apex of the inferior LV is pointing prominently to the right, whereas the leftward pointing superior RV has an underdeveloped apex. Hence, the ventricular mass is predominantly right-sided. Because the D-loop ventricles have twisted so far in the wrong direction, to the left, *L*-TGA is present, and the transposed aortic valve is therefore to the *left* of the transposed pulmonary valve. The presence of *L*-TGA reflects the abnormal *leftward twisting* of these D-loop ventricles.

There was a large VSD of the conoventricular type that was confluent with a VSD of the AV canal type. The mitral valve straddled through the large VSD. The bicameral insertions of the mitral valve, into both the LV and the RV, but mostly into the LV, resulted in congenital mitral regurgitation with left atrial jet lesions. Severe pulmonary outflow tract stenosis was produced by the medial leaflet tissue of both AV valves and by the presence of a unicommissural pulmonary valve.

Other important findings in the heart of this young man included a single coronary artery arising from the right septal sinus of Valsalva of the transposed aortic valve; that is, a single right coronary artery (or absence of the left coronary arterial ostium). He had bilateral Blalock-Taussig anastomoses: left = 1 mm (internal diameter); and right (modified Blalock-Taussig shunt) with a Teflon graft (15.8 mm in length). He had a terminal history of SBE, that is, β-hemolytic streptococci, group B (blood culture). He had a history of headache for 2 weeks (in 1977), with transient right hemiparesis and paresthesia. A cerebellar abscess and hematoma were drained (*S. aureus* and *H. paraphrophilus*). The abnormal leftward twisting of these D-loop ventricles and the presence of a large VSD placed the crest of the muscular ventricular septum beneath the mitral orifice, resulting in mitral straddling and congenital mitral regurgitation.

Congenital Mitral Regurgitation With Truncus Arteriosus

Case 3, a 4½-month-old girl, had truncus arteriosus type A2; that is, there was a large subtruncal VSD (type A) and absence of the aortopulmonary septum (type 2), hence, type A2 in our classification. In the classification of Collett and Edwards, this is truncus arteriosus type III because the origins of the right pulmonary artery and the left pulmonary artery were widely separated. The truncal valve was tricuspid, and there was severe truncal valvar regurgitation. The foramen ovale was patent. Although the mitral valve was normally formed, mitral regurgitation was observed at cardiac catheterization and angiocardiography. Chronic intractable congestive heart failure was present; it was attributed to the patient's large left-to-right shunt and severe truncal valvar regurgitation. Congenital mitral regurgitation was thought to be a relatively minor part of this patient's clinical problem. Mild DiGeorge syndrome was diagnosed clinically. She had a history of neonatal hypocalcemia and her thymus was small. Surgical repair of her truncus arteriosus was undertaken in 1985. Because of severe truncal valvar regurgitation, truncal valvar replacement was included as part of the operative repair, using a no. 17 Bjork-Shiley prosthetic valve. The postoperative course was complicated by bleeding from the truncal closure suture line, leading to death.

Autopsy revealed hypertrophy and enlargement of all cardiac chambers. Severe truncal valvar regurgitation, left ventricular papillary muscle and free wall dysfunction, and enlargement of the mitral annulus were thought to be relevant to this patient's mitral regurgitation, which was regarded as congenital because of its congenital causation (truncus arteriosus). It is important to understand that a *normally formed mitral valve, as in this patient, can regurgitate, if other factors, such as truncus arteriosus, coexist.*

Mitral Regurgitation With Pulmonary Arterial Vascular Obstructive Disease and Pulmonary Veno-occlusive Disease

Case 49, a 13 3/12-year-old girl, was diagnosed as having primary pulmonary hypertension in 1970. Autopsy confirmed this diagnosis, revealing *grade IV Heath-Edwards pulmonary vascular obstructive disease.* For the reader's convenience, permit me to summarize the widely used **Heath-Edwards Classification of hypertensive pulmonary vascular obstructive disease.**

Grade 1. The stage of retention of the fetal type of pulmonary arteries. The media, composed of circularly oriented smooth muscle, is hypertrophied. The *hypertrophied media* is bounded by internal and external elastic laminae. There is no intimal proliferation, and the adventitia is unremarkable.

Grade 2. The stage of medial hypertrophy with intimal cellular proliferation. In addition to *medial hypertrophy* that is limited by internal and external elastic laminae of the small pulmonary arteries and arterioles, there is *intimal cellular proliferation* that narrows and may almost occlude the vascular lumen.

Grade 3. Stage of progressive fibrous vascular occlusion. *The media is hypertrophied. The internal and external elastic laminae are thickened* and can be disrupted by fibrous tissue, as can the media. *The intimal proliferation is now fibrous, and fibroelastic (not cellular).* Arteriolar luminae may be totally, or almost totally, occluded. The media can be considerably thickened by *fascicles (bundles) or muscle running longitudinally,* either exterior or interior to the original medial layer or both exteriorly and interiorly. Stage 3 changes can be seen in association with recanalized thrombi.

Grade 4. The stage of progressive pulmonary arterial generalized dilatation, with the formation of complex dilatation lesions. Small pulmonary arteries and arterioles can have dilated lumina, thin media, and no intimal proliferation. Or the vessel can be dilated, with a thin media, and the lumen can be occluded. Recanalization of occluded lumina by multiple capillary channels may be seen histologically. Wagenvoort, Heath, and Edwards described three different kinds of dilatation lesions in pulmonary vascular obstructive disease grade 4:

1. plexiform lesions;
2. angiomatoid lesions; and
3. veinlike branches (or hypertrophied and usually occluded muscular pulmonary arteries).

Grade 5. Chronic pulmonary arterial dilatation throughout the lung and pulmonary hemosiderosis. Luminal occlusions, vascular dilatations, and pulmonary hemosiderosis, indicating chronic pulmonary arterial and arteriolar obstructions with diapdesis of erythrocytes, red blood cell breakdown, and the abnormal deposition of iron in the pulmonary tissue are the characteristic findings of pulmonary vascular obstructive disease grade 5. These findings indicated the severity and the chronicity of pulmonary vascular obstructive disease.

Grade 6. Fibrinoid necrosis of the media. Inflammatory exudate may involve all layers of the pulmonary arteries and/or arterioles, and the inflammation can vary from mild to severe.

From a practical clinical standpoint in the treatment of patients with congenital heart disease, let us say a large VSD, at Boston Children's Hospital, we thought that pulmonary vascular obstructive disease grades 1 and 2 were operable; that is, the large VSD could be closed surgically. Pulmonary vascular obstructive disease grade 3, with significant luminal narrowing, was borderline, which was very worrying and quite possibly a contraindication to corrective surgery.

Dr. Aldo Castaneda and colleagues decided that operability of patients with congenital heart disease, pulmonary hypertension, and increased pulmonary blood flow could *not* be decided on the basis of lung biopsy. Instead, the patient's clinical and *hemodynamic* status was found to be a better basis upon which to decide whether operation could be safely undertaken or was contraindicated. One of the problems with pulmonary biopsy was the possibility of *sampling error*. A given biopsy might *not* be characteristic of the status of the lungs as a whole. By contrast, cardiopulmonary hemodynamics was thought to be more truly representative of the patient's overall cardiopulmonary physiologic status.

Now, let us return to the discussion of the 13 3/12-year-old girl in Case 49. She had *primary* pulmonary arterial hypertension, with grade 4 pulmonary arterial obstructive disease. Grade 4 pulmonary arterial obstructive disease has always been regarded as a contraindication to shunt or corrective surgery, which she did *not* have. The purpose of the foregoing section was to demonstrate the extreme severity of the changes in grade 4 pulmonary arterial obstructive disease. It will come as no surprise that autopsy revealed right ventricular hypertrophy and enlargement and grossly obvious atherosclerosis of the pulmonary arteries. However, there was a surprise. She also had **pulmonary veno-occlusive disease,** with pseudoangiomatoid collateral circulation in the lungs. *Mild mitral regurgitation* was also found. The mitral valve was normally formed. The mitral leaflets were mildly thickened, and there were small jet lesions of the left atrial endocardium.

The uncertainties concerning this case are as follows:

1. Was the pulmonary veno-occlusive disease in this 13 3/12-year-old girl congenital or acquired? We do not know.
2. Was her primary pulmonary hypertension, with grade 4 changes of pulmonary vascular obstructive disease involving her pulmonary arteries and arterioles congenital or acquired? We do not know. The diagnosis of *primary* pulmonary hypertension means that the pulmonary hypertension was not secondary to any left-to-right shunt.
3. Was the pulmonary arterial hypertension with grade 4 changes of pulmonary arterial obstructive disease secondary to the pulmonary veno-occlusive disease? Again we do not know.
4. Was this patient's mild mitral regurgitation secondary to her pulmonary arterial hypertension or secondary to her pulmonary veno-occlusive disease? We do not know.

In view of our embarrassing ignorance about this case, why am I presenting it?

1. Mitral regurgitation is present. (Therefore I could not omit it.)
2. There was no evidence found of acquired mitral regurgitation. So, we assumed that the mitral regurgitation was congenital. This assumption may be incorrect.
3. This is a very rare case: severe pulmonary venous occlusive disease, with severe pulmonary vascular obstructive disease of the pulmonary arteries and arterioles; that is, severe obstruction of both the pulmonary veins and of the pulmonary arteries and arterioles, without structural congenital heart disease.

Some unknown disease process, such as an autoimmune disease, may have attacked this patient's intima and smooth muscles, leading to pulmonary venous occlusive disease, pulmonary arterial and arteriolar occlusive disease, and mitral valvulitis, resulting in mild mitral regurgitation. If some such disease process, resulting in pulmonary arterial and venous obstruction with mitral regurgitation, is identified in the future, and if the pathogenesis is shown to be postnatal, this case should be deleted from this presentation of *congenital* mitral regurgitation. This patient may have had a disease process resembling rheumatic fever and rheumatic heart disease, rheumatoid arthritis and rheumatoid heart disease, a collagen disease, or other autoimmune disorder. It is my hope that time will tell. Hence, this fascinating and rare case is recorded here.

CONGENITAL MITRAL REGURGITATION WITH HETEROTAXY SYNDROME AND POLYSPLENIA

Case 11, a 3¾-month-old boy, had the polysplenia syndrome with the incomplete form of common AV canal, a cleft anterior leaflet of the mitral valve, and mild mitral regurgitation, which was not his major clinical problem. In somewhat greater detail, he had right-sided polysplenia with nine splenuli in the right upper quadrant adjacent to the greater curvature of his right-sided stomach. The liver was abnormally symmetrical, the right lobe being slightly larger than the left lobe. The IVC was interrupted from the renal veins below to the hepatic segment of the IVC above *(typical of the polysplenia syndrome, but not of the asplenia syndrome)*. Bilaterally bilobed lungs were present *(typical of polysplenia, but not of asplenia)*. Bilateral SVCs were found, with absence of the left innominate vein. The LSVC opened into the roof of the LA because of absence of the coronary sinus septum; the coronary sinus and its right atrial ostium were absent for the same reason (absence of the coronary sinus septum). (Normally, the coronary sinus septum separates the LSVC and the coronary sinus posteriorly from the LA anteriorly.) The hepatic segment of the IVC opened mainly into the RA. A large left hepatic vein opened into the common atrium slightly to the left of the midline. A common atrium was present because of absence of the septum primum (the flap valve of the foramen ovale), with a poorly formed superior limbic band of septum secundum and absence of the inferior limbic band. The cardiac segmental anatomy was {AS,D,S}. This means the set (or combination) of situs ambiguus (A) of the viscera (typical of the polysplenia syndrome, as mentioned earlier) with situs solitus of the atria (S), D-loop ventricles (D), and solitus normally related great arteries (S). Hence, the cardiac segmental anatomy was solitus normal, that is, {S,D,S}, despite the coexistence of visceral heterotaxy with situs ambiguus (A) of the viscera, *typical of the polysplenia syndrome, that is {AS,D,S}*.

It should be assumed that the AV alignments are concordant, that is, solitus normal, because the atrial situs and the ventricular situs are solitus normal, unless the AV alignments are stated to be something other than normal. Similarly, it is assumed that the VA alignments are solitus normal, unless specifically stated to the contrary.

The pulmonary venous connections were normal. The cleft anterior leaflet of the mitral valve showed mild thickening and rolling of the superior cleft margin, indicating mild mitral regurgitation. No VSD was present. *This—the classic form of incompletely common AV canal—is typical of the heterotaxy syndrome with polysplenia but not of the heterotaxy syndrome with asplenia.*

At 36 hours of age (in 1986), necrotizing enterocolitis was diagnosed. At 2 days of age a laparotomy was performed with partial resection of the ascending colon and a colostomy. Resection of the proximal jejunum was also performed because of necrotizing enterocolitis, with a jejunostomy, and a gastrostomy feeding tube was placed. The postoperative course was characterized by continuing congestive heart failure. A PDA was diagnosed and was ligated at 12 days of age. Despite all therapeutic efforts, the postoperative course was slowly downhill, with hypotension leading to anuria and death at 3¾ months of age. Thus, this patient is thought to exemplify **classic neonatal enterocolitis.** What happened? Our best understanding is this. A large common atrium, a regurgitant mitral cleft, a PDA, and no pulmonary outflow tract stenosis were the key findings. When the pulmonary vascular resistance fell soon postnatally, a torrential left-to-right shunt occurred at the atrial and ductal levels. Pulmonary flooding occurred, with critically reduced systemic cardiac output. This resulted in systemic arterial hypotension, leading to ischemic necrosis of the patient's small and large bowel, so-called enterocolitis. (It is not primarily an inflammation. It is ischemic necrosis, followed by inflammation.)

The presence of mild mitral regurgitation via the cleft would not have helped systemic cardiac output. The absence of pulmonary outflow tract obstruction (stenosis or atresia) meant that there was nothing to prevent pulmonary flooding once the pulmonary arteriolar resistance fell, as normally occurs postnatally. Remember what Dr. Jesse Edwards used to say: *"Common atrium is the forgotten form of common AV canal."* The present case illustrates the importance of common atrium in association with common AV canal, even when common AV canal is of the incomplete or partial type, as in this patient.

When a common atrium coexists with a common AV canal, there is much more wrong than an AV septal defect. In this patient, only a partial AV septal defect was present, because there was no VSD of the AV canal type. In this boy, *the atrial septum was missing* (absence of the septum primum and septum secundum), as was the interatrial portion of the AV septum. *The sudden normal fall in this patient's pulmonary arteriolar resistance was one of the most important events resulting in his neonatal ischemic necrosis of the small and large bowel (enterocolitis).*

In congenital heart disease, function (physiology) can sometimes trump structure (anatomy). For example, had this patient's pulmonary vascular resistance remained high in the neonatal period, as it was in utero, then we speculate that ischemic necrosis of the bowel would not have occurred. Had the pulmonary resistance remained high, or had it fallen more slowly, we think that the presence of a common atrium and a PDA would not have been as devastating as they in fact were in this patient.

CONGENITAL MITRAL REGURGITATION WITH HYPOPLASTIC LEFT HEART SYNDROME

Case 13, a 36-hour-(1½ day)-old girl has HLHS. She had HLHS with congenital mitral *regurgitation,* a rare form indeed of HLHS. Typically, HLHS has congenital mitral stenosis or mitral atresia, but not congenital mitral *regurgitation*. This patient was born by cesarean section at 36 weeks gestation in 1986, with a birth weight of 2900 g (6.39 lb), premature by dates, but not by weight. This patient also had an incomplete form of common AV canal with a common atrium. There was a slim strand of inferior limbic band demarcating where the atrial septum should have been, but nothing more. The anterior mitral leaflet was cleft, with thickening and rolling of the free margins of the cleft, indicative of congenital (prenatal) mitral regurgitation.

The tricuspid valve was also "cleft," with an unusually wide gap between the septal and the anterior tricuspid leaflets anterosuperiorly. There was no VSD. The LV was decidedly hypoplastic. Why? There was organic and functional obstruction of the left ventricular outflow tract by a *muscle of Moulaert,* also known as the *anterolateral muscle of the LV*. This muscle arises from the anterolateral papillary muscle group of the LV and then extends superiorly, up almost all the way to the aortic annulus. If prominent, as in this patient, the muscle of Moulaert forms a muscular subaortic stenosis of the left ventricular outflow tract. This is why the LV was "hypoplastic," that is, why it had a small lumen but a thick wall. Severe subaortic muscular left ventricular outflow tract obstruction was present.

Other important findings included preductal coarctation of the aorta (1 mm in internal diameter) and a large but functionally closed ductus arteriosus. This combination of a severe preductal coarctation of the aorta and a functional closed ductus arteriosus is fatal. Circulation below the closed ductus arteriosus—the lower systemic circulation—is very inadequate. There was right ventricular hypertrophy and enlargement. This patient also had atresia of the distal ileum; MCAs were present. So, HLHS with congenital mitral *regurgitation* is possible, if severe left ventricular outflow tract obstruction coexists, as in this patient.

Mitral Regurgitation With a High, Subaortic Ventricular Septal Defect

Case 56, a 20 6/12-year-old young man, died postoperatively in 1971. A heart murmur was first heard soon after birth, and the patient was first seen in the Cardiac Clinic of Children's

Hospital Medical Center in Boston (as our hospital was then known) at 17 months of age (in 1952). Chest x-ray films showed cardiac enlargement with increased pulmonary blood flow, and a clinical diagnosis of VSD was made. (It should be understood that this was before the advent of clinical open heart surgery, before Dr. Walt Lillehei's initiation of open heart surgery using controlled cross-circulation in 1954 and Dr. John Kirklin's introduction of the Mayo-Gibbon heart-lung machine in 1955.) Subsequently, the patient grew and developed normally without cardiovascular symptomatology. However, at age 18 (in 1969), he noticed irregular heartbeats during times of severe anxiety. He was admitted to an outside hospital for 1 week because of this problem and was discharged on tranquilizers. In 1971, just 1 week after his 20th birthday, cardiac catheterization revealed a subaortic VSD with a Qp/Qs ratio (recall that Qp/Qs means pulmonary blood flow/systemic blood flow ratio) of 3/1, pulmonary artery hypertension (2/3 systemic), a mild pulmonary outflow tract gradient (30 mm Hg), and a pulmonary resistance of 1 Woods unit. At 20 6/12 years, he underwent surgical correction of his VSD. During cardiopulmonary bypass, he suffered episodes of severe systemic hypotension. Postoperatively, he could not be weaned from the respirator. Renal failure and severe pneumonia ensued, leading to death 9 days later.

Autopsy revealed a VSD that was high, subaortic, conoventricular (between the conal septum above and the ventricular septum below), and moderate in size (25 × 20 mm). There was mitral regurgitation, with leaflet thickening and a left atrial endocardial jet lesion. The structure of the mitral valve was normal. But the mitral annulus was dilated: 95 mm in circumference, compared with 70 mm in normal controls, 35.7% greater than normal. So, we thought that mitral annular dilatation was one of the causes of his chronic mitral regurgitation. The LV was hypertrophied and enlarged, reflecting its increased flow work secondary to the VSD (Qp/Qs = 3/1). This is also why we thought that this patient's mitral regurgitation should be regarded as *congenital,* because the mitral regurgitation had a congenital basis (the VSD), not a postnatally acquired one.

This patient's postoperative death was related to several factors: incomplete VSD patch closure with a residual VSD (14 × 8 mm); flail tricuspid valve, with the anterior tricuspid leaflet becoming detached from the region of the papillary muscle of the conus; an antemortem right atrial thrombus, thought to be related to indwelling central venous catheter in the SVC; extensive bronchopneumonia, bilateral and alveolar hemorrhages, bilateral, with the lung cultures growing *Pseudomonas aeruginosa, Candida albicans,* and *Streptococcus fecalis* (autopsy performed 2 hours postmortem); myocardial necrosis, recent, with subendocardial hemorrhages of both ventricle and the ventricular septum; pancreatitis; renal infarcts, old and recent, with postoperative azotemia (blood urea nitrogen <300 mg%); adrenocortical hemorrhage, recent, right-sided; and multiple emboli in the cerebrum and cerebellum with multiple infarctions.

As far as mitral regurgitation is concerned, this case indicates that a normally formed mitral valve can become regurgitant, if associated congenital heart disease such as a VSD causes sufficient ventricular enlargement over time and sufficient annular enlargement, such that the mitral leaflets can no longer occlude the enlarged mitral orifice. Other factors such as left ventricular hypertrophy, fibrosis, papillary muscle dysfunction, and coronary emboli may well also play a significant and deleterious role. This case history is a sad and stark picture of where we have come from. It also indicates that mitral regurgitation, while present, was certainly *not* the patient's main clinical problem; rather it was the VSD.

This case history remains very relevant to what is now known as **congenital heart disease in the adult.** Cases like this still exist in the world's poorest countries. **The global management of congenital heart disease** is becoming increasingly more important as a public health problem, one with which we in the wealthier countries will become increasingly involved.

Social Comment

Despite competing nationalists, competing economic systems, competing social and religious ideologies, physicians, biologists, and geneticist know that biologically, all living people are brothers and sisters. We are all members of one and the same human family.

The spread of modern pediatric cardiology and cardiac surgery around the world is an important and growing phenomenon. It seems to me and to many others that we should try to help each other as much as we possibly can. Why? Because we all really are "brothers" and "sisters," members of the same extended, global human family. What better reason could there possibly be? At the very least, we should never forget the ancient medical motto: First do no harm *(primum non nocere).* Physicians really *do* want to help people anywhere and everywhere. This is one of the things that makes medicine the noblest of the great professions.

Other Mitral Valve Anomalies

Now that we have considered the "big three" congenital mitral anomalies in detail, that is, **mitral atresia** (177 autopsied cases, or 5.5% of the 3216 congenital anomalies that constitute the great majority of the database of this study); **congenital mitral stenosis** (224 necropsied cases, or 6.97% of the congenital cardiac anomaly series); and **congenital mitral regurgitation** (216 autopsied cases, or 6.72% of the congenital heart autopsy series) (see Table 14.1), we will briefly describe some of the less common or rare anomalies of the mitral valve that are presented in Table 14.1 but have not been described thus far.

CONGENITAL ABSENCE OF THE MITRAL VALVE LEAFLETS, ALSO KNOWN AS CONGENITALLY UNGUARDED MITRAL ORIFICE

The heart specimen of this patient (C69-88) was sent to us as a consultation in 1969. The patient was a full-term girl with a birth weight of 5 lb 5¼ oz (2416.8 g), the product of an unwanted pregnancy, born to an unmarried 15-year-old black mother. The baby girl died at 42 hours of age.

Autopsy revealed several rare findings: HLHS, with very marked hypoplasia of the LV; hypoplasia of the mitral orifice, with absence of the mitral valve leaflets (also known as congenitally unguarded mitral orifice); an intact ventricular septum;

left ventricular outflow tract atresia; a valve incompetent patent foramen ovale; DORV with noninverted segmental anatomy, that is, DORV {S,D,D}; a subpulmonary conus (infundibulum) with absence of the subaortic conal free wall permitting aortic valvar–to–tricuspid valvar direct fibrous continuity; subaortic outflow tract stenosis, the aortic outflow tract being narrowed between the conal septum anterosuperiorly and the anterior leaflet of the tricuspid valve posteroinferiorly; marked hypoplasia of the aortic valve (internal diameter 2 mm), the aortic valve being tricuspid; marked right ventricular hypertrophy and enlargement; widely patent pulmonary outflow tract, pulmonary valve, and pulmonary artery; hypoplasia of the ascending aorta and aortic arch, with accentuation of the hypoplasia at the aortic isthmus, that is, preductal coarctation of the aorta; and large but closing ductus arteriosus, internal luminal diameter 1 to 2 mm.

The cause of death was thought to be the severe aortic outflow tract obstruction and preductal coarctation of the aorta, plus the large but closing ductus arteriosus. This combination of anomalies would deprive the lower body of adequate aortic blood flow.

The most spectacular finding was absence of the mitral valve leaflets, in association with a truly hypoplastic thin-walled LV. In 1969, we thought that **absence of the mitral valve leaflets (congenitally unguarded mitral orifice) was a newly discovered form of congenital heart disease.** We thought it should be reported. But, we never managed to do so, until now; hence, this book. (There are many undiscovered anomalies that I hope to be able to report in this book.)

Functionally, this case was like mitral atresia, even though the mitral orifice was patent and the mitral leaflets were absent. Why? Because there was left ventricular outflow tract atresia, with an intact ventricular septum. **Submitral atresia** would be more accurate.

The type of DORV that was present is also noteworthy (i.e., rare): DORV with a normal type of conus, subpulmonary with absence of the subaortic conal free wall. This is DORV with an almost normal type of conotruncus. We wondered about reporting the segmental anatomy as DORV {S,D,**"S"**} because the conotruncus is very similar to the solitus (noninverted) normal anatomic type. But, we decided that we could *not* report the segmental anatomy as DORV {S,D,**S**} because DORV with a solitus normal conotruncus is a contraindication in terms. DORV is no kind of normally related great arteries.

However, if someone ever asks you "Is it possible to have DORV with a solitus normal type of conotruncus?" you can look your questioner in the eye and say "Yes." If your questioner then says "But that's impossible!" you should then *not* start mumbling about *miracula naturae*. Instead, you should remind your questioner that DORV is an abnormal relationship between the conotruncus *above,* and the ventricles, ventricular septum, and AV canal *below*. Sometimes, if the *below* part is sufficiently abnormal, then amazing things, such as this case, can happen.

This patient had marked hypoplasia of the LV, a patent but hypoplastic mitral orifice without mitral leaflets, an intact ventricular septum, and left ventricular outflow tract atresia. Our speculation was, and is, that if there had not been left ventricular outflow tract atresia, and if the ventricular septum had not been intact, and if a mitral valve with normal leaflets had formed, there would have been aortic-mitral fibrous continuity with solitus normally related great arteries, that is, {S,D,S} rather than DORV {S,D,D}, which is what we in fact found. Briefly, DORV does not always have an abnormal conotruncus. Remember,

"Sometimes the woe
Can lie below."

Finally, tell your skeptical colleague that DORV with a normal conotruncus, that is, DORV {S,D,"S"}, has a special type of aortic outflow tract stenosis and explain *why*.

To summarize, this very rare case proves several startling facts:

1. It is possible to have a patent mitral orifice with absence of the mitral valve leaflets, also known as congenitally unguarded mitral orifice.
2. It is rarely possible to have DORV with a solitus normal type of conotruncus, that is, with a well-developed subpulmonary muscular conus, and an absent subaortic muscular conal free wall that permits aortic valvar–to–tricuspid valvar direct fibrous continuity. The normal type of aortic-mitral fibrous continuity was impossible because the mitral valve leaflets were absent, and the ventricular septum was intact. Hence, the aorta arose only from the hypertrophied and enlarged RV, and not at all from the very hypoplastic LV.
3. Congenitally unguarded mitral orifice can be associated with submitral atresia because of the association of left ventricular outflow tract atresia and intact ventricular septum.
4. In other words, **HLHS** with marked hypoplasia of the LV rarely can be associated with:
   a. congenitally unguarded mitral orifice (patent mitral orifice with absence of mitral leaflets);
   b. intact ventricular septum;
   c. left ventricular outflow tract atresia, resulting in submitral atresia, despite patency of the mitral orifice and absence of the mitral leaflets;
   d. DORV with a solitus normal type of conotruncus and well-developed subpulmonary conus and absence of the subaortic conal free wall, permitting aortic-tricuspid fibrous continuity;
   e. subaortic stenosis, produced by narrowing of the subaortic outflow tract between the conal septum above and to the right and the tricuspid leaflets below and to the left;
   f. hypoplasia (stenosis) of the aortic valve, ascending aorta, aortic arch, and maximal at the aortic isthmus, resulting in preductal coarctation of the aorta; and right ventricular hypertrophy and enlargement, with a large MPA and branches, and a large PDA.

If the large PDA narrows markedly, or functionally closes normally in the postnatal period, as happened in this patient, death may well result, as occurred at 42 hours of age in this girl. In other words, she was ductus dependent.

Normal development of the conotruncus resulted in subaortic stenosis, aortic hypoplasia, and preductal hypoplasia (coarctation). *The conal septum was located approximately normally.* Consequently, there was little space between the conal septum (to the patient's right) and the muscular ventricular sinus septum (to the patient's left). Normally, this small area is filled by the tricuspid valve leaflets and the membranous portion of the ventricular septum. But in this patient, this small area between the conal septum to the right and the ventricular septum to the left served as the very narrowed subaortic outflow tract; hence, this patient's subaortic stenosis, resulting in a low-flow and thus hypoplastic ascending aorta, aortic arch, and preductal coarctation of the aorta.

ADHERENT MITRAL VALVE RESULTING IN FIBROUS SUBAORTIC STENOSIS

Case 1, a boy who died at 1 8/12 years of age, had the following findings at autopsy. TOF was present with a subaortic VSD, limited inferiorly by the Y of the septal band (as seen from the right ventricular perspective). Pulmonary outflow tract stenosis was severe at the os infundibuli, with intimal fibrous tissue thickening at this site. The pulmonary valve was bicuspid (bicommissural) because the septal commissure was rudimentary. Congenital mitral stenosis was moderately severe, with thickened fibrotic mitral valve leaflets and with obliteration (or failure of formation) of mitral interchordal spaces. *Adherent mitral valve* was also found. The anterior leaflet of the mitral valve had abnormal fibrous tissue attachments to the left ventricular septal surface, producing *severe fibrous subaortic stenosis* approximately 5 mm (0.2 inch) below the aortic valve, and below the level of the VSD. The LV was markedly hypertrophied (wall thickness = 11 to 13 mm, compared with normal controls of 5.5 to 7.5 mm in age- and sex-matched controls, that is, 85% greater than normal). The LV was also markedly enlarged (left ventricular inflow tract length from mitral annulus to the left ventricular apex measured 6.0 cm, compared with normal control of 4.2 cm; i.e., 43% greater than normal). The LA was hypertrophied (wall thickness = 3 mm, compared with 1 mm in normal controls; i.e., 200% greater than normal). There was a jet lesion of the left atrial endocardium, consistent with mitral regurgitation. Hence, this congenitally malformed mitral valve was both stenotic and regurgitant. *Isolation of the LAA* was also present. From within the LA, it was not possible to see into the cavity of the LAA; however, a 1-mm probe did pass into the lumen of the LAA. Right ventricular hypertrophy was marked (wall thickness = 8.5 to 9.0 mm, compared with normal controls of 3 to 3.5 mm; i.e., 169% greater than normal). The RA was also markedly hypertrophied, but otherwise unremarkable (wall thickness = 3 mm, compared with normal controls of 1 mm; i.e., 200% greater than normal).

At 2 months of age, a Waterston anastomosis was performed, a side-to-side anastomosis between the ascending aorta and the right pulmonary artery, 3 × 3 mm in internal diameter. At autopsy, the Waterston anastomosis measured 3.5 mm in internal diameter from the aortic viewpoint. Postoperatively, congestive heart failure appeared. However, because the Waterston anastomosis had *not* enlarged, as the autopsy proved, the development of congestive heart failure was thought *not* to be related to an excessively large Waterston anastomosis. We thought that the unrelieved congenital mitral stenosis and regurgitation, and the unrelieved fibrous left ventricular outflow tract stenosis were the causes of this patient's congestive heart failure. Consequently, in 1971, an attempt was made to surgically resect the subaortic stenosis, and a Brock pulmonary valvotomy was also done. Intraoperative death occurred. This patient also had familial congenital heart disease. His mother had ligation of a PDA when she was 14 years of age.

Comment

When the AV endocardial cushion tissue that normally forms the mitral valve and the AV septum and contributes to the tricuspid valve does not develop normally, a variety of congenital malformations can result. These include three anomalies displayed by this patient: congenital mitral stenosis, congenital mitral regurgitation, and fibrous subaortic stenosis if the fibrous tissue forming the anterior mitral leaflet and the AV septum does not normally get "all tidied up." As in this patient, the results can be a congenitally malformed mitral valve that is both stenotic and regurgitant, and residual ("untidied up") fibrous tissue between the anterior mitral leaflet and the muscular interventricular septum. This results in an adherent mitral valve. The anterior mitral leaflet adheres to the ventricular septum, resulting in fibrous left ventricular outflow tract stenosis.

In this patient with TOF, the subaortic VSD was unusually small because of the adherent mitral valvar fibrous tissue. The VSD measured only 5.4 mm in internal diameter (0.2 inch).

Fibrous left ventricular outflow tract stenosis or atresia is a mitral valve anomaly. That is why it is always fibrous, never muscular. Adherent mitral valve hemodynamically causes left ventricular outflow tract obstruction (stenosis or atresia). This is one of the lessons of this case that is clinically very important. In considerations of mitral valve anomalies, people do not usually think of fibrous left ventricular outflow tract obstruction. They should. It is anomalous mitral valve tissue that is causing the fibrous obstruction.

Case 2, a boy who died at 2 months of age in 1988, had normal segmental anatomy, that is {S,D,S}. Autopsy confirmed the presence of HLHS with aortic atresia that was both valvar and *subvalvar*. Why subvalvar? Because the anterior leaflet of the mitral valve was tightly adherent to the left ventricular septal surface, resulting in subaortic left ventricular outflow tract atresia. The ventricular septum was intact. Right ventricular hypertrophy and enlargement were massive. In contrast, the LV was diminutive.

A modified Norwood procedure was performed at 3 days of age using deep hypothermic circulatory arrest. The ascending aorta and aortic arch were amplified using a pulmonary arterial homograft, 8 mm in length. The distal pulmonary artery was closed with a patch of glutaraldehyde-treated pericardium. A large secundum type of ASD was created surgically, and a modified 4-mm right Blalock-Taussig anastomosis was constructed between the right subclavian and the right pulmonary arteries.

The postoperative clinical picture was characterized by congestive heart failure, low cardiac output, right hemidiaphragmatic paralysis, and right chylothorax. Three days postoperatively, echocardiography suggested coarctation of the aorta, with an estimated gradient of 36 mm Hg. The patient's postoperative course continued to be difficult, and he died at home at 2 months of age.

Autopsy confirmed the foregoing anatomic findings and revealed a coarctation of the aorta between the amplified aortic arch and the descending thoracic aorta (1 to 2 mm in internal diameter). The modified Blalock-Taussig anastomosis measured only 2 mm in internal diameter at the proximal (right subclavian) anastomosis. The 4-mm Gore-Tex conduit was patent (not thrombosed), and precoronary arterial stenosis was not present, that is, the inlet to the coronary arterial compartment was widely patent. Therefore, autopsy revealed the immediate causes of this patient's postoperative death to be severe residual coarctation of the aorta and a moderately narrowed modified Blalock-Taussig anastomosis.

This case illustrates that adherence of the anterior leaflet of the mitral valve to the left ventricular septal surface can produce fibrous subaortic left ventricular outflow tract *atresia,* not just fibrous subaortic stenosis, as in Case 1.

MITRAL DYSPLASIA

Table 14.1 says that we have seen two patients with *mitral dysplasia* in this series of 3216 autopsied cases of congenital heart disease (0.06% of this series). But the question immediately arises, What does *dysplasia* really mean? The dictionary definition of dysplasia is "abnormality of development; in pathology, alteration in size, shape and organization of adult cells." This is Splendid, but very nonspecific. *Plasis* means molding, from *plassein* (Greek). In Medicine, *plassis* is used as combining form to denote development or formation. *Dys* means "bad," in Greek. Hence, *dysplasia* denotes bad (abnormal) development of formation.

Case 1, a boy who died at 1 10/12 years of age, had a very rare finding at autopsy. The mitral valve had a net-like mesh of fibrous strands crisscrossing beneath the mitral orifice. These crisscrossing fibrous strands ran from the free margin of the anterior mitral leaflet to both papillary muscle groups. This crisscrossing submitral fibrous mesh ran through the otherwise normal interpapillary muscle space. This is the first and only case of **submitral mesh** that I have ever seen. I have never heard of this anomaly before seeing this case (in 1981). I consequently think that this may be the first report of a previously unknown form of congenital heart disease.

Other important (but not rare) findings at autopsy included severe preductal coarctation of the aorta, with marked hypoplasia of the transverse aortic arch, and a bicuspid but nonstenotic aortic valve, with absence of the intercoronary commissure.

A large mid-muscular VSD was closed by a 1.5-cm (0.6 inch) Dacron patch. Right ventricular hypertrophy and enlargement were marked. The MPA was enlarged, and a large PDA was also present. At 6 days of age, a subclavian patch aortoplasty of the preductal coarctation of the aorta was performed, with banding of the MPA and ligation and division of the PDA. Postoperatively, the patient did well clinically. However, he was found to have suprasystemic right ventricular pressure and evidence of right ventricular strain electrocardiographically. A decision was made to perform total cardiac correction of his intracardiac defects. Repeat cardiac catheterization revealed that the coarctation gradient was only 10 to 12 mm Hg (down from 25 mm Hg 11 months previously), and the LV was now described as "smallish."

At surgery, in 1981, the mid-muscular VSD was closed through a left ventriculotomy and the MPA band was removed, with Dacron patch augmentation of the MPA. The postoperative period was characterized by agitation and convulsions, leading to death.

Comment

What is the submitral network? My impression was that we were looking at a very rare anomaly of the chordae tendineae of the mitral valve. *I am reminded of one of Dr. Jesse Edwards' jokes.* To get the attention of his listeners, who frequently were tired pediatric cardiology fellows and cardiac surgical residents who had been up and working for most of the previous night, Dr. Edwards would begin by saying, "The mitral valve is just like a woman. The more you study her, the less you understand her." His audience—almost all young men—were now listening hard. Then Jesse would present the riddle of the mitral valve:

"The mitral valve basically has two leaflets, right?"

"Right"

"The chordae tendineae run from each leaflet to both papillary muscles, right?"

"Right"

"So, why is the mitral orifice and the space between the papillary muscles not full of crisscrossing chordae tendineae?" Dr Edwards would ask.

Usually, no one could solve this *riddle of the mitral valve.* Then Dr. Edwards would answer his own question, and later I would find myself doing the same thing. This is the story of the mitral valve tensor apparatus: the chordae tendineae and the papillary muscles.

The anterolateral and posteromedial papillary muscles can be modeled by your left and right hands, respectively, with the fingers of each hand forming facing, concave ovals like the vertices of an ellipse. Each papillary muscle has several heads, represented by your fingers. The chordae tendineae run from the papillary muscle heads to the anterior and posterior mitral leaflets. Each papillary muscle head forms a facing, concave, U-shaped array like the vertices of an ellipse. The papillary muscles are like the major foci of an ellipse. The chordae tendineae resemble the sides of an ellipse (in two dimensions), or the walls of a cone (in three dimensions). The chordae focus down on the papillary muscles, which resemble the major foci of an ellipse. Normally, there are no chordae tendineae within the ellipse, or the cone, because the chordae form the sides of the ellipse or the walls of the cone.

Take your two hands and model the tensor apparatus of the mitral valve in three dimensions. The key to understanding is to realize that the two papillary muscles and their chordae tendineae form facing concave arrays, like the vertices of an ellipse. These facing concavities keep the chordae beneath the mitral annulus, away from the mitral orifice. Hence, the tensor apparatus of the mitral valve normally is elliptical and circumferential, with no chordae tendineae crisscrossing within and beneath the mitral orifice.

Your fifth and fourth fingers are like chordae going to or close to the middle of the anterior mitral leaflet. Your third fingers are like the chordae going to the commissures, anterolateral (left hand) and posteromedial (right hand). Your second (index) fingers and your thumbs represent the chordae tendineae that normally go to the posterior mitral leaflet. Although rather difficult to describe, this is easy to model in three dimensions with your hands. These various heads of the papillary muscles and their attached chordae tendineae are very real and important. For example, absence of the papillary muscle head and chorda (or chordae) to a commissure can result in a commissural cleft or gap, resulting in mitral regurgitation through the poorly anchored portion of the mitral valve.

But the purpose of telling you Dr. Jesse Edwards' joke, and the riddle of the mitral valve and its elliptical solution, is (as no doubt will be obvious by now): Jesse Edwards' joke exists! (He thought it did not.) This case illustrates that rarely it is possible for the mitral chordae tendineae to form a crisscrossing fibrous network beneath the mitral orifice and between the papillary muscles. *This is an anomaly of the mitral tensor apparatus—chordae tendineae and papillary muscles.* Dr. Edwards would point out that the normal absence of a submitral network of chordae tendineae is why it is possible for the surgeon or the pathologist to put his or her finger through a normal mitral orifice.

Was the submitral network of any hemodynamic importance? We thought not. However, if an interventional cardiologist were trying to balloon dilate such a valve, chordal rupture with a flail mitral valve might have resulted. Were a thrombus to form in the LA and then set sail, it might well get trapped by the submitral network. Submitral stenosis might then occur. However, in our patient, no deleterious hemodynamic or surgical sequel occurred. I suggest that this rare anomaly be called **submitral fibrous network.**

Case 2, a 6-month-old girl, had abnormal papillary muscle architecture of the left-sided morphologically LV. A portion of the anterolateral papillary muscle group arose from the left ventricular septal surface. This anomaly of the anterolateral papillary muscle was associated with a cleft in the anterior leaflet of the left-sided mitral valve. This was a *commissural cleft,* not an AV canal type of cleft. In an *AV canal type of cleft,* typically associated with a complete or partial form of common AV canal, the cleft points at the left ventricular septal surface; that is, the plane of the cleft is approximately at right angle (at 90 degrees) relative to the plane of the left ventricular septal surface. However, in a *commissural cleft* the cleft points upward in the direction of a mitral valve commissure. This commissural cleft was the site of mitral regurgitation, observed by two-dimensional echocardiography in 1992, and confirmed at autopsy by a jet lesion in the endocardium of the above-lying atrium. Looking at the mitral valve from the left ventricular apex the commissural cleft pointed upward to approximately 11 o'clock. This unusual form of congenital mitral regurgitation occurred in a rare form of congenital heart disease—so rare that it does not have a generally recognized name.

This segmental anatomic set may be called **AV discordance with VA concordance in visceroatrial situs inversus.** However, this long verbal name may leave you scratching your head in wonder. I think it is easiest and clearest just to spell out the segmental anatomy: **{I,D,S}.** {I,D,S} means the segmental anatomic set or combination of situs inversus of the viscera and atria, {**I**, -, -}, with D-loop ventricles {I,**D**, -}, and with solitus normally related great arteries, {I,D,**S**}. Now, it becomes clear what the long verbal name means specifically. The fact that there is AV discordance with VA concordance—that is, *only one discordance*—is important. This tells you that the systemic and pulmonary venous circulations are *uncorrected* physiologically. In other words, the systemic and pulmonary venous circulations are going to the physiologically wrong destinations: the systemic venous blood stream (the blue blood) is going out the systemic circulation to the body, and the pulmonary venous blood stream (the red blood) is going back to the lungs. This is what happens in typical (physiologically uncorrected) TGA. When there are *two discordances (AV and VA),* the systemic and pulmonary venous circulations are physiologically corrected, associated anomalies permitting, as in physiologically corrected TGA, because the venous blood streams go to the physiologically correct destinations: systemic venous blood stream (blue blood) to the lungs, and pulmonary venous blood stream (red blood) to the body.

Usually, when there is AV discordance ({S,L,-} or {I,D,-}), there also is physiologically corrected TGA (TGA {S,L,L} or TGA {I,D,D}). But not always. Infrequently, the great arteries can be normally related, as in this patient: {I,D,S}.

Because the systemic and pulmonary venous circulations are physiologically uncorrected (only one discordance), what would you like to do therapeutically, if feasible? An atrial switch procedure (Senning or Mustard) would be appropriate, not an arterial switch, because the great arteries are normally related.

In addition to the general floor plan, that is, {I,D,S}, there were additional **associated malformations:**

Mesocardia: Dextrocardia (a predominantly right-sided heart) is normal in situs inversus viscerum, which this patient had. Levocardia (a predominantly left-sided heart) is normal in situs solitus viscerum, that is, when the viscera are not inverted, as in this patient's ventricles (D-loop), and as this patient's infundibuloarterial segment (solitus normally related). Interestingly, this patient's heart was approximately in the middle of the thorax (mesocardia), neither predominantly right-sided (dextrocardia), nor left-sided (levocardia). This anatomic detail was of no clinical significance.

Bilateral superior venae cavae: There was a persistent RSVC, to the coronary sinus, to the morphologically RA that was left-sided, as the segmental anatomy indicates: {**I**, D,S}. There was a very small innominate vein, 2 mm in internal diameter, between the left and right SVCs.

Secundum ASDs: There were two secundum types of ASDs: (1) an enlarged ostium secundum above a deficient septum primum (the flap valve of the foramen ovale), the defect measuring 7 × 4 mm; and (2) a fenestration within septum primum measuring 6 × 4 mm.

Tetralogy of Fallot {I,D,S}. TOF is a very rare form of TOF with two different reasons for cyanosis: (1) a TOF type of conotruncal malformation and (2) AV discordance with VA concordance (only *one* intersegmental discordance that physiologically uncorrected the systemic and pulmonary venous circulations).

Pulmonary infundibular atresia, pulmonary valvar atresia, absence of the main pulmonary, but with confluence of the left and right pulmonary artery branches that were associated with a large overriding aorta, with aortic-mitral direct fibrous continuity. There was a left aortic arch, which is abnormal in situs inversus of the viscera and atria, with otherwise unremarkable branching of the brachiocephalic arteries. However, inappropriate aortic arch sidedness relative to the visceroatrial situs is quite frequent in TOF: that is, *right* aortic arch with valvar atresia, absence of the main pulmonary, but with confluence of the left and right pulmonary artery branches were associated with a large overriding aorta, with aortic-mitral direct fibrous continuity. There was a left aortic arch, which is abnormal in situs inversus of the viscera and atria, with otherwise unremarkable branching of the brachiocephalic arteries. However, inappropriate aortic arch sidedness relative to the visceroatrial situs is quite frequent in TOF: for example, *right* aortic arch with TOF in visceroatrial *situs solitus*; that is, *right* aortic arch with TOF {*S*, D,S}. Hence, this rare patient may be exhibiting the same phenomenon (inappropriate aortic arch sidedness relative to the type of visceroatrial situs); TOF {*I*, D,S} with *left* aortic arch.

This patient may be regarded as having a rare form of *pentalogy* of Fallot, because of the coexistence of two secundum-type ASDs. This anomaly may be regarded as a rare form of *pseudotruncus:* TOF {I,D,S} with atresia of the pulmonary infundibulum and pulmonary valve and absence of the MPA. The term *pseudotruncus,* meaning TOF with pulmonary outflow tract atresia, appears to be becoming obsolete.

A right-sided ductus arteriosus or ductus-like collateral arose from the junction of the right subclavian and right common carotid arteries and ran to the proximal right pulmonary artery. In addition to the mild mitral regurgitation mentioned previously, mild tricuspid regurgitation and mild aortic regurgitation were also documented by two-dimensional echocardiography. (The only valve that did not regurgitate was the pulmonary valve, which was atretic.) Hence, this patient had *polyvalvar disease,* which in turn suggests the possibility of a chromosomal anomaly. However, a karyotype was not performed (in 1992), to the best of our knowledge.

An accessory papillary muscle of the RV arose from the right ventricular free wall. Thus, this patient had abnormal tensor apparatus of both AV valves, with regurgitation or both AV valves. Finally, this patient had *absence of the left coronary ostium and five right coronary arteries* all arising from the right coronary sinus of Valsalva. This right-most coronary ostium supplied the right coronary artery. The left-most coronary ostium supplied the left circumflex coronary artery. The three middle coronary ostia supplied the territory of the anterior descending coronary artery (or arteries). *A right-sided spleen* was present. Visceral heterotaxy with asplenia or polysplenia was definitely excluded.

Why did this patient die? A modified right Blalock-Taussig anastomosis and a central pulmonary arterioplasty to enlarge a stenotic left pulmonary arterial ostium were successfully performed at 4 days of age. At 6 months of age, a repeat cardiac catheterization was performed to further clarify the pathologic anatomy of this rare and complex case. A balloon at the tip of a cardiac catheter ruptured in the LV, releasing carbon dioxide gas into the heart. Hypotension and third-degree heart block ensued, with failure to respond to all resuscitative efforts, leading to death of the patient in the cardiac catheterization laboratory.

The patient is thought to have suffered coronary artery gas (CO_2) embolism. The patient was supine in the catheterization laboratory. All of the coronary arteries arose from the right and *anterior* sinus of Valsalva. Because there was pulmonary infundibular and valvar atresia, all of the gas released into the LV would have gone out into the large, overriding aorta. Gas would also have tended to float upward (ventrally), into the right-sided and most anterior (most ventral) sinus of Valsalva, from which all five coronary arteries arose.

We speculated that, in addition to placing the patient in the Trendelenburg position (head down, feet up), it might also have been helpful to place the patient in a *prone position,* instead of a supine position. Then, the coronary arteries would have been as inferior as possible, perhaps encouraging the CO_2 gas (and ? air) to float upward, away from the coronary arteries. At autopsy, both ventricles had large foci of dark-red discoloration, consistent with acute and terminal myocardial ischemia, secondary to gas (CO_2 and ? air) embolism.

MITRAL VALVE HYPOPLASIA RESULTING HEMODYNAMICALLY IN CONGENITAL MITRAL STENOSIS

We recorded 26 such cases in this series of 3216 patients with congenital heart disease (0.81%; see Table 14.1). Typically, the hypoplastic mitral valve is a structurally normal mitral valve, but in miniature, because the left ventricular inflow tract into which the mitral valve is opening is hypoplastic. Hence, the hypoplasia of the mitral valve appears to be *secondary* to the hypoplasia of the left ventricular inflow tract. Because the primary anomaly is thought to be hypoplasia of the LV, this secondary hypoplasia of the structurally normal but miniature mitral valve will not be discussed further. Its anatomy should be clear.

Mitral Valve Anomaly Causing Left Ventricular Outflow Tract Obstruction: Fibrous Left Ventricular Outflow Tract Stenosis or Atresia

We recorded one case like this that also had a definite mitral valve malformation (0.03%; see Table 14.1). This patient was a 5.75-month-old boy who presented with a fascinating and confusing history, physical examination, and laboratory findings in1967. (This was my second year as Director of the Cardiac Registry at the Boston Children's Hospital and my assistant in doing the cardiac part of this autopsy was a young medical student from Los Angeles named Robert M Freedom, who later achieved eminence as a pediatric cardiologist and angiocardiographer.)

This almost 6-month-old boy was referred from New Hampshire with a chief complaint of many blue spells. He was the product of a full-term pregnancy. His mother had one or two episodes of flu during the first trimester, characterized by fever, hoarseness, and upper respiratory tract infection. Delivery was uncomplicated and his birth weight was 8 lb 5 oz (3.77 kg). No duskiness or cyanosis was noted in the nursery, and the child was discharged home at 5 days of age. At 2 weeks of age, the child was taken to his private physician because of bulging in his right neck. The mother was told that this was secondary to muscle weakness and straining. At 4 weeks of age, while waiting in his physician's waiting room, this patient had an episode that was characterized by marked cyanosis and severe bradycardia. This episode was regarded as a cyanotic spell. He was admitted to a hospital in New Hampshire, where a diagnosis of congestive heart failure was made, and digitalis therapy was initiated. Between 3 weeks and about 5 months of age, the patient was seen by a cardiologist every 10 days to 2 weeks because of repeated spells and congestive heart failure. The patient was maintained on digitalis and had three more hospital admissions, for several days each, because of congestive heart failure. At 5 months of age, the child became very fussy and began eating and sleeping poorly. The mother gave the child morphine suppositories for spells.

Six days before admission to Boston Children's Hospital, the child had a very severe spell characterized by screaming followed by cyanosis, then a stiff appearance, followed by limpness. The child was then seen by a private physician who reassured the mother that there was nothing wrong and sent the baby home. (Remember, this was 1967.) The next day (5 days before admission), the child has two similar spells, more severe than he had ever had before. Four days before admission, the baby had three more spells, after which he remained cyanotic for some time, with apparent apnea. He was then admitted to a private hospital, where he was given oxygen and morphine, with some improvement. Because of his deteriorating clinical condition and because of diagnostic uncertainty, he was transferred to the Children's Hospital Medical Center (as our hospital was called at that time) for evaluation of probable cyanotic congenital heart disease with spells.

Salient findings included a palpable liver edge 3 cm below the right costal margin. Cardiac catheterization and angiocardiography revealed TOF with moderately severe hypoplasia of the MPA. However, other findings included pulmonary arterial hypertension, severe pulmonary venous hypertension, mitral valve dysplasia, and left ventricular outflow tract obstruction were also observed. Because of severe pulmonary venous hypertension, the child underwent the surgical creation of an ASD in the hyperbaric chamber. The patient did poorly postoperatively and expired shortly thereafter. Autopsy confirmed the presence of TOF with relatively mild pulmonary infundibular and valvar stenosis. Congenital mitral stenosis was found with myxomatous leaflets and a paucity of interchordal spaces. The posteromedial papillary muscle was covered with extremely thickened left ventricular endocardium and received thickened chordae tendineae from both mitral leaflets. The anterolateral papillary muscle was markedly hypoplastic, but it too received thickened chordae from both mitral leaflets.

The left ventricular outflow tract was completely occluded by superior and medial extension of leaflet tissue from the anterior (or medial, or aortic) leaflet of the mitral valve. The subaortic VSD was plugged almost completely by fibrous tissue extending medially from the anterior mitral leaflet. However, it was possible to pass a 1-mm probe through this greatly narrowed VSD from the LV into the enlarged aorta that overrides the RV. There was direct aortic-mitral fibrous continuity and a hypoplastic and thus stenotic muscular subpulmonary infundibulum, typical of TOF. The LV had severe EFE, with a thick wall (14 mm in thickness) and a small chamber. The LA had moderate fibroelastosis. There were hypertrophy and enlargement of the LA, the RV, and RA.

Comment. For present purposes, this case again demonstrates that fibrous left ventricular outflow tract obstruction (stenosis or atresia) is caused by redundant, accessory, residual mitral valve fibroelastic tissue that has not been normally "tidied up" (see Table 14.1). This patient demonstrates fibrous subaortic left ventricular outflow tract *atresia,* in association with congenital mitral stenosis. This is really a rare and amazing case because of what it says about **TOF.**

Many modern young pediatric cardiologists have never seen a *blue spell.* This patient, alas, had many blue spells. People tend to think that blue spells are associated with severe pulmonary outflow tract stenosis or with pulmonary outflow tract stenosis that can become severe because of infundibular spasm. In contrast, this patient had pulmonary arterial hypertension and pulmonary venous hypertension. The diagnosis of TOF was not made clinically. I made this diagnosis by looking at the angiocardiograms, before doing the dissection at autopsy, because of the characteristic conotruncal anatomy.

The view in 1967 was that if there was no gradient, there was no tetralogy. It was thought, erroneously, that in TOF, there had to be a gradient on catheter pull-back from the MPA into the RV. However, *when pulmonary artery hypertension coexists, for any reason—congenital or acquired—there can be no pulmonary outflow tract gradient in TOF.*

TOF always has a large, subaortic VSD, right? Not quite. This is another generalization that is usually but not always true in tetralogy. As this patient illustrates, when fibrous subaortic atresia coexists (a mitral valve problem), the VSD can be very small, almost nonexistent.

Tetralogy always has a good-sized LV, without EFE, right? Usually, but not always—not if there is a fibrous subaortic atresia, with an almost intact ventricular septum, as in this patient. Rarely, it is possible for TOF to have HLHS with a small-chambered, thick-walled LV and severe left ventricular EF if there is also fibrous subaortic atresia.

Fibrous subaortic obstruction—stenosis or atresia—is an anomaly of the conus arteriosus or infundibulum, right? No. That's why the obstructive tissue is always fibrous, never muscular. Fibrous subaortic obstruction is an endocardial cushion defect, specifically with aberrant fibroelastosis tissue spanning from the anterior mitral leaflet to the ventricular septum, below the aortic valve. This patient makes the involvement of the mitral valve particularly clear by also having full-blown congenital mitral stenosis.

TOF never presents with blue spells and *congestive heart failure,* right? Wrong. It can, if TOF is also associated with congenital mitral stenosis, left ventricular outflow tract atresia, a highly restrictive VSD, pulmonary venous hypertension, pulmonary arterial hypertension, and HLHS (thick-walled and small-chambered LV, with EFE of the LV and LA), as in this rare patient. Thus, congenital mitral stenosis can cast a very long shadow in TOF, particularly if it is associated with subaortic outflow tract atresia and a highly restrictive VSD. Hence, the view (in 2012 to 2013) is that TOF can still be a difficult surgical problem when it is associated with multiple, unusual, left-sided associated anomalies, as in this rare patient.

MYXOMATOUS MITRAL VALVE

A myxomatous mitral valve was diagnosed in 6 of these 3216 autopsied cases of congenital heart disease (0.19%; see Table 14.1).

Case 1, a 31-day-old boy, was the 3.3-kg product of a 37 weeks gestation to a 33-year-old gravida 3 para 2 mother via normal spontaneous vaginal delivery, complicated by meconium staining of the amniotic fluid. By about 1 hour of postnatal life, he was noted to be tachypneic, cyanotic, and hypoglycemia. There was a maternal family history of renal agenesis (maternal first cousin) and of intellectual disability (maternal uncle). The patient's diagnostic work-up revealed MCAs that were thought to be as follows: pentalogy of Fallot, congestive heart failure, respiratory distress, absence of the right kidney, dysplastic left kidney with proteinuria and hematuria, anal atresia with perineal fistula, overriding sutures of the skull, high-arched palate, low-set ears, hypoplastic testes, sacral dimple, right talipes equinovarus (typical club foot), and left calcaneovalgus deformity. A genetics consult (in 1989) led to the conclusion that this patient's MCAs did not fit into any known syndrome. His karyotype was normal for a male (46XY).

At 10 days of age, the patient underwent anoplasty for anal atresia and perineal fistula. At 18 days of age, a duodenal tube was placed because of feeding problems. At 26 days of age, the patient was intubated and transferred to the Boston Children's Hospital. Echocardiography showed normal segmental anatomy, {S,D,S}; a secundum type of ASD; a conoventricular type of VSD with a left-to-right shunt; and little or no pulmonary outflow tract stenosis. Hence, our diagnostic impression was a conoventricular type of VSD, this is, an Eisenmenger type of VSD, not tetralogy (or pentalogy) of Fallot. The conal septum (parietal band) was displaced mildly in an anterosuperior direction, but not enough to create a significant pulmonary outflow tract gradient. Also, the shunt was left to right, without a demonstrable right-to-left component, and the patient continued to be in congestive heart failure with significant hepatomegaly. The chest radiograph showed interstitial edema.

Cardiac catheterization confirmed that the Qp/Qs ratio was 4:1 and that the pulmonary outflow tract gradient, even with this large left-to-right shunt, was only 14 mm Hg. Although there was a preligamental aortic shelf, there was no gradient across this region, excluding coarctation of the aorta. A large aortopulmonary collateral artery was found, running from the descending thoracic aorta to the left lung. Other significant findings were absence of the right renal artery and a tiny left renal artery.

The next day, the patient was taken back to the Cardiac Catheterization Laboratory in order to embolize and occlude the major aortopulmonary collateral artery to the left lung. After several unsuccessful attempts to enter the collateral artery, apparent dissection of the descending thoracic aorta occurred. Bradycardia, hypotension, transient complete AV block, and metabolic acidosis were treated with cardiopulmonary resuscitation in the catheterization laboratory. Bleeding from the patient's right groin was also difficult to control. Echocardiography after cardiac catheterization revealed irregularity along the posterior border of the upper descending thoracic aorta just distal to the origin of the left subclavian artery. This irregularity extended distally for about 2.0 cm. During the subsequent hours, the patient's clinical status was extremely unstable, with multiple episodes of cardiac arrest. The next day, a second echocardiographic study revealed what was interpreted as a pseudoaneurysm. (A *pseudoaneurysm* is one in which the wall of the structure, in this case the wall of the aorta, is *not* involved; hence, the aneurysm is pseudo. Pseudoaneurysms are also called, more clearly, *pulsating hematomas*—a clinically very serious situation.) The patient died approximately 20 hours after cardiac catheterization. Note that the mitral valve was not mentioned; there was no clinical suspicion that the mitral valve was abnormal.

Salient Autopsy Findings

The aortopulmonary collateral artery to the left lung was relatively small (not large, as had been thought clinically). It originated in the position of the supreme intercostal artery, and its orifice was only slightly larger than that of all of the other intercostal arteries. This explained why it has been so difficult (i.e., impossible) to enter this collateral artery with a catheter. There was a circumferential laceration of the intima and media of the descending thoracic aorta, without perforation of the aortic adventitia. The laceration measured 13 mm in circumference, and the intimal margins were separated by a distance of 5 mm. There was a second smaller laceration of the aortic intima, also oriented circumferentially, 4 mm in length, with no intimal separation, and with no aortic adventitial rupture. Both lacerations were located distal to the origin of the small collateral artery to the left lung.

What is the lesson for catheteers? Major aortopulmonary collateral arteries (MAPCAs) typically are associated with TOF with pulmonary outflow tract atresia or severe stenosis. This patient did not have that. Hence, catheteer beware.

Autopsy revealed a clinically unsuspected anomaly of the mitral valve. There was thickening and myxomatous change of the mitral leaflets. The anterolateral and posteromedial papillary muscles of the mitral valve were fused at their origins. Most of the chordae tendineae attached to the posteromedial papillary muscle group. Although this makes one wonder about congenital mitral stenosis with parachute mitral valve, there was a good sized mitral orifice. Some chordae tendineae did insert into the anterolateral papillary muscle group. No end-diastolic gradient was found at cardiac catheterization between the LA and the LV. So, congenital mitral stenosis was excluded, despite the previously mentioned anatomic findings.

Hence, we concluded that this patient had a myxomatous mitral valve that functioned within normal limits. The mitral valve was a "silent partner" in this patient's very significant congenital heart disease, which in turn was just one part of this patient's familial MCAs. Absence of the right kidney and dysplasia of the left kidney with proteinuria and hematuria is functionally very close to **Potter syndrome,** that is, bilateral renal agenesis.

Case 2 was a 6-week-old girl of Chinese extraction who died in 1986 of a rare infantile form of hypertrophic cardiomyopathy. She also had myxomatous mitral and tricuspid valve leaflets. Although born prematurely at an estimated gestational age of 35 to 36 weeks, her birth weight was 3.8 kg (8.38 lb). After birth, she suffered from neonatal respiratory distress and persistent fetal circulation, with neonatal and persistent hypoglycemia. She was also noted to have macrosomia, hepatomegaly, and spastic quadriparesis. At 6 weeks of age she developed atrial flutter, incomplete heart block, severe acidosis, hypoglycemia, and hypocalcemia. Consequently, she was transferred to Boston Children's Hospital for diagnosis and management. She was stable overnight, but the following morning she developed ventricular tachycardia that progressed to ventricular fibrillation. Resuscitative efforts were unsuccessful, leading to death.

Autopsy revealed hypertrophic cardiomyopathy with massive cardiomegaly. The heart weight was 50 g, compared with a normal heart weight of 18 g. Thus, this patient's heart weight was 178% greater than normal; 50/18 = 2.78/1.0. Marked hypertrophy was found of all four cardiac chambers: right atrial wall thickness = 1 to 3 mm; right ventricular wall thickness = 1.5 to 2.5 mm; left atrial wall thickness = 1.5 to 2.5 mm; left ventricular wall thickness = 12 mm; and ventricular septal thickness = 13 to 15.5 mm. Thus, the ventricular septal thickness/ventricular free wall thickness varied from 13/12 (1.08/1) to 15.5/12 (1.3/1). Hence, asymmetrical hypertrophy of the ventricular septum, compared with the left ventricular free wall, was present.

The ventricular volumes were small, and histologic examination displayed marked ventricular myocardial hypertrophy, with myocardial disarray, typical of hypertrophic cardiomyopathy.

Idiopathic hypertrophic subaortic stenosis was considered to be highly probable, caused by the asymmetrical ventricular septal hypertrophy and perhaps also contributed to by the myxomatous thickening of the anterior mitral leaflet. However, there are no hemodynamic or echocardiographic data with which to assess this postmortem diagnostic impression.

The immediate cause of this patient's death was an observed and documented ventricular tachyarrhythmia: ventricular tachycardia progressing to ventricular fibrillation. The right coronary ostium was absent. But the right coronary artery arose from a large (3 to 4 mm in internal diameter) left anterior descending coronary artery, the right coronary artery passing anteriorly across the right ventricular outflow tract to reach the right AV groove. The left circumflex coronary artery supplied the territory of the posterior descending coronary artery. All coronary arteries were patent. This patient also had a mild form of pectus excavatum.

Comment

This patient had an **infantile form of hypertrophic cardiomyopathy,** clinically much more severe than the familiar adolescent-to-adult form of hypertrophic cardiomyopathy. *The metabolic aspects of this infantile form of hypertrophic cardiomyopathy* were very impressive and important: macrosomia; hypoglycemia; hepatomegaly (181.5 g); pancreatomegaly (6 g); neuromuscular pathologic conditions, including spastic quadriparesis with neurogenic atrophy; mild architectural abnormalities of the cerebral cortex; loose and redundant skin of the lower extremities, different histopathologically from cutis laxa; disordered bone growth, with mild pectus excavatum; and diffuse hypoplasia of lymphoid tissue.

INFANTILE HYPERTROPHIC CARDIOMYOPATHY

Some observers thought this patient might have the Beckwith-Wiedemann syndrome, but this possibility was not supported by the histopathologic findings. As of 1986, none of us had ever seen, or heard of a disease exactly this. So our tentative conclusion was that it perhaps was a newly recognized syndrome. To the best of my knowledge, this is the first time that this case and this disease have been published. More cases and more study of this entity are needed. This autopsy was done by Dr. Gordon Vawter, our Chief of General Pathology at that time, and by Dr. Muller, a general pathology resident. My speculation is that this entity may represent an inborn error of carbohydrate metabolism, as is suggested by this patient's neonatal and persistent hypoglycemia, hepatomegaly, and pancreatomegaly. Metabolically, this entity may be the opposite of type 1 diabetes mellitus, in which the patient produces too little or no insulin. *By contrast, this patient may have been producing too much insulin, suggested by the pancreatomegaly, resulting in hypoglycemia.* One might object, "But I have never heard of a disease that is the *opposite* of type 1 diabetes mellitus." I would agree; neither have I. But that may be because severe and persistent hypoglycemia may not be consistent with a prolonged postnatal life span. This patient died at only 6 weeks of age.

Molecular genetic studies were not performed in an effort to clarify the genetic mutation that may have caused this patient's hypertrophic cardiomyopathy. The myxomatous nature of this patient's mitral (and tricuspid) valves is thought to have been of little or no clinical importance in this case.

Case 3, a girl who died at 12 days of age, also had myxomatous mitral and tricuspid valves. Prominent myxomatous nodules on the free edges of both valves were interpreted as indicating immaturity. But both valves were thought to function probably normally. DORV {S,D,A} was present. In other words, the segmental anatomic set was situs solitus of the viscera and atria {*S*,-,-}, D-loop ventricles {S,*D*,-}, and A-malposition of the great arteries {S,D,*A*}. There was left-sided juxtaposition of the atrial appendages, meaning that both atrial appendages lay to the left of both great arteries.

There were bilateral SVCs. The left SVC drained into the coronary sinus and then to the RA. The left innominate vein was absent. A secundum type of ASD was present. The septum primum was malaligned with the septum secundum, apparently in association with left-sided juxtaposition of the atrial appendages. The AV alignments were concordant. Apart from myxomatous changes of the leaflet margins, the mitral and tricuspid valves were unremarkable. The RV was markedly hypertrophied (free wall 8 mm thick, in the fresh state) and mildly enlarged. The LV was normal, the free wall measuring 4.5 mm in the fresh state. A large VSD was present. The VSD was of the confluent conoventricular type (between the conus above and the ventricular septum below) and the AV canal type (extending behind the septal leaflet of the tricuspid valve). This large VSD was the nonrestrictive left ventricular outflow tract. The conus was subaortic, with pulmonary-tricuspid fibrous continuity. The right ventricular outflow tracts were widely patent toward the aorta and very stenotic toward the MPA. The pulmonary valve was bicuspid with a rudimentary septal commissure, and mildly stenotic. The pulmonary valve and the tricuspid valve were both posterior and inferior. The tricuspid valve contributed importantly to the pulmonary outflow tract stenosis, which was severe. The aortic valve was tricuspid and widely patent. The MPA and branches were mildly hypoplastic. The aorta was of good caliber, with a left arch, a widely patent isthmus, unremarkable brachiocephalic branches, and a right-sided PDA from the base of the innominate artery to the right pulmonary artery. The right coronary artery was dominant, giving origin to a large conus coronary artery that continued supply to apical half of the anterior descending coronary arterial distribution. The right coronary artery also supplied the posterior descending coronary artery distribution. The left coronary artery supplied the left circumflex coronary artery, and a short anterior descending coronary artery that supplied the proximal (upper half) of the anterior coronary artery distribution.

In 1991, at 3 days of age, a modified left-sided Blalock-Taussig shunt was constructed, using a 4-mm Gore-Tex conduit between the proximal left subclavian artery and the left pulmonary artery. Episodes of severe desaturation led to the construction of a central shunt between the ascending aorta and the right pulmonary artery, using a 3.5-mm Gore-Tex conduit at 11 days of age, with clip occlusion of the left-sided modified Blalock-Taussig shunt. However, by this time, generalized edema, systemic hypotension, and increased pulmonary blood flow led to cardiac arrest, with unsuccessful resuscitation at 12 days of age.

Comment

Again, myxomatous changes of the mitral (and tricuspid) valves appeared to be of little or no clinical importance, with death being related to other congenital heart disease, in this case DORV {S,D,A} with left-sided juxtaposition of the atrial appendages, VSD of the confluent conoventricular and AV canal variety, and severe pulmonary outflow tract stenosis. This patient died because of failure of surgical palliation of her severe pulmonary outflow tract stenosis.

Case 4, a man who died at 41 years of age, was referred to us as a pathology consult by our friends and colleagues at the Beth Israel Hospital in Boston. The reasons for this autopsy consult will soon become obvious. As so often, in this case, the basic questions were: What kind of a disease is this? Is this a whole body syndrome, or is this several different diseases? Have we ever seen anything like this case?

This 41-year-old man was admitted to the Beth Israel Hospital in 1991 in status epilepticus. Before admission, he had three successive tonic-clonic seizures without ever recovering consciousness. After intubation and admission, his seizure activity altered to left beating nystagmus with left gaze preference, and intermittent twitching of his right arm. He responded only to pain. A head computerized tomography (CT) suggested dysmorphic ventricles and a corpus callosum abnormality. Other findings included fever (101.9° F or 38.8° C), and a left lower lobe infiltrate on chest film. Antibiotics for bacterial pneumonia were begun.

His medical history was questionable seizures, but not definite. He had a mild intellectual disability, abused alcohol, and had a history of rheumatic fever sometime in the past (exactly when was not established). He had been admitted to Cambridge Hospital for pneumonia 1 year previously. He has multiple pigmented macules over his entire body consistent with café-au-lait spots. Neurofibromatosis was suspected, especially when it was learned that his mother had died of a brain tumor and that one sister had skin findings consistent with neurofibromatosis. Subsequently, MRI revealed that the corpus callosum abnormality was an infiltrating lesion, possibly a low-grade glioma. A cavernous hemangioma or old healed hemorrhage was also found of the right cerebellar hemisphere. A stereotactic needle biopsy of the corpus callosum revealed tissue that was highly suggestive of a low-grade glioma, most likely an oligodendroglioma.

The patient's mental status slowly improved, but he never progressed beyond some spontaneous movements and reflexes. After numerous conferences with family members, he was changed to "do not resuscitate" status. Fever persisted (103° F or 39.4° C), with copious secretions, but with a minimal gag reflex, leading to death on the 25th day in hospital.

My note (earlier) follows the final "official" hospital account of this patient very closely. Please note: *His heart was almost never mentioned.* This is amazing (but understandable), as the autopsy findings revealed pneumonia involving all of the left lung and the right lower lobe. Polyvalvar disease of the heart was present. There was focal myxomatous thickening of the tricuspid valve, that was thought probably to be of little or no functional significance. All tricuspid leaflets displayed nodular thickening, up to 3 mm, especially the thin and delicate chordae tendineae attached. Rolling of the tricuspid leaflet edges was slight.

Moderately marked myxomatous change of the pulmonary valve leaflets was found, with considerable elongation of the pulmonary leaflets (3 cm from the free leaflet margin to the deepest attachment in the sinus of Valsalva). The tricommissural pulmonary valve leaflets showed diffuse myxomatous thickening (up to 1 mm), with rolled leaflet edges. The annulus of the pulmonary valve was approximately 2 cm in internal diameter. We thought that these myxomatous and elongated pulmonary leaflets might have resulted in some degree of pulmonary outflow tract stenosis, but we have no hemodynamic or echocardiographic data with which to assess this speculative possibility.

The mitral valve was markedly myxomatous, with probable mitral valve prolapse, and with evidence of marked mitral regurgitation. The mitral leaflets were myxomatous, with nodular thickening (up to 5 mm thick), very prominent where the thin chordae tendineae attached. The mitral leaflets showed hooding and billowing, with a typically hemorrhoidal appearance as seen from the left atrial aspect. The LA was markedly hypertrophied and enlarged, with diffuse endocardial thickening. The atrial septum displayed a restrictive, but probe-patent foramen ovale. The septum primum (the flap valve of the foramen ovale) bulged into the right atrial cavity. Left ventricular hypertrophy and enlargement were marked. Right ventricular hypertrophy and enlargement were moderate.

This patient had Barlow syndrome, with mitral valve myxomatous change, mitral valve prolapse with hooding, billowing, hemorrhoidal appearance, and marked mitral regurgitation. Rightward aneurysmal bulging of the atrial septum, with hypertrophy and enlargement of the LV, LA, and RV, confirm the massive mitral regurgitation, which was the worst part of this patient's *polyvalvar disease*. Only the aortic valve had a normal appearance.

What should we conclude? This is a case of myxomatous mitral valve in which the myxomatous nature of the mitral valve was of definite clinical importance, with mitral valve prolapse and severe mitral regurgitation, that is, Barlow syndrome. Ironically, perhaps because of the very dramatic and serious clinical presentation of this 41-year-old man in status epilepticus, with a tumor of the corpus callosum (thought to be the basis of the status epilepticus), and pneumonia, attention was focused on these urgent issues and the heart is barely mentioned in the notes available to us. Were the typical mid-to-late-systolic ejection click and the murmur of mitral regurgitation present? We simply do not know. However, it seems important to note that myxomatous mitral valve was *clinically important* only in a middle-aged man (41 years of age), and *in none of our pediatric patients* cited previously in this small series. Geggel and Fyler, in reviewing our experience with mitral valve prolapse at Boston Children's Hospital from 1973 to 2002, reached the following conclusion:

1. Mitral valve prolapse occurs as a primary lesion, and it also occurs in other conditions such as Marfan syndrome, Ehlers-Danlos syndrome, osteogenesis imperfect, pseudoanthoma elasticum, Stickler syndrome, scoliosis, pectus excavatum, asthenic body habitus, straight back syndrome, adults with secundum ASD (abnormal left ventricular geometry created by right ventricular volume overload, or because of reduction in left ventricular cavity size with resolution of mitral valve prolapse postoperatively after occlusion of the secundum ASD in many patients), hyperthyroidism, sickle cell disease, muscular dystrophy, hypomastia, and von Willebrand disease.
2. Mitral valve prolapse is rare in the first decades of life, in the absence of an identifiable cause (listed heretofore).
3. *Myxomatous change of the mitral valve* is thought to be the basis of mitral regurgitation and of mitral valve prolapse. It takes *time* for a myxomatous mitral valve to develop mitral regurgitation and mitral valve prolapse.

Thus, a myxomatous mitral valve may be regarded as a *preregurgitation stage* and as a *preprolapse stage* of the mitral valve.

In other words, a myxomatous valve (AV, or semilunar) may be regarded as a ticking time-bomb. It has not gone off yet (in the pediatric age range), but given enough time (into the adult age range), it will. Myxomatous aortic or truncal valves tend to develop premature fibrosis, calcification, and stenosis.

Returning to our patient, Case 4, it is comforting to know that most patients with mitral valve prolapse have a benign course. *Case 4 definitely had polyvalvar disease with myxomatous changes of the mitral, pulmonary, and tricuspid valves (as above).* Polyvalvar disease is often associated with a chromosomal disorder (e.g., trisomy 18). However, to the best of our knowledge, no study of this patient's karyotype was undertaken.

We also presented the view that this patient had a newly recognized heritable total body metabolic abnormality of connective tissue with multiple expressions involving:

1. *the heart,* with mitral valve regurgitation and prolapse, marked myxomatous change and elongation of the pulmonary valve leaflets, and myxomatous thickening of the tricuspid valve;
2. *the skin,* with pigmented macules over the entire body, consistent with café-au-lait spots, strongly suggestive of neurofibromatosis (sister with neurofibromatosis); and
3. *the brain,* with a low-grade glioma (oligodendroglioma) of the corpus callosum (mother died of a brain tumor).

Thus, in 1991, we realized that this patient had a newly discovered heritable metabolic abnormality of connective tissue involving the heart, the skin, and the brain. Fibrous tissue assumes various forms and appearances in the body:

1. *in the heart,* the AV endocardial cushions that contribute to the mitral and tricuspid valves, and the semilunar endocardial cushions that contribute to the aortic and pulmonary valves;
2. *in the skin,* fibrous and elastic cells are major contributors; and
3. *in the nervous system,* gliomas are a major form of fibrous tissue in the brain and spinal cord.

Case 5 was a girl who died at 16 days of age. She had been born at home, but because of neonatal cyanosis she was admitted to hospital. Echocardiography revealed cardiomegaly, increased pulmonary blood flow, a large RA, a large LA, a prominent pulmonary artery, a small round LV with very poor function, an abnormal wedge-shaped mitral valve, and an aortic valve that appeared small, with thick leaflets and that appeared to be bicuspid.

Cardiac catheterization at 1 day of age also revealed severe aortic insufficiency. The patient was then transferred by air from the Albany Medical Center Hospital in Albany, NY to Boston Children's Hospital. She was intubated and was on a prostaglandin and dopamine infusion. However, transportation was complicated by the loss of the intravenous line supplying dopamine and prostaglandin and also the loss of the arterial line, with some blood loss. She was admitted, appearing cool, pale, mottled, and cyanotic and seemed to be dying.

Echocardiography confirmed the presence of a normal segmental anatomic set of {S,D,S}, with a patent foramen ovale, mild tricuspid regurgitation, moderate mitral regurgitation, some right ventricular dysfunction, a hypoplastic LV one-half to two-thirds normal size, severe left ventricular dysfunction with failure of the LV to generate systemic pressure, a sinus of Valsalva aneurysm involving the right coronary and noncoronary sinuses, a large left aortic arch, large but unremarkable brachiocephalic arteries, a large PDA with predominantly pulmonary artery to aortic flow, an aortic valve annulus of 5 mm in diameter, and an aortic root diameter of 14 mm.

Thus *the diagnostic impression* was HLHS with critical aortic valvar stenosis, left ventricular hypoplasia with severe dysfunction, and with aortic regurgitation and mitral regurgitation resulting in backward flow of blood into the LA and RA. She then developed acute abdominal distention and free intraabdominal air on abdominal x-ray with unstable hemodynamics. Our clinical impression was necrotizing enterocolitis. Emergency laparotomy, with subtotal colectomy and end-ileostomy with mucous fistula, was performed.

Her postoperative course was complicated by the development of congestive heart failure. At 16 days of age, a modified Norwood procedure was performed in an effort to manage her congestive heart failure, but she could not be weaned from cardiopulmonary bypass and she died intraoperatively.

Autopsy revealed hypoplastic and deformed *mitral valve* with a myxomatous, redundant, and prolapsing posterior mitral leaflet. The mitral valve annulus measured 6 mm in diameter. The LA was moderately enlarged and severely hypertrophied. The LV had a small chamber, a thick wall, and left ventricular EFE. The aortic valve was critically stenotic. There were no well-developed commissures; that is, this was an *acommissural* aortic valve. Only ridges were found in the aortic valvar leaflet tissue, suggesting where LC/NC and the RC/LC commissures should have been. There was poststenotic dilatation of the aortic root, and aneurysmal dilatation of the right coronary and noncoronary sinuses of Valsalva. Moderate right atrial hypertrophy and enlargement were found. Right ventricular hypertrophy and enlargement were also moderate. Moderately severe aortic regurgitation appeared following cardiac catheterization. During the modified Norwood procedure, a prosthetic patch was placed over the regurgitant aortic valve, to stop the aortic regurgitation that was thought to be contributing to the patient's congestive heart failure.

Additional postmortem findings included a nontransmural myocardial infarction of the anterior right atrial free wall, infarction of the anterior interatrial septum, infarction of the anterior left ventricular free wall, and an acute infarction of the anterolateral right ventricular free wall.

Comment

How important was the hypoplastic, malformed and myxomatous mitral valve with a redundant and prolapsing posterior mitral leaflet in this 16-day-old girl? Our impression after autopsy was that she had both *congenital mitral stenosis* as part of HLHS with a small-chambered and thick-walled LV *and congenital mitral regurgitation* related to the prolapsing posterior mitral leaflet with chordal elongation, but without chordal rupture. As important as the congenital mitral stenosis and regurgitation were, we thought that *congenital critical aortic valvar stenosis* may have been even more important hemodynamically, as is suggested by the small-chambered and thick-walled LV, the EFE of the LV, and the post-stenotic dilatation of the aortic root and the proximal ascending aorta. (The aortic valve regurgitation was thought to have been secondary to catheter-inflicted tearing of the aortic valve leaflets during cardiac catheterization in 1987.)

We now understand that balloon dilation of congenitally stenotic aortic valves can be complicated by iatrogenic aortic valvar regurgitation, particularly if the stenotic aortic valve leaflets are *not* supported by any commissures. Recall that this hypoplastic and stenotic aortic valve was *acommissural:* no commissures supported and separated the confluent aortic valve leaflets. To stop this iatrogenic aortic regurgitation is why the unusual step was taken during the modified Norwood procedure of patching closed the aortic valvar orifice below the coronary ostia. The modified Norwood procedure was performed technically very well. Why, then, did the patient die intraoperatively? We thought that the answer was because during transportation from Albany, NY, to Boston, MA, both the intravenous line supplying dopamine and prostaglandin, and the arterial line were "lost" (came out), with some blood loss. On admission here, the patient appeared moribund. Various unusual myocardial infarctions were found at autopsy. These, we thought, may well have contributed to our inability to wean this patient from cardiopulmonary bypass after completion of the modified Norwood procedure. (Prostaglandin is essential to keep the PDA patent in patients with HLHS.) Loss of the intravenous line was therefore a very serious therapeutic mishap that occurred during aerial transport of this patient.

To summarize, this patient's mitral valve pathologic condition was *only part* of her HLHS and arguably not the most important part. The congenital aortic valvar stenosis was probably even more severe. Therapeutic mishaps before admission (loss of the venous intravenous line, with cessation of prostaglandin administration probably resulted in narrowing or functional closure of the ductus arteriosus, and loss of the arterial line associated with some degree of blood loss) and after admission (balloon tearing of the markedly stenotic aortic valve that had no supporting aortic valvar commissures, resulting in severe aortic valve regurgitation after diagnostic and therapeutic cardiac catheterization) also may well have been important in leading to a fatal outcome.

Case 6 with a myxomatous mitral valve was a boy with *Hurler syndrome* who died in 1957 at 12 8/12 years of age because of extensive bilateral pneumonia because of *S. aureus* infection. This was *familial Hurler syndrome.* This patient had an older brother and a younger sister, both of whom were afflicted with this genetic mucopolysacharidosis. Interestingly, **type 1 mucopolysaccharidosis (Hurler disease, or gargoylism, or Hurler-Pfaundler disease)** usually is inherited as an autosomal recessive disorder; but this family behaved in a fashion that suggests the possibility of autosomal dominant inheritance, with all three of this mother's children being afflicted. (Admittedly, 3 is a very small series.)

This patient had almost all of the typical features of Hurler syndrome, including dwarfism (height = 116 cm [3 ft 9.7 inches]), characteristic facies (narrowed palpebral fissures, sunken nasal bridge, open mouth, protruding thick tongue, large skull, prominent frontal ridges), kyphosis, inability to extend joints fully, a partly crouched stance with thighs partly flexed and abducted, wide hands, stubby fingers that are partly flexed giving a clawlike appearance, hepatosplenomegaly, widely spaced and peg-shaped teeth, thickened and lardaceous skin that lacks subcutaneous elasticity, thick lips, and generalized hirsutism over the shoulders and back. The pupils were normal and the corneas were clear (not cloudy, as they can be with this disease). Intellectual disability led to his admission to Wrentham State School.

At autopsy, *the tricuspid valve* was thickened and nodular, especially at the valve ring (i.e., the leaflet origins). The chordae tendineae appeared shorter than normal. The mitral valve displayed marked nodularity of its leaflets, and the chordae tendineae were shortened and thickened. However, the LA appeared entirely normal, with no suggestion of mitral stenosis or mitral regurgitation. The prosector was surprised, in view of the very abnormal appearance of the mitral valve, that no heart murmur had been described during life. The brain weight was markedly reduced. Microscopically, the typical abnormal vacuoles were found in many organs, including the liver, spleen, pancreas, heart, blood vessels, brain, and spinal cord. The lungs showed gross and histologic evidence of acute pneumonia and bronchitis. Intraluminal vegetable matter was found histologically in one bronchiole, with adjacent foreign body giant cells. These findings were consistent with the aspiration of food, which may have played a role in the pathogenesis of the pneumonia. *S. aureus* was cultured from the lung.

Etiology. The primary defect in Hurler disease (type 1 mucopolysaccharidosis) is an absence of lysomal α-L-iduronidase in all tissues that results in an accumulation of mucopolysaccharides in parenchymal and mesenchymal tissues and the storage of lipids within neuronal tissues. Parental diagnosis is now possible by measuring α-L-iduronidase in cultured amniotic fluid cells. Type 1 mucopolysaccharidosis, or Hurler disease, is characterized clinically by coarse facies, stiff joints, mental deficiency, and cloudy corneas by 1 or 2 years of age. Our patient was typical, except for the corneas, which were said *not* to be cloudy and the inheritance, with all 3 siblings in this one family being afflicted, raising the question: was this really autosomal recessive inheritance?

Comment

In this series of 6 patients with a myxomatous mitral valve but without a more hemodynamically significant diagnosis (e.g., congenital mitral stenosis, congenital mitral regurgitation), this is the first and only case with a "storage" disease. In our patient, many of the tissues, including the markedly nodular mitral valve leaflets, were stuffed with globules of mucopolysaccharide because of an inborn error of metabolism, absence of α-L-iduronidase. Hence, this patient had a very different kind of myxomatous mitral valve than did our other 5 patients. This observation raises questions about what the myxomatous valve really is and what does *myxomatous* really mean? The dictionary answers this question as "of the nature of a myxoma." The dictionary defines *myxoma* as a benign tumor composed of primitive connective tissue cells and stroma resembling mesenchyme. Myxomas are also called *colloid* tumors, *gelatinous* tumors, or *mucous* tumors. *Mesenchyme* (or *mesenchyma*) is defined as the meshwork of loosely organized embryonic connective tissue in the mesoderm, from which are formed the connective tissues of the body, and also the blood vessels and the lymphatics. A general English dictionary defines a *myxoma* as a benign tumor composed of connective tissue and mucous elements. *Myxo-* and *myx-* indicate mucus or mucus-like material (from Greek *muxa*, "mucus" or "slime"). *What do we mean when we speak of a myxomatous valve?* We mean that the leaflets are abnormally thick and fleshy. Cardiac leaflets start out as cushions, thick little fibroelastic masses of tissue either at the AV or semilunar valve levels. Normally, these AV and semilunar valve cushions thin out greatly and develop into *leaflets* (leaflet = small leaf). When cushions fail to thin out and develop into normally thin leaflets, we assume that the developmental transition from cushion to leaflet is incomplete. We think that abnormally thick and fleshy leaflets are incompletely developed or immature as though they contained too much mucus-like fluid and hence are abnormally thick or cushion-like.

The first 5 cases are considered to have incompletely developed or immature mitral valves. This sixth patient with Hurler syndrome is considered to be basically different, the thickened and nodular mitral valve being stuffed with mucopolysaccharide because of the genetic inborn error of metabolism. The last conclusion that should be mentioned is that myxomatous mitral valves (meaning immature and hence thick and fleshy valve leaflets) are very much more common than the small number of patients in this series (5) would suggest. Many cases of congenital mitral stenosis and congenital mitral regurgitation also have myxomatous mitral valves; but myxomatous mitral valve is not the primary diagnosis in such cases because of the important hemodynamic consequences (stenosis or regurgitation) of the mitral malformation. We only make a primary diagnosis of myxomatous mitral valve when other hemodynamically important sequelae are *not* present. This diagnostic custom means that myxomatous mitral valve is greatly underdiagnosed. Perhaps the mitral valve in Hurler disease and other storage diseases should not be described as "myxomatous" because storage diseases are so different from the results of developmental immaturity (typical myxomatous changes in the mitral and other valves). But this case is included here (not excluded) because this is how the mitral valve in Hurler disease often is described, as it was in our cases. I fully agree that the mitral valve in Hurler syndrome is very different from that in typical so-called myxomatous mitral valve (as earlier).

CONGENITAL MITRAL VALVE PROLAPSE

Mitral valve prolapse is the last of the mitral valve anomalies that was identified in Table 14.1. It was found in 11 of the 3216 autopsied cases of congenital heart disease that form the material basis of this book, constituting 0.34% of this series. But as always, the real questions remain: What really is mitral valve prolapse anatomically? How many different anatomic types are there? In how many different situations does mitral valve prolapse occur? How clinically important is mitral valve prolapse? Does our experience shed any light on therapeutic approaches—those that work versus those that do not?

First, ours is a relatively small series (n = 11). Our experience should be viewed as a contribution to understanding, but not necessarily as the definitive answer to all of these questions.

Sex: Males to females = 5/6 (0.83)

Age at Death or Cardiac Transplantation: Mean, 5 9/12 ± 6 8/12 year*; average, ±1 standard deviation. Range: maximum, 22 7/12 years; minimum, 0 (no postnatal age; Case 9 was an aborted fetus of 21 weeks gestational age); median, 6.0 years.

Anatomic Findings (there were two groups of cases of mitral valve prolapse)**:** isolated, in 2 of 11 (18%); nonisolated, in 9 of 11 (82%).

Isolated mitral valve prolapse is the kind that one reads about in textbooks on adult cardiology. The mitral valve leaflets are redundant and myxomatous, with upward hooding of the leaflet tissue between the insertions of the chordae tendineae. Both leaflets are involved, especially the posterior leaflet. The mitral valve leaflets may be described as floppy. Mitral chordae tendineae may or may not be ruptured, resulting in a flail, or partially flail mitral valve. And mitral regurgitation can be severe. In isolated mitral valve prolapse, this is the patient's main clinical problem. This situation of isolated mitral valve prolapse was found in only about one-fifth of our patients (18%). *Nonisolated mitral valve prolapse* was much more common in our experience (82%). Although mitral valve prolapse was present, other major clinical problems also coexisted and frequently constituted the dominant clinical disability, as will be presented later.

ISOLATED MITRAL VALVE PROLAPSE

Known by many names, including the systolic click-murmur syndrome, Barlow syndrome, billowing mitral cusp syndrome, myxomatous mitral valve syndrome, floppy mitral valve syndrome, and redundant mitral cusp syndrome, isolated mitral valve prolapse syndrome was exemplified by our **Case 8,** a 10-year-old boy who died in 1982. His mitral valve was markedly myxomatous, involving both the leaflets and the chordae tendineae and described as "floppy." He had severe mitral valve prolapse and regurgitation. There was marked upward hooding of the mitral valve leaflets between the insertions of the chordae tendineae. Clinically, he had a honking, loud gurgling, easily heard murmur. Arrhythmias resulted in episodes of dizziness. The patient took frequent naps. He experienced premature ventricular contractions at rest. He complained of chest pains and said that his lungs hurt. He experienced migrating joint pains and occasionally could not walk on his own. No evidence of organic arthritis was found.

The patient's mother and sister also had isolated mitral valve prolapse, which can be inherited as an autosomal dominant trait. (A careful genetic study of this family was not done, to my knowledge. Consequently, I do not want to make any definite genetic diagnosis.)

This patient died a sudden, unexpected, arrhythmic death. So, one can understand why this is regarded as the mitral valve prolapse *syndrome*. *Syndrome* is a Greek word meaning "a running together or concurrence": the honking or gurgling murmur that can often be heard without a stethoscope; the characteristic systolic click-murmur heard on auscultation; the redundant, myxomatous leaflet tissue with systole, and the elongated chordae tendineae; and the ventricular arrhythmias that can lead to a sudden, unexpected, arrhythmic death, as in Case 8. Thus, isolated mitral valve prolapse is indeed a syndrome, with many characteristic signs and symptoms occurring together. It is also the *isolated* mitral valve prolapse syndrome because only the mitral valve was abnormal. The tricuspid, pulmonary, and aortic valves were all within normal limits at autopsy.

Case 11 also had the isolated mitral valve prolapse syndrome. The patient was a 6-year-old girl who underwent successful orthotopic cardiac transplantation in 1992. The explanted native heart specimen had mitral valve prolapse with a hemorrhoidal appearance from the atrial aspect created by the upward hooding of the mitral valve leaflets tissue between the insertions of the chordae tendineae. Upward hooding into the LA was particularly marked of the lateral half of the posterior mitral leaflet adjacent to the anterolateral commissure of the mitral valve. Jet lesions of the endocardium of the posterior wall of the LA were more marked laterally than medially. Left atrial jet lesions were found in all patients with mitral valve prolapse. These left atrial jet lesions may be regarded as proof that mitral regurgitation was present. Left ventricular hypertrophy and enlargement were found, with the left ventricular free wall varying from 8 to 13 mm in thickness. Cardiomegaly was present; the heart weighted 240 g. Apart from isolated mitral valve prolapse, this was a structurally normal heart with normal segmental anatomy, {S,D,S}. This was the only patient in this series who underwent cardiac transplantation and survived. The other 10 cases were all fatalities.

NONISOLATED MITRAL VALVE PROLAPSE

What *congenital mitral valve prolapse* is has been described earlier. But what does *nonisolated* add to it? What does that mean, specifically? As you will see, *nonisolated* means a lot. Often, the conditions with which mitral valve prolapse can be associated are clinically much more important than is the mitral valve prolapse—not always, but often, as we will see. First, here is a list of the associated conditions with which mitral valve prolapse was associated in this series (Table 14.24). Unfortunately, tables like this (see Table 14.24) do not convey what was clinically important. This I shall now attempt to do with brief case descriptions.

Case 1 (see Table 14.24) was a male infant with mitral valve prolapse and idiopathic hypertrophic cardiomyopathy. Left ventricular hypertrophy was marked, involving both the left

TABLE 14.24 Nonisolated Mitral Valve Prolapse (n = 9)

Case No.	Associated Conditions	No. of Cases	% of Group[a]
1	Idiopathic hypertrophic cardiomyopathy	1	11
2	Multiple congenital anomalies	1	11
3	Prematurity, hyaline membranes	1	11
4	Severe congenital aortic stenosis	1	11
5	Double-outlet right ventricle	1	11
6	Trisomy 18, polyvalvar disease	1	11
7 + 10	Marfan syndrome	2	22
9	Polyvalvar disease	1	11

[a]Group = nine cases. Percentages (%) rounded off to the nearest whole number.

ventricular free wall and the ventricular septum. The hypertrophic cardiomyopathy was considered to be concentric, asymmetrical hypertrophy of the ventricular septum not being present.

The mitral valve prolapse was characterized by a redundant posterior leaflet with elongated chordae tendineae. The mitral leaflet margins were thickened and rolled, indicating mitral regurgitation. Left atrial jet lesions confirmed the presence of mitral regurgitation.

His clinical course was characterized by severe, intractable biventricular heart failure with chronic pulmonary congestion and edema, leading to death at 11½ months of age, in 1978.

Autopsy revealed mild left ventricular endocardial sclerosis and left ventricular fibrosis. Left ventricular hypertrophy was confirmed: the left ventricular inflow tract free wall was 11 mm thick (normal age-matched and sex-matched control = 5.5 mm; thus, the left ventricular inflow tract free wall was 100% greater in thickness than normal. The left ventricular outflow tract free wall measured 11.4 mm in thickness (normal control = 8.7 mm thick; thus, the left ventricular outflow tract free wall was 31% greater than normal).

Our impression was that the associated idiopathic hypertrophic cardiomyopathy significantly worsened this patient's clinical course, and was thought to be importantly responsible for the patient's chronic, severe, intractable and ultimately fatal *biventricular* heart failure.

Case 2 (see Table 14.24) was a boy with mitral valve prolapse and MCAs. The trouble with this conventional diagnosis of *MCAs* is that it does not mean anything specific. But what it does mean is that more than one bodily system is anomalous. The diagnosis of this boy may be summarized as lumbar meningomyelocele, closed at birth; asthma with bronchospasm; cerebral palsy with intellectual disability and seizures; hydrocephalus, treated with a ventriculoperitoneal shunt at 1 month of age; denervation of the urinary bladder, leading to contraction of the bladder, augmented with a loop of ileum in 1985; chronic gastroesophageal reflux, treated with a gastrostomy tube; bilateral inguinal hernias, treated with herniorrhaphies; scoliosis, treated with spinal fusion and a Harrington rod; recurrent urinary tract infections with pseudomonas, proteus, and *Escherichia coli;* and mitral valve prolapse, with multiple prolapsing scallops of the posterior leaflet of the mitral valve, and with mild left atrial jet lesions.

This boy suffered a sudden, unexpected death at 8½ years of age in 1986. The immediate cause of his sudden death was uncertain. Our leading hypotheses were aspiration or asthma with bronchospasm. Our impression was that this patient's mitral regurgitation was relatively mild, judging from his mild left atrial jet lesions. His associated abnormalities were thought to have been responsible for his death: gastroesophageal reflux with aspiration, asthma with bronchospasm, or both. It was also not possible to exclude the possibility of a terminal, fatal ventricular arrhythmia, although the first two diagnoses mentioned previously were favored.

Case 3 (see Table 14.24) was a female infant who was born prematurely with an estimated gestational age of 33 weeks (8¼ months) with a birth weight of 1400 g (3 lb 1 oz). Hyaline membrane disease of the lungs developed. Her ductus arteriosus was noted to be closed at 9 days of age. On day 29, she was extubated. Then severe bronchopulmonary dysplasia developed, leading to cor pulmonale. She also had tracheomalacia and recurrent pulmonary infections. An ostium secundum type of ASD was present because of a weblike septum primum with multiple small fenestrations. The patient had mitral valve prolapse with very mild left atrial jet lesions, indicating mild mitral regurgitation. The patient died at 17 months of age, in 1986.

Our impression was that the patient's mitral valve prolapse and mild mitral regurgitation were of little clinical importance. The causes of this patient's death were thought to be prematurity, leading to hyaline membrane disease, leading to severe bronchopulmonary dysplasia, leading to recurrent pulmonary infections and cor pulmonale. The presence of a large secundum ASD would favor "wet" lungs by permitting left-to-right atrial level shunting. This would tend to make the cor pulmonale worse by increasing the pulmonary resistance. Closure of her PDA would deny a decompressing right-to left shunt at the pulmonary arterial level. Closure of the ductus arteriosus by 9 days of age helped to create cor pulmonale (right heart failure). Autopsy also revealed severe, widespread ischemic injury, especially marked in the kidneys and the brain. These ischemic injuries were thought to be due to critically low cardiac output, a fatal degree of heart failure. Thus, in this patient, the causes of death appear to be very largely related to the associated abnormalities, not to the mitral valve prolapse and mild mitral regurgitation. Hence, in *nonisolated* mitral valve prolapse, the *nonisolated* part can be very important—the main clinical problem—whereas in *isolated* mitral valve prolapse, the mitral valve prolapse is essentially always the main clinical problem.

Case 4 (see Table 14.24) was a female infant with critical aortic valvar stenosis. There were no well-developed aortic valvar commissures. Poststenotic dilatation of the aortic root and aneurysmal dilatation of the noncoronary and right coronary sinuses of Valsalva were present. The LV was small-chambered with mild left ventricular hypertrophy and moderately severe EFE of the LV. The mitral valve was hypoplastic, deformed, myxomatous, and redundant. There was prolapse of the posterior leaflet of the mitral valve. The annulus of the mitral valve measured only 6 mm (0.24 inch) in internal diameter. (Draw this out. It's tiny!) The diminutive size of the mitral annulus reflects the diminutive size of the left ventricular inflow tract; that is, the mitral annulus is a measure of the size of the left ventricular inflow tract. The left atrial hypertrophy was marked, and the left ventricular enlargement was moderate.

At 1 day of age, the patient underwent an interventional catheterization to balloon dilate the very stenotic aortic valve. After catheterization, aortic valvar regurgitation appeared. The unsupported aortic leaflets were torn. Recall that there were no well-formed aortic valvar commissures. This was an *acommissural aortic valve.* Iatrogenic aortic regurgitation led to neonatal systemic hypotension, which led to necrotizing enterocolitis. At 2 days of age, a subtotal colectomy, end-ileostomy, and mucous fistula creation were performed. At 15 days of age, a modified Norwood procedure was performed and a patch was placed over the prolapsing and regurgitant mitral valve. The patient died 1 day postoperatively, at 16 days of age, in1987.

Again, this patient illustrates that in *nonisolated* mitral valve prolapse, the nonisolated part may well be the dominant clinical problem and the cause of death, as in Case 4. This is a very important clinical point because in our neonatal and pediatric population, *nonisolated* mitral valve prolapse appears to be very much more common than the *isolated* type of mitral valve prolapse that predominates in adolescent and adult populations.

Case 5 was a young man with DORV. His segmental anatomy was {S,D,D}; there was situs solitus of the viscera and atria {*S*, -,-}, D-loop ventricles {S,*D*,-}, and D-malposition of the great arteries {S,D,*D*}. Briefly, he had DORV {S,D,D}. The muscular conus was subaortic, with pulmonary valve–to–tricuspid valve direct fibrous continuity. He had a stenotic pulmonary outflow tract and a widely patent aortic outflow tract. He also had superoinferior ventricles with a superior RV and an inferior LV. The superior right ventricular sinus (body or inflow tract) was very underdeveloped, whereas the inferior left ventricular sinus was well developed. He almost had a single LV with an infundibular outlet chamber because the right ventricular sinus was so underdeveloped. However, the tricuspid valve connected only with the small superior RV, and the mitral valve connected only with the large inferior LV. Thus, neither DILV nor straddling tricuspid valve was present. *A filigreed tricuspid valve* was present, with multiple fenestrations within the tricuspid valve tissue that varied from less than 1 mm to 4 to 5 mm in diameter. Severe tricuspid regurgitation was present. The tricuspid leaflets were redundant, and severe tricuspid valve prolapse into the RA was present. The mitral valve displayed a hemorrhoidal appearance when viewed from the left atrial aspect. There was marked upward hooding of the interchordal mitral leaflet tissue causing the mitral valve to prolapse into the LA. Mitral regurgitation was present, with thickening and rolling of the free margins of the mitral leaflet tissue. *So, this patient had prolapse of both AV valves!* Two large VSDs were present: a conoventricular defect (20 × 12 mm) and an inlet VSD (35 × 25 mm). The latter VSD was not a VSD of the AV canal type: this defect was not confluent with the tricuspid valve, as are VSDs of the AV canal type. Right atrial hypertrophy and enlargement were very marked, reflecting the severe tricuspid regurgitation.

Duplication of the right ureter was present; hence, this patient had MCAs (meaning that malformations of more than one organ system were present: that is, anomalies of the cardiovascular system and the genitourinary system).

At 6½ months of age, a right Blalock-Tausig shunt was performed because of the pulmonary outflow tract stenosis. A surgical ASD was also created. Why the surgical ASD? I am not sure. Perhaps the thinking was that an ASD would promote right-to-left shunting at the atrial level, so that more of the systemic venous return would reach the large inferior LV, aiding cardiac output. The small superior RV would have been an ineffectual pump. Also, an increased pulmonary venous return to the LA might have functionally narrowed the interatrial communication by moving a well-formed septum primum rightward, tending to narrow or close the interatrial communication. This would deflect more of the systemic venous return away from the patient's only functionally good ventricle, the large LV. Postoperatively, the patient did well. At 9½ years of age, the patient developed SBE caused by a viridans streptococcus. The patient responded well to antibiotic therapy. At 16 5/12 years of age, cardiac catheterization revealed reduced function of both the large inferior LV and the small superior RV. Pump failure was appearing.

In an attempt to reduce the heart's flow work (that had been increased by the Blalock-Taussig shunt and by the tricuspid and mitral regurgitation), a modified Fontan procedure was performed. Tricuspid atresia was created by patch closure of the tricuspid valve. The V was also closed with a patch. The pulmonary valve was closed, and the right Blalock-Taussig shunt was ligated. A conduit was placed between the RA and the right pulmonary artery. The patient's only AV valve was the regurgitating and prolapsing mitral valve.

One year postoperatively at 17 5/12 years of age, it was found that the tricuspid valve had undergone dehiscence. The tricuspid valve patch was replaced with a cloth patch, and pledgetted sutures were used. Postoperatively at 17½ years of age, atrial flutter with 2:1 AV block occurred. Cardioversion succeeded in restoring sinus rhythm. However, by 21½ years of age, the clinical picture of terminal hear failure had appeared. At the time it was described as "biventricular heart failure." It is worth noting that this patient had only *one good ventricle,* the large, inferior LV. The small superior right ventricular sinus (body, or inflow tract—the real RV) was rudimentary. Functionally, this patient had a *single (unpaired) LV with an infundibular outlet chamber and double-outlet from the infundibular outlet chamber* (not really DORV because the right ventricular sinus was rudimentary, almost absent). Note also that a *single LV can occur without double-outlet or common-inlet LV, as in the Lambert heart.*

The Lambert heart, named by Dr. Helen Taussig in honor of Dr. Edward Lambert, described a rare case of single (unpaired) LV with an infundibular outlet chamber that did not have double-inlet or common-inlet LV. Instead, the mitral valve opened into the single LV (as usual). But the tricuspid valve opened into the infundibular outlet chamber (instead of into the single LV, as usual). The Lambert heart taught us that **each cardiovascular variable must be defined primarily in terms of itself, not primarily in terms of any other variable.** For example, absence of the right ventricular sinus, that is, single LV, must be defined primarily in terms of the morphologic anatomy of the ventricular segment, not in terms of the anatomy of the AV canal or junction, which is a different cardiac segment. Dr. Ed Lambert was an excellent pediatric cardiologist and an exemplary human being. It was a privilege to have known him.

To return to our patient: The fact that this patient had only one functional ventricle (the large inferior LV) is one of the reasons that he developed terminal heart failure by 21½ years of age. The findings included chronic edema, protein-losing enteropathy, pleural effusions, ascites, low serum albumin, low serum proteins, and reduced immunoglobulins. Stenosis of the right lower lobe branch of the right pulmonary artery was also found. An attempt to relieve this stenosis by balloon angioplasty failed, and no change in the gradient occurred. Fenestration and dilation of the atrial septal patch were also performed. But inexorable and worsening pump failure led to death at 22 7/12 years of age in 1991. He was the oldest patient in this series of 11 cases with mitral valve prolapse.

Autopsy confirmed that cardiomegaly was massive: the heart weighed 1440 g. Right ventricular hypertrophy was marked: 13 to 15 mm in wall thickness. Left ventricular hypertrophy was similarly marked: 14 to 16 mm in wall thickness. The tricuspid annulus was large, measuring 43 mm in diameter. The mitral annulus was equally large, also measuring 43 mm in diameter. The opening in the atrial septum measured 3 mm in diameter. An opening in the tricuspid valve patch was found that was 15 mm in length. This was an old opening, covered with neopseudointima. The anastomosis of the RA to the right pulmonary artery measured 21 × 11 mm.

This patient illustrates how very important malformations other than mitral valve prolapse with mitral regurgitation can be in such cases: rudimentary right ventricular sinus resulting in single LV, double-outlet infundibular outflow chamber with pulmonary outflow tract stenosis, and tricuspid valve prolapse and regurgitation.

Case 6 was a 6-year-old girl with *trisomy 18*. The karyotype was proved by amniocentesis at 32 weeks gestation. She had a secundum type of ASD because of a deficient septum primum. She also had a conoventricular type of VSD between the conal septum above and the ventricular septum below. She had anterosuperior and leftward malalignment of the conal septum, which was also abnormally short and hypertrophied. There was no right ventricular outflow tract obstruction; hence, TOF was not present. Instead, this was a conoventricular malalignment type of VSD of the Eisenmenger type. *An Eisenmenger type of VSD* has been defined (with a wink) as TOF without pulmonary outflow tract obstruction. In other words, the conal septal malalignment (anteriorly, superiorly, and leftward) is similar to that seen in tetralogy but not as severe; hence, there was no pulmonary outflow tract obstruction. The result is a large subaortic VSD and a large left-to-right shunt at the ventricular level into the pulmonary artery. This often results in heart failure, pulmonary edema, pneumonia, and—if sufficiently chronic—pulmonary vascular obstructive disease, which used to make patients inoperable. She also had a persistent LSVC that drained into the coronary sinus and then to the RA.

Characteristic of trisomy 18, she also had polyvalvar disease. The mitral valve was myxomatous, thickened, redundant, regurgitant, and prolapsed into the LA. The leaflets of the tricuspid valve were also myxomatous, thickened, redundant, regurgitant, and prolapsed into the RA. The pulmonary valve was myxomatous and bicommissural, but was thought not to be malfunctioning. The aortic valve was the only anatomically normal valve.

The patient died at 6 years of age in 1993 with congestive heart failure that was thought to be related to septal defects (an ostium secundum type of ASD and a large subaortic VSD), the absence of pulmonary outflow tract obstruction, and polyvalvar disease (especially mitral and tricuspid valve prolapse and regurgitation). *The finding of polyvalvar disease should diagnostically suggest the possibility of a trisomy,* which should be searched for with a karyotype, as in this girl. *Findings typical of trisomy 18* include normal segmental anatomy, including normally related great arteries, that is, {S,D,S}; persistent LSVC to coronary sinus to RA; a conoventricular malalignment type of VSD; and polyvalvar disease.

Cases 7 and 10 both had *Marfan syndrome* (see Table 14.18). Case 7 was a 6 10/12-year-old girl who died in 1993. Salient findings included mitral valve prolapse and regurgitation with a partially flail mitral valve. Chordae tendineae to the posterior mitral leaflet were spontaneously ruptured close to the anterolateral commissure.

At 6 10/12 years of age, the ruptured chordae were reattached surgically. The postoperative period was complicated by atrial fibrillation that was successfully cardioverted. Moderate mitral regurgitation with marked mitral valve prolapse were found postoperatively, despite the absence of a flail mitral valve leaflet. The cardiac tamponade developed postoperatively. At reoperation, 400 mL of pericardial fluid was removed, with marked clinical improvement. Mitral valve replacement using a 33-mm St. Jude prosthesis was performed. The postoperative period was characterized by severe low cardiac output leading to ventricular tachycardia and fibrillation. Death occurred on the fourth postoperative day, which was 5 days after the first operation.

This patient had many of the other usual features of Marfan syndrome, including mild tricuspid regurgitation, dilated LV and LA, dilated aortic root (27 mm in diameter), subluxation of the ocular lenses, arachnodactyly of fingers and toes, flexion contractures of the extremities, and severe kyphoscoliosis. So this patient definitely had the *nonisolated* form of mitral valve prolapse and regurgitation.

Autopsy revealed that the tricuspid valve prolapse was marked, with elongation (but without rupture) of the tricuspid chordae tendineae. So this patient had *prolapse of both AV valves*. Autopsy confirmed the presence of left atrial hypertrophy and enlargement, the left atrial wall being 3 mm thick in the fresh state. Left ventricular hypertrophy and enlargement were marked, the left ventricular free wall measuring 14 to 20 mm in thickness in the fresh state. Right ventricular hypertrophy and enlargement were mild to moderate, the right ventricular free wall measuring 4 to 8 mm in thickness. Right atrial hypertrophy and enlargement were marked, the right atrial free wall varying from 2 to 6 mm in thickness. There was focal left ventricular endocardial sclerosis and no evidence of left ventricular outflow tract obstruction.

Quantitation

When a cardiac chamber is said to by hypertrophied and enlarged, this means that *compared with normal control heart specimens,* measurements showed that this was the case. The use of normal control heart specimens (age matched, weight matched, and, if desired sex matched) was routine and should be assumed. We did not use tables of normal measurements. We used normal heart specimens. This ensures that measurements of the case and of the control were done in the same way, by the same person.

Case 10, a male infant who died at 10 months and 27 days of age, also had Marfan syndrome (see Table 14.18). He had what is now known as *infantile* Marfan syndrome. He displayed marked hyperextensibility of some of the joints (e.g., of the fingers—metacarpophalangeal), with contractures of some of the large joins (elbows, knees, and ankles). He had bilateral inguinal hernias, treated at 3 weeks of age by bilateral inguinal herniorrhaphies. At 7 weeks of age, he underwent a pyloromyotomy

(Ramstedt operation) for hypertrophic obstructive pyloric stenosis. At 5 months of age, progressive congestive heart failure appeared. Investigation revealed severe mitral regurgitation with marked mitral valve prolapse. The LA was enlarged. Tricuspid regurgitation and tricuspid valve prolapse were also found. Although the aortic root was dilated, there was no aortic valvar regurgitation. Similarly, pulmonary valvar regurgitation was not present. Other findings included severe failure to thrive, arachnodactyly, pectus excavatum, a high-arched palate, a secundum ASD, and eventration of the central fibrous tendon portion of the right leaf of the diaphragm.

At 10 months of age, ventricular arrhythmias appeared: ventricular premature beats, bigeminy, and trigemini. At 10 months and 25 days of age, mitral valve replacement was performed using a No. 19 Hancock prosthesis. Death occurred on the second postoperative day. The native mitral valve was myxomatous, thickened, and redundant. The mitral chordae tendineae were elongated and tortuous, permitting severe mitral valve prolapse.

Autopsy revealed iatrogenic subaortic left ventricular outflow tract narrowing. One of the struts of the mitral valve prosthesis narrowed the left ventricular outflow tract and appeared to cause subaortic stenosis.

ANATOMIC CONSIDERATIONS

Mitral Valve Replacement in Infants

This is an interesting, important, and difficult surgical problem that, to my knowledge, is still unsolved. Mitral valve prostheses typically are *circular*. But the native mitral valve is shaped like a *kidney*, or like a *kidney bean*. The free wall portion of the mitral valve is *convex*, like a circle. But the portion of the mitral valve that is adjacent to the left ventricular outflow tract is *concave*. This mitral concavity is important because the space created by the medial mitral concavity is an important part of the subaortic left ventricular outflow tract. A circular mitral valve prosthesis poses a *double threat* to the left ventricular outflow tract:

1. The annulus of the prosthesis, being circular, can significantly narrow the subaortic left ventricular outflow tract.
2. If the prosthesis has a strut, this strut should not be placed in the left ventricular outflow tract. Instead, the strut should be positioned either in front of or behind the left ventricular outflow tract. This problem of mitral prosthesis–related left ventricular outflow tract stenosis is particularly important in young patients with small hearts; this patient was an infant, younger than 11 months of age. Faced with this problem, surgeons have tried to seat the mitral prosthesis above the native mitral annulus, within the LA. But this does not alter the fact that mitral valve prostheses should be kidney-bean shaped, not circular. It is important to realize that the deep anterior leaflet of the mitral valve is an important component of the left ventricular outflow tract. But many do not realize how important this anatomic fact is surgically, when mitral valve replacement is performed, particularly is infants.

Case 9, an aborted fetus of 21 weeks estimated gestational age, had polyvalvar disease (see Table 14.18). The mitral valve had redundant, myxomatous leaflets that prolapsed into the LA. The tricuspid leaflet tissue was also redundant, and the anterior papillary muscle of the RV was hypoplastic. But the tricuspid valve was not described as prolapsing. The pulmonary valve was bicuspid (bicommissural), with redundant leaflets. The aortic valve appeared normal. Did this fetus have a trisomy? We do not know. This heart specimen was referred to us in 1994 from another institution. No syndrome was diagnosed. Our final diagnostic impression was nonisolated mitral valve prolapse with polyvalvar disease, karyotype unknown.

As mentioned earlier, **nonisolated mitral valve prolapse** can be associated with the findings summarized in Table 14.24, and with the anomalies noted by Geggel and Fyler: Marfan syndrome, Ehlers-Danlos syndrome, osteogenesis imperfecta, pseudoxanthoma elasticum, Stickler syndrome, scoliosis, pectus excavatum, asthenic bodily habitus, straight back syndrome, secundum ASD, hyperthyroidism, sickle cell disease, muscular dystrophy, hypomastia, and von Willebrand disease.

Summary

1. Mitral valve anomalies found in our cardiac pathology database (see Table 14.1).
2. Anatomic classification of mitral atresia, n = 177 (see Table 14.2)
3. Types of relationships between the great arteries associated with mitral atresia (see Table 14.3)
4. Salient anatomic features of mitral atresia, {S,D,S}, intact ventricular septum, and aortic valvar atresia, n = 80 (see Table 14.4)
5. MCAs with mitral atresia, intact ventricular septum, aortic valvar atresia, and {S,D,S} (see Table 14.5)
6. Median ages at death in mitral atresia with normal segmental anatomy, {S,D,S}, or nearly normal segmental anatomy, DORV {S,D,"S"} (see Table 14.6)
7. Salient anatomic features in mitral atresia with DORV {S,D,D/"S"} and VSD (see Table 14.7)
8. Mitral atresia with single RV, absent LV, DORV {S,D,D} and no VSD, n = 7 (see Table 14.8)
9. Median ages at death in mitral atresia of 10 different anatomic types (see Table 14.9)
10. Median ages at death or cardiac transplantation in 18 different anatomic types of mitral atresia (see Table 14.10)
11. Anatomic classification of mitral atresia of Eliot and Edwards et al[69] (see Table 14.11)
12. Anatomic types of congenital mitral stenosis, n = 201 (see Table 14.12)
13. Findings associated with congenital mitral stenosis and HLHS, n = 130 (see Table 14.13)
14. MCAs associated with congenital mitral stenosis and HLHS (see Table 14.14)
15. Ages at death in congenital mitral stenosis: with versus without HLHS (see Table 14.15)
16. Anatomic findings in congenital mitral stenosis without HLHS, n = 48 (see Table 14.16)
17. Typical congenital mitral stenosis, n = 16 (see Table 14.17)
18. Factors causing or associated with congenital mitral regurgitation (n = 108) (see Table 14.18)

19. Anomalies of the tensor apparatus and/or leaflets of the mitral valve in congenital mitral regurgitation, n = 31 (see Table 14.19)
20. Noncardiovascular abnormalities associated with congenital mitral regurgitation, n = 14 (see Table 14.20)
21. Congenital mitral regurgitation caused by, or associated with, severe congenital aortic stenosis or aortic atresia, n = 13 (see Table 14.21)
22. Cardiomyopathy, dilated, and primary EFE
23. Marfan syndrome, with or without other congenital anomalies, infantile and adolescent-adult forms, and Beal syndrome of contractural arachnodactyly without heart disease
24. Congenital mitral regurgitation with Marfan syndrome, n = 11 (see Table 14.22)
25. Congenital mitral regurgitation with TGA {S,D,D}, {S,D,A}, {S,D,L}, and {S,L,L} (see Table 14.23)
26. Congenital mitral regurgitation with hypertrophic obstructive cardiomyopathy, n = 4
27. Congenital mitral regurgitation associated with TOF, n = 4
28. Congenital mitral regurgitation with single LV
29. Congenital mitral regurgitation with congenital aneurysm or dysplasia or the LV
30. Congenital mitral regurgitation with Down syndrome, n = 3
31. Congenital mitral regurgitation with DORV, n = 2
32. Congenital mitral regurgitation with left ventricular outflow tract obstruction
33. Congenital mitral regurgitation with Duchenne muscular hypertrophy
34. Congenital mitral regurgitation with large secundum ASD
35. Congenital mitral regurgitation with straddling mitral valve and crisscross AV relations
36. Congenital mitral regurgitation with truncus arteriosus
37. Congenital mitral regurgitation with pulmonary arterial vascular obstructive disease and with pulmonary veno-occlusive disease
38. Congenital mitral regurgitation with the heterotaxy syndrome of polysplenia
39. Congenital mitral regurgitation with HLHS
40. Mitral regurgitation associated with a high, subaortic VSD
41. Congenital mitral regurgitation caused by congenital absence of the mitral valve leaflets, also known as congenitally unguarded mitral orifice
42. Congenital mitral regurgitation resulting from adherence of the mitral valve to the left ventricular septal surface, also causing fibrous subaortic stenosis, in a patient with TOF: adherent mitral valve
43. Mitral valve dysplasia causing congenital mitral regurgitation: submitral mesh
44. Congenital mitral regurgitation caused by a commissural cleft
45. Congenital mitral regurgitation associated with TOF {I,D,S}
46. Myxomatous mitral valve that functioned normally
47. Mitral valve prolapse associated with congenital mitral regurgitation
48. Hypoplastic, myxomatous, and prolapsing mitral valve with both congenital mitral stenosis and congenital mitral regurgitation
49. Mucopolysaccharidoses such as Hurler syndrome may result in a markedly malformed mitral valve that functions within normal limits
50. Congenital mitral valve prolapse, n = 11
51. Nonisolated mitral valve prolapse, n = 9 (see Table 14.24)
52. Mitral valve replacement in infants: anatomic considerations

REFERENCES

1a. *Dorland's Illustrated Medical Dictionary*. 24th ed. Philadelphia: WB Saunders Co; 1965:1393.

1b. *Webster's New World Dictionary, College Edition*. Nelson, Toronto, Canada: Foster, & Scott, Ltd; 1959:943.

2. Van Praagh R. The segmental approach to diagnosis in congenital heart disease. In: Bergsma D, ed. *Birth Defects: Original Article Series*. 1972;8:4.
3. Van Praagh R, Vlad P. Dextrocardia mesocardia, levocardia. The segmental approach to diagnosis in congenital heart disease. In: Keith JD, Rowe RD, Vlad P, eds. *Heart Disease In Infancy And Childhood*. 3rd ed. New York: Macmillan; 1978:638.
4. Van Praagh R. The segmental approach to understanding complex congenital cardiac lesions. In: Eldredge WJ, Lemole GM, Goldberg H, eds. *Current Problems In Congenital Heart Disease*. New York: Spectrum; 1979:1.
5. Van Praagh R. The segmental approach clarified. *Cardiovasc Intervent Radiol*. 1984;7:320.
6. Van Praagh R, Foran RB, Pasquini L, Sanders SP, Van Praagh S. Rare segmental combinations in congenital heart disease: isolated infundibuloarterial inversion, atrioventricular discordance with ventriculoarterial concordance, and the polysplenia syndrome. *Coeur*. 1988;19:444.
7. Foran RB, Belcourt C, Nanton MA, et al. Isolated infundibuloarterial inversion {S,D,I}: a newly recognized form of congenital heart disease. *Am Heart J*. 1988;116:1337.
8. Van Praagh R. When concordant or discordant atrioventricular alignments predict the ventricular situs wrongly. I. Solitus atria, concordant alignments, and L-loop ventricles. II. Solitus atria, discordant alignments, and D-loop ventricles. *J Am Coll Cardiol*. 1987;10:1278.
9. Van Praagh R. Progress in the understanding or congenital heart disease: double-outlet right ventricle {S,D,L}, definition of transposition of the great arteries, and the illusion of crisscross AV relations. *Texas Heart J*. 1988;15:183.
10. Van Praagh R, Santini F, Geva T. Segmental situs in congenital heart disease: a fundamental concept. *G Ital Cardiol*. 1990;20:246.
11. Santini F, Jonas RA, Sanders SP, Van Praagh R. Tetralogy of Fallot {S,D,I}: successful repair without a conduit. *Ann Thorac Surg*. 1995;59:747.
12. Houyel L, Van Praagh R, Lacour-Gayet F, et al. Transposition of the great arteries {S,D,L}: pathologic anatomy, diagnosis, and surgical management of a newly recognized complex. *J Thorac Cardiovasc Surg*. 1995;110:613.
13. Van Praagh R. Segmental approach to diagnosis. In: Fyler DC, ed. *Nadas' Pediatric Cardiology*. Philadelphia: Hanley & Belfus, Inc; 1992:27.

14. Van Praagh R. Segmental anatomy. In: Sellke FW, del Nido PJ, Swanson SJ, eds. *Sabiston & Spencer Surgery Of The Chest*. Philadelphia: Elsevier Saunders; 2005:1763.
15. Van Praagh R, Corsini I. Cor triatriatum: pathologic anatomy and a consideration of morphogenesis based on 13 postmortem cases and a study of normal development of the pulmonary vein and atrial septum in 83 human embryos. *Am Heart J*. 1969;78:379.
16. Edwards JE, DuShane JW. Thoracic venous anomalies: 1.Vascular connections of the left atrium and the left innominate vein (laevo-atrio-cardinal vein) associated with mitral atresia in premature closure of the foramen ovale. *Arch Pathol*. 1950;49:517.
17. Lucas RV, Lester RG, Lillehei CW, Edwards JE. Mitral atresia with levoatrial cardinal vein, a form of congenital pulmonary venous obstruction. *Am J Cardiol*. 1962;9:607.
18. Waardenburg PJ. A new syndrome combining developmental anomalies of the eyelids, eyebrows and nose root with pigmentary defects of the iris and head hair and with congenital deafness. *Am J Hum Genet*. 1951;3:195.
19. Jones KL. Waardenburg syndrome, types I and II: Lateral displacement of medial canthi, partial albinism, deafness. In: *Smith's Recognizable Patterns of Human Malformation*. 4th ed. Philadelphia: WB Saunders Co, Harcourt Brace Jovanovich, Inc; 1988:208.
20. Van Praagh S, Carrera ME, Sanders SP, Mayer JE, Van Praagh R. Sinus venosus defects: unroofing of the right pulmonary veins – anatomic and echocardiographic findings and surgical treatment. *Am Heart J*. 1994;128:365.
21. Van Praagh R, Ongley PA, Swan HJC. Anatomic types of single or common ventricle in man, morphologic and geometric aspects in sixty autopsied cases. *Am J Cardiol*. 1964;13:367.
22. Van Praagh R, Plett JA, Van Praagh S. Single ventricle: pathology, embryology, terminology, and classification. *Herz*. 1979;4:113.
23. Quero M. Atresia of the left atrioventricular orifice associated with a Holmes heart. *Circulation*. 1970;42:739.
24. Quero M. Coexistence of single ventricle with atresia of one atrioventricular orifice. *Circulation*. 1972;46:794.
25. Robb JS. *Comparative Basic Cardiology*. New York: Grune & Stratton; 1965:129.
26. Van Praagh R, Corwin RD, Dahlquist EH, Freedom RM, Mattioli L, Nebesar RA. Tetralogy of Fallot with severe left ventricular outflow tract obstruction due to anomalous attachment of the mitral valve to the ventricular septum. *Am J Cardiol*. 1970;26:93.
27. Sanders JH, Van Praagh R, Sade RM. Tetralogy of Fallot with discrete fibrous subaortic stenosis. *Chest*. 1976;69:543.
28. Van Praagh R, Bano-Rodrigo A, Smolinsky A, Schuetz TZ, Fyler DC, Van Praagh S. Anatomic variations in congenital valvar, subvalvar, and supravalvar aortic stenosis: a study of 64 postmortem cases. In: Takahashi M, Wells WJ, Lindesmith GG, eds. *Challenges in the Treatment of Congenital Cardiac Anomalies*. Mt Kisco, NY: Futura Publishing Co; 1986:13.
29. Van Praagh S, Carrera ME, Sanders SP, Mayer JE, Van Praagh R. Partial or total direct pulmonary venous drainage to right atrium due to malposition of septum primum: anatomic and echocardiographic findings and surgical treatment: a study based on 36 cases. *Chest*. 1995;107:1488.
30. Melhuish BPP, Van Praagh R. Juxtaposition of the atrial appendages, a sign of severe cyanotic congenital heart disease. *Br Heart J*. 1968;30:269.
31. Van Praagh S, O'Sullivan J, Brili S, Van Praagh R. Juxtaposition of the morphologically left atrial appendage in solitus and inversus atria: a study of 18 postmortem cases. *Am Heart J*. 1996;132:391.
32. Van Praagh S, O'Sullivan J, Brili S, Van Praagh R. Juxtaposition of the morphologically right atrial appendage in solitus and inversus atria: a study of 35 postmortem cases. *Am Heart J*. 1996;132:382.
33. Delisle G, Ando M, Calder AL, et al. Total anomalous pulmonary venous connection: report of 93 autopsied cases with emphasis on diagnostic and surgical considerations. *Am Heart J*. 1976;91:99.
34. Pasquini L, Sanders SP, Parness IA, et al. Conal anatomy in 119 patients with D-loop transposition of the great arteries with ventricular septal defect: an echocardiographic and pathologic study. *J Am Coll Cardiol*. 1993;21:1712.
35. Van Praagh R, O'Connor B, Chacko KA. In: Crupi G, Anderson RH, Parenzan, eds. *The pathologic anatomy of aortic coarctation. Perspectives In Pediatric Cardiology, Vol 2, Pediatric Cardiac Surgery, Part 1*. Mt Kisco, NY: Futura Publishing Co Inc; 1989:261.
36. Van Praagh R, Bernhard WF, Rosenthal A, Parisi LF, Fyler DC. Interrupted aortic arch: surgical treatment. *Am J Cardiol*. 1971;27:200.
37. Van Praagh R, Van Praagh S. The anatomy of common aorticopulmonary trunk (truncus arteriosus communis) and its embryologic implications, a study of 57 necropsied cases. *Am J Cardiol*. 1965;16:406.
38. Calder L, Van Praagh R, Van Praagh S, et al. Truncus arteriosus communis: clinical, angiocardiographic, and pathologic findings in 100 patients. *Am Heart J*. 1976;92:23.
39. Van Praagh R. Classification of Truncus Arteriosus Comunis (TAC). *Am Heart J*. 1976;92:129.
40. Matsuoka R, Van Praagh S, Van Praagh R. Rare types of truncus arteriosus communis. *Circulation*. 1982;66:II–359.
41. Pessotto R, Padalino M, Rubino M, Kadoba K, Buchler JR, Van Praagh R. Straddling tricuspid valve as a sign of ventriculoatrial malalignment: a morphometric study of 19 postmortem cases. *Am Heart J*. 1999;138:1184.
42. Van Praagh R, David I, Wright GB, Van Praagh S. Large RV plus small LV is not single RV. *Circulation*. 1980;61:1057.
43. Lambert EC. Single ventricle with a rudimentary outlet chamber, case report. *Bull Johns Hopkins Hosp*. 1951;88:231.
44. Van Praagh R, Wise JR, Dahl BA, Van Praagh S. Single left ventricle with infundibular outlet chamber and tricuspid valve opening only into outlet chamber in 44-year-old man with thoracoabdominal ectopia cordis without diaphragmatic or pericardial defect. Importance of myocardial morphologic method of chamber identification in congenital heart disease. In: Van Praagh R, Takao A, eds. *Etiology and Morphogenesis of Congenital Heart Disease*. NY: Futura Publishing Co Inc, Mt Kisco; 1980:379.
45. Holmes WF. Case of malformation of the heart. *Trans Med-Chir Soc, Edinburgh*. 1824;1:252.
46. Taussig HB, Bing RJ. Complete transposition of the aorta and a levoposition of the pulmonary artery: clinical, physiological, and pathological findings. *Am Heart J*. 1949;551.
47. Witham AC. Double outlet right ventricle: a partial transposition complex. *Am Heart J*. 1957;53:928.
48. Neufeld HN, DuShane JW, Wood EH, Kirklin JW, Edwards JE. Origin of both great vessels from the right ventricle: I. Without pulmonary stenosis. *Circulation*. 1961;23:399.
49. Neufeld HN, DuShane JW, Edwards JE. Origin of both great vessels from the right ventricle. II. With pulmonary stenosis. *Circulation*. 1961;23:603.

50. Van Praagh R. What is the Taussig-Bing malformation? *Circulation*. 1968;38:445.
51. Lavoie R, Sestier F, Gilbert G, Chameides L, Van Praagh R, Grondin P. Double-outlet right ventricle with left ventricular outflow tract obstruction due to small ventricular septal defect. *Am Heart J*. 1971;82:290.
52. Lev M, Bharati S, Meng L, Liberthson RR, Paul MH, Idriss F. A concept of double-outlet right ventricle. *J Thorac Cardiovasc Surg*. 1972;64:271.
53. Megarity A, Chambers R, Calder AL, Van Praagh S, Van Praagh R. Double-outlet right ventricle with left ventricular-right atrial communication: fibrous obstruction of left ventricular outlet by membranous septum and tricuspid leaflet tissue. *Am Heart J*. 1972;84:242.
54. Zamora R, Moller JH, Edwards JE. Double-outlet right ventricle: anatomic types and associated anomalies. *Chest*. 1975;68:672.
55. Van Praagh R Perez-Trevino C, Reynolds JL, Moes CAF, et al. Double-outlet right ventricle {S,D,L} with subaortic ventricular septal defect and pulmonary stenosis: report of 6 cases. *Am J Cardiol*. 1975;35:42.
56. Van Praagh S, Davidoff A, Chin A, et al. Double-outlet right ventricle: anatomic types and developmental implications based on a study of 101 autopsied cases. *Coeur*. 1982;13:389.
57. Van Praagh R, David I, Van Praagh S. What is a ventricle? The single ventricle trap. *Pediatr Cardiol*. 1982;2:79.
58. Van Praagh S, Kreutzer J, Alday L, Van Praagh R. Systemic and pulmonary venous connections in visceral heterotaxy with emphasis on the diagnosis of the atrial situs: a study of 109 postmortem cases. In: Clark EB, Takao A, eds. *Developmental Cardiology: Morphogenesis and Function*. Mount Kisco, NY: Futura Publishing Co Inc; 1990:671.
59. Van Praagh S. Cardiac malpositions and the heterotaxy syndromes. In: Keane JF, Lock JE, Fyler DC, eds. *Nadas' Pedairic Cardiology*. 2nd ed. Philadelphia: Saunders Elsevier; 2006:675.
60. Van Praagh R, Van Praagh S. Atrial isomerism in the heterotaxy syndromes with asplenia, or polysplenia, or normally formed spleen: an erroneous concept. *Am J Cardiol*. 1990;66:1504.
61. Van Praagh R, Litovsky S. Pathology and embryology of common atrioventricular canal. *Progress Pediatr Cardiol*. 1999;10:115.
62. Van Praagh S, Vangi V, Sul JH, et al. Tricuspid atresia or severe stenosis with partial common atrioventricular canal: anatomic data, clinical profile, and surgical considerations. *J Am Coll Cardiol*. 1991;17:932.
63. Rabinovitch M, Grady S, David I, et al. Compression of intrapulmonary bronchi by abnormally branching pulmonary arteries associated with absent pulmonary valves. *Am J Cardiol*. 1982;50:804.
64. Edwards JE, Rodgers HM. Atresia of the orifice of the mitral valve. *J Tech Methods*. 1947;27:62.
65. Edward JE, DuShane JW. Thoracic venous anomalies: I. Vascular connections of the left atrium and the left innominate vein (laevo-atrio-cardinal vein) associated with mitral atresia in premature closure of the foramen ovale. *Arch Pathol*. 1950;49:517.
66. Friedman S, Murphy L, Ash R. Congenital mitral atresia with hypoplastic non-functioning left heart. *Am J Dis Child*. 1955;90:176.
67. Noonan J, Nadas AS. The hypoplastic left heart syndrome. *Pediatr Clin North Am*. 58 November:1029.
68. Watson DG, Rowe RD, Conen PE, Duckworth JW. Mitral atresia with normal aortic valve. Report of 11 cases and review of the literature. *Pediatrics*. 1960;25:450.
69. Eliot RS, Shone JD, Kanjuh VI, et al. Mitral atresia: a study of 32 cases. *Am Heart J*. 1965;70:6.
70. Abbott ME. Congenital heart disease. In: *Osler and McCrae's Modern Medicine*. Philadelphia: Lea & Febiger; 1927.
71. Van Praagh R, Perez-Treviño C, Lopez-Cuellar M, Baker FW. Transposition of the great arteries with posterior aorta, anterior pulmonary artery, and aortic-mitral fibrous continuity: a new entity. *Circulation*. 1969;40:III–207.
72. Van Praagh R, Perez-Treviño C, Lopez-Cuellar M, et al. Transposition of the great arteries with posterior aorta, anterior pulmonary artery, subpulmonary conus, and fibrous continuity between aortic and atrioventricular valves. *Am J Cardiol*. 1971;28:621.
73. Van Praagh R, Van Praagh S, Vlad P, Keith JD. Anatomic types of congenital dextrocardia, diagnostic and embryologic implications. *Am J Cardiol*. 1964;13:510.
74. Kirklin JW, Pacifico AD, Bargeron LM, Soto B. Cardiac repair in anatomically corrected malposition of the great arteries. *Circulation*. 1973;48:153.
75. Lev M. The pathologic diagnosis of positional variations in cardiac chambers in congenital heart disease. *Lab Invest*. 1954;3:71.
76. Summerell J, Miller C, Persaud V, Talerman A. Congenital mitral atresia. *Br Heart J*. 1968;30:249.
77. Navarro-Lopez F, Marin Garcia J, Zomeño M, Llorian ARC. Mitral atresia and occlusive left atrial thrombus, a case with 11 years of survival. *Br Heart J*. 1969;31:649.
78. Rosenquist GC. Overriding right atrioventricular valve in association with mitral atresia. *Am Heart J*. 1974;87:26.
79. Cabrera A, Azcuma JI, Bilbao F. Single primitive ventricle with D-transposition of the great vessels and atresia of the left A-V valve: Report of a case. *Am Heart J*. 1974;88:225–228.
80. Bjørnstad PG, Michalsen H. Coexistent mitral and aortic valve atresia with intact ventricular septum in sibs. *Br Heart J*. 1974;36:302.
81. Moreno F, Quero M, Perez Diaz L. Mitral atresia with normal aortic valve, a study of eighteen cases and a review of the literature. *Circulation*. 1976;53:1004.
82. Friedman S, Edmunds LH, Saraclar M, Weinstein EM. Mitral atresia with premature closure of foramen ovale, a rare hemodynamic cause for failure of Blalock-Taussig anastomosis to relieve inadequate pulmonary blood flow. *J Thorac Cardiovasc Surg*. 1976;71:118.
83. Ostermeyer J, Körfer R, Bircks W. Mitral atresia with normal-sized ventricles, ventricular septal defect, and dextro-transposition of the great arteries. *J Thorac Cardiovasc Surg*. 1979;77:733.
84. Mickell JJ, Mathews RA, Park SC, et al. Left atrioventricular valve atresia: clinical management. *Circulation*. 1980;61:123.
85. Thiene G, Daliento L, Frescura C, et al. Atresia of left atrioventricular orifice, anatomical investigation in 62 cases. *Br Heart J*. 1981;45:393.
86. Van Praagh R. The importance of ventriculoarterial malalignment in anomalies of the atrioventricular valves, illustrated by "mitral atresia" and congenital mitral stenosis with large left ventricle. In: Doyle EF, Engle MA, Gersony WM, Rashkind WJ, Talner NS, eds. *Pediatric Cardiology, Proceedings of the Second World Congress*. New York: Springer-Verlag; 1986:901.
87. Shinpo H, Van Praagh S, Parness I, Sanders S, Motthan M, Castañeda A. Mitral atresia with a large left ventricle and an underdeveloped or absent right ventricular sinus: clinical profile, anatomic data, and surgical considerations. *J Am Coll Cardiol*. 1992;19:1561.

88. Van Praagh R, Visner MS. The postoperative pathology of congenital heart disease. *Am J Cardiol.* 1976;38:225.
89. Van Praagh S, Kakou-Guikahue M, Kim H-S, Becker J, Alday L, Van Praagh R. Atrial situs in patients with visceral heterotaxy and congenital heart disease: conclusions based on findings in 104 postmortem cases. *Coeur.* 1988;19:483.
90. Van Praagh S, LaCorte M, Fellows KE, et al. Supero-inferior ventricles: anatomic and angiocardiographic findings in ten postmortem cases. In: Van Praagh R, Takao A, eds. *Etiology and Morphogenesis of Congenital Heart Disease.* Mount Kisco, NY: Futura Publishing Co; 1980:317.
91. Weinberg PM, Van Praagh R, Wagner HR, Cuaso CC. *New Form of Crisscross Atrioventricular Relation: An Expanded View of the Meaning of D- and L-loops.* London: World Congress of Pediatric Cardiology; 1980:319.
92. Restivo A, Ho SY, Anderson RH, Cameron H, Wilkinson JL. Absent left atrioventricular connection with right atrium connected to morphologically left ventricular chamber, rudimentary right ventricular chamber, and ventriculoarterial discordance. Problem of mitral versus tricuspid atresia. *Br Heart J.* 1982;48:240.
93. Gittenberger-de Groot AC, Wenink ACG. Mitral atresia, morphological details. *Br Heart J.* 1984;51:252.
94. Starc JJ, Gersony WM. Progressive obstruction of the foramen ovale in patients with left atrioventricular valve atresia. *J Am Coll Cardiol.* 1986;7:1099.
95. Schulze-Neick I, Schneider M, Hausdorf G, Lange PE. Transseptal radiofrequency perforation of the atrial septum in mitral atresia – a new method. *Cardiol Young.* 1993;3:I–93 (abstract 306).
96. Geva T, Santini F, Pear W, Driscoll SG. Cardiac rhabdomyoma, rare cause of fetal death. *Chest.* 1991;99:139.
97. Ruckman RN, Van Praagh R. Anatomic types of congenital mitral stenosis: report of 49 autopsy cases with consideration of diagnosis and surgical implications. *Am J Cardiol.* 1978;42:592.
98. Shone JD, Sellars RD, Anderson RC, Adams PJ, Lillehei CW, Edwards JE. The developmental complex of "parachute mitral valve", supravalvular ring of left atrium, subaortic stenosis, and coarctation of the aorta. *Am J Cardiol.* 1963;11:714.
99. David I, Castañeda AR, Van Praagh R. Potentially parachute mitral valve in common atrioventricular canal: pathologic anatomy and surgical importance. *J Thorac Cardiovasc Surg.* 1982;84:178.
100. Norwood WI, Lang P, Hansen D. Physiologic repair of aortic atresia–hypoplastic left heart syndrome. *N Engl J Med.* 1983;308:23.
101. Bailey L, Concepcion W, Shattuck H, Huang L. Method of heart transplantation for treatment of hypoplastic left heart syndrome. *J Thorac Cardiovasc Surg.* 1986;92(1).
102. Moulaert A. *Ventricular Septal Defects and Anomalies of the Aortic Arch.* Leiden: Drukkerij Luctor et Emergo; 1974:1–125 (MD Thesis).
103. Simpson DP. *Cassell's Latin Dictionary, Latin-English.* English-Latin, New York: Macmillan Publishing Co; 1968:557.
104. Baño-Rodrigo A, Van Praagh S, Trowitzsch E, Van Praagh R. Double-orifice mitral valve: a study of 27 postmortem cases with developmental, diagnostic, and surgical considerations. *Am J Cardiol.* 1988;61:152.
105. Papagiannis J, Van Praagh R, Schwint O, et al. Congenital left ventricular aneurysm: clinical, imaging, pathologic, and surgical findings in severe new cases. *Am Heart J.* 2001;141:491.
106. Van Praagh R, Van Praagh S. Anatomically corrected transposition of the great arteries. *Br Heart J.* 1967;29:112.
107. Watson GH, Miller V. Arteriohepatic dysplasia: Familial pulmonary arterial stenosis with neonatal liver disease. *Arch Dis Child.* 1973;48:459.
108. Alagille D, Odievre M, Gautier M, Dommergues JP. Hepatic ductular hypoplasia associated with characteristic facies, vertebral malformations, retarded physical, mental, and sexual development, and cardiac murmur. *J Pediatr* 1975;86:63–71.
109. Coffin GS, Siris E. Mental retardation with absent fifth fingernail and terminal phalanx. *Am J Dis Child.* 1970;119(5):433–439.
110. Van Praagh R, Durnin RE, Jockin H, et al. Anatomically corrected malposition of the great arteries {S,D,L}. *Circulation.* 1975;51:20.
111. Matsuoka R, Yamamoto Y, Kuroki Y, Matsui I. Phenotypic expression of the trisomic segments in partial trisomy 18. In: Van Praagh R, Takao A, eds. *Etiology and Morphogenesis of Congenital Heart Disease.* Mount Kisco, NY: Futura Publishing Co Inc; 1980:41.
112. Baño-Rodrigo A, Van Praagh S, Trowitzsch E, Hernandez-Latuff P, Van Praagh R. *Double-Orifice Atrioventricular Valves: Pathologic Anatomy in 28 Postmortem Cases, With Diagnosis and Surgical Implications. Pediatric Cardiology.* New York: Springer-Verlag Inc; 1986:915.
113. Greenfield WS: Double mitral valve. *Trans Path Soc London* 76; 27:128.
114. Colan SD. Cardiomyopathies. In: Keane JF, Lock JE, Fyler DC, eds. 2nd ed. Philadelphia: Saunders Elsevier; 2006:415.
115. Geva T, Sanders SP, Diogenes M, Rockenmacher S, Van Praagh R. Two-dimensional and Doppler echocardiographic and pathologic characteristics of the infantile Marfan syndrome. *Am J Cardiol.* 1990;65:1230.
116. Beals RK, Hecht F. Delineation of another heritable disorder of connective tissue. *Am J Bone Joint Surg.* 1971;53:987.
117. Jones KL. Beals syndrome (Beals contractual arachnodactyly syndrome) joint contractions, arachnodactyly, "crumpled" ear. In: *Smith's Recognizable Patterns of Human Malformation.* 4th ed. Philadelphia: WB Saunders Co, Harcout Brace Jovanovich, Inc; 1988:424.
118. Marfan AB. Un cas de déformation congénitale des quatre membres plus prononceé aux extrémités characterisée par l'allongement des os avec un certain degré d'amincissement. *Bull Mem Soc Med Hop (Paris).* 1896;13:220.
119. Jones KL. Marfan syndrome. Arachnodactyly with hyperextensibility, lens subluxation, aortic dilatation. In: *Smith's Recognizable Patterns of Human Malformation.* 4th ed. Philadelphia: WB Saunders Co, Harcourt Brace Jovanovich, Inc; 1988:422.

15

Infundibuloarterial Situs Equations: How Normally and Abnormally Related Great Arteries Are Built and the Importance of Infundibuloarterial Situs Concordance and Discordance

Now that we have considered tricuspid valve anomalies (see Chapter 13), mitral valve anomalies (see Chapter 14), and common atrioventricular (AV) canal (see Chapter 11), we are ready to consider how normally related and abnormally related great arteries are aligned and connected with the underlying ventricles, ventricular septum, AV canal, and AV valves.

In other words, this chapter is about **normally and abnormally related great arteries, *all of them.*** These anomalies are also widely known as **conotruncal malformations,** that is, anomalies of the conus arteriosus (infundibulum) and truncus arteriosus (great arteries). A new, quantitative, symbolic anatomic approach is taken to the understanding of the embryology (morphogenesis) and anatomy of the infundibuloarterial malformations, using **infundibuloarterial equations.**

SOLITUS NORMALLY RELATED GREAT ARTERIES[1]

Solitus normally related great arteries (SNRGAs) means the usual or ordinary type of normally related great arteries, as opposed to the inverted or mirror-image type of normally related great arteries. (*Solitus,* a, um = accustomed, usual, habitual, ordinary, in Latin.)

Following the developmental stages of the cardiogenic crescent and the straight heart tube, a solitus (noninverted) heart normally loops in a rightward direction forming a dextro or D-loop (Fig. 15.1).

Dextro is a combining form meaning right, or relationship to the right (*dexter, dextra, dextrum,* right, on the right side, Latin). Thus, D-loop means a heart tube that has looped to the right (see Fig. 15.1)

The effect of D-loop formation is to make the developing semilunar valves to lie approximately side by side, aortic valve (indicated by coronary ostia) to the right and pulmonary valve (no coronary ostia) to the left (see Fig. 15.1, *dashed lines*).

The preconal mesoderm and the conal myocardium are indicated by parallel, finely hatched lines (see Fig. 15.1). Early after D-loop formation, a bilateral (subaortic and subpulmonary) conus is present. More specifically, both subaortic and subpulmonary conal free walls are present (see Fig. 15.1). Consequently, neither the developing aortic valve nor the developing pulmonary valve is in direct fibrous continuity with either AV valve (the tricuspid valve has three leaflets, and the mitral valve has two leaflets; see Fig. 15.1). Also, both developing great arteries are above the developing right ventricle (RV); that is, the double-outlet right ventricle (DORV) is present at this stage.

KEY TO SYMBOLIC ANATOMY

Development of the muscular subarterial conal free walls may be divided into five grades.

Grade 0 (0) means that the subarterial conal free wall musculature is absent, typically permitting semilunar (aortic or pulmonary)-to-AV (mitral, or tricuspid, or common AV) valvar direct fibrous continuity via an intervalvar fibrosa. Typically, there is no ventriculoarterial (VA) outflow tract obstruction (stenosis or atresia), but this feature is a variable.

Grade 1 (1) means that a very small amount of subarterial conal free wall musculature is present, preventing direct semilunar-AV fibrous continuity. Often, a very small amount of unexpanded, or poorly expanded subarterial conal free wall musculature is associated with total VA outflow tract obstruction (atresia).

Grade 2 (2) development of the subarterial conal free wall means that a small amount of subarterial conal free wall musculature is present, preventing semilunar-AV fibrous continuity, and associated with severe VA outflow tract stenosis.

Grade 3 (3) development of the subarterial conal free wall musculature means that a mildly to moderately subnormal development of the subarterial conal free wall is present. Frequently, this mildly to moderately subnormal conal free wall growth and expansion is associated with mild to moderate VA outflow tract stenosis.

Grade 4 (4) growth and expansion of the subarterial conal free wall is normal development that prevents semilunar-AV fibrous continuity and typically is not associated with VA outflow tract obstruction.

D-loop formation typically carries the developing aortic valve and the subaortic conal free wall to the **right (R)** relative

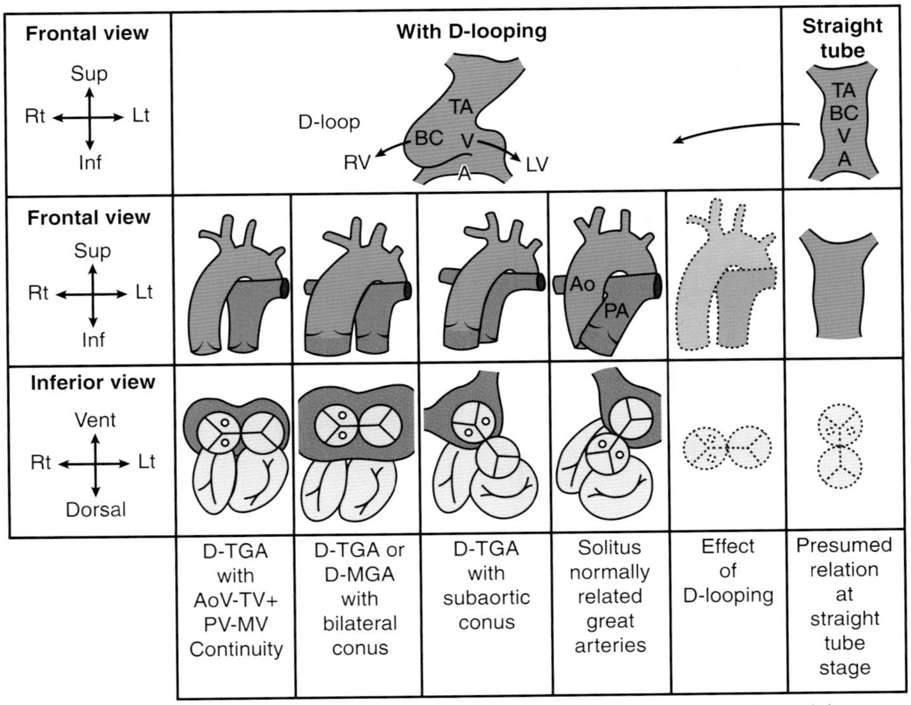

Fig. 15.1 Normal and Abnormal Infundibuloarterial (Conotruncal) Morphogenesis and Anatomy After Bulboventricular D-Loop Formation. *Top row:* A frontal diagrammatic view of the straight heart tube and of the ventricular D-loop that loops convexly to the right (*dextro-* or *D-* is a Latin-based combining form meaning right). Not shown is the earlier cardiogenic crescent of precardiac mesoderm (the primary heart field), the ventrally closely adjacent secondary heart field, or the migratory pathways of the cardiac neural crest cells that contribute to the formation of the straight heart tube and subsequently to the ventricular D-loop. The conventional regional designations are included for general orientation. Cephalocaudally they are: *TA,* truncus arteriosus; *BC,* bulbus cordis; *V,* ventricle; and *A,* atrium. However, as our cinephotomicrography shows, myriads of cells are constantly moving in these areas. Consequently, these labels, when applied to the developing heart, are not static and definite, as anatomic labels later become. Instead, labels applied to developing hearts indicate general, constantly changing regions. These labels are also used *predictively,* meaning this is where this or that structure will, or normally should, develop. For example, the *long arrow* to the right of the straight heart tube means that this is the direction in which the straight heart tube should loop to form a normal D-loop. The *shorter arrow* from the ventricle *(V)* of the D-loop to the left ventricle *(LV)* label means that the morphologically LV normally develops from the ventricle of the ventricular D-loop. *The shorter arrow* from the proximal bulbus cordis to the morphologically right ventricle *(RV)* means that the RV normally develops from the proximal bulbus cordis of a ventricular D-loop. This diagram is also intended to indicate that situs solitus of the ventricles, with a right-sided and right-handed RV and a left-sided and left-handed LV, is associated with ventricular D-loop formation. *Second row from the top:* The great arteries and the subsemilunar conus arteriosus (infundibulum), seen from the front. The conus arteriosus musculature is indicted by *fine parallel hatching. Ao,* Ascending aorta; *PA,* main pulmonary artery *(PA). Dashed lines:* Aorta *(Ao)* to the right, PA to the left; this R-L relationship is thought to be the effect of ventricular D-loop formation. The great arteries are not really separate at this early stage; they are so-diagrammed for conceptual clarity. *Third row from the top:* The semilunar valves, the subsemilunar conus, and the atrioventricular (AV) valves, viewed from below. In this diagram, the developing semilunar and AV valves are shown as separate, for conceptual clarity. At this early stage, these valves are not separate. The aortic valve *(AoV)* is indicated by the coronary ostia. The pulmonary valve *(PV)* is indicted by the absence of coronary ostia. The tricuspid valve is right-sided with three leaflets, and the mitral valve is left-sided with two leaflets, in all four diagrams. These diagrammatic views from below show the presence or absence of semilunar-AV fibrous continuity. *Leftmost column:* For the frontal views, these spatial orientation symbols are superior *(Sup),* inferior *(Inf),* and right *(Rt),* and left *(Lt).* For the inferior views, these symbols are anterior *(Ant)* or ventroposterior *(Post)* or dorsal, and right (Rt) and left (Lt). *Bottom row:* From left to right, the first three labels are as follows: *Label 1:* D-transposition of the great arteries with aortic valve-tricuspid valve and pulmonary valve–mitral valve fibrous continuity. This is a rare form of D-transposition of the great arteries *(TGA). Label 2:* D-TGA or D-malposition of the great arteries *(MGAs)* with bilateral conus (subaortic and subpulmonary). (D-MGA occurs, for example, with the Taussig-Bing type of double-outlet right ventricle [DORV] {S,D,D}.[2,3] D-TGA is shown in this diagram, not DORV.) *Label 3:* D-TGA with subaortic conus and with pulmonary-mitral fibrous continuity. This is the typical form of D-TGA. Everything shown in this diagram is data-based, not hypothetical. (Reproduced with permission from Van Praagh R, Van Praagh S. Isolated ventricular inversion: a consideration of the morphogenesis, definition, and diagnosis of nontransposed and transposed great arteries. *Am J Cardiol.* 1966;17:395-406.)

to the developing pulmonary valve and the subpulmonary conal free wall, which lies to the **left (L)** (see Fig. 15.1).

L-loop formation characteristically carries the developing aortic valve and the subaortic conal free wall to the **left (L)** relative to the developing pulmonary valve and the subpulmonary conal free wall, which lies to the **right (R)** (Fig. 15.2).

In more complex situations, such as **TGA {S,D,L},** TGA {S,D,L} means transposition of the great arteries (TGA) with the segmental anatomic set ({}) of situs solitus (S) of the viscera and atria, ventricular D-loop (D), and L-TGA—the aortic valve and subaortic conal free wall lie to the **left (L)** of the pulmonary valve and subpulmonary conal free wall, which are located to the **right (R).**

Similarly, in **TGA {S,D,A},** the transposed aortic valve and the subaortic conal free wall are directly **anterior (A)** relative to the transposed pulmonary valve and subpulmonary conal free wall, which are directly **posterior (P)** to the aortic valve and subaortic conal free wall.

Thus, we have the segmental anatomic diagnosis, such as
TGA {S,D,**D**} (see Fig. 15.1), or
TGA {S,L,**L**} (see Fig. 15.2).

TGA {S,D,**A**} indicates not only the spatial relationships of the semilunar valves, but also the spatial relationships of the subarterial conal free walls, which usually are **right-left (R-L)** but occasionally can be directly **anteroposterior (AP).**

The combination of the degree of development and the relative spatial location of each subarterial conal free wall makes possible the infundibuloarterial (conotruncal) equations. These equations in turn describe the embryonic morphogenesis and the anatomy of normally and abnormally related great arteries, as will be seen.

SNRGAs result from complete right-left asymmetry in the development of the subarterial conal free walls. The right-sided subaortic infundibular free wall normally undergoes complete resorption (disappearance), and simultaneously the left-sided subpulmonary conal free wall undergoes good expansile growth. Both subarterial conal free wall resorption and growth are thought to be under genetic control, which is now undergoing intense investigation.

With SNRGA (see Fig. 15.1), resorption of the right-sided subaortic conal free wall permits the developing aortic valve to move inferiorly, posteriorly, and leftward and to pass mostly through the interventricular foramen and to come into direct fibrous continuity with the developing mitral valve, above the morphologically left ventricle (LV).

Simultaneously, the left-sided subpulmonary conal free wall undergoes good growth and expansion, elevating the pulmonary valve superiorly, anteriorly, and rightward, above the morphologically RV. The growth and expansion of the subpulmonary conus elevates the pulmonary valve and artery superiorly, getting the pulmonary valve and main pulmonary artery (MPA) out of the way, well above the interventricular foramen, making it possible for the aortic valve and the proximal ascending aorta to be switched from above the RV to above the LV.

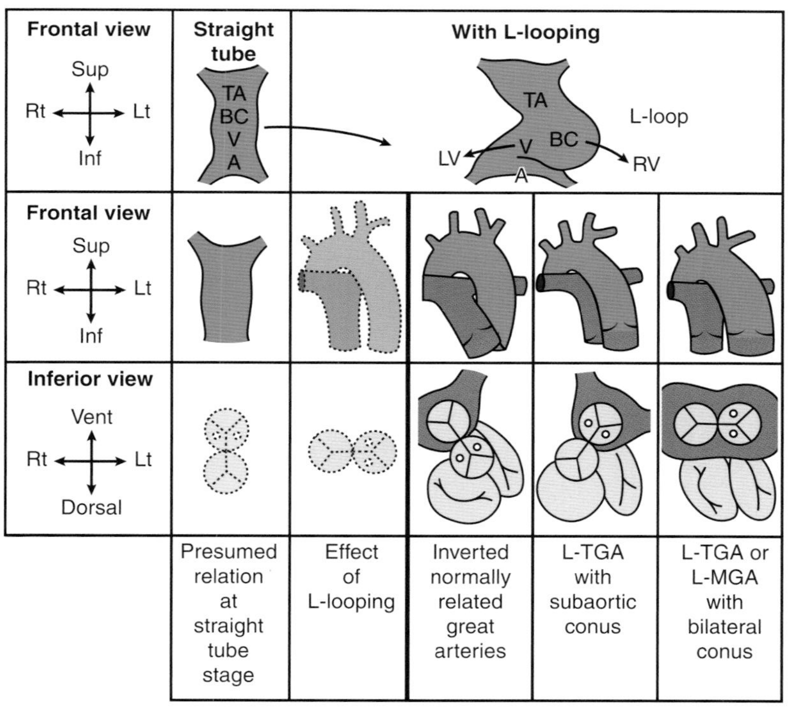

Fig. 15.2 **Normal and Abnormal Infundibuloarterial (Conotruncal) Morphogenesis and Anatomy After Bulboventricular L-Loop Formation.** Organization and abbreviations as in Fig. 15.1. The components of this diagram are real or apparent mirror-images of the corresponding components of Fig. 15.1. (Reproduced with permission from Van Praagh R, Van Praagh S. Isolated ventricular inversion: a consideration of the morphogenesis, definition, and diagnosis of nontransposed and transposed great arteries. *Am J Cardiol.* 1966;17:395-406.)

SNRGAs show how the embryonic aortic switch procedure normally is done. There is only one way of doing it right—with solitus and inversus isomers (see Figs. 15.1 and 15.2, respectively). There are many ways of doing the embryonic aortic switch wrong, and they all result in a conotruncal malformation, as will be seen.

$$\textbf{SNRGA}\ \{\textbf{S, D, S}\} = \textbf{0R} + \textbf{4L}$$

In words, this equation means that after D-loop formation, SNRGAs result from complete resorption of the right-sided subaortic conal free wall plus good development and expansion of the left-sided subpulmonary conal free wall.

INVERTED NORMALLY RELATED GREAT ARTERIES

Inverted normally related great arteries (INRGAs) result from a mirror-image of the "recipe" for SNRGA (see Fig. 15.2):

$$\textbf{INRGA}\ \{\textbf{I, L, I}\} = \textbf{4R} + \textbf{0L}$$

In words, this equation means that after L-loop formation, INRGAs result from good development and expansion of the right-sided subpulmonary conal free wall plus involution of the left-sided subaortic conal free wall (permitting aortic-mitral continuity).

Transposition of the Great Arteries

TGA results from reversed right-left asymmetry in the development of the subarterial conal free walls. *Typical D-TGA* has good development of the right-sided subaortic conal free wall and resorption of the left-sided subpulmonary conal free wall (see Fig. 15.1). Consequently, the D-transposed aorta is elevated superiorly and anteriorly above the RV, and the pulmonary valve and MPA move inferiorly and posteriorly, passing mostly through the interventricular foramen, and the pulmonary valve typically comes into direct fibrous continuity with the mitral valve, above the LV. So in D-TGA, the wrong great artery gets switched from RV to LV: the MPA gets switched instead of the aorta.

The foregoing morphogenesis and pathologic anatomy of typical D-TGA may be expressed in the following equation:

$$\textbf{D} - \textbf{TGA}\ \{\textbf{S, D, D}\} = \textbf{4R} + \textbf{0L}$$

In words, this equation means that after D-loop formation, typical D-TGA results from and is characterized by good development of the right-sided subaortic conal free wall and by involution of the left-sided subpulmonary conal free wall (permitting pulmonary-mitral fibrous continuity). Note that typical D-TGA is characterized by R-L reversal of the subarterial conal free wall development when compared with that of SNRGA: SNRGA {S,D,S} = 0R + 4L.

Thus, typical D-TGA results from conal free wall *inversion* (R-L reversal). In typical D-TGA, this is why the wrong great artery gets switched. *Typical L-TGA* (see Fig. 15.2) is a mirror-image of typical D-TGA (see Fig. 15.1):

$$\textbf{TGA}\ \{\textbf{S, L, L}\} = \textbf{0R} + \textbf{4L}$$

In words, this equation means that after L-loop formation (see Fig. 15.2), the equation or "recipe" for typical L-TGA is right-sided subpulmonary conal free wall resorption and an arterial switch of the MPA through the interventricular foramen from the left-sided RV into the right-sided LV with pulmonary-to-mitral fibrous continuity and good development of the left-sided subaortic conal free wall with elevation of the left-sided aorta superiorly and anteriorly above the left-sided RV.

In typical L-TGA with a left-sided subaortic muscular conus and no right-sided subpulmonary muscular conus, there is R-L reversal of conal free wall development compared with what is normal for a ventricular L-loop (see Fig. 15.2):

$$\text{TGA}\ \{\text{S, L, L}\} = \text{0R} + \text{4L} \text{ whereas}$$

$$\text{INRGA}\ \{\text{I, L, I}\} = \text{4R} + \text{0L}$$

The conus in typical L-TGA has sometimes been described as "inverted for situs inversus." However, the definition of inversion breaks down in visceroatrial situs inversus. As the equation for typical L-TGA indicates, the conal anatomy in typical L-TGA appears the same as that for SNRGAs!

$$TGA\ \{S, L, L\} = 0R + 4L \text{, and}$$

$$SNRGA\ \{S, D, S\}$$

Consequently, we have avoided conal inversion as a general definition of TGA. Conal inversion is accurate in visceroatrial situs solitus. But, in visceroatrial situs inversus, "conal inversion for situs inversus" does not work well because the conal equation for L-TGA is noninverted, the same as in SNRGA.

Instead, it seems clearer to say that TGA results from *reversed* R-L conal free wall asymmetry, bearing in mind what is normal for the situs of the semilunar valves that is present.

Situs in anatomy means the pattern of anatomic organization, that is, solitus (noninverted) or inversus (a mirror-image of solitus).

In L-TGA {S,L,L}, the great arteries are inverted with aorta to the left and pulmonary artery to the right, as the great arterial symbol in the segmental anatomic set indicates:

$$\text{L} - \text{TGA}\ \{\text{S, L, } \textbf{L}\}$$

So the question is: What type of subarterial conus is normal for inverted (L-positioned) great arteries? The answer is the type of conus found with INRGAs:

$$\text{INRGA}\ \{\text{I, L, I}\} = \textbf{4R} + \textbf{0L}$$

The type of conus typically found in L-TGA is:

$$\text{L} - \text{TGA}\ \{\text{S, L, L}\} = \textbf{0R} + \textbf{4L}$$

Therefore, in L-TGA (which is an inverted transposition), the conal situs is R-L reversed compared with the normal conal situs for INRGAs arteries: 0R + 4L (in L-TGA) compared with 4R + 0L (in INRGA). **So, typical L-TGA {S,L,L} has infundibuloarterial (conotruncal) situs discordance (oppositeness).** These **inverted** great arteries have a **noninverted** conal connector. Consequently, the great arteries are abnormally connected and hence are abnormally aligned with the underlying ventricles and AV junction and are abnormally positioned in space (abnormally related).

Infundibuloarterial (conotruncal) anomalies are malformations of right-left conal free wall laterality, as D- and L-TGA exemplify.

A structurally normal heart is characterized by *segmental situs uniformity*. The segmental situs anatomy of the solitus normal heart is {S,D,S}. The three main cardiac segments {atria, ventricles, great arteries} are all in situs solitus. So too are the two connecting segments: the AV canal or junction and the infundibulum or conus arteriosus. The solitus normal heart displays **segmental situs uniformity.** So, too, does the inverted normal heart: {I,L,I}. The three main cardiac segments, {I,L,I}, and the two connecting cardiac segments, the AV valves and the conus arteriosus, are all inverted. Consequently, there is AV concordance and VA concordance, as in situs inversus totalis, because there is **segmental situs uniformity:** all segments are in situs inversus.

But complex congenital heart disease is characterized by segmental situs *nonuniformity*. All of the cardiac segments do not have the same pattern of anatomic organization (situs), either all solitus, or all inversus. **Instead, complex congenital heart disease is characterized by a segmental situs "salad" (mixture), as the infundibuloarterial equations make very clear.**

D-TGA typically is characterized by infundibuloarterial situs discordance (oppositeness). D-TGA {S,D,D} has noninverted great arteries. The aorta is to the right of the pulmonary artery, as the segmental anatomy indicates: TGA {S,D,**D**}.

What kind of subarterial conus is normal for noninverted (D-positioned) great arteries? The kind of conus that is present in the solitus normal heart. What's that?

$$\text{SNRGA}\ \{S, D, S\} = \mathbf{0R} + \mathbf{4L}$$

What kind of conus is found in typical D-TGA?

$$\text{TGA}\ \{S, D, D\} = \mathbf{4R} + \mathbf{0L}$$

So, as we can see, the pattern of anatomic organization of the conus in typical D-TGA **(4R + 0L)** is R-L reversed compared with the solitus normal conus **(0R + 4L).**

Consequently, TGA (both D- and L-) is characterized by infundibuloarterial situs discordance, whereas normally related great arteries (solitus and inversus) have infundibuloarterial situs concordance.

Double-Outlet Right Ventricle

DORV, for example of the Taussig-Bing type,[2,3] has the following equation (see Fig. 15.1):

$$\textbf{Taussig-Bing DORV \{S,D,D\}} = \mathbf{4R} + \mathbf{4L}$$

In words, this equation means that after D-loop formation, there is a well-developed right-sided subaortic conal free wall and a well-developed left-sided subpulmonary conal free wall. Consequently, there is no semilunar-AV fibrous continuity (because of the interposition of the subarterial conal free wall musculature) (see Fig. 15.1). Also, neither great artery has been switched from above the RV to above the LV; hence, persistent DORV is present.

Fig. 15.1 also suggests that a bilateral conus (subaortic and subpulmonary) can be associated not only with DORV {S,D,D} but also with D-TGA with a bilateral conus. Note that the great arteries with DORV may be accurately described as having D-malposition of the great arteries (D-TGA; see Fig. 15.1), not as having D-TGA (because DORV is present, not TGA).

A rare finding is shown in Fig. 15.1: TGA {S,D,D} with a bilaterally deficient conus permitting aortic-tricuspid and pulmonary-mitral fibrous continuity.

Double-Outlet Left Ventricle

Double-outlet left ventricle (DOLV) of the rare Paul type[4] satisfies the following equation:

$$\textbf{Paul DOLV\{S,D,S\}} = \mathbf{0R} + \mathbf{0L}$$

Absence of a right-sided subaortic muscular conus and absence of a left-sided subpulmonary muscular conus permitted right-sided aortic-mitral fibrous continuity and left-sided pulmonary-mitral fibrous continuity. A diminutive conal septum was fibrous, not muscular. The ventricular septum to the right of the aortic valve was intact. The right ventricular outflow tract was atretic. The RV was small-chambered and thick-walled. A fistula connected the RV cavity with the anterior descending coronary arterial branch of a single right coronary artery; the ostium of the left coronary artery was absent. A Blalock-Hanlon atrial septostomy was performed on this boy at 28 months of age because the atrial septum was thought to be restrictive. The patient died at 2 7/12 years of age from chronic congestive heart failure and pneumonitis. This is one of the most rare heart specimens that it has ever been my privilege to study.[4]

CONAL SITUS

There appear to be at least four main anatomic types of conal situs: **situs solitus of the conus,** as in SNRGA {S,D,S} = 0R + 4L (see Fig. 15.1); **situs inversus of the conus**, as in INRGA {I,L,I} = 4R + 0L (see Fig. 15.2); and **situs ambiguus of the conus,** as in DORV of the Taussig-Bing type with a bilateral (subaortic and subpulmonary) conus, that is, DORV {S,D,D} = 4R + 4L; and as in DOLV of the Paul type with bilateral absence of the conal muscular free walls, that is, DOLV {S,D,D} = **0R + 0L**. Hence, there are at least two main anatomic types of conal situs ambiguus: 4R + 4L, as in Taussig-Bing, and 0R + 0L, as in the Paul type of DOLV. Situs ambiguus means uncertain or unknown pattern of anatomic organization that is different from situs solitus and situs inversus. Note that *situs ambiguus* is the correct Latin spelling; *ambiguous* is correct English spelling.

Tetralogy of Fallot

Tetralogy of Fallot (TOF) is a *"subnormality."* The subpulmonary conus arteriosus (infundibulum) is present but underdeveloped, poorly expanded, and hence obstructive (stenotic or atretic).

By contrast, **TGA,** which we have just been considering, is an *abnormality*. Growth and development of the subaortic conal free wall and involution of the subpulmonary conal free wall both are abnormalities of development of the subarterial conal free walls.

Typical TOF, after D-loop formation, satisfies the following equation:

$$\text{TOF} = 0R + 1/2/3L$$

In words, this equation means that typical TOF equals resorption of the right-sided subaortic conal free wall, which in turn permits aortic valve–to–mitral valve direct fibrous continuity, plus underdevelopment of the left-sided subpulmonary conal free wall.

1 *L development* means that the left-sided subpulmonary conus is present, but very poorly developed, very poorly expanded, and hence atretic.
2 *L development* means that the left-sided subpulmonary conus is present, but poorly developed and poorly expanded and hence severely stenotic.
3 *L development* means that the left-sided subpulmonary conus is present, but mildly to moderately underdeveloped and mildly to moderately underexpanded, resulting in mild to moderate pulmonary outflow tract stenosis.

Truncus Arteriosus

Truncus arteriosus type A1[5,6] means that a subsemilunar ventricular septal defect (VSD) is present (type A) and that a remnant of the aorticopulmonary septum is present, with an aorticopulmonary window (APW) or an aorticopulmonary septal defect (type 1). So, truncus arteriosus type A1 has a subsemilunar VSD, a remnant of the aorticopulmonary septum, and an APW.[5,6]

For us, the surprising finding was that if we did not allow ourselves to look at the great arteries, just by examining the RV and LV outflow tracts, we could not tell so-called persistent truncus arteriosus communis from TOF with pulmonary outflow tract atresia (TOF-atresia). The RV outflow tract anatomy in truncus and in TOF-atresia is virtually identical or at least extremely similar.

These observations led us to the hypothesis[5,6] that so-called truncus arteriosus communis type A1 is really TOF with atresia of the RV outflow tract (infundibulum), with partial or complete absence of the pulmonary valve and with an APW.

This hypothesis is thought to explain why we have never seen a case of truncus arteriosus with a six-leaflet semilunar valve as predicted by the classic hypothesis that truncus arteriosus communis is caused by absence of the truncoconal septum. In 79 autopsied cases,[6] the truncal valve was tricuspid and indistinguishable from an aortic valve in 47 cases (61%), bicuspid in 6 (8%) because of underdevelopment or absence of a commissure and quadricuspid in 24 (31%) because of persistence of a pulmonary leaflet remnant, but never the predicted six-leaflet or common semilunar valve.

In 91 cases of truncus arteriosus, a right aortic arch was present in 31 (34%), another finding very similar to TOF.

Truncus arteriosus (TA) type A1 may be represented by the following equation:

$$\text{TA } \{S, D, S\} \text{ type A1} = 0R + 1L + \text{APW}$$

In words, this equation means that after D-loop formation, truncus arteriosus type A1 equals involution of the right-sided subaortic conal free wall (permitting aortic-mitral fibrous continuity) plus atresia of the left-sided subpulmonary infundibulum (similar to TOF-atresia) plus an APW.

Truncus arteriosus {S,D,S} type A2 means that a subsemilunar VSD is present (type A) and that there is no aorticopulmonary septal remnant (type 2). The question is: what is this really? The classic anatomic definition of truncus arteriosus communis (common arterial trunk) is one great artery that arises from the base of the heart and supplies the coronary arteries (at least one), the pulmonary arteries (at least one), and the general systemic circulation. Truncus arteriosus type A2 satisfies this definition.

However, on thinking about this malformation, several questions arise; for example: Why is the aorticopulmonary septum absent? One possibility is because the main pulmonary artery is absent. If this is true, the truncus arteriosus in type A2 is the aorta (only). Hence, there is no aorticopulmonary septal remnant. But then one may wonder whether this possibly can be the aorta only (because the MPA is hypothesized to be absent). Both the right pulmonary artery (RPA) and the left pulmonary artery (LPA) arise from this large artery. Is not a common aortopulmonary trunk more likely? Perhaps. But why is the aorticopulmonary septum absent, if the MPA is really present? Not knowing the answer, one suspends judgment. But the problem does not go away. It just remains there unsolved and waiting for a solution.

Then one day we had a strange and fascinating case. Cardiac catheterization and angiocardiography revealed normal segmental anatomy, that is, {S,D,S}. The right atrium (RA) and RV are normal. Angiocardiography reveals a normal MPA, but with no branches: no RPA and no LPA. The contrast medium passes through a slightly narrowed patent ductus arteriosus and into the descending thoracic aorta.

Study of the left heart shows a normal left atrium (LA) and an unremarkable LV. The aorta arises normally. Then about half way up the ascending aorta, the RPA and the LPA arise from the back of the ascending aorta. I had seen a very similar case of Dr. Alfredo Vizcaino[7] in Mexico City, we had heard of the cases of Beitzke and Shinebourne[8] and of Aotsuka et al[9] of this rare anomaly, and I could not forget about the unsolved mystery of truncus arteriosus type A2.[5,6] These rare cases[7-9] proved that the MPA and branches have a bipartite origin. The MPA can be entirely separate from the RPA and the LPA.

Previously, I had been fortunate enough to study human and comparative embryology in the Department of Embryology of the Carnegie Institution of Washington, which is really in Baltimore, Maryland (close to Washington, D.C.).

To understand cases with a nonbranching MPA, and with both RPA and LPA arising from the dorsal aspect of the ascending aorta, it is helpful to know the following,[7] which is based on the Carnegie Collection of normal human embryos.

1. The pulmonary artery branches originate initially from the ascending aorta, that is, from the aortic sac, at the 4-mm stage (crown-rump length), at 24 to 26 days of age in utero, before the sixth arches have been completely formed.

TABLE 15.1

Infundibuloarterial Equations With Aortic Valve Right and Pulmonary Valve Left	Infundibuloarterial Equations With Aortic Valve Left and Pulmonary Valve Right
1. SNRGA {S,D,S} = 0R + 4L	11. INRGA {I,L,I} = 4R + 0L
2. TOF {S,D,S} with PAt = 0R + 1L	12. ITOF {I,L,I} with PAt = 1R + 0L
3. TOF {S,D,S} with severe PS = 0R + 2L	13. ITOF {I,L,I} with severe PS = 2R + 0L
4. TOF {S,D,S} with mild to moderate PS = 0R + 3L	14. ITOF {I,L,I} with mild/moderate PS = 3R + 0R
5. TA {S,D,S} type A1 = 0R + 1L + APW	15. TGA {S,L,L} = 0R + 4L
6. TA {S,D,S} type A2 = 0R + 1L – MPA	16. DORV {S,L,L} = 2R + 4L
7. TGA {S,D,D} = 4R + 0L	17. TGA {S,D,L} = 2R + 4L
8. DORV {S,D,D}, Taussig Bing = 4R + 4L	
9. DOLV {S,D,D}, Paul type = 0R + 0L	
10. {S,L,S}, isolated ventricular inversion = 0R + 4L	

AoV, Aortic valve; *APW,* aortopulmonary window; *A1,* truncus arteriosus *(TA)* with subsemilunar ventricular septal defect *(VSD)* and an APW; *A2,* TA with VSD and no aortopulmonary septum; *DOLV,* double-outlet left ventricle; *DORV,* double-outlet right ventricle; *{I,L,I},* the set of situs inversus of the atria, L-loop ventricles, and inverted normally related great arteries; *INRGA,* inverted normally related great arteries; *ITOF,* inverted tetralogy of Fallot; *MPA,* main pulmonary artery; *PAt,* pulmonary (outflow tract) atresia; *PS,* pulmonary stenosis; *PV,* pulmonary valve; *{S,D,D},* the set of solitus atria, D-loop ventricles, and solitus normally related great arteries; *{S,D,D},* the set of solitus atria, D-loop ventricles, and D-transposition or D-malposition of the great arteries; *{S,D,L},* the set of solitus atria, D-loop ventricles, and L-transposition or L-malposition of the great arteries: *{S,L,L},* the set of solitus atria, L-loop ventricles, and L-transposition or L-malposition of the great arteries; *{S,L,S},* the set of solitus atria, L-loop ventricles, and solitus normally related great arteries (isolated ventricular inversion); *SNRGA,* solitus normally related great arteries; *TGA,* transposition of the great arteries; *TOF,* tetralogy of Fallot; *0L,* grade zero development (absence) of the subarterial conal free wall on the left side; *0R,* grade 0 development (absence) of the subarterial conal free wall on the right side; 1L, grade 1 development of the subarterial infundibulum (atresia) on the left side; *1R,* grade 1 development (atresia) of the subarterial infundibulum on the right side; *2L,* grade 2 development (severe stenosis) of the subarterial infundibulum on the left side; *2R,* grade 2 development (severe stenosis) of the right-sided subarterial infundibulum; *3L,* grade 3 development (mild to moderate stenosis) of the left-sided subarterial infundibulum; *3R,* grade 3 development (mild to moderate stenosis) of the right-sided subarterial infundibulum; *4L,* grade 4 development (good growth and expansion, no stenosis) of the left-sided subarterial infundibulum; *4R,* grade 4 development (good growth and expansion, no stenosis) of the right-sided subarterial infundibulum; *+,* and; *–,* without.

2. Completion of both sixth arches can occur as early as the 5-mm stage, that is, 26 to 28 days of age in utero. Completion of both sixth arches usually occurs normally by the 6-mm stage, 28 to 30 days after fertilization.
3. As soon as both sixth arches have been completely formed, normally they enlarge considerably and both pulmonary artery branches appear to migrate out onto the sixth arches, where they join with the MPA.
4. Occasionally, the RPA or LPA branch remains arising from the ascending aorta, resulting in "hemitruncus."[10] Only very rarely do both RPA and LPA remain arising from the ascending aorta when the MPA is present (and unbranched).

However, when the MPA is absent, the RPA and the LPA have nowhere to migrate to. Our hypothesis is that this is what happens in so-called truncus arteriosus type A2. Our hypothesis is that so-called truncus arteriosus type A2 is TOF-atresia with *absence* of the MPA. Because the MPA is absent, (1) there is no aortopulmonary septal remnant, because the arterial trunk is the aorta only, and (2) the RPA and the LPA both remain in their starting positions from the ascending aorta, because there is no MPA to migrate on to. In this hypothesis, truncus arteriosus type A1 is a *common* aortopulmonary trunk (truncus arteriosus communis) but truncus arteriosus type A2 is a *solitary* aortic trunk (truncus aorticus solitarius).

In the interests of anatomic accuracy and also wishing to change conventional diagnostic terminology as little as possible, we talk and write about **truncus arteriosus,** not about truncus arteriosus *communis,* because we think that truncus arteriosus type A2 may very well be a solitary aortic (not a common aortopulmonary) trunk.

After D-loop formation, we think that truncus arteriosus type A2 satisfies the following equation:

Truncus arteriosus {*S, D, D*} type A2 = 0R + 1L – MPA

In words, this equation means that after D-loop formation, truncus arteriosus type A2 equals absorption of the right-sided subaortic conal free wall plus left-sided pulmonary infundibular atresia minus the MPA (hence, absence of an aortopulmonary septal remnant and origin of the RPA and the LPA from the aortic sac of the solitary aorta).

Where Are the Great Arteries and the Subarterial Conal Free Walls? In segmental anatomy, the arterial symbol indicates the relative locations of the aorta, subaortic conal free wall, MPA, and subpulmonary conal free wall (**Table 15.**1). For example, in {S,D,**S**}, the aortic valve and the subaortic conal free wall are posterior and to the **right** of the pulmonary valve and the subpulmonary conal free wall.

In {I,L,**I**}, the aortic valve and the subaortic conal free wall are posterior and to the **left** of the pulmonary valve and the subpulmonary conal free wall. In TGA {S,D,**D**}, the aortic valve and the subaortic conal free wall are to the **right** of the pulmonary valve and the subpulmonary conal free wall. In TGA {S,D,**L**}, the aortic valve and the subaortic conal free wall are to the **left** of the pulmonary valve and the subpulmonary conal free wall. In {S,L,**S**}, the aortic valve and the subaortic conal free wall are to the **right** of the pulmonary valve and the subpulmonary conal free wall.

What about TGA {S,D,**A**}? When the aortic valve is directly **anterior** to the pulmonary valve, does this method of analysis and understanding break down? No. Why not? Because it is not really about R-L in the sense of *external* spatial coordinates of right and left. What really matters are *internal* spatial relationships. At the early D-loop stage (see Fig. 15.1), the developing aorta and the subaortic conal free wall are on the greater curvature of the bulboventricular loop, and the developing PA and the subpulmonary conal free wall are on the lesser curvature of the bulboventricular loop. This is true for both the D-loop (see Fig. 15.1) and the L-loop (see Fig. 15.2).

What really matters is that the lesser curvature (the subpulmonary conal free wall) undergoes good growth and expansion, and that simultaneously the greater curvature (the subaortic conal free wall) undergoes involution and disappearance.

These are the internal anatomic relationships relevant to the anatomy of the bulboventricular loop itself that really matter, not the fixed external R-L coordinates that are usually employed because of their descriptive convenience.

These *internal* anatomic relationships are reminiscent of *chirality,* which also is independent of external spatial coordinates (like R-L) and therefore is superior to noninversion and inversion, which are defined in terms of right and left. For example, in crisscross AV relations, both ventricles can be bilateral—both right-sided and left-sided. Consequently, **ventricular noninversion and inversion** break down in this situation because these descriptors are based on the external R-L spatial coordinates. But **chirality** applies accurately because it is based on the right-handed or left-handed anatomy per se, not on external spatial coordinates. So the equation for A-TGA is:

$$\text{TGA}\ \{S, D, A\} = 4A + 0P$$

A stands for anterior, and *P* stands for posterior. But what really matters is that *A* also stands for *subaortic* and *P* also stands for *subpulmonary,* the anatomy per se, independent of external spatial coordinates.

DISCUSSION

There are, of course, many more infundibuloarterial (or conotruncal) equations. Table 15.1 presents some of the more common ones. These equations are intended as a step in the direction of a more quantitative approach to an understanding of the morphogenesis and the anatomy of normally and abnormally related great arteries.

Normally related great arteries show how the embryonic aortic switch procedure should be done. There is only one way of doing it right (correctly), with solitus and inversus isomers (see Eqs. 1 and 11, respectively, in Table 15.1). As noted previously, there are many ways of doing the embryonic aortic switch wrong (incorrectly), and they all result in an infundibuloarterial (or conotruncal) malformation: for example, Eqs. 2 to 9, and 12 to 17 in Table 15.1).

Normally related great arteries (solitus and inversus) result from complete right and left asymmetry in the development of the subarterial conal free walls (see Eqs. 1 and 11, respectively, in Table 15.1). The subaortic conal free wall undergoes involution, permitting the embryonic aortic switch. The subpulmonary conal free wall undergoes good development and expansion, elevating the pulmonary valve and MPA superiorly and anteriorly above the RV, getting the pulmonary valve and the MPA out of the way (i.e., away from the interventricular foramen), thereby facilitating the normal embryonic aortic switch.

The evolution of the RV sinus, body, or inflow tract, which is the lung pump, and ***the evolution of the conus arteriosus or infundibulum*** (described earlier) that performs the embryonic aortic switch procedure are two of the most important cardiovascular evolutionary adaptations in vertebrates that made possible permanent air-breathing and permanent land-living.[11,12]

These were two of the most important cardiovascular evolutionary changes that made it possible for Ordovician and Devonian Age fish to leave the water and to colonize the land, evolving into amniotes, reptiles, birds, and mammals.

The importance of conotruncal malformations in human congenital heart disease indicates that we are still having trouble with our evolutionary adaptations to permanent air-breathing and permanent land-living.

We are walkie-talkie fish—really.[13] An understanding of evolution is just as important as an understanding of pathologic anatomy, cardiovascular embryology, and molecular genetics. Evolution is not just part of the spectrum. Evolution *is* the spectrum.[13] Today, most of our basic research goes down to the level of molecular genetics, where it often stops. My suggestion is: we need to keep going deeper, into nonmammalion evolution.

This study of the conus arteriosus and how it largely determines the anatomy and physiology of normally and abnormally related great arteries (see Table 15.1), strongly suggests that we are watching the natural experiments of how the fish heart evolved into the normal human heart. We may have much to learn from our evolutionary past.

The infundibuloarterial (conotruncal) malformations are anomalies of the conal connector *only;* truncus arteriosus is the only exception (see Table 15.1). Truncus arteriosus is a conal malformation, and there are also anomalies of the great arteries (see Eqs. 5 and 6 in Table 15.1).

In most conotruncal malformations, such as TOF, TGA, DORV, and DOLV, the great arteries per se are normally formed. Most so-called conotruncal malformations are conal (infundibular) malformations, period. The great arteries (truncus) are not malformed. In the conotruncal anomalies, the great arteries are malpositioned because of malformations of the underlying subarterial conus arteriosus on which the great arteries stand.

Abnormally related great arteries, such as TGA and DORV, are not caused by malseptation of the truncoconal septum, as has long been thought. For example, it used to be widely thought that TGA is caused by abnormally straight downgrowth of the truncoconal septum. However, this malseptation hypothesis cannot explain[14] why the free walls of the transposed great arteries are just as abnormally positioned as is the truncoconal septum or why the transposed aortic valve is high, whereas the transposed pulmonary valve is low (see later); or why there is no definite anatomic evidence of abnormality of the aortopulmonary septum in TGA. For example, if you ever see a case of TGA with an aortopulmonary septal defect, you should report it because APWs with TGA are vanishing by rare. If TGA were caused by malseptation of the great arteries and the conus, definite abnormalities of the aortopulmonary septum, such as APW and of the conal septum, such as a conal septal defect, should be relatively common in TGA, which they are not.

Parenthetically, it should be added that some observers have attempted to explain the variation in transposed semilunar valve heights by saying that the conus (infundibulum) is part of the RV, but not part of the LV: hence, the high transposed aortic valve and the low transposed pulmonary valve.

The difficulty with this explanation is that it is anatomically and developmentally wrong: The infundibulum or conus arteriosus is part of the great arterial segment, that is, the **conotruncus,** which is not an intrinsic, inseparable part of the RV. This is why the muscular conus arteriosus can override the ventricular septum to virtually any degree. The conus can be mostly above the RV, or about 50% above the RV and 50% above the LV, or almost entirely above the LV, as in some anatomic types of DOLV, and as in anatomically corrected malposition of the great arteries (ACM). It is a fascinating fact that in the infundibuloarterial anomalies, the great arteries per se are anatomically and developmentally normal, with the exception of truncus arteriosus (see Table 15.1).

As noted earlier the conotruncal anomalies are almost all infundibular or conal anomalies, period. An abnormally straight, nonspiral development of the aorticopulmonary septum is now understood *not* to be the *cause* of the conotruncal malformations. Instead, the abnormally straight aorticopulmonary septum is one of the *effects* of subsemilunar conal free wall malformation.

Anatomically corrected malposition of the great arteries (ACM)[15-17] is not included in Table 15.1. The subsemilunar conus is either bilateral (subaortic and subpulmonary) or subaortic only, in our experience. So ACM, too, is a conal anomaly. But it may be more than just a conal malformation. We do not understand why, in ACM, the infundibulum and great arteries always twist in a direction that is the *opposite* of the direction of ventricular loop formation, as in ACM {S,D,L}, which has AV concordance and VA concordance (the latter by definition). **So ACM can have both a conal malformation and a great arterial positional anomaly.**

The infundibulum or conus arteriosus is the conal connector: how the great arteries connect with the underlying ventricles and AV canal.

The *conotruncus does connect* with the ventricles and the AV valves. But the great arteries (only) do *not* connect with the underlying ventricles and AV canal because of the interposition of the conus arteriosus, which may be well developed (4) or absorbed (0). Instead, the ventricles and the great arteries can be *aligned* in many different ways: normally, or as in TOF (almost normally), or as in TGA, or as DORV, etc.

We make a distinction, in the interests of anatomic and developmental accuracy, between VA *alignments,* and infundibuloarterial (conotruncal) *connections* with the ventricles and AV valves. Abnormally *related* great arteries are abnormally *aligned* and abnormally *connected.*

The conus arteriosus (infundibulum) is a very important connecting segment: **the conus is an independent variable.** The conus arteriosus does not necessarily correspond to the anatomic type of ventricle inferiorly, nor to the anatomic type of the great artery superiorly.

By contrast, **the other important connecting segment—the AV canal and valves—is a dependent variable.** The AV valves correspond to the ventricles of entry or to the type of ventricular loop that is present.

In routine medical and surgical reports, the infundibulum or conus arteriosus should always be described with care: (1) What anatomic type of conus is present? Is it subpulmonary (only), subaortic (only), bilateral (subaortic and subpulmonary), or bilaterally absent or very deficient? (2) Is there semilunar-AV fibrous continuity or separation? Please describe. (3) Are the ventricular outflow tracts normal, stenotic, atretic, or regurgitant? Please describe. It is important to understand that the infundibulum is not "just part of the RV." It is much more interesting than that. The infundibulum is how the great arteries are connected and aligned with the underlying ventricles and AV valves.

When dealing with abnormally related great arteries, remember that "Most of woe lies below." The key to understanding abnormally related great arteries lies below the semilunar valves. That is where the conal connector is located. Understanding the conus helps one to understand the case.

When Dr. Alex Nadas was bringing visitors down to the Cardiac Registry laboratory, he would throw open the door and say in his booming rich Hungarian English, "Welcome to conus country!"

Have you ever wondered what the great arteries are doing? Have you ever spoken to an engineer who said something like this, "Look, why aren't the great arteries straight—pulmonary to the right and aorta to the left? Instead, you say it is normal for them to be all twisted around like that! It would be much more efficient for both great arteries to be *straight*." Fig. 15.3 helps provide an answer to the question, What are the great arteries doing? The short answer is untwisting. The work of Asami,[18] based on normal human embryos, is very informative (see Fig. 15.3). Measurements of the rotation of the semilunar valves relative to the sagittal plane, using a protractor, revealed the following (Table 15.2). At 30 to 32 days of embryonic age, the developing semilunar valvar relationship normally resembles that of **D-TGA**—aortic valve anterior and to the right of the developing pulmonary valve, with only 50 degrees of semilunar dextrorotation. During day 32, dextrorotation continued through 40 degrees more to reach 90 degrees dextrorotation—a side-by-side semilunar interrelationship, reminiscent of that seen with ***the Taussig-Bing type of DORV.***[2,3] During day 33 of embryonic age, dextrorotation at the semilunar valves continued through another 20 degrees to reach 110 degrees dextrorotation, which is reminiscent of that seen with ***TOF.*** By days 34 to 36, dextrorotation continued through 45 degrees more, reaching 155 degrees of dextrorotation relative to the sagittal plane, which is essentially a **normal solitus semilunar interrelationship.**

Fig. 15.3[18] also shows that the **partitioning of the AV canal** normally begins at 34 to 36 days of age in utero in the normal human embryo (Streeter's horizon or stage XVII). However, at 36 to 38 days of age in utero (stage XVIII), there still appears to

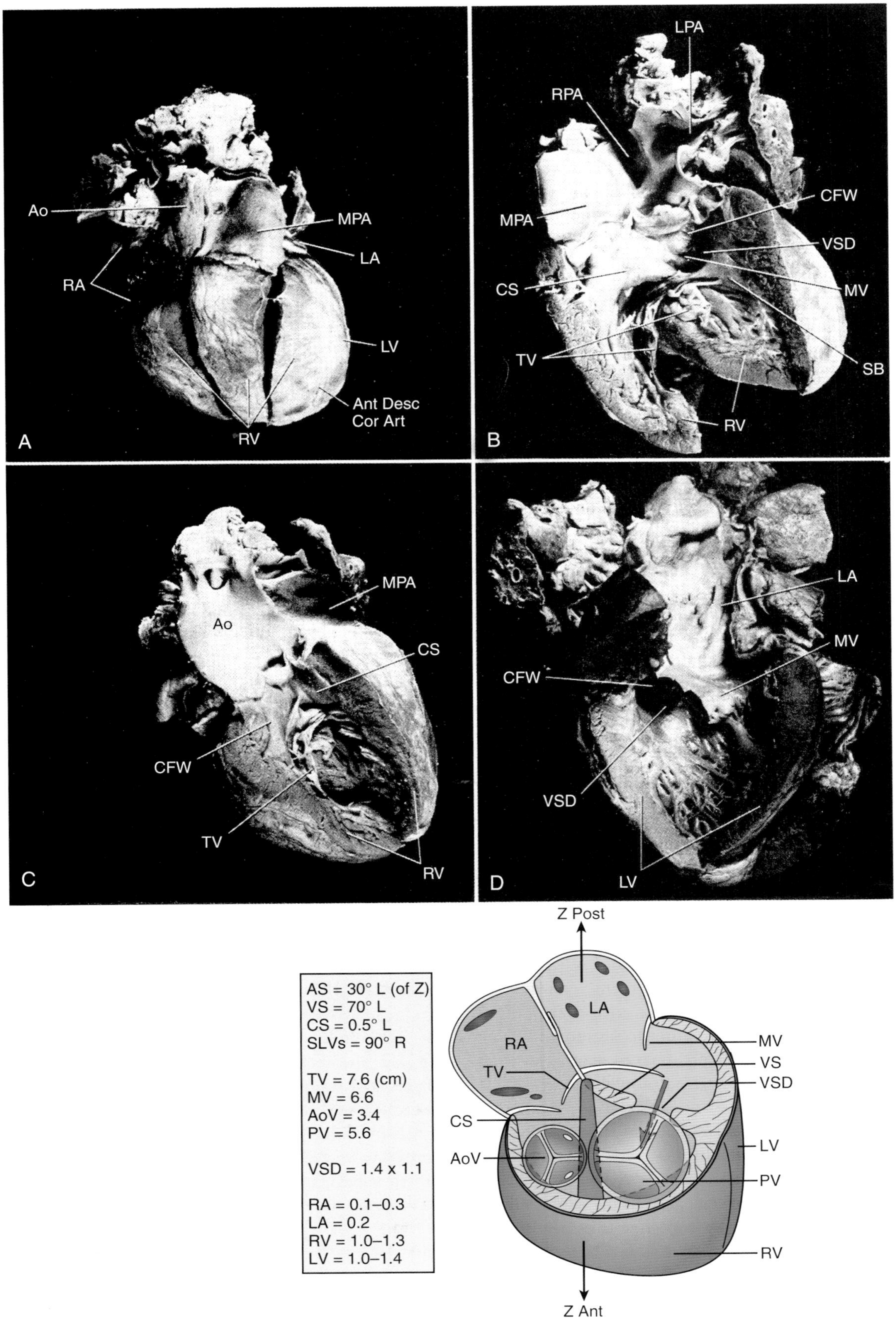
LPA
RPA
Ao
MPA
LA
RA
LV
Ant Desc
Cor Art
RV
A
CFW
VSD
MV
CS
SB
TV
B
MPA
Ao
CS
CFW
TV
RV
C
LA
MV
CFW
VSD
LV
D
Z Post
AS = 30° L (of Z)
VS = 70° L
CS = 0.5° L
SLVs = 90° R
TV = 7.6 (cm)
MV = 6.6
AoV = 3.4
PV = 5.6
VSD = 1.4 x 1.1
RA = 0.1–0.3
LA = 0.2
RV = 1.0–1.3
LV = 1.0–1.4
LA
RA
TV
MV
VS
VSD
CS
AoV
LV
PV
RV
Z Ant

Continued

Fig. 15.3 The Original Taussig-Bing Heart. (A) Exterior frontal view. (B) Opened right ventricle and pulmonary artery. (C) Opened right ventricle and ascending aorta. (D) Opened left atrium and left ventricle. (E) Quantitative geometric drawing of the heart specimen, viewed from above. Septal and semilunar valvar locations are measured relative to the Z axis (sagittal plane) in degrees. Valve measurements are circumferences in centimeters (cm). The subpulmonary ventricular septal defect is indicted by the *arrow* and is measured in cm from the left side which is the effective left ventricular exit. The wall thicknesses are measured in cm. Please see the text for heart description and discussion. *Ant,* Anterior; *Ant Desc Cor Art,* anterior descending coronary artery; *Ao,* aorta; *AS,* atrial septum; *AoV,* aortic valve; *CFW,* conal free wall; *CS,* conal septum; *LA,* left atrium; *LPA,* left pulmonary artery; *LV,* left ventricle; *MPA,* main pulmonary artery; *MV,* mitral valve; *Post,* posterior; *PV,* pulmonary valve; *RA,* right atrium; *R PA,* right pulmonary artery; *RV,* right ventricle; *SB,* septal band; *SLVs,* semilunar valves; *TV,* tricuspid valve; *VS,* muscular ventricular septum; *VSD,* ventricular septal defect. *Semilunar valve-to-atrioventricular valve distances:* (1) AoV-to-TV distance = 8 mm, the height of the subaortic CFW musculature, in C. (2) PV-to-MV distance = 9 mm, the height of the subpulmonary CFW musculature, in B and D. (Reproduced with permission from Van Praagh S, Van Praagh R. What is the Taussig-Bing malformation? *Circulation.* 1968;38:445-449.)

TABLE 15.2 Dextrorotation of the Semilunar Valves of Normal Human Embryos Relative to the Sagittal Plane

Streeter's Stage	Approximate Embryonic Age in Days	Degrees of Dextrorotation of the Semilunar Valves Relative to the Sagittal Plane
XV	30–32	50
XVI_a	32	90
XVI_b	33	110
XVII	34–36	155

From Asami I. Partitioning of the arterial end of the embryonic heart. In: In Van Praagh R, Takao A, eds. *Etiology and Morphogenesis of Congenital Heart Disease.* Mount Kisco, NY: Futura Publishing Co; 1980:51-61.

be a cleft in the anterior mitral leaflet, suggesting that partitioning of the AV canal is still continuing at this age.

The embryonic twisting (dextrorotation) of the great arteries at the semilunar valves (see Fig. 15.3) and subaortic conal free wall resorption are necessary to perform "Mother Nature's" embryonic aortic switch procedure from above the RV to above the LV.

Consequently, after normal cardiogenesis, our fibroelastic great arteries must *untwist* about each other (see Fig. 15.3, embryonic heart at stage XVIII) as they go from the *variable* semilunar spatial aortopulmonary interrelationship proximally at the semilunar valves to the *fixed* aorta–pulmonary artery relationship distally in which the aorta is always ventral (anterior) and cephalad (superior) relative to the pulmonary artery bifurcation. This fixed aorta to pulmonary artery relationship distally is because of the fixed spatial relationship between aortic arches 4 and pulmonary arches 6 (see Fig.15.3).

So this, then, is why the great arteries must normally twist to the right through approximately 150 degrees at the semilunar valve level during embryonic life (from days 30 to 36) and then normally must untwist to left through the same number of degrees throughout their length from the valves below to the aortic arch and pulmonary bifurcation (the aortic arch 4 to 6 junction) above.

Abnormally related great arteries twist much less than normally related great arteries do at the semilunar valve level during cardiac morphogenesis, and consequently abnormally related great arteries have much less untwisting to do after cardiogenesis (see Figs. 15.1 and 15.2).

The infundibuloarterial equations (see Table 15.1) express normal and abnormal infundibuloarterial embryology and anatomy in a way that is brief, clear, and specific. The central importance of infundibular or conal free wall malformation is very different from the classic straight truncoconal septum hypothesis that was thought to cause TGA. For embryologists, geneticists, pediatric cardiologists, and cardiac surgeons, it is helpful to know where the main problem is really located.

Concerning these conotruncal equations (see Table 15.1), it should be understood that subarterial conal free wall developmental **grades 0 to 4** stand for real numbers, that is, measurements (inches, millimeters, centimeters, or other units).

To illustrate how this works, **the original Taussig-Bing heart specimen**[2,3] will be described quantitatively and geometrically (Fig. 15.4).[3] This **quantitative and geometric method of heart description** is applicable to clinical imaging diagnostic studies using angiocardiography, two-dimensional or three-dimensional echocardiography, magnetic resonance imaging, and other modalities. Fig. 15.4E is a quantitative geometric diagram.

The atrial septum lies 30 degrees to the left of the Z axis (the sagittal plane). The ventricular septum lies 70 degrees to the left of the Z axis. The conal septum lies in the sagittal plane. The right side of the conal septum measured 0 degrees relative to the Z axis, and the left side of the conal septum measured 5 degrees to the left of the Z axis.

The semilunar valves measured 90 degrees to the right of the Z axis. The aortic valve lay side-by-side relative to the pulmonary valve, aortic valve to the right. The valve circumferences were:
tricuspid valve, 76 mm;
mitral valve, 66 mm;
aortic valve, 34 mm; and
pulmonary valve, 56 mm.

The VSD was subpulmonary and measured from the LV side 14 × 11 mm in right-left width × superoinferior height, respectively.

Wall thicknesses measured right atrium, 1 to 3 mm; left atrium, 2 mm; right ventricle, 10 to 13 mm; and left ventricle, 10 to 14 mm.

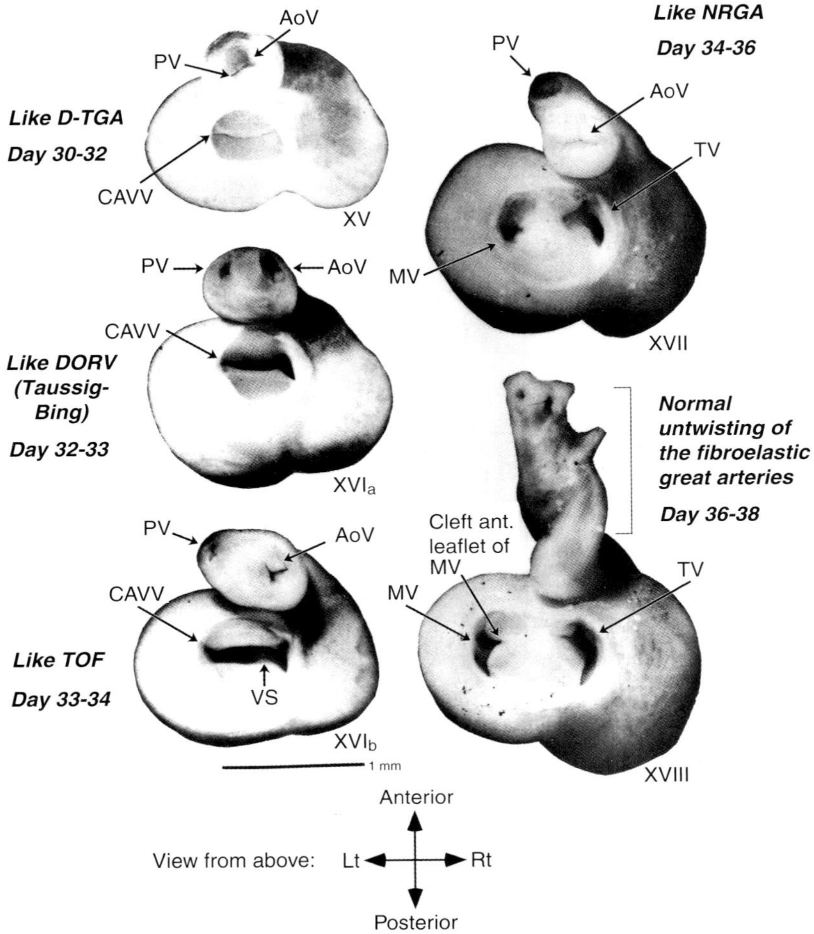

Fig. 15.4 Asami's presentation of normal human cardiac embryos from Streeter's stage XV (30 to 32 days of age in utero) to stage XVIII (36 to 38 days of age since fertilization), dorsal view, that is, view from above. Ventral (anterior) is toward the top of the page, dorsal (posterior) is toward the bottom of the page, right is toward the viewer's right hand, and left is toward the viewer's left hand. The atria have been removed to show the partitioning of the atrioventricular canal. The great arteries have been transected above the developing semilunar valves in stages XV to XVII to show the morphogenetic movements of the developing semilunar valves. The heart at stage 18 has intact, nontransected great arteries to show the normal *untwisting* of the great arteries as they pass from the semilunar valves below to the aortic arch-pulmonary bifurcation above. To convert Streeter's horizons or stages into approximate embryonic ages, multiply the horizon by 2. This gives you the age at the beginning of horizon. Then each horizon (stage) is 2 days long. Thus *horizon 15* gives an approximate embryonic age of 30 to 32 days, from the beginning to the end of the stage. *Horizon XVIa* is the first half of this stage, from day 32 to day 33, that is, day 32 (this 24-hour period). *Horizon XVIb* is the last half of this stage, that is, day 33 (from day 32 to day 34). *Horizon XVII* is day 34 to 36. *Horizon XVIII* is day 36 to 38. The 1-mm marker in our book[18] (Fig. 4-1) measures 30 mm in length. So the degree of magnification equals approximately ×30. *AoV,* Developing aortic valve; *CAVC,* common atrioventricular valve; *MV,* developing mitral valve; *PV,* developing pulmonary valve; *TV,* developing tricuspid valve; *VS,* muscular ventricular septum. *Morphogenetic movements* of developing aortic and pulmonary valves: 30 to 32 days of age in utero (horizon XV), the semilunar interrelation resembles that of *D-TGA*. Day 32 (horizon XVIa), side-by-side semilunar interrelationship resembles that of *DORV*. Day 33 (horizon XVIb), the semilunar interrelationship resembles that of *TOF*. Days 34 to 36 of embryonic life (horizon XVII), the semilunar interretionship resembles that of *solitus normally related great arteries*. The semilunar valves are being carried atop the developing subsemilunar conus arteriosus. (Reproduced with permission from Asami I. Partitioning of the arterial end of the embryonic heart. In: Van Praagh R, Takao A, eds. *Etiology and Morphogenesis of Congenital Heart Disease*. Mount Kisco, NY: Futura Publishing Co; 1980:51-61.)

The subarterial conus was bilateral, that is, subaortic (see Fig. 15.4C) and subpulmonary (see Fig. 15.4B). The subaortic conal free wall (see Fig. 15.4C) measured 8 mm between the aortic valve above and the tricuspid valve below. The subpulmonary conal free wall (see Fig. 15.4B) measured 9 mm between the pulmonary valve above and the mitral valve below.

Thus, the original Taussig-Bing heart had DORV {S,D,D} with a bilateral conus and a subpulmonary VSD. The subaortic conal free wall (aorta to tricuspid valve = 8 mm) and the subpulmonary conal free wall (pulmonary valve to mitral valve = 9 mm) were almost equally well developed and well expanded. The VSD was thought not to be restrictive, and there was no evidence of aortic or pulmonary outflow tract obstruction. The bilaterally well-developed subarterial conal free walls are considered to be the reason for the presence of DORV, because they prevent any semilunar-mitral approximation or direct fibrous continuity.

The lengths of the subsemilunar conal free walls can be measured precisely, permitting morphogenetic understanding.

Historical Note

The first investigator to recognize that TGA is a conal malformation was **Dr. Arthur Keith, in 1909,**[19] before he became **Sir Arthur Keith.** An eminent London anatomist and embryologist, Keith (1866–1955) discovered the sinoatrial node, also known as the **Keith-Flack node.** Martin Flack was a physiologist in London, England. I independently reached the same conclusion in 1966[20] as Keith had in 1909,[19] namely, that TGA is a conal malformation. Later, I discovered the work of Keith, to which I wish to give credit.

SUMMARY

It used to be thought that normally related great arteries result from spiral downgrowth of the truncoconal septum, whereas abnormally related great arteries result from relatively straight, nonspiral downgrowth of this septum.

Anatomic and embryologic data (see Figs. 15.1 to 15.3) have led to a revision of this classic view. The current concept focuses on the development of the subarterial conal free walls (not on the truncoconal septum).

Normally related great arteries are characterized by complete right-left asymmetry in the development of the subarterial conal free walls. With D-loop ventricles, the right-sided subaortic conal free wall musculature normally undergoes complete resorption. It disappears. Absence may be regarded as grade 0 development. In contrast, the left-sided subpulmonary conal free wall musculature normally undergoes good growth and expansile development, which may be symbolized as grade 4 development.

Thus, the usual or solitus form of normally related great arteries (SNRGA) has complete R-L asymmetry of development of the subarterial conal free walls, and may be represented by the following equation:

$$\text{SNRGA}\ \{S, D, S\} = 0R + 4L.$$

After ventricular D-loop formation, both developing great arteries are located side-by-side above the developing RV, developing aorta to the right and developing pulmonary artery to the left.

Involution of the right-sided subaortic conal free wall, thought to be due to apoptosis, causes the developing aorta and aortic valve to move inferiorly, posteriorly, and to pass through the interventricular foramen and to come into direct fibrous continuity with the developing mitral valve, above the LV.

Simultaneously, the left-sided pulmonary artery and valve move superiorly and anteriorly above the RV, the PA being carried aloft by the good expansile growth and development of the left-sided subpulmonary conal free wall. These normal morphogenetic movements of the semilunar valves occur between 30 and 36 days after fertilization in the human embryo (see Fig. 15.3).

Reversed R-L development of the subarterial conal free walls results in transposition of the great arteries (see Fig. 15.1). The aorta is carried aloft above the RV, and the PA is switched into the LV. This reversed R-L development of the subarterial conal free walls that results in typical D-TGA may be expressed as follows:

$$\textbf{TGA}\ \{\textbf{S, D, D}\} = \textbf{4R} + \textbf{0L}$$

There is only one way to do the embryonic aortic switch right (correctly), with solitus and inversus isomers: Eqs. 1 and 11 in Table 15.1.

There are many ways to do the embryonic aortic switch wrong (incorrectly), some of which are shown in Eqs. 2 to 9 and 12 to 17 in Table 15.1.

The normal pattern of complete right-left asymmetry in the development of the subarterial conal free walls (see Eqs. 1 and 11 in Table 15.1), plus the evolution of the RV sinus (body, or inflow tract) which is the lung pump, are the evolutionary cardiovascular keys that made it possible for vertebrates to leave the sea, colonize the land, breath air, and become permanently land-living.

There are many possible patterns of conal development (see Table 15.1), but only one pattern with two isomers (see Eqs. 1 and 11 in Table 15.1) that works physiologically. Evolution of this successful pattern of conal free wall development is one of the reasons why we are here. The physiologically unsuccessful patterns of conal development we regard as conal malformations (see Table 15.1). What we regard as normal was wrought by chance and necessity over an enormous expanse of time.

CONCLUSIONS

1. At the AV junction, assuming that the atria and the ventricles are well developed (not hypoplastic or absent), when there is AV situs concordance, both solitus as in {**S,D,S**} or both inversus as in {**I,L,I**} (Fig. 15.5), then there is AV alignment concordance.
2. At the AV junction, when there is AV situs discordance, both different as in TGA {**S,L,L**} (see Fig. 15.5), then there is AV alignment discordance.

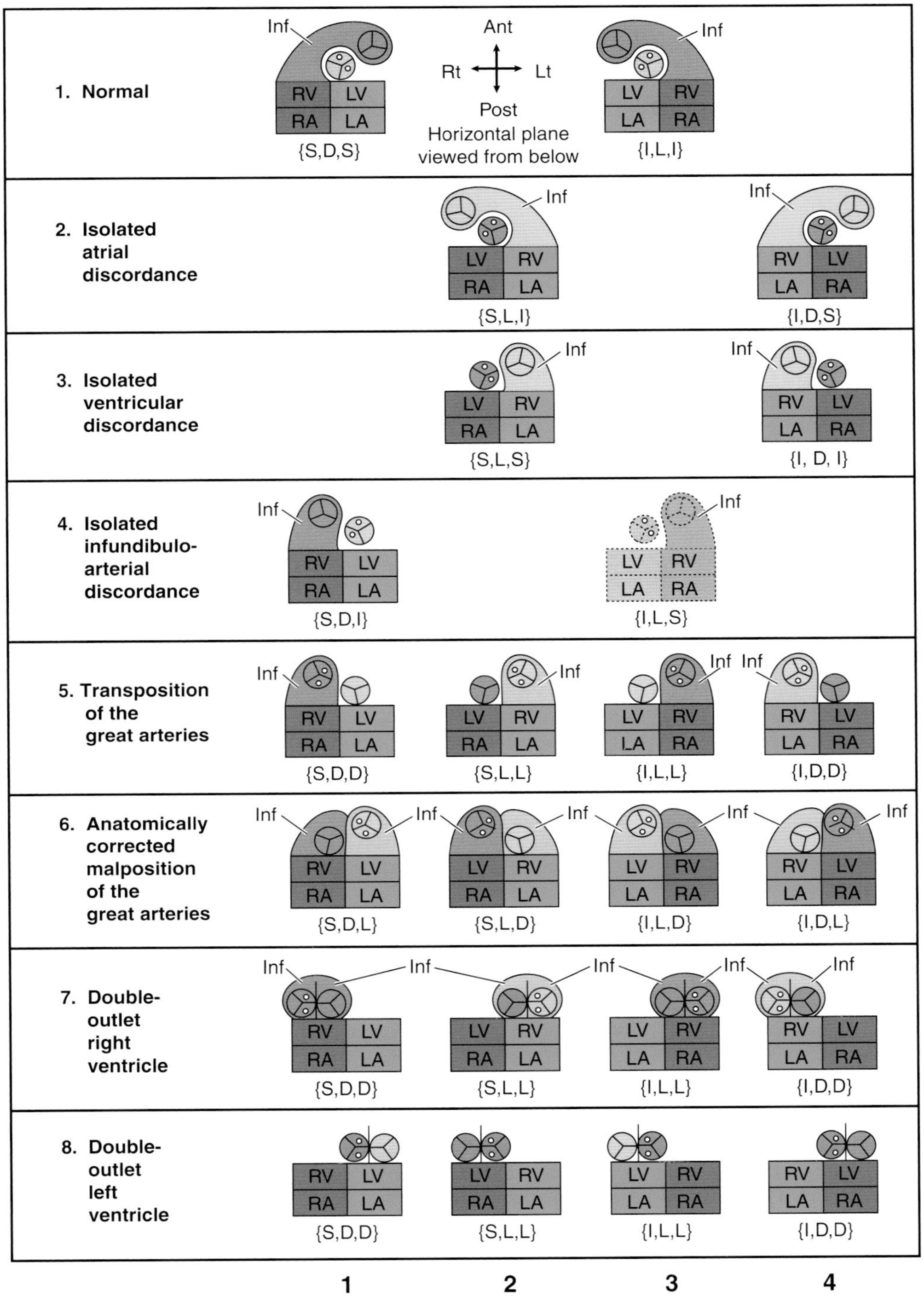

Fig. 15.5 Types of Human Heart in Terms of Segmental Sets, Connections, and Alignments. Heart diagrams are viewed from below, similar to a subxiphoid two-dimensional echocardiogram.

Column 1. All of the heart diagrams have atrioventricular (AV) situs and alignment concordance. The right-sided morphologically right atrium *(RA)* opens into the right-sided morphologically right ventricle *(RV)*, and the left-sided morphologically left atrium *(LA)* opens into the left-sided morphologically left ventricle *(LV)*.

Column 2. All of the heart diagrams have AV situs and alignment discordance. The right-sided RA opens into the right-sided LV and the left-sided LA opens into the left-sided RV.

Column 3. All of the heart diagrams have AV situs and alignment concordance in visceroatrial situs inversus. The left-sided RA opens into the left-sided RV, and the right-sided LA opens into the right-sided LV.

Column 4. All of the heart diagrams have AV situs and alignment discordance in visceroatrial situs inversus. The right-sided LA opens into the right-sided RV, and the left-sided RA opens into the left-sided LV.

Rows 1 to 8 are organized in terms of ventriculoarterial (VA) alignments.

Continued

Fig. 15.5 cont'd **Rows 1 to 4 inclusive** depict VA alignments that are normal (solitus or inversus). **Rows 5 to 8 inclusive** depict VA alignments that are abnormal: transposition of the great arteries (TGA), anatomically corrected malposition of the great arteries (ACM). Braces {} mean "the set of." The main cardiac segments are the atria, the ventricles, and the great arteries. The connecting cardiac segments are the AV junction and the conus arteriosus (subarterial infundibulum). The anatomy of the main cardiac segments may be viewed as sets (combinations) and may be abbreviated as follows:

Normal (row 1): The solitus normal heart is {S,D,S}, meaning situs solitus of the atria, that is, {**S**,-,-}, D-loop (or solitus) ventricles, that is, {S,**D**,-}, and solitus normally related great arteries, that is, {S,D,**S**}. The inversus normal heart is {I,L,I}, meaning situs inversus of the atria, that is, {**I**,-,-} with L-loop (inverted) ventricles, that is, {I,**L**,-}, and inverted normally related great arteries, that is, {I,L,**I**}

Isolated atrial discordance (row 2): Isolated atrial noninversion {S,L,I} means the set of solitus atria, L-loop ventricles, and inverted normally related great arteries. Because there is AV situs and alignment discordance, the systemic and pulmonary venous blood streams are physiologically uncorrected, suggesting that an atrial switch procedure (Senning or Mustard) may be helpful. Isolated atrial inversion {I,D,S} had not been described when this diagram was made; hence, the *broken lines.*

Visceroatrial situs ambiguus (A) of the heterotaxy syndromes is not included because atrial situs ambiguus simply means undiagnosed. Atrial situs ambiguus is not a third type of atrial situs. The concept of **atrial isomerism** is an error.

Isolated ventricular discordance (row 3). **{S,L,S} is isolated ventricular inversion.** The atria are in situs solitus, that is, {**S**,-,-}, L-loop (inverted) ventricles are present, that is, {S,**L**,-}, and solitus normally related great arteries, that is {S,L,**S**} are present. Because there is one intersegmental discordance at the AV level, the systemic and pulmonary venous circulations are physiologically uncorrected, again suggesting that an atrial switch procedure may be helpful.

Isolated ventricular noninversion {I,D,I} means the set of inverted atria {**I**,-,-}, D-loop (noninverted) ventricles, {I,**D**,-}, and inverted normally related great arteries, {I,D,**I**}. Again, one segmental discordance (AV) suggests consideration of an atrial switch procedure.

Isolated ventricular discordance, {S,L,S} and {I,D,I} indicates that the ventricles have looped in one direction and that the infundibuloarterial segment has twisted in the opposite direction. In other words, instead of having a C-shaped or reversed C-shaped bulboventricular loop, the bulboventricular loop is S-shaped or reverse S-shaped.

Isolated infundibuloarterial inversion {S,D,I} means the set of solitus atria {**S**,-,-}, D-loop (solitus) ventricles {S,**D**,-}, and inverted normally related great arteries {S,D,**I**}. AV and VA alignment concordances are present. In {S,**D**,**I**}, it is noteworthy that solitus (noninverted) ventricles eject concordantly into inverted normally related great arteries. In other words, despite VA *situs discordance* (solitus ventricles, and inverted normally related great arteries), VA *alignment concordance* is present. **Thus VA situs concordance is not necessary to have normally related great arteries (VA alignment concordance). {S,L,S} documents the same point: VA situs discordance can occur with VA alignment concordance.**

What is necessary to have normally related great arteries?

Infundibuloarterial situs concordance, both noninverted, or both inverted:

SNRGA {S, D, S} = 0R + 4L

SNRGA requires:

1. a solitus subarterial conus, that is, 0R + 4L, and
2. solitus (noninverted) great arteries, that is, Ao to the right of the MPA.

SNRGA { S, D, S} = **0R + 4L**

INRGA requires (1) an inverted subarterial conus, that is, 4R + 0L, and (2) inverted great arteries, that is, Ao to the left of the MPA.

TGA (row 5) typically is present if the conus is subaortic and the subpulmonary conal free wall typically is absent or poorly developed, and it may be obstructive (stenotic or atretic). In TGA, the infundibuloarterial segment and the ventricular loop both twist in the same direction—both to the right or both to the left. In ACM (row 6), the ventricular loop folds in one direction, and the infundibuloarterial segment twists in the opposite direction, resulting in VA alignment concordance. The conus is malformed, either subaortic only, or bilateral (subaortic and subpulmonary). Although ACM has VA alignment concordance, it has VA situs discordance. Note also that VA alignment concordance is very different from normally related great arteries (solitus or inversus). DORV (row 7) can have a bilateral conus (subaortic and subpulmonary), as in the Taussig-Bing malformation (see Fig. 15.4). A bilateral conus is one form of conal situs ambiguus. DOLV (row 8) rarely can have bilateral absence of the conus, a second form of conal situs ambiguus. The aortic valve is indicated by two coronary ostia. The pulmonary valve is indicated by no coronary ostia. There are many other types of human heart that are not depicted here. The segment-by-segment method of diagnosis applies to them all. (Reproduced with permission from Foran RB, Belcourt C, Nanton MA, et al. Isolated infundibuloarterial inversion {S,D,I}: a newly recognized form of congenital heart disease. *Am Heart J.* 1988;116:1337-1350.)[21]

3. At the VA junction, things are different. VA situs concordance typically is associated with VA alignment concordance, as in {S,**D**,S} and {I,**L**,I} **(see Fig. 15.5, row 1).**
4. But **VA situs discordance** also can be associated with **VA alignment concordance** (normally related great arteries), as in {S,**L**,**S**} (see Fig. 15.5, row 3) and as in {S,**D**,**I**} (see Fig. 15.5, row 4).
5. Anatomically corrected malposition of the great arteries (ACM) (see Fig. 15.5, row 6) has VA alignment concordance, but the great arteries are *not* normally related. The conus is either subaortic (only), or bilateral (subaortic and subpulmonary). By contrast, normally related great arteries (solitus and inversus) have a subpulmonary conus (only) (see Fig. 15.5, rows 1 to 4, inclusive). ACM has VA alignment concordance because in all anatomic types of ACM, the ventricles loop in one direction and the infundibuloarterial segment twists in the opposite direction: ACM {S,D,L}, {S,L,D}, {I,L,D}, and {I,D,L} (see Fig. 15.5, row 6).
6. **What does it take to get normally related great arteries?**
   Infundibuloarterial situs concordance is noninverted subarterial conus and noninverted great arteries or inverted subarterial conus and inverted great arteries. Infundibuloarterial situs concordance is present in {S,D,S} and in {I,L,I}. SNRGA {S,D,S} = 0R + 4L, and INRGA {I,L,I} = 4R + 0L (see Fig. 15.5, row 1). **What about {S,L,S}** (see Fig. 15.5, row 3)? Although the ventricular sinuses are inverted, that is, {S,**L**,S}, the formula for the infundibulum is **0R + 4L** (normal solitus or noninverted subarterial conus). The great arteries are noninverted, with the aorta to the right of the pulmonary artery. So, infundibuloarterial situs concordance (both solitus) is present. **What about {S,D,I}** (see Fig. 15.5, row 4)?

   INRGA {I, L, I} = **4R + 0L**

   In {S,D,I}, although the atria and the ventricles are in situs solitus, that is, {**S**,**D**,I}, what matters for the infundibuloarterial segment is (1) that the infundibular situs (pattern of anatomic organization) is inverted; that is, **4R + 0L,** the same as in {I,L,I}, shown earlier, and in Fig. 15.5, row 4, column 1, and (2) that the great arteries also are inverted, with aorta to the left and MPA to the right. So, in {S,D,I}, there is infundibuloarterial situs concordance (both inverted). Consequently, infundibuloarterial situs concordance (both solitus or both inversus) results in great arteries that are normally connected, normally aligned, and normally related (solitus normal, or inversus normal).
7. What causes transposition of the great arteries?
   The answer is infundibuloarterial situs discordance. In typical D-transposition of the great arteries (TGA), that is, TGA {S,D,D}, the great arteries are noninverted, with the aorta to the right of the pulmonary artery. For noninverted great arteries to be normally connected, normally aligned, and normally spatially related, a noninverted conal connector is needed, as in SNRGA {S,D,S} = **0R + 4L.** But in typical D-TGA (see Fig. 15.5, row 5, column 1), the following infundibuloarterial equation is typical: TGA {S,D,D} = **4R + 0L.** Hence; D-TGA is characterized by subarterial infundibular inversion (R-L reversal); that is, the conal anatomy in D-TGA is the inverted normal type:

   INRGA {I, L, I} = **4R + 0L**

   So typical D-TGA has an inverted conal connector and noninverted great arteries. Infundibuloarterial situs discordance is present. What about congenitally physiologically corrected L-TGA? TGA {S,L,L} = **0R + 4L** (see Fig. 15.5, row 5, column 2). The conus in typical L-TGA is of the normal solitus type:

   SNRGA {S, D, D} = **0R + 4L**

   But in TGA {S,L,**L**}, the great arteries are inverted: the ascending aorta is to the left of the MPA. **So, typical L-TGA also has infundibuloarterial situs discordance**: a *noninverted* (solitus) subarterial infundibulum, with *inverted* great arteries. Hence, infundibuloarterial situs discordance is present: a *noninverted* conal connector with *inverted* great arteries.
8. A bilaterally well-developed conus (subaortic and subpulmonary, as in the Taussig-Bing type of double-outlet right ventricle [DORV]; see Fig. 15.4), and a bilaterally absent conus (no subaortic and no subpulmonary infundibular muscle, as in the Paul type of DOLV) both may be regarded as two different forms of subarterial **conal situs ambiguus** that may be associated with DORV and double-outlet LV, respectively.
9. There is only one normal anatomic type of subarterial conal situs, with solitus and inversus isomers:

   SNRGA {S, D, D} = **0R + 4L**, and INRGA {I, L, I} = **4R + 0L**

   Any other conal anatomic pattern is abnormal and results in a conotruncal (infundibuloarterial) malformation (see Table 15.1).
10. Diagnosing the situs of the subarterial conus (infundibulum), which may be the same as, or different from, that of the ventricular sinuses, is new. These infundibuloarterial equations help delineate the situs of the subarterial conus. There are four anatomic types of subarterial conus:
    a. solitus (noninverted),
    b. inverted (mirror-image of solitus),
    c. bilateral (subaortic and subpulmonary), one type of conal situs ambiguus, and
    d. bilaterally absent (no subaortic and no subpulmonary conal musculature), the other type of conal situs ambiguus.

REFERENCES

1. Van Praagh R. The importance of segmental situs in the diagnosis of congenital heart disease. *Semin Roentgenol.* 1985;20:254–271.
2. Taussig HB, Bing RJ. Complete transposition of the aorta and a levoposition of the pulmonary artery; clinical, physiological, and pathological findings. *Am Heart J.* 1949;37:551–559.
3. Van Praagh R. What is the Taussig-Bing malformation? *Circulation.* 1968;38:445–449.
4. Paul MH, Muster AJ, Sinha SN, Cole RB, Van Praagh R. Double-outlet left ventricle with an intact ventricular septum: clinical and autopsy diagnosis and developmental implications. *Circulation.* 1970;41:129–139.
5. Van Praagh R, Van Praagh S. The anatomy of common aorticopulmonary trunk (truncus arteriosus communis) and its embryologic implications, a study of 57 necropsied cases. *Am J Cardiol.* 1965;16:406–425.
6. Calder L, Van Praagh R, Van Praagh S, et al. Truncus arteriosus communis: clinical, angiocardiographic, and pathologic findings in 100 patients. *Am Heart J.* 1976;92:23–38.
7. Vizcaino A, Campbell J, Litovsky S, Van Praagh R. Single origin of right and left pulmonary artery branches from ascending aorta with nonbranching main pulmonary artery: relevance to a new understanding of truncus arteriosus. *Pediatr Cardiol.* 2002;23:230–234.
8. Beitzke A, Shinebourne EA. Single origin of right and left pulmonary arteries from ascending aorta, with main pulmonary artery from right ventricle. *Br Heart J.* 1980;43:363–365.
9. Aotsuka H, Nagai Y, Saito M, Matsumoto H, Nakamura T. Anomalous origin of both pulmonary arteries from the ascending aorta with a nonbranching main pulmonary artery arising from the right ventricle. *Pediatr Cardiol.* 1990;11:156–158.
10. Penkoske PA, Castañeda AR, Fyler DC, Van Praagh R. Origin of pulmonary artery branch from ascending aorta. Primary surgical repair in infancy. *J Thorac Cardiovasc Surg.* 85:537–545.
11. Van Praagh R. The cardiovascular keys to air-breathing and permanent land-living in vertebrates: the normal human embryonic aortic switch procedure produced by complete right-left asymmetry in the development of the subarterial conal free walls, and the evolution of the right ventricular sinus. *Kardiochirurgia i Torakochirurgia Polska.* 8:1–22. [Polish abstract. Text in English.]
12. Van Praagh R. The evolution of the human heart and its relevance to congenital heart disease. *Kardiochirurgia i Torakochirurgia Polska.* 4:427–431.
13. Shubin N. *Your Inner Fish, A Journey into the 3.5 Billion-Year History of the Human Body.* New York: Vintage Books, a Division of Random House, Inc; 2009:1–237.
14. Van Praagh R. Transposition of the great arteries: history, pathologic anatomy, embryology, etiology, and surgical considerations. *Card Surg: State of the Art Reviews.* 1991;5:7–82.
15. Van Praagh R, Van Praagh S. Anatomically corrected transposition of the great arteries. *Br Heart J.* 1967;29:112–119.
16. Van Praagh R, Durnin RE, Jockin H, et al. Anatomically corrected malposition of the great arteries {S, D, L}. *Circulation.* 1975;51:20–31.
17. Van Praagh R, Van Praagh ADG, Lacour-Gayet F: Anatomically corrected malposition of the great arteries. In: Lacour-Gayet F, Bove EL, Hraska V, et al (Eds). *Surgery of Conotruncal Malformations.* Springer Verlag. 2016; 517–534.
18. Asami I. Partitioning of the arterial end of the embryonic heart. In: Van Praagh R, Takao A, eds. *Etiology and Morphogenesis of Congenital Heart Disease.* Mount Kisco, NY: Futura Publishing Co; 1980:51–61.
19. Keith A. The Hunterian Lectures on malformations of the heart (lecture 2). *Lancet.* 1909;2:433.
20. Van Praagh R, Van Praagh S. Isolated ventricular inversion. A consideration of the morphogenesis, definition, and diagnosis of nontransposed and transposed great arteries. *Am J Cardiol.* 1966;17:395–406.
21. Foran RB, Belcourt C, Nanton MA, et al. Isolated infundibuloarterial inversion {S,D,I}: a newly recognized form of congenital heart disease. *Am Heart J.* 1988;116:1337–1350.

16

Ventricular Septal Defects

In 1989, Dr. John Kirklin asked me how I thought ventricular septal defects (VSDs) should be described, named, and classified. Soto, Ceballos, and Kirklin[1] were just about to publish their best thoughts on this important topic, and Dr. Kirklin asked me and my colleagues[2] to do the same.

COMPONENTS OF THE VENTRICULAR SEPTUM

The four main anatomic components that make up the normal ventricular septum are as follows (Fig. 16.1)[2]:

1. the septum of the atrioventricular (AV) canal (component 1);
2. the muscular ventricular septum, or the ventricular sinus septum (component 2);
3. the septal band, or the proximal conal septum (component 3); and
4. the parietal band, or the distal conal septum (component 4).

Anatomic Types of Ventricular Septal Defect

VSD of the AV Canal Type. The septum of the AV canal (see Fig. 16.1, component 1)[2] is completely absent in *the complete form of common AV canal.*

In *the incomplete form of common AV canal,* the septum of the AV canal is absent above the leaflets of the AV valve(s) but present below the leaflets of the common AV valve. In other words, typically there is no VSD of the AV canal type in the incomplete form of common AV canal. Also typically, there is a cleft in the anterior leaflet of the mitral valve.

The incomplete form of common AV canal is also known as an *ostium primum defect with a cleft anterior mitral leaflet.* Accurately speaking, an ostium primum defect is an incomplete AV septal defect, not an atrial septal defect (ASD). The posterosuperior margin of an ostium primum defect is the anteroinferior margin of the atrial septum. Ostium primum defects have often been called, *inaccurately,* ostium primum *atrial septal* defects because the associated shunt (left to right, or right to left) is above the leaflets of the AV valve(s)—like an ASD. However, it is helpful to know that many different types of shunt occur above the leaflets of the AV valve(s). Ostium primum defects and ASDs are just two of many different anatomic types of abnormal communication that can occur above the AV valve(s).

Straddling tricuspid valve also has a VSD of the AV canal type. Typically, the right ventricular sinus (body or inflow tract) is underdeveloped compared with the left ventricular sinus. Consequently, the muscular ventricular septum (see Fig. 16.1, component 2) is located well to the right of the normally located atrial septum. The muscular ventricular septum lies beneath approximately the middle of the normally located tricuspid orifice. This ventriculoatrial septal malalignment results in a straddling tricuspid valve with biventricular insertions of the tricuspid tensor apparatus, a VSD of the AV canal type between components 1 and 2 (see Fig. 16.1),[2] and often with no septal defect above the level of the AV valves.

A defect in the septum of the AV canal (see Fig. 16.1, component 1) is also known as an **AV septal defect.** AV septal defects occur both with and without common AV canal. An AV septal defect is an integral part of common AV canal, both complete and partial forms.

But an AV septal defect also occurs *without* common AV canal, as in a **Gerbode defect.** There is a left ventricle (LV)–to–right atrium (RA) shunt through a defect in the AV portion of the membranous ventricular septum, predominantly above the tricuspid valve. Megarity et al[3] published a well-documented case of double-outlet right ventricle (DORV) with no VSD and with an LV-to-RA shunt. This patient did not have a common AV canal.

We avoid the term AV septal defect because of its confused usage. Some of our colleagues use this designation when they mean common AV canal. For clarity, we prefer the terms **common AV canal** and **LV-to-RA shunt,** because these terms make their different meanings clear.

We also avoid the designation inlet septal defect because this term is not specific. This term may apply to component 1, or to component 2, or to the component 1-2 junction (see Fig. 16.1). We prefer anatomically specific diagnoses in the interests of accuracy and clarity: defect in the septum of the AV canal, defect in the muscular ventricular septum, or defect at the junction of these two septal components. The latter diagnoses are anatomically accurate and their meanings are clear.

Muscular VSDs. Muscular VSDs are openings in the muscular ventricular septum, also known as the ventricular sinus septum. Muscular VSDs, which is what these defects have long been called, involve component 2 (see Fig. 16.1).

Mid-muscular VSDs are often located at the junction of components 2 and 3 (see Fig. 16.1). From the right ventricular aspect, such apertures are seen slightly above or slightly below the septal band (see Fig. 16.1A, component 3). From the left ventricular

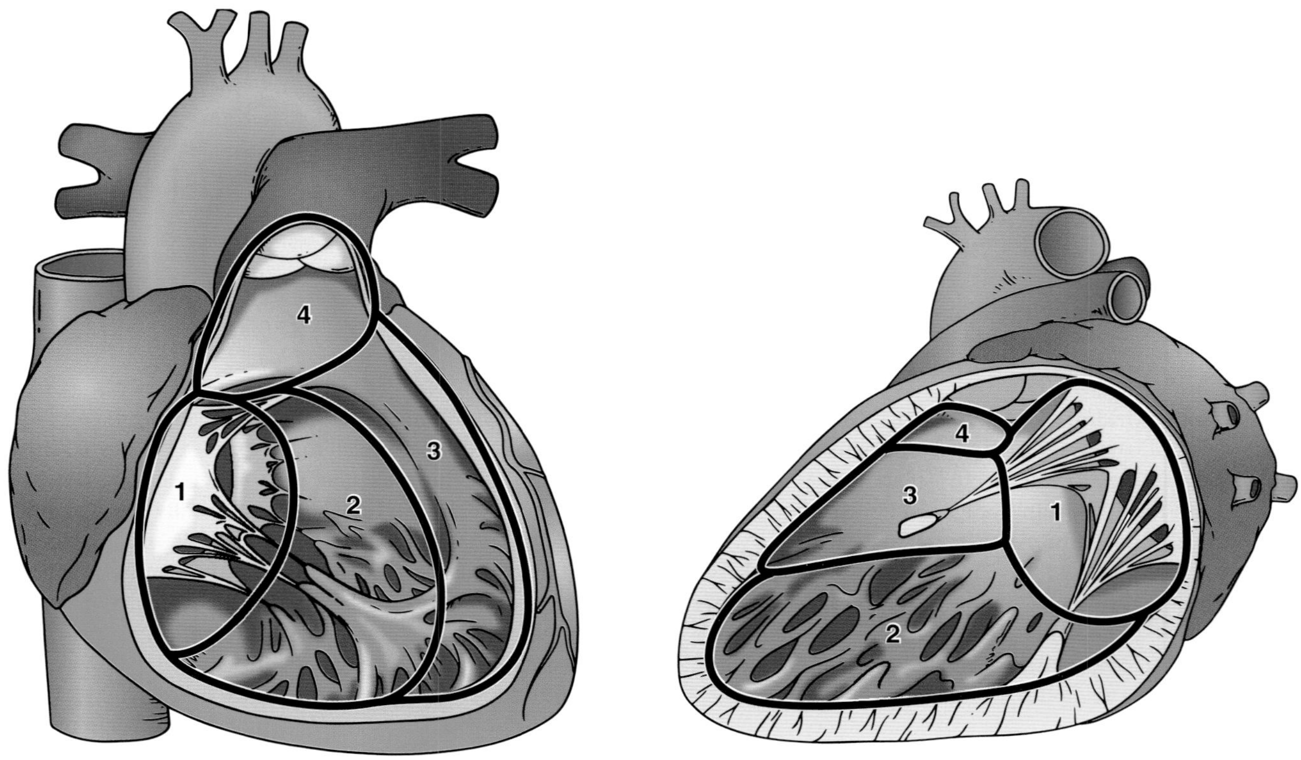

Fig. 16.1 The Four Main Anatomic and Developmental Components of the Interventricular Septum of the Normal Heart. (A) Morphologically right ventricle (RV). (B) Morphologically left ventricle (LV). **Component 1**, septum of the atrioventricular canal. **Component 2**, muscular ventricular septum, or sinus septum. **Component 3**, septal band in A, or proximal infundibular (conal) septum; in B, **component 3** is the proximal conal septum that forms the superior, nontrabeculated portion of the left ventricular septal surface. **Component 4**, the distal or subarterial infundibular septum. **Component 1** is also known as the atrioventricular (AV) septum. **Components 1 and 2** form the right ventricular inflow tract and the left ventricular inflow tract. **Components 3 and 4** form the right ventricular outflow tract and the left ventricular outflow tract. The **moderator band** joins the septal band (component 3) to the anterior papillary muscle of the RV in A. The moderator band is also known as the **septomarginal trabeculation** because it runs from the right ventricular septal surface (septo) to the acute margin of the RV (marginalis). Some of our colleagues use the term septomarginal trabeculation to mean both the septal band and the moderator band. The lower portion of the distal conal septum (component 4) is also known as the **crista suprventricularis** because it forms a supraventricular crest above the right ventricular sinus (component 2). (Reproduced with permission from Van Praagh R, Geva T, Kreutzer J. Ventricular septal defects: how shall we describe, name and classify them? *J Am Coll Cardiol.* 1989;14:1298.)

aspect, mid-muscular VSDs typically are found at the junction of the smooth or nontrabeculated portion of the ventricular septum superiorly (see Fig. 16.1B, component 3)[2] and the finely trabeculated part of the ventricular septum inferiorly (see Fig. 16.1B, component 2). These mid-muscular VSDs are sometimes called *trabecular defects.* Why? Because they are close to the septal band, as noted earlier. Some of our colleagues call the septal band the *trabecular septomarginalis* or the *septomarginal trabeculation.* The term *trabecular septomarginalis* was introduced in 1911 by Tandler for the structure that we now call the moderator band. *Trabecula septomarginalis* (Latin) means "little beam" (*trabecular*) that runs from the septum *(septo)* to the acute margin of the RV *(marginalis).* So, the *trabecular septomarginalis*, or *septomarginal trabeculation,* means the moderator band, not the septal band. But those who revived Tandler's term, *trabecular septomarginalis,* being unfamiliar with Latin, did not understand what Tandler's term really meant. So, they applied *trabecular septomarginalis* and its English equivalent *septomarginal trabeculation* to the septal band and the moderator band.

The foregoing is intended as an explanation, not as a criticism. The history of language is full of similar changes. Indeed, in terminology, the only constant we know is change. But it should be *slow* change, and *necessary* change, to minimize confusion and linguistic errors. What do we think is *necessary* terminologic change?

1. If there is no extant term, the introduction of a designation may be necessary.
2. If the extant term (or terms) is (are) inaccurate, a new and accurate designation may be necessary.

The foregoing explains why mid-muscular VSDs are called trabecular VSDs by some of our colleagues: *trabecular* comes from *trabecula* septomarginalis, or septomarginal *trabeculations,* that is, from the renaming of the septal band by some of our colleagues (see Fig. 16.1A).[2]

Muscular VSDs can be found in many different locations within component 2, and at its junctions with components 1 and/or 3 (see Fig. 16.1). Mid-muscular VSDs do not involve component 3, as seen from the right ventricular aspect (see Fig. 16.1A). Instead, mid-muscular VSDs lie behind and to the left of the septal band.

Ironically, the muscular ventricular septum (see Fig. 16.1A–B, component 2)[2] is trabeculated. The right ventricular septal surface is coarsely trabeculated (see Fig. 16.1A, component 2), whereas the left ventricular surface (see Fig. 16.1B, component 2) is finely trabeculated. Thus, although component 3 is not trabeculated per se (see Fig. 16.1A–B), component 2 is coarsely trabeculated on the right ventricular side and finely trabeculated on the left ventricular side (see Fig. 16.1A–B).[2]

Infundibuloventricular Defects. Infundibuloventricular defects lie between the infundibular (or conal) septum above (see Fig. 16.1A, component 4, and B) and the ventricular septum below (see Fig. 16.1A–B, components 1, 2, and 3).[2] Infundibuloventricular defects are also known as *conoventricular VSDs*. The infundibular or conal septum (see Fig. 16.1A–B component 4) is the "lid" that normally fits on top of and seals the ventricular septal complex[2]:

1. the septum of the AV canal (see Fig. 16.1A–B, component 1), the top of which in the normally formed heart is called the *membranous septum;*
2. the muscular ventricular sinus septum (see Fig. 16.1A–B component 2); and
3. the septal band (see Fig. 16.1A, component 3), and the proximal infundibular or outflow tract septum (see Fig. 16.1B, component 3).[2]

Thus, the ventricular septal complex is a tetralogy: components 1 to 4, inclusive (see Fig. 16.1A–B).[2] To achieve a normal heart, each of these four septal components must be normally formed, normally aligned, and normally connected.

Infundibular Septal Defects. Infundibular septal defects result from an anomaly of, or within, component 4 (see Fig. 16.1A–B).[2] These malformations are also known as conal septal defects.

RELATIVE FREQUENCIES OF THE FOUR ANATOMIC TYPES OF VENTRICULAR SEPTAL DEFECT

The four anatomic types of VSD are:

1. AV canal type of VSD[2] (Dr. Jesse Edwards' term), also known as inlet septal defect[1] (term of Soto et al);
2. muscular VSDs,[2] also known as inlet septal defects or trabecular defects (terms of Soto et al[1]);
3. infundibuloventricular (or conoventricular) VSDs (our terms),[2] also known as infundibuloventricular (or conoventricular) VSD, (terms of Soto et al[1]); and
4. infundibular septal (or conal septal) VSDs (our terms),[2] also known as right ventricular outlet VSDs (term of Soto et al[1]).

The relative frequencies of these four anatomic types of VSD found in 76 patients of Soto, Ceballos, and Kirklin[1] are presented in Table 16.1.

TABLE 16.1 Frequencies of Four Anatomic Types of VSD (n = 76), Soto et al[1]

Anatomic Type of VSD	No. of Cases	Percent of Series
Atrioventricular Canal Type	7	9
Muscular	23	30
Infundibuloventricular	25	33
Infundibular septal	21	28

Why is understanding the four main anatomic and developmental components that normally make up the ventricular septum (see Fig. 16.1) so important? Because VSDs occur within, and/or between, these four main ventricular septal components (see Fig. 16.1). This anatomic and developmental understanding is the key to understanding VSDs.

What is a membranous VSD? Membranous VSDs typically occur toward the top of the membranous septum of the AV canal (see Fig. 16.1A, component 1), just beneath a well-developed and normally located distal conal septum or parietal band (see Fig. 16.1A, component 4). For a VSD to be regarded as membranous, *only* the membranous septum should be abnormal. Everything else should appear to be normal. In particular, the distal conal septum (parietal band) should appear to be normal (see Fig. 16.1A, component 4).

Is the distal infundibular septum (see Fig. 16.1A, component 4) a little hypoplastic or mildly abnormally located? If it is, we do not make the diagnosis of membranous VSD, because such VSDs (with an abnormal parietal band, that is, Fig. 16.1A, component 4) are *more* than membranous. In such cases, we make the diagnosis of an **infundibuloventricular (or conoventricular) VSD.** The diagnosis of infundibuloventricular VSD does *not* imply that the distal conal septum (component 4) is normally formed, whereas the diagnosis of membranous VSD does have this connotation. Membranous VSD implies that the distal conal septum (component 4) is normally formed and that the defect is in the membranous septum only. Frequently, this is not the case. Infundibuloventricular VSDs often have hypoplastic and/or malaligned distal infundibular septa (components 4).

Malalignment infundibuloventricular VSDs often are associated with infundibuloarterial (conotruncal) malformations such as tetralogy of Fallot (TOF), truncus arteriosus, transposition of the great arteries (TGA), DORV, double-outlet left ventricle (DOLV), and anatomically corrected malposition of the great arteries (MPA).

A VSD may or may not be confluent with one or both semilunar valves and/or with one or both AV valves. For example, when a VSD is confluent with the tricuspid valve, such a VSD may be described as *paratricuspid* (*para* = "beside," in Greek), or as *juxtatricuspid* (*juxta* = "beside," in Latin). A VSD can be confluent with the membranous septum. Such VSDs are *paramembranous* (para = **beside, or confluent with, in Greek**).

Some of our colleagues describe such VSDs as *perimembranous*. Unfortunately, this is a semantic error. *Peri* means "around" in Greek. An infundibuloventricular VSD can be confluent with the membranous septum *(paramembranous)*. But such a VSD never surrounds the membranous septum. If the

TABLE 16.2 **Frequencies of the Different Anatomic Types of Ventricular Septal Defect in the Present Study of 3216 Autopsied Cases of Congenital Heart Disease**

Anatomic Type of VSD	No. of Cases	Percent of Series		
Atrioventricular canal type	91	2.83		
Muscular	203	6.31		
Infundibuloventricular	682	(21.21)	851	26.46
Membranous	169	(5.25)		
Infundibular septal	15	0.47		

VSDs, multiple, 128; 3.98%; VSDs, restrictive, 4, 0.12%.

membranous septum were surrounded by a VSD, the membranous septum would be floating freely in space, attached to nothing. No such VSD has ever been documented.

By analogy, the *para*thyroid gland is correctly named, meaning *beside* the thyroid gland. The designation *peri*thyroid gland, meaning "around" the thyroid gland, would be absurd, because there is no such gland. Similarly, the designation *perimembranous* VSD is simply an error in terminology, because there is no such VSD.

Of the 3400 autopsied cases of heart disease in infants and children on which this book is based, 3216 had congenital heart disease (94.59%). The remaining 184 patients had acquired (not congenital) heart disease (5.41%). Of the 3216 patients with congenital heart disease, 1160 had a VSD (36.07%). Of these 1160 patients with a VSD, 128 had multiple VSDs (11.03%).

Table 16.2 needs a little clarification. Membranous VSDs (n = 169) are regarded as a subset of infundibuloventricular VSDs (with a normally developed distal conal septum; see Fig. 16.1A, component 4). Membranous VSDs accounted for 5.25% of the series of congenital heart disease as a whole (n = 3216). The other cases of infundibuloventricular VSD with an abnormally located component 4 (n = 682) composed 21.2% of the series as a whole. Thus, conoventricular or infundibuloventricular VSDs as a whole were found in 26.46% of this series of 3216 cases of congenital heart disease (see Table 16.2). VSDs that were hemodynamically disadvantageously restrictive (not big enough) were found in 4 patients (0.12%; see Table 16.2, footnote).

VSDs of all anatomic types were by far the most common form of congenital heart disease found in this series of 3216 cases of congenital heart disease: 1160 of 3216 = 0.36069, or 36.07%.

LIMITATIONS OF THESE STATISTICS

Even though Table 16.2 is based on a large number of patients with congenital heart disease (3216), these statistics have limits to their accuracy that should be acknowledged:

1. These patients are all autopsied cases, which is both good and bad. The good part is that the diagnoses are accurate, that is, with no clinical guesswork. The bad part is that these cases are all fatalities; thus, these statistics are skewed in the direction of badness (greater severity of disease than in the pediatric population of congenital heart disease as a whole).
2. These statistics (see Table 16.2) are based on the number of patients in which VSD appears in the diagnosis. This means that TOF is omitted because a subaortic, malalignment infundibuloventricular type of VSD is *understood* to be present in TOF and hence is not stated.

If the conoventricular VSDs of our patients with TOF are included in these VSD statistics (see Table 16.2), as they certainly should be, **the number of patients with VSD increases from 1160 (see Table 16.2) + 428 (TOF) to a new total of 1588, which is 49.38% of the whole series of congenital heart disease patients (n = 3216).**

Similarly, if truncus arteriosus communis is included (only 1 of our 111 cases of truncus arteriosus had an intact ventricular septum), then 110 more cases of VSD should be included. **This new final total of cases with a VSD equals 1698, of a total number of 3216 patients with congenital heart disease; that is, 52.8% of our patients had a VSD.** This is a much higher percentage of patients with VSD than is usually found, because TOF and truncus arteriosus are often omitted. Thus, a VSD was present in more than half of our autopsied congenital heart patients: **almost 53%.**

VENTRICULAR SEPTAL DEFECT WITH AND WITHOUT AORTIC INSUFFICIENCY

One of the first questions that Dr. Robert E. Gross, our chief of the Department of Surgery, asked me to try to solve after I joined the staff of Boston Children's Hospital in late 1965 was: **Why do some patients with VSD have aortic insufficiency (AI; aortic regurgitation) whereas others do not?** Dr. Gross suggested that I work with Dr. J. Judson McNamara,[4] one of Dr. Gross's Cardiac surgery residents, who later went on to have a distinguished surgical career in Hawaii.

Nadas et al[5] found that of 756 patients with VSD studied at Boston Children's Hospital between 1948 and 1962, only 34 developed AI (4.5%). Because clinical signs of AI were not discovered during the first year of life in 18 carefully followed patients (protodiastolic blowing murmur and wide pulse pressure), Nadas et al[5] concluded that AI is an *acquired* complication of VSD, *not* a congenital anomaly per se. Similarly, Halloran et al[6] reported 12 patients with VSD and AI; in only one of whom was a diastolic murmur heard within the first year of life, at 6 months of age. In 11 postmortem cases, we found 4 that there are essentially two anatomic types of VSD with AI (Fig. 16.2):

1. with an infundibuloventricular (subcristal) VSD in 7 of 11 (64%); and
2. with an infundibular septal defect (subpulmonary VSD) in 4 of 11 (36%).

When the VSD was of the infundibuloventricular variety, 3 patients had no infundibular outflow tract stenosis (see Fig. 16.2, *left column;* we called this type Ia),[4] and 4 patients had infundibular outflow tract stenosis (see Fig. 16.2, *middle column,* type Ib).[4] When the VSD was of the subpulmonary infundibular septal defect type (see Fig. 16.2, *right column,* type II) as in 4 patients, there was always pulmonary outflow tract stenosis.[4]

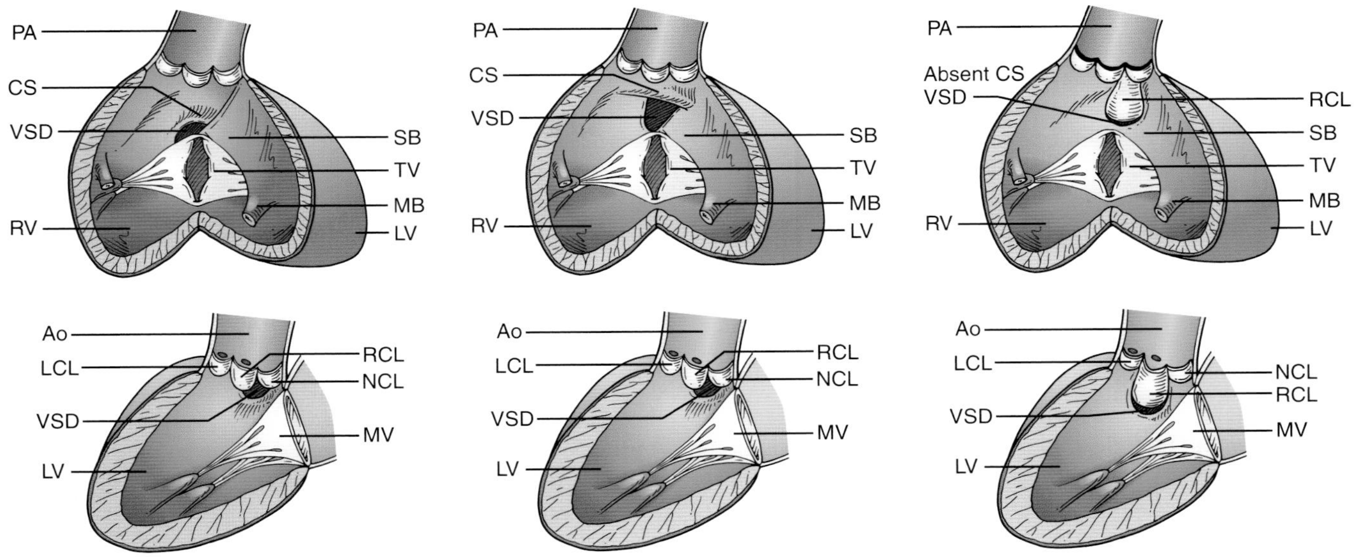

Fig. 16.2 Infundibuloventricular (or Conoventricular) Type of Ventricular Septal Defects *(VSDs)* With Aortic Insufficiency (AI) *(left and center columns)*. The AI is caused by the coexistence of a bicommisural aortic valve, with absence of the right coronary/noncoronary (RC/NC) commissure. The large combined right coronary leaflet *(RCL)* plus noncoronary leaflet *(NCL)* prolapses downward and does not coapt normally with the normal left coronary leaflet *(LCL)*, resulting in AI. The subarterial infundibular (or conal) septum *(CS)* (also known as the infundibular septum and as the parietal band) may be well formed and approximately normally located *(left column, top row)*. Or the CS may be hypoplastic and abnormally located, deviated anteriorly, superiorly, and leftward (CS, *middle column, top row*). Depending on the severity of the subpulmonary infundibular stenosis, there may be right ventricular *(RV)* outflow tract obstruction as in **tetralogy of Fallot:** hemodynamically significant subpulmonary infundibular hypoplasia reflected as stenosis or atresia *(middle column, top row)*. The hypoplastic subpulmonary infundibulum may be secondarily hypertrophied. Or there may be no right ventricular outflow tract obstruction, as in the **Eisenmenger complex:** hemodynamically insignificant subpulmonary infundibular hypoplasia *(middle column, top row)*. An anatomically different type of VSD with AI is depicted in the *right column*. A **conal or infundibular septal defect** is present. The infundibular septum has failed to form, completely or in part. In the infundibular septal defect, the VSD is both subpulmonary and subaortic *(right column)*. The infundibular septal type of VSD is doubly committed, subaortic and subpulmonary. In the infundibuloventricular type of defect, the VSD is subaortic only *(left and middle columns)*. With infundibular septal defects, the aortic valve per se is normally formed: it is tricommissural. However, the infundibular septal defect is located completely beneath the RCL of the aortic valve. Consequently, the RCL of the aortic valve is unsupported below, facilitating downward prolapse of the RCL, with or without herniation of the RCL of the aortic valve into the right ventricular outflow tract. This results in AI, with or without a pulmonary outflow tract gradient. The RCL can reduce the size of the subsemilunar defect, or close it altogether. When an infundibuloventricular type of VSD is associated with a hypoplastic and antero-leftwardly malaligned CS *(middle column)*, the VSD is larger than when there is little or no malalignment of the CS *(left column)*. With CS malalignment *(middle column)*, the VSD lies more beneath the RCL of the aortic valve than it does when the CS is normally located *(left column)*. Thus, it is the *right* coronary leaflet component of a bicuspid aortic valve (RCL + NCL) that tends to prolapse most severely into the left ventricle *(LV)* and to herniate into the right ventricular outflow tract both with an infundibuloventricular VSD *(middle column)* and with an infundibular septal type of VSD *(right column)*. Thus, no matter which type of VSD is present, it typically is the right coronary leaflet of the aortic valve that prolapses and herniates most severely. *Ao,* Ascending aorta; *MB,* moderator band; *MV,* mitral valve; *PA,* main pulmonary artery; *RV,* morphologically right ventricle; *SB,* septal band; *TV,* tricuspid valve; *TSM, Trabecula* septomarginalis, TSM was Tandler's term for the moderator band; *SMT,* septomarginal trabeculation. TSM anglicized by Anderson, who applied SMT to both the septal band and the moderator band. (Reproduced with permission from Van Praagh R, McNamara JJ. Anatomic types of ventricular septal defect with aortic insufficiency. *Am Heart J.* 1968;75:604-619.)

The Essential Facts

When an infundibuloventricular VSD was present (see Fig. 16.2, *left and middle columns*), the aortic valve was often bicommissural (5/7 cases, 71.4%). This means that the aortic valve was often functionally bicuspid, because the number of well-formed aortic commissures equals the number of functional aortic leaflets. The deficient or absent aortic commissure in all 5 cases was the right coronary/noncoronary (RC/NC) commissure. This means that the functionally bicuspid aortic valve had just two functional leaflets: (1) a combined RC plus NC leaflet; and (2) a smaller left coronary (LC) leaflet (see Fig. 16.2, *lower row, left and middle columns*).

During the first year of postnatal life, the combined and poorly supported RC/NC leaflet got stretched (because it lacked RC/NC commissural support). The poorly supported RC/NC leaflet prolapsed downward, into the left ventricular outflow tract. When the large and prolapsing RC/NC leaflet could no longer coapt with the smaller, higher LC leaflet, AI appeared and progressively became more marked.

In the 4 patients with an infundibular (conal) septal type of subpulmonary VSD, the aortic valve was always tricommissural. None had a commissural deficiency or absence (see Fig. 16.2, *right column, lower row*). Instead, these 4 patients had a normally formed RC leaflet that prolapsed inferiorly and herniated partially through the subpulmonary conal septal defect into the right ventricular outflow tract, where it produced pulmonary outflow tract stenosis. Prolapse and herniation of the RC leaflet of the aortic valve also led to lack of aortic leaflet coaptation and AI.

In Fig. 16.2, left ventricular diagrams *(lower row)*, note that in the *left and middle drawings*, the RC/NC commissures are absent, whereas in the *right LV diagram*, all three aortic commissures are well formed. Also note that in Fig. 16.2 diagrams, when a conoventricular VSD is present *(left and middle left ventricular diagrams)*, the missing RC/NC commissure of the aortic valve is located above the *middle* of the conoventricular VSD. In other words, when a conoventricular VSD is present, the VSD lies approximately beneath half of the RC leaflet, and beneath approximately half of the NC leaflet.

But when a conal septal defect is present (see Fig. 16.2, *right diagrams*) the VSD lies beneath the RC leaflet only. This difference in aortic valve and VSD alignment appears to be important. This is why when a subpulmonary conal septal VSD is present, an RC aortic leaflet hernia into the RV outflow tract occurs (see Fig. 16.2, *right diagrams*). However, when a conoventricular VSD is present, an aortic leaflet hernia does not occur. Instead, if AI appears, the problem usually is due to RC/NC aortic commissural deficiency or absence and stretching of the combined RC + NC leaflets.

Is the foregoing explanation of AI with a VSD always true? No. Why not? We[4] had 1 patient with a conoventricular VSD with pulmonary infundibular stenosis and no aortic commissural deficiency who, nonetheless, had prolapse of the RC/NC aortic leaflets with herniation of the RC aortic leaflet into the right ventricular outflow tract, resulting in a right ventricular outflow tract gradient of 13 mm Hg. How do we explain this exception? In our 4 cases with conoventricular VSD and deviation of the parietal band, none had clinical cyanosis. Instead, they resembled mild, acyanotic TOF. But in 1 patient (Case 7),[4] there was enough anterior, superior, and leftward deviation of the parietal band (component 4) to permit prolapse and herniation of a normally formed RC aortic leaflet into the right ventricular outflow tract.

SUMMARY

1. When AI develops in a patient with a conoventricular VSD, the cause of the AI usually is an aortic valve anomaly: absence of an aortic valve commissure.
2. When AI develops in a patient with a subpulmonary conal septal defect, the cause of the AI usually is an RC aortic leaflet hernia, the aortic valve being normally formed.
3. When AI develops in a patient with a conoventricular VSD and a TOF type of infundibular stenosis, if the distal conal septum is deviated sufficiently anteriorly, superiorly, and to the left, a normally formed RC leaflet of the aortic valve occasionally can herniate into the right ventricular outflow tract.
4. Careful diagnosis and early surgical management are necessary to prevent the aortic leaflets being stretched and deformed by prolapse and herniation.
5. Heart specimen photographs are presented in Figs. 16.3 through 16.7.

As noted earlier, when the infundibuloventricular VSD is present (see Fig. 16.2, *left and middle columns*), the VSD is beneath the *posterior half* of the RC leaflet and the anterior half of the NC aortic leaflet. However, when an infundibular septal VSD is present, the VSD is *more anterior.* The VSD typically lies *entirely beneath* the RC aortic leaflet, not just half beneath the RC leaflet. Consequently, when an infundibular septal VSD is present, RC aortic leaflet prolapse downward and herniation into the right ventricular outflow tract is more probable than when an infundibuloventricular VSD is present, *because the VSD is more anterior with a conal septal type of VSD.*

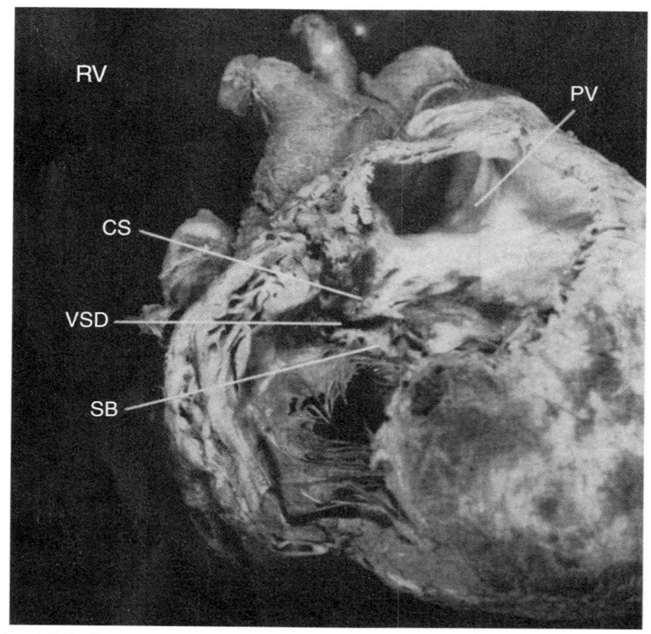

Fig. 16.3 Opened right ventricle *(RV)* showing a small infundibuloventricular type of ventricular septal defect *(VSD)* between a normally located conal septum *(CS)* or infundibular septum above and the septal band *(SB)* and ventricular septum below. There is no right ventricular outflow tract obstruction. The subpulmonary CS is normal, as in Fig. 16.2 *(left column, top row)*. The patient was 3 8/12-year old boy. The VSD measured 4 × 2 mm. The aortic valve was bicommissural because of deficiency of the right coronary-noncoronary (RC/NC) commissure. The RC/NC leaflet prolapsed into the left ventricular cavity, causing aortic insufficiency (or regurgitation). There was no right ventricular outflow tract gradient. The VSD appeared too small to permit herniation of the combined RC leaflet plus the NC leaflet of the aortic valve. This type of defect has also been called a ***membranous VSD*** and a ***subcristal VSD***. *PV,* Pulmonary valve. (Reproduced from Van Praagh R, McNamara JJ. Anatomic types of ventricular septal defect with aortic insufficiency. *Am Heart J.* 1968;75:604-619.)

The exception to this statement is when an infundibuloventricular VSD is associated with marked deviation of the parietal band (component 4) in a leftward, anterior, and superior direction, making the VSD unusually anterior. This is also why a conal septal VSD may be accurately described as a *doubly committed subarterial VSD*. An infundibular septal VSD is both subpulmonary (see Fig. 16.2, *right column, top row*) and subaortic, with downward prolapse and rightward herniation of the RC aortic leaflet (see Fig. 16.2, *right column, bottom row*). However, an infundibuloventricular type of VSD typically is subaortic only (see Fig. 16.2, *left and middle columns*).

Apical Ventricular Septal Defects

Apical muscular VSDs are the most difficult to visualize through the tricuspid valve and the most difficult to close trans-atrially. Consequently, this has left closure of such defects to using a left apical ventriculotomy. The disadvantages of a systemic ventriculotomy and the possible postoperative complication of a left ventricular apical aneurysm led Dr. Stella Van Praagh to start thinking about a more risk-free approach. It was she who conceived of the right ventricular apical infundibulotomy approach.

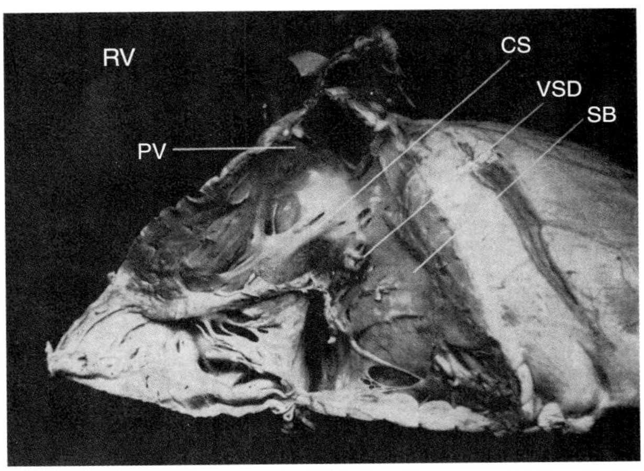

Fig. 16.4 Opened right ventricle *(RV)* showing a small infundibuloventricular type of ventricular septal defect *(VSD)* between an approximately normally located infundibular septum above and a normally located septal band *(SB)* and ventricular septum below. The patient was a 20 7/12-year-old man. The VSD measured only 3 × 2 mm. Note the aneurysm of the membranous septum: see the VSD label. Aneurysms of the membranous septum are thought to be how such conoventricular VSDs can close. Note that the conal septum *(CS)* is unusually far from the tricuspid valve. The CS may be somewhat too short, predisposing to this VSD. "Membranous" VSDs often appear to be more than membranous. This new understanding has spurred the use of other terms such as *paramembranous, juxtamembranous,* and *perimembranous* (which also does not exist, accurately speaking). This patient also had a bicuspid (bicommissural) aortic valve—a rudimentary right coronary/left coronary (RC/LC) commissure. The combined RC/LC leaflet did not prolapse downward (as expected). Instead, the noncoronary aortic leaflet prolapsed, despite the fact that it was supported by two normal-appearing commissures. However, this young man also had a history of subacute bacterial endocarditis and cerebral infarction. We did not know whether subacute bacterial endocarditis played a role in this patient's prolapse of his normally supported NC leaflet. *PV,* pulmonary valve. (Reproduced with permission from Van Praagh R, McNamara JJ. Anatomic types of ventricular septal defect with aortic insufficiency. *Am Heart J.* 1968;75:604-619.)

Dr. Giovanni Stellin,[7] a friend and colleague from Padua, Italy, was so impressed that he tried it, liked it, and published it with us in 2000. Dr. Stella Van Praagh et al[8] published a follow-up in 2002.

The background to this surgical success is as follows. Thanks to Dr. Maurice Lev, we had long understood that the RV has two apices (Fig. 16.8A–B): the right ventricular sinus or inflow tract apex, proximal to the moderator band, and the infundibular or outflow tract apex, distal to the moderator band. The infundibular or outflow tract apex is also known as the infundibular apical recess.

Double-chambered RV shows these two component parts of the RV with great clarity. Many people do not understand that the septal band and the moderator band are apical infundibular structures. They think that the infundibulum begins with the parietal band (component 4). Typically, the apical muscular VSD opens from the left ventricular apex into the infundibular apical recess (the infundibular apex).

The surgery of the right ventricular apical infundibulotomy is presented diagrammatically in Fig. 16.9. The surgical incision is parallel to, and to the right of the distal part of the anterior descending coronary artery. The length of this incision, which extends close to the apex of the heart, varies from 1.5 to 2.5 cm. The apical muscular VSD can extend above and below the moderator band, opening into both the infundibular and the right ventricular sinus apices.

In Fig. 16.10, a heart specimen with an apical muscular VSD is presented. The patient was a 2.5-month-old girl who also had a coarctation of the aorta and a patent ductus arteriosus (PDA). In Fig, 16.10A, the opened right ventricle (RV) is

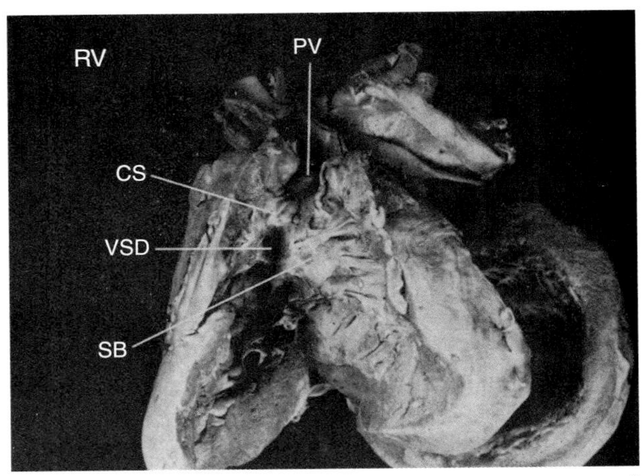

Fig. 16.5 Opened right ventricle *(RV)* showing an anterosuperiorly deviated and shortened conal (infundibular) septum *(CS)*. There is a large conoventricular type of ventricular septal defect *(VSD)* between the malaligned CS above and the normally located septal band *(SB)* below. The VSD measured 13 × 10 mm. The patient was a 7 11/2-year-old boy. The patient had a pulmonary outflow tract gradient of 40 mm Hg and a bicuspid pulmonary valve *(PV)*; his diagnosis was **acyanotic tetralogy of Fallot**. The patient had a bicuspid aortic valve because of a rudimentary right coronary/noncoronary commissure that resulted in aortic insufficiency. This patient's heart was virtually identical to the heart specimens diagrammed in Fig. 16.2, *middle column*. (Reproduced with permission from Van Praagh R, McNamara JJ. Anatomic types of ventricular septal defect with aortic insufficiency. *Am Heart J.* 1968;75:604-619.)

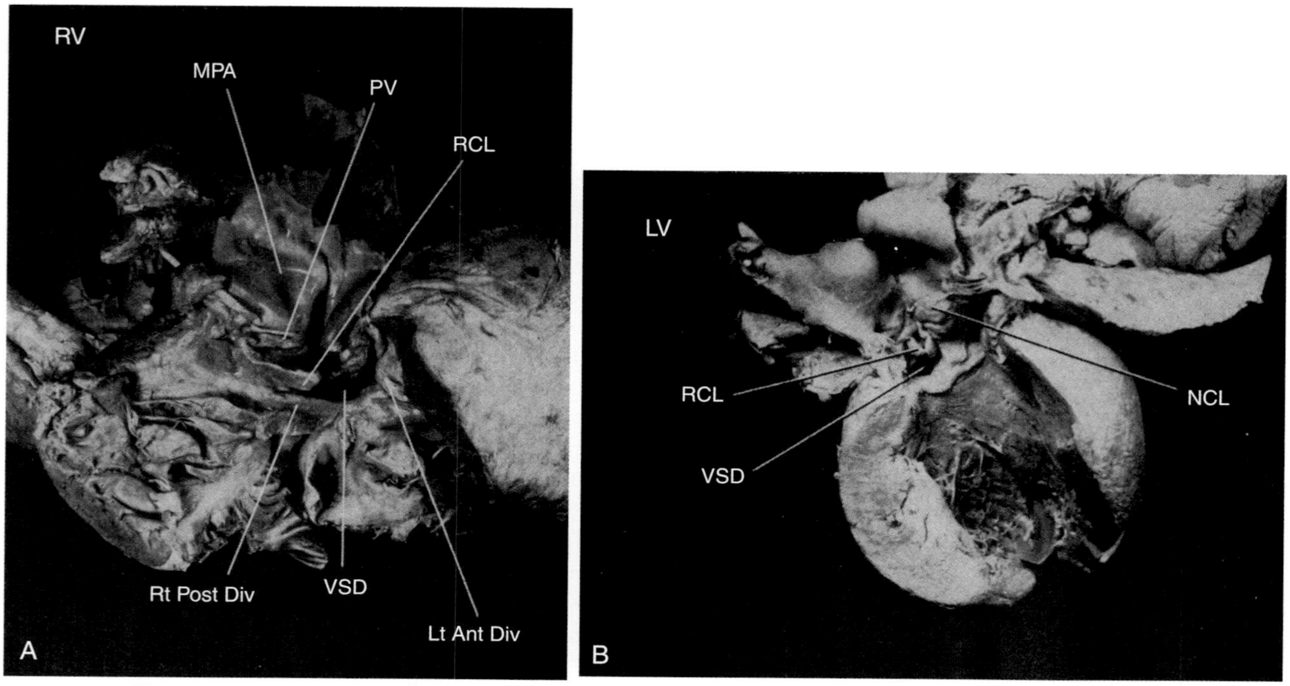

Fig. 16.6 (A) Right ventricle *(RV)* viewed from the front and above. (B) Opened left ventricle *(LV)*. This 13 11/12-year-old boy had a complete conal septal defect, also known as a complete infundibular septal defect. The subarterial ventricular septal defect *(VSD)* was large, measuring 20 × 10 mm. The VSD was both subpulmonary, as seem in A, and subaortic, as seen in B; that is, this VSD was subarterial and doubly committed. The fact that an infundibular septal defect lies beneath both great arteries is also seen in Fig. 16.2, *right column*. In A, one can see that the space above the septal band, normally occupied by the parietal band or distal conal septum, is wide open. The right posterior division *(Rt Post Div)* and the left anterior division *(Lt Ant Div)* of the septal band form the inferior rim of the VSDs. But there is nothing above the septum band until one gets to the pulmonary valve *(PV)* and the main pulmonary artery *(MPA)*. One can also see the right coronary leaflet *(RCL)* of the aortic valve. But the infundibular septum is absent. In B, showing the opened LV and ascending aorta, one can see the RCL and the noncoronary leaflet *(NCL)* of the aortic valve, and the subaortic VSD, but no distal infundibular or outflow tract septum. There was a gradient of 15 mm Hg across the right ventricular outflow tract, measured at cardiac catheterization. The RCL and NCL were both prolapsed at autopsy, and the aortic valvar commissures were normally developed. But we could not tell at autopsy whether the prolapsed RCL had herniated into the RV outflow tract to produce the 15 mm Hg outflow tract gradient. (Reproduced with permission from Van Praagh R, McNamara JJ. Anatomic types of ventricular septal defect with aortic insufficiency. *Am Heart J.* 1968;75:604-619.)

shown. The apical VSD is located between the left ventricular apex and the infundibular apical recess. Fig. 16.10B shows the opened LV and the apical VSD, which is large (25% of the LV's septal length).[9]

We concluded that large apical VSDs can be successfully closed through small right ventricular apical infundibulotomies. This approach, applicable even in small infants, can avoid both pulmonary artery banding and left ventriculotomy. However, extremely large apical VSDs with severe biventricular dysplasia and dysfunction may require cardiac transplantation.

The Story of Ventricular Septal Defects

If you do not know the history of something, you do not really understand it. So this is a story I have to tell you. No one knows the whole story of anything. But I have been reading the medical literature for my whole professional life, taking notes on 5 inch by 8 inch white cards, and keeping them in chronologic order. No one can read everything, of course. But now, more than 60 years later, these white cards have an amazing story to tell: the birth and development of our field, how and when it happened, and who the major players were.

The year **1784** saw the posthumous publication of **Three Cases of Mal-conformation in the Heart,** written by William Hunter[10] (1718–1783), a Scot who was a leading obstetrician of his time in London, England. It should be added that William Hunter was the elder brother of John Hunter, the leading surgeon of his time and the founder of surgical pathology. In William Hunter's paper, Case 3 was a stillborn infant of 6 months gestation who had a VSD and a secundum type of ASD with multiple perforations of the septum primum. This is the earliest report of a VSD that I have in my notes. This report is also remarkable because it contains a clearcut statement of the concepts of evolution, natural selection, and survival of the fittest published 74 years before papers by Darwin and Wallace (1858 to 1860). On page 308, William Hunter wrote:

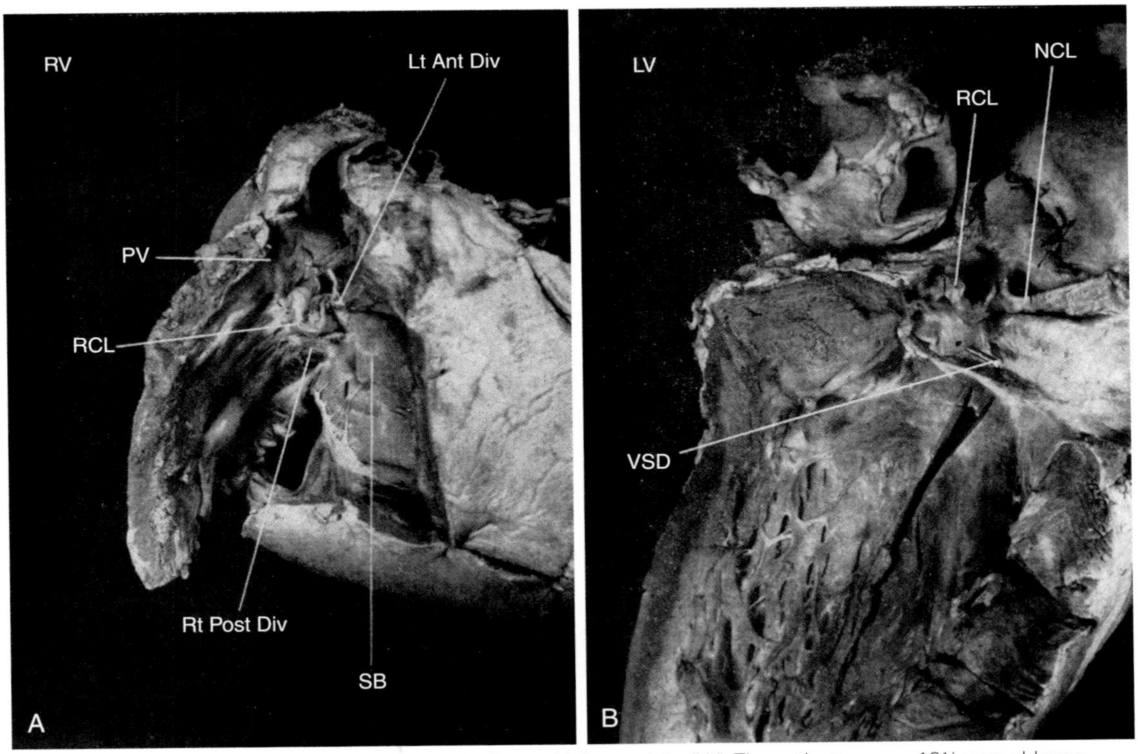

Fig. 16.7 (A) Opened right ventricle *(RV)*. (B) Opened left ventricle *(LV)*. The patient was an 18½-year-old man with a conal septal defect type of ventricular septal defect *(VSD)*. The VSD measured 20 × 10 mm. The aortic valve was tricommissural and tricuspid. The right coronary leaflet of the aortic valve prolapsed into the LV and herniated into the RV outflow tract, resulting in a right ventricular outflow tract gradient of 50 mm Hg. This young man had a history of subacute bacterial endocarditis. He also had a Meckel diverticulum. Histology revealed extensive subendocardial left ventricular myocardial infarction. In A, note that just beneath the pulmonary valve *(PV)*, the infundibular septal defect is filled by the right coronary leaflet *(RCL)* of the aortic valve that has herniated into the subpulmonary right ventricular outflow tract. The inferior rim of the infundibular septal defect is formed by the top of the septal band, that is, by the right posterior division *(Rt Post Div)* and the left anterior division *(Lt Ant Div)* of the septum band. In B, the RCL of the aortic valve can be seen bulging through the infundibular septal defect into the RV outflow tract. The prolapsed and herniated RCL of the aortic valve is essentially absent from its normal location, resulting in aortic regurgitation. The adjacent noncoronary leaflet *(NCL)* of the aortic valve appears uninvolved. *SB*, septal band. (Reproduced with permission from Van Praagh R, McNamara JJ. Anatomic types of ventricular septal defect with aortic insufficiency. *Am Heart J.* 1968;75:604-619.)

As in vegetables too, the parent generally produces a species very like itself; but sometimes a different constitution, whether better or worse. Whatever may happen in a particular instance, or with regard to an individual, the most perfect and sound animal upon the whole, will have the best chance of living to procreate others of his kind: in other words, the best breed will prevail: and the monstrous constitution, and that which is defective, or of such a fabric as necessarily to breed disease, will be cut off. The most perfect constitution will be preserved; it will be most susceptible of love, and the most likely to meet with a warm return of that passion: so that, in every way, the sound constitution will have the preference in procreation, and the defective, weak, or diseased line will be wearing out.

So there it is: evolution by natural selection and survival of the fittest. Am I surprised? No. Why not? Because we[11] have known since 1985 that the concept of evolution by natural selection was understood by **Empedocles** (495–435 BC), an ancient Greek pre-Socratic physicist from Agragas (now Agrigento), Sicily, which at that time was part of Magna Graecia (Great Greece).

To return to Dr. William Hunter, he continued:

If this doctrine were as well known, and as much attended to in our country, with regard to the human species, as it is in breeding up horses and many other animals, personal qualifications would be more attended to in match-making then they generally are. We every day see preference given to rank or birth, or weight of possessions, at the expense of entailing disease of body and mind upon a devoted race doomed to early extinction.

Then, speaking directly to the Society of Physicians in London, Dr. William Hunter wrote:

Your plan, Gentlemen, professes to keep to practical subjects. Some of your readers may look upon this communication as rather philosophical and curious, than practical

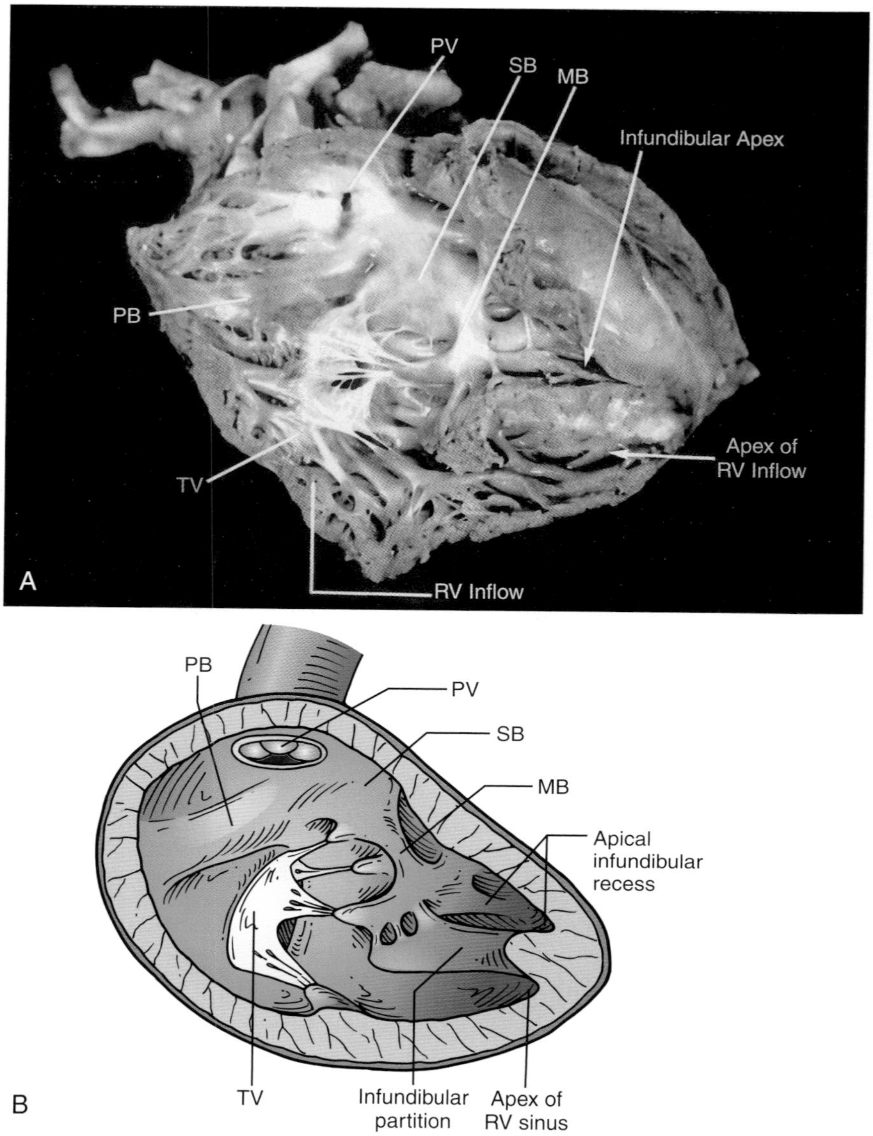

Fig. 16.8 Opened Normal Right Ventricle *(RV)*. (A) Photograph. (B) Explanatory diagram. The infundibulum or conus arteriosus has two parts: a distal or subarterial or parietal band part; and a proximal, or apical, or septal band *(SB)* and moderator band *(MB)* part. Consequently, the RV has two apices. The apex of the right ventricular sinus, body, or inflow tract lies proximal and inferior to the MB. The apex of the infundibulum is distal and superior to the MB and is also known as the infundibular apical recess. Apical muscular ventricular septal defects often run between the left ventricular apex and the infundibular apex. The infundibular apex above and the right ventricular sinus apex below are frequently separated by an infundibulosinus partition. In single left ventricle (LV) with an infundibular outflow chamber, the outlet chamber is formed by the infundibular apical recess. This infundibular myocardium has often been mistaken for RV sinus myocardium, causing confusion regarding single LV, in which the right ventricular sinus typically is absent. The problem is that the apical part of the infundibulum has not been widely understood, and consequently this infundibular apical myocardium has been mistaken for right ventricular sinus myocardium. This, in turn, has led to the mistaken notion that single LV is not really a single LV because a small RV is present (the outlet chamber). However, once one understands that the outlet chamber typically is the proximal part of the infundibulum, and that the right ventricular sinus is absent, then one understands that the LV really is single, because the right ventricular sinus beneath the SB is absent. The "small RV" is really the infundibulum only, without the right ventricular sinus. *PB,* Parietal band; *PV,* pulmonary valve; *TV,* tricuspid valve. (Reproduced with permission from Van Praagh S, Mayer JE, Berman NB, Flanagan ME, Geva T, Van Praagh R. Apical ventricular septal defects: follow-up concerning anatomic and surgical considerations. *Ann Thorac Surg*. 2002;73:48.)

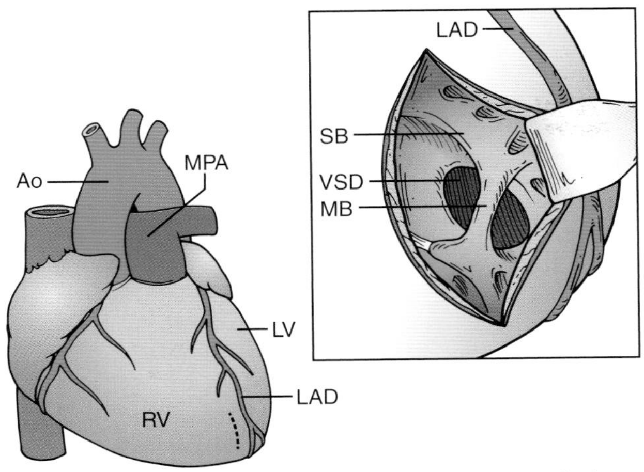

Fig. 16.9 Diagrammatic Presentation of Apical Infundibulotomy. The incision *(dotted line)* is parallel to and to the right of the distal left anterior descending *(LAD)* coronary artery. The incision extends close to the ventricular apex and varies from 15 to 2.5 cm in length. The *inset* shows that the apical muscular ventricular septal defect *(VSD)* opens into the infundibular apical recess distal to the moderator band *(MB)* and in some cases the VSD also opened proximal to the MB into the apex of the right ventricular sinus. *Ao,* Ascending aorta; *LV,* left ventricle; *MPA,* main pulmonary artery; *RV,* right ventricle; *SB,* septal band. (Reproduced with permission from Van Praagh S, Mayer JE, Berman NB, Flanagan ME, Geva T, Van Praagh R. Apical ventricular septal defects: follow-up concerning anatomic and surgical considerations. *Ann Thorac Surg.* 2002;73:48.)

and useful. But though the cure of diseases be the first object of our profession, the knowledge of incurable complaints [such as congenital heart disease] is of much importance to humanity; particularly in restraining us from bleeding, blistering, vomiting, purging, cutting issues, applying caustics: in a word, ***torturing a miserable*** *and incurable human creature.* (Bold words are the author's.)

This was William Hunter's[10] postmortem suggestion to his fellow London medical practitioners in 1784 concerning their medical therapy that he understood often amounted to the torture of patients with incurable disease (such as VSD). Today, few would disagree with William Hunter. How is it possible that **Hunter's** understanding of evolution by natural selection and survival of the fittest (1784),[10] 74 years before Darwin[12] and Wallace (1858), has been forgotten? Or **Empedocles,** whose primacy in this regard is proved by Aristotle's disapproving citation of Empedocles in the Physics.[11,13]

Now, astronomers[14] and astrophysicists know that the concept of evolution applies to the chemistry of our universe, which is about 13.8 billion years old. Shortly after the Big Bang, about 400,000 years later when the universe had cooled enough for the elementary particles to form atoms, these atoms were mostly hydrogen (1 proton in the nucleus), with some helium (2 protons), and a little lithium (3 protons).[14]

What were (and still are) the stars doing, apart from twinkling (an effect of our atmosphere) and adorning our night sky? Large stars, with enormous heat and pressure were, and are, producing the heavier element, in a process known as nuclear fusion or nuclear synthesis. Then, some of these large stars exploded (i.e., they go supernova), seeding interstellar space with the heavy elements found in the Periodic Table. Another method of spreading heavier elements into the interstellar gas is by the stellar wind.[14] The many neutrinos that are passing through you right now are from our solar wind.

Our solar system is now thought to have formed about 4.6 billion years ago, that is, about 9.2 billion years after the beginning of our universe (the so-called Big Bang): 13.8 – 4.6 = 9.2. This 9.2 billion years was a long enough time that enough heavy elements had been formed in the stars and distributed into the interstellar space of our universe so that life as we know it could evolve.[14] We are star dust, the result of the chemical evolution of our universe over the past 13.8 billion years.

When an astronomer or astrophysicist looks at the human body, what does he or she see?[15]

Oxygen	61%	8 protons (in the nucleus)
Carbon	23%	6 protons
Hydrogen	10%	1 proton
Nitrogen	3%	7 protons
Trace elements	3%	Variable

The number of protons in the nucleus is known as the **atomic number.** Life as we know it on Earth is all carbon-based. Are we capable of assessing objectively the overall effects of successful modern treatment of congenital heart disease?

What is the result of successful therapy on our human gene pool, given that molecular genetic abnormalities appear to be the cause of much congenital heart disease?[16] **Are we treating individual patients increasingly more successfully but also polluting the human gene pool**? Sir Brian Barratt-Boyes asked me[16] to consider this question. In his introduction, Sir Brian said, "Now Dr. Van Praagh is going to tell us why we should not be doing, what we are doing." Perhaps, fortunately, I could not do that because we do not have enough relevant data.[16]

Do the children and grandchildren of parents with congenital heart disease have a significantly increased prevalence of congenital heart disease? We still do not know the answer to this very important question. But we must continue to do such studies in order to find out.

Now back to the story of VSDs, as it unfolds over the years. I shall omit papers that have little or nothing "new" to say, in the interests of attempted brevity.

In **1897,** Victor Eisenmenger[17] described what became known as the **Eisenmanger complex,** that is, TOF without pulmonary outflow tract stenosis. There was subpulmonary infundibular underdevelopment, with leftward, anterior, and superior deviation of the parietal band (see Fig. 16.1 distal conal septum, component 4). However, the hypoplasia and deviation of the conal septum were enough to produce a large malalignment type of conoventricular VSD, but not severe enough to produce significant infundibular stenosis.

Dr. Bill Rashkind[17] translated Eisenmenger's paper from German into English. Eisenmenger's patient was a 32-year-old man who had been cyanotic since early childhood. He had

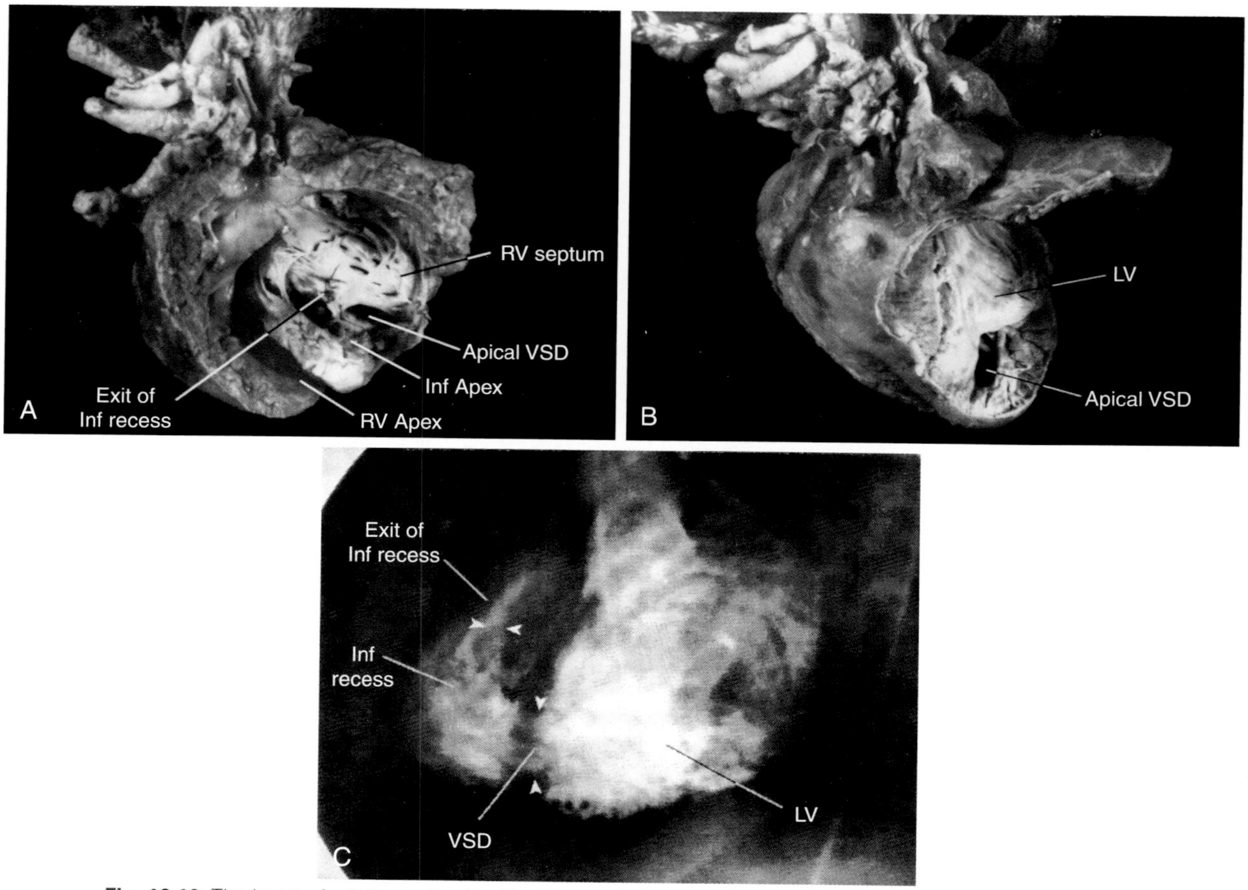

Fig. 16.10 The heart of a 2.5-month-old girl with an apical muscular ventricular septal defect *(VSD)* that measured 40 × 10 mm. The VSD lay between the left ventricular sinus apex and the infundibular apex. The VSD was considered to be relatively large because its maximal dimension equaled 25% of the length of the left ventricular septal surface. (A) Opened right ventricle *(RV)*. (B) Opened left ventricle *(LV)*. (C) Selective left ventricular angiocardiogram, left anterior oblique projection. (A) Apical muscular VSD opens into the infundibular apical recess *(Inf Apex)*. A muscular partition separates the infundibular apex from the right ventricular sinus apex, but the exit from the infundibular apex is nonrestrictive superiorly. (B) Apical muscular VSD from the left ventricular aspect. (C) Documents the apical muscular VSD's superiorinferior dimension (*rightward arrows* with superoinferior orientation). The unobstructed exit from the infundibular apical recess is demarcated by the *leftward, horizontally oriented arrows*. This patient had normal segmental anatomy, that is {S,D,S}, a secundum type of atrial septal defect (ASD), double orifice mitral valve with mild congenital mitral stenosis, coarctation of the aorta, and a patent ductus arteriosus. Before this angiocardiogram was done at 17 days of age, she had the coarctation repair, patent ductus arteriosum ligation, and banding of the main pulmonary artery. (Reproduced with permission from Van Praagh S, Mayer JE, Berman NB, Flanagan ME, Geva T, Van Praagh R. Apical ventricular septal defects: follow-up concerning anatomic and surgical considerations. *Ann Thorac Surg*. 2002;73:48.)

marked digital clubbing and a buzzing systolic murmur over the cardiac apex. S_2 was loud, but P_2 was described as not increased. Autopsy revealed a large subaortic VSD, and what I thought was unrecognized pulmonary vascular obstructive (PVO) disease. The PVO disease was not recognized as such in 1897. On page 180, Dr. Rashkind's translation was as follows: "The slightly dilated pulmonary artery shows endoarteritic thickening on its inner surface, which continues into the main branches of the vessel." I interpreted the latter as lipid streaking and pulmonary atherosclerosis. No pulmonary histology was described.

In **1952,** Drs. Muller and Dammann[18] described and proposed **pulmonary artery banding** to treat malformations of the heart that are characterized by increased pulmonary blood flow. The idea of pulmonary artery banding was to create pulmonary stenosis, thereby reducing pulmonary hypertension and excessive pulmonary blood flow. Their patient was a 3½-month-old boy. Pulmonary artery banding was suggested for single ventricle, VSD, and truncus arteriosus.

In **1955,** Drs. Lillehei, Cohen, Warden, and Varco[19]—the famous Minneapolis–St. Paul team—introduced direct-vision **open-heart surgery** by means of controlled cross circulation. They reported their surgical results in 32 patients with VSDs, TOF, and common AV canal. This report was a bombshell. Open heart surgery had arrived.

In **1955,** Dr. John W. Kirklin et al[20] from the Mayo Clinic in Rochester, Minnesota reported intracardiac surgery in 8 patients with the aid of a **mechanical pump oxygenator** of the Gibbon type. This changed everything. Not only did Kirklin confirm that open heart surgery is possible. He and his team did it in a way, using a mechanical pump-oxygenator, that would prove clinically feasible. Clinical open heart surgery had begun.

In **1956,** Dr. Kirklin et al[21] reported 20 patients with large VSDs who had undergone intracardiac repair with a pump oxygenator. Of these 20 patients, 4 died (a 20% mortality), which was considered low in that era.

In **1960,** Lev[22] did a detailed study of the AV conduction system in hearts with a VSD.

In **1963,** Kirklin, McGoon, et al.[23] used Lev's study to develop surgical techniques to avoid creating heart block during VSD repair.

In **1960,** Morgan, Griffiths, and Blumenthal[24] from Babies' Hospital in New York City published a large study of infants with VSD. Of 125 patients with VSD, 17 developed congestive heart failure (14%). Of the 17 infants with congestive heart failure, 10 died (59%). If congestive heart failure was going to develop, it always did so in the first 6 months of postnatal life.

In **1961,** Neufeld, Titus, DuShane, Burchell, and Edwards[25] from the Mayo Clinic described and named **VSDs of the AV canal type**, based on a study of 15 postmortem cases, because this anatomic type of VSD "usually occupied the position of the ventricular component of the defect in persistent common atrioventricular canal."

They also noted that "the electrocardiographic features were striking. In all cases the mean electrical axis of the QRS lay above the isoelectric point; the vector loop obtained in the frontal plane from the scalar electrocardiogram was directed counterclockwise, and its main mass was above the zero line. In addition, in all cases there were signs of right ventricular overload and in some cases of left ventricular overload as well."[25] These authors proposed that the characteristic counterclockwise and superior frontal plane QRS loop "is the result of congenital displacement of the bundle of His in its relation to the VSD."[25] These authors[25] also noted that this characteristic counterclockwise and superior frontal QRS loop occurred with the common AV canal (*not* present in these cases of *isolated* VSD of the AV canal type). These patients did not have an ostium primum type of septal defect, and they did not have common AV valves. But the presence of an isolated VSD of the AV canal type indicated that this anatomic type of VSD was related to, but different from, common AV canal. This is what these authors meant by calling this anomaly *isolated* VSD of the AV canal type.

I understand and agree with this distinction. We have always regarded VSD of the AV canal type as a **partial form of common AV canal,** often caused by ventriculoatrial malalignment. For example, if the RV is underdeveloped, the muscular ventricular septum may underlie the middle of the tricuspid orifice and the tricuspid valve. This results in a VSD of the AV canal type that is *not* related to an anomaly of the AV canal. The real anomaly is at the ventricular level, not at the AV canal level. A VSD of the AV canal type often appears to be due to **ventriculoatrial malalignment,**[26] not to an anomaly of the AV canal per se. This is why in patients with a VSD of the AV canal type, there is no ostium primum defect and no common AV valve. **Ironically, in VSD of the AV canal type, the basic diagnosis often goes unnoticed and unmentioned: ventriculoatrial malalignment.**[26]

In **1965,** Kidd, Rose, Collins, and Keith[27] from the Hospital For Sick Children in Toronto, Ontario, Canada published a study of the hemodynamics of VSDs in infancy. *Infancy* is defined as the first 12 months of postnatal life. In 151 infants with the diagnosis of isolated VSD who underwent cardiac catheterization before 1 year of age, the salient findings were as follows.[27] A pulmonary-to-systemic flow ratio (Qp/Qs) was greater than 2/1 in 78%. In those with a low flow ratio (Qp/Qs <2/1), the low flow ratio was due to the presence of a small VSD. A low or normal total pulmonary vascular resistance was found in 59%. The total pulmonary vascular resistance was greater than normal in only 25% of patients. Of these 151 patients, 25 were recatheterized subsequently. Of these 25 patients, 3 achieved functional closure (12%).

In the group with low flow and high resistance in the first study, the follow-up study subsequently revealed lower pulmonary resistance. However, 14 of these 25 patients revealed increasing pulmonary vascular resistance at follow-up study (56%). Of these 14 patients, 10 had low or normal pulmonary resistance earlier (71%).

Kidd et al[27] reached the following conclusions. "It is suggested that progressive pulmonary vascular obstruction is a sequel to high flow and low vascular resistance in the pulmonary circulation and is not present from the time of birth. It is proposed that such patients be subjected to serial study in order to define those who are reacting to the pressure-flow stimulus in this way."

In **1965,** Friedman, Mehrizi, and Pusch[28] published a study of multiple muscular VSDs. It was estimated that approximately 10% of VSDs are muscular and that of isolated VSDs, 4% are muscular. Friedman et al[28] reported 7 patients with muscular VSDs; 6 of the 7 died (86% mortality). Their recommendations in 1965 were that if a VSD is suspected, do a left ventricular angiocardiogram, and if multiple VSDs are present, band the main pulmonary artery (MPA).[28]

In **1965,** Barnard and Kennedy[29] published a case of postinfarction VSD. It was apical and muscular, below the septal band. They suggested waiting 5 weeks after the infarction before closing the VSD surgically.

In **1965,** Hoffman and Rudolph[30] published a study of the natural history of VSDs in infancy, based on 62 infants. They estimated the incidence of VSD to be approximately 0.94 in 1000 full-term live births, 4.51 in 1000 premature live births, and 1.35 in 1000 full-term and premature live births. Congestive heart failure occurred in 31 of 62 infants (50%), before 6 months of age in all, much earlier in premature infants than in full-term babies. Spontaneous functional closure occurred in 13 of 36 local infants (36%), but in only 2 of 26 referred infants (8%). For the whole group (local and referred infants), 52% of VSDs closed or became smaller. Only 16% of these infants were seriously affected. Complete closure of VSDs occurred between 7 and 12 months, usually when the VSD was small. But spontaneous closure also "could occur with large defects."

What about pulmonary vascular resistance? "Rise in pulmonary vascular resistance in infancy is not rare when the VSD is big and that, even in these children, the pulmonary vascular resistance does not usually persist at the high level present at birth, but first falls postnatally to normal levels before rising."[30]

In **1965,** Ritter, Feldt, Weidman, and DuShane[31] found that congestive heart failure occurred in infants with VSD between 6 weeks and 6 months in 53 of their 78 cases (68%).

In **1996,** Simmons, Moller, and Edwards[32] published a paper on spontaneous closure of VSD. Assisted by a personal communication from Hoffman and Rudolph, Simmons et al[32] summarized the findings in 40 infants with VSD:

No change in VSD size	11/40, 27.5%
VSD became smaller	19/40, 47.5%
VSD closed	10/40, 25.0%

Simmons et al[32] observed two anatomic types of muscular VSD closure: (1) closure by the septal leaflet of the tricuspid valve and (2) closure by fibrous tissue within the ventricular septum toward the right ventricular side, but not by tricuspid valvar tissue.

In **1966**, Osborn, Hall, Winn, Capper, and Blake[33] reported a fatal complication of pulmonary artery banding. The patient was a male infant who was banded at 5 months of age because of an unsatisfactory response to medical treatment. Cardiac catheterization had shown a 20% left-to-right shunt. Twenty-two months after banding, the infant was found to have developed a thrombus at the band site. The thrombus almost occluded the MPA. The patient died postoperatively. These authors noted that banding removes much of the adventitial circulation at the band site and that banding impedes reestablishment of adventitial circulation to the pulmonary artery wall at the band site. Internally, intimal sclerosis results from the focal narrowing of the MPA. The authors thought that ischemia had occurred involving the inner one-third of the main pulmonary arterial wall at the band site, leading to the occlusive intima thrombus. Osborn et al[33] recommended wide, nonreactive Teflon tape for pulmonary artery banding.

In **1966,** Hoffman and Rudolph[34] published a paper in the general pediatric literature *(Pediatrics)* warning of the dangers of VSDs. Their paper was entitled, "Increasing Pulmonary Vascular Resistance During Infancy in Association With Ventricular Septal Defect." They reported 3 infants with VSD and increasing pulmonary vascular resistance. The point was that elevated pulmonary vascular resistance would make such patients inoperable, and it was therefore essential to have such patients diagnosed accurately and operated on successfully before elevated pulmonary vascular resistance (Rp) would make such patients inoperable. Note also that Hoffman and Rudolph[34] were talking about *infants* needing open-heart surgery in *1966*. These were still early days in open-heart surgery.

Also in **1966,** Rose, Collins, Kidd, and Keith[35] were spreading the word about the importance of VSD in infancy and childhood. Dr. John Keith, the Canadian father of Pediatric Cardiology, and colleagues were publishing another huge and well-documented study based on 407 infants and children with VSD in the general pediatric literature *(Journal of Pediatrics)*. Noncardiologists—pediatricians, neonatologists, obstetricians and gynecologists, radiologists, and pathologists—all had to learn about VSDs in infants and children so that referrals would be made soon enough, diagnoses would be made soon enough, and surgical repair would be done soon enough, so that these otherwise normal infants and children would survive and thrive. That was the challenge in 1966.[35]

In **1966,** Girod, Raghib, Adams, Anderson, Wang, and Edwards[36] published a study of 46 autopsied cases with VSD, focusing on associated cardiac malformations. They studied VSDs that are "not part of a recognized complex" (e.g., TOF or DORV). Why? Because such "associated anomalies" can be very important surgically. Significant surprises at surgery can be fatal.[36]

In **1966,** Gould and Lyon[37] reported the prolapse of a pulmonary leaflet through a VSD; they thought theirs was the first report of this anomaly. The patient was a 37-year-old white man. He had a subpulmonary conal septal defect (their Figure 16.5). The left septal leaflet of the pulmonary valve prolapsed inferiorly and herniated through the subpulmonary conal septal defect, resulting in marked pulmonary insufficiency (regurgitation).

In **1965,** Schrire, Vogelpoel, Beck, Nellen, and Swanepoel[38] from Cape Town, South Africa, presented a paper concerning the clinical spectrum of VSD. Their hemodynamic classification of VSDs was as follows[38]:

$$\text{Type 1}\ \frac{\text{PA systolic pressure}}{\text{Systemic systolic pressure}} < 40\,\%$$

(almost normal PA pressure)

$$\text{Type 2}\ \frac{\text{PA systolic pressure}}{\text{Systemic systolic pressure}} = 40\,\% - 795\,\%$$

(moderate pulmonary hypertension)

(*PA*, Pulmonary artery.)

In **1966,** Reynolds[39] published a case with a subpulmonary conal septal defect (that was called a supracristal VSD), without aortic or pulmonary insufficiency. **"The defect was closed by direct suture."**[39] This is a very important sentence. The subpulmonary conal septal VSD was closed by direct suture, not with a patch. It will be recalled[4] that this type of VSD can be complicated by herniation of a normally formed RC aortic leaflet through a subsemilunar conal septal defect, resulting in significant AI. The way this subsemilunar VSD was closed in Dr. James Reynolds'[39] patient—by direct suture (not with a patch)—is the best way to make this repair, if technically feasible, to prevent the RC leaflet of the aortic valve from herniating through the subsemilunar conal septal defect (see Fig. 16.2, *right column, lower row*). Direct suture closure repair of the conal (infundibular) septal hernia is what the normally formed aortic leaflet needs (normal support from below) to support the aortic valve, before an RC aortic leaflet hernia and stretching occur, resulting in AI.

In **1966,** Williams, Hara, and Bulloch[40] reported a traumatic VSD.

In **1966,** Saab, Burchell, DuShane, and Titus[41] published a paper that focused on muscular VSDs.

In **1967,** Mitchell, Berendes, and Clark[42] suggested the following: "The hypothesis is proposed that the normal time of VSD closure may not be limited to the fourth and fifth postconceptive weeks, but rather may extend, for a minority of patients, throughout pregnancy and into the postpartum period." This is a reasonable way of viewing the rightmost end (the long end) of this distribution curve. This view[42] suggests that spontaneous (medically unassisted) postnatal VSD closure is the rightmost end of the normal VSD closure curve.

In **1967,** Grainger et al[43] published a paper about pulmonary artery banding as treatment for VSD.

In **1967,** Dr. Jesse E. Edwards[44] (one of the great congenital and acquired cardiovascular pathologists of the 20th century; Dr. Maurice Lev was another) published a paper about "unresolved problems" concerning VSDs:

1. Should subpulmonary or subarterial VSDs be called "supracristal" VSDs (his Fig. 16.5)?
2. How could a VSD have subaortic stenosis (see Fig. 16.7)?
3. Should the ventricles be designated hemodynamically, such as "venous" and "arterial" ventricles? Or should the ventricles and the AV valves be named in terms of their morphologic anatomy, as Lev and I were advocating?
4. In classic congenital physiologically corrected TGA, is it permissible to call regurgitation of the left-sided AV valve "mitral" insufficiency? Or should it be called "left-sided tricuspid" insufficiency?

At that time, we (my colleagues and I) thought that the correct answers to these questions were as follows:

1. No. The anatomic meaning of *crista supraventricularis* was confused and erroneous. Initially, it was thought that the crista supraventicularis consisted of the parietal band (component 4) and the septal band (see Fig. 16.1, component 3). Later, study of the conotruncal (infundibuloarterial) anomalies such as TOF, TGA, and DORV made it obvious that the parietal band (component 4) and the septal band (component 3) are two separate structures, not the parietal and septal extensions of one structure, the crista supraventicularis as classically defined and understood. Only the parietal band (component 4) formed a supraventricular crest. The septal band (component 3) did not form a supraventricular crest because, typically, the septal band was attached to the superior right ventricular septal surface. Briefly, the meaning of the crista supraventricularis changed and then collapsed when the crista supraventicularis was understood to be a misconception. So other more accurate anatomic and developmental names were preferred (see Fig. 16.1).
2. How could a VSD have subaortic stenosis? By having a conal septal left shift.
3. Should the ventricles be designated hemodynamically ("venous" ventricle and "arterial" ventricle)? No. We thought that the cardiac chambers (atria and ventricles) should be diagnosed and designated morphologically. The type of blood conveyed by a morphologically RV could be either venous or arterial; the hemodynamics were a variable, whereas a chamber's morphology was a constant.
4. In TGA {S,L,L}, the left-sided AV valve is the tricuspid valve (not the mitral valve). Consequently, we are talking about left-sided tricuspid regurgitation (not about mitral regurgitation).

In **1967,** Anderson, Levy, Naeye, and Tabakin[45] published a case report concerning a 4-year-old girl with a VSD who had developed what the authors regarded as rapidly progressive PVO disease. The authors were shocked. The dangers of a VSD and the risk for becoming inoperable at an early age (4 years) were becoming apparent.

In **1967,** Levin, Spach, Canent, Boineau, Capp, Jain, and Barr[46] published a study of intracardiac pressure-flow dynamics in isolated VSD:

1. When right ventricular pressure is low, shunting is left-to-right throughout the cardiac cycle.
2. But when right ventricular pressure is systemic, the shunt is right-to-left during isovolumic relaxation.

In **1967,** Sigmann, Stern, and Sloan[47] published their results of early surgical correction of large VSDs. In 45 infants who underwent surgery, mortality was 10%. PVO disease was found pathologically as early as 8 months of age, suggesting that surgery in infancy might be required for successful management of patients with VSD.

In **1967,** Tikoff, Schmidt, and Tsagaris[48] published a study of an adult with a large VSD. They found that isoproterenol induced right ventricular infundibular obstruction. They thought their findings suggested that right ventricular infundibular obstruction could be acquired at any time in the history of a patient with VSD. They thought that such obstruction may be intermittent. They also suggested that infundibular obstruction could result in syncope.

In **1968,** Sakakibara and Konno[49] published a paper about the pathologic anatomy of patients with VSD and congenital aneurysm of the sinus of Valsalva, based on 70 cases (55 surgical cases and 15 autopsied cases).

Instead of talking about VSD with AI, as we[4] and others have done, Sakakibara and Konno[49] proposed that these conditions should be understood as VSDs with *aneurysms of the sinuses of Valsalva.* (Readers should be aware that this was a famous Japanese cardiovascular team. Dr. Shigeru Sakakibara was Professor of Cardiac Surgery and Director of the Heart Institute of Japan. Sakakibara discovered and described *double-outlet left ventricle.* Dr. S. Konno was Chief of Staff of the Heart Institute of Japan and Head of the Catheterization Laboratory.) They classified aneurysms of the sinus of Valsalva with VSD into four anatomic types.

In **1968,** Dr. J. I. E. Hoffman[50] published a study of the natural history of VSD. This study found estimated incidence ≈ 20 in 10,000 live births (0.2%) and death before 15 years of age ≈ 10% of VSDs, that is, 2 in 10,000 live births (0.02%). There "should" be about 18 in 10,000 school children with VSD. However, intensive school surveys show only about half of this number, that is, about 9 in 10,000 (0.009%). These findings support the suggestion that there is a high incidence of spontaneous closure of VSDs—perhaps 50%.

In **1968,** Baron, Wolf, Steinfeld, and Van Mierop[51] published a paper concerning the angiocardiographic diagnosis of subpulmonary VSD. In addition, this paper contains many helpful insights concerning the anatomy, embryology, and surgery of subpulmonary and conoventricular VSDs, which comes as no surprise because Ludwig ("Bob") Van Mierop was the senior coauthor. Van Mierop, who was both a cardiac surgeon and an embryologist, says that membranous VSDs can be readily closed by the RA, whereas surgical closure of a subpulmonary VSD requires a right ventriculotomy. Despite his surgical training, Van Mierop spent most of his professional life as a pediatric cardiologist. He was also an excellent artist, as this paper demonstrates. His developmental description merits quotation:

> *As development continues, both the truncus and the conus become divided into two separate channels. The truncus swellings first join in their midportion and with continued growth their line of fusion extends distally toward the aorticopulmonary septum and proximally toward the conus. . . .*
>
> *At first the conus swellings grow slower and lag behind those in the truncus. Fusion begins in the mid region of the conus and extends in both directions. . . .*
>
> *. . . In the adult heart, the line of junction of the two septa is located in the ventricular septum, 1 to 3 mm below the pulmonic valve, but is not demarcated by any gross anatomic landmark.*

Distally, if the conal septal cushions do not fuse with each other, or with truncal septum that extends 1 to 3 mm below the pulmonary valve leaflets, the result is a subpulmonary and a subaortic conal septal defect, that is, a subsemilunar conal septal defect, that typically lies directly beneath the RC leaflet of the normally located aortic valve (see Fig. 16.2).

Proximally, if the conal septal cushions do not fuse completely, in a normal way, the proximal conal septum (the parietal band) is hypoplastic, higher than normal, and also can be deviated anterosuperiorly or in some other direction. This results in a conoventricular type of VSD between the abnormally located conal septum above and the normally located ventricular septum below. We do not call such defects membranous VSDs because there often is much more wrong than an anomaly of the membranous septum. Typically, there is an anomaly of the inferior part of the conal septum that forms the roof of the conoventricular VSD, as seen from the right ventricular perspective.

Conoventricular VSDs and subpulmonary conal septal defects are both conal septal anomalies:

1. Conoventricular VSDs typically are defects of the proximal or inferior conal septum.
2. Subpulmonary VSDs are defects of the distal or superior conal septum.

Van Mierop's[51] diagrams show this beautifully.

In **1968,** Clarkson, Frye, DuShane, Burchell, Wood, and Weidman[52] published a paper on the prognosis of patients with VSD and severe PVO disease.

In **1968,** Rastelli, Ongley, and Titus[53] published a paper about 4 patients with VSD of the AV canal type with straddling tricuspid valve and a mitral valve deformity.

In **1968,** Edgett et al[54] published a case of spontaneous VSD closure after pulmonary artery banding. The patient was a 6-year-old white boy. Banding may have helped promote spontaneous VSD closure.

In 1918, Weber is the first person known to have suspected spontaneous VSD closure. Beyond infancy, 25% of small VSDs will close spontaneously.[54]

In **1968,** Coleman et al[55] from the Royal Hospital for Sick Children in Glascow, Scotland reported their results concerning VSD repair in childhood. In 91 children from 1 to 12 years of age, the mortality rate was 15%. Infundibular stenosis was also present in 18%; I wondered if these patients with infundibular stenosis had TOF, but I could not be sure.

In **1968,** Leachman and Pereyo[56] reported the case of a 2-year-old girl who had a VSD with elevated pulmonary capillary wedge pressure and severe pulmonary arterial hypertension. After surgical VSD closure, her pulmonary vascular resistance decreased significantly, indicating that this is possible. In other words, severe pulmonary arterial hypertension and elevated pulmonary vascular resistance do not always contraindicate VSD closure—a surprising and hopeful finding.

In **1968,** Tandon[57] reported chylothorax after the surgical repair of a VSD in an 8-year-old girl. Treatment involved repeated aspiration and a low-fat, high-protein diet.

In **1969,** Gotsman, Beck, Barnard, and Schrire[58] reported their hemodynamic studies after surgical VSD closure.

In **1969,** Miller et al[59] studied the relationship between hemodynamics in VSD patients and their height and weight. They found "a close association between pulmonary hypertension and poor weight gain."

In **1969,** Hallidie-Smith et al[60] assessed the effects of surgical VSD closure on pulmonary vascular disease. If there were no complicating lesions, surgical VSD closure reduced their mortality rate from 22% to 15%.

In **1969,** Yang et al[61] reported 110 cases of membranous septal aneurysm. Only 2 had a VSD (1.8%). Why do aneurysms of pars membranacea septi (the membranous part of the ventricular septum) matter?

In **1969,** a paper by Varghese et al[62] answers this question. They regard a membranous septal aneurysm as "a method of spontaneous closure of a small [membranous] VSD." The VSD almost did not close. Why not? Often it looks as though the inferior rim of the conal septum (the parietal band) was a bit too far away from the membranous septum; that is, mild hypoplasia of the inferior part of the conal (infundibular) septum. Hence, an aneurysm of the membranous septum suggests that the ventricular septum just barely managed to close and one should look for a small, residual membranous VSD.

In **1969,** Morton et al[63] also reported an aneurysm of the ventricular septum with an aortic valvar malformation in an infant. Thus, aneurysms of the membranous septum and their relationship to membranous VSDs were now being recognized diagnostically and understood as part of the VSD closure process.

In **1969,** Herbert[64] pointed out that some VSDs could be visualized angiocardiographically only in diastole. These VSDs were thought to be muscular. Systole resulted in approximation of the margins of the VSD and functional closure, whereas diastolic relaxation permitted separation of the margins of such VSDs, facilitating their diagnosis.

In **1969,** Scheinman et al[65] reported early repair of an apical muscular VSD caused by nonpenetrating trauma in an 8-year-old boy.

In **1969,** Gonzales-Lavin and Barratt-Boyes[66] reported their surgical experience in patients with VSD and aortic valvar incompetence. In a series of 7 cases, they described VSD closure using the RC leaflet of the aortic valve and homograft aortic valve replacement.

In **1969,** Meng[67] reported a 28-month-old girl with spontaneous closure of a VSD in tricuspid atresia. Hence, VSD closure can be physiologically disadvantageous or disastrous.

In **1969,** Nghiem et al[68] reported spontaneous VSD closure after pulmonary artery banding. Because it was being recognized that this can happen, these authors suggested doing an angiocardiogram before debanding to see if the VSD has closed, to avoid an unnecessary right ventriculotomy.

In **1970,** Pombo et al[69] published 4 cases of aneurysm of the membranous ventricular septum and a VSD. They suggested that the best method of diagnosing these interrelated defects was by selective left ventricular angiocardiography.

In **1970,** Dr. Jane Somerville, Dr. A. Brandao, and Mr. Ronald Ross[70] reported their surgical experience and clinical findings in 20 patients with VSD and aortic regurgitation. They preferred pulmonary homograft replacement of the aortic valve, rather than repair. Of their 20 patients, 2 died (10%), 18 survived (90%), and 17 had a satisfactory result (85%).

In **1970,** Stark, Tyman, and Aberdeen[71] reported their experience with spontaneous VSD closure after pulmonary artery constriction (banding). They recommended reconstruction of the MPA with a pericardial patch.

In **1970,** Ebert, Canent, Spach, and Sabiston[72] reported their experience with VSD closure and prior pulmonary artery banding. The resistance ratio, pulmonary arterial resistance/systemic resistance (Rp/Rs), did not change: after total correction, it was the same as before banding.

In **1970,** Wagner, Ankeney, and Liebman[73] tried to answer an important question: Can one predict how well a patient with a large VSD is likely to do after surgical closure? Their patients had "nonrestrictive" VSDs. "Nonrestrictive" means that they had systemic pressure in the RV. Salient findings are:

1. If the pulmonary arterial mean pressure preoperatively was less than 95 mm Hg, they did well.
2. If the pulmonary arterial pressure preoperatively was greater than 65 mm Hg, mortality was high.

Flows and resistances did not correlate well with surgical results, but mean pulmonary arterial pressures did. This is what the data in their 30 patients showed.

In **1970,** Yokoyama, Takao, and Sakakibara[74] published their findings concerning the natural history and surgical indications in patients with VSD.

In **1970,** Hunt, Formanek, Castañeda, and Moller[75] published a paper concerning 8 patients who had had pulmonary artery banding followed by surgical VSD closure. Pulmonary vascular resistance was normal in 3 (37.5%), moderately increased in 4 (50%), and markedly increased in 1 (12.5%). Mild, acquired pulmonary valvar stenosis was found in 7 of 8 (87.5%). Mild acquired (secondary) infundibular stenosis was observed in 3 of 8 (37.5%). Thus, it seems reasonable to conclude that pulmonary artery constriction (banding) can result in mild secondary (acquired) pulmonary valvar and infundibular stenosis.

In **1970,** Li and Keith[76] found that the incidence of spontaneous VSD closure was about 25%.

In **1971**, Rao and Sissman[77] published a paper about the spontaneous closure of physiologically advantageous VSDs, as in tricuspid atresia and DORV.

In **1970,** Daicoff and Miller[78] proposed that the way to treat patients with VSD and congestive heart failure in infancy was by early repair of the VSD. The ages of their patients were 6 months, 10 months, 11 months, 15 months, 22 months, and 33 months, and all survived. My comment in my private notes was "Bravo!"

In **1970,** Goor, Lillehei, Rees, and Edwards[79] discussed the embryology and anatomic classification of VSDs based on a study of 101 heart specimens with 112 VSDs.

In **1971,** Jarmakani et al[80] found that after VSD closure, left ventricular volume and mass regressed considerably. However, there may be some partially irreversible changes associated with long-term left ventricular hypertrophy.

In **1971,** Lev et al[81] presented the quantitative anatomy of isolated VSD based on 53 cases older than 3 months of age.

In **1971,** Brammel et al[82] presented a clinical and physiologic study of 91 cases of the Eisenmenger syndrome. The Eisenmenger syndrome is defined as a VSD with PVO disease and a right-to-left shunt at the atrial, ventricular, or great arterial level (e.g., with a PDA).

In **1971,** Young and Mark[83] published a paper concerning the fate of the patient with the Eisenmenger syndrome. In 57 patients from 21 months to 58 years, congestive heart failure occurred in 22 of 57 (39%), causing death in 5 patients. Of these 57 patients, 17 died of cardiac causes (30%).

In **1971,** Dr. John W. Kirklin[84] wrote an editorial about pulmonary arterial banding in babies with large VSDs in which he stated that he prefers open repair early. In 1965, Kirklin reported VSD repair between 6 and 12 months of age, with a hospital mortality of 5%.

In **1971,** Campbell[85] presented the natural history of VSD. Salient features are:

1. Spontaneous VSD closure occurs up to the 5th decade of life, that is, 50 years of age;
2. 20% of VSDs have closed by 30 years of age; and
3. 24% of VSDs have closed by 60 years of age.

Closure occurs mainly with small VSDs, which occur in approximately one-third of the total. Hence, about two-thirds of VSDs are large. The overall mortality in large VSDs was 25 of 117 (21.4%). In the first two decades (up to 20 years of age), mortality is 2.2% to 2.9%/year. In the fourth and later decades, mortality is double that.

In **1972,** Coleman et al[86] reported their results of VSD repair after pulmonary artery banding. First they banded the MPA, and then they closed the VSD 3 to 5 years later. The mortality of the second operation was 4 of 15 patients (27%).

In **1972,** Dr. Aldo R. Castañeda became the Chief of Cardiac Surgery at the Boston Children's Hospital, and I can almost hear him saying, "One operation is better than two. No more palliative surgery. Let's fix them whenever they need it, no matter how young they are. No problem." This soon became what we called **the Castañeda doctrine.**

In **1972,** Parisi, Holden, Plauth, and Nadas[87] described **the syndrome of VSD with AI** based on 72 patients (1950–1971). This was the Boston Children's Hospital experience when Dr. Alex Nadas was our Chief of Cardiology and Dr. Robert E. Gross was our Chief of Cardiac Surgery—great pioneers both. The median age at onset of AI was 6.9 years, ranging from 0.1 to 20.5 years. Males were 61%, and females were 39%. The median Qp/Qs was 2.1/1.0, ranging from 1 to 5. AI was moderate or severe in 61%, and there was significant pulmonary outflow tract stenosis in 19%. Three patients developed AI 1.4 to 4.2 years after VSD closure. Surgery was performed in 57% of patients, at an average of 4.3 years after the onset of AI. Mortality was 32% (23/72). Surgical deaths were 16; deaths from congestive heart failure occurred in 6 patients; and the cause of death was unknown in 1. Subacute bacterial endocarditis (SBE) occurred in 12.5% (9/72); 7 of 9 underwent surgery (78%), and 5 of 7 died (71%). This study by Dr. Lucy Parisi et al[87] delineates the natural history of VSD with AI and our therapeutic results in this early time period (1950 to 1971).[88]

In **1972,** Glasser, Cheitlin, McCarty, Haas, Hall, and Mullins[89] published their experience with VSD and AI in 32 cases. Surgery was performed in 62.5% (20/32). In general, the AI was slowly progressive. A pulmonary outflow tract gradient was found in 41% (13/32). This gradient was due to herniation of the RC leaflet of the aortic valve in 6 of 32 patients (19%) (see Fig. 16.2, *right column*). Of the 20 patients who underwent surgery, none had aortic valve replacement. Annuloplasties were done in 6 of 20 (30%), with VSD closure only in 14 of 20 (70%). Of the 14 patients who had VSD closure only, the AI completely disappeared in 3 (21%). The AI was significantly reduced in 4 of 14 (29%). Hence, the AI was significantly reduced in half (7/14, 50%). These authors recommended early VSD closure to prevent progressive AI. These were the same conclusions that we had reached in 1968.

In **1972,** Alpert and Rowe[90] estimated the probability that small VSDs would close spontaneously in the first 5 years of postnatal life. In this clinical study of 52 patients, 30 closed spontaneously (58%).

In **1972,** Steinfeld et al[91] published a paper on the diagnosis of subpulmonary (supracristal) VSD. Elective left ventricular angiocardiography was the diagnostic method of choice at that time.

In **1972,** Collins, Calder, Rose, Kidd, and Keith[92] published a paper on patients with VSD in the first 5 years of life, based on 200 cases. When the Qp/Qs was less than 2/1, patients were asymptomatic and the rate of spontaneous VSD closure was 20%. Most had a Qp/Qs ratio greater than 2/1. At least 15% die in infancy.

In **1973,** Fisher, Brawley, Neill, Donahoo, Haller, Rowe, and Gott[93] published a paper describing severe tricuspid regurgitation after VSD closure.

In **1972,** Rothfeld et al[94] described a patient who had a post-myocardial infarction VSD. Then 17 years later, the patient developed the Eisenmenger syndrome, that is, severe pulmonary hypertension with shunt reversal (right-to-left shunt).

In **1973,** Tandon and Edwards[95] described "aneurysm-like formations" of the membranous ventricular septum.

In **1973,** Kawashima et al[96] from Osaka, Japan described their surgical experience with VSD and AI, based on 35 patients. They had 7 hospital deaths (20%) and 3 late deaths (9%). Since 1968, with 18 consecutive cases, they have had no deaths.

In **1973,** Momma, Mimori, and Takao[97] studied the natural history of pulmonary hypertension with VSD in infancy and childhood. They found progressive pulmonary vascular obstruction in 9 of 33 cases (27%).

In **1973,** under the leadership of Dr. Pierre Corone and et al,[98] an international meeting was held in France that focused on VSD. Numerous excellent papers were published in *Coeur* (NS) in 1973. NS is an abbreviation for Numéro Special (Special Number). The papers were published in French, which I, a native Canadian, can read without difficulty. Unfortunately, *Coeur* (meaning Heart) is no longer being published. In the commentary that follows, I will translate everything into English for the convenience of readers.

Dr. Pierre Corone et al[98] published a paper about the spontaneous evolution of VSDs after the age of 2 years, based on 275 cases. By "spontaneous evolution," these authors mean what we would call natural history. It is also relevant to mention that Dr. Pierre Corone (a good friend) was basically an adult cardiologist very interested in pediatric cardiology. So his understanding of congenital heart disease in the adult was much better than that of most pediatric cardiologists. In his series, no deaths were related to VSDs. In a series of 181 cases, complete VSD closure occurred in 26 patients (14%). In 181 cases, incomplete closure was observed in 23 patients (13%). The average age of delayed spontaneous closure of VSD was 13½ years of age. More than half of these spontaneous VSD closures occurred after the age of 10 years. Large VSDs can also close spontaneously. Infundibular pulmonary outflow tract stenosis was found in 30% of their large VSDs. An increase in pulmonary resistance was found in only 1 patient.

Dr. Gordon Danielson[99] of the Mayo Clinic in Rochester, Minnesota reported that they were not able to reproduce pulmonary hypertension in dogs experimentally.

In **1973,** Dr. Alex Nadas' presentation[100] at a French meeting had to do with operative indications for VSD surgery and the role of pulmonary arterial hypertension. In 170 infants with a large VSD treated medically, cyanosis and a pulmonary artery pressure greater than 75% systemic were thought to be key factors leading to PVO disease.[100] Among 553 infants treated medically and followed for 4 to 8 years, there were 3 deaths (mortality = 0.5%).[100]

Among 46 patients with VSD and pulmonary hypertension, only those who were operated on at younger than 2 years of age had normal pulmonary arterial resistance (Rp). Operation is thought to be imperative when the Qp/Qs is greater than 2/1, and when the pulmonary artery/systemic artery pressure ratio is greater than 1/3. Operation is thought to be debatable when the Qp/Qs ratio is greater than 2/1, and when the pulmonary artery/systemic artery pressure ratio is less than 1/3.[100] Dr.

Nadas said to look for coarctation of the aorta, ASD, or common AV canal. "Debatable" means that the operative indications are unclear, not definite.

Operation for VSD closure is thought to be useless or dangerous when the Qp/Qs ratio is less than 2/1, and the pulmonary artery/systemic artery pressure ratio is greater than 1/3. Operation for VSD closure is unnecessary when the Qp/Qs flow ratio is less than 2/1 and when the pulmonary artery/systemic artery pressure ratio is less than 1/3.[100]

Dr. Richard Bonham-Carter's view from Great Ormond Street Hospital, London, England (p. 372) was *the trial of survival*. Operate only if intensive medical therapy has failed and if the infant's life is in jeopardy. Otherwise, wait and see.

My own view is to remember that there really are no absolute surgical indications for anything. It is all relative. What matters is what one's surgeon can do successfully. Both physicians are right. Each is trying to express what he thinks his surgeon can do successfully at that time.

Dr. Alex Nadas,[100] surgical indications for VSD closure in infants in 1973:

1. Immediate
   - Intractable congestive heart failure
   - Qp/Qs >3/1
   - Pressure in the pulmonary artery/pressure in a systemic artery (PPA/PPS) >0.75
2. With delay of 6 to 12 months
   - Controlled congestive heart failure
   - Failure to thrive
   - Repeated pulmonary infection
   - Persistent hyperkinetic pulmonary artery hypertension
   - PPA, pressure in the pulmonary artery
   - PSA, pressure in a systemic artery

Dr. Nadas' criteria for inoperability of VSDs in 1973:

- Arterial oxygen saturations <90%
- Qp/Qs <1.5/1 and PPA/PSA >0.75
- Peripheral pulmonary stenoses
- Inoperable, associated lesions, for example, mitral atresia

Dr. Dupon's[101] suggestions in 1973 for helping the cardiac surgeon to decide whether to close the VSD:

1. Record the pulmonary artery pressure with the patient breathing room air and with the patient breathing oxygen. If the pulmonary artery pressure falls with oxygen, that is a good sign, suggesting that the patient's elevated pulmonary resistance is labile, not fixed.
2. Test band the MPA, and then measure the distal MPA pressure. If the distal pulmonary artery pressure falls, this suggests that the MPA band will do what it is designed to do, namely, to lower the distal pulmonary artery pressure and flow, thereby lowering the pulmonary arterial resistance (Rp).[101]
3. Digitally obstruct the VSD. If the RV does not "blow up" and start to fail, this is good, suggesting that the pulmonary arterial resistance is low enough that all the right ventricular blood can flow through the lungs, that is, that a right-to-left shunt through the VSD is not physiologically essential. If a right-to-left shunt through the VSD is essential because of a high and fixed pulmonary arterial resistance, then patch closure of the VSD would be fatal.[101]

Mercier et al[102] presented their experience with 160 VSD closures in 1973 at this meeting in France. The pulmonary artery pressure was greater than 60 mm Hg in 91 of these 160 patients (57%). The operative mortality was 13 of 91 (14%). There were 78 survivors, of whom 33 were restudied. A residual shunt was found in one-fourth of these patients, and the pulmonary artery pressure remained high in 10%.

In the discussion that followed Dr. Mercier's presentation,[102] Dr. d'Allaines said that if digital test closure of the VSD is negative, that is, if the pulmonary artery pressure does *not* fall by at least 20%, and if the systemic pressure does not rise significantly, then do NOT close the VSD.

In 42 of 52 patients (81%), the digital test was positive, that is, the pulmonary artery pressure did fall and the systemic pressure did rise. Moreover, after surgical closure of the VSD, the pulmonary artery pressure was the same as it had been with digital test closure of the VSD; in other words, the pulmonary artery pressure obtained after test digital VSD occlusion was the same as the pulmonary artery pressure after surgical VSD closure. So test intraoperative VSD digital occlusion was an accurate predictive test of what the pulmonary artery pressure would be after surgical VSD occlusion. Dr. d'Allaines added that in 4 patients, digital test VSD occlusion was negative (the pulmonary pressure did *not* fall). These VSDs were closed, and all 4 patients died. In 4 other patients, test digital occlusion was negative (the pulmonary pressure did not fall). The VSDs in these 4 patients were not closed, and all 4 patients survived surgery.

Then Dr. Alex Nadas said he thinks that when the pulmonary arterial resistance (Rp) is high (>10 units), it will fall after operation only in those patients who are younger than 1 year of age at the time of surgery (not older than 1 year of age at the time of surgery).

Dr. Gordon Danielson[99] from the (Mayo Clinic) agreed. He added that this is why banding of the pulmonary artery is still being done at major centers, even though it makes mortality at corrective surgery higher. His final sentence was, "Correction is preferable to banding." Dr. Danielson's comment that "this is why banding of the pulmonary artery is still being done at major centers" may require brief explanation. The hope of banding the MPA is that it will reduce or prevent the progressive increase in Pr, thereby making it possible to delay surgical VSD occlusion to later than 1 year of age. Then Dr. Danielson added another important consideration to the conversation: Banding "makes mortality at corrective surgery higher." This is why banding of the pulmonary artery really is not a good idea. As per Dr. Danielson, "Correction is preferable to banding." (Now, in 2021, we know that for VSDs, early correction is the best solution, unless the VSD is likely to close spontaneously.)

Then Dr. Neveux proposed that we should rely on hemodynamic studies, not on surgical explorations with digital tests and test bandings. Neveux dismissed these approaches as "acrobatics" that artifact the circulation. Dr. Danielson said that he agrees entirely with Dr. Neveux. Regarding whether to operate, at the Mayo Clinic they rely on the Rp/Rs. When the Rp/Rs is less than 0.7, they operate. "In effect, we close all whose shunt is predominantly left-to-right. But we have established that when the Rp/Rs > 0.7, 25% will die at surgery, 25% will stay unchanged, 25% will get worse, and 25% are improved. Since we can't tell in advance which 1 of 4 will be benefited, we prefer not to operate on this group at all."

Pernot[103] described the medical management of infants with VSD.

Galey[104] presented a surgical review of VSDs in infancy. He began by saying that VSDs constitute 20% to 30% of all congenital heart disease, that 1 in 1000 live births has a VSD, and that about half are large VSDs with high flows (a large Qp/Qs ratio). His table of banding mortality, based on published data, varied from a high of 23% (Cooley) to a low of 7% (Binet-Langlois), with a mean of 14%.[104] His table of VSD closure mortality in 1973 revealed the following[104]:

Using Extracorporeal Circulation

McGoon, 94 cases	21%
McGoon, last 42 cases	10%
Sloan, 45 cases	20%

Using Profound Hypothermic (Surface)

Horiuschi	61 cases
18%	
Okamoto	62 cases
8%	

Using Extracorporeal Circulation and Profound Surface Hypothermia

Barratt-Boyes, 20 cases,	5%	
(<1 year)	(1 death)	
Subramanian	14 cases	7%
	(1 death)	

Mortality resulting from prior banding at VSD closure was 6% (Subramanian).

Dr. Galey's Conclusions[104]

The only way to avoid the development of PVO disease is to close all VSDs that need closing at younger than 2 years of age.

Guilmet et al[105] presented their experience with VSD and AI. He began by saying that **the first description of VSD with AI was by Pezzi and Laubry in 1921**. This is why the French often call VSD with AI **the syndrome of Pezzi and Laubry.** Guilmet et al[105] presented 2 cases, both treated successfully. They advocated VSD closure and commissuroplasty, not aortic valve replacement.

Cabral pointed out that the VSD can be closed through the aortic valve. Danielson said that his experience involved approximately 30 cases of VSD with AI: one-third had TOF and two-thirds had a simple VSD only. If the AI is minor, they just close the VSD. As far as aortic annuloplasty is concerned, they have obtained a good result in only about half of their cases. Dr. Danielson concluded that if the AI is severe, they presently close the VSD and replace the aortic valve. Dr. Jean Kachaner et al[106] in 1973 presented their experience with 341 infants with VSD, studied between 1957 and 1965. The methods of diagnosis were:

Cardiac catheterization	154	(45%)
Postmortem examination	20	(6%)
To clinical	167	(49%)

The duration of follow-up was: average, 54/12 years, and range, 6 months to 16 5/12 years.

The results were summarized as follows[106]:

Dead	45/341	13%
Unchanged	161/341	47%
Improved	72/341	22%
Worse	7/341	2%
Closed	39/341	11%
Infundibular stenosis	17/341	5%

Surgery was performed in 154 patients; 67 were operated on twice. Of the 45 infants who died, 44 had pulmonary hypertension (98%). Dr. Kachaner said that **the natural history is essentially a function of the type of VSD.**

Groups Ia and Ib: Normal Pulmonary Artery Pressure

History: the same, or improved

Ia: Maladie de Roger

77 cases	6	Operated (8%)
Mortality	0	
Unchanged	55/77	(71%)
Closed	21/77	(27%)
Worse		0
Infundibular stenosis	1/77	(1%)

Group Ib

Left-to-right shunt >1.5
Pulmonary arterial pressure: Normal
n = 51 cases
Surgery in 13 of 51 (25%)
Surgery twice in 4 of 51 (8%)

Dead		1/51	(2%)
Unchanged	12/51	(23%)	
Improved	25/51	(50%)	
Closed	10/51	(19%)	
Worse		3/51	(6%)

Spontaneous closure occurred from 3 months to 9 years of age.
Average age at spontaneous VSD closure was 31 months of age (2 7/12 years).
What does "worse" mean (earlier)? In 3 of 51 patients (6%) the left-to-right shunt increased and the pulmonary artery pressure also increased.

Group IIa[106]

Left-to-right shunt >1.5
Right-to-left shunt = 0
PPA/PSA ratio = 0.2 to 0.66

Clinically, failure to thrive, that is, decreased exercise tolerance, typical murmur, increased P_2,
apical mid-diastolic rumble, cardiomegaly, increased pulmonary vascularity.
n = 103
Surgery in 50/103 (49%)
Operated on twice, 19/103 (18%)
Average follow-up, 6 years

Dead	15/103	(15%)
Same	37/103	(36%)
Better	36/103	(35%)
Closed spontaneously	8/103	(8%)
Infundibular stenosis	7/103	(7%)

In Group IIa, the average age at death was 7 months. Infundibular pulmonary stenosis developed in 7 cases, and in 4 of these 7 cases (57%) the VSD closed spontaneously, resulting in the clinical picture of pulmonary stenosis with an intact ventricular septum.

Review our paper concerning VSD with AI[4] and the related figures. You will see how it is possible for the RC leaflet of the aortic valve to prolapse inferiorly and then herniate through a VSD, thereby functionally closing the VSD and creating a pulmonary infundibular level outflow tract obstruction and gradient, mimicking infundibular pulmonary stenosis. Some such mechanism may explain the previously described four rare cases.

Group IIb[106]

Left-to-right shunt >1.5
Right-to-left shunt ±.
PPA/PSA ratio = 0.66 to 1.0
Clinical: Same as group IIa, except murmur less loud, and P_2 louder
n = 78 cases
Surgery in 64 of 78 (82%)
Surgery performed twice in 37 of 64 (58%)
Average follow-up was 4 8/12 years

Death	24/78	31%
Same	35/78	45%
Improved	11/78	14%
Worse	4/78	5%
Infundibular stenosis	4/78	5%

Average age at death, 11½ months
Spontaneous VSD closure = 0
Patients regarded as worse were moving toward group III, in 4 patients (5%).
Infundibular stenosis was regarded as protective in 4 patients (5%).

Group III[106]

Left-to-right shunt <1.5
Right-to-left shunt present
PPA/PSA ratio = 1
Clinically: Cyanotic
n = 11 cases
Surgical VSD closure, 8/11 (73%)
Surgery performed twice, 3/11 (27%)
Average follow-up, 5 11/12 years

Dead	5/11	(45.5%).
Same	5/11	(45.5%)

Infundibular pulmonary stenosis, 1/11 (9%)
Average age at death, 2 years

Group IV[106]

Developed infundibular pulmonary stenosis
n = 21 cases
Surgery performed in 13 of 21 patients (62%)
Two operations, in 4/13 (31%)
Average follow-up was 5 11/12 years

Dead	0	
Same	17	(80%)
TOF	3/21	(15%)
Pure infundibular pulmonary stenosis with closed VSD	1/21	(5%)

Dr. Jean Kachaner et al[106] presented a large, detailed, and classified natural history of VSD in infants and children. In their Comment, they focused first on mortality rates in the various groups.

Ia	=	0
Ib	=	2%
IIa	=	15%
IIb	=	45%
IV	=	0

They concluded that death is related to the degree of pulmonary hypertension; 80% of the deaths occurred in the first year of life. The overall mortality rate was 13%. Then they considered what leads to improvement. Their conclusion was that improvement occurs when the pulmonary artery pressure is normal or only moderately elevated:
Group Ib became group Ia in 50%.
Group IIa improved in 35%.
Group IIb improved in 14%.
Group III did not improve, except in 1 patient who developed infundibular pulmonary stenosis.

Their over-all conclusion was that patients with VSD tended to improve in 33%, when the pulmonary artery pressure was normal or only moderately elevated. Their most common finding in patients with VSD was that they stayed the same (47%). They found that the development of increasing pulmonary hypertension was uncommon, in only 7 of 341 VSD patients (2%). The development of infundibular pulmonary stenosis occurred in 5%. Of 17 patients with significant pulmonary hypertension (groups IIa and IIb), infundibular pulmonary stenosis developed in 7 (41%). Of these 7 patients, 3 had TOF. In the other 4 patients, the VSD closed spontaneously, resulting in pure infundibular pulmonary stenosis, an uncommon finding.

Recommendations of the Parisian team[106]:

1. When the pulmonary artery pressure is normal, surgery is not needed.
2. If there is pulmonary hypertension with failure of medical management, operate in the first year of life.
3. If there is pulmonary infundibular stenosis, wait.

Pernot et al[107] presented a paper about aneurysm of the membranous septum and its role in spontaneous closure of VSDs.

In **1973,** Freed, Rosenthal, Plauth, and Nadas[108] noted that after banding of the MPA, subaortic stenosis could develop.

In **1973,** Kohno, Kume, Sakakibara, Matsui, Konno, and Sakakibara[109] presented their experience with the surgical management of VSD with pulmonary hypertension.

In **1973,** Schott[110] documented spontaneous VSD closure in adult life, between 23 and 40 years of age.

In **1973,** Galioto, Cooley, El-Said, Mullins, and Sandiford[111] described surgical VSD closure through the aortic valve in 6 patients between 20 months and 66 years of age.

In **1973,** Plass et al[112] described VSD with AI in 8 patients with partial prolapse of the aortic valve. They emphasized that one needs angiocardiograms of both the LV and ascending aorta.

In **1974,** Castleman, Scully, and McNealy[113] presented a clinicopathologic conference of a 57-year-old man with a VSD, PVO disease, thrombosis of the pulmonary arteries, and a right aortic arch.

In **1973,** King, Steeg, and Ellis[114] presented a case of "visualization of VSDs by cardiac ultrasonography." Echocardiography was making its diagnostic debut.

In **1973,** Tatsuno, Konno, Ando, and Sakakibara[115] published a study of the pathogenetic mechanisms leading to prolapsing aortic valve and aortic regurgitation with VSD. They concluded that when a subpulmonary VSD is present, lack of support for the RC sinus of Valsalva of the aortic valve leads to prolapse and herniation of the RC aortic leaflet, resulting in aortic regurgitation. We agree completely (see Fig. 16.2).[4]

At about this time, it was becoming known that a subpulmonary conal septal type of VSD is much more common in Asian populations than in white or African populations.

In **1973,** Maron, Ferrans, and White[116] investigated what they called the unusual evolution of acquired infundibular stenosis in patients with VSD. I thought they were probably dealing with cases of mild TOF in patients who, with increasing age, were developing demonstrable infundibular stenosis. However, the histologic findings of the infundibulum resembled that of idiopathic hypertrophic subaortic stenosis. I did not know what to think about the latter possibility.

In **1973,** Marshall and Josephson[117] described the spontaneous rupture of the interventricular septum in a 74-year-old man who was sawing wood. *Thus, vigorous physical exercise can cause an acquired VSD in an elderly person.*

In **1973,** at Johns Hopkins Hospital in Baltimore, Maryland, Ho, Krovetz, Strife, Brawley, and Rowe[118] assessed the status of their VSD patients postoperatively. They focused on 65 patients who had been operated upon between 1968 and 1971. The total surgical mortality was 10.8%. But the mortality of VSD patients with pulmonary hypertension was more than twice that, at 22%. They commented that auscultation is an excellent diagnostic tool both preoperatively and postoperatively.

In **1973,** Tan, Hashimoto, and Takao[119] presented a patient with **ventriculoradial dysplasia,** which is a familial upper-limb cardiovascular syndrome. Inherited as a mendelian dominant trait, the cardinal features include a short humerus, absence of the radius and thumb, and a VSD.

In **1973,** Armour et al[120] reviewed the functional anatomy of the interventricular septum, which is relevant to the understanding of VSDs. This is shown in our Fig. 16.1.

In **1973,** Mesko, Jones, and Nadas[121] answered the question of whether large VSDs really close after pulmonary artery banding. They found that a left-to-right shunt was greatly reduced in 7 of 55 large VSDs (13%) and a left-to-right shunt disappeared in 3 of 55 large VSDs (5%).

In **1973,** the problems associated with pulmonary artery debanding were considered by Dobell et al.[122]

In **1973,** pulmonary artery banding, followed by VSD repair, were reported by Patel et al[123] from Birmingham, England. Of 54 patients with VSD, the banding mortality was 12%. Of the 20 that underwent subsequent VSD repair and MPA reconstruction, the additional surgical mortality was 30%. They proposed that the second surgical procedure be done as soon as possible. They also advocated that primary VSD repair, not banding, be done over 6 months of age.

Dr. Richard Bonham-Carter[124] of Great Ormond Street Hospital in London, England presented a paper at the VSD meeting in France that was entitled, "The Outcome of 144 Infants with an Isolated VSD Who Were Catheterized Before One Year of Age." The time period was 1960 to 1967, and the patients had congestive heart failure. All were catheterized before banding. Banding was done only if they did not respond to maximal medical management. Since 1967, the Great Ormond Street Hospital team has favored primary VSD closure,[124] rather than banding. Still, they recommend banding for multiple VSDs. Their data are[124]:

Total infants <1 year of age	144	
Deaths, 4 before and 5 after banding	9	(6%)
Banding of main pulmonary artery	44	(30%)
Debanding with VSD closure	30	(21%)
Medical treatment without banding	91	(63%)
Evolution toward spontaneous closure	51	(63%)
Evolution toward PVO	4	(3%)
Evolution toward TOF	5	(3%)

PVO, Pulmonary vascular obstructive disease; *TOF,* tetralogy of Fallot. Their total surgical mortality rate of 6% was very low for this early time period.

In **1973,** Maron et al[125] reported 11 postoperative patients who were 3 to 15 years postoperative. All 11 patients underwent surgery at over 10 years of age. When subjected to intense upright exercise, 5 of the 11 (45%) had cardiac outputs that were less than normal. In view of these findings, these authors suggested the importance of early VSD closure.

In **1973,** Nelson[126] reported a case of what the author called a "subaortic septal perforation" in a 92-year-old woman. I thought the patient probably had a congenital VSD. Autopsy revealed a large aneurysm of the membranous septum, and nine 5-mm conal (infundibular) septal defects containing a dumbbell-shaped thrombus. She had both pulmonary and systemic embolization. In addition, she was hypertensive, hypothyroid, and obese (280 lb). I thought this was an example of congenital heart disease in the adult, a subsemilunar conal septal type of VSD, complicated by a dumbbell-shaped thrombus with both pulmonary and systemic embolism. The author[126] thought the conal septal defect was acquired.

In **1973,** Drs. Trusler, Moes, and Kidd[127] published a surgical aortic valvuloplasty for the repair of the aortic valvar insufficiency that can occur with VSD. They achieved a good result in 12 of 13 patients (92%). Dr. George Trusler's[127] aortic valvuloplasty consists of the following steps: (1) measurement of the elongated margin of the aortic leaflet, (2) fixation of the excessive aortic leaflet to the aortic wall, and (3) commissural reconstruction. These authors[127] stated that this aortic valvuloplasty does not work on bicuspid aortic valves.

In **1974,** Clark et al[128] reported on the management of **traumatic VSD.** In the United States, 150,000 heart injuries/year occur from automobile accidents! They recommend medical management for small VSDs and surgery for large VSDs (>2 cm). A typical large traumatic VSD is a large low defect resulting from blunt chest trauma. Clark et al[128] recommend an apical incision that exposes both ventricular cavities. They place a Dacron patch on the left ventricular septal surface and tie the interrupted, pledgeted sutures on the right ventricular septal surface. The first known description of a traumatic VSD was described by Hewett in 1847. The patient was a 5-year-old boy who had been run over by a horse and carriage.

What are the cardiovascular anomalies that are associated with **radial dysplasia** and how frequent are they? In **1974,** Carroll and Louis[129] reported 53 patients with radial dysplasia, of whom 10 had congenital heart disease (19%):

Dextrocardia	2	(4%)
VSD	2	(4%)
PDA	3	(6%)
Coarctation	2	(4%)
Pulmonary stenosis	1	(2%)

Coarctation, Coarctation of the aorta; *PDA,* patent ductus arteriosus; *VSD,* ventricular septal defect.

Radial dysplasia was associated with VSD in only 4% of cases of radial dysplasia.

In **1974,** Freedom et al[130] presented the natural history of aneurysm of the membranous ventricular septum in childhood, based on 56 cases.

In **1974,** Godman et al[131] presented late postoperative conduction system disturbances after surgical repair of VSD and TOF. Five patients developed late complete heart block, 5 months to 5 years postoperatively.

In **1973,** Subramanian[132] presented the concept of primary, definitive, intracardiac repair of congenital heart disease in infancy, focusing on VSDs.

In **1973,** DuShane and Kirklin[133] considered the late postoperative results in patients with VSD. Their conclusions were as follows. When patients with a large VSD have successful definitive VSD repair before 2 years of age, more than 90% have favorable long-term results, with pulmonary arterial resistance that is normal or only mildly elevated. However, when patients with VSD are more than 2 years of age at the time of surgery, with elevated pulmonary arterial resistance, more than 50% have elevated pulmonary resistance postoperatively and potentially unfavorable long-term results. Therefore, they advocated repair of the VSD before the age of 2 years.[133]

In **1974,** Chung and Manning[134] presented their medical and surgical management of VSD with AI.

In **1974,** Assad-Morell, Tajik, and Giuliani[135] described the echocardiographic diagnosis of membranous septal aneurysm.

In **1974,** Kawashima et al[136] described the fate of pericardium used to close VSDs. In 8 cases, they found that 3 (37.5%) had developed aneurysms.

In **1974,** Katz[137] described a patient with VSD who had acupuncture anesthesia for open heart surgery.

In **1974,** echocardiographic studies were becoming more frequent. For example, Hagan et al[138] described normal septal motion with systole:

1. There is anterior motion of the superior one-third of the ventricular septum during systole.
2. Below a pivot point, there is posterior motion of the inferior two-thirds of the ventricular septum during systole.

With right ventricular volume overload, as with VSD, this paradoxical septal motion is not always present.

In **1974,** Rosenquist and Sweeney[139] described the membranous septum in the normal heart.

In **1974,** Kalmanson et al[140] described the echocardiographic method of diagnosing VSD using directional Doppler ultrasound and the phasic flow velocity patterns of the shunt.

In 1974, there was a meeting in Bergamo, Italy about open heart surgery in infancy that was organized by Dr. Lucio Parenzan and his colleagues. I attended this meeting with Dr. Dominique Metras of Marseille, and with my daughter Helen, who spoke fluent French and Italian.

In **1974,** Wallace[141] presented a paper entitled complete correction of VSD in infancy, based on 143 patients, operated on from 1955 to 1970. The mortality rate was 30 of 143 (21%).

There was no progression of pulmonary vascular obstructive disease if the patient was operated on at younger than 2 years of age. In the discussion that followed, Dr. Marini from Milan said that his mortality rate for VSD closure between 1963 and 1970 was 19%. But between 1968 and 1970, his mortality rate for VSD closure had fallen to 10%. Dr. Subramanian said that his mortality rate for VSD closure, including multiple VSDs, was 6%. Sir Brian Barratt-Boyes said that his VSD mortality in infancy was 1 of 20, that is, 5%. He stressed that VSDs should be closed in infancy. He doubted that the transatrial approach was the right one. Dr. Subramanian then said that he had no mortality in isolated VSD closure and no mortality for MPA banding. Wallace said that his mortality rate for MPA banding was 3 of 8 (37.5%).

In **1974,** Girod et al[142] were advocating the two-stage surgical treatment of large VSDs. They banded 34 patients, with 4 deaths (mortality 12%). They debanded 32 patients and closed the VSD in 32 patients, with only 1 death (mortality 3%). Their total two-stage mortality was 15%.

In **1974,** Griep, French, Shumway, and Baum[143] asked, "Is pulmonary artery banding for VSD obsolete?" Their implicit answer was, Yes. They wrote that there is "no advantage" to banding of the MPA over repair in infancy.

In **1974,** de Leval, Taylor, and Stark[144] advocated primary VSD repair in infancy. They reported 18 infants, operated on from 3 months to 9 months of age, with no mortality.

In **1974,** Friedli, Kidd, Mustard, and Keith[145] reported 57 children with VSD. They reported a mortality rate of 18 of 57 (32%) patients. Late deaths occurred 1 to 7 years postoperatively, due to elevated pulmonary arterial resistance, also known as the Eisenmenger syndrome: 7 of 57 (12%). The total mortality rate was 25 of 57 (44%). Their conclusion[145] was to operate (close or band) before 2 years of age.

In **1974,** Allen, Anderson, Noren, and Moller[146] reported their early VSD experience at the University of Minnesota, from 1954 to 1960, based on 341 patients:

Early mortality, 71/341	(21%)
Later mortality, 30/341	(9%)
Total mortality, 101/341	(30%)

In **1974,** Rosenquist et al[147] pointed out that enlargement of the membranous ventricular septum is an internal stigma (or characteristic) of Down syndrome. I agree.

In **1974,** Pirzada et al[148] published a paper about traumatic VSDs.

In **1974,** Moulaert[149] published a thoughtful and original study of VSDs and anomalies of the aortic arch (his MD thesis). Of particular interest, at least to me, was Dr. Moulaert's description of the anterolateral muscle of the LV, also now known as the muscle of Moulaert. This muscle may be of importance in producing obstruction of the left ventricular inflow tract or obstruction of the left ventricular outflow tract.

In **1974,** Lambert et al[150] published a study of 44 patients with VSD and ventricular septal aneurysm. They were not able to document complete VSD closure in any of their cases. They concluded that if the VSD remains open for a few years, complete closure is unlikely.

In **1975,** Barbero-Marcial et al[151] proposed placing a balloon in the MPA of a 3-month-old girl with a VSD for temporary relief of pulmonary hypertension, followed by banding of the MPA.

In **1975,** Tatsuno et al[152] emphasized the diagnostic importance of aortography in conal septal subarterial VSDs. They pointed out the differences between Asians and whites; that is, Asians are much more prone to conal septal subarterial defects than are whites. They also recommended early surgical closure.

In **1975,** Sapire and Black[153] described the diagnosis of membranous aneurysms associated with VSDs.

In **1975,** Hislop, Haworth, Shinebourne, and Reid[154] described quantitative histologic analysis of pulmonary arterial vessels. They found that pulmonary arterial muscle (1) may regress, resulting in increased pulmonary arterial blood flow, or Qp (group 1); or (2) may not regress, leading to an increase in pulmonary arterial resistance, or Rp (group 2). This was an important increase in the understanding of what controls Qp and Rp.[154]

In **1976,** Hoeffel et al[155] analyzed the radiologic aspects of aneurysms of the membranous septum.

In **1976,** Cordell et al[156] studied left ventricular characteristics after VSD closure in infancy. Their salient findings were:

1. left ventricular end-diastolic (LVED) volume = 255 mL, ± 19% of normal;
2. LV systolic output = 240 mL, ± 19% of normal;
3. LV ejection fraction preoperatively = 100, ± 4% of normal;
4. LV mass was mildly elevated preoperatively = 271, ± 21% of normal; and
5. LV mass decreased significantly postoperatively.

Therefore, they concluded that left ventricular size and function respond well to early operative correction of VSD.[156]

In **1976,** Valdes-Cruz et al[157] described the echocardiographic detection of intracardiac right-to-left shunts after peripheral vein injection.

In **1976,** Graham et al[158] studied right ventricular volume characteristics in 37 patients with VSD. They found that when the left-to-right shunt was large, the right ventricular volume was greater than normal.

In **1976,** Stewart[159] described VSD closure through the aortic valvar orifice. To avoid narrowing the aortic valve annulus, he advised closing the VSD first and then replacing the aortic valve.

In **1977,** Corone et al[160] published a 25-year study of the natural history of VSD, based on 790 untreated patients. Among many interesting and important findings, the incidence of aortic valvar regurgitation was 6.3% and the incidence of bacterial endocarditis was 3.7%.

In **1977,** Nugent et al[161] published a study of membranous septal aneurysm in VSD.

In **1977,** Haworth et al[162] published a quantitative histologic study of the pulmonary arterial circulation in 9 patients with VSD, varying from 3 months to 4 years of age.

In **1977,** Hallidie-Smith et al[163] published a study of the functional status of 27 patients with large VSDs, 6 to 16 years after surgical closure in childhood. All led unrestricted lives. However, with effort, striking pulmonary hypertension developed. Consequently they advocated VSD closure before 1 to 2 years of age.

In **1976,** Vidne et al[164] presented their surgical experience in 29 patients with an aneurysm of the ventricular septum:

1. VSD in 15 of 29 (52%), ASD also present in 5 to 15 (33%);
2. VSD with pulmonary stenosis in 5 of 29 (17%); and
3. with transposition of the greater arteries (TGA) in 9 of 29 cases (31%).

Thus, Vidne, Subramanian et al[164] found surgically that aneurysms of the membranous ventricular septum are not associated only with isolated VSD.

In **1976,** Seybold-Epting, Reul, Hallman, and Cooley[165] published their experience with 90 patients who were treated with pulmonary artery banding followed by VSD repair. They found that this two-stage repair was safe and reliable. Their mortality rate was 8 of 90 patients (9%).

In **1976,** Lewis and Takahashi[166] assessed the volume of left-to-right shunts in children with VSD using echocardiography. They found the left atrium–to–aorta ratio (LA/Ao) to be helpful.

In **1977,** Yasui et al[167] assessed the effects of chronic right bundle branch block (RBBB) after surgical VSD closure. They found that chronic RBBB has a strongly deleterious effect on right ventricular function.

In **1977,** Kawashima et al[168] described the transpulmonary arterial closure of a VSD in 14 patients. In 13 of 14 (93%), the VSD was subpulmonary, and they identified it as supracristal. In 1 of 15 (7%), the VSD was subcristal. Chronic RBBB occurred in 4 of these 14 patients (29%): 3 of these 4 had subpulmonary conal septal defects, and 1 had a conoventricular subcristal type of VSD.

In **1977,** Lincoln, Jamieson, Shinebourne, and Anderson[169] described the trans-atrial repair of VSDs and the importance of the VSD's location. This was a study of 50 patients. The VSD was repaired through the RA in 72%. The incidence of RBBB was 24%. The mortality rate was 4%. The VSD classification was membranous, with membranous with malalignment of the infundibular septum; infundibular; posterior, that is, the AV canal type; and apical muscular.[169]

In **1977,** Hordof, Mellins, Gersony, and Steeg[170] announced the reversibility of chronic obstructive lung disease by repair of VSDs in infancy. Chronic obstructive lung disease was cured by VSD closure in infancy.

In **1977,** Glasser and Baucum[171] described fluttering of the pulmonary valve observed echocardiographically in patients with a subpulmonary VSD.

In **1977,** Bloom et al[172] described the echocardiographic evaluation of left-to-right shunts in VSD and PDA.

In **1977,** Yasui et al[173] presented their concepts in the selection of patients and the timing of surgery for VSD repair. This study was based on 87 patients. Their conclusions were as follows. If the pulmonary/systemic pressure ratio (P_p/P_s) equals 0.5 to 0.8, observe for 8 to 10 months. If no better, operate. If P_p/P_s is 0.8 or greater, operate without delay.

In **1976,** Blackstone, Kirklin, Bradley, DuShane, and Appelbaum[174] presented their results concerning the surgery of large VSDs:

1. For a single VSD, operated at younger than 2 years of age, the hospital mortality rate was 9.1%.
2. For multiple VSDs, the hospital mortality rate was 36.4%.

In **1976,** Taylor, de Leval, and Stark[175] reported their results concerning VSD repair in 31 patients in infancy: operative mortality, 0 of 31; all patients younger than 1 year of age; and late death, 1 of 31 (3%), not related to congenital heart disease. VSD reopened in 2 of 31 (6%). Both underwent successful reoperation. Their conclusion was to close the VSD instead of banding the MPA.

In **1972,** Bersch and Chuaqui[176] published a paper entitled, "On the Formal Genesis of the Eisenmenger Complex," in which they proposed that the Eisenmenger complex (i.e., TOF without pulmonary outflow tract stenosis) is caused by an arrest of bulbar (infundibular) rotation. I agree, but would ask the follow-up question, What causes the arrest of infundibular dextrorotation? We think that the answer is:

1. The right-sided subaortic infundibular free wall undergoes normal, or nearly normal resorption, permitting normal or nearly normal aortomitral fibrous continuity by the intervalvar fibrosa, but with aortic overriding.
2. The left-sided subpulmonary infundibular free wall undergoes subnormal growth and expansion. Consequently, the distal conal septum, that is, component 4 (see Fig. 16.1) or the parietal band, fails to move rightward, posteriorly, and inferiorly to a normal degree. It is an algebraic sum of negative and positive development. The right-sided infundibular free wall resorption (negative development) is appropriately normal. But the left-sided infundibular free wall growth (positive development) is subnormal in TOF. Both the right-sided infundibular free wall resorption and the left-sided infundibular free wall growth (completely asymmetrical right-left infundibular free wall development) are necessary to achieve normally related great arteries. Abnormal left-sided subpulmonary infundibular underdevelopment results in a large, subaortic, conoventricular type of VSD. The distal conal septum is often described as being deviated in a leftward, anterior and superior direction, but not as markedly deviated as in TOF. Consequently, in the Eisenmenger complex, there is no pulmonary outflow tract stenosis. So, the Eisenmenger complex is closely related to the TOF. The Eisenmenger complex may be thought of as acyanotic TOF.

I agree with Bersch and Chuaqui[176] and would add that the reason for the arrested or subnormal bulbar (infundibular) torsion in the Eisenmenger complex appears to be due to hypoplasia or subnormal growth and expansion of the subpulmonary conal (bulbar) free wall and of the conal septum. Why this happens is still unknown, but it is now thought to be one or more molecular genetic abnormalities.

In somewhat greater detail, normal subarterial infundibular development is characterized by complete right-left asymmetry in the development of the infundibular free walls:

1. The right-sided subaortic infundibular free wall normally undergoes complete resorption (it disappears).
2. The left-sided subpulmonary infundibular free wall normally undergoes strong growth and expansion.

In the Eisenmenger complex and the TOF, the previously mentioned left-sided subpulmonary infundibular free wall growth is hypoplastic (subnormal). In the Eisenmenger complex, left-sided subpulmonary infundibular free wall development is subnormal, but nonobstructive. In TOF, left-sided subpulmonary infundibular free wall development is more subnormal and hence is obstructive.

In **1971,** Bersch[177] published a paper on the importance of the bulboauricular flange in the formal genesis of congenital heart defects, with special regard to VSDs. If there is infundibular free wall muscle between a semilunar valve and an AV valve, this musculature may be called a bulboventricular flange. Such flanges are important in the normal and abnormal development of the infundibular connecting segment between the great arteries above and the AV canal and the ventricles below.

In **1972,** Kreinsen and Bersch[178] published a paper illustrating the practical diagnostic and surgical importance of the classification of various different anatomic types of VSD. They published the case of a 7-year-old girl with a large subpulmonary conal septal type of VSD, a large subcristal conoventricular type of VSD, and smaller muscular VSDs in the ventricular septum.

In **1977,** Moreno-Cabral et al[179] published a paper about VSD with AI. They advocated early surgical treatment.

In **1977,** Blount[180] compared patients with VSD at high altitude and at sea level.

In **1977,** Keane, Plauth, and Nadas[181] published a study of VSD with AI in 69 patients. There was a male preponderance: of the 69 patients, 47 were males (68%). AI occurred in 5.5% of patients with VSD. Bacterial endocarditis occurred in 8%.

In **1978**, Kawashima et al[182] published VSD closure without ventriculotomy. He described closure of supracristal subpulmonary VSDs via the pulmonary valve in 31 patients from 4 months to 28 years.

In **1978,** Marino et al[183] presented an echocardiographic study of left ventricular–right atrial communication. They described systolic fluttering of the tricuspid valve.

In **1978**, Eshaghpour et al[184] described tricuspid insufficiency with aneurysm of the ventricular septum.

In **1979,** Snider et al[185] described the evolution of ventricular septal aneurysms by two-dimensional chocardiography.

In **1979,** Ahmad and Hallidie-Smith[186] presented an echocardiographic study of 51 patients with VSD, focusing on their left-to-right shunt and the left ventricular function.

In **1979,** McNicholas, de Leval, Stark, Taylor, and Macartney[187] reported their surgical treatment of VSD in infancy. They focused on primary repair versus pulmonary artery banding and late repair. Their mortality for primary repair was 2.4%. Their mortality for two-stage repair was 19.3%.

In **1979,** Wenink, Oppenheimer-Dekker, and Moulaert[188] published a paper on muscular VSDs. They classified their findings into three types: (1) central, (2) posterior, and (3) marginal.

In **1979,** Allwork[189] published a new translation of the maladie de Roger, first reported in 1879, for the centenary.

In **1978,** Levy, Rosenthal, Miettinen, and Nadas[190] published a paper in which they attempted to determine the factors that lead to growth in patients with VSD. This was a study of 1210 patients. Of these, 793 were described as medical patients, and 194 were described as surgical patients. Successful surgical repair was associated with an increase in weight, but not in height. Factors that were thought to be important regarding failure to thrive included abnormal postnatal hemodynamics, intrauterine factors, genetic factors, and low birth weight.

In **1977,** Quero Jimenez et al[191] reported on VSDs in infancy in Spain. They found that there were 1000 new cases of VSD per year in Spain. (This paper is in Spanish.)

In **1979,** Hobbins, Izukawa, Radford, Williams, and Trusler[192] reported their postoperative conduction system disturbances in VSD patients. Using an atrial approach, complete RBBB occurred in 13 of 39 patients (33.3%). Using a trans–right-ventricular approach, their incidence of complete RBBB had been 15 of 19 (78.9%).

In **1979,** Allwork and Anderson[193] studied the developmental anatomy of the membranous part of the ventricular septum in the human heart.

In **1979,** Wise and Wilson[194] presented angiographic documentation of spontaneous closure of a subcristal conoventricular VSD in a 33-year-old woman.

In **1978,** Pham et al[195] compared the right atrial ultrastructure in VSD and in common AV canal (endocardial cushion defect).

In **1979,** Riggs et al[196] studied VSD in infancy using echocardiography and vector cardiography.

In **1978,** McNicholas, Bowman, Hayes, Edie, and Malm[197] considered the surgical management of VSD in infants. Their conclusion was that primary intracardiac repair is the procedure of choice.

In **1978,** Oh et al[198] presented the possible role of pulmonary hyperinflation in the management of VSD. Salient findings were:

1. With pulmonary hyperinflation, mean age at cardiac catheterization was less.
2. The mean age at operation was less.
3. The mean Qp/Qs was greater.
4. The mean P_{PA}/P_{Ao} was greater than with normal pulmonary inflation
5. The pulmonary resistance (Rp) was the same for both groups (pulmonary hyperinflation, and pulmonary normal inflation).
6. Pulmonary hyperinflation was returned to pulmonary normal inflation within 1 month of VSD closure in 35 of 44 patients (79.5%).
7. Pulmonary hyperinflation may lead to progressive lung disease.
8. Pulmonary hyperinflation is another indication for early surgical correction of VSD.

Pulmonary hyperinflation may lead to pulmonary emphysema. I think pulmonary hyperinflation is unnecessary and should be avoided because of its potentially destructive effects on newborn alveoli.

In **1979,** Castañeda and Norwood[199] described surgical closure of VSDs in infancy using the technique of deep hypothermia and circulatory arrest.

In **1978,** Fox, Patel, Graham, Taylor, Stark, de Leval, and Macartney[200] compared single and multiple VSDs clinically and hemodynamically. There were single VSDs in 52 patients and multiple VSDs in 40 patients. Salient findings were:

Findings	Single VSD	Multiple VSDs
Left axis deviation (ECG)	10%	40%
Total mortality	4%	20%
Banding mortality	0%	8%
Subsequent VSD closure mortality	0%	27%
Mortality when repaired beyond 1 year	0%	18%

ECG, Electrocardiogram; *VSD,* ventricular septal defect.

In **1979,** Alpert, Cook, Varghese, and Rowe[201] presented a 10-year follow-up study of spontaneous closure of small VSDs:

1. In 50 infants, the VSD closed spontaneously in 34 patients (68%).
2. By 10 years of age, 75% of small VSDs will close spontaneously.
3. For small muscular VSDs, 83% will close spontaneously.

In **1978,** Mirro[202] reported the management of VSD in the adult, based on a 20-year-old white man with clinical evaluations by Drs. Alexander Nadas and S. Gilbert Blount, Jr.

In **1979,** the diagnosis of VSD was described by two-dimensional echocardiography by Meltzer et al.[203]

In **1978,** Midwall et al[204] studied left-to-right shunt flow and pulmonary hemodynamics in a 28-year-old woman in labor. She had an uncorrected VSD and pulmonary hypertension. With uterine contractions, the mother's Qp/Qs decreased from 1.6 to 1.05. With the use of forceps and bearing down, the Qp/Qs declined.

These authors[204] recommended high concentrations of oxygen for the mother in labor, epidural anesthesia (not general anesthesia), and serial blood gases to monitor changes in Qp/Qs.

In **1979,** Lester et al[205] assessed the diagnostic value of the ratio of left atria to aortic root (LA/Ao) for estimating the left-to-right shunt in VSDs. Arcilla et al[205] (Dr. Rene Arcilla was the senior author) found that the LA/Ao ratio is *not* an accurate estimate of the left-to-right shunt in VSDs.

In **1979,** Aziz, Cole, and Paul[206] presented the echocardiographic features of supracristal subpulmonary conal septal defect with prolapsing aortic valve leaflet.

In **1980,** Arciniegas et al[207] reported their results in surgically closing VSDs in the first 12 months of life. In 52 infants, their operative mortality was 7.6%.

In **1980,** Tharion et al[208] reported their experience with the transpulmonary arterial repair of supracristal subpulmonary VSDs in 5 patients, from 2 months to 2 years of age.

In **1980,** James K. Kirklin, Castañeda, Keane, Fellows, and Norwood[209] reported their experience in the surgical management of 29 patients with multiple VSDs:

1. isolated VSDs, with mortality of 1 in 19 (5.2%);
2. TOF, with mortality of 0 in 5 (0%);
3. TGA, with mortality of 1 in 2 (50%);
4. complete form of common AV canal, with mortality of 1 in 2 (50%); and
5. common atrium, with mortality of 1 in 1 (100%).

The overall hospital mortality was 4 of 29 patients (14%).

In **1980,** Rizzoli, Blackstone, Kirklin, Pacifico, and Bargeron[210] presented incremental risk factors in hospital mortality rate after surgical repair of VSD, based on 312 patients.

In **1980,** Milo, Ho, Wilkinson, and Anderson[211] presented the surgical anatomy and AV conduction tissues of hearts with isolated VSDs.

In **1980,** Gussenhoven et al[212] presented the echocardiographic findings in membranous aneurysms of the ventricular septum.

In **1980,** Bierman, Fellows, and Williams[213] presented the two-dimensional echocardiographic diagnosis of VSDs in infants using the subxiphoid approach.

In **1980,** Alam et al[214] described tricuspid valve fluttering as an echocardiographic sign of a VSD.

In **1980,** Nesje[215] presented systolic time intervals in isolated VSD in the adult. When there is a significant left-to-right shunt, the left ventricular preejection period (PEP) is prolonged, and the left ventricular ejection time (LVET) is shortened. If the PEP/LVET ratio is normal, or if the LVET is normal, a Qp/Qs ratio of 1.4 or greater may be excluded.

In **1980,** Soto et al[216] presented a classification of VSDs.

In **1980,** Kratz et al[217] presented a case of systemic thromboembolism in a 17-year-old black man who had suffered an auto accident. He had a traumatic VSD, and the systemic thromboembolism was thought to have come from his VSD patch.

In **1980,** Silverman, Snider, and Rudolph[218] presented an evaluation of pulmonary hypertension in children with a VSD by means of M-mode echocardiography. Their conclusion was that one needs cardiac catheterization for accurate assessment.

In **1981,** Sethia and Cotter[219] published an unusual cause of a mediastinal mass: a giant aneurysm of the membranous septum in a 36-year-old man.

In **1981,** Canale et al[220] considered factors affecting cross-sectional imaging of membranous or conoventricular VSDs. They call these "perimembranous" VSDs; the difficulty is that there is no such thing as a perimembranous VSD, that is, a defect that extends all around the membranous septum. *Peri* means "around" in Greek.

In **1981,** Green et al[221] described axial cineangiography for the evaluation of VSDs of the AV canal type, which they call posterior VSDs. Muscular VSDs of the inlet portion of the muscular ventricular septum also can be very posterior. I thought the authors were talking about VSDs of the AV canal type, but their axial approach also would be good for posterior muscular VSDs.

In **1981,** Griffiths et al[222] presented the surgical repair of muscular VSDs by a left ventriculotomy. In 2000[7] and 2002,[9] we published a method of muscular VSD closure by a *right ventricular* apical infundibulotomy that we think is better than a *left* ventriculotomy approach.

In **1981,** Dickinson, Arnold, and Wilkinson[223] presented their experience with VSD in children born in Liverpool, England from 1960 to 1969. There were 385 patients. The spontaneous VSD closure rate was 31%. They concluded that only 15% of isolated VSDs were likely to need surgical closure.

In **1981,** Wenink, Oppenheimer-Dekker, and Moulaert[224] published a book entitled, *The Ventricular Septum of the Heart.* This 17-chapter work dealt with the myocardial architecture of the ventricular septum, ventricular septal geometry, development of the ventricular septum, comparative anatomy, ventricular septum defects, two-dimensional echocardiographic localization of VSDs, phonocardiographic follow-up of VSDs, spontaneous closure or decrease in size of VSD in tricuspid atresia with normally related great arteries, the ventricular septum in the common AV canal (which they call an AV defect), echocardiography and angiocardiography in common AV canal, straddling and overriding AV valves, straddling tricuspid valve, straddling mitral valve, classification of ventricular septal anatomy, single ventricle, ventricular septum, and echocardiography in a single ventricle.

In **1981,** Cheatham, Latson, and Gutgesell[225] assessed the accuracy of two-dimensional echocardiography in the diagnosis of VSD in infancy. They concluded that two-dimensional echo detected about three-fourths of the VSDs that were large enough to need cardiac catheterization.

In **1981,** Karpawich, Duff, Mullins, Cooley, and McNamara[226] published a study of VSD with AI. They concluded that often one can defer surgery until after 5 years of age.

In **1982,** Fisher, Snider, Silverman, and Stanger[227] presented a paper on VSD with silent, discrete, subaortic stenosis.

In **1982,** LaCorte et al[228] presented the angiocardiographic and echocardiographic features of a VSD of the AV canal type associated with a cleft mitral valve.

In **1982,** Fellows, Westerman, and Keane[229] presented the angiocardiography features of multiple VSDs in infants. Of those patients with VSD, the VSDs were multiple in 15%. Of those with multiple VSDs, D-TGA was associated in 19% and TOF was present in 7%. A correct diagnosis was made in 86% of these patients.

In **1982,** Smallhorn, Sutherland, Anderson, and Macartney[230] presented the cross-sectional echocardiographic assessment of conditions in which the AV valve leaflets attach to the atrial septum at the same level.

In **1982,** Wenink and Gittenberger de Groot[231] published a paper about ventricular septation and their proposed terminology. (This paper is in French.)

In **1982,** Beekman, Rocchini, and Rosenthal[232] studied the effects of hydralazine in infants with large VSDs. Hydralazine reduces systemic resistance, that is, it is a systemic afterload reducer; 0.2 mcg/kg was administered at cardiac catheterization. The hemodynamic effects were most pronounced 35 minutes after the administration of hydralazine: Qp/Qs was reduced by 24%. Systemic resistance (Rs) fell by 9.5 units to 13.9 units. Systemic flow (Q) was increased.

In **1982,** Shore, Smallhorn, Stark, Lincoln, and de Leval[233] reported 13 patients with VSD and discrete left ventricular outflow tract narrowing. TOF coexisted in 2, and TOF with completely common AV canal was found in 1. A fibromuscular subaortic shelf was excised in 11 of these 13 patients (85%). These authors advocated excision of the discrete subaortic fibromuscular shelf at the time of VSD closure, even if there is no preoperative gradient at that time.

In **1982,** Sutherland, Godman, Smallhorn, Guiterras, Anderson, and Hunter[234] presented a two-dimensional echocardiographic-anatomic correlation and classification of VSDs in children. They classified VSDs as follows:

1. perimembranous inlet,
2. perimembranous outlet,
3. muscular inlet,
4. single trabecular,
5. muscular outlet, and
6. doubly committed subarterial.

By "perimembranous," these authors meant confluent with the membranous septum. *Para*membranous would have been a more accurate adjective because *para* means "to," "at," or "beside" in Greek. *Peri* means "around" in Greek. Used accurately, *peri-* and *para-* have very different meanings. For example, if a patient has had a mitral valve replacement, postoperative assessment might reveal a paravalvar leak, that is, a leak beside the mitral valve replacement—a complication that could readily be repaired. By contrast, a perivalvar leak—a leak all around the mitral valve replacement—would be a disaster, a surgical emergency. In the designation, the *para*thyroid glands, *para* is used correctly: beside the thyroid gland. *Peri*thyroid glands would have a very different meaning, that is, that these glands surrounded the thyroid gland (incorrect meaning).

Used accurately, *perimembranous* VSD would mean that the VSD surrounded the membranous septum. The membranous septum would be floating in space, attached to nothing, because the VSD surrounds the membranous septum.

The decline in the teaching of Latin and Greek in the West is becoming evident in our scientific terminology. Fortunately, I studied Latin in high school for 6 years (grades 9 to 13, inclusive, in Canada), and Dr. Stella Zacharioudaki-Van Praagh, my wife, was Greek. She was conversant with ancient Greek, Byzantine Greek, and (of course) modern Greek.

In **1982,** Lister, Hellenbrand, Kleinman, and Talner[235] studied the physiologic effects of increasing hemoglobin concentration on left-to-right shunting in infants with VSDs. Their findings were as follows. When the hemoglobin went up, the systemic resistance increased. When the pulmonary resistance increased, the left-to-right decreased. Normally, the postnatal decline of hemoglobin is associated with the normal postnatal drop in pulmonary resistance.

In **1982,** Wenink and Gittenberger de Groot[231] proposed the following terminology for the ventricular septum. "primary septum" for the septal band, "inlet septum," for the sinus septum, and "outlet septum" for the infundibular or conal septum.

In **1983,** Beerman et al[236] studied the natural history of VSDs associated with aneurysms of the membranous septum. They concluded that membranous septal aneurysms are not as predictive of VSD closure as had previously been thought.

In **1983,** Anderson, Lenox, and Zuberbuhler[237] studied the mechanisms of closure of conoventricular VSDs (which they called "perimembranous" VSDs) in 69 unoperated heart specimens. They concluded that only rarely are VSDs closed by so-called aneurysms of the membranous septum. Instead, membranous conoventricular VSDs usually are closed by tricuspid valve tissue. I agree with these authors in the following sense: The membranous portion of the ventricular septum lies at the anterosuperior commissure of the tricuspid valve, between the anterior and the septal leaflets of the tricuspid valve. Normally, therefore, the membranous portion of the ventricular septum is within the tricuspid valve; that is, the membranous septum is formed by tricuspid valve tissue. Another way of saying this is as follows. The membranous septum is formed by AV endocardial cushion tissue at the rightmost side of the interventricular foramen (or VSD), which is where the tricuspid valve formally forms. Consequently, the membranous septum may normally be seen as part of the tricuspid valve, between the anterior and septal tricuspid valve leaflets.

What used to be called a "membranous" VSD is now seldom so called, because people have come to realize that most so-called "membranous" VSDs are not really membranous defects.

Typically, the infundibular (or conal) septum is not normally located. The infundibular septum may be a bit too short, it may be deviated slightly anteriorly and superiorly to the left, or it may be deviated abnormally somewhat to the right. This is why we[2] and Kirklin[1] prefer to call such defects **conoventricular**—between the conal (or infundibular) septum above, and the ventricular septum below. In other words, membranous VSDs usually are not defects of the membranous septum only. That is why others have been searching for a better term, such as perimembranous, *paramembranous,* or *juxtamembranous.* The latter two terms have the correct meanings, whereas perimembranous does not (as earlier).

In **1983,** Grenadier et al[238] reported the echocardiographic diagnosis of *left ventricular–right atrial communication.* AV septal defects from LV to RA are often referred to as Gerbode defects (1958). The first LV-to-RA defect was reported in 1838 by Thurman.

In **1983,** Bisset and Hirschfeld[239] described severe pulmonary hypertension associated with a small VSD.

In **1983,** Anderson, Lenox, and Zuberbuhler[240] described the morphology of VSDs that are associated with coarctation of the aorta.

In **1983,** Smallhorn, Anderson, and Macartney[241] described VSDs associated with coarctation of the aorta, diagnosed by cross-sectional echocardiography.

In **1983,** Capelli, Andrade, and Somerville[242] presented their classification of the sites of VSDs as visualized by two-dimensional echocardiography: inlet, which we call VSD of the AV canal type; subvalvar, subtricuspid, subaortic, subarterial doubly committed subpulmonary; and muscular, outlet central apical. What do we think of this classification?[242] Their *inlet* VSD is what we call VSD of the AV canal type, which is above the scooped-out crest of the muscular ventricular septum. The problem is that a muscular VSD in the proximal or inflow portion of the ventricular septum also has been called an *inlet* VSD. Also, is the subtricuspid VSD the same as, or different from, their *inlet* VSD? Note also that there is no *inlet* defect under muscular VSD.

In **1983,** Burrows, Fellows, and Keane[243] published a paper about the cineangiography of left ventricular–to–right atrial shunt, based on 9 cases. They said that their patient has a "perimembranous VSD." I have stated previously what we think about "perimembranous," so no further comment on this adjective shall be made here. But did these patients really have a VSD? Remember that VSD is short for interventricular septal defect (IVSD). LV-to-RA shunt has a defect in the AV portion of the membranous septum, not in the interventricular portion of the membranous septum. Accurately defined, a *membranous VSD* is a defect in the *interventricular* portion of the membranous septum, not in the AV portion of the membranous septum.

From a practical standpoint, LV-to-RA communications are often right at the tricuspid annulus. These defects often go right through the tricuspid valve's septal origin, with most of the shunt from the LV going into the RA. However, I think these authors[242] were wise not to call this communication an AV membranous septal defect, even though it is, because AV septal defect strongly suggests a common AV canal, which was *not* present. LV-to-RA communication or shunt is a preferable term, because it does not invite diagnostic confusion. **LV-to-RA communication is a small AV septal defect without a common AV valve.**

In **1983,** Doty and McGoon[244] described their surgical results of closing conoventricular VSDs (that they called "perimembranous").

In **1983,** Peter, Bowyer, and Jones[245] described right and left ventricular response to exercise, in patients with ASDs and VSDs, by radionuclide analysis. They found that cardiac output was increased only by heart rate. Right ventricular function was the major determinant of total cardiac output during exercise in patients with a VSD, or an ASD, and a left-to-right shunt.

In **1983,** Aziz, Memon, Rehman, and Rehman[246] studied VSD and its hemodynamic correlates in Pakistan.

In **1983,** Otterstad et al[247] studied the clinical and hemodynamic findings in isolated VSDs in adults. They concluded that regardless of symptoms, VSD in the adult should be viewed as potentially serious.

In **1983,** Vogel, Freedom, Brand, Trusler, Williams, and Rowe[248] published their findings in VSD with subaortic stenosis in 41 patients: coarctation of the aorta in 12 (29%), mitral valve anomalies in 4 (10%), right-sided obstruction in 6 (15%), TOF in 4 (10%), and pulmonary stenosis in 1 (2%). What was the anatomic nature of the subaortic stenosis? Findings (n = 41) were fibrous diaphragm, 31 (76%); muscular narrowing, 4 (10%); protruding tricuspid leaflet, 2 (5%); hypertrophic cardiomyopathy, 2 (5%); anterolateral twist, 1 (2%); and redundant tissue tag, 1 (2%).

In **1983,** Yeager, Freed, Norwood, and Castañeda[249] reported our results from Boston Children's Hospital on the primary closure of VSD in 128 patients who underwent surgery at younger than 1 year of age:

Hospital mortality	7.8%
Late mortality	2.3%
Total mortality	10.1%

In **1984,** Dajee, Benson, and Laks[250] reported an improved method of pulmonary artery banding in patients with VSD.

In **1984,** Blieden and Moller[251] reported an 18-year-old young man with a small VSD and severe pulmonary hypertension.

In **1984,** de Leval[252] reported trans-atrial VSD closure in infancy. In closing a conoventricular "perimembranous" VSD from the right atrium, he buttressed the VSD patch with a strip of autologous pericardium.

In **1985,** Soto et al[253] reported their experience in the radiologic diagnosis of VSD.

In **1985,** Becker and Anderson[254] presented their classification of VSDs.

In **1985,** Hagler, Edwards, Seward, and Tajik[255] presented their standardized nomenclature for VSDs in two-dimensional echocardiography.

In **1985,** Vincent, Lang, Chipman, and Castañeda[256] presented their assessment of the patient's hemodynamic status in the intensive care unit, immediately after VSD closure.

In **1984,** Johnson et al[257] presented a method of detecting and quantifying right ventricular outflow tract obstruction secondary to an aneurysm of the membranous ventricular septum in a 5½-year-old boy. They used a combination of two-dimensional echocardiography and continuous-wave Doppler ultrasound.

In **1985,** Marx, Allen, and Goldberg[258] presented a noninvasive method of estimating systolic pulmonary artery pressure in pediatric patients with VSDs by Doppler echocardiography. Doppler can closely estimate pulmonary artery pressure.

In **1985,** Newman[259] considered the cause of VSDs, using an epidemiologic approach, and concluded that VSDs often occur as random errors in development. Therefore, the author said VSDs are not preventable and parents are not responsible for their children's VSDs.

In **1986,** Lillehei, Varco, Cohen, Warden, Patton, and Moller[260] reported a 30-year follow-up of the first open-heart repairs of VSD, AV communis, and TOF using extracorporeal circulation by cross-circulation. From March 26, 1954 to July 19, 1955, the surgical team of Lillehei, Varco, Cohen and Warden operated on 45 patients using cross-circulation in Minneapolis, Minnesota. Their results were as follows[260]:

1. They operated on 27 patients with VSD, more than half of whom were infants. Hospital deaths, 8 of 27 (30%). Late deaths, 2 of 27 (7%).
2. Completely common AV canal, 5 patients. Hospital deaths, 3 of 5 (60%).
3. TOF, 10 patients. Hospital mortality, 5 of 10 (50%).

This heroic and skillful act by Clarence Walton Lillehei and his colleagues was very important in establishing clinical open heart surgery in patients with complex congenital heart disease. What happened in Minneapolis and in Rochester, Minnesota (John Webster Kirklin) inspired many young physicians to devote their professional lives to the field of congenital disease (I was just one among many.)

In **1986,** Leung et al[261] presented an echocardiographic study of LV-to-RA shunting.

In **1986,** Ramaciotti, Keren, and Silverman[262] published a paper pointing out the importance of membranous aneurysms in the natural history of isolated "perimembranous" (conoventricular) VSDs.

In **1987,** Kusuhara et al[263] pointed out the usefulness of electromagnetic blood flow measurement (flowmetry) in the intraoperative evaluation of aortic regurgitation with VSD.

In **1987,** Moene et al[264] reported the anatomic characteristics of VSDs associated with coarctation of the aorta, based on a study of 45 heart specimens.

In **1986,** Didier and Higgins[265] presented the diagnosis and localization of VSDs by gated magnetic resonance imaging (MRI).

In **1986,** Moene et al[266] presented VSDs with normally connected and with transposed great arteries.

In **1987,** Hisatomi et al[267] presented a study of VSD with AI based on 76 patients.

In **1986,** Johnson et al[268] reported a VSD with a mobile tricuspid valve pouch that mimicked TOF.

In **1986,** van de Wal et al[269] published a rare complication of VSD closure—a dissecting aneurysm of the ventricular septum.

In **1988,** Kakou et al[270] published the anatomic types of VSD found in Abidjan, Côte d'Ivoire (Ivory Coast) Africa. (The paper is in French). In 158 diagnosed patients, 75 of whom were operated upon (47%), the anatomic types of VSD were membranous, 77.3%; infundibular, 18.6%; posterior, 2.6%; and muscular, 1.3%.

In **1988,** Baker et al[271] published a revised version of their two-dimensional echocardiographic diagnosis of VSDs.

In **1986,** Lue et al[272] published a study of VSD in Chinese patients with aortic valve prolapse and aortic regurgitation.

In **1985,** Capelli, Marantz, Micheli, Rodriguez Coronel, Kreutzer, Becú, and Berri,[273] from Buenos Aires, Argentina, published a two-dimensional echocardiographic study based on 100 patients "who survived heart failure in the first year" of life. Of these 100 patients, 26 required surgery: subaortic VSD, 16; doubly committed subarterial, 5; and inlet defects, 5.

In **1987,** Kawashima et al[274] presented an improved technique for closure VSDs when ventricular inversion (ventricular L-loop) is present. They advocated putting the VSD sutures in radially, into the morphologically right ventricular side, which is positionally left-sided, from the morphologically left ventricular side, which is positionally right-sided.

In **1987,** Matsuoka et al[275] reported the plasma atrial natriuretic peptide levels in patients with VSD.

In **1988,** Parsons et al[276] reported the diagnosis of VSDs in infants with MRI. MRI is clearer than two dimensional echocardiography, they said.

In **1988,** Yamaki et al[277] presented a paper at the meeting in Bergamo, Italy about the indications for surgery in patients with VSD, or with PDA, and pulmonary hypertension. They suggest that in such cases, the indication for surgery should be based on lung biopsy. They presented their index of pulmonary vascular disease. For example, they found that the upper limits for successful surgery in non-Down patients was 2.1, and in Down syndrome was 2.2. When these indices were adhered to, 25 of 26 patients (96%) underwent successful surgery. There were no late deaths. Of these 25 cases, 6 (24%) had Heath-Edwards changes of grade 4 or more. They concluded that a lung biopsy should be carried out when the pulmonary resistance (R_p) is greater than 8 units/M^2 and R_p does not decrease to less than 4 units/M^2 with oxygen or tolazoline.

In **1988,** at the meeting in Bergamo, Italy, Shore, Rigby, Anderson, and Lincoln[278] proposed that VSDs could be closed surgically without prior cardiac catheterization and angiocardiography. They said that echocardiography alone usually is adequate to show additional defects such as a PDA or a muscular VSD.

In **1988,** at Bergamo, Maehara, Blackstone, Kirklin, Kirklin, Pacifico, and Colvin[279] assessed the results of the Trusler operation for VSD and aortic incompetence. Their conclusion was that the results were good but relief was not certain.

In **1988,** at Bergamo, Daenen and Lesaffre[280] from Leuven, Belgium reported that their mortality rate for VSD closure in infancy was 12.3%.

In **1988,** at Bergamo, Zielinsky et al[281] discussed the surgical management of VSD with subaortic stenosis. They advocated that in addition to closing the VSD, one should also excise the subaortic fibrous membrane to avoid the postoperative appearance of subaortic fibrous stenosis.

In **1988,** at the Bergamo meeting, Alexi-Meskhishvili, Nikoljuk, Popov, and Zajtcev[282] made a presentation entitled

is an AV septal defect. **A membranous defect** is a hole in the interventricular portion of the membranous septum between the LV and the RV (IVSD).

In **1996,** Chaturvedi, Shore, Yacoub, and Redington[370] reported the intraoperative closure of an apical VSD using a modified Rashkind double umbrella.

In **1997,** Carotti et al[371] reported the primary surgical repair of isolated VSD in infancy, guided by echocardiography, without cardiac catheterization, and without angiocardiography, in 96 patients.

In **1997,** Yacoub, Khan, Stavri, Shinebourne, and Radley-Smith[372] reported on their experience with the anatomic correction of the syndrome of prolapsing RC aortic leaflet, dilatation of the sinus of Valsalva, and VSD. Yacoub used a transaortic approach, pledgetted mattress sutures, and autogenous pericardium to close the VSD. He plicated the RC aortic sinus and corrected the outward and downward displacement of the aortic annulus. Yacoub had been using this surgical approach since 1981 (for the previous 16 years). Aortic regurgitation was abolished in 16 of 46 patients (35%), and was improved in the rest (65%).

In **1999,** Niwa, Perloff, Kaplan, Child, and Miner[373] studied the Eisenmenger syndrome in adults. As opposed to the Eisenmenger *complex* (TOF without pulmonary outflow tract stenosis), the Eisenmenger *syndrome* means pulmonary vascular obstructive disease with right-to-left shunting, in congenital anomalies with initially increased pulmonary arterial blood flow (>Qp) such as VSD, truncus arteriosus, and a single ventricle, without pulmonary outflow tract stenosis. Based on 77 adult patients, the authors found that their mortality rate was 35%, with sudden death in 63% of these fatalities. The immediate causes of death included intrapulmonary hemorrhage, rupture of the MPA, rupture of the ascending aorta, or rupture of a bronchial artery. These patients also had vasospastic cerebral infarction. There were no tachyarrhythmic sudden deaths. This is the fate of adults with untreated congenital heart disease with initially excessive Qp.

In **1999,** Macé et al[374] described "Swiss cheese" muscular VSDs and their surgical closure with a single patch using intermediate fixations.

In **1999,** Kalra et al[375] from New Delhi reported that transcatheter device closure of paramembranous and muscular VSDs with Rashkind double-umbrella devices was safe and effective.

In **1998,** Eriksson, Cooper, Rosenbaum, and Ruckman[376] reported the familial occurrence of a congenital aneurysm of the *muscular* ventricular septum. (Note that this is an aneurysm of the *muscular* ventricular septum, *not* of the *membranous* ventricular septum.) Two brothers and their father were involved. There was marked thinning of the muscular ventricular septum, with paradoxical motion of the septum.

In **1999,** Thanopoulos et al[377] reported their experience with closing VSDs, mostly muscular, using a transcatheter approach with the Amplatzer VSD occluded in children. Their 6 patients were from 3 to 10 years of age. A mid-muscular VSD was present in 5, and 1 patient had a subpulmonary VSD. Occlusion was successful in all 6 patients. Transient complete left bundle branch block (LBBB) occurred in 2 of 6 patients (33%). (A subpulmonary VSD ordinarily is not classified as a muscular VSD, as it was in this report.)

In **2000,** Black et al[378] described the repair of multiple VSDs in 8 patients using the septal obliteration technique.

In **2000,** Stellin, Padalino, Milanesi, Rubino, Casaratto, Van Praagh, and Van Praagh[7] described surgical closure of apical VSDs by a right ventricular apical infundibulotomy. **This is Dr. Stella Van Praagh's operation.** Dr. Stella explained it to our good friend Dr. Giovanni Stellin when he was visiting the Cardiac Registry of Boston Children's Hospital. Dr. Stellin liked it so much that when he went home to Padova, he tried it. He found that it worked well and was clearly superior to the conventional *left* ventricular apical surgical approach. Hence, Dr. Giovanni Stellin decided he had to write a paper about this new surgical approach to closing apical muscular VSDs. This is the real back story of this publication.[7]

Here are a few of the key points. Make a short incision to the right of the left anterior descending coronary artery, just above the ventricular apex. You are making an incision into the infundibular apex, which is anterior and superior to the moderator band. The apex of the right ventricular sinus is posterior and inferior to the moderator band. So yes, the RV has two apices, as mentioned previously: (1) the apex of the right ventricular sinus, body, or inflow tract, which is proximal to and posteroinferior to the moderator band; and (2) the apex of the infundibulum or conus arteriosus, which is distal to and anterosuperior to the moderator band. Typically, muscular apical VSDs open from the left ventricular apex into the infundibular apex, anterosuperiorly to the moderator band. Exposure typically is excellent. One can see the complete margins of the apical VSD. Patching the defect is quick and easy. Postoperatively, there is no left ventricular apical aneurysm to worry about.

Closing an apical VSD with a transcatheter approach or with a trans–right-atrial surgical approach is usually difficult because apical muscular VSDs are hard to reach using a trans-tricuspid approach because these defects are "hiding" behind and beyond the moderator band. By contrast, an apical infundibulotomy provides excellent and safe access to the typical apical muscular VSD.[7,8]

In **1998,** Kardon et al[379] presented new observations and insights concerning three-dimensional echocardiography of VSDs, based on experimental and clinical studies. Dr. Gerald Marx, the senior author on this study, is our expert on three-dimensional echocardiography.

In **1997,** Batista et al[380] described successful reversal of pulmonary hypertension in the Eisenmenger complex. The patient was a 19-year-old woman with a VSD and ASD. She had grade IV PVO disease. Her MPA was banded to increase her right-to-left shunt, decrease her aortic saturation, decrease her pulmonary arterial saturation, and reduce her pulmonary arterial blood pressure. One year later, pulmonary biopsy showed total regression of pulmonary vascular obstructive disease. The VSD and ASD were closed and the MPA was debanded. Catheterization was performed 1 week postoperatively. The pulmonary artery pressure was 50% of systemic. The authors' hypothesis was that the regression of PVO is due to lower pulmonary arterial oxygen saturation and lower pulmonary artery blood pressure. These authors subsequently did the same things to 6 more patients, with similar positive results. They concluded that pulmonary artery banding to increase the right-to-left shunt, lower aortic and pulmonary oxygen saturation, and reduce pulmonary arterial blood pressure is a desirable alternative to heart and lung transplantation.[380]

I thought that what Batista et al[380] did was brilliant and a very promising approach to the surgical management of older untreated VSD patients and others with the Eisenmenger syndrome. Corroboration is needed. Their banding of the MPA reversed all of the hemodynamic factors that produced the PVO disease:

1. It lowered pulmonary arterial blood pressure.
2. It lowered pulmonary arterial blood flow.
3 It reduced the pulmonary arterial oxygenation.

From a practical clinical standpoint, we try to close all significant VSDs within the first year of life, to prevent and to avoid PVO. However, for patients who did not receive early VSD occlusion, the Batista approach[380] merits serious consideration.

In **1998,** Lin et al[381] proposed minimally invasive cardiac surgical techniques for closing VSDs, in 14 patients with an average age of 8.9 ± 5.5 years. (Note that these patients were older than our current desired age of younger than 1 year.) Key components of this minimally invasive technique included a left anterior minithoracotomy, video-assisted endoscopy, femorofemoral bypass, continuous coronary perfusion, hypothermic fibrillatory arrest, pericardiotomy, and right ventricular outflow tract entry. All VSDs were successfully closed surgically, with no residual shunts.

In **1999,** Seddio, Reddy, McElhinney, Tworetsky, Silverman, and Hanley[382] considered multiple VSDs: How and when should they be repaired? They advocated repair without ventriculotomy, and without banding of the MPA.

In **1999,** Merrick et al[383] surveyed the management of VSDs in the United Kingdom.

In **1998,** Kaneko et al[384] described right ventricular outflow tract obstruction by a tricuspid pouch in a 5-year-old girl with a VSD. These findings confirm that the membranous septum is really part of the tricuspid valve—between the anterior and the septal leaflets—and that when the membranous septum becomes aneurysmal, it can form an obstructive pouch in the right ventricular outflow tract.

In **2001,** Lun et al[385] studied conal septal defects resulting in subarterial (subpulmonary and subaortic) VSD. In a series of 214 patients, they found that prolapse of the RC leaflet of the aortic valve and aortic valve regurgitation both increased with age.

Age	Prolapse (%)	Aortic Regurgitation (%)
1 year	8	3
5 years	30	24
10 years	64	45
15 years	83	64

Their conclusions were:

1. Subarterial VSDs greater 5 mm should be closed as early as possible to prevent aortic leaflet prolapse and aortic regurgitation.
2. Aysmptomatic patients with small defects, less than 5 mm, may be managed conservatively.

In **1999,** Sim et al[386] reported the outcome of surgical closure of doubly-committed subarterial infundibular septal defect. They found that if surgical closure is done before the onset of aortic valve deformity, progressive aortic regurgitation may be prevented. But when aortic valve repair is done after the development of aortic valvar deformity, then progressive aortic regurgitation is not always prevented.

In **2001,** Okubo et al[387] from the Hospital for Sick Children in Toronto (Dr. Bill Williams, senior author) presented their experience with intraoperative device closure of muscular VSDs in 14 patients. They advocated intraoperative device closure because it avoids ventriculotomy and it avoids the division of intracardiac muscle bands. Their mortality rates were early, 2 of 14; and late, 1 of 14; total, 3 of 14 (21%).

In **1998,** Kitagawa, Durham, Mosca, and Bove[388] presented their techniques and results in the surgical management of multiple VSDs, based on 33 patients. They found that a right atrial approach was optimal for most muscular VSDs, except for apical muscular VSDs, for which they recommended a *left* ventriculotomy. (This paper was published in 1998, 2 years before the paper by Stellin et al[7] and 4 years before the paper by Dr. Stella Van Praagh et al[8] in 2002.)

In **1997,** Grünenfelder, Kiaffas, Bartram, Herlong, and Van Praagh[389] presented a rare case of patch repair of a subarterial infundibular septal defect in which the patch bulged into the left ventricular outflow tract, causing severe left ventricular outflow tract obstruction.

In **1997,** Komai et al[390] presented their strategy for the surgical management of doubly committed subarterial infundibular septal defect. Early operation with minimal observation period is essential to prevent aortic regurgitation. They advocated that if even a tiny amount of aortic regurgitation is detected, operate immediately.[390]

In **2001,** Amin et al[391] published a paper entitled "Intraoperative Closure of Muscular VSDs Without Cardiopulmonary Bypass: Preliminary Results of Periventricular Approach." This paper is about the use of the Amplatzer muscular VSD device, which was successful in all of their cases.

In **2001,** Le et al[392] reported transcatheter occlusion of a subaortic VSD using a nitinol coil. The authors explain that umbrella devices do not work well for the occlusion of conoventricular VSDs because of the proximity of the aortic valve above and the tricuspid valve leaflets below. Instead of an umbrella device, the authors used a retrievable nitinol double-disk coil. These nitinol double-disk coils are available in up to 5-mm diameter, and they are thought to be promising for the occlusion of infundibuloventricular VSDs.

In **2002,** Dr. Stella Van Praagh et al[8] provided follow-up data concerning anatomic and surgical considerations about apical VSD closure: extremely large apical VSDs with severe biventricular dysplasia may require cardiac transplantation and large apical VSDs can be closed through a small apical infundibulotomy, thereby avoiding MPA banding, and left ventriculotomy with the risk for left ventricular apical aneurysm postoperatively.

I would like to acknowledge a debt of gratitude to Dr. Maurice Lev, with whom I had the pleasure and privilege of working for 2 years (1964 and 1965) concerning the pathologic anatomy of congenital heart disease. One of the many things I learned was that the infundibulum (conus arteriosus) consists not only of the infundibular septum and the parietal band distally, but also of the septal band, the moderator band, and the infundibular apical recess proximally.

Many people think that the infundibulum is the distal part only—the part that is obstructively hypoplastic in TOF. They do not know that the septal band, the moderator band, and the infundibular apex (anterior to the moderator band) are also the proximal parts of the infundibulum.

Double-chambered RV is an important example of the foregoing understanding. The right ventricular inflow tract (right ventricular sinus) and outflow tract (the proximal or apical part of the infundibulum) are separated at about the middle of the RV by an obstructive wall (often called a high take off of the moderator band). This understanding is very relevant to the understanding of **single LV with an infundibular outlet chamber.**

If you do not know that the septal and moderator bands are proximal *infundibular* structures, you are very likely to look at the outlet chamber associated with single LV and conclude that the outlet chamber is really a hypoplastic RV (which is incorrect). You are very likely also to conclude that this type of heart really is not a single ventricle. The big LV plus the small RV is not a single ventricle. *This has actually happened.* But, if you know what Dr. Lev taught me, you will recognize that the outlet chamber is the proximal part of the infundibulum, and that the right ventricular sinus (inflow tract) really is absent. Then you will understand that this type of heart really is single LV because the right ventricular inflow tract (the right ventricular sinus) is absent.

In congenital heart disease, anything that is true is likely to be important, somehow, somewhere. Understanding that there is an infundibular apex, just in front of the moderator band, is basic to doing an apical infundibulotomy and patching the apical muscular VSD that typically opens into the infundibular apex.

Why does an apical muscular VSD typically run from the LV apex into the infundibular apex? I do not know why. For the moment, at least, I remember what Dr. Edward Lambert used to say about mysteries like this, "It's just one of those dirty little facts." Hopefully, one day we will know. Dr. Edward Lambert was the Chief of Cardiology at the Buffalo Children's Hospital. He was Dr. Stella's first employer. He had been trained at Johns Hopkins Hospital by Dr. Helen Taussig, as Dr. Stella and I also were.

In **2002,** Tsang, Hsia, Yates, and Anderson[393] published a paper with an intriguing title, "Surgical Repair of Supposedly Multiple Defects Within the Apical Part of the Muscular Ventricular Septum." The authors said that two of their cases could not be closed using a transcatheter interventional approach. Consequently, they used a "modified apical right ventriculotomy." They used Dr. Stella Van Praagh's operation.[7,8]

In **2002,** Cheung et al[394] focused on the impact of preoperative aortic leaflet prolapse on the long-term outcome after surgical closure of subarterial infundibular VSD. They recommended early surgical closure. They also said that aortic valvuloplasty is not needed for mild to moderate aortic RC leaflet prolapse.

In **2002,** Gabriel et al[395] assessed the long-term outlook of patients with VSD who were considered not to require surgical closure in childhood. These authors conclude that surgical closure of VSD in childhood is not required:

- if the left-to-right shunt is less than 50%,
- if there are no signs of left ventricular volume overload,
- if the pulmonary artery pressure is not elevated,
- if there are no symptoms related to VSD, and
- if there are no symptoms related to aortic insufficiency.

In **2002,** Yamagishi et al[396] proposed that the atrial septum around the fossa ovalis (I think they mean septum primum) is an ideal patch for the typical VSD. The ASD so-created is closed by direct suture.

In **2002,** Tsai et al[397] found that after VSD repair, many serum growth factor levels improved in infants, including insulin-like growth factor 1 (IGF-1), IGF-3, and human growth hormone.

In **2002,** Vaidyanathan et al[398] described the outcome of VSD repair in a developing country, in Kerala, India. They concluded that poor nutritional status, preoperative pneumonia, and the patients' ages do not increase mortality after VSD repair.

In **2002,** Puchalski, Brook, and Silverman[399] published simplified echocardiographic criteria for decision making in conoventricular ("perimembranous") VSD in childhood:

1. In infants younger than 3 months of age, when the maximal VSD diameter is 5 mm or less, such a VSD is likely to close or to be hemodynamically insignificant.
2. When the maximum VSD diameter is 6.5 mm or greater, such a VSD most likely will require closure.

In **2002,** Fukuda et al[400] stated that shallow stitching close to the rim of the VSD eliminates injury to the right bundle branch of the conduction system. These authors found that when they used shallow stitches close to the rim of the VSD, their incidence of complete RBBB was only 6.3%, compared with 43.8% when they used deeper stitches further from the rim.

From an anatomic standpoint, I would add that one can often see the right bundle branch (RBB). It is a thin, whitish, linear streak. The RBB appears close to and often a bit under the right posterior division of the septal band. Then the RBB runs inferiorly downward on the septal band, close to the inferior rim of the septal band and parallel to it, heading for the moderator band, which carries the RBB to the anterior papillary muscle of the RV and then on to the right ventricular free wall. My point is that because one can *see* the RBBB (because of its whitish glycogen content), it then becomes much easier to avoid spearing the RBB with a surgical needle and then transecting the RBB with a suture.

It is often assumed, erroneously, that the right and left bundle branches of the AV conduction system are grossly invisible. Once you know exactly where they are, then you can see them. Visualization of the RBB intraoperatively aids atraumatic suture placement.

In **2003,** Ootaki et al[401] described the "sandwich technique" for occluding trabecular (i.e., muscular) VSDs surgically. In 11 patients, the authors introduced 8- to 10-mm circulator polyester patches through the mitral valve into the LV, and through the tricuspid valve into the RV. The right-sided patch was placed over a 3-0 Nespolen suture. A 3-French catheter was placed through the muscular VSD. Finally, the suture was tied firmly, sandwiching the septum between the two felt patches. The results were as follows: no shunt, 3 of 11 (27%); minimal shunt, 5 of 11 (45%); and mild to moderate shunt, 3 of 11 (27%). (Minimal shunt means tiny shunt, with Qp/Qs = 1.)

In **2003,** Sivakumar et al[402] published a paper about the closure of muscular VSDs, aided by en face reconstruction and pictorial representation. The authors thought that a diagram was a better guide than were different classifications and confusing terminology.

In **2003,** Thanopoulos et al[403] published their experience with transcatheter closure of infundibuloventricular ("perimembranous") VSDs using the Amplatzer asymmetrical VSD occluder. This preliminary experience in children was based on 10 patients. The VSDs varied from 2 to 8 mm in maximal dimension. The devices varied from 4 to 8 mm in maximal dimension. The results were as follows: no shunt, 9 of 10 (90%); and trivial shunt that disappeared at 3-month follow-up in 1 of 10 (10%). Transient complete (LBBB) occurred in 3 of 10 (30%).

In **2003,** Maile et al[404] reported detachment of the anterior leaflet of the tricuspid valve to expose infundibuloventricular ("perimembranous") VSDs. In this series of 49 patients, the VSD exposure was described as excellent. Detaching the anterior tricuspid leaflet was found to be better than detaching the septal tricuspid leaflet. The authors used a Gore-Tex patch and a continuous suture.

In **2003,** Zhao et al[405] reported that tricuspid valve detachment does facilitate VSD closure.

In **2003,** Aeba et al[406] confirmed that liberal use of tricuspid valve detachment does indeed facilitate trans-atrial VSD closure. These authors pronounced tricuspid valve detachment to be safe and effective. They said it improves speed and reliability. This study was based on 87 patients with isolated VSD, of the infundibuloventricular and AV canal types. Tricuspid detachment resulted in shorter bypass times: on average, 59 minutes versus 67 minutes.

In **2003,** Partin[407] published a fascinating article on **Victor Eisenmenger** (1864–1932). His article was entitled, "The Evolution of Eisenmenger's Eponymic Enshrinement." Victor Eisenmenger was born in Vienna, Austria, of German parents, in 1864. He is described as having been in poor health. He published his famous paper describing what is now called the Eisenmenger complex when he was 33 years of age in 1897.

Eisenmenger was court physician to the royal Hapsburg family and physician to Archduke Franz Ferdinand, who had pulmonary tuberculosis. As almost everyone now knows, but few really understood, how Archduke Franz Ferdinand and his wife Countess Sophie Chotek were assassinated at Sarajevo on June 28, 1914, triggering the Great War—World War I, which was continued a generation later as World War II. I shall never forget, on or about September 3, 1939, listening to the radio at home in Toronto, Canada, with my family when King George VI of Great Britain announced that a state of war existed between Great Britain and Nazi Germany. I was 9 years old, and my brother Ian was 7. We thought it was very exciting. Then I looked up at my Dad, a native Englishman. With infinite sadness he said, "The Great War has been resumed."

Now, here we are in the early 21st century, survivors of the bloodiest century in the history of the Earth. What happened at Sarajevo in 1914? Briefly, it was an accident. The background may be summarized as follows. Archduke Franz Ferdinand was next in succession to be Emperor of Austria. He was also King of Hungary. His wife Sophie Chotek was merely a Countess, far below her husband in aristocratic rank. She was not allowed to appear with her husband at most public events, except military affairs. Franz loved Sophie and deeply resented the aristocratic absurdities.

Bosnia and Hercegovina were recent Habsburg acquisitions. Formerly Turkish and the scene of many rebellions, they had been annexed by the Habsburgs in 1908, 6 years previously. Some of the southern Slavs, Serbs, or Croats were resentful at having been taken over by the Habsburgs.

So, when a visit to Sarajevo by the Archduke was announced, about 6 high-school-aged boys decided they would try to kill the Archduke. They received encouragement and weapons from a Serb secret society. The day of their visit to Sarajevo was the anniversary of their wedding day. Franz took Sophia along for love and because it was a military occasion. So on June 28, 1914, the Archduke and his wife drove into Sarajevo. One of the young conspirators failed to draw his revolver. Another felt sorry for Countess Sophie and went home. A third threw his bomb and missed. The Archduke reached the town hall. But he was angry because this special drive for his wife had been spoiled. He decided to drive straight out of town. But his chauffeur was not told. He took a wrong turn. Then he stopped the car and reversed. One of the schoolboy conspirators, Gavrilo Princip, saw to his amazement Archduke Franz Ferdinand and his wife Countess Sophie sitting in a stopped car. So he ran over to the car, stepped on the running board, and killed the Archduke with one shot. With a second shot, he hit Countess Sophie, who died almost immediately.

I said this double assassination was an accident because it probably would not have happened had the chauffeur not taken a wrong turn, requiring him to stop and turn around. And the chauffeur left the car stopped because he did not realize that the Archduke was angry and wanted to leave. The Archduke and his wife appeared to have no one close to the car to protect them. So, this is how Dr. Victor Eisenmenger's most important patients, the Archduke Franz Ferdinand and his beloved wife Countess Sophie, died.[407]

Dr. Maude Abbott defined the Eisenmenger complex (and the TOF). In **1951,** Dr. Paul Wood introduced the concept of the Eisenmenger *syndrome:* PVO, with shunt reversal (right-to-left). In **1847,** the Eisenmenger complex was first described by Dalrymple.

The Eisenmenger syndrome (PVO) is what happens to the Eisenmenger complex (TOF without pulmonary outflow tract obstruction) when the it is not treated appropriately: the complex becomes the syndrome. All, or most of the literature that we have been reviewing is designed to prevent the development of the Eisenmenger syndrome.

In **2003,** Bacha et al[408] described device closure of muscular VSDs using the Amplatzer muscular VSD occluding device. Based on 6 patients, their technique was described as safe and effective, with no cardiopulmonary bypass needed.

In **2004,** Gott and Shumway[409] published a paper entitled, "Cross-Circulation: A Milestone in Cardiac Surgery." **This was an inspiring historical paper.**

In March **1954,** C. Walton Lillehei and his team performed their first VSD repair using cross-circulation. (This was 3 months before I graduated from the Faculty of Medicine, University of Toronto.) The patient was 1 year old. The VSD was closed without a patch during 19 minutes of cross-circulatory support. The patient developed pneumonia and died on the 11th postoperative day.[409] One week later, Lillehei and his team successfully closed a VSD in a 4-year-old boy, using the same technique.[409] From March 1954 to May 1955, Lillehei and his team operated on 45 children using cross-circulation. **They were the first to successfully repair VSD, TOF, and common AV canal.**[409] Their survival rate for these 45 patients was 62% (discharged from hospital). At follow-up 30 years later, 49% were alive and well.[409]

On July 14, **1954,** Dr. Clarence Crafood successfully removed an atrial myxoma using a disk oxygenator developed by Dr. Åke Senning. The next surgical group to successfully repair congenital heart disease using a Mayo-Gibbon screen oxygenator was the Mayo Clinic in Rochester, Minnesota, led by Dr. John Webster Kirklin, beginning on May 22, 1955.

In **1955,** only two centers in the world were doing open heart surgery—in Minneapolis-St. Paul and Rochester, Minnesota. Lillehei in Minneapolis-St. Paul started open heart surgery first, using cross-circulation. Kirklin in Rochester made open surgery a clinical reality with the use of the Gibbon-Mayo heart-lung machine.[20,21]

In **2004,** Holzer et al,[410] for the Amplatzer Muscular VSD Investigators, reported the immediate and mid-term results for this US registry:
successful implantation, 72 of 83 (87%);
multiple devices used, 17 of 83 (20.5%);
procedure-related complications, 8 of 75 (11%);
procedure-related deaths, 2 of 75 (3%);
24-hour postprocedure complete closure 34 of 72 (47%);
6 months, complete closure, 32 of 46 (70%); and
12 months, complete closure, 24/26 (92%).
These authors[410] concluded that the closure rate was excellent, that the mortality was low, and that the procedure was safe and effective.

In **2004,** Bhatt et al[411] considered the problem of how best to manage infants with large unrepaired VSDs and respiratory infection requiring mechanical ventilation. The authors found that medical and surgical management should both be done during the same hospitalization. In a series of 18 such infants, 12 had VSD closure (67%). Of the 12 who were repaired, 11 were discharged (92%).[411]

In **2005,** Novick et al[412] published a paper entitled "Flap Valve Double Patch Closure of VSDs in Children With Increased Pulmonary Vascular Resistance." In a series of 91 patients, these authors advocated closure of large VSDs with elevated pulmonary vascular resistance (10.5 ± 4.9 Wood units) with a fenestrated VSD patch that can open from right to left. The early mortality was 7 of 91 (8%). Total mortality was 14 of 91 (15%). The median patient age was 4.0 ± 3.1 years.[412]

In the discussion after the presentation,[412] Dr. Randas Batista from Curitiba, Brazil said, What causes high resistance in the lungs is high oxygen content of the pulmonary arterial blood, not high blood flow in the pulmonary arteries. Therefore, the MPA should be banded to increase the right-to-left shunt through the VSD, thereby lowering the oxygen content of the blood in the MPA and its branches. Within 2 years, Batista reported the "irreversible" lung lesions were cured. Then he debanded the MPA and closed the VSD. He has done 23 cases in this way. (See Dr. Batista's[380] earlier description of this technique.)

In **2004,** Knauth, Lock, Perry, McElhinney, Gauvreau, Landzberg, Rome, Hellenbrand, Ruiz, and Jenkins[413] published their experience of transcatheter device closure of VSDs, both congenital and postoperative residual. Their mortality was 1 of 170 (0.59%). Surgical device removal was required in 8%.[413]

In **2005,** Carminati et al[414] reported their results with transcatheter VSD occlusion using Amplatzer septal occluders. This study was based on 122 cases: paramembranous, 87; muscular 30; and postsurgical repair of infundibuloventricular (paramembranous) defects, 5. The mean age at occlusion was 15 years, ranging from 6 months to 64 years. The mean VSD diameter was 7 mm, ranging from 4 to 16 mm. The device size was 1 to 2 mm larger than the maximal VSD dimension. Amplatzer membranous devices were deployed in 72 patients and Amplatzer muscular devices in 47. Satisfactory device implantation was accomplished in 119 of 122 (97.5%). Tiny residual flow was observed immediately after the procedure in 50%. Residual shunt after 24 hours was 19%, and residual shunt after 6 months was 4%. Minimal aortic regurgitation was present in 3 of 122 (2%). Device embolization occurred in 3 of 122 (2%). The device was retrieved successfully in all 3, and device reimplantation was successful in all three. Transient LBBB occurred in 2 patients. Transient first-degree AV block was found in 1 patient. In membranous VSD patients, complete AV block occurred acutely (within 48 hours of the procedure) in 3 patients; treated with a pacemaker in 1. Late complete heart block occurred in 2 patients, 5 months and 12 months after the procedure. Complete heart block occurred in 5 of 122 patients (4%). Complete heart block occurred in 5 of 87 paramembranous VSDs (6%). The mortality was 0. At mid-term follow-up complete VSD closure was achieved in 96%. The authors conclude that greater experience and long-term follow-up are needed.[413]

My concern is with the AV conduction system, which is vulnerable to device trauma. Surgical VSD closure in expert hands may prove to be safer for the conduction system. Time will tell.

In **2006,** Robinson et al[415] published a paper about cardiac conduction disturbances after transcatheter device closure of muscular VSDs using the Amplatzer occluder. This study was based on 27 patients: single muscular VSD, 16; Swiss cheese septum, 5; multiple muscular VSDs, 9; and post–myocardial infarction muscular VSDs, 3.

Permanent changes (ECG) were observed in 3 procedures (10%), involving 3 patients (11%). Complete RBBB occurred in 1 patient, and left anterior hemiblock occurred in 2 patients. **Transient changes** (ECG documented) occurred with 2 procedures (7%) in 2 patients (7%). Transient second-degree AV block occurred in 1. Transient left anterior hemiblock occurred in 1 patient. After the procedure, 13 of 16 had ectopy (81%); 11 had isolated premature contractions for less than 1% of 24 hours; and 4 had nonsustained ventricular tachycardia. Subsequently, all were asymptomatic.[414]

In **2007,** Meadows, Pigula, Lock, and Marshall[416] focused on transcatheter creation and enlargement of VSDs for the relief of ventricular hypertension. In DORV authors[416] proposed the creation or enlargement of physiologically restrictive VSDs using a transcatheter approach to create a decompressing VSD in the midventricular septum. We reported the *surgical* enlargement of a restrictive VSD in DORV in 1971 (Lavoie et al).[417]

In **2010,** Xing et al[418] reported a minimally invasive perventricular device closure of infundibuloventricular ("perimembranous") VSDs without cardiopulmonary bypass. This was a multicenter experience and mid-term follow-up of 408 patients, who varied from 5 months to 15 years in age. The success rate for VSD occlusion was 96.3%. Open cardiac repair was done in 3.7%. The authors concluded that this is a simple, effective, relatively safe technique with trans-esophageal echocardiographic guidance. They used concentric and eccentric occluders.[418]

In **2010,** Zuo et al[419] from China reported their experience with transcatheter occlusion for infundibuloventricular ("perimembranous") VSDs using the Amplatzer membranous VSD occluder in 301 patients. Their mean age was 9.8 years, and their mean weight was 32 kg (70.5 lb). Successful VSD occlusion was achieved in 294 of 301 patients (97.6%). The mortality rate was zero. Complications were as follows. Aortic regurgitation occurred in 11 of 301 (3.7%). Two required occluder retrieval. Tricuspid regurgitation occurred in 16 of 301 (5.4%). Hemolysis was found in 2 of 301 (0.7%). Complete AV block occurred in 17 of 301 (5.6%). Early complete AV block occurred in 15 and late complete AV block in 3, with early and late complete AV block in 1. Of 15 early complete AV blocks, block was transient in 12 and prolonged (>2 weeks) in 3. Surgery was performed in 3, and postoperative sinus rhythm occurred in all. Late complete AV block occurred in 3, and these patients were treated with a pacemaker. The authors[419] concluded that the VSD closure rate was high (97.6%). However, they also stated that a major concern was the complication of complete AV block.[419] I strongly agree with the latter concern. AV conduction systemic trauma, particularly with paramembranous VSD occluders, may be the Achilles heel of transcatheter VSD occlusion. However, only time will tell.

Maladie de Roger. Why do our French friends and colleagues sometimes refer to a VSD as a *maladie de Roger?* Because Henri Louis Roger (1809–1891), a surgeon in Paris, wrote a well-known paper on VSD in 1879.[420] VSDs have occasionally been described in English as *Roger's disease,* or as *Roger's syndrome.*

VENTRAL SEPTAL DEFECTS AS PARTS OF A CONOTRUNCAL MALFORMATION

So far, this chapter has been concerned with relatively isolated VSDs. However, VSDs often are not isolated. Indeed, VSDs are integral parts of almost all infundibuloarterial (or conotruncal) anomalies such as **TOF, truncus arteriosus, TGA, DORV, DOLV, and anatomically corrected MPA.**

In **2016,** Francois Lacour-Gayet et al[421] published a cardiac surgical textbook entitled ***Surgery of Conotruncal Malformations*** in which the anatomy, diagnosis, and surgery, including that of associated VSDs are presented in detail.

The associated VSDs mentioned previously are considered in association with the infundibuloarterial anomalies of which they are a part, in the appropriate chapters of the present book.

REFERENCES

1. Soto S, Ceballos R, Kirklin JW. Ventricular septal defects: a surgical viewpoint. *J Am Coll Cardiol.* 1989;14:1291.
2. Van Praagh R, Geva T, Kreutzer J. Ventricular septal defects: how shall we describe, name and classify them? *J Am Coll Cardiol.* 1989;14:1298.
3. Megarity A, Chambers R, Calder AL, Van Praagh S, Van Praagh R. Double-outlet right ventricle with left ventricular-right atrial communication: fibrous obstruction of left ventricular outlet by membranous septum and tricuspid leaflet tissue. *Am Heart J.* 1972;84:242.
4. Van Praagh R, McNamara JJ. Anatomic types of ventricular septal defect with aortic insufficiency. *Am Heart J.* 1968;75:604–619.
5. Nadas AS, Thilenius OG, LaFarge CG, Hauk AJ. Ventricular septal defect with aortic regurgitation. Medical and pathologic aspects. *Circulation.* 1964;29:862.
6. Halloran KH, Talner NS, Brown MJ. A study of ventricular septal defect associated with aortic insufficiency. *Am Heart J.* 1965;69:320.
7. Stellin G, Padalino M, Milanesi O, et al. Surgical closure of apical ventricular septal defects through a right ventricular apical infundibulotomy. *Ann Thorac Surg.* 2000;69:597.
8. Van Praagh S, Mayer JE, Berman NB, Flanagan ME, Geva T, Van Praagh R. Apical ventricular septal defects: follow-up concerning anatomic and surgical considerations. *Ann Thorac Surg.* 2002;73:48.
9. Wollenek G, Wyse R, Sullivan I, Elliott M, de Leval M, Stark J. Closure of muscular ventricular septal defects through a left ventriculotomy. *Eur J Cardio Thorac Surg.* 1996;10:595.
10. Hunter W. Three cases of mal-conformation in the heart. Medical Observations and Inquiries, Society of Physicians in London. vol. 6. T Cadell publisher; 1784:291–417.
11. Van Praagh R. *Survival. A New Approach from the Life Sciences to the Major Problem of Our Time.* Phoenix, Arizona: Falcon Press; 1985.
12. Darwin C. *The Origin of the Species.* New York: New American Library, Mentor Books originally published in 1859; 1958.
13. Aristotle. *The Physics, Volume IV, Books I-IV, with English Translation by PW Wickstead and FM Cornford.* London and Cambridge: W Heinemann, Ltd, Harvard University Pressthe Loeb Classical Library; 1970:168.

14. Frebel A. *Searching for the Oldest Stars, Ancient Relics from the Early Universe. Translated by AM Hentschell.* Princeton and Oxford: Princeton University Press; 2015.
15. Frebel A. *Op. cit.: Carbon, Hydrogen, Oxygen, Phosphorous, Sulfur, and Nitrogen-The Elements of Life, Translated by AM Hentschell.* Princeton and Oxford: Princeton University Press; 2015:238.
16. Van Praagh R. Genetic implications of successful treatment of congenital heart disease. In: Barratt-Boyes BG, Neutze JM, Harris EA, eds. *Heart Disease in Infancy.* Edinburgh and London: Churchill and Livingstone; 1973:331.
17. Eisenmenger V. Die angeborenen Defecte der Kammerscheidewand des Herzens. *Z kiln Med.* 1897;32:1. Translated in Rashkind WT: Congenital Heart Disease 1982, Hutchinson Ross Publishing Company, Benchmark Papers in Human Physiology 1982; 16:176.
18. Muller WH, Dammann JF. The treatment of certain congenital malformations of the heart by the creation of pulmonic stenosis to reduce pulmonary blood flow, a preliminary report. *Surg Gynecol Obstet.* 1952;95:213.
19. Lillehei CW, Cohen M, Warden HE, Varco RL. The direct-vision intracardiac correction of congenital anomalies by controlled cross circulation. Result in thirty-two patients with ventricular septal defects, tetralogy of Fallot, and atrioventricularis communis defects. *Surgery.* 1955;38:11.
20. Kirklin JW, DuShane JW, Patrick RT, et al. Intracardiac surgery with the aid of a mechanical pump-oxygenator system (Gibbon type): report of eight cases. *Mayo Clin Proc.* 1955;30:201.
21. DuShane JW, Kirklin JW, Patrick RT, et al. Ventricular septal defects with pulmonary hypertension. Surgical treatment by means of a mechanical pump-oxygenator. *J Am Med Assoc.* 1956;160:950.
22. Lev M. The architecture of the conduction system in congenital heart disease. III. Ventricular septal defect. *Arch Path.* 1960;70:529.
23. Kirklin JW, McGoon DC, DuShane JW. Indications for repair of ventricular septal defects. *Am J Cardiol.* 1963;12:75.
24. Morgan BC, Griffiths SP, Blumenthal S:I. Congestive heart failure in infancy. *Pediatrics.* 1960;25:54.
25. Neufeld HN, Titus JL, DuShane JW, Burchell HB, Edwards JE. Isolated ventricular septal defect of the persistent common atrioventricular canal type. *Circulation.* 1961;23:685.
26. Van Praagh R. *The Importance of Ventriculoatrial Malalignment in Anomalies of the Atrioventricular Valves, Illustrated by "Mitral Atresia" and Congenital Mitral Stenosis with Large Left Ventricle, Pediatric Cardiology.* New York: Springer-Verlag Inc; 1986:901–903.
27. Kidd L, Rose V, Collins G, Keith JD. The hemodynamics in ventricular septal defect in childhood. *Am Heart J.* 1966;70:732.
28. Friedman WF, Mehrizi A, Pusch AL. Multiple muscular ventricular septal defects. *Circulation.* 1965;32:35.
29. Barnard PM, Kennedy JH. Post infarction ventricular septal defect. *Circulation.* 1965;32:76.
30. Hoffman JIE, Rudolph AM. The natural history of ventricular septal defects in infancy. *Am J Cardiol.* 1965;16:634.
31. Ritter DG, Feldt RH, Weidman WH, DuShane JW. Ventricular septal defect. *Circulation.* 1965;32:42.
32. Simmons RL, Moller JH, Edwards JE. Anatomic evidence for spontaneous closure of ventricular septal defect. *Circulation.* 1966;34:38.
33. Osborn JR, Hall RJ, Winn DF, Capper RS, Blake HA. An unusual late complication of pulmonary artery banding. *Circulation.* 1966;34:61.
34. Hoffman JIE, Rudolph AM. Increasing pulmonary vascular resistance during infancy in association with ventricular septal defect. *Pediatrics.* 1966;38:220.
35. Rose V, Collins G, Kidd L, Keith J. Clinico-hemodynamic correlations in ventricular septal defect in childhood. *J Pediat.* 1966;69:359.
36. Girod DA, Raghib G, Adams P, Anderson RC, Wang Y, Edwards JE. Cardiac malformations associated with ventricular septal defect. *Am J Cardiol.* 1966;17:73.
37. Gould L, Lyon AF. Prolapse of the pulmonary valve through a ventricular septal defect. *Am J Cardiol.* 1966;18:127.
38. Schrire V, Vogelpoel L, Beck W, Nellen M, Swanepoel A. Ventricular septal defect: the clinical spectrum. *Br Heart J.* 1965;27:813.
39. Reynolds JL. Supracristal ventricular septal defect. *Am J Cardiol.* 1966;18:610.
40. Williams GD, Hara M, Bullock R. Traumatic ventricular septal defect. *Am J Cardiol.* 1966;18:907.
41. Saab NG, Burchell HB, DuShane JW, Titus JL. Muscular ventricular septal defects. *Am J Cardiol.* 1966;18:713.
42. Mitchell SC, Berendes HW, Clark WM. The normal closure of the ventricular septum. *Am Heart J.* 1967;73:334.
43. Grainger RG, Nagle RE, Pawidapha C, et al. Pulmonary artery banding for ventricular septal defect. *Br Heart J.* 1967;29:289.
44. Edwards JE. Ventricular septal defect. Unresolved problems. *Am J Cardiol.* 1967;19:832.
45. Anderson RA, Levy AM, Naeye RL, Tabakin BS. Rapidly progressing pulmonary vascular obstructive disease. Association with ventricular septal defects during early childhood. *Am J Cardiol.* 1967;19:854.
46. Levin AR, Spach MS, Canent RV, Jain V, Barr RC, et al. Intracardiac pressure-flow dynamics in isolated ventricular septal defects. *Circulation.* 1967;35:430.
47. Sigmann JM, Stern AM, Sloan HE. Early surgical correction of large ventricular septal defects. *Pediatrics.* 1967;39:4.
48. Tikoff G, Schmidt AM, Tsagaris T. Isoproterenol-induced right ventricular infundibular obstruction. Study in adult with a large ventricular septal defect. *Am J Cardiol.* 1967;20:173.
49. Sakakibara S, Konno S. Congenital aneurysm of the sinus of Valsalva associated with ventricular septal defect. Anatomical aspects. *Am Heart J.* 1968;75:595.
50. Hoffman JIE. Natural history of congenital heart disease. Problems in its assessment with special reference to ventricular septal defects. *Circulation.* 1968;37:97.
51. Baron MG, Wolf BS, Steinfeld L, Van Mierop LHS. Angiocardiographic diagnosis of subpulmonary ventricular septal defect. *Am J Roentgenol.* 1968;103:93.
52. Clarkson PM, Frye RL, DuShane JW, Burchell HB, Wood EH, Weidman WH. Prognosis for patients with ventricular septal defect and severe pulmonary vascular obstructive disease. *Circulation.* 1968;38:129.
53. Rastelli GC, Ongley PA, Titus JL. Ventricular septal defect of atrioventricular canal type with straddling right atrioventricular valve and mitral valve deformity. *Circulation.* 1968;37:16.
54. Edgett JW, Nelson WP, Hall RJ, Jahnke EJ, Aaby GV. Spontaneous closure of a ventricular septal defect after banding of the pulmonary artery. *Am J Cardiol.* 1968;22:729.
55. Coleman EN, Reid JM, Inall JA, Stevenson JG. Ventricular septal defect repair in childhood. *Br Heart J.* 1968;30:845.
56. Leachman RD, Pereyo JA. Decrease in pulmonary vascular resistance following surgical closure of a ventricular septal defect associated with elevated capillary wedge pressure and severe pulmonary arterial hypertension. *Am Heart J.* 1968;76:816.

57. Tandon RK. Chylothorax after repair of ventricular septal defect. *J Thorac Cardiovasc Surg*. 1968;56:378.
58. Gotsman MS, Beck W, Barnard CN, Schrire V. Hemodynamic studies after repair of ventricular septal defect. *Br Heart J*. 1969;31:63.
59. Miller RH, Schiebler GL, Grumbar P, Krovetz LJ. Relation of hemodynamics to height and weight percentiles in children with ventricular septal defects. *Am Heart J*. 1969;78:523.
60. Hallidie-Smith KA, Hollman A, Cleland WP, Bentall HH, Goodwin JF. Effects of surgical closure of ventricular septal defects upon pulmonary vascular disease. *Br Heart J*. 1969;31:246.
61. Yang SS, Maranhao V, Ablaza SGG, Morse DP, Goldberg H. Aneurysm of the membranous portion of the ventricular septum. *Am J Cardiol*. 1969;23:83.
62. Varghese PJ, Izukawa T, Celermajer J, Simon A, Rowe RD. Aneurysm of the membranous ventricular septum. A method of spontaneous closure of small ventricular septal defect. *Am J Cardiol*. 1969;24:531.
63. Morton P, Murtagh JG, O'Hara MD. Aneurysm of interventricular septum with aortic valve malformation in an infant. *Br Heart J*. 1969;31:807.
64. Herbert WH. Hydrogen-detected ventricular septal defects. *Br Heart J*. 1969;31:766.
65. Scheinman JI, Kelminson LL, Vogel JHK, Rosenkrantz JG. Early repair of ventricular septal defect due to nonpenetrating trauma. *J Pediat*. 1969;74:406.
66. Gonzales-Lavin L, Barratt-Boyes BG. Surgical considerations in the treatment of ventricular septal defect associated with aortic valvular incompetence. *J Thorac Cardiovasc Surg*. 1969;57:422.
67. Meng CCL. Spontaneous closure of ventricular septal defect in tricuspid atresia. *J Pediat*. 1969;75:697.
68. Ngheim QX, Harris LC, Tyson KRT. Spontaneous closure of a ventricular septal defect after pulmonary artery banding. *Pediat*. 1969;75:694.
69. Pombo E, Pilapil VR, Lehan PH. Aneurysm of the membranous ventricular septum. *Am Heart J*. 1970;79:188.
70. Somerville J, Brandao A, Ross DN. Aortic regurgitation with ventricular septal defect. Surgical management and clinical features. *Circulation*. 1970;41:317.
71. Stark J, Tynan M, Aberdeen E. Spontaneous closure of ventricular septal defect following pulmonary artery constriction (banding). *Am Heart J*. 1970;79:548.
72. Ebert PA, Canent RV, Spach MS, Sabiston DC. Late cardiodynamics following correction of ventricular septal defects with previous pulmonary artery banding. *J Thorac Cardiovasc Surg*. 1970;60:516.
73. Wagner RB, Ankeney JL, Liebman J. Correlation of mean pulmonary arterial pressure with results of surgery for nonrestrictive ventricular septal defects. *J Thorac Cardiovasc Surg*. 1970;60:510.
74. Yokoyama M, Takao A, Sakakibara S. Natural history and surgical indications of ventricular septal defect. *Am Heart J*. 1970;80:597.
75. Hunt CE, Formanek G, Castañeda A, Moller JH. Closure of ventricular septal defect and removal of pulmonary arterial band. Results in eight children. *Am J Cardiol*. 1970;26:345.
76. Li MD, Keith JD. Spontaneous closure of ventricular septal defect. *Am Heart J*. 1970;80:432.
77. Rao PS, Sissman NJ. Spontaneous closure of physiologically advantageous ventricular septal defects. *Circulation*. 1971;43:83.
78. Daicoff GR, Miller RH. Congestive heart failure in infancy treated by early repair of ventricular septal defect. *Circulation*. 1970;41(suppl II):110.
79. Goor DA, Lillehei CW, Rees R, Edwards JE. Isolated ventricular septal defect. Developmental basis for various types and presentation of classification. *Chest*. 1970;58:468.
80. Jarmakani JMM, Graham TP, Canent RV, Capp MP. The effect of corrective surgery on left heart volume and mass in children with ventricular septal defect. *Am J Cardiol*. 1971;27:254.
81. Lev M, Joseph RH, Rimoldi HJA, Paiva R, Arcilla RA. The quantitative anatomy of isolated ventricular septal defect. *Am Heart J*. 1971;81:315.
82. Brammel HL, Vogel JHK, Pryor R, Blount SG. The Eisenmenger syndrome, a clinical and physiologic reappraisal. *Am J Cardiol*. 1971;28:679.
83. Young D, Mark H. Fate of the patient with the Eisenmenger syndrome. *Am J Cardiol*. 1971;28:658.
84. Kirklin JW. Pulmonary arterial banding in babies with large ventricular septal defects. *Circulation*. 1971;43:321.
85. Campbell M. Natural history of ventricular septal defect. *Br Heart J*. 1971;33:246.
86. Coleman EN, Reid JM, Barclay RS, Stevenson JG. Ventricular septal defect repair after pulmonary artery banding. *Br Heart J*. 1972;34:134.
87. Parisi LF, Holden AM, Plauth WH, Nadas AS. Syndrome of ventricular septal defect with aortic insufficiency. *Am J Cardiol*. 1972;29:284.
88. Mesko ZG, Jones JE, Nadas AS. Diminution and closure of large ventricular septal defects after pulmonary artery banding. *Am J Cardiol*. 1972;29:280.
89. Glasser SP, Cheitlin MD, McCarty RJ, Haas JH, Hall RJ, Mullins CE. Thirty-two cases of interventricular septal defect and aortic insufficiency: clinical, hemodynamic, and surgical features. *Am J Cardiol*. 1972;29:265.
90. Alpert B, Rowe RD. Spontaneous closure of small ventricular defects. Probability rates in the first 5 years of life. *Am J Cardiol*. 1972;29:250.
91. Steinfeld L, Dimich I, Park SG, Baron MG. Clinical diagnosis of isolated subpulmonary (supracristal) ventricular septal defect. *Am J Cardiol*. 1972;30:19.
92. Collins G, Calder L, Rose V, Kidd L, Keith JD. Ventricular septal defect: clinical and hemodynamic changes in the first five years of life. *Am Heart J*. 1972;84:695.
93. Fisher RD, Brawley RK, Neill CA, et al. Severe tricuspid regurgitation after repair of ventricular septal defect. *J Thorac Cardiovasc Surg*. 1973;65:702.
94. Rothfeld EL, Zucker IR, Parsonnet V. Postinfarction ventricular septal defect and the Eisenmenger syndrome. *Chest*. 1972;62:224.
95. Tandon R, Edwards JE. Aneurysmlike formations in relation to membranous ventricular septum. *Circulation*. 1973;47:1089.
96. Kawashima Y, Danno M, Shimizu Y, et al. Ventricular septal defect associated with aortic insufficiency. Anatomic classification and method of operation. *Circulation*. 1973;47:1057.
97. Momma K, Mimori S, Takao A. Natural history of ventricular septal defects with pulmonary hypertension in infancy and childhood: a serial catheterization study. *Bull Heart Inst Japan*. 1973;13(57).
98. Corone P, Guérin F, Gaudeau S, Doyon F, Ruet JC. Evolution spontanée des communications interventriculaires apres deux ans. *Coeur*. 1973;NS: 368.

99. Danielson GK. *CIV Avec Hypertension Pulmonaire*. Expermentation Animale Coeur; 1973;NS:373.
100. Nadas AS. Indications operatoires dans les CIV en function de l'hypertension arterialle pulmonaires. *Coeur*. 1973;NS:374.
101. Dupon H. Arguments per-operatoires pour fermer les CIV avec hypertension pulmonaire. *Coeur*. 1973;NS; 376.
102. Mercier JN, Thibert M, Dander B. Controle hemodynamique des communications interventriculaires opérees (à propos de 33 observations). *Coeur*. 1973;NS: 380.
103. Pernot C. Traitement medical des communications interventriculaires mal tolerées du nourisson. *Coeur*. 1973;NS: 389.
104. Galey JJ. Traitement chirurgical des communications interventriculaires mal tolerées du nourissons. *Coeur*. 1973;NS:397.
105. Guilmet D, Gandjakhch I, Brunet A, Cron J-P, Gontard F. Communication interventriculaire avec insuffisance aortique. *Coeur*. 1973;NS: 407.
106. Kachaner J, Ivanczak F, Thibert M, Gautier M, Loth P. Histoire naturelle des communications interventriculaires du nourrison. Étude longitudinale de 341 cas. *Coeur*. 1973;NS: 353.
107. Pernot C, Tridon P, Hoeffel JC, Picard L, Henry M. L'anévrysme du septum membraneux. Son rôle dans la fermeture spontanée de certaines communications interventriculaires. *Coeur*. 1973;4:41.
108. Freed MD, Rosenthal A, Plauth WH, Nadas AS. Development of subaortic stenosis after pulmonary artery banding. *Circulation*. 1973;48:III–7.
109. Kohno R, Kume H, Sakakibara T, Matsui M, Konno S, Sakakibara S: Operative results and surgical treatment of cases of ventricular septal defect associated with pulmonary hypertension, *Bull Heart Inst Japan* 14:59, 1972–1973.
110. Schott GD. Documentation of spontaneous functional closure of a ventricular septal defect during adult life. *Br Heart J*. 1973;35:1214.
111. Galioto FM, Cooley DA, El-Said G, Mullins CE, Sandiford FM. Closure of ventricular septal defect through the aortic valve. *Chest*. 1973;64:683.
112. Plass R, Münster W, Ivanov S, Stürmer U. Angiocardiographic diagnosis of aortic insufficiency in cases of ventricular septal defect associated with partial prolapse of the aortic valve. *Cardiology*. 1973;58:257.
113. Castleman B, Scully RE, McNealy BU. Case records of the Massachusetts General Hospital. Weekly clinicopathological exercises. Case 3, 1974. *New Engl J Med*. 1974;290:216.
114. King DL, Steeg CN, Ellis K. Visualization of ventricular septal defects by cardiac ultrasonography. *Circulation*. 1973;48:1215.
115. Tatsuno K, Konno S, Ando M, Sakakibara S. Pathogenetic mechanisms of prolapsing aortic valve and aortic regurgitation associated with ventricular septal defect. Anatomical, angiographic, and surgical considerations. *Circulation*. 1973;48:1028.
116. Maron BJ, Ferrans VJ, White RI. Unusual evolution of acquired infundibular stenosis in patients with ventricular septal defect. Clinical and morphologic observations. *Circulation*. 1973;48:1092.
117. Marshall RM, Josephson C. Spontaneous rupture of the interventricular septum in an elderly man. *Hopkins Med J*. 1973;133:161.
118. Ho CS, Krovetz LJ, Strife JL, Brawley RK, Rowe RD. Postoperative assessment of residual defects following cardiac surgery in infants and children. II. Ventricular septal defects. *Hopkins Med J*. 1973;133:278.
119. Tan KT, Hashimoto A, Takao A. Ventriculo-radial dysplasia: a familial upper-limb cardiovascular syndrome, *Bull Heart Inst Japan* 14:109, 1972–1973.
120. Armour JA, Lippincott DB, Randall WC. Functional anatomy of the interventricular septum. *Cardiology*. 1973;58:65.
121. Mesko ZG, Jonas JE, Nadas AS. Diminution and closure of large ventricular septal defects after pulmonary artery banding. *Circulation*. 1973;48:847.
122. Dobell ARC, Murphy DA, Poirier NL, Gibbons JE. The pulmonary artery after debanding. *J Thorac Cardiovasc Surg*. 1973;65:32.
123. Patel RG, Ihenacho HNC, Abrams LD, et al. Pulmonary artery banding and subsequent repair in ventricular septal defect. *Br Heart J*. 1973;35:651.
124. Bonham-Carter RE. Devenir de 144 enfants atteints d'une CIV isolée et catheterizés avant l'age d'un an. *Coeur NS*. 1972;366.
125. Maron BJ, Redwood DR, Hirschfeld JW, Goldstein RE, Morrow AG, Epstein SE. Postoperative assessment of patients with ventricular septal defect and pulmonary hypertension. Response to intense upright exercise. *Circulation*. 1973;48:864.
126. Nelson CS. Subaortic septal perforation associated with pulmonary and systemic embolism. *Chest*. 1973;64:534.
127. Trusler GA, Moes CAF, Kidd BSL. Repair of ventricular septal defect with aortic insufficiency. *J Thorac Cardiovasc Surg*. 1973;66:394.
128. Clark TA, Corcoran FH, Baker WP, Mills M. Early repair of traumatic ventricular septal defect. *J Thorac Cardiovasc Surg*. 1974;67:121.
129. Carroll RE, Louis DS. Anomalies associated with radial dysplasia. *J Pediat*. 1974;84:409.
130. Freedom RM, White RD, Pieroni DR, Varghese PJ, Krovetz LJ, Rowe RD. The natural history of the so-called aneurysm of the membranous ventricular septum in childhood. *Circulation*. 1974;49:375.
131. Godman MJ, Roberts NK, Izukawa T. Late postoperative conduction disturbances after repair of ventricular septal defect and tetralogy of Fallot. Analysis by His bundle recordings. *Circulation*. 1974;49:214.
132. Subramanian S. Primary definitive intracardiac operations in infants: ventricular septal defects. In: Kirklin JW, ed. *Advances in Cardiovascular Surgery*. New York: Grune and Stratton; 1973:141.
133. DuShane JW, Kirklin JW. Late results of the repair of ventricular septal defect on pulmonary vascular disease. In: Kirklin JW, ed. *Advances in Cardiovascular Surgery*. New York: Grune and Stratton; 1973:9.
134. Chung KJ, Manning JA. Ventricular septal defect associated with aortic insufficiency: medical and surgical management. *Am Heart J*. 1974;87:435.
135. Assad-Morell JL, Tajik AJ, Giuliani ER. Aneurysm of membranous interventricular septum. Echocardiographic features. *Mayo Clin Proc*. 1974;49:164.
136. Kawashima Y, Nakano S, Kato M, Danno M, Sato K, Manabe H. Fate of pericardium utilized for the closure of ventricular septal defect. Postoperative ventricular septal aneurysm. *J Thorac Cardiovasc Surg*. 1974;68:209.
137. Katz AM. Acupuncture anesthesia for open heart surgery. A case report. *Am J Cardiol*. 1974;34:250.
138. Hagan AD, Francis GS, Sahn DJ, Karliner JS, Friedman WF, O'Rourke RA. Ultrasound evaluation of systolic anterior septal motion in patients with and without right ventricular volume overload. *Circulation*. 1974;50:248.
139. Rosenquist GC, Sweeney LT. The membranous ventricular septum in the normal heart. *Hopkins Med J*. 1974;135(9).

140. Kalmanson D, Aigueperse J, Veyrat C, Cornec C, Chiche P. Non-invasive technique for diagnosing congenital and acquired ventricular septal defects using directional Doppler ultrasound. correlations with phasic flow velocity patterns of the shunt. *Br Heart J*. 1974;36:428.
141. Wallace R. Complete correction of ventricular septal defect in infancy. In: Parenzan L, Carcassone M, eds. *Open Heart Surgery in Infancy*. Milano: Sapil; 1974:191.
142. Girod DA, Hurwitz RA, King H, Jolly W. Recent results of two-stage surgical treatment of large ventricular septal defect. *Circulation*. 1974;50:II–9.
143. Griep E, French JW, Shumway NE, Baum D. Is pulmonary artery banding for ventricular septal defect obsolete? *Circulation*. 1974;50:II–14.
144. de Leval M, Taylor JFN, Stark J. Primary repair of ventricular septal defect in infancy. *Br Heart J*. 1974;36:400.
145. Friedli B, Kidd BSL, Mustard WT, Keith JD. Ventricular septal defect with increased pulmonary vascular resistance. Late results of surgical closure. *Am J Cardiol*. 1974;33:403.
146. Allen HD, Anderson RC, Noren GR, Moller JH. Postoperative follow-up of patients with ventricular septal defect. *Circulation*. 1974;50:465.
147. Rosenquist GC, Sweeney LJ, Amsel J, McAllister HA. Enlargement of the membranous ventricular septum: an internal stigma of Down's syndrome. *J Pediat*. 1974;85:490.
148. Pirzada FA, McDowell JW, Cohen EM, Saini VK, Berger RL. Traumatic ventricular septal defect. *New Engl J Med*. 1974;291:892.
149. Moulaert AJMG. *Ventricular Septal Defects and Anomalies of the Aortic Arch*. Leiden: Luctor et Emergo (MD thesis); 1974.
150. Lambert ME, Widlansky S, Franken EA, Hurwitz R, Nielson R, Nasser WK. Natural history of ventricular septal defects associated with ventricular septal aneurysms. *Am Heart J*. 1974;88:566.
151. Barbero-Marcial M, Verginelli G, Arie S, Atik E, Macruz R, Zerbini EJ. Intrapulmonary balloon for temporary relief of pulmonary hypertension. *J Thorac Cardiovasc Surg*. 1975;69:942.
152. Tatsuno K, Ando M, Takao A, Hatsune K, Konno S. Diagnostic importance of aortography in conal ventricular septal defect. *Am Heart J*. 1975;89:171.
153. Sapire DW, Black IFS. Echocardiographic detection of aneurysms of the interventricular septum associated with ventricular septal defect, a method of noninvasive diagnosis and follow-up. *Am J Cardiol*. 1975;36:797.
154. Hislop A, Haworth SG, Shinebourne EA, Reid L. Quantitative structural analysis of pulmonary vessels in isolated ventricular septal defect in infancy. *Br Heart J*. 1975;37:1014.
155. Hoeffel JC, Henry M, Flizot M, Luceri R, Pernot C. Radiologic patterns of aneurysms of the membranous septum. *Am Heart J*. 1976;91:450.
156. Cordell D, Graham TP, Atwood GF, Boerth RC, Boucek RJ, Bender HW. Left heart volume characteristics following ventricular septal defect closure in infancy. *Circulation*. 1976;54:294.
157. Valdes-Cruz LM, Pieroni DR, Roland J-MA, Varghese PJ. Echocardiographic detection of intracardiac right-to-left shunts following peripheral vein injection. *Circulation*. 1976;54:558.
158. Graham TP, Atwood GF, Boucek RJ, Cordell D, Boerth RC. Right ventricular volume characteristics in ventricular septal defect. *Circulation*. 1976;54:800.
159. Stewart S. Closure of a ventricular septal defect through the aortic valve. A note of caution regarding resultant narrowing of the aortic valve annulus. *Chest*. 1976;70:311.
160. Corone P, Doyon F, Gaudeau S, et al. Natural history of ventricular septal defect, a study involving 790 cases. *Circulation*. 1977;55:908.
161. Nugent EW, Freedom RM, Rowe RD, Wagner HR, Rees JK. Aneurysm of the membranous septum in ventricular septal defect. *Circulation*. 1977;56:I–82.
162. Haworth SG, Sauer U, Bühlmeyer K, Reid L. Development of the pulmonary circulation in ventricular septal defect: a quantitative structural study. *Am J Cardiol*. 1977;40:781.
163. Hallidie-Smith KA, Wilson RSE, Hart A, Zeidifard E. Functional status of patients with large ventricular septal defect and pulmonary vascular disease 6 to 16 years after surgical closure of their defect in childhood. *Br Heart J*. 1977;39:1093.
164. Vidne BA, Chiariello L, Wagner H, Subramanian S. Aneurysm of the membranous ventricular septum. Surgical considerations and experience in 29 cases. *J Thorac Cardiovasc Surg*. 1976;71:402.
165. Seybold-Epting W, Reul GJ, Hallman GL, Cooley D. Repair of ventricular septal defect after pulmonary artery banding. *J Thorac Cardiovasc Surg*. 1976;71:392.
166. Lewis AB, Takahashi M. Echocardiographic assessment of left-to-right shunt volume in children with ventricular septal defect. *Circulation*. 1976;54:78.
167. Yasui H, Takeda Y, Yamauchi S, et al. The deleterious effects of surgically induced complete right bundle branch block on long-term follow-up results of closure of ventricular septal defect. *J Thorac Cardiovasc Surg*. 1976;74:210.
168. Kawashima Y, Fujita T, Mori T, Ihara K, Manabe H. Transpulmonary arterial closure of ventricular septal defect. *J Thorac Cardiovasc Surg*. 1977;74:191.
169. Lincoln C, Jamieson S, Shinebourne E, Anderson RH. Transatrial repair of ventricular septal defects with reference to their anatomic classification. *J Thorac Cardiovasc Surg*. 1977;74:183.
170. Hordof AJ, Mellins RB, Gersony WM, Steeg CN. Reversibility of chronic obstructive lung disease in infants following repair of ventricular septal defect. *J Pediat*. 1977;90:187.
171. Glasser SP, Baucum RW. Pulmonary valve fluttering in subpulmonic ventricular septal defect. *Am Heart J*. 1977;94:3.
172. Bloom KR, Rodrigues L, Swan EM. Echocardiographic evaluation of left-to-right shunt in ventricular septal defect and persistent ductus arteriosus. *Br Heart J*. 1977;39:260.
173. Yasui H, Yoshitoshi M, Miyamoto AT, Kato H, Takeda Y, Tomoike H. Ventricular septal defect: selection of patients and timing for surgery. *Am Heart J*. 1977;93:40.
174. Blackstone EH, Kirklin JW, Bradley EL, DuShane JW, Appelbaum A. Optimal age and results in repair of large ventricular septal defects. *J Thorac Cardiovasc Surg*. 1976;72:661.
175. Taylor JFN, de Leval M, Stark J. Repair of ventricular septal defects in infancy. *Br Heart J*. 1976;38:535.
176. Bersch W, Chuaqui JB. On the formal genesis of the Eisenmenger complex. *Virchows Arch Abt A Path Anat*. 1972;356:307.
177. Bersch W. On the importance of the bulboauricular flange for the formal genesis of congenital heart defects with special regard to the ventricular septum defects. *Virchows Arch Abt A Path Anat*. 1971;354:252.
178. Kreinsen U, Bersch W. Applying a classification principle of ventricular septal defects to a case with several defects of the interventricular septum. *Virchows Arch Abt A Path Anat*. 1972;355:290.
179. Moreno-Cabral RJ, Mamiya RT, Nakamura FF, Brainard SC, McNamara JJ. Ventricular septal defect and aortic insufficiency. Surgical treatment. *J Thorac Cardiovasc Surg*. 1977;73:358.

180. Blount SG. Comparison of patients with ventricular septal defect at high altitude and sea level. *Circulation*. 1977;56:I–79.
181. Keane JF, Plauth WH, Nadas AS. Ventricular septal defect with aortic regurgitation. *Circulation*. 1977;56:I–72.
182. Kawashima Y, Mori T, Yagihara T, Ihara K, Hasimoto S. Vol 1. Tokyo: VII World Congress of Cardiology; 1978:243.
183. Marino P, Dander B, Salazzari GC, Perini GP, Poppi A. *Left Ventricular-Right Atrial Communication, an Echocardiographic Study*. Vol 1. Tokyo: VII World Congress of Cardiology; 1978:232.
184. Eshaghpour E, Kawai N, Linhart JW. Tricuspid insufficiency associated with aneurysm of the ventricular septum. *Pediatrics*. 1978;61:586.
185. Snider AR, Silverman NH, Schiller NB, Ports TA. Echocardiographic evaluation of ventricular septal aneurysms. *Circulation*. 1979;59:920.
186. Ahmad M, Hallidie-Smith KA. Assessment of left-to-right shunt and left ventricular function in isolated ventricular septal defect. Echocardiographic study. *Br Heart J*. 1979;41:147.
187. McNicholas K, de Leval M, Stark J, Taylor JFN, Macartney FJ. Surgical treatment of ventricular septal defect in infancy. Primary repair versus banding of pulmonary artery and later repair. *Br Heart J*. 1979;41:133.
188. Wenink ACG, Oppenheimer-Dekker A, Moulaert AJ. Muscular ventricular septal defects: a reappraisal of the anatomy. *Am J Cardiol*. 1979;43:259.
189. Allwork SP, de Roger M. A new translation for the centenary. *Am Heart J*. 1879;98(307):1979.
190. Levy RJ, Rosenthal A, Miettinen OS, Nadas AS. Determinants of growth in patients with ventricular septal defect. *Circulation*. 1978;57:793.
191. Quero Jimenez M, Gonzalez Dieguez C, Herraiz Sarachago I. Communicaciones interventriculares en el lactante. *Bol Soc Pediat Madrid*. 1977;23:125.
192. Hobbins SM, Izukawa T, Radford DJ, Williams WG, Trusler GA. Conduction disturbances after surgical correction of ventricular septal defect by the atrial approach. *Br Heart J*. 1979;41:289.
193. Allwork SP, Anderson RH. Developmental anatomy of the membranous part of the ventricular septum in the human heart. *Br Heart J*. 1979;41:275.
194. Wise JR, Wilson WS. Angiographic documentation of spontaneous closure of ventricular septal defect in an adult. *Chest*. 1979;75:90.
195. Pham TD, Wit AL, Hordof AJ, Malm JR, Fenoglio JJ. Right atrial ultrastructure in congenital heart disease. 1. Comparison of ventricular septal defect and endocardial cushion defect. *Am J Cardiol*. 1978;42:973.
196. Riggs T, Mehta S, Hirschfeld S, Borkat G, Liebman J. Ventricular septal defect in infancy: a combined vectorgraphic and echocardiographic study. *Circulation*. 1979;59:385.
197. McNicholas KW, Bowman FO, Hayes CJ, Edie RN, Malm JR. Surgical management of ventricular septal defects in infants. *J Thorac Cardiovasc Surg*. 1978;75:346.
198. Oh KS, Park SC, Galvis AG, Young LW, Neches WH, Zuberbuhler JR. Pulmonary hyperinflation in ventricular septal defect. *J Thorac Cardiovasc Surg*. 1978;76:706.
199. Castañeda AR, Norwood WI. Closure of ventricular septal defects in infancy: deep hypothermic circulatory arrest technic. In: *Modern Technics in Surgery. Cardiac/Thoracic Surgery*. Vol 1. Mt Kisco, NY: Futura Publishing Company; 1979:1.
200. Fox KM, Patel RG, Graham GR, et al. Multiple and single ventricular septal defect, a clinical and haemodynamic comparison. *Br Heart J*. 1978;40:141.
201. Alpert BS, Cook DH, Varghese P, Rowe RD. Spontaneous closure of small ventricular septal defects: ten-year follow-up. *Pediatrics*. 1979;63:204.
202. Mirro MJ. Management of ventricular septal defects in adults. Clinical evaluations by Alexander S Nadas, MD and S Gilbert Blount Jr MD. *Chest*. 1978;74:293.
203. Meltzer RS, Schwartz J, French J, Popp R. Ventricular septal defect noted by two-dimensional echocardiography. *Chest*. 1979;76:455.
204. Midwall J, Jaffin H, Herman MV, Kupersmith J. Shunt flow and pulmonary hemodynamics during labor and delivery in the Eisenmenger syndrome. *Am J Cardiol*. 1978;42:299.
205. Lester LA, Vitullo D, Sodt P, Hutcheon N, Arcilla R. An evaluation of the left atrial/aortic root ratio in children with ventricular septal defect. *Circulation*. 1979;60:364.
206. Aziz KU, Cole RB, Paul MH. Echocardiographic features of supracristal ventricular septal defect with prolapsed aortic valve leaflet. *Am J Cardiol*. 1979;43:854.
207. Arciniegas E, Faraooki ZQ, Hakimi M, Perry EL, Green EW. Surgical closure of ventricular septal defect during the first twelve months of life. *J Thorac Cardiovasc Surg*. 1980;80:921.
208. Tharion J, Cartmill TB, Johnson DC, Celermajer JM. Transpulmonary arterial repair of supracristal ventricular septal defects in infancy. *J Thorac Cardiovasc Surg*. 1980;80:948.
209. Kirklin JK, Castañeda AR, Keane JF, Fellows KE, Norwood WI. Surgical management of multiple ventricular septal defects. *J Thorac Cardiovasc Surg*. 1980;80:485.
210. Rizzoli G, Blackstone EH, Kirklin JW, Pacifico AD, Bargeron LM. Incremental risk factors in hospital mortality rate after repair of ventricular septal defect. *J Thorac Cardiovasc Surg*. 1980;80:494.
211. Milo S, Ho SY, Wilkinson JL, Anderson RH. Surgical anatomy and atrioventricular conduction tissues of hearts with isolated ventricular septal defects. *J Thorac Cardiovasc Surg*. 1980;79:244.
212. Gussenhoven WJ, te Riele JAM, Scherpenzeel W, Roelandt J. Echocardiographic pattern in an aneurysm of the membranous interventricular septum. *Chest*. 1980;77:541.
213. Bierman FZ, Fellows K, Williams RG. Prospective identification of ventricular septal defects in infancy using subxiphoid two-dimensional echocardiography. *Circulation*. 1980;62:807.
214. Alam M, Folger GM, Goldstein S. Tricuspid valve fluttering, echocardiographic feature of ventricular septal defect. *Chest*. 1980;77:517.
215. Nesje OA. Systolic time intervals in isolated ventricular septal defect in the adult. *Circulation*. 1980;62:609.
216. Soto B, Becker AE, Moulaert AJ, Lie JJ, Anderson RH. Classification of ventricular septal defects. *Br Heart J*. 1980;43:332.
217. Kratz JM, Usher BW, Sade RM, Gaddy JE. Systemic thromboembolism from a ventricular septal patch. *Chest*. 1980;78:774.
218. Silverman NH, Snider AR, Rudolph AM. Evaluation of pulmonary hypertension by M-mode echocardiography in children with ventricular septal defect. *Circulation*. 1980;61:1125.
219. Sethia B, Cotter L. Giant aneurysm of membranous septum. Unusual cause of mediastinal mass. *Br Heart J*. 1981;46:107.
220. Canale JM, Sahn DJ, Allen HD, Goldberg SJ, Valdes-Cruz LM, Ovitt TW. Factors affecting real-time cross-sectional echocardiographic imaging of perimembranous ventricular septal defects. *Circulation*. 1981;63:689.
221. Green CE, Elliott LP, Bargeron LM. Axial cineangiographic evaluation of the posterior ventricular septal defect. *Am J Cardiol*. 1981;48:331. [posterior VSD = VSD of the AV canal type.]

222. Griffiths SP, Turi GK, Ellis K, Krongrad E, et al. Muscular ventricular septal defects repaired with left ventriculotomy. *Am J Cardiol.* 1981;48:877.
223. Dickinson DF, Arnold R, Wilkinson JL. Ventricular septal defect in children born in Liverpool 1960 to 1969. *Br Heart J.* 1981;46:47.
224. Wenink ACG, Oppenheimer-Dekker A, Moulaert AJ, eds. *The Ventricular Septum of the Heart.* The Hague, Boston: Leiden University Press; 1981.
225. Cheatham JP, Latson LA, Gutgesell HP. Ventricular septal defect in infancy. Detection with two-dimensional echocardiography. *Am J Cardiol.* 1981;47:85.
226. Karpawich PP, Duff DF, Mullins CE, Cooley DA, McNamara DG. Ventricular septal defect with associated aortic valve insufficiency. Progression of insufficiency and operative results in young children. *J Thorac Cardiovasc Surg.* 1981;82:182.
227. Fisher DJ, Snider AR, Silverman NH, Stanger P. Ventricular septal defect with silent discrete subaortic stenosis. *Ped Cardiol.* 1982;2:265.
228. LaCorte MA, Cooper RS, Kauffman SL, Schiller MS, Golinko RJ, Griepp RP. Atrioventricular canal ventricular septal defect with cleft mitral valve, angiographic and echocardiographic features. *Ped Cardiol.* 1982;2:289.
229. Fellows KE, Westerman GR, Keane JF. Angiocardiography of multiple ventricular septal defects in infancy. *Circulation.* 1982;66:1094.
230. Smallhorn JF, Sutherland GR, Anderson RH, Macartney FJ. Cross-sectional echocardiographic assessment of conditions with atrioventricular valve leaflets attached to the atrial septum at the same level. *Br Heart J.* 1982;48:331.
231. Wenink CAG, Gittenberger de Groot CA. Cloisonnement ventriculaire. Terminologie proposée. *Coeur.* 1982;13:467.
232. Beekman RH, Rocchini AP, Rosenthal A. Hemodynamic effects of hydralazine in infants with a large ventricular septal defect. *Circulation.* 1982;65:523.
233. Shore DF, Smallhorn J, Stark J, Lincoln C, de Leval MR. Left ventricular outflow tract obstruction coexisting with ventricular septal defect. *Br Heart J.* 1982;48:421.
234. Sutherland GR, Godman MJ, Smallhorn JF, Guiterras P, Anderson RH, Hunter S. Ventricular septal defects. Two-dimensional echocardiographic and morphologic correlations. *Br Heart J.* 1982;47:316.
235. Lister G, Hellenbrand WE, Kleinman CS, Talner NS. Physiologic effects of increasing hemoglobin concentration in left-to-right shunting in infants with ventricular septal defects. *New Engl J Med.* 1982;306:502.
236. Beerman LB, Park SC, Fischer DR, et al. Natural history of ventricular septal defects associated with aneurysm of the membranous septum. *Circulation.* 1983;68:III–396.
237. Anderson RH, Lenox CC, Zuberbuhler JR. Mechanisms of closure of perimembranous ventricular septal defect. *Am J Cardiol.* 1983;52:341.
238. Grenadier E, Shem-Tov A, Motro M, Palant A. Echocardiographic diagnosis of left ventricular-right atrial communication. *Am Heart J.* 1983;106:407.
239. Bisset GS, Hirschfeld SS. Severe pulmonary hypertension associated with a small ventricular septal defect. *Circulation.* 1983;67:470.
240. Anderson RH, Lenox CC, Zuberbuhler JR. Morphology of ventricular septal defect associated with coarctation of aorta. *Br Heart J.* 1983;50:176.
241. Smallhorn JF, Anderson RH, Macartney FJ. Morphological characterization of ventricular septal defects associated with coarctation of aorta by cross-sectional echocardiography. *Br Heart J.* 1983;49:485.
242. Capelli H, Andrade JL, Somerville J. Classification of the site of ventricular septal defect by 2-dimensional echocardiography. *Am J Cardiol.* 1983;51:1474.
243. Burrows PE, Fellows KE, Keane JF. Cineangiography of the perimembranous ventricular septal defect with left ventricular – right atrial shunt. *J Am Coll Cardiol.* 1983;1:1129.
244. Doty DB, McGoon DC. Closure of perimembranous ventricular septal defect. *J Thorac Cardiovasc Surg.* 1983;85:781.
245. Peter CA, Bowyer K, Jones RH. Radionuclide analysis of right and left ventricular response to exercise in patients with atrial and ventricular septal defects. *Am Heart J.* 1983;105:428.
246. Aziz K-U, Memon AD, Rehman M, Rehman F. Ventricular septal defect and its hemodynamic correlates. *Pakistan Heart J.* 1983;16:50.
247. Otterstad JE, Nitter-Hauge S, Myhre E. Isolated ventricular septal defect in adults. Clinical and haemodynamic findings. *Br Heart J.* 1983;50:343.
248. Vogel M, Freedom RM, Brand A, Trusler GA, Williams WG, Rowe RD. Ventricular septal defect and subaortic stenosis: an analysis of 41 patients. *Am J Cardiol.* 1983;52:1258.
249. Yeager SB, Freed MD, Norwood WI, Castañeda AR. Primary closure of ventricular septal defects in infancy. *Circulation.* 1983;68:III–210.
250. Dajee H, Benson LH, Laks H. An improved method of pulmonary artery banding. *Ann Thorac Surg.* 1984;37:254.
251. Blieden LC, Moller JH. Small ventricular septal defect associated with severe pulmonary hypertension. *Br Heart J.* 1984;52:117.
252. de Leval M. Transatrial closure of perimembranous ventricular septal defect in infancy. *J Thorac Cardiovasc Surg.* 1984;87:640.
253. Soto B, Bargeron LM, Diethelm E. Ventricular septal defect. *Seminars in Roentgenol.* 1985;20:200.
254. Becker AE, Anderson RH. Classification of ventricular septal defects—a matter of precision. *Heart Ves.* 1985;1:120.
255. Hagler DJ, Edwards WD, Seward JB, Tajik AJ. Standardized nomenclature of the ventricular septum and ventricular septal defects, with applications for two-dimensional echocardiography. *Mayo Clin Proc.* 1985;60:741.
256. Vincent RN, Lang P, Chipman CW, Castañeda AR. Assessment of hemodynamic status in the intensive care unit immediately after closure of ventricular septal defect. *Am J Cardiol.* 1985;55:526.
257. Johnson GL, Kwan OL, Cottrill CM, De Maria AN. Detection and quantitation of right ventricular outlet obstruction secondary to aneurysm of the membranous ventricular septum by combined two-dimensional echocardiography: continuous-wave Doppler ultrasound. *Am J Cardiol.* 1985;53:1477.
258. Marx GR, Allen HD, Goldberg SJ. Doppler echocardiographic estimation of systolic pulmonary artery pressure in pediatric patients with interventricular communications. *J Am Coll Cardiol.* 1985;6:1132.
259. Newman TB. Etiology of ventricular septal defects: an epidemiologic approach. *Pediatrics.* 1985;76:741.
260. Lillehei CW, Varco RL, Cohen M, Warden HE, Patton C, Moller JH. The first open-heart repairs of ventricular septal defect, atrioventricular communis, and tetralogy of Fallot using extracorporeal circulation by cross-circulation: a 30-year follow-up. *Ann Thor Surg.* 1986;41:4.

261. Leung MP, Mok CK, Lo RNS, Lau KC. An echocardiographic study of perimembranous ventricular septal defect with left ventricular to right atrial shunting. *Br Heart J*. 1986;55:45.
262. Ramaciotti C, Keren A, Silverman NH. Importance of (perimembranous) ventricular septal aneurysm in the natural history of isolated perimembranous ventricular septal defect. *Am J Cardiol*. 1986;57:268.
263. Kusuhara K, Miki S, Ueda Y, Ohkita Y, Tahata T, Komeda M. Usefulness of electromagnetic flowmetry in intraoperative evaluation of aortic regurgitation associated with ventricular septal defect. *Am J Cardiol*. 1987;59:1152.
264. Moene RJ, Gittenberger-de Groot AC, Oppenheimer-Dekker A, Bartelings MM. Anatomic characteristics of ventricular septal defect associated with coarctation of the aorta. *Am J Cardiol*. 1987;59:952.
265. Didier D, Higgins CB. Identification and localization of ventricular septal defect by gated magnetic resonance imaging. *Am J Cardiol*. 1986;57:1363.
266. Moene RJ, Oppenheimer-Dekker A, Bartelings MM, Wenink AC, Gittenberger-de Groot AC. Ventricular septal defect with normally connected and with transposed great arteries. *Am J Cardiol*. 1986;58:627.
267. Hisatomi K, Kosuga K, Isomura T, Akagawa H, Ohishi K, Koga M. Ventricular septal defect associated with aortic regurgitation. *Ann Thorac Surg*. 1987;43:363.
268. Johnson GL, O'Connor WN, Verble SM, Cottrill CM, Noonan JA. Ventricular septal defect with mobile tricuspid valve pouch mimicking tetralogy of Fallot. *Pediatr Cardiol*. 1986;7:53.
269. van de Wal HJCM, Daniëls O, Lacquet LK. Dissecting ventricular septal aneurysm after open-heart surgery. *Pediatric Cardiol*. 1986;6:319.
270. Guikahue Kakou M, Chauvet J, Dyemkouma F, et al. Les forms anatomo-pathologiques des communications interventriculaires en Afrique Noire. Étude de 75 cas opéreś a Abidjan. *Cardiologie Tropicale*. 1988;14(5).
271. Baker ET, Leung MP, Anderson RH, Fischer DR, Zuberbuhler JR. The cross sectional anatomy of ventricular septal defects; a reappraisal. *Br Heart J*. 1988;59:339.
272. Lue HC, Sung TC, Hou SH, et al. Ventricular septal defect in Chinese with aortic valve prolapse and aortic regurgitation. *Heart Ves*. 1986;2:111–116.
273. Capelli H, Marantz P, Micheli D, et al. Types of ventricular septal defect present in patients who survived heart failure in the first year. A two-dimensional echocardiographic study. *Rev Latina de Card Inf*. 1985;1:292.
274. Kawashima Y, Hashimoto S, Miyamoto K, Hirose H, Nagai I, Kadoba K. An improved technique for the closure of ventricular septal defect in ventricular inversion. *Ann Thorac Surg*. 1987;43:107.
275. Matsuoka S, Kurahashi Y, Tomimatsu H, et al. Plasma atrial natriuretic peptide levels in patients with ventricular septal defect. *J Pediatr*. 1987;110:578.
276. Parsons JM, Baker EJ, Ladusans EJ, Ayton V, Tynan MJ. Magnetic resonance imaging of ventricular septal defects in infants. *Bergamo Meeting*. 1988:21 (abstract book).
277. Yamaki S, Hanada K, Mohri H. Indications for surgery based on lung biopsy in cases of ventricular septal defect and/or patent ductus arteriosus with pulmonary hypertension. *Bergamo meeting*. 1988:21 (abstract book).
278. Shore DF, Rigby ML, Anderson RH, Lincoln C. Surgical closure of ventricular septal defects without cardiac catheterization and angiocardiography. *Bergamo Meeting*. 1988:22 (abstract book).
279. Maehara T, Blackstone EH, Kirklin JW, Kirklin JK, Pacifico AD, Colvin E. The results of the Trusler operation for ventricular septal defect and aortic valvar incompetence. *Bergamo Meeting*. 1988:22 (abstract book).
280. Daenen W, Lesaffre E. Factors influencing results after closure of ventricular septal defect in infancy. *Bergamo Meeting*. 1988:23 (abstract book).
281. Zielinsky P, Rossi MB, Rossi FRI, et al. Surgical-angiographic-echocardiographic correlation in subaortic stenosis associated with ventricular septal defect. *Bergamo Meeting*. 1988:24. Abstracts.
282. Alexi-Meskhishvili V, Nikoljuk A, Popov S, Zajtcev L. Closure of ventricular septal defect in infancy with a xenopericardial patch. *Bergamo Meeting*. 1988:24 (abstract book).
283. Sakornpant P, Athapaisalsarudee S: *Transpulmonary closure of ventricular septal defect*. Bergamo meeting, p 25 (abstract).
284. Neirotti R, Campos M, Quaglio M, Vazquez J. Surgical treatment of ventricular septal defect. *Bergamo Meeting*. 1988:25 (abstract book).
285. Moe DG, Guntheroth WG. Spontaneous closure of uncomplicated ventricular septal defect. *Am J Cardiol*. 1987;60:674.
286. Lock JE, Block PC, McKay RG, Baim DS, Keane JF. Transcatheter closure of ventricular septal defects. *Circulation*. 1988;78:361.
287. Lue HC, Takao A, eds. *Subpulmonary Ventricular Septal Defect*. New York: Springer Verlag; 1983.
288. Leung MP, Beerman LB, Siewers RD, Bahnson HT, Zuberbuhler JR. Long term follow-up after aortic valvuloplasty and defect closure in ventricular septal defect with aortic regurgitation. *Am J Cardiol*. 1987;60:890.
289. Neutze JM, Ishikawa T, Clarkson PM, Calder AL, Barratt-Boyes BG, Kerr AR. Assessment and follow-up of patients with ventricular septal defect and elevated pulmonary vascular resistance. *Am J Cardiol*. 1989;63:327.
290. Ellis JH, Moodie DS, Sterba R, Gill CC. Ventricular septal defect in the adult: natural and unnatural history. *Am Heart J*. 1987;114:115.
291. Kurokawa S, Takahashi M, Katoh Y, Muramatsu J, Kikawada R. Noninvasive evaluation of the ratio of pulmonary to systemic flow in ventricular septal defect by means of Doppler two-dimensional echocardiography. *Am Heart J*. 1988;16:1033.
292. Huhta JC, Edwards ED, Danielson GK, Feldt RH. Abnormalities of the tricuspid valve in complete transposition of the great arteries with ventricular septal defect. *J Thorac Cardiovasc Surg*. 1982;83:569.
293. de Leval MR, Pozzi M, Starnes V, et al. Surgical management of doubly committed subarterial ventricular septal defects. *Circulation*. 1988;78:III–40.
294. Schmidt KG, Cassidy SC, Silverman NH, Stanger P. Doubly committed subarterial ventricular septal defects: echocardiographic features and surgical implications. *J Am Coll Cardiol*. 1988;12:1538.
295. Hornberger LK, Sahn DJ, Krabill KA, et al. Elucidation of the natural history of ventricular septal defects by serial Doppler color flow mapping studies. *J Am Coll Cardiol*. 1989;13:1111.
296. Williams WG. Doppler color flow mapping and prediction of ventricular septal defect outcome. *J Am Coll Cardiol*. 1989;13:1119.
297. Helmcke F, de Sousa A, Nanda NC, et al. Two-dimensional and color Doppler assessment of ventricular septal defect of congenital origin. *Am J Cardiol*. 1989;63:1112.
298. McDaniel N, Gutgesell HP, Nolan SP, Kron IL. Repair of large muscular ventricular septal defects in infants employing left ventriculotomy. *Ann Thor Surg*. 1989;47:593.

299. Sharif DS, Huhta JC, Marantz P, Hawkins HK, Yoon GY. Two-dimensional echocardiographic determination of ventricular septal defect size: correlation with autopsy. *Am Heart J.* 1989;117:1333.
300. Bush HS, Perin E, Massumi A, Klima T, Hall RJ. Detection of thombus in an aneurysm of the ventricular septum. *Am J Cardiol.* 1989;63:1533.
301. Sutherland GR, Smyllie JH, Ogilvie BC, Keeton BR. Colour flow imaging in the diagnosis of multiple ventricular septal defects. *Br Heart J.* 1989;62:43.
302. Cassidy SC, Van Hare GF, Silverman NH. The probability of detecting a subaortic ridge in children with ventricular septal defect or coarctation of the aorta. *Am J Cardiol.* 1990;66:505.
303. Farrú-Albohaire O, Arcil G, Hernández I. An association between left axis deviation and an aneurysmal defect in children with a perimembranous ventricular septal defect. *Br Heart J.* 1990;64:146.
304. Baker EJ, Ayton V, Smith MA, et al. Magnetic resonance imaging at a high field strength of ventricular septal defects in infants. *Br Heart J.* 1989;62:305.
305. Shaw NJ, Godman MJ, Hayes A, Sutherland GR. Superior QRS axis in ventricular septal defect. *Br Heart J.* 1989;62:281.
306. Boone JW, Vincent RN, Dooley KJ, Williams WH. Ventricular septal defect closure without aortic valve plication in patients with aortic valve prolapse. *Am J Cardiol.* 1990;65:1271.
307. Rhodes LA, Keane JF, Keane JP, et al. Long follow-up (to 43 years) of ventricular septal defect with audible aortic regurgitation. *Am J Cardiol.* 1990;66:340.
308. Chauvaud S, Serraf A, Mihaileanu S, et al. Ventricular septal defect associated with aortic valve incompetence: results of two surgical managements. *Ann Thor Surg.* 1990;49:875.
309. Schwarz SM, Gewitz MH, See CC, et al. Enteral nutrition in infants with congenital heart disease and growth failure. *Pediatrics.* 1990;86:368.
310. Houyel L, Vaksmann G, Fournier A, Davignon A. Ventricular arrhythmias after correction of ventricular septal defects: importance of surgical approach. *J Am Coll Cardiol.* 1990;16:1224.
311. Sommer RJ, Golinko RJ, Ritter SB. Intracardiac shunting in children with ventricular septal defect: evaluation with Doppler color flow mapping. *J Am Coll Cardiol.* 1990;16:1437.
312. Stümper O, Fraser AG, Elzenga N, et al. Assessment of ventricular septal defect closure by intraoperative epicardial ultrasound. *J Am Coll Cardiol.* 1990;16:1672.
313. Faxon DP, O'Gara PT. A 67-year-old man with a ventricular septal defect and progressive dyspnea. *N Engl J Med.* 1991;324:831.
314. Bridges NH, Perry SB, Keane JF, et al. Preoperative transcatheter closure of congenital muscular ventricular septal defects. *N Engl J Med.* 1991;324:1312.
315. Linker DT, Rossvoll O, Chapman JV, Angelsen BAJ. Sensitivity and speed of colour Doppler flow mapping compared with continuous wave Doppler for the detection of ventricular septal defects. *Br Heart J.* 1991;65:201.
316. Chen M-R, Rigby ML, Redington AN. Familial aneurysms of the interventricular septum. *Br Heart J.* 1991;65:104.
317. Weintraub RG, Menahem S. Early surgical closure of a large ventricular septal defect: influence of long-term growth. *J Am Coll Cardiol.* 1991;18:552.
318. Kimball TR, Daniels SR, Meyer RA, Hannon DW, Khoury P, Schwartz DC. Relation of symptoms to contractility and defect size in infants with ventricular septal defect. *Am J Cardiol.* 1991;67:1097.
319. Hitchcock JF, Suijker WJL, Ksiezycka E, et al. Management of ventricular septal defect with associated aortic incompetence. *Ann Thor Surg.* 1991;52:70.
320. Backer CL, Idriss FS, Zales VR, et al. Surgical management of the conal (supracristal) ventricular septal defect. *J Thorac Cardiovasc Surg.* 1991;102:288.
321. Moises VA, Maciel BC, Hornberger LK, et al. A new method for noninvasive estimation of ventricular septal defect shunt flow by Doppler color flow mapping: imaging of the laminar flow convergence region on the left septal surface. *J Am Coll Cardiol.* 1991;18:824.
322. Chin AJ, Alboliras ET, Barber G, et al. Prospective detection by Doppler color flow imaging of additional defects in infants with a large ventricular septal defect. *J Am Coll Cardiol.* 1990;15:1637.
323. Meijboom F, Szatmari A, Utens E, Bos E, Hess J. Long-term follow-up after surgical closure of ventricular septal defect in childhood. *Cardiol Young.* 1993;I–104.
324. Termignon JL, Leca F, Karam J, et al. Surgical treatment of multiple ventricular septal defects using a biological glue. *Cardiol Young.* 1993;3:I–99 (abstract 327).
325. Seguchi M, Nakazawa M, Momma K. Significance of vascular action of digitalis in determining left-to-right shunts in infants with large ventricular septal defect. *Cardiol Young.* 1993;3:I–90.
326. Oberhansli I, Mermillod B, Favre H, Friedli B. Alpha-atrial natriuretic factor secretion in patients with ventricular septal defects and pulmonary hypertension, or from tetralogy of Fallot. *Cardiol Young.* 1993;3:I–88.
327. Rigby M, Redington A. Primary transcatheter closure of perimembranous ventricular septal defects. *Cardiol Young.* 1993;3:I–38.
328. Khoury W, Leca F, Mounet F, Vouhé P, Tamisier D. Single homograft aortic cusp replacement for aortic insufficiency and ventricular septal defect. *Cardiol Young.* 1993;3:I–14.
329. Rychik J, Lieb DR, Jacobs ML, Norwood WI, Chin AJ. Acute changes in left ventricular geometry following removal of volume overload. *Cardiol Young.* 1993;3:I–12.
330. Ludomirsky A, Tani L, Murphy DJ, Huhta JC. Usefulness of color-flow Doppler in diagnosing and in differentiating supracristal ventricular septal defect from right ventricular outflow tract obstruction. *Am J Cardiol.* 1991;67:194.
331. Ouellette Y, Rosenberg H, Joubert G, Li M, Dayton S. Mid-diastolic flow murmur in large ventricular septal defects is not caused by increased flow velocity across the mitral valve. *Cardiol Young.* 1993;3:I–144 (abstract 508).
332. Ruygrok P, Fenwick J, Calder L, Wilson N. Minor progression of aortic regurgitation in patients with ventricular septal defect and mild aortic deformity, *Cardiol Young* 3:1, 1993 (abstract 510).
333. Colloridi V, Ventriglia F, Bastianon V, et al. Natural history of ventricular septal defects by serial color-flow Doppler echocardiographic studies. *Cardiol Young.* 1993;3:I–140 (abstract 492).
334. Chang CH, Hsieh HC, Lin PJ, et al. Surgical correction of subarterial ventricular septal defect can prevent progression of aortic insufficiency. *Cardiol Young.* 1993;3:I–140 (abstract 491).
335. Brauner R, Birk E, Sahar G, Blieden L, Vidne B. Surgical results of defect closure and aortic valvuloplasty in ventricular septal defect with aortic valve prolapse. *Cardiol Young.* 1993;3:I (abstract 489).
336. Fishberger SB, Bridges ND, Keane JF, et al. Intraoperative device closure of ventricular septal defects. *Circulation.* 1993;88(part 2):205.

337. Serraf A, Lacour-Gayet F, Bruniaux J, et al. Surgical management of isolated multiple ventricular septal defects. Logical approach in 130 cases. *J Thorac Cardiovasc Surg*. 1992;103:437.
338. Hiraishi S, Agata Y, Nowatari M, et al. Incidence and natural course of trabecular ventricular septal defect: two-dimensional echocardiography and color Doppler flow imaging study. *J Pediatr*. 1992;120:409.
339. Backer CL, Winters RC, Zales VR, et al. Restrictive ventricular septal defect. How small is too small to close? *Ann Thorac Surg*. 1993;56:104.
340. Van der Velde ME, Sanders SP, Keane JF, Perry SB, Lock JE. Transesophageal echocardiographic guidance of transcatheter ventricular septal defect closure. *J Am Coll Cardiol*. 1994;23:1660.
341. Moller JH, Patton C, Varco RL, Lillehei CW. Late results (30 to 35 years) after operative closure of isolated ventricular septal defect from 1954 to 1960. *Am J Cardiol*. 1991;68:1491.
342. Hardin JT, Muskett AD, Carter CE, Martin TC, Spray TL. Primary surgical closure of large ventricular septal defects in small infants. *Ann Thorac Surg*. 1992;53:397.
343. Rivera JM, Siu SC, Handschumacher MD, et al. Three-dimensional reconstruction of ventricular septal defects: validation studies and in vivo feasibility. *J Am Coll Cardiol*. 1994;23:201.
344. Trusler GA, Williams WG, Smallhorn JF, Freedom RM. Late results after repair of aortic insufficiency associated with ventricular septal defect. *J Thorac Cardiovasc Surg*. 1992;103:276.
345. Kumar A, Van Mierop LHS, Epstein ML. Pathogenetic implications of muscular ventricular septal defect in Holt-Oram syndrome. *Am J Cardiol*. 1992;73:993.
346. Sapin SO, Junkel PA, Wong AL, Simandle KG. The congenital isolated apical ventricular septal defect. *Pediatrics*. 1994;93:516.
347. O'Fallon WM, Weidman WH, eds. Long-term follow-up of congenital aortic stenosis, pulmonary stenosis, and ventricular septal defect. Report from the second joint study on the natural history of congenital heart defects (NHS-2). *Circulation*. 1993;87:I-1-I-126.
348. Leca F, Karam J, Vouhé PR, et al. Surgical treatment of multiple ventricular septal defects using a biologic glue. *J Thorac Cardiovasc Surg*. 1994;107:96.
349. Burke R, Michielon G, Wernovsky G. Video-assisted cardioscopy in congenital heart operations. *Ann Thor Surg*. 1994;58:864.
350. Idriss FS, Muster AJ, Paul MH, Backer CL, Mavroudis C. Ventricular septal defect with tricuspid pouch with and without transposition. Anatomic and surgical considerations. *J Thorac Cardiovasc Surg*. 1992;103:52.
351. Rigby ML, Redington AN. Primary transcatheter umbrella closure of perimembranous ventricular septal defect. *Br Heart J*. 1994;72:368.
352. Orie J, Flotta D, Sherman FS. To be or not to be a VSD. *Am J Cardiol*. 1994;74:1284.
353. Wu M-H, Wu J-M, Chang CI, et al. Implication of aneurysmal transformation in isolated perimembranous ventricular septal defect. *Am J Cardiol*. 1993;72:596.
354. Rychik J, Norwood WI, Chin AJ. Doppler color flow mapping assessment of residual shunt after closure of large ventricular septal defects. *Circulation*. 1991;84(suppl III):III-153.
355. Mehta AV, Chidambaram B. Ventricular septal defect in the first year of life. *Am J Cardiol*. 1992;70:364.
356. Van den Heuvel F, Timmers T, Hess J. Morphological, haemodynamic, and clinical variables as predictors for management of isolated ventricular septal defect. *Br Heart J*. 1995;73:49.
357. Gheen KM, Reeves JT. Effects of size of ventricular septal defect and age on pulmonary hemodynamics at sea level. *Am J Cardiol*. 1995;75:66.
358. Ramaciotti C, Vetter JM, Bornemeier RA, Chin AJ. Prevalence, relation to spontaneous closure, and association of muscular ventricular septal defects with other cardiac defects. *Am J Cardiol*. 1995;75:61.
359. Bonhoeffer P, Fabbrocini M, Lecompte Y, et al. Infundibular septal defect with severe aortic regurgitation: a new surgical approach. *Ann Thorac Surg*. 1992;53:851.
360. Sadamatsu K, Harasawa Y, Ozono K, et al. A rare case of large ventricular septal defect with minimal pulmonary vascular obstructive changes in a 41-year-old woman. *Heart Ves*. 1995;10:218.
361. von Segesser LK, Fasnacht MS, Vogt PR, Genoni M, Arbenz U, Turina MI. Prevention of residual ventricular septal defects with fibrin sealant. *Ann Thorac Surg*. 1995;60:511.
362. Roguin N, Du Z-D, Barak M, Nasser N, Herschkowitz S, Milgram E. High prevalence of muscular ventricular septal defects in neonates. *J Am Coll Cardiol*. 1995;26:1545.
363. Vogel M, Rigby ML, Shore D. 3-dimensional echocardiography of ventricular septal defects before and after transcatheter closure with a modified Rashkind umbrella. *Circulation*. 1995;92:(suppl I):647.
364. Shirali GS, Smith EO, Geva T. Quantitation of echocardiographic predictors of outcome in infants with isolated ventricular septal defect. *Am Heart J*. 1995;130:1228.
365. Leung MP, Chan K-t, Chiu C, Yung T-c, Mok C-k. Intraoperative TEE assessment of ventricular septal defect with aortic regurgitation. *Ann Thor Surg*. 1996;61:854.
366. Sarris GE, Dillon T, Murphy D, Mee RBB. Delayed presentation and repair of isolated traumatic ventricular septal defect. *Ann Thor Surg*. 1996;62:1194.
367. Kumar K, Lock JE, Geva T. Ventricular septal defects between the left ventricle and the right ventricular infundibulum. Diagnostic and interventional considerations. *Circulation*. 1997;95:1207. [The title of their abstract in Pediatrics 1996; 98:suppl 521 was perhaps better: Ventricular septal defects between the left ventricular and infundibular apices.]
368. Sideris EB, Walsh KP, Haddad JL, Chen C-R, Ren SG, Kulkarni H. Occlusion of congenital ventricular septal defects by the buttoned device. *Heart*. 1997;77:276.
369. Michel C, Rabinovitch MA, Huynh T. Gerbode's defect associated with acute sinus node dysfunction as a complication of infective endocarditis. *Heart*. 1996;76:379.
370. Chaturvedi RR, Shore DF, Yacoub M, Redington AN. Intraoperative apical ventricular septal defect closure using a modified Rashkind double umbrella. *Heart*. 1996;76:367.
371. Carotti A, Marino B, Bevilacqua M, et al. Primary repair of isolated ventricular septal defect in infancy guided by echocardiography. *Am J Cardiol*. 1997;79:1498.
372. Yacoub MH, Khan H, Stavri G, Shinebourne E, Radley-Smith R. Anatomic correction of the syndrome of prolapsing right coronary cusp, dilatation of the sinus of Valsalva, and ventricular septal defect. *J Thorac Cardiovasc Surg*. 1997;113:253.
373. Niwa K, Perloff JK, Kaplan S, Child JS, Miner PD. Eisenmenger syndrome in adults: ventricular septal defect, truncus arteriosus, univentricular heart. *J Am Coll Cardiol*. 1999;34:223.
374. Macé L, Dervanian P, Le Bret E, et al. "Swiss cheese" septal defects: surgical closure using a single patch with intermediate fixings. *Ann Thor Surg*. 1999;67:1754.

375. Kalra GS, Verma PK, Dhall A, Singh S, Arora R. Transcatheter device closure of ventricular septal defects: immediate results and intermediate-term follow-up. *Am Heart J.* 1999;138:339.
376. Eriksson H, Cooper SM, Rosenbaum KN, Ruckman RN. Familial occurrence of congenital aneurysm of the muscular interventricular septum. *Pediatr Cardiol.* 1998;19:249.
377. Thanopoulos VD, Tsaousis GS, Konstadopoulou GN, Zarayelyan AG. Transcatheter closure of muscular ventricular septal defects with the Amplatzer ventricular septal defect occluder: initial clinical applications in children. *J Am Coll Cardiol.* 1999;33:1395.
378. Black MD, Shukla V, Rao V, Smallhorn JF, Freedom RM. Repair of isolated multiple ventricular septal defects: the septal obliteration technique. *Ann Thor Surg.* 2000;70:106.
379. Kardon RE, Cao QL, Masani N, et al. New insights and observations in three-dimensional echocardiographic visualization of ventricular septal defects. Experimental and clinical studies. *Circulation.* 1998;98:1307.
380. Batista RJV, Santos JLV, Takeshita N, al E. Successful reversal of pulmonary hypertension in Eisenmenger complex. *Arq Bras Cardiol.* 1997;68:279.
381. Lin PJ, Chang CH, Chu JJ, et al. Minimally invasive cardiac surgical techniques in the closure of ventricular septal defect: an alternative approach. *Ann Thor Surg.* 1998;65:165.
382. Seddio F, Reddy VM, McElhinney DB, Tworetsky W, Silverman NH, Hanley FL. Multiple ventricular septal defects: how and when should they be repaired? *J Thorac Cardiovasc Surg.* 1999;117:134.
383. Merrick AF, Lal M, Anderson RH, Shore DF. Management of ventricular septal defect: a survey of practice in the United Kingdom. *Ann Thor Surg.* 1999;68:9831.
384. Kaneko Y, Okabe H, Nagata N, Kanemoto S, Yamada S. Right ventricular obstruction by tricuspid pouch in simple ventricular septal defect. *Ann Thor Surg.* 1998;65:550.
385. Lun K-s, Li H, Leung MP, et al. Analysis of indications for surgical closure of subarterial ventricular septal defect without associated aortic cusp prolapse and aortic regurgitation. *Am J Cardiol.* 2001;87:1266.
386. Sim EKW, Grignani RT, Dip IB, et al. Outcome of surgical closure of doubly committed subarterial ventricular septal defect. *Ann Thor Surg.* 1999;67:736.
387. Okubo M, Benson LN, Nykanen D, et al. Outcomes of intraoperative device closure of muscular ventricular septal defects. *Ann Thor Surg.* 2001;72:416.
388. Kitagawa T, Durham LA, Mosca RS, Bove EL. Techniques and results in the management of multiple ventricular septal defects. *J Thorac Cardiovasc Surg.* 1998;115:848.
389. Grünenfelder J, Kiaffas M, Bartram U, Herlong R, Van Praagh R. Patch repair of subsemilunar conal septal defect resulting in severe left ventricular outflow tract obstruction. *Am J Cardiol.* 1997;80:1256.
390. Komai H, Naito Y, Fujiwara K, Noguchi Y, Nishimura Y, Uemura S. Surgical strategy for doubly committed subarterial ventricular septal defect with aortic cusp prolapse. *Ann Thor Surg.* 1997;64:1146.
391. Amin Z, Gu X, Berry JM, Titus JL, Gidding SS, Rocchini AP. Perventricular closure of ventricular septal defects without cardiopulmonary bypass. *Ann Thor Surg.* 1999;68:149.
392. Le T-P, Freudenthal F, Sievert H, Vaessen P, Grabitz R. Transcatheter occlusion of subaortic ventricular septal defect using a nitinol coil: initial clinical results. *Circulation.* 2001;104(suppl II):593.
393. Tsang VT, Hsia T-Y, Yates RWM, Anderson RH. Surgical repair of supposedly multiple defects within the apical part of the muscular ventricular septum. *Ann Thor Surg.* 2002;73:58.
394. Cheung W-f, Chiu CSW, Yung T-c, Chan AKT. Impact of preoperative aortic cusp prolapse on long term outcome after surgical closure of subarterial ventricular septal defect. *Ann Thorac Surg.* 2002;73:622.
395. Gabriel HM, Heger M, Innerhofer P, et al. Long-term outcome of patients with ventricular septal defect considered not to require surgical closure during childhood. *J Am Coll Cardiol.* 2002;39:1066.
396. Yamagishi M, Shuntoh K, Takahashi A, Shinkawa T, Miyazaki T, Kitamura N. Atrial septum around the fossa ovalis: an ideal patch for the ventricular septal defect. *J Thorac Cardiovasc Surg.* 2002;123:999.
397. Tsai T-P, Yu J-M, Wu Y-L, Huang C-Y, Chen F-L. Change of serum growth factors in infants with isolated ventricular septal defect undergoing surgical repair. *Ann Thor Surg.* 2002;73:1765.
398. Vaidyanathan B, Roth SJ, Rao S, Gauvreau K, Shivaprakasha K, Kumar K. Outcome of ventricular septal defect repair in a developing country. *J Pediatr.* 2002;140:736.
399. Puchalski MD, Brook MM, Silverman NH. Simplified echocardiographic criteria for decision making in perimembranous ventricular septal defect in childhood. *Am J Cardiol.* 2002;90:569.
400. Fukuda T, Suzuki T, Kashima I, Sato M, Morikawa Y. Shallow stitching close to the rim of the ventricular septal defect eliminates injury to the right bundle branch. *Ann Thor Surg.* 2002;75:550.
401. Ootaki Y, Yamaguchi M, Yoshimura N, Oka S, Yoshida M, Hasegawa T. Surgical management of trabecular ventricular septal defects: the sandwich technique. *J Thorac Cardiovasc Surg.* 2003;125:508.
402. Sivakumar K, Anil SR, Rao SG, Shivaprakash K, Kumar RK. Closure of muscular ventricular septal defects guided by en face reconstruction and pictorial representation. *Ann Thor Surg.* 2003;76:158.
403. Thanopoulos BD, Tsaousis GS, Karanasios E, Eleftherakis NG, Paphitis C. Transcatheter closure of perimembranous ventricular septal defects with the Amplatzer asymmetric ventricular septal defect occluder: preliminary experience in children. *Heart.* 2003;89:918.
404. Maile S, Kadner A, Turina I, Prêtre R. Detachment of the anterior leaflet of the tricuspid valve to expose perimembranous ventricular septal defects. *Ann Thorac Surg.* 2003;75:944.
405. Zhao J, Li J, Wei X, Zhao B, Sun W. Tricuspid valve detachment in closure of congenital ventricular septal defect. *Texas Heart Inst J.* 2003;30:38.
406. Aeba R, Katogi T, Hashizume K, et al. Liberal use of tricuspid valve detachment for transatrial ventricular septal defect closure. *Ann Thorac Surg.* 2003;76:1073.
407. Partin C. The evolution of Eisenmenger's eponymic enshrinement. *Am J Cardiol.* 2003;92:1187.
408. Bacha EA, Cao Q-L, Starr JP, Waight D, Ebeid MR, Hijazi ZM. Perventricular device closure of muscular ventricular septal defects on the beating heart: technique and results. *J Thorac Cardiovasc Surg.* 2003;126:1718.
409. Gott VL, Shumway NE. Cross-circulation: a milestone in cardiac surgery. *J Thorac Cardiovasc Surg.* 2004;127:617.
410. Holzer R, Balzer D, Cao Q-L, Lock K, Hijazi ZM. For the Amplatzer muscular ventricular septal defect investigators. *J Am Coll Cardiol.* 2004;43:1257.

411. Bhatt M, Roth SJ, Kumar RK, et al. Management of infants with large, unrepaired ventricular septal defects and respiratory infection requiring mechanical ventilation. *J Thorac Cardiovasc Surg.* 2004;127:1466.
412. Novick WM, Sandoval N, Lazorhysynets VV, et al. Flap valve double patch closure of ventricular septal defects in children with increased pulmonary vascular resistance. *Ann Thorac Surg.* 2005;79:21.
413. Knauth AL, Lock JE, Perry SB, et al. Transcatheter device closure of congenital and postoperative residual ventricular septal defects. *Circulation.* 2004;110:501.
414. Carminati M, Butera G, Chessa M, Drago M, Negura D, Piazza L. Transcatheter closure of congenital ventricular septal defect with Amplatzer septal occluders. *Am J Cardiol.* 2005;96(suppl):52L.
415. Robinson JD, Zimmerman FJ, De Loera O, Heitschmidt M, Hijazi ZM. Cardiac conduction disturbances seen after transcatheter device closure of muscular ventricular septal defects with the Amplatzer occluder. *Am J Cardiol.* 2006;97:558.
416. Meadows J, Pigula F, Lock J, Marshall A. Transcatheter creation and enlargement of ventricular septal defects for relief of ventricular hypertension. *J Thorac Cardiovasc Surg.* 2007;133:912.
417. Lavoie R, Sestier F, Gilbert G, Chameides L, Van Praagh R, Grondin P. Double outlet right ventricle with left ventricular outflow obstruction due to small ventricular septal defect. *Am Heart J.* 1971;82:290.
418. Xing Q, Pan S, An Q, et al. Minimally invasive perventricular device closure of perimembranous ventricular septal defect without cardiopulmonary bypass: multicenter experienced and mid-term follow-up. *J Thorac Cardiovasc Surg.* 2010;139:1409.
419. Zuo J, Xie J, Yi W, et al. Results of transcatheter closure of perimembranous ventricular septal defect. *Am J Cardiol.* 2010;106:1034.
420. Roger H: Recherches cliniques sur la communication congénitale des deux coeurs, par inocclusion du septum interventriculaire. *Bull Acad de Méd, Paris* 8:1074 and 11891879.
421. Lacour-Gayet F, Bove EL, Hraška V, Morell VO, Spray TL, eds. *Surgery of Conotruncal Anomalies.* Switzerland, Cham Heidelberg New York Dordrecht London: Springer International Publishing AG; 2016.

17

Single Ventricle

Single ventricle means that one ventricular sinus, body, or inflow tract is present; in other words, one ventricular sinus, body, or inflow tract is absent.

In **single LV (morphologically left ventricle),** the right ventricular sinus is absent (component 2, Fig. 17.1A).

In **single RV (morphologically right ventricle),** the left ventricular sinus is absent (component 2, see Fig. 17.1B).

In single LV, the most common form of single ventricle occurring in about 74% of cases,[1,2] there is an infundibular outlet chamber (component 3, see Fig. 17.1A).

The infundibular outlet chamber which is characteristic of single LV is shown in Figs. 17.2, 17.3, and 17.4.

In single RV with absence of the left ventricular sinus (about 26% of cases)[2] even though the infundibulum is present, it does not look like an infundibular *outlet chamber*. Why not? With single LV, the infundibulum looks like an outlet *chamber* because the infundibulum has an inlet constriction or narrowing that is produced by displacement of the ventricular septum. When the right ventricular sinus is absent, the ventricular septum is displaced in that direction—toward the location of the absent right ventricular sinus. This is similar to the shift of the mediastinum in the direction of a small or absent lung.

This "right ventriculad" shift of the ventricular septum brings the crest of the muscular ventricular septum abnormally close beneath the inferior rim of the infundibular septum, creating the appearance of an inlet narrowing leading into the infundibulum. The inlet narrowing makes the subarterial infundibulum look like a chamber—a diagnostically helpful appearance. An outlet chamber appearance strongly suggests a single LV with an infundibular outlet chamber. By contrast, with single RV, because of an absent left ventricular sinus, the ventricular septum moves away from beneath the infundibular septum. The ventricular septal remnant moves "left ventriculad," posteriorly and to the left with a ventricular D-loop, or posteriorly and to the right with a ventricular L-loop. Consequently, there is no inlet constriction leading into the infundibular or outlet part of the heart: no inlet constriction and no outlet chamber appearance.

The premorphologic definition of single or common ventricle used to be as follows. Single or common ventricle is present if both atrioventricular (AV) valves or a common AV valve open into the same ventricular chamber.[2,3]

Lambert[4] reported a case of single ventricle with a rudimentary outlet chamber in 1951 in which the tricuspid valve opened predominantly into the outlet chamber. In other words, we knew in the early 1960s that single ventricle with an infundibular outlet chamber did not necessarily have double-inlet single ventricle. In other words, we knew that the premorphologic definition of single ventricle was not always accurate.

When I speak of the *premorphologic definition* of single or common ventricle I mean that before 1964[2] the morphologic anatomy of single or common ventricle was not understood. That is why Dr. Jeremy Swan, my boss in the Cardiac Catheterization Laboratory at the Mayo Clinic in Rochester, Minnesota, gave me this as a research project in 1960 to 1961. I was his fellow in the Catheterization Laboratory for 1 year, a high privilege. Before this time, I had been an Assistant Resident in Pathology in 1956 to 1957 at Boston Children's Hospital, between my junior and senior years as a Resident in Pediatrics. During my year of training in Pathology, I had fortunately learned of the work of Dr. Maurice Lev[5] in Chicago in which he introduced the morphologic anatomic approach to the diagnosis of the cardiac chambers by means of the morphologic anatomy of their septal surfaces, not in terms of their relative positions, such as right-sided or left-sided.

I expanded Lev's[5] approach by including the morphologic anatomy of the septal surfaces **and of the free wall surfaces.** Both were specific, different, and diagnostically very helpful.[2] Then it became obvious that using the AV valves to diagnose the presence or absence of single ventricle was a violation of logic, in the following sense. Using one variable (the AV valves) to diagnose the status of another, different variable (the presence or absence of single ventricle) was a violation of logic in the sense that each variable should be diagnosed primarily in terms of itself, not in terms of some other, different variable. **The principle that each variable should be diagnosed primarily in terms of itself,** if possible, not in terms of some other different variable, is important and has widespread applicability. In addition to cases like Dr. Edward Lambert's,[4,6] later we would also learn that the type of ventricular loop

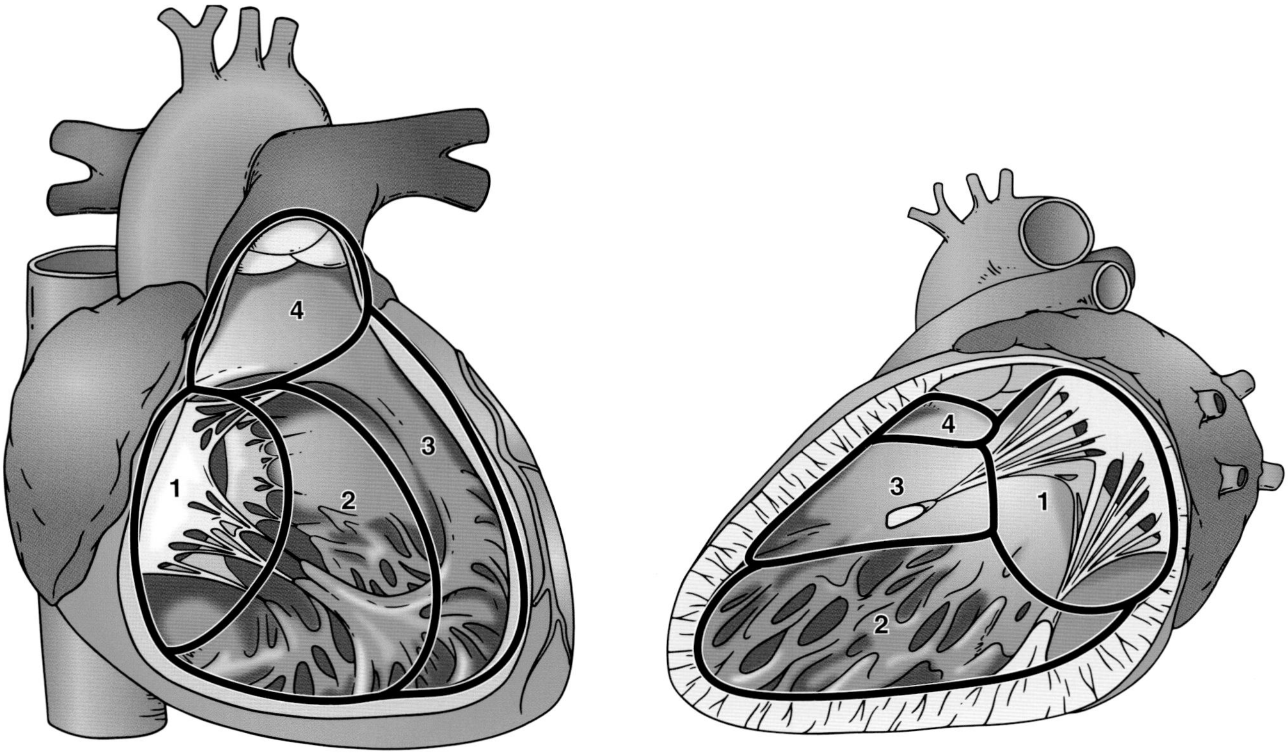

Fig. 17.1 (A) The normal right ventricular (RV) septal surface. (B) The normal left ventricle (LV) of septal surface. The ventricular septum and the free walls of both ventricles are composed of four anatomic and developmental components. **Component *1*** is the atrioventricular (AV) canal and the AV valves. **Component *2*** is the sinus, body, or inflow tract and the main pumping portion of the RV and LV. **Component *3*** is the proximal or apical portion of the infundibulum or conus arteriosus. In the RV, component 3 is called the **septal band,** and its apical extension to the anterior papillary muscle of the RV is known as the **moderator band.** In the LV, component 3 is the smooth, nontrabeculated superior portion of the left ventricular septal surface. The inferior part of the left ventricular septal surface is finely trabeculated and is part of component 2. **Component *4*** is the distal or subarterial part of the infundibulum or conus arteriosus. From the RV aspect, component 4 is known as the **infundibular or conal septum.** Its right ventricular free wall extension is called the **parietal band.** The septal band is so designated because it forms the upper part of the RV septal surface. The parietal band is also known as the crista supraventricularis, or supraventricular crest, because it normally forms a crest above the RV sinus. Normally, component 4 makes a small contribution to the top of the left ventricular septal surface. **Single LV** results from absence of the right ventricular sinus (component 2). But components 3 and 4 are present. That is why single LV (absence of component 2) has an infundibular outlet chamber—because components 3 and 4 are present. Also, the muscular ventricular septum is displaced toward the location of the absent right ventricular sinus: in a rightward and anterior direction with a ventricular D-loop, or in a leftward and anterior (ventral) direction with a ventricular L-loop. This displacement of the ventricular septum places the crest of the muscular ventricular septum beneath the opening leading into the infundibular outlet chamber. In turn, the crest of the displaced muscular ventricular septum narrows the opening leading into the infundibulum, making the infundibulum look like an outlet *chamber*. This somewhat narrowed opening leading from the single LV into the infundibulum is called the **bulboventricular foramen, or the infundibuloventricular foramen. Single RV** is absence of the LV sinus (component 2). The ventricular septum is displaced toward the location of the absent LV sinus, posteriorly and to the left with a ventricular D-loop or posteriorly and to the right with a ventricular L-loop. Because the ventricular septal remnant is displaced *posteriorly, not anteriorly*, there is no narrowing of the outflow tract leading from the single RV into the infundibulum. Consequently, the infundibulum in single RV does not look like an outlet *chamber* because there is no inlet narrowing by the displaced ventricular septal remnant. (Reproduced with permission from Van Praagh R, Geva T, Kreutzer J. Ventricular septal defects: how shall we describe, name, and classify them? *J Am Coll Cardiol.* 1989;14:1298.[11])

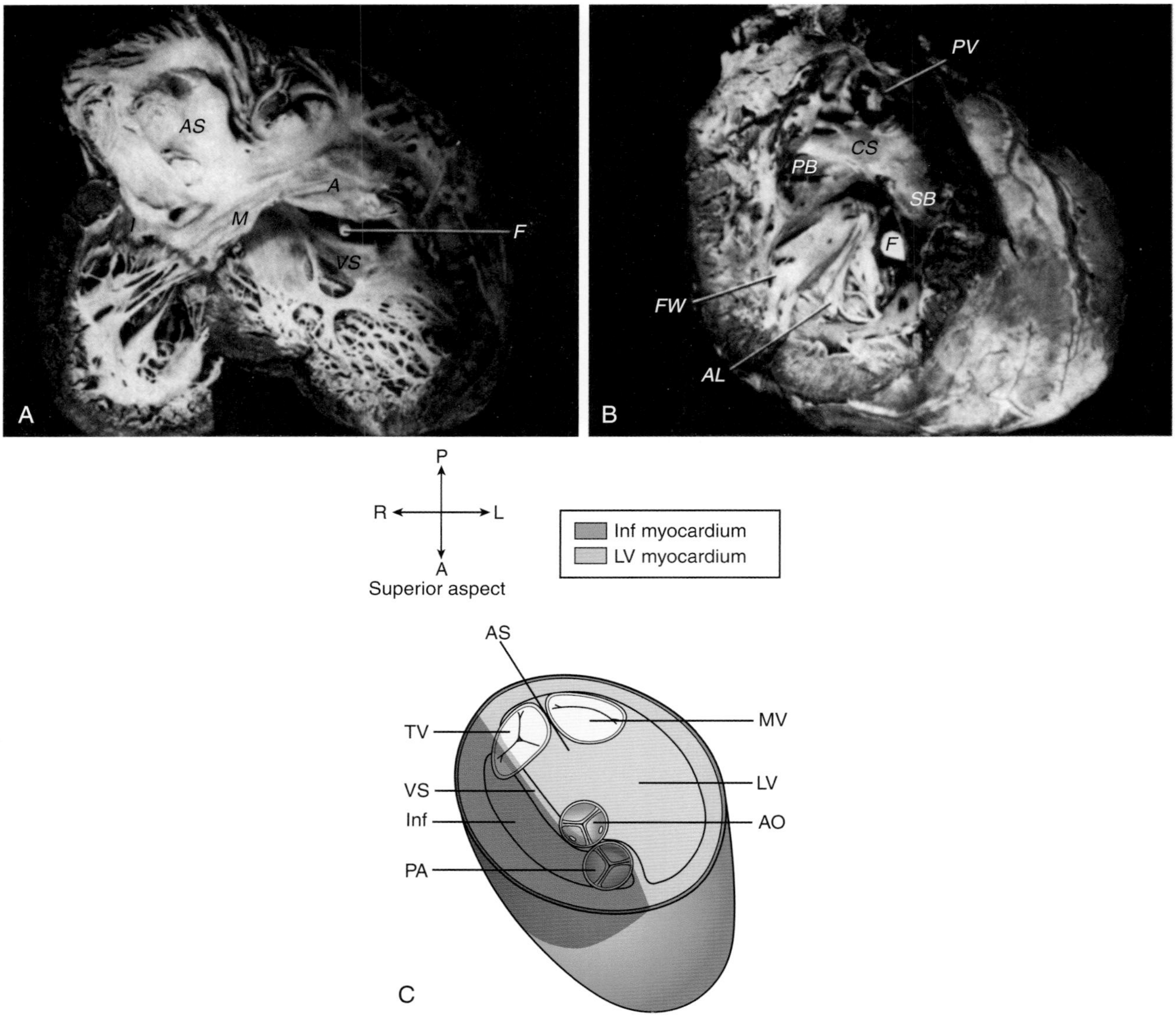

Fig. 17.2 Holmes Heart With Single Left Ventricle *(LV),* Infundibular Outlet Chamber, and Normally Related Great Arteries (i.e., a Normal Anatomic Type of Infundibulum and Great Arteries). The segmental anatomy is normal: {S,D,S}; that is, each segment is in situs solitus. (A) The opened right atrium, tricuspid valve *(TV),* and single LV. A probe is seen passing from the single LV through the infundibuloventricular foramen into the infundibular outlet chamber. (B) The opened subpulmonary infundibular outlet chamber. A probe passes through a normally located pulmonary valve *(PV).* A probe passes through a widely patent infundibuloventricular foramen *(F).* Note that what normally should be the right ventricular sinus septal surface (below F) is extremely shallow, that is, extremely undeveloped or absent. (C) The geometric diagram shows a single LV; no right ventricular sinus, a subpulmonary infundibular outlet chamber *(Inf);* rightward and anterior displacement of the ventricular septum *(VS);* a normally located atrial septum *(AS)* angulated 35 degrees to the left of the sagittal plane; a normally angulated VS, 40 degrees to the left of the sagittal plane; double-inlet left ventricle (DILV), the TV with bicameral insertions, barely into the outlet chamber, with thickened tricuspid leaflet margins indicating tricuspid regurgitation; and mitral valve *(MV)* unremarkable; semilunar valves normally related, displaying 150 degrees of dextrorotation relative to the sagittal plane; and no evidence of outflow tract obstruction or regurgitation. *A* and *M,* Anterior and medial leaflets of the TV; *AL,* anterior leaflet; *AO,* aorta; *CS,* conal septum or crista supraventricularis; *PA,* pulmonary artery; *PB,* parietal band; *SB,* septal band; *FW,* free wall of the infundibular outlet chamber. (Reproduced with permission from Van Praagh R, Plett JA, Van Praagh S. Single ventricle: pathology, embryology, terminology, and classification. *Herz.* 1979;4:113; and Van Praagh R, Ongley PA, Swan HJC. Anatomic types of single or common ventricle in man: morphologic and geometric aspects of 60 necropsied cases. *Am J Cardiol.* 1964;13:367.[1,2])

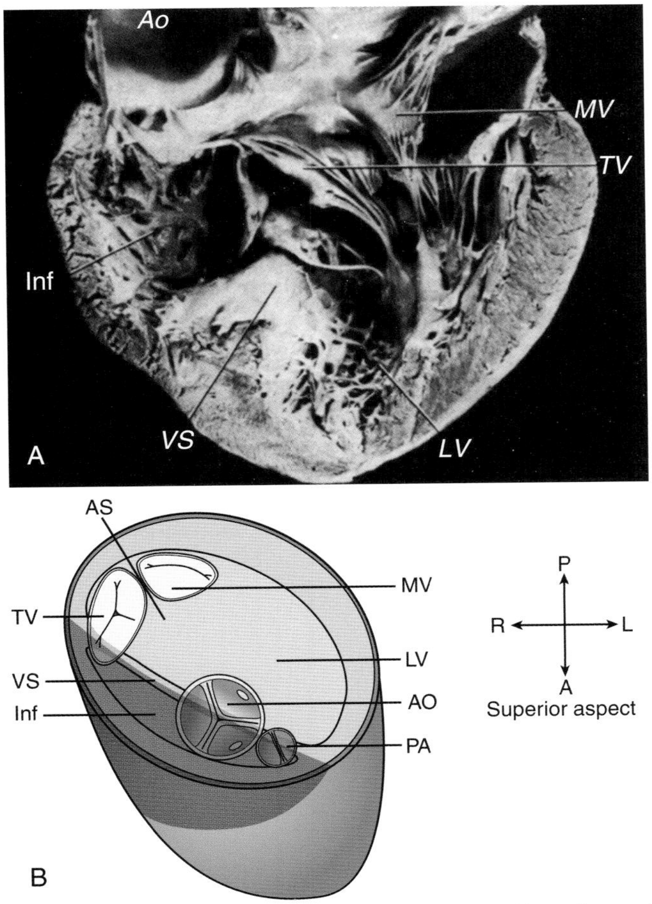

Fig. 17.3 Holmes Heart With Pulmonary Outflow Tract Stenosis, That Is, Single Left Ventricle *(LV)* Because of Absence of the Right Ventricular Sinus, With an Infundibular Outlet Chamber and Normally Related Great Arteries. The great arteries are normally related to each other and to the LV, but not to the right ventricular sinus that is absent. The segmental anatomy is normal, that is, {S,D,S}. (A) Note that the left ventricular septal surface is well developed, but what normally should be the right ventricular septal surface is absent. The ventricular septum *(VS)* is displaced to the right and anteriorly. Consequently the infundibulum looks like an outlet chamber. There is double-inlet left ventricle, with the tricuspid valve *(TV)* straddling the VS to insert a small amount into the outlet chamber. The bicameral insertions of the TV were associated with tricuspid regurgitation, indicated by thickening and rolling of the free margins of the tricuspid leaflets. Note that the medial leaflets of the regurgitant TV and of the normal mitral valve are indirect fibrous continuity. The atrioventricular (AV) valves are not separated by the ventricular septum because the VS is displaced abnormally to the right and anteriorly. Note the direct fibrous continuity between the aortic valve and both AV valves, which is normal with normally related great arteries. (B) Note that the valve of the pulmonary artery *(PA)* is hypoplastic and bicuspid. Relative to the sagittal plane, the atrial septal angle is 30 degrees to the left (normal) and the ventricular septal angle is 60 degrees to the left (a bit greater than normal). *AO* and *Ao,* Aorta; *AS,* atrial septum; *Inf,* infundibular; *MV,* mitral valve. (Reproduced with permission from Van Praagh R, Plett JA, Van Praagh S. Single ventricle: pathology, embryology, terminology, and classification. *Herz.* 1979;4:113. Van Praagh R, Ongley PA, Swan HJC. Anatomic types of single or common ventricle in man: morphologic and geometric aspects of 60 necropsied cases. *Am J Cardiol.* 1964;13:367.[1,2])

(D- or L-) should be diagnosed specifically in terms of itself, not in terms of whether the AV alignments and connections are concordant or discordant[7]:

1. When the atria are in situs solitus and the AV alignments ("connections") are concordant, L-loop ventricles can be present, not the expected D-loop ventricles.
2. When the atria are in situs solitus and the AV alignments are discordant, D-loop ventricles can be present, not the expected L-loop ventricles.

In other words, to avoid diagnostic errors, the ventricular situs must be diagnosed specifically per se, not in terms of a different variable.

Before morphologic anatomic understanding, single ventricle used to be called *common ventricle,* based on the impression that single ventricle is a huge ventricular septal defect (VSD), that is, absence of the ventricular septum. Does common ventricle occur? The answer is yes, but it is rare (Fig. 17.5A–B).[2] In our last large study of single ventricle,[1] we found no cases of common ventricle.

SINGLE LEFT VENTRICLE WITH INFUNDIBULAR OUTLET CHAMBER

Six different anatomic types of single LV with infundibular outlet chamber were found (Table 17.1). Single LV with an infundibular outlet chamber and a segmental situs set of solitus atria, ventricular D-loop, and solitus normally related great arteries were found in only 1 case (3% of this series as a whole).

Single LV with normally related great arteries is known as a **Holmes heart,** named in honor of Andrew F. Holmes, the first dean of McGill's medical school in Montreal, Canada, who described the first known case of this infrequent anomaly in 1824.[8] Maude Abbott (1869–1940), who was the curator of the McGill Medical Museum, found this unlabeled heart specimen in 1900, sitting in a bottle of formalin. William Osler (1849–1919) remembered this heart specimen well and told young Maude Abbott that it had first been published in 1824 by Andrew Fernando Holmes (1797–1860).[9] Dr. Abbott located Holmes' publication. It was the Holmes heart, Dr. Holmes' paper of 1824, and William Osler (later to become Sir William) that recruited Maude Abbott into the field of congenital heart disease and led to her becoming the leading world authority of her time in our field. Abbott[10] republished the Holmes heart in 1901 because no such case had been published after 1824. She thought that the Holmes heart might be unique. We now know that single LV with an infundibular outlet chamber and solitus normally related great arteries is infrequent to rare but not unique.

Anatomic type 6 (see Table 17.1, single LV) also has solitus normally related, but with ventricular inversion: single LV with infundibular outlet chamber and **{S,L,S}** segmental anatomy is **isolated inversion of the ventricular loop** (Fig. 17.6)**.** The atria are in situs solitus, {S,-,-}. The great arteries are solitus normally related, {-,-,S}. But a ventricular L-loop is present, {-,L,-}.

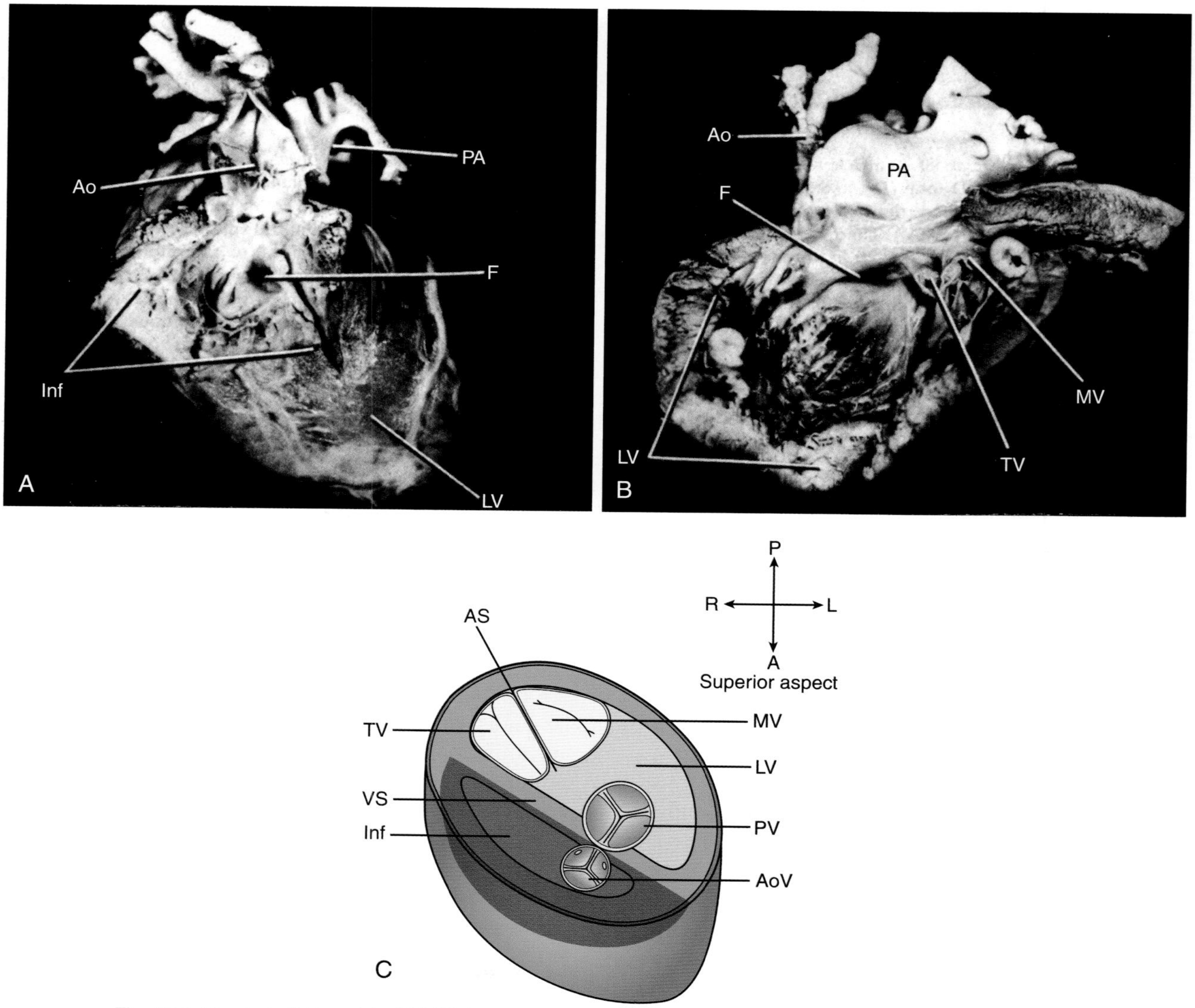

Fig. 17.4 **Single Left Ventricle *(LV)* With an Infundibular Outlet Chamber and Transposition of the Great Arteries {S,D,D}.** (A) Opened infundibular outlet chamber *(Inf)* and the D-transposed ascending aorta *(Ao)*. The infundibuloventricular foramen *(F)* is obstructively small, resulting in subaortic stenosis, hypoplasia of the aortic valve, and ascending Ao, and atresia of the aortic isthmus. The infundibuloventricular foramen lies between the infundibular septum above and the displaced ventricular septum below. This foramen is not called a ventricular septal defect (VSD) because VSD is short for interventricular septal defect (IVSD). To have an IVSD, two ventricles must be present. But in single ventricle, only one ventricle is present. So accurately speaking, these communications are called infundibuloventricular foramina, not VSDs. (B) The opened single LV is seen, with double-inlet LV by both the tricuspid valve *(TV)* and the mitral valve *(MV)*. The restrictive infundibuloventricular foramen, the hypoplastic ascending D-transposed Ao, and the dilated transposed pulmonary artery *(PA)* are seen. (C) The diagram shows absence of the right ventricular sinus beneath the infundibular outlet chamber, the rightward and anterior displacement of the ventricular septal *(VS)* remnant, and double-inlet single LV. In this case, the TV inserted only into the LV, without straddling of the TV into the Inf. The cardiac geometry was as follows: relative to the sagittal plane, the atrial septal angle was 30 degrees left, the ventricular septal angle was 60 degrees left, and the dextrorotation at the semilunar valves was only 30 degrees right (normal is 150 degrees right). The RV is the anterior ventricle. The LV is the posterior ventricle. Absence of the RV sinus results in **anterior displacement** of muscular VS, bringing the muscular VS close to and beneath the infundibular septum that lies between the semilunar valves. This resulted in a restrictively small infundibuloventricular defect (IVD) in this case. Absence of the LV sinus results in **posterior displacement** of the muscular VS, away from the infundibular septum that is anterior. This results in no narrowing of the inlet into the subarterial infundibulum produced by approximation of the muscular VS crest and the infundibular septal crest. Hence, in this patient, absence of the anterior right ventricular sinus is associated with an infundibular outlet chamber appearance, whereas absence of the left ventricular sinus typically has no such association. *AoV,* Aortic valve; *PV,* pulmonary valve. (Reproduced with permission from Van Praagh R, Plett JA, Van Praagh S. Single ventricle: pathology, embryology, terminology, and classification. *Herz.* 1979; 4:113; and Van Praagh R, Ongley PA, Swan HJC. Anatomic types of single or common ventricle in man: morphologic and geometric aspects of 60 necropsied cases. *Am J Cardiol.* 1964;13:367.[1,2])

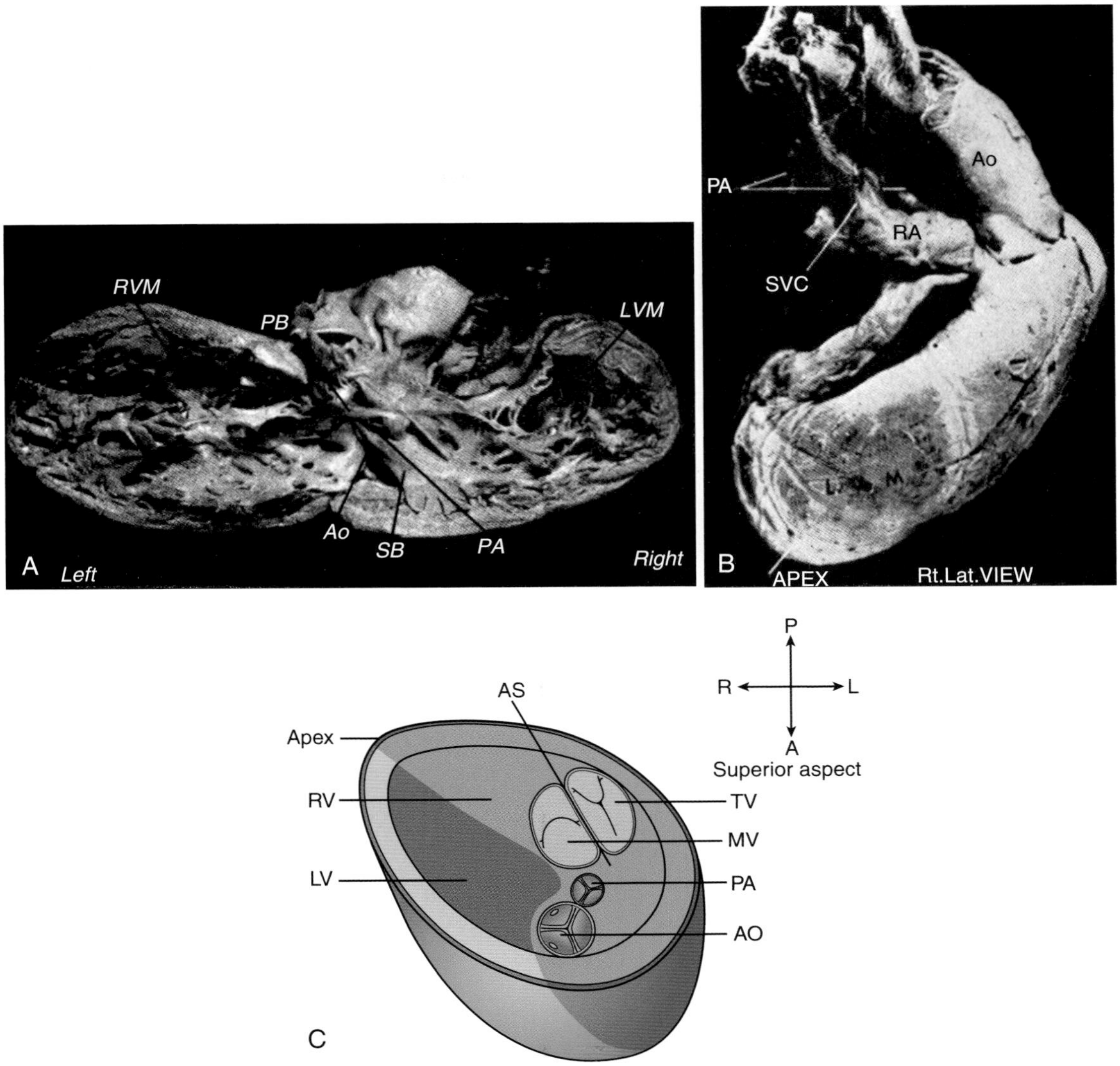

Fig. 17.5 Does common ventricle exist? Is it possible for the free walls of the right ventricular sinus and the left ventricular sinus to be present, but with absence of the muscular ventricular septum, and consequently the right ventricular sinus and the left ventricular sinus are in common (not separated)? We think the answer is probably yes, but, if so, common ventricle must be very rare. In this patient, dextrocardia was present because the ventricular apex pointed rightward and posteriorly. (A) View of the interior of the ventricular part of the heart as seen from the ventricular apex. The right-sided free wall myocardium is finely trabeculated, consistent with left ventricular myocardium *(LVM)*. The left-sided ventricular free wall is more coarsely trabeculated, consistent with right ventricular myocardium *(RVM)*. (B) Right lateral view of the exterior of this extremely malformed tubular heart, with the ventricular apex pointing posteriorly and rightward. (C) Geometric diagram. The atria were in situs solitus, that is, {S,-,-}. The ventricular segment may well have had an L-loop, as is suggested by inversion of the tricuspid valve *(TV)* and the mitral valve *(MV)*; and the RVM *(stippled)* is left-sided and the LVM is right-sided. Hence, the segmental anatomy appears, so far, to be {S,L,-}. The great arteries are in D-malposition, with 30-degree dextrorotation of the semilunar valves. Hence the segmental anatomy appears to be {S,L,D}. A coronary artery arises anomalously from the anterior nonseptal sinus of Valsalva of the aortic valve *(Ao)*. The pulmonary valve is tricuspid, but hypoplastic, indicating pulmonary outflow tract stenosis. Double-inlet RV and double-outlet RV appear to be present in C, but absence of the ventricular septum makes these diagnoses less certain and less meaningful than usual. The diagnosis appears to be common ventricle (absence of the interventricular septum) with dextrocardia (ventricular apex pointing rightward and posteriorly), with double-outlet RV {S,L,D}, with pulmonary outflow tract stenosis, and with an anomalous coronary arterial origin from the anterior nonseptal aortic sinus of Valsalva. *AO,* Aorta; *AS,* atrial septum; *LV,* left ventricle; *PB,* parietal band; *RtLat,* right lateral; *RV,* right ventricle; *SB,* septal band; *SVC,* superior vena cava. Note that this case is not included in the database of this chapter (see Table 17.1) for several reasons: (1) I am not certain that the previously mentioned diagnosis is entirely correct. (2) This chapter is about single ventricle, not about common ventricle. These are two very different anomalies. (3) Previously, it was widely assumed that single ventricle is common ventricle, that is, that single ventricle is "a huge VSD." This premorphologic assumption is not supported by morphologic anatomic data. I have not seen a case of common ventricle in the Cardiac Registry, the Cardiac Pathology Laboratory, of Boston Children's Hospital (1965 to 2002). (Reproduced with permission from Van Praagh R, Ongley PA, Swan HJC. Anatomic types of single or common ventricle in man: morphologic and geometric aspects of 60 necropsied cases. *Am J Cardiol.* 1964;13:367.[2])

TABLE 17.1 Our Findings in 31 Postmortem Cases of Single Ventricle (Table 17.1)[1]

Anatomic Types of Single Ventricle	No. of Cases (n = 31)	% of Series
Single Left Ventricle		
1. Single LV {S,D,S}	1	3
2. Single LV TGA {S,D,D}	6	19
3. Single LV TGA {S,D,L}	2	7
4. Single LV TGA {S,L,L}	12	39
5. Single LV TGA {S,L,D}	1	3
6. Single LV {S,L,S}	1	3
Subtotal	23	74
Single Right Ventricle		
1. Single RV DORV {S,D,D}	2	7
2. Single RV DORV {I,L,I}	1	3
3. Single RV TGA {A,D,D} and asplenia	1	3
4. Single RV DORV {A,D,D} and asplenia	3	10
5. Single RV TGA {A,L,L} and asplenia	1	3
Subtotal	8	26

DORV, Double-outlet right ventricle; *LV,* left ventricle; *RV,* right ventricular; *TGA,* transposition of the great arteries.

However, apart from these 2 patients with solitus normally related great arteries, {S,D,**S**} and {S,L,**S**} (see Table 17.1), the other 21 cases of single LV have transposition of the great arteries (TGA; see Table 17.1). Considering just single LV (n = 23), solitus normally related great arteries occurred in only 2 (9%), whereas TGA occurred in 21 of 23 (91%).

By far the most common anatomic type of single ventricle in our study was single LV with an infundibular outlet chamber and TGA {S,L,L} that occurred in 12 of 31 cases in the series as a whole (39%; see Table 17.1). In single LV, the incidence of TGA {S,L,L} was 12 of 23 (91%).

Single LV with infundibular outlet chamber is shown pictorially in Figs. 17.7 and 17.8.

Stenosis of the inlet into the subaortic infundibular outlet chamber in single LV with TGA {S,L,L} anatomy is shown in Fig. 17.9.

Atresia of the inlet into the subaortic infundibular outlet chamber with aortic valvar atresia is shown in Fig. 17.10.

The importance of **additional associated malformations** is illustrated by the case of single LV with infundibular outlet chamber and TGA {S,L,L} anatomy (Fig. 17.11). In addition to subaortic stenosis of the bulboventricular foramen leading into the subaortic infundibular outlet chamber, this patient also has left-sided tricuspid stenosis (see Fig. 17.11). Similarly, single LV with TGA {S,D,D} can have severe left-sided mitral stenosis (Fig. 17.12).[11]

The AV valves are a dependent variable. The situs of the AV valves corresponds to the situs of the ventricular loop into which the AV valves open. By contrast, **the situs of the atria, of the ventricular sinuses, and of the subarterial infundibulum are independent variables.**

Note that in patients with single LV and an infundibular outlet chamber, the viscera and atria always were in situs solitus (see Table 17.1). That is not the case with single RV, as we will see.

SINGLE RIGHT VENTRICLE

The 8 cases of single RV (see Table 17.1) are fascinating. That 6 of these 8 cases **(75%)** have double-outlet right ventricle (DORV) is no surprise (see Table 17.1). But how can 2 of these 8 cases (25%; see Table 17.1) of "single" RV have TGA? Because a small or tiny LV is present (Fig. 17.13). Such cases *anatomically* are not *single* RVs; in fact they are *biventricular* hearts with a large RV and a diminutive LV (see Fig. 17.13). But *functionally,* they are single RVs in the sense that only one good ventricular pumping chamber is present, and that is what matters clinically and surgically.

Ventricular sinus (inflow tract and main pumping portion) development is a spectrum. Consequently, a diminutive right ventricular sinus can be present in so-called "single" LV. But remember that the right ventricular sinus develops below the *infundibular ring,* which is formed by the *septal band* (component 3, see Fig. 17.1), the *moderator band* (continuous with component 3 apically), and the *parietal band* (the free wall extension of component 4, see Fig. 17.1). The infundibular ring may be regarded as the "mother" of the RV sinus or inflow tract that normally develops beneath the infundibular or conal ring. Consequently, a distinction exists between an *anatomically* single LV or RV and a *functionally* single LV or RV.

How is it possible to have a single RV with the following segmental anatomy: **DORV** {I,L,**I**}? Many people think that DORV is an abnormal relationship between the great arteries and the ventricular sinuses and the AV valves in which the subarterial infundibulum and the great arteries are malformed. Usually this is the case, but not always. Rarely it is possible to have a single RV with inverted normally related great arteries, as in DORV {I,L,I} (Fig. 17.14). This is a mirror image of a Holmes heart that has single LV with solitus normally related great arteries, that is, single LV {S,D,S} (see Fig. 17.2).

In DORV {I,L,I} with single RV (see Fig. 17.14), the infundibuloarterial anatomy is as in inverted tetralogy of Fallot (TOF) with a right-sided, anterior, stenotic subpulmonary infundibulum and a left-sided, posterior, widely patent aortic valve that is in direct fibrous continuity with the anterosuperior leaflet of a common AV valve that opened only into the inverted (left-handed) RV because the presumably inverted LV was absent.

RETHINKING BASIC DEFINITIONS

Single ventricle forces one to rethink some of our basic definitions. Is it really possible to have solitus normally related great arteries with single LV, as in the Holmes heart, that is, {S,L,**S**} with single LV? When the right ventricular sinus is absent, but the infundibuloarterial (conotruncal) segment is solitus normal, the ventriculoarterial (VA) alignments cannot be normal because the right ventricular sinus (component 2) is absent.

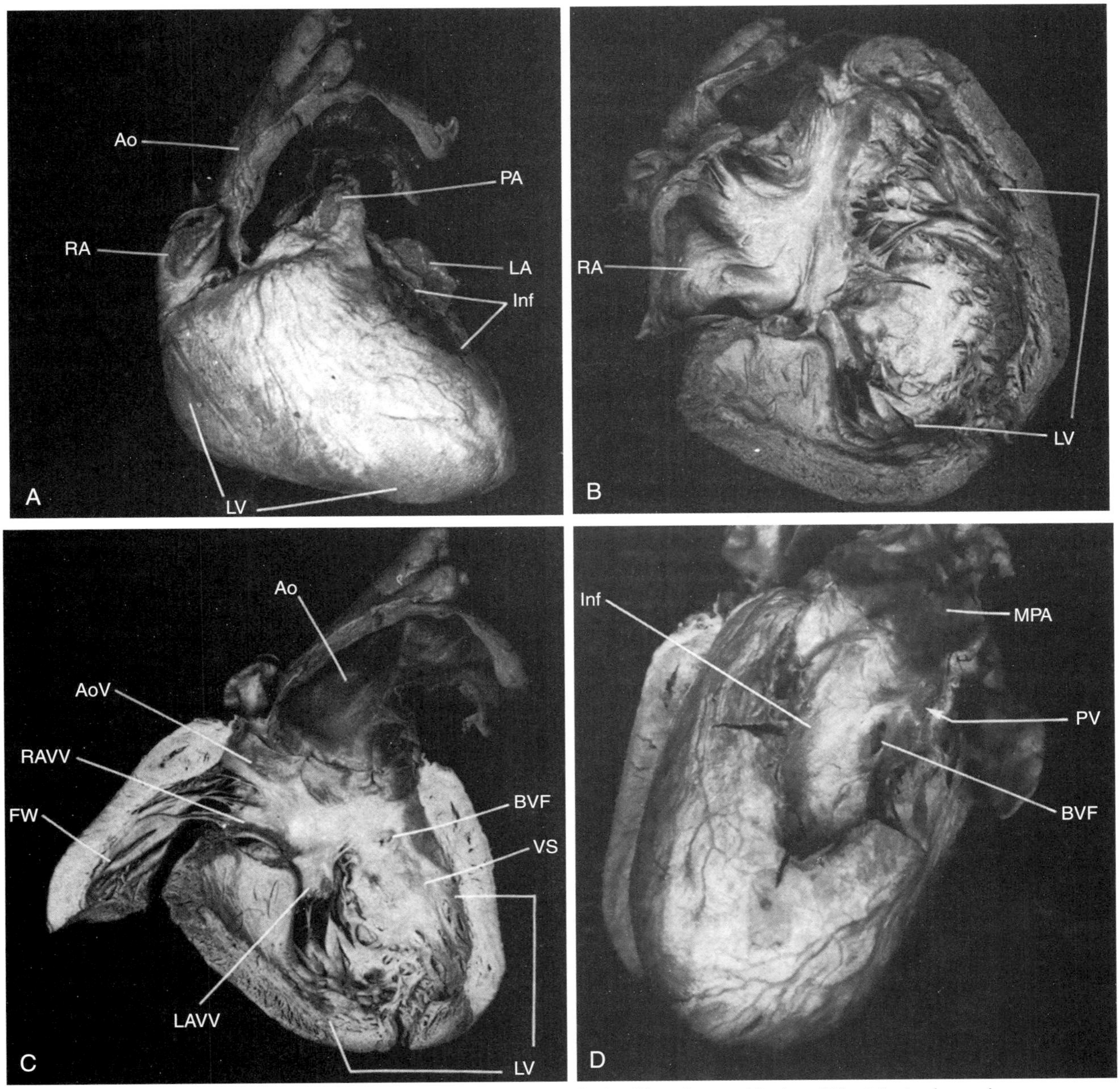

Fig. 17.6 Single Left Ventricle *(LV)* With Infundibular Outlet Chamber and Isolated Ventricular Inversion {S,L,S}. (A) The external frontal view of the heart and great arteries. (B) Right atrium *(RA)* opening through the right-sided mitral valve into the single LV inflow tract (LV). (C) Double-inlet LV with a right-sided mitral valve *(RAVV)* in fibrous continuity with a left-sided tricuspid valve *(LAVV),* and an inverted or right-handed LV opening into a solitus or noninverted ascending aorta *(Ao).* The bulboventricular foramen *(BVF)* is sealed, resulting in subpulmonary outflow tract atresia. There is direct fibrous continuity between the aortic valve *(AoV)* above and both atrioventricular (AV) valves below. In A, it is seen that the main pulmonary artery *(MPA)* is anterior and to the left of the ascending aorta, suggestive of solitus normally related great arteries. In C this is confirmed by the absence of subaortic infundibular free wall *(FW)* myocardium that permits aortic-AV valvar direct fibrous continuity, which is typical of solitus normally related great arteries. (D) The subpulmonary infundibular outlet chamber *(Inf),* which is left-sided and well developed, relative to the right-sided and resorbed subaortic infundibulum. The infundibuloarterial situs equation of this heart is SNRGA {S,L,S} = OR + 4L.[14] OR means grade 0 development of the right-sided (R) subaortic infundibular free wall and (+) good development (grade 4) of the left-sided (L) subpulmonary infundibular free wall. OR + 4L is the formula or "recipe" for solitus normally related great arteries: SNRGA {S,D,S} = OR + 4L.[14] Thus, in {S,L,S} the infundibular situs and the great arterial situs both are in situs solitus (normal). Hence, infundibuloarterial situs concordance (both solitus) is present. Infundibuloarterial situs concordance is characteristic of normally related great arteries (both solitus and inversus).[14] (Reproduced with permission from Van Praagh R, Plett JA, Van Praagh S. Single ventricle: pathology, embryology, terminology, and classification. *Herz.* 1979;4:113.[1])

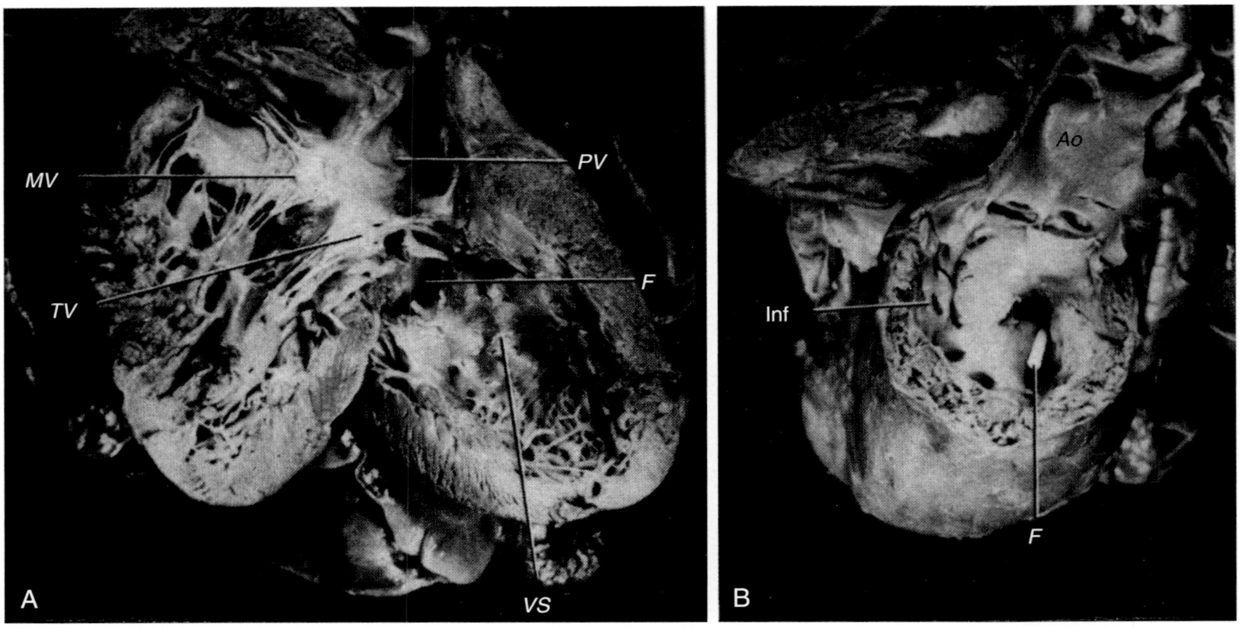

Fig. 17.7 The Most Common Anatomic Type of Single Left Ventricle (LV) (Absent Right Ventricular Sinus) With Infundibular Outlet Chamber Also Has Transposition of the Great Arteries {S,L,L}. (A) Inverted single LV with double-inlet LV. The mitral valve *(MV)* was right-sided, the tricuspid valve *(TV)* was left-sided, and the transposed pulmonary valve *(PV)* was in direct fibrous continuity with both the MV and the TV. The outflow tract into the transposed pulmonary artery was widely patent, but the infundibuloventricular foramen *(F)* was restrictive, producing subaortic stenosis. (B) Subaortic infundibular outlet chamber beneath the L-transposed aorta is seen. There is a probe in the stenotic F. There is no left-sided RV sinus beneath the infundibulum *(Inf)*. In A, the ventricular septal remnant *(VS)* is displaced anteriorly and leftward, toward the location of the absent right ventricular sinus. This anterior and leftward displacement of the ventricular septum brings the crest of the muscular VS close to and beneath the infundibular septum (in B, above the probe), producing a stenotic infundibuloventricular foramen. The left-sided TV in A inserted into the crest of the muscular VS, contributing to the stenotic infundibuloventricular foramen. (Reproduced with permission from Van Praagh R, Plett JA, Van Praagh S. Single ventricle: pathology, embryology, terminology, and classification. *Herz.* 1979;4:113.[1])

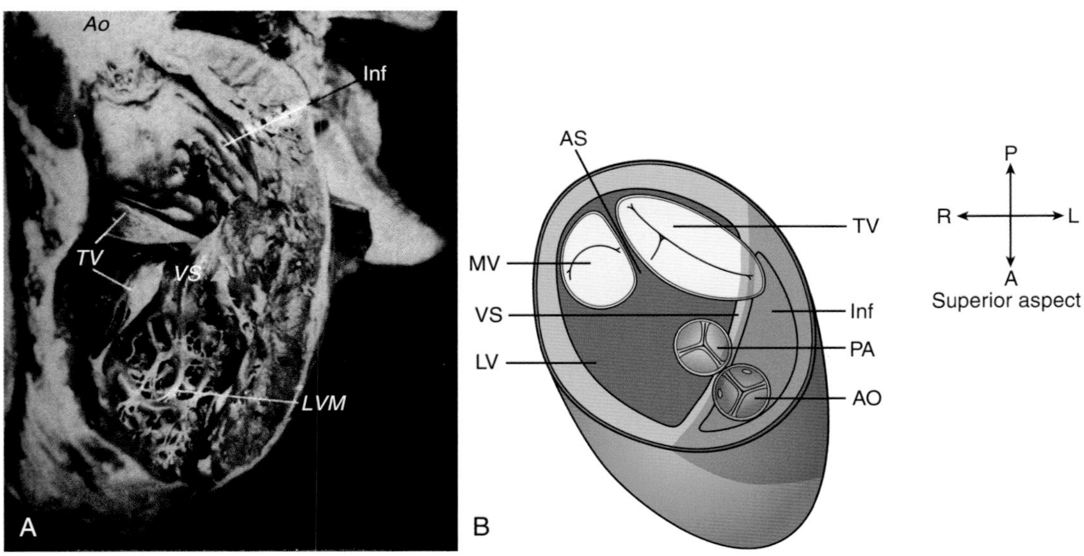

Fig. 17.8 Another Case of Transposition of the Great Arteries {S,L,L} With Single Left Ventricle and a Subaortic Infundibular Outlet Chamber *(Inf).* (A) The left-sided tricuspid valve *(TV)* straddles the crest of the muscular ventricular septum *(VS)* and inserts into the Inf outlet chamber. (B) The atrial septum *(AS)* is 30 degrees to the left of the anteroposterior (AP) plane (normal in visceroatrial situs solitus). The VS remnant is 20 degrees to the right of the AP plane. The semilunar valves display 40-degree rotation to the left of the AP plane. (A) Note that the left ventricular myocardium *(LVM)* displays trabeculae carneae that are numerous, fine, and oblique, whereas the trabeculations of the Inf are coarse, few, and straight (parallel). *AO* and *Ao,* Aorta; *LV,* left ventricle; *MV,* mitral valve. (Reproduced with permission from Van Praagh R, Plett JA, Van Praagh S. Single ventricle: pathology, embryology, terminology, and classification. *Herz.* 1979;4:113.[1])

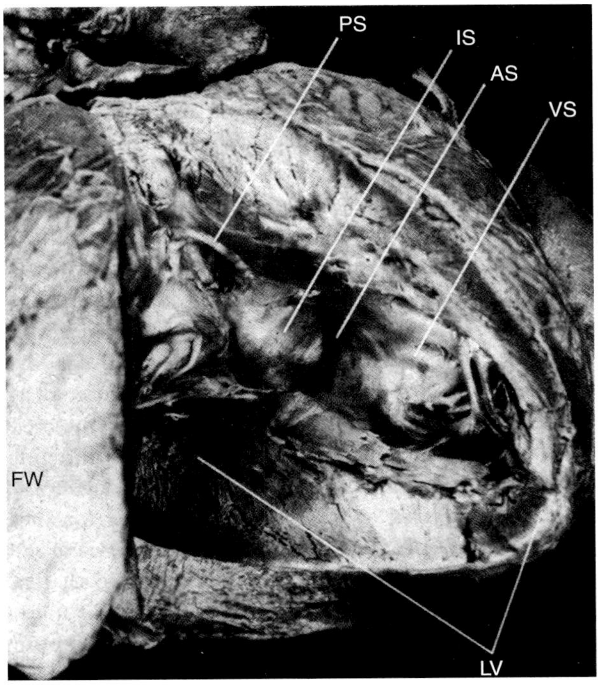

Fig. 17.9 Single Left Ventricle *(LV)* With Infundibular Outlet Chamber and Transposition of the Great Arteries {S,L,L}. There was stenosis of both aortic and pulmonary outflow tracts in this 6 11/12-year-old boy. The infundibuloventricular foramen was markedly narrowed, resulting in severe subaortic stenosis *(AS)*. The hypertrophied infundibular septum *(IS)* above, and the hypertrophied ventricular septum *(VS)* below the defect led to progressive narrowing of the defect leading into the infundibular outlet chamber, from which the L-transposed aorta originated. The hypertrophied IS also resulted in pulmonary outflow tract stenosis and in hypertrophy of the single LV from which the transposed pulmonary artery originated. *FW*, Free wall. (Reproduced with permission from Van Praagh R, Plett JA, Van Praagh S. Single ventricle: pathology, embryology, terminology, and classification. *Herz.* 1979;4:113.[1])

Thus, the infundibuloarterial segments are solitus normal, but the VA alignments are not normal because the RV sinus (component 2) is absent. Thus, situs solitus of the infundibulum and situs solitus of the great arteries are really associated with solitus normally related great arteries, *only if both the right ventricular sinus and the left ventricular sinus also develop normally,* which does not happen with the Holmes heart.

Similarly, is it really possible for inverted normally related great arteries to be present with DORV, as in single RV with DORV {I,L,**I**}? Again, the answer is no, because the left ventricular sinus is absent. Even though the infundibulum and the great arteries are in situs inversus, the VA alignments are really normally inverted only if the right ventricular sinus and the left ventricular sinus are both normally developed, which does not happen with single RV (or absent LV). Thus, the third element of the segmental anatomy indicates the situs of the infundibulum and the situs of the great arteries: single RV with DORV {I,L,**I**}. But it is what is *outside* the segmental anatomic set (indicated by braces) that indicates what the VA alignments and the associated malformations really are: single RV with DORV {I,L,I}.

Single Right Ventricle With Double-Outlet Right Ventricle {I,L,I}

In other words, the situs of the segmental anatomy of the atria, the ventricles, and the great arteries is enclosed by braces { }, meaning "the set or combination of"; what is outside the braces indicates the VA alignments and the associated malformations.

For reasons that are still unknown, the most common form of single ventricle is single LV with an infundibular outlet chamber and TGA {S,L,L} (39%; see Table 17.1). Again, we may ask, is it really possible to have TGA with single LV (i.e., with absence of the right ventricular sinus)? The obvious answer is no. But we tend to regard the infundibulum as a "right ventricular structure" because normally, the infundibulum is mostly connected with the right ventricular sinus.

We know that the infundibulum is the connecting segment between the great arteries above, and the ventricles and the AV canal below. In other words, we know that the infundibulum is not really the right ventricular sinus. But the infundibulum is "right ventriculoid" enough so that when the aorta arises from the right ventriculoid infundibulum and the pulmonary artery originates from the LV, we can call that TGA and people will understand, as in single LV with **TGA** {S,L,L} (see Table 17.1).

All of the foregoing needs to be understood and accepted when dealing with single ventricle. We have long understood that the terminology associated with single ventricle may occasionally stretch logic in the interests of clinical communication. It should come as no great surprise that when one ventricular sinus is absent, such hearts do not and cannot function as biventricular hearts do. This is why single ventricle is such an important cardiac malformation. Single ventricle changes VA alignments.

CARDIAC GEOMETRY

The anatomy of single ventricle invites one to do a little cardiac geometry. One can measure the angulation of the atrial septum relative to the sagittal plane. The normal **atrial septal angle** is about 30 degrees to the left. The normal **ventricular septal angle** is approximately 40 to 50 degrees to the left. The normal **semilunar valvar rotation** is about 150 degrees to the right, that is, 150 degrees dextrorotation.

In single LV, the ventricular septal remnant is often abnormally angulated and is always abnormally displaced, as the cardiac diagrams show: see Figs. 17.2C, 17.3B, 17.4C, and 17.5B. Single RV hearts are also clarified by geometric diagrams, as in Fig. 17.15. Common ventricle is depicted geometrically in Fig. 17.5.

The point is that geometric analysis can be applied clinically to invasive and noninvasive diagnostic investigations. As the aforementioned geometric diagrams illustrate, with **single LV** and an infundibular outlet chamber, angulation and displacement of the ventricular septal remnant explain why there is **double-inlet LV** (DILV) or **common inlet LV.** In single LV, the left ventricular sinus septal surface is well developed, but the

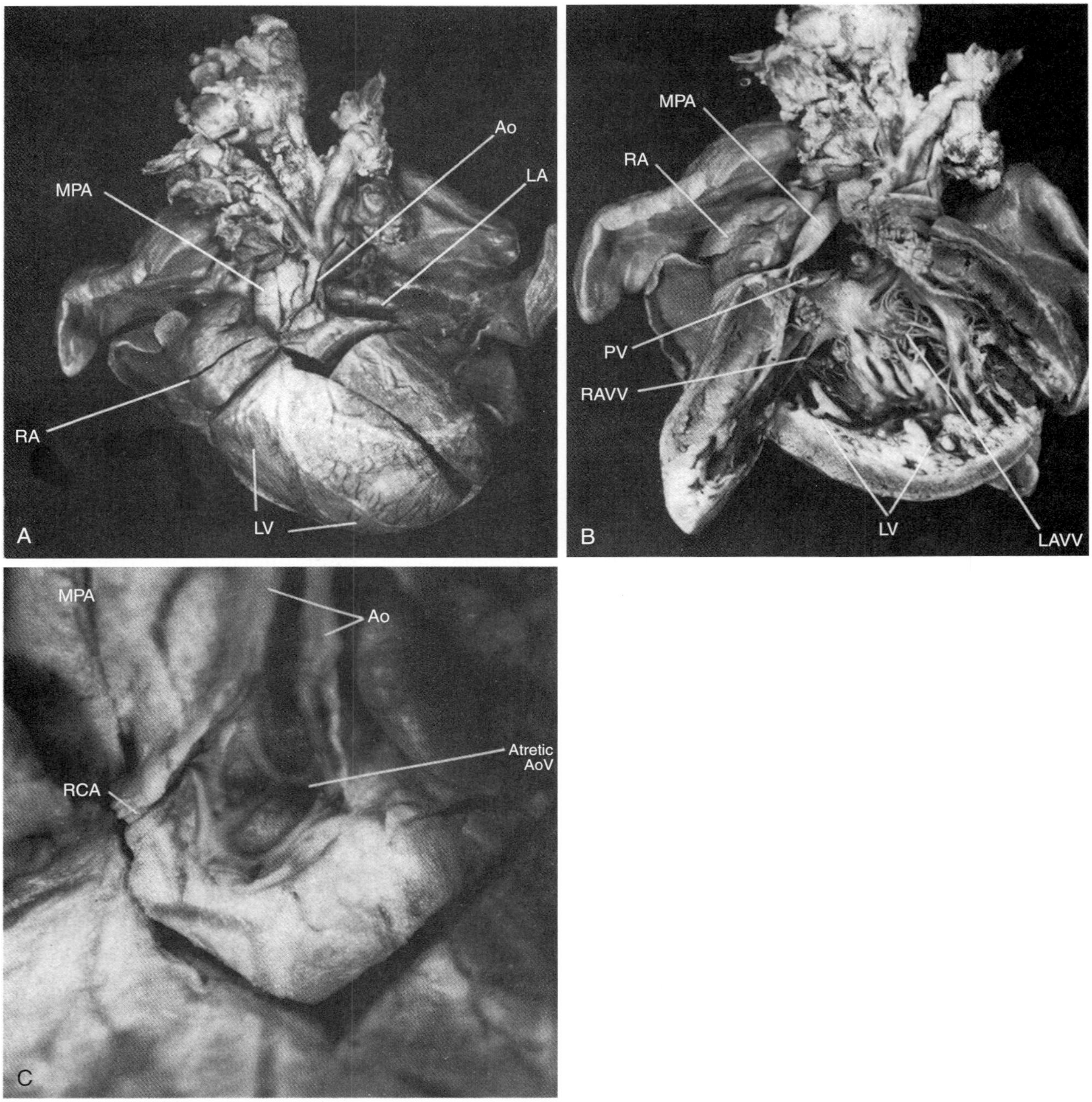

Fig. 17.10 A Rare Case of Single Left Ventricle *(LV)* With Transposition of the Great Arteries (TGA) {S,L,L} With an Intact Ventricular Septum, That Is, With No Infundibuloventricular Foramen. Although there is a leftward and anterior infundibulum beneath an L-transposed aorta, the infundibulum has no lumen; it is *not* an infundibular outlet *chamber*. And the L-transposed aortic valve is atretic. Aortic valvar atresia is rare in patients with TGA, D- or L-. Figs. 17.9 and 17.10 clearly indicate that single LV is not a huge ventricular septal defect between a large LV and a rudimentary right ventricle (RV). The foramen can be so small as to constitute subaortic stenosis or atresia. And the subaortic infundibulum is just that—the subaortic infundibulum, not a rudimentary RV. The right ventricular sinus is absent. That is why the LV is single. (A) Frontal view of the heart and lungs. The atria are in situs solitus, with the right atrium *(RA)* to the right and the left atrium *(LA)* to the left. The single LV is right-sided. The very hypoplastic ascending aorta *(Ao)* is anterior and to the left of the dilated main pulmonary artery *(MPA)*. (B) Opened single LV, the transposed MPA, and double-inlet LV. The mitral valve (right AV valve *[RAVV]*) is to the right, the tricuspid valve (left AV valve *[LAVV]*) is to the left, and both AV valves are in direct fibrous continuity with the pulmonary valve *(PV)*. (C) Closeup of the potential tricuspid (tricommissural) but atretic aortic valve *(AoV)*, the hypoplastic ascending aorta, and the ostium of the right coronary artery *(RCA)* that supplies the anterior descending coronary artery—appropriate for a ventricular L-loop (ventricular inversion). (Reproduced with permission from Van Praagh R, Plett JA, Van Praagh S. Single ventricle: pathology, embryology, terminology, and classification. *Herz.* 1979;4:113.[1])

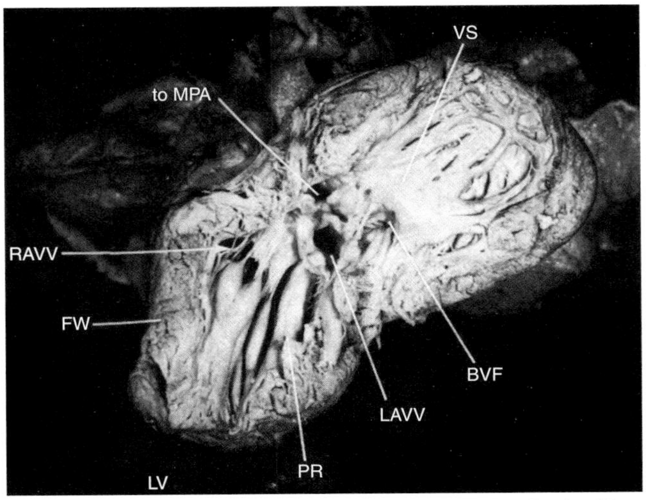

Fig. 17.11 Single Left Ventricle *(LV)* With Infundibular Outlet Chamber and Transposition of the Great Arteries {S,L,L}. Frontal view of the opened single LV. The left ventricular septal surface *(VS)* is abnormally located anteriorly and to the left. The left ventricular free wall *(FW)* is abnormally located posteriorly and to the right. There is double-inlet LV with a widely patent right atrioventricular (AV) ("mitral") valve and a stenotic left atrioventricular ("tricuspid") valve. The interventricular foramen was restrictively small, constituting subaortic stenosis but without preductal coarctation of the aorta. Note the prominent posterior ridge *(PR)* between the chordal insertions and papillary muscles of both AV valves. Both AV valves insert superiorly into this prominent PR, which is in fact a medial papillary muscle, with morphologically left ventricular myocardium on both sides of the PR. Consequently, this PR is not a ventricular septal remnant. Instead, the PR is a prominent medial papillary muscle shared by both incoming AV valves. An omphalocele was also present. Hence, this patient had multiple congenital anomalies, that is, malformations of more than one body system. *BVF,* Bulboventricular foramen; *LAVV,* left atrioventricular valve; *MPA,* main pulmonary artery; *RAVV,* right atrioventricular valve. (Reproduced with permission from Van Praagh R, Plett JA, Van Praagh S. Single ventricle: pathology, embryology, terminology, and classification. *Herz.* 1979;4:113.[1])

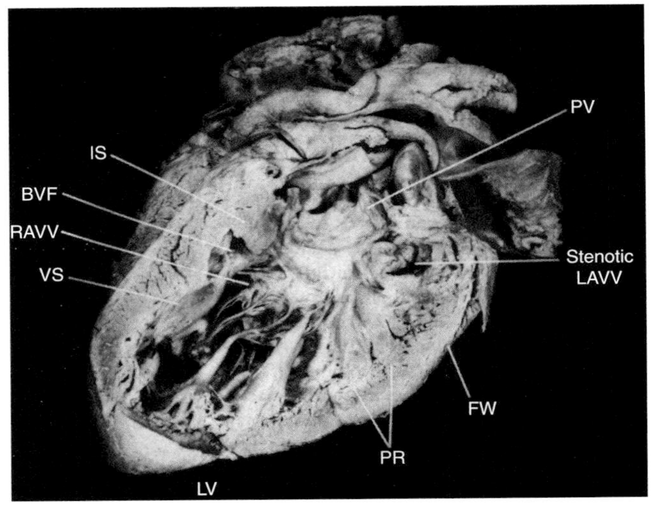

Fig. 17.12 Single Left Ventricle *(LV)* With an Infundibular Outlet Chamber and Transposition of the Great Arteries {S,D,D} in the Heart of a 9-Year-Old Boy Who Also Had Severe Stenosis of the Left Atrioventricular (AV) or Mitral Valve *(LAVV).* The ostium was small and the leaflets were thick, myxomatous, and gnarled. The valve inserted directly into the left ventricular free wall *(FW)* without intervening chordae tendineae or papillary muscles. Thus, it is important to know that in double-inlet single LV, the AV valves may not be normal in form or function. *BVF,* Bulboventricular foramen; *IS,* infundibular septum; *PR,* posterior ridge; *PV,* pulmonary valve; *RAVV,* right atrioventricular valve; *VS,* ventricular septum. (Reproduced with permission from Van Praagh R, Plett JA, Van Praagh S. Single ventricle: pathology, embryology, terminology, and classification. *Herz.* 1979;4:113.[1])

right ventricular sinus septal surface (beneath the septal band) is absent.

In **single RV,** the location of the ventricular septal remnant is less obvious. The right ventricular sinus septal surface beneath the septal band is well developed, but the left ventricular sinus septal surface is absent. This inference is confirmed by biventricular hearts with a large RV and a diminutive LV (see Fig. 17.13). When hearts are biventricular, rather than univentricular, even if the LV is tiny, the location of the angulated and displaced ventricular septum is obvious. The abnormal location of the ventricular septal remnant, when the LV is grossly absent or extremely hypoplastic, explains why there is associated **DIRV** or **common inlet RV.**

In single LV and single RV, the abnormal location of the ventricular septal remnant is determined by aplasia or extreme hypoplasia of the adjacent ventricular sinus (right or left ventricular). This is not a primary malformation of the ventricular septum per se. Nor is this a primary malformation of the AV canal or of the AV valves. Instead, the abnormal locations of the ventricular septum and the abnormal alignments and connections of the AV valves appear to be *secondary effects* of ventricular sinus absence or marked hypoplasia.

Another striking observation that emerges from Table 17.1 is that single LV with an infundibular outlet chamber is a malformation of the ventricular loop and often of the infundibuloarterial segment, but the situs of the viscera and the situs of the atria typically are normal; that is, both are in situs solitus.

By contrast, with single RV, visceroatrial situs solitus occurred in only 2 of 8 cases (25%). Visceroatrial situs inversus was found in 1 of 8 patients (12.5%). In the majority of our patients with single RV, there was visceroatrial situs ambiguus with the heterotaxy syndrome and congenital asplenia, in 5 of 8 patients (62.5%).

In other words, single LV typically (in 100% of our cases) is an isolated cardiac anomaly in which other body systems are not involved, whereas single RV is often part of a whole body syndromic anomaly, the heterotaxy syndrome with asplenia (in 62.5% of our cases) and with situs inversus totalis is an additional 12.5%. Thus, in 75% of our cases, single RV was part of a whole body situs anomaly—the asplenia syndrome, or situs inversus totalis.

STATISTICS

Single LV with an infundibular outlet chamber occurred in 81 of 3216 autopsied cases of congenital heart disease in the cardiac pathology database of Boston Children's Hospital (2.52%) between 1962 and 1996. **Single RV** occurred in 28 of

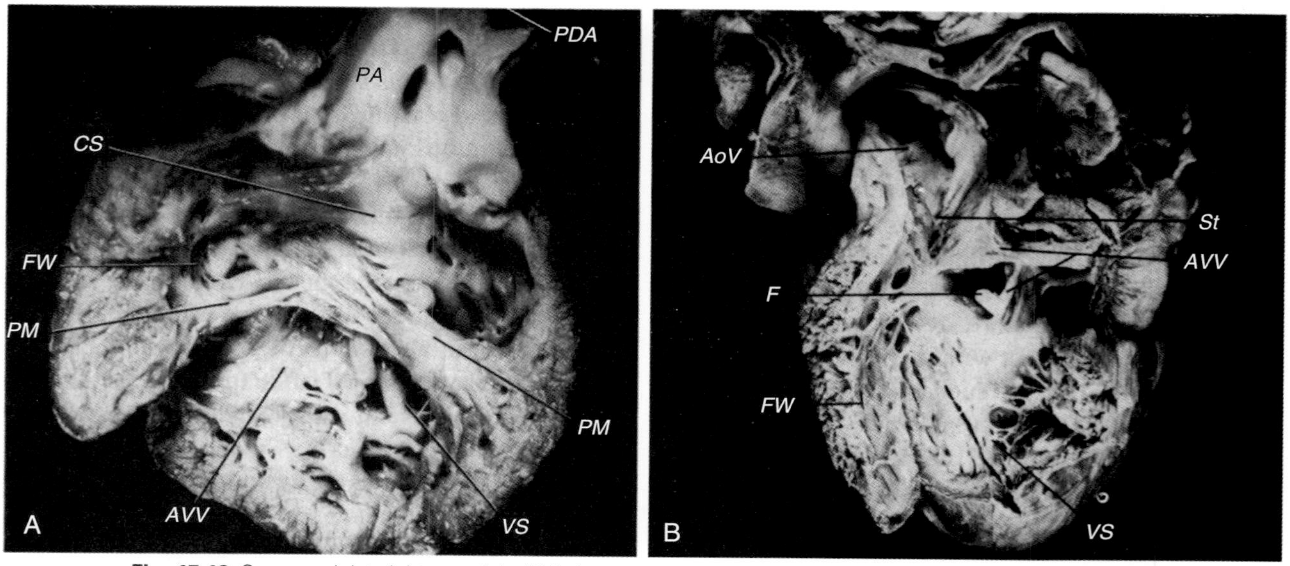

Fig. 17.13 Common-inlet right ventricle (RV) does not necessarily mean that single RV is present. In this patient with normal segmental anatomy, that is, {S,D,S}, the common atrioventricular (AV) valve *(AVV)* opens almost entirely into the hypertrophied and enlarged RV. Nonetheless, a diminutive left ventricle (LV) is present. To diagnose accurately whether a single ventricle is present, one must examine the ventricular part of the heart, not the alignments and connections of the AV valve or valves. (A) Common AV valve *(AVV)* opening almost entirely into a large RV. (B) Common AV valve opening minimally into a diminutive LV. *AoV,* Aortic valve; *CS,* conal septum; *F,* infundibuloventricular foramen; *FW,* free wall; *PA,* pulmonary artery; *PDA,* patent ductus arteriosus; *PM,* papillary muscle; *St,* stenosis; *VS,* ventricular septum. (Reproduced with permission from Van Praagh R, Plett JA, Van Praagh S. Single ventricle: pathology, embryology, terminology, and classification. *Herz.* 1979;4:113.[1])

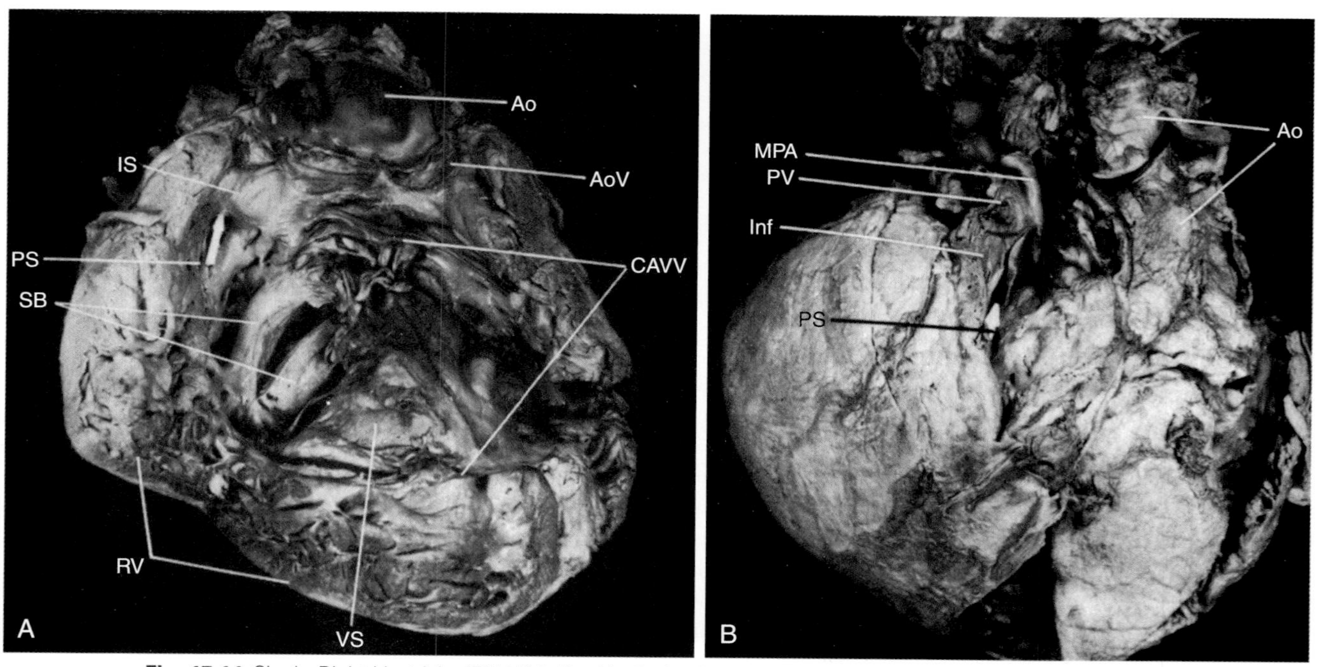

Fig. 17.14 Single Right Ventricle *(RV)* With Double-Outlet Right Ventricle (DORV) {I,L,I} and Polysplenia. This rare case indicates that it is possible to have inverted normally related great arteries with single RV (i.e., absence of the left ventricular sinus). Normally related great arteries do not happen only with single left ventricle, as in the Holmes heart. Rarely, inverted normally related great arteries can happen with single RV, as in this case. The infundibulum and great arteries were like inverted tetralogy of Fallot. The stenotic pulmonary outflow tract lay to the right of the widely patent aortic outflow tract. Infundibular pulmonary stenosis was severe. There was direct fibrous continuity between the right coronary and noncoronary leaflets of the aortic valve *(AoV)* and the superior leaflet of the common atrioventricular valve *(CAVV)*. The pulmonary valve *(PV)* was bicuspid because of rudimentary development of the left septal–nonseptal commissure. (A) Frontal view of the single RV, which is left-handed (inverted). The pulmonary infundibular stenosis *(PS)* is severe. (B) The severely stenotic pulmonary outflow tract to the right, and the widely patent aortic outflow tract to the left are seen. *Ao,* Aorta; *Inf,* infundibulum; *IS,* infundibular septum; *MPA,* main pulmonary artery; *SB,* septal band; *VS,* ventricular septum. (Reproduced with permission from Van Praagh R, Plett JA, Van Praagh S. Single ventricle: pathology, embryology, terminology, and classification. *Herz.* 1979;4:113.[1])

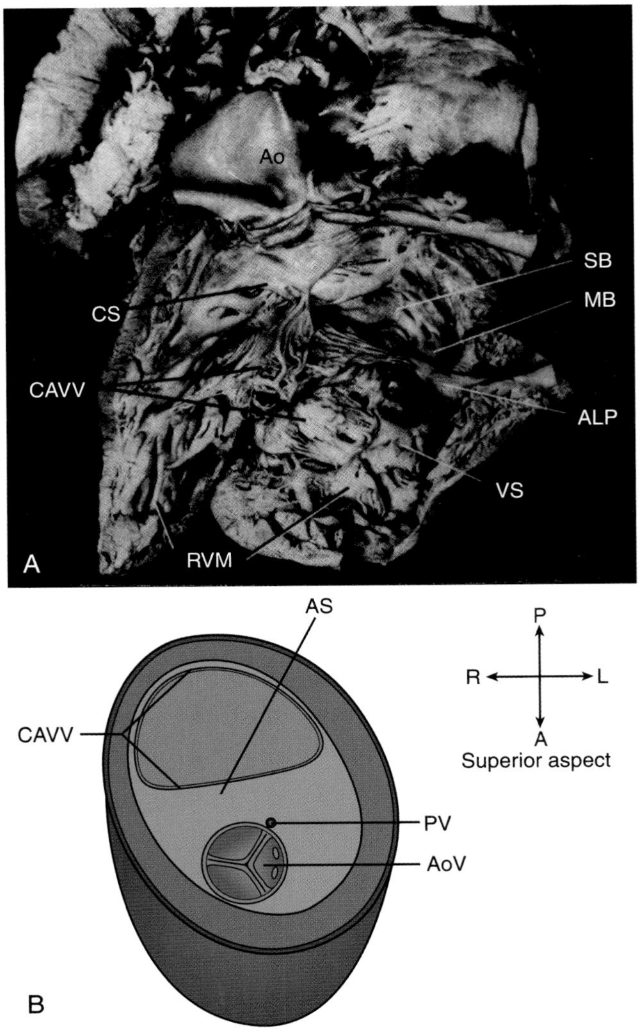

Fig. 17.15 Single Right Ventricle (RV), That Is, Absence of Left Ventricular Sinus, With Double-Outlet Right Ventricle (DORV) {I,D,D}. DORV with situs inversus (I) of viscera and atria, discordant ventricular D-loop (D), and D-malposition of the great arteries (D) were present. There was pulmonary outflow tract atresia. We made the diagnosis of DORV, despite the presence of pulmonary outflow tract atresia, because DORV is short for origin of both great arteries above the right ventricle, which does not specify the patency, or otherwise, of the great arteries. (A) Opened RV and aorta *(Ao)*. (B) Geometric diagram. (A) A common atrioventricular valve *(CAVV)* opens into the right ventricular sinus. The right ventricular septal surface *(VS)* and the RV free wall both display the coarse trabeculation of right ventricular myocardium *(RVM)*. The RV is right-handed, indicating that a ventricular D-loop is present, that is, a solitus RV is seen. (B) The atrial septum *(AS)* is 30 degrees to the right of the sagittal plane, which is normal in situs inversus. No left ventricular sinus myocardium was identified by a careful search. Common-inlet RV is seen, the CAVV opening only into the single RV. The aortic valve displays only 30 degrees of dextrorotation relative to the sagittal plane; this is very subnormal, with 150 degrees dextrorotation being normal, as in Fig. 17.2C. A well-developed subaortic infundibulum is seen, with wide separation of the aortic valve above and the CAVV below. *ALP*, Anterolateral papillary muscle; *AoV*, aortic valve; *CS*, conal septum; *MB*, moderator band; *PV*, pulmonary valve; *SB*, septal band. (Reproduced with permission from Van Praagh R, Plett JA, Van Praagh S. Single ventricle: pathology, embryology, terminology, and classification. *Herz*. 1979;4:113.[1])

3216 (0.87%) autopsied cases of congenital heart disease in the database between 1961 and 1998. What is wrong with these statistics? Well, as Dr. Richard Bonham Carter of Great Ormond Street Hospital in London England used to say, "There are lies, damn lies, and statistics." In other words, statistics should be approached with interested skepticism. For example, it should be understood that tricuspid atresia (n = 111 cases) and mitral atresia (n = 183 cases) have been arbitrarily excluded from the category of single ventricle, even though tricuspid atresia has at least a functionally single LV and mitral atresia usually has a functionally single RV.

Why has it become customary to exclude tricuspid atresia and mitral atresia from the diagnostic category of single ventricle? I think it was probably because tricuspid atresia and mitral atresia were described and classified before single ventricle—without AV valve atresia—had been understood. By the early 1960s, people thought they understood tricuspid and mitral atresia. But they also knew that there were other cases that only had one ventricle, that could not be "blamed on" tricuspid or mitral atresia because they had two patent AV valves, or a common AV valve. These other cases were called single or common ventricle. So what? Well, this means that hearts with only one good pumping ventricle are much more common than the previously mentioned statistics suggest. **Functionally single LV** with absent right ventricular sinus and two AV valves or a common AV valve, and cases with tricuspid atresia occurred in 192 of 3216 cases (5.97%). **Functionally single RV** with absent left ventricular sinus and with two AV valves or a common AV valve and cases with mitral atresia occurred in 211 of 3216 cases (6.56%).

THE MORPHOLOGIC ANATOMIC KEY TO THE DIAGNOSTIC UNDERSTANDING OF SINGLE VENTRICLE

The diagnostic key to understanding the morphologic anatomy of single ventricle was the spongiosum heart (Fig. 17.16). This patient had situs inversus totalis {I,L,I} with inverted TOF and common AV canal. This patient also had differentiation of the ventricular stratum spongiosum, which forms the ventricular trabeculations. But the stratum spongiosum (the spongy layer) had failed to undergo normal resorption. Consequently, the differences between left ventricular trabeculations that are numerous, fine, and oblique (A) and right ventricular trabeculations that are fewer and much coarser (B) are unusually clear. Also, the trabeculations of the septal surface and of the internal free wall of each ventricle were characteristic and different. Hence, it was possible to use the morphologic anatomy of the ventricular septum *and of the free wall* to understand single ventricle diagnostically.[1-3]

How can one be sure that the prominent posterior ridge between the two entering AV valves in typical single LV is not a ventricular septal remnant (Fig. 17.17)**?** Look on either side of the posterior ridge and you will see finely trabeculated typical left ventricular myocardium on both sides of the structure, and both AV valves insert into it superiorly. Large papillary muscles are typical of the morphologically LV.

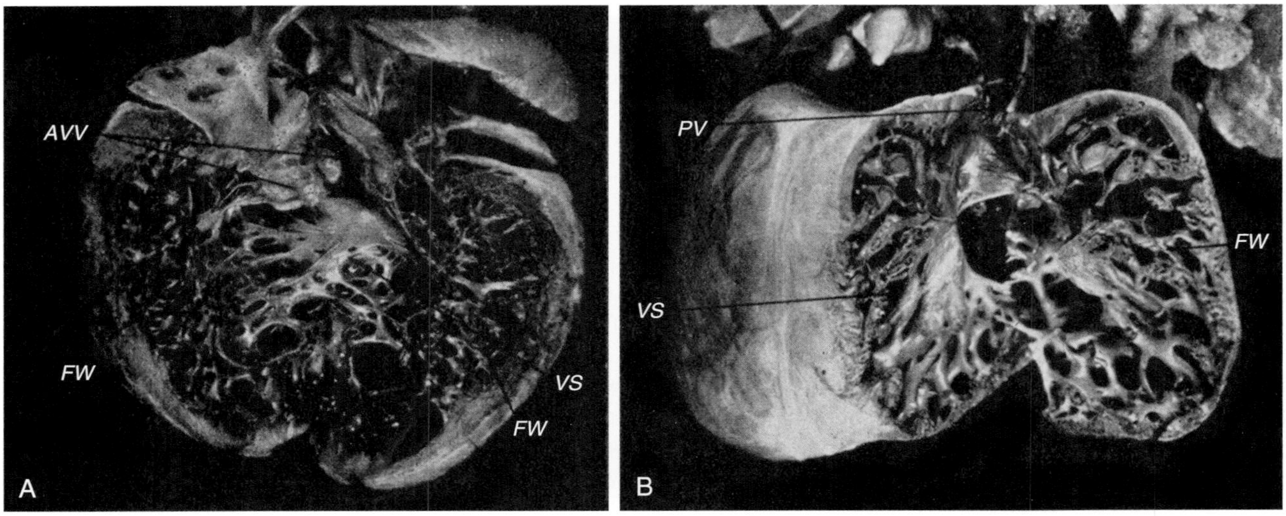

Fig. 17.16 Failure of resorption of stratum spongiosum (the spongy layer) that makes the trabeculations of left ventricular myocardium (A) and of right ventricular myocardium (B) is seen. This patient had situs inversus totalis, inverted tetralogy of Fallot, and common atrioventricular canal. Note that the trabeculations of the left ventricle (in A) are numerous, fine, and oblique, whereas the trabeculations of the right ventricle (in B) are fewer and much coarser. The morphologic anatomy of the septal surface and of the internal free wall of both ventricles are specific and very different. Consequently, both the septal surfaces and the free walls *(FW)* may be used for diagnostic purposes. *AVV,* Atrioventricular valve; *PV,* pulmonary valve; *VS,* ventricular septum. (Reproduced with permission from Van Praagh R, Plett JA, Van Praagh S. Single ventricle: pathology, embryology, terminology, and classification. *Herz.* 1979;4:113.[1,2])

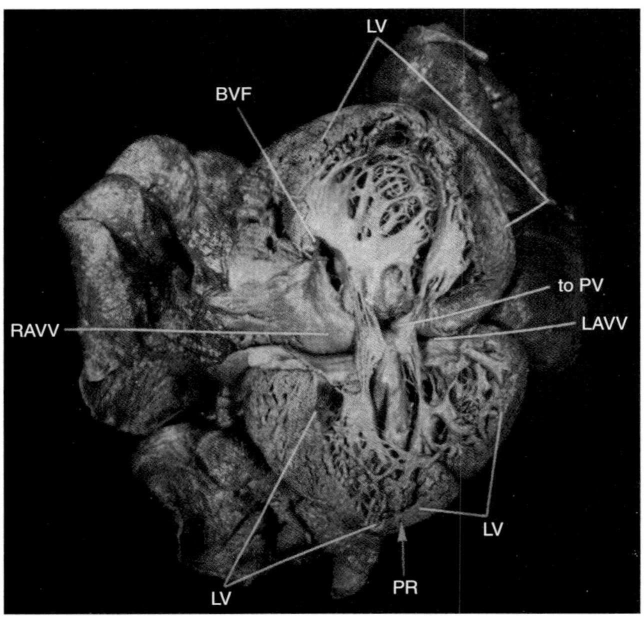

Fig. 17.17 Single Left Ventricle *(LV)* With Infundibular Outlet Chamber and Transposition of the Great Arteries {S,D,D}. The left ventricular septum of the opened single LV is reflected superiorly, and the left ventricular free wall is reflected inferiorly. Looking at the free wall, note that the posterior ridge *(PR)* lies between the two entering atrioventricular (AV) valves, and beneath the transposed pulmonary valve *(PV)* that arises from the single LV. Left ventricular myocardium with numerous, fine, oblique trabeculations lie on both sides of the posterior ridge. This ridge also receives chordal attachments superiorly from both AV valves. This posterior ridge is a medial papillary muscle of the LV. *BVF,* Bulboventricular foramen; *LAVV,* left atrioventricular valve; *RAVV,* right atrioventricular valve. (Reproduced with permission from Van Praagh R, Plett JA, Van Praagh S. Single ventricle. Pathology, embryology, terminology, and classification. *Herz.* 1979;4:113.[1])

THE INFUNDIBULAR APEX AND THE RIGHT VENTRICULAR SINUS APEX

Lack of understanding of the infundibular apex and of the right ventricular sinus apex (Fig. 17.18) has led to confusion and controversy concerning single LV. I had the great good fortune to work for several years (1963 to 1965) with Dr. Maurice Lev in Chicago doing only congenial cardiac pathology. Dr. Lev is the father of morphologic understanding of the heart, and this is where I learned that the normal RV has two apices, an infundibular apex and a sinus apex (see Fig. 17.18). This led to Dr. Stella Van Praagh's **apical infundibulotomy operation** for closing apical muscular VSDs.[12] Earlier, this understanding of the infundibular apex helped us understand single LV with an infundibular outlet chamber.[1-3]

If one does not understand that there is an apical infundibulum, when one looks into the outlet chamber that typically accompanies DILV, one sees a small amount of coarsely trabeculated myocardium in the outlet chamber. At this point, one is likely to think, "I see a small amount of right ventricular myocardium in the outlet chamber. This must be a rudimentary RV. *Single* LV really is not present, because a small and deformed RV is also present. This is really a biventricular heart with a big LV and a small RV. So, let's call it DILV, or functionally single LV because anatomically single LV really is not present." We think that this interpretation is wrong. But how can we convince our contrary-minded friends and colleagues that the "rudimentary RV" interpretation is incorrect? Well, an understanding that both ventricles are normally composed of four different components (see Fig. 17.1A) may well help.

But perhaps **double-chambered RV** may be the most persuasive natural experiment. A moderator band–like structure

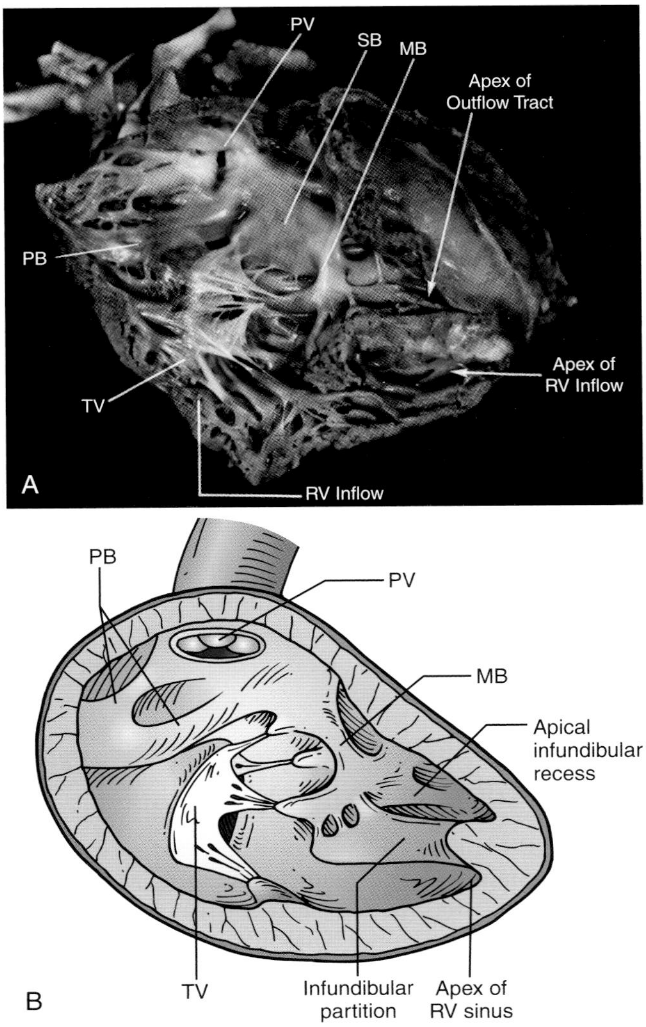

Fig. 17.18 The right ventricle *(RV)* has two apexes, an inflow tract or right ventricular sinus apex below and an outflow tract or infundibular apex above. The two apexes are partially separated by an infundibulo-sinus partition. (A) Photo. (B) Diagram. (A) One can see that the outflow tract apex does contain some coarse, parallel trabeculations. These findings are normal for the infundibular apical recess. *MB,* Moderator band; *PB,* parietal band; *PV,* pulmonary valve; *SB,* septal band; *TV,* tricuspid valve. (Reproduced with permission from Van Praagh S, Mayer JE, Berman NB, Flanagan MF, Geva T, Van Praagh R. Apical ventricular septal defects: follow-up concerning anatomic and surgical considerations. *Ann Thorac Surg.* 2002;73:48.[12])

takes off high from the septal band and divides the RV into an inlet or sinus chamber and an outlet or infundibular chamber, with stenosis in the mid-RV caused by narrowing between the moderator band–like wall below and the normal infundibular septum above. This anomaly, known as double-chambered RV, clearly separates and demarcates what is the RV sinus (the inflow tract chamber) and what is the infundibulum (the outflow tract chamber). Double-chambered RV should teach one what the infundibulum really is.

When one examines the outlet chamber morphologically, one finds that the outlet chamber is the proximal or apical component of the infundibulum (component 3, Fig. 17.1A). It looks normal. In single LV, the reason that the outlet chamber is often described as "a rudimentary RV" is that the "RV" appears abnormally small. In fact, the infundibulum is of normal size, but the right ventricular sinus is absent.

DIAGNOSTIC AND SURGICAL CONSIDERATIONS

The diagnostic and surgical management of patients with a single ventricle, who usually also have a conotruncal malformation, was considered in 2016 by Constantine Mavroudis.[13]

REFERENCES

1. Van Praagh R, Plett JA, Van Praagh S. Single ventricle. Pathology, embryology, terminology, and classification. *Herz.* 1979;4:113.
2. Van Praagh R, Ongley PA, Swan HJC. Anatomic types of single or common ventricle in man. Morphologic and geometric aspects of 60 necropsied cases. *Am J Cardiol.* 1964;13:367.
3. Van Praagh R, Van Praagh S, Vlad P, Keith JD. Diagnosis of the anatomic types of single or common ventricle. *Am J Cardiol.* 1965;15:345.
4. Lambert EC. Single ventricle with a rudimentary outlet chamber. Case report. Johns Hopkins Hosp. *Bull.* 1951;88:231.
5. Lev M. Pathologic diagnosis of positional variations in cardiac chambers in congenital heart disease. *Lab Invest.* 1954;3:71.
6. Van Praagh R, Wise JR, Dahl BA, Van Praagh S. Single left ventricle with infundibular outlet chamber and tricuspid valve opening into outlet chamber in a 44-year-old man with thoracoabdominal ectopia cordis without diaphragmatic or pericardial defect: importance of myocardial morphologic method of chamber identification in congenital heart disease. In: Van Praagh R, Takao A, eds. *Etiology and Morphogenesis of Congenital Heart Disease.* Mt Kisco, New York: Futura Publishing Co; 1980:379.
7. Van Praagh R. When concordant or discordant atrioventricular alignments predict the ventricular situs wrongly. I. Solitus atria, concordant alignments, and L-loop ventricles. II. Solitus atria, discordant alignments, and D-loop ventricles. *J Am Coll Cardiol.* 1987;10:1278.
8. Holmes WF. Case of malformation of the heart. *Trans Med-Chir Soc Edinburgh.* 1824;1:252.
9. Dobell ARC, Van Praagh R. The Holmes heart: historical associations and pathologic anatomy. *Am Heart J.* 1996;132:437.
10. Abbott ME. Unique case of malformation of the heart. Defect of the interventricular septum, rudimentary right ventricle, patent foramen ovale, great dilatation of the right auricle and right auricular appendix. *Montreal Med J.* 1901;30:522.
11. Van Praagh R, Geva T, Kreutzer J. Ventricular septal defects: how shall we describe, name, and classify them? *J Am Coll Cardiol.* 1989;14:1298.
12. Van Praagh S, Mayer JE, Berman NB, Flanagan MF, Geva T, Van Praagh R. Apical ventricular septal defects: follow-up concerning anatomic and surgical considerations. *Ann Thorac Surg.* 2002;73:48.
13. Mavroudis C. Single ventricle repair for conotruncal anomalies. In: Lacour-Gayet F, Bove EL, Hraška V, Morell VO, Spray TL, eds. *Surgery of Conotruncal Anomalies.* Cham Heidelberg New York, Dordrecht London: Springer International Publishing AG Switzerland; 2016;597.
14. Van Praagh R. What determines whether the great arteries are normally or abnormally related? *Am J Cardiol.* 2016;118:1390.

18

Superoinferior Ventricles

The malformation known as superoinferior (SI) ventricles is characterized typically by a superior morphologically right ventricle (RV), an inferior morphologically left ventricle (LV), and a relatively horizontal ventricular septum (VS).[1] Rarely, the LV can be superior and the RV can be inferior.[2]

Our Cardiac Pathology database indicates that we have seen and studied 22 cases of SI ventricles out of a total series of 3216 autopsied cases of congenital heart disease (0.68%). Of these 22 cases, 21 had a superior RV and an inferior LV (0.65% of the total series), whereas only 1 patient had a superior LV and an inferior RV (0.03%).

This chapter is based primarily on our 11 published cases.[1,2]

Sex: Males 9, females 2; males 82%, females 18%; males-to-females = 9/2 (4.5/1). Thus, a strong male preponderance was found in this small series.

Age at Death: Mean, 982 days (2.69 years) ± 2572 days (7.05 years), minimum 7 days, maximum 23 10/12 years.

SEGMENTAL ANATOMY[3-6]

Double-outlet right ventricle (DORV) was the most common diagnosis, with 6 of 11 (54.55%). The variations in DORV segmental anatomy were: DORV {S,L,D} in 3; DORV {S,D,D} in 2; and DORV {S,L,L} in 1.

Transposition of the great arteries (TGA) was second in frequency, with 4 of 11 (36.36%). The variations in TGA segmental anatomy were: TGA {S,D,L} in 3 and TGA {S,L,L} in 1.

Solitus normally related great arteries with isolated ventricular inversion was the least frequent segmental anatomic set: {S,L,S} in 1 in 11 (9.09%).

These findings are summarized in Table 18.1.[3-6]

STATUS OF THE ATRIOVENTRICULAR VALVES

The atrioventricular (AV) valves were morphologically **normal** in only 3 of 11 cases (27%); all 3 patients had AV valves that were in situs solitus. The AV valves were malformed in 8 of these 11 cases of SI ventricles (73%). Specifically, the AV valvar anomalies were as follows:

The mitral valve (MV) overrode the VS in 2 patients. The MV was left-sided with a ventricular D-loop (solitus ventricular situs) in 1 case, and the MV was right-sided with a ventricular L-loop (inverted ventricular situs) in 1 case.

The MV (left-sided) was cleft in 1 patient.

The MV (right-sided) was atretic in 1 case.

The left-sided tricuspid valve (TV) obstructed the ventricular septal defect (VSD) in 1 patient with {S,L,S}.

A left-sided TV had Ebstein anomaly with tricuspid stenosis and tricuspid regurgitation in 1 case.

Both inverted AV valves overrode the VS in 1 patient.

Why is the frequency of AV valvar anomalies so high (73%) in these cases of SI ventricles? We think that the answer, at least in part, is because the ventricular malformations frequently result in significant ventriculoatrial malalignments.

Ventricular Situs. In these 11 patients with SI ventricles, a ventricular D-loop (solitus organizational pattern) was present in 5 (45%) and a ventricular L-loop (inversus organizational pattern) was found in 6 (55%). So no predilection for either type of ventricular situs was apparent.

TYPICAL SUPEROINFERIOR VENTRICLES WITH A SMALL SUPERIOR RIGHT VENTRICLE

All 10 patients (100%) had a small-chambered superior right ventricular sinus, body, or inflow tract, that is, hypoplasia of the true RV. This was the only anatomic constant that all 10 cases of SI ventricles with a small RV had in common[1]; all other findings were anatomic variables. The LV was always well developed.[1]

DEVELOPMENTAL HYPOTHESIS

These observations concerning SI ventricles with a small superior RV and a well-developed inferior LV led to the following developmental and anatomic hypothesis.[3-6] SI ventricles with a small superior right ventricular sinus and a well-developed inferior LV is closely related to single LV with an infundibular outlet chamber and absence of the right ventricular sinus. When the right ventricular sinus is absent, the subarterial chamber is composed of the infundibulum only. But when a small right ventricular sinus develops beneath the infundibular ring composed of the septal band, the moderator band, the infundibular septum, and the parietal band, the subarterial chamber enlarges and cardiac loop formation begins.

Initially, the developing right ventricular sinus is above the left ventricular sinus. Consequently, the VS is approximately horizontal. But as the right ventricular sinus develops, it starts to descend anteriorly on the right (D-loop formation), or anteriorly on the left (L-loop formation). With descent of the right ventricular sinus on the right, or on the left, the spatial orientation of the VS normally changes from horizontal to approximately vertical. But not in typical SI ventricles. The VS remains approximately horizontal, and the hypoplastic right ventricular

TABLE 18.1 Anatomic Types of Superoinferior Ventricles

Anatomic Types	No. of Cases n = 11	% of Series*
1. With DORV {S,L,D}	3	27
2. With DORV {S,D,D}	2	18
3. With DORV {S,L,L}	1	9
4. With TGA {S,D,L}	3	27
5. With TGA {S,L,L}	1	9
6. With NRGA {S,L,S}	1	9

*Statistics rounded off to the nearest whole number.

sinus remains superior and undescended. **Cardiac loop formation does not occur, or it remains very incomplete.**

If any of the foregoing concepts are unfamiliar, please look them up elsewhere in this book: straight heart tube, D-loop formation, L-loop formation, chirality for diagnosing atrial and ventricular situs, the four components that make up the normal RV and LV. Reiteration is avoided here for brevity.[3-6]

As will be seen, SI ventricles with a small superior *LV* is a very different malformation.[2]

DEGREES OF RIGHT VENTRICULAR SINUS UNDERDEVELOPMENT

In these 10 cases,[1] right ventricular sinus underdevelopment was described as follows: mild, 2; moderate, 3; severe, 4; and normal development, 1.

Anatomic Types of Ventricular Septal Defect[1]

In these 10 cases of typical SI ventricles with small superior RV, the anatomic types of VSD were VSD of the AV canal type, 6 (large 5, medium 1); membranous, subpulmonary, small, 1; infundibuloventricular, subpulmonary, large, 2; and infundibular septal defect, small 1.

ANATOMIC TYPES OF INFUNDIBULUM

The anatomic types of infundibulum found in these 10 typical cases of SI ventricles were as follows:

1. Bilateral (subaortic and subpulmonary), 6
   DORV {S,L,D}, 3
   DORV {S,D,D}, 2
   TGA {S,L,L}, 1
2. Subaortic, 3
   TGA {S,D,L}, 3
3. Subpulmonary, 1
   {S,L,S}, 1

The most common type of infundibulum was bilateral (60%), found in DORV in 5 of 6, and also observed in 1 patient with TGA. The second most frequent type of infundibulum was subaortic (30%), found only in 3 cases of TGA. The least frequent type of infundibulum found in SI ventricles with a small superior right ventricular sinus was noted in 10%, in a patient with solitus normally related great arteries with isolated ventricular inversion {S,L,S}.

Given that the type of relationship between the great arteries is largely determined by infundibuloarterial situs concordance or discordance,[3,4] the types of relationships between the great arteries observed in these 10 cases of SI ventricles[1] are as expected.

All of these cases have infundibuloarterial situs nonconcordance, except for {S,L,S} with a subpulmonary infundibulum (situs solitus) and solitus normally related great arteries.[3,4] Hence, infundibuloarterial situs concordance is present (both the subarterial infundibulum and the great arteries are in situs solitus). Please see Chapter 15 for more information concerning infundibuloarterial situs equations.

Figures of SI ventricles with a small superior RV are presented in Figs. 18.1 to 18.10 inclusive.

SUPEROINFERIOR VENTRICLES WITH A SMALL SUPERIOR LEFT VENTRICLE AND A LARGE INFERIOR RIGHT VENTRICLE

In 2003, Porras, Kratz, Loukas, van Doesburg, Davignon, and Van Praagh[2] reported a newly discovered form of congenital heart disease, that is, SI ventricles with a small superior LV and a large inferior RV. The patient was a 2½-year-old boy from Sainte-Justine Hospital in Montreal, Quebec, Canada. He was full-term. On the first day of postnatal life he was noted to be cyanotic with a heart murmur.

Investigation revealed **dextrocardia, DORV {S,L,L}, right-sided mitral atresia, left-sided tricuspid regurgitation, a small and superior right-sided morphologically LV, a large and inferior left-sided morphologically RV, a large infundibuloventricular type of VSD, and pulmonary outflow tract stenosis.**

The subpulmonary infundibulum was hypoplastic, and the pulmonary artery and branches were small. The subaortic infundibulum was well developed, with a widely patent aortic outflow tract, a dilated ascending aorta, a left aortic arch, and a small patent ductus arteriosus. The arterial saturation was 69%. Cyanosis became progressively more marked, clubbing developed, and shortness of breath appeared. Consequently, at 2½ years of age, a right-sided Blalock-Taussig anastomosis and an atrial septal resection were undertaken. A classic right Blalock-Taussig shunt was performed uneventfully. However, on opening the pericardium, supraventricular tachycardia developed, leading to ventricular tachycardia followed by intractable ventricular fibrillation, resulting in intraoperative death. **Autopsy** findings were summarized earlier and are presented in Figs. 18.11 and 18.12.

THE MORPHOGENESIS OF SUPEROINFERIOR VENTRICLES

What really is the anomaly known as SI ventricles? My hypothesis is as follows. There are two different anatomic types of SI ventricles:

1. with a small superior right ventricular sinus (Figs. 18.1 to 18.10); and
2. with a small superior left ventricular sinus (Figs. 18.11 and 18.12).

text continues after figure 18.9

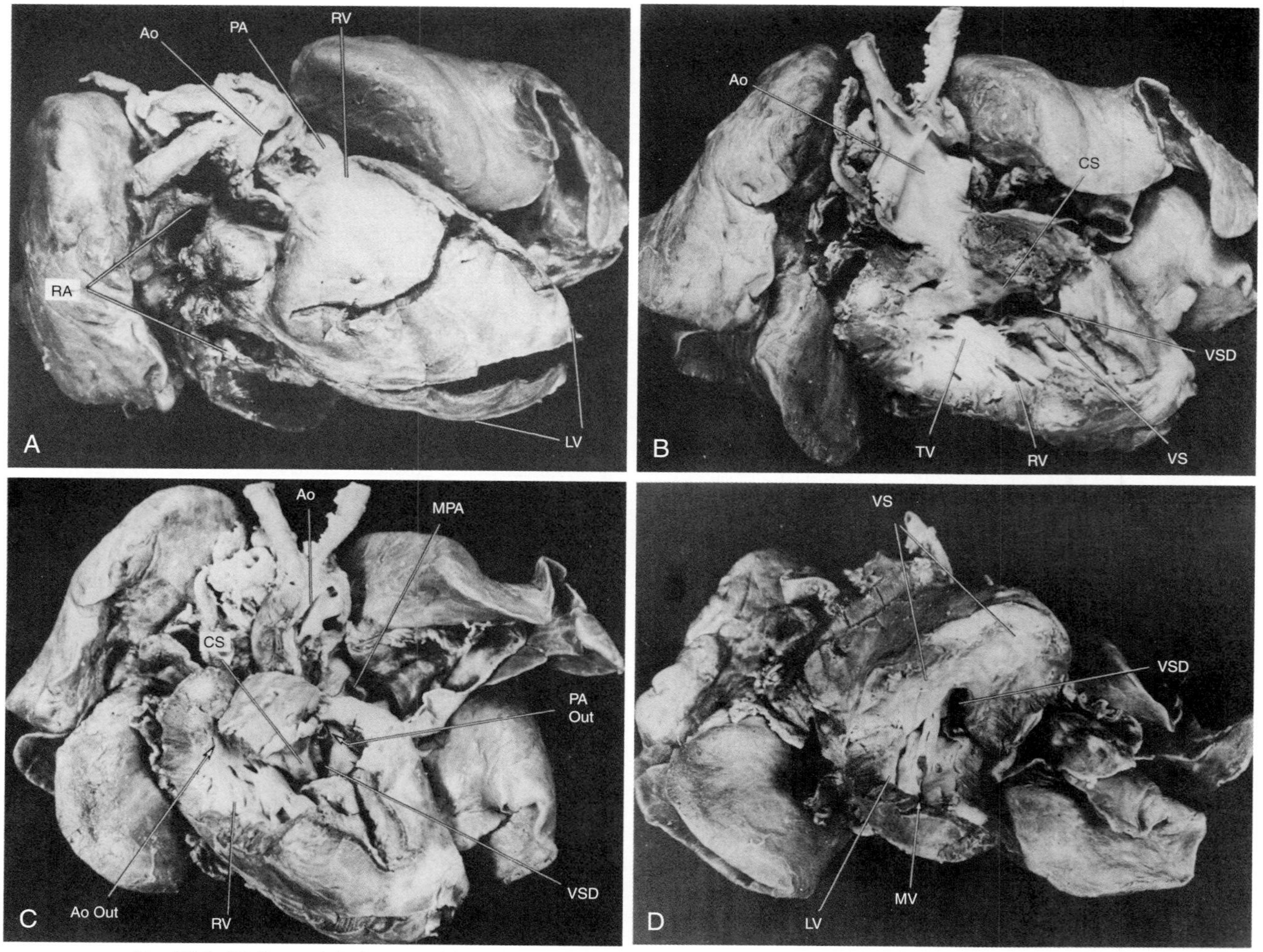

Fig. 18.1 (A) Superoinferior ventricles with double-outlet right ventricle (DORV) {S,D,D} external frontal view of the heart and lungs. The morphologically right atrium *(RA)* is right-sided. The morphologically right ventricle *(RV)* is right-sided, superior, and small. The morphologically left ventricle *(LV)* is left-sided, inferior, and large. Both great arteries appear to arise from the superior RV, the aorta *(Ao)* to the right of the pulmonary artery *(PA)*. (B) The right ventricular inflow tract, and the outflow tract of the aorta. The aortic valve (unlabeled) and the underlying tricuspid valve *(TV)* are widely separated by a well-developed muscular subaortic infundibulum or conus. There is an infundibuloventricular type of ventricular septal defect *(VSD)* between the inferior rim of the conal septum *(CS)* above, and the superior rim of the ventricular septum *(VS)* and the septal band below. (C) Right ventricular inflow tract showing aortic outflow tract *(Ao Out)* to the right of the CS and the pulmonary outflow tract *(PA Out)* to the left of the CS. A bilateral conus (both subaortic and subpulmonary) is present, indicating that neither subarterial infundibular free wall has undergone involution. The CS lies to the right of the ventricular septum and septal band. This rightward malalignment of the infundibulum and great arteries (the conotruncus) relative to the ventricles and VS is characteristic of DORV. Both the Ao and the main pulmonary artery *(MPA)* arise *from* the infundibulum, *above* the small and superior RV. Cases of DORV like this make it clear that the great arteries really do *not* arise *from* the ventricles. The Ao and the MPA really arise *from* the infundibulum, which is *above* the ventricular sinuses. This is why **infundibular development** is basic to understanding ventriculoarterial alignments and connections.[3] The conus is the connector between the ventricles and the great arteries. (D) The large opened LV, viewed from the front and below. Note the approximately horizontal left VS surface superiorly and the hypertrophied left ventricular free wall inferiorly. The mitral valve *(MV)* has a cleft anterior leaflet that attaches abnormally to the crest of the VS. The only outlet from the large inferior LV is the unobstructive VSD. (Reproduced with permission from Van Praagh S, LaCorte M, Fellows KE. Supero-inferior ventricles: anatomic and angiocardiographic findings in ten post-mortem cases. In Van Praagh R and Takao A, eds. *Etiology and Morphogenesis of Congenital Heart Disease*. Mount Kisco, NY: Futura Publishing Co; 1980:317.)

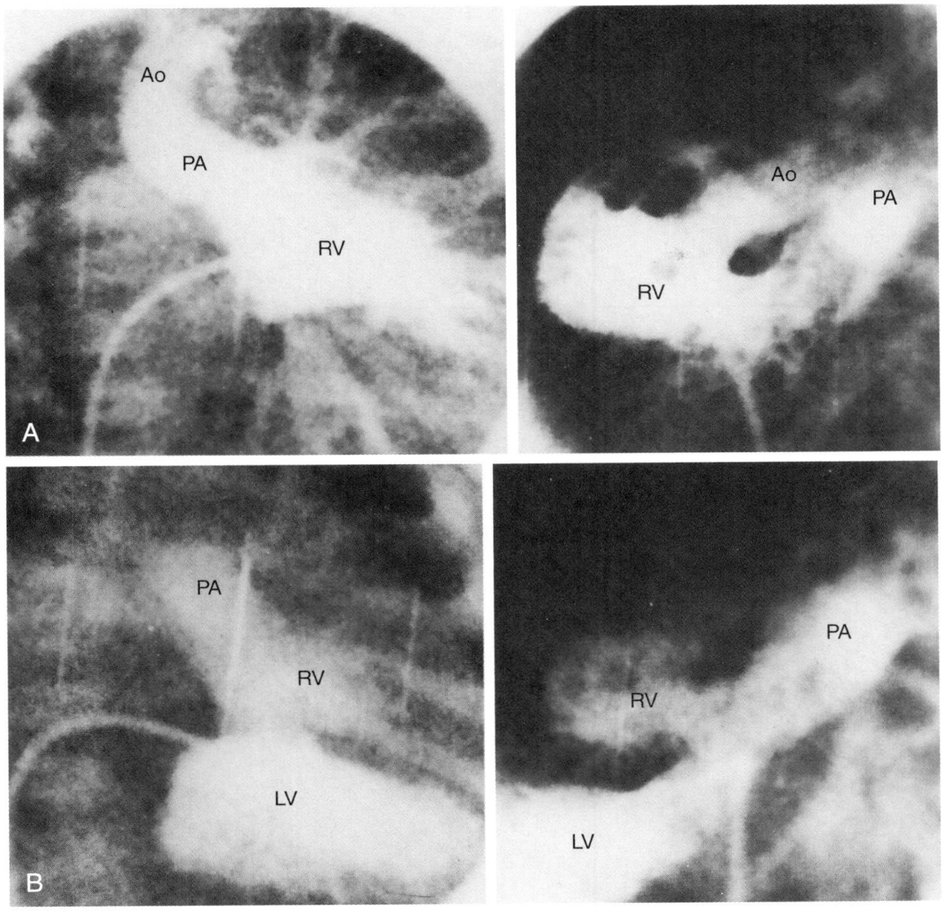

Fig. 18.2 (A) The *upper panel* is a selective right ventricular biplane cineangiocardiogram; *left* is a posteroanterior projection, and *right* is a simultaneous left lateral projection. (B) Is a selective biplane left ventricular cineangiocardiogram; *left* is a posteroanterior projection and *right* is a simultaneous left lateral projection. These angiocardiograms are of the patient shown in Fig. 18.1, a 5-month-old boy. Note that the morphologically right ventricle *(RV)* is superior and small compared with morphologically left ventricle *(LV)*, which is inferior and large. The ventricular septum is approximately horizontal, best seen in *panel B, right*, indicating the presence of superoinferior ventricles **(unlooped ventricles)**. *Ao*, Aorta; *PA*, pulmonary artery. (Reproduced with permission from Van Praagh S, LaCorte M, Fellows KE. Supero-inferior ventricles: anatomic and angiocardiographic findings in ten post-mortem cases. In Van Praagh R and Takao A, eds. *Etiology and Morphogenesis of Congenital Heart Disease*. Mount Kisco, NY: Futura Publishing Co; 1980:317.)

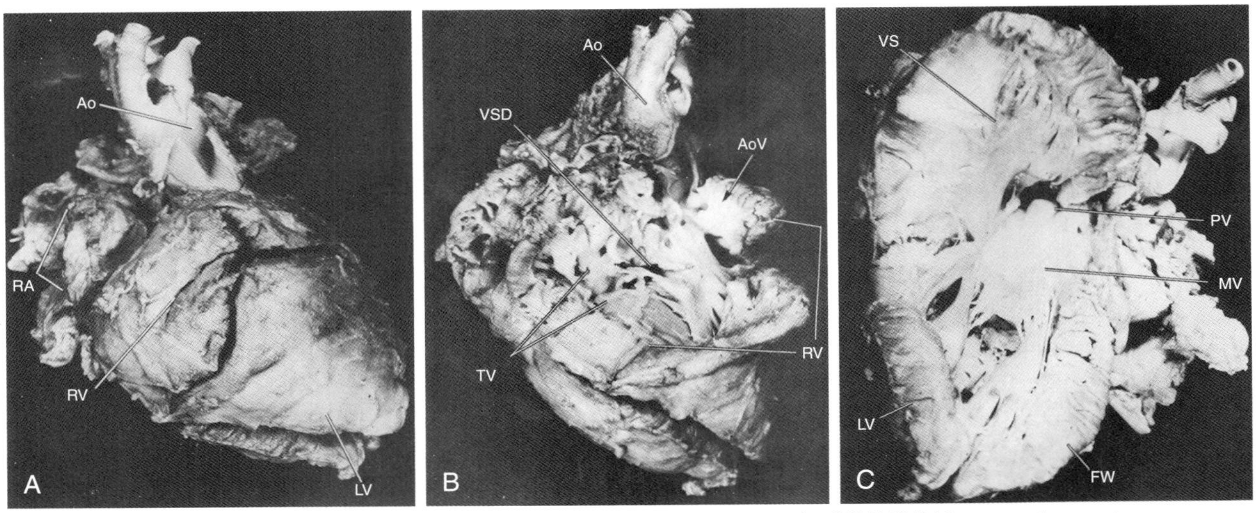

Fig. 18.3 (A) Superoinferior ventricles with transposition of the great arteries (TGA) {S,D,L}, as seen in an external frontal view. The right atrium *(RA)* is right-sided. The right ventricle *(RV)* is small, superior, and right-sided. The left ventricle *(LV)* is large, inferior, and left-sided. The L-transposed aorta *(Ao)* is anterior and to the *left* of the transposed pulmonary artery (not well seen in this view). Their patient was a 4-month-old boy. (B) The opened

Continued

Fig. 18.3 cont'd RV receives the tricuspid valve *(TV)*. The RV is small, superior, and right-sided. A small infundibuloventricular ventricular septal defect *(VSD)* is seen. The aortic valve *(AoV)* is quite far to the left. (C) The opened LV is seen from the front. The ventricular septum *(VS)* is superior and approximately horizontal. The left ventricular free wall *(FW)* is inferior and hypertrophied. The mitral valve *(MV)* is abnormally inferior, and the TV in Fig. 18.3B is abnormally superior. There is direct fibrous continuity between the transposed pulmonary valve *(PV)* and the MV. A subaortic infundibulum is present, typical of TGA. The heart is "lying on its back," that is, lying on its LV FW. When the heart is rotated approximately 90 degrees counterclockwise, its spatial orientation becomes much more normal. (Reproduced with permission from Van Praagh S, LaCorte M, Fellows KE. Supero-inferior ventricles: anatomic and angiocardiographic findings in ten post-mortem cases. In Van Praagh R, Takao A, eds. *Etiology and Morphogenesis of Congenital Heart Disease*. Mount Kisco, NY: Futura Publishing Co; 1980:317.)

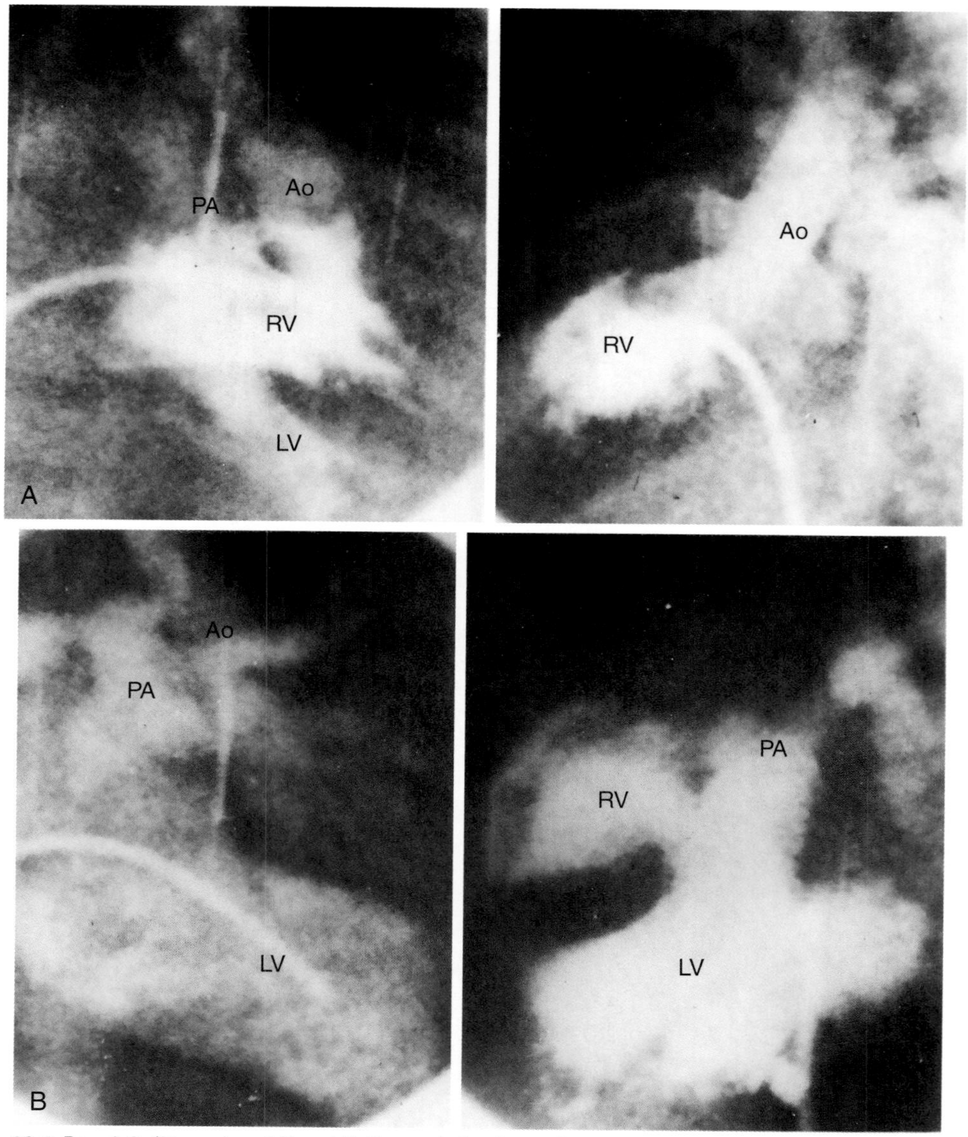

Fig. 18.4 Panel A *(Upper)* and Panel B *(Lower)*. **Angiocardiograms of Superoinferior Ventricles With Transposition of the Great Arteries {S,D,L}, in the Patient in Fig. 18.3.** (A) Selective right ventricular *(RV)* injection posteroanterior and left lateral projections. (B) Selective left ventricular injection, posteroanterior and left lateral projections. (A) Note how high the tricuspid valve is (catheter course). The aorta *(Ao)* is clearly to the left of the pulmonary artery *(PA)*. The right atrium opens into the right ventricle (RV) (catheter course), indicating atrial situs solitus and a concordant alignment with the superior, right-sided, and small RV. (B) The fact that the left ventricle *(LV)* is much larger than the RV becomes obvious. The ventricular septum is approximately horizontal. Banding of the PA is evident (in B, *right*). (Reproduced with permission from Van Praagh S, LaCorte M, Fellows KE. Supero-inferior ventricles: anatomic and angiocardiographic findings in ten post-mortem cases. In Van Praagh R, Takao A, eds. *Etiology and Morphogenesis of Congenital Heart Disease*. Mount Kisco, NY: Futura Publishing Co; 1980:317.)

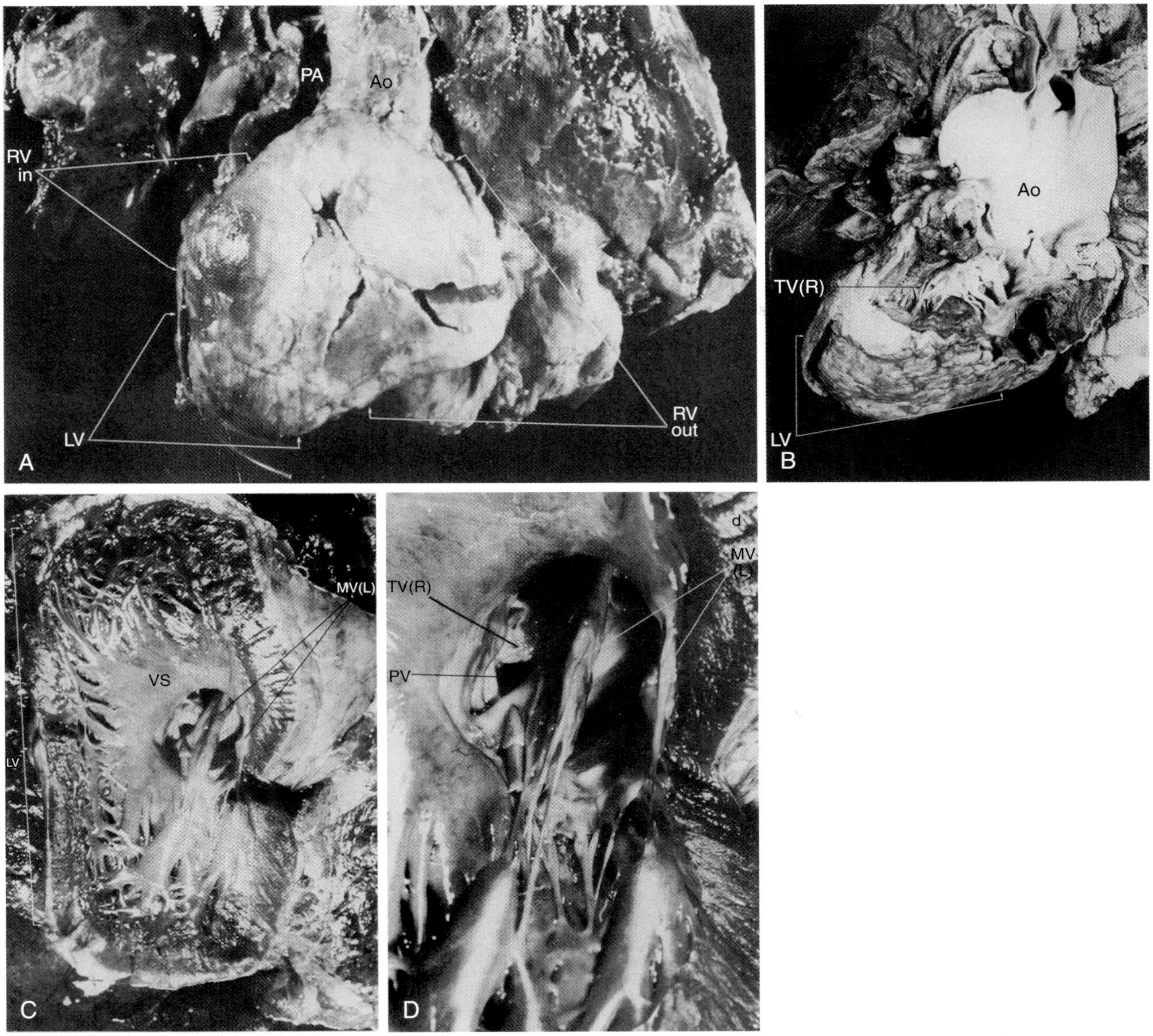

Fig. 18.5 **Superoinferior Ventricles With Crisscross Atrioventricular (AV) Relations, Transposition of the Great Arteries (TGAs) {S,D,L}, and Dextrocardia.** This is the heart of a 23 10/12- year-old man. (A) The external frontal view of the heart. The locations of several subatrial chambers are indicated by demarcating labels. Dextrocardia means that the heart was predominantly right-sided. Superoinferior ventricles indicates that the right ventricular sinus *(RV in)* is superior to the left ventricle *(LV)*. Crisscross AV relations indicates that the AV inflow tracts are abnormally angulated relative to each other (approximately 130 degrees). Normally, the AV inflow tracts are approximately parallel to each other. The AV inflow tract angle normally equals 10 degrees or less. This AV angle in this patient is huge (130 degrees) and very abnormal. The right atrial (RA) to RV inflow tract vector is directed from right superiorly to left inferiorly. *RV out* means the infundibulum or RV outflow tract. The left AV inflow tract vector runs from left superiorly to right inferiorly. The ventricular inflow tracts begin normally beneath the AV valves, RV to the right and superiorly and LV to the left and a bit inferiorly, as in a normal ventricular D-loop. But then, as one proceeds toward the ventricular apices, **the ventricles twist in the wrong direction: to the left, instead of to the right.** Abnormal axial rotation of the ventricular loop in a clockwise direction, to the left (as viewed from the front), appears to explain why the infundibulum (RV out) is left-sided and unusually inferior, why *L*-TGA is present (not *D*-TGA), and why the left ventricular apex is right-sided and inferior (not left-sided and inferior), resulting in dextrocardia. D-loop AV alignments and connections were established, and then the ventricles twisted the wrong way for a D-loop—to the left. This wrong-way twisting of solitus (D-loop) ventricles to the left, typically with hypoplasia of the RV, results in marked angulation of the AV inflow tracts, known as crisscross AV relations, in which the RV starts on the right, but then twists to the left. And the LV starts on the left, but then twists to the right. So the AV inflow tracts head in opposite directions. They crisscross. The same thing can happen, in mirror-image, to L-loop ventricles. They start as inverted ventricles and then apically they twist (or get twisted) to the right. Crisscross AV relations result when the ventricles twist in the wrong direction for their situs: when D-loops twist leftward, and when L-loops twist rightward: **contra-situs twisting results in crisscross AV relations.** (B) A right-sided tricuspid valve, or *TV(R)*, opened into a small, superior, right-sided RV. A large, inferior LV lay beneath, its apex pointing rightward. A large L-transposed aorta *(Ao)* originated above the small RV. The muscular subaortic conus was regarded as deficient for TGA. There was aortic valve–TV fibrous continuity. (C) The opened morphologically LV, seen from the front. A large ventricular septal defect of the AV canal type is present. A cleft regurgitant, left-sided mitral valve, or *MV(L)* overrode the ventricular septum *(VS)*.

Continued

Fig. 18.5 cont'd (D) A close-up shows the cleft anterior leaflet as from the MV. Note the thickening and rolling of the leaflet margins of the MV cleft, indicating mitral regurgitation. An *arrowhead* points to the pulmonary valve *(PV)*, which was bicuspid. There was subvalvar pulmonary outflow tract stenosis. The right-sided tricuspid valve (TV[R]) is also seen crowding the stenotic left ventricular pulmonary outflow tract. *PA*, Pulmonary artery. (Reproduced with permission from Van Praagh S, LaCorte M, Fellows KE. Supero-inferior ventricles: anatomic and angiocardiographic findings in ten post-mortem cases. In Van Praagh R, Takao A, eds. *Etiology and Morphogenesis of Congenital Heart Disease*. Futura Publishing Co: Mount Kisco, NY; 1980:317.)

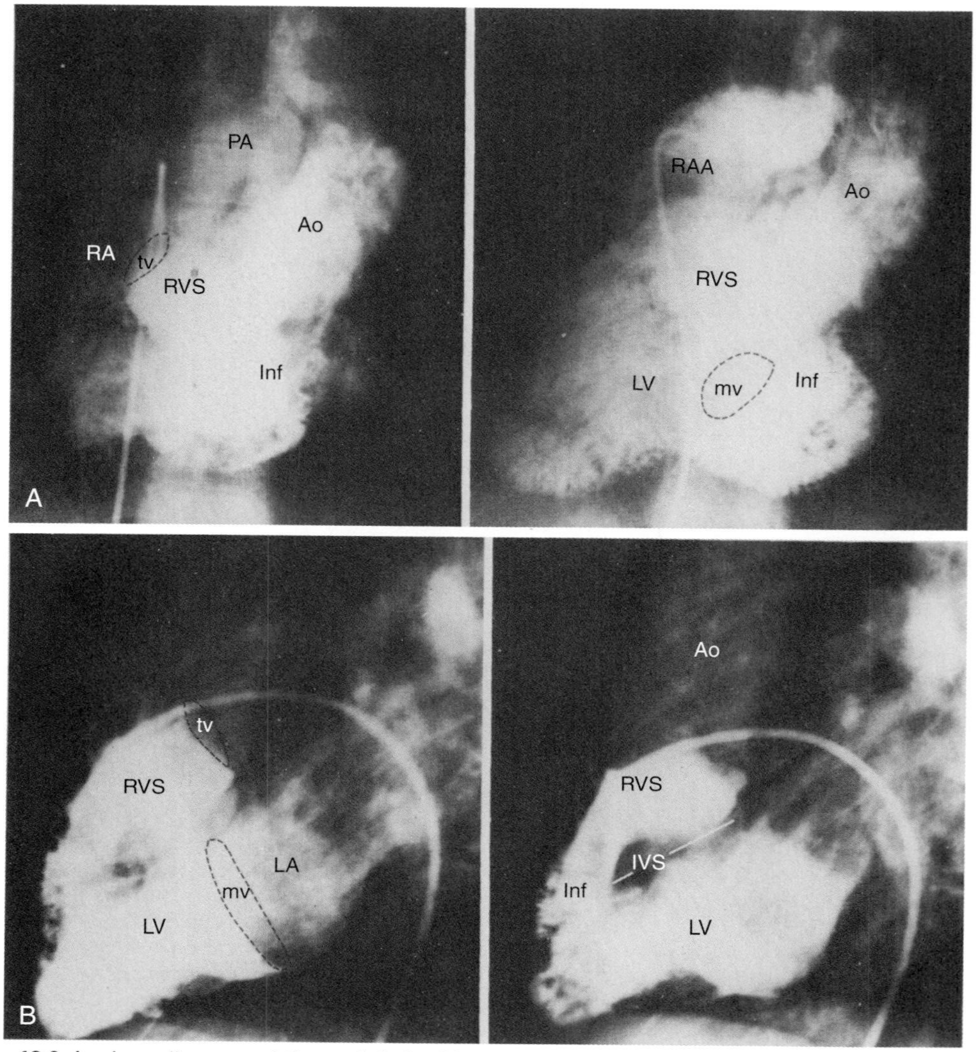

Fig. 18.6 Angiocardiogram of Superoinferior Ventricles, With Crisscross Atrioventricular Relations, Dextrocardia, and Transposition of the Great Arteries (TGA) {S,D,L}. *Panel A* shows posteroanterior projections. *Panel B* shows left lateral projections. In *panel A*, the right ventricular sinus *(RVS)* is seen to be small, right-sided, and superior relative to the large inferior left ventricle *(LV)*, establishing the diagnosis of superoinferior ventricles. The tricuspid valve *(tv)* is very superior and right-sided (B *left* and A *left*). The catheter retracted into the right atrial appendage *(RAA)*. The catheter course from the right-sided right atrium *(RA)* into the RV sinus indicates the presence of a ventricular D-loop (solitus ventricles). But the presence of the infundibulum *(Inf)* to the patient's left and inferiorly *(panel A right)* indicates that the ventricular D-loop has undergone abnormal rotation to the patient's left *(panel A, right)*. The right-sided location of the left ventricular apex *(panel A right)* also indicates that abnormal rotation of the ventricles to the patient's left has occurred. In the posteroanterior projection *(panel A)*, there appears to be a large angle between the RA-to-RV inflow tract and the LA-to-LV inflow tract (approximately 90 degrees); that is, crisscross atrioventricular relations appears to be present. The presence of L-malposition of the great arteries between the leftward aorta *(Ao)* and the rightward pulmonary artery *(PA)* is seen *(in panel A left)*. Whether the ventriculoarterial alignments are those of L-TGA, or of double-outlet LV are not clearly apparent in these films. What they do show clearly is superoinferior ventricles with wrong-way twisting of the ventricles (crisscross heart). *IVS*, interventricular septum; *LA*, left atrium; *mv*, mitral valve. (Reproduced with permission from Van Praagh S, LaCorte M, Fellows KE. Supero-inferior ventricles: anatomic and angiocardiographic findings in ten post-mortem cases. In Van Praagh R, Takao A, eds. *Etiology and Morphogenesis of Congenital Heart Disease*. Futura Publishing Co: Mount Kisco, NY; 1980:317.)

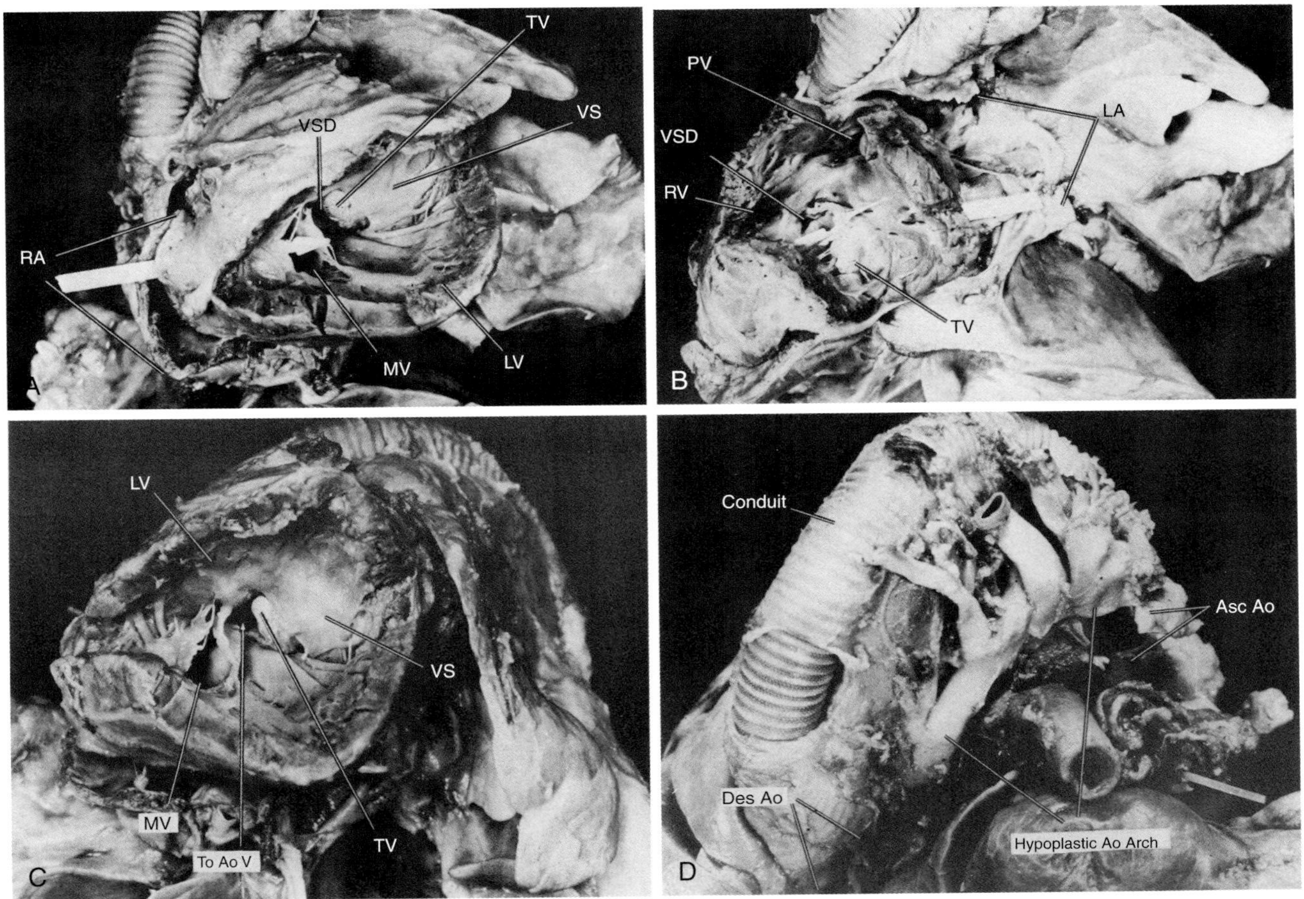

Fig. 18.7 Superoinferior Ventricles With Isolated Ventricular Inversion {S,L,S}. As the segmental anatomy indicates, this 8.5-month-old boy had visceroatrial situs solitus {S,-,-} discordant L-loop ventricles or ventricular inversion {S,L, -}, and solitus normally related great arteries {S,L,S}. The segmental anatomy also may be rendered as **NRGA {S,L,S}**. NRGA is short for normally related great arteries, and the segmental anatomy indicates which kind of normally related great arteries—solitus or inversus—is present: {S,L,S}. (A) The right-sided right atrium *(RA)* opens through an inferior and right-sided mitral valve *(MV)* into a well-developed and inferior left ventricle (LV). A *white arrow* from RA to LV demarcates this discordant atrioventricular (AV) alignment. An AV canal type of ventricular septal defect *(VSD)* was present. The mitral valve *(MV)* was cleft. The left-sided tricuspid valve *(TV)* bulged into the aortic outflow tract and contributed to subaortic outflow tract stenosis. There was aortic valve–to–mitral valve direct fibrous continuity (not seen in this photo). The left ventricular septal surface *(VS)* was approximately horizontal, typical of superoinferior ventricles. (B) The left-sided left atrium *(LA)* opening through a left-sided TV into a right ventricle *(RV)* that is high, small, left-sided, and left-handed. A VSD of the AV canal type is present. The pulmonary artery originates above the RV. Between the pulmonary valve (PV) above and the TV and the VSD below, a well-developed left-sided subpulmonary infundibulum is seen. (C) Opened LV, the right-sided mitral inflow tract, and the obstructed aortic outflow tract leading to the aortic valve *(to AoV)* between the MV to the right and the encroaching TV to the left. (D) The hypoplastic ascending aorta *(Asc Ao),* aortic arch, and aortic isthmus, related to the subaortic outflow tract stenosis. There was also a patent ductus arteriosus. **The infundibuloarterial situs equation**[3] is:

$$\text{NRGAS,L,S} = 0.\text{R} + 4\text{L}$$

The situs of the infundibulum (0R + 4L) is the situs formula of the infundibulum of solitus normally related great arteries. The situs of the great arteries is also solitus. So there is infundibular and great arterial situs concordance: both are in situs solitus. The infundibulum and the great arteries are both solitus, even though the ventricular sinuses (inflow tracts or pumps) are inverted. When there is infundibuloarterial situs concordance (both solitus or both inversus), the great arteries are normally related (solitus or inversus). When there is infundibuloarterial situs discordance, the great arteries are abnormally related.[3] Hemodynamically, if one cardiac segment is discordant, the systemic and pulmonary arterial circulations are physiologically uncorrected. Such patients need a switch procedure. In {S,L,S}, the *ventricles* are discordant. Hemodynamically, such patients need an atrial switch operation (a Senning or a Mustard operation). Preoperatively, the circulations are physiologically uncorrected: RA → LV → Ao and LA → RV → PA. Postoperatively, the circulations are physiologically corrected: RA → LA → RV → PA and LA → RA → LV → Ao. Usually, it is the subarterial infundibular segment that is discordant,[3] not the ventricular sinus segment. (Reproduced with permission from Van Praagh S, LaCorte M, Fellows KE. Supero-inferior ventricles: anatomic and angiocardiographic findings in ten post-mortem cases. In Van Praagh R, Takao A, eds. *Etiology and Morphogenesis of Congenital Heart Disease*. Futura Publishing Co: Mount Kisco, NY; 1980:317.)

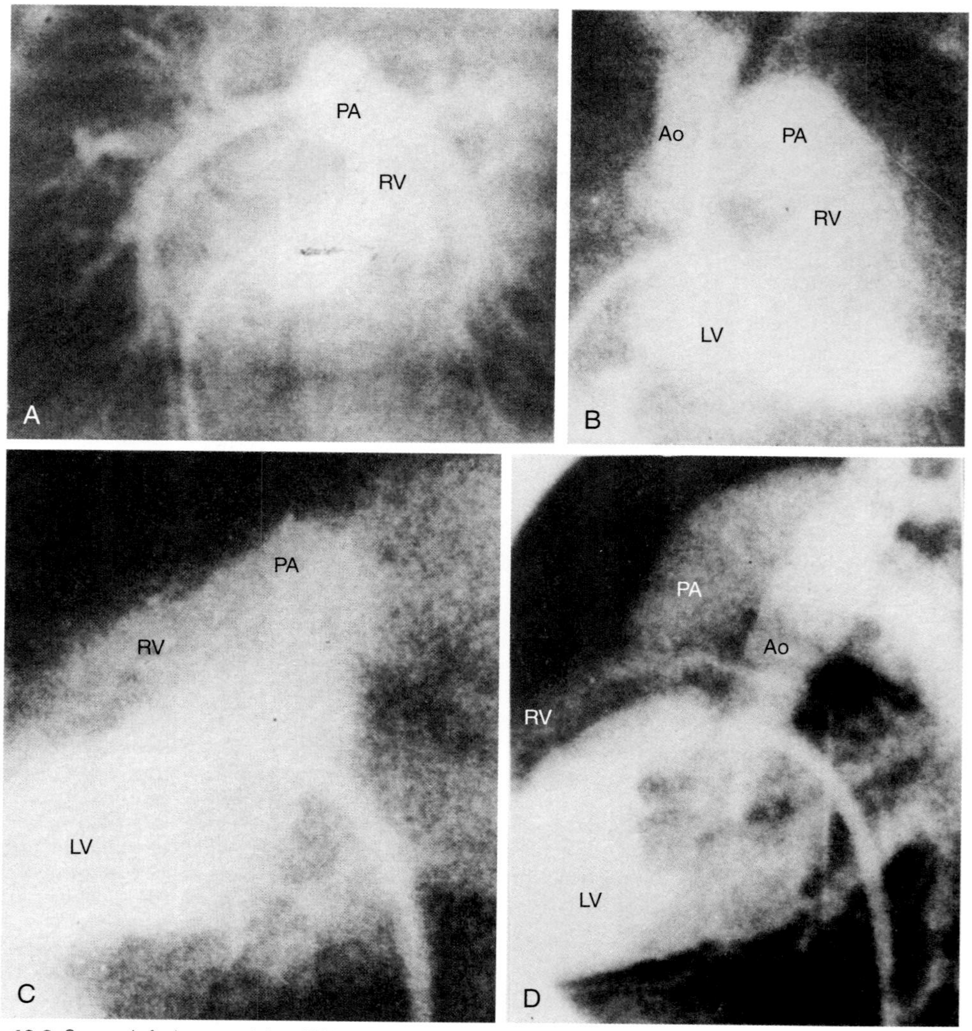

Fig. 18.8 Superoinferior ventricles (SIVs) with isolated ventricular inversion, i.e., IVI {S,L,S}. A and B are posteroanterior projections, and C and D are simultaneous left lateral projections of this cineangiocardiogram. The condition of SIVs is seen in B, C, and D, where a small morphologically right ventricle (RV) is superior to the large morphologically left ventricle (LV). The catheter is located in the right-sided inferior vena cava and right atrium (unlabeled), (A), indicating visceroatrial situs solitus: {S,-,-}. The RV is to the left of the LV, (B), indicating ventricular inversion or ventricular L-loop: {S,L,-}. The ascending aorta (Ao) lies to the right of and inferior to the main pulmonary artery (PA), (B), indicating solitus normally related great arteries: {S,L,S}. A subpulmonary infundibulum is present (D). Hence the diagnosis is: superoinferior ventricles, with a small superior RC, and large inferior LV, with isolated ventricular inversion IVI {S,L,S}, and ventricular septal defect (VSD).

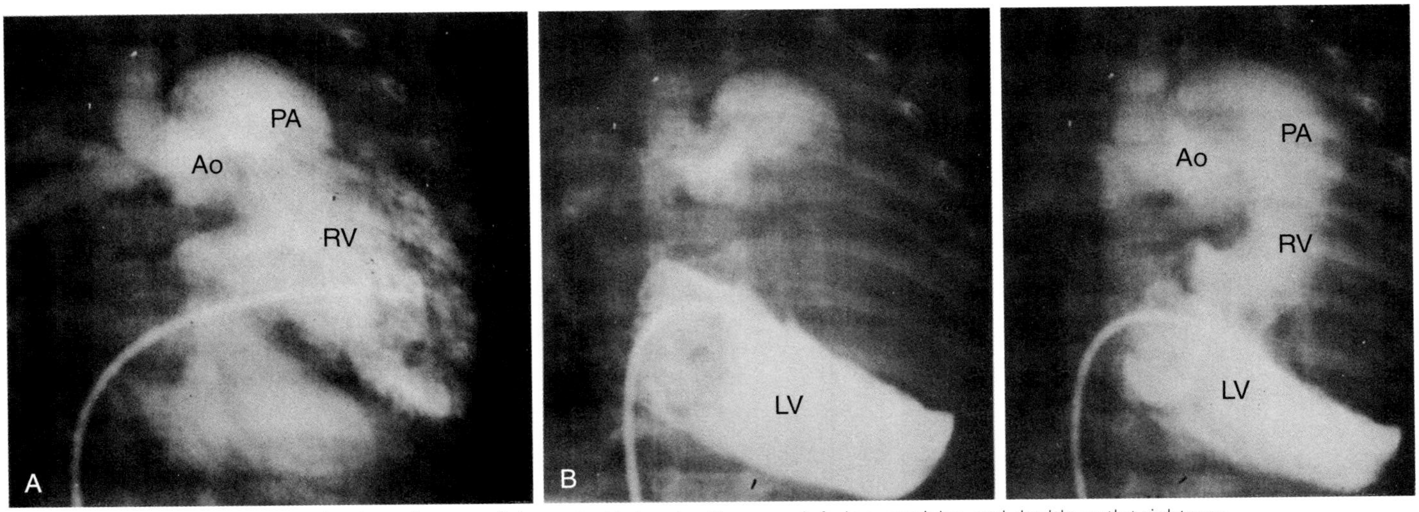

Fig. 18.9 (A) Angiocardiogram of the patient's heart with superoinferior ventricles and double-outlet right ventricle DORV {S,L,D}, the same patient as in Fig. 18.8. This is a selective right ventricular injection, viewed in a posteroanterior projection. The patient was a 15.5-month-old boy. The catheter course is typical of visceroatrial situs solitus. The morphologically right ventricle *(RV)* was left-sided, superior, and quite well developed. The left ventricle (LV; unlabeled) was right-sided, inferior, and well developed. The ventricular septum is oblique, approximately 40 degrees below the horizontal, not horizontal, apparently because the RV has grown and expanded. (B) Selective left ventricular injection, viewed in posteroanterior projections. *The left image* shows the catheter passing through the inferior and right-sided mitral valve (unlabeled) into a well developed, inferior, and right-sided *LV*. The plane of the left ventricular septal surface is oblique, that is, more horizontal than normal. The right image shows the ventricular septal defect, with contrast flowing into the left-sided and superior RV and into the D-malposed great arteries in this patient with DORV {S,L,D}. *Ao,* Aorta; *PA,* pulmonary artery. (Reproduced with permission from Van Praagh S, LaCorte M, Fellows KE. Supero-inferior ventricles: anatomic and angiocardiographic findings in ten post-mortem cases. In Van Praagh R, Takao A, eds. *Etiology and Morphogenesis of Congenital Heart Disease*. Futura Publishing Co: Mount Kisco, NY; 1980:317.)

When the right ventricular sinus is superior and small, D-loop formation and L-loop formation fail to occur, resulting in persistence of a straight heart tube with a superior small RV, an inferior large LV, and an approximately horizontal VS. This is the most common form of SI ventricles, that occurs with both solitus (normally D-loop) and inversus (normally L-loop) straight heart tubes. **So, SI ventricles with a small superior right ventricular sinus is the no looping type of SI ventricles.**

However, SI ventricles with a small superior LV sinus is the hyperlooping type of SI ventricles. Looking at the diagram (see Fig. 18.12E), the VS appears to have undergone about 170 degrees of levorotation (clockwise rotation) as viewed from the front. The VS starts in the straight tube stage in a horizontal orientation with the developing RV above and with the developing LV below. Normal L-rotation (clockwise rotation as seen from the front) goes through about 90 degrees leftward rotation. This brings the VS to an approximately vertical orientation, with the RV to the left and with the LV to the right (i.e., typical ventricular inversion).

When the right-sided LV is small and essentially nonfunctional, the left-sided RV can keep on growing. And L-looping can then become excessive. The VS can continue its clockwise L-rotation as seen from the front. Why? Because the left-sided right ventricular sinus is the only functional ventricular sinus this patient has. Clockwise L-rotation continues and finally stops at about 170 degrees leftward rotation. This flips the ventricles. The small LV is now superior, and the large RV now extends beneath the VS.

The smallness of the right-sided LV and the coexistence of right-sided mitral atresia appear basic to the morphogenesis of this rare form of SI ventricles with a small superior LV (see Figs. 18.11 and 18.12). Thus, there are two anatomic types of SI ventricles: the no-looping type and the hyperlooping type. And in both, the RV appears to be importantly involved:

1. In the more common type of SI ventricles with a superior and hypoplastic right ventricular sinus, ventricular loop formation (D-loop or L-loop) fails to occur. The ventricular straight tube stage persists, apparently because of marked hypoplasia of the right ventricular sinus.
2. In the rare type of SI ventricles with a hypoplastic and superior left ventricular sinus and a large inferior right ventricular sinus, excessive ventricular loop formation appears to have occurred, because of hypertrophy and enlargement of the RV and hypoplasia of the LV and mitral atresia.

Thus, the right ventricular sinus appears to be the "prime mover":

1. When the right ventricular sinus is present but very hypoplastic, there is no movement (no ventricular looping).
2. When the right ventricular sinus is hypertrophied and enlarged, and the left ventricular sinus is markedly hypoplastic but present, movement can be excessive (ventricular hyperlooping).

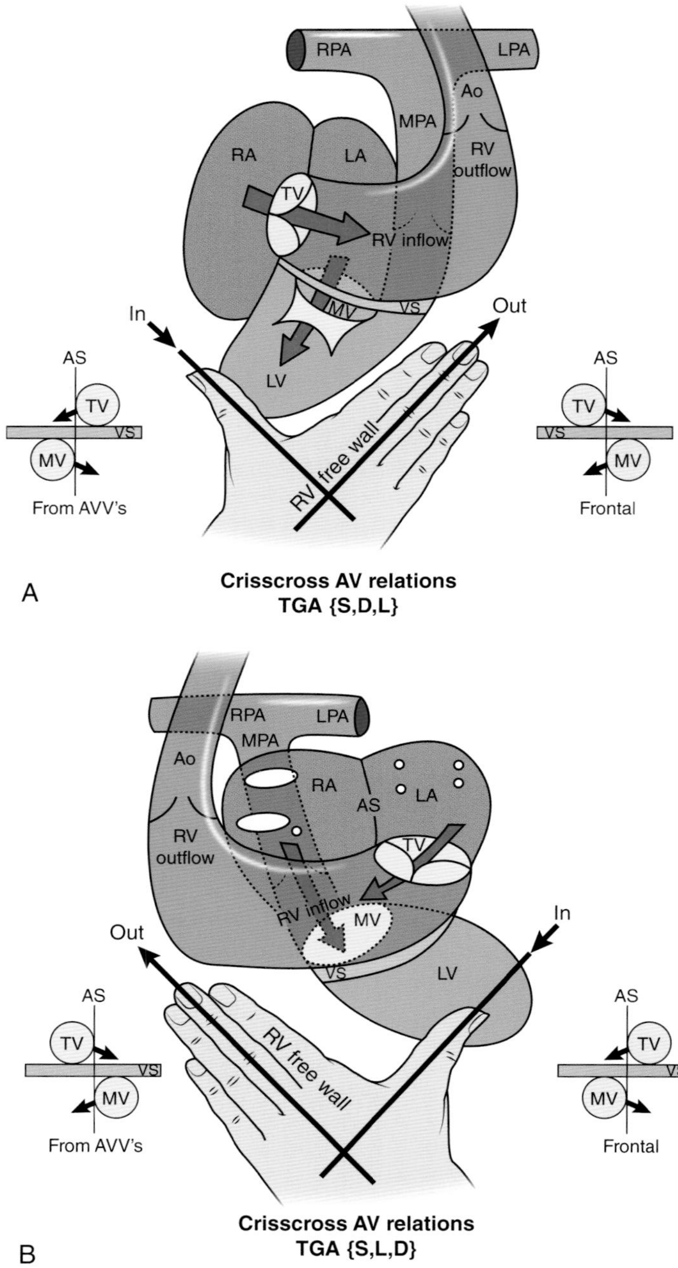

Fig. 18.10 (A) Transposition of the great arteries (TGA) {S,D,L} with superoinferior ventricles and crisscross atrioventricular *(AV)* relations. The atria are in situs solitus, morphologically right atrium *(RA)* to the right and morphologically left atrium *(LA)* to the left. A ventricular D-loop (solitus loop) is present. The systemic venous blood flows from the RA, through the tricuspid valve *(TV)* into the right ventricular *(RV)* sinus, body, or inflow tract (horizontal right-to-left *arrow*). The pulmonary venous blood flows from the left atrium *(LA)* through the mitral valve *(MV)* into the morphologically left ventricle *(LV)*. The right ventricular sinus is underdeveloped, and the LV is well developed. The ventricular septum *(VS)* is approximately horizontal. The atrial septum *(AS)* is approximately vertical. The angle between the plane of the VS and the plane of the atrial septum is approximately 90 degrees. The pulmonary venous blood flow passes from the LA through the MV into the large LV (*arrow* directed inferiorly, anteriorly and rightward. The prominent apex of the LV points rightward, creating the appearance of **dextrocardia.** The superior small RV and the inferior large LV together constitute **superoinferior ventricles.** The marked angulation of the AV inflow tract directions is **crisscross AV relations.** The right ventricular outflow tract is the infundibulum or conus arteriosus. L-transposition of the great arteries is present. The aortic valve and ascending aorta *(Ao)* lie to the left of the pulmonary valve and main pulmonary artery

Fig. 18.10 cont'd *(MPA).* So L-TGA is not necessarily physiologically corrected TGA. This is why one needs to know *all* of the segmental anatomy: TGA {S,D,L}, including the AV alignments (concordant in this case) and the ventriculoarterial (VA) alignments (L-TGA in this patient). **With D-loop (solitus) ventricles, the RV is right handed.** One's thumb represents the right ventricular inflow tract *(In).* The fingers represent the right ventricular outflow tract *(Out).* The palm of the right hand represents the right ventricular septum, and the dorsum of the right hand represents the right ventricular free wall. **Chirality** or handedness is a fundamental characteristic of matter that applies to stereoisomers. (Greek, *kheir,* "hand"). **The D-loop or solitus RV is right handed.** (B) TGA {S,L,D} with superoinferior ventricles, that is, RV above, LV below, and approximately horizontal ventricular septum (VS), with crisscross AV relations, and a left handed RV. The atria are in situs solitus, with right atrium (RA) to the right, left atrium (LA) to the left, and with an approximately vertical atrial septum (AS). L-loop (inverted) ventricles are present. The RV is high, small and it is aligned and connected with the left-sided LA via a high and left-sided tricuspid valve (TV). The pulmonary venous inflow is oriented from posteriorly on the left to anteriorly on the right, as the almost horizontal LA inflow arrow indicates. The systemic venous inflow comes from posteriorly on the right, that is, the RA and passes almost vertically through an inferior MV into an inferior and large LV. Thus, when viewed from the front and above, the left atrial and right atrial venous inflow streams appear to crisscross, making an angle of approximately 90 degrees with each other. In fact, these two entering venous blood streams seldom really intermingle, unless one or both AV valves straddle the VS. So, crisscrossing AV inflow tract venous blood streams is usually just an appearance, without actual mixing of the blood streams. D-TGA is present, which may suggest that physiologically uncorrected TGA is present. But not in this case. This is congenitally physiologically corrected TGA. Again, this is why one needs to know the complete segmental anatomy and the AV and VA alignments. The L-loop (inverted) RV is left handed. The thumb of one's left hand represents the inverted RV inflow tract or sinus (In). The fingers of the left hand represent the inverted RV outflow tract (Out). The palm of one's left hand represents the septum of the inverted RV. And the dorsum of the left hand represents the free wall of the inverted RV. One's right and left hands are stereoisomers, as are ventricular D-loops and L-loops in situs solitus totalis and in situs inversus totalis, respectively. This is why chirality applies to the ventricles. **The D-loop (noninverted) LV is left handed. The L-loop (inverted) LV is right handed.** Chirality also applies to the atria, but is seldom needed there diagnostically. Chirality is needed when the standard definition of noninversion and inversion break down. For example: *When there is only ventricle.* No other ventricle is present. How can I tell if this is right, or left, nonnverted or inverted? *Answer:* Look at it. Apply morphology and chirality. *When ventricles are both right-sided and left-sided? Answer:* The same. Look at it. Apply morphology and chirality. *LPA,* Left pulmonary artery; *RPA,* right pulmonary artery. (Reproduced with permission from R. Van Praagh.)

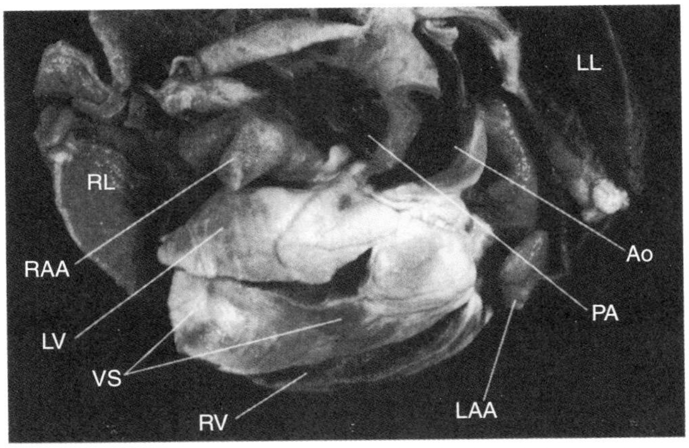

Fig. 18.11 Superoinferior ventricles with superior left ventricle *(LV)* and inferior right ventricle *(RV).* The heart and lungs of a 2½-year-old boy with dextrocardia, viewed from the front. The patient also had double-outlet right ventricle {S,L,L}, mitral atresia (right-sided), hypoplasia of the superior LV, hypertrophy and enlargement of the inferior RV, and a horizontal ventricular septum *(VS). Ao,* Aorta; *LAA,* left atrial appendage; *LL,* left lung; *PA,* pulmonary artery; *RAA,* right atrial appendage; *RL,* right lung. (Reproduced with permission from Porras D, Kratz C, Loukas M, van Doesburg NH, Davignon A, Van Praagh R. Superoinferior ventricles with superior left ventricle and inferior right ventricle: a newly recognized form of congenital heart disease. *Pediatr Cardiol.* 2003;24:604.)

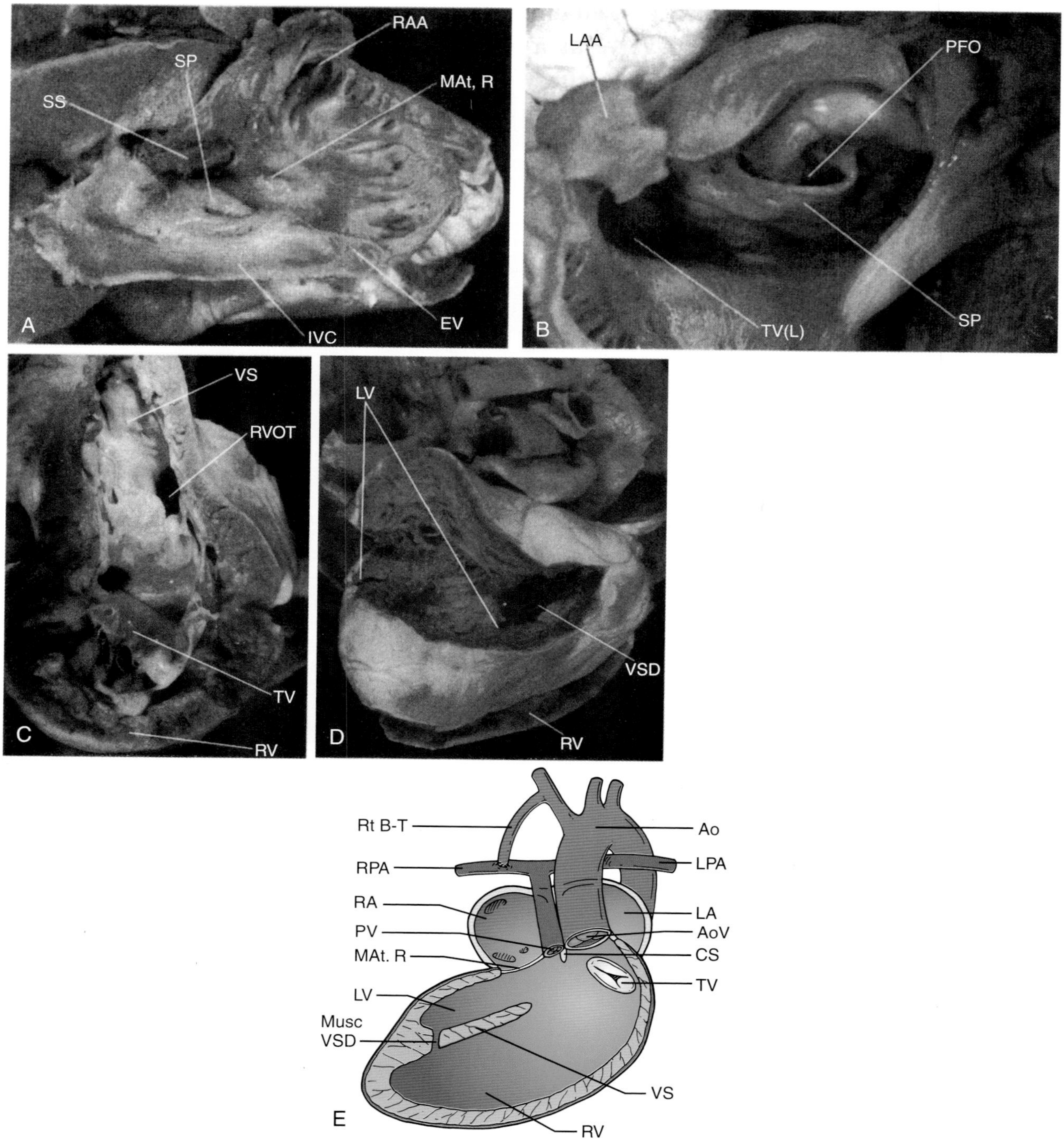

Fig. 18.12 (A) The opened right atrium reveals right-sided mitral atresia *(MAt, R)*, the inferior vena cava *(IVC)*, the Eustachian valve *(EV)* of the IVC, septum primum *(SP)*, septum secundum *(SS)*, and the right atrial appendage *(RAA)*. (B) The opened left atrium *(LA)* shows a patent foramen ovale *(PFO)* with a thickened and muscularized SP, and a left-sided tricuspid valve *(TV[L])*. There is a prominent left atrial jet lesion above the TV, indicating tricuspid regurgitation. (C) The opened inferior right ventricle *(RV)*, which is hypertrophied and enlarged, the regurgitant tricuspid valve *(TV)*, the ventricular septum *(VS)*, and the right ventricular outflow tract *(RVOT)* leading to both great arteries. (D) The opened superior LV showing the ventral septal defect *(VSD)* and the inferior RV. (E) Diagram showing DORV {S,L,L} with right-sided mitral atresia, left-sided regurgitant TV, hypoplastic superior left ventricle *(LV)*, hypertrophied and enlarged inferior RV, a unique form of superoinferior ventricles (superior LV and inferior RV), a large infundibuloventricular type of VSD, marked hypoplasia of the conal (infundibular) septum *(CS)*, approximately a 90-degree angulation between the planes of the CS and the VS, a unicommissural and severely stenotic pulmonary valvar *(PV)* stenosis, and a right-sided Blalock-Taussig anastomosis *(Rt B-T)*. There was a muscular VSD at the base of the muscular VS. A bilateral (subaortic and subpulmonary) infundibulum was present. Both coronary ostia were eccentric, that is,

(Fig. 18.12 cont'd) abnormally close to aortic valvar commissures (see the aortic annulus, with a magnifying glass if necessary). The right-sided coronary ostium was just to the right of and posterior to the aortic septal commissure. The left-sided aortic ostium was just to the left of, and slightly anterior to, the left septal–nonseptal aortic commissure. We thought that the eccentric coronary ostia were not clinically significant. *Ao,* Aorta; *AoV,* aortic valve; *LAA,* left atrial appendage; *LPA,* left pulmonary artery; *Musc VSD,* muscular ventral septal defect; *RA,* right atrium; *RPA,* right pulmonary artery. (Reproduced with permission from Porras D, Kratz C, Loukas M, van Doesburg NH, Davignon A, Van Praagh R. Superoinferior ventricles with superior left ventricle and inferior right ventricle: a newly recognized form of congenital heart disease. *Pediatr Cardiol.* 2003;24:604.)

Single LV with an infundibular outlet chamber appears to be closely related to the common type of SI ventricles with a superior hypoplastic right ventricular sinus. Single LV has absence of the right ventricular sinus (not just hypoplasia of the right ventricular sinus). When the right ventricular sinus is absent (in single LV), the appearance of a horizontal VS with SI ventricles does not occur. But when a hyperplastic right ventricular sinus is present, the appearance of SI ventricles occurs.

Animals such as fish that normally have only one ventricle, such as sharks, have hearts at the straight tube stage: single ventricle below, and conus arteriosus above.[5] Biologists often describe such hearts as having four chambers: sinus venosus, atrium, ventricle, and conus arteriosus.

It is enlightening to appreciate that animals that normally have two ventricles, such as the higher reptiles (crocodiles and alligators), birds, and mammals, have *looped* ventricular hearts (D-loops or L-loops), not *straight* tubular hearts. Again, **it is the evolution and the development of the morphologically RV that creates the ventricular loop (D- or L-).**

Human single LV with an infundibular outlet chamber closely resembles the normal fish heart with a single ventricle below and a conus arteriosus above.

SI ventricles with a large inferior LV, a small superior RV, and a horizontal VS resembles the early stage in the evolution and development of a biventricular heart. A small morphologically RV is present superiorly, but it has not as yet enlarged and descended on the right side to lie beside the much older systemic ventricle of our phylum Chordata, thereby forming a ventricular loop. This is how the lung pump became the morphologically RV and the systemic pump became the morphologically LV—because of D-loop formation. The human anomaly of SI ventricles is an interesting glimpse into how the fish heart would eventually become our heart, over some 500 million years, from the Ordovician period to about 200,000 years ago when modern humans are now thought to have evolved. Although the timing of our evolution is still the subject of research, there is now no doubt that we are recently evolved. We are "modern."[3,5,6]

D-loop formation explains why the coarsely trabeculated pulmonary ventricle typically is the *RV* and why the finely trabeculated systemic ventricle typically is the *LV*. But what does *ventricle* really mean? What is its etymology? *Venter* is Latin for "belly." *Ventriculus,* the diminutive of *venter,* means "little belly." *Ventricle* came into Middle English from Old French, from Latin *ventriculus*. French has had a major impact on English, thanks in no small part to a Norman duke, William, who invaded England in 1066 and defeated Harold of Wessex at the Battle of Hastings. Before the year was out, William the Conqueror had been proclaimed King of England. Historians typically describe this event as the Norman Conquest of England, which is correct. But it is also helpful to understand that the Normans were French-speaking Scandinavians. The Normans were *les homes du nord, les Normands (Northmann),* Scandinavian. So *ventricle* comes to us from Latin, via French (one form of modern Latin), and delivered by French-speaking Scandinavians.

REFERENCES

1. Van Praagh S, LaCorte M, Fellows KE. Supero-inferior ventricles: anatomic and angiocardiographic findings in ten post-mortem cases. In: Van Praagh R, Takao A, eds. *Etiology and Morphogenesis of Congenital Heart Disease*. New York: Futura Publishing Co; 1980:317. Mount Kisco.
2. Porras D, Kratz C, Loukas M, van Doesburg NH, Davignon A, Van Praagh R. Superoinferior ventricles with superior left ventricle and inferior right ventricle: a newly recognized form of congenital heart disease. *Pediatr Cardiol.* 2003;24:604.
3. Van Praagh R. What determines whether the great arteries are normally or abnormally related? *Am J Cardiol.* 2016;118:1390.
4. Van Praagh R. Definition of conotruncal anomalies. In: Lacour-Gayet F, Bove EL, Hraška V, Morell VO, Spray TL, eds. *Surgery of Conotruncal Anomalies*. Springer International Publishing; 2016:1.
5. Robb JS. The heart in chordates. In: *Comparative Basic Cardiology*. 1965:41.
6. Van Praagh R. Chapter 106: Segmental anatomy. In: Sellke FW, del Nido PJ, Swanson SJ, eds. *Sabiston & Spencer. Surgery of the Chest*. 8th ed. Philadelphia: Saunders Elsevier; 2010:1651.

19

Anomalous Infundibular Muscle Bundles

Also Known as Anomalous Muscle Bundles of the Right Ventricle and as Double-Chambered Right Ventricle

What are anomalous muscle bundles of the right ventricle, also known as double-chambered right ventricle?

As will be seen, these malformations really are **anomalous infundibular muscle bundles.**

STATISTICS

In the Congenital Cardiac Pathology Database of Boston Children's Hospital, the diagnosis of anomalous muscle bundles of the right ventricle was made in 33 postmortem patients.

The diagnosis of double-chambered right ventricle was made in 17 of our postmortem congenital heart patients.

These two diagnoses were made in a total of 50 of 3216 autopsied patients with congenital heart disease (1.55%).

Gender: males, 9; females, 10; males/females, 0.9. The gender was not known by us in one consultation. No gender predominance was found.

Age at death: mean, 5.2 years; standard deviation, ±13.1 years; minimum, 1 day; maximum, 55 years. The age at death was not known by us in one consultation.

TERMINOLOGY

I have used the terminology of Lev, Edwards, and the American school. But other designations are used by some of our friends and colleagues. Hence, a few words of explanation are given here to facilitate widespread comprehension.

When introduced, *trabecula septomarginalis* meant the moderator band: *trabecula* (little beam) *septomarginalis* (from the septum to the acute margin of the right ventricle). But since *trabecula septomarginalis* is Latin, some of our colleagues translated it into English: *septomarginal trabeculation*. We think that's fine; we have no quarrel with English.

But the problem is: the meaning of this term has changed. Now, some of our colleagues use *septomarginal trabeculation* to mean both septal band and moderator band.

As will be seen, in dealing with anomalous muscle bundles of the right ventricle, it is helpful to be able to designate the *septal band* and the *moderator band* separately and clearly, and to avoid the confusion in usage that has now occurred to the meaning of septomarginal trabeculation.

FINDINGS

The normal morphologically and segmentally right ventricle (Fig. 19.1A) and left ventricle (Fig. 19.1B) are presented diagrammatically in this figure.

A random sample of 20 autopsied cases of anomalous muscle bundles (AMB) of the right ventricle (RV) revealed the following:

We did not encounter a case of AMB of the right RV in which this anomaly occurred as an isolated malformation; it was always associated with other anomalies.

AMB of the RV can be associated not only with malformation of the *proximal* infundibulum, that is, **the obstructive moderator band type** (Fig. 19.1A). It can also be associated with malformation of the *distal* infundibulum, that is, **the obstructive parietal band type** (Fig. 19.1A).

C83-162 was a 2½-year-old boy with **double-outlet right ventricle (DORV) {S,D,D}.** He had an incomplete bilateral conus, that is, a complete subpulmonary conus, and an incomplete subaortic conus. There was a "tongue" of fibrous tissue between the aortic valve and the tricuspid valve. The left ventricular pressure measured at cardiac catheterization was 132/13 mm Hg, which was 46 mm Hg suprasystemic. The ventricular septal defect (VSD) was obstructive. Inferior atrioventricular endocardial cushion tissue produced the obstruction. The VSD was of the atrioventricular endocardial cushion type. The pulmonary outflow tract was also stenotic; the pulmonary outflow tract gradient was 40 mm Hg and the pulmonary artery pressure was 41/28 mm Hg, with a mean pulmonary arterial pressure of 32 mm Hg. Thus, despite the pulmonary outflow tract stenosis, there was mild pulmonary arterial hypertension.

In this patient, anomalous *distal* infundibular muscle bundles of the parietal band type (component 4, Fig. 19.1A) separated the RV sinus (component 2, Fig. 19.1A) from the infundibular outflow tract (components 3 and 4, Fig. 19.1A).

In this study of 20 autopsied cases of AMB of the RV, this was the only case in which *the distal, subarterial, parietal band part of the infundibulum (component 4, Fig. 19.1A) was involved (5%).* In all other patients (95%), it was the proximal part of the infundibulum—the septal band and the moderator band—that was involved.

In this patient, there were three sites of obstruction:

1. at the VSD, obstructing the left ventricle (LV) outflow tract;
2. between the RV sinus and the infundibulum, caused by the distal infundibular muscle bundles—the parietal band type of AMB of the RV; and
3. the pulmonary outflow tract.

It will be recalled that this patient had DORV {S,D,D} with a bilateral conus (subaortic and subpulmonary), but that the muscular subaortic conus was incomplete, with a "tongue" of fibrous tissue connecting the aortic and tricuspid valves. We think that this conal anatomy represents an early stage in the normal demuscularization or involution of the subaortic infundibular free wall musculature, known as apoptosis. Normally, demuscularization or involution of the subaortic infundibular free wall happens more extensively, permitting normal aortic-mitral and aortic-tricuspid fibrous continuity with normally related great arteries.

DORV was present in 3 of these 20 patients with AMB of the RV (15%).

C89-176 was another fascinating patient with AMB of the RV and DORV.[1] This patient had DORV {S,D,D} and a subpulmonary infundibulum. There was no subaortic infundibular

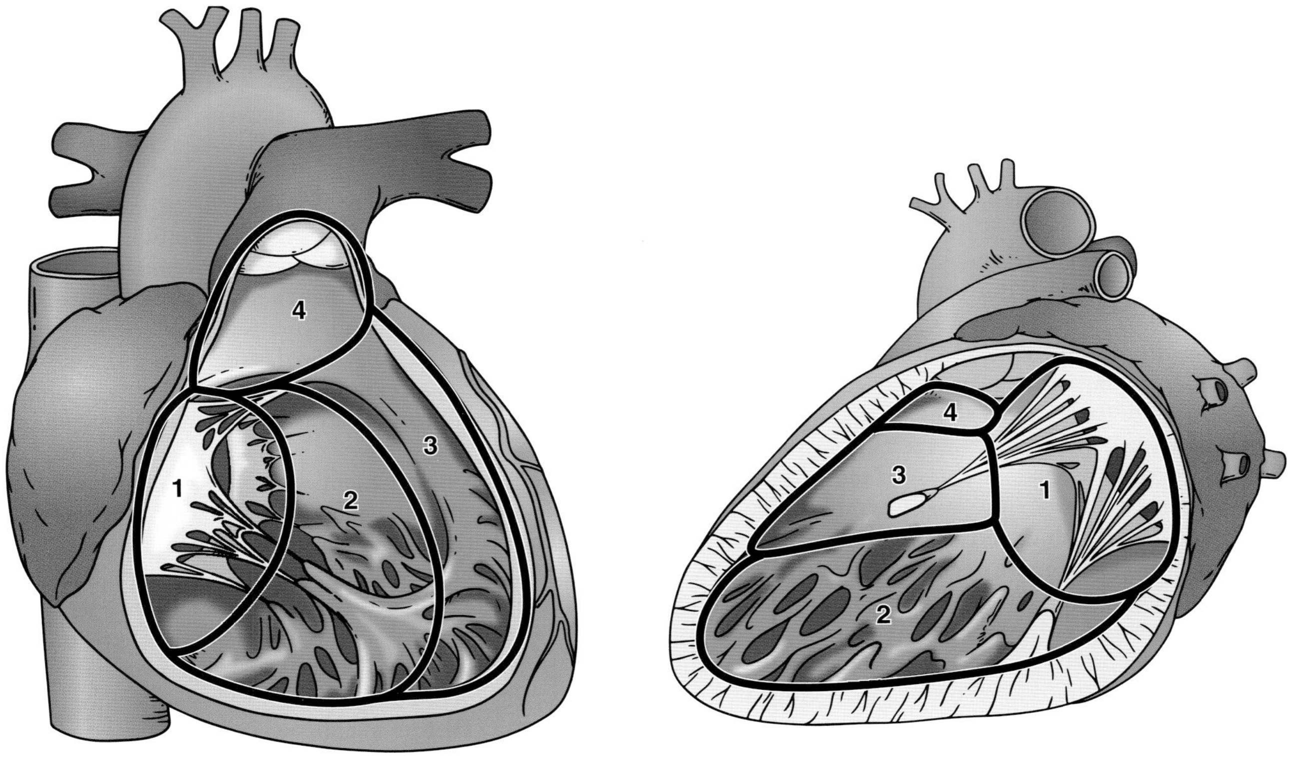

A B

Fig. 19.1 (A) Normal morphologically right ventricle (RV). (B) Normal morphologically left ventricle (LV). The four anatomic and developmental components that make up each ventricle: *1,* the atrioventricular canal or junction; *2,* the ventricular sinuses, inflow tracts, main pumping portions; *3,* the septal band in RV, continuous with the small low moderator band (unlabeled), leading to the anterior papillary muscle of the RV. The septal band and the moderator band are the inferior, or proximal or apical part of the infundibulum (conus arteriosus). In the LV, component 3 is the superior nontrabeculated portion of the ventricular septum that is continuous with component 3 in the RV and is considered to represent the proximal infundibulum. Component *4* is the superior, distal, subarterial part of the infundibulum in both RV and LV. The most common type of anomalous muscle bundles of the RV is a high or "fetal" takeoff of a prominent moderator band from the septal band. This can create a wall between the RV sinus (component 2) behind the moderator band, and the infundibular apical recess (component 3) in front of the abnormally high and prominent moderator band, resulting in stenosis of the proximal infundibular ostium—between component 2 and component 3. If the infundibular septum (component 4) is abnormally located, too close above the high moderator band, then this approximation of the high moderator band below and the malaligned infundibular septum above can together greatly narrow the outflow tract from the RV sinus (component 2) into the inferior infundibulum (component 3). Infundibular septal malalignment is common with tetralogy of Fallot, double-outlet right ventricle, and D-transposition of the great arteries (Table 19.1). (Reproduced with permission from Van Praagh R, Geva T, Kreutzer J. Ventricular septal defects: how shall we describe, name, and classify them? *J Am Coll Cardiol* 1989;14:1298.[7])

free wall, which permitted aortic valve–to–tricuspid valve direct fibrous continuity.

This heart was like the original Taussig-Bing heart,[2,3] except that there was no subaortic infundibular free wall in the present AMB case. The VSD was subpulmonary. The double-chambered RV (DCRV) muscle bundles between the RV sinus to the right and the infundibulum to the left were very restrictive. The proximal os infundibuli had one slit-like opening and two barely probe patent ostia. There was subaortic stenosis between the infundibular septum anteriorly and the tricuspid leaflets posteriorly. In other words, the infundibular septum was much too close to the tricuspid valve, producing significant subaortic outflow tract stenosis. The result was hypoplasia of the ascending aorta, tubular hypoplasia of the aortic arch, and a juxtaductal coarctation of the aorta. Thus, DCRV was part of complex congenital heart disease.

Tetralogy of Fallot (TOF) occurred in 4 of these 20 patients (20%) with AMB of the RV. Three patients had the usual solitus segmental anatomy, {S,D,S}. But one patient had inverted TOF with inverted segmental anatomy, {I,L,I}, and also with dextrocardia. All had a high takeoff of the moderator band from the septal band, that is, the proximal infundibular or moderator band type of AMB of the RV (Fig. 19.1A).

Multiple congenital anomalies occurred in 4 patients with AMB of the RV (20%), three of which were noteworthy: the polysplenia syndrome in 1, trisomy 13 in 1 patient with TOF {S,D,S}, and parachute mitral valve with no congenital mitral stenosis in 1.

Congenital absence of tricuspid valve leaflets, also known as congenitally unguarded tricuspid orifice, occurred in one patient with AMB of the RV (5%).

C73-311, a 4-week-old girl with normal segmental anatomy, that is, {S,D,S}, had congenital absence of the tricuspid valve leaflets, hypoplasia of the RV sinus, and Uhl's disease of the RV sinus free wall. The RV sinus did not communicate with the infundibulum. This is a rare case of double-chambered RV with complete separation of the RV sinus and the proximal infundibular chamber. In other words, there is *atresia of the proximal os infundibuli pulmonalis* (atresia of the proximal ostium leading into the subpulmonary infundibulum).

There was aortic-mitral fibrous continuity, and the left ventricular–to–aortic outflow tract was normal.

There was no right ventricular–to–pulmonary artery outflow tract, as above. But there was an outflow tract from the LV, through the subaortic VSD, into the subpulmonary infundibulum and through a normal appearing pulmonary valve. The main pulmonary artery and branches were mildly hypoplastic.

The functional part of this heart was similar to a Holmes heart:[4] a single LV {S,D,S}. The differences are as follows: the RV sinus has appeared, but the tricuspid leaflets have not appeared; the RV free wall myocardium is absent or very deficient (Uhl's disease); and the RV sinus does not communicate with the *proximal* part of the infundibulum, which was not identified (absent). The LV opens into the *distal* or subarterial part of the infundibulum, as it does in single LV with an infundibular outlet chamber and normally related great arteries {S,D,S}—the Holmes heart.[4]

These observations suggest that more attention needs to be focused on anomalies of the *proximal* part of the infundibulum, which is often malformed in AMB of the RV. The *distal* part of the infundibulum is involved in abnormally related great arteries.[5]

A79-105, a 3-month-old girl, had **congenital absence of the pulmonary valve leaflets.** She had pulmonary annular stenosis. She had marked dilation of the main pulmonary artery, right pulmonary artery, and left pulmonary artery. There was associated anterior flattening of the trachea and bronchi. She also had a VSD of the infundibuloventral type that was subaortic in location. Her anomalous muscle bundle of the right ventricle was a high takeoff of a prominent moderator band from the septal band.

This patient did *not* have TOF. This negative finding is mentioned specifically because absence of pulmonary leaflets has been associated with TOF. Rarely, we have seen absence of pulmonary valve leaflets in TGA {S,D,S}.

Pulmonary atresia with intact ventricular septum occurred in two patients (A71-60 and A70-6). Extremely severe pulmonary valvar stenosis with an intact ventricular septum occurred in one additional patient (A82-61). All three cases had high, prominent moderator bands.

Truncus arteriosus type A2[6] occurred in a 7-day-old girl (A88-44). Type A means that a VSD is present. Type 2 means that there is no aortopulmonary septal remnant present. AMB of the RV was present, namely, a high takeoff of the moderator band from the septal band. This patient also had a completely common atrioventricular canal, type A of Rastelli, an interrupted inferior vena cava, a small right ventricle, a thick myxomatous bicuspid truncal valve, and absence of the right superior vena cava.

In addition, this patient with truncus arteriosus also had *multiple congenital anomalies with a normal karyotype:* dysmorphic facies with a broad flat nasal bridge, right microtia, right hemifacial microsomia, anteverted nares, retrognathia, pectus excavatum, short sternum, webbed neck, two-vessel umbilical cord, 13 ribs bilaterally, bifid upper thoracic vertebrae, umbilical hernia, clinodactyly, and hypoplasia of the left lobe of the thymus.

TGA {S,D,D} with a large muscular VSD and a patent ductus arteriosus were found in a 4-month-old girl (A90-137). This patient had typical AMB of the RV, namely, a high takeoff of the moderator band from the septal band. There was hypoplasia of the aortic arch and aortic isthmus. Was this aortic hypoplasia secondary to her AMB of the RV? We were not sure.

Severe aortic valvar stenosis was found in a 55-year-old man (MR 15). He had a congenitally bicuspid aortic valve with marked underdevelopment of the right coronary–left coronary commissure. He also had typical AMB of the RV with a high takeoff of the moderator band from the septal band. We thought that his right ventricular AMB was of no clinical importance.

DISCUSSION

Accurately speaking, anomalous muscle bundles of the right ventricle is really anomalous muscle bundles of the infundibulum.

There are two main anatomic types:

1. anomalous muscles of the inferior infundibulum, involving a high takeoff of the moderator band from the septal band (Fig. 19.1A); and
2. anomalous muscle bundles of the superior infundibulum, involving the distal conal septum and the parietal band (Fig. 19.1A).

In a patient with solitus or D-loop ventricles, anomalous infundibular muscles, both inferiorly and superiorly, tend to separate the right ventricular sinus (component 2) from the outflow tract (components 3 and 4) (Fig. 19.1A). Consequently, anomalous infundibular muscle bundles at the junction of the RV sinus (component 2) and the proximal infundibulum (component 3) and the distal infundibulum (component 4) can produce stenosis or rarely atresia at these component junctions (Fig. 19.1A). The result can be obstruction at approximately the mid-RV, halfway between the tricuspid valve and the semilunar valve, creating the appearance of a double-chambered RV.

TABLE 19.1 Types of Congenital Heart Disease Associated With Anomalous Muscle Bundles of the Right Ventricle (n = 20)

Anomaly	No. of Patients	% of Series
1. Tetralogy of Fallot	4	20
2. Double-outlet RV	3	15
3. Pulmonary atresia with IVS	2	10
4. Extreme PS with IVS	1	5
5. Aortic stenosis, valvar	1	5
6. TGA {S,D,D}	1	5
7. Truncus arteriosus	1	5
8. Absence of TV leaflets	1	5
9. VSD with valvar PS	1	5
10. Absence of PV leaflets	1	5
11. Multiple congenital anomalies	4	20

IVS, Intact ventricular septum; *PS*, pulmonary stenosis; *RV*, morphologically right ventricle; *TGA {S,D,D}*, transposition of the great arteries with solitus atria, D-loop (solitus) ventricles, and D-transposition; *TV*, tricuspid valve; *VSD*, ventricular septal defect.

CONCLUSIONS

The salient findings of this study are as follows:

1. Anomalous muscle bundles of the right ventricle are really anomalous muscle bundles of the infundibulum.
2. The inferior infundibulum (septal and moderator bands), the superior infundibulum (the infundibular septum and the parietal band), or both, may be involved in anomalous muscle bundles of the right ventricle.
3. Anomalous muscle bundles of the right ventricle usually involves the inferior infundibulum, typically resulting in a high takeoff of the moderator band from the septal band (95% in this study). Involvement of the distal or subarterial infundibulum (the parietal band type) was infrequent (5%).
4. The physiologic consequences of anomalous muscle bundles of the right ventricle were variable. They could result in stenosis in approximately the mid-RV, or rarely in atresia, or occasionally in no demonstrable obstruction.
5. The obstruction, whether demonstrable or not, typically occurs at the junction of the right ventricular sinus (component 2) and the proximal infundibulum (component 3) (Fig. 19.1A). Typically, anomalous muscle bundles of the RV may produce stenosis at the proximal ostium of the infundibulum.
6. We did not encounter anomalous muscle bundles of the right ventricle as an isolated anomaly.
7. Anomalous muscle bundles of the right ventricle typically occurs with many different anatomic types of congenital heart disease, and with multiple noncardiovascular malformations (Table 19.1).

REFERENCES

1. Alday L, Wagner HR, Vlad P, Paul MH, Van Praagh R. Right ventricular aorta and biventricular pulmonary artery: new entity with aortic-tricuspid fibrous continuity. *Circulation*. 1969:39–40. supplement III-34.
2. Taussig HB, Bing RJ. Complete transposition of aorta and levoposition of pulmonary artery. *Am Heart J*. 1949;37:551.
3. Van Praagh R. What is the Taussign-Bing malformation? *Circulation*. 1968;38:445.
4. Dobell ARC, Van Praagh R. The Holmes heart: historical associations and pathologic anatomy. *Am Heart J*. 1996;132:437.
5. Van Praagh R. What determines whether the great arteries are normally or abnormally related? *Am J Cardiol*. 2016;118:1390.
6. Van Praagh R, Van Praagh S. The anatomy of common aorticopulmonary trunk (truncusarteriosus communis) and its embryologic implications, a study of 57 necropsied cases. *Am J Cardiol*. 1965;16:406.
7. Van Praagh R, Geva T, Kreutzer J. Ventricular septal defects: how shall we describe, name, and classify them? *J Am Coll Cardiol*. 1989;14:1298.

20

Tetralogy of Fallot

The anomaly now known as the tetralogy of Fallot (TOF) was first described, insofar as is known, by **Niels Stensen** in 1671.[1] He was also known in Latin as Nicolaus Steno.

Stensen (1638–1686) was a Danish anatomist and naturalist from Copenhagen. He is said to have given up his medical career for the church, becoming the Bishop of Titiopolis in 1667. However, he remained a devoted anatomist. Four years later, in 1671, he published the first known case of tetralogy.[1] His other famous paper about the anatomy and function of the parotid duct—**Stensen's duct**—did not appear until 1682. He also described the principles leading to the formation of the Earth's crust and the occurrence of fossils. Thus, Stensen was a bishop and an anatomist, with the expertise and the wide-ranging interests of a 17th-century naturalist.

Stensen's Case.[1,2] Stensen's patient was a malformed fetus. The gestational age was neither stated nor estimated. The salient findings were as follows: a cleft palate; right-sided hare lip; all fingers of the left hand were united by a common skin fold; the third finger of the left hand was shortest; the left thumb was free—not united with the left fingers; the sternum was split; the heart, liver, spleen, right kidney, and most of the intestines were outside of the thorax and abdomen; these organs were uncovered; the lungs were in the thorax; the kidneys were lobulated; and the adrenals were large and triangular.

Thus, this fetus had ectopia cordis, thoracic and abdominal—with ectopy of much more than the heart. The diaphragm and the brain were not described.

Regarding the heart, the pulmonary artery was much narrower than the aorta. The ductus arteriosus was absent. There was a subaortic ventricular septal defect (VSD) and an overriding aorta.

I think that this fetus with multiple congenital anomalies including ectopia cordis probably did have what we now call tetralogy of Fallot with pulmonary outflow tract atresia.

EARLY PRE-FALLOT REPORTS

Edouard Sandifort (1742–1814), a Dutch physician, described a patient with tetralogy in 1777.[3] Known as "the blue boy," this patient died at 12 4⁄12 years of age. Clinically, he had been thought to have asthma. However, his parents suggested an autopsy, which revealed a congenitally malformed heart. The heart description sounded like tetralogy. Again there was no ductus arteriosus or ligamentum arteriosum. Sandifort thought that the congenital heart malformation of the blue boy[3] resembled that of Stensen's patient.[1,2]

William Hunter (1718–1783) was the elder brother of his more famous young brother John, who was an eminent surgeon. William Hunter was a Scottish physician from the University of Glasgow, who moved to London where he became a leading obstetrician and obstetrical anatomist. In 1784, three cases of congenital heart disease were published 1 year following the author's death. Hunter's Case 2 was a 13-year-old boy with tetralogy and blue spells.[4]

Numerous other case reports followed over the next century.[5-13] (The references cited are not a complete list.)

What, then, was so special about the serialized reports of Etienne-Louis Arthur Fallot (Fig. 20.1) in *Marseille Médical* of 1888? Parenthetically, his friends called him Arthur, which is how he signed his published work.[14] Just listen to a literal translation of his first sentence:[14,15]

> *One of the happy hazards which comes sometimes to procure for the clinician precious occasions to instruct himself, has in the space of several years, made to pass beneath our eyes three cases of a rare and curious malady, on the pathologic anatomy of which reigns, even in the informed medical public, grave errors and singular incertitudes, we have had the occasion to observe during their life and at autopsy following their death, three subjects afflicted with the malady called cardiac cyanosis, and it would be according to us, much more correct to designate exclusively under the name of the blue malady.*

In Fallot's late-19th-century prose, I hear similarities with the elegance and charm of Charles Dickens and Sir Arthur Conan Doyle.

But there was much more to Fallot than elegance and charm. There was also substance and clinical relevance.

He described **the tetralogy,** the four anatomic features that occurred together in his three patients:

1. pulmonary outflow tract obstruction, stenosis, or atresia;
2. a subaortic VSD;
3. aortic overriding; and
4. right ventricular hypertrophy.

He emphasized that cyanosis was not caused by a patent foramen ovale, as many had supposed.

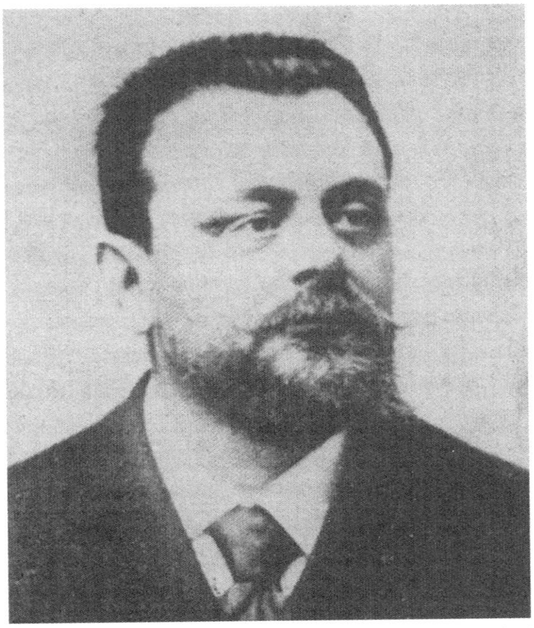

Fig. 20.1 Etienne-Louis Arthur Fallot (1850–1911) realized that four anatomic anomalies are interrelated and form one entity, that together cause cyanotic congenital heart disease. These four interrelated malformations that occur together in a nonrandom way are (1) pulmonary outflow tract obstruction (stenosis or atresia), (2) ventricular septal defect, (3) aortic overriding, and (4) right ventricular hypertrophy. Thus, Fallot made two discoveries: (1) *anatomic,* understanding the anatomic tetralogy; and (2) *physiologic,* realizing that the anatomic tetralogy physiologically caused cyanosis (and that isolated patent foramen ovale was not the cause of cyanosis, as many observers thought at that time). (Reprinted with permission from Van Praagh R. Etienne-Louis Arthur Fallot and his tetralogy: a new translation of Fallot's summary and a modern reassessment of this anomaly. *Eur J Cardiothorac Surg* 1989;3:381–386.)

Fallot proposed that these four interrelated malformations were caused by an intrauterine pathologic process involving the pulmonary valve and the subpulmonary infundibulum. In other words, Fallot understood that one pathologic process underlay this nonrandom and interrelated tetrad of anomalies.

Fallot called this group of four malformations *la maladie bleue*[14] (the blue malady).

It was Maude Abbott[16] of Montreal, Canada who coined the term *tetralogy of Fallot* in 1924.

Thus, in 1888, Fallot understood that this tetralogy was basically just one anomaly involving the pulmonary valve and the subpulmonary infundibulum—not four unrelated malformations that occurred together only by chance.

We independently reached a very similar conclusion in 1970.[17] We proposed that the TOF results from underdevelopment of the subpulmonary infundibulum in three dimensions (Figs. 20.2 to 20.8).[18] The classical tetralogy consists of the sequelae of an underdeveloped, low-volume, and hence obstructive subpulmonary infundibulum. The pulmonary valve is the "back door" of the subpulmonary infundibulum. This helps to explain why the pulmonary valve is frequently, but not universally, involved in right ventricular outflow tract obstruction. By contrast, the subpulmonary infundibulum is always abnormal in TOF.

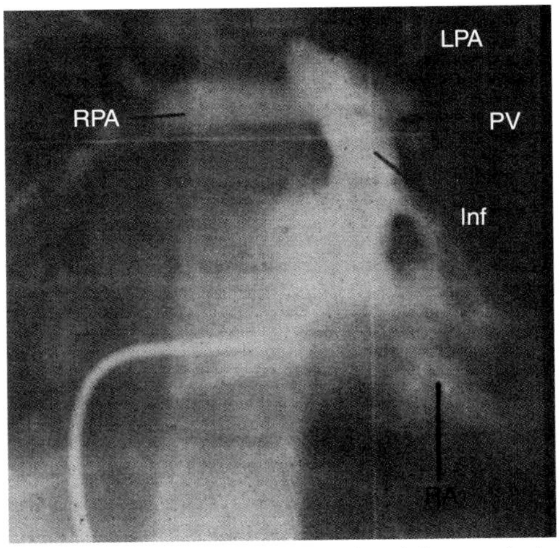

Fig. 20.2 Typical tetralogy of Fallot, selective right ventricular angiocardiogram, posteroanterior projection. The subpulmonary infundibulum *(Inf)* has a smaller volume than normal. The main pulmonary artery distal to the pulmonary valve *(PV),* the right pulmonary artery *(RPA),* and the left pulmonary artery *(LPA)* all are smaller than normal. (Reproduced with permission from Van Praagh R. The first Stella Van Praagh memorial lecture: the history and anatomy of tetralogy of Fallot, *Semin Thorac Cardiovasc Surg Ann* 2009;12:19.[18])

Hence, the tetralogy of Fallot is basically the "monology of Stensen." The tetralogy is really just one anomaly (a monology), that is, three-dimensional underdevelopment of the subpulmonary infundibulum and the sequelae thereof, that was first described by Stensen.[1]

The concept of the monology of Stensen is intended to deepen morphogenetic and anatomic understanding. We are not trying to change diagnostic terminology.

Compare the normal morphologically right ventricle (Fig. 20.9) with the right ventricle in TOF (Figs. 20.2 to 20.8). Normally, the subpulmonary infundibulum forms a conal septum (or an infundibular septum) that flows into the parietal band (Fig. 20.9). The infundibular septum and parietal band form a crista supraventricularis (or supraventricular crest) that arches over the septal band, the ventricular septum, the tricuspid valve, and the right ventricular sinus (body, or inflow tract) (Fig. 20.9). Normally, the subpulmonary infundibulum fills the space above the septal band, the ventricular sinus septum, and the tricuspid valve (Fig. 20.9).

But abnormally, when the subpulmonary infundibulum is hypoplastic in three dimensions, the space above the septal band and the ventricular septum remains wide open (Figs. 20.3 to 20.8), resulting in a subaortic VSD. The subpulmonary infundibular septum remains abnormally leftward, anterior, and superior. In other words, the subpulmonary infundibular septum fails to move normally in a rightward, posterior, and inferior direction.

This results not only in a large subaortic VSD, in a typical case. It also results in subpulmonary infundibular outflow tract obstruction because the infundibular septum, the "floor" of the infundibular outflow tract, is abnormally close to the infundibular free wall, the "roof" of the infundibular outflow tract. Hypoplasia of the subpulmonary infundibulum in three

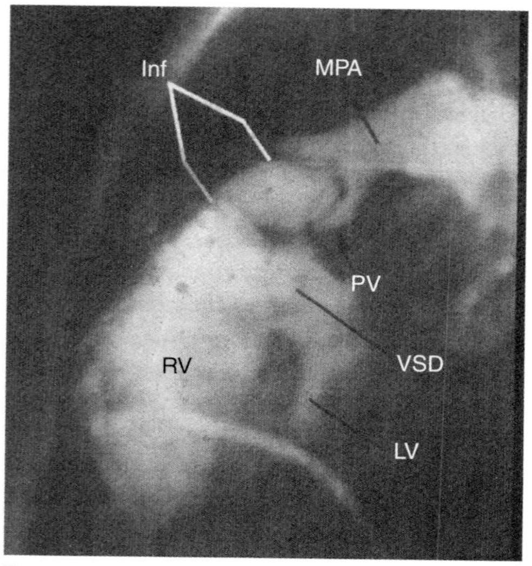

Fig. 20.3 Typical tetralogy of Fallot, selective right ventricular angiocardiogram, left lateral projection, simultaneous with Fig. 20.2. The subpulmonary infundibulum *(Inf)* has a smaller volume than normal. The infundibular septum (unlabeled) is hypoplastic and malaligned anterosuperiorly, narrowing the inlet into the infundibulum and producing subpulmonary infundibular stenosis. The pulmonary valve *(PV)* appears thickened and stenotic. The main pulmonary *(MPA)* is smaller than normal. The anterosuperior malalignment and the hypoplasia of the infundibular septum results in a large open space above the muscular ventricular septum between the right ventricle *(RV)* and the left ventricle *(LV)*. This wide-open space, this ventricular septal defect *(VSD)*, permits right-to-left shunting of contrast from the RV into the LV. This is an **infundibuloventricular type of VSD**, between the infundibular septum above and the ventricular septum below. This type of VSD is sometimes also called a **malalignment VSD** because it is caused by the malalignment and hypoplasia of the infundibular septum. Dr. Aldo Castañeda encountered cases of TOF with absence of the infundibular septum when operating as a guest surgeon in Mexico City. Since then we have referred to this infrequent subset as the "Mexican type of TOF." Infundibular septal defects are known to be more frequent in Asiatic populations than in Caucasian or Negroid populations. American "Indians" are thought to have discovered America during the last Ice Age 10,000 to 12,000 years ago, via the Bering Land Bridge, when the sea level was much lower than it is today, because so much more water was ice than pertains today. Thus, in TOF, the infundibular septum is not always of normal length. (Reproduced with permission from Van Praagh R. The first Stella Van Praagh memorial lecture: the history and anatomy of tetralogy of Fallot, *Semin Thorac Cardiovasc Surg Ann* 2009;12:19.[18])

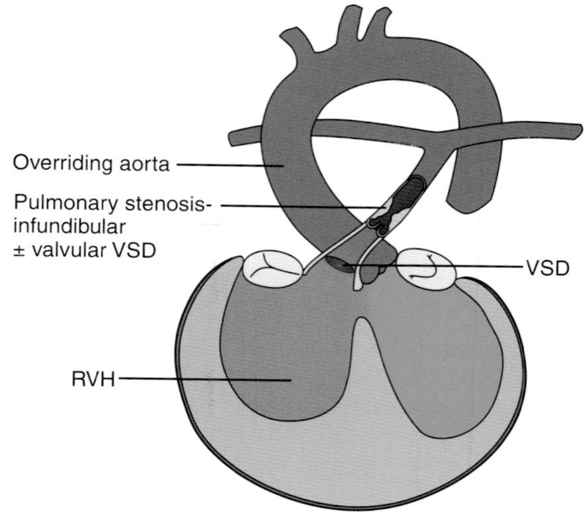

Fig. 20.4 Diagram of typical TOF characterized by (1) pulmonary outflow tract stenosis that is always infundibular, and may or may not be valvar; (2) ventricular septal defect *(VSD)*; (3) aortic overriding; and (4) right ventricular hypertrophy *(RVH)*. TOF is basically the monology of Stensen, just one malformation—a low-volume subpulmonary infundibulum first described by Stensen[1] in 1671, and three of its sequelae. (Reproduced with permission from Van Praagh R. The first Stella Van Praagh memorial lecture: the history and anatomy of tetralogy of Fallot, *Semin Thorac Cardiovasc Surg Ann* 2009;12:19.[18])

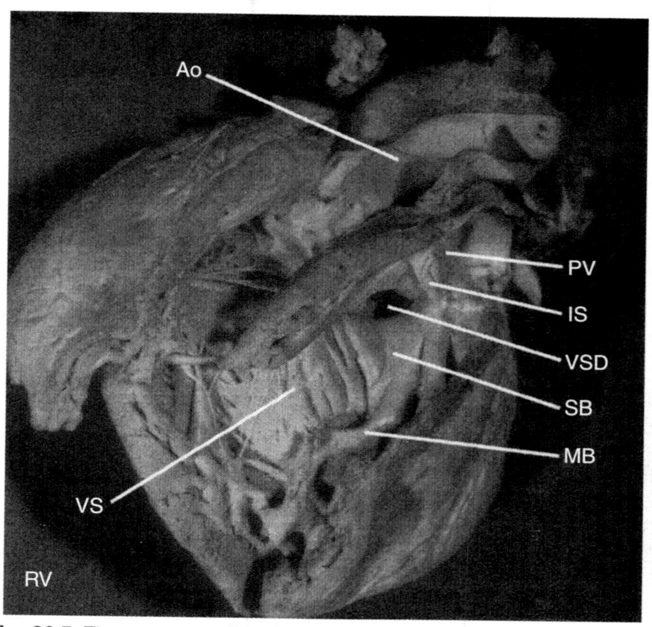

Fig. 20.5 The anatomy of typical TOF showing the opened right ventricle *(RV)* and the pulmonary outflow tract. The infundibular septum *(IS)* is hypoplastic and it intersects the left anterior division of the top of the septal band *(SB)*. The infundibular septum is malaligned anterosuperiorly, leaving a large space above the septal band and ventricular septum *(VS)* and below the aortic valve, namely, the ventricular septal defect *(VSD)*. The pulmonary valve *(PV)* is stenotic and bicuspid. The moderator band *(MB)* flows out of the bottom of the septal band. The ascending aorta *(Ao)* is enlarged. This is a view of the stenotic pulmonary outflow tract in typical TOF. (Reproduced with permission from Van Praagh R. The first Stella Van Praagh memorial lecture: the history and anatomy of tetralogy of Fallot, *Semin Thorac Cardiovasc Surg Ann* 2009;12:19.[18])

dimensions (3D) results in a low-volume and hence obstructive subpulmonary infundibulum that is either stenotic (Figs. 20.2 to 20.7) or atretic (Fig. 20.8).

The low-volume, obstructive subpulmonary infundibulum results in right-to-left shunting through the large VSD into the left ventricle and the aorta, resulting in cyanosis in untreated patients with TOF (Fig. 20.3). This is why in 1777 Sandifort's[3] patient, "the blue boy," was blue, and why in 1888, Fallot[14] wanted to call the anomaly that he was describing the blue disease ("la maladie bleue"). However, by 1924, it was clear to Abbott[16] that this tetralogy was not the only blue disease; hence Abbott's proposal: the tetralogy of Fallot. Abbott was also aware of transposition of the great arteries.

The understanding that TOF is only one malformation and its sequelae has important diagnostic and surgical consequences.

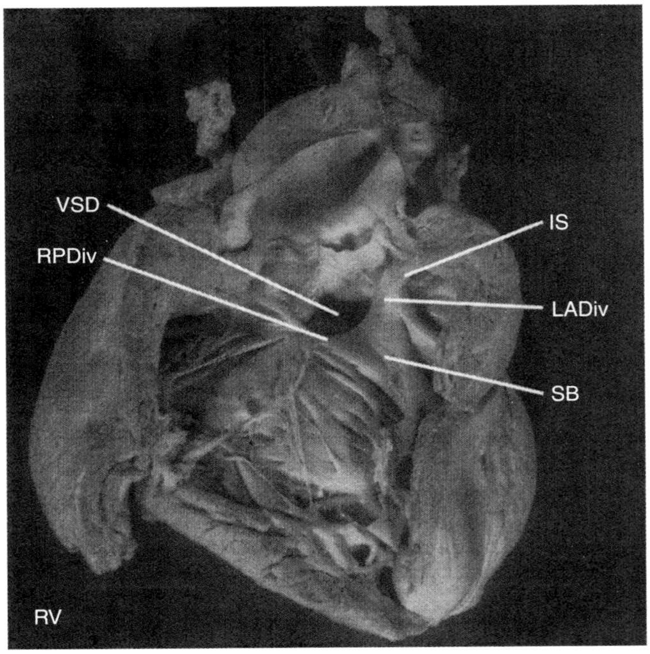

Fig. 20.6 The anatomy of typical TOF showing the aortic outflow tract from the same opened *RV* shown in Fig. 20.5. Note how hypoplastic the infundibular septum *(IS)* is. The IS intersects with the left anterior division *(LADiv)* of the "Y" of the septal band *(SB)*. The right posterior division *(RPDiv)* of the SB is also well seen. The space above the SB is wide open, forming a large subaortic ventricular septal defect *(VSD)*. The top of the SB forms the inferior rim of the VSD as seen from the RV. Normally, the IS fills the space that in TOF is the VSD. Because the RPDiv of the SB is slender, the VSD is confluent with the anterior and septal leaflets of the tricuspid valve. Hence, this VSD may be described as paramembranous or juxtamembranous, meaning "beside" or "close to" the membranous tissue of the tricuspid valve. *Para*membranous is derived from Greek, and *juxta*membranous is derived from Latin. Perimembranous VSDs do not exist. *Peri*membranous is derived from Greek, *peri* meaning around. There is no VSD that is all around the membranous septum. If there were, the membranous septum would be floating freely in space, attached to nothing. When the RPDiv of the SB is prominent and muscular (the muscle of Lancisi, also known as the muscle of Lushka), then the VSD is not confluent with the membranous tissue of the tricuspid valve. Such VSDs may be described as not paramembranous, or as not juxtamembranous. The right bundle branch of the atrioventricular conduction system enters the right ventricle just beneath the RPDiv and then runs down the SB close to its inferior margin. The right bundle branch of the conduction system then continues on to the moderator band to reach the anterior papillary muscle and the right ventricular free wall. When the muscle of Lancisi (RPDiv) is thin and delicate, as in this heart, it offers little or no protection to the underlying right bundle branch of the conduction system during surgical patch closure of the "lower angle" of the VSD. This is why many surgeons place their sutures into the membranous tricuspid tissue at this point, rather than into the ventricular septal myocardium, in order to avoid surgically induced right bundle branch block. (Reproduced with permission from Van Praagh R. The first Stella Van Praagh memorial lecture: the history and anatomy of tetralogy of Fallot, *Semin Thorac Cardiovasc Surg Ann* 2009;12:19.[18])

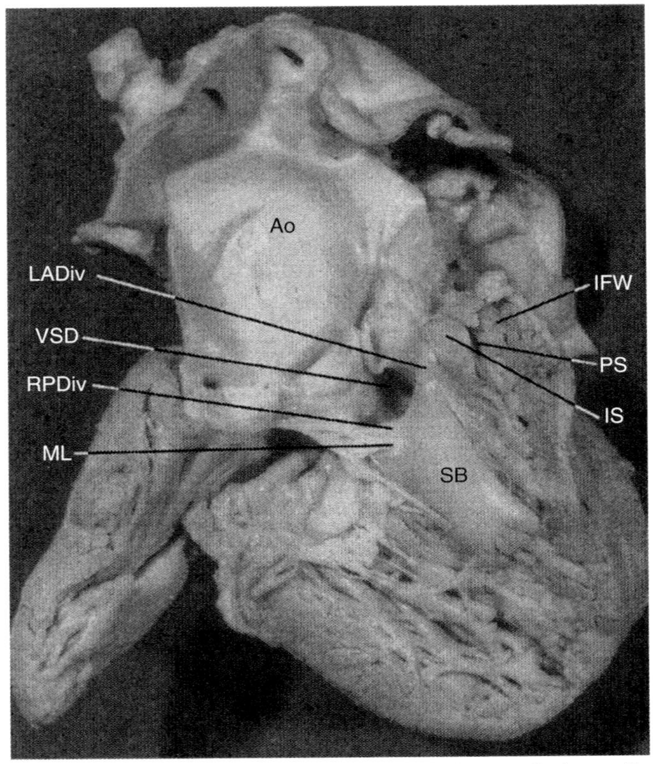

Fig. 20.7 The anatomy of TOF with severe right ventricular outflow tract stenosis. Note how close the infundibular septum *(IS)* is to the infundibular free wall *(IFW)*, greatly reducing he lumen of the subpulmonary infundibulum, resulting in severe pulmonary outflow tract stenosis *(PS)*. The infundibular septum intersects the ventricular septum anterior to the left anterior division *(LADiv)* of the septal band *(SB)*, indicating that the failure of infundibular expansile growth is even greater than that seen in Fig. 20.6. Consequently, the degree of infundibular PS is greater than that seen in Fig. 20.6. The right posterior division *(RPDiv)* of the septal band (SB) is very thin and delicate; consequently the *VSD* is paramembranous. The ascending aorta *(Ao)* is huge, indicating that it is carrying most of the right ventricular output, plus all of the left ventricular output. *ML*, Muscle of Lancisi or muscle of Lushka. (Reproduced with permission from Van Praagh R. The first Stella Van Praagh memorial lecture: the history and anatomy of tetralogy of Fallot, *Semin Thorac Cardiovasc Surg Ann* 2009;12:19.[18])

Diagnostically, it was appreciated that if a patient has a high pulmonary artery wedge pressure indicating left atrial hypertension (for example, because of cor triatriatum, or congenital mitral stenosis), it is nonetheless possible to make the diagnosis of TOF.[17] It used to be thought that if there were no demonstrable gradient on catheter pull-back from the main pulmonary artery into the right ventricle, TOF could not be present. "No pull-back gradient, no TOF" used to be a cath lab dictum. But we learned that left atrial obstruction could produce pulmonary artery hypertension that in turn could *mask* significant infundibular obstruction, that is, that could mask the coexistence of TOF.

When pulmonary hypertension coexists for any reason (congenital or acquired), how does one make the diagnosis of coexistent TOF?

The answer is almost absurdly simple: Look at the subpulmonary infundibulum (angiocardiographically, or by any accurate noninvasive technique). Is the infundibulum hypoplastic and obstructive-looking, or not?

The importance of understanding that the TOF basically is the monology of Stensen (obstructive hypoplasia of the subpulmonary infundibulum and its sequelae) is even more important surgically than diagnostically. Gone was the

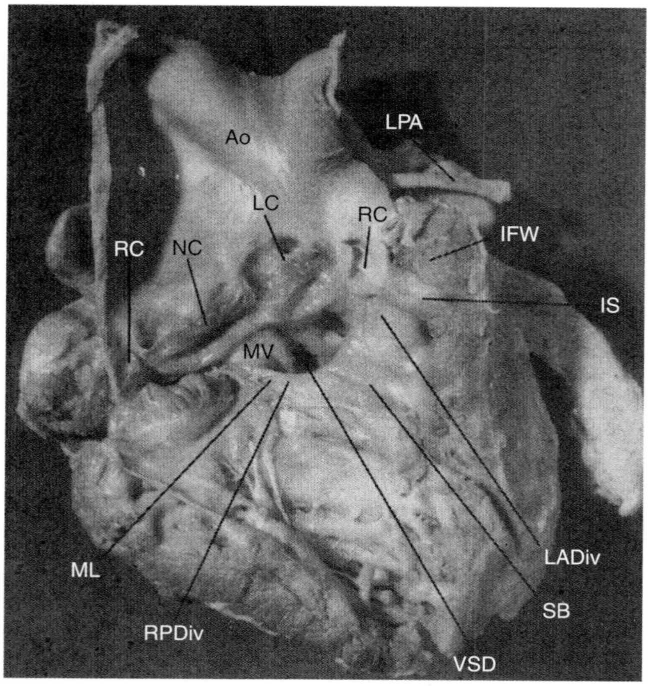

Fig. 20.8 TOF with right ventricular outflow tract atresia. The opened right ventricle reveals that the infundibular septum *(IS)* and the infundibular free wall *(IFW)* are fused. There is no patent infundibular lumen. The ventricular septal defect *(VSD)* is as big as it can be. The superior part of the septal band *(SB)* forms the inferior rim of the VSD, extending from the left anterior division *(LADiv)* of the SB anteriorly to the right posterior division *(RPDiv)* of the SB and the muscle of Lancisi posteriorly. The left pulmonary artery *(LPA)* is diminutive, whereas the ascending aorta *(Ao)* is huge. One can see the three leaflets of the overriding aortic valve: right coronary leaflet *(RC)*, left coronary leaflet *(LC)*, and noncoronary leaflet *(NC)*. One can also see the mitral valve *(MV)*. Aortic-mitral direct fibrous continuity is present, which is typical of TOF. However, the AoV-MV fibrous continuity is subnormal. This aortic-mitral continuity is mostly between the left coronary leaflet of the aortic valve and the anterior leaflet of the mitral valve. With completely normally related great arteries, the aortic-mitral continuity is between the noncoronary and the left coronary leaflets of the aortic valve approximately equally, and the anterior mitral leaflet. But in this case of TOF with severe underdevelopment of the subpulmonary infundibulum (pulmonary infundibular and pulmonary valvar atresia), the aortic-mitral fibrous continuity is mostly between the left coronary aortic leaflet and the anterior mitral leaflet because the aortic valve is mildly dextroposed (aortic overriding) and the pulmonary valve is reciprocally mildly levoposed, so TOF has *almost* normally related great arteries. If the pulmonary valve overrides above the LV, we call this *double-outlet left ventricle (DOLV) of the TOF type*—because there typically is infundibular and valvar PS, a subaortic VSD, and aortic-mitral fibrous continuity. (Reproduced with permission from Van Praagh R. The first Stella Van Praagh memorial lecture: the history and anatomy of tetralogy of Fallot, *Semin Thorac Cardiovasc Surg Ann* 2009;12:19.[18])

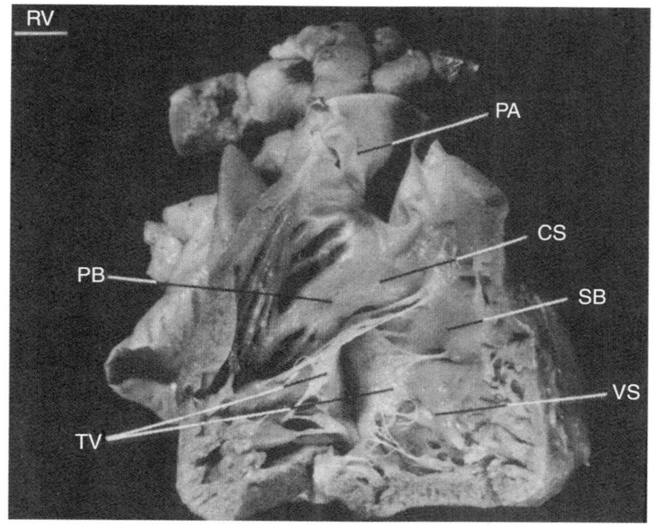

Fig. 20.9 The anatomically normal right ventricle *(RV)* reveals several major differences on comparison with TOF (Figs. 20.4 to 20.8). The space above the septal band *(SB)* normally is filled by the infundibular septum, also known as the conal septum *(CS)*. The infundibular septum normally extends out on to the right ventricular free wall as the parietal band *(PB)*. Normally, the subpulmonary infundibulum, the pulmonary valve, and the main pulmonary artery *(PA)* are well developed, well expanded, and nonobstructive. *TV*, Tricuspid valve; *VS*, ventricular septum. (Reproduced with permission from Van Praagh R. The first Stella Van Praagh memorial lecture: the history and anatomy of tetralogy of Fallot, *Semin Thorac Cardiovasc Surg Ann* 2009;12:19.[18])

old-fashioned repair of TOF. It began with a long, low, J-shaped or hockey-stick–shaped right ventriculotomy, to provide good visualization of the VSD. This was followed by extensive myocardial resection of the parietal band and of the septal band, with thinning of the right ventricular free wall. Much of this septal and free wall myocardial resection was proximal or upstream to the infundibular and valvar and pulmonary arterial obstructions. This old-fashioned surgical approach to the repair of TOF often led to low cardiac output and death postoperatively. The thinned right ventricular free wall often became a paradoxing right ventricular outflow tract aneurysm. The causes of death were right ventricular iatrogenic infarction, or unrelieved right ventricular outflow tract obstruction because of fear of transannular patches, or both.

Once the foregoing[17,18] was understood, our surgical approach was transformed and our results improved dramatically.[19] The infundibulotomy became as short as possible. Right ventricular myocardial resection was essentially abandoned altogether. Castañeda and his colleagues,[19] who led this surgical transformation, found that in young infants with TOF, there really is very little muscle to excise. If one operates early enough, secondary postnatal myocardial right ventricular hypertrophy has not as yet occurred. The use of transannular patches without myocardial resection achieved absence of right ventricular outflow tract obstruction with minimal right ventricular trauma.

With this new surgical approach,[19] we realized that TOF could be successfully repaired at any postnatal age—in the newborn period (the first 30 days), or in infancy (the first year of life).

This new therapeutic approach became known as **the Castañeda doctrine:**

1. Repair TOF whenever the patient needs it, in the newborn period if necessary.
2. One operation is better than two. Avoid palliative surgery such as Blalock-Taussig shunts, whenever possible.

HOW COMMON IS TETRALOGY OF FALLOT?

In a series of 2965 patients selected at random in the cardiac pathology database of the Cardiac Registry of Boston Children's Hospital and Harvard Medical School, there were 407 cases of TOF (14%) (Table 20.1).[18] TOF was the fifth most common type of congenital heart disease in our cardiac pathology database, right behind transposition of the great arteries (442 cases, 15%, Table 20.1).[18]

WHAT ARE THE SITUS OF THE MAIN CARDIAC SEGMENTS IN TOF?

Are the atria, the ventricles, and the great arteries always in situs solitus (i.e., normal, noninverted anatomic organizational patterns) in TOF? Almost always, but not always (Table 20.2).

In 100 randomly selected autopsied cases of TOF, the segmental anatomy was {S,D,S} in 97 cases (97%, Table 20.2), meaning that the atria were in situs solitus {**S**,-,-}, D-loop or solitus ventricles were present {S,**D**,-}, and solitus normally related great arteries {S,D,**S**} were present. The normal solitus heart is shown diagrammatically in Fig. 20.10, row 1, column 1.[20] In the normal segmental situs set, {S,D,S}, there is atrioventricular (AV) *situs concordance* (sameness), and there is ventriculoarterial (VA) *situs concordance*. AV and VA *alignment concordance* are assumed to be present (Fig. 20.10, row 1, column 1) unless it is specifically stated that this is not the case. For example, if straddling tricuspid valve or double-inlet left ventricle is present, such abnormalities of AV alignment must be stated specifically.

Thus, **TOF {S,D,S}** is the most familiar and by far the most common anatomic type of TOF, found in 97% of our series (Table 20.2).[18]

TOF in situs inversus totalis, that is, **TOF {I,L,I}**, was found in 1% of our random series (Table 20.2) (Fig. 20.10, row 1, column 3). TOF {I,L,I} means TOF with inverted atria, that is, TOF {**I**,-,-}, with L-loop or inverted ventricles, that is, TOF {I,**L**,-}, and with inverted normally related great arteries, that is, TOF {I,L,**I**}.

The least familiar anatomic type of TOF found in our unselected postmortem series of 100 cases of TOF was TOF **{I,D,S}**, in 2% (Table 20.2). Until recently, I did not know that we had ever seen this rare segmental combination (Fig. 20.10, row 2, column 4).

As the segmental anatomy indicates, this rare type of TOF occurs in patients with visceroatrial situs inversus, that is, TOF {**I**,-,-}, but with discordant D-loop or solitus ventricles, that is, TOF {I,**D**,-}, and with solitus normally related great arteries, that is, TOF {I,D,**S**}.

How absolutely fascinating! Most patients with {I,D,-} situs anatomy have D-transposition of the great arteries. Had the great arterial situs been D-, then these two patients might well have had TGA {I,D,**D**}, that is, congenital physiologically corrected TGA in situs inversus. **Why did this not happen?**

As I learned recently,[20] the type of relationship between the great arteries is determined by the subarterial infundibular situs and by the great arterial situs. **When the infundibular situs and the great arterial situs are concordant (the same), both solitus or both inversus, then the great arteries are normally related—solitus normally related or inversus normally related.**

But if the infundibular situs (pattern of anatomic organization) and the great arterial situs are discordant (different), then the great arteries are abnormally related.

In TOF {I,D,S}, the infundibuloarterial situs equation may be: **TOF {I,D,S} = 0R + 2L.** This IA situs equation says:

TOF {I,D,S} equals (=) complete resorption (0) of the right-sided (R) subaortic infundibular free wall, the aortic valve being right-sided in solitus normally related great arteries (S) and (+) with moderate underdevelopment (grade 2) of the left-sided (L) subpulmonary infundibulum. Infundibular development, right-sided and left-sided, is graded from grade 0 (absent) to grade 4 (normally well developed and expanded).

The right side of the equation is the infundibular situs "recipe" or formula for the great arteries. The left side of the equation indicates the type of relationship between the great arteries that is present.

TOF {I,D,S} (Fig. 20.10, row 2, column 4) is noteworthy because, in addition to TOF of solitus normally related great arteries, that is, **TOF** {I,D,**S**}, there is also one segmental situs discordance at the atrioventricular level, that is, TOF {**I,D**,S}. One segmental situs discordance physiologically uncorrects

TABLE 20.1 Autopsied Cases of Congenital Heart Disease: The Top 15 Anatomic Types (*n* = 2965 patients)

	No.	%
1. Ventricular septal defect	1077	36
2. Atrial septal defect, secundum	745	25
3. Patent ductus arteriosus (>2 weeks)	557	19
4. Transposition of the great arteries	442	15
5. Tetralogy of Fallot	407	14
6. Aortic stenosis	358	12
7. Coarctation of the aorta	356	12
8. Persistent left superior vena cava	345	12
9. Completely common arterioventricular canal	343	12
10. Pulmonary stenosis	304	10
11. Bicuspid aortic valve	240	8
12. Bicuspid pulmonary valve	238	8
13. Double-outlet right ventricle	233	8
14. Anomalous pulmonary venous return	223	8
15. Aortic atresia, valvar	207	7

Percentages are all rounded to the nearest whole number. This table lists 5852 congenital heart malformations that occurred in 2965 patients; many patients had more than one cardiac anomaly.

TABLE 20.2 Situs of the Main Cardiac Segments {Atria, Ventricles, Great Arteries} in Tetralogy of Fallot (*n* = 100)

{S,D,S}	97
{I,D,S}	2
{I,L,I}	1

D-loop ventricles are solitus ventricles. L-loop ventricles are inversus (inverted) ventricles. Situs is a fourth declension masculine Latin noun. The plural is situs (or sitūs).

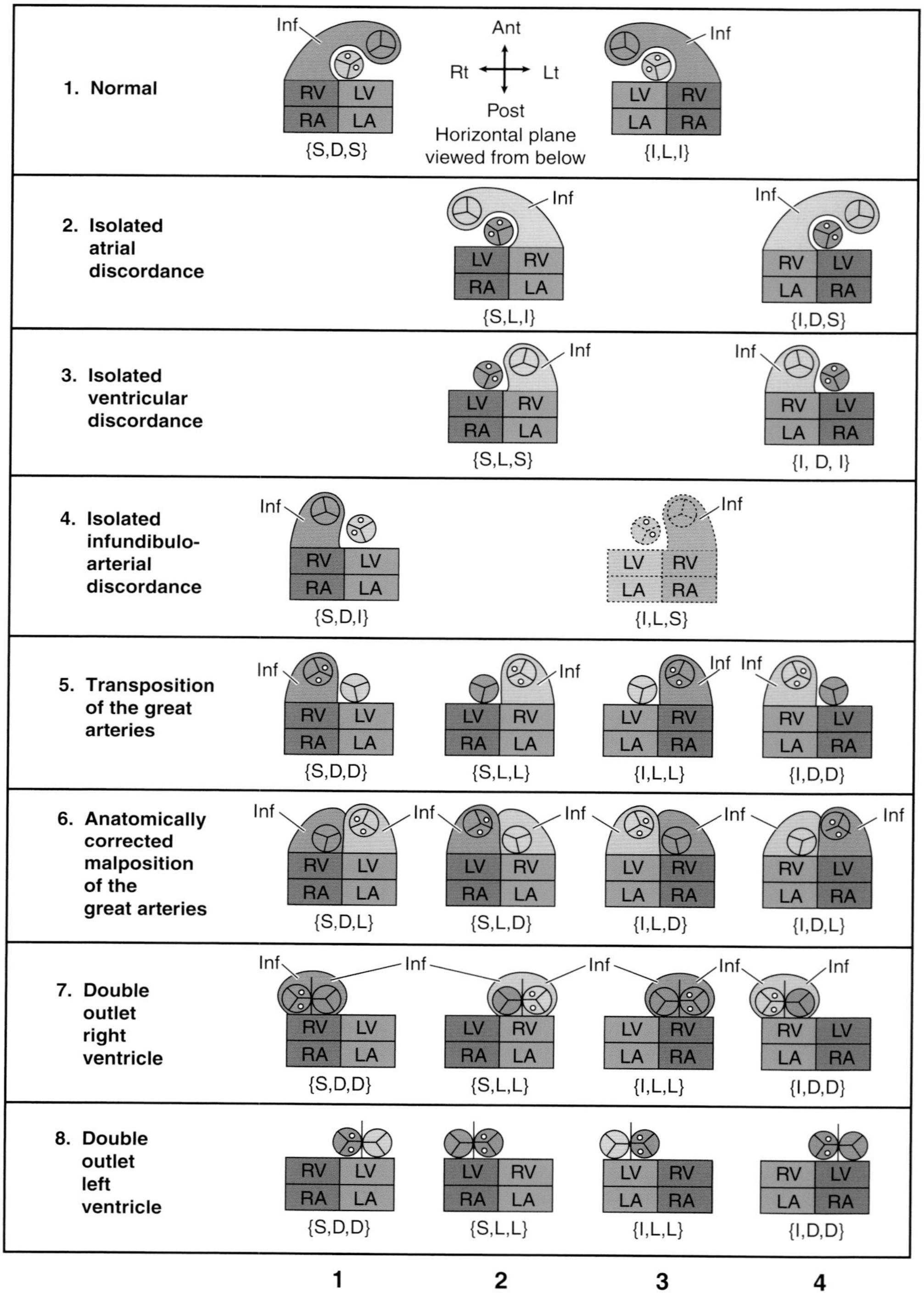

Fig. 20.10 The segmental anatomy of some forms, but not all forms, of congenital heart disease. The cardiac diagrams are viewed from below, similar to a subxiphoid two-dimensional echocardiogram. In a randomly selected series of 100 postmortem cases of TOF, three different segmental sets were found (Table 20.2): (1) TOF {S,D,S} in 97% (row 1, column 1); (2) TOF {I,D,S} in 2% (row 2, column 4); and (3) TOF {I,L,I} in 1% (row 1, column 3). Since TOF has essentially normally related great arteries (solitus and inversus), and since there are many other segmental sets with normally related great arteries, solitus and inversus (rows 1 to 4), other anatomic sets with TOF may well be discovered in the future. Normally related great arteries (rows 1 to 4) have infundibuloarterial situs concordance (sameness).[20] Abnormally related great arteries (rows 5 to 8) have infundibuloarterial situs discordance (difference).[20] **TOF has infundibuloarterial situs concordance and hypoplasia of the subpulmonary infundibulum.** (Reproduced with permission from Van Praagh R. What determines whether the great arteries are normally or abnormally related? *Am J Cardiol* 2016;118:1390.[20])

the systemic venous and the pulmonary venous circulations. **Consequently, from a surgical standpoint, in addition to repairing the TOF, an inverted atrial switch procedure (a Senning or a Mustard procedure) is also necessary.**

Preoperatively, in TOF {I,D,S} (Fig. 20.10, row 2, column 4), the systemic venous bloodstream (blue blood) flows into the left-sided right atrium (RA), then into the left-sided left ventricle (LV), and then into the left-sided aorta, resulting in cyanosis. The pulmonary venous bloodstream (red blood) flows into the right-sided left atrium (LA), then into the right-sided right ventricle (RV), and then into the right-sided pulmonary artery and back to the lungs.

In TOF, the degree of underdevelopment of the subpulmonary infundibulum is variable, which may be expressed as follows:

1. TOF {S,D,S} = 0R + 1L

We use **grade 1** to mean atresia of the subpulmonary infundibulum, as in Fig. 20.8.

2. TOF {S,D,S} = 0R + 2L

Grade 2 indicates severe right ventricular outflow tract stenosis, as in Fig. 20.7.

3. TOF {S,D,S} = 0R + 3L

Grade 3 indicates mild to moderate right ventricular outflow tract (infundibular ± pulmonary valvar) stenosis, as in Figs. 20.2 and 20.3.

4. SNRGA{S,D,S} = 0R + 4L

Grade 4 indicates normal subpulmonary infundibular growth and expansion.

For more information concerning infundibuloarterial situs equations, see Chapter 15.

TOF always has infundibuloarterial situs concordance (both solitus, or both inversus) (Table 20.2), as the segmental anatomy also confirms, that is, {-,-,S} or {-,-,I}.

This means that TOF is not really a conotruncal (or infundibuloarterial) malformation. In TOF, there is always aortic-mitral direct fibrous continuity. And the pulmonary arteries are hypoplastic because they do not receive a normal volume of blood per unit of time; but the pulmonary arteries are not primarily malformed. The pulmonary arteries are hypoplastic because of subpulmonary stenosis and a typically large subaortic infundibuloventricular type of malalignment VSD that facilitates right-to-left shunting.

TOF (or "the monology of Stensen") is infundibular hypoplasia in three dimensions, resulting in a low-volume, stenotic subpulmonary infundibulum. All of the other anatomic features of typical TOF are secondary to subpulmonary infundibular hypoplasia.

One of the other anatomic features of the TOF that is routinely ignored in classical accounts of the TOF is the abnormal location of the pulmonary valve. Just as the aortic valve is too right-sided, too anterior, and too superior in typical TOF, the pulmonary valve is *reciprocally* too left-sided, too posterior, and too inferior.

Why is the abnormal location of the pulmonary valve in TOF routinely ignored? Because the pulmonary valve in TOF nonetheless communicates with and arises above the LV (except in patients with pulmonary outflow tract atresia).

SURGICAL REPAIR

In **TOF {S,D,S}** and in **TOF {I,L,I}** (Fig. 20.10, row 1, columns 1 and 3), the tasks are to eliminate the right ventricular outflow tract obstruction and to close the VSD. Our best surgeons also take great care to minimize right ventricular myocardial trauma, to preserve the coronary arteries, to avoid trauma to the atrioventricular conduction system, and to spare the aortic valve.[18-22]

But in **TOF {I,D,S}**, as noted above, in addition to TOF, the surgeon also has one intersegmental situs discordance to manage, at the AV level (Fig. 20.10, row 2, column 4). One intersegmental situs discordance physiologically uncorrects the systemic and pulmonary circulations, necessitating an atrial switch procedure, an inverted Senning or Mustard procedure.

TOF {S,D,I} was a previously unknown form of TOF that was discovered and reported by Foran and colleagues[21] in 1988 and was successfully repaired by Santini and colleagues[22] in 1995. As the segmental anatomy indicates, the rare feature of this type of TOF is that the infundibulum and great arteries are inverted (or in mirror-image) compared with the usual type of TOF. Compare Figs. 20.11 to 20.13 with Fig. 20.14. In Figs. 20.11 and 20.13, the main pulmonary artery lies to the right of the ascending aorta. Normally, the main pulmonary artery lies to the left of the ascending aorta (Fig. 20.14).[18]

In a left lateral projection of a selective right ventricular injection, the right coronary artery is seen (Fig. 20.12). It is very important that the medical team understand that in TOF {S,D,I}, the right coronary artery always runs across the pulmonary outflow tract, from left to right. Why? Because the aorta, from which the right coronary artery arises, lies to the left of the main pulmonary artery. To reach the right atrioventricular groove, the right coronary artery runs across the infundibular outflow tract—exactly where the surgeon would like to place his ventriculotomy.

So, in TOF {S,D,I}, the right coronary artery is always "in the way." In an 8-month-old girl, Santini, Jonas, Sanders, and Van Praagh[22] reported a successful correction of TOF {S,D,I} *without a conduit*. Instead, careful myocardial resection beneath the right coronary artery was employed.

The infundibuloarterial situs equation in TGA {S,D,I} is: TGA {S,D,I} = 1R or 2R + 0L.

The infundibular "recipe" is of the inverted type. INRGA {I,L,I} = 4R + 0L. But the right-sided subpulmonary infundibulum is hypoplastic in TOF; hence grade 1 or 2 in the foregoing equation (1R or 2R + 0L).

TOF {S,D,I} is interesting in another way. The segmental anatomy shows that it is possible to have segmental **situs** discordance, that is, TOF {S,**D,I**}, with segmental **alignment** concordance, that is, **solitus** or D-loop ventricles eject concordantly into **inverted** normally related great arteries—because the great arteries are normally related, although inverted (Fig. 20.10, row 4, column 1). Hence, TOF {S,D,I} has ventriculoarterial *situs* discordance, without ventriculoarterial *alignment* discordance.

Some of our friends and colleagues talk about atrioventricular (AV) and ventriculoarterial (VA) **connections** concordance

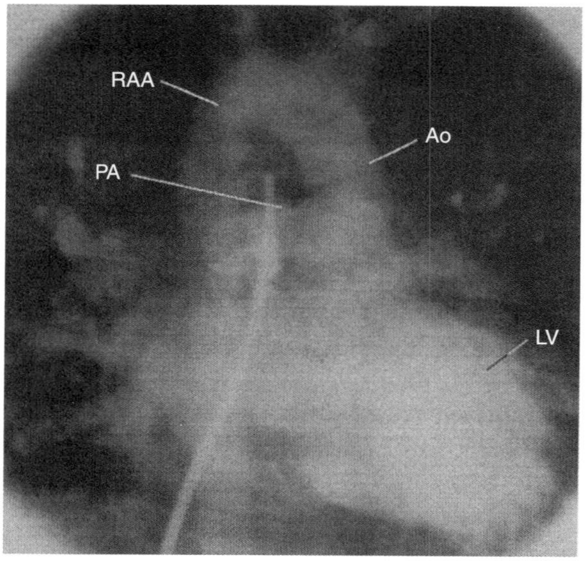

Fig. 20.11 Angiocardiography in TOF {S,D,I},[22] posteroanterior projection. This rare segmental anatomic set is presented diagrammatically in Fig. 20.10, row 4, column 1. Note that the catheter in the pulmonary artery *(PA)* is to the *right* of the aortic valve and the ascending aorta *(Ao)*, because the infundibulum and the great arteries are both inverted, with hypoplasia (stenosis) of the right-sided subpulmonary infundibulum and with the sequelae thereof (inverted TOF with noninverted atria and ventricles). Infundibuloarterial inversion with atrioventricular noninversion is important diagnostically and surgically because the right coronary artery runs from the left-sided aorta in a rightward direction—right across the stenotic right-sided pulmonary outflow tract in order to reach the right-sided atrioventricular groove. So the right coronary artery is always "in the way" in TOF {S,D,I}, running right across the area where the surgeon wants to do an infundibulotomy to open up the stenotic pulmonary outflow tract. This is why Drs. Jonas and Santini[22] were pleased to be able to manage the pulmonary outflow tract obstruction with careful myocardial resection beneath the right coronary artery, rather than jumping the right coronary artery with a pulmonary outflow tract conduit. Thus, in TOF {S,D,I}, it is important that the surgical team be aware that the right coronary artery runs across the obstructed pulmonary outflow tract, so that inadvertent transection of the right coronary artery can be avoided. This patient also had a right aortic arch *(RAA)*. *LV*, Left ventricle. (Reprinted with permission from Santini F, Jonas RA, Sanders S, Van Praagh R. Tetralogy of Fallot {S,D,I}: successful repair without a conduit, *Ann Thorac Surg* 1995;59:747.)

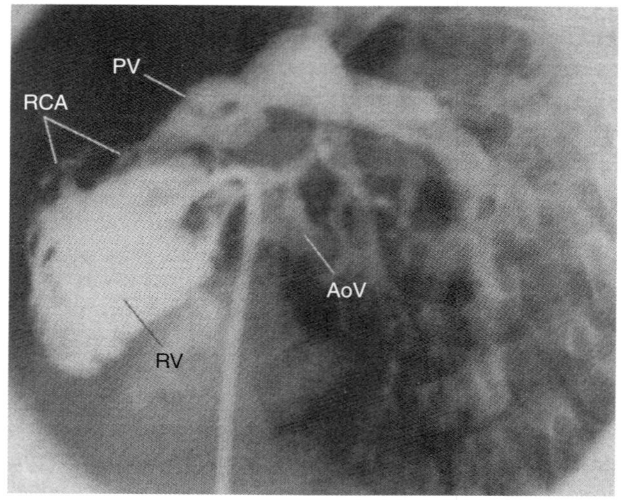

Fig. 20.12 Angiocardiography in TOF {S,D,I}, selective right ventricular *(RV)* injection, left lateral projection. This is the patient of Santini and colleagues,[22] the same patient as in Fig. 20.11. One can see the right coronary artery *(RCA)* coursing across the infundibulo–right ventricular junction. The stenotic infundibulum, the pulmonary valve *(PV)*, and the aortic valve *(AoV)* are also seen. The course of the RCA in front of the os infundibula and in front of the RV free wall is a very important surgical observation (as in Fig. 20.11 legend). (Reprinted with permission from Santini F, Jonas RA, Sanders S, Van Praagh R. Tetralogy of Fallot {S,D,I}: successful repair without a conduit, *Ann Thorac Surg* 1995;59:747.)

and discordance. We prefer AV and VA **alignments** concordance and discordance, for anatomic accuracy. The main cardiac segments (atria, ventricles, and great arteries) normally do not connect with each other because of the interposition of the connecting cardiac segments (the AV canal or junction, and the infundibulum or conus arteriosus).

ASSOCIATED MALFORMATIONS

In TOF, associated malformations can be of decisive importance to surgical outcomes: cor triatriatum,[17] pulmonary sequestration,[17] left ventricular outflow tract obstruction caused by adherence of the mitral valve to the left ventricular septal surface,[23] discrete fibrous subaortic stenosis,[24] obstructive VSD,[25] aortic valvar stenosis,[26] and absence of pulmonary valve leaflets.[27]

I was so impressed by the importance of associated malformations, which were often surgical "surprises," that a

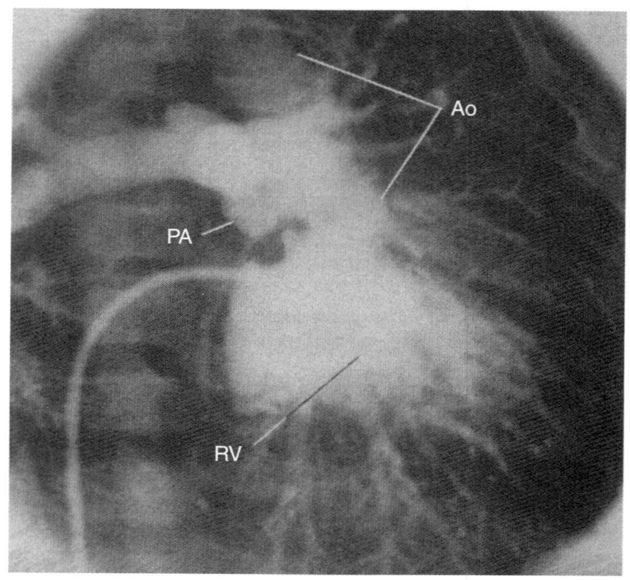

Fig. 20.13 Angiocardiography in TOF {S,D,I}, selective right ventricular *(RV)* injection, posteroanterior projection. This is TOF with atrioventricular noninversion and with infundibuloarterial inversion. The viscera and atria are in situs solitus (noninversion), as the catheter position indicates. There is atrioventricular alignment concordance, as the catheter course from the right atrium (unlabeled) into the right ventricle *(RV)* indicates. This is a solitus (noninverted, right-handed) RV. By contrast, the infundibulum and the great arteries are inverted, the pulmonary artery *(PA)* being right-sided relative to the aorta *(Ao)*. (Reprinted with permission from Santini F, Jonas RA, Sanders S, Van Praagh R. Tetralogy of Fallot {S,D,I}: successful repair without a conduit, *Ann Thorac Surg* 1995;59:747.)

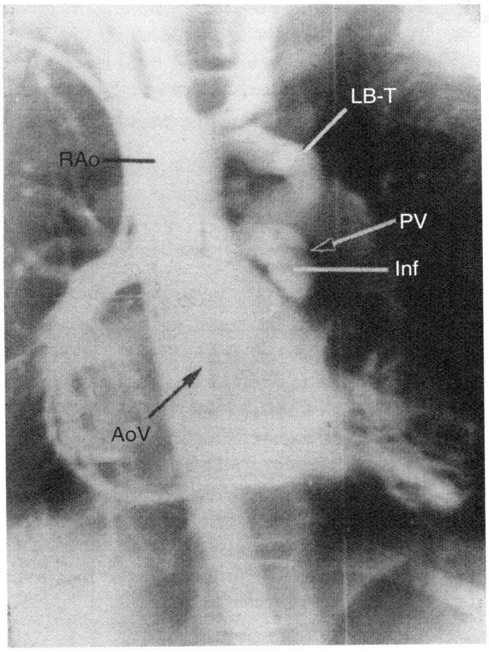

Fig. 20.14 Angiocardiography in typical TOF {S,D,S}, selective right ventricular injection, posteroanterior projection. The infundibulum and the great arteries are both noninverted (in situs solitus). The subpulmonary infundibulum *(Inf)* and the pulmonary valve *(PV)* are both *left-sided* relative to the aortic valve *(AoV)*. There is also a right aortic arch *(RAo)* and a left-sided Blalock-Taussig *(LB-T)* anastomosis, that is, left subclavian artery to left pulmonary artery end-to-side anastomosis. (Reproduced with permission from Van Praagh R. The first Stella Van Praagh memorial lecture: the history and anatomy of tetralogy of Fallot, *Semin Thorac Cardiovasc Surg Ann* 2009;12:19.[18])

study of associated malformations in TOF patients was performed in 100 randomly selected cases[18] from the 1980s and the 1990s. There were 10 fetuses. The ages at postnatal death in 90 patients were as follows: median 6.75 months, ranging from 6.5 hours to 48 years. There were 48 males, 47 females, and 5 were unknown. The findings are presented in order of descending frequency. This is "the big picture" of TOF, how TOF really is. Numbers of cases and percentages are the same.

Pulmonary stenosis	63
Pulmonary atresia	37
Secundum atrial septal defect (common atrium 5)	35
Multiple congenital anomalies	29
Right aortic arch	28
Aortopulmonary collateral arteries	26
Persistent left or right SVC (LSVC 15, RSVC 1)	16
Patent ductus arteriosus	13
Absent ductus arteriosus	12
Completely common atrioventricular canal (type A1, type C6, NOS 2)	9
Down syndrome (familial 2)	8
Aberrant right or left subclavian artery	8
Anomalous muscle bundles of the right ventricle	8
Absent pulmonary valvar leaflets syndrome	6
Restrictive ventricular septal defect	5
Additional muscular ventricular septal defects	5
Ectopia cordis (complete thoracic 1, thoracoabdominal 3)	4
Familial congenital heart disease	4
Myxomatous aortic valve	4
Aortic regurgitation	4
Bicuspid aortic valve	3
Coronary sinus septal defect	3
Single left coronary artery	3
Trisomy 18	2
Tricuspid stenosis	2
Parachute mitral valve	2
Superior vena cava to left atrium because of unroofed coronary sinus	2
Chromosomal anomalies	2
Twins	2
Conjoined twins	1
Aortic stenosis, valvar	1
Partially anomalous pulmonary venous connection	1
Turner syndrome	1
Noonan syndrome	1
Kleinfelter syndrome	1
Thick-walled and small-chambered right ventricle with restrictive ventricular septal defect	1
Sinusoids between right ventricle and right coronary artery with restrictive ventricular septal defect	1
Small anterolateral papillary muscle group of left ventricle	1
Dextrocardia	1
Mesocardia	1
Heterotaxy with polysplenia syndrome	1
Quadricuspid aortic valve	1
Vascular ring formed by right aortic arch, aberrant left subclavian artery, and left-sided patent ductus arteriosus	1
Intussusception of left atrial appendage, that is, inside-out appendages producing supramitral stenosis	1
Congenital mitral stenosis	1
Absence of infundibular septum	1
Hypertrophy of infundibular septum	1
Visceroatrial situs discordance, that is, {IS,D,S}	1
Absence of main pulmonary artery, of right and left pulmonary artery branches, and of right and left ductus arteriosi*	1

**Ductus* is a fourth declension masculine Latin noun. The plural is *ductus*, or *ductūs*.
LSVC, Left superior vena cava; *NOS*, not otherwise specified; *RSVC*, right superior vena cava.

Thus, concerning patients with TOF, a careful search should be made preoperatively for associated malformations, in order to minimize surgical "surprises" and to achieve optimal surgical outcomes.

MORPHOMETRIC STUDY OF TOF IN THE NEONATAL PERIOD[18]

A morphometric study was done of unoperated patients with TOF who died in the first month of life, prior to the development of acquired, secondary postnatal changes. These measurements and calculations were compared with the findings in normal, age-matched control hearts. The measurements, calculations, and comparisons were as follows:

1. the infundibular cross-sectional area;
2. the pulmonary valvar area;
3. the main pulmonary artery cross-sectional area; and
4. the infundibular volume.

This morphometric study was done by Drs. Keishi Kadoba, Maurizio Rubino, and Renzo Pessotto—cardiac surgeons all, when it was our privilege to have them as Fellows in the Cardiac Registry.

In all four categories, the findings in neonatal TOF were significantly less than in the normal control hearts: $p < 0.01$ for all measurements (Fig. 20.15).

These morphometric findings confirm the concept that TOF is underdevelopment or hypoplasia of the subpulmonary infundibulum in three dimensions or volumetrically (Fig. 20.15, rightmost study), with numerous important sequelae such as an abnormally small pulmonary valvar cross-sectional area, and a significant reduction in the main pulmonary arterial cross-sectional area (Fig. 20.15). Other sequelae of the subpulmonary infundibular hypoplasia include right ventricular outflow tract hemodynamic obstruction (stenosis or atresia), ventricular septal defect (Figs. 20.3 to 20.8), right-to-left shunting through the ventricular septal defect (Fig. 20.3), and postnatally acquired right ventricular hypertrophy.

And let us always remember the possibility of numerous significant associated malformations, as listed above.

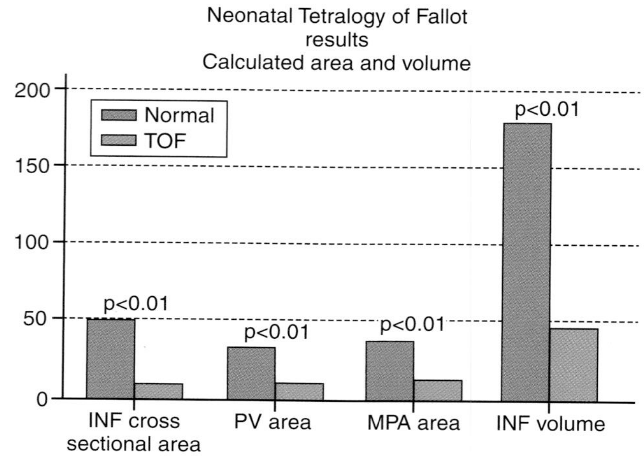

Fig. 20.15 Knowing that right ventricular hypertrophy is a *postnatally* acquired finding in TOF, the question arises, What are the truly congenital anomalies, present at birth, in TOF? In an effort to answer this question, a morphometric study was done of 16 postmortem cases of TOF in the neonatal period. The TOF data were statistically compared with age-matched normal controls. The following anatomic features were studied: infundibular cross-sectional area; pulmonary valve area; main pulmonary artery cross-sectional area; and infundibular volume. Morphometry showed that all four of these anatomic features were statistically significantly smaller in neonatal TOF patients than in normal controls: $p < 0.01$ for all anatomic features. (Reproduced with permission from Van Praagh R. The first Stella Van Praagh memorial lecture: the history and anatomy of tetralogy of Fallot, *Semin Thorac Cardiovasc Surg Ann* 2009;12:19.[18])

WHO WAS DR. ARTHUR FALLOT AND WHAT DID HE HOPE TO ACCOMPLISH WITH HIS PUBLICATIONS IN 1888?[14,15]

Born at Sète on the French coast of the Mediterranean on September 20, 1850, Arthur Fallot studied medicine at the École de Médicine of Marseille. Following graduation, he became an intern at the Hospital of Marseille and he passed a competitive examination known as the Concours de Médecine des Hôpitaux in 1883.

In 1886, Fallot taught pathologic anatomy, which may have helped him to do his monograph on tetralogy only 2 years later, in 1888.

In 1888, Fallot was appointed Professor of Hygiene and Legal Medicine, a post which he held until his death in 1911, at 61 years of age.

Fallot was a respected and experienced clinician who served as Chef de Clinique (Chief of the Clinic) at the Hôtel-Dieu Hospital in Marseille and as Chef de Service (Chief of Service) of l'Hôpital de la Conception, Marseille.

Fallot made no pretense about being the first to describe this form of congenital heart disease. Quite the contrary. Fallot referred to and summarized the first known case of Stensen[1] in 1671, the second known case of Sandifort[3] in 1777, the case of Hunter[4] in 1784, and many more.

Fallot[14] also writes on his page 348,

> ***It is sufficient to go over the observations of Hunter, Sandifort, Duncan, and Pallois, etc to find indicated here, in a fashion most clear and detailed, our pathologic anatomic tetralogy: stenosis of the pulmonary artery, interventricular communication, hypertrophy of the right ventricle, and deviation of the aorta to the right. One asks oneself why a group of facts so numerous and of such demonstrable value has not already become established in science.*** *[My bolding.]*

Just listen to that! Fallot is essentially universally credited with describing this classical tetrad. But Fallot is saying, No, I didn't first describe the tetralogy. It's well described by many earlier observers, who did not understand what they were seeing. Then he asks the inevitable question: Why not? How can this be? Then Fallot answers his own question:

> *Above all, one has trouble in comprehending how, despite the opinion of Gintrac, Senior, and of Cruveilhier, it has been possible for this belief, so profoundly erroneous, to be born, to grow, and to develop to the point of becoming almost universal: the belief that blue disease is linked to the failure of the hole of Botallo to close. [The hole of Botallo is the foramen ovale.]*

In other words, Fallot thought that the reason that the significance of this tetralogy of pathologic anatomic findings had not been understood was that cardiac cyanosis was widely thought to be caused by persistent patency of the foramen ovale.

Thus, we see that Fallot may not have been the first observer to describe the tetralogy, but he was the first to *understand* the tetralogy. Fallot was the first to understand that this anatomic tetralogy was a cause of cardiac *cyanosis*.

I think that Fallot deserves the credit for two discoveries:

1. **His anatomic discovery** was the realization that these four findings were different parts of one interrelated anatomic entity.
2. **His physiologic discovery** was the cause of cardiac cyanosis, which we now call right-to-left shunting at the ventricular level, and that cyanosis is not caused by a patent foramen ovale at the atrial level.

FALLOT'S CONCLUSIONS[15] (1888)

The following lines will summarize briefly the conclusions that we believe may be drawn from this study:

1. Up to the present time clinicians have considered the precise diagnosis of the anatomic lesions of blue disease as an almost insurmountable problem and have hardly been able to mention it except in the form of an altogether vague and uncertain hypothesis. Based on the observations we have gathered, it turns out that, on the contrary, blue disease, especially in the adult, is the result of a small number of cardiac malformations that are perfectly well defined.
2. Of these cardiac malformations there is one that surpasses all others in frequency. We have encountered it in nearly 74% of our observations, and this is therefore the malformation that the clinician should see because the chances then of making an error in diagnosis will be relatively infrequent.
3. This malformation constitutes a veritable pathological anatomic pattern that is represented by the following tetralogy: (1) stenosis of the pulmonary artery; (2) ventricular septal defect; (3) deviation to the right of the origin of the aorta; (4) hypertrophy almost always concentric, of the right ventricle. To this may be added, but in an entirely accessory fashion, failure of the hole of Botallo to close (the foramen ovale).
4. At present, one could not attribute blue disease to persistent patency of the hole of Botallo (patency of the foramen ovale) without putting oneself in opposition to the immense majority of the facts observed. Communication of the atria, when it exists alone without any other associated cardiac lesions, does not produce cyanosis.
5. From the historical point of view, authors in the last century and at the beginning of this one made quite a few observations on blue disease. The majority show very clearly the existence of the various cardiac lesions previously mentioned.
6. Finally, from the point of view of pathogenesis, the theory that regards the interventricular communication as a simple phenomenon belonging to the group of atavistic anomalies is based only on a superficial and inexact interpretation of the facts. The incompletely developed septum of the subject afflicted with the blue malady can in no way be considered as analogous to the false septum of vertebrates with communicating ventricles. It appears much more logical and more in conformity with the laws of physiology to regard the entire series of cardiac alterations enumerated as a consequence of stenosis of the pulmonary artery. As for the cause of this stenosis, we think that it should be attributed not to simple arrest of development, but rather to a pathological process developing during intrauterine life at the level of the pulmonary valve leaflets and the infundibulum that is contiguous with them.*

*I did the translation from French to English. As a native Canadian I studied French for 7 years at high school and university.

WHY IS THE TETRALOGY OF FALLOT REALLY THE MONOLOGY OF STENSEN?

Why are these four malformations (the classical tetrad) really just one thing?[14,17] To understand, one must comprehend **the morphogenesis of TOF.**

Ventricular D-loop formation in humans begins about 21 days after fertilization. At this stage, both developing great arteries are above the developing right ventricle. The aorta (Ao) is to the right and the main pulmonary artery (PA) is to the left. Normally and in TOF, the right-sided subaortic infundibular free wall undergoes resorption. It disappears because of apoptosis (programmed cell death).

Simultaneously, the left-sided subpulmonary infundibular free wall normally undergoes good expansile growth.

Normally, the subarterial infundibular free walls undergo totally asymmetric free wall development: The right-sided subaortic infundibular free wall disappears; and the left-sided subpulmonary infundibular free wall grows well and expands.

So, what happens?

Because the subaortic infundibular free wall is disappearing, the aortic valve sinks inferiorly and posteriorly. The aortic valve passes mostly through the ventricular septal defect and comes into direct fibrous continuity with the developing mitral valve via the intervalvar fibrosa. **This is the normal embryonic aortic switch procedure.** This is why with normally related great arteries and in TOF, there is aortic valve (AoV)–mitral valve (MV) direct fibrous continuity.

But in TOF, the left-sided subpulmonary infundibulum is underdeveloped. This is the "monology," the one thing that the TOF really is.

Normally, the pulmonary valve (PV) is carried superiorly, anteriorly, and to the right above the right ventricle. Normally, the morphogenetic movements of the semilunar valves are opposites, reciprocals of each other. Normally, the AoV moves inferiorly, posteriorly, and leftward, whereas the PV moves superiorly, anteriorly, and rightward.

But not in TOF. Because the left-sided subpulmonary infundibulum is hypoplastic in three dimensions, the volume of the subpulmonary infundibulum is subnormal and hence obstructive. The smallness of the subpulmonary infundibulum results in a subaortic ventricular septal defect, aortic valvar overriding, and postnatal right ventricular hypertrophy.

Not noted by Fallot, the PV in TOF is also malpositioned: the PV is abnormally left-sided, posterior, and inferior—because the subpulmonary infundibulum is hypoplastic.

The abnormal locations of the PV and of the AoV are reciprocals of each other.

The relations between the great arteries in TOF are not quite normal. The AoV-MV fibrous continuity in TOF is often subnormal (Fig. 20.16). The noncoronary–left coronary (NC-LC) commissure of the aortic valve normally is above the middle of the anterior mitral leaflet. But in TOF, the NC-LC commissure of the aortic valve is often further to the right, above the ventricular septum (Fig. 20.16).

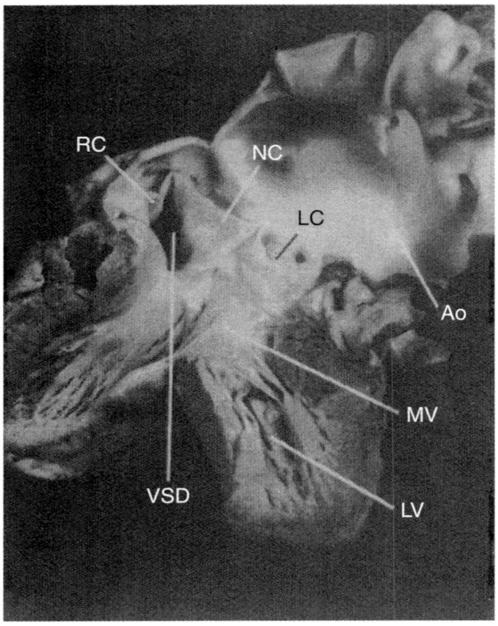

Fig. 20.16 In TOF, aortic-mitral approximation is often subnormal. In the normal heart, the commissure between the noncoronary *(NC)* and the left coronary *(LC)* leaflets of the aortic valve is located above the middle of the anterior leaflet of the mitral valve *(MV)*. But in TOF, the NC-LC commissure is often shifted to the right, and is located above the interventricular septum. Thus, in TOF, the aorta *(Ao)* is often mildly dextroposed, compared with the normal heart. Hence, in TOF, there is aortic overriding, because the aortic valve is a bit too right-sided, anterior, and superior. Reciprocally, in TOF, the pulmonary valve is somewhat too left-sided, posterior, and inferior. The inference appears to be that in order to achieve completely normally related great arteries, one needs not only resorption of the right-sided subaortic infundibular free wall, but also normal growth and expansion of the left-sided subpulmonary infundibulum. *LV*, Left ventricle; *RC*, right coronary leaflet of the aortic valve; *VSD*, ventricular septal defect. (Reproduced with permission from Van Praagh R. The first Stella Van Praagh memorial lecture: the history and anatomy of tetralogy of Fallot, *Semin Thorac Cardiovasc Surg Ann* 2009;12:19.[18])

Thus, completely normally related great arteries depends on normal morphogenesis of *both* halves of the subarterial infundibulum: resorption of the right-sided subaortic infundibular free wall, *and* good growth and expansion of the left-sided subpulmonary infundibular free wall.

Once you understand the morphogenesis of TOF, then you can understand how one malformation, hypoplasia of the subpulmonary infundibulum, can have multiple nonrandom interrelated effects, that is, an interrelated tetralogy of cardiac malformations.

INFUNDIBULOARTERIAL SITUS EQUATIONS AND TETRALOGY OF FALLOT[20]

Solitus normally related great arteries:
1. SNRGA {S,D,S} = 0R + 4L (Fig. 20.14)

Inverted normally related great arteries:
2. INRGA {I,L,I} = 4R + 0L

Tetralogy of Fallot:
3. TOF {S,D,S} = 0R + 1L (tet-atresia, Fig. 20.8)
4. TOF {S,D,S} = 0R + 2L (severe stenosis, Fig. 20.7)
5. TOF {S,D,S} = 0R + 3L (mild to moderate stenosis, Figs. 20.5 and 20.6)

IS TOF RELATED TO OTHER TYPES OF CONGENITAL HEART DISEASE?

Truncus arteriosus:[28-30]
6. TA {S,D,S} = 0R + 1L + APW (truncus type A1; APW, aortopulmonary window)
7. TA {S,D,S} = 0R + 1L + MPA (truncus type A2; MPA, main pulmonary artery)

Double-outlet left ventricle (DOLV):
8. DOLV {S,D,S} = 0R + 2L (DOLV of TOF type)

EXPLANATION OF INFUNDIBULOARTERIAL SITUS EQUATIONS

As you know, equations are just symbolic sentences.
1. SNRGA {S,D,S} = 0R + 4L

Equation 1 says solitus normally related great arteries with the set of solitus atria {**S**,-,-}, D-loop or solitus ventricles {S,**D**,-}, and solitus normally related great arteries {S,D,**S**} equals/is (=) zero development (**0**) of the right-sided (**R**) subaortic infundibular free wall and (+) grade 4 or normal development (**4**) of the left-sided (**L**) subpulmonary infundibular free wall.

How are you supposed to know that the right-sided infundibular free wall is **subaortic** and that the left-sided infundibular free wall is **subpulmonary**?

Because with solitus normally related great arteries, indicated by {S,D,**S**}, the aortic valve is relatively right-sided and the pulmonary valve is relatively left-sided.

So now, let's have another look at equation 1:

It says that SNRGA with the familiar segmental anatomy is/equals/results from complete absorption of the right-sided subaortic infundibular free wall and normal growth and expansion of the left-sided subpulmonary infundibular free wall. Briefly,

$$\text{SNRGA} = 0\text{R} + 4\text{L}$$

The type of relationship between the great arteries is stated to the left of the equals sign.

The "recipe" or formula for that type of relationship between the great arteries is indicated to the right of the equals sign.

Since this is an equation, it is bidirectional. It can be read in the usual way from left-to-right. And it can be read "backwards," from right-to-left.

Reading equation 1 from right-to-left indicates how SNRGA are made: **0R + 4L.**

Equation 2 for **inverted normally related great arteries** is a mirror-image of equation 1:

$$\text{INRGA }\{\text{I,L,I}\} = 4\text{R} + 0\text{L}$$

Tetralogy of Fallot is represented by equations 3, 4, and 5. The recipe for TOF with pulmonary outflow tract atresia is **0R + 1L**. Equation 3 is: TOF {S,D,S} = 0R + 1L (Fig. 20.8).

Equation 4 is: TOF {S,D,S} = 0% + 2L. 2L indicates severe stenosis (Fig. 20.7).

Equation 5 is: TOF {S,D,S} = 0% + 3L. 3L denotes mild to moderate pulmonary outflow tract stenosis, as in Figs. 20.5 and 20.6. SNRGA {S,D,S} = 0R + 4L. 4L is normal.

TRUNCUS ARTERIOSUS[28-30]

We think that truncus arteriosus type A1 is related to TOF, but with pulmonary outflow tract absence plus an aortopulmonary window–(septal defect): **TA {S,D,S} = 0R + 0L + APW.**

We think that truncus arteriosus type A2 is related to TOF with pulmonary outflow tract absence or agenesis plus absence of the main pulmonary artery (MPA). The pulmonary arterial branches remain in their starting positions, arising from the ascending aorta (the aortic sac). Normally, the pulmonary arterial branches migrate on to the MPA. But in truncus arteriosus type A2, there is no MPA to migrate onto.

$$\text{TA } \{S,D,S\} = 0R + 0L - \text{MPA}$$

Thus, in typical TOF, the great arteries are not primarily malformed. The hypoplasia, atresia, or absence of the MPA appears to be secondary to pulmonary outflow tract obstruction.

But when there is absence of the subpulmonary infundibulum, of the pulmonary valve, and of the MPA, with unmigrated pulmonary artery branches arising from the aortic sac, this is what we have been calling truncus arteriosus type A2.

The main point I seek to make is that so-called truncus arteriosus (types A1 and A2) appears to be closely related to TOF with pulmonary outflow tract atresia. Truncus arteriosus communis, as classically conceived, is, we think erroneous, that is, nonexistent. Please see the chapter on absence of the subpulmonary infundibulum.

The point that we have just recently understood about so-called truncus arteriosus communis type A2 is the following: The MPA is absent. Only the right pulmonary arterial branch (RPA) and the left pulmonary arterial branch (LPA) are present, arising unmigrated from the aortic sac. **Since the MPA is absent, truncus type A2 is a solitary aortic trunk, not a common aortopulmonary trunk (or truncus arteriosus communis persistens).**

The anatomic "common denominator" of what we all have been calling truncus arteriosus communis appears to be absence of the subpulmonary infundibulum (and its sequelae). The large aorta types of "truncus arteriosus" (types A1, A2+, A3) appear to be closely related anatomically and developmentally to TOF. "Truncus" type A4 is less clear. "Truncus" types A1, A2, and A3 appear to be "extreme TOF," that is, like TOF only worse.

DOUBLE-OUTLET LEFT VENTRICLE[31]

Rarely, DOLV of the TOF type can occur. There is aortic-mitral fibrous continuity. And the MPA arises above the LV, with a short and stenotic subpulmonary infundibulum.

The abnormal location of the pulmonary valve in TOF is routinely overlooked, or not described. Just as the aortic valve is abnormally right-sided, anterior, and superior in TOF, that is, aortic overriding, the pulmonary valve is reciprocally abnormally left-sided, posterior, and inferior. The highly stenotic or atretic MPA can be located right on top of the ventricular septum. **Rarely, the pulmonary artery can "override" and arise above the LV, resulting in the tetralogy of Fallot type of DOLV.**

This type of DOLV also appears to be closely related to TOF anatomically and developmentally, with pulmonary outflow tract stenosis, underdeveloped subpulmonary infundibulum, VSD, and aortic-mitral fibrous continuity.

REFERENCES

1. Stenonis DN. Anatomicus Rogij Hafniensis, Embryo monstro affinis Parisiis dissectus. In: Bartholin T: Acta medica et philosophica, *Hafniencia* 1671–1672:1:202 (in Latin).
2. Niels Stensens. Beskrivelse af det forste publicerede Tiflaelde af "Fallots Tetrade". *Nord Med.* 1942;16:3550. (Abstract in English.)
3. Sandifort E. *Observationes anatomico-pathologicae. Lugduni Batavorum, apud PVD Eyk et D Vygh, 1777.* Caput Primum, De rarismo cordis vitio, plates I, II, and III:1–38.
4. Hunter W. *Three Cases of Mal-Conformation in the Heart. Medical Observations and Inquiries, Soc of Physicians in London.* Vol. 6. London: T Cadell; 1784;291–417 (Case 2, pp 303–304).
5. Pulteney R. An account of an extraordinary conformation of the heart, London: medical transactions. *Coll Phys.* 1785;3:339.
6. Abernethy J. An essay on the nature of the matter perspired and absorbed from the skin, *London: Surgical and Physiological Essays* Part II;1793:157.
7. Bell J. Of malconformations of the heart, and other causes, preventing the due oxidation of the blood. *Anatom Human Body.* 1797;2:201 (Edinburgh: Anatomy of the heart and arteries).
8. Dorsey JS. Case and dissection of a blue female child. *New Engl J Med and Surg.* 1812;1:69. [First reported American case.]
9. Farre JR: Pathological researches, Essay 1. *London: Longman, Hurst, Rees, Orme, Brown.* 1814:1.
10. Thaxter R. Case of malformation of heart. *N Engl J Med Surg.* 1816;5:228.
11. Peacock TB. *On Malformations Etc of the Human Heart with Original Cases.* Vol. 28. London: John Churchill; 1858;75, 130, 139.
12. Peacock TB. Malformation of the heart. Atresia of the orifice of the pulmonary artery. Aorta communicating with both ventricles. *Trans Path Soc London.* 1869;20:61.
13. Widmann O. A case of pulmonary artery stenosis. *Med Rev.* 1881;20:469 (in Polish).
14. Fallot A. Contribution à l'anatomie pathalogique de la maladie bleue (cyanose cardiaque). *Marseille Med.* 1888;25(77):138, 207, 270, 341, 403.
15. Van Praagh R. Etienne-Louis Arthur Fallot and his tetralogy. A new translation of Fallot's summary and a modern reassessment of this anomaly. *Eur J Cardio Thorac Surg.* 1989;3:381.
16. Abbott ME, Dawson WT. The clinical classification of congenital cardiac disease, with remarks upon its pathological anatomy, diagnosis, and treatment. *Internat Clin.* 1924;4:156.
17. Van Praagh R, Van Praagh S, Nebesar RA, Muster AJ, Sinha SN, Paul MH. Tetralogy of Fallot: underdevelopment of the pulmonary infundibulum and its sequelae. Report of a case with cor triatriatum and pulmonary sequestration. *Am J Cardiol.* 1970;26:25.
18. Van Praagh R. The first Stella Van Praagh memorial lecture: the history and anatomy of tetralogy of Fallot. *Semin Thorac Cardiovasc Surg Ann.* 2009;12:19.

19. Castañeda AR, Jonas RA, Mayer JE, Lang P, Freed MD. Repair of tetralogy of Fallot in infancy. In: Doyle EF, Engle MA, Gersony WM, Rashkind WJ, Talner NS, eds. *Pediatric Cardiology. Proceedings of the Second World Congress. Berlin Heidelberg*. New York: Springer; 1985:491.
20. Van Praagh R. What determines whether the great arteries are normally or abnormally related? *Am J Cardiol.* 2016;118:1390.
21. Foran RB, Belcourt C, Nanton MA, et al. Isolated infundibuloarterial inversion {S, D, I}: a newly recognized form of congenital heart disease. *Am Heart J.* 1988;116:1337.
22. Santini F, Jonas RA, Sanders S, Van Praagh R. Tetralogy of Fallot {S,D,I}: successful repair without a conduit. *Ann Thorac Surg.* 1995;59:747.
23. Van Praagh R, Corwin RD, Dahlquist EH, Freedom RM, Mattioli L, Nebesar RA. Tetralogy of Fallot with severe left ventricular outflow tract obstruction due to anomalous attachment of the mitral valve to the ventricular septum. *Am J Cardiol.* 1970;26:93.
24. Sanders JH, Van Praagh R, Sade RM. Tetralogy of Fallot with discrete fibrous subaortic stenosis. *Chest.* 1976;69:543.
25. Flanagan MF, Foran RB, Sanders SP, Jonas R, Van Praagh R. Tetralogy of Fallot with obstruction of the ventricular septal defect: spectrum of echocardiographic findings. *J Am Coll Cardiol.* 1988;11:386.
26. Ghez OY, Chetaille PM, Campbell BJ, Van Praagh R, Metras D. Tetralogy of Fallot with aortic valvular stenosis: surgical correction in one case. *Ann Thorac Surg.* 2002;73:967.
27. Rabinovitch M, Grady S, David I, et al. Compression of intrapulmonary bronchi by abnormally branching pulmonary arteries associated with absent pulmonary valves. *Am J Cardiol.* 1982;50:804.
28. Van Praagh R, Van Praagh S. The anatomy of common aorticopulmonary trunk (truncus arteriosus communis) and its embryologic implications, a study of 57 necropsied cases. *Am J Cardiol.* 1965;16:406.
29. Calder L, Van Praagh R, Van Praagh S, et al. Truncus arteriosus communis: clinical, angiocardiographic, and pathologic findings in 100 patients. *Am Heart J.* 1976;92:23.
30. Vizcaino A, Campbell J, Litovsky S, Van Praagh R. Single origin of right and left pulmonary artery branches from ascending aorta with nonbranching main pulmonary artery: relevance to a new understanding of truncus arteriosus. *Pediatr Cardiol.* 2002;23:230.
31. Van Praagh R, Weinberg PM. Double outlet left ventricle. In: Moss AJ, Adams FH, Emmanouilides GC, eds. *Heart Disease in Infants, Children, and Adolescents*. 2nd ed. Baltimore: Williams and Wilkins; 1977:367.

21

Absence of the Subpulmonary Infundibulum With Its Sequelae Has Been Misinterpreted as Common Aortopulmonary Trunk

As classically conceived,[1-6] truncus arteriosus communis (common aortopulmonary trunk) seems not to exist.

The classical embryologic conception[1-6] is that the truncoconal septum has failed to grow downward from the aortic arch 4–pulmonary arch 6 junction. This results in a failure of septation (or separation) of the ascending aorta and main pulmonary artery, of the aortic and pulmonary valves, and of the subarterial pulmonary and aortic outflow tracts.

The anatomic definition of so-called "truncus arteriosus communis" is as follows: one great artery that arises from the base of the heart and gives rise to the coronary arteries (at least one), to the pulmonary branches (at last one), and to the systemic arteries.

Classification. In 1965, based on a study of 57 autopsied cases, we endeavored to classify "truncus arteriosus communis" ("TAC") (Fig. 21.1).[7] We used this classification in later studies[8-10] (Fig. 21.2).

In "TAC" type A1, type A indicates that a subarterial ventricular septal defect (VSD) is present, and type 1 indicates the presence of an aortopulmonary septal remnant, and a small low aortopulmonary septal defect (or anteroposterior [AP] window) (Fig. 21.1). Note also that there is a large aorta and a relatively small main pulmonary artery.

The subpulmonary infundibulum, normally above the septal band, is *absent* (Fig. 21.3).

If the classical nonseptation hypothesis were correct, one would expect to find an infundibular septal defect (not subpulmonary infundibular absence). The pulmonary valve also was absent, also not consistent with a failure of septation (Fig. 21.3). The semilunar valve had three moderately thick leaflets, indistinguishable from an aortic valve (also inconsistent with the nonseptation embryologic hypothesis).

In "TAC" type A1, the appearance of the right ventricle (RV) outflow tract (Fig. 21.3) was very similar to the appearance of the RV outflow tract in tetralogy of Fallot (TOF) with subpulmonary infundibular atresia (Fig. 21.4). In fact, we could not reliably tell one from the other, unless we looked at the great arteries. One is comparing infundibular *stenosis* and *atresia* in TOF (Fig. 21.4) with infundibular *absence* in TAC type A1 (Fig. 21.3).

This extreme similarity between "TAC" type A1 and TOF-atresia strongly suggests that these two anomalies are closely related developmentally and anatomically.

"TAC" type A2 (Fig. 21.1 and Fig. 21.5) has no aortopulmonary septal remnant, and both pulmonary artery branches arise from the posterior surface of the arterial trunk.

Note that again the subpulmonary infundibulum beneath the semilunar valve and above the septal band is *absent*.

In "TAC" type A1 (Fig. 21.3), note that the width of the arterial trunk *below* the origins of the pulmonary artery branches is wider than *above* the pulmonary artery branches. In "TAC" type A2 (Fig. 21.5), the width of the arterial trunk below and above the origins of the pulmonary artery branches is the same. In "TAC" type A1 (Fig. 21.3), the arterial trunk is wider below the pulmonary arteries than above them because in type A1, a small main pulmonary artery is present, whereas in type A2, there is no anatomic evidence to support the presence of a main pulmonary artery.

Nonetheless, in type A2, it has long been suspected that because the pulmonary artery branches both arise from the arterial trunk, the main pulmonary artery "must" be there too, despite the absence of supporting anatomic evidence.

In the early 2000s, Dr. Alfredo Vizcaino from the Department of Cardiology of the Hospital Infantil de Mexico, in Mexico City, brought us a fascinating case in consultation (Fig. 21.6) that we published in 2002.[11] The heart was normal, except that the right pulmonary artery (RPA) and the left pulmonary artery (LPA) arose from a single origin (the aortic sac) on the dorsal surface of the ascending thoracic aorta. The other rare finding was a normal sized main pulmonary artery (MPA), with no branches, that emptied through a patent ductus arteriosus into the descending thoracic aorta (Fig. 21.6).

Beitzke and Shinebourne[12] published such a case in 1980, and Aotsuka and colleagues[13] published a second such case in 1990. But it was Vizcaino's case,[11] the third known example of this anomaly, and the first that we had examined personally, that really opened our eyes.

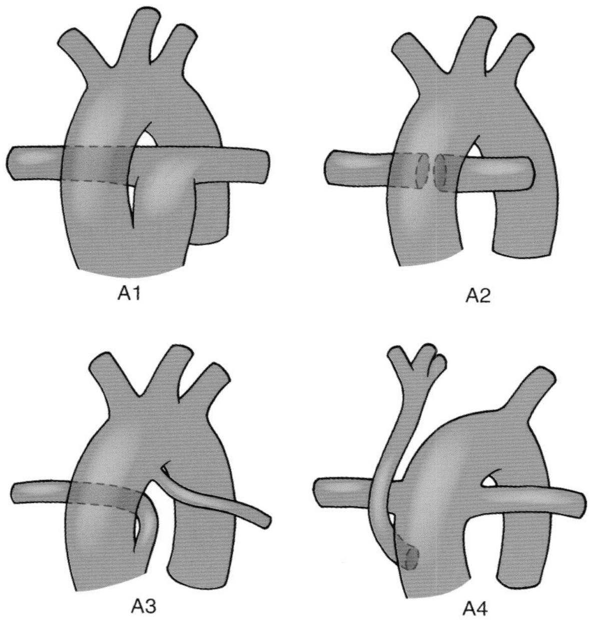

Fig. 21.1 Absence of the subpulmonary infundibulum and associated anomalies. *Type A* means that a subarterial ventricular septal defect is present. *Type A1* indicates that a small main pulmonary artery (MPA) is present with a low aortopulmonary (AP) septal defect and a remnant of the AP septum. *Type A2* means that the MPA is absent and that both pulmonary artery branches arise from the aortic sac on the dorsal surface of the ascending aorta. *Type A3* is the same as type A2, except that one pulmonary branch is absent, the left in this case. Collateral arteries supply the lung without a pulmonary artery branch. *Type A4* has a hypoplastic ascending aorta, an interrupted aortic arch, and a large MPA, large pulmonary arterial branches, and a large ductus arteriosus. We used to think,[1-4] as did many others,[5-10] that such hearts had truncus arteriosus communis. But now we have realized that truncus arteriosus, as classically conceived, probably does not exist. See the text. (Reproduced with permission from Calder L, Van Praagh R, Van Praagh S, et al. Truncus arteriosus communis: clinical, angiocardiographic, and pathologic findings in 100 patients, *Am Heart J* 1976;92:23.[8])

We realized that the normal pulmonary artery and its right and left branches have a bipartite origin:

1. MPA from the truncus arteriosus; and
2. both right and left pulmonary artery branches from the aortic sac[14] on the dorsal surface of the ascending thoracic aorta (Fig. 21.6).

The RPA and the LPA arise initially from the aortic sac of the ascending aorta at the 4-mm stage (24 to 26 days after conception in utero), before the sixth embryonic arterial arches have completely formed.[14]

Completion of both right and left sixth embryonic arches can occur as early as the 5-mm stage (26 to 28 days of age), and usually has occurred by the 6-mm stage (28 to 30 days of age).[14]

As soon as both right and left sixth arches have been completely formed, normally they enlarge considerably and both pulmonary artery branches migrate out on to the sixth arches and join the MPA part of the truncus arteriosus.

But if the ventral part of both sixth arches fails to form, this prevents migration of both the RPA and the LPA.[15]

Another hypothesis is that there may be abnormal growth of the wall of the aortic sac, preventing formation of the sixth arches.[15]

It has long been known embryologically that the RPA and the LPA initially arise from the aortic sac on the posterior aspect of the ascending aorta.[14] The anatomic finding of origin of both pulmonary arterial branches from the posterior surface of the ascending aorta with a nonbranching MPA[11-13] proves that the aforementioned embryologic understanding[14] is correct.

In Vizcaino's case,[11] why did the right and left pulmonary artery branches remain in their original unmigrated origins from the aortic sac?

We hypothesize that the embryonic ventral sixth arches failed to develop. Vizcaino's patient[11] was a 2-day-old female infant, with a birth weight of 2200 grams, who had visceral heterotaxy with polysplenia and multiple congenital anomalies. For whatever reason, the right and left pulmonary artery branches did remain in their initial, unmigrated positions, both arising from the aortic sac (Fig. 21.6).

In Vizcaino's patient,[11] why was the unbranched MPA of such good, normal size?

Because the heart was otherwise normally formed. There was no pulmonary outflow tract stenosis and no VSD (Fig. 21.6).

Given that we think that **the diagnosis of "TAC" type A2** is wrong, what is the **correct diagnosis** (Fig. 21.5)?

Revised diagnosis:

Absence of the subpulmonary infundibulum
Absence of the pulmonary valve
Absence of the MPA
Subaortic VSD
Origin of unmigrated pulmonary artery branches from aortic sac
Absent ductus arteriosus

This case, too, is like a tetralogy of Fallot, only worse. (That's what I mean by *extreme* tetralogy of Fallot.) The pulmonary artery branches are in their original unmigrated positions. Since the MPA was absent, the pulmonary artery branches had nowhere to migrate to.

"TAC" type A2 (Fig. 21.5) is a **solitary aortic trunk** (truncus aorticus solitarius), not a common aortopulmonary trunk, because the subpulmonary infundibulum, the pulmonary valve, the MPA, and the ductus arteriosus are all absent in this 1-month-old boy.

What is so-called "TAC" type A3 (Fig. 21.1)?

It is the same as type A2, except that one pulmonary artery branch is missing. So, type A3 is **a solitary aortic trunk** (not a common aortopulmonary trunk), with absence of a pulmonary artery branch. A patent ductus arteriosus supplied the left lung in one case.[1] The patient was a 3-week-old boy. He had a pulmonary leaflet remnant in a quadricuspid semilunar valve with right coronary, left coronary, noncoronary, and pulmonary leaflets. We thought that aortic stenosis and insufficiency were probable. There was right ureterovesical stenosis with right hydroureter and right hydronephrosis.

In so-called "TAC" type A4 (Fig. 21.7), a large MPA arises from the base of the heart, the pulmonary arterial branches are large, and the ductus arteriosus is large, but closing. The

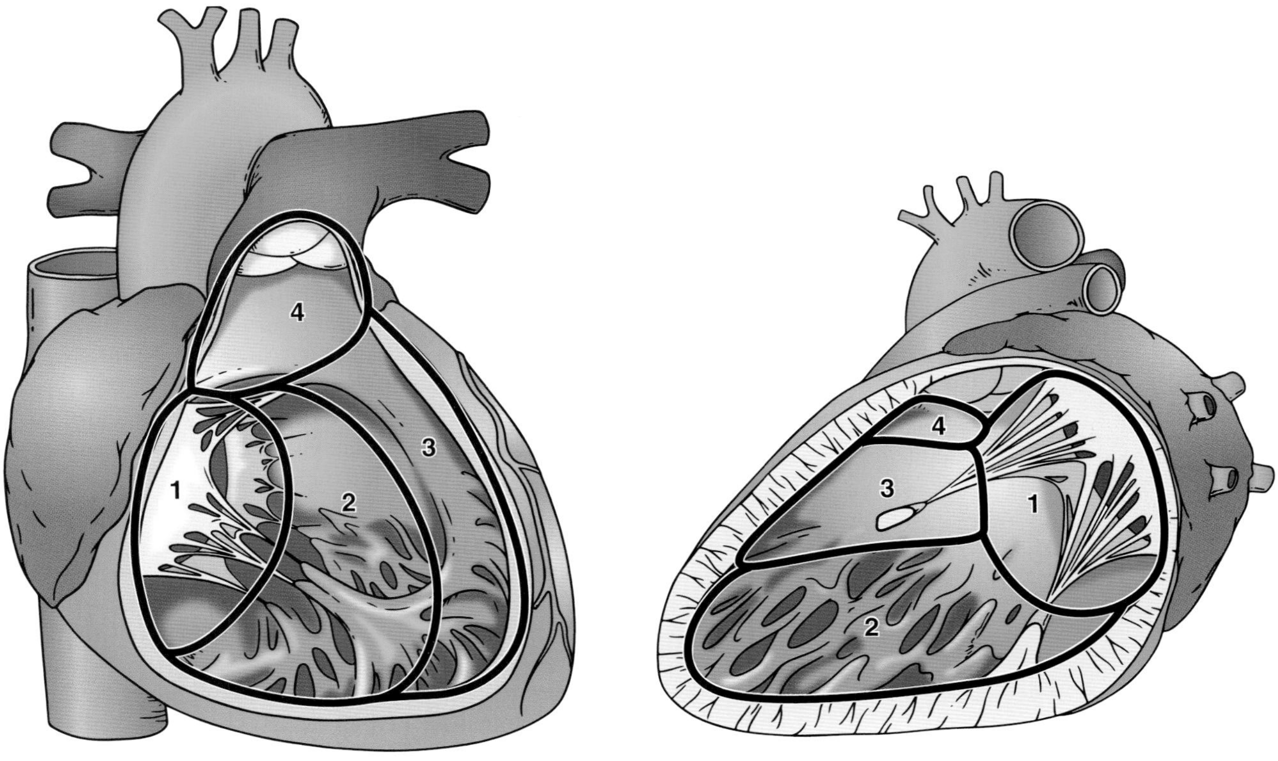

Fig. 21.2 What is the subpulmonary infundibulum that appears to be absent in so-called truncus arteriosus communis? Perhaps the best way to make this clear is to review the segmental composition of the normal human heart. (A) is a diagram of the morphologically right ventricle (RV). (B) is a diagram of the morphologically left ventricle (LV). The normal human heart is composed of four segments, i.e., developmental and anatomic components: *segment 1* is the atrioventricular canal or junction; *segment 2* is the ventricular sinus, or body, or inflow tract, coarsely trabeculated on the RV side and finely trabeculated on the LV side; *segment 3* is the proximal or apical part of the infundibulum or outflow tract, on the RV side known as the septal band that apically is continuous with the moderator band, and on the LV side is the smooth nontrabeculated part of the upper LV septal surface; and *segment 4* is the subpulmonary part of the infundibulum or outflow tract, which has both septal and free-wall parts bilaterally. This is the subarterial infundibulum that is absent in "truncus arteriosus communis:" segment 4. (Reproduced with permission from Van Praagh R. What determines whether the great arteries are normally or abnormally related? *Am J Cardiol* 2016;118:1390.[18])

ascending aorta is small, about the caliber of the RPA. The ascending aorta arises well above the semilunar valve, at about the height of the RPA. The ascending aorta looks like a small branch arising from the right side of the MPA. The isthmus of the aortic arch is interrupted (absent).

A large VSD is present, between the semilunar valve above and the septal band and ventricular septum below. Since the right posterior division of the septal band is prominent, the VSD is not confluent with the tricuspid valve; that is, the VSD is not paramembranous.

The subpulmonary infundibulum is absent. The semilunar valve is tricuspid, and the leaflets are markedly thick, fleshy, soft, and polypoid.

Is this a common aortopulmonary trunk? I would say no for the following reasons:

1. The subpulmonary infundibulum is absent. If the failure-of-septation hypothesis were correct, an infundibular septal defect "should" be present; but it is not.
2. The semilunar valve is tricuspid. It does not appear to be in common with another semilunar valve, as is required by the failure-of-fusion hypothesis.
3. The great artery that arises from the base of this heart looks like a large MPA. It does not look like a common aortopulmonary trunk. Instead, it looks like a large MPA, from which the small ascending aorta arises at about the level of the pulmonary artery branches, well above the semilunar valve.

ABSENCE OF THE INFUNDIBULUM AND ITS SEQUELAE

Absence of the subpulmonary infundibulum has important cardiovascular anatomic sequelae: (1) subarterial VSD; (2) partial or complete absence of the pulmonary valve leaflets; (3) aortopulmonary septal defect (AP window); (4) small or absent MPA; (5) unmigrated pulmonary artery branches, both originating from the aortic sac; and (6) reciprocal development of

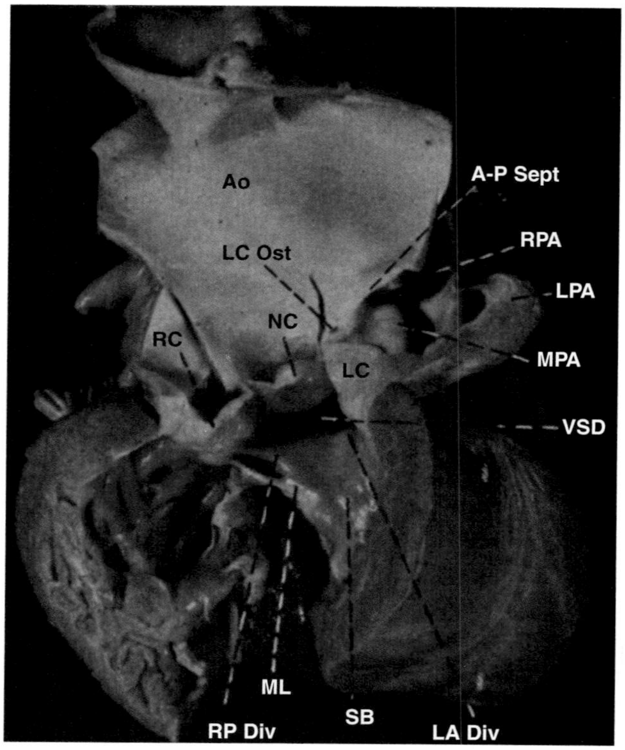

Fig. 21.3 Absence of the subpulmonary infundibulum type A1. This is the heart of a 4.75-month-old boy. A ventricular septal defect *(VSD)* is located between the aortic valve above and the septal band *(SB)* and the ventricular septum below. Normally the subpulmonary infundibulum is located beneath the pulmonary valve and above the septal band. But in this case, the pulmonary valve is absent and there is nothing above the septal band. The three aortic leaflets are moderately thick: right coronary leaflet *(RC)*, the noncoronary leaflet *(NC)*, and the left coronary leaflet *(LC)*. The ascending aorta *(Ao)* with a right aortic arch is large. The main pulmonary artery *(MPA)* is relatively small. The left pulmonary artery *(LPA)* and the right pulmonary artery *(RPA)* are also seen. The aortopulmonary septum *(A-P Sept)* is defective. The ascending Ao and the MPA are not completely separated because of the presence of a low AP window. From the right ventricular aspect, the inferior rim of the subaortic VSD is formed by the top of the septal band that extends from its left anterior division *(LA Div)* to its right posterior division *(RP Div)*. *ML,* Muscle of Lancisi, or muscle of Lushka, or papillary muscle of the conus. Absence of the subpulmonary infundibulum is thought to be developmentally responsible for absence of the pulmonary valve, for the low AP window, and for the VSD. (Reproduced with permission from Van Praagh R, Van Praagh S. The anatomy of common aorticopulmonary trunk [truncus arteriosus communis] and its embryologic implications, a study of 57 necropsy cases, *Am J Cardiol* 1965;16:406.[7])

the great arteries: large aorta, with small or absent MPA; and large MPA and ductus arteriosus, with small ascending aorta and interrupted or obstructively small aortic arch. In embryologic terms, this is large aortic arch 4, with small or absent pulmonary arch 6; and large pulmonary arch 6, with small or absent aortic arch 4.

The associated anatomic features of absence of the subpulmonary infundibulum are summarized in the classification (Fig. 21.1) and are presented photographically (Figs. 21.3, 21.5, and 21.7).

Infundibular absence (IA) and associated cardiovascular anomalies tell a story of progression. IA type A1 is the mildest form. The MPA is present, at least in part. The RPA and the LPA both have migrated from the aortic sac and are confluent with the MPA.

IA type A2 is more severe. The MPA is absent, and the RPA and LPA have not migrated from the aortic sac because the MPA is absent.

IA type A3 is even more severe because a pulmonary artery branch, in our series the LPA, is absent.

In **IA type A4,** the great arteries are reciprocals of types A1, A2, and A3: large MPA instead of large ascending aorta (Ao). *IA type A4, in terms of natural history, is the worst form of all: the median age at death was only 1 week.* Why? Because the aortic arch is interrupted or severely small, and the ductus arteriosus conveys almost all of the blood to the lower body. This means that any inexperienced caregiver, by giving oxygen that tends to close the ductus, may kill the baby.

OTHER FINDINGS

Other important findings in 57 autopsied cases with absence of the subpulmonary infundibulum[1] may be summarized as follows:

Gender: males, 27; females, 27; and unknown, 3. There was no predominance of either sex.

Ages at death: for the series as a whole,[1] mean 2.5 months; range, 1.5 hours to 3.4 years; and median, 5 weeks.

For each of the anatomic types of absent subpulmonary infundibulum (Fig. 21.1), the median ages at death were as follows:

type A1, 6 weeks;
type A2, 8½ weeks;
type A3, 3 weeks (1 case);
type A4, 1 week.

Thus, absence of the subpulmonary infundibulum and the characteristic associated anomalies (Figs. 21.1, 21.3, 21.5, and 21.7) are highly lethal forms of congenital heart disease.

The frequencies of the anatomic types of subpulmonary IA with associated anomalies were as follows ($n = 57$):[1]

type A1, 47%;
type A2, 28%;
type A3, 2%; and
type A4, 23%.

Thus, the large aorta type, with small or absent MPA and ductus arteriosus, occurred in 77%.

The large main pulmonary type, with small aorta and interrupted or obstructively small aortic arch, occurred in 23%.

Segmental anatomy: Normal in all, that is, {S,D,S}.

Heart location: All had levocardia, that is, left-sided hearts (100%).

Veins: All cardiac veins—superior and inferior venae cavae, coronary sinus, and pulmonary veins—were normal in 86% (49 of 57 cases). A persistent left superior vena cava drained through the coronary sinus into the right atrium in 12% (7 patients). In 1 of these, there was membranous atresia of the right atrial ostium of the coronary sinus, associated with a small opening between the coronary sinus and the left atrium (i.e., a small coronary sinus septal defect).

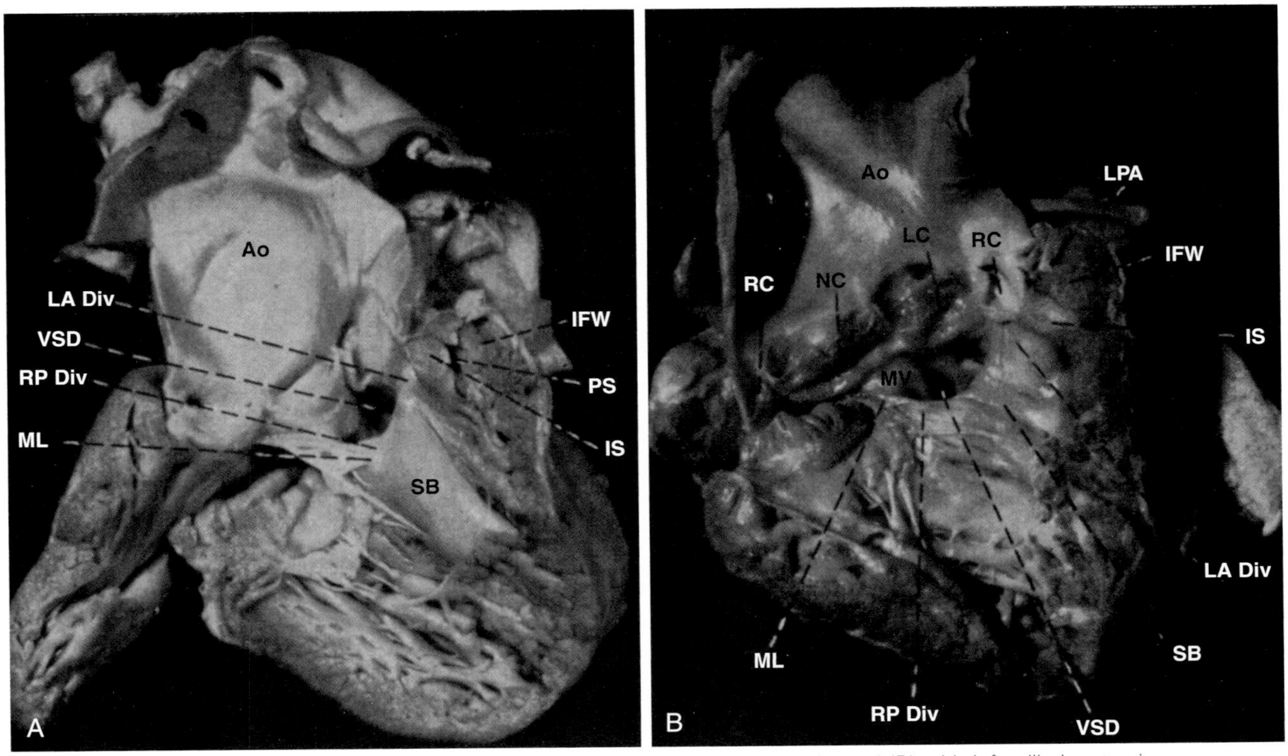

Fig. 21.4 Tetralogy of Fallot (TOF): (A) with severe infundibular stenosis, and (B) with infundibular atresia, opened right ventricular views. The subpulmonary infundibulum in TOF is present, but hypoplastic in A and hence hemodynamically stenotic, or in B even more hypoplastic with no lumen and hence atretic. But in Fig. 21.3, the infundibulum is *absent*. However, the appearance of the infundibulum in TOF with subpulmonary infundibular atresia (Fig. 21.4B), and in these cases with infundibular absence (Fig. 21.3), is very similar. This is why we think these patients with infundibular absence (types A1, A2, and A3, in Fig. 21.1) are closely related to tetralogy of Fallot (Fig. 21.4). (Reproduced with permission from Van Praagh R, Van Praagh S. The anatomy of common aorticopulmonary trunk [truncus arteriosus communis] and its embryologic implications, a study of 57 necropsy cases, *Am J Cardiol* 1965;16:406.[7])

The pulmonary veins were normal in all but 1 patient (2%) in whom a right upper lobe pulmonary vein drained into the right superior vena cava.

Atrial septum: The atrial septum had a patent foramen ovale in 90% (51 cases), which appeared valve competent in 67% (38 cases), but valve incompetent in 23% (13 cases); that is, a secundum type of atrial septal defect was present in almost one-quarter of these patients (23%). The foramen ovale was sealed in only 7% (4 cases). Artifact prevented accurate assessment of the atrial septum in 3% (2 cases).

Atrioventricular valves: Normal in 97% (55 patients). One patient had a common atrioventricular valve, and one had congenital mitral stenosis.

Ventricular septum: All had a subarterial VSD between the great artery (aorta or MPA) above, and the ventricular septum and the septal band below (Figs. 21.5 and 21.6), with no other pathology of the ventricular septum.

Semilunar valve leaflets: The most frequent leaflet number was three leaflets in 67% (38 cases). Second in frequency was four leaflets in 24% (14 cases). Least frequent was two leaflets in 7% (4 cases). Artifact made the leaflet number uncertain in 2% (1 case).

We were not able to relate the leaflet number to any other variable, such as the anatomic type of subpulmonary IA and associated cardiovascular malformations, and so on.

When the semilunar valve was tricuspid, the three leaflets were always of approximately the same length from commissure to commissure. The tricuspid truncal valve was anatomically indistinguishable from the aortic valve.

When the semilunar valve was quadricuspid, we often found three aortic leaflets of approximately the same size, and one pulmonary leaflet that was longer (commissure to commissure) and taller than the three aortic leaflets.

In type A1, it sometimes looked as though a relatively large pulmonary leaflet could occlude, or greatly narrow, the AP window. If so, such quadricuspid semilunar valves in type A1 might produce a form of pulmonary valvar stenosis during systole, which permitted pulmonary blood flow during diastole—when the large pulmonary leaflet component of the four-leaflet valve would not occlude the AP window component in type A1.

We never observed a "truncal" valve with five or six leaflets.

A bicuspid semilunar valve resulted from commissural underdevelopment or absence involving one (or more) commissure(s).

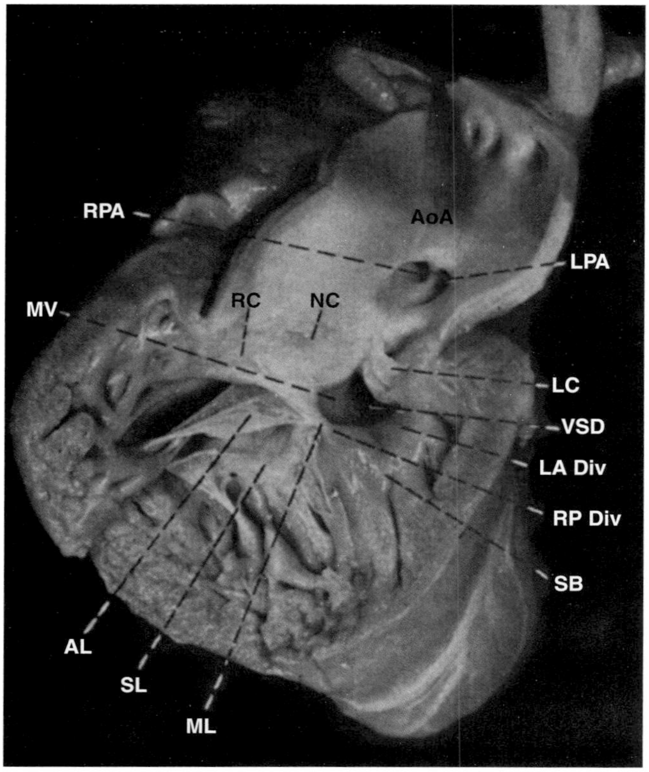

Fig. 21.5 Absence of the infundibulum type A2. This was the heart of a 1-year-old boy. Note that there is no suggestion of a subarterial infundibulum beneath the three-leaflet aortic valve, or above the septal band, or elsewhere. The unmigrated right pulmonary artery *(RPA)* and the unmigrated left pulmonary artery *(LPA)* both arise from the aortic sac on the dorsal surface of the ascending aorta. The main pulmonary artery (MPA) is absent. That is thought to be why the RPA and LPA have not migrated from the aortic sac. Normally, the RPA and the LPA migrate from the aortic sac to the MPA. But when the MPA is absent, the RPA and the LPA have nowhere to migrate to. Absence of the subpulmonary infundibulum is considered developmentally responsible for absence of the pulmonary valve, absence of the main pulmonary artery, and nonmigration of the pulmonary artery branches. What is the basic difference between type A1 and type A2? *Hypothesis:* Both have absence of the subpulmonary infundibulum. Type A1 has an anteroposterior (AP) window, facilitating blood flow in the MPA. Type A2 did not have an AP window. Hence, no blood flow in the MPA, leading to hypoplasia, then atresia, then involution (disappearance) of the MPA. Or the MPA may never have formed. (Reproduced with permission from Van Praagh R, Van Praagh S. The anatomy of common aorticopulmonary trunk [truncus arteriosus communis] and its embryologic implications, a study of 57 necropsy cases, *Am J Cardiol* 1965;16:406.[7])

The circumference of the semilunar valve equaled that of a normal aortic valve or pulmonary valve, but never equaled the sum of the normal aortic valve plus the normal pulmonary valve. We worked with age-matched normal control heart specimens.[1]

Coronary ostial anomalies: These were found in almost half of the cases: 49% (28 cases):

1. the right coronary ostium above the normally noncoronary leaflet in 19% (11 cases);
2. high left coronary ostium in 9% (5 cases);
3. left coronary ostium above or within the left coronary–noncoronary commissure in 7% (4 cases);

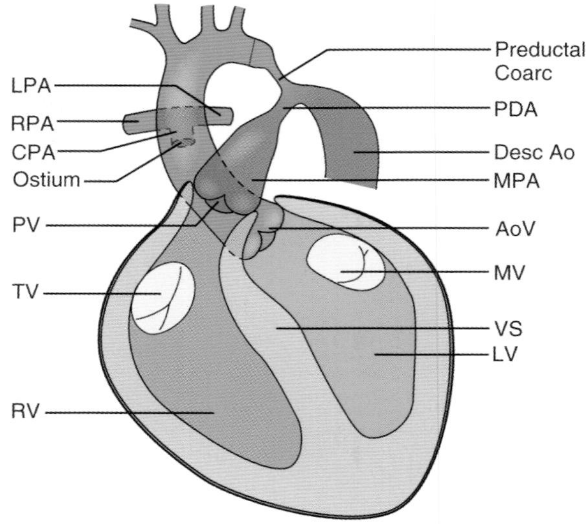

Fig. 21.6 Origin of the right pulmonary artery *(RPA)* and the left pulmonary artery *(LPA)* from the aortic sac of the ascending aorta, and origin of a nonbranching main pulmonary artery *(MPA)* from the right ventricle *(RV)*. This rare anomaly shows that initially, the RPA and the LPA normally arise from the aortic sac, which we called the common pulmonary artery *(CPA)*. When the ventral sixth aortic arches develop by 26 to 30 days of age in utero, the RPA and LPA then migrate out on the sixth arches and become confluent with the MPA. But if the sixth aortic arches fail to develop, then the RPA and the LPA cannot migrate to the MPA. This results in unmigrated RPA and LPA still arising from the aortic sac, and an MPA with no branches. The circulation in this case of Vizcaino[11] is similar to that in the absent infundibulum type A2 patient (Fig. 21.5), with one important difference: In this case (Fig. 21.6), the pulmonary blood flow was normal (no pulmonary outflow tract obstruction, and no VSD). But in the infundibular absence type A2 case (Fig. 21.5), there was no qP (pulmonary blood flow) because the MPA was absent. Dr. Vizcaino's case[11] (Fig. 21.6) made it possible to understand the anatomy of absent infundibulum type A2 (Fig. 21.5). In the case of Vizcaino, the segmental anatomy was normal, i.e., {S,D,S}. The great arteries were solitus normally related. But the associated anomalies resulted in a rare form of **partial transposition of the circulations.** Because the MPA had no pulmonary artery branches and because there was preductal coarctation of the aorta, the lower body was perfused with unoxygenated systemic venous blood. The RPA and the LPA in Vizcaino's case perfused the lungs with oxygenated blood (as in typical D-transposition of the great arteries). The upper body was perfused with oxygenated blood. Differential cyanosis was not described (upper versus lower body). The danger of giving a baby with type A4 anomalies oxygen merits mention. Oxygen tends to make the ductus arteriosus close, depriving the lower body of adequate circulation. The left ventricle *(LV)* would not have been able to alleviate this situation because of the coexistence of preductal coarctation. (Reproduced with permission from Vizcaino A, Campbell J, Litovsky S, Van Praagh R. Single origin of right and left pulmonary artery branches from ascending aorta with nonbranching main pulmonary artery: relevance to a new understanding of truncus arteriosus, *Pediatr Cardiol* 2002;23:230.[11])

4. absent left coronary ostium in 5% (3 cases), resulting in so-called "single" right coronary artery;
5. high right coronary ostium in 5% (3 cases);
6. left coronary ostium above the normally noncoronary leaflet in 5% (3 cases);
7. stenosis of the left coronary ostium in 5% (3 cases);
8. right coronary ostium above the right coronary–noncoronary commissure in 2% (1 case);

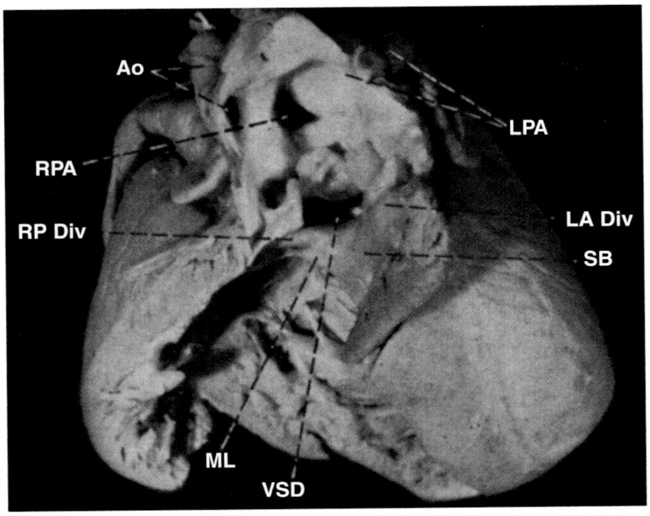

Fig. 21.7 Absence of the subpulmonary infundibulum type A4. A large main pulmonary artery arises from the base of the heart. The subarterial ventricular septal defect *(VSD)* is well seen immediately beneath the semilunar valve that has three leaflets: the left coronary leaflet, a combined noncoronary and right coronary leaflet (with a poorly developed noncoronary–right coronary commissure), and a pulmonary leaflet. The semilunar leaflets are markedly thickened, fleshy, soft, and polypoid. Note that there is no subpulmonary infundibulum between the semilunar valve above and the left anterior division *(LA Div)* of the septal band *(SB)* below. The right pulmonary artery *(RPA)* and the left pulmonary artery *(LPA)* are enlarged. The small ascending aorta *(Ao)* arises well above the semilunar valve. The Ao is about the same size as the RPA. The aortic arch is interrupted. The ductus arteriosus is large and appeared to be closing in this 5-day-old boy. The right coronary ostium is high, above the poorly developed right coronary–noncoronary commissure. Absence of the subpulmonary infundibulum is associated with both types of reciprocal development of the great arteries: (a) large aorta, and small or absent main pulmonary artery and ductus arteriosus in types A1, A2, and A3; and (b) large main pulmonary artery and ductus arteriosus, with small or interrupted aortic arch in type A4, exemplified by this case. (Reproduced with permission from Van Praagh R, Van Praagh S. The anatomy of common aorticopulmonary trunk [truncus arteriosus communis] and its embryologic implications, a study of 57 necropsy cases, *Am J Cardiol* 1965;16:406.[7])

9. abnormally low left coronary ostium, deep in its sinus of Valsalva, in 2% (1 case); and
10. left coronary ostium above the normally right coronary–left coronary commissure in 2% (1 case).

Abnormal locations of the coronary ostia are also frequent in tetralogy of Fallot.[16]

In view of their frequently anomalous locations, the coronary ostia were of limited value in identifying the semilunar leaflets.

Leaflet identification was often assisted by the mitral valve. The deep anterior leaflet of the mitral valve was in direct fibrous continuity with the noncoronary and left coronary semilunar (aortic) valve leaflets. Hence, the mitral valve helped to identify the semilunar leaflets when the locations of the coronary ostia were anomalous and potentially misleading.

Anomalies of the pulmonary artery branches: The LPA was absent in 2% (1 patient), and stenotic in 4% (2 other patients). The ostium of the RPA was often much lower than the ostium of the LPA.

Aortic arch: A left aortic arch was present in 58% (33 cases), a right aortic arch in 21% (12 cases), and was unknown in 2% (1 patient).

The aortic arch was absent (interrupted) in 19% (11 cases). The interrupted aortic arch was replaced functionally by a large patent ductus arteriosus in all such patients. In developmental terms, the interrupted fourth (aortic) arch was replaced by a large sixth (ductal) arch in conveying blood to the lower body.

Considering only the 45 patients in whom an aortic arch was present, a right aortic arch was present in 27% (12 cases), which is similar to the incidence of right aortic arch in tetralogy of Fallot (25% to 30%).[16]

Ductus arteriosus: The arterial duct was absent (no vestige found) in 49% (28 patients). The ductus was ligamentous in 21% (12 patients), and it was patent in 30% (17 patients).

Of the 44 patients with a large aorta, the ductus arteriosus was patent in only 9% (4 patients). But in these few cases, the patent ductus arteriosus was small. From a developmental viewpoint, these 44 cases with a large aorta and a small or absent ductus arteriosus had a well-developed embryonic fourth or aortic arch, and a poorly developed or absent embryonic sixth or ductal arch.

Conversely, in the 13 patients with a large MPA and a large ductus arteriosus, the ascending aorta was hypoplastic and the aortic arch was hypoplastic or interrupted. From a developmental standpoint, these patients had a well-developed pulmonary and ductal or sixth embryonic arterial arch, and a poorly developed fourth or aortic arterial arch.

Absence of the subpulmonary infundibulum is associated with reciprocal development of the great arteries. As noted above, a well-developed aorta with a poorly developed MPA and ductus arteriosus is much more common (77%)[1] than is the reverse, a well-developed MPA and ductus arteriosus with a poorly developed ascending aorta and an interrupted or hypoplastic aortic arch (23%). The probably genetic etiology and the morphogenesis of this reciprocal development of the great arteries in association with subarterial IA are unknown at the present time. Also unknown is why the large aortic types of reciprocal development (types A1, A2, and A3) are more than three times as common as the large MPA type (type A4): 3.35 to 1.00.[1]

Associated noncardiovascular anomalies usually did *not* occur with subpulmonary IA and associated cardiovascular anomalies (types A1, A2, A3, and A4).[1] In 54 patients, no noncardiovascular anomaly was found in 42 (78%). In 12 cases (22%), a noncardiovascular anomaly was present. In 3 patients (5%), this information was unknown by us.

In 1986, we published a paper[9] about rare forms of "truncus arteriosus communis" that was based on the classical definition of TAC that we now know is wrong, as indicated above. Consequently, the findings of this study[9] should be ignored and will not be commented on further here.

When was it realized that truncus arteriosus communis persistens does not exist, that it's a misconception, an error?

Speaking for myself, I think it was 1987. The first sentence of an editorial[10] that I was invited to write in that year reads as follows:

"Truncus arteriosus is a fascinating and mysterious anomaly, at least in part because, as classically conceived, it appears not to exist."

Now, some 30 years later (in 2017), I would say, "Yes, exactly right."

To the best of my knowledge, no other investigator has said the same thing.

I wrote this chapter for several reasons:

1. First of all, it is important for pediatric cardiologists, congenital heart surgeons, and others to realize that truncus arteriosus communis persistens, as classically conceived, defined, and classified, really does not exist.
2. Even though these malformations have been misunderstood (misinterpreted), these hearts do exist. So what are the correct anatomic diagnoses?
3. The majority of these cases with absence of the subpulmonary infundibulum have associated cardiovascular anomalies that closely resemble "extreme" tetralogy of Fallot, that is, anatomic types A1, A2, and A3—the large aorta type. Hence, I thought this chapter should follow the chapter on typical tetralogy of Fallot.
4. Absent distal or subpulmonary infundibulum type A2 (Fig. 21.5) is "the fooler." Unless you understand Fig. 21.6, you can't understand Fig. 21.5. Figure 21.5 looks like it fulfills the conventional definition of truncus arteriosus communis. You have to know that you are looking at **the aortic sac** from which both *unmigrated* pulmonary artery branches arise because the MPA is *absent*—and the pulmonary artery branches have nowhere to migrate to. All of this proves that in Fig. 21.5, you are looking at a *solitary aortic trunk,* not a common aortopulmonary trunk. To understand the foregoing, it is very helpful to have seen Vizcaino's heart specimen (Fig. 21.6), or Beitzke and Shinebourne's case,[12] or Aotsuka and colleagues' case.[13]

Is the subpulmonary infundibulum (or conus) *truly absent* in so-called "truncus arteriosus communis" ("TAC"), or only *apparently absent*? I hypothesize that the answer may prove to be: apparently absent (not truly totally absent). Why?

In so-called "TAC," the pulmonary valve region is not in direct fibrous continuity with the mitral valve, whereas the aortic valve region is (Fig. 21.3). This suggests that the subaortic infundibular free wall has undergone normal programmed cell death (apoptosis); hence aortic-mitral fibrous continuity in "TAC." These observations also suggest that there may well have been some subpulmonary infundibular development. Otherwise, there might have been aortic-mitral and pulmonary-mitral direct fibrous continuity, as rarely occurs in the Paul type of double-outlet left ventricle, but that one does not find in "TAC" type A1 (Fig. 21.3).

Consequently, the data suggest that *apparent* absence of the subpulmonary infundibulum and its sequelae are what "truncus arteriosus communis" really is. I am using *absence* in its gross, surgical sense. Grossly, one cannot exclude the possibility that some subpulmonary infundibular cells may be present histologically (Box 21.1).

So-called common arterial trunk is absence of the subpulmonary infundibulum and its sequelae. Many of the sequelae are what one would expect, such as the following:

1. partial or complete absence of the pulmonary valve; and
2. small or absent MPA and ductus arteriosus. This is what one finds in absence of the subpulmonary infundibulum with associated cardiovascular malformation types A1, A2, and A3 (Figs. 21.1, 21.3, 21.5, and 21.7).

BOX 21.1 Infundibuloarterial Situs Equations

The degree of gross development and the localization of development of the subarterial infundibulum can be expressed precisely and briefly by these equations (see Chapter 15).

Degree of development, assessed grossly, varies from well developed (grade 4) to absent (grade 0).

Location of development may be left sided (L) or right sided (R).

The location of each great artery is indicated by the segmental situs anatomy.

A few examples will make this clear:

Solitus normally related great arteries:

1. **SNRGA {S,D,*S*} = 0R + 4L**

Inversus normally related great arteries:

2. **INRGA {I,L,*I*} = 4R + 0L**

Tetralogy of Fallot (TOF) with *mild* pulmonary outflow tract stenosis:

3. **TOF {S,D,S} = 0R + *3*L**

TOF with *moderate to severe* pulmonary outflow tract stenosis:

4. **TOF {S,D,S} = 0R + *2*L**

TOF with pulmonary outflow tract *atresia:*

5. **TOF {S,D,S} = 0R + *1*L**

The problem posed by so-called truncus arteriosus communis is that the development of the subpulmonary infundibulum appears to be less than in TOF with infundibular atresia, i.e., <1L, but more than absent, i.e., >0L. Consequently, the equation suggested for "truncus arteriosus communis" basically is:

6. **"TAC" {S,D,S} = 0R + *0.5*L**

Subpulmonary infundibular atresia has various degrees of infundibular hypoplasia, >0 but <1. If this degree of precision ever becomes important, it could be expressed as varying from *0.1*L to *0.9*L. At the present time, *0.5*L means: less well developed than in typical TOF with infundibular atresia, but greater than zero.

Thus, the infundibuloarterial situs equation for "TAC" type A1 is:

7. **"TAC" {S,D,S} = 0R + 0.5L + APW**

The infundibuloarterial situs equation for "TAC" type A2 is:

8. **"TAC" {S,D,S} = 0R + 0.5L – MPA**

The infundibuloarterial situs equation for "TAC" type A4 is:

9. **"TAC" {S,D,S} = 0R + 0.5L + IAA**

TAC may well have absence of the subpulmonary infundibulum: 0R + 0L. *APW,* Aortopulmonary window; *IAA,* interrupted aortic arch; *MPA,* main pulmonary artery.

However, absent subpulmonary infundibulum with associated cardiovascular malformations type A4 (Figs. 21.1 and 21.7) is counterintuitive: large MPA and ductus arteriosus, with small ascending aorta and interrupted or obstructively small aortic arch.

How and why did type A4 happen? I really don't know. Perhaps the blood was directed predominantly toward embryonic aortic arch 6 and away from aortic arch 4 by the thick and myxomatous semilunar leaflets (Fig. 21.7). Or perhaps there is a molecular genetic reason for this unexpected type A4 anatomy.

What made it possible to recognize that the conventional view of truncus arteriosus communis is wrong?

Several things:

1. *Absence* of the subpulmonary infundibulum. If the classical view was right, there should have been an infundibular septal defect, that is, failure of the right-sided and left-sided

infundibular cushions to fuse with each other—not absence of the subpulmonary infundibulum (septum and free walls).

2. The cases of Vizcaino (Fig. 21.6),[11] Beitzke,[12] and Aotsuka[13] were very helpful in understanding types A2 and A3. In particular, Vizcaino's case, which I was privileged to examine in person,[11] prompted me to recall the aortic sac[14] from which both the RPA and the LPA originate. I learned what unmigrated RPA and LPA are, and why they do not migrate. I learned that IA, with absence of the MPA (Fig. 21.5), and Vizcaino's case are very similar. The big and eye-catching difference is that Vizcaino's case (Fig. 21.6) has a normal-sized MPA with no branches because there was no pulmonary outflow tract obstruction and no VSD; whereas our case (Fig. 21.5) had absence of the infundibulum with no infundibular outflow tract and no MPA. Because our patient of so-called "TAC" type A2 has no MPA, it cannot be regarded as a common aortopulmonary trunk. Also, our patient's great artery has an aortic sac, from which the unmigrated RPA and LPA arise. **The aortic sac proves that our patient has a solitary aortic trunk, not a common (undivided) aortopulmonary trunk.**

One cannot have an undivided aortopulmonary trunk if the MPA is absent. The pulmonary artery branches did not migrate from the aortic sac because there was nowhere to migrate to—because the MPA was absent. It is not surprising that in some cases the MPA is absent when the subpulmonary infundibulum is absent and when the pulmonary valve is partially or totally absent.

Vizcaino's case[11] also teaches that the normal pulmonary artery system has bipartite origins: the MPA from the truncus arteriosus, and the RPA and LPA from the aortic sac.

The classical definition of truncus arteriosus communis, cited above, does not distinguish between the pulmonary trunk (the MPA) and the pulmonary branches (the RPA and LPA).

The malformations associated with IA and with pulmonary valvar absence (complete or partial) are as follows:

type A1, AP window;
type A2, absent MPA and unmigrated RPA and LPA;
type A3, absent MPA and absent LPA or RPA; and
type A4, hypoplastic ascending aorta and interrupted or obstructive aortic arch.

I think that investigators—all of us—failed to understand types A2 and A3. But the cases of Beitzke and Shinebourne,[12] Aotsuka and colleagues,[13] and Vizcaino and colleagues[11] (Fig. 21.6) now facilitate comprehension.

Absence of the subarterial infundibulum typically is associated with a large subarterial VSD and reciprocal development of the great arteries:

1. large aorta with small or absent MPA and ductus arteriosus (types A1, A2, and A3); or
2. large MPA and ductus arteriosus, with a small ascending aorta and an interrupted or obstructively small aortic arch (type A4).

The blood of the biventricular outputs will flow predominantly into the aorta, or predominantly into the pulmonary artery, depending on which has the lower resistance. This preferential blood flow is made possible by absence of the infundibular septum. Preferential great arterial blood flow (aorta or pulmonary artery) creates the appearance of reciprocal great arterial development (large aorta, types A1, A2, and A3, or large main pulmonary, type A4).

In other words, one of the functions of the infundibular septum in normal heart development is to prevent preferential blood flow into either great artery. Preferential blood flow into one great artery creates the appearance of reciprocal development of the great arteries that is so prominent when the infundibular septum is absent.

Double-outlet left ventricle (DOLV):[17] Is it possible to have absence of the infundibulum beneath *both* great arteries with nothing else wrong? Yes, DOLV! Rarely is it possible to have no distal subvalvar infundibulum, both semiaortic valves present, and both great arteries being present. See Chapter 24 for additional information on DOLV.

Subpulmonary Infundibular Absence

This is what "TAC" really is. TOF is subpulmonary infundibular hypoplasia or underdevelopment (0 + 3, 0 + 2, 0 + 1), but not absence (0 + 0). "TAC" is "**pretetragology of Fallot,**" i.e., absence of an RV outflow tract to the lungs. The development of an RV outflow tract to the lungs is a crucially important evolutionary adaptation to land-living and air breathing when we first started coming ashore.

So, TOF and "TAC" are closely related evolutionary failures (Chapters 20 and 21).

REFERENCES

1. Abbott ME. Absence or rudimentary development of aortic septum. In: Osler W, McCrae T, Funk EH, eds. *Modern Medicine.* vol. 4. Philadelphia: Lea & Febiger; 1927:707.
2. Feller A. Zur Kenntnis der angeborenen Herzkrankheiten. 1. Truncus arteriosus communis persistens und seine fornale Enststehung. Virchows. *Arch path Anat.* 1931;279:869.
3. Humphreys EM. Truncus arteriosus communis persistens. Criteria for identification of the common arterial trunk, with report of a case with four semilunar cusps. *Arch Path.* 1932;14:671.
4. Roos A. Persistent truncus arteriosus communis. Report of a case with four semilunar cusps and aortic arch on the right side. *Am J Dis Child.* 1935;50:966.
5. Lev M, Saphir O. Truncus arteriosus communis persistens. *J Pediat.* 1942;20:74.
6. Collett RW, Edwards JE. Persistent truncus arteriosus: a classification according to anatomic types. *S Clin North America.* 1949;29:1245.
7. Van Praagh R, Van Praagh S. The anatomy of common aorticopulmonary trunk (truncus arteriosus communis) and its embryologic implications, a study of 57 necropsy cases. *Am J Cardiol.* 1965;16:406.
8. Calder L, Van Praagh R, Van Praagh S, et al. Truncus arteriosus communis: clinical, angiocardiographic, and pathologic findings in 100 patients. *Am Heart J.* 1976;92:23.
9. Van Praagh R, Matsuoka R, Van Praagh S. Anatomic variations in truncus arteriosus. In: Takahashi M, Wells WJ, Lindesmith GG, eds. *Challenges in the Treatment of Congenital Cardiac Anomalies.* Mt. Kisko: Futura Publ Co; 1986:199.
10. Van Praagh R. Truncus arteriosus: what is it really and how should it be classified? *Eur J Cardio Thorac Surg.* 1987;1:65.

11. Vizcaino A, Campbell J, Litovsky S, Van Praagh R. Single origin of right and left pulmonary artery branches from ascending aorta with nonbranching main pulmonary artery: relevance to a new understanding of truncus arteriosus. *Pediatr Cardiol.* 2002;23:230.
12. Beitzke A, Shinebourne EA. Single origin of right and left pulmonary arteries from ascending aorta, with main pulmonary artery from right ventricle. *Br Heart J.* 1980;43:363.
13. Aotsuka H, Nagai Y, Saito M, Matsumoto H, Nakamura T. Anomalous origin of both pulmonary arteries from the ascending aorta with a nonbranching main pulmonary artery arising from the right ventricle. *Pediatr Cardiol.* 1990;11:156.
14. Congdon ED. Transformation of the aortic-arch system during the development of the human embryo. *Contrib Embryol.* 1922;14:47.
15. Penkoskie PA, Castañeda AR, Fyler DC, Van Praagh R. Origin of pulmonary artery branch from ascending aorta. Primary surgical repair in infancy. *J Thorac Cardiovasc Surg.* 1983;85:537.
16. Keith JD, Rowe RD, Vlad P. *Heart Disease in Infancy and Childhood.* New York: Macmillan Co; 1958:521.
17. Paul MH, Muster AJ, Sinha SN, Cole RB, Van Praagh R. Double-outlet left ventricle with an intact ventricular septum: clinical and autopsy diagnosis and developmental implications. *Circulation.* 1970;41:129.
18. Van Praagh R. What determines whether the great arteries are normally or abnormally related? *Am J Cardiol.* 2016;118:1390.

22

Transposition of the Great Arteries

What determines whether the great arteries are normally or abnormally related?[1] That really is the basic question.

The answer is thought to be as follows:

When the situs (or pattern of anatomic organization) of the subarterial infundibulum and of the great arteries are both the same (both solitus, or both inversus), then the aorta and the main pulmonary artery are normally related (solitus normally related, or inversus normally related, Figs. 22.1 and 22.2).

In solitus normally related great arteries (SNRGA) (Fig. 22.1, third column from the right), the left-sided subpulmonary infundibulum is normally well developed (grade 4 development), and the right-sided subaortic infundibular development is absent (grade 0 development). Thus, the situs of solitus normal infundibular development is **0R + 4L** (Fig. 22.1).

The solitus normal situs of the great arteries is **right-sided aorta** and **left-sided main pulmonary artery** (Fig. 22.1).

Thus, the infundibuloarterial situs equation of solitus normally related great arteries is:

$$\text{SNRGA } \{S,D,S\} = 0R + 4L^{1,2} \qquad (1)$$

In inverted (or inversus) normally related great arteries, that is, INRGA {I,L,I} (Fig. 22.2, third column from the right), **a well developed (grade 4) subpulmonary infundibulum is right-sided** and a resorbed and hence **absent (grade 0) subaortic infundibular free wall is left-sided.**

Hence, the infundibuloarterial situs equation in INRGA is:

$$\text{INRGA } \{1,L,I\} = 4R + 0L \qquad (2)$$

Both SNRGA and INRGA have infundibuloarterial situs concordance: both the infundibulum and the great arteries are in situs solitus (equation 1), or both the infundibulum and the great arteries are in situs inversus (equation 2).

Equations 1 and 2 are mirror-images.

Equations 1 and 2 are the normal frames of reference, against which all other abnormal forms of infundibuloarterial situs development can be judged and understood.

Equations are bidirectional symbolic sentences. When read in the usual direction from left-to-right, these equations describe the anatomic pattern (or situs) of the infundibulum and of the type of great arteries being described.

But when read "backward," from right-to-left, these equations become "recipes," describing how this or that type of relationship between the great arteries developed.

Why is that so?

Because, as will be seen, almost all anomalies that are regarded as malformations of the great arteries are really anomalies of the subarterial infundibulum. In other words, typically the great arteries *per se* are normally formed.

Abnormally related great arteries typically have infundibuloarterial situs discordance. The situs of the infundibulum and the situs of the great arteries are not the same.

TRANSPOSITION OF THE GREAT ARTERIES

Classical complete, physiologically uncorrected, D-transposition of the great arteries (D-TGA) may be represented as follows:

$$\text{TGA } \{S,D,D\} = 4R + 0L^{1} \qquad (3)$$

Typical D-TGA is presented diagrammatically in Fig. 22.1, fourth column from the right. Equation 3 says: transposition of the great arteries (TGA) with the segmental situs set of {} solitus atria {S,-,-},concordant D-loop or solitus ventricles {S,**D**,-}, and D-TGA or solitus TGA {S,D,**D**} is or equals (=) a well-developed (grade 4) right-sided (R) subaortic infundibulum (4R) and an absent (grade 0) left-sided (L) subpulmonary muscular infundibulum (0L). D-TGA means that the transposed aortic valve lies to the right, *dextro,* or D (Latin) relative to the transposed pulmonary valve. **Transposition** of the great arteries means that both great arteries are placed across the ventricular septum and consequently arise above the morphologically inappropriate ventricles: ascending aorta (Ao) above the morphologically right ventricle (RV), and main pulmonary artery (MPA) above the morphologically left ventricle (*trans,* across, and *positio,* a placing or putting).

$$\text{TGA } \{S,L,L\} = 0R + 4L \qquad (4)$$

Equation 4 says: TGA with the set of solitus atria {S,-,-}, discordant L-loop or inverted ventricles {S,**L**,-}, and L-TGA {S,L,L} is (or equals) absence of the right-sided subpulmonary infundibulum (0R) and (+) a well-developed left-sided subaortic infundibulum (4L). L-TGA means that the transposed aortic valve is to the left, *levo,* or *L* (Latin) relative to the transposed pulmonary valve.

INFUNDIBULOARTERIAL SITUS ANALYSIS

Typical D-TGA (equation 3) shows infundibuloarterial (IA) situs discordance:

$$\text{TGA } \{S,D,\mathbf{D}\} = \mathbf{4R + 0L} \qquad (3)$$

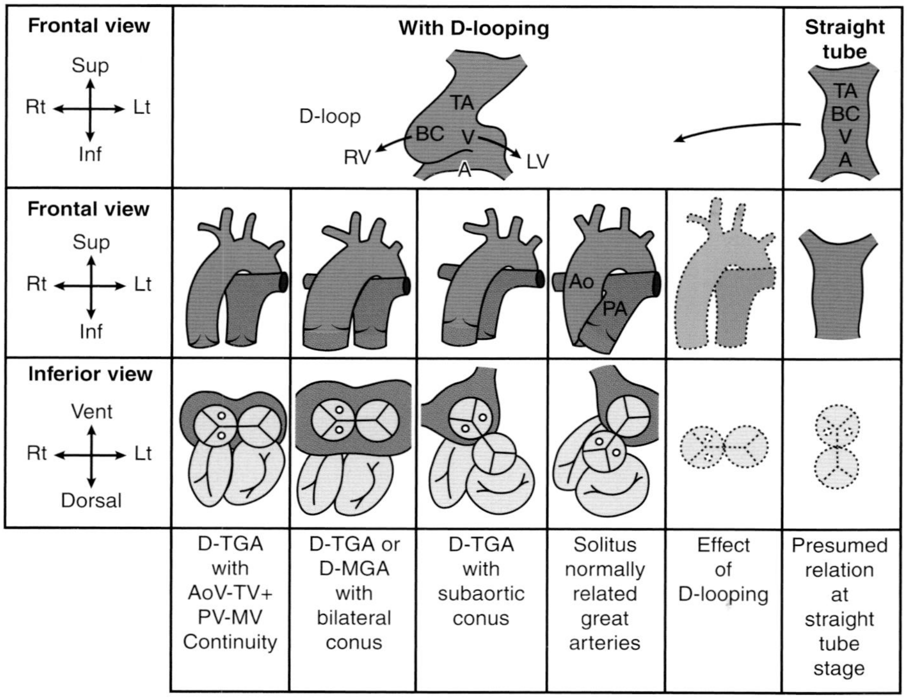

Fig. 22.1 Normal and abnormal anatomy and development of the solitus (or noninverted) heart in the human embryo, presented diagrammatically. *Top row:* The straight heart tube at 20 days of age in utero normally loops convexly to the right, forming a dextro- or D-loop, starting at 21 days of age in the human embryo. The various segments of the developing normal heart are the truncus arteriosus *(TA),* where the great arteries will form; the bulbus cordis *(BC),* where the infundibulum and morphologically right ventricle *(RV)* will form; the ventricle *(V)* of the bulboventricular loop where the morphologically left ventricle *(LV)* will form; and the atrium *(A)* where the morphologically right and left atria (*RA* and *LA*) will develop. *Second row from the top:* The aorta *(Ao)* and the pulmonary artery *(PA),* seen from the front. The subarterial infundibulum is shown in brown. *Third row from the top:* Semilunar valves, infundibulum, and atrioventricular valves as viewed from below, as in a subxiphoid two-dimensional echocardiogram. Broken lines indicate that the semilunar valves and the aorta are not two separate structures at this early stage; they are shown as such to facilitate understanding. The aortic valve *(AoV)* is indicated by the coronary ostia. The pulmonary valve *(PV)* has no coronary ostia. The mitral valve *(MV)* has 2 leaflets and the tricuspid valve *(TV)* has 3 leaflets. *The bottom row* states what the various columns depict. *The rightmost column* depicts the straight tube (or preloop) stage in which the developing aortic valve is thought to be anterior (ventral) to the developing pulmonary valve, which is thought to be posterior (dorsal). *Second column from the right* shows the effect of D-loop formation on the great arteries: The aortic valve and the ascending aorta are carried to the right of the pulmonary valve and the main pulmonary artery. *Third column from the right:* Normally, the right-sided subaortic infundibular free wall involutes (disappears), while simultaneously the left-sided subpulmonary infundibular free wall develops well. Consequently, the developing AoV sinks inferiorly, posteriorly, and leftward and passes through the interventricular foramen, and comes into direct fibrous continuity with the developing MV via the intervalvar fibrosa. This is **the normal embryonic aortic switch** in which the AoV goes from above the developing RV to above the developing LV. Reciprocally, the developing PV is carried superiorly, anteriorly, and rightward above the developing RV, and away from the interventricular foramen, facilitating the aortic switch maneuver. These normal and opposite developmental processes and morphometric movements may be expressed by the following equation: **SNRGA** {**S,D,S**} = **0R + 4L.** The infundibular + arterial situs combination is solitus + solitus. Thus, infundibuloarterial situs concordance (sameness) is present. *The fourth column from the right* shows typical D-TGA with a well-developed right-sided subaortic infundibulum, and a resorbed left-sided subpulmonary infundibular free wall. Involution or disappearance of the left-sided subpulmonary infundibular free wall is thought to be due to apoptosis (genetically programmed cell death). Involution of the subpulmonary infundibular free wall causes the PV to move inferiorly, posteriorly, and leftward, passing from above the developing RV to above the developing LV, by going through the interventricular foramen and coming into direct fibrous continuity with the developing MV via an intervalvar fibrosa. Reciprocally, the aortic valve, sitting atop a well-developed right-sided subaortic infundibulum, is carried superiorly and anteriorly above the developing RV. Thus, in typical D-TGA, the wrong great artery (the PA) gets transposed from above the RV to above the LV because of inverted development of the subarterial connecting segment. This may be expressed as follows: **TGA** {**S,D,D**} = **4R + 0L** so the infundibuloarterial (IA) situs combination is inversus + solitus. Thus IA situs discordance (difference) is present. The anatomic pattern (situs) of the infundibular connector (inversus) and the situs of the great arteries (solitus) are not the same. Because the anatomic pattern of the infundibular connector is "backward," the "pipes" (great arteries) get connected to the ventricles "backward." All plumbers know that the structural type of the connector and the structural type of the pipes being connected must be the same; otherwise, the connection won't work. *The fifth column to the right* presents the problem of the bilateral infundibulum, i.e., when neither the right-sided subaortic infundibular free wall nor the left-sided subpulmonary infundibular free wall undergoes involution. When both the subaortic infundibulum and the subpulmonary infundibulum are approximately equally well developed, as in the Taussig-Bing malformation, then both the Ao and the PA remain high above the RV, resulting in double-outlet right ventricle (DORV), as in the following equation: **DORV** {**S,D,D**} = **4R + 4L.** The IA situs analysis is ambiguus + solitus. Since the infundibular situs and the great arterial situs are different, IA situs discordance (difference) is present. D malposition of the great arteries (D-MGA) is typical in the Taussig-Bing type of DORV. If the subpulmonary infundibulum is present, but much less well developed than the subaortic infundibulum, then D-TGA can be present, but *without* PV-MV fibrous continuity, as in Fig. 22.1: TGA {S,D,D} = 4R + 2L. The IA situs combination is ambiguus + solitus, i.e., discordant. **IA situs ambiguus** is any IA situs combination that is neither solitus (0R + 4L) nor inversus (4R + 0L), nor a variation of these two. For example, in tetralogy of Fallot {S,D,S}, the IA situs equation can be TOF {S,D,D} = 0R + 2L. This IA situs combination is closely related to the solitus normal IA situs combination (0R + 4L) and hence is not regarded as an ambiguous combination. **To be an ambiguus IA situs combination,** either the infundibular situs or the arterial situs must be in situs ambiguus.

Fig. 22.1, cont'd Many cases of D-TGA have a bilateral conus, often with pulmonary outflow tract stenosis or atresia. In *the sixth column to the right*, a rare case of D-TGA is included with AoV-TV and PV-MV direct fibrous continuity because both the right-sided subaortic infundibular free wall and the left-sided subpulmonary infundibular free wall were focally absent, rarely permitting AoV-TV and PV-MV fibrous continuity. The IA situs equation in this rare case is TGA {S,D,D} = 0R + 0L. A note should be included indicating that the absence of each conus (subaortic and subpulmonary) was focal, not total. Double-outlet left ventricle (DOLV) was not included in this diagram because we had not seen a case of DOLV when this diagram was made. **Geometry:** D-loop formation results in approximately 90° of dextrorotation of the semilunar valves relative to the sagittal (or anteroposterior) plane. Rotation at the semilunar valves relative to the sagittal plane in solitus normally related great arteries equals approximately 150° of dextrorotation. This means that the normally *totally asymmetrical* development of the subaortic and the subpulmonary infundibular free walls increases the normal dextrorotation at the semilunar valves by approximately 60°: 150° − 90° = 60°. In typical D-TGA, dextrorotation at the semilunar valves is much less than normal: about 40° dextrorotation at the semilunar valves relative to the sagittal plane. If D-loop formation of the ventricles is normal, as it typically is (90° dextrorotation at the valves), the finding of only 40° D-rotation at the valves in typical D-TGA suggests that inverted development of the infundibulum results in 50° of *levorotation* at the semilunar valves in typical D-TGA: 90° dextrorotation (D-loop formation) plus 50° levorotation (infundibular inversion) equals 40° dextrorotation at the semilunar valves in D-TGA. Since the aortic arch is anterior to the pulmonary bifurcation at the aortic arch 4/pulmonary arch 6 junction, with the Ao-PA relationship = 0°, this means that in typical D-TGA, the Ao and PA have to undergo only about 40° levorotation as they go from the semilunar valves proximally (40° dextrorotation) to the Ao-PA relationship distally at the arch 4/6 junction (0° rotation). This is why in typical D-TGA, the transposed Ao and PA appear to be almost parallel, because they have so little untwisting to do (about 40° levorotation) compared with solitus normally related great arteries (about 150° levorotation) as they untwist from the valves proximally to the aortic arch/PA bifurcation distally. In this diagram, the transposed great arteries have only about as much untwisting to do as do normally related great arteries: 40°/150° = 0.27. Or, put another way, these transposed great arteries have only about 27% as much untwisting to do as do solitus normally related great arteries. Although we often speak of normally related great arteries as being "twisted around each other," it is helpful to realize that the normal Ao and PA are *untwisting* about each other. The great arteries normally have to undo the dextrorotation that was put into the bulboventricular loop by D-loop formation (90° dextrorotation) and by asymmetrical subarterial infundibular free wall development (60° dextrorotation), i.e., a total of about 150° dextrorotation, that must be taken out of the system by about 150° of levorotation by the great arteries. That's why the ascending Ao and the PA are fibroelastic—so they can untwist. That is also why the conus arteriosus (which means arterial cone, Latin) or infundibulum (funnel, Latin) retreated from the arterial arches (as in sharks) to a subsemilunar valvar position. If our great arteries were "muscle bound," as in sharks, they could not untwist. The shark heart, with only one ventricle, is a straight, untwisted pump. But higher reptiles (crocodiles and alligators), mammals, and birds have two ventricles. So our tubular heart had to twist (usually to the right) to develop a lung pump (our RV). But if a twist is put into a tubular heart to make a second ventricle (our RV), the twist has to be taken out of the tubular heart system somewhere, and that's what the normal ascending Ao and the PA are doing, by untwisting about each other. Our great arteries are more than passive conduits. They are also structural engineers. Our fibroelastic great arteries, by untwisting about each other in a leftward or clockwise direction as seen from below, take the dextral torsion out of the normal ventricular D-looping (about 90°), and the dextral torsion out of normally asymmetrical development of the infundibulum (about 60°). That is why normally related great arteries untwist through about 150° of leftward or clockwise rotation (as seen from below) as they go from the semilunar valves proximally to the aortic arch and ligamentum arteriosum distally. (Modified and reproduced with permission from Van Praagh R, Van Praagh S. Isolated ventricular inversion, a consideration of the morphogenesis, definition, and diagnosis of nontransposed and transposed great arteries. *Am J Cardiol* 1966;17:395e406.)

The infundibular situs **(4R + 0L)** in typical D-TGA is the same as the infundibular situs in situs inversus totalis:

$$\text{INRGA } \{I,L,I\} = \mathbf{4R + 0L} \qquad (2)$$

In typical D-TGA, the infundibular situs is inverted **(4R + 0L)**, but the great arteries are not inverted. D-TGA is noninverted or solitus TGA, that is, TGA without right-left reversal. The aortic valve is to the right of the pulmonary valve, which is normal in situs solitus.

So, as equation 3 indicates, **typical D-TGA is isolated infundibular inversion.**

Equation 4 indicates that classical physiologically corrected TGA is isolated infundibular noninversion and great arterial inversion.

Terminology

We avoided the term "complete" TGA (meaning D-TGA), because both D-TGA and L-TGA are complete: both great arteries are completely transposed or placed across the ventricular septum in both D-TGA and L-TGA.

We avoided the designation "partial" TGA because of its nonspecificity. There are two types of "partial" TGA: double-outlet right ventricle (DORV) and double-outlet left ventricle (DOLV).

We avoided the designations "physiologically uncorrected" and "physiologically corrected" TGA because there are different anatomic types, and because they are so frequently inaccurate physiologically because of associated malformations.

We avoided "noninverted" and "inverted" TGA because these terms mean one thing in visceroatrial situs solitus, the opposite thing in visceroatrial situs inversus, and nothing in visceroatrial situs ambiguus with the heterotaxy syndromes of asplenia, polysplenia, and right-sided spleen. If you don't know what the visceroatrial situs is you can't make the diagnosis of noninverted or inverted TGA because the visceroatrial situs is the frame of reference.

The only diagnostic approach that always works well is the **segmental approach** (Fig. 22.3). The anatomy of each of the three main cardiac segments, that is, {atria, ventricles, and great arteries}, is diagnosed specifically. The anatomy of each of the two connecting cardiac segments—the atrioventricular canal or junction, and the infundibulum or conus—is also diagnosed specifically. Finally, all clinically and surgically important associated anomalies are included.

The infundibuloarterial (IA) situs equations[1] are relatively new. They were developed in 2015 and 2016, and they are tabulated here for the reader's convenience.

History

The anomaly now known as transposition of the great arteries was first described by **Matthew Baillie** of London, England, in 1797 (Fig. 22.4).[1,2] He called it "a very singular malformation of the heart."

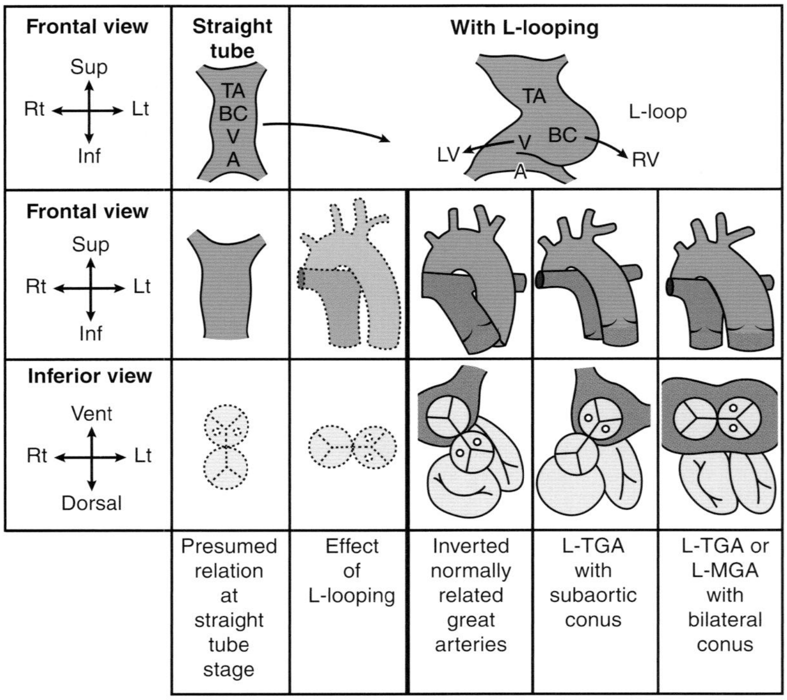

Fig. 22.2 This figure is a mirror image of Fig. 22.1. The straight heart tube in this figure *(leftmost column)* is assumed to be a mirror-image of the straight heart tube in Fig. 22.1. L-loop formation *(top row)* carries the developing aortic valve 90° to the left of the pulmonary valve *(second column from the left).* Inverted normally related great arteries are depicted in the *third column from the left.* The infundibuloarterial (IA) situs equation is **INRGA {1,L,I} = 4R + 0L.** The IA situs combination is inversus + inversus (concordant). In the *fourth column to the right,* L-TGA is depicted. This diagram could apply to physiologically uncorrected TGA in visceroatrial situs inversus, i.e., TGA {I,L,L}, or to physiologically corrected TGA in visceroatrial situs solitus, i.e., TGA {S,L,L}. In either case, the IA situs equation is TGA {1,L,L} = 0R + 4L, or TGA {S,L,L} = 0R + 4L. The IA situs combination is solitus infundibulum + inverted great arteries, i.e., a discordant IA situs combination, which is why the great arteries are transposed. In the *fifth column to the right,* a bilateral infundibulum (subaortic and subpulmonary) is depicted. This can occur with left-sided double-outlet right ventricle (DORV) {I,L,L} or with TGA {S,L,L}. In either case, the IA situs equation is, for example, DORV {I,L,L} = 4R + 4L. Hence, the IA situs combination is ambiguus + inversus, hence discordant. When the infundibular (or great arterial) situs is neither solitus nor inversus, it is ambiguus. Geometrically, inverted normally related great arteries *(column 3)* have rotated approximately 150° to the left relative to the sagittal plane. L-TGA has undergone much less levorotation at the semilunar valves, in this case approximately 33° levorotation *(fourth column from the left).* When the subaortic and the subpulmonary infundibular musculature is approximately the same bilaterally, then the rotation at the semilunar valves is not influenced by infundibular development. The rotational effects of right-sided versus left-sided infundibular growth, being equal, cancel each other. Hence, the rotational effect at the semilunar valves is that of ventricular looping only. In L-TGA, there are two rotational effects at the semilunar valves: (1) levorotation because of ventricular L-looping; and (2) rotation in the opposite direction, to the right (dextrorotation), because of left-sided infundibular growth and right-sided infundibular resorption (60° or less). **This is why the transposed aortic valve typically is anterior to the transposed pulmonary valve, because in TGA there are two opposite rotational vectors:** (1) in the direction of ventricular looping, say 90° to the right, and (2) in the *opposite* direction to the left because of infundibular development, say 50° to the left. The result is 90° − 50° = 40° rotation to the right of the sagittal (anteroposterior) plane, a typical D-TGA, as in Fig. 22.1. **In normally related great arteries (solitus and inversus), there is only one direction of rotation,** the effect of ventricular looping and the effect of infundibular development both causing rotation in the *same* direction at the semilunar valve level. In other words, normally, the direction of ventricular looping and the sidedness of infundibular resorption must both be the same (both right-sided or both left-sided). If the direction of ventricular looping and the sidedness of infundibular resorption are opposites, TGA results. Contralateral infundibular development reverses semilunar rotation, prevents the normal embryonic aortic switch, and results in the abnormal pulmonary arterial switch. (Modified and reproduced with permission from Van Praagh R, Van Praagh S. Isolated ventricular inversion, a consideration of the morphogenesis, definition, and diagnosis of nontransposed and transposed great arteries. *Am J Cardiol* 1966;17:395e406.)

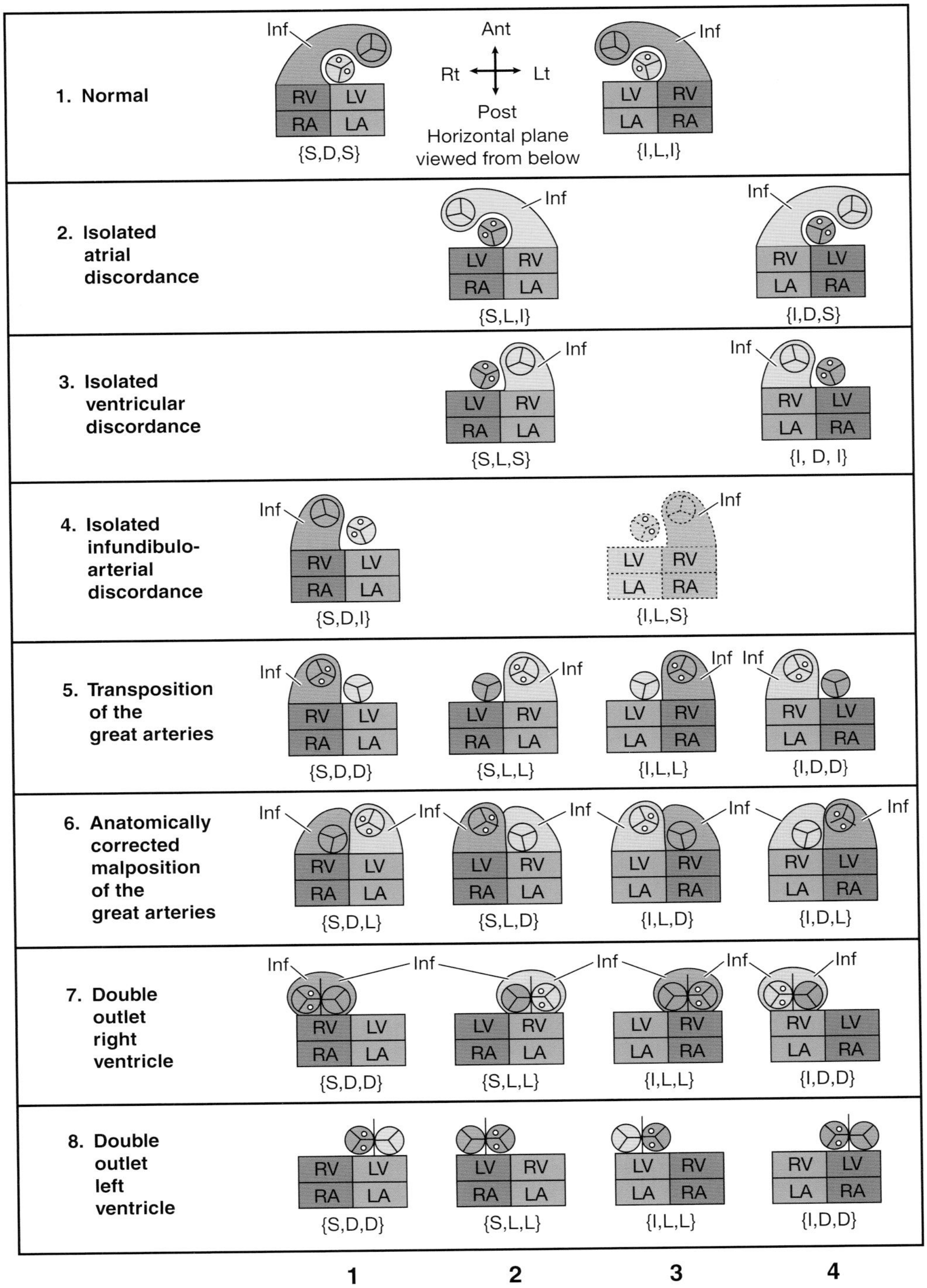

Fig. 22.3 Types of human heart in terms of segmental sets, alignments, and connections. Braces {} mean the set (or combination) of. The three main cardiac segments are {atria, ventricles, great arteries}. The two connecting cardiac segments are {the atrioventricular canal or junction, infundibulum or conus arteriosus}. Thus, there are five cardiac segments. Set theory facilitates multivariate analysis. Cardiac chambers are identified and named morphologically, not positionally. The heart diagrams are viewed from below. *Inf,* Infundibulum. The columns are arranged in terms of their atrioventricular *(AV)* concordance or discordance. Column 1 has AV concordance. The morphologically right atrium *(RA)* opens into the morphologically right ventricle *(RV),* and the morphologically left atrium *(LA)* opens into the morphologically left ventricle *(LV).* Column 2 has atrioventricular discordance. RA opens into LV, and LA opens into RV. Columns 1 and 2 have visceroatrial situs solitus with a right-sided RA and a left-sided LA. Columns 3 and 4 have visceroatrial situs inversus. Column 3 has AV concordance, while column 4 has AV discordance. Rows 1 to 4 have normally related great arteries (ventriculoarterial concordance). Rows 5 to 8 have various types of ventriculoarterial discordance: transposition of the great arteries (row 5); anatomically corrected malposition of the great arteries (row 6); double-outlet right ventricle (row 7); and double-outlet left ventricle (row 8). This figure does not depict all of the types of heart that exist. Instead, it illustrates how the segmental approach to the diagnosis and classification of congenital heart disease works. (Reproduced with permission from Van Praagh R. What determines whether the great arteries are normally or abnormally related? *Am J Cardiol* 2016;118:1390.)

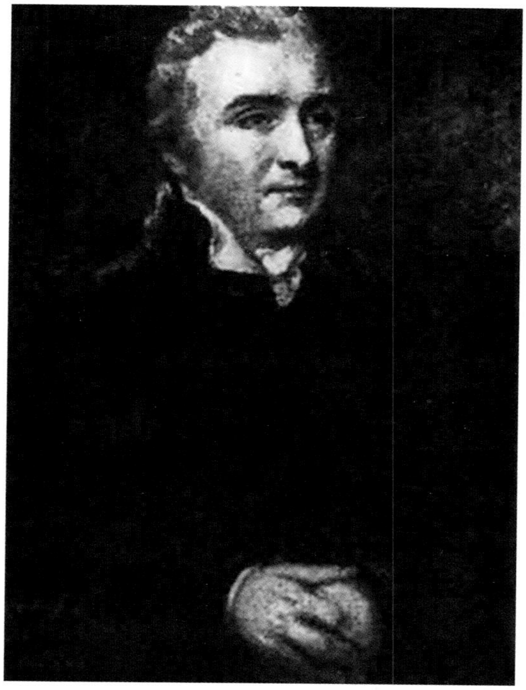

Fig. 22.4 Matthew Baillie (1761–1823) of London, England, the discoverer of transposition of the great arteries in 1797. Baillie was a nephew of John Hunter, the leading surgeon of his time. Both Baillie and Hunter were Scots from Lanarkshire who practiced in London. Baillie practiced at St. George's Hospital, served as physician to King George III during his last illness, and wrote a book titled *Morbid Anatomy of Some of the Most Important Parts of the Human Body* in 1793. This was the first book to treat pathology systematically, as in a modem textbook. Baillie correlated clinical medicine and pathologic anatomy, and consequently he is regarded as one of the founding fathers of pathology. His important medical findings were numerous and included emphysema of the lungs, situs inversus totalis with dextrocardia (1788), the association between rheumatic disease and valvar lesions of the heart (1797), and much more. (Reproduced with permission from Van Praagh R. What determines whether the great arteries are normally or abnormally related? *Am J Cardiol* 2016;118:1390.)

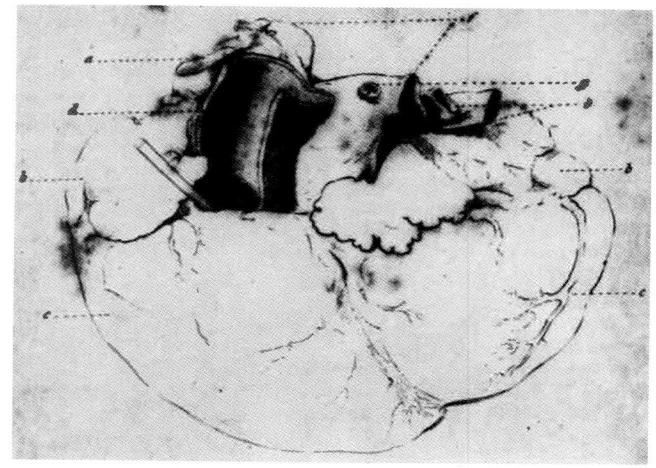

Fig. 22.5 Drawing of John Farre's heart specimen. He coined the term "transposition of the aorta and pulmonary artery." *a,* Superior vena cava; *b,* right atrium; *c,* right ventricle; *d,* transposed aorta; *e,* coronary artery; *f,* pulmonary artery branches; *g,* patent ductus arteriosus. (From Van Praagh R. What determines whether the great arteries are normally or abnormally related? *Am J Cardiol* 2016;118:1390 with permission.)

The second case of this anomaly was described by **Langstaff** in 1811; he also called it "a singular malformation of the heart."[2] He is referred to as Mr. Langstaff, suggesting that he may have been a barber-surgeon.

The third known case was published by **John Richard Farre** of London in 1814 (Fig. 22.5). It was he who coined the term "transposition" of the aorta and the pulmonary artery. Farre used the term "transposition" of the great arteries literally: **trans** = across, and **positio** = placement. The ventricular septum was the structure across which the great arteries were placed in transposition of the great arteries (TGA). Farre meant that the aorta arose from the right ventricle and that the pulmonary artery originated from the left ventricle. Farre did not mention that the transposed aortic valve was anterior to the transposed pulmonary valve, although it probably was. But that is not what Farre meant by his designation transposition of the great arteries.

In 1844, **Sir Richard Quain** proposed that transposition of the great arteries is caused by *straight* downgrowth of the truncoconal septum (Fig. 22.6). Normally, the aortopulmonary and

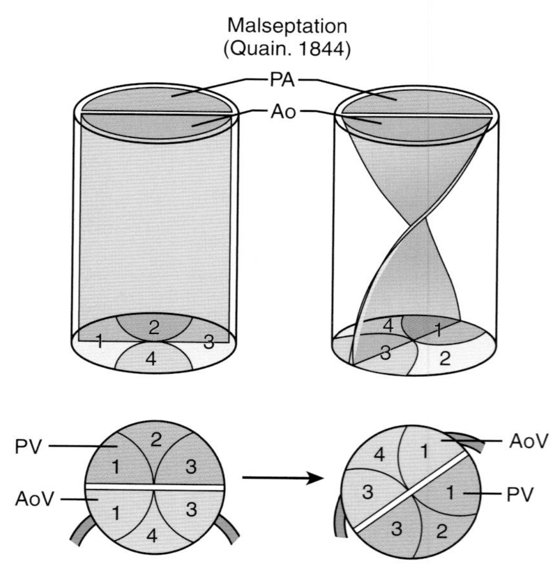

Fig. 22.6 Straight development of the aortopulmonary septum was proposed by Sir Richard Quain in 1844 (cited by Peacock in 1858). Quain thought that if the aortopulmonary septum were to grow down straight, i.e., in a nonspiral fashion, from the aortic arch 4/pulmonary arch 6 junction distally, then proximally at the semilunar valve level, the aortic valve and the coronary arteries would be anterior, and the pulmonary valve (with no coronary arteries) would be posterior, thereby explaining the morphogenesis of transposition of the great arteries *(left diagram).* If the aorta-pulmonary septum grows down in the normal spiral fashion, then the great arteries are normally related. Thus, Quain's concept was a malseptation hypothesis: a straight anteroposterior septum, instead of a spiral septum. *Ao,* Aorta; *AoV,* aortic valve; *PA,* pulmonary artery; *PV,* pulmonary valve. The numbers on the developing semilunar leaflets are the conventional numbers used to identify the leaflets in all stages of rotation. (Reproduced with permission from Van Praagh R. What determines whether the great arteries are normally or abnormally related? *Am J Cardiol* 2016;118:1390.)

infundibular septum grow down in a *spiral* fashion. Quain's straight septum hypothesis endeavored to explain why the great arteries are parallel or straight in TGA, and do not spiral around each other normally. Quain's very influential straight truncoconal septum hypothesis is referred to by Thomas Bevill Peacock (1858).[2]

In 1875, **Carl von Rokitansky** of Vienna (Fig. 22.6) reported the malformation that would become known as congenital physiologically corrected transposition of the great arteries (Fig. 22.3, row 5, column 2).[1] Thus, as of 1875, two anatomic types of TGA were known. Von Rokitansky called them **anomalous transposition,** as described by Baillie, Langstaff, Farre, and others (Fig. 22.3, row 5, column 1), and **corrected transposition,** described by himself.

In 1898, **Hermann Vierordt** of Tübingen, Germany, described **partial transposition.** Only the aorta is transposed into the right ventricle. Since the early 1960s, this type of malformation has been known as **double-outlet right ventricle.**

Since Vierordt had discovered **partial** transposition of the great arteries, he renamed **anomalous** transposition of von Rokitansky **complete** transposition of the great arteries. In 1909, **Sir Arthur Keith**[2] figured out and published what we think typical D-TGA really is: **infundibular inversion** (Fig. 22.7). In typical TGA, the right-sided subaortic part of the infundibulum develops well, and the left-sided subpulmonary part of the infundibulum involutes (disappears)—instead of vice versa, which is normal.

Then what happened? Nothing. It seemed that no one understood. Not until 1967—58 years later—when a Canadian, Keith (Dr. John D. Keith, Chief of Cardiology at the Hospital for Sick Children in Toronto, Canada) asked one of his fellows in Pediatric Cardiology (me) and Dr. Peter Vlad to write a new chapter on TGA for the next edition of their book.

Then, when we had finished our work on TGA and had realized that TGA is an infundibular malformation, someone suggested that we really should look at a paper by Arthur Keith that was published in 1909, and that I was unaware of. I was amazed to discover that Arthur Keith[3] in 1909 had reached the same conclusions that we did in 1967.[4] This is why I have always given Arthur Keith credit for this discovery.

Now, we must return to the early years of the 20th century, when three different anatomic types of transposition of the great arteries were known: (1) **complete,** (2) **partial,** and (3) **corrected.** This is how TGA was presented in 1915 by **Maude Abbott** of Montreal, Canada. Abbott's diagrams of normally related great arteries, true or complete TGA, and corrected TGA are presented in Fig. 22.8.

In 1923, **Alexander Spitzer**[5,6] of Vienna reclassified TGA into eight types[2] (Fig. 22.9). Spitzer's theory is not supported by the morphologic anatomy and hence will not be considered in detail. For example, in his type III TGA, he says that the true ventricular septum has disappeared; hence the dotted line in the middle of the left-sided ventricle. Spitzer says that the apparent ventricular septum is a hugely hypertrophied crista supraventricularis.

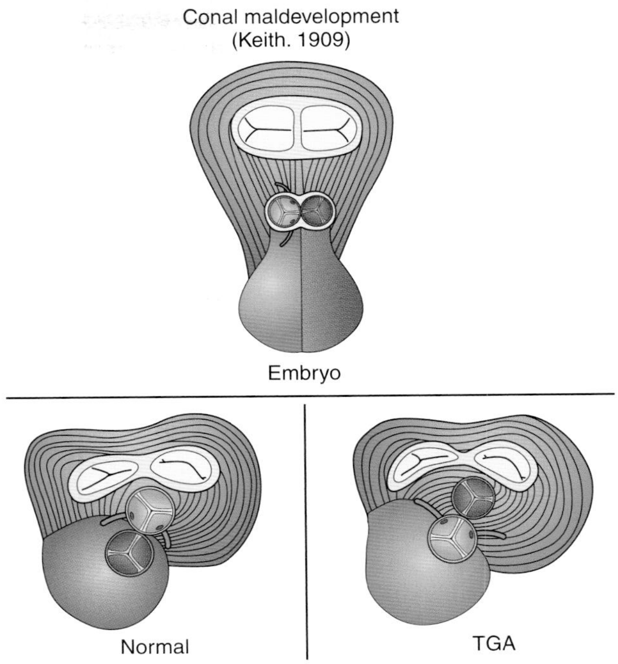

Fig. 22.7 Sir Arthur Keith (1866–1955), of Aberdeen, Scotland, came to London to work as an anatomist and embryologist. Virtually all accounts correctly state that while working with Flack in 1907, Keith discovered the sinoatrial node, the pacemaker of the human heart. But almost no account states that 2 years later, in 1909, Keith discovered the correct morphogenesis of transposition of the great arteries *(TGA)* in humans. He observed that in TGA, the right-sided subaortic part of the infundibulum (or conus arteriosus) grows and expands *(red),* whereas the left-sided subpulmonary part of the infundibulum *(blue)* involutes (disappears). Keith realized that the opposite is what happens normally resulting in normally related great arteries. Note that Keith shows the normal pulmonary valve as being anterior and to the *right* of the normal aortic valve. This was a common preangiocardiographic error. Although counterintuitive, the normal pulmonary valve is anterior, superior, and to the *left* of the normal aortic valve. (Reproduced with permission from Van Praagh R. What determines whether the great arteries are normally or abnormally related? *Am J Cardiol* 2016;118:1390.)

Why?

So that the *transposed* pulmonary valve is located above the *right* ventricular myocardium, not the *left* ventricular myocardium.[7]

Why?

Because there is no animal known in which the pulmonary artery arises naturally above the left ventricle.

In his atavistic theory, the pulmonary artery "must" arise above the *right* ventricle. But in typical D-TGA, the transposed pulmonary artery in fact does originate above the morphologically *left* ventricle, not above the right ventricle.

In 1927, **Abbott** defined TGA as an alteration of the position of the great arteries relative to each other, or relative to the ventricles from which they arise.[2]

In 1937, **Maurice Lev and Otto Saphir,**[8] who had translated Spitzer's phylogenetic hypothesis from German into English, defined TGA in a fashion similar to Abbott's definition. But by the late 1930s, this meant that TGA was defined as almost any abnormality in the spatial relationship between the great

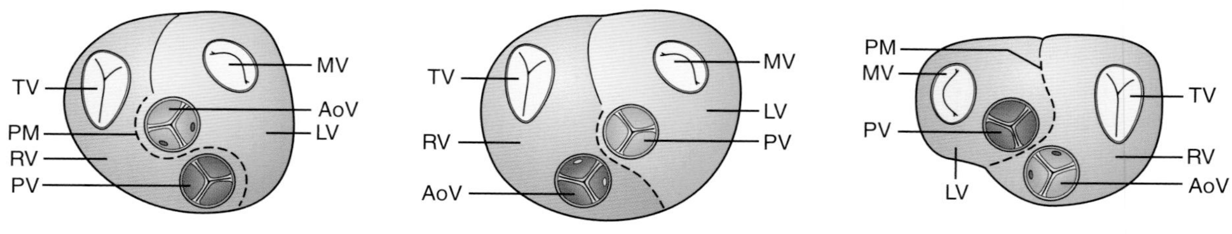

Fig. 22.8 Abbott's diagram in 1915 of the normal relation between the great arteries, true complete transposition, and corrected transposition. Note that Abbott omitted partial transposition (Vierordt, 1898), that is now called double-outlet right ventricle. *AoV,* Aortic valve; *LV,* morphologically left ventricle; *MV,* mitral valve; *PM,* pars membranacea septi; *RV,* morphologically right ventricle; *TV,* tricuspid valve. (Reproduced with permission from Van Praagh R. What determines whether the great arteries are normally or abnormally related? *Am J Cardiol* 2016;118:1390.)

arteries themselves, and/or between the great arteries and the ventricles. **Thus, TGA meant almost anything and everything, clearly an untenable situation.**

In 1939, **Harris and Farber**[9] of Boston tried to assess Spitzer's work on TGA.[2] They accepted Spitzer's most important insight, namely, the importance of segmental inversions (Fig. 22.10). Harris and Farber tacitly excluded Spitzer's type I TGA (overriding aorta), type II TGA (double-outlet right ventricle), and type IV TGA (double-inlet single LV with infundibular outlet chamber and D-TGA). Harris and Farber played solitus inversus permutations with the atria, the ventricles, and the great arteries. They emerged with eight theoretical types of crossed TGA, and they succeeded in reintroducing a semblance of order and comprehensibility into the field.

In 1956, **Cardell** of London accepted Harris and Farber's classification of TGA, but reorganized it into **four physiologically uncorrected forms** (Fig. 22.11, A1, A2, A3, and A4) and into **four physiologically corrected forms** (Fig. 22.11, B1, B2, B3, and B4).

In the physiologically uncorrected forms, the morphologically right atrium (RA) and the aorta are ipsilateral (same-sided). In the physiologically corrected types, the morphologically left atrium (LA) and the aorta are ipsilateral.

I graduated from the Faculty of Medicine of the University of Toronto, Canada, in 1954. So, Cardell's classification of TGA (Fig. 22.11) was "state of the art" in my early years of postgraduate training to become a pediatric cardiologist. Cardell's classification was anatomically precise and physiologically meaningful. But could it be improved? Little did I know that I would try to answer this question.

Although Cardell's classification of TGA (Fig. 22.11) was a considerable improvement, it was difficult to use clinically. The eight different combinations of atria, ventricles, and great arteries were almost impossible to memorize, and the anatomic types (A1 to A4 and B1 to B4) were meaningless. So, unless one kept a copy of this classification in one's pocket, one could not use it.

I realized that we needed a diagnostic approach and a classification that could be *understood,* and that did not have to be memorized. My first big study was based on 60 autopsied cases of single or common ventricle.[10] In addition to an understanding of morphologic anatomy (what is a morphologically right atrium, left atrium, right ventricle, left ventricle), one also needs to understand the various cardiac segments or compartments: the main cardiac segments are the atria, the ventricles, and the great arteries; and the connecting cardiac segments are the atrioventricular canal or junction, and the infundibulum or conus arteriosus.

Presented diagrammatically, **the situs of the viscera and atria** in 60 autopsied cases of single or common ventricule[10] is shown in Fig. 22.12.

The situs and the malformations of the ventricular segment are presented in Fig. 22.13 and in Table 22.1. For example, absence of the RV sinus resulting in single LV with an infundibular outlet chamber occurred in 47 of 60 cases (78%). Ventricular D-loops (solitus ventricular loops) occurred in 20 of 47 cases (43%), and ventricular L-loops (inverted ventricular loops) were found in 27 of 47 cases (57%) (Fig. 22.13).[10]

The situs and malformations of the great arteries are shown in Fig. 22.14. There were nine **Holmes hearts** (15%), that is, solitus normally related great arteries with single LV. The incidences of D-TGA (42%) and L-TGA (43%) were almost the same. But don't forget that when this study was done (published in 1964),[10] transposition of the great arteries was still being used in the old imprecise way. This means that the 3 patients with single RV (absence of the LV sinus) (5%), the 4 patients with a rudimentary or absent ventricular septum (7%), and the 6 patients with morphologically unidentified ventricular myocardium (10%) would all have been considered to have some type of TGA (D- or L-). Thus, the diagnosis of TGA may well have been imprecise in 13 of 60 patients with single or common ventricle (22%).[10]

The type of data analysis that we knew how to do in the early 1960s[4,10] was good for **univariate analysis,** for example, that single LV, due to absence of the RV sinus, was by far the commonest type of single ventricle (78%).[10] But by about 1980, we

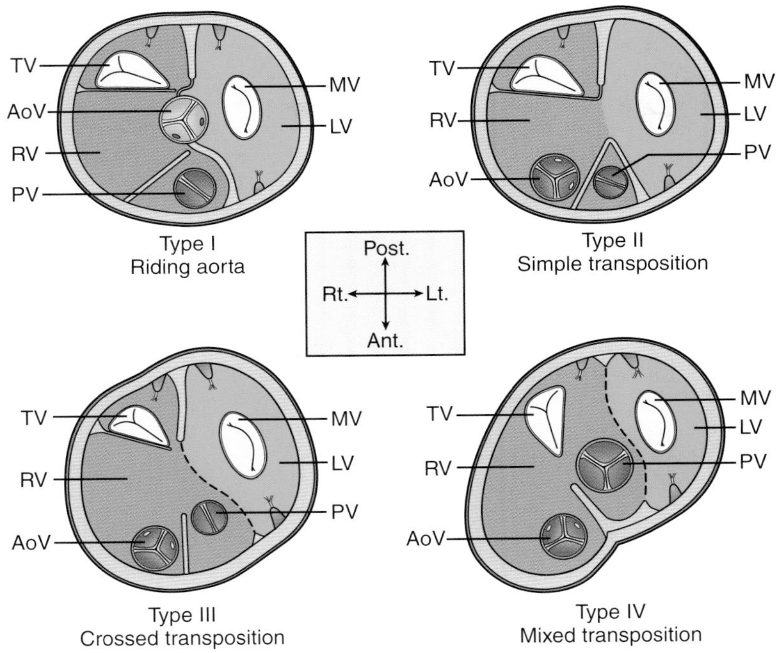

Fig. 22.9 Spitzer's classification of transposition of the great arteries (1923): type I, riding aorta, what we now call an overriding aorta; type II, simple transposition, what we now call double-outlet right ventricle (DORV); type III, crossed transposition; and type IV, mixed transposition. Regarding type I, no other investigator, to my knowledge, has ever called an overriding aorta a form of TGA. Type II is what we call DORV with pulmonary stenosis (PS). Regarding type III, the *dotted line* indicates where Spitzer thought the ventricular septum had disappeared. The vanished ventricular septum runs to the left of the pulmonary valve. Consequently, the bicuspid pulmonary valve arises above the right ventricle *(RV)*, not above the left ventricle *(LV)*, Spitzer says. This assertion is contrary to morphologic anatomic fact. There is no animal known in which the pulmonary artery normally arises above the LV, as it does in typical D-TGA. This morphologic anatomic fact is fatal for Spitzer's atavistic theory: In typical D-TGA, the transposed PV does arise above the LV, not above the RV, as Spitzer illustrates. Type IV Spitzer calls *mixed* TGA, by which he means that not only is the outlet (the aorta and the pulmonary artery) transposed, but so too the inlet (the tricuspid and the mitral valve) is also transposed. But note the dotted line, i.e., the ventricular septum that has disappeared so that the transposed pulmonary valve can arise above RV myocardium, as it must in any atavistic hypothesis. Accepting Spitzer's dotted line, then the inlet is not transposed. The tricuspid valve opens into the RV, not into the LV. If there is not double-inlet LV, then what Spitzer is showing is not mixed TGA. In conclusion, Spitzer's atavistic hypothesis is not supported by the morphologic anatomy of the subpulmonary LV in TGA. (Reproduced with permission from Van Praagh R. What determines whether the great arteries are normally or abnormally related? *Am J Cardiol* 2016;118:1390.)

had learned how to use set theory, which made it possible to do multivariate analysis.

In our later study of single ventricle,[11] TGA occurred in 23 of 31 cases (74%). DORV was found in 6 of 31 cases (74%). DORV was found in 6 of 31 cases of single ventricle (19%). Normally related great arteries occurred in only 2 patients (6%).

CHIRALITY OR HANDEDNESS

Chirality or handedness is a helpful way of diagnosing the situs of the atria, or of the ventricles in potentially confusing situations. Your hands are isomers.

A D-loop or solitus RV is right-handed (Fig. 22.15).[12] Your thumb represents the RV inflow tract. Your fingers represent the RV outflow tract. The palm of your right hand stands for the right ventricular septal surface. The dorsum of your right hand represents the RV free wall.

Conversely, your left hand is like an L-loop or an inversus RV (Fig. 22.16).[13] Your left thumb is like the inflow tract of an inverted RV. The fingers of your left hand are like the outflow tract of an L-loop RV. The palm of your left hand symbolizes the septal surface of an inverted RV. The dorsum of your left hand represents the free wall of an inverted RV.

In crisscross atrioventricular (AV) relations, the AV inflow tracts can be very angulated relative to each other. Note the arrows in Figs. 22.15 and 22.16. Both ventricles can be bilateral.

If only one ventricle is present, you can tell which ventricle is present, and which is absent: **Apply the morphologic method of diagnosis.**

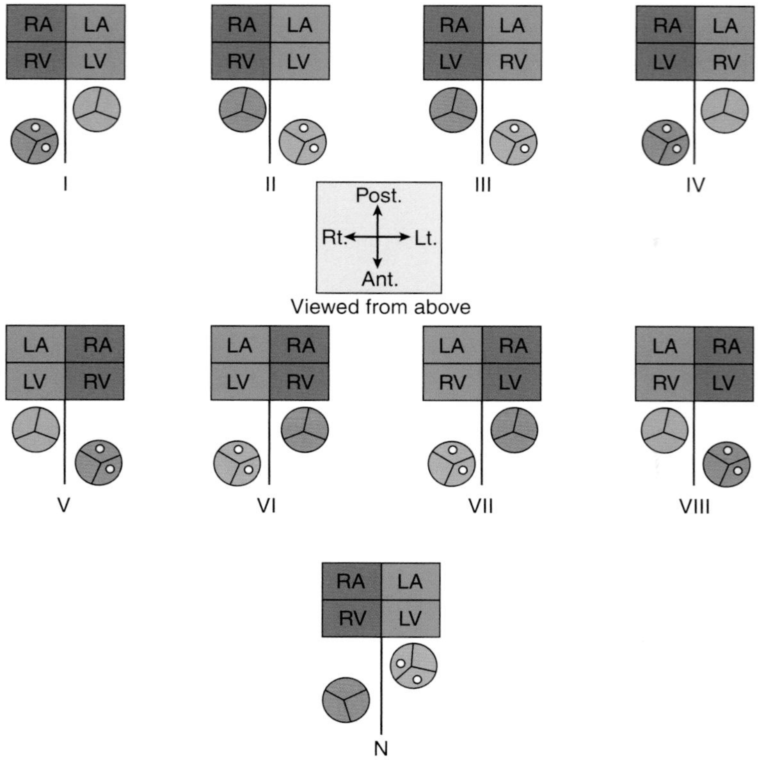

Fig. 22.10 Harris and Farber's classification of transposition of the great arteries (TGA) in 1939. Note that these authors did not include overriding aorta or partial transposition (double-outlet right ventricle) in their classification of TGA, only complete TGA in which both the aorta and the pulmonary artery were transposed. Their types I to IV included all possible combinations of atria, ventricles, and great arteries in visceroatrial situs solitus. Their types V to VIII included all possible combinations of atria, ventricles, and great arteries in visceroatrial situs inversus. Their types II, IV, VI, and VIII they called *anatomically corrected transposition of the great arteries* because both great arteries had been abnormally placed across the ventricular septum with anterior aorta and posterior pulmonary artery. Nonetheless, each great artery was placed above the morphologically appropriate ventricle: A above LV, and P above RV. Hence, these transpositions were regarded as *anatomically* corrected. Their classification proves that Harris and Farber understood the *morphologically* right ventricle, as opposed to the *positionally* right ventricle. Similarly these authors understood the difference between the *morphologically* left ventricle and the *positionally* left ventricle. These investigators also understood that their type II was *physiologically* corrected TGA in visceroatrial situs solitus, and that their type VII was *physiologically* corrected TGA. In congenital physiologically corrected TGA, there is atrioarterial alignment concordance because of a canceling double discordance at both the atrioventricular and the ventriculoarterial alignments. (Reproduced with permission from Van Praagh R. What determines whether the great arteries are normally or abnormally related? *Am J Cardiol* 2016;118:1390.)

You can also tell whether a ventricular D-loop (solitus) or a ventricular L-loop (inversus) is present. Use **chirality.** Handedness works just as well for the LV as for the RV. The solitus (D-loop) LV is left-handed. The inverted (L-loop) LV is right-handed.

Chirality works well for the atria too. The solitus RA is right-handed and the solitus LA is left-handed. The inverted RA is left-handed and the inverted LA is right-handed.

ERRORS: BILATERALLY RIGHT ATRIA AND BILATERALLY LEFT ATRIA

We think that the concept of bilaterally right atria (RA), or bilaterally right atrial appendages (RAA), is anatomically erroneous. Similarly, the concept of bilaterally left atria (LA), or bilaterally left atrial appendages (LAA), is also anatomically erroneous. First of all, bilaterally RA have never been accurately documented, that is, a right-sided RA and a left-sided RA, both receiving an inferior vena cava, both receiving a coronary sinus ostium, and both having a septal surface displaying the superior limbic band of septum secundum.

Similarly, bilaterally LA have never been accurately documented, that is, a left-sided and a right-sided atrium, both receiving four pulmonary veins and both displaying septum primum on its septal surface.

The proponents of these erroneous concepts call them right atrial *isomerism* or left atrial *isomerism*. When confined to the

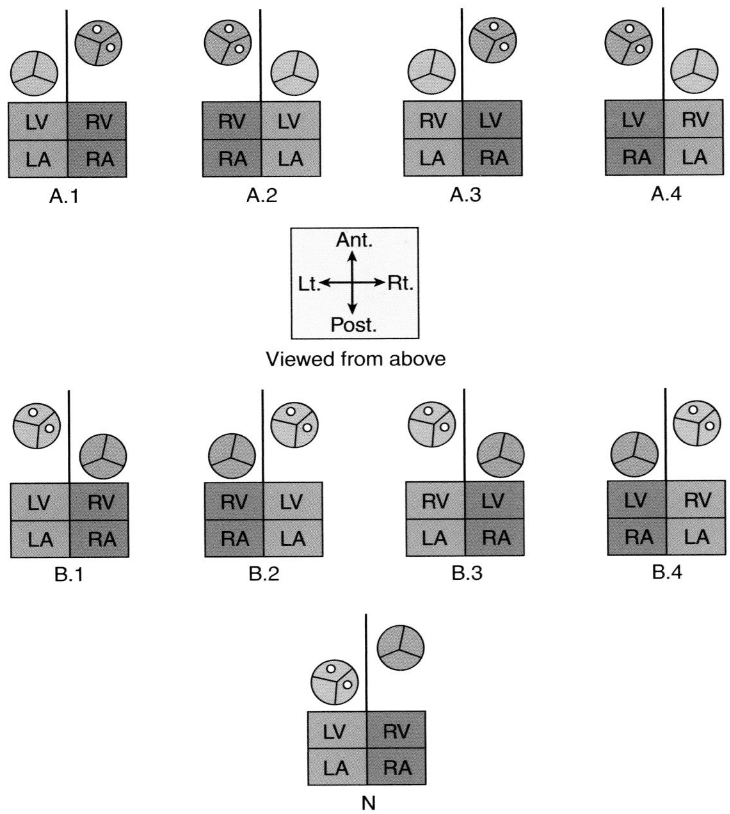

Fig. 22.11 Cardell's classification in 1956 of transposition of the great arteries into four physiologically uncorrected types (*A.1* to *A.4*) and four physiologically corrected types (*B.1* to *B4*). He also included a diagram of the normal heart *(N)*. The spatial orientation of these diagrams is a bit unusual. It is as though the reader were looking downward at his own heart. The view is from above; anterior is toward the top of the page; posterior is toward the bottom of he page; right is toward the reader's right hand; and left is toward the reader's left hand. Cardell's classification is Harris and Farber's classification, reorganized in terms of physiologic uncorrection (types A.1 to A.4) and physiologic correction (types B.1 to B.4). (Reproduced with permission from Van Praagh R. What determines whether the great arteries are normally or abnormally related? *Am J Cardiol* 2016;118:1390.)

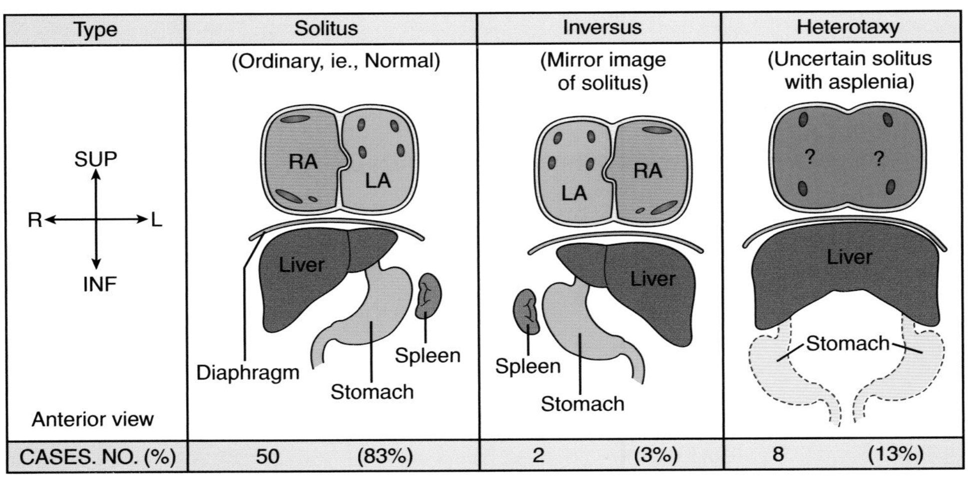

Fig. 22.12 The two types of visceroatrial situs: situs solitus, the normal or noninverted pattern of visceroatrial organization; and situs inversus, the mirror-image pattern of anatomic organization. Visceroatrial heterotaxy is *not* a third type of situs. Instead, heterotaxy means that the pattern of anatomic organization is other than, or different from, that seen in situs solitus or in situs inversus: *heteros*, other, different, Greek; and *taxis*, arrangement, Greek. In clinical practice, visceroatrial heterotaxy (or heterotaxia) means that the type of visceroatrial situs is not diagnosed. In the study of 60 autopsied cases of single and common ventricle (also known as univentricular heart) from which these data were taken, situs solitus of the viscera and atria were present in 83.3%, situs inversus was found in 3.3%, and visceroatrial heterotaxy (uncertain or unknown situs) with the asplenia syndrome occurred in 13.3%. (Reproduced with permission from Van Praagh R. What determines whether the great arteries are normally or abnormally related? *Am J Cardiol* 2016;118:1390.)

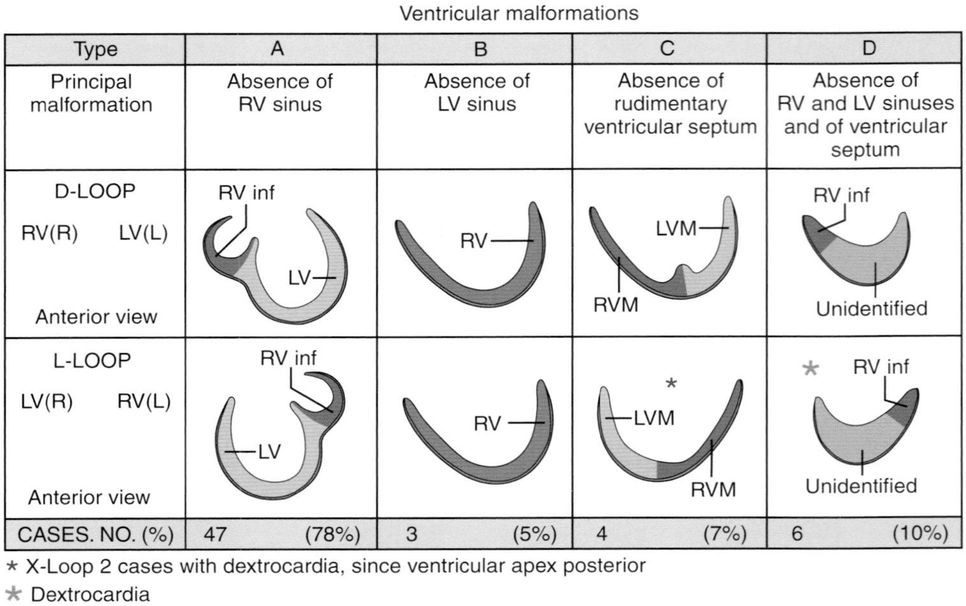

Fig. 22.13 Our first attempt in 1964 to understand the pathologic anatomy of single and common ventricle, based on 60 autopsied cases. By far the most common anatomic type was single morphologically left ventricle *(LV)* with an infundibular outlet chamber *(RV inf)*, caused by absence of the right ventricular sinus or inflow tract (78%). Single morphologically right ventricle, due to absence of the LV sinus, was found in only 5% of cases. A common ventricle, caused by absence or only rudimentary development of the ventricular septum, was identified in 7%. Unidentified ventricular myocardium was encountered in 10%. All of these 60 cases had double-inlet or common-inlet into an apparently single or common ventricle. In other words, tricuspid atresia and mitral atresia were excluded. Why? Because in 1964, we thought we understood tricuspid and mitral atresia. But there were other cases in which both atrioventricular *(AV)* valves or a common AV valve opened into a "single" or "common" ventricle. In cases with double-inlet or common-inlet "single" ventricle, one could not blame the apparent presence of only one ventricle on tricuspid or mitral atresia—because *two* AV valves or a *common* AV valve were present in these cases. So what is going on in these cases? This was essentially the questions that led to my first project in 1964 in pediatric cardiology, in the Catheter Laboratory at the Mayo Clinic in Rochester, Minnesota. A later study of single ventricle in 1979 revealed only two anatomic types: (1) single LV in 74% and (2) single RV in 26%. Since we came to the Boston Children's Hospital in October 1965, we have never seen a case of absence of the ventricular septum or unidentified ventricular myocardium.[6] I think that either such cases are very rare, or they were part of our "learning curve" (early errors). (Reproduced with permission from Van Praagh R, Ongley PA, Swan HJC. Anatomic types of single or common ventricle in man, morphologic and geometric aspects of 60 necropsied cases. *Am J Cardiol* 1964;13:510.)

TABLE 22.1 Infundibuloarterial Situs Equations

1. SNRGA {S,D,S} = 0R + 4L
2. INRGA {1,L,I} = 4R + 0L
3. TGA {S,D,D} = 4R + 0L
4. TGA {S,L,L} = 0R + 4L

INRGA, Inverted normally related great arteries; *SNRGA,* solitus normally related great arteries; *TGA,* transposition of the great arteries.

atrial appendages, these concepts have been called right atrial appendage *isomerism* and left atrial appendage *isomerism.* We think that atrial appendage "isomerism" is a conceptual error. When two complex structures are regarded as isomers (or mirror-images), all parts of one structure must be mirror-images of corresponding components of the other structure. The molecules of D-glucose and L-glucose will illustrate this point:

D-Glucose	**L-Glucose**
C-HO	C-HO
I	I
H-C-OH	HO-C-H
I	I
HO-C-H	H-C-OH
I	I
H-C-OH	HO-C-H
I	I
H-C-OH	HO-C-H
I	I
CH_2OH	CH_2OH

If only two hydroxyl groups (OH) were mirror-images, but nothing else was, then nobody would regard these two molecules as isomers. Partial isomerism (like appendages only) is a conceptual error.

Visceroatrial heterotaxy with the asplenia syndrome has often been regarded as having "bilateral right-sidedness."

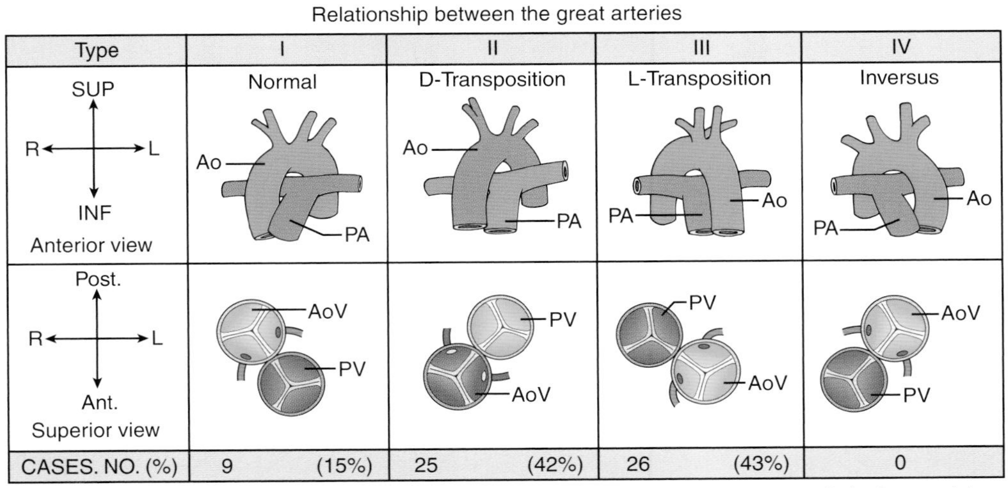

Fig. 22.14 Types of relationship between the great arteries in 60 postmortem cases of single ventricle, as understood in 1964. All of the abnormal relationships between the great arteries were diagnosed as *transpositions,* D- or L-. The D- or L-part is accurate, but the "transposition" part is not. It was not until about 1970 that we started diagnosing the ventriculoarterial (VA) alignments with literal accuracy: TGA = VA discordance (RV to Ao, and LV to PA); DORV = RV to Ao and RV to PA; DOLV = LV to Ao and LV to PA, etc. The diagnosis of "TGA" was inaccurate in 3 patients with single RV, probably inaccurate in the 4 cases with absence of the ventricular septum, and inaccurate in the 6 patients with unidentified ventricular myocardium. Hence, the diagnosis of "transposition" of the great arteries in our 1964 paper[5] was probably inaccurate in 13 of 60 cases (22%). In our 1979 paper on single ventricle,[6] in which the ventriculoarterial alignments were described accurately, the great arterial findings were as follows: In single LV (n = 23), {S,D,S} = 4%; {S,L,S} = 4%; TGA {S,D,D} = 26%; TGA {S,D,L} = 9%; TGA {S,L,L} = 52%; and TGA {S,L,D} = 4%. In single RV (n = 8), DORV {S,D,D} = 25%; DORV {I,L,I} = 12.5%; DORV {A,D,D} with asplenia = 37.5%; TGA {A,D,D} with diminutive LV and asplenia = 12.5%; and TGA {A,L,L} with diminutive LV and asplenia = 12.5%. (Reproduced with permission from Van Praagh R. What determines whether the great arteries are normally or abnormally related? *Am J Cardiol* 2016;118:1390.)

While this is a good mnemonic, it is not accurate anatomy. For example, the liver may have large right and left lobes, suggesting that the liver has large ("rightish") lobes, bilaterally. But then look underneath at the porta hepatis, and you will soon discover whether the patient has a solitus or an inversus liver. The "bilaterally right-sided" mnemonic is intended to help you to think of the heterotaxy syndrome with asplenia.

Visceroatrial heterotaxy with bilateral left-sidedness is a similar mnemonic that is intended to remind you of **the visceroatrial heterotaxy syndrome with "bilateral left-sidedness" and the polysplenia syndrome. Remember these mnemonics, but don't believe them.**

Alignments and Connections

The atria and the ventricles can be *aligned* in many different ways (Fig. 22.3). But the atria and the ventricles normally do not connect tissue-to-tissue because of the interposition of the AV canal or junction.

Similarly, the ventricles and the great arteries can be aligned in many different ways (Fig. 22.3), but they do not connect tissue-to-tissue because of the interposition of the subarterial infundibulum or conus arteriosus, which may be well developed or resorbed (an intervalvar fibrosa).

Thus, the main cardiac segments {atria, ventricles, great arteries} may be aligned in many different ways, but they do not connect.

The connecting cardiac segments—the AV canal or junction, and the infundibulum or conus arteriosus—*connect* the main cardiac segments together.

Alignments and *connections* are both important concepts that should be used accurately. We shouldn't say "the AV *connections* are concordant or discordant" when we mean that the AV *alignments* are concordant or discordant. **Only alignments** can be concordant or discordant because only alignments look forward, in an anterograde or blood-flow direction: atria to ventricles to great arteries.

By contrast, **connections** look forward (anterograde) and backward (retrograde). The AV junction and the infundibulum are like the ancient Roman god **Janus,** who gives us January. Janus, the double-headed god of doorways, looked both forward and backward simultaneously. **Alignments** apply to the main cardiac segments {atria, ventricles, great arteries} that only look forward (anterograde). **Connections** apply to the connecting segments {AV and ventriculoarterial (VA) junctions} that look both forward and backward.

Pathologic Anatomy of TGA

The Second Henry Ford Hospital International Symposium on Cardiac Surgery was held in Detroit in 1975. Dr. Aldo Castaneda and I attended from Boston Children's Hospital. Aldo said to me, "Ricardo, you've got to go to this meeting. It will be very good. I attended the first one, and that's why I went into cardiac surgery." So attend I did, and they put me on the program.

Dr. Jesse Edwards, whom I had gotten to know well at the Mayo Clinic in Rochester, Minnesota, during 1960–1961—when I had the privilege of spending a whole year as one of Dr. Jeremy

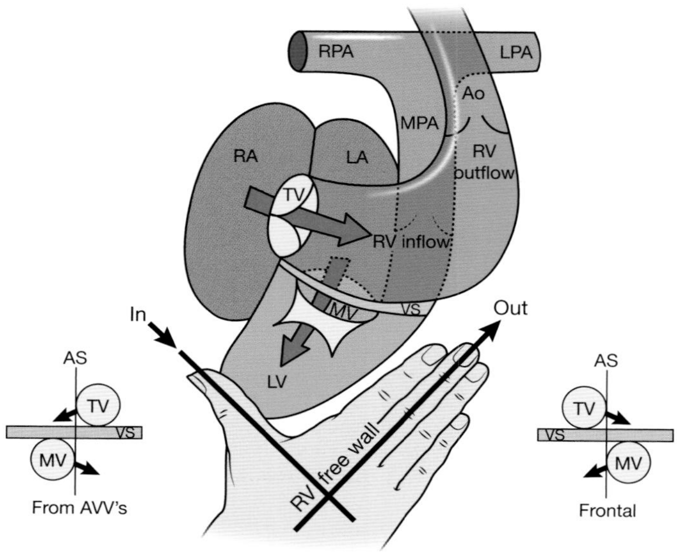

Crisscross AV relations
TGA {S,D,L}

Fig. 22.15 The D-loop morphologically right ventricle *(RV)* is right-handed. Figuratively speaking, the thumb of one's right hand represents the RV inflow tract *(In)*, fitting through the tricuspid valve *(TV)*. The fingers of the right hand go into the RV outflow tract *(Out)*. The palm of only the right hand faces the RV septal surface, and the dorsum of only the right hand faces the RV free wall surface. *Crisscross AV relations* means that the atrioventricular inflow tract vectors are markedly angulated *(arrows)*. Normally, they are approximately parallel. The ventricular septum *(VS)* is approximately horizontal. The TV is superior and to the right. The mitral valve *(MV)* is inferior and to the left. The viscera and atria are in situs solitus, i.e., {S,-,-}. The morphologically right atrium *(RA)* is right-sided and right-handed. Figuratively, the thumb of the right hand fits into the right superior vena cava; and the fingers of one's right hand go into the right atrial appendage. The palm of only one's right hand faces the right atrial septal surface, and the dorsum of only one's right hand faces the right atrial free wall surface. **Chirality or handedness** applies to all of the cardiac chambers. TGA {S,D,L} is present. The AV alignments are concordant: RA to RV, and LA to LV. The RV to great arterial alignments are discordant: RV to aorta *(Ao)*, and LV to main pulmonary artery *(MPA)*. So, TGA is present. It's L-TGA, because the aortic valve and the ascending Ao are to the left of the pulmonary valve and the MPA. Cases like this can be diagnostically confusing. The RV and the LV are both bilateral. The RV starts on the right side but then goes leftward. The LV starts on the left and then goes rightward. How do we know that D-loop ventricles are present? L-TGA is usually associated with a ventricular L-loop. The answer is: Look at the ventricles and apply chirality. If the RV is right-handed, it's a D-loop. If the LV is left-handed, it's a D-loop. Looking at the LV, if only the palm of the left hand can face the septal surface, and only the dorsum of the left hand can be adjacent to the LV free wall, it's a D-loop. **Summary:** In D-loop or solitus or noninverted ventricles, the RV is right-handed and the LV is left-handed. (Reproduced with permission from Van Praagh R. What determines whether the great arteries are normally or abnormally related? *Am J Cardiol* 2016;118:1390.)

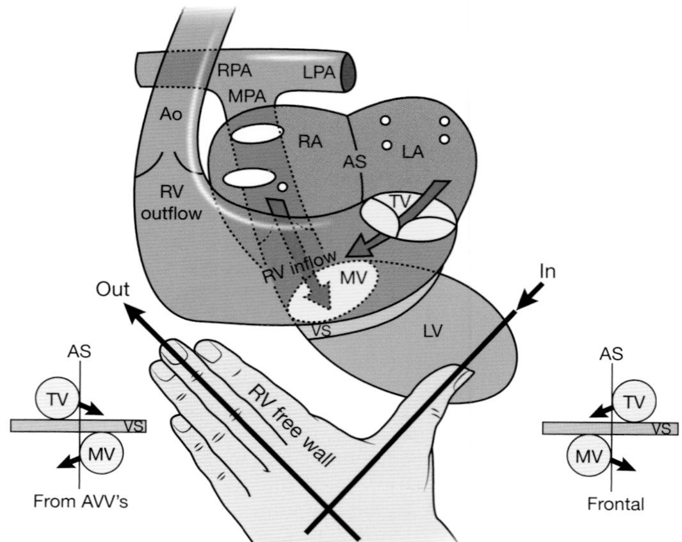

Crisscross AV relations
TGA {S,L,D}

Fig. 22.16 The L-loop morphologically right ventricle *(RV)* is left-handed. With the thumb of the left hand through the left-sided tricuspid valve *(TV)*, and the fingers of the left hand in the RV outflow tract, the palm of only the left hand faces the RV septal surface, and the dorsum of only the left hand faces the RV free wall. Just as physiologically uncorrected TGA {S,D,**L**} is shown in Fig. 22.15, so too physiologically corrected TGA {S,L,**D**} is presented here. The great arteries in both cases are unusually located because of the malposition of the underlying ventricles. *Crisscross AV relations* is another reflection of the underlying ventricular malposition. **Summary:** In L-loop or inverted ventricles, the RV is left-handed and the LV is right-handed. (Reproduced with permission from Van Praagh R. What determines whether the great arteries are normally or abnormally related? *Am J Cardiol* 2016;118:1390.)

Swan's fellows in the Cardiac Catheterization Laboratory—asked me to make a presentation on the pathologic anatomy of the transposition complexes. He privately asked me, "How many transposition complexes are there, and what are they?" I suspected that that might be an impossible question to answer, but I volunteered to try.

First, I had to decide, What is a *complex*? The word is defined as "consisting of interconnected or interwoven parts; composite, compound."[2] It is derived from *complectere*, to entwine: *com-*, together, + *plectere*, to twine or braid (Latin). *Complexus* means an embrace (Latin). As Dr. Maurice Lev put it, "Congenital anomalies of the heart have a tendency to group themselves into patterns or complexes."[2] I had the privilege to work with Dr. Lev as his fellow in congenital cardiac pathology at the Congenital Heart Disease Research and Training Center in Chicago from 1963 to 1965.

By 1974–1975, I was the Director of the Cardiac Registry—the congenital cardiac pathology and embryology laboratory of Boston Children's Hospital—since October 1965. The Cardiac Registry was part of the Departments of Cardiology, Pathology, and Cardiac Surgery.

In our lab, we decided that the first task was to discover what the main types of TGA are, and what their relative frequencies are in our congenital cardiac pathology database (Fig. 22.17).

In a study of 243 autopsied cases of TGA, **6 main anatomic types** were found (Fig. 22.17):

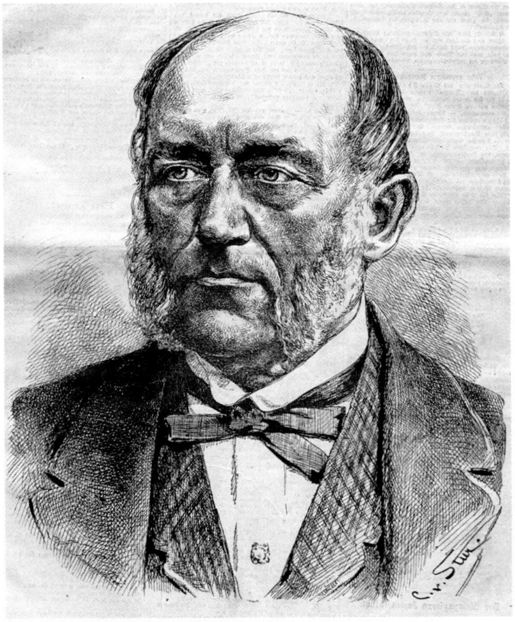

Fig. 22.17 Carl von Rokitansky (1804–1878) of Vienna, the discoverer in 1875 of congenital physiologically corrected transposition of the great arteries {S,L,L}. Rudolph Virchow (1821–1902) of Berlin, the eminent German founder of cellular pathology, regarded his jolly Viennese rival von Rokitansky as the ablest descriptive pathologist of his time.

TABLE 22.2 Types of Single Ventricle

Types of Single Ventricle	n = 31	% of Series
Single Left Ventricle		
1. Single LV {S,D,S}	1	3
2. Single LV with TGA {S,D,D}	6	19
3. Single LV with TGA {S,D,L}	2	7
4. Single LV with TGA {S,L,L}	12	39
5. Single LV with TGA {S,L,D}	1	3
6. Single LV with {S,L,S}	1	3
Single Right Ventricle		
1. Single RV with DORV {S,D,D}	2	7
2. Single RV with DORV {I,L,I}	1	3
3. Single RV with TGA {A,D,D} and asplenia	1	3
4. Single RV with DORV {A,D,D} and asplenia	3	10
5. Single RV with TGA {A,L,L} and asplenia	1	3

DORV, Double-outlet right ventricle; *LV*, left ventricle; *RV*, right ventricle; *TGA*, transposition of the great arteries.
Van Praagh R, Plett JA, Van Praagh S. Single ventricle: pathology, embryology, terminology, and classification, *Herz* 1979;4:113.

1. **Physiologically uncorrected TGA in visceroatrial situs solitus** occurred in 193 of 243 patients (79.4%) (Table 22.2). Most had TGA {S,D,D} in 186 of 193 cases (96.4%). But 1 case had TGA {S,D,A} (1/193 = 0.5%), and 6 patients had TGA {S,D,L} (6/193 = 3.1%). Thus, TGA {S,D,D/A/L} occurred in 193/243 patients (79.4%). TGA {S,D,**D**} or D-TGA indicates that the transposed aortic valve lies to the right (**dextro-** or **D-**) relative to the transposed pulmonary valve.

TABLE 22.3 TGA With D-Loop Ventricles (*n* = 200)

TGA Complexes	No. of Cases	% of Series
Infundibulum + Great Arteries		
1. TGA {S,D,D} with IVS	89	44.5
2. TGA {S,D,D} with IVS + PS	5	2.5
3. TGA {S,D,D} with VSD	38	19.0
4. TGA {S,D,D/A}* with VSD + PS	17	8.5
5. TGA {S,D,D} with VSD + PAt	4	2.0
6. TGA {S,D,D} with VSD + Preduct Coarc	10	5.0
7. TGA {S,D,L}	6	3.0
Infundibuloarterial + Ventricular + AV Canal		
8. TGA {S,D,D} with TAt	6	3.0
9. TGA {S,D,D} with Straddling TV	5	2.5
10. TGA {S,D,D} with DILV + Single LV	6	3.0
11. TGA {S,D,D} with DICV huge VSD		0.5
12. TGA {S,D,D/A}* with MAt	6	3.0
Infundibuloarterial		
13. TGA {1,D,D} with VSD + PAt	1	0.5
Infundibuloarterial + Ventricular + AV Canal + Atrial + Visceral		
14. TGA {A,D,D} with Asplenia	5	2.5
15. TGA {A,D,D} with Polysplenia	1	0.5

*Including one case with TGA {S,D,A}.
AV, Atrioventricular; *DICV*, double-inlet common ventricle; *DILV*, double-inlet left ventricle; *IVS*, intact ventricular septum; *LV*, morphologically left ventricle; *MAt*, mitral atresia; *PAt*, pulmonary atresia; *Preduct Coarc*, preductal coarctation; *PS*, pulmonary stenosis; *TAt*, tricuspid atresia; *TV*, tricuspid valve; *VSD*, ventricular septal defect.
From Van Praagh R. Transposition of the great arteries: history, pathologic anatomy, embryology, etiology, and surgical considerations. *Cardiac Surgery: State of the Art Reviews*, vol 5, Philadelphia, 1991, Hanley & Belfus, Figure 17.

Physiologically uncorrected or complete TGA in visceroatrial situs solitus is not always D-TGA. It can be A-TGA or L-TGA (Fig. 22.17). This is why one needs to know the anatomic type of all three of the main cardiac segment, that is, {atria, ventricles, and great arteries}. One diagnostically also needs to know the status of the AV and the VA alignments. The intersegmental alignments can be concordant (appropriate or normal), discordant (the opposite of normal), double-inlet, double-outlet, stenotic, atretic, regurgitant, or absent.

The anatomic details concerning TGA are presented in Table 22.1, Table 22.3, and Table 22.4.

Physiologic uncorrection of the systemic and pulmonary venous circulations[14] is produced by one intersegmental discordance, as in TGA {S,D,D/A/L}. In physiologically uncorrected TGA, the one intersegmental discordance occurs at the VA alignment, because of malformation of the infundibular connecting segment.

When the muscular subaortic infundibular free wall remains well developed (Figs. 22.7 and 22.8), instead of normally undergoing resorption, the subaortic infundibulum prevents the aortic valve from moving inferiorly and posteriorly and coming into direct fibrous continuity with the mitral valve. Instead, the

TABLE 22.4 Anatomic Types of L-Loop TGA (*n* = 43)

	TGA Complexes	No. of Cases	% of Series
Infundibuloarterial:			
1.	TGA {I,L,L} with IVS		2.3
2.	TGA {I,L,D}		2.3
3.	TGA {S,L,L} with IVS	4	9.3
Infundibuloarterial + Ventricular:			
4.	TGA {S,L,L} with VSD	3	7.0
5.	TGA {S,L,L} with VSD + PS	2	4.7
6.	TGA {S,L,L} with VSD +PAt		2.3
7.	TGA {S,L,D}	3	7.0
Infundibuloarterial + Ventricular + AV Canal:			
8.	TGA {S,L,L} with IVS, Ao At, Ebstein's + Uhl's		2.3
9.	TGA {S,L,L} with TAt (L)	3	7.0
10.	TGA {S,L,L} with TS (L)		2.3
11.	TGA {S,L,L} with straddling TV (L)	3	7.0
12.	TGA {S,L,L} with DILV + single LV (R)	12	27.9
13.	TGA {S,L,L} with DIRV (L)		2.3
14.	TGA {S,L,L} with MAt (R)	3	7.0
15.	TGA {S,L,L} with MS (R)	1	2.3
Infundibuloarterial + Ventricular + AV Canal + Atrial + Visceral:			
16.	TGA {A,L,L} with Asplenia	2	4.7
17.	TGA {A,L,L} with Polysplenia		2.3

Ao At, Aortic atresia; *AV,* atrioventricular; *DILV,* double-inlet left ventricle; *DIRV,* double-inlet right ventricle; *IVS,* intact ventricular septum; *(L),* left-sided; *LV,* morphologically left ventricle; *MAt,* mitral atresia; *MS,* mitral stenosis; *PAt,* pulmonary atresia; *PS,* pulmonary stenosis; *(R),* right-sided; *TAt,* tricuspid atresia; *TGA,* transposition of the great arteries; *TS,* tricuspid stenosis; *TV,* tricuspid valve; *VSD,* ventricular septal defect.

Modified from Van Praagh R, Plett JA, Van Praagh S. Single ventricle: pathology, embryology, terminology, and classification, *Herz* 1979;4: 113, and Van Praagh R, Weinberg PM, Calder AL, Buckley LFP, Van Praagh S. The transposition complexes: How many are there? In Davila JC (ed): Second Henry Ford Hospital International Symposium on Cardiac Surgery. New York, 1977, Appleton-Century-Crofts, pp 207–213; with permission.

subaortic infundibulum holds the aortic valve high above the RV.

The subpulmonary infundibular free wall undergoes resorption, instead of growing well (which is normal). The disappearance of the subpulmonary infundibular free wall permits the pulmonary valve to move inferiorly and posteriorly and to come into direct fibrous continuity with the mitral valve (Figs. 22.7 and 22.8). Thus, inverted development of the subarterial infundibulum results in inverted morphogenetic movements of the semilunar valves, causing TGA.

2. **Congenital physiologically corrected TGA in visceroatrial situs solitus** occurred in 36 of 243 patients (15.6%). Most had TGA {S,L,L} (35/38, 92%). However, 3 of 38 had TGA {S,L,D} (8%).[14]

In physiologically corrected TGA, there are two intersegmental discordances or switching errors, at both the AV alignments and at the VA alignments. In theory, two right-left switching errors should cancel each other. Usually, however, associated malformations undo the theoretical physiologic corrections of the systemic and pulmonary venous circulations.

We usually leave out the words. For example, we usually do not say or write: "physiologically uncorrected TGA in visceroatrial situs solitus." Instead, we simply say and write: TGA {S,D,D}, or TGA {S,D,A}, or TGA {S,D,L} (Fig. 22.18).

Why?

Because it's briefer, it's more specific, and what the words say is obvious from the segmental anatomy, making the words redundant and unnecessary.

The rare segmental sets, such as TGA {S,D,A}, TGA {S,D,L}, TGA {S,L,A}, and TGA {S,L,D}, usually appear to have an unusual semilunar spatial interrelationship because of a ventricular loop malposition.

Thus the usual segmental set, such as TGA {S,D,D} and TGA {S,L,L}, is used for writing infundibuloarterial (IA) situs equations.

For TGA {S,D,D}, the IA situs equation is TGA {S,D,D} = 4R + 0L. The infundibular situs formula or "recipe" is inverted, and the great arterial situs is solitus. Thus, IA situs analysis in typical D-TGA reveals infundibular inversion with noninverted great arteries, that is, IA situs discordance (oppositeness). Thus, typical D-TGA is isolated infundibular inversion.

Typical L-TGA, that is, TGA {S,L,L}, is the reverse. The IA situs equation for typical L-TGA is TGA {S,L,L} = 0R + 4L. The formula for the infundibulum is solitus normal, but the great arteries are inverted: solitus with inversion is IA situs discordance.

So, both D-TGA and L-TGA have IA situs discordances of opposite types: inverted-solitus; and solitus-inverted, respectively.

Figure 22.17 reveals that the third and fourth main anatomic types of TGA are physiologically uncorrected TGA in visceroatrial situs inversus, and congenital physiologically corrected TGA in visceroatrial situs inversus.

3. **Anatomically, physiologically uncorrected TGA in visceroatrial situs inversus**[14] was TGA {I,L,L} in 1 of 243 patients (0.4%), and was TGA {I,L,D} in 1 (0.4%). In TGA {I,L,L}, IA situs analysis is solitus-inversus, that is, discordant (abnormal). (We use *inversus* and *inverted* interchangeably.)
4. **Anatomically, congenitally physiologically corrected TGA in visceroatrial situs inversus**[12] was TGA {I,D,D} in 1 of 243 patients (0.4%). Situs inversus of the viscera and atria was the most infrequent type of visceroatrial situs found in this study: 223 of 243 patients (1.2%).[12] In TGA {I,D,D}, the infundibular situs and the great arterial situs are inversus and solitus respectively, that is, discordant (abnormal).
5. **TGA in the heterotaxy syndromes with asplenia or polysplenia and with visceroatrial situs ambiguous,**[14] the anatomy was TGA {A,D,D} in 6 patients (2.5%).
6. **TGA in the heterotaxy syndromes with asplenia or polysplenia and with visceroatrial situs ambiguus,**[14] the specific anatomy was TGA {A,L,L} in 3 of 243 autopsied cases of TGA (1.2%).

Situs ambiguus occurred in 9 of these 243 patients (3.7%). Situs ambiguus means that the situs or pattern of anatomic

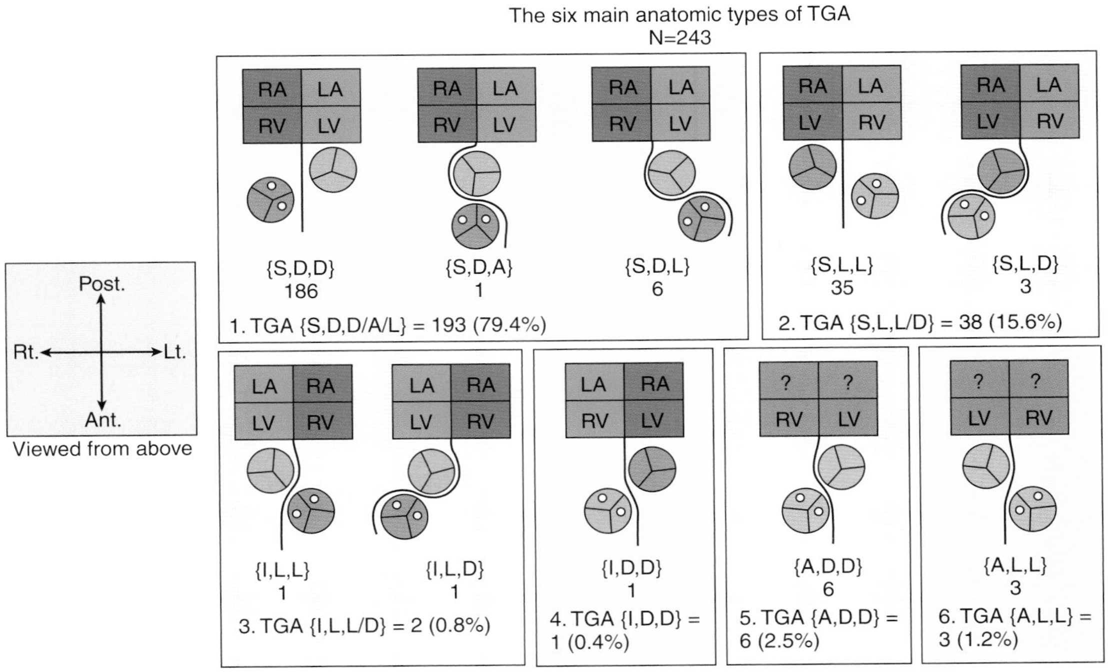

Fig. 22.18 The six main anatomic types of transposition of the great arteries *(TGA)* found in 243 postmortem cases: (l) Physiologically uncorrected TGA in visceroatrial situs solitus occurred in 193 of 243 cases (79.4%). (2) Congenital physiologically corrected TGA in visceroatrial situs solitus was found in 15.6% of 243 cases. (3) Physiologically uncorrected TGA in visceroatrial situs inversus occurred in 0.8%. (4) Congenital physiologically corrected TGA in visceroatrial situs inversus was found in 0.4%. (5) D-loop TGA in visceroatrial situs ambiguus occurred in 2.5%. (6) L-loop TGA in visceroatrial situs ambiguus was present in 1.2%. In physiologically uncorrected TGA in visceroatrial situs solitus, we found three subsets or anatomic subtypes: TGA {S,D,D} in 186/243 cases (76.5%), TGA {S,D,A} in 1/243 patients (0.4%), and TGA {S,D,L} in 6/243 cases (2.5%). In congenital physiologically corrected TGA, there were two subsets or anatomic subtypes: TGA {S,L,L} in 35/243 patients (14.4%); and TGA {S,L,D} in 3/243 cases (1.2%). In physiologically uncorrected TGA in visceroatrial situs inversus, there were two subsets or anatomic subtypes: TGA {I,L,L} in 1/243 patients (0.4%, and TGA {I,L,D} in 1/243 0.4%. In congenital physiologically corrected TGA in visceroatrial situs inversus, there was only one subset or anatomic subtype: TGA {I,D,D} in 1/243 patients (0.4%). When TGA was associated with visceroatrial situs ambiguus and a heterotaxy syndrome with D-loop ventricles, there was only one set or anatomic type (and no subsets or anatomic subtypes); TGA {A,D,D} in 6/243 cases (2.5%). When TGA was associated with visceroatrial situs ambiguus and a heterotaxy syndrome and L-loop ventricles, there was only one set or anatomic type (and no subset or anatomic subtype) in 3 of 243 patients (1.2%). In other larger series, additional anatomic subtypes of TGA may well be found. (Reproduced with permission from Van Praagh R. What determines whether the great arteries are normally or abnormally related? *Am J Cardiol* 2016;118:1390.)

organization of the viscera and atria is uncertain, or unknown, that is, not diagnosed. This also means that one cannot diagnose a case of TGA as *physiologically uncorrected,* or as *physiologically corrected* when the visceroatrial situs is unknown—because the visceroatrial situs is the frame of reference concerning physiologic uncorrection versus physiologic correction of the systemic and pulmonary venous circulations.

In the heterotaxy syndromes of congenital asplenia and polysplenia, IA situs analysis is as above. In TGA {A,D,D}, IA situs analysis was inversus-solitus; and in TGA {A,L,L}, IA situs analysis was typically solitus-inversus.

Thus, the classical physiologically uncorrected/corrected classification of TGA breaks down in the heterotaxy syndromes, because of visceroatrial situs ambiguus. The only diagnostic method that always works is the **segmental approach**[15,16] that is used (Fig. 22.17) in this book. Thus we have established that there are six main anatomic types of TGA.[7] But it must also be emphasized that, almost certainly, there are more anatomic subtypes than are summarized in Fig. 22.17, because this study was based on only 243 autopsied cases.

To obtain the most accurate data concerning the anatomic types of TGA, we must go into the Cardiac Pathology Database (Table 22.5).

TGA {A(1),D,D} means that there was atrial situs ambiguus, but we thought that the atria probably were in situs inversus, but we were not certain. TGA {A(S),L,L} means that the atria were in situs ambiguus, but we thought that the atria probably were in situs solitus, but we were not sure.

TGA {A(IS),L,L} means that the atria were in situs ambiguus, but the viscera were in situs inversus and we thought the atria probably were in situs solitus. Thus, the larger series of TGA (database = 475 cases) revealed 17 different subsets of TGA, whereas the paper[12] (based on 243 cases) contained only 10 TGA subsets. It goes without saying that even larger studies (>475 cases) may contain more than 17 anatomic types of TGA.

TABLE 22.5 Anatomic Types of TGA Found in Our Cardiac Pathology Database ($n = 475$)

Anatomic Types of TGA	No. of Cases	% of Series
I. TGA in Visceroatrial Situs Solitus		
1. TGA {S,D,D}	338	71
2. TGA {S,D,D} with subpulmonary inferior + posterior Ao	2	0.4
3. TGA {S,D,D} with bilateral inferior + posterior Ao		0.2
4. TGA {S,D,L}	18	3.8
5. TGA {S,L,A}	2	0.4
6. TGA {S,L,D}	6	1.3
7. TGA {S,L,L}	84	17.7
II. TGA in Visceroatrial Situs Inversus		
8. TGA {I,L,L}	4	0.8
9. TGA {I,L,D}	1	0.2
10. TGA {1,D,L}	1	0.2
11. TGA {I,D,D}	3	0.6
12. TGA {I,D,A}	1	0.2
III. TGA in Visceroatrial Situs Ambiguus		
13. TGA {A(I),D,D}	4	0.8
14. TGA {A,L,D}	1	0.2
15. TGA {A(I),L,L}	1	0.2
16. TGA {A(S),L,L}	3	0.6
17. TGA {A(IS),L,L}	1	0.2

Ao, Aorta; *TGA,* transposition of the great arteries.

TABLE 22.6 Significant Differences Between D-Loop TGA and L-Loop TGA

Differences	TGA With D-Loop Ventricles $n = 200$		TGA With L-Loop Ventricles $n = 43$		
	No.	%	No.	%	*p* Value
1. Inf + GAs	170	85	2	4.7	<.001
2. Intact VS	94	47	6	14	<.0001
3. Inf + GA + Vent + AVC	24	12	25	58	<.0001
4. Single LV	6	3	12	28	<.00004

AVC, Atrioventricular canal; *GAs,* great arteries; *Inf,* infundibulum; *LV,* morphologically left ventricle; *TGA,* transposition of the great arteries; *Vent,* ventricles; *VS,* ventricular septum.

Incidence of TGA. Since this book represents a detailed study of 3216 autopsied cases of congenital heart disease, the incidence or frequency of TGA in this study was 475 of 3216 cases (14.8%). Acquired (not congenital) heart disease occurred in 184 cases, bringing the total cases studied to 3400.

The Transposition Complexes. A complex in congenital heart disease consists of the following:

1. the segmental situs set, such as {S,D,D};
2. segmental malalignments, such as TGA; and
3. associated malformations, such as VSD, or pulmonary outflow tract stenosis, and so on.

Abbreviations are the same as in Table 22.3, except as follows: *Ao At,* aortic atresia; *(L),* left-sided; *MS,* mitral stenosis; *(R),* right-sided; *TS,* tricuspid stenosis.

In 200 autopsied cases of D-loop TGA, 15 different complexes were found (Table 22.3). In 43 autopsied cases of L-loop TGA, 17 different complexes were identified (Table 22.4). The question arises: **Are there any significant differences between TGA with D-loop (solitus) ventricles and TGA with L-loop (inversus) ventricles?**

Comparison of Tables 22.3 and 22.4 reveals four differences that are statistically highly significant (Table 22.6). The statistically significant differences between D-loop TGA and L-loop TGA were as follows (Fig. 22.6):

1. Anomalies were largely confined to the infundibulum and the great arteries in D-loop TGA (85%), but not in L-loop TGA (4.7%) ($p < 0.0001$).
2. The ventricular septum was much more likely to be intact in D-loop TGA (47%) than in L-loop TGA (14%) ($p < 0.0001$).
3. In addition to malformations of the infundibulum and great arteries, anomalies of the ventricles and of the atrioventricular canal were much more likely to be present in L-loop TGA (58%) than in D-loop TGA (12%) ($p < 0.0001$). This makes sense because "typical" L-TGA, that is, TGA {S,L,L}—congenital physiologically corrected TGA—is not only a malformation of the great arteries, it is also inversion of the atrioventricular valves and of the ventricles relative to the viscera and the atria.
4. Single morphologically left ventricle with double-inlet LV and with an infundibular outlet chamber were much more likely to be associated with L-loop TGA (28%) then with D-loop TGA (3%) ($p = 0.00004$).

In addition to ventricular inversion, the phylogenetically younger ventricle, the morphologically right ventricle (RV), fails to develop. Phylogenetically, the RV is only about 36% as old as is the LV.[17]

CORONARY ARTERIES IN TGA

The six most common types of coronary artery anatomy in D-TGA in the surgical experience of Castaneda and colleagues[18] are presented diagrammatically in Fig. 22.19. **Intramural left coronary artery** is presented diagrammatically in Fig. 22.20.

The variations in the origins and courses of the coronary arteries in TGA (Figs. 22.19 and 22.20) have acquired a new surgical importance because of the arterial switch procedure for physiologically uncorrected TGA and for the Taussig-Bing type of double-outlet right ventricle (DORV).[18]

The intramural left coronary artery (Fig. 22.20) is one of the most difficult coronary anomalies to manage successfully.[19] The anomalous left coronary artery (LCA) arises from the right and posterior septal sinus of Valsalva of the aortic valve, much too close to the septal commissure. Then the LCA runs intramurally, within the aortic wall, between the aortic valve and the pulmonary valve. The abnormal intramural course of the left coronary artery is *stenotic,* and that is a surgical problem. In fact, when this surgical problem was first identified, it was regarded as a contraindication for the arterial switch operation.

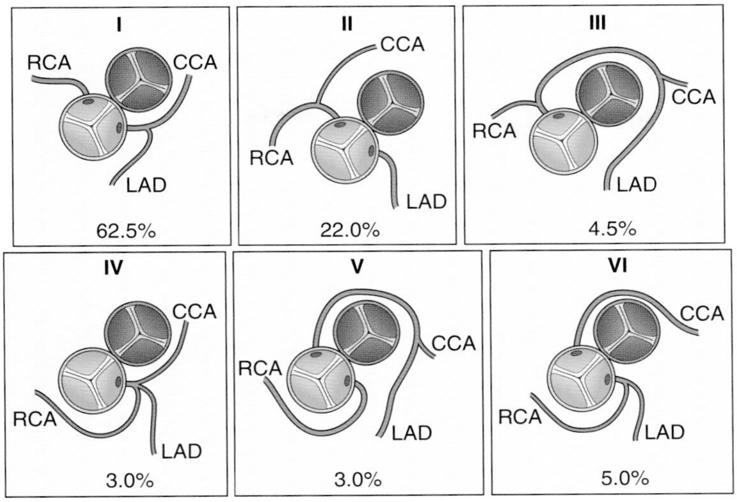

Fig. 22.19 The six most common types of coronary artery anatomy in D-TGA in this surgical experience of Castaneda and colleagues in 1989. *CCA,* Circumflex coronary artery; *LAD,* left anterior descending; *RCA,* right coronary artery. (Reproduced with permission from Van Praagh R. What determines whether the great arteries are normally or abnormally related? *Am J Cardiol* 2016;118:1390.)

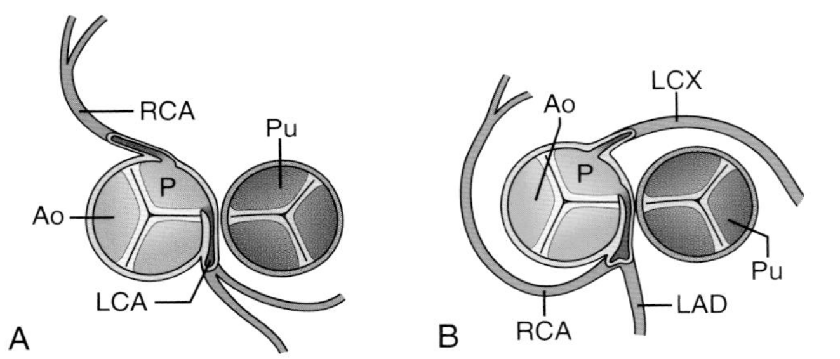

Fig. 22.20 Intramural left coronary artery. (A) The right coronary artery *(RCA)* arises normally from the right-sided and posterior *(P)* septal sinus of Valsalva. However, the left coronary artery *(LCA)* does not arise normally. Instead, the LCA also originates from the right and posterior sinus of Valsalva, abnormally close to the septal commissure. Then the LCA runs between the valve of the aorta *(Ao)* and the valve of the pulmonary artery *(Pu),* within the wall of the aorta. Typically, the abnormally located ostium of the LCA and its intramural course are both stenotic. This can be a surgical dilemma when transferring the LCA as part of the arterial switch procedure for D-TGA. In (B), the LAD and the RCA both arise from the posterior and right-sided septal sinus of Valsalva. Thus, both the LAD and the RCA share a common and stenotic origin. The left circumflex *(LCX)* originates from the right and posterior aortic sinus of Valsalva (instead of from the left and anterior sinus of Valsalva, which is usual). The LCX runs behind the pulmonary valve, instead of in front of it. (Reproduced with permission from Van Praagh R. What determines whether the great arteries are normally or abnormally related? *Am J Cardiol* 2016;118:1390.)

MORPHOGENESIS OF TGA

Figure 22.21 summarizes the four main hypotheses concerning the embryonic morphogenesis of TGA:

1. **The straight aortopulmonary septum and infundibular septum hypothesis** was first proposed (to our knowledge) by Sir Richard Quain[20] in 1844, and was subsequently accepted by many authors. We think the straight arterioinfundibular hypothesis is wrong for several reasons:
   (1) The free walls of the great arteries are just as abnormal as the aortopulmonary septum is; that is, the abnormality in TGA is not confined to the septum. The coronary arterial ostia—the first branches of the aortic free walls—are very different in normally related great arteries and in TGA. In other words, TGA is an anomaly of both the aortopulmonary septum and of the aortic and pulmonary free walls, not of the aortopulmonary septum only, as the variable locations of the coronary ostia in various types of TGA indicate.
   (2) Definite evidence of abnormality of the aortopulmonary (AP) septum, such as aortopulmonary septal defect, is rare in TGA. If TGA were an anomaly of the AP septum, anatomic evidence of AP septal malformation should be common, not vanishingly rare.
   (3) The straight septum hypothesis cannot explain the variations in semilunar valve heights in TGA and in other infundibuloarterial malformations.
2. **Infundibular maldevelopment.** Sir Arthur Keith[21] was the first to propose, in 1909, that TGA results from malformation of the subarterial infundibulum (or conus arteriosus): that is, persistence and development of the subaortic infundibulum, and involution and disappearance of the subpulmonary infundibulum. Note that Keith thought that with normally related great arteries, the pulmonary valve is anterior, superior, and to the *right* of the aortic valve—a common preangiocardiographic error. In 1967, Van Praagh, Vlad, and Keith[4] independently reached the same conclusion that Sir Arthur Keith had reached 58 years earlier, in 1909.
3. **Atavism.** Alexander Spitzer of Vienna proposed an atavistic hypothesis to explain human TGA in 1923.[5,6] He suggested that TGA in humans results from a phylogenetic regression or atavism back to the higher reptilian stage of crocodiles and alligators. Such higher reptiles normally have a right ventricular aorta and a left ventricular aorta. Spitzer proposed that

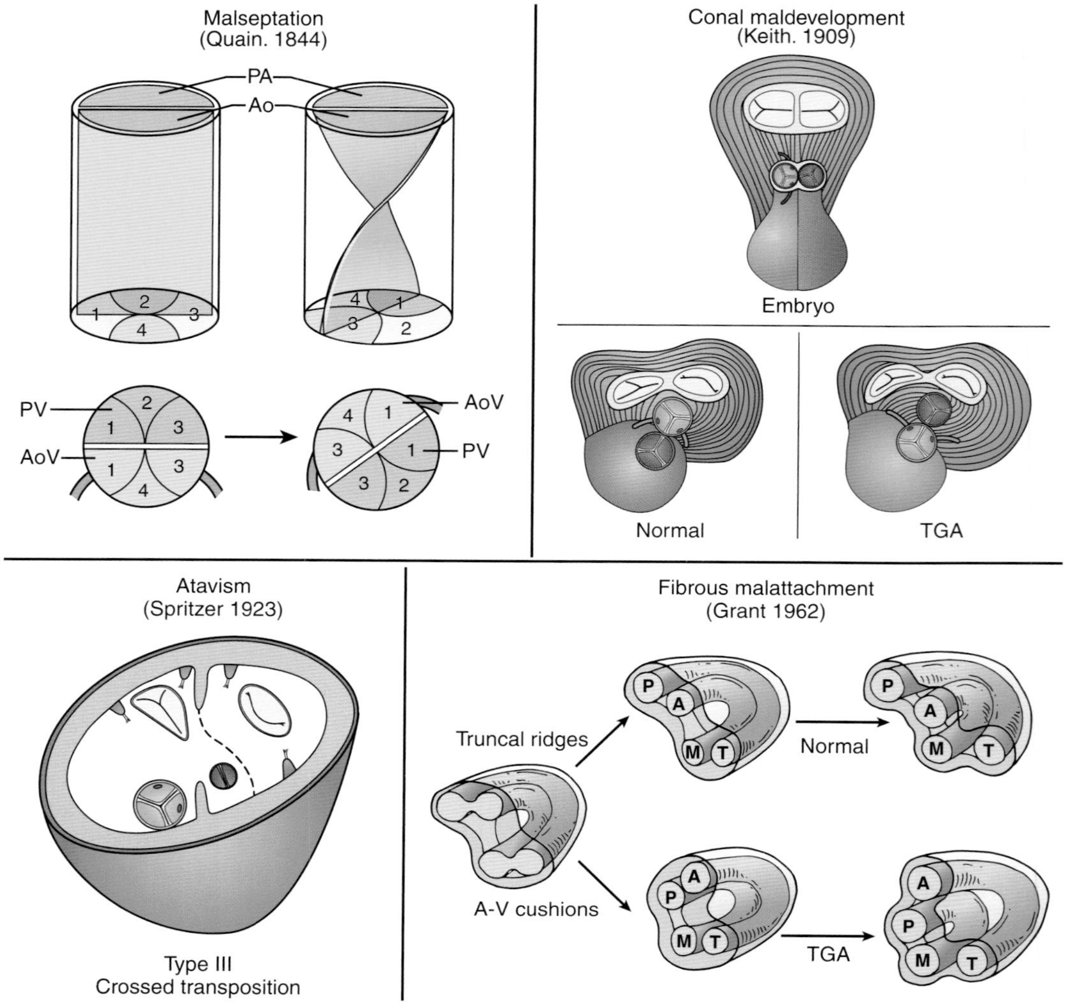

Fig. 22.21 The four main theories concerning the morphogenesis of transposition of the great arteries. Each of these concepts has been presented in the text and will not be reiterated here. All four theories are brought together here for the reader's convenience. (Reproduced with permission from Van Praagh R. What determines whether the great arteries are normally or abnormally related? *Am J Cardiol* 2016;118:1390.)

in human TGA, the higher reptilian right ventricular aorta persists, and that the higher reptilian left ventricular aorta disappears, or involutes. So, Spitzer's atavistic hypothesis could explain the right ventricular aorta in human TGA.

But the atavistic hypothesis broke down when Spitzer tried to explain the human transposed pulmonary artery. Spitzer knew that in all known animals, the pulmonary artery normally arises above the right ventricle (RV), never above the left ventricle (LV).

So, in typical D-TGA, Spitzer said that the apparent ventricular septum disappears: note the dotted line (Fig. 22.21, bottom left). Spitzer said that the apparent ventricular septum is a hugely hypertrophied crista supraventricularis, not the true ventricular septum that has disappeared, along with the right ventricular aorta of higher reptiles.

Therefore, said Spitzer, the transposed pulmonary artery in typical TGA arises above morphologically right ventricular myocardium (RV), not above left ventricular myocardium (LV).

The problem is that, in fact, the human transposed pulmonary artery in typical D-TGA arises above the LV, not above the RV as Spitzer's atavistic hypothesis requires. The ventricular septum in typical D-TGA does *not* disappear. Spitzer's hypothesis of devolution (reversed evolution) mesmerized a medical generation.[6,8,9] However, his phylogenetic hypothesis is not supported by the *morphologic anatomy* of the LV, and of the subpulmonary ventricular myocardium in typical D-TGA, which is only LV myocardium. Consequently, Spitzer's atavistic hypothesis is considered to be incorrect.[12]

4. **Semilunar-mitral fibrous malattachment.** Grant[22] proposed in 1962 that normally, there is a fibrous tract of low growth potential between the aortic valve (AoV) and the mitral valve (MV) that tethers the aortic valve to the mitral valve via an intervalvar fibrosa. Consequently, the LV ejects into the aorta. The pulmonary valve, not being tethered, grows and develops above the RV. Normally, the RV ejects into the aorta. Grant proposed that abnormally, this fibrous tract of low growth potential is shifted to the left, consequently tethering the pulmonary valve (PV) to the mitral valve and allowing the untethered aortic valve to develop above the RV.

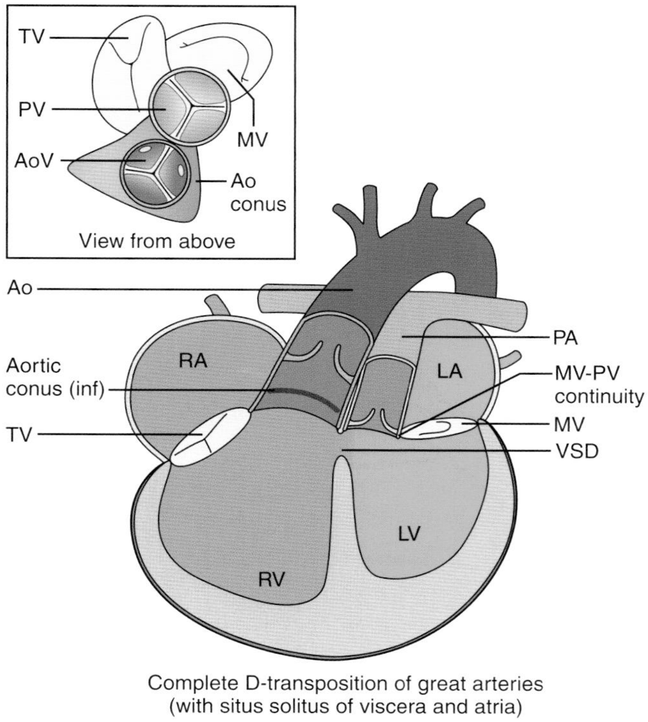

Fig. 22.22 Diagram of typical D-transposition of the great arteries {S,D,D}. When this diagram was made, this type of D-TGA was often called *complete* TGA, as opposed to *partial* TGA, which is now called double-outlet right ventricle (DORV). *Complete* TGA meant physiologically uncorrected TGA in which both great arteries are placed completely across the ventricular septum, Ao above the RV and PA above the LV. However, congenital physiologically corrected TGA {S,L,L} is also a complete TGA. Consequently, *complete* TGA is now seldom used because of its lack of specificity. Anatomically, the viscera and atria are in situs solitus, i.e., {S,-,-}. The morphologically right atrium *(RA)* is right-sided and right-handed. The morphologically left atrium *(LA)* is left-sided and left-handed. A ventricular D-loop is present, i.e., {S,*D*,-}. The morphologically right ventricle *(RV)* is right-sided and right-handed (Fig. 22.15). The morphologically left ventricle *(LV)* is left-sided and left-handed. The atrioventricular *(AV)* connecting segment connects the atria with the ventricles. The tricuspid valve *(TV)* connects the RA and the RV. The mitral valve *(MV)* connects the LA and the LV. The AV alignments are concordant (appropriate): RA to RV and LA to LV. The infundibular or conal connecting segment connects the ventricles with the great arteries. The infundibulum *(inf)* is inverted: well developed beneath the right-sided transposed aortic valve; and absent beneath the left-sided transposed pulmonary valve. The well-developed muscular subaortic infundibulum widely separates the transposed aortic valve above from the AV valves below. The subpulmonary infundibular free wall has undergone resorption and hence is absent, permitting pulmonary valve–MV direct fibrous continuity via an intervalvar fibrosa. As the *inset* shows, the transposed pulmonary valve *(PV)* is often in fibrous continuity also with the TV. An infundibuloventricular type of ventricular septal defect *(VSD)* is present between the infundibular septum above and the muscular interventricular septum below. Because the PV is lower than the aortic valve *(AoV)*, the VSD is subpulmonary. The ventriculoarterial (VA) alignments are discordant: RV to Ao, and LV to PA because the great arteries are transposed. The great arteries are transposed because the situs of the infundibulum and the situs of the great arteries are discordant (different). The infundibulum is inverted, and the great arteries are noninverted (solitus). The infundibuloarterial (IA) situs equation of typical D-TGA {S,D,D} is TGA {S,D,D} = **4R + 0L**. The IA situs equation of solitus normally related great arteries is SNRGA {S,D,S} = 0R + 4L. The expression to the right of the equals sign (=) is the formula of the infundibular connector. With solitus normally related great arteries {S,D,S}, the solitus infundibular situs formula is **0R + 4L**, as above. But in D-TGA {S,D,D}, the transposed great arteries are still in situs solitus. The aortic valve is to the right of the pulmonary valve. But the infundibulum is inverted: **4R + 0L**. This is the same infundibular situs formula as in situs inversus totalis: INRGA {1,L,I} = **4R + 0L**. If the patterns of anatomic organization (the situs) of the infundibular connector and the situs of the great arteries being connected are both the same (both solitus, or both inversus), then the great arteries can be connected normally. Otherwise, they cannot. (Reproduced with permission from Van Praagh R. What determines whether the great arteries are normally or abnormally related? *Am J Cardiol* 2016;118:1390.)

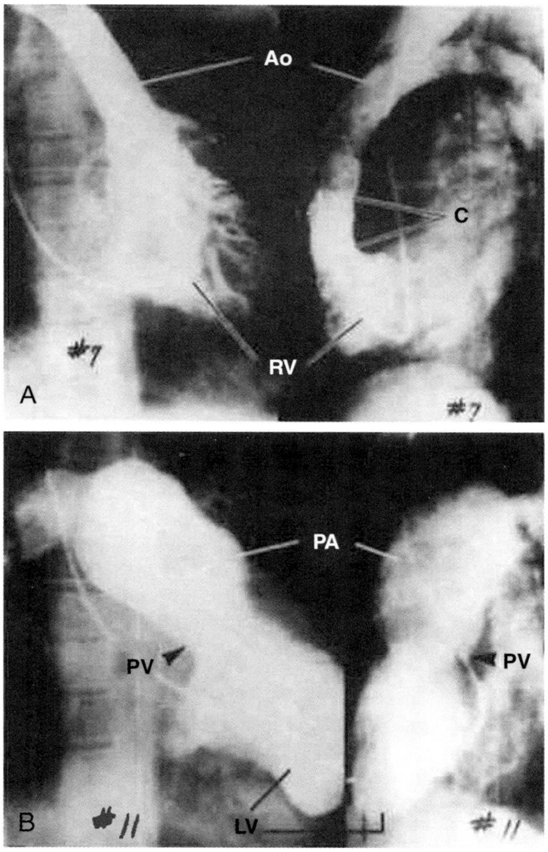

Fig. 22.23 Angiocardiography of typical D-TGA. (A) Selective right ventricular *(RV)* injection in the posteroanterior projection *(left panel)*, and simultaneously in the left lateral projection *(right panel)*. Note the course right ventricular trabeculations and the prominent subaortic conus *(C)* or infundibulum beneath the D-transposed aorta *(Ao)*. (B) Selective left ventricular *(LV)* injection showing the transposed pulmonary artery *(PA)*. The pulmonary valve *(PV)* is low and posterior, in fibrous contiguity with the mitral valve. The LV is so finely trabeculated that it appears almost untrabeculated. (Reproduced with permission from Van Praagh R. What determines whether the great arteries are normally or abnormally related? *Am J Cardiol* 2016;118:1390.)

Thus, Grant[22] proposed that AoV-MV tethering causes normally related great arteries and that PV-MV tethering causes TGA. I think that this hypothesis is essentially half right. Grant's hypothesis is a recognition of the morphogenetic importance of semilunar valve–mitral valve fibrous continuity via an

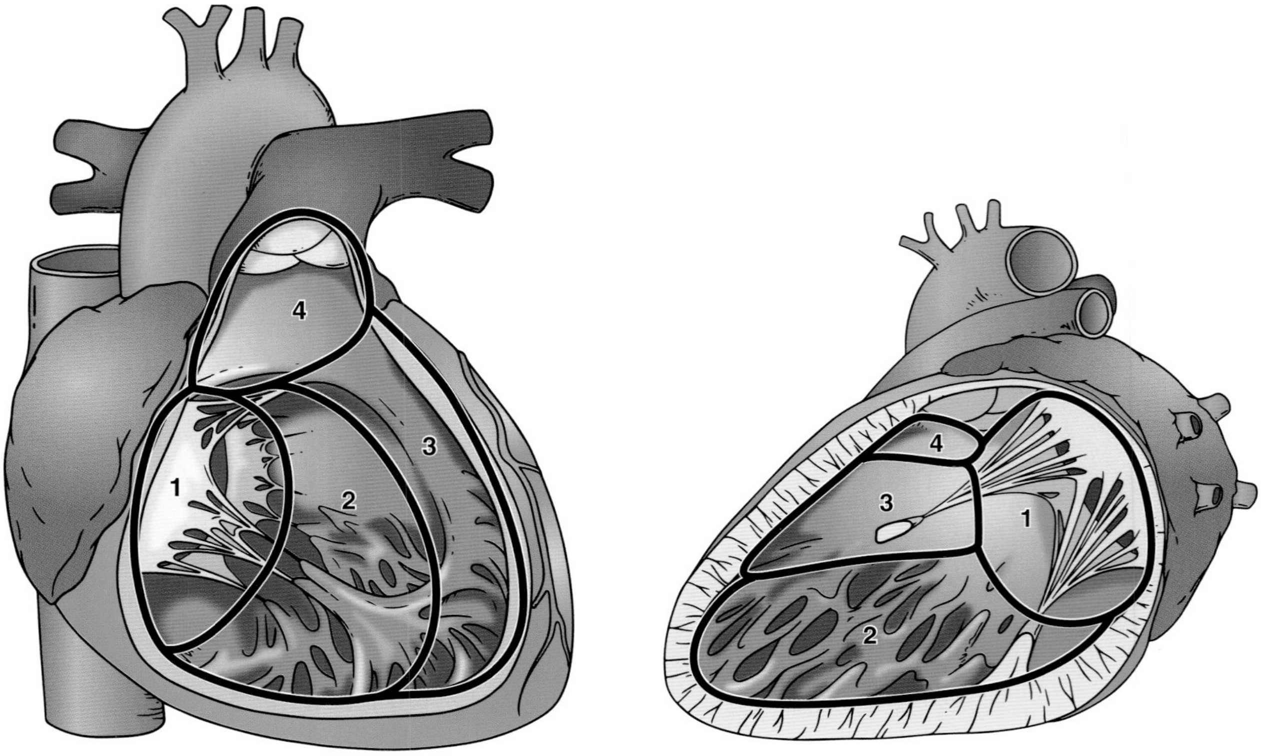

Fig. 22.24 The four main components of the morphologically right ventricle (A) and of the morphologically left ventricle (B). *Component 1* is the atrioventricular canal or junction. *Component 2* is the trabeculated sinus, or body, or inflow tract of both ventricles. *Component 3* in the RV is the septal band. It extends into the moderator band that runs from the septal band to the anterior papillary muscle of the RV. In the LV, *component 3* is the smooth, nontrabeculated part of the left ventricular septal surface. Component 3 is regarded as the proximal or apical part of the infundibulum. The RV has two apices: the *RV sinus apex* is behind or posterior to the moderator band. The *infundibular apex* is in front of or anterior to the moderator band. *Component 4* is the distal or subarterial part of the infundibulum. This is the subarterial infundibulum with which we are mainly concerned in this chapter. (Reproduced with permission from Van Praagh R. What determines whether the great arteries are normally or abnormally related? *Am J Cardiol* 2016;118:1390.)

intervalvar fibrosa: AoV-MV fibrous continuity normally; and PV-MV fibrous continuity in typical TGA.

Our hypothesis[4,7] recognizes the importance of subarterial infundibular *growth,* and of subarterial infundibular *hypoplasia* or *absence* caused by infundibular involution (apoptosis, or programmed cell death). In other words, ours is a hypothesis of subarterial infundibular *development,* with the understanding that development can be *positive* or *negative: grades 0, 1, 2, 3, 4.* Grant's hypothesis[22] was very important in 1962 because it focused attention on the importance of semilunar-mitral continuity and discontinuity.

So, what is TGA really? Figure 22.21 suggests that TGA is an infundibular (or canal) malformation. Is that correct? Believe it or not, the answer is: no, that is not completely true. In TGA {S,D,D}, TGA results from isolated infundibular inversion: TGA {S,D,D} = **4R + 0L.**

The infundibulum is well developed (grade 4) on the right side (R) beneath the aorta {-,-,D}, and the infundibulum is absent (grade 0) on the left side (L) beneath the pulmonary artery. The infundibulum in D-TGA is presented diagrammatically in Fig. 22.1, fourth column from the right. The infundibuloarterial situs analysis is presented in typical D-TGA in equation 3 (previous paragraph and at the beginning of this chapter). The infundibuloarterial situs combination in typical D-TGA (4R + 0L) is the same as in situs inversus totalis (4R + 0L, equation 2). Thus typical D-TGA does indeed have isolated infundibular inversion, as Sir Arthur Keith understood in 1909.

But congenital physiologically corrected TGA {S,L,L} has a solitus normal type of infundibulum, not an abnormal malformed infundibular situs: Fig. 22.2, second column to the right. Infundibuloarterial situs analysis in TGA {S,L,L} is given in equation 4: TGA {S,L,L} = **0R + 4L.**

The infundibular formula for TGA {S,**L**,L} is the same as for solitus normally related great arteries in equation 1: SNRGA {S,D,S} = **0R + 4L.** Thus, classical congenital physiologically corrected TGA does *not* have a malformed infundibulum.

So, what then is TGA really? As was stated at the beginning of this chapter, infundibuloarterial situs concordance (sameness) typically results in solitus or inversus normally related great arteries; and infundibuloarterial situs discordance (oppositeness) typically results in transposition of the great arteries.

Thus, TGA is infundibuloarterial situs discordance (difference). However, some clarification is necessary at this point:

1. By *typical* TGA, I mean TGA with a well-developed subaortic infundibular free wall, and an absent subpulmonary infundibular free wall. Typical TGA has aortic-tricuspid discontinuity, and pulmonary-mitral fibrous continuity. Typical D-TGA, that is, TGA {S,D,D}, has an *inverted* infundibulum and *solitus* great arteries. So, in typical D-TGA, there is infundibuloarterial situs *oppositeness.* IA situs oppositeness is one form of IA situs *discordance.* But there are other forms of IA situs discordance.
2. For example, TGA can have a *bilateral* infundibulum, both subaortic and subpulmonary. A bilateral infundibulum (e.g., **4R, 2L**) is anatomically different from a solitus infundibulum (**0R, 4L**), and different from an inversus infundibulum (**4R, 0L**). Consequently, a *bilaterally present* infundibulum is considered to be in *situs ambiguus,* that is, uncertain or unknown pattern of anatomic organization.

Thus, IA situs discordance includes IA situs oppositeness and IA situs ambiguus combinations.

DIAGRAMS AND PHOTOGRAPHS

Diagrams and photographs will help to deepen one's understanding of TGA. The examination of heart specimens is the best teacher because only heart specimens are real and three-dimensional.

Figure 22.22 is a **diagram of typical D-TGA, that is, TGA {S,D,D}.** D-TGA used to be called *complete* TGA, meaning physiologically uncorrected TGA, as opposed to *corrected* TGA, meaning physiologically (not surgically) corrected TGA. But then it was understood that both physiologically uncorrected and corrected TGAs are complete TGAs, that is, both great arteries are placed completely across the ventricular septum. Then *complete* TGA fell into disuse because of its anatomic nonspecificity. By contrast, *D-, L-,* and *A-*TGA are anatomically specific. Each of these terms means only one thing:

D-TGA, the transposed aortic valve is to the right (dextro-, or D, Latin) relative to the transposed pulmonary valve.

L-TGA, the transposed aortic valve is to the left (levo-, or L-, Latin) relative to the transposed pulmonary valve.

A-TGA, the transposed aortic valve is directly anterior (antero, - or A-, Latin) relative to the pulmonary valve.

As you can see, the atria are in situs solitus. D-loop (solitus) ventricles are present. D-TGA is present. The atrioventricular alignments are concordant. The ventriculoarterial alignments are discordant (transposed). A well-developed subaortic infundibulum is present, preventing aortic valve–atrioventricular valve direct fibrous continuity. There is no infundibulum beneath the transposed pulmonary valve, permitting pulmonary valve–mitral valve direct fibrous continuity. The inset shows that there was also pulmonary-tricuspid fibrous continuity. The VSD is subpulmonary because the subpulmonary infundibulum has been resorbed, whereas the subaortic infundibulum is well developed. The VSD is of the **infundibuloventricular type** because it is limited superiorly by the infundibular septum and inferiorly by the ventricular septum. Pulmonary-mitral contiguity and direct fibrous continuity are made possible by involution (disappearance) of the subpulmonary infundibular free wall.

The infundibuloarterial situs analysis is 4R + 0L, which is inverted, whereas the great arteries are solitus or noninverted because the aortic valve is to the right of the pulmonary valve. D-TGA is solitus TGA or noninverted TGA (Fig. 22.23).

Angiocardiography in typical D-TGA, that is, TGA {S,D,D}. Part (A) shows right ventricular *(RV)* injection in the posteroanterior projection *(left panel)* and left lateral projection *(right panel).* Note the well-developed subaortic infundibulum or conus *(C),* best seen in the left lateral projection, that separates the transposed aortic valve above from the coarsely trabeculated RV below. Part (B) shows left ventricular *(LV)* injection in the posteroanterior projection *(left panel)* and in the left lateral projection *(right panel).* There is no subpulmonary muscular conus beneath the transposed pulmonary valve *(PV).* Consequently, the PV is "sitting on" the mitral valve; that is, pulmonary-mitral contiguity and direct fibrous continuity are present. Note the finely trabeculated architecture of the LV. The great arteries arise from the infundibulum or conus arteriosus, which may be well developed, as beneath the aortic valve in this case of TGA, or involuted, as beneath this PV. The great arteries really do not arise from the RV and the LV sinuses or inflow tracts, which are the main pumping portions.

The four components that make up the normal human morphologically right ventricle (RV) and the normal human morphologically left ventricle (LV) are presented diagrammatically in Fig. 22.24:

1. Component 1 is the atrioventricular canal or junction.
2. Component 2 is composed of the ventricular sinuses.

Components 1 and 2 make up the right and left ventricular inflow tracts.

3. **Component 3** is the proximal or apical infundibulum or conus. In the RV, component 3 is the septal band and the moderator band. In the LV, component 3 is the superior, *nontrabeculated* portion of the ventricular septum.

The inferior or apical part of the left ventricular septal surface, that is *finely trabeculated,* is part of component 2. Midseptal muscular VSDs occur between finely trabeculated component 2 below and nontrabeculated component 3 above.

The RV, viewed as a composite whole, has two apices:

1. The RV sinus apex is behind and below the moderator band.
2. The infundibular apex is anterior and superior to the moderator band.

Some of our colleagues refer to the septal band and the moderator band as **the septomarginal trabeculation.** The background is that in 1911, Tandler proposed the term *trabecula septomarginalis* for the term moderator band. *Trabecula septomarginalis* (Latin) means little beam running from the ventricular septum to the acute margin of the heart. So this term means the moderator band, but not the septal band. Our British colleagues did not understand this, they told me. But knowing this term was Latin, they decided it should be translated into

English; hence they Anglicized this term to *septomarginal trabeculation,* a perfectly good translation.

We continue to use the original terms *septal band* and *moderator band* for two reasons:

1. Usage has not confused their meanings.
2. It is useful to be able to distinguish between the septal band and the moderator band, because they are two different structures.

D-TGA involves anomalies of component 4, the subarterial infundibulum (Fig. 22.24). But classical congenital physiologically corrected L-TGA, that is, TGA {S,L,L}, is *not* a malformation of subarterial infundibular component 4. TGA is different from most other forms of congenital heart disease that typically are anomalies of one or more specific anatomic structures. But TGA is a relationships diagnosis, the relationship between the situs of the subarterial infundibular connector, and the situs of the great arteries that are being connected:

1. In typical D-TGA, that is, in TGA {S,D,D}, the situs of the infundibulum is inverted, but the situs of the great arteries is noninverted (solitus).
2. But in typical L-TGA, that is, in TGA {S,L,L}, the situs of the infundibulum is noninverted (solitus), and the situs of the great arteries is inverted. So, one could conclude that in D-TGA, that is, TGA {S,D,D}, only the infundibulum is malformed (inverted). But in L-TGA, that is, TGA {S,L,L}, the great arteries and the ventricles are both malformed (inverted).

In L-TGA, we think one can discount the morphogenetic importance of ventricular L-loop formation because of isolated ventricular inversion {S,L,S} (Fig. 22.3, row 3, column 2). In other words, ventricular L-loop formation is not always associated with L-TGA, as {S,L,S} illustrates. Thus, TGA is considered to be a relationship diagnosis, that is, an infundibuloarterial (IA) situs discordance (difference), with two opposite anatomic IA situs types: (1) inversus-solitus as in TGA {S,D,D}, and (2) solitus-inversus, as in TGA {S,L,L} (as above).

Infundibuloarterial situs concordance or discordance is a newly recognized basic principle. But it really is not unfamiliar or arcane. Every plumber knows this principle. If the type of connector is not the same as the type of pipes being connected, then the pipes will not be properly connected. In other words, the concept of *situs,* that is, the pattern of anatomic organization of the various cardiac segments, is of great importance in the understanding of congenital heart disease.[23] Complex congenital heart disease is often a segmental situs "salad" or mixture (Fig. 22.3, rows 2 to 8 inclusive). By contrast, the normal heart—solitus or inversus—is characterized by segmental situs uniformity, with all cardiac segments in situs solitus, or all segments in situs inversus (Fig. 22.3, row 1).

TGA {S,D,D} with a subaortic infundibulum and an intact ventricular septum is shown in Fig. 22.25. Note the well-developed subaortic infundibulum (or conus) that fills the space above the septal band. The involution of the subpulmonary infundibular free wall permits pulmonary valve–mitral valve fibrous continuity. A very small membranous VSD is seen in the opened LV of a patient with D-TGA (Fig. 22.26). A moderate-sized infundibuloventricular type of VSD is seen in a patient with D-TGA between the infundibular septum (or conal septum) above and the ventricular septum below (Fig. 22.27). A relatively large infundibuloventricular type of VSD, without pulmonary outflow tract stenosis, is seen in Fig. 22.28.

An infundibuloventricular VSD in D-TGA with posterior infundibular septal malalignment causing pulmonary outflow tract stenosis is shown in Fig. 22.29. The geometry of pulmonary outflow tract obstruction and VSD location in D-TGA is presented in Fig. 22.30. When the posterior angle between the infundibular septum (or parietal band) and the ventricular septum is acute (relatively small, about 30° in the figure), then there is no pulmonary outflow tract obstruction and the VSD is subpulmonary *(arrow).* But when the angle between the infundibular septum and the ventricular septum is large (about 90° in the figure), then the infundibular septum can contribute to severe pulmonary outflow tract stenosis or atresia because a large infundibuloventricular septal angle often is associated with posterior infundibular septal malalignment. Also, the VSD becomes subaortic *(arrow),* rather than subpulmonary—depending on how large the infundibuloseptal angle is and how much posterior infundibular septal malalignment there is.

Anterior and rightward malalignment of the infundibular septum in D-TGA, with aortic outflow tract stenosis, is shown in Fig. 22.31. The subaortic infundibulum was smaller than is usually seen in D-TGA. The transposed aortic valve was smaller than normal. The ascending aorta and the aortic arch were hypoplastic. And there was interruption of the aortic arch distal to the left subclavian artery (type A aortic arch interruption).

An aneurysm of the membranous septum produced severe subpulmonary stenosis in a patient with D-TGA (Fig. 22.32). The aneurysm was large, firm, immediately subpulmonary, and highly occlusive. Because of the highly obstructive membranous aneurysm, this patient could not be weaned from the pump-oxygenator. The surgeon thought there was a myxoma below the pulmonary valve.

Isolated pulmonary valvar stenosis can occur in D-TGA with an intact ventricular septum (Fig. 22.33).

A VSD of the AV canal type in D-TGA is shown in Fig. 22.34. **A muscular VSD** is also seen behind and below the septal band. **A straddling tricuspid valve with a VSD of the atrioventricular canal type** is seen in a patient with TGA {S,D,D} (Fig. 22.35). **A large muscular ventricular septal defect (VSD)** is presented in a patient with TGA {S,D,D} in Fig. 22.36.

Classical congenital physiologically corrected TGA {S,**L,L**} is shown in Fig. 22.37. Part (A) shows the left-sided, inverted morphologically right ventricle, the left-sided tricuspid valve, and the left-sided L-transposed aorta sitting atop a well-developed left-sided subaortic muscular infundibulum that widely separates the aortic valve from the tricuspid valve. Part (B) shows the right-sided inverted morphologically left ventricle, the right-sided pulmonary valve–mitral valve fibrous continuity, and the subpulmonary VSD. In part (A), the RV is left-handed. In part (B), the LV is right-handed. As the segmental anatomy indicates, there is discordance between the atrial segment and the ventricular segment, that is, {S,**L**,-}, and there also is discordance between the

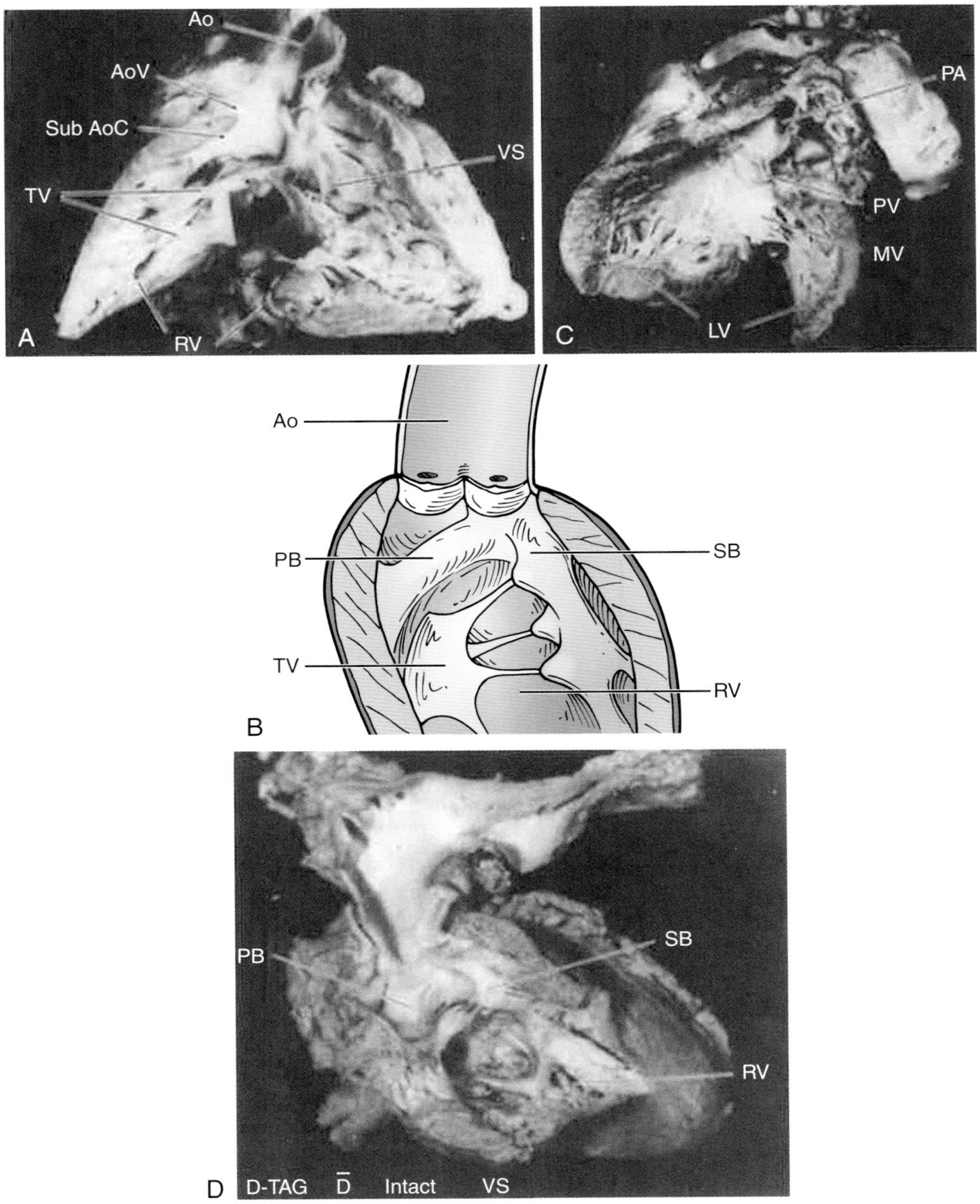

Fig. 22.25 TGA {S,D,D} with subaortic infundibulum and intact ventricular septum. (A) Opened morphologically right ventricle *(RV)* and D-transposed aorta *(Ao)*. The subaortic conus *(Sub AoC)* or infundibulum separates the transposed aortic valve above *(AoV)* from the tricuspid valve *(TV)*. The ventricular septum *(VS)* is intact. (B) The subaortic conus or infundibulum is also known as the parietal band *(PB)* because it sweeps out on to the right ventricular parietal wall or free wall. Note that the parietal band (component 4, Fig. 22.24) perfectly fills the potential space above the septal band *(SB)* (component 3, Fig. 22.24). VSDs between the parietal band and the septal band are **intraconal VSDs or intrainfundibular VSDs** because they occur between the distal subarterial part of the infundibulum and the proximal or apical part of the infundibulum, i.e., between components 4 and 3, Fig. 22.24. (C) The opened morphologically left ventricle *(LV)* and the transposed pulmonary artery *(PA)*. Note the pulmonary valve (PV)–mitral valve (MV) direct fibrous continuity and the intact ventricular septum. In the photographic part of (B), note the perfect union of the PB and the SB, which is why the ventricular septum is intact. The infundibular septum (PB) often is imperfectly aligned with the SB and the ventricular septum, which is why VSDs are so common at this site. We call such defects **infundibuloventricular VSDs.** The infundibular septum can be malaligned in almost any direction causing not only a VSD, but also pulmonary outflow tract stenosis (leftward and posterior malalignment), or aortic outflow tract stenosis and interrupted aortic arch (rightward malalignment). Such infundibuloventricular VSDs are also called **malalignment VSDs.** (Reproduced with permission from Van Praagh R. What determines whether the great arteries are normally or abnormally related? *Am J Cardiol* 2016;118:1390.)

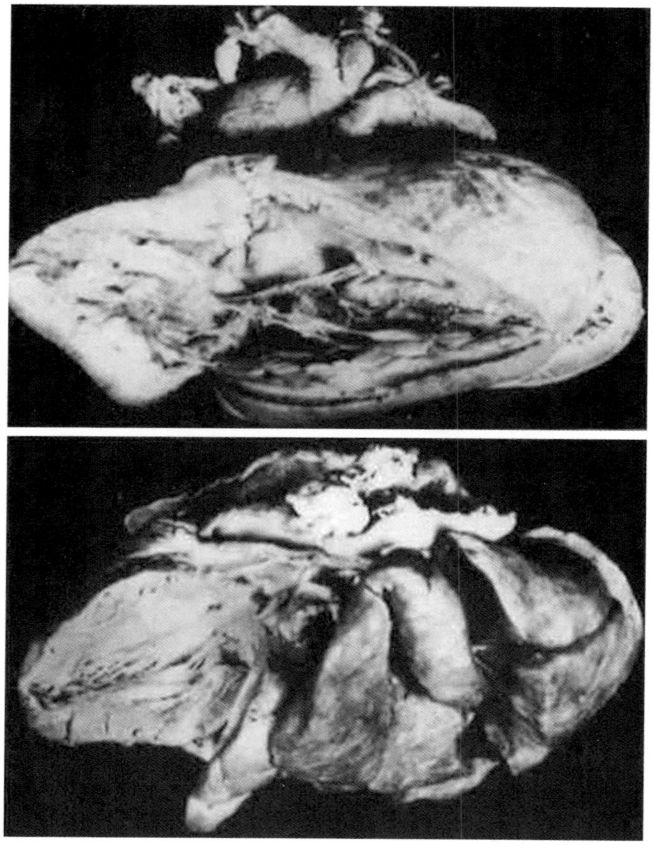

Fig. 22.26 VSDs in D-TGA can be tiny, invisible from the right ventricular aspect *(top)*, and barely seen from the left ventricular aspect *(bottom)*, below the transposed pulmonary valve. (Reproduced with permission from Van Praagh R. What determines whether the great arteries are normally or abnormally related? *Am J Cardiol* 2016;118:1390.)

ventricular segment and the great arterial segment, that is, **TGA {-,L,L}.** This double discordance (atrioventricular and ventriculoarterial) physiologically corrects the destinations of the systemic and pulmonary venous circulations, as long as associated malformations (such as VSD and pulmonary stenosis) do not uncorrect the potentially physiologically corrected atrioarterial alignments. In TGA {S,L,L}, the right atrium and the pulmonary artery are ipsilateral—both are right-sided; and the left atrium and the aorta are ipsilateral—both are left-sided.

By contrast with congenital physiologically corrected TGA {S,L,L} which has intersegmental **double discordance,** physiologically uncorrected TGA {S,D,D} has a **single alignment discordance** between the ventricles and the great arteries, that is, **TGA {S,D,D}. TGA is a ventriculoarterial (VA) discordance.** In turn, VA discordance in TGA {S,D,D} is caused by **infundibular inversion,** which in turn is caused by **infundibuloarterial situs discordance of the inversus-solitus type.**

Segmental discordance between main cardiac segments—atria, ventricles, great arteries—is usually caused by infundibular connecting segment–great arterial main segment discordance, apparently because the infundibular connecting segment is an **independent variable.**

The AV canal or junction acts like a **dependent variable,** corresponding to the situs of the ventricles of entry, not to the situs of the atria of exit.

The cardiac segments that appear to be independent variables are the atria, the ventricular sinuses (or inflow tracts), and the distal or subarterial infundibulum.

Rarely, a main cardiac segment—and not the infundibulum (a connecting segment)—appears to be responsible for segmental discordance, for example, isolated ventricular inversion

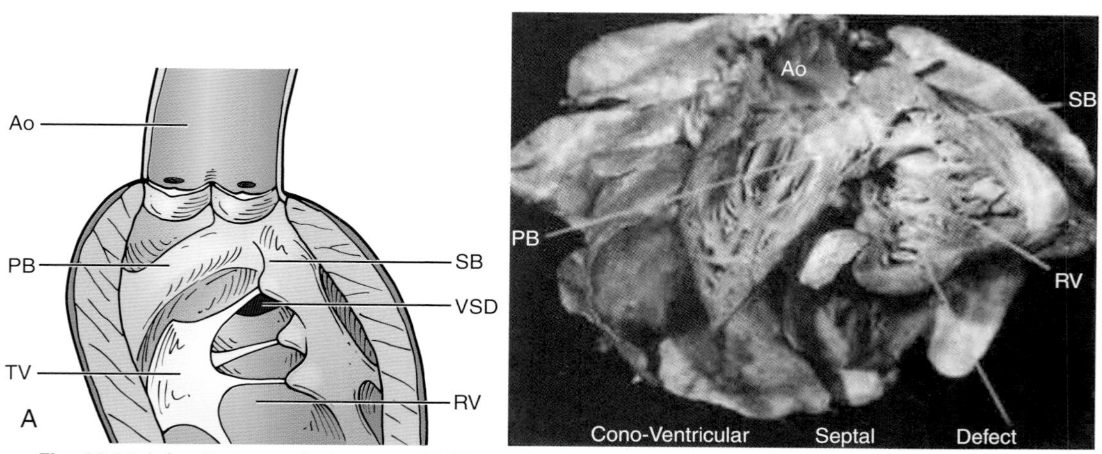

Fig. 22.27 Infundibuloventricular type of VSD in TGA {S,D,D} between the infundibular septum or parietal band *(PB)* above and the ventricular septum below. The defect, also known as a conoventricular type of VSD, is confluent with the tricuspid valve *(TV)*. Consequently, the VSD is described as paramembranous or as juxtamembranous, or as paratricuspid, or as juxtatricuspid. *Para,* beside (Greek); *juxta,* beside (Latin). (Reproduced with permission from Van Praagh R. What determines whether the great arteries are normally or abnormally related? *Am J Cardiol* 2016;118:1390.)

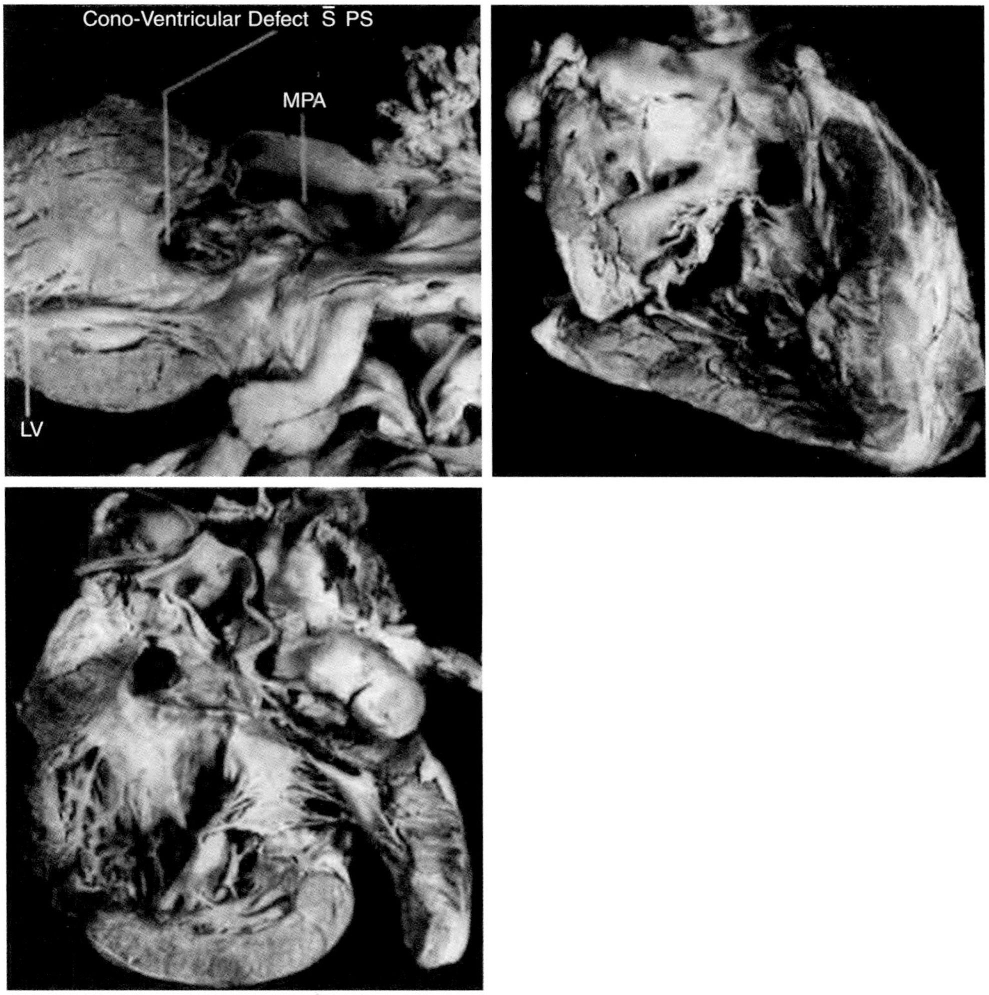

Fig. 22.28 *Left upper:* D-TGA with a large infundibuloventricular VSD, opened left ventricle *(LV),* and transposed main pulmonary artery *(MPA).* The large MPA indicates that there was no pulmonary stenosis. Note the direct fibrous continuity between the transposed pulmonary valve and the anterior mitral leaflet, indicating resorption of the transposed subpulmonary infundibular free wall, which is typical of D-TGA. *Right upper and left lower:* D-TGA with a VSD that is both subaortic and subpulmonary. How is that possible? The opened right ventricular view *(upper right)* shows posterior malalignment of the infundibular septum. The VSD is in front of (anterior to) the infundibular septum, above the septal band, and immediately subaortic—because of posterior malalignment of the infundibular septum (component 4), which is rare. The opened left ventricle *(lower left)* shows the same heart specimen as in the upper right photo. The VSD is also immediately subpulmonary. There is no pulmonary outflow tract obstruction, and pulmonary-mitral fibrous continuity is present. We think that all of these findings can be explained by hypoplasia of the central portion of the infundibular septum above the muscular interventricular septum. (Reproduced with permission from Van Praagh R. What determines whether the great arteries are normally or abnormally related? *Am J Cardiol* 2016;118:1390.)

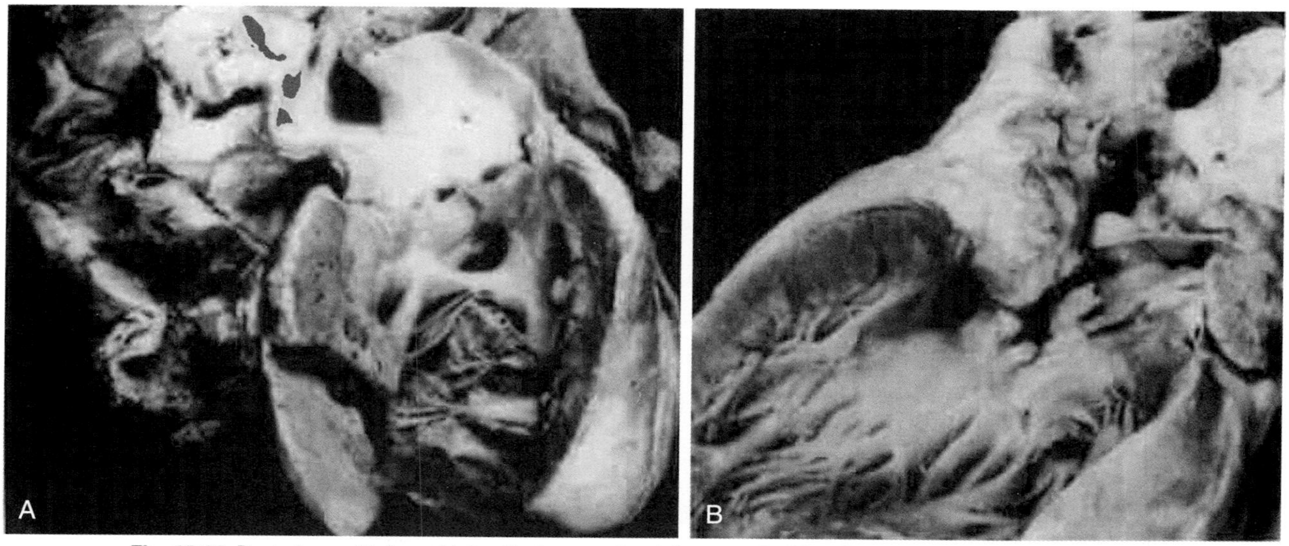

Fig. 22.29 Posterior and leftward infundibular septal malalignment in TGA {S,D,D}. (A) The opened right ventricle and D-transposed aorta reveal what appears to be a subaortic VSD. To the unwary eye, the appearance might suggest an infundibular septal defect. However, being familiar with the four main components that make up both ventricles (Fig. 22.24), one should recognize the "Y" of the septal band, the top of the septal band being formed by its left anterior and right posterior divisions, giving the septal band as a whole a "Y" shape. But even from the right ventricular side, one can see—through the VSD—a small, leftwardly displaced infundibular septum. Note that the VSD, in addition to being subaortic, is also not paramembranous, being separated from the tricuspid valve by an unusually prominent right posterior division of the septal band. (B) The opened left ventricle and transposed pulmonary artery reveals the hypoplastic and posteriorly malaligned infundibular septum that forms the anterior wall of the stenotic subpulmonary outflow tract. The anterior mitral leaflet forms the posterior wall of the stenotic subpulmonary outflow tract. There is direct fibrous continuity between the hypoplastic (stenotic) pulmonary valve and the anterior mitral leaflet. (Reproduced with permission from Van Praagh R. What determines whether the great arteries are normally or abnormally related? *Am J Cardiol* 2016;118:1390.)

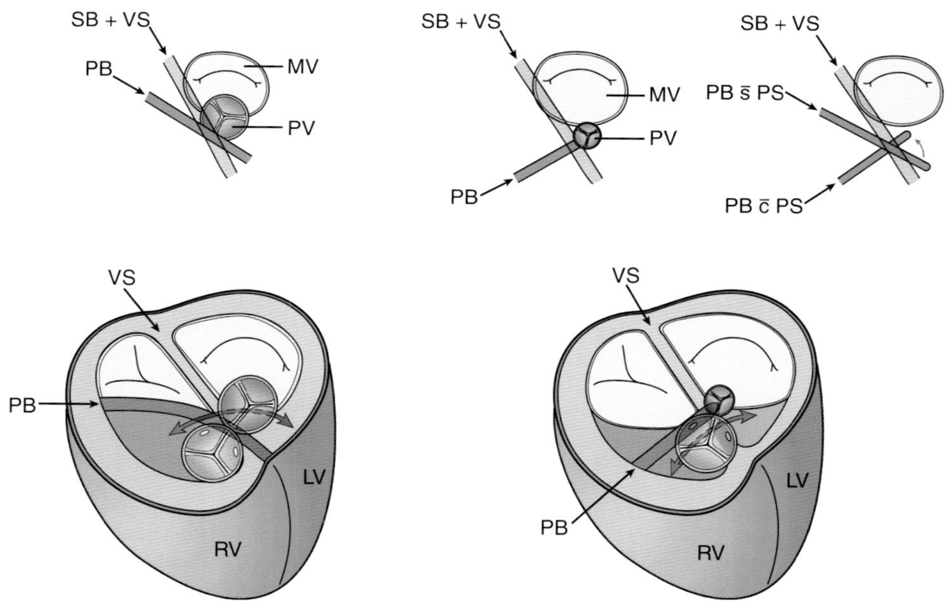

Fig. 22.30 **Geometry of pulmonary outflow tract obstruction and ventricular septal defect location.** When TGA {S,D,D} has an infundibuloventricular type of ventricular septal defect *(VSD)* that is subpulmonary *(arrow)*, the angle between the infundibular septum or parietal band *(PB)* and the septal band and ventricular septum *(SB + VS)* is acute (small), about 30°. But when the infundibuloventricular septal angle is large, about 90°, then this malaligned infundibular septum (PB) can compress the subpulmonary outflow tract, resulting in pulmonary outflow tract stenosis or atresia, and the VSD becomes subaortic *(arrow)*, not subpulmonary. **From the standpoint of the pulmonary outflow tract, this is the geometry of posterior infundibular septal malalignment, as in Fig. 22.29.** (Reproduced with permission from Van Praagh R. What determines whether the great arteries are normally or abnormally related? *Am J Cardiol* 2016;118:1390.)

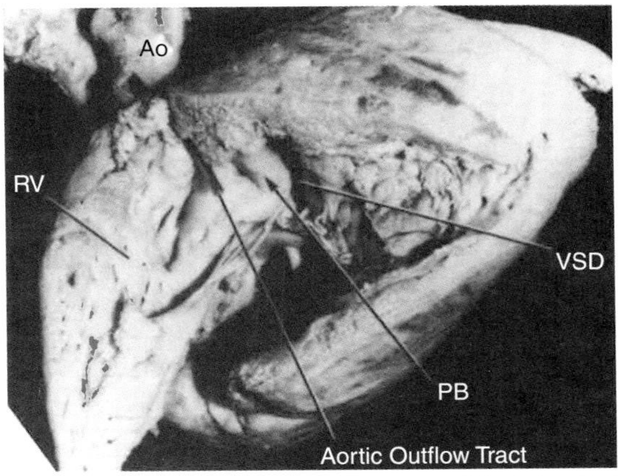

Fig. 22.31 Anterior and rightward malalignment of the infundibular septum or parietal band *(PB)* with TGA {S,D,D} and interrupted aortic arch distal to the left subclavian artery (type A). The opened right ventricle *(RV)* leads to a D-transposed aorta *(Ao)*. The infundibular septum *(PB)* is displaced abnormally anteriorly and to the right. The left surface of the PB is aligned with the right surface of the ventricular septum. This rightward malalignment of the infundibular septum results in a malalignment type of infundibuloventricular VSD. The right-shifted infundibular septum is associated with an unusually small subaortic infundibulum, a small aortic annulus, a hypoplastic ascending aorta, and interrupted aortic arch type A. **It should be understood that when we are talking about infundibular septal malalignment, the infundibular septal malalignment is a proxy for malalignment of the entire infundibuloarterial part of the heart.** We are *not* talking about isolated malalignment of the infundibular septum only. (Reproduced with permission from Van Praagh R. What determines whether the great arteries are normally or abnormally related? *Am J Cardiol* 2016;118:1390.)

{S,L,S}[24] (Fig. 22.3, row 3, column 2). In isolated ventricular inversion, the single segmental discordance involves the ventricular segment, that is, {S,**L**,S}, a main segment, not the infundibulum, a connecting segment. This single discordance causes physiologic uncorrection of the venous circulations because the right atrium and the aorta are both ipsilateral (right-sided), and the left atrium and the pulmonary artery are both ipsilateral (both left-sided) (Fig. 22.3).[24] In {S,L,S}, this single discordance should be treated with an *atrial* switch procedure surgically (a Mustard or Senning procedure, not an *arterial* switch procedure), because in {S,L,S}, the ventriculoarterial alignments and connections are normal.

Transposition of the great arteries in the IV/IV mouse is shown in Fig. 22.38. This is thought to be a good model of human D-TGA. Part (A) shows the right heart, sagittal section, left lateral view. Part (B) shows the left heart, sagittal section, left lateral view. In part (A), note that the inferior vena cava drains into the right atrium, that opens into the right ventricle, that ejects into a D-transposed aorta. In particular, note the well-developed subaortic infundibulum that separates the transposed aortic valve above from the tricuspid valve below. In part (B), note that the transposed pulmonary valve is in direct fibrous continuity with the mitral valve.[2]

The iv/iv mouse is homozygous for a gene causing situs inversus.[25] Figure 22.38 was the first time that an animal model, very similar to human D-TGA, was produced. Anatomically, we have concluded that **human D-TGA is isolated infundibular inversion.** Therefore, it is perhaps not surprising that a good

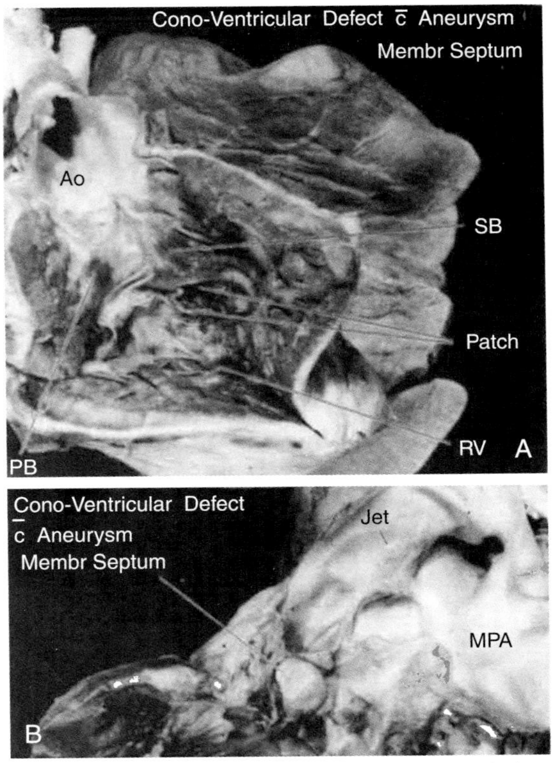

Fig. 22.32 Aneurysm of the membranous septum producing severe subpulmonary stenosis. (A) Opened right ventricle *(RV)* of D-TGA. A conoventricular or infundibuloventricular type of VSD was occluded with a patch. (B) The opened left ventricle *(LV)* and transposed main pulmonary artery *(MPA)*. Immediately beneath the transposed pulmonary valve is a large, firm, highly occlusive mass—a large aneurysm of the membranous septum. There is a jet lesion in the MPA. In the early 1970s, this patient underwent a Mustard procedure and a VSD patch closure at another institution. Because of this large and highly obstructive membranous aneurysm, the patient could not be weaned from the pump-oxygenator. The surgeon initially thought there was a myxoma below the pulmonary valve. (Reproduced with permission from Van Praagh R. What determines whether the great arteries are normally or abnormally related? *Am J Cardiol* 2016;118:1390.)

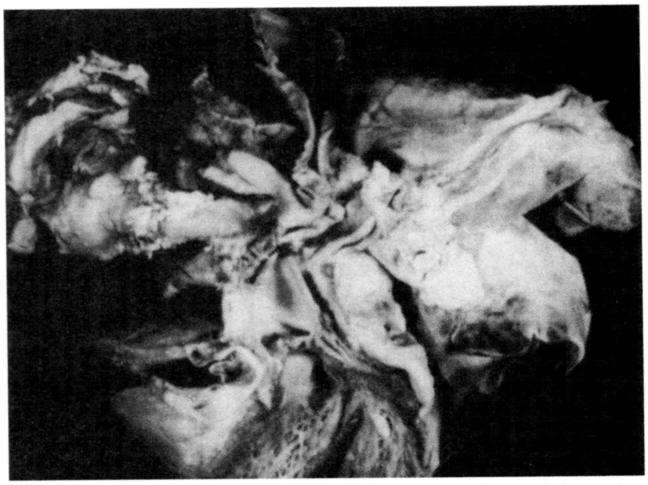

Fig. 22.33 Isolated pulmonary valvar stenosis in TGA {S,D,D} with an intact ventricular septum. View of the opened LV, transposed pulmonary artery, and the stenotic pulmonary valve. (Reproduced with permission from Van Praagh R. What determines whether the great arteries are normally or abnormally related? *Am J Cardiol* 2016;118:1390.)

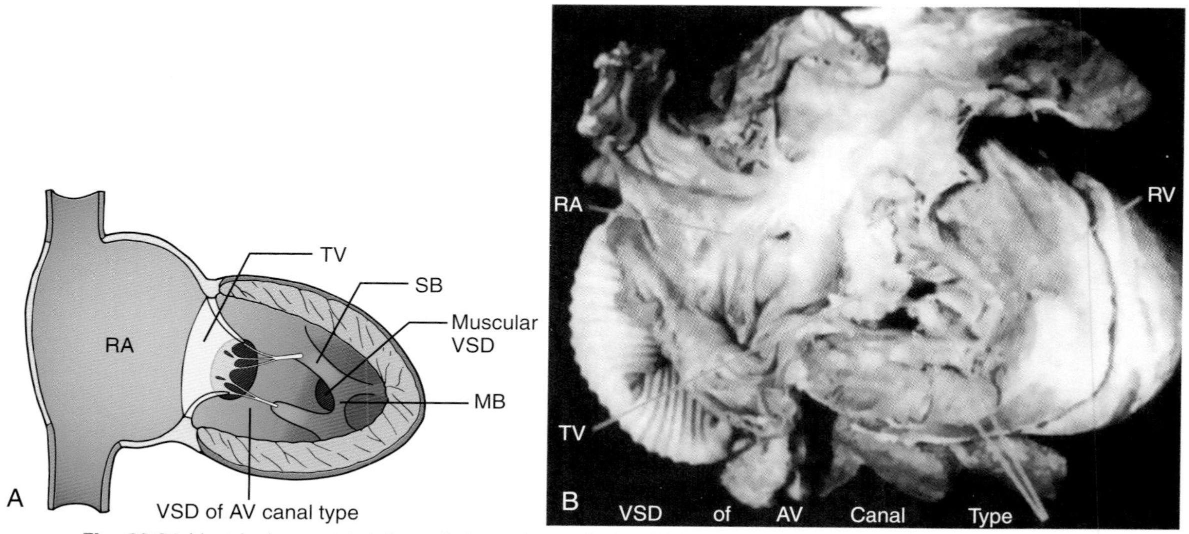

Fig. 22.34 Ventricular septal defect of the atrioventricular *(AV)* canal type shown diagrammatically *(A)* and photographically *(B)*. This type of VSD is located beneath the septal leaflet of the tricuspid valve *(TV)* and is confluent with the origin of this leaflet; i.e., no septal musculature between this VSD and the origin of the septal leaflet of the TV. If the VSD is not confluent with the origin of the septal leaflet of the TV, such a defect is a muscular VSD in the ventricular septum, not a VSD of the AV canal type. This VSD of the AV canal type was "isolated" in the following sense: A common AV valve was not present, and no ostium primum defect was present. A muscular VSD is shown peeking out beneath the septal band (A). Such midmuscular VSDs often are located between the finely trabeculated left ventricular septal surface inferiorly (component 2) and the nontrabeculated left ventricular septal surface superiorly (component 3) (Fig. 22.24, LV). (Reproduced with permission from Van Praagh R. What determines whether the great arteries are normally or abnormally related? *Am J Cardiol* 2016;118:1390.)

animal example of human D-TGA (Fig. 22.38)[26,27] should be found in a mammalian model of situs inversus.[25] We hope that these insights and findings will help to further elucidate the molecular genetic etiology of human TGA.

The morphogenetic movements of solitus normally related great arteries and in D-TGA are presented in Fig. 22.39.

TGA With Posterior Aorta, Anterior Pulmonary Artery, Subpulmonary Infundibulum, and Aortic-Atrioventricular Fibrous Continuity[28]

By about 1970 we knew that TGA did not always have an anterior aortic valve and a posterior pulmonary valve, as in typical D-TGA (Fig. 22.39), not if there was a subpulmonary infundibulum and little or no subaortic infundibulum[28] (Fig. 22.40). Indeed, such cases support **the differential infundibular development hypothesis** concerning the morphogenesis of normally and abnormally related great arteries that has been presented (Figs. 22.1, 22.2, and 22.3). Growth of the subpulmonary infundibulum can elevate the pulmonary valve superiorly and protrude the pulmonary valve anteriorly relative to the aortic valve, if there is no growth or resorption of the subaortic infundibulum.[28] Thus, the presence of a posterior aortic valve and an anterior pulmonary valve does not exclude the diagnosis of TGA. **TGA is defined** as ventriculoarterial alignment discordance: RV to aorta and LV to pulmonary artery. **The aortic valve in TGA** can be anterior, beside, or posterior relative to the pulmonary valve. **The infundibulum in TGA** can be subaortic (in 92%),[28] or subaortic and subpulmonary (in 8%),[29] or subpulmonary and deficient (rare, as in TGA with posterior aorta, Fig. 22.40).

TGA is a malposition of the great arteries. Malpositions of the great arteries (MGA) include:

1. transposition of the great arteries (TGA);
2. double-outlet right ventricle (DORV);
3. double-outlet left ventricle (DOLV); and
4. anatomically corrected malposition of the great arteries (ACMGA).

In TGA, we have already seen that the subarterial infundibulum usually is *subaortic* (92%), and occasionally is *subaortic and subpulmonary* (8%).[28] Rarely, the infundibulum can be *subpulmonary and deficient* in TGA with posterior aorta (much less than 1%)[28] (Fig. 22.41).

This raises the question: What about the fourth logically predictable possibility? Is it possible for there to be absence of the subarterial infundibula, that is, no subaortic infundibulum and no subpulmonary infundibulum? And if so, what happens then?

The answer is: yes, it is rarely possible for there to be absence of both the subaortic and the subpulmonary halves of the infundibulum. As will be seen, this rare anomaly occurs in the Paul type of DOLV.[30]

For further consideration of the embryonic great arterial switches, see Chapter 26. TGA is one example of a general principle. The question becomes: What is the infundibulum really doing?

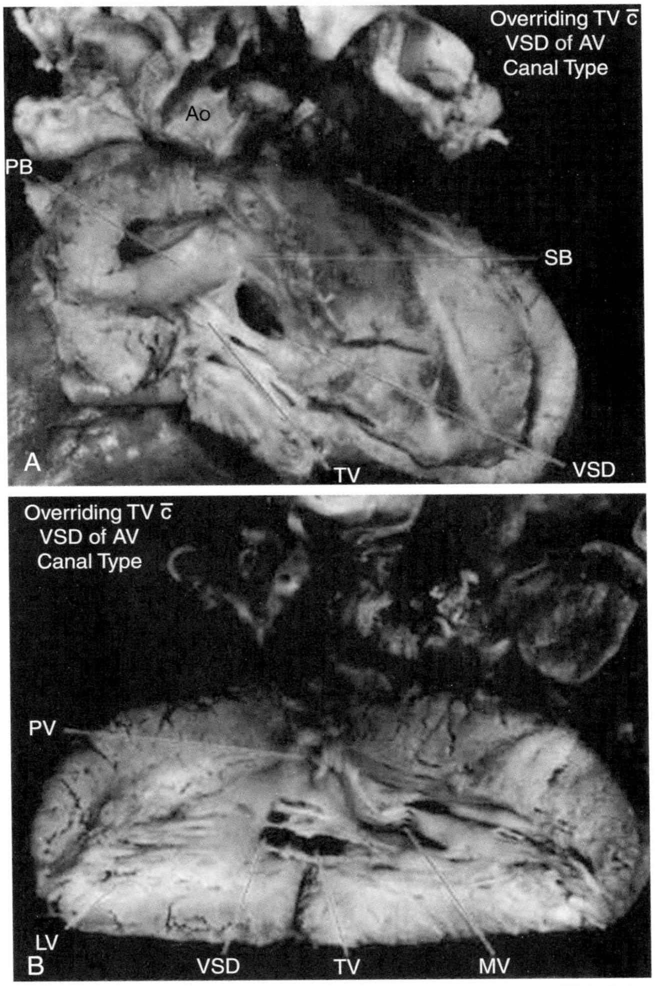

Fig. 22.35 (A) Straddling tricuspid valve *(TV)* with ventricular septal defect *(VSD)* of the atrioventricular *(AV)* canal type in TGA {S,D,D}. The VSD is medial to the TV, not superior to the TV where most infundibuloventricular VSDs are located, nor anterior to the TV where most muscular VSDs are found. The infundibular septum or parietal band *(PB)*, the septal band *(SB)*, and the D-transposed aorta *(Ao)* are also seen. (B) The opened left ventricle *(LV)* shows the transposed pulmonary valve *(PV)*, which is in direct fibrous continuity with the mitral valve *(MV)*. The MV inserts only into the anterolateral papillary muscle group of the LV. In (A), the RV sinus is moderately underdeveloped, and the ventricular septum is right-shifted relative to the normally located atrial septum. This right shift of the ventricular loop (not just of the ventricular septum) is thought to be the morphogenetic basis of straddling tricuspid valve because it results in ventriculoatrial malalignment. Note that the insertions of the tricuspid valve are biventricular, whereas those of the mitral valve are into the LV only. Indeed, **parachute mitral valve** is present: all mitral chordae tendineae insert into only one papillary muscle, the anterolateral papillary muscle of the LV. If congenital mitral stenosis was present we were not aware of it. We think that when straddling tricuspid valve is present, one should consider the possibility of parachute mitral valve with congenital mitral stenosis. When these photos were made, the condition presented here was called *overriding* tricuspid valve. Later, however, a useful distinction was introduced, I think by Dr. Maurice Lev. When only the annulus of an AV valve overrides the ventricular septum, but the chordae tendineae and the papillary muscles remain appropriate for the AV valve (tensor apparatus of the TV to the RV only, and tensor apparatus of the mitral valve to the LV only), then this situation is designated **overriding (of the annulus only) of the AV valve.** But when the tensor apparatus of an AV valve is biventricular, then this situation is diagnosed as **straddling of the AV valve.** We favor this distinction because the surgical management is different, depending on whether or not the tensor apparatus straddles the ventricular septum. (Reproduced with permission from Van Praagh R. What determines whether the great arteries are normally or abnormally related? *Am J Cardiol* 2016;118:1390.)

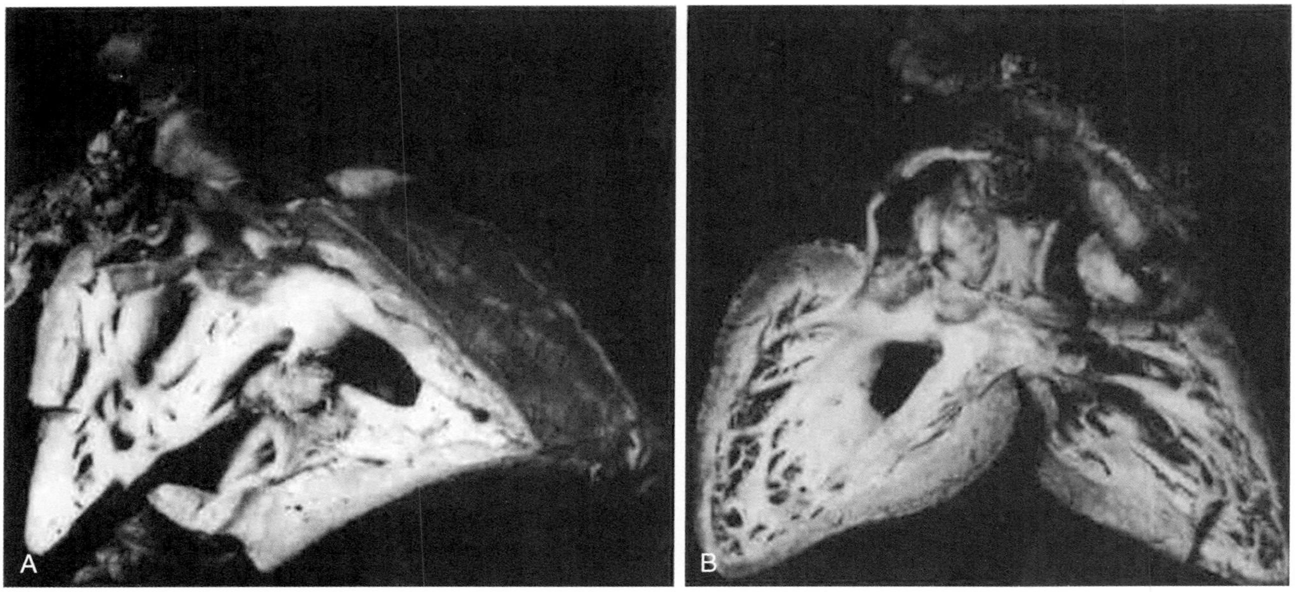

Fig. 22.36 Muscular VSD in TGA {S,D,D}. (A) Opened right ventricle and D-transposed aorta showing a large muscular VSD anterior to the tricuspid valve. (B) Opened left ventricle and transposed pulmonary artery showing the large muscular VSD below the infundibular septum. (Reproduced with permission from Van Praagh R. What determines whether the great arteries are normally or abnormally related? *Am J Cardiol* 2016;118:1390.)

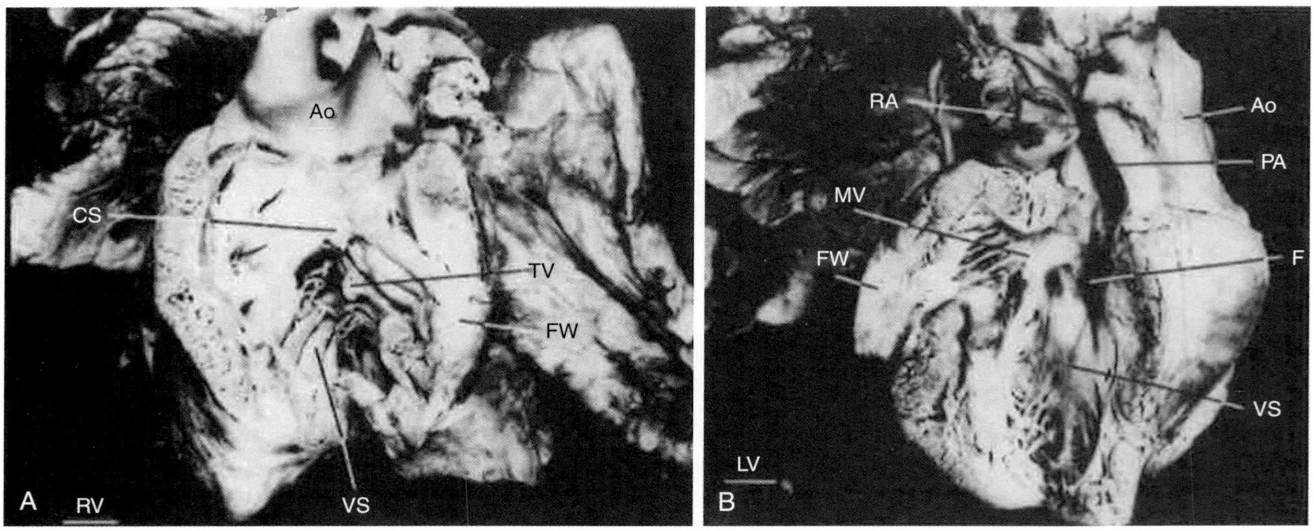

Fig. 22.37 Congenital physiologically corrected TGA {S,L,L}. (A) Opened left-sided morphologically right ventricle *(RV)* and L-transposed aorta *(Ao)*. Note the well-developed muscular subaortic infundibular septum or conal septum *(CS)* that widely separates the aortic valve above from the left-sided tricuspid valve *(TV)* below. The ventricular septum, into which the TV inserts, is right-sided, the free wall of the RV is left-sided. This left-sided RV is left-handed (Fig. 22.17), i.e., inverted. (B) The opened right-sided morphologically left ventricle *(LV)* and transposed pulmonary artery. Note that the right-sided morphologically right atrium *(RA)* opens through the right-sided mitral valve *(MV)* into the right-sided LV that is right-handed. There is atrioventricular *(AV)* alignment discordance (RA to LV). There is also ventriculoarterial *(VA)* alignment discordance (LV to PA). So there is *double discordance,* AV and VA, which should cancel each other physiologically, lack of associated malformations permitting. The only associated malformation is a subpulmonary infundibuloventricular type of VSD *(F)*. The double discordance means that the RA and the PA are ipsilateral (both right-sided), and the LA and the Ao are also both ipsilateral (both left-sided). There is pulmonary-mitral direct fibrous continuity. The sinoatrial node is located normally, to the right of the entry of the right superior vena cava into the right atrium. **But the course of the atrioventricular conduction system or His bundle typically is as follows:** The AV bundle runs from the RA into the right-sided LV posteriorly and just to the right of the transposed pulmonary artery. Then the conduction system runs anteriorly and just to the right of the pulmonary annulus. Then the conduction system proceeds anteriorly, above a VSD, if a VSD is present, and then downward in front of a VSD, if present. Then the left bundle branches of the conduction system fan downward and right laterally, heading for the left ventricular papillary muscles and the left ventricular free wall. The right bundle branch passes through the VSD to enter the left-sided RV. The delineation of the course of the atrioventricular conduction system in congenital physiologically corrected TGA {S,D,D} was one of Dr. Robert Henry Anderson's greatest achievements. (Reproduced with permission from Van Praagh R. What determines whether the great arteries are normally or abnormally related? *Am J Cardiol* 2016;118:1390.)

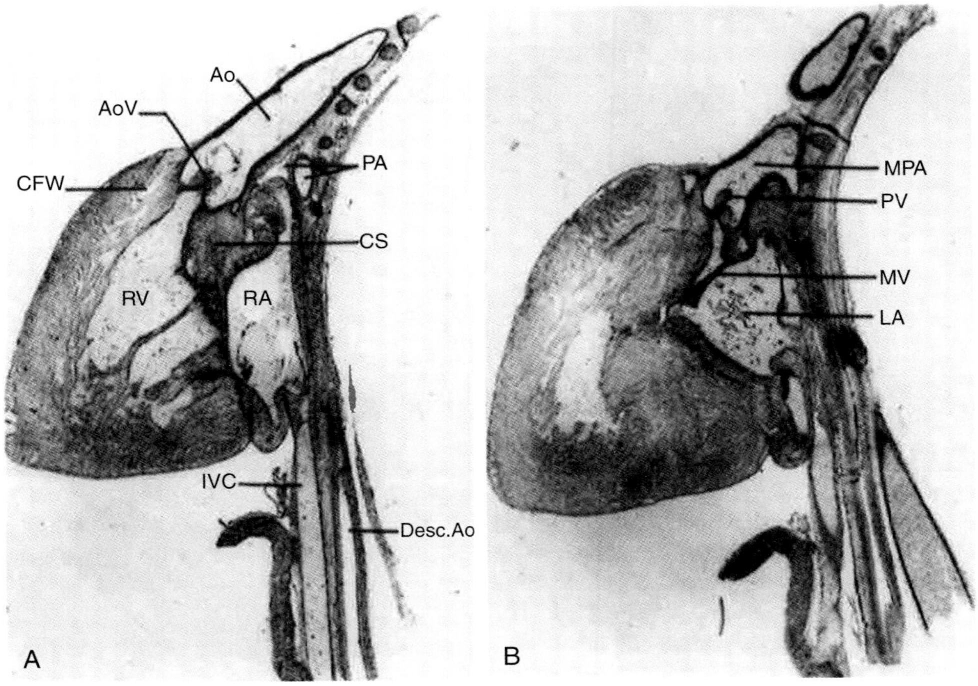

Fig. 22.38 D-transposition of the great arteries in the iv/iv mouse that is homozygous for the situs inversus gene iv. (A) Right heart, sagittal section, left lateral view. The inferior vena cava *(IVC)* returns to the morphologically right atrium *(RA)*. The RA opens through the tricuspid valve (unlabeled) into the morphologically right ventricle *(RV)*. The RV opens into the D-transposed ascending aorta *(Ao)*. A well-developed infundibular septum *(CS)* and infundibular (or conal) free wall *(CFW)* are seen. (B) Left heart, sagittal section, left lateral view. Note the left atrium *(LA)*, the mitral valve *(MV)*, the pulmonary valve *(PV)*, and the main pulmonary artery *(MPA)*. There is PV-MV continuity. This mammalian model of human D-TGA is an excellent model, with a well-developed right-sided subaortic infundibulum and pulmonary-mitral fibrous continuity. Since typical human D-TGA has infundibular inversion, it is perhaps not surprising to find an excellent animal model of human D-TGA in a mammal that is homozygous for the situs inversus gene, the iv/iv mouse. Much of complex congenital heart disease appears to be a segmental situs "salad" (a mixture), as the infundibuloarterial situs equations illustrate (Table 22.1). In other words, complex congenital heart disease is characterized by a lack of situs solitus in all cardiac segments. Thus, the etiology of complex congenital heart disease appears to be a lack of genetic control of segmental situs. (Stained with PAS, original magnification ×70.) (Reproduced with permission from Van Praagh R. What determines whether the great arteries are normally or abnormally related? *Am J Cardiol* 2016;118:1390.)

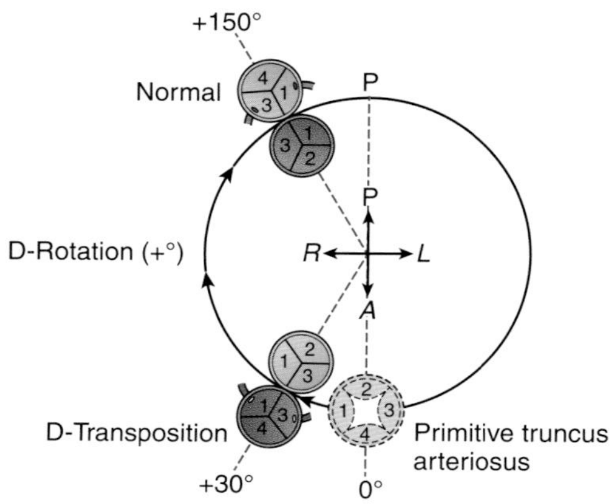

Fig. 22.39 Development of the semilunar valves, seen from above, in solitus normally related great arteries *(Normal)* and in D-TGA *(D-Transposition)*. The endocardial cushions, from which the semilunar valves develop, are numbered conventionally. The semilunar valves undergo rotation to the right *(D-Rotation)* relative to the anteroposterior *(AP)* plane. Ventricular loop formation results is about 90° dextrorotation, aortic valve to the right and pulmonary valve to the left, side by side. For example, in the Taussig-Bing heart (see DORV), ventricular D-loop formation was normal, and the development of the right-sided subaortic infundibulum and of the left-sided subpulmonary infundibulum was approximately equal, canceling each other as far as morphogenetic movements of both semilunar valves were concerned. Whenever subaortic and subpulmonary infundibular development is the same, the rotation at the great arterial level is approximately 90°, i.e., no AP morphogenetic movement. Unequal development of the subarterial free walls can change this side-by-side (+90° D-rotation) relationship. Normally, the development of the subarterial infundibular free walls is completely asymmetrical. The right-sided subaortic infundibular free wall involutes (disappears), and the left-sided subpulmonary infundibular free wall grows and expands. One of the effects of this asymmetric infundibular free wall development is to increase the D-rotation of the semilunar valves from a side-by-side (+90°) relationship to an approximately 150° dextrorotation, i.e., 60° more dextrorotation. But if the development of the subarterial infundibular free walls is inverted, as in D-TGA, with growth and expansion of the right-sided subaortic infundibular free wall and resorption (disappearance) of the left-sided subpulmonary infundibular free wall, then some *leftward* rotation can occur at the semilunar valves, reducing the dextrorotation from about 90° to about 30°, because of about 60° of levorotation in the wrong direction. *Infundibular inversion,* the basic malformation in D-TGA, is clearly expressed in infundibuloarterial situs equations. SNRGA {S,D,S} = *0R + 4L,* and TGA {S,D,D} = *4R + 0L*. Note also that septal leaflets 1 and 3 are left-sided and right-sided with solitus normally related great arteries, but are right-sided and left-sided, respectively, in typical D-TGA. Nonseptal leaflets 2 and 4 are normally predominantly left-sided and right-sided, respectively, both normally and in D-TGA. Considered as a whole, the aortic and pulmonary valves in D- TGA are considered to be noninverted or solitus. In visceroatrial situs solitus, the aortic valve is right-sided, which it is in typical D-TGA, and the pulmonary valve is left-sided, as it is in typical D-TGA. Hence, the semilunar valves in D-TGA are considered to be noninverted or solitus, despite the fact that septal leaflets 1 and 3 are right-left reversed in D-TGA, compared with normal.

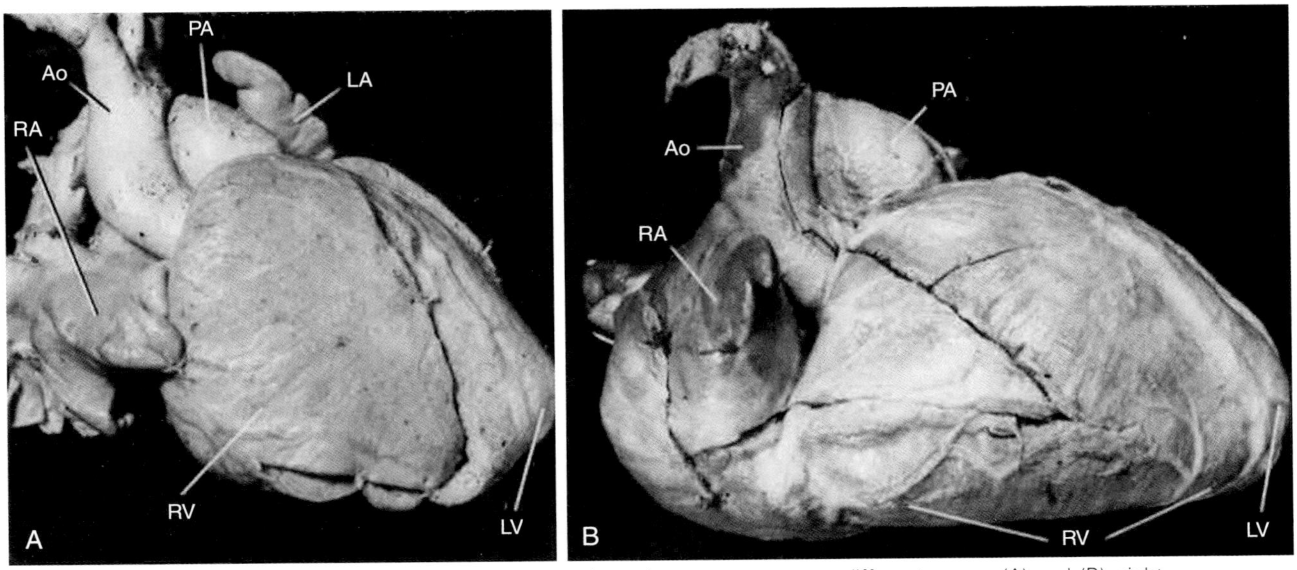

Fig. 22.40 TGA with posterior aorta and anterior pulmonary artery, two different cases, (A) and (B), right lateral views. The great arteries untwist about each other to an almost normal degree. The aorticopulmonary septum is spiral, not straight. *Ao,* Transposed aorta; *LA,* solitus morphologically left atrium; *LV,* solitus or D-loop morphologically left ventricle; *PA,* transposed pulmonary artery; *RA,* solitus morphologically right atrium; *RV,* solitus or D-loop morphologically right ventricle. (Reproduced with permission from Van Praagh R, Perez-Treviilo C, Lopez-Cuellar M, Baker FW, Zuberbuhler JR, Quero M, Perez VM, Moreno F, Van Praagh S. Transposition of the great arteries with posterior aorta, anterior pulmonary artery, subpulmonary conus, and fibrous continuity between aortic and atrioventricular valves. *Am J Cardiol* 1971;28:621.)

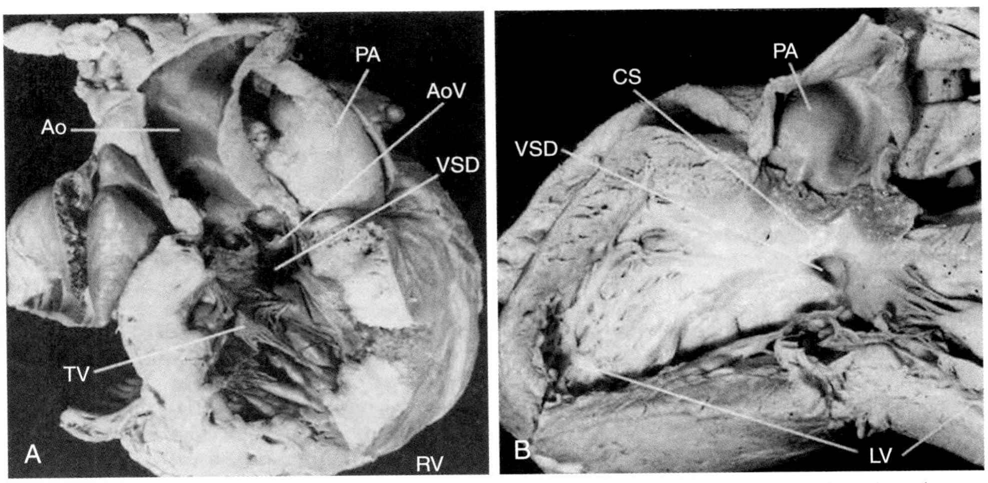

Fig. 22.41 (A) Opened right ventricle *(RV)* and D-transposed ascending aorta *(Ao)*. Note how low the transposed aortic valve *(AoV)* is. The ventricular septal defect *(VSD)* is immediately subaortic and the aortic valve is in direct fibrous continuity with the tricuspid valve *(TV)*; both are due to absence of subaortic infundibular musculature. The transposed main pulmonary artery *(PA)* is markedly anterior to the transposed ascending Ao. (B) Opened left ventricle *(LV)* and transposed pulmonary artery *(PA)*. The transposed pulmonary valve is separated from the ventricular septal defect *(VSD)* by a small amount of subpulmonary infundibular myocardium. Thus, pulmonary-mitral fibrous continuity is *not* present. *CS,* Conal (infundibular) septum. (Reproduced with permission from Van Praagh R, Perez-Treviilo C, Lopez-Cuellar M, Baker FW, Zuberbuhler JR, Quero M, Perez VM, Moreno F, Van Praagh S. Transposition of the great arteries with posterior aorta, anterior pulmonary artery, subpulmonary conus, and fibrous continuity between aortic and atrioventricular valves. *Am J Cardiol* 1971;28:621.)

REFERENCES

1. Van Praagh R. What determines whether the great arteries are normally or abnormally related? *Am J Cardiol.* 2016;118:1390.
2. Van Praagh R. *Transposition of the Great Arteries: History, Pathologic Anatomy, Embryology, Etiology, and Surgical Considerations. Cardiac Surgery: State of the Art Reviews.* Vol. 5. Philadelphia: Hanley & Belfus, Inc; 1991:7.
3. Keith A. The Hunterian lectures on malformations of the heart. *Lancet.* 1909:433.
4. Van Praagh R, Vlad P, Keith JD. Complete transposition of the great arteries. In: Keith JD, Rowe RD, Vlad P, eds. *Heart Disease in Infancy and Childhood.* 2nd ed. New York: Macmillan; 1967:682.
5. Spitzer A. Uber den Bauplan des normalen und missbildeten Herzens. Versuch einer phylogenetischen Theorie. *Virchows Arch F Path Anat.* 1923;243:81.
6. Spitzer A. *The Architecture of Normal and Malformed Hearts: A Phylogenetic Theory of Their Development, with a Summary and Analysis of the Theory by M Lev and A Vass.* Springfield, IL: Charles C Thomas; 1951.
7. Reference 1, Idem, Figure 20.
8. Lev M. Saphir 0: transposition of the large vessels. *J Technical Methods Bull Int Assoc Medical Museums.* 1937;17:126.
9. Harris JS, Farber S. Transposition of the great cardiac vessels with special reference to the phylogenetic theory of Spitzer. *Arch Pathol.* 1939;28:427.
10. Van Praagh R, Ongley PA, Swan HJC. Anatomic types of single or common ventricle in man, morphologic and geometric aspects of 60 necropsied cases. *Am J Cardiol.* 1964;13:510.
11. Van Praagh R, Plett JA, Van Praagh S. Single ventricle: pathology, embryology, terminology, and classification. *Herz.* 1979;4:113.
12. Reference 1, Idem, Figure 17.
13. Reference 1, Idem, Figure 18.
14. Reference 1, Idem, Figure 19.
15. Van Praagh R. The segmental approach to diagnosis in congenital heart disease. In: Bergsma D, ed. *Birth Defects: Original Article Series.* Vol 8. 1972:4.
16. Van Praagh R. Chapter 106: Segmental anatomy. In: Sellke FW, del Nido PJ, Swanson SJ, eds. *Sabiston & Spencer, Surgery of the Chest.* 8th ed. Philadelphia: Saunders Elsevier; 2010:1651.
17. Van Praagh R. The evolution of the right ventricle and its relation to the surgical management of congenital heart disease. *Rev Argentina Cardiol.* 1995;63:417.
18. Castaneda AR, Mayer JE, Jonas RA, Wemovsky G, DiDonato R. Transposition of the great arteries: the arterial switch operation. *Cardiol Clin.* 1989;7:369.
19. Gittenberger-de Groot AC, Sauer U, Quaeguebeur J. Aortic intramural coronary artery in three hearts with transposition of the great arteries. *J Thorac Cardiovasc Surg.* 1986;91:566.
20. Quain R. Cited by Peacock TB: *On malformations, etc. of the human heart, with original cases.* London, Churchill; 1858, p. 116. Birmingham, Alabama, The Classics of Medicine Library, 1981, Gryphon Editions Limited.
21. Keith A, Reference 3, Idem, Figure 41.
22. Grant RP. The morphogenesis of transposition of the great vessels. *Circulation.* 1962;26:819.
23. Van Praagh R, Leidenfrost RD, Matsuoka R, Truman AT, Lee SK, Van Praagh S. Segmental situs in congenital heart disease: relevance to diagnosis, pathology, embryology, and etiology. In: Nora JJ, Takao A, eds. *Congenital Heart Disease: Causes and Processes.* Mt Kisco, New York: Futura Publ Co; 1984:173.
24. Van Praagh R, Van Praagh S. Isolated ventricular inversion, a consideration of the morphogenesis, definition, and diagnosis of nontransposed and transposed great arteries. *Am J Cardiol.* 1966;17:395.
25. Layton WM. Random determination of a developmental process. Reversal of normal visceral asymmetry in the mouse. *J Hered.* 1976;67:336.
26. Layton WM. Heart malformations in mice homozygous for a gene causing situs inversus. In: Bergsma D, ed. *Abnormal Cardiac Morphogenesis. Birth Defects: Original Article Series.* Vol 14. 1978:277.
27. Van Praagh R, Layton WM, Van Praagh S. The morphogenesis of normal and abnormal relations between the great arteries and the ventricles: pathologic and experimental data. In: Van Praagh R, Takao A, eds. *Etiology and Morphogenesis of Congenital Heart Disease.* Mount Kisco, NY: Futura Publishing Co; 1980:271.
28. Van Praagh R, Perez-Treviilo C, Lõpez-Cuellar M, et al. Transposition of the great arteries with posterior aorta, anterior pulmonary artery, subpulmonary conus, and fibrous continuity between aortic and atrioventricular valves. *Am J Cardiol.* 1971;28:621.
29. Sebastian A. *A Dictionary of the History of Medicine.* New York, London: Parthenon Publishing Group; 1999.
30. Paul MH, Muster AJ, Sinha SN, Cole RB, Van Praagh R: Double-outlet left ventricle with an intact ventricular septum. Clinical and autopsy diagnosis and developmental implications. *Circulation* 41: 129.
31. Taussig HB, Bing RJ. Complete transposition of aorta and levoposition of pulmonary artery. *Am Heart J.* 1949;37:551.
32. Van Praagh R. What is the Taussig-Bing malformation? *Circulation.* 1968;38:445.

SUGGESTED READINGS

For investigators who might like to have access to all of the references on which this chapter is based, here they are:

1. Baillie M. *Morbid Anatomy of Some of the Most Important Parts of the Human Body, J Johnson and G. Nicol.* London; 1793:38.
2. Garrison FH. *An Introduction to the History of Medicine, with Medical Chronology, Suggestions for Study and Bibliographic Data.* 4th ed. Philadelphia and London: W.B. Saunders Co.; 1929:355.
3. Van Praagh R. Transposition des gros vaisseaux: definition, historique et correlations anatomoradiologiques. *Coeur.* 1973;4:207.
4. Langstaff MR. Case of a singular malformation of the heart. *Med Review (London).* 1811;4:88.
5. Farre JR. *Pathological Researches.* Essay 1. On Malformations of the Human Heart: illustrated by numerous cases and 5 plates, containing 14 figures; and preceded by some observations on the method of improving the diagnostic part of medicine. London, Longman, Hurst, Rees, Orme, and Brown p 28, 1814.
6. Kirklin JW, Pacifico AD, Bargeron LM, Soto B. Cardiac repair in anatomically corrected malposition of the great arteries. *Circulation.* 1973;48:154.
7. Von Rokitansky CF. *Die Defecte der Scheidewande des Herzens.* Vienna: W. Braumi.iller; 1875:83.
8. Vierordt H. Die angeborenen herzkrankheiten. In: *Nothnagel's Spec Path Therapie.* 1898.
9. Abbott ME. Congenital cardiac diseases. In: Osler W, McCrae T, eds. *Modern Medicine.* Philadelphia: Lea & Febiger; 1915:323. Ch. X.
10. Spitzer A. Uber den Bauplan des normalen und missbildeten Herzens. Versuch einer phylogenetischen Theorie. *Virchows Arch Path Anat.* 1923;243:81.

11. Spitzer A. *The Architecture of Normal and Malformed Hearts: a phylogenetic theory of their development, with a summary and analysis of the theory by M. Lev and A. Vass*. Springfield, IL: Charles C Thomas; 1951.
12. Abbott ME. Transposition or reversed torsion of the arterial trunks. In: Osler W, McCrae T, eds. *Modern Medicine: Its Theory and Practice*. Vol 4. Philadelphia: Lea & Febiger; 1927:716.
13. Lev M. Saphir 0: transposition of the large vessels. *J Technical Methods Bull Int Assoc MedMuseums*. 1937;17:126.
14. Harris JS, Farber S. Transposition of the great cardiac vessels with special reference to the phylogenetic theory of Spitzer. *Arch Pathol*. 1939;28:427.
15. Cardell BS. Corrected transposition of the great vessels. *Br Heart J*. 1956;18:186.
16. Taussig HB, Bing RJ. Complete transposition of the aorta and a levoposition of the pulmonary artery. Clinical, physiological, and pathological findings. *Am Heart J*. 1949;37:551.
17. Lev M, Volk BW. The pathologic anatomy of the Taussig-Bing heart: riding pulmonary artery: report of a case. *Bull Int Assoc Med Museums*. 1950;31:54.
18. Braun K, de Vries A, Feingold DS, et al. Complete dextroposition of the aorta, pulmonary stenosis, interventricular septal defect, and patent foramen ovale. *Am Heart J*. 1952;43:773.
19. Witham WC. Double outlet right ventricle, a partial transposition complex. *Am Heart J*. 1957;53:928.
20. Neufeld HN, DuShane JW, Wood EH, et al. Origin of both great vessels from the right ventricle. I. Without pulmonary stenosis. *Circulation*. 1961;23:399.
21. Neufeld HN, DuShane JW, Edwards JE. Origin of both great vessels from the right ventricle. II. With pulmonary stenosis. *Circulation*. 1961;23:603.
22. Neufeld HN, Lucas RV, Lester RG, et al. Origin of both great vessels from the right ventricle without pulmonary stenosis. *Br Heart J*. 1962;24:393.
23. Van Praagh R, Ongley PA, Swan HJC. Anatomic types of single or common ventricle in man, morphologic and geometric aspects of sixty autopsied cases. *Am J Cardiol*. 1964;13:367.
24. Van Praagh R, Van Praagh S, Vlad P, Keith JD. Anatomic types of congenital dextrocardia, diagnostic and embryologic implications. *Am J Cardiol*. 1964;13:1510.
25. Van Praagh R, Van Praagh S, Vlad P, Keith JD. Diagnosis of the anatomic types of single or common ventricle. *Am J Cardiol*. 1965;15:345.
26. Van Praagh R, Van Praagh S, Vlad P, Keith JD. Diagnosis of the anatomic types of congenital dextrocardia. *Am J Cardiol*. 1965;15:234.
27. Tandler J. The development of the heart. In: Keibel F, Mall FP, eds. *Manual of Human Embryology*. Vol 2. Philadelphia: J B Lip pincott Co; 1912:534.
28. Mall FP. On the development of the human heart. *Am J Anat*. 1912;13:249.
29. Robertson JI. The development of the heart and vascular system in Lepidosiren paradoxa. *Q J Micros Sci*. 1913;59:53.
30. Von Schulte HW. The fusion of the cardiac anlages and the formation of the cardiac loop in the cat (felis domestica). *Am J Anat*. 1916;20:45.
31. Wang C-C. The earliest stages of development of the blood vessels and of the heart in ferret embryos. *J Anat*. 1917;52:137.
32. Waterston D. The development of the heart in man. *Trans Roy Soc Edinburgh*, 52 (pt II) 257, 1918–1919.
33. Murray HA. The development of the cardiac loop in the rabbit, with special reference to the bulboventricular groove and origin of the interventricular septum. *Am J Anat*. 1919;26:29.
34. O'Donoghue CH: The blood vascular system of the tuatara, Sphenodon punctatus. *Phil Trans Roy Soc London* 210 (B):175, 1920-1921.
35. Yoshinaga T. A contribution to the early development of the heart in mammalia, with special reference to the Guinea pig. *Anat Rec*. 1921;21:239.
36. Patten BM. The formation of the cardiac loop in the chick. *Am J Anat*. 1922;30:373.
37. Watson KM. The origin of the heart and blood vessels in Felis Domestica. *J Anat*. 1924;58:105.
38. Copenhaver WM. Experiments on the development of the heart of amblystoma punctatum. *J Exp Zool*. 1926;43:321.
39. Davis CL. Development of the human heart from its first appearance to the stage found in embryos of 20 paired somites. Carnegie Inst Washington Publ 380. *Contrib Embryol*. 1927;19:245.
40. Girgis A. A further contribution on the development of the heart in the rabbit. *Proc Zool Soc*. 1933:421. London.
41. Goss CM. Double heart produced experimentally in rat embryos. *J Exp Zool*. 1935;72:33.
42. Streeter GL. Developmental horizons in human embryos. Description of age groups XV, XVI, XVII and VXIII. *Contrib Embrol*. 1948;32:133.
43. Keith A. *Human Embryology and Morphology*. Baltimore: Williams & Wilkins; 1948:427.
44. Butler JK. An experimental analysis of cardiac loop formation in the chick. Thesis for MA, University ofTexas, August 31, 1952. Presented to the faculty of the Graduate School of the University of Texas in partial fulfillment of the requirements of the degree of Master of Arts, University of Texas.
45. Wilens S. The migration of heart mesoderm and associated areas in Amblystoma punctatum. *J Exp Zool*. 1955;129:579.
46. DelaCruz M, DaRocha JP. An ontogenetic theory for the explanation of congenital malformations involving the truncus and conus. *Am Heart J*. 1956;51:782.
47. DeHaan RL. Cardia bifida and the development of pacemaker function in the early chick heart. *Dev Biol*. 1959;1:586.
48. Lewis FT, Abbott ME. Reversed torsion of the ventricular bend of the embryonic heart in the explanation of certain forms of cardiac anomaly. *Int Assoc Med Museums Bull*. 1916;6:111.
49. DelaCruz MV, Anselmi G, Cisneros F, et al. An embryologic explanation for the corrected transposition of the great vessels: additional description of the main anatomic features of this malformation and its varieties. *Am Heart J*. 1959;57:104.
50. Layton WM. Random determination of a developmental process. Reversal of normal visceral asymmetry in the mouse. *J Hered*. 1976;67:336.
51. Layton WM. Heart malformations in mice homozygous for a gene causing situs inversus. In: Bergsma D, ed. *Abnormal Cardiac Morphogenesis. Birth Defects: Original Article Series*. Vol 14. 1978:277.
52. Van Praagh R, Layton WM, Van Praagh S. The morphogenesis of normal and abnormal relations between the great arteries and the ventricles: pathologic and experimental data. In: Van Praagh R, Takao A, eds. *Etiology and Morphogenesis of Congenital Heart Disease*. Mount Kisco, NY: Futura Publishing Co.; 1980:271.
53. Layton WM, Manasek FJ. Cardiac looping in early iv/iv mouse embryos. In: Van Praagh R, Takao A, eds. *Etiology and Morphogenesis of Congenital Heart Disease*. Mount Kisco, NY: Futura Publishing Co.; 1980:109.
54. Okamoto N, Satow Y, Hidaka N, Akimoto N. Anomalous development of the conotruncus in neutron-irradiated rats. In: Van Praagh R, Takao A, eds. *Etiology and Morphogenesis of Congenital Heart Disease*. Mount Kisco, NY: Futura Publishing Co.; 1980:195.

55. Van Praagh R, Van Praagh S. Anatomically corrected transposition of the great arteries. *Br Heart J.* 1967;29:112.
56. Sakakibara S, Takao A, Arai T, et al. Both great vessels arising from the left ventricle (double outlet left ventricle) origin of both great vessels from the left ventricle. *Bull Heart Inst Japan.* 1967:66.
57. Paul MH, Muster AJ, Sinha SN, Cole RB, Van Praagh R. Double-outlet left ventricle: report of an autopsy case with an intact ventricular septum and consideration of its developmental implications. *Circulation.* 1970;41:129.
58. Melhuish BPP, Van Praagh R. Juxtaposition of the atrial appendages, a sign of severe cyanotic congenital heart disease. *Br Heart J.* 1968;30:269.
59. Van Praagh R. The segmental approach to diagnosis of congenital heart disease. In: Bergsma D, ed. *Birth Defects: Original Article Series.* Vol 8. 1972:4.
60. Van Praagh R, Perez-Trevifio C, Reynolds JL, et al. Double-outlet right ventricle {S,D,L} with subaortic ventricular septal defect and pulmonary stenosis: report of six cases. *Am J Cardiol.* 1975;35:42.
61. Foran RB, Belcourt C, Nanton MA, et al. Isolated infundibuloarterial inversion {S,D,I}: a newly recognized form of congenital heart disease. *Am Heart J.* 1988;116:1337.
62. Van Praagh R, Perez-Trevifio C, Lopez-Cuellar M, et al. Transposition of the great arteries with posterior aorta, anterior pulmonary artery, subpulmonary conus, and fibrous continuity between aortic and atrioventricular valves. *Am J Cardiol.* 1971;28:621.
63. Shineboume EA, Macartney FJ, Anderson RH. Sequential chamber localization—logical approach to diagnosis in congenital heart disease. *Br Heart J.* 1976;38:327.
64. Tynan MJ, Becker AE, Macartney FJ, et al. Nomenclature and classification of congenital heart disease. *Br Heart J.* 1979;41:544.
65. Stanger P, Rudolph AM, Edwards JE. Cardiac malpositions. An overview based on study of sixty-five necropsy specimens. *Circulation.* 1977;56:159.
66. Calcaterra G, Anderson RH, Lau KC, Shineboume EA. Dextrocardia—value of segmental analysis in its categorization. *Br Heart J.* 1979;42:497.
67. Ando M, Satomi G, Takao A. Atresia of tricuspid or mitral orifice: anatomic spectrum and morphogenetic hypothesis. In: Van Praagh R, Takao A, eds. *Etiology and Morphogenesis of Congenital Heart Disease.* Mount Kisco, NY: Futura Publishing Co.; 1980:421.
68. Rao PS. Systematic approach to differential diagnosis. *Am Heart J.* 1981;102:389.
69. Otero Coto E, Quero Jimenez M. Approximacion segmentaria al diagnostico y clasificacion de las cardiopatias congenitas. Fundamentos y utilidad. *Rev Esp Cardiol.* 1977;30:557.
70. Weinberg PM. Systematic approach to diagnosis and coding of pediatric cardiac disease. *Pediatr Cardiol.* 1986;7:35.
71. Weinberg PM, Van Praagh R, Wagner HR, Cuaso CC. *New Form of Criss-Cross Atrioventricular Relation: An Expanded View of the Meaning of D- and L-Loops.* London: World Congress of Paediatric Cardiology; 1980. Abstract No. 319.
72. Van Praagh R, David I, Gordon D, Wright GB, Van Praagh S. Ventricular diagnosis and designation. In: Godman MJ, ed. *Paediatric Cardiology.* Vol 4. London: Churchill Livingstone; 1981:153.
73. Van Praagh R, Weinberg PM, Foran RB, Smith SD, Van Praagh S. Malpositions of the heart. In: Adams FH, Emmanouilides GC, Riemenschneider TA, eds. *Moss' Heart Disease in Infants, Children, and Adolescents.* 4th ed. Baltimore: Williams & Wilkins; 1989:530.
74. Van Praagh S, LaCorte M, Fellows KE, et al. Superoinferior ventricles, anatomic and angiocardiographic findings in 10 postmortem cases. In: Van Praagh R, Takao A, eds. *Etiology and Morphogenesis of Congenital Heart Disease.* Mount Kisco, NY: Futura Publishing Co.; 1980:317.
75. Wagner HR, Alday LE, Vlad P. Juxtaposition of the atrial appendages: a report of six necropsied cases. *Circulation.* 1970;42:157.
76. Anderson RH, Smith A, Wilkinson JL. Disharmony between atrioventricular connections and segmental combinations, unusual variants of "crisscross" hearts. *J Am Coll Cardiol.* 1987;10:1273.
77. Van Praagh R. When concordant or discordant atrioventricular alignments predict the ventricular situs wrongly. I. Solitus atria, concordant alignments, and L-loop ventricles. II. Solitus atria, discordant alignments, and D-loop ventricles. *J Am Coll Cardiol.* 1987;10:1278.
78. Soto S, Ceballos R, Kirklin JW. Ventricular septal defects: a surgical viewpoint. *J Am Coll Cardiol.* 1989;14:1291.
79. Van Praagh S, Kreutzer J, Alday L, Van Praagh R. Systemic and pulmonary venous connections in visceral heterotaxy, with emphasis on the diagnosis of the atrial situs: a study of 109 postmortem cases. In: Clark EB, Takao A, eds. *Developmental Cardiology: Morphogenesis and Function.* Mt Kisco: Futura Publishing Co.; 1990:671.
80. Van Praagh R, Weinberg PM, Calder AL, Buckley LFP, Van Praagh S. The transposition complexes: how many are there? In: Davila JC, ed. *Second Henry Ford Hospital International Symposium on Cardiac Surgery.* New York: Appleton-Century-Crofts; 1977:207.
81. Morris W, ed. *The American Heritage Dictionary of the English Language.* Boston: Houghton Mifflin Co.; 1976:272.
82. Simpson DP. *Cassell's Latin Dictionary, Latin-English, English-Latin.* New York: Macmillan Publishing Co.; 1968:123.
83. Lev M. *Autopsy Diagnosis of Congenitally Malformed Hearts.* Springfield, IL: Charles C Thomas; 1953:71.
84. Lev M. Pathologic diagnosis and positional variations in cardiac chambers in congenital heart disease. *Lab Invest.* 1954;3:71.
85. Van Praagh R, Geva T, Kreutzer J. Ventricular septal defects: how shall we describe, name, and classify them? *J Am Coll Cardiol.* 1989;14:1298.
86. Van Praagh R, Bernhard WF, Rosenthal A, Parisi LF, Fyler DC. Interrupted aortic arch: surgical treatment. *Am J Cardiol.* 1971;27:200.
87. Castaneda AR, Mayer JE, Jonas RA, et al. Transposition of the great arteries: the arterial switch operation. *Cardiol Clin.* 1989;7:369.
88. Gittenberger-de Groot AC, Sauer U, Quaegebeur J. Aortic intramural coronary artery in three hearts with transposition of the great arteries. *J Thorac Cardiovasc Surg.* 1986;91:566.
89. Quain R: Cited in Peacock TB: On malformations, etc. of the human heart, with original cases. London, Churchill, 1858, p. 116. Birmingham, Alabama, The Classics of Medicine Library 1981, Gryphon Editions Limited.
90. Keith A. The Hunterian lectures on malformations of the heart. *Lancet.* 1909;14:433. August.
91. Grant RP. The morphogenesis of transposition of the great vessels. *Circulation.* 1962;26:819.
92. Van Praagh R, Van Praagh S. Isolated ventricular inversion, a consideration of the morphogenesis, definition, and diagnosis of non-transposed and transposed great arteries. *Am J Cardiol.* 1966;17:395.
93. Van Praagh R, Vlad P, Keith JD. Complete transposition of the great arteries. In: Keith JD, Rowe RD, Vlad P, eds. *Heart Disease in Infancy and Childhood.* 2nd ed. New York: Macmillan; 1967:682.

94. Brueckner M, D'Eustachio P, Horwich AL. Linkage mapping of a mouse gene, iv, that controls left-right asymmetry of the heart and viscera. *Proc Natl Acad Sci USA*. 1989;86:5035.
95. Paul MH. Transposition of the great arteries. In: Moss AJ, Adams FH, eds. *Heart Disease in Infants, Children, and Adolescents*. Baltimore: Williams & Wilkins; 1968:527.
96. Paul MH. D-transposition of the great arteries. In: Moss AJ, Adams FH, Emmanouilides GC, eds. *Heart Disease in Infants, Children, and Adolescents*. 2nd ed. Baltimore: Williams & Wilkins; 1977:301.
97. Paul MH. Transposition of the great arteries. In: Adams FH, Emmanouilides GC, eds. *Moss' Heart Disease in Infants, Children, and Adolescents*. 3rd ed. Baltimore: Williams & Wilkins; 1983:296.
98. Paul MH. Complete transpositions of the great arteries. In: Adams FH, Emmanouilides GC, Riemenschneider TA, eds. *Moss' Heart Disease in Infants, Children, and Adolescents*. 4th ed. Baltimore: Williams & Wilkins; 1989:371.
99. Segall HN. *Pioneers of Cardiology in Canada, 1820-1970: The Genesis of Canadian Cardiology*. Willowdale, Ontario, Canada: Hounslow Press; 1988:248.

23

Double-Outlet Right Ventricle

Double-outlet right ventricle (DORV) is what Vierordt[1] called *partial* transposition of the great arteries (TGA) in 1898, meaning that only the aorta was transposed from the left ventricle (LV) to the right ventricle (RV). Vierordt[1] also renamed von Rokitansky's[2] *anomalous* transposition *complete* transposition, as opposed to his *partial* transposition. In 1923, Spitzer[3] renamed Vierordt's *partial* transposition *simple* transposition.

Around 1960, Dr. Jesse Edwards et al[4] decided that more anatomically specific diagnostic terminology would be advantageous. So they introduced *origin of both great arteries from the RV.*

Eight years earlier, in 1952, Braun, de Vries, Feingold, Ehrenfeld, Feldman, and Schorr[5] from Jerusalem, Israel wrote concerning a 19-year-old man with Down syndrome, "Thus the right ventricle serves as a 'double outlet ventricle'. According to the classification of Lev and Volk, this malformation is a type of partial transposition of the Fallot type." (Right. Lev and Volk were using Vierordt's term and concept of partial transposition.) To the best of my knowledge, Braun et al[5] in 1952 used *double outlet* referring to the RV for the first time.

In 1957, A. Calhoun Witham[6] entitled his paper "Double Outlet Right Ventricle, A Partial Transposition Complex." This is how DORV was introduced.

In the spring of 1984, Dr. Aldo Ricardo Castañeda asked me to make a presentation on DORV to the Society of Pediatric Cardiovascular Surgery that was going to meet at the Boston Children's Hospital on May 5 and 6. My colleagues thought this was an excellent suggestion because almost nobody really understands DORV, not even the so-called experts! My colleagues were serious. They were saying, If you doubt that, just ask your favorite expert how many anatomic types of DORV exist? At this point, the expert is very likely to start mumbling, "Almost infinite . . . an impossible question . . . no one knows."

My dear wife, Dr. Stella Van Praagh (who died in 2006), having studied DORV for years,[7] used to say, "DORV is all of congenital heart disease. Each case must be diagnosed individually and completely, so that one can make the wisest decisions concerning management." As the reader will see, what Dr. Stella said is literally true. Almost any form of congenital heart disease that one can imagine occurs with DORV. That is why DORV is so difficult to classify satisfactorily.

DEFINITION AND DIFFERENTIAL DIAGNOSIS

DORV is present when both great arteries are aligned entirely or predominantly with the morphologically RV.[4,7-14] Both great arteries do not arise *from* the right ventricular sinus. Instead, both great arteries arise from the infundibulum (or conus arteriosus), which may be a well-developed muscular structure or resorbed and merely an intervalvar fibrosa. In the normal heart, the subpulmonary infundibulum is a well-developed muscular structure, whereas the subaortic infundibular free wall has been resorbed by apoptosis (programmed cell death) and consequently is reduced to the aortic-mitral intervalvar fibrosa. *Infundibulum* means funnel (Latin). *Conus* means cone (Latin). *Infundibulum* is the *inside* look at the ventriculoarterial (VA) connecting segment, most often used in anatomic descriptions. *Conus,* or *conus arteriosus,* is the outside appearance of the VA connecting segment, often used in embryologic descriptions. I use *infundibulum* and *conus* interchangeably, but prefer *infundibulum* for anatomic description.

In DORV, the great arteries do not always arise *above* the RV. For example, in superoinferior ventricles with RV superior to the LV, DORV is the most common type of VA alignment, in our experience.[15] The RV and the semilunar valves are almost in the same horizontal plane. The great arteries are often *beside* the RV, not above the RV. However, the great arteries are *aligned* predominantly or exclusively with the RV.

As far as **differential diagnosis** is concerned, we make the diagnosis of *tetralogy of Fallot (TOF),* for example, if there is aortic valve–mitral valve direct fibrous continuity. Even if there is a lot of aortic overriding, we do not call such cases DORV. Similarly, if there is pulmonary valve–mitral valve direct fibrous continuity, we call such cases *transposition of the great arteries (TGA),* not DORV, even if there is a lot of overriding of the pulmonary valve and artery.

Why? Because the degree of semilunar valvar overriding is a criterion that does not always work. In solitus normally related great arteries, for example, the aortic valve does not sit predominantly above the LV cavity. Instead, the normal aortic valve is mostly above the ventricular septum, to the right of the LV cavity. Similarly, the normally located pulmonary valve is not located predominantly above the RV cavity. Instead, the normal pulmonary valve is located predominantly to the left of the RV cavity, mostly above the infundibular septum. Consequently, we do not use the 50% rule, which does not apply well to normally related great arteries. This does not mean that we have given up on measuring the degree of overriding of the great arteries.

Instead, this means that we are interested in what aortic-mitral and pulmonary-mitral fibrous continuity really mean. **Aortic-mitral fibrous continuity** means that the normal embryonic aortic switch procedure has been performed more or less successfully. In turn, this also means that one should not make the diagnosis of DORV because DORV means that the embryonic aortic switch has *not* been done, hence DORV.

Pulmonary valve–mitral valve fibrous continuity means that the abnormal embryonic transposed pulmonary arterial switch has been performed. Hence, the diagnosis of DORV is not accurate. Thus, it is important to understand the biological meaning of these embryonic arterial switch procedures. If an embryonic arterial switch has been performed, DORV is no longer present.

Diagnoses should be specific and mutually exclusive. For example, the diagnosis should be TOF, **or** DORV, not TOF **and** DORV. Similarly, the diagnosis should be DORV **or** TGA, not DORV **with** (and) TGA. This is a basic principle of classification.

FINDINGS

DORV With Subpulmonary VSD (n = 11)		
1.	DORV {S,D,D} with bilateral infundibulum, subpulmonary infundibuloventricular VSD, and no outflow obstruction	3
2.	DORV {S,D,D} with bilateral infundibulum, subpulmonary infundibuloventricular plus the AV canal–type VSD, and no outflow obstruction	1
3.	DORV {S,D,D} with bilateral infundibulum, subpulmonary infundibuloventricular VSD, and AS	3
4.	DORV {S,D,D} with bilateral infundibulum, subpulmonary infundibuloventricular plus AV canal type of VSD, and AS	1
5.	DORV {S,D,D} with bilateral infundibulum, subpulmonary infundibuloventricular VSD, uncommitted muscular VSD, and AS	2
6.	DORV {S,D,D} with subaortic infundibulum, subpulmonary infundibuloventricular VSD, and AS	1

AS, Aortic stenosis; *AV*, atrioventricular; *VSD*, ventricular septal defect.

DORV With Uncommitted VSD (n = 11)		
1.	DORV {S,D,D} with bilateral infundibulum, uncommitted infundibuloventricular VSD, and PS	6
2.	DORV {S,D,D} with bilateral infundibulum, uncommitted infundibuloventricular VSD, AS, and PS	1
3.	DORV {S,D,L} with bilateral infundibulum, uncommitted infundibuloventricular VSD, and PS	1
4.	DORV {S,D,D} with subaortic infundibulum, uncommitted muscular VSD, and PS	1
5.	DORV {S,L,L} with bilateral infundibulum, uncommitted infundibuloventricular VSD, and PS	1
6.	DORV {S,L,D} with bilateral infundibulum, uncommitted infundibuloventricular VSD, and no outflow obstruction	1

AS, Aortic stenosis (valvar); *AV*, atrioventricular; *bilateral infundibulum*, subaortic and subpulmonary infundibulum; *DORV*, double-outlet right ventricle; *infundibuloventricular*, between the infundibular and the ventricular septa; *PS*, pulmonary stenosis (valvar); *{S,D,D}*, the set of situs solitus of the viscera and atria, concordant D-loop (solitus) ventricles, and D-malposition of the great arteries, that is, aortic valve to the right (*dextro-*, or D- relative to the pulmonary valve), D-malposition of the great arteries being solitus or noninverted malposition of the great arteries; *{S,D,L}*, the set of solitus (noninverted) visceroatrial situs, concordant D-loop (solitus) ventricles, and L-malposition of the great arteries, that is, aortic valve to the left (*levo-* or L-, Latin) relative to the pulmonary valve, L-malposition being inverted (mirror-image) malposition of the great arteries; *{S,L,L}*, the set of situs solitus of the viscera and atria, discordant L-loop (inverted) ventricles, and L-malposition of the great arteries, that is, aortic valve to the left (*levo-*, or L-, Latin) relative to the pulmonary valve; *{S,L,D}*, the set or segmental situs combination of solitus viscera and atria, discordant L-loop (inverted) ventricles, and D-malposition of the semilunar valves, that is, with the malposed aortic valve to the right (*dextro-* or D-, Latin) relative to the malposed pulmonary valve; *uncommitted*, meaning that the ventricular septal defect (VSD) is neither subaortic nor subpulmonary.

DORV with malformations mainly involving the infundibular and the great arterial segments (**Group 1**) are summarized in Table 23.1. There are 17 different anatomic types of DORV in Table 23.1, involving about one-third of this series: 32 of 101 patients (32%). These are the least complex cases of DORV. As will soon be seen, there are two more complex groups of DORV:

Group II patients with DORV have malformations not only of the infundibulum and great arteries, but also of the atrioventricular (AV) valves and the ventricles (n = 42 cases).

TABLE 23.1 How Many Anatomic Types of DORV Are There and What Are They? (n = 101 Patients)[7]

Group I: DORV with anomalies of the infundibulum and great arteries only (n = 32/101 patients [32%])		
DORV With Subaortic VSD (n = 10)		
1.	DORV {S,D,D} with bilateral infundibulum, subaortic infundibuloventricular VSD, and no outflow tract stenosis	1
2.	DORV {S,D,D} with bilateral infundibum, subaortic infundibuloventricular VSD, and PS	5
3.	DORV {S,D,D} with bilateral infundibulum, subaortic infundibuloventricular VSD, and AS	2
4.	DORV {S,D,L} with bilateral infundibulum, subaortic infundibuloventricular VSD and mild PS	1
5.	DORV {S,D,L} with bilateral infundibulum, subaortic infundibuloventricular VSD, uncommitted muscular VSD, and AS	1

AS, Aortic stenosis; *PS*, pulmonary stenosis; *VSD*, ventricular septal defect.

Data from Van Praagh S, Davidoff A, Chin A, Shiel FS, Reynolds J, Van Praagh R. Double-outlet right ventricle: anatomic types and developmental implications based on a study of 101 autopsied cases. *Coeur.* 1982;13:389.

Group III patients with DORV have anomalies of all five cardiac segments: viscera and atria, AV valves, ventricles, infundibulum, and great arteries (n = 27: asplenia 17 and polysplenia 10).

DORV With Subpulmonary VSD (5 of 42 Cases)

1.	DORV {S,D,D} with subaortic infundibulum, subpulmonary infundibuloventricular VSD, no outflow obstruction, and straddling MV	1
2.	DORV {S,D,D} with subaortic infundibulum, subpulmonary infundibuloventricular VSD, PS, and straddling MV	2
3.	DORV {S,D,D} with subaortic infundibulum, subpulmonary infundibuloventricular VSD, uncommitted muscular VSD, and straddling MV	1
4.	DORV {S,L,D} with subaortic infundibulum, subpulmonary infundibuloventricular VSD, PS, Ebstein anomaly of TV, and straddling MV	1

MV, Mitral valve; *PS,* pulmonary stenosis; *TV,* tricuspid valve; *VSD,* ventricular septal defect.

DORV With Uncommitted VSD (20 of 42 Cases)

1.	DORV {S,D,D} with bilateral infundibulum, uncommitted muscular VSD, no outflow obstruction, MAt	1
2.	DORV {S,D,D} with subaortic infundibulum, uncommitted VSD of the AV canal type, no outflow obstruction, MAt	1
3.	DORV {S,D,D} with subaortic infundibulum, uncommitted muscular VSD, MAt, AS	1
4.	DORV {S,D,D} with subpulmonary infundibulum, uncommitted muscular VSD, no outflow obstruction, MAt	1
5.	DORV {I,D,D} with bilateral infundibulum, uncommitted VSD of the AV canal type, PS, and MAt	1
6.	DORV {S,D,D} with bilateral infundibulum, uncommitted infundibuloventricular VSD, no outflow obstruction, straddling MV	1
7.	DORV {S,D,L} with subaortic infundibulum, uncommitted infundibuloventricular VSD, PS, severe TS, and straddling MV	1
8.	DORV {S,D,D) with subpulmonary infundibulum, uncommitted VSD of the AV canal type, AS, straddling TV	1
9.	DORV {S,D,D} with bilateral infundibulum, uncommitted VSD of the AV canal type, PS, straddling TV, and MS	1
10.	DORV {S,L,L} with subaortic infundibulum, uncommitted VSD of AV canal type, PS, double-inlet RV	1
11.	DORV {S,D,D} with bilateral infundibulum, uncommitted VSD of the AV canal type, no outflow obstruction, MAt, and straddling TV	1
12.	DORV {S,D,D} with bilateral infundibulum, uncommitted VSD of the AV canal type, common AV valve, no outflow obstruction	1
13.	DORV {S,D,D} with subpulmonary infundibulum, uncommitted VSD of the AV canal type, common AV canal with MS, no outflow obstruction	1
14.	DORV {S,D,D} with subpulmonary infundibulum, uncommitted VSD of the AV canal type, common AV canal, and PS	1
15.	DORV {S,D,D} with subpulmonary infundibulum, uncommitted AV canal VSD, common AV canal with MS, and AS	1
16.	DORV {S,L,L}, bilateral infundibulum, uncommitted AV canal VSD, common AV canal, PS	1
17.	DORV {S,L,L} with subaortic infundibular, uncommitted AV canal VSD, common AV canal, AS	1
18.	DORV {S,L,D} with subaortic infundibulum, uncommitted AV canal VSD, common AV canal, no outflow obstruction	1
19.	DORV {I,D,D} with bilateral infundibulum, uncommitted AV canal VSD, common AV canal, and PS	1
20.	DORV {I,D,L} with bilateral infundibulum, uncommitted AV canal VSD, common AV canal, PS	1

AS, Aortic stenosis; *AV,* atrioventricular; *MAt,* mitral atresia; *MS,* mitral stenosis; *MV,* mitral valve; *PS,* pulmonary stenosis; *RV,* right ventricle; *TV,* tricuspid valve; *VSD,* ventricular septal defect.

DORV With Intact Ventricular Septum (8 of 42 Cases)

1.	DORV {S,D,D} with bilateral infundibulum, no VSD, PS, MAt	3
2.	DORV {S,D,D} with subpulmonary infundibulum, no VSD, no outflow obstruction, MS	1
3.	DORV {S,D,D} with subpulmonary infundibulum, no VSD, AS, MAt	1
4.	DORV with subpulmonary infundibulum, no VSD, AS, absence of MV leaflets with small MV orifice, that is, MS	1
5.	DORV {S,L,L} with bilateral infundibulum, no VSD, PS, MAt (R)	1
6.	DORV {S,L,L} with bilateral infundibulum no VSD, PS, MS (R)	1

AS, Aortic stenosis; *{I, D, D},* the segmental situs set of inversus atria, discordant D-loop (solitus) ventricles, and D-malposition (noninverted or solitus malposition) of the great arteries; *{I, D, L},* the segmental situs set of inversus atria, discordant D-loop or solitus ventricles, and L-malposition of the great arteries; *LV,* morphologically left ventricle; *MAt,* mitral atresia; *MAt (R),* mitral atresia, right-sided; *MS,* mitral stenosis; *MS (R),* mitral stenosis, right-sided; *MV,* mitral valve; *RV,* morphologically right ventricle; *TAt,* tricuspid atresia; *TS,* tricuspid stenosis; *TV,* tricuspid valve.

Group I DORV contains malformations of one connecting segment and one main cardiac segment: infundibulum and great arteries, respectively.

Group II DORV contains anomalies of two connecting segments and two main segments: infundibulum and great arteries, and AV valves and ventricles.

Group III DORV contains malformations in all five cardiac segments: viscera and atria, AV valves, ventricles, infundibulum, and great arteries, because group III DORV involves the heterotaxy syndromes of congenital asplenia and polysplenia (Table 23.2).

DORV With Asplenia and No VSD (4 of 17 Cases)

1.	DORV {A,D,D} with asplenia, bilateral infundibulum, no VSD, no outflow obstruction, common AV canal (RV type)	1
2.	DORV {A,D,D} with asplenia, bilateral infundibulum, no VSD, PS, common AV canal (RV type)	2
3.	DORV {A,L,L} with asplenia, bilateral infundibulum, no VSD, PS, common AV canal (RV type)	1

AV, Atrioventricular; *PS,* pulmonary stenosis; *RV,* right ventricle; *VSD,* ventricular septal defect.

DORV With Polysplenia and Subaortic VSD (2 of 10 Cases)

1.	DORV {A(S),D,D} with polysplenia, subpulmonary infundibulum, subaortic infundibuloventricular VSD, PS, and divided AV valves	2

AV, Atrioventricular; *PS,* pulmonary stenosis; *VSD,* ventricular septal defect.

TABLE 23.2 Group III DORV With Asplenia and Uncommitted Ventral Septal Defect (13 of 17 Cases)

1.	DORV {A(I),L,A} with asplenia, bilateral infundibulum, uncommitted infundibuloventricular VSD, PS, AV valves divided	1
2.	DORV {A,D,D} with asplenia, bilateral infundibulum, uncommitted AV canal VSD, common AV canal (RV type), and PS	3
3.	DORV {A,D,D} with asplenia, bilateral infundibulum, uncommitted AV canal VSD, common AV canal (RV type), PAt	1
4.	DORV {A,D,D} with asplenia, bilateral infundibulum, uncommitted AV canal VSD, common AV canal (LV type)	2
5.	DORV {A,D,D} with asplenia, bilateral infundibulum, uncommitted AV canal VSD, common AV canal (balanced type), PS	1
6.	DORV {A,L,L} with asplenia, bilateral infundibulum, uncommitted AV canal VSD, common AV canal (LV type), PS	2
7.	DORV {A,L,L} with asplenia, bilateral infundibulum, uncommitted AV canal VSD, common AV canal (balanced), PS	1
8.	DORV {A,L,L} with asplenia, bilateral infundibulum, uncommitted AV canal VSD, common AV canal (balanced), PAt	1
9.	DORV {A,L,L} with asplenia, bilateral infundibulum, uncommitted AV canal VSD, common AV canal (RV type), PAt	1

AV, Atrioventricular; *LV,* left ventricle; *PAt,* pulmonary atresia; *PS,* pulmonary stenosis; *RV,* right ventricle; *VSD,* ventricular septal defect.

DORV With Polysplenia and Uncommitted VSD (4 of 10 Cases)

1.	DORV {A(S),D,D} with polysplenia, bilateral infundibulum, uncommitted infundibuloventricular VSD, PS, MV hypoplasia (MS)	1
2.	DORV {A(S),D,D} with polysplenia, subpulmonary infundibulum, uncommitted VSD of the AV canal type, common AV canal (RV types), and AS	2
3.	DORV {A(I),L,L} with polysplenia, subpulmonary infundibulum, uncommitted VSD of the AV canal type, common AV canal (balanced type), no outflow obstruction	1

AS, Aortic stenosis; *AV,* atrioventricular; *MS,* mitral stenosis; *MV,* mitral valve; *PS,* pulmonary stenosis; *RV,* right ventricle; *VSD,* ventricular septal defect.

DORV With Polysplenia and No VSD (4 of 10 Cases)

1.	DORV {A(S),D,D} with polysplenia, subpulmonary infundibulum, no VSD, common AV canal (RV type), and AS	1
2.	DORV {A(S),D,D} with polysplenia, subpulmonary infundibulum, no VSD, PS, common AV canal (RV type)	1
3.	DORV {A(S),D,D} with polysplenia, subpulmonary infundibulum, no VSD, AS, absence of MV and LA	1
4.	DORV {A(I),L,L} with polysplenia, subpulmonary infundibulum, no VSD, PS, common AV valve (RV type)	1

{A,D,D}, The segmental situs set, that we often just call the segmental anatomy, of situs ambiguus of the viscera and atria, D-loop ventricles, and D-malposition of the great arteries; *{A(I),L,A},* the segmental situs set of situs ambiguus of the viscera and atria (probably situs inversus), L-loop ventricles, and antero-malposition or A-malposition of the great arteries in which the aortic valve is directly anterior to the pulmonary valve; *{A(I),L,L},* the segmental situs set of situs ambiguus of the viscera and the atria (probably situs inversus), L-loop ventricles, and L-malposition of the great arteries; *{A,L,L},* the segmental situs set of visceroatrial situs ambiguus L-loop (inverted) ventricles, and L-malposition (inverted malposition) of the great arteries. A common AV valve is regarded as **balanced** if it opens approximately equally into both ventricles, of the **left ventricular type** if the common AV valve opens predominantly into the morphologically left ventricle, and of **the right ventricular type** if the common AV valve opens predominantly into the morphologically right ventricle. *AS,* Aortic stenosis; *{A(S),D,D},* the segmental situs set or combination of situs ambiguus of the viscera and atria (probably situs solitus), D-loop ventricles, and D-malposition of the great arteries; *AV,* atrioventricular; *LA,* left atrium; *MV,* mitral valve; *PS,* pulmonary stenosis; *VSD,* ventral septal defect.

The locations of the VSD relative to the great arteries in this series of DORV as a whole are summarized in Table 23.3.

DISCUSSION

So, how many different anatomic types of DORV are there? In 101 autopsied patients with DORV, we found 73 different subsets or subtypes (Tables 23.1, 23.2, and 23.4). Do we think that 73 anatomic types of DORV is the correct number? No. Why

TABLE 23.3 Summary of the Ventricular Septal Defect Relative to the Great Arteries in This Series of DORV as a Whole

VSD Locations	DORV as a Whole	Subaortic	Subpulmonary	Uncommitted	Absent
Group I DORV,	N = 32	10	11	11	0
Group II DORV,	N = 42	9	5	20	8
Group III, asplenia,	N = 17	0	0	13	4
Group III, polysplenia, N = 10	2	0	4	4	
Totals	N = 101	21	16	48	16

VSD, Ventral septal defect.

TABLE 23.4 Group II DORV With Malformation of the Infundibulum, Great Arteries, Atrioventricular Valves, and Ventricles (n = 42)

DORV With Subaortic VSD (9 of 42 Cases)	
1. DORV {S,D,D} with subpulmonary infundibulum, subaortic infundibuloventricular VSD, no outflow tract obstruction, and MAt	1
2. DORV {S,D,D} with subpulmonary infundibulum, subaortic infundibuloventricular VSD, PS, MAt	2
3. DORV {S,D,L} with bilateral infundibulum, subaortic infundibuloventricular VSD, PS, and straddling MV	1
4. DORV {S,L,D} with subpulmonary infundibulum, subaortic infundibuloventricular VSD, PS, Ebstein anomaly of TV, and straddling MV	1
5. DORV {S,D,D} with bilateral infundibulum, subaortic infundibuloventricular VSD, PS, and tricuspid atresia (TAt)	1
6. DORV {S,D,D} with subpulmonary infundibulum, subaortic infundibuloventriclular plus AV canal VSD, PS, common AV canal	3

AV, Atrioventricular; *MAt*, mitral atresia; *MV*, mitral valve; *PS*, pulmonary stenosis; *TAt*, tricuspid atresia; *TV*, tricuspid valve; *VSD*, ventricular septal defect.

not? We strongly suspect that in a larger series of DORV, additional anatomic types of DORV will be found. But this study[7] is regarded as a good first approximation.

Table 23.3 concerning VSD locations in the series as a whole is fascinating. Because this series was based on 101 autopsied cases, the number of cases and the percentage of the series are essentially the same.

Groups I, II, and III: A Segmental Classification

Group I DORV involves patients with malformations of the infundibulum (the connecting segment) and the great arteries (the main segment). DORV with infundibuloarterial anomalies only used to be regarded as "typical" DORV. But these cases make up only about one-third of this total series (32%) (see Table 23.3). Within group I, the VSD was subaortic in 10 of 32 (31%), subpulmonary in 11 of 32 (34%), and uncommitted in 11 of 32 (34%) (see Table 23.3).

Group II DORV was the largest group (42%). Group II means that there were malformations not only of the infundibulum and the great arteries but also of the AV valves and the ventricles. Of these 42 group II DORV cases, anomalies of the AV valves were mitral atresia, 14 of 42 (33%); common AV canal, 12 of 42 (29%); straddling mitral valve, 10 of 42 (24%); congenital mitral stenosis, 6 of 42 (14%); straddling tricuspid valve, 2 of 42 (5%); tricuspid atresia, 1 of 42 (2%); and double-inlet RV, 1 of 42 (2%). Intact ventricular septum was found in 7 of 42 (17%).

Returning to group I DORV, the type of infundibulum was bilateral (subaortic and subpulmonary) in 30 of 32 cases (94%), and was described as subaortic (only) in 2 of 32 cases (6%).

We expected the infundibulum to be bilateral in this anatomic type of DORV, indicating that neither the subaortic nor the subpulmonary infundibular free wall had undergone involution and therefore that neither great artery had undergone an embryonic arterial switch, resulting in DORV. But we were surprised to find that 2 cases had a subaortic infundibulum only, suggesting that the pulmonary artery had (or should have) undergone an embryonic pulmonary arterial switch, but for unknown reasons had not. Thus, in terms of the infundibular anatomy, 94% had bilateral infundibula, as expected, resulting in DORV. Our reaction was that this is good but not perfect. Mysteries remain.

In group I DORV, what anatomic types of segmental situs sets were present? These were {S,D,D}, 27 of 32 (84%); {S,D,L}, 3 of 32 (9%); {S,L,L}, 1 of 32 (3%); and {S,L,D}, 1 of 32 (3%). Thus, the most common segmental anatomic set was {S,D,D} in 84% of group I DORV, in which all three main segments were in situs solitus (noninverted).

Second in frequency was {S,D,L} in 9% of group I DORV. Our impression in these cases was that the aortic valve lay to the left of the pulmonary valve, that is, {S,D,**L**}, because of some degree of malrotation of the ventricular loop that carried the aortic valve more leftward than usual. We thought that these L-malposed great arteries probably were only *apparently* inverted, *not* truly inverted. (However, we are not certain that this interpretation is correct.) In either case, L-malposition of the great arteries is anatomically accurate.

The least frequent segmental anatomic sets in group I DORV were {S,L,L} and {S,L,D}, in 3% each. In group I DORV {S,L,L}, we think that the ventricular and the great arterial segments are both inverted. But in DORV {S,L,D}, we are not sure that the D-malposed great arteries are really in situs solitus (noninverted). The rightward location of the aortic valve could be due to a malposition of the L-loop ventricles. So these D-malposed great arteries may really be inverted and rightwardly malpositioned great arteries (speculation).

It is not always easy to make the diagnosis of inversion versus noninversion when malposition may also be present. The purely descriptive D-, L-, and A-malposition or transposition system does not force the diagnosing physician to try to make the differential diagnosis between true versus apparent inversion or noninversion.

Returning to Group II DORV (Table 23.4) **(n = 42):** The anatomic types of infundibulum in group II DORV are *very different* from those in group I DORV. In group II DORV, the anatomic types of infundibulum were as follows: subpulmonary, 15 of 42 (36%); bilateral, 16 of 42 (38%); and subaortic, 11 of 42 (26%).

You may now be thinking, "How is this possible? For example, a normal subpulmonary infundibulum in more than one-third (36%) of patients with group II DORV? Doesn't this mean that more than one-third of these cases with DORV have a normal infundibulum and normal great arteries?" Exactly right. But these patients with type II DORV are teaching us the importance of anomalies of the AV valves and ventricles. For example, 15 of these patients had a normal subpulmonary infundibulum and normally formed great arteries. But they also had mitral atresia, 5 of 15; Ebstein anomaly of the tricuspid valve and straddling mitral valve, 1 of 15; common AV canal, 4 of 15; straddling tricuspid valve, 1 of 15; common AV canal with mitral stenosis, 1 of 15; congenital mitral stenosis, 2 of 15; and absence of the mitral valve leaflets with a small mitral orifice, 1 of 15.

When the morphologically LV is small, tiny, or absent, both great arteries may arise above the morphologically RV.

DORV is not an infundibuloarterial malformation only. DORV is an abnormal VA alignment. Hence, the AV valves, the ventricles, and the ventricular septum are important in DORV.

The segmental situs sets in group II DORV were as follows (see Table 23.4):

DORV {S,D,D}	29/42	69%
DORV {S,D,L}	3/42	7%
DORV {S,L,L}	5/42	12%
DORV {S,L,D}	2/42	5%
DORV {I,D,D}	2/42	5%
DORV {I,D,L)	1/42	2%

INFUNDIBULUM IN GROUP III DOUBLE-OUTLET RIGHT VENTRICLE

In the 17 cases of group III DORV with **asplenia,** the anatomic type of infundibulum was bilateral in 17 of 17 (100%). In the 10 cases of group III DORV with **polysplenia,** the anatomic types of infundibulum were subpulmonary, 9 of 10 (90%), and bilateral, 1 of 10 (10%).

{A (S), D, D}	8/27	30%
{A,D,D}	10/27	37%
{A(I),L,L}	2/27	7%
{A,L,L}	6/27	22%
{A(I),L,A}	1/27	4.0%

The location of VSDs in DORV (n = 101) is summarized in Table 23.3. The incidence of **subaortic VSDs** was as follows:

Group I	DORV	31%
Group II	DORV	21%
Group III	Asplenia	0%
Group III	Polysplenia	20%

The low frequency of subaortic VSDs in the heterotaxy syndromes of asplenia (0%) and polysplenia (20%) is noteworthy. The incidence of subpulmonary VSD was as follows:

Group I	DORV	11%
Group II	DORV	5%
Group III	Asplenia	0%
Group III	Polysplenia	0%

The absence of a subpulmonary VSD in the asplenia and polysplenia syndromes is noteworthy. The incidence of **uncommitted VSDs** was as follows:

Group I	DORV	11%
Group II	DORV	20%
Group III	DORV, asplenia	13%
Group III	DORV, polysplenia	4%

Absence of a VSD was as follows:

Group I	DORV	0%
Group II	DORV	8%
Group III	DORV, asplenia	4%
Group III	DORV, polysplenia	4%

CLASSIFICATION OF DOUBLE-OUTLET RIGHT VENTRICLE

A practical, working, abbreviated **classification of DORV based on the VSD location** is suggested as follows (see Table 23.3, n = 101):

DORV with subaortic VSD	21%
DORV with subpulmonary VSD	16%
DORV with uncommitted VSD	48%
DORV with no VSD	16%

A more detailed classification that we have found useful is based on the segmental groups that are involved.

Group I is characterized by malformations of the infundibulum and great arteries.

Group II has involvement of the infundibulum and great arteries and of the AV valves and ventricles.

Group III has malformations involving the infundibulum and great arteries, the AV valves and the ventricles, the viscera and the atria, and the heterotaxy syndromes of asplenia and polysplenia.

The next section has to do with some of the fascinating personal encounters that I have had with DORV.

THE TAUSSIG-BING MALFORMATION

In the mid-1960s, Dr. Patrick Ongley asked me to write an editorial for *Circulation* to clarify the question: What really is the Taussig-Bing malformation?[16] In 1949, Dr. Helen B. Taussig and Dr. Richard J. Bing had published a paper entitled **"Complete Transposition of Aorta and Levoposition of Pulmonary Artery."**[16] In 1950, Lev and Volk[17] published a paper calling this malformation **the Taussig-Bing heart.** They recognized that this was the first published case of partial transposition with a subpulmonary VSD. (It will be recalled that *partial transposition* was Vierordt's term, introduced in 1898, for what we now call DORV: *partial* transposition, because only the aorta was transposed from the LV to the RV.) All previously known cases of partial transposition had a subaortic VSD, not a subpulmonary VSD as in Taussig and Bing's case.[16]

Then, over the next 10 to 15 years, usage became confused. Is the Taussig-Bing malformation a form of DORV or is it really TGA with an overriding main pulmonary artery (MPA)? In other words, how much does the MPA override the ventricular septum?

The suggestion was that, if possible, I should reexamine the original heart specimen of Taussig and Bing and document the findings with photographs and a precise diagram. With the kind permission of Dr. Helen Taussig, and with the assistance of Dr. Catherine Neill and Dr. Ali Mehrizi at Johns Hopkins Hospital in Baltimore, that is what happened (Fig. 23.1).[8]

The original Taussig-Bing heart[8,16] has DORV {S,D,D} with a bilateral infundibulum and a subpulmonary VSD. The pulmonary valve overrides the ventricular septum, but does not override the left ventricular cavity at all (see Fig. 23.1E).

The bilateral infundibulum (subaortic and subpulmonary) was located above the right-sided and anterior morphologically RV. The great arteries were side-by-side, aorta (Ao) to the right and MPA to the left (see Fig. 23.1A and E). The subaortic infundibular (or conal) muscular free wall separated the aortic valve (AoV) above from the tricuspid valve (TV) below by 8 mm (see Fig. 23.1C). The left-sided subpulmonary muscular infundibular free wall was 9 mm in height, separating the pulmonary valve (PV) above from the mitral valve (MV) below (Fig. 23.1B, D, and E). In other words, the subpulmonary infundibular free wall was slightly taller (9 mm) than was the subaortic infundibular free wall (8 mm). But the subarterial infundibular free walls were very similar: both were well developed, well expanded, and nonobstructive. The distal or subarterial infundibular (or conal) septum was 20 mm in length (or height) (see Fig. 23.1B, C, and E).

The cardiac septal and semilunar geometry (see Fig. 23.1E) was as follows:

The atrial septum (AS) lay 30 degrees to the left of the Z axis (or anteroposterior plane) (normal).

The ventricular septum (VS) was 70 degrees to the left of the AP plane (normal).

The infundibular septum or conal septum (CS) measured 0 degrees on its right surface relative to the AP plane (i.e., parallel with the AP plane); and on its left surface, the measurement was 5 degrees to the left of the AP plane. So the subarterial infundibular septum was essentially sagittal, in the AP plane (abnormal).

The semilunar valves, relative to the AP plane, measured 90 degrees to the right, which is why the great arteries are side-by-side (90 degrees dextrorotation of the aortic valve and the pulmonary valve relative to the AP plane is subnormal; normal semilunar dextrorotation is about 150 degrees).

Right atrial free wall was 1 to 2 mm thick.

Left atrial free wall was 2 mm thick.

Right ventricular free wall was 10 to 13 mm thick (hypertrophied).

Left ventricular free wall was 10 to 14 mm thick.

The tricuspid valve was 76 mm in circumference.

The mitral valve was 66 mm in circumference.

The aortic valve was 34 mm in circumference.

The pulmonary valve measured 56 mm in circumference.

The subpulmonary VSD measured 14 mm × 11 mm (horizontally × vertically).

MORPHOGENESIS

The Taussig-Bing malformation[8,16] is an excellent example of what we have been calling **group I DORV,** that is, a malformation of the infundibulum and great arteries only, resulting in DORV, without anomalies of the AV valves and ventricles (group II) and without malformations of the viscera and atria (group III).

In the Taussig-Bing malformation, ventricular D-loop formation has been completed normally (see Fig. 23.1). The problem in the Taussig-Bing malformation is that both the subaortic part of the muscular infundibulum and the subpulmonary part of the muscular infundibulum have developed *symmetrically.* Both the subaortic infundibulum and the subpulmonary infundibulum are almost identical. As noted previously, the subaortic infundibular muscular free wall was 8 mm tall, and the subpulmonary infundibular muscular free wall was 9 mm tall. Good, approximately symmetrical development of both subarterial infundibular free walls prevents both great arteries from undergoing the embryonic arterial switch process.

Normally, the development of the subarterial infundibular free walls is **totally asymmetrical.** The subaortic infundibular free wall normally undergoes complete involution, thought to be due to apoptosis (genetically programmed cell death). This is what fails to happen in the Taussig-Bing malformation. The subaortic infundibular free wall fails to involute (disappear); therefore, the aortic valve cannot move inferiorly and posteriorly, pass through the interventricular foramen, and come into direct fibrous continuity with the developing mitral valve via the intervalvar fibrosa. In other words, the normal embryonic aortic switch process cannot occur in the Taussig-Bing malformation because of the persistence of a well-developed subaortic infundibular free wall that should have been removed by apoptosis. This can be expressed clearly and briefly by **infundibuloarterial situs equations.** The normal equation is SNRGA {S,D,S} = 0R + 4L.

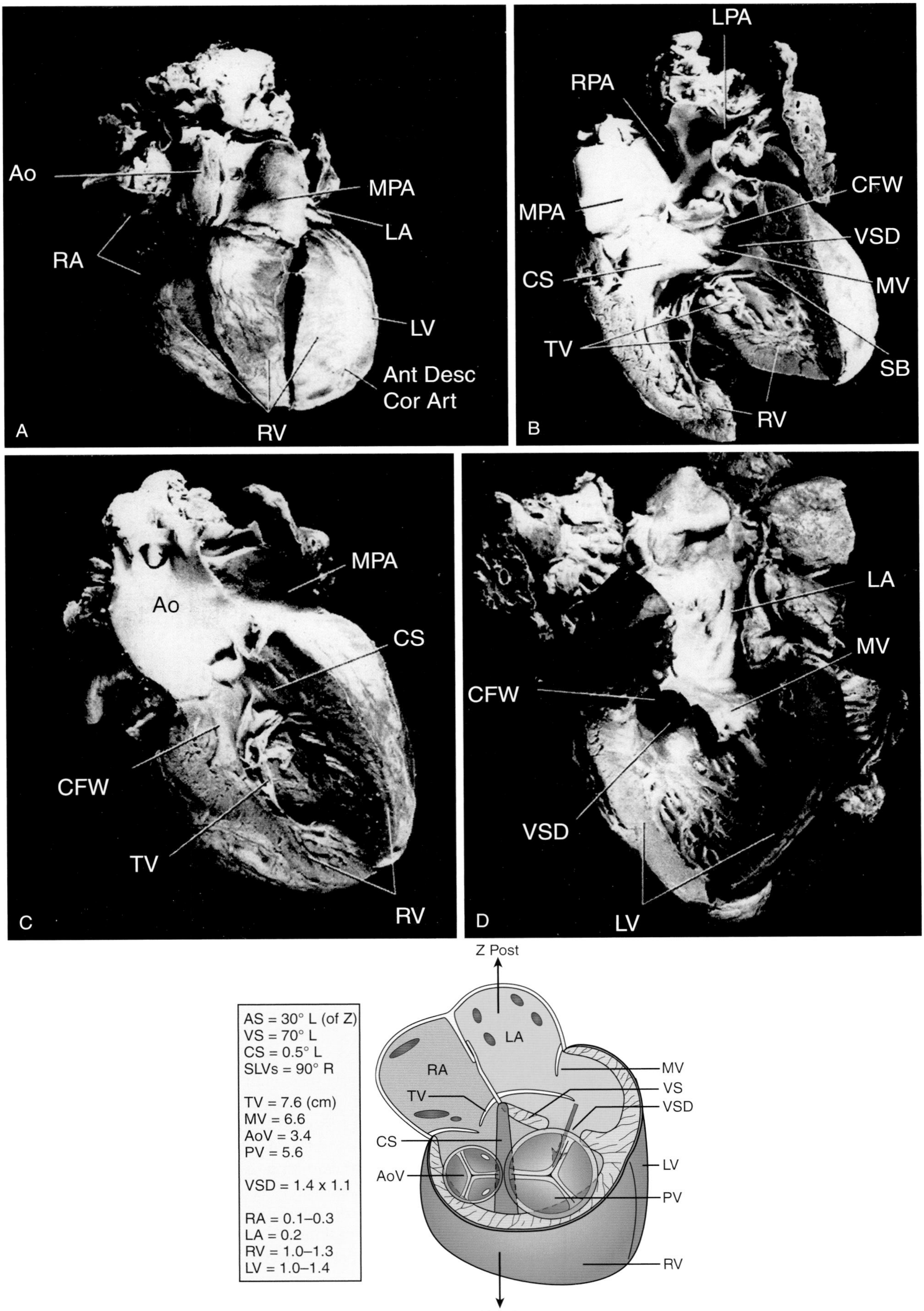

Ao
MPA
LA
RA
LV
Ant Desc
Cor Art
RV
A
LPA
RPA
CFW
MPA
VSD
CS
MV
TV
SB
RV
B
MPA
Ao
CS
CFW
TV
RV
C
LA
MV
CFW
VSD
LV
D
Z Post
AS = 30° L (of Z)
VS = 70° L
CS = 0.5° L
SLVs = 90° R
TV = 7.6 (cm)
MV = 6.6
AoV = 3.4
PV = 5.6
VSD = 1.4 x 1.1
RA = 0.1–0.3
LA = 0.2
RV = 1.0–1.3
LV = 1.0–1.4
LA
RA
TV
MV
VS
VSD
CS
AoV
LV
PV
RV
Z Ant

Continued

Fig. 23.1 The original Taussig-Bing heart.[8,16] (A) Exterior, frontal view. (B) Opened right ventricle *(RV)* and pulmonary outflow tract. (C) Opened right ventricle (RV) and aortic outflow tract. (D) Opened left atrium *(LA)* and left ventricle *(LV)*. (E) Geometric horizontal plane diagram. Photos are described in the text. The subaortic infundibular free wall in C, from aortic valve *(AoV)* above to tricuspid valve *(TV)* below, is 8 mm in height. The subpulmonary infundibular free wall, in D from pulmonary valve *(PV)* above to mitral valve *(MV)* below, is 9 mm in height. In E, the PV overrides the ventricular septum *(VS)*, but does not override the left ventricular cavity at all. Hence, the Taussig-Bing malformation is a form of double-outlet right ventricle. The cardiac septal and semilunar geometry is measured relative to the Z axis (or the anteroposterior plane). The atrial septal angle is 30 degrees to the left of the Z axis (i.e., 30 degrees L). The ventricular septal angle is 70 degrees L. The infundibular (or conal) septum is 0 degrees on the right side and 5 degrees L on the left side. The semilunar valvar angle is 90 degrees R (assuming the aortic valve *[AO/Ao]* is directly anterior to the pulmonary valve before semilunar valvar rotation). The wall thicknesses and valve circumferences are measured in centimeters. The ventral septal defect *(VSD)* measures 1.4 cm (horizontal dimension) by 1.1 cm (vertical dimension) from the left ventricular aspect, the VSD being the outlet from the LV. The infundibular septum measures 2.0 cm in height. *Ant,* Anterior; *Ant Desc Cor Art,* anterior descending coronary artery; *AS,* atrial septum; *CFW,* conal (or infundibular) free wall; *CS,* distal or subarterial conal septum; *LPA,* left pulmonary artery; *MPA,* main pulmonary artery; *Post,* posterior; *PV,* pulmonary valve; *RA,* right atrium; *RPA,* right pulmonary artery; *SB,* septal band or proximal infundibular septum; *SLVs,* semilunar valves. (Reproduced with permission from Van Praagh R. What is the Taussig-Bing malformation? *Circulation.* 1968;38:445.)

Normally, there is no subaortic infundibular free wall on the right side beneath the aorta (0R) and there is a well-developed (grade 4) infundibular free wall beneath the pulmonary artery on the left (4L). Note that subarterial infundibular free wall development normally is totally asymmetrical: grade 0 on the right, and grade 4 (standing for 100% of normal) on the left.

The equation in Taussig-Bing is DORV {S,D,D} = 4R + 4L. The infundibular situs beneath the right-sided aorta is grade 4 (standing for 100% of possible development) and beneath the left-sided pulmonary artery is also 100% of possible development. So, in the Taussig-Bing malformation, infundibular development is bilaterally symmetrical, whereas normally infundibular development is 100% bilaterally asymmetrical.

THE INFUNDIBULOARTERIAL SITUS EQUATIONS

1. Solitus normally related great arteries: SNRGA {S,D,S} = 0R + 4L
2. Inversus normally related great arteries: INRGA {I,L,I} = 4R + 0L
3. Taussig-Bing type of DORV: DORV {S,D,D, = 4R + 4L

Because the infundibuloarterial situs formula in the Taussig-Bing malformation (4R + 4L) is different from that of solitus normally related great arteries (0R + 4L) and is also different from that of inversus normally related great arteries (4R + 0L); therefore, the infundibuloarterial situs combination in the Taussig-Bing malformation is regarded as ambiguus (Latin spelling) or ambiguous (English spelling).

WHEN THE VSD IS TOO SMALL

In DORV, what do you do when the VSD is too small and obstructs the left ventricular outlet?[9] In 1971, Lavoie et al[9] presented the following solution in a 5-year-old white boy at the Montreal Heart Institute. At operation, Dr. Pierre Grondin confirmed that the aorta and the pulmonary artery both originated above the right ventricle. The VSD was obstructively small and slit-like. From the right ventricular aspect, the VSD measured 6 × 2 mm and the VSD was much closer to the aortic valve than to the pulmonary valve. A short cuff of subaortic infundibular muscle separated the aortic valve from the small VSD.

Excision of the subaortic infundibular muscle was carried out. This raised the "roof" of the VSD, thereby enlarging the defect that served as the only left ventricular outflow tract. The enlarged VSD then measured 25 × 30 mm. The VSD was then closed with a Teflon patch that was sutured to the right of the aortic annulus.

Virtually normal hemodynamics were achieved: LV, 105 mm Hg; ascending aorta, 100 mm Hg; and RV, 35 mm Hg. Seventeen months postoperatively, cardiac catheterization revealed no left ventricular outflow tract gradient.

We published[9] another similar autopsied case, a 9-month-old female infant, with a similar type of DORV with an obstructive VSD, to document this crucially important anatomic aspect. At the Hartford Hospital in Hartford, Connecticut, selective right ventricular cineangiocardiography (Fig. 23.2) revealed DORV {S,D,D} with a bilateral infundibulum or conus, subaortic and subpulmonary. The great arteries were side-by-side, aorta to the right and pulmonary artery to the left. Subpulmonary infundibular stenosis is seen at the os infundibuli pulmonalis (at the ostium of the subpulmonary infundibulum).

The catheter was advanced from the RV through a VSD into the LV. At this point, the heart slowed markedly. The catheteer thought that the VSD could be very small and that the catheter could be largely or completely obstructing the left ventricular outflow tract. The catheter was quickly withdrawn, and cardiac function was restored. The operating room was readied for the creation of an atrial septal defect (in 1971). But before the operation could be started, cardiac arrest occurred and resuscitation was not possible.

Autopsy confirmed the presence of DORV {S,D,D} with a bilateral infundibulum, and revealed massive left ventricular hypertrophy and enlargement (Fig. 23.3A). The VSD measured only 3 × 3 mm (very small). There was a jet lesion just to the right of this highly obstructive VSD. The VSD was of the

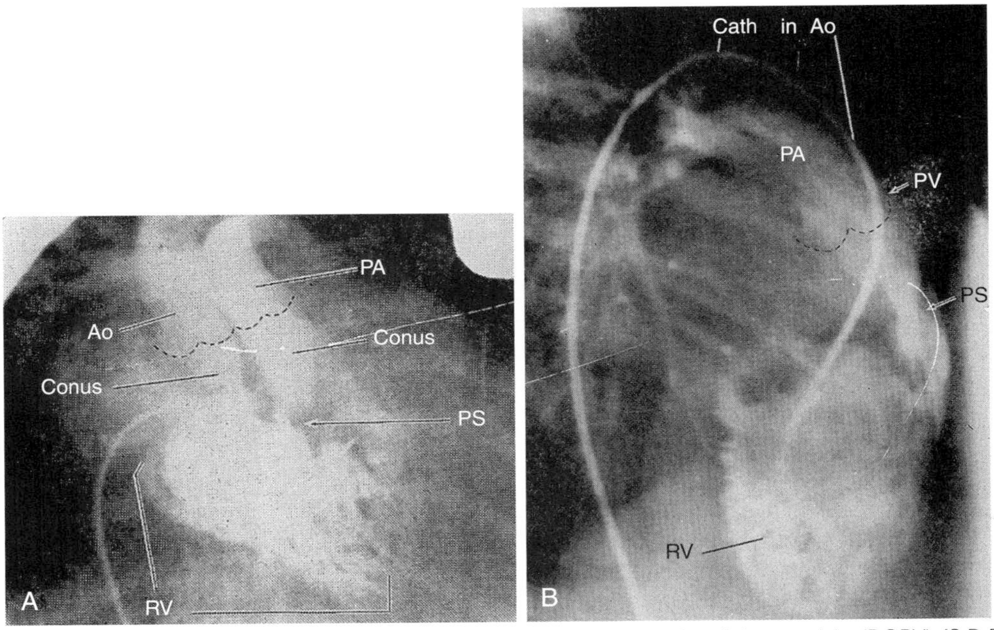

Fig. 23.2 Selective right ventricular cineangiocardiogram of double-outlet right ventricle (DORV) {S,D,D} with bilateral infundibulum (or conus). (A) Posteroanterior projection. (B) Right lateral projection. Note the infundibular pulmonary stenosis *(PS)* at the os infundibuli pulmonalis, the ostium leading into the subpulmonary infundibulum. *Ao,* Aorta; *Cath,* catheter; *PA,* pulmonary valve; *PV,* pulmonary valve; *RV,* right ventricle. (Reproduced with permission from Lavoie R, Sestier R, Gilbert G, Chameides L, Van Praagh R, and Grondin P. Double-outlet right ventricle with left ventricular outflow tract obstruction due to small ventricular septal defect. *Am Heart J.* 1971;82:290.)

infundibuloventricular type, between the subarterial infundibular septum above and the ventricular septum and septal band below (see Fig. 23.3B). The subpulmonary stenosis was also very small (3 × 4 mm) (see Fig. 23.3C).

DOUBLE-OUTLET RIGHT VENTRICLE WITH INTACT VENTRICULAR SEPTUM AND LEFT VENTRICLE–TO–RIGHT ATRIUM SHUNT

In 1972, Megarity et al[10] reported the first known case of DORV with an intact ventricular septum and an LV-to-RA communication (Fig. 23.4A). On external inspection, right ventricular hypertrophy and left ventricular hypertrophy were evident (see Fig. 23.4A). DORV {S,D,D} was apparent. The MPA was enlarged, and the ascending aorta was mildly hypoplastic.

The opened right atrium (RA), tricuspid valve, and RV (see Fig. 23.4B) revealed the right atrial opening of a left ventricular–to–right atrial communication within the superior commissure of the tricuspid valve between the anterior and septal leaflets. This opening measured 1.5 mm in diameter and was surrounded by thickened, firm tricuspid valvar fibrous tissue. This opening was located within the fibrous AV septum, that is, within the atrial portion of the AV membranous septum.

The opened right ventricular outflow tract revealed DORV (see Fig. 23.4C). Beneath the aortopulmonary septum, there was no infundibular septum. Consequently the aortic valve and the pulmonary valve were in fibrous continuity. The pulmonary valve was separated from the tricuspid valve by the septal band (which is the proximal or apical part of the infundibulum). Beneath the aortic valve, there was a 3-mm-tall (superoinferior dimension) cuff of infundibular muscle that separated the aortic valve above from the tricuspid valve below.

However, when the subaortic muscular cuff was incised vertically, we discovered that the aortic valve and the tricuspid valve were in fibrous continuity behind this 3-mm-tall cuff of subaortic infundibular muscle (see Fig. 23.4D). We were not sure how to interpret this finding. Perhaps the process of subaortic infundibular free wall demuscularization by apoptosis was incomplete and was occurring from left to right (hypothesis). The subarterial infundibular malformation was most unusual: absence of the distal or subarterial infundibular septum; absence of the parietal band extending out on to the right ventricular parietal or free wall; but with a small cuff of infundibular muscle between the aortic and tricuspid valves that, nonetheless, were in fibrous continuity on their leftward or septal side. The small subaortic cuff of muscle was associated with subaortic stenosis and hypoplasia of the aortic arch. This rare infundibular malformation was associated with DORV with an intact ventricular septum and an LV-to-RA shunt.

The opened left atrium (LA), mitral valve, and LV (see Fig. 23.4E) are shown. The LA was hypertrophied but not enlarged. The mitral valve and papillary muscles were mildly hypoplastic. The LV was hypertrophied and enlarged.

The left ventricular outflow tract (see Fig. 23.4F) showed severe fibrous obstruction by endocardial cushion tissue of the AV valves. This severe fibrous left ventricular outflow tract obstruction appears to explain how it was possible to have

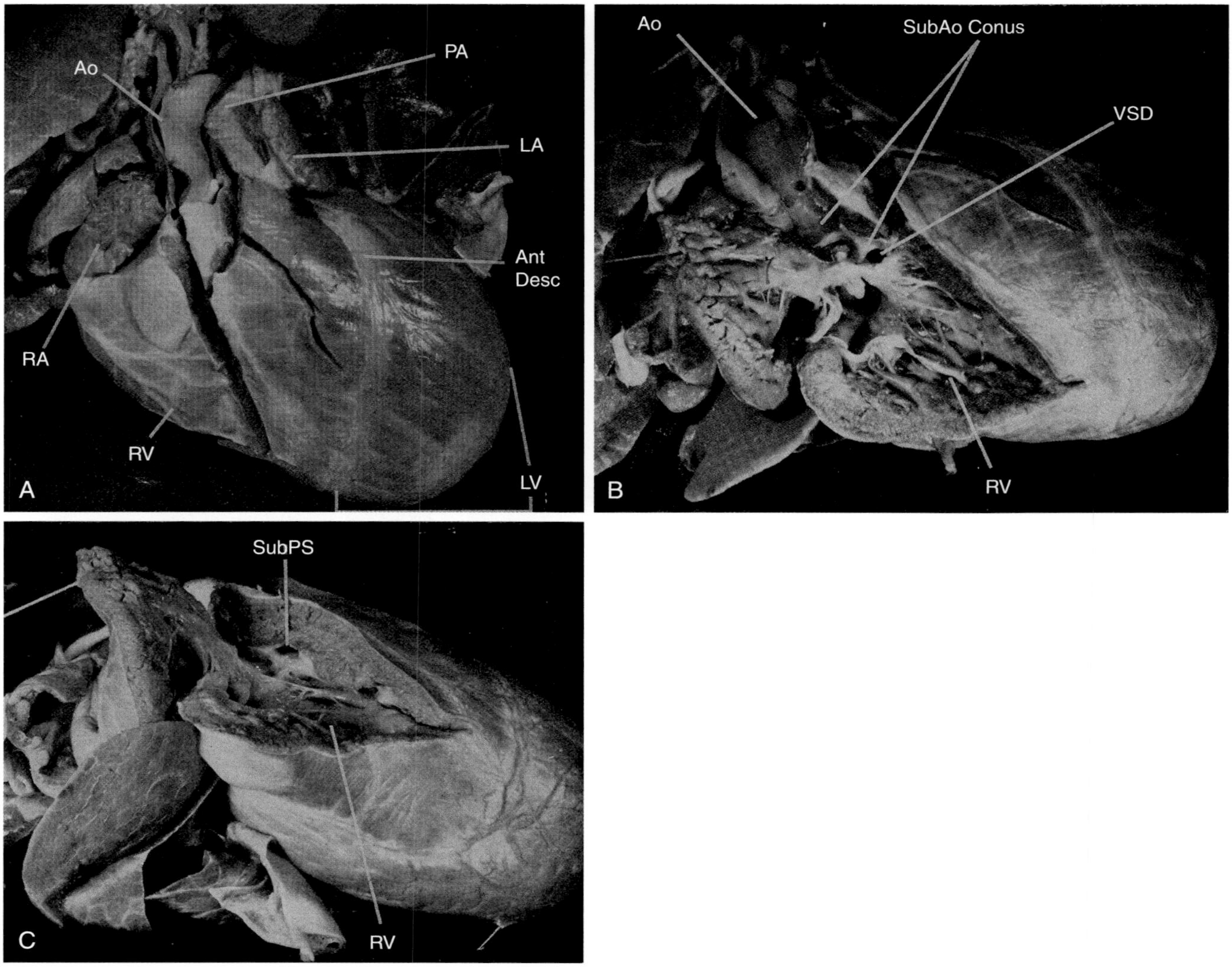

Fig. 23.3 Double-outlet right ventricle {S,D,D} with bilateral infundibulum (same patient as in Fig. 23.2). (A) Both great arteries arise to the right of the ventricular septum, indicated by the anterior descending coronary artery *(Ant Desc)*, accurately confirming double-outlet ventricle. The aorta *(Ao)* and the pulmonary artery *(PA)* both arise at approximately the same height and side-by-side, accurately suggesting the possibility of a bilateral infundibulum. Much more left ventricle *(LV)* is more visible in this frontal view than normal, accurately indicating marked left ventricular hypertrophy and enlargement. (B) Opened right ventricle *(RV)* showing obstructively small ventricular septal defect *(VSD)*, measuring 3 × 3 mm. The VSD is neither subaortic nor subpulmonary. Instead, it is beneath and between both semilunar valves. The subsemilunar infundibulum lowers the "roof" on this infundibuloventricular VSD. There was a jet lesion to the right of this stenotic VSD. (C) The opened RV, showing the stenotic os leading into the subpulmonary infundibulum that measures 3 × 4 mm, resulting in severe pulmonary infundibular stenosis. *LA*, Left atrium; *RA*, right atrium; *SubAo*, subaortic; *SubPS*, subpulmonary stenosis. (Reproduced with permission from Lavoie R, Sestier R, Gilbert G, Chameides L, Van Praagh R, and Grondin P. Double-outlet right ventricle with left ventricular outflow tract obstruction due to small ventricular septal defect. *Am Heart J.* 1971;82:290.)

absence of the subarterial infundibular septum, with an intact ventricular septum—that is, no VSD! It is amazing that this little boy lived for 35 postnatal days, given that his LV-to-RA shunt was only 1.5 mm in diameter, his fossa ovalis was sealed at the atrial level, and we found no other way for oxygenated blood to get from the left heart into the right heart. For example, he did not have a coronary sinus septal defect between his LA and his coronary sinus. No wonder he was found to have cyanosis, tachypnea, and splenomegaly immediately after birth, with a systemic oxygen saturation of only 30%.

Double-Outlet Right Ventricle {S,D,L} With Subaortic Ventricular Septal Defect, Bilateral Infundibulum, and Pulmonary Stenosis

In 1975, we published 6 such cases because of the importance of understanding the surgical anatomy (Fig. 23.5). External inspection (see Fig. 23.5A) strongly suggests the correct diagnosis, without incising anything. Levocardia, left-sided heart, is present. The viscera and atria are in situs solitus (S); the morphologically RA is right-sided.

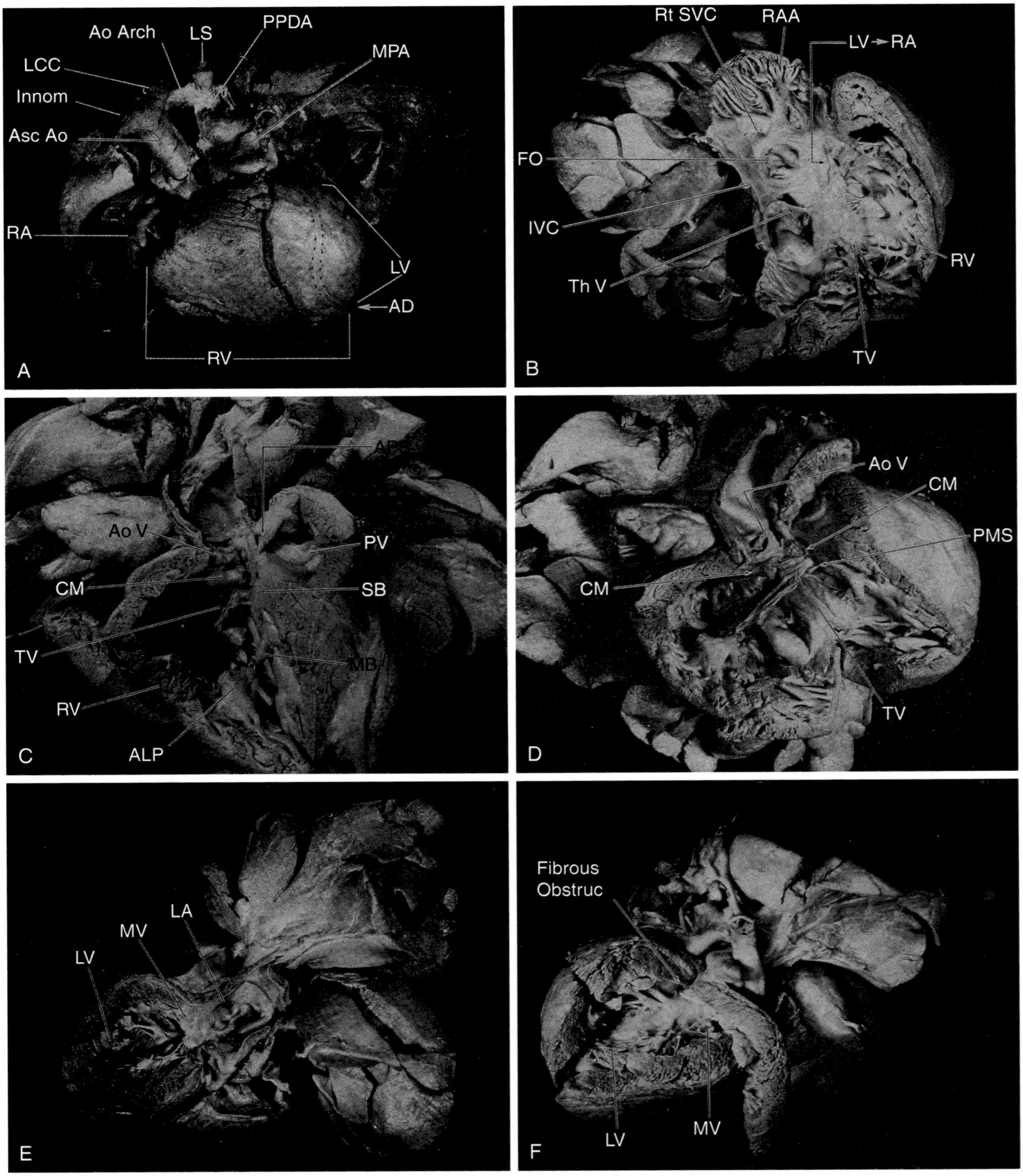

Fig. 23.4 Double-outlet right ventricle with left ventricular–to–right atrial communication. (A) External frontal view of the heart and lungs. Right ventricular hypertrophy is accurately suggested: right ventricle *(RV)* forms ventricular apex. Left ventricular hypertrophy is also accurately suggested by the sigmoid course of the left anterior descending coronary artery *(AD)*. The main pulmonary artery *(MPA)* is enlarged, and the ascending aorta *(Asc Ao)* is mildly hypoplastic. Distal to the innominate *(Innom)* and left common carotid *(LCC)* arteries, the aortic arch *(Ao Arch)* is moderately to markedly hypoplastic. Distal to the left subclavian *(LS)* artery, the functionally closed but probe patent ductus arteriosus *(PPDA)* is seen. The right atrium *(RA)* is hypertrophied. (B) Opened RA, tricuspid valve *(TV)*, and right ventricular inflow tract *(RV)*. The right atrial appendage *(RAA)* and the RV are hypertrophied and enlarged. The right superior vena cava *(Rt SVC)* is markedly hypoplastic, admitting a 1-mm probe snugly. The foramen ovale is sealed; that is, a fossa ovalis *(FO)* is present, unusual in

Continued

a 35-day-old patient (a white boy). Anterior to the FO is the right atrial opening of the LV-to-RA communication that measures only 1.5 mm in diameter and is surrounded by thickened, firm tricuspid valvar tissue. This opening is located within the superior and anterior commissure of the TV, at the junction of the anterior and septal tricuspid valve leaflets. This tiny opening is the only outlet from the left side of the heart. The tricuspid valve was enlarged (circumference, 55 mm/normal, 33 mm). The Thebesian valve *(ThV)* partly covers the markedly enlarged ostium of the coronary sinus that receives a persistent left superior vena cava. (C) The opened right ventricular outflow tract. Both great arteries arise from the RV outflow tract, aortic valve *(AoV)* to the right and pulmonary valve *(PV)* to the left. There is no distal or subarterial infundibular septum beneath the aortopulmonary septum. Hence, the AoV and the PV are in fibrous continuity. Beneath the AoV there is a 3-mm-tall band of infundibular muscle, measured in the vertical dimension, between the AoV above and the tricuspid valve *(TV)* below. In the horizontal dimension, this small band of infundibular muscle runs from the ventricular septum to the right ventricular free wall, probably producing subaortic infundibular stenosis. (D) Division of this subaortic band of infundibular muscle *(CM)* revealed fibrous tissue to the left of the infundibular muscle, with aortic valve–to–tricuspid valve fibrous continuity. No VSD was found. The LV-to-RA defect is within the pars membranacea septi *(PMS)*; that is, the LV-RA communication lies within the membranous septum. (E) The opened left atrium *(LA)*, mitral valve *(MV)*, and left ventricle *(LV)*. The LA is hypertrophied, but not enlarged. The MV is mildly hypoplastic, as are the papillary muscles. The LV is otherwise hypertrophied and enlarged. (F) The outflow tract of the LV reveals fibrous obstruction *(fibrous Obstruc)*. *ALP,* Anterolateral papillary muscle; *MB,* moderator band; *SB,* septal band. (Reproduced with permission from Megarity AL, Chambers RG, Calder AL, Van Praagh S, Van Praagh R. Double-outlet right ventricle with left ventricular-right atrial communication: fibrous obstruction of left ventricular outlet by membranous septum and tricuspid leaflet tissue. *Am Heart J.* 1972;84:242.)

The coronary arterial distribution indicates that D-loop (solitus) ventricles are present (D). Note the marginal branch of the right coronary artery running along the acute margin of the RV. The right coronary artery gives off three large visible branches:

1. the anterior descending coronary artery, furthest to the left;
2. one or more preventricular branches supplying the right ventricular free wall, somewhat to the right; and
3. the usual right coronary artery running to the right and into the AV groove between the RA and the RV.

A *"Sherlock Holmes"* point: If ever you see the anterior descending coronary artery arising from the *right* coronary artery in a patient with D-loop (solitus) ventricles, you should say to yourself, or out loud, "The left coronary ostium is probably absent. This is what is often called single right coronary artery." The great arteries are in L-malposition. The ascending aorta is anterior and to the left of the pulmonary artery. The pulmonary artery is posterior and to the right relative to the aorta. The MPA is smaller than the ascending aorta, correctly suggesting that pulmonary outflow tract stenosis is probably present. Both great arteries arise to the right of the ventricular septum. The location of the ventricular septum is indicated by the location of the anterior descending coronary artery. So, again you say to yourself, "DORV is probably present." Now you have a tentative diagnosis that is probably highly accurate, based only on external inspection without incising anything.

Double-Outlet Right Ventricle {S,D,L} With Pulmonary Stenosis

Opening the RV (see Fig. 23.5B and C) you discover that the VSD is subaortic, that a bilateral infundibulum is present (both subaortic and subpulmonary), and that mild pulmonary infundibular and valvar stenosis were present. The mitral valve straddled the ventricular septum mildly and inserted slightly though the VSD and into the RV anterosuperiorly. Although the RV was hypertrophied and enlarged (see Fig. 23.5A–C), the LV was of normal dimensions (see Fig. 23.5D). The cardiac dimensions and geometry of this 5-month-old boy are presented in Fig. 23.5E. The pulmonary valve was mildly hypoplastic and bicuspid because the septal commissure was not present.

A second *"Sherlock Holmes"* point: From a surgical viewpoint, in Fig. 23.5A, note that the right coronary artery runs right across the pulmonary outflow tract, slightly below the pulmonary valve. Because there is pulmonary outflow tract stenosis, the surgeon might want to make an incision from the RV into the MPA (as in TOF). However, this would transect the right coronary artery, a major mistake that one should not make. Instead, one should "jump" the right coronary artery with a conduit from the RV to the pulmonary artery. Or, if possible, one should excise the restrictive subpulmonary infundibular myocardium, with or without pulmonary valvotomy, to surgically abolish the pulmonary outflow tract stenosis.

Regarding Sherlock Holmes, many do not know that Sir Arthur Conan Doyle (1859–1930) was a Scottish physician, born in Edinburgh, who earned his MB in 1881 and his MD in 1885 from Edinburgh University. He was practicing as a physician in Southsea when he published *A Study In Scarlet* in 1887, his first novel about Sherlock Holmes. Doyle began practicing medicine in 1882. He started writing while waiting for patients who never came. Ultimately, Sherlock Holmes appeared in 56 short stories and three other novels. Dr. Doyle fascinated millions of readers who delighted in Holmes' ability to solve crimes by an amazing use of observation and reason (deduction and induction). Readers thought this was fiction. But Doyle understood that the fascination of Sherlock Holmes was his use of the **medical method** of making accurate diagnoses, based on extremely careful observation and brilliant cerebration, without almost all of the technology that modern physicians rely on today. Even now, with a bit of luck, medical diagnosticians may become Sherlock Holmes, thanks to the inspiration of Dr. Arthur Conan Doyle.

Dr. Watson, Sherlock Holmes' assistant, has now morphed into IBM's famous Watson, the artificial intelligence system that won the *Jeopardy!* television game show in 2011 by beating

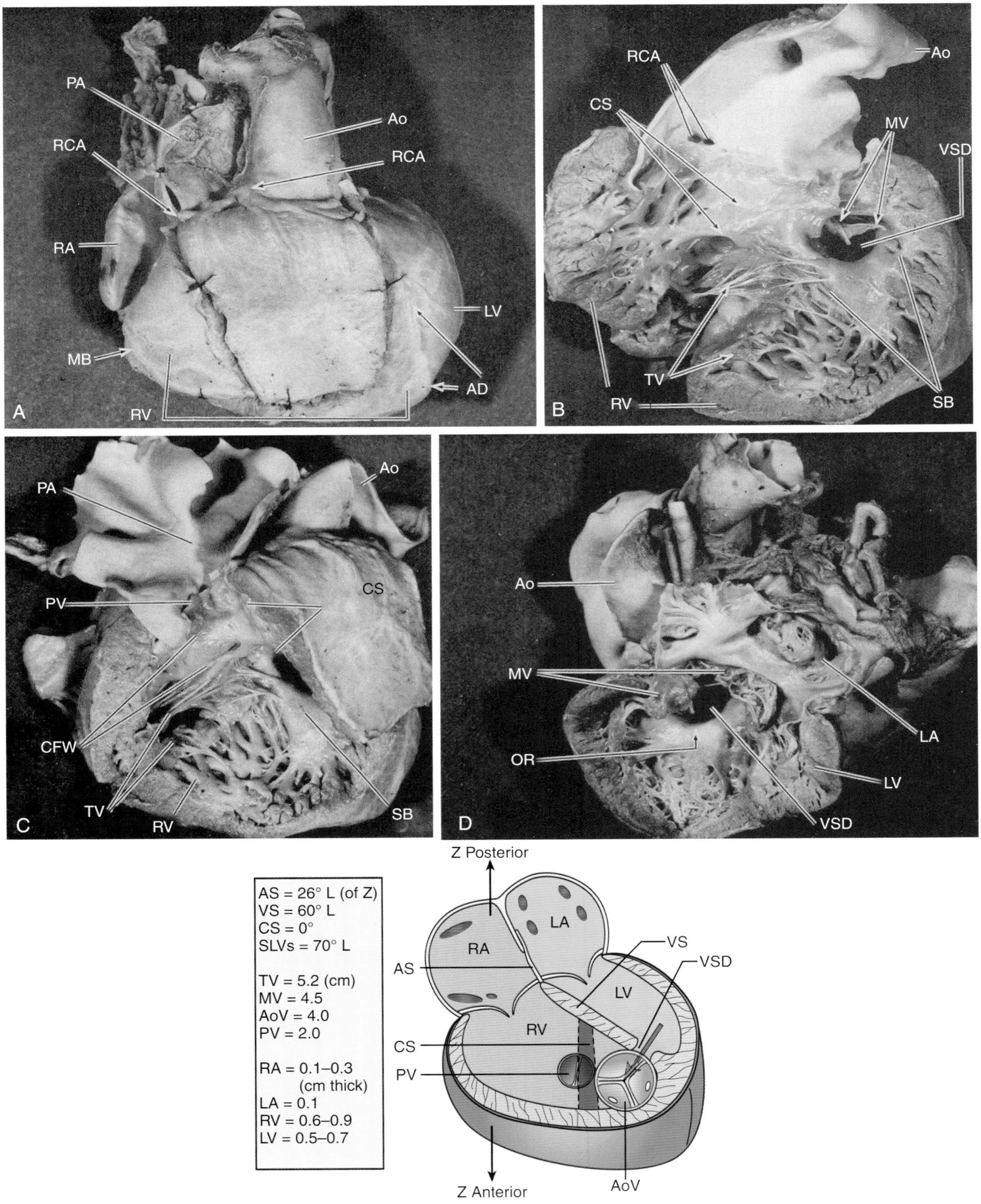

Fig. 23.5 Double-outlet right ventricle (DORV) {S, D, L} with subaortic ventricular septal defect *(VSD)* and pulmonary stenosis. (A) External frontal view. The morphologically right atrium *(RA)* is right-sided, in visceroatrial situs solitus, that is, {S,-,-}. The morphologically right ventricle *(RV)* is right-sided and right-handed, and the morphologically left ventricle *(LV)* is left-sided and left-handed, indicating that D-loop or solitus ventricles are present; that is, {S,D,-}. The great arteries are in L-malposition (or inverted), the aorta to the left *(Ao)*, and the

Continued

pulmonary artery *(PA)* to the right, that is, {S,D,L}. The PA is distinctly smaller than the aorta, correctly suggesting that pulmonary stenosis is present. Both great arteries arise to the right of the ventricular septum, accurately suggested by their rightward location relative to the location of the anterior descending coronary artery *(AD)*. Hence, the segmental anatomic diagnosis is **DORV {S,D,L}**. (B) The opened RV shows that the VSD is subaortic, that mitral valve *(MV)* is slightly straddling into the RV, and that the muscular subaortic infundibulum *(CS)* is well developed and left-sided, separating the aortic valve *(AoV)* above from the tricuspid valve *(TV)* below. (B) Aortic outflow tract from the RV. (C) The outflow tract from the RV to the PA, with mild pulmonary outflow tract stenosis and a well-developed right-sided subpulmonary muscular infundibulum separating the pulmonary valve above *(PV)* from the TV below. (D) The opened left atrium *(LA)*, MV, and LV. The mild straddling of the MV is seen. The VSD is the only outlet from the LV. (E) Horizontal plane geometric diagram of the heart. The septal and the semilunar valvar geometry are measured relative to the Z axis (the anteroposterior plane). The valve circumferences and the wall thicknesses are measured in centimeters. The pulmonary valve is stenotic and bicuspid (absence of the septal commissure.) *AS*, Aortic stenosis; *CFW*, conal free wall; *MB*, moderator band; *RCA*, right coronary artery; *SB*, septal band; *SLVs*, semilunar valves. (Reproduced with permission from Van Praagh R, Pérez-Treviño C, Reynolds JL, Moes CAF, Keith JD, Roy DL, Belcourt C, Weinberg PM, Parisi LF. Double-outlet right ventricle {S, D, L} with subaortic ventricular septal defect and pulmonary stenosis: report of six cases. *Am J Cardiol*. 1975;35:42.)

two human former champions. Many humans now think that artificial intelligence and machine learning will soon outperform human cognitive abilities, leading us all into a new world with superhumans[18] (time of writing, 2017). As always, time will tell.

HISTORY

The earliest definite report of DORV of which I am aware is that of J. Abernathy[19] in 1793. The VSD was subaortic. Pulmonary stenosis was present.

SUMMARY OF DOUBLE-OUTLET RIGHT VENTRICLE

Groups

Group I: Anomalies mainly of infundibulum and great arteries
Group II: Malformations of infundibulum and great arteries and of AV valves and ventricles
Group III: Anomalies of infundibulum and great arteries, AV valves and ventricles, and viscera and atria (the heterotaxy syndromes)

Anatomic Types

n = 101 cases. Number of cases equals percent of series.

1. Group	I	DORV with subaortic VSD = 10 cases
2. Group	I	DORV with subpulmonary VSD = 11 cases
3. Group	I	DORV with uncommitted VSD = 11 cases
4. Group	II	DORV with subaortic VSD = 9 cases
5. Group	II	DORV with subpulmonary VSD = 5 cases
6. Group	II	DORV with uncommitted VSD = 20 cases
7. Group	II	DORV with no VSD = 8 cases
8. Group	III	DORV with asplenia and uncommitted VSD = 13 cases
9. Group	III	DORV with asplenia and no VSD = 4 cases
10. Group	III	DORV with polysplenia and subaortic VSD = 2 cases
11. Group	III	DORV with polysplenia and uncommitted VSD = 4 cases
12. Group	III	DORV with polysplenia and no VSD = 4 cases

VSD, Ventricular septal defect.

Putting Groups I, II, and III Together (No. + %)		
1.	DORV with subaortic VSD	21
2.	DORV with subpulmonary VSD	16
3.	DORV with uncommitted VSD	48
	Asplenia	13
	Polysplenia	4
4.	DORV with no VSD	16
	Asplenia	4
	Polysplenia	4

VSD, Ventricular septal defect.

DETAILED ANATOMIC TYPES OF DOUBLE-OUTLET RIGHT VENTRICLE (N = 73)

When specific detailed anatomic information is desired concerning any of the 73 anatomic types of DORV found in this study of 101 postmortem cases,[7] please see the Findings section of this chapter.

Why is DORV perhaps the most complex form of congenital heart disease? Typically, DORV appears to represent a developmental arrest before the embryonic arterial switch procedure has occurred (aortic valve to mitral valve = NRGA, or pulmonary valve to mitral valve = TGA).

DORV is the normal starting position for both developing great arteries, and it appears to correspond to Streeter's horizon 11, with an estimated embryonic age since ovulation of only 22 to 24 days. If DORV persists, many other primitive features may also persist, accounting for the high frequency of so-called associated malformations with DORV (groups II and III). "Pure" (isolated) DORV is group I. Associated malformations, that is, other early developmental features, account for groups II and III. DORV may be an isolated congenital cardiovascular anomaly (groups I and II) or it can be part of a whole bodily form of malformation: the heterotaxy syndromes of asplenia and polysplenia. The statement was made that no great artery arises from the left ventricle.

REFERENCES

1. Vierordt H. Die angeborenen Herzkrankheiten, In: *Nothnagel's Spec Path Therapie. Vol* 1, 1898.
2. Von Rokitansky CF. Die Defecte der Scheidewande des Herzens, *Vienna, W Braumüller*. vol. 83, 1875.
3. Spitzer A. Über den Bauplan des normalen und missbildeten Herzens. Versuch einer phylogenetischen Theorie. *Virchows Arch F Path Anat*. 1923;243:81. [Spitzer A: The Architecture of Normal and Malformed Hearts: A Phylogenetic Theory Of Their Development, with a Summary and Analysis of the Theory by M Lev and A Vass, Springfield IL, Charles C Thomas, 1951.]
4. Neufeld HN, DuShane JW, Wood EH, Kirklin JW, Edwards JE. Origin of both great vessels from the right ventricle. I. Without pulmonary stenosis. *Circulation*. 1961;23:399.
5. Braun K, de Vries A, Feingold DS, Ehrenfeld NE, Feldman J, Schorr S. Complete dextroposition of the aorta, pulmonary stenosis, interventricular septal defect, and patent foramen ovale. *Am Heart J*. 1952;43:773.
6. Witham AC. Double outlet right ventricle, a partial transposition complex. *Am Heart J*. 1957;53:928.
7. Van Praagh S, Davidoff A, Chin A, Shiel FS, Reynolds J, Van Praagh R. Double- outlet right ventricle: anatomic types and developmental implications based on a study of 101 autopsied cases. *Coeur*. 1982;13:389.
8. Van Praagh R. What is the Taussig-Bing malformation? *Circulation*. 1968;38:445.
9. Lavoie R, Sestier R, Gilbert G, Chameides L, Van Praagh R, Grondin P. Double-outlet right ventricle with left ventricular outflow tract obstruction due to small ventricular septal defect. *Am Heart J*. 1971;82:290.
10. Megarity AL, Chambers RG, Calder AL, Van Praagh S, Van Praagh R. Double-outlet right ventricle with left ventricular-right atrial communication: fibrous obstruction of left ventricular outlet by membranous septum and tricuspid leaflet tissue. *Am Heart J*. 1972;84:242.
11. Van Praagh R, Pérez-Treviño C, Reynolds JL, et al. Double-outlet right ventricle {S, D, L} with subaortic ventricular septal defect and pulmonary stenosis. Report of six cases. *Am J Cardiol*. 1975;35:42.
12. Neufeld HN, DuShane JW, Edwards JE. Origin of both great vessels from the right ventricle. II. With pulmonary stenosis. *Circulation*. 1961;23:603.
13. Neufeld HN, Lucas RV, Lester RG, Adams P, Anderson RC, Edwards JE. Origin of both great vessels from the right ventricle without pulmonary stenosis. *Br Heart J*. 1962;24:393.
14. Lev M, Bharati S, Meng CCL, Liberthson RR, Paul MH, Idriss F. A concept of double-outlet right ventricle. *J Thorac Cardiovasc Surg*. 1972;64:271.
15. Van Praagh S, LaCorte M, Fellows KE, et al. Superoinferior ventricles, anatomic and angiocardiographic findings in 10 postmortem cases. In: Van Praagh R, Takao A, eds. *Etiology and Morphogenesis of Congenital Heart Disease*. Mt Kisco, New York: Futura Publishing Co; 1980:317.
16. Taussig HB, Bing RJ. Complete transposition of aorta and levoposition of pulmonary artery. *Am Heart J*. 1949;37:551.
17. Lev M, Volk BW. Pathologic anatomy of Taussig-Bing heart: riding pulmonary artery. Report of case. *Bull Internat Assoc Med Museums*. 1950;31:54.
18. Harari YN. *Homo Deus, A Brief History of Tomorrow*. New York: Harper Collins Publishers; 2017:318.
19. Abernathy J. *Surgical and Physiological Essays, Part II*. London: James Evans Publisher; 1793:162.

24

Double-Outlet Left Ventricle

Most pediatric cardiologists and congenital heart surgeons have never seen a patient with double-outlet left ventricle (DOLV). It is that rare. How rare is that? Well, in our cardiac pathology database on which this book is based (n = 3216 cases of congenital heart disease, mostly between 1966 and 2002, the approximately 36 years when I was the director of the Cardiac Registry), there were 14 cases of DOLV (0.44%) of the total series. However, of these 14 cases, 8 were consults from other medical centers. Consequently, for Boston Children's Hospital, only 6 cases of DOLV came to autopsy over this 36-year period, that is, on average, only 1 case every 6 years. As far as the cardiac pathology database is concerned, DOLV = 6 of 3216 cases = 0.001865, or 0.1865% (or 0.19%).

WHY IS DOUBLE-OULET LEFT VENTRICLE SO RARE?

At least part of the answer is that because DOLV is not part of the normal development of the cardiovascular system. Many forms of congenital heart disease appear to be arrests of normal cardiovascular development, such as double-outlet RV (DORV). But DOLV is *not* part of normal development. Something abnormal has to happen for DOLV to occur, as will be seen.

Definition

DOLV is present[1,2] when both great arteries arise entirely or predominantly above the morphologically left ventricle (LV). In this definition, "arise entirely or predominantly above the morphologically left ventricle" means "are *aligned* entirely or predominantly *with* the morphologically left ventricle," no matter what the spatial orientation of the great arteries and the ventricles relative to fixed external spatial coordinates (superior-inferior, right-left, and anterior-posterior) may be (Fig. 24.1).

The great arteries do not arise *from* the ventricles. The great arteries arise *from* the infundibulum, be it well developed or resorbed to an intervalvar fibrosa. This is why we say that the great arteries typically arise *above* the ventricles, *not from* the ventricles.

The clinical relevance of the rarity of DOLV is that when this anomaly occurs, pediatric cardiologists and cardiac surgeons may well be confronted by a malformation that they have never seen or heard of before. The task of this chapter is to prepare physicians as well as possible for this challenge.

WHAT DOLV IS NOT

DOLV has been reported[3] when both great arteries arise from the left-sided ventricle, but the left-sided ventricle was the morphologically right ventricle (RV) because ventricular inversion (L-loop formation) was present. Diagnostically, it is important to distinguish between a *positionally* left-sided ventricle and a *morphologically* LV. One of Dr. Maurice Lev's most important papers,[4] published in 1954, presented the distinction between the morphologic anatomic diagnosis of the various cardiac chambers, which is a constant, and the spatial locations of the various cardiac chambers, which is a variable in congenital heart disease. This distinction—morphologic anatomic diagnosis versus spatial location—is the basis of accurate diagnosis in complex congenital heart disease. That is why this is one of the all-time greatest papers[4] ever written about congenital heart disease.

The diagnosis of DOLV also has been made in a patient with normally related great arteries and a large infundibular septal defect.[5] How could expert cardiovascular surgeons make the diagnosis of DOLV during surgery on such a patient?

They were right, of course. When a large infundibular septal defect is present, it is possible—particularly if you are a cardiac surgeon or a pathologist—to look downward through an open and normally located pulmonary valve into the LV. Most people do not know that their pulmonary valve is located above their LV. This anatomic fact is normally concealed by a normally developed infundibular septum. But when the infundibular septum is absent, what may be called a form of DOLV is surprisingly present. Would we call it that? No. Why not? How can you call normally related great arteries DOLV? The primary abnormal diagnosis in cases such as this is infundibular (conal) septal defect. The great arteries are normally related. Nonetheless, the observations of the surgeons and their cardiologists were correct, and illuminating.[5]

ANATOMIC TYPES OF DOUBLE-OUTLET LEFT VENTRICLE

The first well-documented case of DOLV, to my knowledge, was that of Paul, Muster, Sinha, Cole, and Van Praagh,[1] reported in 1970. The patient was a 2 7/12-year-old white boy. His clinical and autopsy-proved diagnosis was DOLV {S,D,D} with bilateral absence of the infundibulum, that is, no subaortic and no subpulmonary muscular infundibulum, aortic-mitral and pulmonary-mitral direct fibrous continuity, intact ventricular septum, thick-walled and small-chambered RV with infundibular atresia, severe endocardial fibroelastosis of the apical half of the RV. No great artery arose from the RV. There was a fistula between the right ventricular apex and the anterior descending coronary artery. Both atria and the LV were hypertrophied and

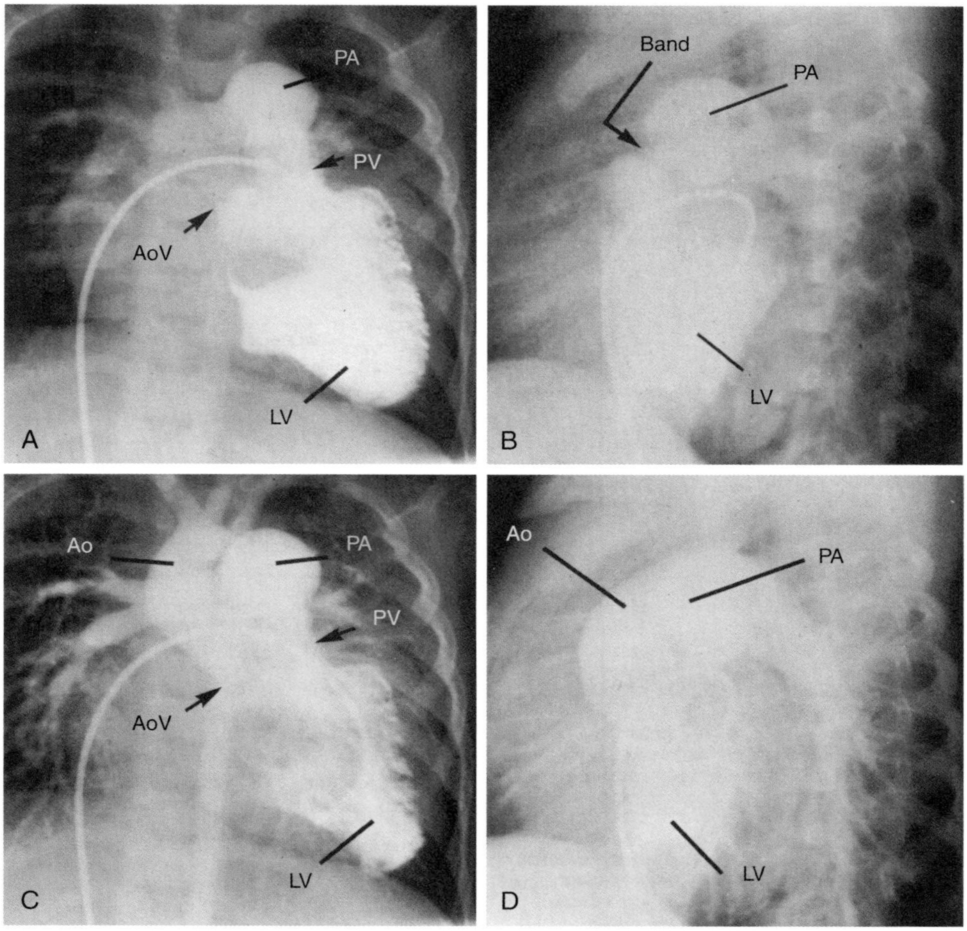

Fig. 24.1 Selective left ventricular angiocardiograms in the patient of Paul et al,[1] the first clinically diagnosed and autopsy confirmed case of direct-outlet left ventricle (DOLV). (A and B) Simultaneous posteroanterior and left lateral projections. Although the pulmonary artery *(PA)* has been banded (in B), contrast enters the pulmonary artery first. The aortic valve *(AoV)* and the pulmonary valve *(PV)* are both located above the left ventricle *(LV),* and the AoV and the PV are located in approximately the same horizontal plane, AoV to the right. (C) Note that there is no evidence of a ventricular septal defect. (C and D) Slightly lateral posteroanterior and left lateral projections, respectively, showing a well-opacified aorta *(Ao).* The Ao and the PA are side-by-side, Ao to the right, and both above the LV. (Reproduced with permission from Paul MH, Muster AJ, Sinha SN, Cole RB, Van Praagh R. Double-outlet left ventricle with an intact ventricular septum: clinical and autopsy diagnosis and developmental implications. *Circulation.* 1970;41:129.[1])

enlarged. The left coronary ostium was absent, resulting in so-called single right coronary artery.

Salient clinical features included cardiomegaly on the posteroanterior chest radiograph at 6 months of age (Fig. 24.2), with a cardiothoracic ratio of 61% and increased pulmonary vascularity. Electrocardiography (Fig. 24.3) revealed biatrial enlargement, mainly right, and increasing biventricular hypertrophy with strain.

He was in chronic congestive heart failure. Cardiac catheterization at 6 months of age revealed increased pulmonary blood flow (Qp/Q_s = 3.5/1), following which the main pulmonary artery was banded. Repeat cardiac catheterization at 25 months of age revealed that the pressure in the small-chambered and thick-walled RV with an atretic outflow tract and no VSD was 220/20 mm Hg. The right atrial a wave was 17 mm Hg, the v wave was 11 mm Hg, the left ventricular pressure was 95/9 mm Hg, and the aortic saturation was 90%.

Selective left ventricular angiocardiography showed a large LV; the pulmonary artery was banded, but filled before the aorta. Both great arteries arose above the left-sided and posterior LV. The aortic valve was to the right of the pulmonary valve, and both valves were at approximately the same horizontal level. There was no ventricular septal defect (VSD).

Selective right ventricular angiocardiography showed that the RV was small-chambered. There was no tricuspid regurgitation, despite the fact that the cardiac catheter passed through the tricuspid valve. A fistula from the right ventricular apex connected with the anterior descending coronary artery. Contrast flowed from the RV cavity through the fistula into the anterior "ascending" coronary artery, all the way up to the origin of the single right coronary artery. Contrast also flowed into the right coronary artery and into the circumflex coronary (Circ) artery. This was an example of marked perfusion of ventricular myocardium by unoxygenated blood from the RV. There was infundibular outflow tract atresia. The only outflow tract from this very hypertensive RV (220/20 mm Hg) was by the apical fistula.

This heart displayed complete infundibuloarterial dissociation. The infundibulum was associated with the RV; infundibular atresia is why there was no patent RV outflow tract.

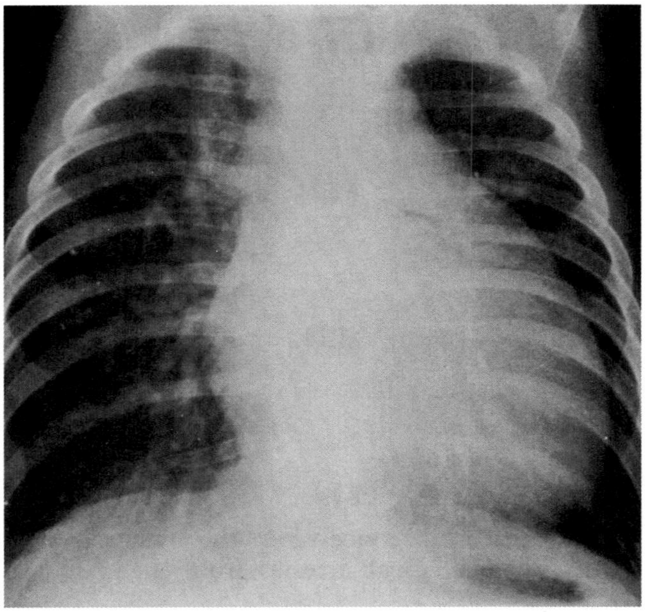

Fig. 24.2 Posteroanterior chest radiograph at 6 months of age, patient of Paul et al,[1] showing cardiomegaly (cardiothoracic ratio, 61%) and increased pulmonary vascularity. (Reproduced with permission from Paul MH, Muster AJ, Sinha SN, Cole RB, Van Praagh R. Double-outlet left ventricle with an intact ventricular septum: clinical and autopsy diagnosis and developmental implications. *Circulation.* 1970;41:129.)

Both great arteries were located above the LV. As will be seen, there was no muscular infundibulum beneath either great artery.

This is total infundibuloarterial dissociation: the infundibulum is right ventricular, and both great arteries are left ventricular. This is the first time I have ever seen complete dissociation or separation of the muscular infundibulum (or conus arteriosus) from both great arteries.

The pathologic anatomy of the Paul type[1] of DOLV is presented photographically in Fig. 24.4. Viewed externally from the front (see Fig. 24.4A), it is obvious that the LV is very large and that the RV is small. The LV does not just form the ventricular apex. The junction between the LV and the RV, marked by the anterior descending coronary artery (not labeled), *bisects* the anterior ventricular surface; that is, much more LV is seen from the front than ever occurs normally. Both the aorta *(Ao)* and the pulmonary artery *(PA)* are large, indicating that there is no aortic or pulmonary outflow tract stenosis.

The opened right atrium *(RA)* (see Fig. 24.4B) shows that the patent foramen ovale *(PFO)* was small and potentially obstructive; but the surgically created atrial septal defect *(Surg ASD)* was of good size. The exterior surface of the RV confirms that the RV is small-chambered.

Viewed from above (see Fig. 24.4C), the tricuspid valve *(TV)* is seen to be small, again confirming that the RV, into which the TV opens, is small-chambered.

The opened right atrium *(RA)*, tricuspid valve *(TV)*, and right ventricle *(RV)* (see Fig. 24.4D) show hypertrophy and enlargement of the RA, hypoplasia and stenosis of the TV, and a thick-walled and small-chambered RV with endocardial fibroelastosis *(EFE)* of the apical portion of the RV. The septal band *(SB)* is also seen.

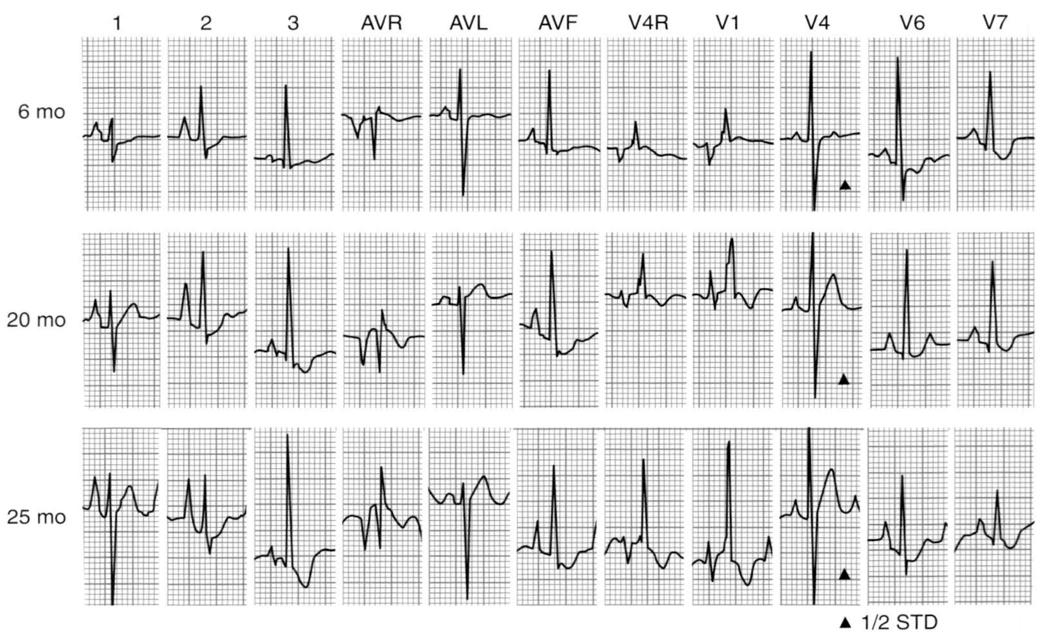

Fig. 24.3 Electrocardiograms of the patient of Paul et al[1] at 6 months (mo), 20 months, and 25 months of age showing evidence of biatrial enlargement, mainly right, and biventricular hypertrophy with strain. (Reproduced with permission from Paul MH, Muster AJ, Sinha SN, Cole RB, Van Praagh R. Double-outlet left ventricle with an intact ventricular septum: clinical and autopsy diagnosis and developmental implications. *Circulation.* 1970;41:129.)

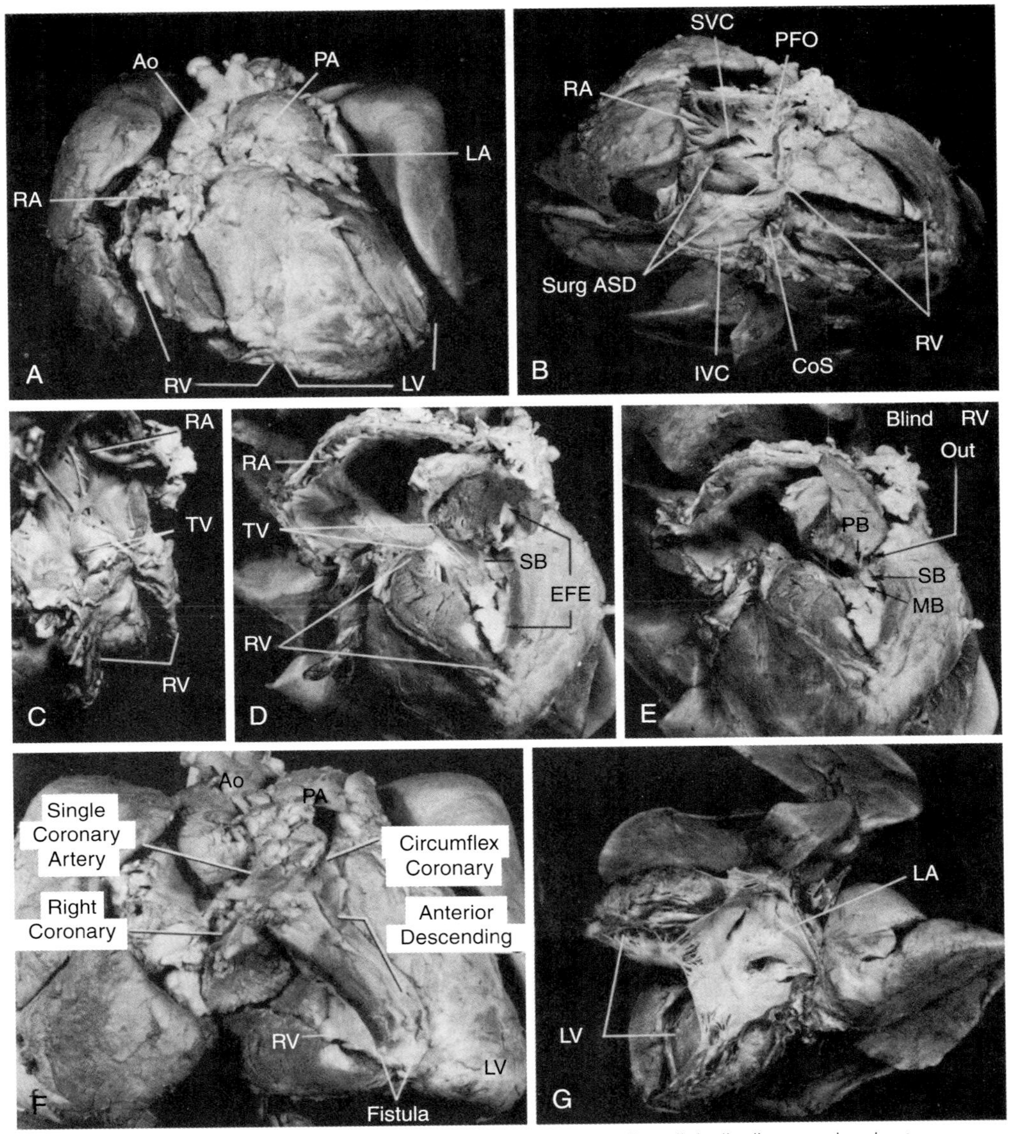

Fig. 24.4 Dr. Milton H. Paul's case of double-outlet left ventricle, the first clinically diagnosed and autopsy proved case of DOLV. (A) The morphologically right atrium *(RA)* is right-sided. The morphologically left atrium *(LA)* is left-sided. The morphologically right ventricle *(RV)* is right-sided and appears unusually small. The morphologically left ventricle *(LV)* is left-sided and it appears much larger than normal. The anterior descending coronary artery between the RV and the LV approximately bisects the anterior ventricular surface of the heart, indicating that the RV is unusually small, or that the LV is unusually large, or both. The pulmonary artery *(PA)* appears dilated. The aorta *(Ao)* is of normal size, with a left aortic arch. (B) The opened RA, right lateral view, showing the opened inferior vena cava *(IVC)*, the orifice of the superior vena cava *(SVC)*, the patent foramen ovale *(PFO)*, the ostium of the coronary sinus *(CoS)*, and the wide-open surgically created atrial septal defect *(Surg ASD)*—a Blalock-Hanlon procedure at 28 months of age. The RA is markedly hypertrophied, 4 to 7 mm thick, and enlarged. The surgically created ASD measured 20 × 14 mm. (C) The tricuspid valve *(TV)*, viewed from above, has a very hypoplastic orifice that measures 8 mm in circumference. The tricuspid leaflets and chordae tendineae are miniature, but otherwise normally formed. The degree of hypoplasia of the tricuspid valve appears appropriate to the smallness of the right ventricular cavity. (D) Opened RA (TV and RV). The RV is thick-walled (7 to 15 mm in thickness) and small-chambered with severe endocardial fibroelastosis *(EFE)* of the apical portion of the RV sinus. (E) The opened atretic infundibular outflow tract *(Blind RV Out)* with diminutive infundibular septum band *(SB)* and parietal band *(PB)*, and moderator band *(MB)*. The ventricular septum is intact. No great artery arises from the infundibulum above the RV. (F) The heart and lungs, viewed from the front, showing the opened coronary arteries. From the apex of the opened RV, a fistula communicates with the anterior descending coronary artery *(Anterior Descending)*. The single right coronary artery *(Single Coronary Artery)* also gives rise to the right coronary artery *(Right Coronary)* and to the left circumflex coronary artery *(Circumflex Coronary)*. The lumen of the fistula was narrowed at the endocardial surface of the RV by the marked EFE. Here, the lumen of the fistula barely accommodated a 1-mm probe. It looked as though the fistula was undergoing occlusion by the EFE. (G) A left lateral view of the opened LA, mitral valve *(MV)*, and the left ventricular inflow tract. In the left atrial septal surface, the upper opening is the PFO, and the lower larger opening is the surgically created ASD (a Blalock-Hanlon procedure).

Continued

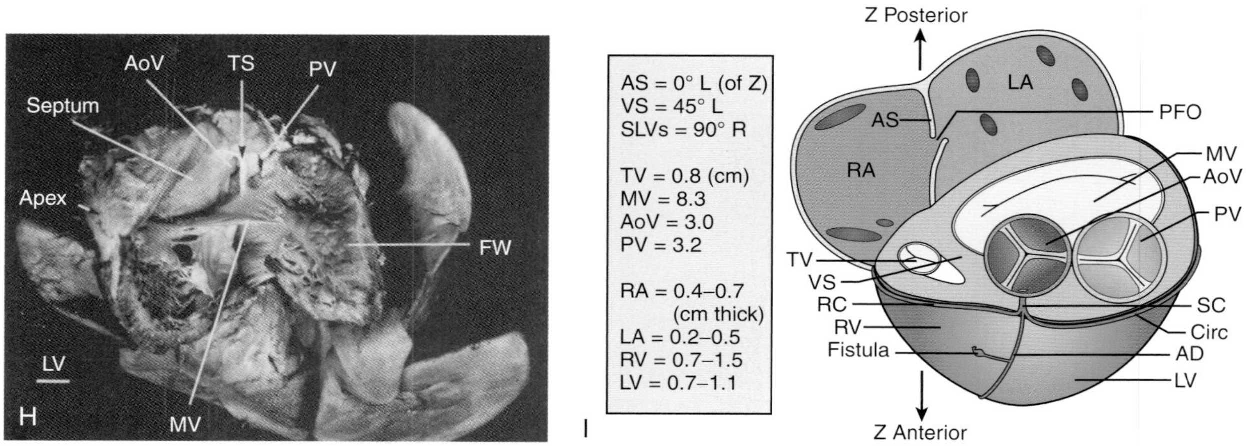

Fig. 24.4, cont'd (H) An apical view of the opened LV showing the intact ventricular septum *(Septum)*, the left ventricular free wall *(FW)*, the left ventricular apex *(Apex)*, the unobstructed outflow tracts to the aortic valve *(AoV)* to the right, and to the pulmonary valve *(PV)* to the left, the fibroelastic truncal (or aortopulmonary) septum *(TS)* between the AoV and the PV, and the direct fibrous continuity between the AoV and the anterior leaflet of the MV, and between the PV and anterior leaflet of the MV. The absence of subarterial infundibular muscle was confirmed by 111 serial histologic sections between the semilunar valves above and the anterior leaflet of the MV below. (I) A geometric horizontal plane diagram of the heart. The atrial septum *(AS)* was in the anteroposterior plane or Z axis. The atrial septal angle was 0 degrees relative to the Z axis. The ventricular septal *(VS)* angle was 45 degrees to the left of Z. The semilunar valve angle was 90 degrees to the right of Z. The valve circumferences were TV, 8 mm; MV, 83 mm; AoV, 30 mm; and PV, 32 mm. FW thicknesses were RA, 4 to 7 mm; LA, 2 to 5 mm; RV, 7 to 15 mm; and LV, 7 to 11 mm. A fistula connects the apex of the RV cavity with the anterior descending *(AD)* branch of the single coronary *(SC)* artery. The SC artery was the anterior coronary artery, which normally would have been the right coronary artery. The posterior coronary arterial ostium, which normally would have been the left coronary arterial ostium, was absent. "Single coronary artery" really means that one coronary arterial *ostium* is absent. All of the *branches* of both coronary arteries typically are present. Both the AoV and the PV are in direct fibrous continuity with the MV. The atretic infundibulum is above the RV, and both great arteries are above the LV. There is **total anatomic dissociation of the infundibulum (in E) from the great arteries (in H)**, a rare anomaly. *SLV,* Single left ventricle. (Reproduced with permission from Paul MH, Muster AJ, Sinha SN, Cole RB, Van Praagh R. Double-outlet left ventricle with an intact ventricular septum: clinical and autopsy diagnosis and developmental implications. *Circulation*. 1970;41:129.)

The opened right ventricular infundibulum (see Fig. 24.4E) shows that there is infundibular atresia *(Blind RV Out)*. The parietal band (PB), the septal band *(SB)*, and the moderator band *(MB)* are identified.

The opened coronary arteries are shown in Fig. 24.4F. The single right coronary artery gives origin to the right coronary artery, the anterior descending coronary artery, and the left circumflex coronary artery. The left coronary ostium was absent. A fistula connects the apex of the RV with the anterior descending coronary artery, as is seen in Fig. 24.5.

The opened left atrium *(LA)*, mitral valve (not labeled), and left ventricular inflow tract *(LV)* are shown in Fig, 24.4G).

A view of the opened LV from the apex shows (see Fig. 24.4H) the intact ventricular septum, the unopened aortic valve *(AoV)*, the unopened pulmonary valve *(PV)*, the truncal septum *(TS)*, or aortopulmonary septum that extended 3 mm below the semilunar valves and demarcated the separation between the aortic and the pulmonary outflow tracts. There was aortic-mitral direct fibrous continuity and pulmonary-mitral fibrous continuity between both semilunar valves above (AoV and PV) and the anterior leaflet of the mitral valve *(MV)* below. There was no infundibular musculature beneath either semilunar valve, or in the fibroelastic truncal septum *(TS)*, either grossly or histologically.

More than 1000 serial sections were done of the tissue between both semilunar valves and the anterior mitral leaflet and of the 3 mm septum *(TS)* extending down between and beneath the semilunar valves, searching microscopically for infundibular musculature. None was found grossly or histologically. Consequently, there was direct fibrous continuity between the aortic and mitral valves and between the pulmonary and mitral valves. The 3 mm septum *(TS)* was identified as the aortopulmonary (or truncal) septum, not as a remnant of the infundibular (or conal) septum.

A geometric horizontal plane diagram of this heart specimen is presented in Fig. 24.4I. Cardiac geometry (measured in degrees relative to the Z axis or anteroposterior plane): The atrial septum *(AS)* measured 0 degrees; hence, the atrial septum lay in the anteroposterior plane. The ventricular septum *(VS)* was 45 degrees to the left of the sagittal plane. The semilunar valves were rotated 90 degrees to the right relative to the anteroposterior plane. Consequently, the semilunar valves were side-by-side, with the aortic valve to the right of the pulmonary valve.

Valve circumferences, in centimeters, are given in the middle of the *left panel:* tricuspid valve, 0.8 cm; mitral valve, 8.3 cm; aortic valve, 3.0 cm; and pulmonary valve, 3.2 cm. The circumference of the hypoplastic tricuspid valve was only 9.6% of that

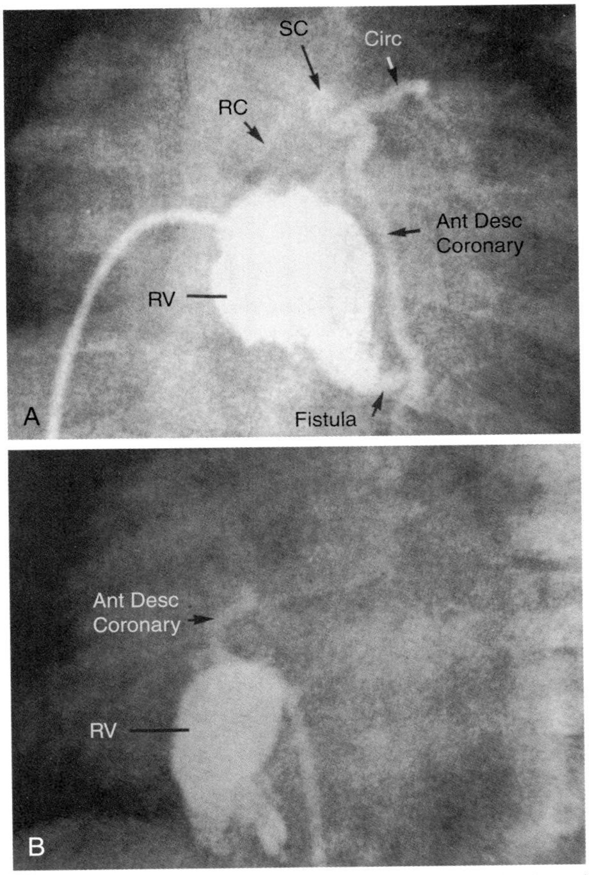

Fig. 24.5 Selective right ventricular injection, patient of Paul et al.[1] (A) Posteroanterior projection. (B) simultaneous left lateral projection. The right ventricle *(RV)* is small-chambered, with no great arterial outflow tract, that is, apparent infundibular atresia, and no ventricular septal defect. There is a fistula from the RV apex that communicates with the anterior descending coronary artery *(Ant Desc Coronary)*. Surprisingly, the contrast went in a retrograde direction *up* the anterior descending coronary artery to the ostium of the single right coronary ostium *(SC)*, and contrast also opacified the right coronary artery *(RC)* and the left circumflex coronary artery *(Circ)*. (Reproduced with permission from Paul MH, Muster AJ, Sinha SN, Cole RB, Van Praagh R. Double-outlet left ventricle with an intact ventricular septum: clinical and autopsy diagnosis and developmental implications. *Circulation.* 1970;41:129.[1])

of the mitral valve. The pulmonary valve's circumference was 6.7% greater than that of the aortic valve.

Thicknesses of the atrial and ventricular free walls are given, in centimeters, in the bottom third of the left panel of Fig. 24.4I: The right atrium *(RA)* varied from 0.4 to 0.7 cm in thickness. The left atrial *(LA)* free wall thickness varied from 0.2 to 0.5 cm. The right ventricular *(RV)* free wall thickness varied from 0.7 to 1.5 cm. The left ventricular *(LV)* free wall thickness varied from 0.7 to 1.1 cm.

DISCUSSION

This was our first encounter with DOLV and it taught us a lot.

The Paul type of DOLV[1] is the opposite of the Taussig-Bing malformation.[6] In the Taussig-Bing anomaly, the right-sided subaortic infundibulum and the left-sided subpulmonary infundibulum both remain well developed, which prevents any embryonic arterial switch from above the RV to above the LV. Neither the aorta, nor the pulmonary artery can be switched and come into close proximity with the mitral valve because of the subvalvar well-developed infundibula. Consequently, in the Taussig-Bing malformation, both the aorta and the pulmonary artery remain unswitched. This results in DORV, with both great arteries side-by-side, aortic valve to the right, pulmonary valve to the left, both semilunar valves at about the same height, both sitting high on the well-developed subvalvar infundibula, and both anterior above the anterior and right-sided RV.

What happens in the Paul type of DOLV[1] is the opposite. Both the subaortic and the subpulmonary infundibula undergo resorption (or fail to form). Because there is no subaortic and no subpulmonary infundibulum, both great arteries can sink inferiorly and posteriorly. Both semilunar valves pass through the interventricular foramen and come into direct fibrous continuity with the mitral valve. So now the semilunar valves sit side-by-side, aortic valve to the right, pulmonary valve to the left, and both valves at about the same height—both equally low and both equally posterior, above the posterior and left-sided LV. Thus, in the Paul type of DOLV, a double embryonic arterial switch is performed because there is no infundibulum beneath either great artery.

But the infundibulum is not absent; for reasons unknown, the infundibulum has become detached from beneath both great arteries. There is enough infundibulum to close the interventricular foramen; hence, there is no VSD. But this *ectopic infundibulum* remains above the anterior and right-sided RV, with no great artery for attachment. So, the ectopic, isolated right ventricular infundibulum fuses with itself, resulting in right ventricular outflow tract atresia.

Based on the anatomic findings, this appears to be what happened developmentally to produce the rare Paul type of DOLV.[1]

Note that when the subarterial infundibular development is bilaterally symmetrical, equally well developed (Taussig-Bing) or equally poorly developed (Paul), in both cases the semilunar valves are side-by-side (90-degree dextrorotation, the effect of D-loop formation only) and at about the same height, because of the bilateral symmetry of the subaorta and the sub–pulmonary artery infundibular development.

Growth and resorption of the subarterial infundibular free walls are *both* important in determining embryonic morphogenetic movements of the great arteries. This is why we speak of subarterial infundibular free wall *development*. Development includes both growth and resorption.

By 1970,[1] we knew that there are five important cardiac segments, that is, that from a developmental and an anatomic standpoint, the heart is a "five-story house":

1. the viscera and atria;
2. the atrioventricular canal or junction;
3. the ventricular loop;
4. the infundibulum or conus arteriosus; and
5. the great arteries or truncus arteriosus.

Another way of putting it is that there are three *main* cardiac segments {viscera and atria, ventricles, great arteries} and there are two *connecting* cardiac segments—the atrioventricular canal or junction and the infundibulum or conus arteriosus.

The atrioventricular (AV) canal or junction appears to be a **dependent variable.** The morphology of the AV canal typically corresponds to that of the ventricles of entry, not to that of the atria of exit.

The other four cardiac segments appear to be **independent variables.** For example, the subarterial infundibulum can be beneath either great artery or beneath neither great artery (as we have just seen[1]). Similarly, the subarterial infundibulum can be above either ventricle or above both ventricles.

The above described case of Dr. Milton H. Paul et al[1] was the first clinically diagnosed and autopsy-proved case of DOLV.

It is now my privilege to present to you a summary of what is now known about DOLV, based on 109 well-documented cases, representing 26 different anatomic types of patients with DOLV.

Given the rarity of DOLV mentioned in the introduction, you may well wonder, "How is it possible to present such a large series of this truly rare form of congenital heart disease?" The answer is friends and colleagues worldwide. When Drs. Forrest H. Adams, George C. Emmanouilides, and Thomas A. Riemenschneider, the editors of the fourth edition of *Moss' Heart Disease in Infants, Children, and Adolescents,* which was published in 1989 asked me and my colleagues to write a chapter for the upcoming edition of their book, I decided to try to do so, with the help of friends and colleagues.[2] In fact, the book story began with their third edition, which was published in 1977. Dr. Arthur J. Moss and I were at a meeting together. I was telling Dr. Moss about Dr. Milt Paul's case of DOLV. As soon as I had finished, with a huge smile, Dr. Moss said, "Thank you for agreeing to write this up as a chapter for our book!" So that is how this much larger study really began. Before presenting the data, I would like to thank the many friends and colleagues who made this large study possible: Alan B. Gazzaniga, MD, Donald R. Sperling, MD, and Marshall Rowen, MD, Medical Center, University of California, Irvine, and Children's Hospital and St. Joseph's Hospital, Orange, CA; Teruo Izukawa, MD, Hospital for Sick Children, Toronto, Canada; Billy Hightower, MD, and Jerry D. Jordan, MD, Mobile General Hospital, Mobile, AL; A. Louise Calder, MD, Peter W. T. Brandt, MD, Sir Brian G. Barratt-Boyes, MD, and John M. Neutze, MD, Green Lane Hospital, Auckland, New Zealand; K. Diane Vaughan, MD, and Neil Finer, MD, Royal Alexandra Hospital, Edmonton, Canada; William W. Miller, MD, and Arthur G. Weinberg, MD, Children's Medical Center of Dallas, Dallas, TX; Ina Bhan, MD, Marshall B. Kreidberg, MD, and M. A. Ali Khan, MD, New England Medical Center Hospital, Boston, MA; Carlos Lozano-Sainz; MD, Joaquin Simon-Lamuela, MD, José M. Revuelta, MD, and José M. Arqué, MD, Clinical Infantil "Francisco Franco," Barcelona, Spain; Dominique Metras, MD, Hôpital de Treichville, Abidjan, Ivory Coast, Africa; Manuel Quero Jimenez, MD, Ciudad Sanitaria de la Seguridad Social "La Paz," Madrid, Spain; Milton H. Paul, MD, and Alex J. Muster, MD, Children's Memorial Hospital, Chicago, IL; and Kareem Minhas, MD.

ANATOMIC TYPES OF DOUBLE-OUTLET LEFT VENTRICLE

Table 24.1 summarizes the anatomic findings in 109 patients with DOLV that may be divided into 26 different anatomic types. Thus, in 109 autopsied cases of DOLV, 26 different anatomic types of DOLV were found (Table 24.1 and Fig. 24.6). Now we shall analyze the data.

ONE GOOD VENTRICLE HEART

One of the more surprising findings was that more than half of the 26 anatomic types of DOLV had only one anatomically normal ventricle, always the LV: 14 of 26 anatomic types of DOLV (54%) (see Table 24.1). The other 12 anatomic types of DOLV did have two normal appearing ventricles (46%).

One normal-appearing-ventricle heart with DOLV included the following (see Table 24.1):

1. tricuspid atresia, 20 cases;
2. Ebstein's anomaly, 3 cases;
3. double-inlet single LV, with absence of the right ventricular sinus or inflow tract, 3 cases;
4. common-inlet single LV, with absence of the right ventricular sinus, 1 case;
5. mitral atresia with large LV, and with absence of the right ventricular sinus, 1 case (0.9%); and
6. thick-walled, small-chambered RV with infundibular outflow tract atresia and intact ventricular septum, 1 case (0.9%).

SEGMENTAL ANATOMY

Nine different kinds of segmental anatomy were found in these 109 cases of DOLV (see Table 24.1):

1. DOLV {S,D,D} in 67 cases (61%);
2. DOLV {S,D,L} in 30 cases (28%);
3. DOLV {S,L,L}, 4 cases (4%);
4. DOLV {I,L,L}, 2 cases (2%);
5. DOLV {I,D,D}, 2 cases (2%);
6. DOLV {I,L,D}, 1 case (1%);
7. DOLV {S,D,A}, 1 case (1%);
8. DOLV {S,D,L (I)}, 1 case (1%); and
9. DOLV {A,?D,L}, 1 case (1%).

Thus, DOLV is characterized by considerable segmental anatomic variability.

INFUNDIBULUM

The anatomic types of subarterial infundibulum (or conus arteriosus), in order of decreasing frequency, were as follows:
bilateral absence, 8 of 26 (31%);
bilateral presence, 6 of 26 (23%);
short subpulmonary, 6 of 26 (23%); and
short subaortic, 6 of 26 (23%).

Bilateral absence of the infundibulum means no subpulmonary and subaortic infundibulum. **Bilateral presence of the infundibulum** means that both the subpulmonary infundibulum and the subaortic infundibulum are present.

EMBRYONIC MORPHOGENETIC MOVEMENTS OF THE GREAT ARTERIES

Now it is time to take another very careful look at the diagrams of Fig. 24.6, which were drawn with care from heart specimens, bearing in mind the following principles:

1. A well-developed muscular subsemilunar infundibulum prevents the embryonic arterial switch, as in the Taussig-Bing malformation.[6,7]

TABLE 24.1 Anatomic Types of Double-Outlet Left Ventricle (n = 109)

Two Functional Ventricles and Subaortic VSD

Anatomic Types

1. DOLV {S,D,D} with short subpulmonary infundibulum, subaortic VSD, no PS: 2 cases (1.8%), Fig. 24.6 (1).
2. DOLV {S,D,D} with short subpulmonary infundibulum, subaortic VSD, PS: 29 cases (26.6%), Fig. 24.6 (2).
3. DOLV {S,D,D} with bilaterally absent infundibulum, subaortic VSD, aortic stenosis, preductal coarctation: 4 cases (3.7%), Fig. 24.6 (3).
4. DOLV {S,D,L} with short subaortic infundibulum, subaortic VSD, PS: 18 cases (16.5%), Fig. 24.6 (4).

Two Ventricles, Subpulmonary VSD

5. DOLV {S,D,D} with short subpulmonary infundibulum, subpulmonary VSD, no PS, no AS: 1 case (0.9%), Fig. 24.6 (5).
6. DOLV {S,D,D}with short subpulmonary infundibulum, subpulmonary VSD, PS: 2 cases (1.8%), Fig. 24.6 (6).
7. DOLV {S,D,D} with short subpulmonary infundibulum, subpulmonary VSD, AS: 8 cases (7.3%), Fig. 24.6 (7).

Two Ventricles, Doubly Committed VSD

8. DOLV {S,D,D} with bilaterally absent infundibulum, double committed VSD, no PS, ± AS: 7 cases (6.4%), Fig. 24.6 (8).

Two Ventricles, Subaortic VSD, Situs Inversus

9. DOLV {I,L,L} with short subpulmonary infundibulum, subaortic VSD, PS: 2 Cases (1.8%), Fig. 24.6 (9).
10. DOLV {I,L,D} with subaortic infundibulum, subaortic VSD, PS: 1 case (0.9%), Fig. 24.6 (10).

Two Ventricles, Subaortic VSD, Atrioventricular Discordance

11. DOLV {S,L,L} with subaortic infundibulum, subaortic VSD, ± PS, ± pulmonary atresia: 4 cases (3.7%), Fig. 24.6 (11).
12. DOLV {I,D,D} with bilateral absence of the infundibulum, subaortic VSD, PS: 2 (1.8%), Fig. 24.6 (12).

One Well-Developed Ventricle, Intact Ventricular Septum

13. DOLV {S,D,D} with absence of the infundibulum beneath both great arteries, no VSD, no PS, no AS, imperforate infundibulum above thick-walled and small-chambered RV with RV outflow tract atresia, fistula between hypertensive RV and left anterior descending coronary artery, absent left coronary ostium resulting in "single" right coronary artery, left ventricular hypertrophy and enlargement: 1 case (0.9%), Fig. 24.6 (13).

One Ventricle, Subaortic Defect

14. DOLV {S,D,D} with subaortic and subpulmonary infundibula, tricuspid atresia with absence of the RV sinus or inflow tract and with an IOC, subaortic defect between IOC and LV, no PS, no AS: 3 (2.8%), Fig. 24.6 (14).
15. DOLV {S,D,D} with bilaterally absent infundibulum, tricuspid atresia, subaortic defect between the IOC and the LV, PS, atretic proximal left pulmonary artery: 1 case (0.9%), Fig. 24.6 (15).
16. DOLV {S,D,A} with subaortic infundibulum, tricuspid atresia, subaortic defect, no PS, no AS: 1 case (0.9%), Fig. 24.6 (16).
17. DOLV {S,D,L} with subaortic infundibulum, tricuspid atresia, subaortic defect between the IOC and the LV, ± PS: 10 cases (9.2%), Fig. 24.6 (17).

One Ventricle, Subpulmonary Defect

18. DOLV {S,D,D} with bilateral absence of the infundibulum, tricuspid atresia, subpulmonary defect between the IOC and the LV, ± AS, preductal coarctation, ± PDA: 3 cases (2.8%), Fig. 24.6 (18).

One Ventricle, Noncommitted Defect

19. DOLV {S,D,L} with bilateral infundibulum, tricuspid atresia, noncommitted muscular defect, PS: 1 case (0.9%), Fig. 24.6 (19).
20. DOLV {S,DL(I)} with bilaterally absent infundibulum, tricuspid atresia, noncommitted defect between IOC and LV, PS: 1 case (0.9%), Fig. 24.6 (20).

One Functional Ventricle, the LV, and Ebstein Anomaly

21. DOLV {S,D,D} with bilaterally absent infundibulum, Ebstein anomaly of the tricuspid valve and RV, subaortic VSD, PS: 1 case (0.9%), Fig. 24.6 (21).
22. DOLV {S,D,D} with bilateral infundibulum, Ebstein anomaly, subpulmonary VSD, AS, preductal coarctation, PDA: 1 case (0.9%), Fig. 24.6 (22).
23. DOLV {S,D,L} with bilateral infundibulum, Ebstein anomaly, subpulmonary VSD, no PS, subvalvar AS, preductal coarctation, PDA, mild mitral stenosis, well-developed LV: 1 case (0.9%), Fig. 24.6 (23).

Single LV With Mitral Atresia

24. DOLV {S,D,D} with bilateral infundibulum, mitral atresia, large LV, absent RV sinus with IOC, subaortic defect, subvalvar AS, preductal coarctation: 1 case (0.9%), Fig. 24.6 (24).

Double-Inlet Single LV

25. DOLV {S,D,D} with subaortic infundibulum, double-inlet single LV, absent RV sinus with IOC, subaortic defect, ± cleft mitral valve: 3 cases (2.5%), Fig. 24.6 (25).

Asplenia Syndrome With Single LV

26. DOLV {A,?D,L} with bilateral infundibulum, heterotaxy syndrome with visceroatrial situs ambiguus and asplenia, common atrium, common AV valve, common-inlet single LV, absence of right ventricular sinus with infundibular outlet chamber (IOC), PS: 1 case (0.9%), Fig. 24.6 (26).

AS, Atrial stenosis; *DOLV,* double-outlet left ventricle; *IOC,* infundibular outlet chamber; *LV,* left ventricle; *PS,* pulmonary stenosis; *RV,* right ventricle; *VSD,* ventricular septal defect.

2. Marked hypoplasia or absence of the muscular subsemilunar infundibulum permits the embryonic arterial switch from above the RV to above the LV. In Fig. 24.6 (1), the subaortic infundibulum is absent; so the aorta *(Ao)* is normally switched. The subpulmonary infundibulum is very short (hypoplastic), so the pulmonary artery *(PA)* is also switched into the LV.

In Fig. 24.6 (2), the same is true, except that the very hypoplastic subpulmonary infundibulum is also stenotic. Fig. 24.6 (3), there is bilateral absence of both subarterial infundibula. So both great arteries are switched into the LV. In Fig. 24.6 (4), there was no subpulmonary infundibulum; consequently there was pulmonary-to-mitral fibrous continuity. There was also pulmonary outflow tract stenosis. The short and deficient subaortic infundibulum narrowly separated the L-malposed aortic valve from the mitral valve, resulting in DOLV, and also narrowed the subpulmonary outflow tract and the pulmonary annulus, resulting in pulmonary outflow tract stenosis.

Even more interesting are Figs. 24.6 (5, 6, and 7). As you will see, I recorded each of these types of DOLV as having a subpulmonary infundibulum, which is correct. But look at these subpulmonary infundibula. They are all low. They are not subvalvar. There is nothing beneath these pulmonary valve leaflets. The infundibular septum is usually described as being composed of proximal, middle, and distal conal cushions. The proximal conal cushions (the lowest ones) are present. But the middle and definitely the distal (or uppermost) conal cushions are absent.

Hence, these partial subpulmonary infundibula also may be viewed as having **distal, subpulmonary infundibular septal defects.** Absence of subvalvar infundibular tissue facilitates pulmonary–mitral fibrous continuity, which in turn results in DOLV as long as the aorta is normal. So, a subpulmonary VSD is a distal conal septal defect, that is, a partial infundibular septal defect.

Fig. 24.6 (8) depicts bilateral (subaortic and subpulmonary) infundibular absence that permits embryonic arterial switches of both great arteries, resulting in DOLV. Fig. 24.6 (9) shows a very short and stenotic subpulmonary infundibulum that narrowly separates the pulmonary valve from the mitral valve. There is no subaortic infundibulum, hence aortic-mitral fibrous continuity. Thus, both great arteries were switched into the LV. Fig. 24.6 (10) has a short subaortic conus and no subpulmonary infundibulum. Consequently, the pulmonary artery has been switched into the LV and there is pulmonary-mitral fibrous

Text continues on page 935

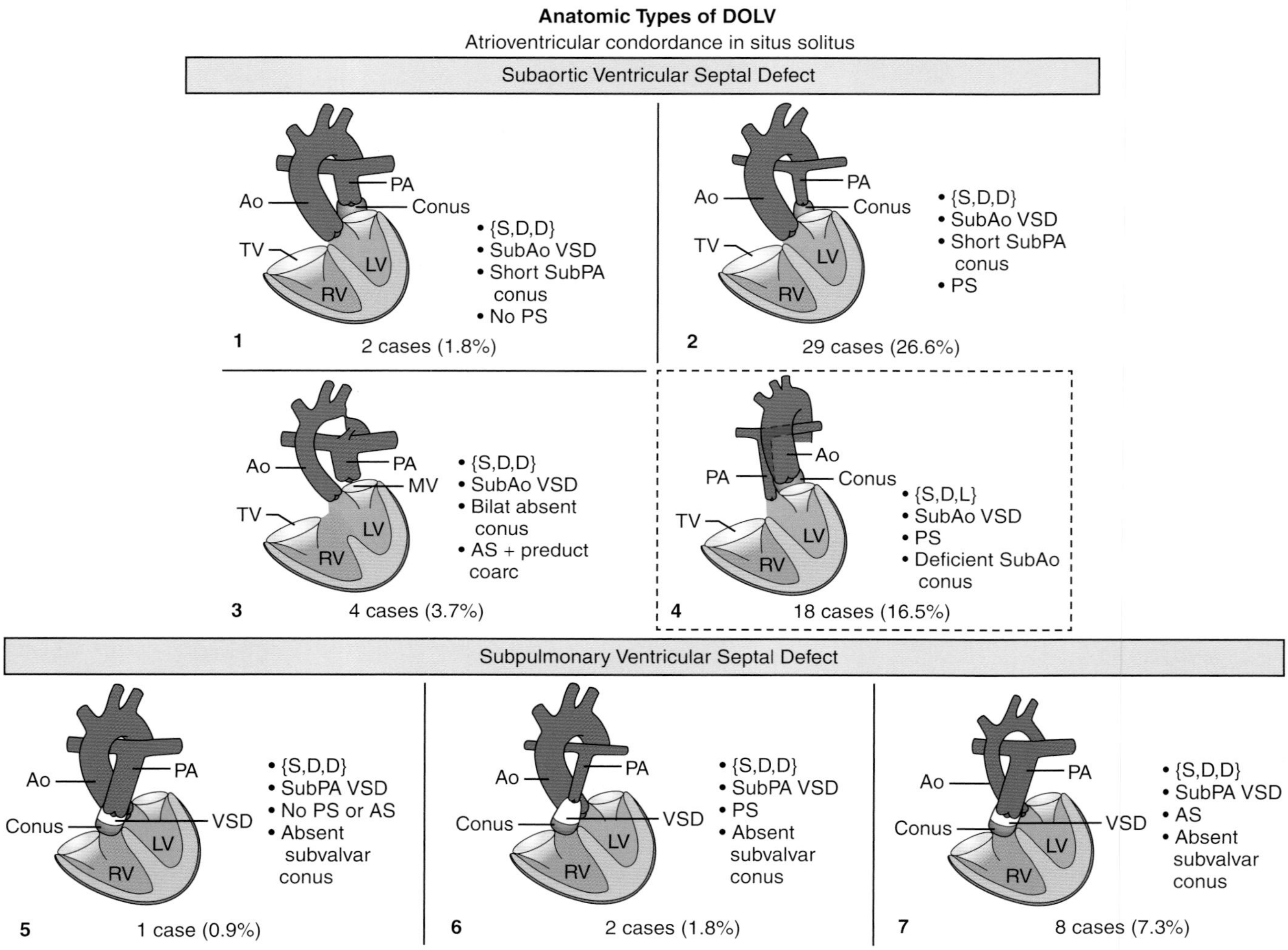

Fig. 24.6 (A–D) Diagrams of 26 different anatomic types of direct-outlet left ventricle (DOLV) found in 109 cases[2] are presented. The diagrams are self-explanatory. Each anatomic type of DOLV is also presented and discussed in Tables 24.1 and 24.2. The first 12 anatomic types of DOLV have two well-developed ventricles (types 1 to 12 inclusive). The last 14 anatomic types of DOLV have only one well-developed ventricle, always the left ventricle *(LV)* (types 13 to 26, inclusive). *Ao,* Aorta; *Bilat,* bilateral; *AS,* atrial septum; *CA,* common atrium; *Coarc,* coarctation; *Inf,* inferior; *IOC,* infundibular outlet chamber; *GAs,* great arteries; *LA,* left atrium; *LV,* left ventricle; *MS,* mitral stenosis; *MV,* mitral valve; *PA,* pulmonary artery; *P At,* pulmonary atresia; *PDA,* patent ductus arteriosus; *PS,* pulmonary stenosis; *SubAo,* subaortic; *SubPA,* subpulmonary (valvar); *Subvalv,* subvalvar; *RA,* right atrium; *RV,* right ventricle; *TV,* tricuspid valve; *TV At,* tricuspid valve atresia; *VS,* ventricular septum; *VSD,* ventricle septal defect. (Reproduced with permission from Van Praagh R, Weinberg PM, Srebro JP. Double-outlet left ventricle. In: Adams FH, Emmanouilides GC, Riemenschneider TA, eds. *Moss' Heart Disease in Infants, Children, and Adolescents.* 4th ed. Baltimore, MD: Williams & Wilkins; 1989;461.)

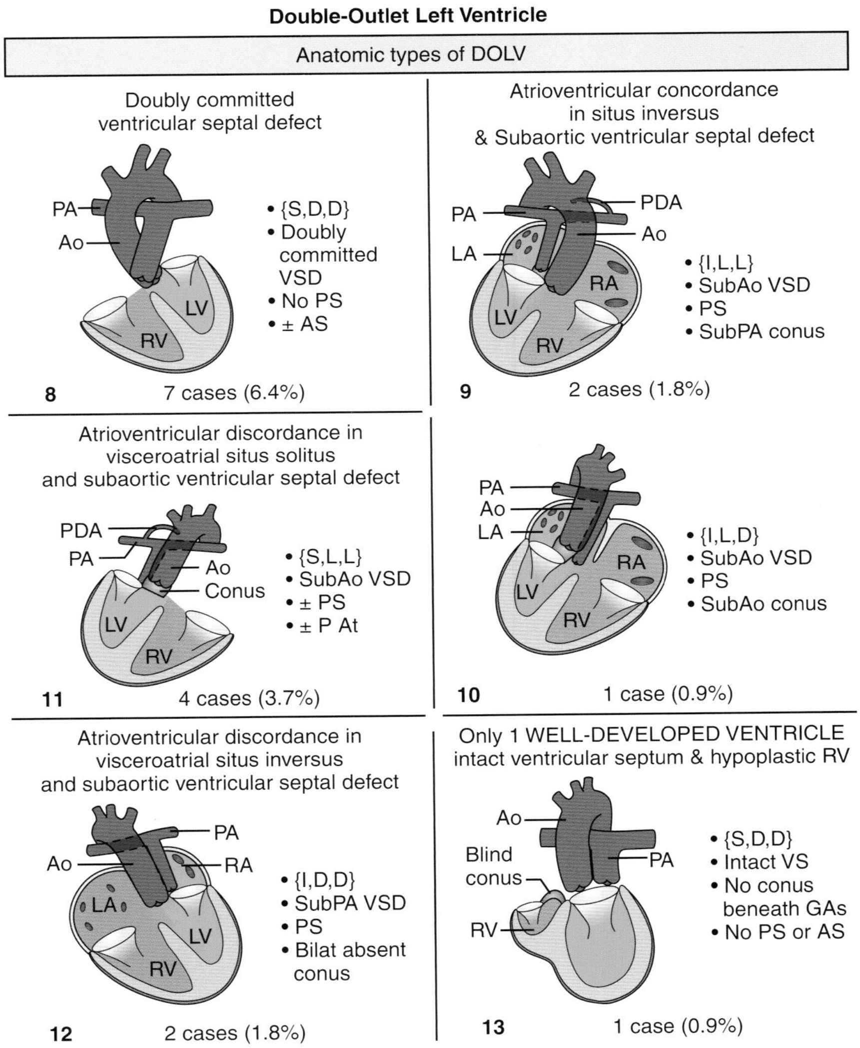

Fig. 24.6, cont'd

(Continued)

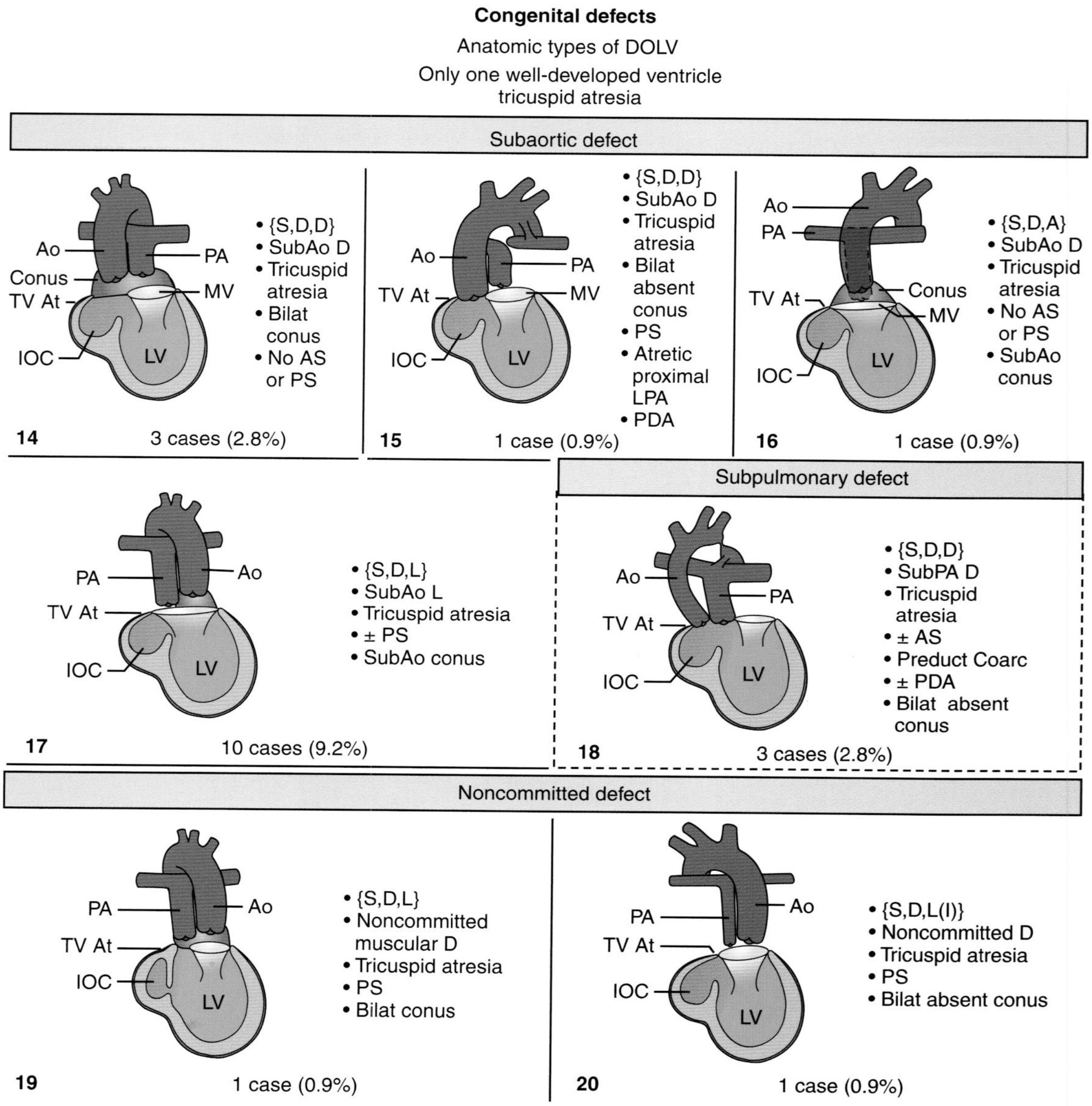

Fig. 24.6, cont'd

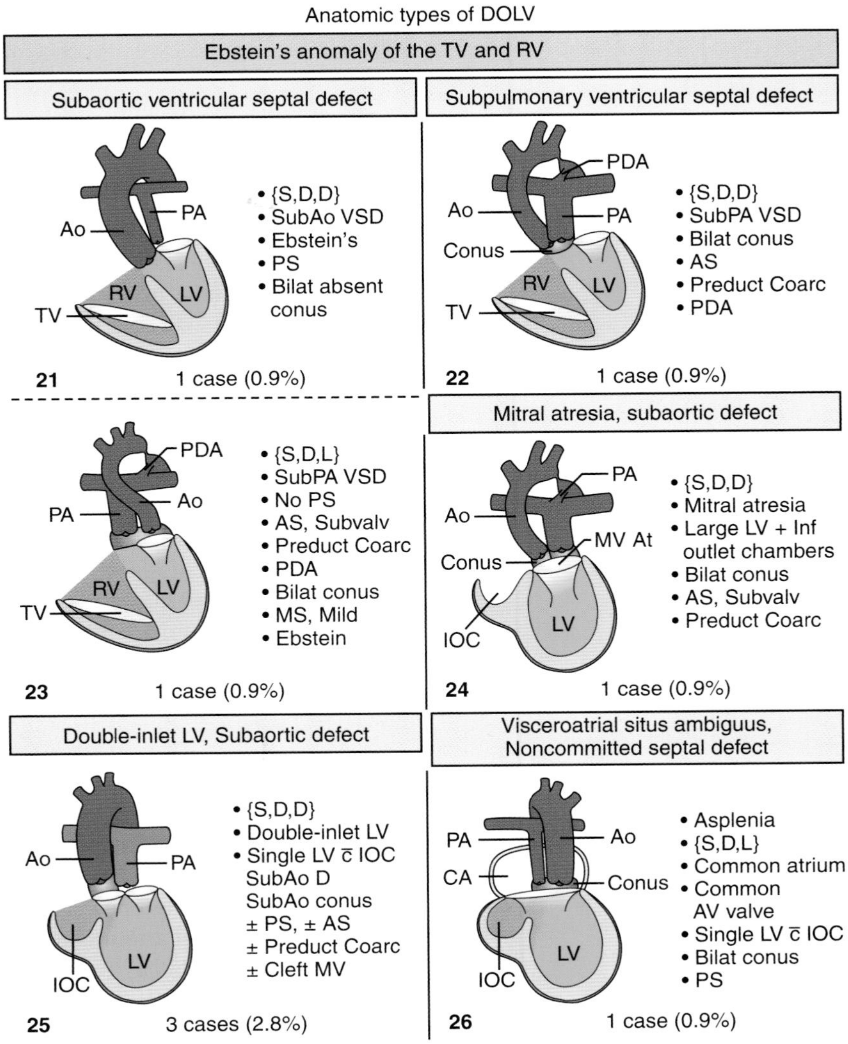

Fig. 24.6, cont'd

continuity. The D-malposed aortic valve is narrowly separated from the mitral valve. Hence, DOLV is present.

The function of the subarterial infundibulum is to block or to facilitate the embryonic arterial switch procedure. The Taussig-Bing malformation illustrates what happens when both the subaortic infundibulum and the subpulmonary infundibulum both remain well developed, and resorption of neither infundibular free wall occurs. The persistence of a well-developed subaortic infundibular free wall blocks the embryonic aortic switch. The persistence of a well-developed subpulmonary infundibular free wall prevents the embryonic pulmonary arterial switch. The persistence of a well-developed subsemilunar infundibular free wall blocks semilunar valve–to–mitral valve spatial approximation. Hence, the Taussig-Bing malformation is characterized by DORV because both great arteries are prevented from undergoing an embryonic arterial switch. By contrast, in DOLV, both great arteries undergo an embryonic RV to LV switch because both subarterial infundibular free walls are absent, or very poorly developed, thereby facilitating a double great arterial switch.

These principles are exemplified by all of the DOLV diagrams (see Table 24.1). Subsemilunar infundibular free wall development may be quantified as follows:

Absent	Grade 0
Very poorly developed	Grade 1
Poorly developed	Grade 2
Mildly underdeveloped	Grade 3
Well developed	Grade 4

Table 24.2 suggests that when two well-developed ventricles are present, (anatomic types 1 to 12, inclusive), *infundibular* development is very important in the morphogenesis of DOLV, as explained earlier.

But when two well-developed ventricles are *not* present (anatomic types 13 to 26 inclusive), then *ventricular* factors become much more important in the anatomy and morphogenesis of DOLV. In the one good ventricle group, the average grade of infundibular development was 3.43: 48/14

TABLE 24.2 Development of Infundibulum in Double-Outlet Left Ventricle

Diagram Number	Infundibular Development	SubAo	SubPA
1		0	2
2		0	1
3		0	0
4		2	0
5		0	0
6		0	0
7		0	0
8		0	0
9		0	1
10		2	0
11		1	0
12		1	0
13	Small RV	0	0
14	TAt	4	4
15	TAt	0	0
16	TAt	4	0
17	TAt	3	0
18	TAt	0	0
19	TAt	3	3
20	TAt	0	0
21	Ebstein	0	0
22	Ebstein	2	2
23	Ebstein	3	3
24	MAt, large LV	3	3
25	DILV	3	0
26	Asplenia	4	4

DILV, Double-inlet left ventricle; *LV,* left ventricle; *MAt,* mitral atresia; *RV,* right ventricle; *SubAo,* subaortic; *SubPA,* subpulmonary valvar; *TAt,* tricuspid atresia.

= 3.43 (see Table 24.2). When two good ventricles were present, the average grade of infundibular development was 0.83.

$$\frac{10}{12} = 0.83$$

$$\frac{3.48}{83} = 4.13$$

In other words, when two good ventricles were not present, but DOLV was present, the average grade of infundibular development was more than four times as high (4.13/1.0) as when two good ventricles were associated with DOLV. In other words, when the RV sinus was hypoplastic or absent (as with tricuspid atresia, or double-inlet single LV), or when the RV sinus was dysplastic (as with Ebstein anomaly), then a diagnosis of DOLV is more likely to be made for ventricular reasons than because the infundibulum was very hypoplastic or absent. These are two different anatomic types of DOLV (see Table 24.1).

DISCUSSION

DOLV is a rare group of anomalies. The first clinically diagnosed and autopsy proved case was published by Paul et al[1] in 1970. The findings in 109 cases of DOLV[2] are presented (see Table 24.1), diagrammed (see Fig. 24.6), and discussed (see Table 24.2).

The importance of embryonic great arterial switches is emphasized. By 22 to 24 days after conception, ventricular D-loop formation normally has occurred. Both developing great arteries are located above the developing RV, aorta to the right and pulmonary artery to the left. Normally, the subaortic infundibular free wall undergoes involution. It disappears, it is thought, because of apoptosis (programmed cell death). The aortic valve moves inferiorly, posteriorly, and leftward. It passes through the interventricular foramen and comes into direct fibrous continuity with the mitral valve via the intervalvar fibrosa. The ascending aorta has been switched from above the RV to above the left ventricular cavity and above the muscular interventricular septum.

The subpulmonary infundibular free wall normally persists, grows, and develops. The left-sided subpulmonary valve, sitting atop the left-sided half of the infundibulum, moves superiorly, anteriorly, and rightward, above the RV. Normally, only the aorta is switched. The pulmonary artery is not. The normal morphogenetic movements of the semilunar valves are reciprocals: the aortic valve moves inferiorly, posteriorly, and leftward; the pulmonary valve moves superiorly, anteriorly, and rightward. The normal morphogenetic movements of the pulmonary artery not only keep the pulmonary artery above the RV. They also move the pulmonary valve and the pulmonary artery away from the interventricular foramen, getting the pulmonary artery "out of the way," thereby facilitating the aortic switch.

When two well-developed ventricles are present, DOLV can occur if both great arteries are switched, that is, if not only the subaortic infundibular free wall is resorbed completely or almost completely but also if the subpulmonary infundibular free wall also is resorbed completely or almost completely. Then both great arteries undergo the same morphogenetic movements that, normally, only the aorta does. A double great arterial switch occurs—aorta and main pulmonary artery—resulting in DOLV.

Thus, when two well-developed ventricles are present, DOLV can occur from infundibular maldevelopment: complete or nearly complete resorption of the subaortic and of the subpulmonary infundibular free wall myocardium (see Table 24.1, anatomic types 1 to 12, inclusive).

However, when two well-developed ventricles are *not* present (see Table 24.1, anatomic types 13 to 26 inclusive), which may involve the presence of tricuspid atresia, Ebstein anomaly, or single LV, the diagnosis of DOLV can be made accurately when an LV is the only normal ventricle the patient has.

Thus, when two well-developed ventricles are present, the diagnosis of DOLV typically is made for "infundibular reasons" that lead to an embryonic switch of both great arteries.

However, when the LV is the only normal ventricle that the patient has, because the RV is hypoplastic, dysplastic, or absent, then the diagnosis of DOLV can be made accurately for "ventricular reasons" that have nothing to do with infundibular free wall involution.

We are learning a lot about the infundibulum. We have known for a long time that one of the functions of the infundibulum (or conus arteriosus) is to connect the great arteries with the underlying ventricles and AV canal. That is why we refer to the infundibulum as a **connecting segment.**

But there is so much more to it than that.[8] **Infundibular development** decides whether the great arteries will be normally related.[9] The infundibulum is one of the *prime movers* of the great arteries. (Ventricular loop formation is another.) Infundibular development decides whether a great artery will be switched in embryo, or not. **The infundibulum is the embryonic "switch master":**

1. Aorta, switch; pulmonary artery, no switch. That is normally related great arteries.
2. Ao, no switch; PA, switch. That is transposition of the great arteries (TGA).
3. Ao, no switch, PA, no switch. That is the Taussig-Bing type of DORV.
4. Ao, switch; and PA, switch. That is DOLV. And so on.

Clinically, we still do not routinely and specifically diagnose the anatomic type of infundibulum that is present in every case. We should, in view of the enormous anatomic and embryologic importance of the infundibulum.

DOLV is just one example of how important it is to understand the functions of the infundibulum. In normally related great arteries, tetralogy of Fallot (TOF), TGA, DORV, and anatomically corrected malposition of the great arteries, the infundibulum plays other critically important roles.

How is it possible for the infundibulum to play so many important and different roles in cardiogenesis? It helps to understand that we are dealing with the cardiovascular keys to permanent air-breathing and land-living—with the epochal transition from aquatic to terrestrial living for vertebrates.[8]

One of the key cardiovascular evolutionary achievements was total right-left asymmetry in the development of the infundibulum or conus cordis. The right-sided subaortic infundibular free wall underwent total involution or resorption; it disappeared. The left-sided subpulmonary infundibular free wall grew and expanded well: SNRGA {S,D,S} = 0R + 4L.

This total asymmetry in the normal development of the subarterial infundibular free walls of the great arteries made possible the embryonic aortic RV-to-LV switch, and prevented the pulmonary arterial switch, thereby crossing the systemic venous and the pulmonary venous circulations and obtaining an optimal physiologic result.

The second key cardiovascular evolutionary adaptation to permanent air-breathing and land-living was the evolution of the morphologically right ventricular sinus (body or inflow tract) as the lung pump.

The foregoing list of conotruncal (or infundibuloarterial) anomalies indicates that we are still having trouble with our evolutionary adaptation to permanent air-breathing and land-living. Only the normal complete right-left infundibular developmental asymmetry works successfully: **0R + 4L,** which means grade zero development beneath the right-sided aorta and grade 4 development (normally good development) beneath the left-sided pulmonary artery.

All infundibuloarterial anomalies have a different infundibular developmental and anatomic formula:

$$\text{TOF }\{S,D,S\} = 0R + 1L \quad \textbf{Equation 24.1}$$

$$= 0R + 2L$$

$$= 0R + 3L$$

$$\text{TGA }\{S,D,D\} = 4R + 0L \quad \textbf{Equation 24.2}$$

$$\text{DORV }\{S,D,D\} = 4R + 4L \quad \textbf{Equation 24.3}$$

$$\text{DOLV }\{S,D,D\} = 0R + 0L, \text{ etc.}$$

Equation 24.4

None of the foregoing infundibuloarterial malformations has the same anatomic formula as solitus normally related great arteries (SNRGA) do: SNRGA {S,D,S} = 0R + 4L.

We have finally understood what the functions of the subarterial infundibulum are:

1. When the muscular subarterial infundibular free wall is well developed, the function of the infundibulum is to elevate the semilunar valve and great artery, to hold the great artery above the RV, and to prevent the embryonic switch of this great artery to the mitral valve and the LV. Examples are the normal pulmonary artery and the transposed aorta.
2. When the muscular subarterial infundibular free wall is resorbed and therefore absent, the function of the infundibulum is to lower the great artery and switch the great artery from above the RV to above the LV and to come into fibrous continuity with the mitral valve. Examples include the normally related aorta, and the transposed pulmonary artery.

Stated as briefly as possible, the presence of a well-developed subarterial infundibulum blocks the embryonic arterial switch; whereas the absence of a subarterial infundibulum facilitates the embryonic arterial switch.

It follows that DOLV with bilateral absence of the subarterial infundibulum, as in anatomic types 3, 5, 6, 7, and 8 (see Table 24.1 and Fig. 24.6) are anatomic and developmental opposites of the Taussig-Bing type of DORV. Please compare these two equations:

$$\text{DOLV }\{S,D,D\} = 0R + 0L, \text{ and}$$

Equation 24.3

$$\text{DORV }\{S,D,D\} = 4R + 4L$$

Equation 24.4

The evolutionary "trick" that Mother Nature (our genome) had to master is not an easy "trick" to perform: SNRGA {S,D,S} = 0R + RL.

The right and left halves of the subarterial infundibulum have to develop in opposite ways. The right half has to involute (disappear), and the left half has to develop well. So, the development of the subarterial infundibulum is normally characterized by complete right-left asymmetry[8,9]: SNRGA {S,D,S} = 0R + 4L.

TOF is a **subnormality,** that is, underdevelopment of the subpulmonary infundibulum, of variable degrees, as is indicated in the foregoing equations. In TOF, the great arteries are essentially (almost) normally related. But most of the other infundibuloarterial malformations, such as TGA, DORV, and DOLV are **developmental anomalies of infundibular R-L asymmetry.** There is only one way for the infundibulum to develop normally, including its mirror-image isomer: INRGA {I,L,I} = 4R + 0L.

But there are many ways for the normal R-L infundibular asymmetry to develop incorrectly. It is easy to do it wrong. There is only one way to do it right. The genetic instructions for the construction of a completely right-left asymmetrical infundibulum must be correct, and their execution must be error-free. Opposite development of different parts of one structure is not a simple developmental task. This appears to be why there are so many different types of infundibuloarterial anomalies. DOLV is one of the rarest, but is highly instructive.

DOLV has helped us understand what the functions of the subarterial infundibulum really are:

1. A well-developed subarterial infundibulum separates a semilunar valve above from the AV canal and mitral valve below, blocking an embryonic great arterial switch from above the RV to above the LV.
2. Absence of a subarterial infundibulum facilitates a great arterial switch from above the RV to above the LV.

Thus, the subarterial infundibulum is the great arterial "switch master." Infundibular *development* includes both *growth* and *involution*. The sequelae of normal and abnormal infundibular development are normally and abnormally related great arteries. The embryonic great arterial switches are important morphogenetic movement mechanisms, as DOLV illustrates. Indeed, DOLV is the only form of congenital heart disease in which both great arteries can get switched.

MECHANISMS RESULTING IN DOUBLE-OUTLET LEFT VENTRICLE

1. Marked underdevelopment or absence of infundibular musculature beneath the semilunar valves of the great arteries facilitate an embryonic double great arterial switch, resulting in DOLV.
2. The persistence of a well-developed subarterial infundibulum blocks and prevents an embryonic great arterial switch.
3. Atresia, dysplasia, or absence of the right ventricular sinus (body or inflow tract) also appears to predispose to DOLV.
4. Both subarterial infundibular absence or marked hypoplasia, and severe right ventricular pathologic conditions can coexist, resulting in DOLV. The data of this study[2] support these suggestions.

Of the 12 anatomic types of DOLV with two well-developed ventricles (see Fig. 24.6 and Tables 24.1 and 24.2), the infundibular anatomy was as follows:

1. bilateral absence, 6 of 12 (50%);
2. very deficient subpulmonary infundibulum and absent subaortic infundibulum, 3 of 12 (25%); and
3. very deficient subaortic infundibulum and absent subpulmonary infundibulum, 3 of 12 (25%).

Of the 14 anatomic types of DOLV with severe right ventricular pathology, the infundibular anatomy was quite different:

1. bilateral absence, 5 of 14 (36%);
2. bilateral presence, 6 of 14 (43%); and
3. subaortic, 3 of 14 (21%).

In these 14 patients with DOLV, the ventricular pathology was as follows:

1. tricuspid atresia, 7 of 14 (50%);
2. Ebstein anomaly, 3 of 14 (21%);
3. mitral atresia with a large LV, 9 of 14 (7%);
4. single LV, 3 of 14 (21%).

Another factor that appeared to predispose to DOLV when combined with severe RV pathologic conditions was D-loop (solitus) ventricles with L-malposition (inversion) of the great arteries, that is, DOLV {S/A,**D,L**} in 5 of 14 (36%). **L**-malposition of the infundibulum and great arteries with **D**-loop ventricles with right ventricular sinus atresia, dysplasia, or absence make it more likely that both great arteries will be located above the only well-developed ventricle, the LV. **L**-malposition of the great arteries swings both great arteries over the LV when D-loop ventricles are present, particularly when the right ventricular sinus is absent, or atretic, or dysplastic. In this situation, both great arteries are left-sided; the LV is left-sided, and there is little or no RV present. So neither great artery can arise above the RV, which increases the probability of DOLV. Hence, mechanisms resulting in DOLV are both infundibular and ventricular. There was also 1 patient who had congenital asplenia and the heterotaxy syndrome, a multisystem disorder: DOLV {**A**,D,L}.

For me, the most exciting part of this study has been the very recent realization of what the subarterial infundibulum is really doing. We have known for a long time that the infundibulum connects the ventricles with the great arteries, and that abnormal infundibular connections result in abnormally related great arteries. Now, thanks to DOLV (see Fig. 24.6), we understand *how* the infundibulum is doing it:

1. A well-developed infundibulum beneath a great artery blocks and prevents an embryonic great arterial switch from happening to the overlying great artery.
2. When there is no (or very little) infundibulum beneath a great artery, such a great artery can undergo an embryonic great arterial switch from above the RV to above the LV.
3. Briefly, DOLV may be viewed as a series of natural experiments concerning embryonic great arterial switchability that illustrate an important general principle:
   a. present, no switch; and
   b. absent, switch.

This principle of infundibular development is not as binary as the foregoing may sound. Small amounts of infundibulum can be present, and DOLV occurs nonetheless, as we have seen. Where is the cutoff? How much infundibulum must be present to prevent a great arterial embryonic switch? How little infundibulum needs to be present to permit a great arterial embryonic switch? I do not know the answers to these questions.

The foregoing are general principles that apply to the extremes of subarterial infundibular development: well-developed or absent. Refinements could be made. DOLV has given us a much better understanding of what the infundibulum is really doing, and how it is doing it. The foregoing is relevant to normal and abnormal morphogenetic movements.

REFERENCES

1. Paul MH, Muster AJ, Sinha SN, Cole RB, Van Praagh R. Double-outlet left ventricle with an intact ventricular septum. Clinical and autopsy diagnosis and developmental implications. *Circulation.* 1970;41:129.
2. Van Praagh R, Weinberg PM, Srebro JP. Double-outlet left ventricle. In: Adams FH, Emmanouilides GC, Riemenschneider TA, eds. *Moss' Heart Disease in Infants, Children, and Adolescents.* 4th ed. Baltimore: Williams & Wilkins; 1989:461.
3. Fragoyannis S, Kardalinos A. Transposition of the great vessels, both arising from the left ventricle (juxtaposition of pulmonary artery): tricuspid atresia, atrial septal defect and ventricular septal defect. *Am J Cardiol.* 1962;10:601.
4. Lev M. Pathologic diagnosis of positional variations in cardiac chambers in congenital heart disease. *Lab Invest.* 1954;3:71.
5. Sakakibara S, Takao A, Arai T, Hashimoto A, Nogi M. Both great vessels arising from the left ventricle (double outlet left ventricle) (origin of both great vessels from the left ventricle). *Bull Heart Inst Japan.* 1967:66.
6. Taussig HB, Bing RJ. Complete transposition of the aorta and a levoposition of the pulmonary artery. *Am Heart J.* 1949;37:551.
7. Van Praagh R. What is the Taussig-Bing malformation? *Circulation.* 1968;38:445.
8. Van Praagh R. The cardiovascular keys to air-breathing and permanent land-living in vertebrates: the normal human embryonic aortic switch procedure produced by complete right-left asymmetry in the development of the subaterial conal free walls, and the evolution of the right ventricular sinus. *Kardiochirurgia i Torakochirurgia Polska.* 2011;8:1.
9. Van Praagh R. What determines whether the great arteries are normally or abnormally related? *Am J Cardiol.* 2016;118:1390.

25

Anatomically Corrected Malposition of the Great Arteries

Anatomically corrected malposition of the great arteries is defined as malposition of the great arteries in which both great arteries nevertheless arise above the morphologically appropriate ventricles, aorta above the morphologically left ventricle (LV), and pulmonary artery above the morphologically right ventricle (RV). Such cases have been regarded as errors of observation (Lochte,[1] 1898), as inexplicable variations of nature (Geipel,[2] 1903), as embryologically impossible and hence nonexistent (Van Mierop and Wiglesworth,[3] 1963), and as probably nonexistent (Van Praagh and Van Praagh,[4] 1964).

But shortly thereafter, we encountered three autopsied cases that proved that anatomically corrected malposition of the great arteries (ACMGA) does indeed exist.[5] The anomaly now known as ACMGA was first described in 1895 by Théremin (his case 47). In 1939, Harris and Farber[6] named this malformation "anatomically corrected transposition," but they did not present any case of this rare anomaly.

Why anatomically correct *transposition*? you may wonder. Before 1971, *transposition* of the great arteries was defined, very broadly, as any anomaly of the great arteries between the great arteries themselves, and/or between the great arteries and the ventricles, or the ventricular septum, or the atrioventricular (AV) valves. So, before about 1971, virtually any positional anomaly of the great arteries was called a *transposition* of the great arteries; hence Harris and Farber's[6] anatomically corrected *transposition* of the great arteries.

In 1971, we[7] proposed that transposition of the great arteries (TGA) be used in its literal and original sense: *trans,* "across" and *positio,* "a placing" (Latin), the ventricular septum being the frame of reference. This is what Farre meant when he introduced the term *transposition* of the aorta and pulmonary artery in 1814.[8] Both great arteries are placed across the ventricular septum, and so both arise above the wrong ventricles. By 1970, this very broad usage of *transposition* was becoming obsolete. Clear, accurate terminology was needed, not only for TGA, but also for double-outlet RV (DORV), for double-outlet LV (DOLV), and for ACMGA. In ACMGA, TGA is not present, by definition. In ACMGA, neither great artery is transposed, accurately speaking.

WHAT CAUSES ANATOMICALLY CORRECTED MALPOSITION OF THE GREAT ARTERIES?

The answer is surprisingly simple. The ventricles loop in one direction, say to the right; and the subarterial infundibulum and the great arteries twist in the opposite direction, to the left. Opposite directions of torsion of the ventricular segment, relative to the infundibular and the great arterial segments, result in ACMGA. (What developmentally causes these opposite morphogenetic movements is unknown at the present time.)

However, at the level of cardiac anatomy, it may safely be said that **cardiac geometry** facilitates diagnostic understanding. Fig. 25.1 summarizes some normal cardiovascular anatomic geometry and other important diagnostic concepts.

Now let us consider a case of ACMGA (Fig. 25.2).[5] This patient was 2 years and 20 days of age. She died during a surgical attempt to relieve her pulmonary outflow tract stenosis. Autopsy revealed dextrocardia, situs solitus of the viscera and atria with a normal spleen, left-sided juxtaposition of the atrial appendages (both to the left of the great arteries), tricuspid atresia, a large secundum type of atrial septal defect, a ventricular D-loop (right-handed morphologically RV to the right of a left-handed morphologically LV), a small infundibuloventricular type of ventricular septal defect (VSD) between the infundibulum above and the ventricular septum below, a bilateral infundibulum (subaortic and subpulmonary), infundibular and valvar pulmonary outflow tract stenosis with a thickened, bicuspid pulmonary valve, and L-malposition of the great arteries (L-malposed aortic valve to the left of the malposed pulmonary valve). The malposed aortic valve was located above the LV, and the malposed pulmonary valve was above the RV. So, ACMGA was present. The diagnosis was ACMGA {S,D,L} with a bilateral infundibulum (subaortic and subpulmonary), tricuspid atresia, and pulmonary outflow tract stenosis. There was a probe-patent ductus arteriosus and a right aortic arch.

Cardiac geometry makes this diagnosis much more precise. The following measurements are projected on the horizontal plane and are expressed relative to the Z axis (the anteroposterior line):

- Atrial septal angle ≈ 60 degrees left (normal ≈ 30 degrees left; see Fig. 25.2)
- Ventricular septal angle ≈ 60 degrees right (normal ≈ 35 to 40 degrees left)
- **AV septal angle** ≈ 120 degrees[a] (normal ≈ 5 to 10 degrees)
- **Infundibular septal angle** ≈ 65 degrees right (normal ≈ 65 degrees right)

[a]The AV septal angle = the difference between the atrial and the ventricular septal angles.

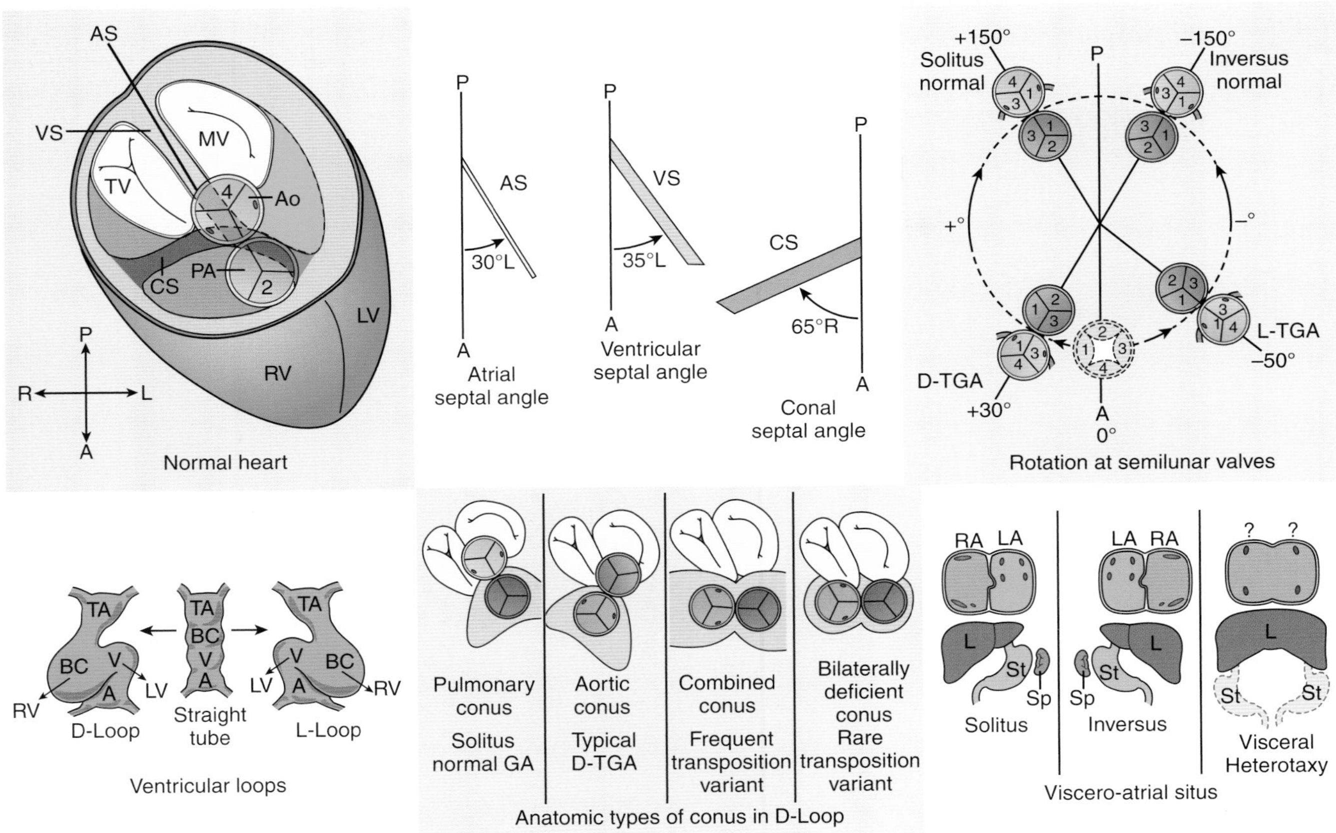

Fig. 25.1 Basic concepts and cardiovascular geometry. **Types of visceroatrial situs:** situs solitus (normal), with liver and morphologically right atrium *(RA)* right-sided, and with stomach *(St)*, spleen *(Sp)*, and morphologically left atrium *(LA)* left-sided; situs inversus (mirror-image of situs solitus), with liver and RA left-sided, and with stomach, spleen, and LA right-sided; and situs ambiguus (ambiguous, uncertain, or unknown type of situs or pattern of anatomic organization). The stomach can be left-sided or right-sided. The spleen can be absent (asplenia), polysplenia can be present, or the spleen can be present, but right-sided. The liver can appear to be bilaterally symmetrical. The situs of the atria can be uncertain or undiagnosable (? ?). These are some of the features of the heterotaxy syndromes. Visceroatrial situs ambiguus is not a third anatomic type of visceroatrial situs. Visceroatrial situs ambiguus just means that the anatomic type of visceroatrial situs is undiagnosed; all cases of visceroatrial situs ambiguus are not necessarily the same. There are only two types of visceroatrial situs, solitus and inversus, not three. Types of ventricular situs: There are two anatomic types of ventricular situs: D-loop ventricles or situs solitus ventricles, and L-loop ventricles or situs inversus ventricles. The straight heart tube normally loops to the right, beginning about 20 days of age after fertilization. D-loop formation (dextro- or D- means right, Latin) places the bulbus cordis *(BC)*, from which the morphologically right ventricle *(RV)* develops, to the right of the ventricle *(V)* from which the morphologically left ventricle *(LV)* develops. L-loop formation (levo- or L- means left, Latin) places the BC, from which the morphologically RV develops, to the left of the ventricle, from which the morphologically LV develops. Thus, the bulboventricular D-loop forms D-loop or solitus RV and LV. The bulboventricular L-loop forms L-loop or inversus RV and LV. The D-loop or solitus RV is right-handed, and the D-loop or solitus LV is left-handed. The L-loop or inverted RV is left-handed, and the L-loop or inverted LV is right-handed. Chirality, or handedness, is diagnostically helpful when bulboventricular D-loops or L-loops have undergone malrotation of any kind. The truncus arteriosus *(TA)* is the region from which the fibroelastic great arteries develop. The distal BC is the region where the infundibulum or conus arteriosus develops. The proximal BC is the region where the right ventricular sinus or inflow tract develops. A is the undivided atrial region at the straight tube or preloop stage. These conventional labels should all be taken with a grain of salt. At this early embryonic stage (20 to 24 days of age), our cinephotomicrography in chick embryos shows myriad cells on the march—streaming into the developing heart. Investigators now think that it is too early for static labels. However, these labels do predict future development quite accurately. Some of the rotations of the great arteries at the semilunar valves are shown, as well as how to measure these rotations. The four different anatomic types of infundibulum are depicted: *(1)* subpulmonary, which is normal; *(2)* subaortic, often with transposition of the great arteries (TGA); *(3)* bilaterally present (subaortic and subpulmonary), often with double-outlet RV DORV and TGA; and *(4)* bilaterally absent or very deficient, can occur with double-outlet LV (DOLV). In normal cardiovascular geometry, relative to the Z axis, or the anteroposterior line, projected on the horizontal plane: the normal atrial septal angle ≈ 30 degrees left; the normal ventricular septal angle ≈ 35 degrees L; the normal infundibular (conal) septal angle ≈ 65 degrees right; the solitus normal rotation at the semilunar valves ≈ 150 degrees right; the inverted normal rotation at the semilunar valves ≈ 150 degrees to the left; D-transpositions of the great arteries *(D-TGA)*, L-transpositions of the great arteries *(L-TGA)*, and other malpositions of the great arteries have rotations at the semilunar valves that are typically much less than normal. Geometric diagram of a normal heart, measured from above and projected on the horizontal plane. *A*, anterior; *Ao*, aorta; *AS*, atrial septum; *CS*, conal septum; *GA*, great artery; *MV*, mitral valve; *P*, posterior; *PA*, pulmonary artery; *R*, right; *TV*, tricuspid valve; *VS*, ventricular septum. (Reproduced with permission from Van Praagh R, Van Praagh S. Anatomically corrected transposition of the great arteries. *Br Heart J*. 1967;29:112.[5])

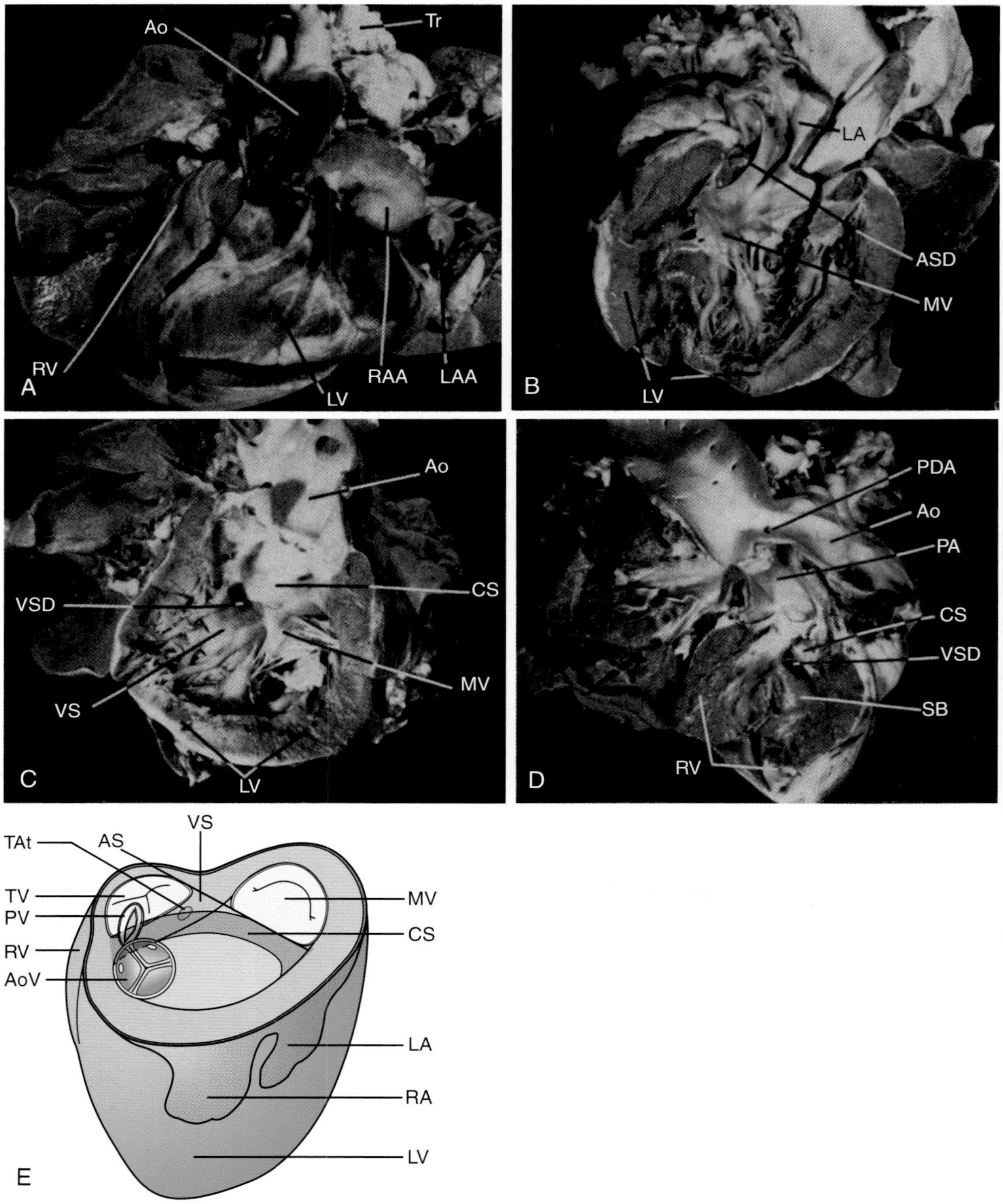

Fig. 25.2 Anatomically corrected malposition of the great arteries (ACMGA) with visceroatrial situs solitus, D-loop ventricles, L-malposition of the great arteries. Briefly, the segmental anatomy is ACMGA {S, D, L}. (A) Exterior anteroposterior view showing dextrocardia, a small right ventricle *(RV)*, a large left ventricle *(LV)*, left juxtaposition of the atrial appendages with the right atrial appendage *(RAA)* and the left atrial appendage *(LAA)* both lying to the left of the anterior aorta *(Ao)*. (B) Opened left atrium *(LA)*, mitral valve *(MV)*, and LV inflow tract. Note the large secundum type of atrial septal defect *(ASD)*. (C) Opened LV outflow tract and ascending aorta. The MV appeared normal. The infundibuloventricular type of ventricular septal defect *(VSD)* was small and lay between the infundibular (conal) septum *(CS)* above and the ventricular septum *(VS)* below. The infundibular septum was prominent and separated the aortic valve *(AoV)* from the mitral valve. There was ventriculoarterial alignment concordance, but the L-malposed aorta was abnormally related to the D-loop LV. (D) The opened RV and small main pulmonary artery *(PA)*. Posterior and inferior to the septal band *(SB)*, the RV inflow tract is very underdeveloped, as is typical of tricuspid atresia *(TAt)*. The pulmonary valve *(PV)* is bicuspid. (E) Geometric diagram of the heart, viewed from above, projected on the horizontal plane. Measurements relative to the Z axis (the anteroposterior plane): atrial septal angle ≈ 60 degrees left; ventricular septal angle ≈ 60 degrees right; infundibular septal angle ≈ 65 degrees right; and rotation at semilunar valves ≈ 20 degrees left. *AS,* Atrial septum; *PDA,* patent ductus arteriosus; *RA,* right atrium; *Tr,* trachea. (Reproduced with permission from Van Praagh R, Van Praagh S. Anatomically corrected transposition of the great arteries. *Br Heart J.* 1967;29:112.[5])

- Infundibuloventricular septal angle[b] ≈ 5 degrees[1] (normal ≈ 100 degrees)
- Rotation at the semilunar valves ≈ 20 degrees left (normal ≈ 150 degrees right)

Because all of these geometric measurements can now be made noninvasively, my task is to show why they are diagnostically and surgically helpful. The abnormally large atrial septal angle is related to **left-sided juxtaposition of the atrial appendages (Lt JAA).** Lt JAA in turn indicates that the right atrial appendage (RAA) is still in its early embryonic location to the left of the great arteries, which is normal at an embryonic age of less than 24 days of age in utero. But between 24 and 27 days of age, the RAA moves to the right of the great arteries—to its normal, definitive postnatal location. In somewhat greater detail, ventricular loop formation is a **"two-step dance."** With normal D-loop formation, first you loop to the right (step 1). Then you swing to the left (step 2)—from dextrocardia, through mesocardia, to levocardia. If step 2 is not performed well, one is left with dextrocardia (as in this patient) or mesocardia. And the great arteries are not carried far enough to the left. So the great arteries remain to the right of both atrial appendages, resulting in Lt JAA. So Lt JAA indicates subnormal ventricular D-looping.

If this left-to-right shift in the location of the RAA fails to occur, this strongly suggests that there is a major malformation at the ventricular level.[8-10] Left-sided juxtaposition of the RAA is strongly associated with right-heart pathologic conditions, and this patient has tricuspid atresia and a diminutive RV (see Fig. 25.2D–E).

The angle between the atrial septum and the ventricular septum (the AV septal angle) is enormous (120 degrees), documenting that there is a major malalignment between the atria and the ventricles. This *ventriculoatrial malalignment* placed the ventricular septum immediately beneath the expected site of the tricuspid valve, apparently resulting in *tricuspid atresia.* The very right-sided location of the ventricular septum (60 degrees right) and the large LV correlate with *dextrocardia* (see Fig. 25.2A, C). The L-malposition of the aortic valve (20 degrees left) plus the malformed ventricular D-loop support the diagnosis of anatomically corrected malposition (ACM).

Thus, cardiovascular geometry provides a new level of spatial diagnostic precision that can be used clinically by noninvasive diagnostic imaging.

ACMGA also occurs in patients with L-loop ventricles (ventricular inversion), as the next case illustrates. This baby boy (Fig. 25.3)[5] died at 4 weeks and 5 days of age from congestive heart failure. Autopsy revealed levocardia (left-sided heart), situs solitus of the viscera and atria, a ventricular L-loop (morphologically RV left-sided, levo- or L-, and left-handed, and morphologically LV right-sided and right-handed), a bilateral infundibulum (subaortic and subpulmonary, with no semilunar–AV valvar fibrous continuity), and with D-malposition of the great arteries, malposed aortic valve to the right, dextro- or D-, of the malposed pulmonary valve. The malposed aortic valve was above the morphologically LV, and the malposed pulmonary valve was above the morphologically right ventricle. Hence, anatomically corrected malposition of the great arteries (ACMGA) was present. The diagnosis was ACMGA {S,L,D} with a bilateral infundibulum and a slit-like infundibuloventricular type of VSD (between the infundibular septum above and the ventricular septum below) (see Fig. 25.3).

In terms of the segmental alignments, there was AV discordance with ventriculoarterial (VA) concordance. As you know, one alignment discordance physiologically uncorrects the circulations, whereas two alignment discordances physiologically correct the circulations, absence of associated malformations permitting.

This patient had *anatomically* corrected, but *physiologically* uncorrected malposition of the great arteries. **Cardiac geometry:** atrial septal angle ≈ 50 degrees left (approximately normal—a bit bigger than usual); ventricular septal angle ≈ 60 degrees left (very abnormal for inverted or L-loop ventricles; should be about 35 degrees right; that is, 95 degrees too far to the left); infundibular (or conal) septal angle ≈ 50 degrees L; and rotation at semilunar valves ≈ 80 degrees right. **Why did this patient have ACMGA?** Because the ventricles looped to the *left* (L-loop), but the great arteries twisted in the opposite direction, to the *right* (80 degrees right) (see Fig. 25.3D).[5]

This is a basic principle. All cases of ACMGA display opposite directions of twisting of the ventricular loop and of the infundibulum and great arteries. These *opposite* directions of ventricular and infundibuloarterial torsion explain the embryonic morphogenetic movements that result in ACMGA, and these opposite torsions explain why ACMGA is so rare.

Almost always, ventricular and infundibuloarterial twistings occur in the *same* direction: both to the *right* in visceroatrial situs solitus, or both to the *left* in visceroatrial situs inversus. But in ACMGA, the directions of ventricular and infundibuloarterial twists are in *opposite* directions. In Fig. 25.2, the directions of ventricular and infundibuloarterial twistings are *right* and *left,* respectively, as the diagnosis indicates: ACMGA {S,**D**,**L**}. In Fig. 25.3, the directions of ventricular and infundibuloarterial torsions are *left* and *right,* respectively, as the diagnosis indicates: ACMGA {S,**L**,**D**}.

ANATOMIC TYPES OF ANATOMICALLY CORRECTED MALPOSITION OF THE GREAT ARTERIES

Six anatomic types of ACMGA are presented diagrammatically in Fig. 25.4[11]:

1. ACMGA {S,D,L},
2. ACMGA {S,L,D},
3. ACMGA {I,L,D},
4. ACMGA {I,D,L},
5. ACMGA {A,D,L}, and
6. ACMGA {A,L,D}.

There are two different kinds of VA concordance:

1. normally related great arteries, solitus or inversus; and
2. ACMGA.

[b]Infundibuloventricular septal angle ≈ the difference between the infundibular and the ventricular septal angles.

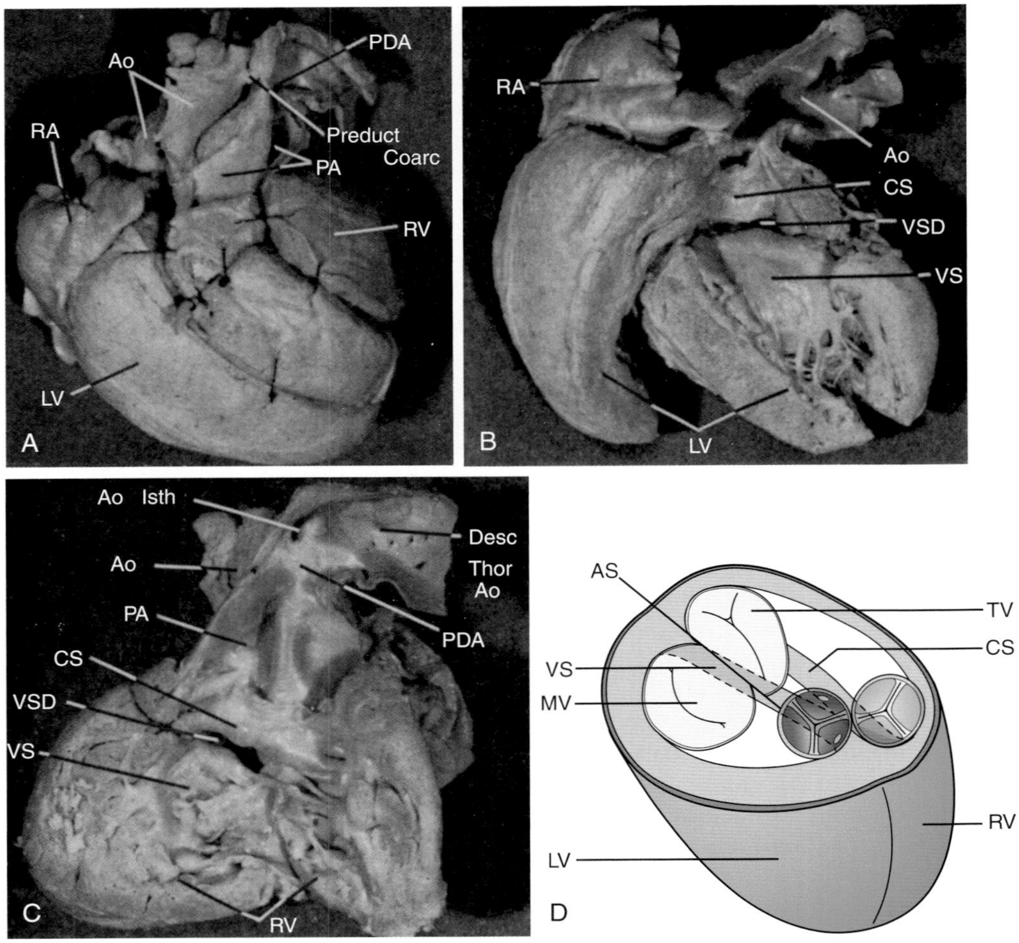

Fig. 25.3 Anatomically corrected malposition of the great arteries (ACMGA) {S,L,D}, that is, ACMGA with the segmental situs set of visceroatrial situs solitus, L-loop (or situs inversus) of the ventricles, and D-malposition (or solitus malposition) of the great arteries. (A) External frontal view of the heart. The right atrium *(RA)* is right-sided, indicating visceroatrial situs solitus. The left atrium is not seen in this view. The morphologically right ventricle *(RV)* is left-sided and superior, and the morphologically left ventricle *(LV)* is right-sided and inferior, indicating that L-loop (or inverted) ventricles are present. D-malposition (solitus or noninverted malposition) of the great arteries is present, with a small ascending aorta *(Ao)* to the right, with a preductal coarctation of the aorta *(Preduct Coarc)*, and an enlarged main pulmonary artery *(PA)* to the left. The aorta appears to arise to the right of the anterior descending coronary artery (not labeled). The PA appears to originate to the left of the anterior descending coronary artery. Thus, careful external inspection indicates the diagnosis accurately, even in rare forms of congenital heart. This is a helpful game for congenital heart surgeons to learn how to play. It helps to answer an important question: Did the cardiologists get it right this time? In successful cases, the surgeon, not the pathologist, is the final diagnostician. (B) The opened right-sided LV and ascending right-sided aorta. Note the smooth superior septal surface and the finely trabeculated apical septal surface, typical of the morphologically LV. (C) The opened left-sided RV and main PA. The left pulmonary artery is absent. The patent ductus arteriosus *(PDA)* is widely patent. Note how small the aortic isthmus *(Ao Isth)* is, where the aortic arch opens through a preductal coarctation into the descending thoracic aorta *(Desc Thor Ao)*. (D) Geometric diagram of this case of ACMGA {S,L,D}: atrial septal angle ≈ 50 degrees left; ventricular septal angle ≈ 60 degrees left; infundibular septal angle ≈ 50 degrees left; rotation at semilunar valves ≈ 80 degrees right. *AS,* Arial septum; *CS,* conal septum; *MV,* mitral valve; *TV,* tricuspid valve; *VS,* ventricular septum; *VSD,* ventricular septal defect. (Reproduced with permission from Van Praagh R, Van Praagh S. Anatomically corrected transposition of the great arteries. *Br Heart J.* 1967;29:112.[5])

In ACMGA, you know that there is VA concordance, by definition. So, to quickly figure out whether *physiologically* corrected malposition is present, just look at the AV alignment. If the AV alignments are concordant, as in ACMGA {**S**,**D**,L}, the circulations are physiologically corrected. If the AV alignments are discordant, as in ACMGA {**S**,**L**,D}, the circulations are physiologically uncorrected.

In ACMGA, why do the ventricles and the great arteries twist in opposite directions? Because VA situs discordance is present. Examples include ACMGA {S,D,L}, with D-loop or *solitus* ventricles that loop to the right, and L-malposition or *inverted* malposition of the great arteries that twist to the left.

In ACMGA {S,**L**,**D**}, L-loop or *inverted* ventricles that loop to the left coexist with D-malposition or solitus malposition of the

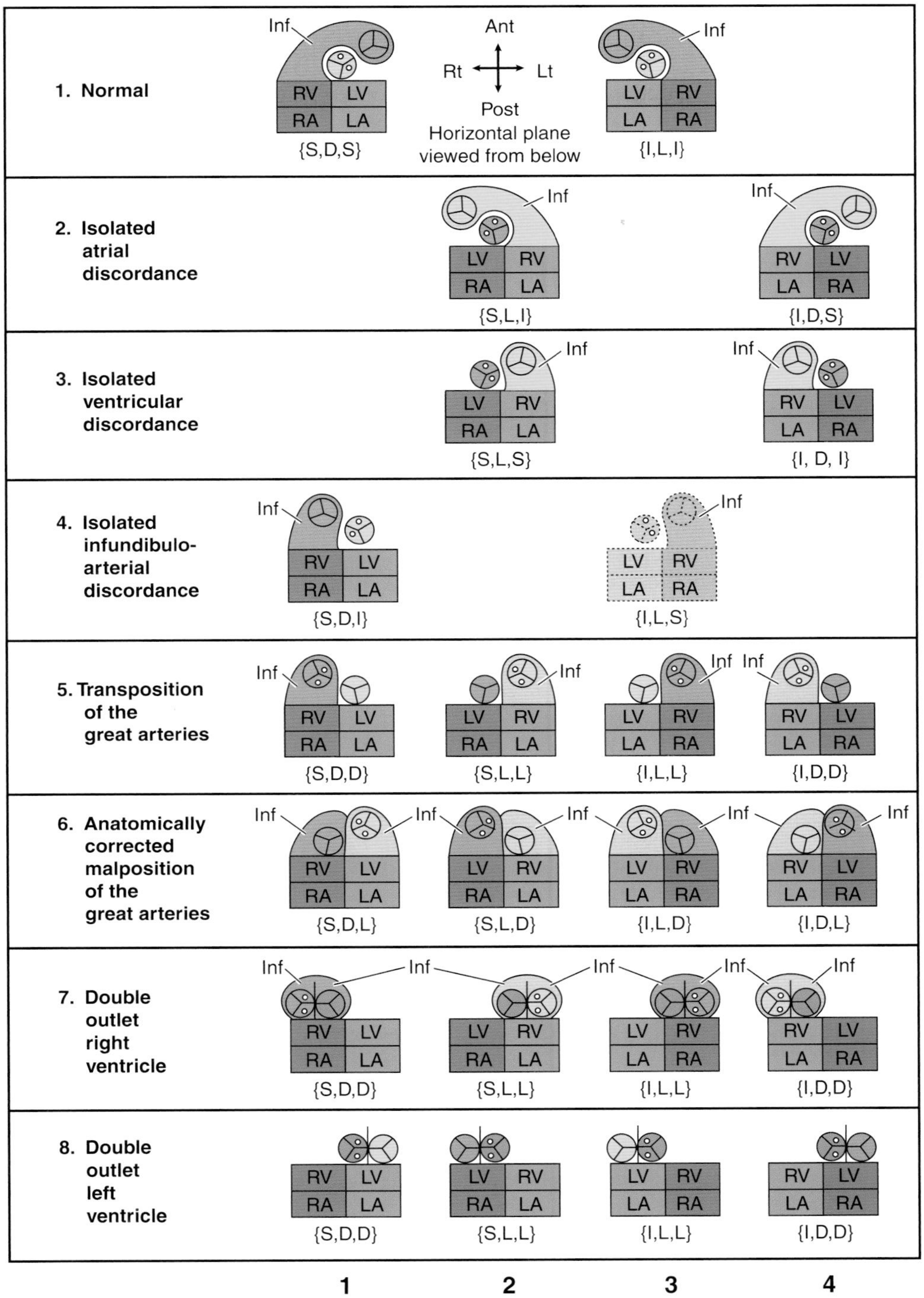

Fig. 25.4 Anatomic types of anatomically corrected malposition of the great arteries (ACMGA). (1) ACMGA {S,D,L}; (2) ACMGA {S,L,D}; (3) ACMGA {I,L,D}; (4) ACMGA {I,D,L}; (5) ACMGA {A,D,L}; and (6) ACMGA {A,L,D}. In all anatomic types of ACM, the ventricles loop in one direction, and the infundibulum and the great arteries twist in the opposite direction. When there is visceroatrial situs solitus or situs inversus, and when there is **atrioventricular (AV) concordance**, then ACMGA also has physiologically corrected malposition of the great arteries (PCM); hence, surgical management involves the repair of associated malformations only, such as ventricular septal defect (VSD) closure. However, when **AV discordance** is present, the circulations are **physiologically uncorrected.** Consequently, an atrial switch procedure is also needed surgically: a Senning or a Mustard procedure. When the patient has visceroatrial situs ambiguus (A), one may well be dealing with one of the **heterotaxy syndromes** characterized by congenital asplenia, or polysplenia, or with a normal but right-sided spleen. For example, the **asplenia syndrome** often has common AV canal, and pulmonary outflow tract stenosis or atresia, in other words more challenging associated malformations. The circulations are less likely to be "physiologically corrected." (Reproduced with permission, from Van Praagh R, Van Praagh ADG, Lacour- Gayet F. Anatomically corrected malposition of the great arteries. In: Lacour-Gayet F, Bove EL, Hraška V, Morell VO, Spray TL, eds. *Surgery of Conotruncal Anomalies*. Cham, Switzerland: Springer International Publishing AG; 2016:517.[11])

great arteries that rotate to the right. **So, the brief answer to the question of why ACMGA appears to be VA situs discordance (difference).** Typical D-TGA and typical L-TGA both have VA situs *concordance (sameness):* both solitus or both inversus. (Not VA situs discordance.)

ACMGA also has infundibuloarterial situs discordance similar to TGA and DORV. ACMGA has double segmental situs discordance: VA and infundibuloarterial.

SURGERY OF ANATOMICALLY CORRECTED MALPOSITION OF THE GREAT ARTERIES

A review of the literature that we performed in 2016 indicated that in patients with ACMGA and AV concordance, that is, in ACMGA {S,D,L}, the surgical results have been satisfactory. Surgery was limited to the repair of associated lesions, including VSD repair,[12-14] and relief of left ventricular outflow tract obstruction.[15,16] Hypoplasia of one ventricle is frequent and would indicate a Fontan type of surgical procedure. Lt JAA is frequent with ACMGA (see Fig. 25.2) and may modify surgical techniques because of the small size of the right atrium (RA). The Senning procedure would be challenging and would need enlargement of the pulmonary venous channel—the "knee" of the Senning—using a flap of autologous pericardium, as described by Senning.[17] A Mustard procedure, performed during the third week of life as reported by Bailey et al[18] for D-TGA, is another good surgical option.

In 2016, we found no publications on the repair of ACMGA with AV alignment discordance, such as ACMGA {S,L,D}[11] (see Fig. 25.3). We proposed that if a patient had an intact ventricular septum, a prostaglandin infusion and a balloon atrial septostomy also could be helpful. If a patient had a VSD, we thought that congestive heart failure and pulmonary hypertension could be major management problems.[11]

DIFFERENTIAL DIAGNOSIS

Entities that might be confused with ACMGA {S,D,L} include:

1. **{S,D,I}, that is, isolated infundibuloarterial inversion,** that was discovered and described by Foran et al.[19] The difference between ACMGA {S,D,**L**} and {S,D,**I**}[19] is that in {S,D,**I**}, the great arteries are inverted normally related; that is, the aorta was left-sided, but posterior and inferior with aortic-mitral fibrous continuity, whereas in ACMGA {S,D,**L**} the aorta is left-sided, but anterior and superior, sitting on a subaortic muscular infundibulum.
2. **DORV {S,D,L}**[20] versus ACMGA {S,D,L}: In DORV {S,D,L}, both great arteries originate from the right-sided RV, whereas in ACM {S,D,L} the aorta arises from the left-sided LV.

ORIGINAL SOURCES

For those who may be interested in researching original sources, the question arises, How many papers have I authored or coauthored concerning ACMGA? The answer is four,[5,11,20,21] before this chapter.

WHO FIRST DISCOVERED AND DESCRIBED ANATOMICALLY CORRECTED MALPOSITION OF THE GREAT ARTERIES?

To the best of my knowledge, the first investigator to discover and describe the anomaly now known as ACGMA was **E. Théremin.**[22] His work was published in 1895 in Paris, France: case 47 in his study of congenital heart disease, on page 83. Théremin's study, entitled **Etudes sur les Affections Congénitales du Coeur,** has been largely forgotten, at least in the anglophone world—a misfortune that I am trying to remedy.

SUMMARY

All six anatomic types of ACMGA (see Fig. 25.4) have VA situs discordance and infundibuloarterial situs discordance. AV situs discordance is present in two of the four anatomic types in which this diagnosis can be made. In two types with visceroatrial situs ambiguus in the heterotaxy syndromes, the diagnosis of AV situs may be undiagnosable.

VA situs discordance (difference) and infundibuloarterial situs discordance (difference), that is, **double segmental situs discordance,** are typical of these rare anomalies.

INFUNDIBULOARTERIAL SITUS EQUATIONS

For information concerning infundibuloarterial situs equations, please see Chapter 15. Examples of these equations in ACMGA follow:

$$ACMGA\{S,\ D,\ L\} = 0R + 4L \qquad \textbf{Equation 25.1}$$

In ACMGA, the VA alignments are concordant (physiologically appropriate) because the ventricles and the great arteries have twisted in opposite directions: the ventricles have twisted to the right (D-loop), but the infundibulum and great arteries have twisted to the left, L-malposition, that is, {S,**D**,**L**}. **Mother Nature has done an arterial switch procedure!**

Although the VA alignments are physiologically appropriate, the great arteries are not normally related, as infundibuloarterial situs analysis indicates: The infundibular situs is solitus normal (0R+ 4L); but the great arteries are inverted (L-malposition). So the infundibuloarterial situs analysis is discordant: solitus, inversus, that is, discordant (different). Thus, the infundibular connector and the great arterial "pipes" are of structurally opposite types: a solitus infundibular connector and inversus (mirror-image) pipes.

ACMGA {S,D,L} is physiologically corrected because the RA and the malposed pulmonary artery are both right-sided, and the LA and the malposed aorta are both left-sided. **ACMGA {S,L,D} = 4R + 4L** is a physiologically uncorrected type of ACMGA because the normally located RA and the D-malposed aorta are ipsilateral—both right-sided, and the normally located LA and the malposed pulmonary artery are ipsilateral—both left-sided.

Infundibular situs is ambiguus (4R + 4L), and the great arterial situs is solitus (D-malposition). Hence, the infundibuloarterial situs combination is ambiguus, solitus, that is, unknown, normal, and therefore discordant (different) and abnormal structurally and physiologically.

REFERENCES

1. Lochte EHT. Ein Fall von Situs viscerum irregularis, nebst einem Beitrag zur Lehre von der Transposition der arteriellen grossen Gefässtämme des Herzens. *Beitr Path Anat.* 1898;24:187.
2. Geipel P. Weitere Beiträge zum Situs transversus und zur Lehre von der Transpositionen der grossen Gefässe der Herzens. *Arch Kinderheik.* 1903;35:112.
3. Van Mierop LHS, Wiglesworth FW. Pathogenesis of transposition complexes: 3. True transposition of the great vessels. *Am J Cardiol.* 1963;12:233.
4. Van Praagh R, Van Praagh S. Isolated ventricular inversion with a consideration of the morphogenesis, definition, and diagnosis of non-transposed and transposed great arteries. *Am J Cardiol.* 1966;17:395.
5. Van Praagh R, Van Praagh S. Anatomically corrected transposition of the great arteries. *Br Heart J.* 1967;29:112.
6. Harris JS, Farber S. Transposition of the great cardiac vessels with special reference to the phylogenetic theory of Spitzer. *Arch Pathol.* 1939;28:427.
7. Van Praagh R, Pérez-Treviño C, Lopez-Cuellar M, et al. Transposition of the great arteries with posterior aorta, anterior pulmonary artery, subpulmonary conus, and fibrous continuity between aortic and atrioventricular valves. *Am J Cardiol.* 1971;28:621.
8. Melhuish BPP, Van Praagh R. Juxtaposition of the atrial appendages, a sign of severe cyanotic congenital heart disease. *Br Heart J.* 1968;30:269.
9. Van Praagh S, O'Sullivan J, Brili S, Van Praagh R. Juxtaposition of the morphologically right atrial appendage in solitus and inversus atria: a study of 35 postmortem cases. *Am Heart J.* 1996;132:382.
10. Van Praagh S, O'Sullivan J, Brili S, Van Praagh R. Juxtaposition of the morphologically left atrial appendage in solitus and inversus atria: a study of 18 postmortem cases. *Am Heart J.* 1996;132:391.
11. Van Praagh R, Van Praagh ADG, Lacour- Gayet F. Anatomically corrected malposition of the great arteries. In: Lacour-Gayet F, Bove EL, Hraška V, Morell VO, Spray TL, eds. *Surgery of Conotruncal Anomalies.* Cham Heidelberg New York Dordrecht London: Springer International Publishing AG Switzerland; 2016:517.
12. Miyamura H, Tsuchida S, Matsukawa T, Eguchi S, Takeuchi Y. Surgical experience with anatomically corrected malposition of the great arteries without subpulmonary conus. *Chest.* 1982;82:115.
13. Tsuchida K, Fujiwara T, Ishihara S, Kurosawa H, Imai Y. Intracardiac repair in anatomically corrected malposition of the great arteries {S, D, L}: report on 2 successful repair. *Nihon Kyobu Geka Gakkai Zasshi.* 1989;37:760.
14. Rittenhouse EA, Tenckhoff L, Kawabori I, et al. Surgical repair of anatomically corrected malposition of the great arteries. *Ann Thorac Surg.* 1986;42:220.
15. Sridhar A, Subramanyan R, Verma S, Abraham S. Anatomically corrected malposition of great arteries. *Ann Pediatr Cardiol.* 2010;3:187.
16. Colli AM, de Leval M, Somerville J. Anatomically corrected malposition of the great arteries: diagnostic difficulties and surgical repair of associated lesions. *Am J Cardiol.* 1985;55:1367.
17. Senning A. Correction of transposition of the great arteries. *Ann Surg.* 1975;182:287.
18. Alonso de Begona J, Kawauchi M, Fullerton D, Razzouk AJ, Gundry SR, Bailey LL. The Mustard procedure for correction of simple transposition of the great arteries before 1 month of age. *J Thorac Cardiovasc Surg.* 1992;104:1218.
19. Foran RB, Belcourt C, Nanton MA, et al. Isolated infundibuloarterial inversion {S, D, I}: a newly recognized form of congenital heart disease. *Am Heart J.* 1988;116:1337.
20. Van Praagh R, Pérez-Treviño C, Reynolds JL, et al. Double-outlet right ventricle {S, D, L} with subaortic ventricular septal defect and pulmonary stenosis: report of 6 cases. *Am J Cardiol.* 1975;35:42.
21. Van Praagh R. The story of anatomically corrected malposition of the great arteries. *Chest.* 1976;69:2.
22. Théremin E. *Etudes sur les Affections Congénitales du Coeur.* Paris: Asselin and Houzeau; 1895:83.

26

What Prevents and What Permits the Embryonic Great Arterial Switch?

BASIC PRINCIPLES

1. When the situs (or pattern of anatomic organization) of the subarterial infundibulum and the situs of the great arteries are the same (concordant), the great arteries are normally related.
2. When the situs of the subarterial infundibulum and the situs of the great arteries are different (discordant), the great arteries are abnormally related.
3. A well-developed subarterial muscular infundibulum prevents the embryonic great arterial switch from above the morphologically right ventricle (RV) to above the morphologically left ventricle (LV).
4. Absence of a subarterial muscular infundibulum permits an embryonic great arterial switch from above the RV to above the LV. So the subarterial infundibulum is the embryonic great arterial "switch master."

Segmental situs equations, including the situs of the subarterial infundibulum and the situs of the great arteries, help clarify infundibuloarterial situs comparison, which in turn determines whether the great arteries are normally or abnormally related.

Synergy also helps to explain the normal and abnormal relationships between the great arteries, as we shall see.

TYPES OF SITUS

In anatomy, there are two types of situs, or patterns of anatomic organization:

1. **situs solitus,** the normal or usual pattern; and
2. **situs inversus,** a mirror-image, characterized by right-left reversal, but without superoinferior or anteroposterior change.

Situs ambiguus is not a third type of situs. It means that the pattern of anatomic organization is ambiguous or uncertain and is therefore not diagnosed. Situs ambiguus is different from situs solitus and situs inversus. There is more than one anatomic type of situs ambiguus, as we shall see.

GRADING INFUNDIBULAR DEVELOPMENT

The development of the subarterial infundibular free wall is highly variable and may be graded as follows:

Grade 0	Absent
Grade 1	Severely underdeveloped
Grade 2	Moderately underdeveloped
Grade 3	Mildly underdeveloped
Grade 4	Normally developed.

SITUS EQUATIONS

Equations based on the situs of the cardiac segments clarify and simplify the understanding of congenital heart disease.[1] In this chapter, emphasis is placed on the situs of the subarterial infundibulum and on the situs of the great arteries because these are the keys to understanding normally and abnormally related great arteries.

$$SNRGA\ \{S,D,S\} = 0R + 4L \quad \textbf{Equation 26.1}$$

Equation 26.1, read from left to right, says: solitus normally related great arteries with the set of solitus atria, D-loop (solitus) ventricular, and solitus normally related great arteries equals zero development of the right-sided subaortic infundibular free wall plus a well-developed left-sided subpulmonary infundibular free wall.

In these subarterial infundibular situs equations, the formula or recipe for the infundibular situs lies to the right of the equal sign: **0R + 4L;** and the situs of the great arteries is indicated by the third element of the segmental anatomy immediately to the left of the equal sign: {-,-,**S**} = the infundibuloarterial situs combination:

1. The situs of the infundibulum is solitus normal, that is, 0R + 4L.
2. The situs of the great arteries also is solitus normal, that is, {-,-,S}.

So, the infundibuloarterial situs combination is solitus normal–solitus normal, which is same–same, that is, concordant or normal. Why normal? Because the infundibular connector and the great arteries being connected are both of the same normal anatomic type. Both are in situs solitus. Plumbers know this. The connector and the pipes being connected must be of the same type. Otherwise, the pipes cannot be connected normally.

These same points can be made diagrammatically (Fig. 26.1). In the solitus (noninverted) heart, as seen from the front, the aortic valve is to the *right* and the pulmonary valve is to the *left*. So in Equation 26.1, you know that normally, the right-sided semilunar valve is the aortic valve, and the left-sided semilunar valve is the pulmonic valve (see Fig. 26.1).

The effect of D-loop formation is thought to produce about 90-degree dextrorotation at the semilunar valve level relative to the sagittal plane (see Fig. 26.1, *second column from the right*). Looking at the diagrams of solitus normally related great arteries (see Fig. 26.1, *third column from the right*), you can see the formula of the normal solitus subarterial infundibulum. There is no subaortic infundibular free-wall muscle, remote from the infundibular septum. This subaortic infundibular free-wall muscle has disappeared because of **apoptosis** (programmed

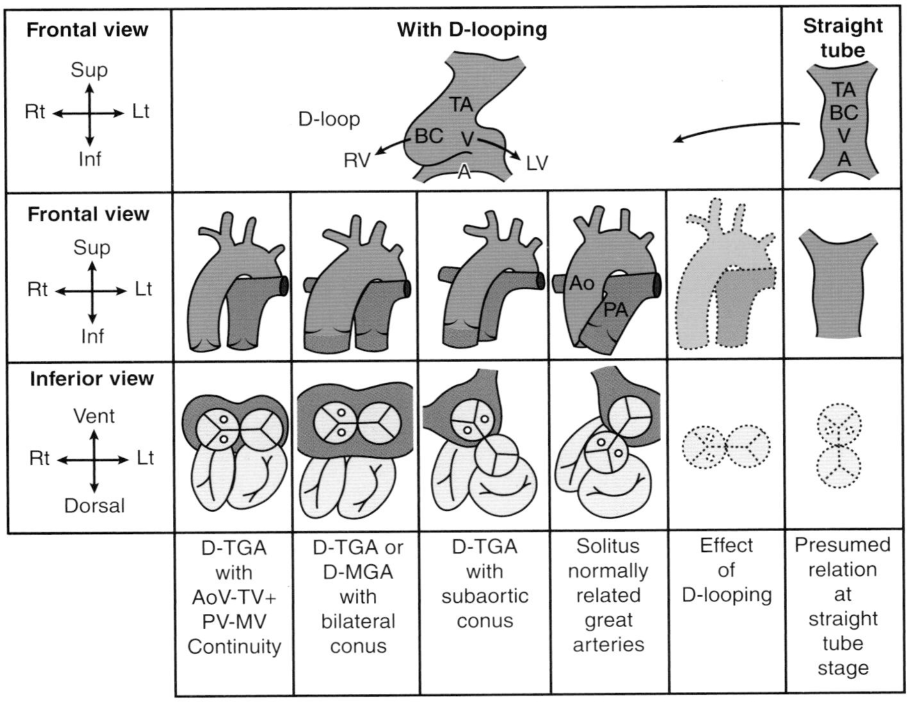

Fig. 26.1 Normal and abnormal development and anatomy of the situs solitus (noninverted) human heart, presented diagrammatically. *A,* Undivided atrium; *Ao,* aorta; *AoV-TV,* aortic valve–tricuspid valve; *BC,* bulbus cordis; *Inf,* inferior; *Lt,* left; *LV,* morphologically left ventricle; *MGA,* malposition of the great arteries; *MV,* mitral valve; *PA,* pulmonary artery; *PV,* pulmonary valve; *Rt,* right; *RV,* morphologically right ventricle; *Sup,* superior, *TA,* truncus arteriosus; *TGA,* transposition of the great arteries; *V,* ventricle of bulboventricular tube or loop; *Vent,* ventral. (Modified and reproduced with permission from Van Praagh R, Van Praagh S. Isolated ventricular inversion, a consideration of the morphogenesis, definition, and diagnosis of nontransposed and transposed great arteries. *Am J Cardiol.* 1966;17:395e406.)

cell death), which in turn makes possible aortic-mitral fibrous continuity via the intervalvar fibrosa in the LV, and often aortic-tricuspid fibrous continuity via the membranous ventricular septum. In contrast, the left-sided subpulmonary infundibular free wall develops well above the RV.

The normal infundibular situs solitus, that is, 0R + 4L, contains another "secret." 0R means not only that there is no subaortic infundibular free-wall muscle because of apoptosis. **0R also means that the right-sided aorta has undergone an embryonic switch from above the RV to above the LV.** Here is how this is thought to work:

1. A well-developed subarterial infundibulum is thought to block or prevent an embryonic great arterial switch. A subarterial infundibulum acts as a platform on which a great artery stands and is held high.
2. When there is no subarterial muscular platform, a great artery can move inferiorly, posteriorly, and leftward. Passing through the interventricular foramen, the great artery becomes left ventricular. **So, the subarterial infundibulum may be regarded as the embryonic great arterial switch master.**

Whenever the subaortic infundibulum is absent, as in the solitus normal heart—**0R** + 4L—one should expect that the aorta has been switched from RV to LV in utero.

In *Homo sapiens,* the normal human embryonic aortic switch is produced by complete right-left asymmetry in the development of the subarterial infundibular free walls between 38 and 45 days of age in utero[2]:

$$\text{SNRGA}\ \{S,D,S\} = 0R + 4L$$

Equation 26.2 is inverted normally related great arteries.

$$\textit{INGRA}\ \{I,L,I\} = 4R + 0L \quad \textbf{Equation 26.2}$$

This Equation 26.2 and Figure 26.2 (third column from the left) represent inverted normally related great arteries. In words, this equation says: Inverted normally related great arteries with the set of situs inversus of the atria, situs inversus of the ventricles (ventricular L-loop), and inverted normally related great arteries equals a well-developed, right-sided subpulmonary infundibular free wall plus absence of a left-sided subaortic infundibular free wall.

The infundibular situs is the inverted normal: **4R + 0L.** The great arterial situs is the inverted normal: {-,-,**I**}. Thus, the infundibular situs—great arterial situs combination is inverted normal; that is, concordant or the same, which is normal in situs inversus totalis.

The inverted infundibular situs in Equation 26.2 to the right of the equal sign (4R + 0L) tells you the switch—no switch story. In situs inversus totalis, the right-sided great artery normally is the pulmonary artery (Fig. 26.2, *third column from the left*), and there is a well-developed (grade 4) infundibulum beneath the main pulmonary artery (MPA). Knowing that a well-developed subarterial infundibulum blocks the embryonic great arterial

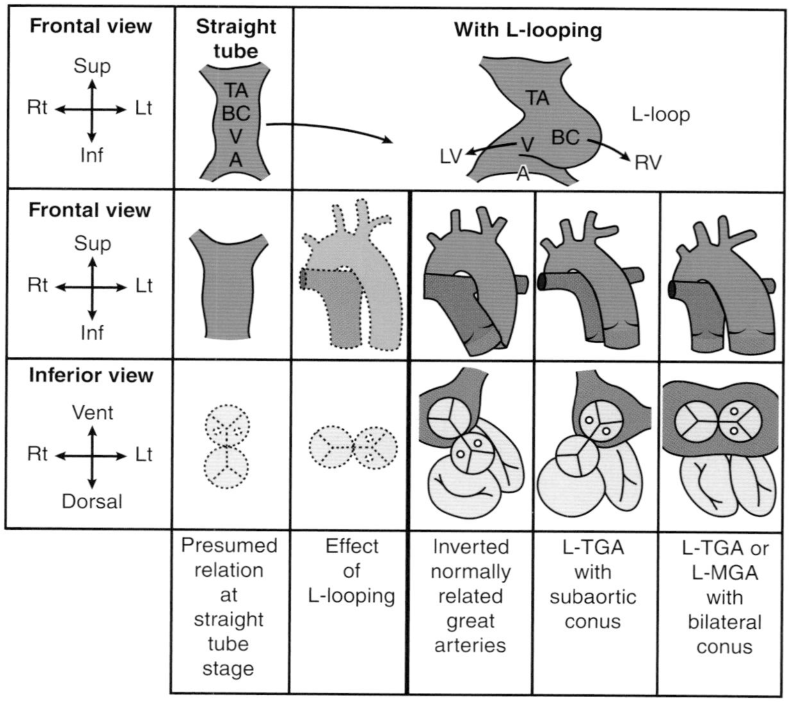

Fig. 26.2 Normal and abnormal development and anatomy of the situs inversus human heart. *A,* Undivided atrium; *BC,* bulbus cordis; *Inf,* inferior; *L-,* levo- (left, Latin), as in L-looping; *L-MGA,* L-malposition of the great arteries; *Lt,* left; *L-TGA,* L-transposition of the great arteries; *LV,* morphologically left ventricle; *Rt,* right; *RV,* morphologically right ventricle; *Sup,* superior, *TA,* truncus arteriosus; *V,* ventricle of bulboventricular tube or loop; *Vent,* ventral. (Reproduced with permission from Van Praagh R. What determines whether the great arteries are normally or abnormally related? *Am J Cardiol.* 2026;118:1390.)

switch, you realize that the pulmonary artery has not been switched and is still high above the left-sided morphologically right ventricle (RV). This is what **4R** tells you.

What about **0**? You know that in situs inversus totalis, the left-sided great artery is the aorta (see Fig. 26.2, *column 3 from the left*). And you also know that when there is no infundibular muscle beneath the aortic valvar free wall, this is a precondition for a great arterial switch. So you correctly conclude that the aorta has been switched from above the left-sided RV to above the right-sided LV.

Equations 26.3, 26.4, and 26.5 describe tetralogy of Fallot, with variable degrees of right ventricular outflow tract obstruction.

$$TOF\ \{S,D,S\} = 0R + 1L \qquad \textbf{Equation 26.3}$$

$$TOF\ \{S,D,S\} = 0R + 2L \qquad \textbf{Equation 26.4}$$

$$TOF\ \{S,D,S\} = 0R + 3L \qquad \textbf{Equation 26.5}$$

Tetralogy of Fallot (TOF) with the set of solitus atria, solitus (D-loop) ventricles, and solitus normally related great arteries typically has no infundibular muscle beneath the right-sided aortic valve. But the degree of hypoplasia and hence of obstruction of the left-sided subpulmonary infundibulum is highly variable:

1L indicates very severe obstruction.
2L means severe stenosis.
3L denotes mild to moderate stenosis.

As far as now known, the TOF was first described in 1671 by Niels Stensen,[3] not by Arthur Fallot[4] in 1888.

Morphometry has revealed that right ventricular hypertrophy is not present at birth in "TOF."[5] Right ventricular hypertrophy is a postnatally acquired sequelea.[5]

In 1970, we proposed[6] that the TOF is, in fact, just one malformation and its sequelae. The one malformation[6] is hypoplasia of the subpulmonary infundibulum, which leads to pulmonary outflow tract obstruction (stenosis or atresia), a typically large subaortic ventricular septal defect (VSD), aortic overriding, and right ventricular hypertrophy (postnatally).

So, TOF might well be called **the monology of Stensen.** However, out of deference to common usage and in the interests of widespread comprehension, I shall continue to call this anomaly (or these anomalies) the tetralogy of Fallot.

What comes after TOF? What is closely related to TOF? We used to call it **truncus arteriosus communis type A2.**[7] But now we have realized that the diagnosis of persistent common arterial trunk is wrong because the MPA can be absent. Abbott[8] introduced the concept of a common (undivided) great arterial trunk in 1927. She thought this anomaly was "absence or rudimentary development of [the] aortic septum." The concept of common aortopulmonary trunk also included the ideas that the semilunar valves and the infundibular septum are in common, because that is what the anatomy seemed to show.[9-13] This was our interpretation in 1965.[7]

But about 36 years later, in 2001, Dr. Alfredo Vizcaino, a pediatric cardiologist, friend, and colleague brought us a rare case in consultation from the Hospital Infantil de Mexico, Mexico City, Mexico that opened my eyes (Fig. 26.3).[14] The specimen

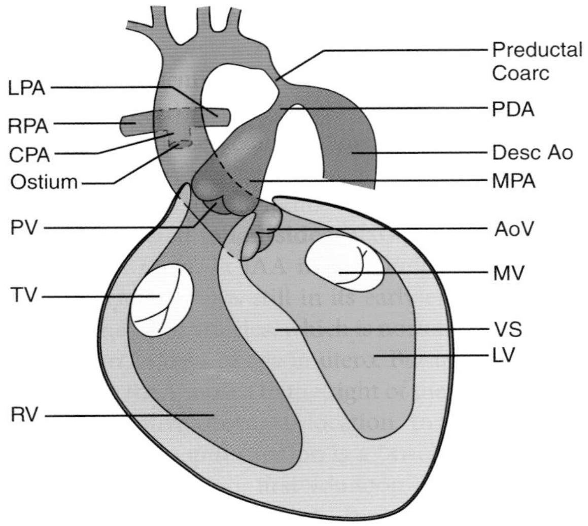

Fig. 26.3 The main pulmonary artery *(MPA)* has no branches. The right pulmonary artery *(RPA)* and the left pulmonary artery *(LPA)* both arise from the dorsal surface of the ascending aorta via a single ostium that opens into a short common pulmonary artery *(CPA)*, also known as the aortic sac. The RPA and the LPA arise from the aortic sac. This is their starting location. Normally, the RPA and the LPA then migrate on the sixth aortic arches and become confluent with the MPA. The sixth aortic arches were not identified in this case. This rare heart specimen confirms the concept that the pulmonary arterial system consists of three separate components: (1) the branches arising from the aortic sac; (2) the sixth aortic arches on which the RPA and the LPA migrate from the aorta to the MPA, and (3) the MPA. This patient had multiple congenital anomalies (see text). The diagnosis is absence or dysfunction of the sixth aortic arches, resulting in unmigrated RPA and LPA and a PA without branches. *AoV,* Aortic valve, *Coarc,* coarctation; *Desc Ao,* descending aorta; *PDA,* patent ductus arteriosus; *TV,* tricuspid valve; *VS,* ventricular septum. (Reproduced with permission from Vizcaino A, Campbell J, Litovsky S, Van Praagh R. Single origin of right and left pulmonary artery branches from ascending aorta with nonbranching main pulmonary artery: relevance to a new understanding of truncus arteriosus. *Pediatr Cardiol.* 2002;23:230.)

of heart and lungs was that of a 2-day-old female infant who weighed 2200 g. A complete autopsy showed that the segmental cardiac anatomy was normal: {S,D,S}. The atrioventricular (AV) and ventriculoarterial (VA) alignments were normal. The septum primum was almost absent, resulting in a common atrium.

The MPA was of good size (9 mm in external diameter). But it gave origin to no pulmonary artery branches. The only outlet from the MPA was a patent ductus arteriosus (internal diameter 3 to 4 mm) that opened into the descending thoracic aorta (external diameter 9 mm). The ventricular septum was intact, and both ventricular outflow tracts were unremarkable. The right pulmonary artery (RPA) and left pulmonary artery (LPA) branches both originated from the aortic sac on the dorsal surface of the ascending aorta via a single ostium (internal diameter 3 mm). This ostium led into a short common pulmonary artery that then bifurcated into right and LPA branches. The opening into the short common pulmonary artery lay 8 mm above an unremarkable aortic valve and 7 mm below an unremarkable appearing innominate artery. The common pulmonary artery proceeded posteriorly for 5 mm and then bifurcated into the RPA and LPA branches, as noted earlier. The common pulmonary artery measured 4 mm in external diameter. The RPA and left LPA branches both measured 3 mm in external diameter.

This patient had a heterotaxy syndrome with polysplenia. There were two small splenuli, each weighing 1.5 g. Both lungs were bilobed. Both right and left mainstem bronchi were hypoarterial. The liver was bilaterally symmetrical, and the gallbladder was absent. The inferior vena cava was interrupted. An enlarged azygos vein drained into the right superior vena cava. There was also marked congenital stenosis of the lower trachea, with complete tracheal rings. Severe airway stenosis also involved the carina and the proximal mainstem bronchi, with luminal narrowing to a diameter of less than 1 mm. The aortic arch was left-sided, with marked tubular hypoplasia and severe preductal coarctation (internal diameter 1 mm) (see Fig. 26.3).[14] Biventricular hypertrophy and enlargement were also present.

Additional associated congenital anomalies included tracheomalacia, stomach in the right upper quadrant, atresia of the first portion of the duodenum with annular pancreas, intestinal malrotation with cecum and appendix in the left upper quadrant, horseshoe kidneys, agenesis of the ovaries and fallopian tubes, atresia of the inferior one-third of the urinary bladder, atresia of the inferior one-third of the vagina, absence of the urethral meatus, and absence of the hymen and clitoris. Although this patient had the heterotaxy syndrome with polysplenia, she also had additional severe malformations, some of which were consistent with the XO Turner syndrome. Unfortunately, the karyotype was not done.

How were we to interpret Dr. Vizcaino's amazing case? A normal MPA, but with no branches! And with the pulmonary artery branches arising from the posterior wall of the ascending aorta!

Fortunately I remembered a paper by Congdon[15] that had been published in 1922 from the Contributions to Embryology of the Carnegie Institution of Washington, where I had studied their embryology collections and had done experimental embryology in 1966. I was well aware that this was an excellent source of highly reliable embryologic information. Congdon[15] found that the RPA and LPA branches originate from the aortic sac on the dorsal surface of the ascending aorta at the 4-mm stage, when the human embryo is 24 to 26 days of age in utero, before the embryonic sixth arches have completely formed. Completion of both sixth aortic arches can occur as early as the 5-mm stage, 26 to 28 days of age in utero. Completion of both sixth aortic arches usually occurs by the 6-mm stage, at 28 to 30 days of age in utero. As soon as both sixth arches have been completely formed, they normally enlarge considerably, and both pulmonary artery branches migrate on the sixth arches and unite with the MPA. Thus, the normal pulmonary arterial system has a tripartite origin:

1. The pulmonary artery branches arise from the aortic sac.
2. The MPA originates from the truncus arteriosus.
3. The RPA and LPA migrate on the ventral sixth aortic arches from the aortic sac to become confluent with the MPA at about 28 to 30 days of age in the normal human embryo.

Our interpretations of the foregoing data are as follows:

1. In Vizcaino's[14] very rare case (see Fig. 26.3) with multiple congenital anomalies, the sixth aortic arches did not form normally. Consequently, the RPA and the LPA could not

migrate and become confluent with the normally formed MPA. **Consequently, the RPA and the LPA are unmigrated (see Fig. 26.3).**[14]

2. In our case of so-called truncus arteriosus communis (Fig. 26.4),[3] the RPA and the LPA are still in their starting, premigration locations, arising from the aortic sac, because the RPA and the LPA have nowhere to migrate to—the MPA is absent. There is no vestige of the aortopulmonary septum because the MPA is absent. So, too, are the subpulmonary infundibulum and the pulmonary valve. Fig. 26.4[3] shows a solitary aorta with absence of the MPA, and unmigrated RPA and LPA.

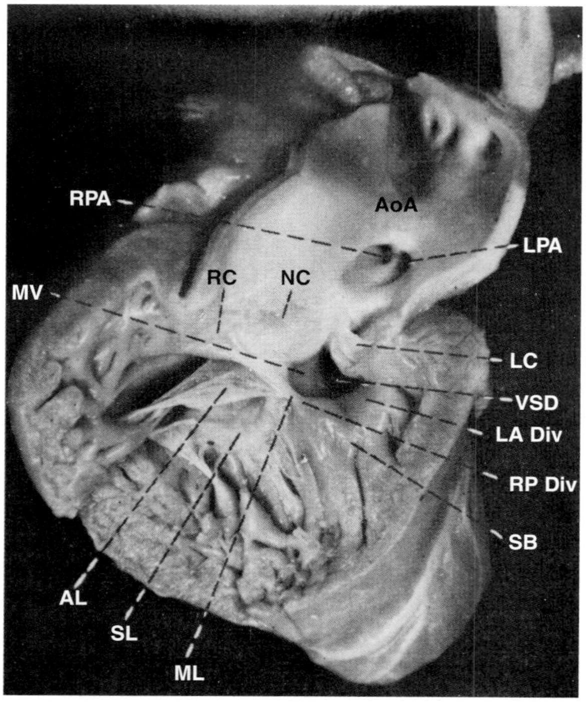

Fig. 26.4 We and many others used to regard this kind of case as having truncus arteriosus communis, our type A2[7] in 1965. This was well before we came to understand the aortic sac as the site of origin of the pulmonary artery branches (about 2001).[14] The heart presented in Fig. 26.3 was what opened my eyes. The above heart has a typical aortic sac giving rise to unmigrated pulmonary artery branches. The subpulmonary infundibulum, the pulmonary valve, and the main pulmonary artery are all absent. The right pulmonary artery *(RPA)* and the left pulmonary artery *(LPA)* are unmigrated, perhaps because they have nowhere to migrate to, because the main pulmonary artery is absent. The large subaortic ventricular septal defect is caused by absence of the subpulmonary infundibulum. The diagnosis is absence of the pulmonary outflow tract, that is, absence of the subpulmonary infundibulum, pulmonary valve, main pulmonary artery, and unmigrated pulmonary artery branches arising from the aortic sac. Is this pre-tetralogy of Fallot (TOF)? TOF is progressively more severe infundibular hypoplasia. But in TOF, the worst infundibular hypoplasia ever gets is infundibular atresia. But never infundibular *absence*. And not just infundibular absence. The whole pulmonary outflow tract is absent. *AoA,* Aortic arch; *AL,* anterior leaflet (of the tricuspid valve); *LA Div,* left anterior division (of top of septal band); LC, left coronary (leaflet of aortic valve); *ML,* muscle of Lancisi; *MV,* mitral valve; *NC,* noncoronary leaflet (of aortic valve); *RC,* right coronary (leaflet of aortic valve); *RP Div,* right posterior division of the top of the septal band; *SB,* septal band; *SL,* septal leaflet (of tricuspid valve); *VSD,* ventricular septal defect. (Reproduced with permission from Van Praagh R, Van Praagh S. The anatomy of common aorticopulmonary trunk (truncus arteriosus communis) and its embryologic implications, a study of 57 necropsy cases. *Am J Cardiol.* 1965;16:406.)

By 2002, we understood that the normal pulmonary arterial system is a three-component system[14]:

1. the truncus arteriosus (arterial trunk) supplies the MPA:
2. the aortic sac is where the RPA and LPA branches originate; and
3. the sixth aortic arches are the third component that is necessary to connect component one (the MPA) and component two (the RPA and LPA branches). This is what Vizcaino's case[14] taught us, confirming what Congdon[15] had published in 1922.

We also realized that it is impossible to have a common (undivided) aortopulmonary trunk if the subpulmonary infundibulum, the pulmonary valve, and the MPA are all *absent*. These data mean that we are dealing with a *solitary* aortic trunk (see Fig. 26.4), not with a *common* (undivided) aortopulmonary trunk. This also means that cases of truncus arteriosus communis persisens (persistent common arterial trunk)[3,11-16] need to be reinterpreted, which we have been doing previously[14] and are endeavoring to do here.

How could we all have been so wrong? My best assessment is as follows. We did not know about, or had forgotten about, Congdon's[15] work in 1922, that is, that the RPA and the LPA originate from the aortic sac and then have to migrate on the sixth aortic arches to connect with the MPA. Congdon[15] knew that the normal pulmonary arteries were a three-part system, which he described. Later investigators[2-13]—the rest of us—seem to have assumed that the pulmonary arteries are one structure. We assumed that because the RPA and the LPA branches are present (see Fig. 26.4), the MPA "must" be present, even though there is no vestige of the aortopulmonary septum that would support the presence of an MPA in our type A2. We used to think that absence of aortopulmonary septation was the malformation. We did not know that the RPA and LPA could be present and that the MPA could be absent, because the pulmonary arteries are a composite three-part system. We did not know that the presence of the RPA and LPA arising from the aortic sac implies nothing, of necessity, concerning the MPA component of the arterial trunk (the truncus arteriosus).

We did not understand the silent testimony of the unmigrated RPA and LPA arising from the aortic sac. The most obvious "messages" being sent by the unmigrated RPA and LPA are:

1. the MPA is absent, that is, there is nowhere for the RPA and the LPA to migrate to; or
2. the sixth aortic arches—the transport system for the RPA and the LPA—are absent, or nonfunctional; or
3. both 1 and 2.

Thus, the presence of *unmigrated* RPA and LPA supports the possibility that the MPA is absent. Because we now know that the pulmonary arteries normally are a three-component system, the presence of unmigrated RPA and LPA does *not* suggest that the MPA must be present, when there is no anatomic evidence that this is the case.

Why have I spent so much time on so-called truncus arteriosus communis type A2?[7] Because it is perhaps the best example of "absence of [the] aortic septum,"[8] including absence of septation at the level of the semilunar valves and infundibular septum.[9-13] **It is now clear that this classic concept of persistent common aortopulmonary trunk was, and is, a mistake; thus, I propose that this erroneous diagnosis be discontinued, in the interests of anatomic and developmental accuracy.** It must be added that it is rarely possible for there to be **almost total absence of the aortopulmonary septum,** with normal separated semilunar valves and with an intact ventricular septum (Fig. 26.5).[7] I have never seen a case like this. This photograph was sent to me by Professor J. W. A. Duckworth, Professor of Anatomy, University of Toronto, Ontario, Canada. This is the heart of a 42-year-old white woman who dies of unrecognized pulmonary tuberculosis. The heart specimen is from the Department of Anatomy of the University of Edinburgh, Scotland.

The heart could be diagnosed as truncus arteriosus communis, without anatomic inaccuracy, because the ascending aorta and the MPA both are present and both are unseparated (or in common) because of a huge, almost total aortopulmonary septal defect (or window). Only the semilunar valves are separated and normally formed. What is the accurate diagnosis of our so-called truncus arteriosus communis type A2 (see Fig. 26.4)?[7] In 2019, our diagnosis is absence of the subpulmonary infundibulum, absence of the pulmonary valve, and absence of the MPA.

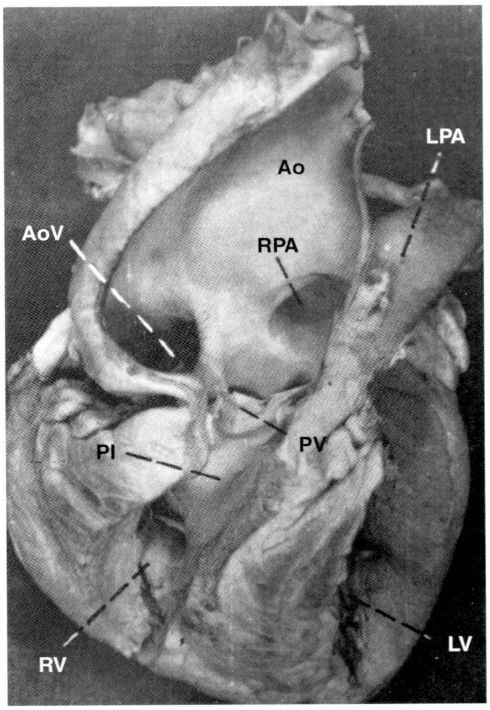

Fig. 26.5 Almost total aortopulmonary septal defect, except for separate and divided pulmonary valve *(PV)* and aortic valve *(AoV)*, and an intact ventricular septum separating the right ventricle *(RV)* and the left ventricle *(LV)*. It seems wise to call this type of very rare case a virtually total aortopulmonary septal defect, which does not suggest involvement of the semilunar valves, whereas the term *truncus arteriosus* suggests that the semilunar valves may be in common. I have never examined a case like this. This photograph was kindly sent to us by Prof. J. W. A. Duckworth, Professor of Anatomy, University of Toronto, Canada. This heart specimen actually came from the Department of Anatomy, University of Edinburgh, Scotland. The patient was a 42-year-old white woman who died of unrecognized pulmonary tuberculosis. *Ao,* Aorta; *LPA,* left pulmonary artery; *PI,* pulmonary infundibulum; *RPA,* right pulmonary artery. (Reproduced with permission from Van Praagh R, Van Praagh S. The anatomy of common aorticopulmonary trunk (truncus arteriosus communis) and its embryologic implications, a study of 57 necropsy cases. *Am J Cardiol.* 1965;16:406.)

Unmigrated RPA and LPA branches arising from the aortic sac {S,D,05S}, that is, the set of situs solitus atria, situs solitus (D-loop) ventricles, situs solitus aorta with absence of the pulmonary valve and MPA (as earlier), and subaortic VSD because of absence of the subpulmonary infundibulum.

But, what is the "big-picture" diagnosis of type A2?[7] This is **pre-TOF, and pre–situs solitus normally related great arteries.** All of those structures are absent that must be developed to create TOF and/or SNRGA. The lung pump (the RV inflow tract) is present, but the lung pump's outflow tract is absent. **The whole right ventricular outflow tract is absent.** That is the correct diagnosis, we now think.

Reexaming our 1965 paper on truncus arteriosus communis,[7] my thoughts some 54 years later are as follows:

Type A1[7]**:** The aortopulmonary windows were low and small. The aortopulmonary septum was fairly well developed, not "absent or rudimentary," as Abbott[8] described.

Types A2 and A3: Described earlier.

Type A4: The great artery arising from the base of the heart looks like the MPA (Fig. 26.6). No vestige of the aortopulmonary septum was found. The small aorta arises as a side branch of the MPA. Immediately to its left, at the same height and of the same size is the ostium of the RPA. To the left is the ostium of the LPA. Finally, to the left and above is the ostium of a large and probably closing patent ductus arteriosus. The isthmus of the aortic arch is interrupted. Thus, the aortic valve and the ascending aorta appeared to be absent. A small aortic arch arose to the right of the ostium of the RPA. The small aortic arch was interrupted at the aortic isthmus. So, this 5-day-old boy had an arterial arch that was formed by a large but closing ductus arteriosus.

This may be a newly recognized form of congenital heart disease (see Fig. 26.6)[7]**:** absence of the aortic valve, absence of the ascending aorta, small aortic arch arising as a branch from the distal end of the MPA, with interrupted aortic arch and a large closing ductus arteriosus.

Now you can see why I am advocating that the diagnosis of truncus arteriosus communis be phased out. The diagnosis of truncus arteriosus communis does not apply well to any of the anatomic types: A1, A2, A3, or A4.[7,16] The diagnosis of truncus arteriosus communis does not apply perfectly to almost total absence of the aortopulmonary septum because, in this very rare anomaly (see Fig. 26.5),[7] the semilunar valves are divided and normally formed, and there is no VSD. Nonetheless, this very rare anomaly—that I personally have never examined—does have a common aortopulmonary trunk in the sense that the ascending aorta and the MPA both are present, and both great arteries are in common (or unseparated) because of the presence of a huge aortopulmonary septal defect that is complete,

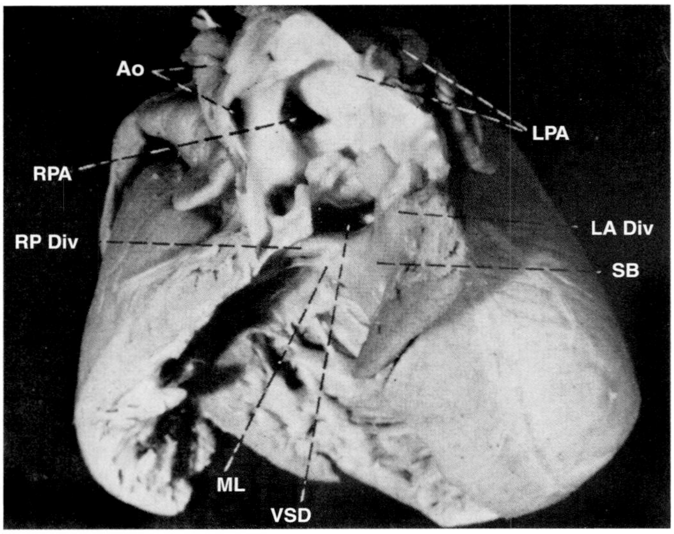

Fig. 26.6 "Truncus arteriosus communis" type A4.[7] The great artery arising from the base of the heart looks like a main pulmonary artery (MPA). Three semilunar leaflets are thick, fleshy, and soft. A large subvalvar ventricular septal defect *(VSD)* is present. No remnant of the aortopulmonary septum is found. The aortic valve and ascending aorta appear to be absent. The large MPA has large right pulmonary artery *(RPA)* and left pulmonary artery *(LPA)* branches and a large and apparently closing patent ductus arteriosus. To the right of the ostium leading into the large RPA, at the same level, there is a similar-sized ostium leading into a small aortic arch, which is interrupted at the aortic isthmus. This anomaly does not appear to be the large absence of the aortopulmonary septum envisioned by Abbott.[8] Instead, this malformation is now thought to be absence of the ascending aorta, with an interrupted aortic arch being a small branch at the end of a large MPA. Absence of the MPA has long been recognized as a cardiovascular malformation. *But absence of the ascending aorta is a newly recognized cardiovascular malformation,* its existence having been previously disguised by our erroneous understanding of "truncus arteriosus communis." *Ao,* Aorta; *LA Div,* left anterior division of the septal band; *RP Div,* right posterior division of the septal band; *SB,* septal band. (Reproduced with permission from Van Praagh R, Van Praagh S. The anatomy of common aorticopulmonary trunk (truncus arteriosus communis) and its embryologic implications, a study of 57 necropsy cases. *Am J Cardiol.* 1965;16:406.)

except between the semilunar valves, which are separate and normally formed, and there is no VSD. So, in this sense, truncus arteriosus communis does exist. But most of the cases to which all of us have been assigning this diagnosis of *truncus arteriosus communis* are misdiagnoses.

$$TGA\ S,\ D,\ D = 4R + 0L \quad \textbf{Equation 26.6}$$

Equation 26.6 represents typical physiologically uncorrected transposition of the great arteries (TGA). **In words, Equation 26.6 says:** transposition of the great arteries with the set of situs solitus of the atria, solitus (or D-loop) ventricles, and solitus (or D-) transposition of the great arteries equals a well-developed right-sided subaortic infundibulum plus absence of left-sided subpulmonary infundibulum.

D-TGA is presented diagrammatically in Fig. 26.1 *(fourth column from the right).* Note that the infundibulum (or conus arteriosus) is right-sided and subaortic. The subaortic infundibular free wall (remote from the aortopulmonary septum) is well developed. The transposed aortic valve is separated by the infundibulum from the tricuspid valve. There is no subpulmonary infundibular free-wall myocardium. Consequently, the transposed pulmonary valve is in direct fibrous continuity with the mitral valve, often via an intervalvar fibrosa. D-TGA is also diagrammed in Fig. 26.7 *(row 5, column 1).* The AV alignments are appropriate (concordant or normal): right atrium (RA) to RV, and left atrium (LA) to LV. However, the VA alignments are inappropriate (discordant or abnormal): RV to aorta and LV to pulmonary artery.

One intersegmental discordance (at the VA level) physiologically uncorrects the systemic and pulmonary venous circulations. The transposed aorta receives deoxygenated systemic venous blood because the RA and the aorta are ipsilateral (both right-sided). Hence, such patients are cyanotic (see Fig. 26.7).

The transposed pulmonary artery and the LA are both left-sided. Consequently the pulmonary artery is receiving oxygenated blood (see Fig. 26.7). Postnatal survival depends on left-to-right and right-to-left shunting of blood.

Equation 26.6 reveals what D-TGA really is. Infundibuloarterial situs analysis shows that the situs of the subarterial infundibulum (4R + 0L) is different from that of normal situs solitus (0R + 4L).

In D-TGA, the situs of the transposed great arteries is solitus TGA. D-TGA is solitus TGA because the transposed aortic valve is to the right of the transposed pulmonary valve, which is normal in situs solitus (Equation 26.1), not inverted (Equation 26.2). Thus, in typical D-TGA (Equation 26.6), the infundibuloarterial situs combination is discordant-concordant (abnormal). In D-TGA, the situs of the infundibulum (4R – 0L) is a mirror-image of the situs of the solitus normal infundibulum (0R + 4L) (Equation 26.1). Typical D-TGA, as in Equation 26.6, is isolated infundibular inversion, or mirror imagery (right-left reversal, without superoinferior, or anteroposterior change). In D-TGA, the great arteries are normal per se. D-TGA is an infundibular malformation, not a great arterial anomaly.

$$TGA\ S,\ L,\ L = 0R + 4L \quad \textbf{Equation 26.7}$$

This is the classic form of congenitally physiologically corrected TGA. L-loop formation of the bulboventricular loop places the MPA to the right of the ascending aorta (see Fig. 26.2). **Equation 26.7 says:** TGA with the set of situs solitus of the atria, discordant situs inversus of the ventricles (ventricular L-loop), and inverted (L-) TGA equals no right-sided subpulmonary free-wall myocardium plus a well-developed left-sided subaortic infundibular free wall (see Fig. 26.2, *fourth column from the right*).

The segmental alignments largely determine physiology (see Fig. 26.7, *row 5, column 2*). The right-sided deoxygenated system's venous return: RA → LV → PA. Both the systemic venous pathway and the pulmonary venous pathway have two segmental discordances, at the AV junction and at the VA junction (see Fig. 26.7).

One segmental discordance, as in Equation 6, physiologically uncorrects the circulations, resulting in central cyanosis. **Two segmental discordances,** as in Equation 26.7, may cancel each other, theoretically correcting the circulations. However, associated malformations, such as pulmonary stenosis or atresia

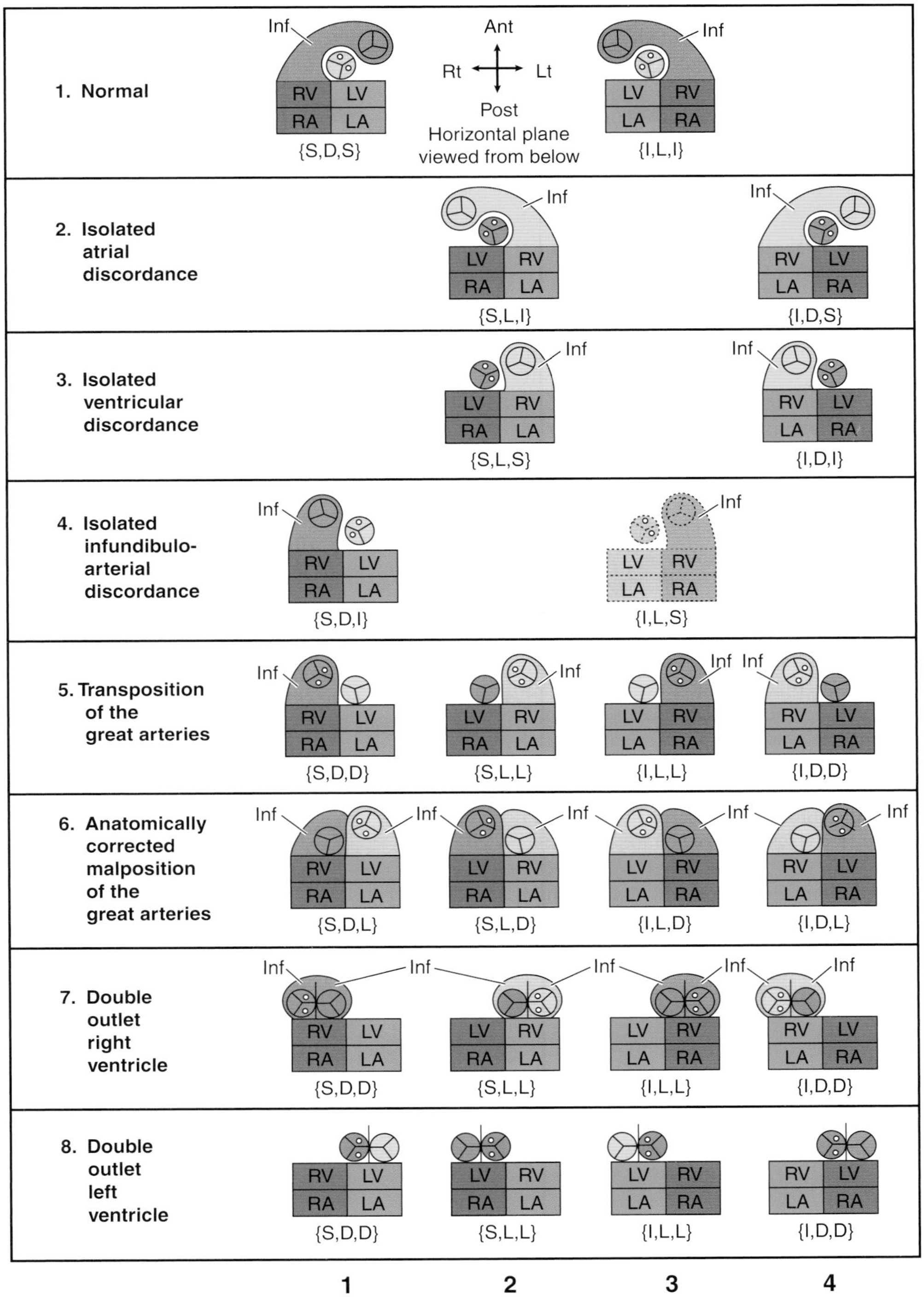

Fig. 26.7 Types of human heart, viewed from below, in terms of the morphologic anatomy of the cardiac chambers, the infundibulum, and the great arteries, the segmental sets of {atria, ventricles, and great arteries}, and the atrioventricular (AV) alignments and the ventriculoarterial (VA) alignments. *Column 1* has AV alignment concordance. *Column 2* has AV alignment discordance in visceroatrial situs solitus. *Column 3* has AV alignment concordance. *Column 4* has AV alignment discordance in visceroatrial situs inversus. *Rows 1 to 4* have VA alignment concordance, that is, normally aligned great arteries. *Rows 5, 7, and 8* have VA alignment discordance: transposition of the great arteries, double-outlet right ventricle, and double-outlet left ventricle. *Row 6*, anatomically corrected malposition of the great arteries, has VA alignment concordance with abnormally related great arteries (e.g., aorta anterior to pulmonary artery). Diagrams drawn with *dashed lines* mean malformation(s) not reported when this diagram was made. *Ant*, Anterior; *{I,L,I}*, the set of inverted atria, L-loop (inverted) ventricles, and inverted normally related great arteries; *Inf*, infundibulum; *LA*, morphologically left atrium; *Lt*, left; *LV*, morphologically left ventricle; *RA*, morphologically right atrium, *RV*, morphologically right ventricle; *{S,D,S}*, the set of solitus atria, D-loop (solitus) ventricles, and solitus normally related great arteries. Aorta indicated by coronary ostia; pulmonary artery, no coronary ostia. All other diagrams are similarly self-explanatory. (Reproduced with permission from Van Praagh R. What determines whether the great arteries are normally or abnormally related? *Am J Cardiol.* 2016;118:1390.)

with a VSD, frequently prevent physiologic correction of the circulations.

TGA {S,D,D} has isolated infundibular inversion: 4R + 0L. This is the same infundibular situs as in Equation 26.2 for situs inversus totalis. TGA {I,L,L} (see Fig. 26.7, *row 5, column 3*), typically has isolated infundibular noninversion (0R + 4L), the same as in Equation 26.1. In L-TGA the infundibulum is solitus normal. Therefore, TGA cannot be defined as an infundibulum malformation. Instead, the only definition of TGA that always applies accurately is as follows: TGA is infundibuloarterial situs discordance (difference) with VA alignment discordance (inappropriateness).

Please note that we speak of AV *alignments* (not connections) and VA *alignments* (not connections) in the interests of anatomic accuracy. The atria and the ventricles normally do not connect, except at the AV bundle of His, because of the interposition of the AV canal or junction that separates the atria from the ventricles. Similarly, the ventricles and the great arteries normally do not connect, because of the infundibulum or conus arteriosus that separates the ventricles and the great arteries. The main cardiac segments (atria, ventricles, and great arteries) are separated by the connecting cardiac segments (the AV canal, and the infundibulum or conus arteriosus). **The AV canal behaves like a dependent variable. But the infundibulum appears to be an independent variable,** controlled neither by the ventricles below nor by the great arteries above, as this chapter illustrates.

$$DORV\ S,\ D,\ D = 4R + 4L \quad \textbf{Equation 26.8}$$

Equation 26.8 represents double-outlet right ventricle (DORV) of the Taussig-Bing type.[17,18] **Equation 26.8 says:** DORV with the set of solitus atria, solitus (D-loop) ventricles, and solitus (D-) malposition of the great arteries equals a well-developed right-sided subaortic infundibular free wall plus a well-developed left-sided subpulmonary infundibular free wall. The infundibular septum was also well developed. A well-developed bilateral infundibulum is diagrammed in Fig. 26.1 *(fifth column from the left)*. The bilateral infundibulum prevents semilunar valvar–AV valvar fibrous continuity. The Taussig-Bing type of DORV is diagrammed in Fig. 26.7 *(row 7, column 1)*. The subpulmonary VSD (i.e., the interventricular foramen) is not depicted.

Apoptosis, genetically programmed cell death, is now thought to be an important mechanism leading to normal and abnormal morphogenesis of the great arteries:

1. Normally, the right-sided subaortic infundibular free wall undergoes "resorption" as a result of apoptosis: **0R** + 4L, Equation 26.1. Resorption of the right-sided subaortic infundibular free wall permits or facilitates the embryonic aortic switch from above the RV to above the LV and into fibrous continuity with the mitral valve via the aortic-mitral intervalvar fibrosa, the remains of the resorbed subaortic infundibular free wall.
2. In typical D-TGA, the pattern of apoptosis is right-left reversed ("inverted"): 4R + **0L** (Equation 26.6). Thus, in D-TGA, the wrong infundibular free wall gets resorbed by left-sided subpulmonary infundibular free-wall apoptosis. So the wrong great artery, the pulmonary artery, gets embryonically right-left switched from above the RV to above the LV and into fibrous continuity with the mitral valve. And the wrong great artery, the aorta, gets held above the RV by the unresorbed right-sided subaortic infundibular free-wall myocardium. **D-TGA** is one example of what the infundibulum is really doing:
   a. Resorption of the subarterial infundibular free wall by apoptosis permits or facilitates the embryonic great arterial switch from above the RV to above the LV and into fibrous continuity with the mitral valve.
   b. Failure of resorption of the subarterial infundibular free wall, presumably because of a failure of apoptosis or other resorptive mechanism(s), prevents the great arterial switch from RV to LV, and results in such a great artery (or arteries) remaining above the RV. We will see that these are the functions of the subarterial infundibular free walls: resorption permits a switch, and no resorption prevents a switch.
3. DORV of the Taussig-Bing type[17,18] has a well-developed right-sided subaortic infundibular free wall, and a well-developed left-sided subpulmonary infundibular free wall: **4R + 4L,** Equation 26.8. The bilaterally well-developed infundibular free walls prevented both great arteries from undergoing an embryonic RV-to-LV great arterial switch, resulting in DORV.

DOUBLE-OUTLET LEFT VENTRICLE OF THE PAUL TYPE[19]

$$DOLV\ S,\ D,\ D = 0R + 0L \quad \textbf{Equation 26.9}$$

Equation 26.9 says: Double-outlet left ventricle with the set of solitus atria, solitus (D-loop) ventricles, and solitus (D-) malposition of the great arteries equals absence of right-sided subaortic infundibular free-wall myocardium plus absence of left-sided subpulmonary infundibular free-wall myocardium.[19] The infundibular septum was also membranous. There was aortic-mitral and pulmonary-mitral direct fibrous continuity. This anatomic type of DOLV[6] is presented diagrammatically in Fig. 26.7 *(row 8, column 1)*.

Again we see the subarterial infundibular free walls acting as the great arterial "switch master." Rarely, when there is no subarterial infundibular free-wall myocardium beneath either great artery, both great arteries can be switched in embryonic life from the RV to the LV, resulting in DOLV (see Chapter 24).

Anatomically corrected malposition of the great arteries (ACMGA) means that the great arteries are malpositioned, but that nonetheless they arise above the anatomically appropriate ventricles—the aorta above the LV and the pulmonary artery above the RV. This is what *anatomically corrected* malposition means. But how is that possible? The "secret" of ACMGA is that the ventricular sinuses loop in one direction, say to the right, but the infundibulum and the great arteries twist in the opposite direction, to the left. And the infundibulum may or may not be malformed.

$$ACMGA\ \{S,D,L\} = 0R + 4L \quad \textbf{Equation 26.10}$$

Equation 26.10 says: Anatomically corrected malposition of the great arteries with the set of solitus atria, *solitus* (D-loop) ventricles, and *inverted* (L-) malposition of the great arteries equals absence of right-sided subpulmonary infundibular free-wall myocardium plus a well-developed left-sided subaortic infundibular free-wall myocardium. Infundibuloarterial situs analysis reveals that the infundibular situs is solitus normal, the same as Equation 26.1: 0R + 4L. But the great arterial situs is inverted: {-,-,L}. Hence, the infundibuloarterial situs combination is solitus normal-inverted abnormal, that is, discordant (abnormal) (see Fig. 26.7, *row 6, column 1*). (Inverted normal is {-,-,I}.)

The ventricles looped to the right: {-,D,-}. But the infundibulum and great arteries twisted to the left: {-,-,L}, resulting in ACMGA (see Fig. 26.7, *row 6, column 1*). ACMGA {S,D,L} is physiologically corrected, lack of associated malformations permitting. The LA and the aorta both are left-sided, and the RA and the pulmonary artery both are right-sided. So, this type of ACMGA is corrected both anatomically and physiologically (see Fig. 26.7, *row 6, column 1*).

$$ACMGA\ S,\ L,\ D = 4R + 4L \quad \textbf{Equation 26.11}$$

In words, **Equation 26.11 says:** ACMGA with the set of solitus atria, *inverted (L-loop)* ventricles, and *solitus (D-)* malposition of the great arteries equals a well-developed right-sided subaortic infundibular free wall plus a well-developed left-sided subpulmonary infundibular free wall. The infundibular situs is ambiguus (uncertain or unknown): 4R + 4L (different from solitus normal, Equation 26.1): 0R + 4L. Also different from inversus normal, Equation 26.2: 4R + 0L. The great arterial situs is solitus abnormal {-,-,D}. (Solitus normal is S.) Hence, the infundibuloarterial situs combination is: ambiguus-solitus abnormal, which is discordant (abnormal).

The VA contralaterality is characteristic of ACMGA: {-,L,D}. The inverted ventricles looped to the *left,* and the noninverted malposed great arteries twisted to the *right.* This anatomic type of ACMGA {S,L,D} is physiologically uncorrected (Fig. 26.8, *row 6, column 2*): the RA and the aorta are both right-sided and the LA and the pulmonary artery are both left-sided.

SYNERGY

Why is the transposed aorta typically anterior to the transposed pulmonary artery? Normal solitus ventricular (D-loop) formation is associated with approximately 90 degrees dextrorotation at the semilunar valves relative to the sagittal (or anteroposterior) plane: 0 to 90 degrees D-rotation (see Fig. 26.8).

Normal solitus infundibular development (0R + 4L, Equation 26.1) is associated with another approximately 60-degree D-rotation: 90- to 150-degree D-rotation (see Fig. 26.8). Inverted normal ventricular (L-loop) formation is associated with about 90 degrees of levorotation at the semilunar valves relative to the AP plane: 0 to 90-degree L-rotation (see Fig. 26.8). Inverted normal infundibular development is associated with another approximately 60 degrees of L-rotation: from 90 to 150 degrees of L-rotation (see Fig. 26.8). As a convenience, D-rotation may be expressed in positive degrees, for example, 90 degrees + 60 degrees = 150 degrees. L-rotation may be expressed in negative degrees, for example, −90 degrees + (−60 degrees) = −150 degrees.

Thus, both solitus and inversus normally related great arteries have two rotational "engines." In the solitus normal heart, both rotational engines generate D-rotation. In the inverted normal heart, both rotational engines generate L-rotation. But in each normal heart, are both rotational forces in the *same* direction? But in D-TGA, the two rotational engines are working *against* each other.

$$TGA\ S,D,D = 4R + 0L$$

The infundibular situs, 4R + 0L, is inverted normal (as in Equation 26.2), but the great arterial situs is solitus abnormal, {-,-,D}. So, the infundibuloarterial situs comparison is inversus-solitus, which is situs discordant, that is, abnormal, typical of D-TGA: **isolated infundibular inversion.** But, one can also extend the analysis to include the morphogenetic movements of the great arteries. Again, the equation is: TGA {S,**D**,D} = **4R + 0L.** The equation indicates the presence of solitus (D-loop) ventricles (90 degrees dextrorotation) and an inverted infundibulum (60 degrees levorotation). The expected final rotation at the semilunar valves equals approximately 30 degrees dextrorotation: 90 degrees + (−60 degrees) = 30 degrees. This is an example of **synergy,** which is derived from *synergia* (Latin), from Greek, *syn,* together + *ergon,* work. The correlated action or cooperation on the part of two or more structures or drugs. When two or more forces act together normally (e.g., 90 degrees + 60 degrees = 150 degrees D-rotation in normally related great arteries), this may be called normal or positive synergy. When two or more forces act against each other abnormally, this may be called **pathologic or negative synergy** (e.g., 90 degrees − 60 degrees = 30 degrees dextrorotation in D-TGA).

EVOLUTION

The evolutionary history of the human heart is highly relevant to the understanding of congenital heart disease.[20] Our phylum Chordata goes back to ancient **fish** of the Ordovician and upper Devonian periods, 500 million to 345 million years ago. These fish had a single ventricle from which our morphologically LV is derived. **Amphibia** evolved 345 million to 325 million years ago during the Carboniferous period. These amphibians had lungs and so could breathe air. But they had no RV. Some amphibians evolved into fully terrestrial animals, the **Amniota.** These animals had an amniotic sac filled with amniotic fluid in which the embryo and fetus could float, like our fish ancestors. Some amniotes evolved into reptiles. Others evolved into birds, which are feathered reptiles like *archaeopteryx.* Still others evolved into mammals, which are furry or hairy reptiles. Mammals evolved during the Jurassic period, about 180 million years ago. Although fish and amphibians do not have a morphologically RV, higher reptiles (crocodiles and alligators), birds, and mammals normally all do. The RV is comparatively "recently" evolved, being only about 36% as old as the LV: 180 million years versus at least 500 million years, respectively.

Most human congenital heart disease consists of anomalies of one or more of the four components (Fig. 26.9) that make up the RV. Malformations of the LV are comparatively infrequent. Congenital heart disease is the most common anomaly in liveborn infants: 0.8%. It accounts for more than 20% of all spontaneous abortions and is responsible for 10% of all still births.

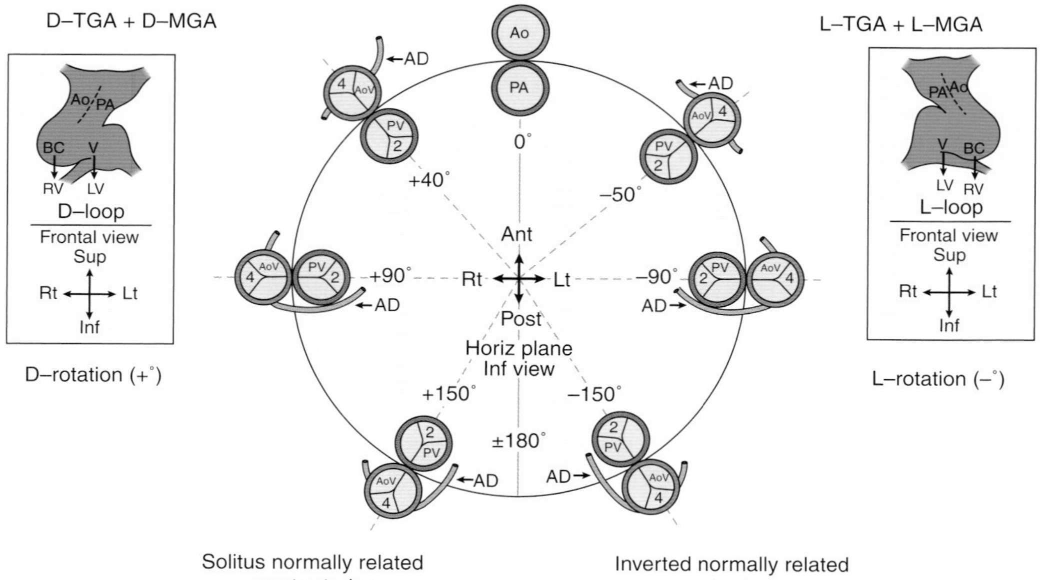

Fig. 26.8 The morphogenetic movements of the semilunar valves and the roles of synergy. The D-loop (or solitus) normal heart normally undergoes approximately 150 degrees of dextrorotation relative to the sagittal plane. D-loop formation is associated with about 90 degrees of this rightward rotation, causing the semilunar valves to be side-by-side, aortic valve *(AoV)* to the right pulmonary valve and pulmonary valve *(PV)* to the left, as in the Taussig-Bing malformation. Double-outlet right ventricle is present, with a well-developed infundibulum bilaterally (4R + 4L, Equation 26.8). Normally, the right-sided subaortic infundibular free wall involutes (disappears) because of apoptosis (programmed cell death). This converts the infundibulum to the normal situs solitus type (0R + 4L, Equation 26.1), which facilitates the embryonic aortic switch from right ventricle *(RV)* to left ventricle *(LV)* and also is associated with another approximately 60 degrees of D-rotation at the semilunar valve level. The "normal" inverted (L-loop) heart is mirror-image of the solitus (D-loop) heart. L-loop formation is associated with about 90 degrees of L-rotation at the semilunar valves, and inverted infundibular development (4R + 0L, Equation 26.2) is associated with another approximately 60 degrees L-rotation (–90 degrees to –150 degrees). Thus, it takes the synergy (or working together) of two intrauterine forces to achieve the 150-degree D-rotation or L-rotation to achieve normally related great arteries, solitus or inversus: (1) the ventricular loop force (90 degrees) and (2) the infundibular development force (60 degrees). Now remember that typical D-transposition of the great arteries *(D-TGA)* results from infundibular inversion (4R + 0L, Equation 26.6) and is associated with ≈ 60 degrees of L-rotation. Thus, D-TGA is associated with 90-degree D-rotation + (–60 degrees) L-rotation ≈ 30 degrees D-rotation. That is why the transposed aorta typically is anterior to the transposed pulmonary artery. There are two kinds of synergy: (1) *positive synergy,* that operates in a positive or healthful direction; and (2) *negative synergy,* that operates in in a negative and disease-producing way (biologic sabotage). The infundibular formulas found in the equations to the right of the equal sign indicate the direction of great arterial rotation. For example: 0R + 4L (Equation 26.1) means there is no infundibular muscle beneath the right-sided aorta and there is a well-developed infundibulum beneath the left-sided pulmonary artery. The well-developed subpulmonary infundibulum is like a raft or a float. The pulmonary artery cannot sink. But the right-sided aorta has no muscle holding it up. It can, and does sink and switch. Left side stays high and right side sinks. That is D-rotation. The reverse is L-rotation. *AD,* anterior descending coronary artery; *Ao,* aorta; *BC,* bulbus cordis; *Inf,* interior; *Horiz,* horizontal; *Lt,* left; *MGA,* malposition of the great arteries; *PA,* pulmonary artery; *Post,* posterior; *Rt,* right; *Sup,* superior. (Reproduced with permission from Van Praagh R. What determines whether the great arteries are normally or abnormally related? *Am J Cardiol.* 2016;118:1390.)

Thus, we are still having trouble with our major cardiovascular evolutionary adaptations to air-breathing and permanent land-living. This study of the infundibuloarterial malformations shows that there is only one way of doing it right (Equation 26.1 and its mirror-image isomer, Equation 26.2). And there are many ways of doing it wrong (Equations 26.3 to 26.11, inclusive, and Fig. 26.7).

Equation Summary

1. SNRGA {S,D,S} = 0R + 4L
2. INRGA {I,L,I} = 4R + 0L
3. TOF {S,D,S} = 0R + 1L
4. TOF {S,D,S} = 0R + 2L
5. TOF {S,D,S} = 0R + 3L
6. TGA {S,D,D} = 4R + 0L
7. TGA {S,L,L} = 0R + 4L
8. DORV {S,D,S} = 4R + 4L
9. DOLV {S,D,D} = 0R + 0L
10. ACMGA {S,D,L} = 0R + 4L
11. ACMGA {S,L,D} = 4R + 4L

ACMGA, Anatomically corrected malposition of the great arteries; *DOLV,* double-outlet left ventricle; *DORV,* double-outlet right ventricle; *INRGA,* inverted normally related great arteries; *SNRGA,* solitus normally related great arteries; *TGA,* transposition of the great arteries; *TOF,* tetralogy of Fallot.

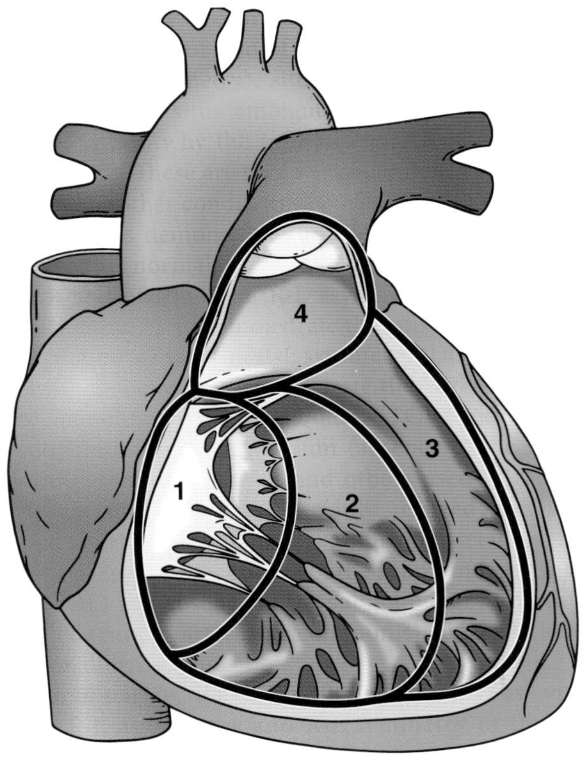

A

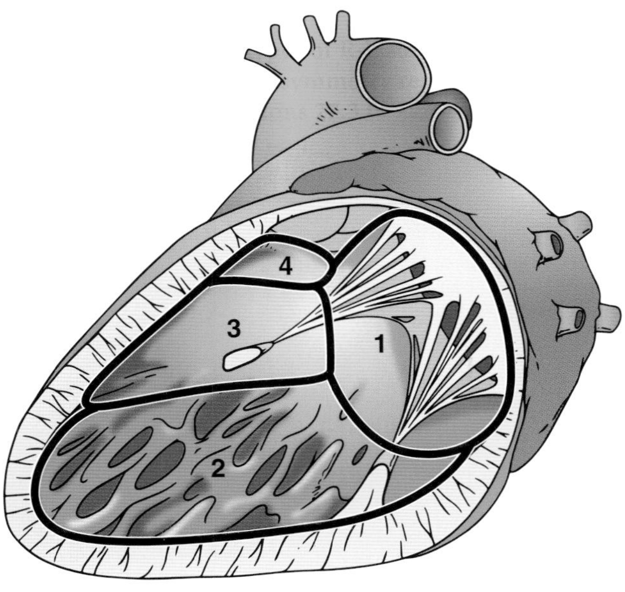

B

Fig. 26.9 The four segments that make up the morphologically right ventricle (RV) (A) and the morphologically left ventricle (LV) (B). Beginning with the RV, *segment 1* is the atrioventricular (AV) canal or junction. *Segment 2* is the RV sinus, body, or inflow tract. *Segments 1 and 2* make up the RV inflow tract. *Segment 2* is the lung pump. *Segment 3* is the proximal or apical portion of the infundibulum. *Segment 4* is the distal or subarterial part of the infundibulum. This is the infundibulum that this chapter has been all about. This structure is also known as the conus arteriosus and as the parietal band. The component parts of the LV and of the RV are very similar, as the component numbers indicate. Most of the anomalies of the great arteries are primarily anomalies of the subarterial infundibulum *(Segment 4)*. (Reproduced with permission from Van Praagh R, Geva T, Kreutzer J. Ventricular septal defects: how shall we describe, name and classify them? *J Am Coll Cardiol.* 1989;14:1298.)

BIOPHYSICS

Modern physicists have discovered that science is not a description of immutable things. Instead, it is a study of events, of happenings, of becomings, of change.[21] Embryologists and many other developmental biologists will have no trouble understanding this view point.

We have long been told that mathematics is the language of science, and we biologists have long been a bit embarrassed that so many of our verbal descriptions lack mathematical equivalents. An equation is not a static thing. It is a process, a statement of change: This + That = Something else.

This chapter is a contribution to the algebra and the geometry of the infundibuloarterial anomalies of the human heart. These anomalies are, almost = 4, primary malformations of the subarterial infundibulum that have important secondary effects on the great arteries.

APOPTOSIS

Normally and abnormally related great arteries result form normally and abnormally located apoptosis, which means "falling off," from *apo,* off, + *ptosis,* fall, (Greek). Apoptosis is a morphologic pattern of cell death affecting single cells. It is characterized as cell shrinkage, condensation of chromatin, cytoplasmic blebs, fragmentation into membrane-bound apoptotic bodies that are eliminated by phagocytosis. *Apoptosis is often called programmed cell death, that is, normal or physiologic cell death,* as opposed to abnormal or pathologic cell death, which is not part of the normal developmental program. **The location of the apoptosis determines whether the great arteries are normally or abnormally related:**

1. Apoptosis beneath aortic free wall
   0R + 4L, as in Equation 26.1,
   4R + 0L, as in Equation 26.2.
   O = Apoptosis site and the site of great arterial switching.
   Aorta switched into LV in SNRGA (Equation 26.1) and in INRGA (Equation 26.2).
   Pulmonary artery held above the RV by subpulmonary infundibulum in both Equations 26.1 and 26.2.
2. Apoptosis beneath left-sided pulmonary artery
   Pulmonary artery is switched into LV.
   Aorta remains above RV.
   The result is TGA, D, and L.
3. No apoptosis, right-sided or left-sided.
   Result is no switch, that is,
   DORV, Taussig-Bing type.
4. Bilateral apoptosis, subaortic and subpulmonary. The result is DOLV, Paul type.

CONCLUSIONS

1. Normally related great arteries include solitus and inversus forms:
   a. SNRGA {S,D,S} = 0R + 4L
   b. INRGA {I,L,I} = 4R + 0L
   c. TOF {S,D,S} = 0R + 3L/2L/1L

TOF is variable hypoplasia of the subpulmonary infundibulum with *almost* normally related great arteries.

2. Truncus arteriosus communis, very frequently, is a misdiagnosis. For example, truncus arteriosus communis type A2 is absence of the subpulmonary infundibulum, absence of the pulmonary valve, and absence of the MPA.
3. Abnormally located apoptosis (programmed cell death) creates different anatomic types of subarterial infundibulopathy. Normally, apoptosis is subaortic, facilitating the aortic switch from the RV to the LV. But abnormally located apoptosis can result in TGA, DORV, and DOLV. Thus, normally and abnormally related great arteries are created by at least two mechanisms:
   a. subarterial infundibulum prevents a switch, and
   b. normal and abnormal apoptosis creates the arterial switch.

REFERENCES

1. Van Praagh R. What determines whether the great arteries are normally or abnormally related? *Am J Cardiol.* 2016;118:1390.
2. Van Praagh R. The cardiovascular keys to air-breathing and permanent land-living in vertebrates: the normal human embryonic aortic switch procedure produced by complete right-left asymmetry in the development of the subarterial conal free walls, and the evolution of the right ventricular sinus. *Kardiochirurgia I Torakochirurgia Polska.* 2010;8:1. 2011.
3. Stenonis DN. Embryo monstro affinis Parisii dissectus. In: Bartholini T, editors. *Acta Medica et Philosophice Hafniensia*, Petrus Haubold, Copenhagen vol. 1; 202, 1671-1672 (in Latin).
4. Fallot A. Contribution à lànatomie patchologique de la maladie bleue, *Marseille-Médical* 25:77, 138, 207, 270, 341, 403, 1888.
5. Van Praagh R. The first Stella Van Praagh memorial lecture: the history and anatomy of tetralogy of Fallot. *Semin Thorac Cardiovasc Surg Pediatr Card Surg Annu.* 2009;2:19.
6. Van Praagh R, Van Praagh S, Nebesar RA, Muster AJ, Sinha SN, Paul MH. Tetralogy of Fallot: underdevelopment of the pulmonary infundibulum and its sequelae. *Am J Cardiol.* 1970;26:25.
7. Van Praagh R, Van Praagh S. The anatomy of common aorticopulmonary trunk (truncus arteriosus communis) and its embryologic implications, a study of 57 necropsy cases. *Am J Cardiol.* 1965;16:406.
8. Abbott ME. Absence or rudimentary development of aortic septum. In: Osler W, McCrae T, Funk EH, eds. *Modern Medicine.* vol. 4. Philadelphia: Lea + Febiger; 1927:707.
9. Feller A. Zur Kenntnis der angeborenen Herzkrankheiten. 1. Truncus arteriosus communis persistens und seine formale Entstehung. *Virchows Arch Path Anat.* 1931;279:869.
10. Humphreys EM. Truncus arteriosus communis persistens. Criteria for identification of the common arterial trunk, with report of a case with four semilunar cusps. *Arch Path.* 1932;14:671.
11. Roos A. Persistent truncus arteriosus communis. Report of a case with four semilunar cusps and aortic arch on the right side. *Am J Dis Child.* 1935;50:966.
12. Lev M, Saphir O. Truncus arteriosus communis persistens. *J Pediat.* 1942;20:74.
13. Collett RW, Edwards JE. Persistent truncus arteriosus: a classification according to anatomic types. *S Clin North America.* 1949;29:1245.
14. Vizcaino A, Campbell J, Litovsky S, Van Praagh R. Single origin of right and left pulmonary artery branches from ascending aorta with nonbranching main pulmonary artery: relevance to a new understanding of truncus arteriosus. *Pediatr Cardiol.* 2002;23:230.
15. Congdon ED. Transformation of the aortic-arch system during the development of the human embryo. *Contrib Embryol.* 1922;14:47.
16. Calder L, Van Praagh R, Van Praagh S, et al. Truncus arteriosus communis: clinical, angiocardiographic, and pathologic findings in 100 patients. *Am Heart J.* 1976;92:23.
17. Taussig HB, Bing RJ. Complete transposition of the aorta and a levoposition of the pulmonary artery, clinical, physiological, and pathological findings. *Am Heart J.* 1949;37:551.
18. Van Praagh R. What is the Taussig-Bing malformation? *Circulation.* 1968;38:445.
19. Paul MH, Muster AJ, Sinha SN, Cole RB, Van Praagh R. Double-outlet left ventricle with an intact ventricular septum: clinical and autopsy diagnosis and developmental implications. *Circulation.* 1970;41:129.
20. Van Praagh R. The evolution of the human heart and its relevance to congenital heart disease. *Kardiochirurgia i Torakochirurgia Polska.* 2011;41:427.
21. Rovelli C. *The Order of Time.* New York, NY: Riverhead Books; 2018.

27

Infundibuloarterial Situs Equations and Analysis

There is so much that is new in Chapters 22 to 26, it may be helpful to summarize and to integrate this new understanding. The abbreviations, references, and implicit figures in this summary are the same as in Chapters 22 to 26 and will not be reiterated here.

INFUNDIBULOARTERIAL SITUS CONCORDANCE AND DISCORDANCE

1. If the situs (pattern of anatomic organization) of the infundibulum and the situs of the great arteries are the same (concordant), the great arteries are normally related (solitus normally related, or inversus normally related).
2. If the situs of the infundibulum and the situs of the great arteries are different (discordant), the great arteries are abnormally related.

Relationships between the great arteries that have infundibuloarterial situs concordance and hence normally related great arteries include:

Solitus normally related great arteries (SNRGA):

SNRGA {S,D,S} = 0R + 4L

Equation 27.1

Inverted normally related great arteries (INRGA):

INRGA {I,L,I} = 4R + 0L **Equation 27.2**

Tetralogy of Fallot (TOF):

TOF {S,D,S} = 0R + 1L (TOF – atresia)

Equation 27.3

TOF {S,D,S} = 0R + 2L
(TOF – severe pulmonary stenosis [PS])

Equation 27.4

TOF {S,D,S} = 0R + 3L
(TOF–mild/moderate PS) **Equation 27.5**

TOF is a hypoplastic, obstructive subpulmonary infundibulum and its sequelae.

Absent subpulmonary infundibulum (AOSPI) and its sequelae, formerly misinterpreted as truncus arteriosus communis (TAC):

AOSPI {S,D,–} = 0R + (–L)
+ APSD (TAC) (type A1)

Equation 27.6

AOSPI {S,D,–} = 0R + (–L) + (–PV)
+ (–MPA) (TAC) (type A2)

Equation 27.7

The third element in the segmental situs set, a horizontal dash, that is { , ,−L} indicates absence of a subarterial muscular infundibulum, both right-sided and left-sided: = 0R + (-L). In Equation 27.6 there is an aortopulmonary window (APW) or aortopulmonary septal defect (APSD).

In Equation 27.7, there is absence of the main pulmonary artery (MPA). Absence of the MPA is fatal to the idea of truncus arteriosus communis. If the MPA is absent, truncus arteriosus communis cannot be present because truncus arteriosus communis means a very large APW. Hence, if the MPA is absent, there can be no APW.

The symbol zero (0) means that there is no subarterial infundibular muscle. Zero means that there is subarterial fibrous tissue. By contrast, the symbol (–) means that the subarterial region is absent, with no muscle and no fibrous tissue. Consequently, the symbols zero and dash have very different meanings. Zero (0) means subarterial fibrous tissue, whereas dash (–) means no subarterial fibrous tissue or muscular tissue, that is, subarterial tissue is absent. For example, there is no subarterial infundibular muscular tissue and there is no subarterial fibrous tissue such as an intervalvar fibrosa.

TOF and AOSPI appear to be interrelated anomalies. TOF is *hypoplasia* of the subpulmonary infundibulum, whereas AOSPI is *absence* of the subpulmonary infundibulum (septum and free wall). The foregoing seven infundibular malformations (Equations 27.1 to 27.7) all have infundibuloarterial **situs concordance** with essentially normally related great arteries in all except Equation 27.7, in which the MPA is absent (type A2).

AOAPS {S,D,S} = 0R + 4L + (–APS)

Equation 27.8

The following six equations have different anatomic types of infundibuloarterial **situs discordance,** resulting in different anatomic types of abnormally related great arteries.

D-Transposition of the great arteries (D-TGA), physiologically uncorrected:

$$\text{TGA } \{S,D,D\} = 4R + 0L \quad \text{Equation 27.9}$$

L-TGA, physiologically corrected:

$$\text{TGA } \{S,L,L\} = 0R + 4L \quad \text{Equation 27.10}$$

Double-outlet right ventricle (DORV), Taussig-Bing type:

$$\text{DORV } \{S,D,D\} = 4R + 4L \quad \text{Equation 27.11}$$

Double-outlet left ventricle (DOLV), Paul type:

$$\text{DOLV } \{S,D,D\} = 0R + 0L \quad \text{Equations 27.12}$$

Anatomically corrected malposition of the great arteries (ACMGA):

$$\text{ACMGA } \{S,D,L\} = 0R + 4L \quad \text{Equation 27.13}$$

$$\text{ACMGA } \{S,L,D\} = 4R + 4L \quad \text{Equation 27.14}$$

$$\text{IVI } \{S,L,S\} = 0R + 4L + \text{VSD} + \text{L - loopventricles} \quad \text{Equation 27.15}$$

These are the *most basic* equations. Many more could be written to reflect variations in visceroatrial situs (situs inversus, and situs ambiguus) and variations in infundibular development (e.g., TGA {S,D,D} = 4R + 2L with PS), and associated malformations (e.g., ventricular septal defect [VSD]).

THE LAWS OF THE GREAT ARTERIES

Equations 27.1 to 27.15 illustrate the laws of the great arteries, which, in words, are as follows:

1. A well-developed subpulmonary infundibular free wall and absence of a subaortic infundibular free wall result in (cause) normally related great arteries, solitus (Equation 27.1) and inversus or inverted (Equation 27.2).
2. Underdevelopment of the subpulmonary infundibulum causes TOF with variable right ventricular outflow tract obstruction (Equations 27.3, 27.4, and 27.5).
3. Absence of the subpulmonary infundibulum (septum and free wall) causes what we used to call truncus arteriosus communis (a widespread misinterpretation) (Equations 27.6 and 27.7).
4. Isolated absence of the aortopulmonary septum, a rare anomaly that I have never seen in person (Equation 27.8).
5. A well-developed subaortic infundibular free wall and absence of a subpulmonary infundibular free wall (or a relative small subpulmonary infundibular free wall) causes D-TGA and L-TGA (Equations 27.9 and 27.10).
6. Bilaterally well-developed infundibular free walls, subaortic and subpulmonary, result in DORV of the Taussig-Bing type (Equation 27.11).
7. Bilateral absence of the subarterial infundibular musculature, both subaortic and subpulmonary, results in DOLV of the Paul type (Equation 27.12).
8. When the ventricular sinuses or inflow tracts loop in one direction, say to the right, and the subarterial infundibulum and the great arteries twist in the opposite direction, to the left, and the situs of the subarterial infundibulum is different from the situs of the great arteries, this results in ACMGA (Equations 27.13 and 27.14). Because the ventricles and the great arteries twist in opposite directions, these abnormally related and malposed great arteries end up arising from the morphologically appropriate ventricles—aorta arising from the morphologically left ventricle (LV) and pulmonary artery originating from the morphologically right ventricle (RV). Hence, these malposed great arteries are anatomically corrected (Equations 27.13 and 27.14), that is, with ventriculoarterial (VA) alignment concordance. In Equation 27.13, the great arteries were also physiologically corrected. In Equation 27.14, the systemic and pulmonary circulations were physiologically uncorrected.

VENTRICULOARTERIAL ALIGNMENT CONCORDANCE

Note that there are two very different anatomic types of VA alignment concordance: (1) with solitus and inversus normally related great arteries (Equations 27.1 and 27.2); and (2) with anatomically corrected malposition of the great arteries (ACMGA), as in Equations 27.13 and 27.14. ACMGA is rarely possible because the ventricles loop in one direction, and the infundibulum and great arteries twist in the opposite direction.

Normally related great arteries have infundibuloarterial situs concordance, as in Equations 27.1 and 27.2. ACMGA has infundibuloarterial situs discordance, as in Equations 27.13 and 27.14.

Note also normally and abnormally developed great arteries (Equations 27.1 to 27.15) display variations in the development of the subarterial infundibular *free walls.* Variations in the aortopulmonary septum (spiral/straight) are secondary effects.

MORPHOGENETIC MOVEMENTS OF THE GREAT ARTERIES

The laws or rules governing the development of normal and abnormal great arteries are regarded as fundamental (earlier). Doing infundibuloarterial situs analysis and comparing the results with solitus normal (Equation 27.1) or with inversus normal (Equation 27.2) can be diagnostically helpful. **But**

what is responsible for normal and abnormal morphogenetic movements of the great arteries?

THE INFUNDIBULUM

Following ventricular D-loop formation at about 21 to 22 days of age in the human embryo, both developing great arteries are located above the developing morphologically RV. This is the starting position for both the aorta to the right and for the pulmonary artery to the left. What can happen then?

1. The right-sided subaortic infundibular free wall involutes or disappears because of **apoptosis** (programmed cell death) leading to the embryonic aortic switch from above the RV to above the LV and into fibrous continuity with the mitral valve. The left-sided subpulmonary infundibulum grows and expands, keeping the pulmonary valve above the RV and preventing an embryonic switch of the pulmonary artery. The result of these totally asymmetrical developments of the right-sided subaortic and left-sided subpulmonary infundibula is solitus normally related great arteries, symbolized in Equation 27.1 as 0R + 4L. Inverted normally related great arteries develop in the same way, but in mirror-image, and are symbolized in Equation 27.2 as 4R +0L. *Grade 4* (or 4+) development of the subarterial infundibular free wall means good (strong) development. *Grade 0* development means absent (no) development. Intermediate grades of development: *grade 1,* very severe under development with outflow tract atresia; *grade 2,* severe stenosis; and *grade 3,* mild to moderate stenosis. These intermediate grades of infundibular development are often useful, for example, in TOF (Equations 27.3, 27.4, and 27.5).
2. Or the development of the subarterial infundibulum can be inverted (right-left switched), resulting in D-TGA, as in Equation 27.9, that is, 4R + 0L, which is the same pattern as in situs inversus totalis (Equation 27.2). The left-sided pulmonary artery with no subpulmonary infundibular free wall gets switched into the LV, typically with pulmonary-mitral fibrous continuity, and the right-sided aorta, sitting on a well-developed subaortic infundibulum, remains above the RV and is not switched into the LV. **So isolated infundibular inversion is basically what typical D-TGA is (Equation 27.8).**

   Typical physiologically corrected L-TGA, that is, TGA {S,L,L} = 0R + 4L, develops in mirror-image relative to typical D-TGA. In typical L-TGA (Equation 27.10), the infundibulum is of the solitus normal pattern, that is, 0R + 4L, which is the same as the solitus normal pattern (in Equation 27.1). So just as typical D-TGA is basically isolated infundibular inversion (Equation 27.9), typical L-TGA is basically isolated infundibular noninversion, with Equation 27.10 of L-TGA being a mirror-image of Equation 27.9 of D-TGA at the all-important infundibular level. Both D-TGA and L-TGA have infundibuloarterial situs oppositeness (one form of infundibuloarterial situs discordance): D-TGA has infundibular inversion and great arterial noninversion. L-TGA has infundibular noninversion (situs solitus) with great arterial inversion.

   D-TGA is noninverted or solitus TGA, because of infundibular inversion. L-TGA is inverted TGA, caused by infundibular noninversion or situs solitus.

   The reason we do not use *solitus* TGA (D-TGA) and *inversus* TGA (L-TGA) routinely is that these designations are meaningless in visceroatrial situs ambiguus with asplenia and/or polysplenia, in which the type of visceroatrial situs can be uncertain or unknown. D- and L-TGA are always applicable, clear, and brief. However, it is important to understand solitus and inversus terminology because of the importance of segmental mirror-imagery in congenital heart disease.
3. Or the subarterial infundibular free walls can both be developed—subaortic and subpulmonary. If both are well developed, the result can be DORV of the Taussig-Bing type. The presence of a well-developed subaortic infundibulum and a well-developed subpulmonary infundibulum prevents both an embryonic aortic switch and an embryonic pulmonary switch into the morphologically LV. Consequently, both great arteries are held above the RV, resulting in DORV with a subpulmonary VSD.
4. Rarely, there can be no subaortic infundibulum and no subpulmonary muscular infundibulum, permitting or facilitating an embryonic switch of both great arteries from above the RV into the LV, resulting in DOLV of the Paul type.

In ACMGA, why do the ventricles loop in one direction and the infundibulum and the great arteries rotate in the opposite direction? In Equation 27.13, the ventricles loop to the right (D-loop) but the subarterial infundibulum and the great arteries rotate to the left (L-malposition of the great arteries): ACMGA {S,**D**,**L**} = 0R + 4L. An answer to this question is because ACMGA is characterized by VA situs discordance (or mismatch) and by **infundibuloarterial situs discordance (or mismatch).** Thus, ACMGA is characterized by **double segmental situs discordance**: VA and infundibuloarterial.

The VA situs discordance (solitus or D-loop ventricles, and inverted or L-malposition of the great arteries) is why the ventricles loop to the *right* and the infundibulum and the great arteries twist to the *left*.

The infundibuloarterial situs discordance is why the relationship between the semilunar valves is so abnormal. In Equation 27.13, the formula for the subarterial infundibulum is 0R + 4L—a solitus normal infundibulum—the same as in Equation 27.1. But the great arteries are in inverted malposition (L-malposition).

Most infundibuloarterial anomalies typically have only one intersegmental situs mismatch between the infundibulum and the great arteries, but not between the situs of the ventricles and the situs of the great arteries: typical D-TGA, typical L-TGA, the Taussig-Bing type of DORV, and the Paul type of DOLV (see equations).

But ACMGA typically has *two* intersegmental situs mismatches, VA and infundibuloarterial. Equation 27.13 is just one example of ACMGA. There are six different anatomic types of

ACMGA, which are presented in Chapter 25. ACMGA exemplifies the view that **complex congenital heart disease is a segmental situs "salad" (or mixture).** In normally formed hearts, all of the cardiac segments have the same situs (or pattern of anatomic organization): all are in situs solitus (noninverted), or all are in situs inversus (a mirror-image of situs solitus).

It was in considering all of the foregoing patterns that what the infundibulum is really doing finally became clear.

INFUNDIBULAR FUNCTIONS

1. It has long been clear that the subarterial infundibulum is a very important *connecting segment* between the ventricles below and the great arteries above.
2. It has also been understood for some time that most of the anomalies of the great arteries are basically *anomalies of the subarterial infundibulum* (or conus arteriosus) on which the great arteries stand. The great arteries per se are almost always normally formed. The only exception is absence of the subpulmonary infundibulum (Equations 27.6 and 27.7), that we and others used to call truncus arteriosus communis (a widespread misinterpretation that probably does not exist as classically conceived). In AOSPI, the great arterial pathologic conditions of anatomic types A1 and A2 appear to be secondary to, or associated with, absence of the subpulmonary infundibulum and absence of the pulmonary valve.
3. The new understanding has to do with the control of the embryonic great arterial switch procedure:
   a. When a well-developed subarterial infundibulum is present, this infundibulum typically prevents an embryonic great arterial switch from above the RV sinus to above the LV sinus. Examples include the normal pulmonary artery (in situs solitus and in situs inversus); the transposed aorta, D- and L-; and both great arteries in DORV of the Taussig-Bing type.
   b. When there is no great subarterial infundibular free wall, this infundibular myocardial absence permits or facilitates great arterial switches from above the RV to above the LV. Examples include the normal aorta, solitus and inversus; the transposed pulmonary artery, in typical D-TGA and in typical L-TGA; and beneath both great arteries in DOLV of the Paul type.

In addition to infundibular development (as earlier), other factors influence VA alignments, including unusual ventricular loop formation and contrary ventricular torsions, such as crisscross atrioventricular relations (a solitus or ventricular *D*-loop that twists to the *left;* or an inversus or ventricular *L*-loop that twists to the *right*); and ACMGA (Equation 27.13), in which the ventricles loop in one direction (say to the right), and the infundibulum and the great arteries rotate in the opposite direction (to the left).

So yes, there are many factors that influence VA alignments. However, the opposite roles of sub–great arterial infundibular free-wall presence and absence were unknown to us until very recently.

Infundibular Anatomic Opposites

Solitus normally related great arteries: 0R + 4L (Equation 27.1) and typical D-TGA: 4R + 0L (Equation 27.9).

Infundibular Anatomic Sameness

Taussig-Bing DORV: 4R + 4L (Equation 27.11) and Paul DOLV: 0R + 0L (Equation 27.12).

INTERMEDIATE CASES

There are intermediate cases. Sometimes a great artery gets switched embryonically, even though there is a relatively small amount of subarterial infundibular free-wall musculature present. In biology, findings typically are a relative continuum; seldom are they present-versus-absent absolutes, with no intermediate findings. The existence of intermediate cases is to be expected. Their existence does not deny the reality of different groups.

Instead, the question becomes precisely how much subarterial infundibular free-wall myocardium is needed to block embryonic great arterial switches. The answer remains to be determined.

LABORATORY DIAGNOSIS OF THE INFUNDIBULUM

The anatomic type of the subarterial infundibulum should be diagnosed routinely in every case of congenital heart disease. Why do we not do that? Why is the subarterial infundibulum so often the forgotten cardiac segment? Perhaps because many regard the subarterial infundibulum as an unchanging and integral part of the RV. Consequently, when one has diagnosed the status of the RV sinus or inflow tract (D-loop/L-loop, solitus/inverted RV, right-handed/left-handed RV), that diagnosis is assumed to cover the RV outflow tract also, and that is all one needs to know.

This view is incorrect. The RV sinus and the subarterial infundibulum belong to different cardiac segments. The RV sinus and the RV outflow tract (subarterial infundibulum) are not different parts of one structure; they are two different structures. The normal subarterial infundibulum and the infundibulum in typical D-TGA are not the same structure. They are two very different structures. They are, in fact, mirror-images. Anomalies of the great arteries are widely thought of as, well, anomalies of the great arteries—that most of them basically are not. Consequently, diagnostic attention is focused on the great arteries, not on the subarterial infundibulum, on which the great arteries stand, that is the more basic problem.

Many do not know that there are **four different anatomic types of subarterial infundibulum** that pediatric cardiologists, pediatric cardiac surgeons, radiologists, pathologists, and nurses should be diagnosing and understanding:

1. Subpulmonary infundibulum with no subaortic infundibulum that causes normally related great arteries;
2. Subaortic infundibulum with no subpulmonary infundibulum that causes TGA;
3. **Subaortic and subpulmonary infundibulum,** that causes DORV, and also TGA; and
4. **No subaortic and no subpulmonary infundibulum** that results in DOLV.

Each of these four different anatomic types of subarterial infundibulum has a solitus (or a noninverted) and an inverted (or a mirror-image) isomer. In these four different anatomic types of infundibulum (subpulmonary, subaortic, bilaterally present, and bilaterally absent), what is *not* present is every bit as important as what is present. Absence of subarterial infundibular free wall permits or facilitates the embryonic great arterial switches from above the RV to above the LV; whereas the presence of a well-developed subarterial infundibulum blocks or prevents embryonic great arterial switches.

Both the presence and the absence of subarterial infundibulum are equally important, and opposite in effect, concerning whether an embryonic great arterial switch from RV to LV will, or will not, occur. **This is the subarterial infundibular free-wall development theory.** *Development* includes both growth and expansion, and absorption or involution leading to disappearance.

EVOLUTION AND HUMAN CONGENITAL HEART DISEASE

To understand infundibuloarterial anomalies in depth, one needs context, and that context is an understanding of vertebrate evolution.[1,2]

Our phylum Chordata goes back to the ancient fish of the Ordovician and upper Devonian periods, 500 million to 345 million years ago. These fish had a single ventricle, from which our morphologically LV is derived. Amphibia evolved 345 to 325 million years ago during the Carboniferous period. Amphibia had lungs and so could breathe air, but they had no RV. Some amphibia evolved into fully terrestrial animals called the Amniota, because they had an amniotic sac, filled with amniotic fluid, in which their embryos and fetuses could float, like our aquatic ancestors. Some amniotes evolved into reptiles. Other amniotes evolved into birds, which are feathered reptiles (e.g., *archaeopteryx*). Still other amniotes evolved into mammals that are furry or hairy reptiles. Mammals evolved during the Jurassic period, about 180 million years ago. Fish and amphibia do not have a RV. But higher reptiles (crocodiles and alligators), birds, and mammals normally do. The mammalian RV is comparatively recently evolved—"only" about 180 million years ago, compared with the LV that is at least 500 million years ago—going back to Ordovician fish, before our vertebrate ancestors had started coming ashore. Thus, the more recently evolved mammalian RV is only about 36% as old as the LV. Hence, it is not surprising that most human congenital heart disease consists of anomalies of one or more of the components that make up the human RV. By comparison, anomalies of the human LV are relatively much less frequent.

Congenital heart disease is the most common malformation in live-born infants (0.8%, or 8 per thousand). Congenital heart disease accounts for 10% of all still births and for more than 20% of all spontaneous abortions. Thus, we are still having significant trouble with our major cardiovascular evolutionary adaptations to air-breathing and permanent land-living:

1. the development of an RV sinus or inflow tract, to serve as a lung pump;
2. the embryonic aortic switch procedure, to move the ascending aorta from above the RV to above the LV, with which this chapter has been primarily concerned; and
3. septation, to separate the systemic and pulmonary circulations.

Just think what a complex and delicate process it is that we have been considering. This process is often called **the crossing of the circulations** because, when viewed from a left lateral projection, normally related great arteries appear to cross each other, whereas in typical D-TGA, the great arteries are more or less parallel or uncrossed. I have been calling this process **the normal embryonic aortic switch.**

No matter what you call it, this process is amazing. After ventricular D-loop formation, the great arteries are side-by-side above the RV sinus, aorta to the right, MPA to the left, and subarterial infundibular free walls beneath both great arteries, very similar to the Taussig-Bing type of DORV.

Then, because of **complete right-left asymmetry** in the development of the subarterial infundibular free walls, the right-sided subaortic infundibular free wall undergoes absorption or involution, it is thought because of **apoptosis (genetically programmed cell death).** Simultaneously, the left-sided subpulmonary infundibular free wall undergoes strong, normal growth.

These opposite developments of the right-sided subaortic infundibular free wall (disappearance) and left-sided subpulmonary infundibulum (growth) initiate opposite (reciprocal) morphogenetic movements of the ascending aorta and of the MPA. The aorta moves posteriorly, leftward, and inferiorly. The MPA moves anteriorly, rightward, and superiorly. The aorta passes through the interventricular foramen (the normal embryonic VSD), into the LV, and into fibrous continuity with the mitral valve. The pulmonary artery remains above the RV. This is the normal aortic switch (Equation 27.1). The inverted or mirror-image isomer is presented in Equation 27.2.

Equations 27.3 to 27.15 are thought to represent failed, random, evolutionary, natural "experiments." There is only one way to do the aortic switch right (correctly) (Equations 27.1 and 27.2). These are thought to represent *successful,* random, evolutionary, natural "experiments." There are many ways to do the aortic switch wrong (incorrectly) (Equations 27.3 to 27.14).

Just think, normal **complete right-left asymmetry** causes the subaortic right half of the subarterial infundibulum to disappear and the subpulmonary left half of the subarterial infundibulum to grow strongly. No wonder developmental errors are relatively frequent. In TOF, the left-sided subpulmonary infundibulum is **obstructively hypoplastic** (Equations 27.3 to 27.5). The left-sided subpulmonary infundibulum can be **absent** (Equations 27.6 and 27.7).

The development of the left-sided subpulmonary infundibular free wall and of the right-sided subaortic infundibular free wall can be **R-L reversed,** resulting in typical D-TGA (Equation 27.9).

When the great arteries are inverted (aorta to the left and pulmonary artery to the right), the development of the subarterial infundibular free walls can be noninverted (or solitus).

This infundibuloarterial situs oppositeness results in congenital physiologically corrected L-TGA. The infundibuloarterial situs oppositeness in D-TGA (Equation 27.9) and in L-TGA (Equation 27.10) are mirror-images.

The left-sided subpulmonary infundibular free wall and the right-sided subaortic infundibular free wall can **both remain well developed,** neither disappearing. Consequently, neither great artery can undergo an embryonic switch, resulting in DORV. In terms of situs, this type of subarterial infundibular free wall is one form of infundibular situs ambiguus: the left-sided subpulmonary infundibular free wall is as in infundibular situs solitus. But the right-sided subarterial infundibular free wall resembles infundibular situs inversus. Because the subpulmonary and the subaortic infundibula are different from both the solitus infundibulum (Equation 27.1) and the inversus infundibulum (Equation 27.2), the bilateral infundibulum is regarded as one form of infundibular situs ambiguus (Equation 27.11).

Remember that infundibular situs ambiguus is not a specific type of infundibular situs. Situs ambiguus means that the situs is ambiguous (English spelling), that is, uncertain or unknown (not diagnosed). **Rarely, the infundibulum can be bilaterally absent:** no left-sided subpulmonary infundibulum and no right-sided subaortic infundibulum, resulting in DOLV. A bilaterally absent subarterial infundibulum (Equation 27.12) is another form of infundibular situs ambiguous—neither a solitus, nor an inversus infundibulum (neither Equation 27.1 nor Equation 27.2).

Would you ever think it possible that two great arteries that look like L-TGA—with aorta anterior and to the left of the pulmonary artery—could originate from morphologically appropriate ventricles, with the aorta arising from the LV and the pulmonary artery originating from the RV? I know this sounds impossible, but that does happen in ACMGA (Equation 27.13). How? The ventricles loop in one direction, say to the right, and the infundibulum and great arteries twist in the opposite direction, to the left (Equation 27.13).

RIGHT-LEFT ASYMMETRY

Right-left asymmetry in the development of the subarterial infundibular free walls is the key to the morphogenetic movements of the great arteries in:

1. Solitus normally related great arteries (Equation 1);
2. Inverted normally related great arteries (Equation 2);
3. Typical D-transposition of the great arteries (Equation 9); and
4. Typical L-transposition of the great arteries (Equation 10).

Whole-body situs is also a matter of R-L asymmetry:

1. In visceroatrial situs solitus, the right lung is trilobed and the left lung is bilobed, the heart is left-sided, the morphologically right atrium (RA) is right-sided, the morphologically left atrium (LA) is left-sided, the liver is predominantly right-sided, the spleen is left-sided, the stomach is left-sided, and the appendix is right-sided.

All of the previously mentioned organ locations in situs solitus are R-L reversed in situs inversus. R-L visceroatrial asymmetry is *normal* in humans. R-L visceroatrial symmetry also can be *abnormal* in humans. The heterotaxy syndromes with asplenia, or polysplenia, or with a right-sided spleen often have abnormally symmetrical viscera. **The heterotaxy syndromes have subnormal R-L asymmetry.**

Molecular genetic evidence suggests that one or more mutations in the Nodal cascade may be important in **anomalies of R-L asymmetry** such as L-TGA and D-TGA and the heterotaxy syndromes.[1,2] However, much remains to be learned concerning molecular genetics.

EMBRYONIC ARTERIAL SWITCHES FROM RIGHT VENTRICLE TO LEFT VENTRICLE

1. Right-sided aorta, solitus normally related great arteries, Equation 27.1;
2. Left-sided aorta, inverted normally related great arteries, Equation 27.2;
3. Right-sided aorta, TOF, Equations 27.3, 27.4, and 27.5;
4. Right-sided aorta, absent subpulmonary infundibulum (truncus arteriosus communis), Equations 27.6 and 27.7;
5. Right-sided aorta, absent aortopulmonary septum, Equation 8;
6. Left-sided pulmonary artery, typical D-TGA, Equation 27.9;
7. Right-sided pulmonary artery, typical L-TGA, Equation 27.10;
8. Both right-sided aorta and left-sided pulmonary artery, DOLV, Equation 27.11;
9. Right-sided pulmonary artery, ACMGA {S,D,L}, Equation 27.13; and
10. But what is happening in Equation 27.13, ACMGA {S,L,D} = 4R + 4L, Equation 27.14?

The great arteries are in D-malposition, that is, aorta to the right and PA to the left: {S,L,**D**}. The right-sided subaortic infundibular free wall is well developed (4R), preventing an embryonic aortic switch. The left-sided subpulmonary infundibular free wall also is well developed (4L), preventing an embryonic pulmonary artery switch. But ACMGA is present. How can that have happened? We think that the arterial switch mechanism is excluded. We think that **malrotation of the heart tube is the right answer.** The ventricular inflow tracts looped to the *left:* {S,**L**,D}, placing the RV to the left and the LV to the right. But then the infundibulum and the great arteries twisted to the *right*: {S,L,**D**}. This placed the right-sided aorta over the right-sided LV, and the left-sided pulmonary artery over the left-sided RV, resulting in ACMGA {S,L,D} = 4R + 4L.

Opposite torsions at the ventricles, in this case to the left, and at the infundibular and great arterial levels, in this case to the right, is always present in ACMGA.

Any great artery associated with zero (0) subarterial infundibular free-wall development was R-L switched when an embryo. The equations contain much information and help in data analysis. **Right-left asymmetry is one of the laws of life.**

It applies not only to normal subarterial infundibular free-wall development but also of whole bodily situs: situs solitus (normal R-L asymmetry), situs inversus (mirror-image R-L asymmetry), and situs ambiguus (subnormal R-L asymmetry). This is also why the infundibuloarterial situs equations are important. These are the laws of cardiovascular R-L asymmetry and of other conditions as well. The infundibuloarterial situs equations demonstrate the effects of normal R-L asymmetry (solitus normally related great arteries and its inverted isomer), and of abnormal R-L asymmetry (D- and L-TGA). These equations also demonstrate the effects of the absence of R-L asymmetry, that is, of R-L symmetry (DORV and DOLV). Finally, these equations demonstrate the effects of hypoplasia of the subpulmonary infundibulum (TOF) and of aplasia of the subpulmonary infundibulum (absence of the subpulmonary infundibulum, that we and others used to call truncus arteriosus communis). We recently realized that so-called truncus arteriosus communis is a misinterpretation that may not exist or is rare. Hypoplasia of the subpulmonary infundibulum (TOF) and absence of the subpulmonary infundibulum (so-called truncus arteriosus communis) appear to be closely related malformations.

To summarize, the infundibuloarterial situs equations express R-L asymmetry and R-L symmetry of the subarterial infundibular free walls. Only one type of R-L subarterial infundibular free-wall asymmetry results in normally related great arteries (Equation 27.1) and its mirror-image isomer (Equation 27.2). All other types of R-L subarterial infundibular free-wall asymmetry and symmetry result in abnormally related great arteries (Equations 27.3 to 27.14).

THE PROBABLE IMPORTANCE OF APOPTOSIS

The normal and abnormal subarterial infundibular development may well be due to normal and abnormal apoptosis. Apoptosis means "a falling off" (Greek), from *apo*off + *ptosis* fall. Apoptosis is defined as a morphologic pattern of cell death affecting single cells, indicated by shrinkage of the cell, condensation of chromatin, formation of cytoplasmic blebs, and fragmentation of the cell into membrane-bound apoptotic bodies that are eliminated by phagocytosis.[3] It is a mechanism for cell deletion. Apoptosis is often a synonym for *programmed cell death.* Apoptosis is a *physiologic* regulation of cell populations (not a *pathologic* form of cell death). This chapter shows the important physiologic results of normally located apoptosis (Equations 27.1 and 27.2) and the pathologic results of abnormally apoptosis (Equations 27.8, 27.9, 27.10, and 27.11).

REFERENCES

1. Van Praagh R. The evolution of the human heart and its relevance to congenital heart disease. *Kardiochirurgiai Torakochirurgia Polska*. 2011;4:427.
2. Van Praagh R. The cardiovascular keys to air-breathing and permanent land-living in vertebrates: the normal human embryonic aortic switch procedure produced by complete right-left asymmetry in the development of the subarterialconal free walls, and the evolution of the right ventricular sinus. *Kardiochirurgiai Torakochirurgia Polska*. 2011;8:1.
3. Anderson DM. *Dorland's Illustrated Medical Dictionary*. Philadelphia, London, Toronto, Montreal, Sydney, Tokyo: W. B. Saunders Company; 1994:115–116.

28

The Cardiac Conduction System

THE SINOATRIAL NODE

The sinoatrial node (SAN) is the pacemaker of the human heart (Fig. 28.1). **In visceroatrial situs solitus,** the normal pattern of anatomic organization of the viscera and atria, the SAN normally is located to the right of the superior vena cava (SVC; see Fig. 28.1, *left upper diagram*). The SAN is located in the sulcus terminalis (the terminal sulcus), a shallow sulcus or depression that marks the termination of the right horn of the sinus venosus—the smooth venous tissue that includes the terminations of the SVC and the inferior vena cava (IVC). The sulcus terminalis also marks the beginning of the free wall of the right atrium (RA) with its characteristic musculi pectinati (pectinate muscles). *Pecten* is a Latin noun meaning "comb." The pectinate muscles of the right atrial appendage (RAA) are remarkably parallel, like the teeth of a comb. The SAN is also known as the **sinus node** because it is located in the right horn of the sinus venosus (venous sinus). However, the pacemaker is immediately adjacent to the RA; hence **sinoatrial node.**

The *sulcus terminalis* externally, where the SAN is located, and the *crista terminalis* (terminal crest) internally both mark the junction of the right horn of the sinus venosus with the RA. The SAN is an invisible subepicardial structure. That is why you have to know where the SAN is, because you cannot see the SAN with the naked eye. This is also why the SAN was not discovered until 1907 by **Sir Arthur Keith**[1] (1866–1955), while he was working with Martin Flack (1882–1931). Keith was an anatomist and anthropologist, a Scot from Aberdeen, who made many important contributions. For example, he was the first to understand that typical D-transposition of the great arteries (TGA) is caused by infundibular inversion.[2]

In visceroatrial situs inversus, the location of the SAN is a mirror-image of its location in visceroatrial situs solitus (see Fig. 28.1, *upper right diagram*), that is, to the left of the entering SVC, in the left horn of the sinus venosus.

In the heterotaxy syndrome with visceroatrial situs ambiguus and asplenia (see Fig. 28.1, *left lower diagram*), there often are bilateral SVCs and bilateral SANs.

In the heterotaxy syndrome with visceroatrial situs ambiguus and polysplenia (see Fig. 28.1, *right lower diagram*), the SAN can be absent or difficult to locate.

Heterotaxy is derived from two Greek words. *Heteros* means "other or different." *Taxis* means "arrangement." **The heterotaxy syndromes** with asplenia, polysplenia, or a right-sided spleen mean that the situs—the pattern of anatomic organization of the viscera and atria—is different from situs solitus (normal) and from situs inversus (the mirror-image of normal).

Ambiguus is a Latin word meaning "uncertain or going about"; from *ambigere,* "to wander about." In anatomy, *ambiguus* has the connotations of uncertain, unknown, undiagnosed. This is what we mean when we use these terms. Others have a different interpretation. In the heterotaxy syndrome with asplenia, they talk about bilaterally right atria (right atrial isomerism) or about bilaterally RAAs (RAA isomerism). In the heterotaxy syndrome with polysplenia, they talk about bilaterally left atria (left atrial isomerism) or about bilaterally left atrial appendages (LAA isomerism).

We think that the concept of atrial level mirror-imagery (isomerism) is anatomically incorrect.[3] Why? Because bilaterally right atria (RAs) and bilaterally left atria (LAs) have never been documented anatomically, accurately speaking.

Bilaterally RA would have to have bilateral IVCs, bilateral SVCs, bilateral coronary sinus ostia, bilateral superior limbic bands of septum secundum, and a SAN bilaterally. No such case has ever been documented.[3] **Bilaterally LA** would have to have a septum primum bilaterally, four pulmonary veins bilaterally, and no SAN bilaterally. Again, no such case has ever been documented in a single individual.[3] (Siamese twins are excluded.)

Our friends and colleagues concede these points. But then they may retreat to **atrial appendage isomerism.** We agree that in the **asplenia syndrome** both atrial appendages often are broad, triangular, and bilaterally "rightish" in appearance. Similarly, in the **polysplenia syndrome,** we agree that the atrial appendages both often appear small and narrow, that is, bilaterally "leftish." We think that the appearances of the atrial appendages—bilaterally "rightish" in asplenia and bilaterally "leftish" in polysplenia—are for hemodynamic reasons.

In asplenia the IVC typically is intact and the atrial septum is often poorly formed because of the presence of common atrioventricular (AV) canal. Consequently, the full systemic venous return often can flow into *both* atrial appendages, distending both, making both atrial appendages appear like RAAs.

In polysplenia, the IVC often is interrupted—absent between the renal veins and the hepatic veins. The blood flow of the hepatic and suprahepatic IVC is much less than normal, that is, no subhepatic systemic venous return. The systemic venous blood returns to the heart via the azygos vein and by the SVC.

So the systemic venous return flows into the atrial level predominantly in a superior-to-inferior direction, passing *behind*

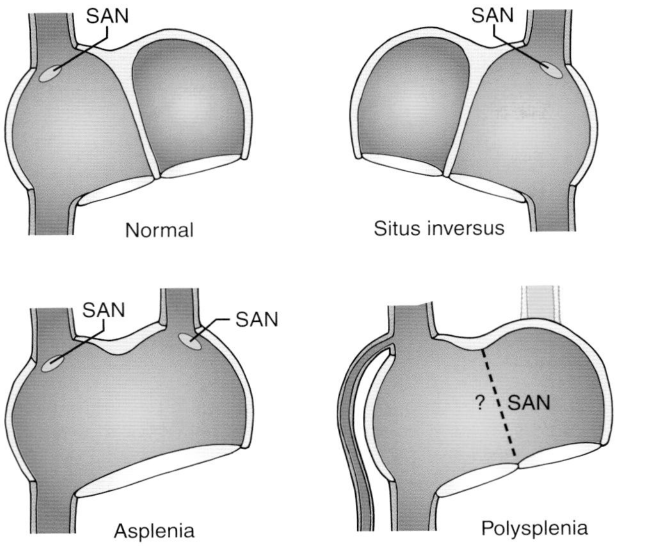

Fig. 28.1 **Where is the sinoatrial node** ***(SAN)*****?** This is a reasonable question because to the unaided and uninformed eye, the SAN is invisible. Normally, **in visceroatrial situs solitus,** the SAN lies to the right of the superior vena cava (SVC) where it enters the right atrium *(upper left diagram)*. The SAN is also called the **sinus node** because it is located in the smooth venous tissue that is confluent with the SVC inferior venae cava (IVC). This smooth (nontrabeculated) venous tissue is the right horn of the *sinus venosus* (venous sinus). Hence, the pacemaker is often called the **sinus node,** because that is where it is located—in the right horn of the sinus venosus. The pacemaker is in a shallow depression, the sulcus terminalis (the terminal sulcus). This is where the sinus venosus ends and where the trabeculated right atrial appendage begins. So the SAN is immediately adjacent to the right atrial appendage. Consequently, the pacemaker's most widely used name is the **sinoatrial node.** The "head" of the SAN is laterally and to the right of the SVC, in the sulcus terminalis. The "body" of the SAN may extend downward in the sulcus terminalis toward the IVC. **In viceroatrial situs inversus** *(right upper diagram)*, the SAN is inverted (right-left switched). The SAN is to the left of the left-sided SVC. In the heterotaxy syndrome with congenital asplenia *(left lower diagram)*, there can be bilateral SVCs with bilateral SANs. In the heterotaxy syndrome with polysplenia *(right lower diagram)*, the SAN can be absent, or difficult to find. (Reproduced with permission from Mullin MP, Van Praagh R, Walsh EP. Development and anatomy of the cardiac conducting system. In: Walsh EP, Saul JP, Triedman JK, eds. *Cardiac Arrhythmias in Children and Young Adults with Congenital Heart Disease.* Philadelphia, PA: Lippincott Williams & Wilkins; 2001:3.[5])

(dorsal to) the atrial appendages, and failing to dilate the atrial appendages, which therefore are bilaterally undistended and bilaterally "leftish" in appearance.[3]

But what about the SAN data? Remember that the SAN is often just called the **sinus node,** not the sinoatrial node. **The SAN tells you where the sinus venosus and SAN are located. It does not necessarily tell you that all of the other features of the RA are there also.** So, a bilateral SAN does not mean that the RA is bilateral. Instead, it only means that the sinus venosus and the SAN are bilateral.[3] Similarly, bilateral absence of the SAN means bilateral absence of the SAN, not that a LA is bilateral.[3]

It also should be mentioned that **"partial" isomerism** is a conceptual error, such as isomerism of the right or LAAs only. Consider D-glucose and L-glucose. These are real isomers.

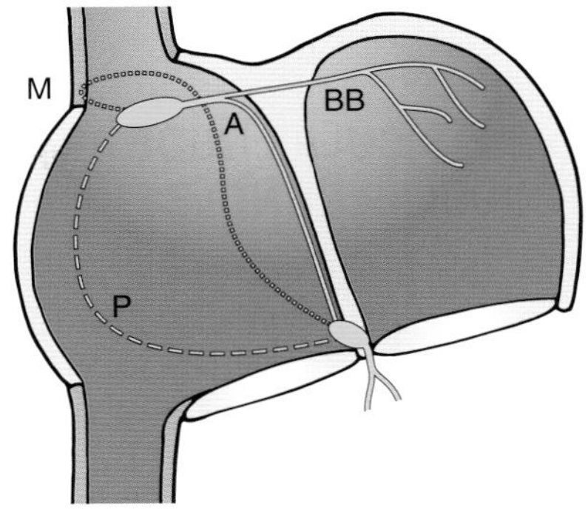

Fig. 28.2 **Diagrammatic presentation of the three internodal conduction pathways and of the interatrial conduction pathway.** The three internodal conduction pathways from the sinoatrial node (close to the superior vena cava) to the atrioventricular node (close to the tricuspid valve) are: the anterior *(A)* internodal pathway, the middle *(M)* internodal pathway, and the posterior *(P)* internodal pathway. The interatrial conduction pathway from the right atrium to the left atrium is the Bachmann bundle *(BB)*. (Reproduced with permission from Anderson RH, Arnold R, Wilkinson JL. The conducting system in congenitally corrected transposition. *Lancet* 1973;1:1286.[13])

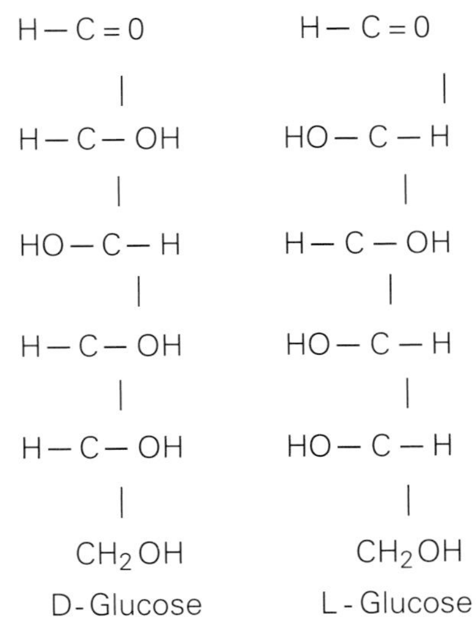

Isomerism applies to complex structures such as the atria (see Fig. 28.1, *left upper and right upper diagrams*), and like D-glucose and L-glucose molecules, in which *all* asymmetrical groups are mirror-images. There are four asymmetrical groups. If only one or two asymmetrical groups were mirror-images, but the other asymmetrical groups were not mirror-images, these two molecules would not be mirror-images (isomers).[3] Isomerism is an all-or-nothing phenomenon. "Partial" isomerism—of the appendages only, but not the whole atria—is a mistake.[3] Mirror-imagery (isomerism) applies to the whole structures, like the whole D- and L-glucose molecules, not to just some, but not all, of the asymmetrical parts of these molecules, or of other structures such as cardiac atria.

THE INTERNODAL AND INTERATRIAL CONDUCTION PATHWAYS

There are three internodal conduction pathways[4] (Fig. 28.2)[5] between the SAN and the AVN: the anterior, middle, and posterior internodal pathways. There is one interatrial conduction pathway between the RA and the LA: the Bachmann bundle.

THE ATRIOVENTRICULAR NODE AND THE ATRIOVENTRICULAR BUNDLE

Now that we have briefly considered the variable locations of the SAN in visceroatrial situs solitus, in visceroatrial situs inversus, and in visceroatria situs ambiguus (see Fig. 28.1), it is now time to consider the variations in the location of the AVN and the AVB.

Where is the AVN? *Mentally,* draw a line between the right atrial ostium of the coronary sinus and a point slightly below the anteroseptal commissure of the tricuspid valve adjacent to the atrial septum. I say draw this line *mentally,* not with a sucker in the operating room, because a sucker can get stuck on this line, and pulling it off this line can damage the invisible AVN and/or the invisible AVB. For convenient brevity, we call this line *the coronary sinus–membranous septum line.* Others use the *triangle of Koch* to localize the invisible AVN and AV (or His) bundle. The triangle of Koch is formed by (1) the origin of the septal leaflet of the tricuspid valve, (2) the Thebesian valve of the coronary sinus, and (3) the Eustachian valve of the IVC and its anterior extension, the tendon of Todaro. The AVN is close to the apex of the triangle of Koch.

Because the Thebesian valve of the coronary sinus and the Eustachian valve of the IVC are variable in their morphology and can be absent, and because the tendon of Todaro is difficult to visualize grossly (but is well seen histologically), we prefer to use the coronary sinus–membranous septum line to localize the AVN and the AVB.

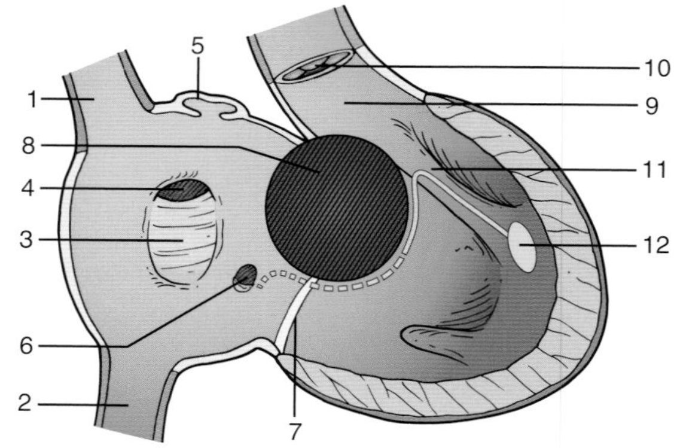

Fig. 28.3 Diagrammatic presentation of the atrioventricular (AV) conduction system in common AV canal, right lateral view of right atrium and right ventricle. *1,* superior vena cava; *2,* inferior vena cava; *3,* limbus of foramen ovale (superior limbic band); *4,* patent foramen ovale; *5,* cut edge of right atrial appendage; *6,* right atrial ostium of coronary sinus; *7,* base of tricuspid valve; *8,* defect in the septum of the AV canal (between the atrial septum posteriorly and superiorly and the ventricular septum anteriorly and inferiorly), that is, an AV septal defect (AVSD); *9,* infundibulum; *10,* base of pulmonary valve; *11,* muscle of Lancisi, or muscle of Lushka, or papillary muscle of the conus (or infundibulum), beneath which the right bundle branch of the conduction system appears; and *12,* transection of the moderator band. The AV bundle runs inferiorly and anteriorly relative to the AVSD, and the top (crest) of the muscular ventricular septum is "scooped out" (concave). (Reproduced with permission from Titus JL. Normal anatomy of the human cardiac conduction system. *Mayo Clin Proc.* 1973;48:24.[11])

HISTORICAL NOTE

Wilhelm His, Jr. (1863–1934) described the AVB in 1893; it is now widely known as the His bundle, or the AVB of His.[6] Born in Basel, Switzerland, he moved to Leipzig, Germany as a child. He became a German citizen and a physician. In 1907, he became the director of the first medical clinic at the Charité Hospital in Berlin. He served in the army in World War I, during which he saw and described trench fever. He had a long-standing interest in gout and diet.

Walter Karl Koch[7] (1880–1962) was a German physician from Berlin. He was a cardiologist, surgeon, and pathologist who described the triangle of Koch in which the AVN is sometimes referred to as Koch's node.

Adam Christian Thebesius[8] (1686–1732) was a German anatomist who worked at Leiden, the Netherlands. He described the small veins of the heart, the Thebesian veins. He also described the coronary sinus and its valve, the Thebesian valve, in 1708.

Bartolomeo Eustachio[9] (1524–1574) was a professor in Rome at the Collegia della Sapienza. In 1552, he completed a superb set of anatomical plates, Tabulae Anatomicae, drawn by himself. These plates remained unprinted in the Papal Library for 162 years. Finally, Pope Clement XI presented the engraved plates to his physician Lancisi. On the advice of Morgagni, Lancisi published these plates with his own notes in 1714. They were the first anatomic plates on copper. These plates were more accurate in delineation than those of Vesalius. These plates revealed that Eustachius (Latin spelling of his name) had discovered the Eustachian valve of the IVC, the Eustachian tube, the thoracic duct, the adrenal glands in 1563 and the abducens (sixth) cranial nerve. Eustachio (Italian spelling of his name) also described the origins of the optic nerves, the cochlea, the pulmonary veins, and the muscles of the throat and neck. He also gave the first correct picture of the uterus, and he wrote the best description of his time of the structure of the teeth, giving the nerve and blood supply in 1563. Eustachio is regarded as a genius of discovery.

Francesco Todaro[10] (1839–1918) was an Italian physician who described the Todaro tendon.

THE ATRIOVENTRICULAR NODE AND ATRIOVENTRICULAR BUNDLE CONTINUED

In 1958, Maurice Lev,[11] who was one of my teachers and an outstanding investigator of the conduction system in congenital heart disease, published a paper concerning the conduction system in common AV canal (Fig. 28.3). In a right lateral view of the opened RA, common AV valve, and right ventricle (RV), many of the most important anatomic details are shown, including the ostium of the coronary sinus, the posteroinferior AVN, the penetrating portion of the AVB, and the branching portion of the AVB.

In 1973, Jack Titus[12] published a study of the normal human cardiac conduction system (Fig. 28.4). This is a left posterolateral

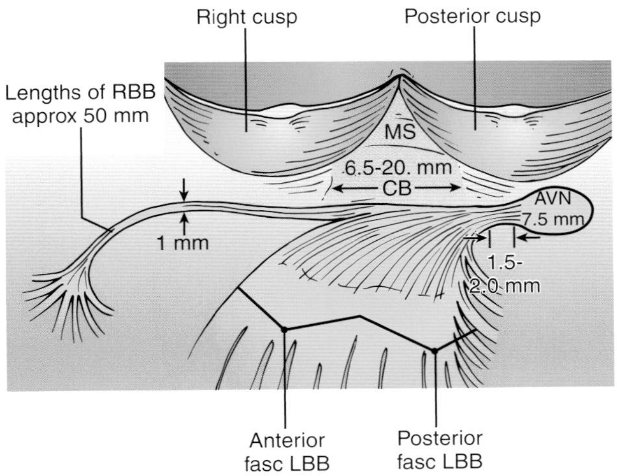

Fig. 28.4 Diagrammatic presentation of the normal atrioventricular (AV) conduction system, left posterolateral view. In the average adult, the AV node *(AVN)* measured 7.5 mm in length. Then the AV bundle (AVB) began. The first 1.5 to 2.0 mm were unbranched. This portion of the AV bundle penetrates from the atrial level to the ventricular level. Branching occurs at the ventricular level: the posterior fascicle *(fasc)* or posterior left bundle branch *(LBB);* the anterior fascicle or the anterior LBB; and the right bundle branch *(RBB)* that was 1 mm wide (diameter) and about 50 mm in length. The normal branching AVB ran beneath the membranous septum and beneath the right coronary and noncoronary leaflets of the normally located aortic valve. The membranous septum and the branching AVB varied between 6.5 and 20 mm in length. *MS,* membranous septum. (Reproduced with permission, from Mullin MP, Van Praagh R, Walsh EP. Development and anatomy of the cardiac conducting system. In: Walsh EP, Saul JP, Triedman JK, eds. *Cardiac Arrhythmias in Children and Young Adults with Congenital Heart Disease.* Philadelphia, PA: Lippincott Williams & Wilkins; 2001:3.[12])

view. Titus found that in the average adult, the AVN measures 7.5 mm in length. Then the AVB begins. The first 1.5 to 2.0 mm are unbranched. This unbranched portion of the AVB penetrates from the atrial level to the ventricular level. Branching occurs at the ventricular level. The left posterior bundle branch travels to the posteromedial papillary muscle group of the left ventricle (LV). The left anterior bundle branch runs to the anterolateral papillary muscle group of the LV. Some fascicles of the left bundle branch (LBB) travel down the left ventricular septal surface between the anterior and posterior LBBs. The right bundle branch (RBB) is 1 mm wide (diameter) and about 50 mm in length.

The normal branching AVB runs immediately beneath the membranous septum, and beneath the right coronary and noncoronary leaflets of the normal aortic valve. The membranous septum and the branching AVB vary between 6.5 and 20 mm in length.

SURGICAL RELEVANCE

Now you can see how misplaced surgical sutures (or devices) can produce various kinds of iatrogenic heart block:

1. If the misplaced suture is superficial, the result can be **RBB block (RBBB).**
2. If the misplaced suture is deeper, the result can be **RBBB and left anterior hemiblock.**
3. If the misplaced surgical suture is even deeper, the result can be **complete heart block.** These are some of the reasons why a good understanding of the conduction system is so important in the interventional transcatheter management and in the surgical management of congenital heart disease.

THE COMMUNICATING ATRIOVENTRICULAR NODE

Many studies have confirmed that the **communicating AVN** usually is located posteroinferiorly, quite close to the right atrial ostium of the coronary sinus (see Fig. 28.3). By *communicating* AVN we mean an AVN that is confluent with the AVB and its branches. As we shall soon see, there is such a thing as a *noncommunicating* AVN, that is, an AVN that communicates with nothing.

THE COURSE OF THE ATRIOVENTRICULAR BUNDLE

Many studies have confirmed that the branching portion of the AVB usually runs beneath (or inferior to) (1) the membranous portion of the ventricular septum normally, as in Fig. 28.4; or (2) inferior to the usual type of ventricular septal defect (VSD) between the infundibular septum above and the ventricular septum below (an infundibuloventricular type of VSD, as in tetralogy of Fallot); or (3) inferior to an AV septal defect, as in the complete form of common AV canal (see Fig. 28.3).

Why are the LBBs so much bigger than the RBB? The LBB enters the LV first and massively. The RBB enters the RV second, as a single, slim bundle (see Fig. 28.4). Why is there such a difference between the LBB and the RBB of the conduction system? It is hard to answer questions like this. But it is worth remembering that the RV is only about 36% as old phylogenetically as is the LV—180 million years (RV) as opposed to at least 500 million years (LV). And, of course, the LV is the systemic pump, whereas the RV is the lung pump. Fish and amphibia do not have an RV, whereas higher reptiles (such as alligators and crocodiles), birds, and mammals normally all do. Thus, in the evolution of our phylum Chordata (the Chordates), the RV and the RBB are Johnnies-come-lately compared with the LV and the LBB (see Fig. 28.3). The two fascicles, or radiations, of the LBB—the superior (or anterior) and the inferior (or posterior)—are clearly shown (see Fig. 28.3).

THE ATRIOVENTRICULAR CONDUCTION SYSTEM IN TRANSPOSITION OF THE GREAT ARTERIES {S,L,L}

One of the most important form of congenital heart disease with AV situs discordance is congenital physiologically corrected TGA {S,L,L}. To the best of my knowledge, the location of the AV conduction system in TGA {S,L,L} was first figured out correctly and presented comprehensibly in 1973 and 1974 by Robert Anderson et al[13,14] (Figs. 28.5 through 28.9), a great achievement.

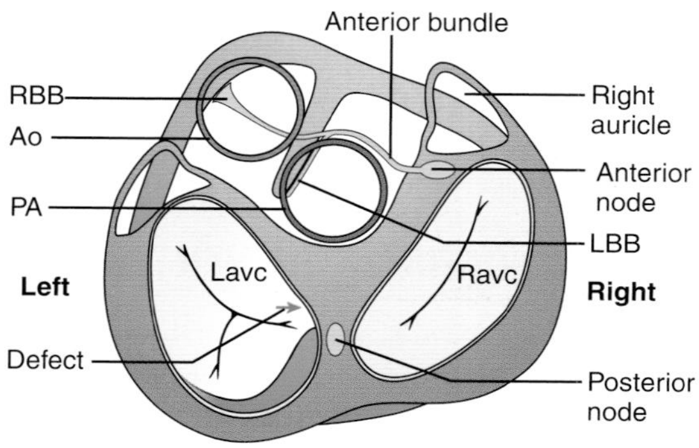

Fig. 28.5 Congenital physiologically corrected transposition of the great arteries in visceroatrial situs solitus, that is, transposition of the great arteries (TGA) {S,L,L}, diagrammatic presentation viewed from above showing the atrioventricular (AV) conduction system. The normal AV node (AVN) is posterior *(Posterior node)*, but it does not connect with either bundle branch; that is, the posterior AVN is noncommunicating. The anterior AVN is communicating; it does connect with the left bundle branch *(LBB)* and with the right bundle branch *(RBB)* of the AV conduction system. The anterior AVN is located in the medial wall of the right atrium *(Right auricle)*. The anterior AVN lies to the right of the transposed pulmonary artery *(PA)* that originates from the right-sided morphologically left ventricle (LV). The right-sided AV valve is a bicuspid mitral valve because the morphology of the AV valves corresponds to that of the ventricle of entry, not to that of the atrium of exit. Thus, the right-sided AV connection *(Ravc)* between the right-sided right atrium and the right-sided LV is via a right-sided mitral valve. Similarly, the left-sided AV connection *(Lavc)* between the left-sided left atrium and the left-sided morphologically right ventricle is via a left-sided trileaflet tricuspid valve. The transposed aorta *(Ao)* is anterior and to the left of the transposed PA. A subpulmonary ventricular septal defect is present *(Defect)*. The anterior AVN gives off an anterior AV bundle (AVB) that runs anteriorly relative to the transposed PA. Then the anterior AVB gives off the LBB that heads down into the right-sided LV. At about the same level, the anterior AVB also branches into the RBB that continues leftward into the left-sided right ventricle. (Reproduced with permission from Anderson RH, Becker AE, Arnold R, Wilkinson JL. The conduction tissues in congenitally corrected transposition. *Circulation*. 1974;50:911.[13])

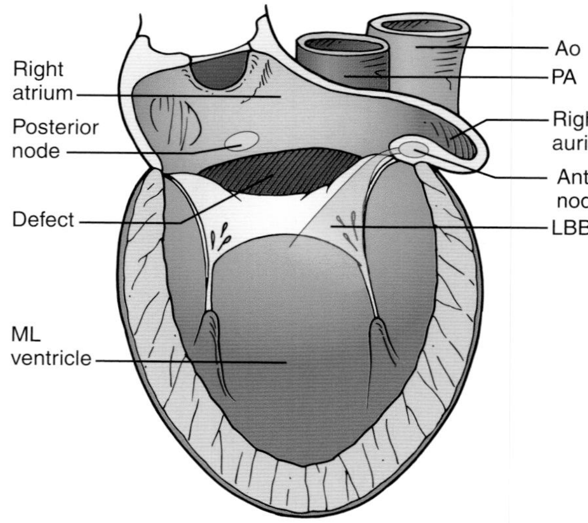

Fig. 28.6 Transposition of the great arteries (TGA) {S,L,L}, right lateral diagrammatic view of the right-sided morphologically right atrium (RA) and of the right-sided morphologically left ventricle *(ML ventricle)* showing the atrioventricular (AV) conduction system and a ventricular septal defect *(Defect)*. The normal AV node (AVN) is present and posterior *(Posterior node)*, but it does not communicate with the AV bundle (AVB) or bundle branches. The normal posterior AVN is hypoplastic and has no known function. A second AVN is present. It is anterior *(Anterior node)*. The anterior AVN is located in the medial wall of the RA. It is to the right of the transposed pulmonary valve and slightly posterior to the pulmonary valve. The anterior AVN is the communicating AVN that connects with the AVB. In turn, the AVB connects with the left and right bundle branches. Here one can see that the anterior AVN and AVB connect with the right-sided left bundle branch *(LBB)* that flows into the right-sided left ventricle. Just as the AV valves correspond to the ventricles of entry, not to the atria of exit, so too the LV and RV bundle branches of the conduction system correspond to the ventricles of entry, not to the atria of exit. These are basic principles. The transposed aorta *(Ao)* is anterior and to the left of the transposed pulmonary artery *(PA)*; that is, L-TGA is present. This heart diagram is drawn in the *vertical heart position* (ventricular apex pointing downward). This is the correct cardiac position for many adults. However, infants and children usually have a *horizontal heart position* (ventricular apex pointing horizontally). As drawn in the vertical heart position, the AVB runs in the *anterior* rim of the VSD. Now rotate this diagram 90 degrees counterclockwise, putting this heart diagram into a horizontal heart position, and you will see that the AV bundle is running in the *horizontal or superior rim of the VSD*. In the normal heart, and in most forms of congenital heart disease, there is a posterior communicating AVN, not an anterior communicating AVN as in TGA {S,L,L}. In most forms of congenital heart disease, the AVB runs in the *posteroinferior* rim of the VSD, not in the *anterosuperior* rim of the VSD, as in TGA {S,L,L}. Thus congenital physiologically corrected L-TGA typically has anomalies of the AVN and AVB that are associated with AV situs discordance: TGA {S,L,L}, that is, solitus atria and inverted (L-loop) ventricles. (Reproduced with permission from Anderson RH, Becker AE, Arnold R, Wilkinson JL. The conduction tissues in congenitally corrected transposition. *Circulation*. 1974;50:911.[13])

The normal posterior AVN does not communicate with the AVB (see Figs. 28.7 and 28.9). Instead, the communicating AVN is *anterior*, to the right of and slightly posterior relative to the transposed pulmonary valve. Then the conduction tissue goes anteriorly in front of the pulmonary valve and down into the right-sided LV (see Fig. 28.8).

In TGA {S,L,L} the communicating AVN is anterior compared with the normal noncommunicating posterior AVN (see Figs. 28.5 and 28.7); this is why the AVB runs *anteriorly* relative to the transposed pulmonary valve (see Fig. 28.8). When a VSD is present, the AVB runs in the *superior or anterior rim of the VSD* (see Fig. 28.9). In other words, classic congenital physiologically corrected TGA {S,L,L} has **AV situs discordance:** {**S**,**L**,-}, that is, solitus (noninverted) atria {**S**,-,-}, but with inversus (mirror-image) ventricles, {S,**L**,-}. So the ventricles do not fit the atria.

In typical complete physiologically uncorrected D-TGA {S,D,D}, there is **AV situs concordance,** that is, {**S**,**D**,-} solitus atria {**S**,-,-} with D-loop or solitus ventricles {S,**D**,-}. So, the ventricles fit the atria. Both the atria and the ventricles are in situs solitus (normal anatomic patterns). So in TGA {S,D,D}, the normal *posterior* AVN communicates with the AVB. The AVB runs *posteriorly and inferiorly* relative to the transposed pulmonary valve, and *posteriorly and inferiorly* relative to a VSD, if present. Thus, in TGA {S,L,L}, apparently because of the presence of AV situs discordance, the AVN and the AVB are malformed:

1. The AVN is anterior (instead of posterior).
2. The AVB runs anteriorly to the pulmonary valve (instead of posteriorly to the pulmonary valve).

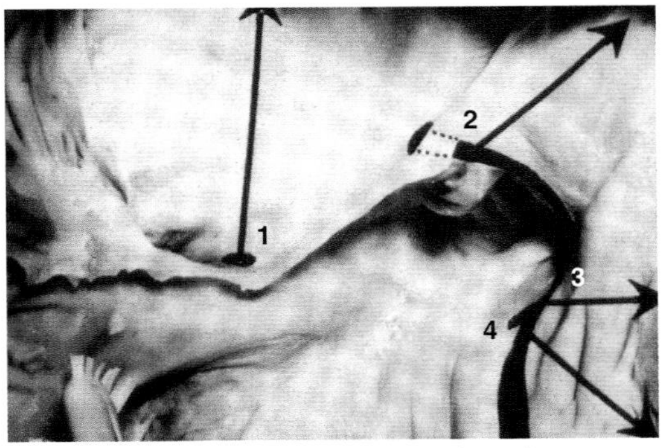

Fig. 28.7 Transposition of the great arteries {S,L,L}, right lateral view of right-sided right atrium and of right-sided left ventricle. Right-sided mitral valve has been excised to permit a better view of the atrioventricular (AV) conduction system. *1,* The location of the normal posterior AV node (AVN) that is hypoplastic and noncommunicating. The posterior AVN is slightly anterior to the right atrial ostium of the coronary sinus. *2,* The location of the abnormal anterior AVN, to the right of the transposed pulmonary valve. From 2 to 3 is a *black line* indicating the location of the AV bundle (AVB) that runs to the right of and anterior to the transposed pulmonary valve. *2,* Indicates where the abnormal AVB penetrates from the atrial to the ventricular level. *3,* Indicates where the AVB branches. *4,* Depicts where the right-sided left bundle branch descends down the left ventricular septal surface into the right-sided left ventricle. (Reproduced with permission from Anderson RH, Arnold R, Wilkinson JL. The conducting system in congenitally corrected transposition. *Lancet.* 1973;1:1286.[14])

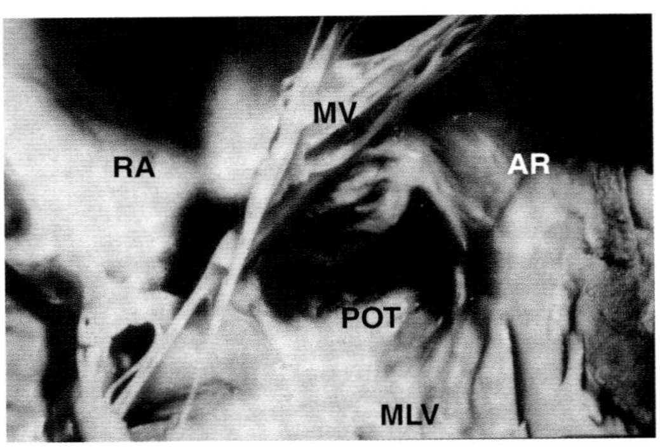

Fig. 28.8 Transposition of the great arteries (TGA) {S,L,L}, photo showing right-sided right atrium *(RA),* right-sided mitral valve *(MV),* right-sided morphologically left ventricle *(MLV),* and pulmonary outflow tract *(POT)* of right-sided transposed pulmonary artery (PA). Because there is a double alignment discordance in TGA {S,L,L}, at the atrioventricular (AV*) and ventriculoarterial (VA**) levels, RA and the PA are ipsilateral. Both are right-sided. Similarly, the left atrium (LA) and the aorta are both ipsilateral; that is, both are left-sided. Consequently, TGA {S,L,L} is congenitally physiologically corrected because of the ipsilaterality of the RA and PA (both right-sided) and of the left atrium (LA) and aorta (both left-sided), as long as associated malformations (such as pulmonary stenosis or atresia with a ventricular septal defect [VSD]) do not spoil the potential physiologic correction of the systemic venous and the pulmonary venous circulations. This same photo is used in the next figure to delineate the abnormal course of the AV conduction system in classic corrected TGA {S,L,L}. (Reproduced with permission from Anderson RH, Arnold R, Wilkinson JL. The conducting system in congenitally corrected transposition. *Lancet.* 1973;1:1286.[14])

3. If a subpulmonary VSD is present, the conduction system runs in the superoanterior rim of the VSD (instead of in the posteroinferior rim of the VSD).

However, despite the AV situs discordance, the RBB and LBB do go to the morphologically appropriate ventricles, despite their contralaterality: LBB to the right-sided LV, and RBB to the left-sided RV.

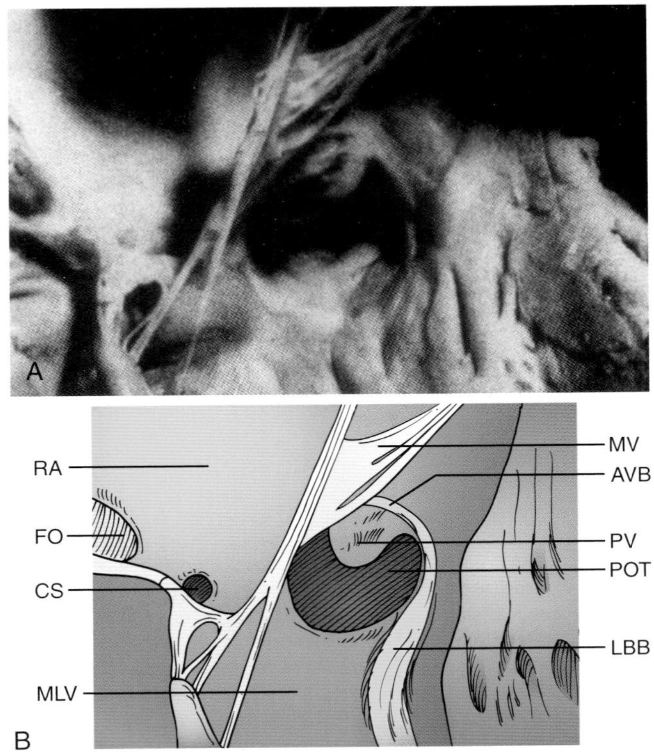

Fig. 28.9 The upper half of this figure is the same photograph as in Fig. 28.8, except that in the A there are no labels. (B) Labeled diagram of the conduction system and of other anatomic structures. The conduction system is shown as a *thick black line.* The anterior atrioventricular node (AVN) is not shown in the right *AV, atrioventricular, ventriculoarterial (**VA) atrium, although it is depicted in Figs. 28.5, 28.6, and 28.7. After penetrating to the ventricular level, the *AV* bundle *(AVB)* runs to the right of and then anteriorly to the pulmonary outflow tract *(POT).* Then the AVB gives off the left bundle branch *(LBB),* which then runs down into the right-sided morphologically left ventricle *(MLV). CS,* Coronary sinus; *FO,* foramen ovale. The right bundle branch, which runs leftward, is not shown in this figure, but is shown in Fig. 28.5. *PV,* Pulmonary valve. (Reproduced with permission from Anderson RH, Arnold R, Wilkinson JL. The conducting system in congenitally corrected transposition. *Lancet.* 1973;1:1286.[14])

These anomalies of the AV and the AVB look like an attempt by "Mother Nature" to avoid AV noncommunication resulting in heart block because of AV situs discordance, that is, {S,L,-}. However, TGA {S,L,L} does have an increased tendency to develop heart block (12%).[15]

Do hearts with AV situs discordance always have these anomalies of the AVN and His bundle? We think the answer to this question is usually, but not always. For example, in 1977, Dick, Van Praagh, Rudd, Folkerth, and Castañeda[16] published a study of the electrophysiologic delineation of the AV conduction system in two patients at surgery with TGA {I,D,D}, that is, congenital physiologically corrected TGA in visceroatrial situs inversus. AV situs discordance was present in both cases: {**I,D,**D}, that is, situs inversus of the atria, with situs solitus (D-loop) of the ventricles.

However, the intraoperative electrophysiologic study revealed a "normal" course of both the intraatrial and intraventricular

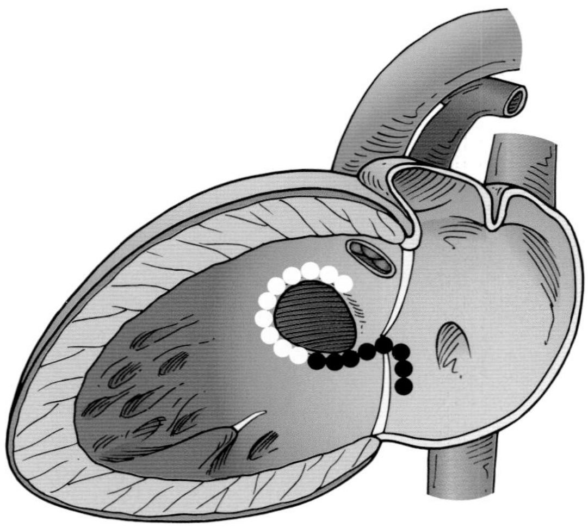

Fig. 28.10 Transposition of the great arteries (TGA) {I,D,D}, that is, congenitally corrected TGA in visceroatrial situs inversus, with atrioventricular (AV) situs discordance: {I,D,-}, that is, with atrial inversion and ventricular noninversion. Despite the presence of AV situs discordance, the communicating AV node was posterior (normal), and the conduction system ran posteriorly and inferiorly relative to the ventricular septal defect (VSD) (normal). The diagram shows a left-sided morphologically right atrium, a left-sided morphologically left ventricle, a VSD, and D-TGA with pulmonary stenosis. The *black circles* show where the exploring electrode probe at surgery recorded specialized AV conduction tissue. The *white circles* show areas where no specialized electrograms were recorded. (Reproduced with permission from Dick M, Van Praagh R, Rudd M, Folkerth T, Castañeda A. Electrophysiologic delineation of the specialized atrioventricular conduction system in two patients with corrected transposition of the great arteries in situs inversus {I, D, D}. *Circulation.* 1977;55:896.[16])

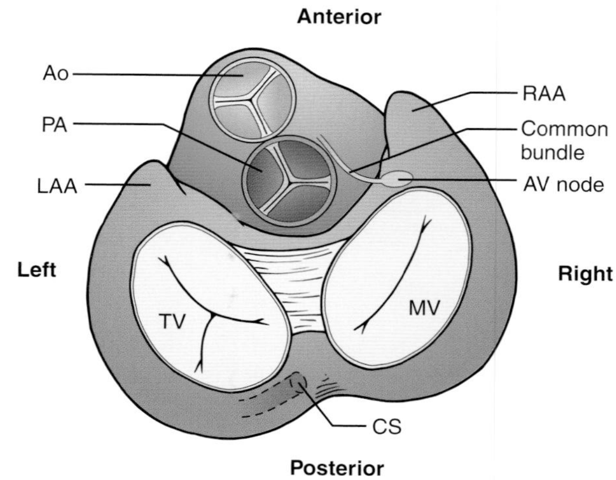

Fig. 28.11 Transposition of the great arteries (TGA) {S, L, L}, showing the salient features from an electrophysiologic perspective. There is an anterior communicating atrioventricular node (AVN). There is no communicating AVN posteriorly, close to the right atrial ostium of the coronary sinus *(CS)*. The common AV bundle runs to the right of and anteriorly relative to the pulmonary valve. Diagram of TGA{S,L,L} from above. *Ao,* Aorta; *LAA,* left atrial appendage; *MV,* mitral valve; *PA,* pulmonary artery; *RAA,* right atrial appendage; *TV,* tricuspid valve. (Reproduced with permission from Mullin MP, Van Praagh R, Walsh EP. Development and anatomy of the cardiac conducting system. In: Walsh EP, Saul JP, Triedman JK, eds. *Cardiac Arrhythmias in Children and Young Adults with Congenital Heart Disease.* Philadelphia, PA: Lippincott Williams & Wilkins; 2001:3.[5])

portions of the specialized conduction system. In 1 patient, specialized AV conduction tissue was found in the RA close to the coronary sinus (Fig. 28.10), indicating the presence of a *posterior* AVN, *not* an *anterior* AVN as in TGA {S,L,L}. The specialized AV conduction tissue was recorded along the *posteroinferior* margin of the VSD in both patients (see Fig. 28.10), *not* along the *anterosuperior* margin of the VSD, as in TGA {S,L,L}. Thus, AV situs discordance occurs with an abnormal AVN and His bundle as in TGA {**S**,**L**,L} and with a normal AVN and His bundle as in TGA {**I**,**D**,D}.

Hence, AV situs discordance may not be the cause of an abnormal AVN and an abnormal AVB, as has been widely assumed, based on the findings in TGA {S,L,L}. Another possible interpretation was proposed by Dick et al[16]:

1. When the discordant ventricles are an L-loop (inverted), as in TGA {S,**L**,L}, the AVN and AVB are abnormal (Fig. 28.11).
2. When the discordant ventricles are a D-loop (noninverted or solitus), then the AVN and His bundle are normal.

More experience is needed to see whether this hypothesis is true.

IS THE CARDIAC CONDUCTION SYSTEM INVISIBLE TO THE NAKED EYE?

The answer is yes and no:

Yes, the invisible components of the conduction system are the SAN, the three internodal pathways, the Bachmann bundle, the AVN, and the AVB. That is why you have to know where these important structures are, particularly if you are a cardiac surgeon.

No, the LBB and RBB are visible to the experienced naked eye.

The RBB emerges just beneath the muscle of Lancisi (i.e., the muscle of Lushka, the papillary muscle of the conus). The RBB is about 1-mm wide. In the fresh state (as in the operating room), it is yellow-white in color because the RBB is surrounded by glycogen. The RBB looks like a thin, yellow-white line as it runs down the septal band, close to the inferior margin of the septal band, heading for the moderator band, the anterior papillary muscle of the RV, and then arborizing as the Purkinje network in the RV free wall. The RBB is visible only on the septal band. In the fixed state (e.g., 10% formalin solution), the RBB becomes invisible because the glycogen is no longer present.

The LBBs are visible to the experienced eye on the left ventricular septal surface (Fig. 28.12). This slide was given to me by Dr. Alexi Sinev of Moscow, the Soviet Union, when he visited our laboratory in 1977. Dr. Sinev outlined the LBBs of the AV conduction system using short black horse hairs. With only a very little practice, it becomes easy to identify the anterior and posterior radiations of the LBB.

LITERATURE REVIEW

In 1963, James[4] described the connecting pathways between the SAN and the AVN and between the RA and LA in the human heart (see Fig. 28.2).

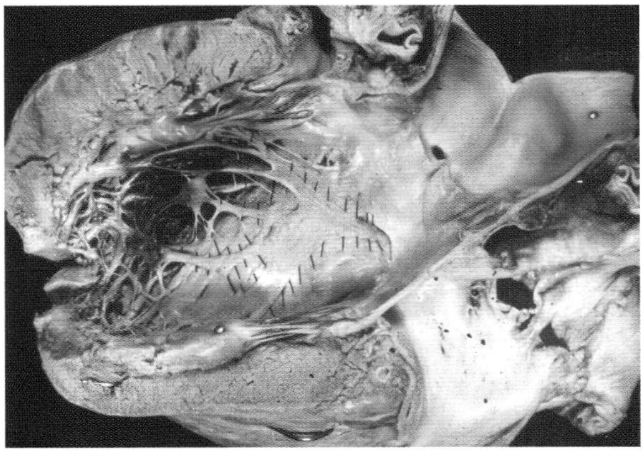

Fig. 28.12 With a little practice, one can learn to see the left bundle branch (LBB) of the atrioventricular (AV) cardiac conduction system and its many sub-branches, with the naked unaided eye. This slide was given to me by Dr. Alexi Sinev of Moscow, the Soviet Union, in 1977 when he visited our laboratory. It shows an opened normal left ventricle. Dr Sinev outlined the LBB of the AV conduction system using short black horse hairs. Soon, you do not need any help to see the right and the LBBs. **The right bundle branch (RBB)** emerges just beneath the papillary muscle of the conus (the muscle of Lancisi or Lushka). In the fresh state (in the operating room, i.e., not formalin fixed), the RBB is surrounded by glycogen. So it looks like a little linear yellow-white streak that runs down the septal band, close to the inferior rim of the septal band. The RBB is going straight down to the moderate band. Because the RBB is easily visible with the naked eye, it also is readily avoidable surgically. **The practical surgical point is to avoid iatrogenic RBB block.** A practical diagnostic problem is that a right ventriculotomy often produces a RBB pattern in the surface electrocardiogram. But if the surgeons are sure that they did not produce real RBB, everyone can be reassured that real RBB transection did not occur, and that the electrocardiogram is only reflecting the effects of right ventriculotomy, not RBB transection. This question can, if necessary, be settled electrophysiologically; but usually electrophysiologic study is unnecessary because experienced surgical teams know how to avoid surgical RBB transection. **The LBB and the RBB both are visible to the naked eye.** (Courtesy Dr. Alexi Sinev, Moscow.)

In 1965, Clarke[17] described the arterial blood supply of the conducting system of the human heart. Of 50 SANs, 35 were supplied by the right coronary artery (RCA) (70%). Of 50 AVNs, 45 were supplied by the RCA (90%). That is why the RCA is sometimes called "the artery of sudden death." The author concluded that there is extensive arterial and capillary supply to the SAN, to the AVN, and to the AVB.

In 1966, Lev et al[18] published the case of a patient with systemic scleroderma and complete heart block. Serial section study revealed that the AV conduction system had been replaced by fibrosis.

In 1967, Hudson[19] described the surgical pathologic conditions of the conduction system of the heart.

In 1967, Verhaeghe and van der Hauwaert[20] presented a study of the arterial blood supply of the human SAN.

In 1968, Merideth and Titus[21] reported on the anatomic atrial connections between the SAN and the AVN. They confirmed the existence of the three pathways from the SAN to the AVN found by James[4] in 1963.

In 1968, Lev[22] reported on the conduction system in congenital heart disease.

In 1968, James and Sherf[23] presented a paper on the ultrastructure of the human AVN. They found no anatomic syncytium and four different cell types:

1. simple rounded cells, identical to the P cells of the SAN;
2. slender transitional cells, by much the most numerous; and at the nodal margins
3. Purkinje; and
4. ordinary myocardium.

In 1969, Matoušek and Posner[24] published a paper entitled **"Purkyně's (Purkinje's) Muscle Fibres in the Heart."** The year 1969 was the 100th anniversary of the death of **Jan Evangelista Purkyně** (1787–1869). Jan is short for Johannes, which is John in English. His given names mean John Evangelist. **So, he was named for the Christian St. John the Evangelist.**[25] Perhaps because of the influence of Goethe, Purkyně was appointed professor of physiology and pathology at the University of Breslau (now Wroclaw) in western Poland in 1823. **Purkyně** was the Polish version of his name; and **Purkinje** was the German rendition of his name, with which we are more familiar. In 1850, Purkinje was called to Praha (Prague) to be the Chairman of the Department of Physiology. Regarded as a genius by his colleagues, much of his best work was done in Breslau.

In 1821, he found that **deaf mutes can hear through the bones of the skull,** a discovery that contributed to the study of deafness in mutes.

In 1832, Purkinje classified fingerprints.

In 1839, having observed the living substance in eggs and embryos, Purkinje was the first to call it **protoplasm.**

Purkinje founded laboratory training as an integral part of German university teaching. He developed a physiologic laboratory in his own house in Breslau in 1824. The work done by the master and his students was of such a high quality that the Prussian government finally established a Physiologic Institute for Prof. Purkinje at Breslau in 1842.

In 1844, Purkinje proposed **microdissection.** Purkinje was the first microscopist to use a microtome, Canada balsam, glacial acetic acid, potassium bichromate, and the Drummond lime light, in 1839. Purkinje invented modern medical microscopic histology. It was after that technologic advance—the development of microscopic slides—that he **discovered and described the Purkinje fibers of cardiac myocardium in 1839.**[25]

In 1970, James[26] described the fetal and postnatal development of the cardiac conduction system.

In the interests of brevity, only a few more papers will be cited individually. The world's medical literature is an almost infinite source of ever-expanding information.

In 1975, Bharati and Lev[27] described the course of the conduction system in single LV with an inverted (L-) ventricular loop and inverted (L-) TGA.

In 1976, Janse, Anderson, van Capelle, and Durrer[28] published a combined electrophysiologic and anatomic study of the human fetal heart. **They found no support for the internodal tracts of James.**[4]

In 1978, Wenink[29] published a study of the embryology of the conducting system.

In 1980, Bharati, Rosen, Steinfield, Miller, and Lev[30] published a study of 3 cases of corrected transposition with VSD and ventricular preexcitation. All had Ebstein malformation of the left-sided tricuspid valve. **Kent bundle sites** were found inferior to and to the left of the left-sided tricuspid valve. These Kent bundles bypassed the AV conduction system, causing ventricular preexcitation.

In 1983, Brodman, Fisher, Mitsudo, Kim, and Matos[31] published a paper entitled **"Kent Pathways Visualized In Situ and Removed at Operation."** In 2 patients, left free-wall accessory Kent bundles were found in the coronary sulcus fat and were removed. The average widest dimension was 1.8 mm.

In 1983, SAN coronary arteries were studied angiographically by Kyriakidis et al[32] in 309 patients. The findings were as follows: from the RCA in 59%, from the left coronary artery (LCA) in 38%, and from both in 3%. When the SAN artery arose from the left circumflex artery, there was a posterior SAN artery in 27% (and in 10.5% of the whole series).

In 1983, Thorgeirsson and Liebman[33] reported the case of a **21-month-old boy who had a mesothelioma of the AVN.** This is a rare cause of supra-His block, arrhythmias, and sudden death.

The AVB is often called **the bundle of His.** But who was His, and what did he really discover? **Wilhelm His, Jr.**[6] (1863–1934), as was mentioned previously, was born in Basel, Switzerland, but his family moved to Leipzig, Germany when he was a child. He became a physician and served as the director of the first medical clinic at Berlin's Charité Hospital in 1907. His became a German citizen and served in the army during World War I, during which he described trench fever.

In 1893, His discovered the AVB of the human cardiac conduction system, which is therefore now often called the bundle of His.[6]

Fascinating to relate, the same narrow bundle of specialized cardiac muscle **was discovered a little earlier by Stanley Kent in 1892–1893.**[25] So who was Stanley Kent? **Albert Frank Stanley Kent**[25] (1863–1958) was an English physiologist from Torrey, Wiltshire, who graduated in natural sciences from Magdalen College, Oxford in 1886. He did much research on the mammalian heart, and in 1892–1893 he discovered the AVB, now known as **the bundle of Kent,** and also known as the bundle of His. Kent helped to found the Radiology Department at St. Thomas' Hospital, London. He served as the first professor of physiology at University College, Bristol in 1890.

We have told the "human history" of the AVN and AVB, but not of the **SAN. Sir Arthur Keith**[1] (1866–1955) was an anatomist and anthropologist from Aberdeen, Scotland, who studied medicine at Marischal College, University of Aberdeen. He discovered the SAN of the heart in 1907, while working with Martin Flack (1882–1931).

In 1908, Keith was appointed Curator of the Museum at the Royal College of Surgeons in London. In 1909, in his Hunterian Lecture on the human heart, Keith[2] was the first to state that typical D-TGA is infundibular inversion,[2] not a great arterial malformation. Some of his many publications include *Human Embryology and Morphology* (1902), and *The Antiquity of Man* (1915).[25]

It is often said that we stand on the shoulders of giants.[a] As far as the conduction system of the human heart is concerned, we have just met four of the giants: **Arthur Keith, Jan Evangelista Purkinje, Stanley Kent, and Wilhelm His, Jr.**[1,25]

[a]If I have seen further (than you and Descartes), it is by standing on the shoulders of giants.

Sir Isaac Newton. Letter to Robert Hooke, February 5, 1675–1676.

In 1984, Allen and Doherty[34] reported the case of a 54-year-old man who died suddenly with amyloidosis of the cardiac conduction system that was thought to be secondary to bilateral basilar bronchiectasis.

In 1984, Daliento, Nava, Fasoli, Mazzucco, and Thiene[35] reported the association of myomatous dysplasia of the tricuspid and mitral valve with anomalies of the conduction system. The AVN was on the left side of the atrial septum. There was an accessory nodoventricular pathway to the left side of the ventricular septum. The membranous septum and the central fibrous body were hypoplastic. These findings occurred in two siblings who also had an atrial septal defect.

Accessory conduction fibers can also arise from the AVB, as was reported by Lev, Leffler, Langendorf, and Pick[36] in 1966. Their patient had ventricular preexcitation (Wolff-Parkinson-White syndrome) that terminated in complete AV block. Copious **Mahaim fibers from the AVB to the posterior muscular ventricular septum were thought to explain the delta wave. This was the first case in which Mahaim fibers were shown to be responsible for the AV conduction in the WPW syndrome.**[36]

In 1984, Rossi, Montella, Frescura, and Thiene[37] reported a case of congenital AV block in a patient with the heterotaxy syndrome and congenital asplenia. This patient was found to have congenital atrionodal discontinuity. There were two AVNs, but neither connected with atrial myocardium.

In 1985, Litsey, Noonan, O'Connor, Cottrill, and Mitchell[38] published a paper about **maternal connective tissue disease causing congenital heart block.** Immunoglobulin was demonstrated in the infant's cardiac tissue.

In 1986, Bharati and Lev[39] reported on the status of the conduction system of patients who **died suddenly and unexpectedly many years after the surgical repair** of their congenital heart disease.

In 1988, Ishibashi-Ueda, Yutani, Imakita, Kanzaki, Utsu, and Chiba[40] published an autopsied case of a newborn infant with congenital complete heart block who was born to a mother with systemic lupus erythematosus. The infant died 10 hours after birth. Autopsy revealed hematoxylin bodies in the AVN, in the central fibrous body, and in the fibrous skeleton of the heart. The authors concluded that **immunoglobulin G (IgG) (or immune complexes) had crossed from the placenta into the infant's circulation. Deposition into the AV conduction system had led to congenital AV block.**

In 1990, Case and Gillette[41] published a study entitled "Conduction System Disease in a Child with Long QT Syndrome."

Sudden infant death syndrome (SIDS) has long been an enigma. In 1968, James[42] published a paper entitled: "Sudden Death in Babies: New Observations in the Heart." James found **focal degeneration of the left bundle in SIDS and in normal hearts.** If future studies of SIDS babies were to confirm the existence of focal degenerative lesions of the AV conduction system, the mystery of these sudden deaths might well be solved. The current problem is that routine autopsies of SIDS patients typically reveal nothing significant. Why? Perhaps because serial histologic-section study of the AV conduction system typically is not done. The general pediatric pathologist who usually is in charge of SIDS autopsies thinks that congenital heart disease is not present because no congenital anomaly is grossly visible. So SIDS cases typically are not referred to a cardiac pathologist, and no serial section study of the cardiac conduction system is done. This may be why SIDS remains a mystery. James' study[42] (1968) suggests that **serial-section study of the conduction should be routine in SIDS autopsies, until we know whether or not James' findings[42] in SIDS are typical.**

In 1989, Behan, Behan, Reid, Doig, and Gairns[43] published **family studies of congenital heart block associated with Ro antibody.** Their hypothesis was as follows:

1. Mother gets a viral infection.
2. This leads to maternal autoantibody production.
3. Virus crosses the placenta and damages the fetal heart.
4. Maternal antibody then crosses the placenta and is deposited in the fetal heart.

This hypothesis seeks to explain how and why the maternal viral antibody is found in the fetal heart.[43]

In 1991, Randall, Wurster, Duff, O'Toole, and Wehrmacher[44] described surgical interruption of postganglionic innervation of the SAN region. **The major parasympathetic postganglionic projections to the SAN in the dog heart are by way of the right atrial free wall and therefore are vulnerable to surgical right atriotomy incisions.** This one is for the surgeons and the electrophysiologists.

In 1991, Racker[45] reported sinoventricular transmission in the dog heart of the superior atrionodal bundle and of the proximal AVB of James.[11]

In 1991, Bharati, Moskowitz, Scheinman, Estes, and Lev[46] reported on the anatomic substrate of junctional tachycardias and its importance in ablative procedures.

In 1991, Anderson and Ho[47] reported on the **morphologic substrates of pediatric cardiac arrhythmias.**

In 1993, Nakagawa, Thompson, Terracio, and Borg[48] reported on the developmental anatomy of HNK-1 immunoreactivity in the embryonic rat heart that showed codistribution with early conduction tissue.

In 1992, Holman, Kirklin, Epstein, Plumb, and Kay[49] presented **a quantitative morphometric analysis of the surgical anatomy of the Wolff-Parkinson-White syndrome.**

In 1993, Wang, Kragel, Friedlander, and Cheng[50] reported the case of a 44-year-old black woman who died suddenly and unexpectedly of cardiac arrest. **Autopsy revealed a granular cell tumor of the SAN. A granular cell tumor is benign, and most often occurs in the tongue. She died of unexpected cardiac arrest.**

In 1993, Chow, Chow, Anderson, and Gosling[51] reported a study of **the innervation of the human cardiac conduction system at birth.**

In 1991, Dick, O'Connor, Serwer, LeRoy, and Armstrong[52] reported that **the use of radiofrequency current to ablate accessory connections in children is effective and safe.**

In 1992, McGuire, Johnson, Robotin, Richards, Uther, and Ross[53] reported **the dimensions of the triangle of Koch** in humans. Although often helpful in locating the invisible AVN, we have found that the triangle of Koch can be poorly defined or absent. For example, when the right leaflet of the sinoatrial valve (the right leaflet of the valve of the IVC) is absent, a method that almost always works is as follows:

1. Find the right atrial ostium of the coronary sinus.
2. Find the inferior rim of the membranous septum, or the membranous VSD (where the AVB penetrates to reach the ventricles).
3. ***Mentally* draw a straight line from the coronary sinus ostium to the inferior rim of the membranous septum. That is where the invisible AVN and proximal AVB are located.** (Do not draw the coronary sinus–to–membranous septum line on the right atrial endocardium with an instrument, in particular, *not* with a sucker—to avoid injuring the AVN and AVB.)

In 1993, Burke, Subramanian, Smialek, and Virmani[54] reported nonatherosclerotic narrowing of the AVN artery and sudden death.

In 1994, Dean, Ho, Rowland, Mann, and Anderson[55] published a paper about the clinical anatomy of the AV junctions.

In 1994, Sealy[56] reported on the surgical anatomy of accessory connections of AV conduction.

In 1995, Martinez-Leon, Garcia-Civera, Sanjuan, and Otero-Coto[57] reported the case of a 34-year-old man with WPW in whom a Kent bundle was visualized in situ at operation after an unsuccessful radiofrequency ablation. This Kent bundle was subepicardial and was superficial to the RCA. The authors thought that the location of the Kent bundle, very superficial, outside the RCA, may have been why the attempted radiofrequency ablation failed.

In 1996, James, St. Martin, Willis, and Lohr[58] proposed apoptosis as a possible cause of gradual development of complete heart block and fatal arrhythmias associated with absence of the AVN, SAN, and intermodal pathways.

In 1996, Holdaway, Hernandez, Mohanty, and Topaz[59] reported on an anomalous SAN artery originating from the left main coronary artery.

In 1996, Diamandakis, Shutte, and Lamb[60] cloned, sequenced, and mapped the human phospholemman gene. This gene is located on chromosome 19 (exact location to be determined). This gene causes isolated cardiac conduction system disease, and it behaves as though autosomal dominant.

In 1999, Blom, Gittenberger-de Groot, De Ruiter, Poelmann, Mentink, and Ottenkamp[61] published a study of the development of the cardiac conduction tissue in human embryos using HNK-1 antigen expression. The authors think that their study may provide an understanding of abnormal atrial automaticity. They also demonstrated James' three intermodal tracts.[11]

In 1998, Suarez-Mier and Gamallo[62] studied the conduction system in 347 human hearts. The title of their paper was "Atrioventricular Node Fetal Dispersion and His Bundle Fragmentation of the Cardiac Conduction System in Sudden Cardiac Death." The title suggests that fetal dispersion of the AVN and fragmentation of the AVB caused sudden cardiac death. And that may well be true. However, these authors did things right. They had a control group: patients of similar ages, but who did *not* have a sudden cardiac death. Their findings in the control group were eye-opening:

1. Persistent fetal dispersion of the AVN was higher in the control group (40.81%) than in the sudden death group.
2. Fragmentation of the His bundle was also higher in the control group (47.67%).

What Did the Authors Conclude?

1. Persistent fetal dispersion of the AVN and fragmentation of the His bundle can be normal variants.
2. Persistent fetal dispersion of the AVN and/or fragmentation of the His bundle should not be regarded as the cause of sudden death unless there are also documented electrocardiographic abnormalities.

This is a **HUGE WARNING**[62] to pathologists who do serial section studies of the conduction system in cases of sudden death WITHOUT AGE-MATCHED NORMAL CONTROLS and WITHOUT ELECTROCARDIOGRAPHIC DATA.

This makes the task of accurate interpretation of perinatal and pediatric serial section data of the conduction system more difficult.

In 2000, Chauvin, Shah, Haïssaguerre, Marcellin, and Brechenmacher[63] published a study about the anatomic basis of connections between the coronary sinus musculature and the LA atrium in humans. This study is relevant to ablation to cure atrial fibrillation. In case you are having trouble understanding this, the following few words may help: The *right* horn of the sinus venosus, immediately adjacent to the right atrial musculature, is where the normal SAN is located.

A hypothesis is that the *left* sinus horn, that is, the coronary sinus, which is immediately adjacent to the left atrial musculature, may be electrically stimulating the LA. In other words, the left sinus horn (the coronary sinus) may be acting like an abnormal, rapidly firing, ectopic, left-sided SAN.

If so, the authors propose a laterally displaced ablation line—to the left of the coronary sinus, or a similarly placed left atriotomy. Either should be an effective form of therapy for atrial fibrillation, by blocking the abnormal stimuli from the coronary sinus (the left sinus horn).

In 2000, Racker and Kadish[64] published a detailed histologic study of the AV conduction system in three dimensions (three orthogonal planes). The parts of the AV conduction system, from proximally to distally, are as follows:

1. **The lateral atrionodal bundle** runs posteroinferiorly to the coronary sinus.
2. **The medial atrionodal bundle** runs between the coronary sinus and the IVC. Then the lateral and the medial atrionodal bundles flow together, forming
3. **the proximal AVB.** Then just before the proximal AVB reaches the AVN,
4. **the superior atrionodal bundle** joins the proximal AVB, which then flows into the
5. **AVN.** Note that all three internodal tracts (atrionodal bundles) have been accounted for: (1) the lateral, (2) the medial, and (3) the superior. The proximal AVB is where all three atrionodal bundles run together before flowing into the AVN.
6. **The distal AVB** is what "everybody" calls the AV or His bundle. In other words, the three internodal tracts and the proximal AVB have now been accepted into the standard description of the cardiac conduction system by most experts. Then the distal AVB flows into
7. the bundle branches.

The authors' title[54] states that the proximal AVB, the AVN, and the distal AVB are distinct anatomic structures with unique histologic features and innervation. Specifically, some of the authors' findings:

1. In the conduction system, the myocardium is aggregated into fascicles containing approximately eight myofibers.
2. Within fascicles, myofibers are coiled or spiraled about each other.
3. Spiraling is most compact in the proximal AVB.
4. Collagen encases individual fascicles.
5. In the proximal AVB, the fascicles are in parallel array.
6. In the AVN, fascicles are interwoven.
7. In the distal AVB, the fascicles are in parallel array.
8. Collagen septation constitutes natural barriers within the conduction system and between the conduction system and the surrounding myocardium.[64]

In 1988, Abuin and Nieponice[65] published a paper about the treatment of hypertrophic obstructive cardiomyopathy by injecting alcohol into ventricular septal branch arteries. However, the authors found that **the first ventricular septal branch of the left anterior descending (LAD) coronary artery supplies the AVN, the His bundle, and the RBB of the AV conduction system.** So the message of their paper was: Do *not* inject alcohol into the first ventricular septal branch of the LAD.[65]

In 1998, Abuin and Nieponice[66] published a paper entitled "New Findings on the Origin of the Blood Supply to the AV Node: Clinical and Surgical Significance." The **Kugel artery** supplied the AVN in 40% of their cases. The Kugel artery is also known as the circle of Vieussens that connects the RCA and the LCA, just below the aortic root. Kugel artery has several perforating branches, one of which goes to the AVN. The proximity of the aortic root to Kugel artery is surgically important.

The right descending superior artery supplied the AVN in 70% of their cases. The right descending superior artery is an atrial artery that runs anteriorly to the foramen ovale.

The AVN artery and the first septal branch of the left anterior descending coronary artery also supply the AVN.[66]

In 2002, Angelini, Moreolo, Ruffatti, Milanesi, and Thiene[67] reported **calcification of the AVN in a fetus with congenital complete heart block.** At 18 weeks gestation, the fetus had lymphocytic, fetal, autoimmune myocarditis, with calcification of the AVN that was detectable by two-dimensional echocardiography.[68]

In 2003, Lemery, Guiraudon, and Veinot[68] reported an anatomic description of the Bachmann bundle and its relation to the atrial septum.

In 2004, Lemery, Soucie, Martin, Tang, Green, and Healey[69] reported a study in humans of biatrial electrical coupling. They found that electrical coupling of the RA and the LA is predominantly provided by muscular connections of the Bachmann bundle and the coronary sinus. In sinus rhythm, conduction over the Bachmann bundle at a mean rate of 23 ± 15 ms provides nearly synchronous biatrial activation. The atrial septum (the limbus and the fossa ovalis) typically is not involved in contralateral conduction in normal sinus rhythm or in atrial pacing.

In 2004, Sternick, Timmermans, Sosa, Cruz, Rodriguez, Fagundes, Gerken, and Wellens[70] published a paper on **the electrocardiogram during sinus rhythm and tachycardia in patients with Mahaim fibers.** They emphasized the importance of an rS pattern in lead III. This study was based on 33 patients with tachycardia and anterograde conduction. The patients were mostly young adults (median age was 24 ± 10 years), and they were predominantly female (20/33, 60.61%).

During tachycardia, a LBB-like QRS pattern was observed with left axis deviation. An rS pattern in lead III was observed in 6% of controls. WPW patients were excluded from this study, as were other patients with short AV accessory pathways.

These authors[70] **stated that Mahaim fibers are slowly conducting accessory pathways that reach into the right ventricle, and that often play a role in tachycardia.**

REFERENCES

1. Keith A, Sebastian A. *A Dictionary of the History of Medicine.* Pearl River, NY: The Parthenon Publishing Group Inc; 1999:441.
2. Keith A. The Hunterian lectures on malformations of the heart. *Lancet August.* 1909;14:433.
3. Van Praagh R, Van Praagh S. Atrial isomerism in the heterotaxy syndromes with asplenia, or polysplenia, or normally formed spleen: an erroneous concept. *Am J Cardiol.* 1999;66:1504.
4. James TN. The connecting pathways between the sinus node and the A-V node and between the right and the left atrium in the human heart. *Am Heart J.* 1963;66:498.
5. Mullin MP, Van Praagh R, Walsh EP. Development and anatomy of the cardiac conducting system. In: Walsh EP, Saul JP, Triedman JK, eds. *Cardiac Arrhythmias in Children and Young Adults with Congenital Heart Disease.* Philadelphia: Lippincott Williams & Wilkins; 2001. p3.
6. His Jr W, Sebastian A. *A Dictionary of the History of Medicine.* Pearl River, NY: The Parthenon Publishing Group Inc; 1999:394.
7. Koch WK, Koch T, Sebastian A. *A Dictionary of the History of Medicine.* Pearl River, NY: The Parthenon Publishing Group Inc; 1999:448.
8. Thebesius, Adam C, Sebastian A. *A Dictionary of the History of Medicine.* Pearl River, NY: The Parthenon Publishing Group Inc; 1999:708.
9. Eustachio B, Sebastian A. *A Dictionary of the History of Medicine.* Pearl River, NY: The Parthenon Publishing Group Inc; 1999:298.
10. Todaro F. *Todaro's Tendon, in Dorland's Illustrated Medical Dictionary.* 29th ed. Philadelphia: WB Saunders; 1994:1846.
11. Lev M. The architecture of the conduction system in congenital heart disease: I. Common atrioventricular orifice. *AMA Arch Path.* 1958;65:174.
12. Titus JL. Normal anatomy of the human cardiac conduction system. *Mayo Clin Proc.* 1973;48(24).
13. Anderson RH, Arnold R, Wilkinson JL. The conducting system in congenitally corrected transposition. *Lancet.* 1973;1:1286.
14. Anderson RH, Becker AE, Arnold R, Wilkinson JL. The conduction tissues in congenitally corrected transposition. *Circulation.* 1974;50:911.
15. Friedberg DZ, Nadas AS. The clinical profile of patients with congenital corrected transposition of the great arteries. A study of 60 cases. *N Engl J Med.* 1970;282:1053.
16. Dick M, Van Praagh R, Rudd M, Folkerth T, Castañeda A. Electrophysiologic delineation of the specialized atrioventricular conduction system in two patients with corrected transposition of the great arteries in situs inversus {I, D, D}. *Circulation.* 1977;55:896.
17. Clarke JA. An x-ray microscopic study of the arterial supply of the conducting system of the human heart. *Brit Heart J.* 1965;27:879.
18. Lev M, Landowne M, Matchar JC, Wagner JA. Systemic scleroderma with complete heart block. Report of a case with comprehensive study of the conduction system. *Am Heart J.* 1966;72(13).
19. Hudson REB. Surgical pathology of the conducting system of the heart. *Brit Heart J.* 1967;29:646.
20. Verhaeghe L, van der Hauwaert L. Arterial blood supply of the human sinus node. *Brit Heart J.* 1967;29:801.
21. Merideth J, Titus JL. The anatomic atrial connections between sinus and A-V node. *Circulation.* 1968;37:566.
22. Lev M. Conduction system in congenital heart disease. *Am J Cardiol.* 1968;21:619.
23. James TN, Sherf L. Ultra structure of the human atrioventricular node. *Circulation.* 1968;37:1049.
24. Matoušek M, Posner E. Purkyně's (Purkinje's) muscle fibers in the heart. *Brit Heart J.* 1969;31:718.
25. Garrison FH: An Introduction to the History of Medicine, WB Saunders Company. 4th ed., Philadelphia, 1929, Johannes Evangelista Purkinje, p 459; Wilhelm His, Jr, p 686; Stanley Kent, p 686; Sir Arthur Keith, p 521.
26. James TN. Cardiac conduction system: fetal and postnatal development. *Am J Cardiol.* 1970;25:213.
27. Bharati S, Lev M. The course of the conduction system in single ventricle with inverted (L-) loop and inverted (L-) transposition. *Circulation.* 1975;51:723.
28. Janse MJ, Anderson RH, van Capelle FJL, Durrer D. A combined electrophysiological and anatomical study of the human fetal heart. *Am Heart J.* 1976;91:556.
29. Wenink ACG. Embryology of the conducting system. In: Van Mierop LHS, Oppenheimer-Dekker A, Bruins CLDC, eds. *Embryology and Teratology of the Heart and Great Arteries.* Leiden: University Press; 1978:p3.
30. Bharati S, Rosen K, Steinfield L, Miller RA, Lev M. The anatomic substrate for preexcitation in corrected transposition. *Circulation.* 1980;62:831.
31. Brodman R, Fisher J, Mitsudo S, Kim SG, Matos J. Kent pathways visualized in situ and removed at operation. *Am J Cardiol.* 1983;51:1457.
32. Kyriakidis MK, Kourouklis CB, Papaioannou JT, Christakos SG, Spanos GP, Avgoustakis DG. Sinus node coronary arteries studied with angiography. *Am J Cardiol.* 1983;51:749.
33. Thorgeirsson G, Liebman J. Mesothelioma of the AV node. *Ped Cardiol.* 1983;4:219.
34. Allen DC, Doherty CC. Sudden death in a patient with amyloidosis of the cardiac conduction system. *Brit Heart J.* 1984;51:233.
35. Daliento L, Nava A, Fasoli G, Mazzucco A, Thiene G. Dysplasia of the atrioventricular valves associated with conduction system anomalies. *Brit Heart J.* 1984;51:243.
36. Lev M, Leffler WB, Langendorf R, Pick A. Anatomic findings in a case of ventricular pre-excitation (WPW) terminating in complete block. *Circulation.* 1966;34:718.
37. Rossi L, Montella S, Frescura C, Thiene G. Congenital atrioventricular block in right atrial isomerism (asplenia), a case due to atrionodal discontinuity. *Chest.* 1984;85:578.

38. Litsey SE, Noonan JA, O'Connor WN, Cottrill CM, Mitchell B. Maternal connective tissue disease and congenital heart block. Demonstration of immunoglobulin in cardiac tissue. *New Engl J Med.* 1985;312:98.
39. Bharati S, Lev M. Conduction system in cases of sudden death in congenital heart disease many years after surgical correction. *Chest.* 1986;90:861.
40. Ishibashi-Ueda H, Yutani C, Imakita M, Kanzaki T, Utsu M, Chiba Y. An autopsy case of congenital complete heart block in a newly born of a mother with systemic lupus erythematosus. *Pediatr Cardiol.* 1988;9(157).
41. Case CL, Gillette PC. Conduction system disease in a child with long QT syndrome. *Am Heart J.* 1990;120:984.
42. James TN. Sudden death in babies: new observations in the heart. *Am J Cardiol.* 1968;22:479.
43. Behan WMH, Behan PO, Reid JM, Doig W, Gairns J. Family studies of congenital heart block associated with Ro antibody. *Brit Heart J.* 1989;62:320.
44. Randall WC, Wurster RD, Duff M, O'Toole MF, Wehrmacher W. Surgical interruption of postganglionic innervation of the sinoatrial nodal region. *J Thorac Cardiovasc Surg.* 1991;101:66.
45. Racker DK. Sinoventricular transmission in 10m M K^+ by canine atrioventricular nodal inputs, superior atrionodal bundle and proximal atrionodal bundle. *Circulation.* 1991;23:1738.
46. Bharati S, Moskowitz WB, Scheinman M, Estes NAM, Lev M. Junctional tachycardias: anatomic substrate and its significance in ablative procedures. *J Am Coll Cardiol.* 1991;18:179.
47. Anderson RH, Ho S. The morphologic substrates for pediatric arrhythmias. *Cardiol Young.* 1991;1:159.
48. Nakagawa M, Thompson RP, Terracio L, Borg TK. Developmental anatomy of HNK-1 immunoreactivity in the embryonic rat heart—co-distribution with early conduction tissue. *Cardiol Young.* 1993;3(I-125). abstract 433.
49. Holman WL, Kirklin JK, Epstein AE, Plumb VJ, Kay GN. Wolff-Parkinson-White syndrome, a quantitative morphometric analysis of surgical anatomy. *J Thorac Cardiovasc Surg.* 1992;104:802.
50. Wang J, Kragel AH, Friedlander ER, Cheng JT. Granular cell tumor of the sinus node. *Am J Cardiol.* 1993;71:490.
51. Chow LT-c, Chow SS-m, Anderson RH, Gosling JA. Innervation of the human cardiac conduction system at birth. *Brit Heart J.* 1993;69:430.
52. Dick M, O'Connor BK, Serwer GA, LeRoy S, Armstrong B. Use of radiofrequency current to ablate accessory connections in children. *Circulation.* 1991;84:2318.
53. McGuire MA, Johnson DC, Robotin M, Richards DA, Uther JB, Ross DL. Dimensions of the triangle of Koch in humans. *Am J Cardiol.* 1992;70:829.
54. Burke AP, Subramanian R, Smialek J, Virmani R. Nonatherosclerotic narrowing of the atrioventricular node artery and sudden death. *J Am Coll Cardiol.* 1993;21:117.
55. Dean JW, Ho SY, Rowland E, Mann J, Anderson RH. Clinical anatomy of the atrioventricular junctions. *J Am Coll Cardiol.* 1994;24:1725.
56. Sealy WC. Surgical anatomy of accessory connections of atrioventricular conduction. *Ann Thorac Surgery.* 1994;57:1675.
57. Martinez-Leon J, Garcia-Civera R, Sanjuan R, Otero-Coto E. Kent bundle visualized in situ at operation after unsuccessful radiofrequency ablation. *Ann Thorac Surg.* 1995;59:218.
58. James TN, St. Martin E, Willis PW, Lohr TO. Apoptosis as a possible cause of gradual development of complete heart block and fatal arrhythmias associated with absence of the AV node, sinus node and intermodal pathways. *Circulation.* 1996;93:1424.
59. Holdaway B, Hernandez E, Mohanty PK, Topaz O. Anomalous sinus node artery originating from the left main coronary artery. *Am Heart J.* 1996;132:449.
60. Diamandakis VM, Schutte BC, Lamb FS. Cloning, sequencing, and mapping the human phospholemman gene. *Pediatrics.* 1996;1–98(suppl 526). abstract 6.
61. Blom NA, Gittenberger-de Groot AC, De Ruiter MC, Poelmann RE, Mentink MMT, Ottenkamp J. Development of the cardiac conduction tissue in human embryos using HNK-1 antigen expression. Possible relevance for understanding of abnormal atrial automaticity. *Circulation.* 1999;99:800.
62. Suarez-Mier MP, Gamallo C. Atrioventricular node fetal dispersion and His bundle fragmentation of the cardiac conduction system in sudden cardiac death. *J Am Coll Cardiol.* 1998;32:1885.
63. Chauvin M, Shah DC, Haïssaguerre M, Marcellin L, Brechenmacher C. The anatomic basis of connections between the coronary sinus musculature and the left atrium in humans. *Circulation.* 2000;101:647.
64. Racker DK, Kadish AH. Proximal atrioventricular bundle, atrioventricular node, and distal atrioventricular bundle are distinct anatomic structures with unique histological characteristics and innervation. *Circulation.* 2000;101:1049.
65. Abuin G, Nieponice A. The first septal artery supplies the atrioventricular node. *Texas Heart Inst J.* 1998;25:318.
66. Abuin G, Nieponice A. New findings on the origin of the blood supply to the atrioventricular node, clinical and surgical significance. *Texas Heart Inst.* 1998;25:113.
67. Angelini A, Moreolo GS, Ruffatti A, Milanesi O, Thiene G. Calcification of the atrioventricular node in a fetus affected by congenital complete heart block. *Circulation.* 2002;105:1254.
68. Lemery R, Guiraudon G, Veinot JP. Anatomic description of Bachmann's bundle and its relation to the atrial septum. *Am J Cardiol.* 2003;91:1482.
69. Lemery R, Soucie L, Martin B, Tang ASL, Green M, Healey J. Human study of biatrial electrical coupling. Determinants of endocardial septal activation and conduction over interatrial connections. *Circulation.* 2004;110:2083.
70. Sternick EB, Timmermans C, Sosa E, et al. The electrocardiogram during sinus rhythm and tachycardia in patients with Mahaim fibers. The importance of an "rS" pattern in lead III. *J Am Coll Cardiol.* 2004;44:1626.

29

The Heterotaxy Syndromes

Asplenia, Polysplenia, and With Normally Formed but Right-Sided Spleen

WHAT ARE THE HETEROTAXY SYNDROMES?

Heterotaxy is derived from two Greek words: heteros, "other," and taxis, "arrangement." Hence, heterotaxy is an arrangement of the viscera that is other than normal (situs solitus) or its mirror image (situs inversus).

Although there is now much literature relevant to the understanding of the heterotaxy syndromes(s),[1-133] from very early in their recognition and delineation, anomalies of the spleen were identified as important markers of these syndromes,[5] namely, congenital asplenia[15] and congenital polysplenia.[6]

Later it was realized that visceral heterotaxy (scrambling of the situs) could also occur with a normally formed spleen. Consequently, the heterotaxy syndromes cannot be satisfactorily designated in terms of asplenia or polysplenia (because the spleen can be normally formed).

Thus, as the title of this chapter indicates, there are three different types of heterotaxy syndrome in terms of the status of the spleen: (1) the heterotaxy syndrome with asplenia; (2) the heterotaxy syndrome with polysplenia; and (3) the heterotaxy syndrome with a normally formed, but often right sided, spleen.

Other efforts have been made to characterize these syndromes in terms of bilateral right-sidedness (right isomerism) and bilateral left-sidedness (left isomerism).[6-8] The asplenia syndrome was said, as a teaching mnemonic, to have bilateral right-sidedness: a bilaterally symmetrical liver, with a large lobe on both right and left sides; the inferior vena cava (IVC) was almost always intact (not interrupted), this being a right-sided feature; bilateral superior venae cavae (SVCs) (an SVC bilaterally also may be regarded as a bilaterally right-sided feature); the lungs are often bilaterally trilobed; both bronchi frequently eparterial; and both atrial appendages often being abnormally broad and triangular (resembling right atrial appendages bilaterally).

Conversely, the polysplenia syndrome may be regarded as having bilateral left-sidedness (left isomerism)[7,8]; the lungs are often bilaterally bilobed; both bronchi are frequently hyparterial; the pulmonary veins may be ipsilateral, with the right veins draining into the right-sided atrium and the left veins draining into the left-sided atrium, suggesting that the left atrium (LA) is present bilaterally; the tips of the atrial appendages are often long and thin, like pointing fingers, resembling left atrial appendages bilaterally; and the gallbladder can be absent (absence of the gallbladder being remembered as a bilaterally left-sided feature because the gallbladder normally is a right-sided structure).

Initially, we thought these were wonderful and helpful mnemonics (memory aids), until we realized that some of our friends and colleagues thought them literal. Some people thought that the right atrium (RA) really could be bilateral, and that the LA also really could be bilateral. It was at this juncture that we started whispering into influential ears that right atrial "isomerism" and left atrial "isomerism" were just memory aids, not accurate anatomy. We were telling any who would listen that bilaterally RAs and bilaterally LAs in fact have never been documented.

Accurately speaking, we said, for the morphologically RA to be bilateral, there would have to be an IVC bilaterally, a coronary sinus bilaterally, a SVC bilaterally, a septum secundum with superior and inferior limbic band bilaterally, and a broad triangular atrial appendage bilaterally. This situation has never been documented in a single human being (conjoined twins excluded).

Accurately speaking, we added, for the morphologically left atrium to be bilateral, there would have to be four pulmonary veins bilaterally, septum primum bilaterally, and a long, thin, finger-like appendage bilaterally. Again, this situation has never been documented in a single human being (conjoined twins excluded).

To their credit, our colleagues listened, pondered, and agreed. However, some of them then retreated from atrial "isomerism" (an untenable position), to atrial *appendage* isomerism. Again, we whispered in influential ears that this position also is untenable, both factually[9] and conceptually.[10]

Factually, one does not always have a large triangular atrial appendage bilaterally in the asplenia syndrome; nor does one always have a long thin atrial appendage bilaterally in the polysplenia syndrome,[9] as will be documented subsequently.

Conceptually, the idea of partial atrial isomerism—involving the atrial appendages only or the pectinate muscles only—is not isomerism.[10] By analogy, consider the molecules of 0-glucose and L-glucose, which really are isomers. These molecules are isomers because each of the asymmetrical atoms in L-glucose is a mirror-image of the corresponding asymmetrical atoms in 0-glucose. If a molecule had only a few atoms that were mirror images of those in 0-glucose, such a molecule would not be considered a "partial" isomer of 0-glucose. Isomerism must involve the whole structure (the whole atrium, or the whole molecule). Partial isomerism is a contradiction in terms. Isomerism is binary: either it is present or it is not present. Conceptually and logically, isomerism cannot be partial. Or to put in another way, "partial" isomerism (appendages only or pectinate muscles only) is not isomerism.

At a less abstract level, consider a patient with right sided polysplenia. The left-sided IVC was interrupted. A large left-sided azygos vein connected with a left-sided SVC that drained into the left-sided atrium. The suprahepatic segment of the IVC also connected with the left-sided atrium, as did the coronary sinus.

The left-sided atrium had septum secundum's superior and inferior limbic bands on its septal surface. The right-sided atrium received all of the pulmonary veins, and the septal surface of the right-sided atrium displayed a well-formed septum primum. The appendage of the left-sided atrium was broad, triangular, and anterior, whereas the appendage of the right-sided atrium was long, thin, and posterior.

This case was actually presented to one of us (RVP) at an international symposium in Tokyo. One final detail: The left-sided atrial appendage (that was broad, triangular, and anterior) also had at its tip a long, thin, projecting point.

WHAT WAS THE ATRIAL SITUS?

We replied with no hesitation: situs inversus. But what about the finger-like tip of this right atrial appendage (RAA)? True, this part of the left-sided atrial appendage looks a little "leftish," but it is not really the left atrial appendage (LAA). (The morphologically LAA was right-sided in this patient with visceroatrial situs inversus.) To insist that this pointed tip of the left-sided atrial appendage really is the LAA would be to state that this morphologically RA is a composite structure consisting mostly of the morphologically RA, but having an atrial appendage tip consisting of morphologically LAA.

Briefly, we think that the latter interpretation is both erroneous and absurd. To insist on LAA isomerism (literally) is to assert that this left-sided *morphologically RA* really does have the tip of its appendage composed of morphologically LAA myocardium. The assertion that this left-sided atrium really is composed of both right and left atrial myocardium is to say that it is a chimera. (In Greek mythology, Chimera was a fire-breathing female monster usually represented as a composite of a lion, a goat, and a serpent.) We think that such a composite atrium, literally composed of both morphologically right and left atrial myocardium, is highly improbable (and amusing). (We cannot imagine how one could literally have a morphologically RA, with the tip of its appendage composed of morphologically left atrial myocardium. Biologically, we think this is a joke. We hope that you too will see how funny this concept of atrial appendage isomerism really is.)

The foregoing, then, are the main reasons why we are presenting these cases as follows: (1) as the heterotaxy syndromes, because visceral heterotaxy is the only accurate anatomic common denominator (the spleen is not always abnormally formed); and (2) bearing in mind the status of the spleen—asplenia, or polysplenia, or occasionally with a normally formed spleen. Not only do the asplenia and the polysplenia syndromes have statistically significant anatomic differences (as will be shown), but also the clinical importance of the status of the spleen merits emphasis concerning susceptibility to fulminating and rapidly fatal infection by encapsulated gram-negative coliform bacilli during the first 6 months of life and by encapsulated gram-positive bacteria— mainly pneumococcus—thereafter.[11] Another advantage of this approach is avoidance of the assertion that either right or left atrial isomerism or atrial appendage isomerism is present, thereby sidestepping these morphologic anatomic and conceptual errors.

The Essence of the Heterotaxy Syndromes

To the best of our present understanding, what is the essence of the heterotaxy syndromes? We think that the brief answer is anomalies of the visceral asymmetry and of midline associated defects. As will be seen, abnormalities of asymmetry do not necessarily mean the presence of visceral symmetry.

WHAT STRUCTURES ARE INVOLVED?

Normally asymmetrical structures are typically involved: bronchi, lungs, liver, stomach, spleen, pancreas, gastrointestinal (GI) tract, IVC, SVC, azygos vein, coronary sinus, pulmonary veins, septum primum, septum secundum, atrioventricular (AV) valves, ventricles, conus arteriosus, great arteries, and the aortic arch. These normally asymmetrical structures do not necessarily become symmetrical in the heterotaxy syndromes, although they often do become less asymmetrical than normal.

How Many Kinds of Atrial Situs are There?

We think that there are really only two kinds of atrial situs: situs solitus (normal) and situs inversus (its mirror image). Atrial situs ambiguus is not a specific anatomic type of atrial situs. Atrial situs ambiguus only means that the basic type of atrial situs is undiagnosed.

The importance of realizing that the concept of atrial-level "isomerism" is erroneous in that this understanding then facilitates the diagnosis of the types of atrial situs (solitus or inversus) in the heterotaxy syndromes. It should be noted that lung isomerism does indeed exist.

Although "bilateral right-sidedness" or "right isomerism" and "bilateral left-sidedness" or "left isomerism" are helpful teaching mnemonics for the asplenia syndrome and the polysplenia syndrome, respectively, they should not be regarded as accurate morphologic anatomy.

WHAT IS THE MORPHOLOGICALLY RIGHT ATRIUM?

As is presented in Chapter 3, the key gross anatomic features are the IVC, the ostium of the coronary sinus, the septum secundum (superior and inferior limbic bands), and a large, triangular, anterior atrial appendage.

The key to diagnosing the atrial situs is to figure out which is the morphologically right atrium (RA). The connection of the IVC is a very highly reliable diagnostic marker of the RA. The IVC works even with interruption of the IVC, which is sometimes called absence of the IVC, because the suprahepatic segment of the IVC that connects with and identifies the RA is always present. The ostium of the coronary sinus is not always present; it can be atretic, or unidentifiable (absent), as is frequent with common AV canal because of associated unroofing of the coronary sinus. But when the ostium of the coronary sinus is present, it too is a highly reliable diagnostic marker of the RA, as is the large triangular anterior atrial appendage.

WHAT IS THE MORPHOLOGICALLY LEFT ATRIUM?

The morphologically LA is the other atrium, which has a small, finger-like, posterior atrial appendage. Typically (but not always), the LA has a septum primum—the flap valve of the foramen ovale—on its septal surface, and, normally, it receives the pulmonary veins.

WHEN CAN WE NOT DIAGNOSE THE ATRIAL SITUS?

We cannot diagnose the atrial situs with confidence when the IVC and the atrial appendages appear to tell two different stories: for example, when the IVC is right-sided, and the large triangular atrial appendage is left sided, or vice versa. A right-sided IVC suggests visceroatrial situs solitus; but a left-sided morphologically right atrial appendage suggests atrial situs inversus. Which should one believe, the IVC or the appendages? From the scientific standpoint, we are not sure how to answer this question. From the practical hemodynamic standpoint, there is no doubt that the connections of the great veins (e.g., the IVC) are more important than the shape of the atrial appendages.

Consequently, we make the diagnosis of **atrial situs ambiguus** when we are not sure whether the atrial situs is solitus or inversus. Note that atrial situs ambiguus is not a specific third type of atrial situs. It may be a "scrambled" atrial situs solitus or a "scrambled" atrial situs inversus. Atrial situs ambiguus means nothing more.

Septum Primum Can Be Malpositioned

The septum primum—the flap valve of the foramen ovale—can be displaced into the morphologically LA.[15] Then septum primum can lie to the left of the right pulmonary veins (Fig. 29.1),[15] resulting in partially anomalous pulmonary venous drainage into the RA, also known as **ipsilateral pulmonary veins,** which are quite frequent in the heterotaxy syndrome with polysplenia. Ipsilateral pulmonary veins means that the pulmonary veins are same-sided (Latin: *ipse,* "self," *latus,* "side").

The right pulmonary veins drain into the right-sided atrium, and the left pulmonary veins drain into the left-sided atrium. This is part of the mnemonic that characterizes the polysplenia syndrome—"bilateral left-sidedness": the presence of pulmonary veins entering both atria is somewhat suggestive of a LA bilaterally (not really, but as an aide memoire).

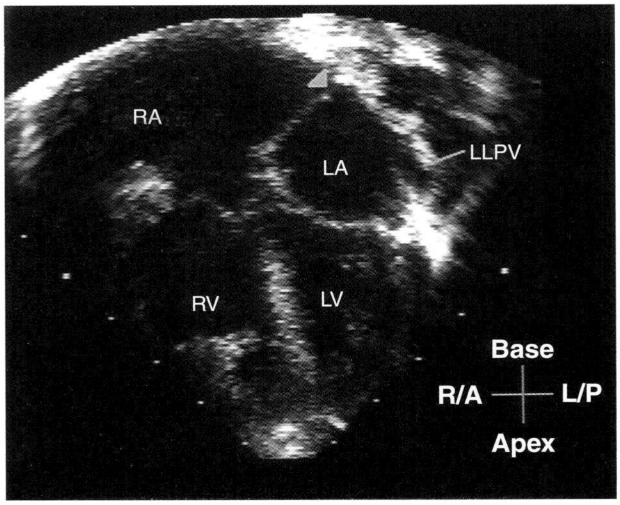

Fig. 29.1 Malposition of septum primum into left atrium. Apical four-chamber two-dimensional echocardiogram of a living 3 9/12-year-old girl with visceral heterotaxy, interruption of the inferior vena cava, an enlarged right azygos vein to the right superior vena cava, normal segmental anatomy {S,D,S}, and probable polysplenia (status of spleen not documented). Note that the atrial septum (septum primum) is displaced markedly leftward, where it attaches to posterior atrial wall between left pulmonary veins (*LLPV,* left lower pulmonary vein) and right pulmonary veins (unlabeled), resulting in ipsilateral pulmonary veins. *Arrowhead* indicates small septum primum malposition defect between malposed septum primum and posterior left atrial wall. The angle between normally located ventricular septum and leftwardly malpositioned septum primum equals 60 degrees. Normally, planes of ventricular and atrial septa are parallel; normal ventriculoatrial septal angle equals 0 degrees in this view. Malpositioned septum primum, verified surgically, was resected and replaced with normally positioned pericardial septum to right of right pulmonary veins. *LA,* Morphologically left atrium; *L/P,* left and posterior; *LV,* morphologically left ventricle; *RA,* morphologically right atrium; *R/A,* right and anterior; *RV,* morphologically right ventricle. (Reproduced with permission from Van Praagh S, Carrera ME, Sanders S, Mayer JE, Van Praagh R. Partial or total direct pulmonary venous drainage to right atrium due to malposition of septum primum, anatomic and echocardiographic findings and surgical treatment: a study based on 36 cases. *Chest.* 1995;107:1488.[15])

Displacement of the septum primum to the left of the right pulmonary veins is, we think, what produces so-called ipsilateral pulmonary veins. The septum primum can be malaligned further to the left, lying to the left of the left pulmonary veins (Fig. 29.2),[15] resulting in **totally anomalous pulmonary venous drainage (TAPVD) into the RA.** Such marked leftward malalignment of the septum primum may erroneously suggest a common atrium with a supramitral stenosing membrane (see Fig. 29.2).

Understanding of the pathologic anatomy of leftwardly displaced septum primum (Figs. 29.1 to 29.3) suggests its appropriate *surgical management:* excision of the malaligned septum primum and construction of a normally positioned atrial septum.[15] Malalignment of the septum primum is associated with a newly recognized type of atrial septal defect (ASD): a septum primum malposition ASD.[15,46,153] Malposition of the septum primum into the morphologically LA is associated with leftward malalignment in visceroatrial situs solitus, and with rightward malalignment in visceroatrial situs inversus.[15]

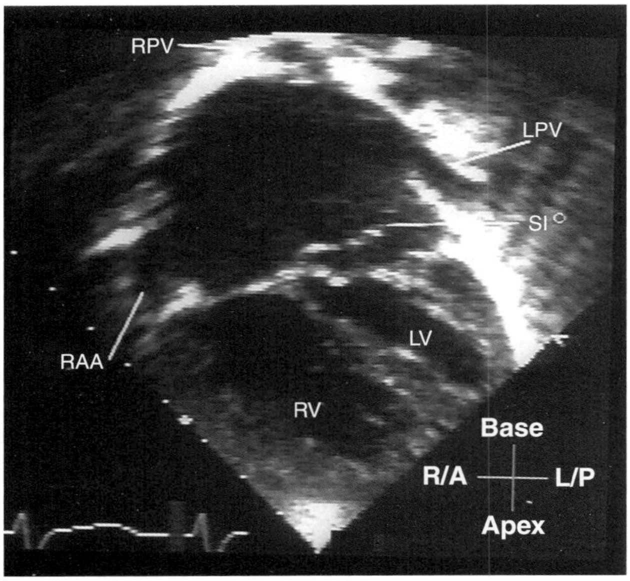

Fig. 29.2 Malposition of septum primum into left atrium. Apical four-chamber view, 2½-year-old girl with heterotaxy, probable polysplenia, interrupted inferior vena cava, enlarged right azygos vein, retroaortic innominate vein, ectopic right atrial pacemaker, tetralogy of Fallot {S,D,S}, and right aortic arch. Note that the septum primum *(SI°)* is markedly malpositioned leftward, attaching to left atrial free wall just above left atrial appendage, to left of both left pulmonary veins *(LPV)* and right pulmonary veins *(RPV)*, resulting in totally anomalous pulmonary venous drainage to right atrium (*RAA*, right atrial appendage). Leftwardly malpositioned septum primum makes an angle of 120 degrees relative to normally located ventricular septum. In addition to atrial septum primum malposition defect between septum primum and left atrial wall, there were also multiple small fenestrations in the septum primum that appeared to function as stenotic supramitral membrane. At surgical repair, the previously mentioned findings were confirmed and the malpositioned septum primum was excised and replaced with normally positioned pericardial patch to the right of the normally connected right pulmonary veins. *L/P*, Left and posterior; *LV*, morphologically left ventricle; *R/A*, right and anterior; *RV*, morphologically right ventricle. (Reproduced with permission from Van Praagh S, Carrera ME, Sanders S, Mayer JE, Van Praagh R. Partial or total direct pulmonary venous drainage to right atrium due to malposition of septum primum, anatomic and echocardiographic findings and surgical treatment: a study based on 36 cases. *Chest*. 1995;107:1488995.[15])

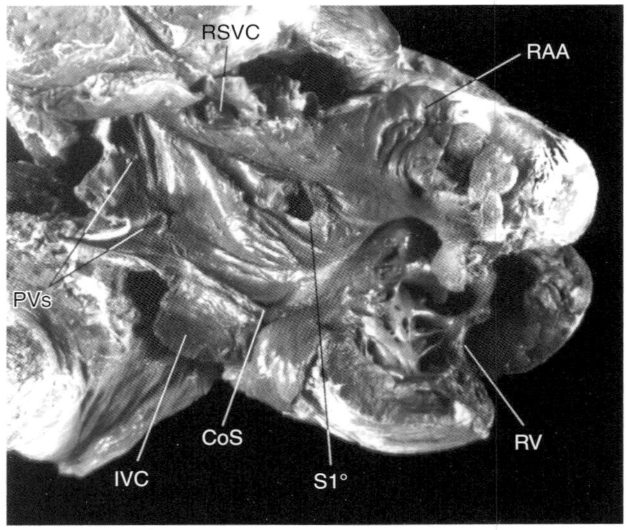

Fig. 29.3 Malposition of septum primum into left atrium. Opened right atrium (*RAA*, right atrial appendage), tricuspid valve, and right ventricle *(RV)* of a 7 $\frac{2}{12}$-year-old girl with totally anomalous pulmonary venous drainage into the RA. The septum primum *(SI°)* is displaced to the left of all pulmonary veins *(PVs)*. The septum primum is much more easily seen from the RA than is normally the case. The superior limbic band of septum secundum is virtually absent. Hence, the superior attachments of the septum primum are not covered from the right atrial perspective, as they usually are. The space between the leftwardly displaced septum primum below and the left atrial wall above is a septum primum malposition type of atrial septal defect (ASD). This type of ASD is similar to an ostium secundum ASD, except that the septum primum is very leftwardly malpositioned and the superior limbic band of septum secundum is poorly formed or absent. Note that pulmonary veins connect normally relative to right and left horns of sinus venosus: inferior vena cava *(IVC)* and right superior vena cava *(RSVC)* lie to the right of the pulmonary veins, and the ostium of coronary sinus *(CoS)* and the ligament of Marshall (not seen) lie below and to left of the pulmonary veins, respectively. Hence, there is totally anomalous pulmonary venous drainage into the right atrium, despite normal pulmonary venous connections, because of leftward malposition of the septum primum to left of left pulmonary veins. (Reproduced with permission from Van Praagh S, Carrera ME, Sanders S, Mayer JE, Van Praagh R. Partial or total direct pulmonary venous drainage to right atrium due to malposition of septum primum, anatomic and echocardiographic findings and surgical treatment: a study based on 36 cases. *Chest*. 1995;107:1488.[15])

Whenever the pulmonary veins connect at the atrial level (except with the sinus), we think that the pulmonary veins are normally connected, because the relationships of the pulmonary veins with the sinus venosus are normal. The pulmonary veins connect within a horseshoe of sinus venosus tissue, typically composed of the right horn of the sinus venosus to the right (the medial venous part of the morphologically RA), and the left horn of the sinus venosus to the left and below (the persistent left SVC or the ligament of Marshall to the left, and the coronary sinus below). (The normal development of the sinus venosus and the pulmonary veins is presented diagrammatically in Fig. 29.4.)

The realization that these partially or totally anomalously draining pulmonary veins are normally connected relative to both the right and left sinus horns, but not relative to the leftwardly malpositioned septum primum, leads us to realize the important distinction that exists between anomalous pulmonary venous *drainage* and anomalous pulmonary venous *connection*. In these cases (see Figs. 29.1 and 29.2), normally connected pulmonary veins drain anomalously because of malposition of the septum primum into the LA.

From the anatomic standpoint, the septum primum can be clearly seen from the right atrial view, because the superior limbic band of septum secundum is very deficient or absent (see Fig. 29.3).[15] Indeed, our understanding of septum primum malposition and its importance began with a question from Dr. Luis Alday of Cordoba, Argentina: In a case of polysplenia with all pulmonary veins draining into the RA, why is the septum primum so well seen from within the *right* atrium? Normally, the septum primum is well seen only from within the *left* atrium. This question led to a surprising voyage of discovery.[15]

In our experience, septum primum malposition has occurred predominantly in patients with the heterotaxy syndrome with

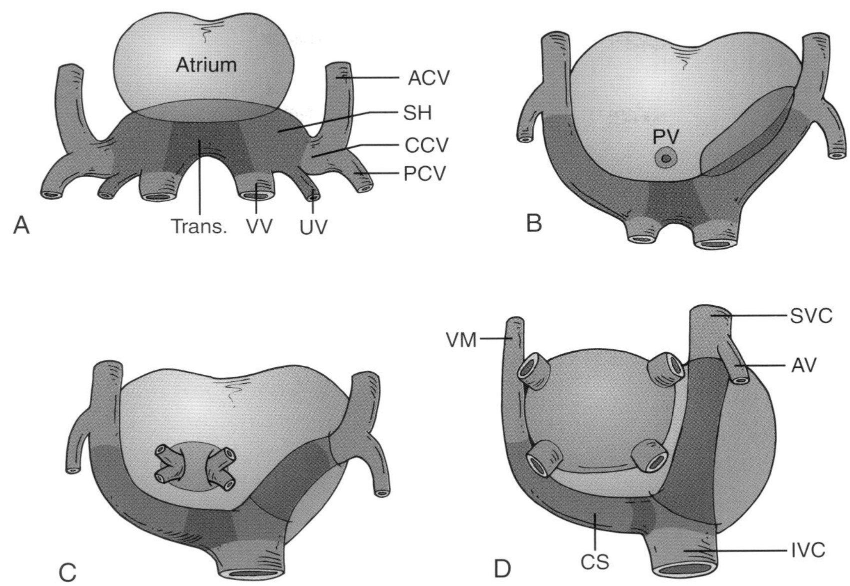

Fig. 29.4 Diagrammatic presentation of the sinus venosus, posterior view, in human embryos of various ages: *A*, 3-mm crown rump length; *B*, 5 mm; *C*, 12 mm; *D*, newborn. *ACV*, Anterior cardinal vein; *AV*, azygos vein; *CCV*, common cardinal vein; *CS*, coronary sinus; *IVC*, inferior vena cava; *PCV*, posterior cardinal vein; *PV*, pulmonary vein; *SH*, sinus horn; *SVC*, superior vena cava; *Trans.*, transverse portion of sinus venosus; *UV*, umbilical vein; *VM*, vein of Marshall; *VV*, vitelline vein. (From Van Mierop LHS, Wigglesworth FW. Isomerism of the cardiac atria in the asplenia syndrome. *Lab Invest*. 1962;11:1303, ©US-Canadian Academy of Pathology, with permission.)

polysplenia but can occur, rarely, in association with asplenia or with a right-sided but otherwise normally formed spleen.[15]

The following study of the heterotaxy syndromes was first presented in part at the meeting of the American Heart Association in Dallas, Texas, November 8, 1998, and has not been published previously. In the interests of clarity and brevity, the findings are presented mainly in tables and figures (Table 29.1)

TABLE 29.1 Material (n = 168)

Status of the Spleen	No. of Patients	% of Series
1. Asplenia	95	57
2. Polysplenia	68	40
3. Right-sided spleen	5	3

Findings of Heterotaxy Syndrome With Asplenia

Sex: Males-to-females, 56/38 (1.5/1)

Age at Death: Mean, 22.3 ± 56 months; range, 0 (fetuses) to 35.7 years; and median, 34 days.

Lobation of the Lungs

The lobation of the lungs in 74 postmortem cases of the heterotaxy syndrome with asplenia is summarized in Table 29.2.

Although the pattern of bilaterally trilobed lungs was, as expected, by far the most common pattern of lung lobation found in these 74 postmortem cases of asplenia syndrome (84%), eight other patterns were also found (Table 29.2). Hence, bilaterally trilobed lungs was by no means the only pattern of lung lobation associated with asplenia.

TABLE 29.2 Heterotaxy Syndrome With Asplenia: Lobation of the Lungs (n = 74)

Findings	No. of Patients	% of Series[a]
1. Bilaterally trilobed	62	84
2. Bilaterally quadrilobed	4	5
3. Bilaterally bilobed	1	1
4. Bilaterally unilobed	1	1
5. 4 lobes Rt, 3 lobes Lt	1	1
6. 2 lobes Rt, 3 lobes Lt (Inverted)	2	3
7. 3 lobes Rt, 5 lobes Lt	1	1
8. 7 lobes Rt, 8 lobes Lt	1	1
9. Agenesis Rt, Unilobed Lt	1	1

[a]Percentages rounded off to nearest whole number.
Lt, Left; *Rt*, right.

Types of Relationship Between the Great Arteries

The types of relationship between the great arteries—or, more accurately speaking—the types of ventriculoarterial alignment, are summarized in Table 29.3.

Double-outlet right ventricle (DORV) was by far the more common type of ventriculoarterial (VA) alignment (67%) in these 95 postmortem cases of asplenia syndrome. Transposition of the great arteries (TGA) was a distant second (22%). Third in prevalence were normally related great arteries (9%). Least frequent was anatomically corrected malposition (ACM) of the great arteries (1%). (See Chapter 32 for information concerning anatomically corrected malposition, a rare and hence unfamiliar anomaly.)

Double-Outlet Right Ventricle With Asplenia

The segmental anatomy of the 64 patients with DORV and asplenia is summarized in Table 29.4. In Table 29.4, it is noteworthy that DORV with D-loop ventricles was almost twice as common as DORV with L-loop ventricles: 66% versus 34%, respectively.

The atria were in situs solitus in 25 of 64 cases (39%), in situs inversus in 22 of 64 patients (34% which is a very high percentage), and in atria situs ambiguus (undiagnosed atrial situs) in 17 of 64 cases (27%). Hence, we thought it was possible to diagnose the basic type of atrial situs in 73% of these cases of the heterotaxy syndrome with asplenia.

DORV with D-loop ventricles displayed D-malposition of the great arteries (aortic valve to the right, dextro- or D- relative to the pulmonary valve) in 38 of 42 cases (90%) (see Table 29.4), L malposition of the great arteries in 3 of 42 patients (7%), and a solitus normally related great arteries type of conotruncus: DORV {I,D,"S"} in 1 of 42 cases (2%) (percentages rounded off to the nearest whole number).

One may well ask, What do we mean by solitus normally related great arteries in a case of DORV? Is that not a contradiction in terms? This, of course, is a good, logical question. Briefly, the answer is that a solitus normal type of infundibulum and great arteries can indeed be present with a VA alignment of DORV, as follows: The aortic valve is rightward, posterior, and inferior relative to the pulmonary valve. A subpulmonary conus is present, with aortic AV valvar direct fibrous continuity. The ventricular septum is displaced abnormally leftward, in association with an abnormal small morphologically LV. The resulting VA alignment is DORV. It is important to understand that DORV is not always the result of a conotruncal (really, an infundibular) malformation. An anomaly of the ventricles, ventricular septum, and AV valves also can result in DORV. With L-loop ventricles, DORV in the asplenia syndrome had L malposition of the great arteries (aortic valve levo- or L relative to the pulmonary valve) in 19 of 22 cases (86%), A-malposition of the great arteries (aortic valve antero- or A relative to the pulmonary valve) in 2 of 22 patients (9%), and D malposition of the great arteries in 1 of 22 cases (5%).

One of the advantages of segmental set analysis, as shown in Table 29.4, is that it makes possible not only univariate analysis, as earlier (type of atrial situs, type of ventricular loop, and type of semilunar interrelationship), but it also facilitates multivariate analysis, that is, the various segmental combinations or sets that occurred. The most common segmental combination was DORV {S,D,D}, which was found in 15 of 64 patients (23%), that is, DORV with the segmental set of situs ambiguus (A) of the viscera with situs solitus (S) of the atria, concordant 0-loop ventricles (D), and D-malposition of the great arteries (D) (see Table 29.4). Second in frequency was DORV {I,D,D}, which occurred in 13 of 64 patients (20%), that is, DORV with the segmental set of visceral situs ambiguus (A), atrial situs inversus (I), discordant D-loop ventricles (D), and D-malposition of the great arteries (D). Third in prevalence was DORV {A,D,D}, which occurred in 10 of 64 patients (16%), that is, DORV with the segmental situs set of visceroatrial situs ambiguus (A) (the atrial situs being undiagnosed), D-loop ventricles (D), and D malposition of the great arteries (D). We hope that the meaning of the other eight segmental combinations will be self-evident in Table 29.4. (For those who may not be familiar with segmental anatomy, please see Chapter 4.)

WHAT DOES DOUBLE-OUTLET RIGHT VENTRICLE WITH ASPLENIA LOOK LIKE?

We shall present 3 cases photographically in an effort to answer this question. (It should be understood that by far the best way to learn the morphologic anatomy of DORV with asplenia—or indeed of any other form of complex congenital heart disease—is to study heart specimens personally, as is readily possible in the Cardiac Registry laboratory of Children's Hospital in Boston and in similar laboratories elsewhere. Any photograph, no matter how good, reduces three-dimensional reality to two dimensions.)

TABLE 29.3 Types of Relationship Between the Great Arteries

Types of Ventriculoarterial AlignmentTypes	No. of Patients (n = 95)	% of Series
1. Double-outlet right ventricle	64	67
2. Transposition of the great arteries	21	22
3. Normally related great arteries	9	9
4. Anatomically corrected malposition of the great arteries	1	1

TABLE 29.4 Double-Outlet Right Ventricle With Asplenia

Segmental Anatomy	No. of Patients (n = 64)	% of DORV[a]
I. D-Loop DORV	42	66
1. DORV {S,D,D}	15	23
2. DORV {A,D,D}	10	16
3. DORV {S,D,L}	2	3
4. DORV {A,D,L}	1	2
5. DORV {I,D,L}	13	20
6. DORV {I,D,"S"}	1	2
II. L-Loop DORV	22	34
1. DORV {S,L,L}	8	12
2. DORV {I,L,L}	5	8
3. DORV {A,L,L}	6	9
4. DORV {I,L,A}	2	3
5. DORV {I,L,D}	1	2

[a]Percentages rounded off to nearest whole number.

Fig. 29.5 shows the exterior of the heart and left lung, viewed from the front. The patient was a 3 2⁄12-year-old girl (A69-61) with visceral heterotaxy, asplenia, DORV {S,D,D}, bilateral conus (subaortic and subpulmonary), with severe subpulmonary stenosis. Note that the morphologically RAA is large, broad, triangular, and anterior, whereas the LAA is much smaller, finger-like, and posterior. The hypertrophic morphologically RV is right-sided, whereas the hypertrophic morphologically left ventricle (LV) lies to the left of the anterior descending coronary artery and the great cardiac vein that demarcate the interventricular septum. Both great arteries arise above the RV (to the right of the plane of the ventricular septum; hence, the diagnosis of DORV can be strongly suspected based on external inspection), the large ascending aorta lying anterior and to the right of the much smaller main pulmonary artery (MPA). The right superior vena cava (RSVC) receives all of the pulmonary veins, with totally anomalous pulmonary venous connection (TAPVC) being present. The RSVC connected normally with the right-sided RA; thus, TAPVD was present. A large persistent left superior vena cava (LSVC) drained into the left-sided LA because of the characteristic

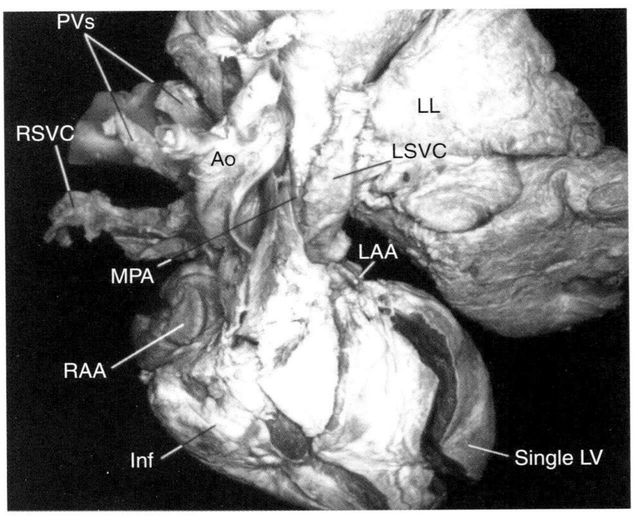

Fig. 29.5 Heterotaxy syndrome with asplenia. The right-sided right atrial appendage *(RAA)* is large, broad, and triangular. The left atrial appendage *(LAA)* is much smaller and finger-like. The inferior vena cava connected with the right-sided right atrium, as did the right superior vena cava *(RSVC)*. A persistent left superior vena cava *(LSVC)* drained into the coronary sinus that was unroofed and hence drained into the left atrium. The atria were in situs solitus; right atrial isomerism or RAA isomerism was not present. This 3 2⁄12-year-old girl had double-outlet from an infundibular outlet chamber {S,D,D} with single left ventricle *(LV)*, common atrioventricular canal opening only into the single LV, bilateral conus (subaortic and subpulmonary), with pulmonary infundibular and valvar stenosis and TAPVC with all pulmonary veins *(PVs)* to RSVC. *Ao.* Aorta; *LL,* left lung; *MPA,* main pulmonary artery. (Reproduced with permission from Van Praagh S, Santini F, Sanders SP. Cardiac malpositions with special emphasis on visceral heterotaxy (asplenia and polysplenia syndromes). In: Fyler DC, ed. *Nadas' Pediatric Cardiology.* Philadelphia, PA: Hanley & Belfus; 1992:589.13.)

coexistence of a large coronary sinus septal defect, also known as unroofing of the coronary sinus, which therefore has no discrete right atrial ostium and thus appears to be absent. The left innominate vein was absent, typical of bilateral SVCs. The left lung and the right lung were both trilobed, and both bronchi were eparterial.

The relations between the bronchi and the pulmonary artery branches require explanation (Fig. 29.6). Normally, the right mainstem bronchus is short and broad, giving off the right upper lobe bronchus a relatively short distance below the carina. By contrast, the left mainstem bronchus is relatively long, thin, and sway backed because the upper lobe bronchus originates relatively further down the mainstem bronchus, farther away from the carina. Consequently, the right mainstem bronchus normally is the eparterial bronchus (in Greek, *epi,* "on or upon") because this bronchus is above the level of the right pulmonary artery, whereas the long, thin, left mainstem bronchus passes all the way beneath the left pulmonary artery before giving off its upper lobe bronchus. Hence, the left mainstem bronchus normally is the hyparterial bronchus (Greek, *hypo,* "under") (see Fig. 29.6, *top*). Fig. 29.7 shows the frontal P wave axis in asplenia.

In the heterotaxy syndrome with asplenia, both lungs typically are trilobed, as in Fig. 29.6. Hence, the upper lobe had the larger, more anterior, triangular atrial appendage. All of the pulmonary veins connected with a common atrium to the left of a subdividing atrial strand that was interpreted as the inferior limbic band of septum secundum. All of the pulmonary veins connected with this left-sided atrium by a common orifice; that is, incomplete incorporation of the common pulmonary vein was present. The left-sided atrial appendage was smaller, more finger-like, and posterior relative to the right-sided atrial appendage. In view of the venous connections (the IVC and the common pulmonary vein) and the shapes of the atrial appendages, the diagnosis of situs solitus of the atria was made.

As is seen in Fig. 29.8A–B, a completely common AV canal (CCAVC), type C of Rastelli, was present. A large ventricular septal defect (VSD) of the AV canal type was confluent with the common atrium; that is, there was a large and complete AV septal defect (complete absence of the AV septum that normally subdivides the common AV canal, thereby normally producing a divided AV canal consisting of separate mitral and tricuspid canals). The complete AV septal defect was associated with a huge secundum type of ASD (absence of the septum primum, with a poorly formed superior and inferior limbic bands of septum secundum). This combination of a complete AV septal defect plus a huge secundum type of ASD together produced a common (essentially undivided) atrium.

The common AV valve is balanced; that is, it opens approximately equally into the right-sided and hypertrophied morphologically RV (see Fig. 29.8A) and into the left-sided and hypertrophied morphologically LV (see Fig. 29.8B). The RV is right-handed (see Fig 29.8A) and the LV is left-handed (see Fig. 29.8B); hence D-loop ventricles are

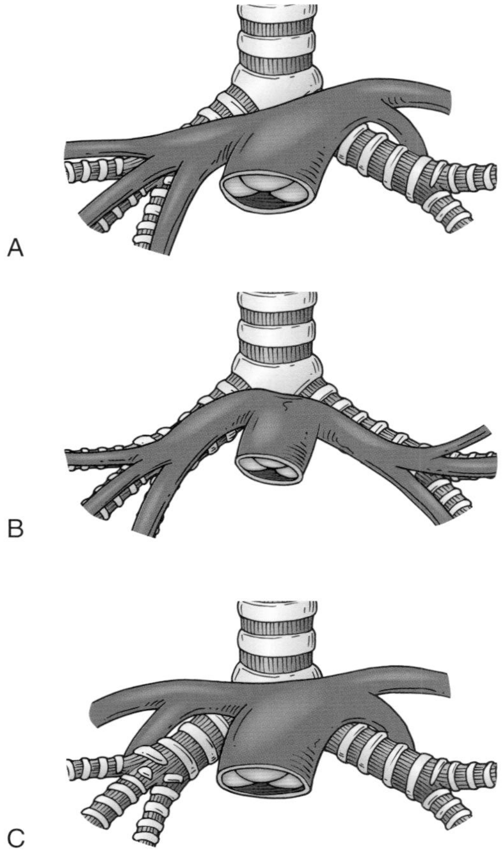

Fig. 29.6 **Diagrammatic representation of the relationship between the mainstem bronchi and the pulmonary artery branches,** anterior view. (A) Normal relationship. The beginning of the right mainstem bronchus is at a higher level than is the beginning of the right pulmonary artery. Normally, therefore, the right mainstem bronchus is short, broad, and eparterial (higher than) the right pulmonary artery. The right mainstem bronchus does not swoop under the right pulmonary artery. The right upper lobe bronchus branches off early and often remains entirely above the level of the right pulmonary artery. By contrast, the left mainstem bronchus is long, narrow, and passes under the left pulmonary artery; hence, the left mainstem bronchus normally is hyparterial (below the level of the left pulmonary artery). The left upper lobe bronchus does not branch off until the bronchus has passed under the left pulmonary artery. (B) Bilaterally eparterial bronchi, typically with asplenia and bilaterally trilobed lungs. Both bronchi begin higher than either pulmonary artery, and neither bronchus swoops under a pulmonary artery. (C) Bilaterally hyparterial bronchi, typically with polysplenia and bilaterally bilobed lungs. Both bronchi swoop under the pulmonary arterial branches. (Reproduced with permission from Van Praagh S, Santini F, Sanders SP. Cardiac malpositions with special emphasis on visceral heterotaxy (asplenia and polysplenia syndromes). In: Fyler DC, ed. *Nadas' Pediatric Cardiology*. Philadelphia, PA: Hanley & Belfus; 1992:589.13.[15])

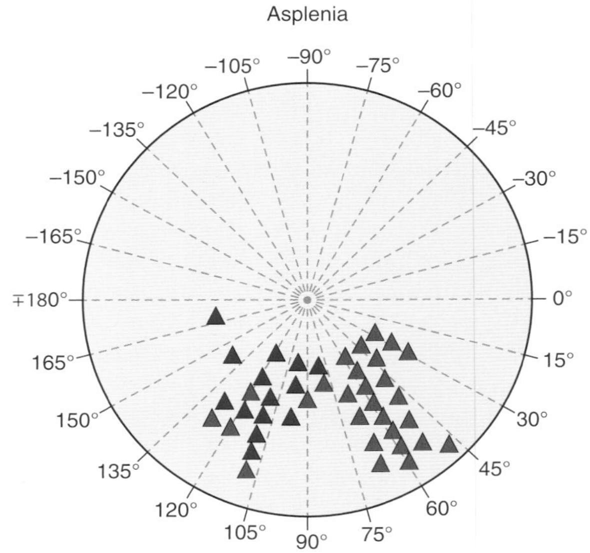

Fig. 29.7 The frontal P wave axis in asplenia. *Blue triangles* indicate atrial situs solitus. *Red triangles* denote atrial situs inversus. Among the 28 patients with atrial situs solitus, 24 (86%) had the expected P axis between 30 and 90 degrees. Among the 14 patients with atrial situs inversus, 13 (92%) had expected P axis between 90 and 150 degrees. (Reproduced with permission from Van Praagh S, Santini F, Sanders SP. Cardiac malpositions with special emphasis on visceral heterotaxy (asplenia and polysplenia syndromes). In: Fyler DC, ed. *Nadas' Pediatric Cardiology*. Philadelphia, PA: Hanley & Belfus; 1992:589.13.[15])

present, both in terms of the relative spatial positions of the ventricles, and in terms of the ventricular situs (pattern of anatomic organization), which is well expressed and easily diagnosed in terms of ventricular chirality or handedness, as mentioned earlier.

Both great arteries originate above the morphologically RV; hence, DORV is present. A bilateral muscular conus arteriosus is present. The subaortic part of the conus is well developed, well expanded, and nonobstructive. There is aortic-AV fibrous discontinuity, produced by the interposition of the large subaortic conus.

There is severe pulmonary outflow tract stenosis (see Fig 29.8A). Note the tight stenosis of the subpulmonary os infundibuli. The pulmonary infundibular stenosis has a punched-out appearance, typical of asplenia. The presence of a stenotic subpulmonary infundibulum prevents pulmonary-AV fibrous continuity.

This VSD of the AV canal type is remote from both semilunar valves, being separated from the aortic valve by a large and well-developed subaortic conus, and separated from the small pulmonary valve by a tightly stenotic subpulmonary infundibulum. Such VSDs are also described as *noncommitted*, meaning that the VSD is not confluent with (not committed to) either semilunar valve. From a hemodynamic standpoint, however, this VSD of the AV canal type is much more subaortic than subpulmonary because of the presence of severe subpulmonary infundibular stenosis and pulmonary valvar stenosis.

In DORV, it should be understood that subaortic, or subpulmonary, or doubly committed or noncommitted VSDs are not anatomic types of VSD. In other words, all noncommitted VSDs are not AV canal type defects. They can be muscular VSDs. They also can be conoventricular VSDs, but with a well-developed subaortic and subpulmonary conus. Hence, the relationship of the VSD to the semilunar valves is very important hemodynamically and surgically in DORV (and

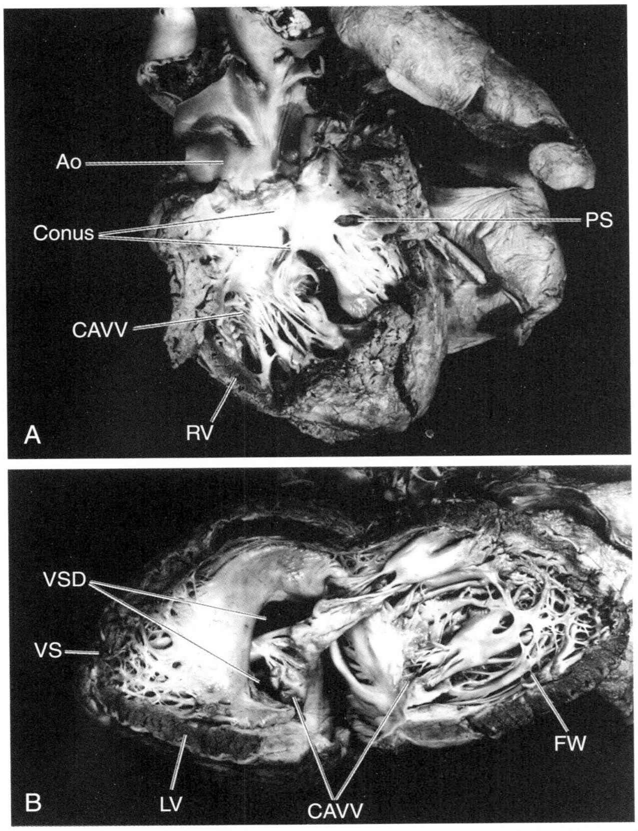

Fig. 29.8 The heterotaxy syndrome with asplenia and double-outlet right ventricle (DORV) {S,D,D}. This is the heart of a 4 9/12-year-old girl (A70-91) with levocardia. The inferior vena cava was left sided below the liver, where it switched to the right and entered the right-sided atrium, which had the larger and more anterior appendage. All the pulmonary veins entered the common atrium to the left of the inferior limbic band—a subdividing atrial strand. Thus, solitus atria were associated with D-loop ventricles and DORV with D-malposition of the great arteries. (A) The opened right ventricle *(RV)* shows a well-developed muscular subaortic conus, no aortic outflow tract obstruction, and a "punched-out" type of severe pulmonary outflow tract stenosis *(PS)* typical of the asplenia syndrome. (B) The interior of the left ventricle *(LV)* reveals the presence of a complete form of common atrioventricular canal. *Ao,* Aorta; *CAVV,* common atrioventricular valve; *FW,* free wall; *VS,* ventricular septum; *VSD,* ventricular septal defect. (Reproduced with permission from Van Praagh S, Santini F, Sanders SP. Cardiac malpositions with special emphasis on visceral heterotaxy (asplenia and polysplenia syndromes). In: Fyler DC, ed. *Nadas' Pediatric Cardiology.* Philadelphia, PA: Hanley & Belfus; 1992:589.13.[15])

other so-called conotruncal anomalies), but these hemodynamic descriptions are not the same thing as anatomic types of VSD.

Looking at the LV (see Fig. 29.8B), one sees that there are two well-developed and well-spaced left ventricular papillary muscle groups, thereby excluding potentially parachute mitral valve. In other words, after surgical repair of the common AV canal, one would not end up with a parachute mitral valve, with all chordae tendineae inserting into one focus (typically, into the anterolateral or superior papillary muscle group of the LV).

Diagnosis 0 (see Fig. 29.8A–B): The heterotaxy syndrome with asplenia, DORV {S,D,D}, TAPVC to the RSVC, common atrium, CCAVC (type C), bilateral conus, and severe pulmonary outflow tract stenosis (infundibular and valvar). This is a typical case of the asplenia syndrome.

In Fig. 29.9 we present the heart specimen of a 3 3/12-year old boy with the heterotaxy syndrome with asplenia and DORV (MR 43). Fig. 29.9A is a right lateral view of the morphologically RA, the common AV canal, and a single RV. Note that the right-sided atrium has a broad triangular appendage and receives the IVC and SVC. The left-sided atrial appendage was smaller and more posterior (not shown). Hence, we made the diagnosis of situs solitus of the atria. There was TAPVC to the junction of the RSVC with the RA.

The coronary sinus septum was absent; that is, a large coronary sinus septal defect was present, resulting in unroofing of the coronary sinus. Consequently, a persistent LSVC drained directly into the LA, and there was no right atrial ostium of the coronary sinus, making it look as though the coronary sinus were absent. (We think that the posterior wall of the coronary sinus, that is, the posterior wall of the left sinus horn, is present, with only the anterior wall of the coronary sinus—the so-called coronary sinus septum—being absent.) The left innominate vein was absent, as is usual with bilateral SVCs.

A large secundum type of ASD is seen above and behind the inferior limbic band (Fig. 29.9A). A prominent ostium primum type of ASD is present in front of and below the inferior limbic band. Common AV canal is present, the common AV valve underlying both the RA and LA and opening into the single RV. Common-inlet RV is present, not double inlet right ventricle, because only one AV valve (a common AV valve) is present. No vestige of a morphologically LV could be identified (despite multiple incisions in the appropriate location). Hence, a single morphologically RV is present, meaning that no morphologically LV could be identified. However, we cannot exclude the possibility of the existence microscopically of some left ventricular myocardial cells. Instead, what we mean is that, despite an intensive and careful search, no remnant whatsoever of the LV was found. Because the LV is absent (unidentifiable), there can be no VSD, which is really an interventricular septal defect.

Hence, the question arises: *Is this a complete form* or *a partial form of common AV canal?* No VSD of the AV canal type can be present (because the LV is missing); thus, we do not know how to answer this question. We think that this anomaly—common inlet into a single RV—exposes one of the weaknesses in the classification of common AV canal: With a primum type of ASD, when there is a VSD of the AV canal type, we conventionally call this a *complete* form of common AV canal; but when there is no VSD of the AV canal type, we make the diagnosis of a *partial* form of common AV canal. However, in the present anomaly (common-inlet single RV), the point is that the usual classification of common AV canal breaks down, because the usual classification assumes the presence of an identifiable ventricular septum, which then makes it possible to determine the presence or absence of a VSD of the AV canal type.

It is because of this problem that we made the diagnosis of common AV canal (not otherwise qualified); we avoided making the diagnosis either of complete or partial common AV canal because we do not know which is anatomically accurate.

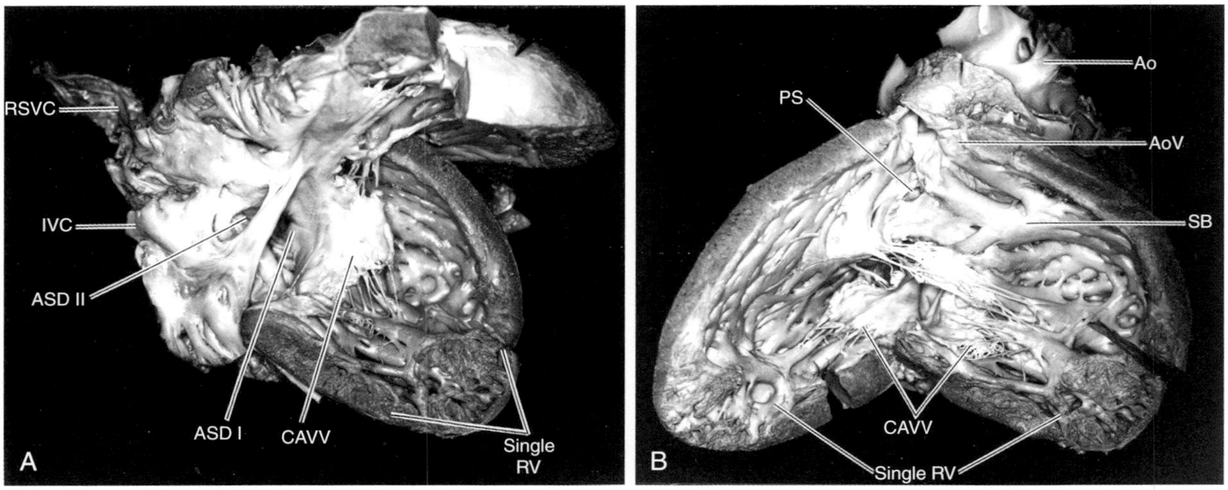

Fig. 29.9 The heterotaxy syndrome with asplenia and single right ventricle *(RV).* This is the heart of a 3 $^{3}/_{12}$-year-old boy (MR 43). (A) Right lateral view of opened, right-sided, morphologically right atrium (RA), common atrioventricular canal, and single morphologically RV. The RA receives the inferior vena cava *(IVC)* and the right superior vena cava *(RSVC).* There is a large ostium secundum type of atrial septal defect *(ASD II),* which is superior and posterior to the inferior limbic band. Anterior and inferior to the inferior limbic band is an ostium primum type of atrial septal defect *(ASD I).* The common atrioventricular valve *(CAVV)* underlies both atria, and there is a common-inlet single RV. The CAVV is present in view of the coexistence of ASD I and CAVV. There was totally anomalous pulmonary venous connection (TAPVC) to the junction of the RSVC with the RA. The coronary sinus septum was absent. Consequently, the left superior vena cava was unroofed and drained into the left atrium. (B) Anterior view of opened single RV. The septal band *(SB)* is superior and left-sided, indicating that a right-handed D-loop RV is present. The right ventricular sinus (inflow tract) septal surface is located directly beneath the SB. The moderator band is very left-sided, inferior, and flows into the left-sided anterior papillary muscle group. Note the coarse right ventricular style trabeculations everywhere. The aortic valve *(AoV)* is large, unobstructed, anterior, and somewhat to the left of the stenotic pulmonary valve. A bilateral conus is present, and there is tight, subpulmonary, infundibular stenosis *(PS).* Both great arteries arise above this single RV per force (the LV being absent). This patient has DORV {S,D,L}. *Ao,* Aorta. (Reproduced with permission from Van Praagh S, Santini F, Sanders SP. Cardiac malpositions with special emphasis on visceral heterotaxy (asplenia and polysplenia syndromes). In: Fyler DC, ed. *Nadas' Pediatric Cardiology*. Philadelphia, PA: Hanley & Belfus; 1992:589.13.[15])

In Fig. 29.9B, we present an anterior view of this opened single RV. Note the coarse right ventricular type of trabeculae carneae everywhere. Again, the common AV valve can be seen opening from both atria into this single RV.

Note that the septal band is located anteriorly, superiorly, and to the left relative to the entering common AV valve. The myocardium beneath the septal band is the right ventricular sinus (or inflow tract) septal surface. The right ventricular free wall lies toward the reader's left side. This is a right-handed, noninverted, D-loop type of RV. Note that the moderator band lies far toward the viewer's right side, where it flows into the prominent anterior papillary muscle group of this single RV.

DORV is present, with both great arteries arising *per force* above this single RV. We say *above* the single RV intentionally, not *from* the single RV. Accurately speaking, the great arteries arise from the conus arteriosus, not directly from either ventricular sinus—in this case, not directly from the right ventricular sinus. The conus arteriosus is part of the conotruncal cardiac segment; that is, the conus "belongs to" the great arteries. The conus is how the great arteries connect with the ventricular sinuses. The conus is part of the ventricular outflow tracts (the conotruncus), not part of the ventricular inflow tracts (the sinuses or pumping portions). Consequently, we prefer, in the interests of accuracy, to say that both great arteries arise above the RV (not from the RV). We think that the best way to achieve clarity and to avoid confusion is to be as accurate as possible. A bilateral conus is present. The large unobstructed aortic outflow tract and aortic valve lie anteriorly and slightly to the left of the tightly stenotic pulmonary outflow tract, which has both infundibular and valvar stenosis. Note that, once again, the tightly stenotic pulmonary os infundibulum looks "punched out." Indeed, it is reminiscent of a conal septal defect.

Diagnosis (see Fig 29.9A–B): Heterotaxy syndrome with asplenia with DORV {S,D,L}, bilateral SVCs, absent left innominate vein, unroofing of the coronary sinus (the LSVC draining into the LA and the right atrial ostium of the coronary sinus being absent), TAPVC to the right superior vena septal defect, common AV valve, common-inlet RV, single RV (no remnant of the LV being found), bilateral conus, and severe pulmonary outflow tract stenosis (infundibular and valvar).

Heterotaxy Syndrome With Asplenia and Transposition of the Great Arteries

Of our 95 patients with the heterotaxy syndrome and asplenia, 21 (22%) had TGA (see Table 29.3). What kinds of TGA were associated with the asplenia syndrome? Their segmental anatomy and prevalences are summarized in Table 29.5.

TABLE 29.5 Transposition of the Great Arteries in Heterotaxy Syndrome With Asplenia

Segmental Anatomy	No. of Patients (n = 21)	% of TGA[a]
I. D-Loop TGA	14	67
1. TGA {S,D,D}	6	29
2. TGA {I,D,D}	4	19
3. TGA {A,D,D}	4	19
II. L-Loop TGA	7	33
1. TGA {S,L,L}	2	10
2. TGA {I,S,L,L}[b]	1	5
3. TGA {I,L,L}	1	5
4. TGA {A,L,L}	1	5
5. TGA {S,L,D}	1	5
6. TGA {A,L,D}	1	5

[a]Percentages rounded off to nearest whole number.
[b]Visceral situs inversus (I) with atrial situs solitus (S).

TABLE 29.6 Anatomic Types of Transposition of the Great Arteries (TGA) With Asplenia

Uncorrected TGA (n = 7)
1. TGA {S,D,D} in 6
2. TGA {I,L,L} in 1

Corrected TGA (n = 8)
1. TGA {I,D,D} in 4
2. TGA {S,L,L} in 2
3. TGA {I,S,L, 1} in 1[a]
4. TGA {S, 1, D} in 1

[a]Visceral situs inversus (I) with atrial situs solitus (S).

TABLE 29.7 Ventriculoarterial Concordance With Asplenia

Segmental Anatomy	No. of Patients (n = 10)	% of VAC
I. D-Loop VAC	6	60
1. {S,D,S}	5	50
2. ACM {I,D,L}	1	10
II. 1-Loop VAC	4	40
1. {I,L,I}	1	10
2. {A,L,I}	2	20
3. {S,L,S}	1	10

VAC, Ventriculoarterial concordance.

In these 21 patients with TGA in the asplenia syndrome, despite the presence of visceral heterotaxy (situs ambiguus), it was possible to diagnose the atrial situs with confidence in 15 cases (71%) (see Table 29.5). The atrial situs could not be diagnosed (it remained ambiguous) in 6 patients (29%). Asplenia and TGA represents a new and improved level of understanding of these complex cases. Unless one understands the atrial situs, one cannot really understand the heart diagnostically.

In the 15 patients with TGA in whom the atrial situs could be diagnosed, **physiologically uncorrected (complete) TGA** was present in 7 patients (47%) and **physiologically corrected TGA** was found in 8 cases (53%). In the series of TGA as a whole (n = 21), TGA could not be diagnosed as physiologically uncorrected or corrected in 6 (29%), because the atrial situs remained unknown. In these 15 patients with TGA and asplenia, **congenitally physiologically uncorrected** TGA occurred in two different anatomic types (Table 29.6).

For brevity and convenience, we often omit "congenitally physiologically," thinking that this will be understood. However, if there is any risk that physiologically uncorrected or corrected TGA could be misunderstood for *surgically* uncorrected or corrected TGA, we include the adverb "congenitally," in the interests of clarity.

In physiologically uncorrected TGA, there is **atrioventricular concordance,** either {S,D,-} or {I,L,-}. In **physiologically corrected TGA,** there is AV discordance, either {S,L,-} or {I,D,-}. Both D-TGA and L-TGA can be physiologically uncorrected or corrected. To determine which, establish the presence of AV concordance or discordance, respectively.

What is really new about Tab1e 29.5 is that, to our knowledge, this is the first time that the majority of cases of TGA in the asplenia syndrome have been classified as physiologically uncorrected or corrected (time of writing February 1, 1999). This, in turn, is why the concepts of atrial situs ambiguus, atrial isomerism, and atrial appendage isomerism need to be understood, rather than believed. Understanding "opens the door" to the diagnosis of the atrial situs in many (but not all) cases of asplenia, leading to a more complete understanding of this form of complex congenital heart disease.

Ventriculoarterial Concordance With Asplenia

Although DORV is by far the most common type of VA alignment in the asplenia syndrome (67%), followed by TGA (22%), infrequently it is possible for VA concordance to occur (10%) either in the form of **normally related great arteries,** as in 9 of 95 cases (9%), or in the form of **ACM of the great arteries,** as in 1 of 95 cases (1%) (see Table 29.3). These cases of asplenia with VA concordance are presented in greater detail in Table 29.7.

Of these 10 patients with asplenia and VA concordance, the atrial situs was diagnosed in 8 (80%). Of the 9 patients with normally related great arteries, solitus normally related great arteries were present in 6 (67%), and inversus normally related great arteries were found in 3 (33%).

Isolated ventricular inversion[18] was present in 1 patient (see Table 29.7): {S,L,S}. Solitus atria {S,-,-} were associated with L-loop ventricles {-,L,-} and solitus normally related great arteries {-,-,S}. Only the ventricles were inverted; hence, the name of this rare anomaly. Because there is only one intersegmental discordance (at the AV alignment), the circulations are physiologically uncorrected. Consequently, an atrial switch operation (Senning or Mustard procedure) is needed to produce physiologic and anatomic repair. Although the meaning of physiologic repair should be clear (systemic venous return to the pulmonary artery, and pulmonary venous return to the aorta), one may wonder, What does an anatomic repair mean? If one ends up with the morphologically LV supplying the aorta, and with the morphologically RV ejecting into the pulmonary artery—as one does, by definition, in {S,L,S}—one has an anatomic repair: the morphologically appropriate ventricle ejects into the appropriate great artery; that is, the morphologically LV ejects into the aorta, and the morphologically RV ejects into the pulmonary artery.

ACM of the great arteries, such as ACM {I,D,L} (see Table 29.7), means that the great arteries are malposed, but despite this fact, each malposed great artery nonetheless originates above the morphologically appropriate ventricle: aorta above the morphologically left ventricle, and pulmonary artery above the morphologically right ventricle (i.e., VA alignment concordance is present). Let's think about this case of ACM {I,D,L}. There is only one intersegmental discordance, at the AV alignment. So you know that the systemic and pulmonary circulations are physiologically uncorrected. Consequently, such a patient should have an atrial switch operation, if feasible. You should end up with a physiologic repair (because of the atrial switch) and an anatomic repair (because of the nature ACM). Thus ACM of the great arteries may be congenitally physiologically corrected or congenitally physiologically uncorrected, as in this patient.

As is always the case, to the best of our present knowledge, the ventricles have looped in one direction (D-loop), whereas the infundibulum and great arteries have twisted in the opposite direction (L-malposition of the great arteries). This rare situation may explain why ACM is so uncommon: the ventricles and the great arteries have to twist in opposite directions to result in the VA alignment of ACM.[19,20]

It is noteworthy that VA concordance is not synonymous with normally related great arteries because ACM also has VA concordance.

The Conus in Asplenia. The anatomic types of conus arteriosus found in association with 94 postmortem cases of the heterotaxy syndrome with asplenia are summarized in Table 29.8.

Although a bilateral conus (subaortic and subpulmonary) is by far the most common type of infundibulum found in the asplenia syndrome, often in association with DORV (Figs. 29.8 and 29.9), the conus can be subaortic (only) with pulmonary-AV fibrous continuity, typically with TGA; or the conus can be subpulmonary (only) with aortic-AV fibrous continuity and normally related great arteries.

The Superior Vena(e) Cava(e) With Asplenia

The anatomic status of the SVC(s) in the heterotaxy syndrome with asplenia is summarized, based on 72 postmortem cases, in Table 29.9.

Bilateral SVCs was by far the most common pattern found in association with asplenia (65%). RSVC (only) was a distant second in prevalence (24%), and LSVC (only) was least frequent (11%).

Inferior Vena Cava With Asplenia

The anatomic status of the IVC in 76 postmortem cases of the heterotaxy syndrome with asplenia is presented in Table 29.10. Several points are noteworthy (see Table 29.10):

TABLE 29.8 The Conus in Asplenia

Finding	No. of Cases (n = 94)	% of Series[a]
1. Bilateral conus (subaortic and subpulmonary)	56	60
2. Subaortic conus (only)	25	27
3. Subpulmonary conus (only)	13	14

[a]Percentages rounded off to the nearest whole number.

TABLE 29.9 The Superior Vena(e) Cava(e) With Asplenia

Finding	No. of Patients (n = 72)	% of Series
1. Bilateral SVC	47	65
2. RSVC only	17	24
3. LSVC only	8	11

LSVC, Left SVC; *RSVC*, right SVC; *SVC*, superior vena cava.

TABLE 29.10 The Inferior Vena Cava With Asplenia

Findings	No. of Patients (n = 76)	% of Series[a]
1. Right-sided IVC	24	32
2. Left-sided IVC	28	37
3. Rt-to-Lt switching of IVC	7	9
4. Lt-to-Rt switching of IVC	11	14
5. Midline IVC	2	3
6. Interruption of IVC	2	3
7. 2 IVCs below the liver	1	1
8. IVC to unroofed CoS to LA	1	1

[a]Percentages rounded off to the nearest whole number.
CoS, Coronary sinus; *IVC*, inferior vena cava; *LA*, morphologically left atrium; *Lt*, left; *Rt*, right.

1. A left-sided IVC was even more common than a right-sided IVC (37% versus 32%, respectively).
2. Almost one-quarter of our cases (23%) had lateral switching of the IVC, left-to-right being slightly more common than right-to-left (14% versus 9%, respectively). The morphogenesis of lateral shifting of the IVC by the intersubcardinal anastomosis is explained in Chapter 6.
3. The IVC can even be midline in the asplenia syndrome (3%).
4. Although interruption of the IVC is common with polysplenia, such interruption is rare with asplenia but does occur (3%).
5. Although there can rarely be two IVCs below the liver (1%), to our knowledge the IVC is never completely bilateral, below and above the liver, with the two IVCs connecting separately at the atrial level. We have seen a very rare and fascinating case (a patient of Drs. Stephen Sanders and John Murphy from Genolier, Switzerland), who was studied angiocardiographically. There were two separate IVCs, both of which connected with a subatrial venous sinus before entering a common atrium by

TABLE 29.11 Pulmonary Veins With Asplenia

Findings	No. of Patients (n = 93)	% of Series[a]
1. Totally anomalous pulmonary venous connection	64	69
2. Partially anomalous pulmonary venous connection	5	5
3. Normally connected with left atrium	24	26

[a]Percentages rounded off to the nearest whole number.

TABLE 29.12 Totally Anomalous Pulmonary Venous Connection in the Heterotaxy Syndrome With Asplenia

Findings	No. of Patients (n = 64)	% of Series[a] (n = 93)
Totally anomalous PVC	64	69
1. Supracardiac	37	40
2. Cardiac	9	10
3. Infracardiac	14	15
4. Mixed	4	4

[a]Percentages rounded off to nearest whole number.
PVC, Pulmonary venous connection.

an apparently single venous connection. Hence, this patient almost has two separate and complete IVCs.

6. The IVC never connects directly with the morphologically LA, to the best of our present knowledge. However, the IVC can drain into the LA in several different ways (see Chapter 6), one of which is to connect with a coronary sinus that is unroofed, permitting the IVC to drain into the LA, as in 1 of these patients (1%).

Pulmonary Veins in Asplenia Syndrome

The status of the pulmonary veins in 93 postmortem cases of the heterotaxy syndrome with asplenia may be summarized as follows. The pulmonary veins were anomalously connected in almost three-quarters of these patients with asplenia (74%), TAPVC being the rule (69%), and partially anomalous pulmonary venous connection being the exception (5%). Normally connected pulmonary veins were found in 26% (Table 29.11). (We were surprised that the proportion of normally connected pulmonary veins in asplenia was this high, slightly more than one-quarter.)

What anatomic types of **TAPVC** occurred in the asplenia syndrome?[14] The findings are summarized in Table 29.12. The most common form of TAPVC in the asplenia syndrome was the supracardiac type (40%), followed by the infracardiac type (15%), then the cardiac form (10%), and finally by the mixed variety (4%). (Again, these findings surprised us, we having previously thought that the infracardiac type was the most common with asplenia. Thus, we learned that our previous impression had been wrong.)

TABLE 29.13 Supracardiac TAPVC With Asplenia

Findings	No. of Patients (n = 37)	% of Series[a] (n = 93)
Supracardiac TAPVC	37	40
1. To RSVC	21	23
2. To LSVC	12	13
3. "Snowman" pathway	3	3
4. To SVC-RA junction	1	1

LSVC, Left superior vena cava; *RA*, morphologically right atrium; *RSVC*, right superior vena cava; *SVC*, superior vena cava; *TAPVC*, totally anomalous pulmonary venous connection.
[a]Percentages rounded off to nearest whole number.

TABLE 29.14 Cardiac Type of TAPVC With Asplenia

Findings	No. of Patients (n = 9)	% of Series[a] (n = 93)
To RA	9	10

RA, Morphologically right atrium; *TAPVC*, totally anomalous pulmonary venous connection.
[a]Percentage rounded off to nearest whole number.

TABLE 29.15 Infracardiac TAPVC in Asplenia

Findings	No. of Patients (n = 14)	% of Series[a] (n = 93)
To ductus venosus	14	15

[a]Percentage rounded off to nearest whole number.
TAPVC, Totally anomalous pulmonary venous connection.

What types of supracardiac TAPVC were associated with asplenia? The answer is summarized in Table 29.13. It is noteworthy that in the heterotaxy syndrome with asplenia, the supracardiac type of TAPVC usually was not of the classic "snowman" variety, that is, from the horizontal vein connecting the right pulmonary hilum with the left pulmonary hilum, then by a vertical vein to the left innominate vein, and thence to the RSVC and the RA.21. The "snowman" variety of supracardiac TAPVC occurred in only 3% of this series of asplenic patients (see Table 29.13).

The most common type was to the RSVC (23%), followed by to the LSVC (13%) (see Table 29.13). The least frequent form in this series was to the SVC-to-RA junction (1%) (see Table 29.13). What did the cardiac type of TAPVC involve? See Table 29.14.

All cases of TAPVC of the cardiac type in the asplenia syndrome connected with the morphologically RA, never with the coronary sinus. Delisle et al[21] concluded that this type of TAPVC is characteristic of the asplenia syndrome, rarely if ever occurring in patients without visceral heterotaxy. What were the specific anatomic details of the infracardiac type of TAPVC in the asplenia syndrome? These findings are presented in Table 29.15.

All 14 cases of the infracardiac type of TAPVC with asplenia had a paraesophageal vein that went below the diaphragm and connected with the ductus venosus, constituting 15% of

TABLE 29.16 Mixed TAPVC With Asplenia

Findings	No. of Patients (n = 8)	% of Series[a] (n = 93)
Mixed TAPVC	4	4
1. To RSVC and to RA	1	1
2. To RA and to "snowman" pathway	1	1
3. To azygos vein and to RVC	1	1
4. To RSVC and to LSVC	1	1

[a]Percentages rounded off to nearest whole number.
LSVC, Left superior vena cava; *RA*, right atrium; *RSVC*, right superior vena cava; *RVC*, right vena cava; *TAPVC*, totally anomalous pulmonary venous connection.

TABLE 29.17 Partially Anomalous Pulmonary Venous Connection With Asplenia

Findings	No. of Patients (n = 5)	% of Series[a] (n = 93)
Partially APVC	5	5
1. Ipsilateral pulmonary veins	3	3
2. To RSVC and to LA	1	1
3. Mixed, to RSVC and to LA	1	1

[a]Percentages rounded off to nearest whole number.
APVC, Anonymous pulmonary venous connection; *LA*, left atrium; RSVC, right superior vena cava.

the series as a whole. None of our cases of the infracardiac type connected with any other intraabdominal vein. All cases were thought to have obstruction of the anomalous pulmonary venous pathway because of acute angulation of the paraesophageal vertical vein with the ductus venosus.[21] The findings in mixed TAPVC with asplenia are summarized in Table 29.16.

The findings in partially anomalous pulmonary venous connection with asplenia are summarized in Table 29.17.

1. Our interpretation of ipsilateral pulmonary veins, that is, that it may well represent malposition of the septum primum to the left of the right pulmonary veins (see Fig. 29.1), has been mentioned previously and hence will not be reiterated here.
2. Pattern 2 in Table 29.17 indicates that the right upper lobe pulmonary vein connected with the RSVC, whereas all of the other pulmonary veins connected normally with the LA.
3. But what does pattern 3 (see Table 29.17) mean? All of the right pulmonary veins connected with the RSVC, whereas all of the left pulmonary veins connected with the LA. Hence, this patient with partially anomalous pulmonary venous connection also has mixed partially anomalous pulmonary venous connection because all of the pulmonary venous blood from each lung connects with different structures: the right lung's pulmonary veins to the RSVC and the left lung's pulmonary veins to LA.

The status of the atrial septum in the heterotaxy syndrome with asplenia is summarized in Table 29.18.

In these 95 postmortem patients with the asplenia syndrome, the atrial septum was normally formed (with a patent foramen ovale) in only 2%. A common atrium with a largely or totally absent atrial septum was the most frequent finding (72%). Second in frequency was the combination of a secundum ASD with a primum ASD (the latter being part of a common AV canal), this combination of secundum and primum ASDs being found in 18% of our asplenia patients. Third in frequency was a primum ASD only (without a secundum ASD), in 5%. Fourth was a secundum type of atrial septal defect (2%). Also at a 2% prevalence was a normally formed atrial septum, with a patent foramen ovale as the only finding.

TABLE 29.18 Atrial Septum With Asplenia

Findings	No. of Patients (n = 95)	% of Series[a] (n = 95)
1. Common atrium	68	72
2. ASD II and I	17	18
3. ASD I only (no ASD II)	5	5
4. ASD II only	2	2
5. PFO only	2	2
6. Single RA (LA and atrial septum absent)	1	1

[a]Percentages rounded off to nearest whole number.
ASD I, Atrial septal defect of the ostium primum type; *ASD II*, atrial septal defect of the ostium secundum type; *LA*, morphologically left atrium; *PFO*, patent foramen ovale; *RA*, morphologically right atrium.

TABLE 29.19 The Atrioventricular Valves With Asplenia

Findings	No. of Patients	% of Series[a] (n = 95)
1. Common atrioventricular canal	91	96
a. Completely common AVC	77	81
b. Partially common AVC	14	15
2. Normal atrioventricular valves	4	4

[a]Percentages rounded off to nearest whole number.
AVC, Atrioventricular canal.

Least in frequency (1%) was single RA, that is, absence of the morphologically LA and interatrial septum. This is an exceedingly rare malformation, a virtually unknown form of congenital heart disease.

The anatomic status of the **AV valves** in 95 postmortem patients with the heterotaxy syndrome and asplenia is summarized in Table 29.19.

Common AV canal was present in almost all (96%), the complete form being much more frequent than the partial form (81% versus 15%, respectively). Although the AV valves can be normally formed in the asplenia syndrome, this was very infrequent (4%).

What was the complete form of common AV canal like in our cases of the asplenia syndrome? Salient data are presented in Table 29.20.

TABLE 29.20 Complete Form of CAVC With Asplenia

Findings	No. of Patients (n = 77)	% of Series[a] (n = 95)
I. Completely common AVC	77	81
1. Balanced CCAVC	34	36
2. RV type of CCAVC	32	34
3. LV type of CCAVC	11	12

[a]Percentages rounded off to nearest whole number.
AVC, Atrioventricular canal; *CCAVC,* completely common atrioventricular canal; *LV,* morphologically left ventricular; *RV,* morphologically right ventricle.

The **balanced type** of CCAVC was the most common form (36%). "Balanced" means that the common AV valve opens approximately equally into the morphologically LV and RV. This in turn means that both ventricles are approximately equally well developed.

The **right ventricular type** of CCAVC was a close second in frequency (34%). The right ventricular type means that the common AV valve is "unbalanced" toward the morphologically RV, opening mainly into this ventricle. What this really means is that the morphologically RV is large and well developed, whereas the morphologically LV is small and poorly developed.

The common AV canal and the common AV valve really are not "unbalanced" toward the RV. Instead, the right ventricular type of complete common AV canal (CCAVC) means that the LV is small and hence the muscular interventricular septum has shifted toward the side of the small LV. In turn, this is why the common AV valve opens predominantly into the morphologically RV (because the left ventricle is small). Hence, it is the ventricles that are unbalanced, not the AV canal nor the common AV valve.

The **left ventricular type** of CCAVC was the least frequent type found in association with the asplenia syndrome (12%) (see Table 29.20). Again, the "left ventricular" type means that a large LV and a small RV are present, and consequently the common AV valve opens predominantly into the large LV.

Hence, these findings (see Table 29.20) accurately indicate that the LV is often underdeveloped in the asplenia syndrome; hence, the high prevalence of the right ventricular type of CCAVC (34%). These findings also indicate that underdevelopment of the RV is much less frequent; hence, the much lower frequency of the left ventricular type (12%) compared with the right ventricular type (34%).

The foregoing understanding is very relevant to surgical repair. If either ventricle is markedly underdeveloped (this is what the unbalanced types of common AV canal mean), a single ventricle type of repair may well be more feasible than a biventricular repair. We prefer the term CCAVC to complete common AV canal, and we similarly prefer partially common atrioventricular canal to partial common AV canal. Why? Because grammatically, an adverb (completely or partially) is required to modify an adjective (common). Complete common AV canal and partial common AV canal are grammatically incorrect. (We sometimes feel like founding a Society for the Preservation of the Adverb.) Similarly, it should be morphologically RV (not morphologic RV) and morphologically LV (not morphologic LV) for the same reason. An adverb (morphologically) is required to modify an adjective (right or left).

TABLE 29.21 Partial Form of Common AV Canal With Asplenia

Findings	No. of Patients (n = 14)	% of Series[a] (n = 95)
Partially common AV canal	14	15
1. ASD I + cleft MV	6	6
2. With mitral atresia	3	3
3. With tricuspid atresia	3	3
4. With hypoplastic LV (RV type)	2	2

[a]Percentages rounded off to nearest whole number.
ASD I, Ostium primum type of atrial septal defect; *AV,* atrioventricular; *LV,* morphologically left ventricle; *MV,* mitral valve; *RV,* morphologically right ventricle.

What were the salient features of **the partial form of common AV canal with asplenia**? These data are summarized in Table 29.21.

The most frequent type of partially common AV canal associated with asplenia was an ostium primum type of ASD with a cleft mitral valve (6%), the classic partial form of common AV canal. But the other types were infrequent to rare and decidedly less familiar. None had a VSD of the AV canal type (making them partial forms of common AV canal). But, in addition to that, 3 patients had mitral atresia (3%), 3 had tricuspid atresia (3%), and 2 had a hypoplastic LV (2%) and hence were regarded as partial forms of common AV canal of the RV type.

Hence, the LV and RV types of common atrioventricular canal apply to both the complete and partial forms because ventricular hypoplasia can occur with both.

The anatomic status of **the morphologically RV with asplenia** is summarized in Table 29.22.

Biventricular hypertrophy and enlargement was the most commonest finding, but this occurred in only slightly more than one-quarter of these 95 patients with asplenia (28%; see Table 29.22). This means that only slightly less than three-quarters of these patients (72%) did not have two well-developed ventricles—a very important fact from the surgical perspective.

The second most common finding concerning the RV in asplenia was single RV, that is, absence of the morphologically LV (20%) (see Fig. 29.9). (We were surprised by this very high prevalence of single RV. Good and experienced morphologists have told us that they have never seen single RV, that is, total demonstrable absence of the morphologically LV. All we could say at the time was, "Well, it really does occur." Perhaps what we should have said is, "Go study asplenia.") Third in frequency was underdevelopment of the right ventricular sinus (19%). Fourth was functionally single RV, meaning that a diminutive but functionally useless LV was present, in 18% of these asplenia patients. From the hemodynamic and surgical viewpoints, this means that a functionally single RV (i.e., LV absent or diminutive) occurred in 38% of these cases—a remarkably high proportion. Fifth in prevalence was single LV (i.e., absence of the

TABLE 29.22 The RV in the Asplenia Syndrome

Findings	No. of Patients	% of Series[a] (n = 95)
1. RVH and E, LVH and E	27	28
2. Single RV (LV absent)	19	20
3. Underdeveloped RV sinus	18	19
4. Functionally single RV (LV very hypoplastic)	17	18
5. Single LV (RV sinus absent) with roc	5	5
6. Normal RV	4	4
7. Dysplastic RV sinus with atretic Ebstein anomaly and CAVC	2	2
8. RVH and E with CAVC, mitral atresia, and hypoplastic LV	1	1
9. Atretic RV sinus, tricuspid atresia (without CAVC)	1	1
10. RVH & E, mitral atresia (without CAVC)	1	1

[a]Percentages rounded off to nearest whole number.
CAVC, Common atrioventricular canal; *roc,* rudimentary outlet chamber; *LV,* morphologically left ventricle; *LVH & E,* left ventricular hypertrophy and enlargement; *RV,* morphologically right ventricle; *RVH & E,* right ventricular hypertrophy and enlargement.

TABLE 29.23 The LV in the Asplenia Syndrome

Findings	No. of Patients	% of Series[a] (n = 95)
1. LVH and E	27	28
2. LV absent (single RV)	19	20
3. LV hypoplasia, extreme	17	18
4. LV hypoplasia, mild to moderate	13	14
5. LV normal	10	11
6. Single LV (RV sinus absent) with roc	5	5
7. Single papillary muscle with LV hypoplastic (3) or WNL (1)	4	4

[a]Percentages rounded off to nearest whole number.
ROC, rudimentary outlet chamber; *LV,* morphologically left ventricle; *LVH and E,* left ventricular hypertrophy and enlargement; *RV,* morphologically right ventricle; *WNL,* within normal limits.

TABLE 29.24 Pulmonary Outflow Tract in Asplenia

Findings	No. of Cases	% of Series[a] (n = 95)
1. Pulmonary outflow tract stenosis	45	47
2. Pulmonary outflow tract atresia	40	42
3. No pulmonary outflow tract obstruction	10	11

[a]Percentages rounded off to nearest whole number.

right ventricular sinus, inflow tract, or main pumping portion) in 5%. A morphologically normal RV, without hypertrophy, enlargement, or other abnormality, was found in only 4% of these asplenic patients.

The remaining 5% of patients had functionally univentricular hearts:

1. common AV canal with an atretic Ebstein malformation of its right ventricular component, and an Ebstein type of right ventricular dysplasia (2%); and
2. common AV canal with mitral atresia (i.e., atresia of its mitral component), with left ventricular hypoplasia (1%); tricuspid atresia with an atretic right ventricular sinus, with a divided AV canal (as opposed to an undivided or common AV canal) in 1%; and mitral atresia with a divided (not a common) AV canal (1%).

The foregoing results mean that a **functionally single ventricle** was present in 46 of these 95 asplenic patients (48%) (see Table 29.22). A **functionally single RV** was found in 38 of 95 cases (40%) and a **functionally single LV** in 8 of 95 patients (8%).

The anatomic status of **the morphologically LV in asplenia** is presented in Table 29.23.

The most common finding concerning the morphologically LV in 95 cases of the asplenia syndrome was hypertrophy and enlargement (28%). Second in frequency was left ventricular absence (20%), followed by extreme hypoplasia (18%), followed by mild to moderate hypoplasia (14%). The left ventricle was judged entirely normal in only 11% of cases. Single LV as a result of absence of the right ventricular sinus, with only an infundibular outlet chamber present, occurred in 5% of these patients. These data confirm those concerning the RV (see Table 29.22), namely, that the prevalence of functionally single ventricle was very high: 41 of 95 patients (43%). Even if one does not include obstructive anomalies of the AV valves, functionally single RV was present in 36 of 95 patients (38%), while functionally single LV occurred in 5 of 95 cases (5%). Moreover, mild to moderate left ventricular hypoplasia occurred in an additional 16 patients (17%) (see Table 29.23). The anatomic status of the pulmonary outflow tract in the heterotaxy syndrome with asplenia is summarized in Table 29.24.

To any experienced pediatric cardiologist or cardiac surgeon, this high frequency of pulmonary outflow tract obstruction (89%) will come as no surprise. Pulmonary outflow tract stenosis (47%) was slightly more common than pulmonary outflow tract atresia (42%). The **nature of the pulmonary outflow tract stenosis** is analyzed in Table 29.25.

When pulmonary outflow tract stenosis was present, it almost always involved both the subvalvar and the valvar levels (89%). However, when only one level was involved, it was always subvalvar pulmonary stenosis only (11%), never valvar pulmonary stenosis only (0%). **Asplenia without pulmonary outflow obstruction, but with aortic outflow tract obstruction** is an unusual situation (Table 29.26).

In asplenia, when there was no pulmonary outflow tract obstruction (10 patients, 11%; see Table 29.24), there was aortic outflow tract obstruction in more than half of those cases (6 patients; Table 29.26), that is, in 60% of the group without pulmonary outflow tract obstruction. These patients without pulmonary outflow obstruction and with aortic outflow obstruction either had aortic outflow tract stenosis (3 patients, 30% of the group with no aortic outflow obstruction) or aortic outflow tract atresia (3 patients, 30% of the group with no pulmonary outflow obstruction) (see Table 29.26). These cases

TABLE 29.25 Pulmonary Outflow Tract Stenosis in Asplenia

Findings	No. of Patients (n = 45)	% of Series[a] (n = 95)
1. Subvalvar and valvar PS	40	89
2. Subvalvar PS with normal PV	5	11

[a]Percentages rounded off to nearest whole number.
PS, Pulmonary stenosis; *PV*, pulmonary valve.

TABLE 29.26 Aortic Outflow Tract in Asplenia

Findings	No. of Cases (n = 90)	% of Series (n = 90)
1. No obstruction	84	93
2. Aortic outflow tract stenosis	3	3
3. Aortic outflow tract atresia	3	3

tended to have unusual segmental sets: Patients with aortic outflow tract stenosis:

1. The first patient had **{I,D,S}**, that is, situs inversus of the viscera and atria, discordant 0-loop ventricles, and solitus normally related great arteries. The circulations were congenitally physiologically uncorrected because there was only one intersegmental discordance. Therapeutically, one would like to do an atrial switch, if otherwise feasible. {I,D,S} is so rare that it has no generally recognized conventional name. {I,D,S} is one of five known anatomic types of **AV discordance with VA concordance.**[22] One might call this anomaly **AV discordance with VA concordance {I,D,S},** meaning AV discordance with VA concordance of the {I,D,S} type. But perhaps the simplest and the clearest approach is just to spell out the segments in words: **inverted atria with noninverted (D-loop) ventricles and noninverted normally related great arteries.**
2. The second patient without pulmonary outflow obstruction and with aortic stenosis had {A,L,I}, meaning visceroatrial situs ambiguus (with asplenia), L-loop ventricles, and inverted normally related great arteries. Again, this rare anomaly has no generally recognized conventional name. We suggest expressing the segmental symbols in words, as earlier.
3. The third patient with no pulmonary outflow tract obstruction and with aortic outflow tract stenosis had **DORV {A(I),D,D}, that is, DORV with the segmental combination of situs ambiguus of the viscera with situs inversus of the atria, discordant D-loop ventricles, and D malposition of the great arteries.** Again, this is not a familiar form of DORV; it has no conventional name, and, consequently, calling it by its three main segmental components (as earlier) may be a satisfactory designation.

Patients With Aortic Outflow Tract Atresia

In patients with aortic atresia, the atresia is not always at the valvar level, but also can be subvalvar. Hence, aortic outflow tract atresia is used intentionally.

TABLE 29.27 Asplenia Without Pulmonary Outflow Tract Obstruction and With Aortic Outflow Tract Obstruction

Findings	No. of Cases (n = 6)	% of Series[a] (n = 95)
1. Aortic outflow tract stenosis[b]	3	3
2. Aortic outflow tract atresia[c]	3	3

[a]Percentages rounded off to nearest whole number.
[b]{I,D,S}, {A,L,I}, DORV {I,D,D}.
[c]{S,L,I}, {I,L,I}, DORV {I,L,D}.

1. Patient 1 (see Table 29.26, footnote) had {S,L,I}, that is, situs solitus of the viscera and atria, discordant L-loop ventricles, and inverted normally related great arteries. This is another rare form of congenital heart disease with AV discordance and VA concordance.[22,126]
2. Patient 2 with aortic atresia had inverted normal segmental anatomy: {I,L,I}, that is, situs inversus of the viscera and atria, concordant L-loop ventricles, and inverted normally related great arteries.
3. Patient 3 with asplenia, no pulmonary outflow tract obstruction, and aortic atresia had **DORV {I,L,D}, that is, DORV with situs inversus of the atria, concordant L-loop ventricles, and D-malposition of the great arteries** (instead of L-malposition of the great arteries, which is more usual with L-loop ventricles). Again, this is a rare and unfamiliar form of DORV. The anatomic status of the aortic outflow tract in the asplenia syndrome is summarized in Table 29.27.

Thus, a wide-open aortic outflow tract is the rule in asplenia (93%). Note that there are no cases with both aortic and pulmonary outflow tract obstruction (see Tables 29.24 to 29.27). One may speculate that if such cases exist, they may lead to intrauterine death because significant obstruction of both the aortic and the pulmonary outflow tracts very probably would lead to heart failure with embryonic or fetal demise.

Heterotaxy Syndrome With Polysplenia Sex Ratio: Males-to-females, 31/35 (0.89/1).

Age at Death: Mean, 52 ± 89.2 months, ranging from 0 (fetal demise) to 29.7 years, with a median of 4 months of age.

The **relations between the great arteries in the heterotaxy syndrome with polysplenia** are presented in Table 29.28.

Although normally related great arteries are the rule in the polysplenia syndrome (70%), the question remains: What kinds of normally related great arteries were present (Table 29.29)?

Tetralogy of Fallot (TOF): Present in 10 of 47 polysplenic patients (21%), being solitus (noninverted) tetralogy in 7 (15%) and inverted tetralogy in 3 (6%).

D-loop ventricles: Present in 39 of 47 patients (83%), being concordant in 36 of 39 cases (92%), and discordant in 3 of 39 (8%).

L-loop ventricles: Found in 8 of 47 patients (17%), being concordant in 5 of 8 cases (62.5%), discordant in 2 of 8 (25%), and indeterminate in 1 (12.5%).

The atrial situs was solitus: Present in 38 of 47 patients (81%), inverted in 8 of 47 cases (17%), and in situs ambiguus in 1 (2%).

TABLE 29.28 Relations Between Great Arteries in Polysplenia

Types of Ventriculoarterial Alignment	No. of Patients	% of Series[a] (n = 67)
1. Normally related great arteries	47	70
2. Double-outlet right ventricle	16	24
3. Transposition of the great arteries	4	6

[a]Percentages rounded off to nearest whole number.

The visceral situs was solitus: Present in 34 of 47 patients (72%), ambiguus in 8 of 47 (17%), and inversus in 5 of 47 (11%).

Visceroatrial discordance: Present in 2 of 47 polysplenic patients (4%). Both had situs inversus of the abdominal viscera with situs solitus of the atria: {IS,D,S} (see Table 29.29).

Segmental alignment discordances: Occurred only between the atrial and the ventricular segments in 4 of 47 patients (8.5%), 2 cases having {S,L,-} and 2 having {I,D,-}. Because the great arteries always were normally related, VA alignment discordance could not occur, by definition, in these 47 patients (see Table 29.29).

Segmental situs discordance (not alignment discordance): Occurred between the ventricular and the great arteries segments in 2 of 47 patients (4%). Both had {-,L,S}: {S,L,S} in 1 and {I,L,S} in the other. Because the VA alignments were normal, the VA situs discordance had no deleterious hemodynamic consequences.

The total known prevalence of segmental situs discordance in these 47 polysplenia patients was 8 (17%): {I,S,-,-} in 2; {S,L,-} in 2; {I,D,-} in 2; and {-,L,S} in 2. The heterotaxy syndromes of asplenia and of polysplenia both are characterized by high prevalences of intersegmental situs discordances. These segmental situs inconsistencies or mismatches lead to much of the complexity of the heterotaxy syndromes (see Table 29.29).

Concerning VA alignments (often called the relationships between the great arteries) in the heterotaxy syndrome with polysplenia, far behind normally related great arteries (70%) came DORV (24%) (Table 29.30). The various anatomic types of **DORV with polysplenia** are summarized in Table 29.30.

Atrial situs: Solitus in 10 of 16 (62.5%); inversus in 6 of 16 (37.5%); and indeterminate (ambiguus) in none.

Visceroatrial situs discordance: Situs inversus of the abdominal viscera with situs solitus of the atria, that is, {I,S,-,} occurred in 1 of these 16 polysplenic patients (6%) and loop in 7 of 16 (44%).

AV concordance: Present in 13 of 16 polysplenia patients with DORV (81%). The segmental anatomy was {S,D,-} in 8 and {I,L,-} in 5.

AV discordance: Present in 3 of 16 patients (19%). The segmental anatomy was {S,L,-} in 2 and {I,D,-} in 1.

Semilunar interrelationship: D-malposition of the great arteries was present in 10 of 16 patients (62.5%) and L-malposition of the great arteries in 6 of 16 (37.5%).

VA situs concordance: Present in 15 of 16 patients (94%). The segmental anatomy was {-,D,D} in 9 patients, and {-,L,L} in 6.

TABLE 29.29 Types of Normally Related Great Arteries in the Polysplenia Syndrome

Findings	No. of Cases	% of Series[a] (n = 47)
1. {S,D,S}	29	62
2. TOF {S,D,S}	5	11
3. {I,D,S}	2	4
4. TOF {I,L,I}	2	4
5. {I,L,S}	2	4
6. TOF {I,S,D,S}	1	2
7. {I,S,D,S}	1	2
8. {S,L,S}	1	2
9. TOF {S,L,I}	1	2
10. {I,L,I}	1	2
11. TOF {I,D,S}	1	2
12. {A,L,I}	1	2

[a]Percentages rounded to nearest whole number.
TOF, Tetralogy of Fallot.
Segmental symbols from 1 to 12, inclusive:
1. Situs solitus of viscera and atria, D-loop ventricles, solitus normally related great arteries
2. TOF {S,D,S}
3. Situs inversus of viscera and atria, D-loop ventricles, solitus normally related great arteries
4. TOF with situs inversus of the atria, L loop ventricles, and inverted normally related great arteries
5. Situs inversus of the atria, L-loop ventricles, solitus normally related great arteries
6. TOF with situs inversus of the abdominal viscera and situs solitus of the atria, D-loop ventricles, solitus normally related great arteries
7. Situs inversus of the abdominal viscera and situs solitus of the atria, D-loop ventricles, solitus normally related great arteries
8. Situs solitus of the atria, L-loop ventricles, solitus normally related great arteries
9. TOF with situs solitus of the atria, L-loop ventricles, inverted normally related great arteries
10. Situs inversus of the atria, L-loop ventricles, inverted normally related great arteries
11. TOF with atrial situs inversus, D-loop ventricles, solitus normally related great arteries
12. Situs ambiguus of the atria, L-loop ventricles, inverted normally related great arteries

Braces, i.e., { }, mean the set of types of normally related great arteries.
In 47 postmortem cases of polysplenia, the great arteries were solitus normally related in 42 (89%) and inverted normally related in 5 (11%).

TABLE 29.30 Double-Outlet Right Ventricle with Polysplenia

Findings		No. of Patients	% of Series[a] (n = 16)
1. DORV	{S,D,D}	7	44
2. DORV	{I,S,D,D}	1	6
3. DORV	{S,L,L}	2	12.5
4. DORV	{I,L,L}	4	25
5. DORV	{I,L,D}	1	6
6. DORV	{I,D,D}	1	6

[a]Percentages rounded off to nearest whole number.

TABLE 29.31 TGA With Polysplenia

Findings		No. of Patients	% of Series[a] (n = 4)
1. TGA	{S,D,D}	1	25
2. TGA	{S,L,L}	2	50
3. TGA	{I,D,D}	1	25

TGA, Transposition of the great arteries.
[a]Percentages rounded off to nearest whole number.

TABLE 29.32 The Conus With Polysplenia

Findings	No. of Patients	% of Series[a] (n = 66)
1. Subpulmonary (only)	59	89
2. Bilateral (subaortic and subpulmonary)	6	9
3. Bilaterally deficient	1	2

[a]Percentages rounded off to nearest whole number.

VA situs discordance: Present in 1 of 16 patients (6%). The segmental anatomy was {-,L,D}. The combination {-,D,L} did not occur in this small series.

TGA was the least frequent type of VA alignment found in association with the heterotaxy syndrome with polysplenia (6%; see Table 29.28). **The anatomic types of TGA associated with polysplenia** are summarized in Table 29.31.

Only 1 patient had congenitally physiologically uncorrected (complete) TGA {S,D,D}. The other 3 patients had congenitally physiologically corrected transposition, the segmental anatomy being TGA {S,L,L} in 2 and TGA {I,D,D} in 1.

The anatomy of the **conus with polysplenia** is presented in Table 29.32. The high prevalence of a subpulmonary conus (89%) correlates with the high prevalence of normally related great arteries that is characteristic of the polysplenia syndrome. Note the absence of a well-developed subaortic conus (only) (see Table 29.32). We have never found a well-developed subaortic conus with pulmonary-AV valvar fibrous continuity in association with polysplenia; in other words, the typical transposition type of conus seems not to occur with polysplenia.

A bilateral (subaortic and subpulmonary) conus (9%) often is associated with DORV. A bilaterally deficient conus (2%) means that both the subaortic conal musculature and the subpulmonary conal musculature are sufficiently deficient so as to permit aortic continuity.

Lobation of the lungs in the polysplenia syndrome is summarized in Table 29.33. In 58 postmortem patients with polysplenia, the lungs were bilaterally bilobed in more than half (57%). However, 5 other patterns were found in the remaining 43% of patients.

The anatomic status of the SVC with polysplenia is presented in Table 29.34. The SVC may be regarded as having been "normal" (*usual* may be more accurate) in 38 of 67 patients (57%), including not only the 30 cases with a RSVC only, but also including the 8 patients in situs inversus with a LSVC only. However, in the 29 patients with bilateral SVCs as clearly abnormal (43%).

TABLE 29.33 Lung Lobation In Polysplenia

Findings	No. of Cases	% of Series[a] (n = 58)
I. Bilaterally bilobed	33	57
2. Normal: 3 Rt, 2 Lt	13	22
3. Inverted: 2 Rt, 3 Lt	6	10
4. Bilaterally unilobed	3	5
5. Bilaterally trilobed	2	3
6. Agenesis RL, unilobed LL	1	2

[a]Percentages rounded off to nearest whole numbers.
Lt, Left; *RL,* right lobe; *Rt,* right.

TABLE 29.34 SVC With Polysplenia

Findings	No. of Patients	% of Series[a] (n = 67)
1. Normal: RSVC only	30	45
2. Bilateral SVC	29	43
3. Inverted: LSVC only in situs inversus	8	12

[a]Percentages rounded off to nearest whole number.
LSVC, Left superior vena cava; *RSVC,* right superior vena cava; *bilateral SVC,* bilateral superior venaes cavaes.

TABLE 29.35 IVC With Polysplenia and Visceral Heterotaxy

Findings	No. of Patients	% of Series[a] (n = 54)
1. Interruption of the IVC	42	78
2. Right IVC	6	11
3. Left IVC	5	9
4. Left IVC switching to right	1	2

[a]Percentages rounded off to nearest whole number.
IVC, Inferior vena cava.

The anatomic status of the **IVC with polysplenia** is summarized in Table 29.35. Interruption of the IVC from the renal veins below to the hepatic veins above is characteristic of the polysplenia syndrome (78%; see Table 29.35). An enlarged azygos vein(s), often called an "azygos extension" returned the systemic venous blood from the lower body to the SVC(s) (Fig. 29.10). In the remaining 22% of polysplenic patients, the systemic venous blood returned to the heart by a noninterrupted IVC that was right-sided (11%) or left-sided (9%) or that switched from left to right (2%) (see Table 29.35).

The anatomic status of the pulmonary veins in the heterotaxy syndrome with polysplenia is presented in Table 29.36. In the polysplenia syndrome, the pulmonary veins usually were normally connected (63%). Anomalous pulmonary venous drainage occurred in 37%, either being totally anomalous (22%) or partially anomalous (15%). Ipsilateral pulmonary veins (right pulmonary veins to the right-sided atrium and left pulmonary veins to the left-sided atrium) occurred in only 9% (see Table 29.36). Ipsilateral pulmonary veins have been thought by some to lend credence to the view that in the polysplenia syndrome,

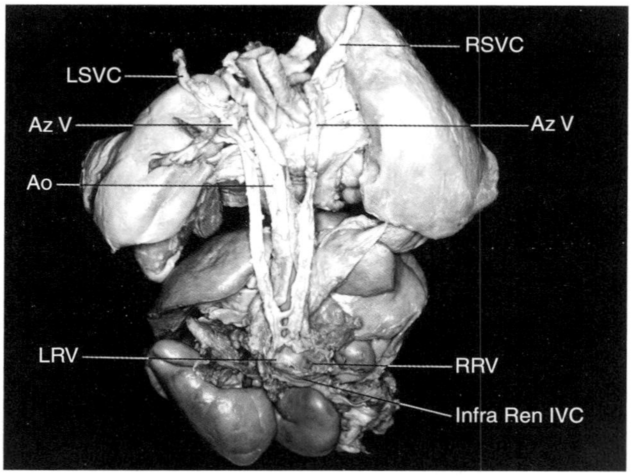

Fig. 29.10 **The heterotaxy syndrome with left-sided polysplenia.** The heart, lungs, liver, and kidneys of this 6 ½-month-old boy (A73-17) are shown from behind. There is interruption of the right-sided inferior vena cava (IVC). The right-sided infrarenal IVC *(Infra Ren IVC)* proceeds up to the interrenal anastomosis between the right renal vein *(RRV)* and the left renal vein *(LRV)*. This interrenal venous anastomosis is derived from the intersubcardinal plexus. From the superior and right-sided portion of the interrenal venous anastomosis, the renal-to hepatic segment of the normal IVC is missing. Instead, bilateral azygos veins *(Az V)* originate from the interrenal anastomosis and proceed cephalad. The right Az V connects with the right superior vena cava *(RSVC)*, which enters the right-sided right atrium (RA) directly. The left-sided Az V connects with the left superior vena cava (LSVC), which connected with the coronary sinus and drained normally into the RA. All of the pulmonary veins also drained into the right sided morphologically RA. Our hypothesis is that leftward malposition of this multiply fenestrated septum primum made possible the totally anomalous pulmonary venous drainage of these normally connected pulmonary veins. The fenestrations of septum primum facilitated entry of blood into left atrium to the left of the malpositioned septum primum. The atrioventricular canal was normally divided. *Ao,* Aorta. (Reproduced with permission from Van Praagh S, Santini F, Sanders SP. Cardiac malpositions with special emphasis on visceral heterotaxy (asplenia and polysplenia syndromes). In: Fyler DC, ed. *Nadas' Pediatric Cardiology.* Philadelphia, PA: Hanley & Belfus; 1992:589.13.[15])

the morphologically LA, or only its appendage, is bilateral. The low incidence of ipsilateral pulmonary veins is noteworthy in several respects: (1) With a prevalence of only 9%, ipsilateral pulmonary veins are hardly characteristic of the polysplenia syndrome. (2) Ipsilateral pulmonary veins have been used to support the concept of left atrial isomerism, or LAA isomerism, that we think is erroneous.[8,9,13,14] From a factual perspective, this low prevalence of ipsilateral pulmonary veins (9%) does not support the hypothesis that left atrial isomerism or LAA isomerism is typical of the polysplenia syndrome, because 91% of these patients did not have ipsilateral pulmonary veins. The anatomic status of the **atrial septum in polysplenia** is summarized in Table 29.36.

In these 68 postmortem patients with the polysplenia syndrome, the atrial septum was normally formed in only 22% (intact, 9%, and patent foramen ovale, 13%). Hence, the atrial septum was malformed in 78% (Table 29.37). Septum primum malposition defect (6%) is shown echocardiographically in Figs. 29.1 and 29.2. The anatomic status of the AV valves with polysplenia is summarized in Table 29.38.

TABLE 29.36 Pulmonary Veins With Polysplenia

Findings	No. of Patients	% of Series[a] (n = 65)
1. Normally connected with LA	41	63
2. Totally anomalous PVD	14	22
a. To RA	12	18
b. Rt to RA, Lt to CoS	2	3
3. Partially anomalous PVD	10	15
a. Ipsilateral	6	9
b. Rt to ductus venosus	1	2
4. Scimitar syndrome	1	2
5. Rt to RA	2	3

[a]Percentages rounded off to nearest whole number.
CoS, Coronary sinus; *LA,* left atrium; *Lt,* left; *PVD,* pulmonary venous drainage; *RA,* right atrium.

TABLE 29.37 Atrial Septum With Polysplenia

Findings	No. of Cases	% of Series[a] (n = 68)
1. Common atrium	22	32
2. ASD II	21	31
a. ASD II + ASD I	1	1
b. ASD II + CSSD	1	1
3. PFO	9	13
4. ASD I	6	9
5 Intact	6	9
6 Septum I malposition defect	4	6

[a]Percentages rounded off to nearest whole number.
ASD I, Atrial septal defect of ostium primum type; *ASD II,* atrial septal defect of ostium secundum type; *CSSD,* coronary sinus septal defect; *PFO,* patent foramen ovale; *Septum I,* septum primum.

It is of interest to note that in these 67 postmortem patients with the heterotaxy syndrome with polysplenia, normally formed AV valves were more frequent than was common AV canal (55% versus 45%, respectively). However, when common AV canal was present, the complete form was more frequent than the partial form (33% versus 12%, respectively).

The anatomic status of the morphologically **RV in the heterotaxy syndrome with polysplenia** is summarized in Table 29.39.

Right ventricular hypertrophy and enlargement was by far the most common finding (59%). In our laboratory it is routine to compare the measurements of the ventricles with those of normal control heart specimens matched for age, body weight, and, if advantageous, for sex. We think that one should not make statements concerning hypertrophy, enlargement, normalcy, or hypoplasia of cardiovascular structures without measuring normal control heart specimens at the same time that one is measuring a case of heart disease. We do not use tables of normal data, to ensure the case and the controls are measured in the same way, at the same time, by the same observer.

TABLE 29.38 Atrioventricular Valves With Polysplenia

Findings	No. of Patients	% of Series[a] (n = 67)
1. Common AV canal	30	45
a. Complete form	22	33
b. Partial form	8	12
2. Normal AV valves	37	55

[a]Percentages rounded off to nearest whole number.
AV, Atrioventricular.

TABLE 29.39 Right Ventricle with Polysplenia

Findings	No. of Cases	% of Series[a] (n = 58)
1. RVH + E	34	59
2. Normal RV	9	16
3. RVH	7	12
4. Hypoplastic RV sinus	5	9
5. Absent RV sinus (single LV)	2	3
6. Single RV (absent LV sinus)	1	2

[a]Percentages rounded off to nearest whole number.
LV, Morphologically left ventricle; *RV*, morphologically right ventricle; *RVH + E*, right ventricular hypertrophy and enlargement.

In order of decreasing frequency after right ventricular hypertrophy and enlargement, the findings were as follows: normal RV (16%); right ventricular hypertrophy, without enlargement (12%); hypoplasia of the RV, meaning of the right ventricular sinus, also known as the right ventricular body or inflow tract, that is, the main pumping portion, as opposed to the right ventricular infundibulum, conus, or outflow tract (9%); absence of the RV, meaning absence of the right ventricular sinus, understanding that the infundibulum belongs to the great arteries, that is, it is part of the conotruncal segment—absence of the RV resulting in single LV with an infundibular outlet chamber (3%); and single RV, because of the absence of the LV, meaning absence of the left ventricular sinus, resulting in single RV, typically without a discrete infundibular outlet chamber, although the infundibulum is always present above the right ventricular sinus, but usually does not look like a separate chamber (2%). The foregoing is the understanding implicit in Table 29.39.

The anatomic status of the morphologically **LV with polysplenia** is presented in Table 29.40. Underdevelopment of the morphologically LV was quite frequent in the polysplenia syndrome (in 24/64 patients, or 37.5%): hypoplasia in 23 cases (36%), and absence in 1 (2%). One of these patients (A78-92), with a normal-sized LV had an extraordinarily rare finding: superoinferior ventricles with an *inferior* and *anterior* RV and a *superior* and *posterior* LV. (With superoinferior ventricles, the reverse is almost always present, that is, a superior right ventricle and an inferior left ventricle.)[23] The segmental set was also rare: {I,D,S}. In words, this of course means the set or combination of atrial situs inversus, discordant D-loop ventricles, and solitus normally related great arteries. This is one of the five known types of AV discordance with VA concordance.[22] We have seen only one other postmortem case of superoinferior ventricles in which the RV was *inferior* and the LV was *superior*.

TABLE 29.40 Left Ventricle With Polysplenia

Findings	No. of Cases	% of Series[a] (n = 64)
1. Normal LV[b]	24	37.5
2. Hypoplastic LV	23	36
3. LVH + E	14	22
4. Single LV (RV sinus absent)	2	3
5. Single RV (LV sinus absent)	1	2

[a]Percentages rounded off to nearest whole number.
[b]One patient (A78-92) with superoinferior ventricles of rare type: LV superior and RV inferior.
LV, Left ventricle; *LVH and E*, left ventricular hypertrophy and enlargement; *RV*, right ventricle.

TABLE 29.41 Pulmonary Outflow Tract With Polysplenia

Findings	No. of Cases	% of Series[a] (n = 67)
1. No obstruction	42	63
2. Pulmonary outflow tract stenosis	21	31
3. Pulmonary outflow tract atresia	4	6

[a]Percentages rounded off to nearest whole number.

TABLE 29.42 Aortic Outflow Tract With Polysplenia

Findings	No. of Cases	% of Series[a] (n = 63)
1. No obstruction[b]	56	89
2. Aortic outflow tract stenosis	5	8
3. Aortic outflow tract atresia	2	3

[a]Percentages rounded off to nearest whole number.
[b]Bicuspid aortic valve in 8 cases (13%).

The anatomic status of the **pulmonary outflow tract with polysplenia** is summarized in Table 29.41. The majority of these 67 polysplenic patients had no pulmonary outflow tract obstruction (63%). However, pulmonary outflow tract obstruction was present in 37% of patients: stenosis in 31% and atresia in 6%. The anatomic status of the **aortic outflow tract with polysplenia** is presented in Table 29.42. Although the aortic outflow tract in polysplenia typically was widely patent, aortic outflow tract stenosis (8%) and aortic valvar atresia (3%) both occurred.

WHAT DOES THE HEART IN THE HETEROTAXY SYNDROME WITH POLYSPLENIA LOOK LIKE?

Fig. 29.10 is a posterior view of the heart, lungs, liver, and kidneys of a 6.5-month-old boy with the heterotaxy syndrome and left-sided polysplenia (A73-17). There is interruption of the

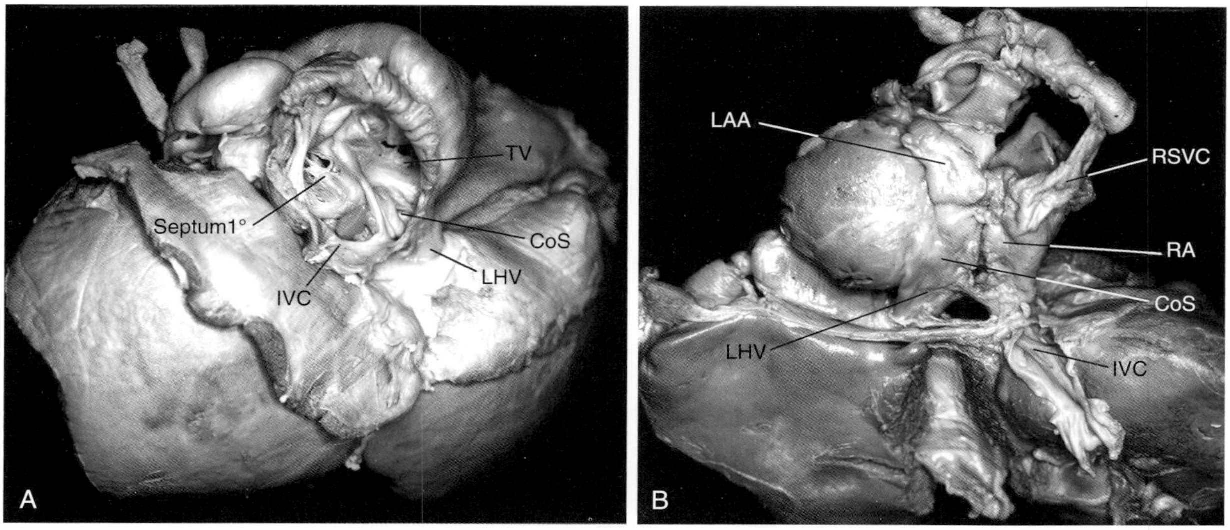

Fig. 29.11 Heterotaxy syndrome with left-sided polysplenia, tetralogy of Fallot {S,D,S}, and tracheal agenesis. This specimen consists of the heart, diaphragm, and liver of a 2 day-old white male infant (A76-121). (A) The interior of the right-sided morphologically right atrium *(RA)*. Note how well the septum primum *(Septum 1°)* is seen from the right atrial view. Septum 1° is somewhat deficient and contains several small fenestrations. The inferior vena cava *(IVC)* connects normally with the RA *(arrowhead)*, as does the coronary sinus *(CoS)*. The atrioventricular canal is normally divided (not in common) and the tricuspid valve *(TV)* is unremarkable. The left hepatic vein *(LHV)* also enters the RA at the site of the orifice of the CoS. Note the extensive pectination of the broad, triangular, and anterior right atrial appendage (to the right of, and superior to the TV). (B) The posterior view of this specimen. In this case of polysplenia, the IVC is not interrupted. The LHV connects with the CoS at its ostium, and drains normally into the RA. (Reproduced with permission from Van Praagh S, Santini F, Sanders SP. Cardiac malpositions with special emphasis on visceral heterotaxy (asplenia and polysplenia syndromes). In: Fyler DC, ed. *Nadas' Pediatric Cardiology.* Philadelphia, PA: Hanley & Belfus; 1992:589.13.[15])

right-sided IVC. Note that bilateral azygos veins connect with bilateral SVCs. The RSVC enters the RA directly, whereas the LSVC connects with an enlarged coronary sinus and drains normally into the right-sided morphologically RA. All of the pulmonary veins also drain into the RA. Multiple fenestrations in the septum primum and a moderate-sized membranous VSD allowed blood to enter the left-sided morphologically LA and LV, respectively. The AV valves are normally divided (not in common), and the great arteries are normally related; hence, the segmental set in {S,D,S}. This is a dramatic demonstration of interruption of the IVC with polysplenia because bilateral enlarged azygos veins are unusual. As a rule, there is only one enlarged azygos vein (often called an "azygos extension"), which can be right- or left-sided.

Fig. 29.11 shows the heart and liver of a 2-day-old white male infant (A76-121) with the heterotaxy syndrome, left-sided polysplenia, TOF {S,D,S}, and tracheal agenesis. Fig. 29.11A shows the interior of the right-sided morphologically RA. Note that both the uninterrupted IVC and the coronary sinus connect with the RA. The septum primum is unusually easy to see from this right atrial aspect, this being characteristic of the polysplenia syndrome, we think because the superior limbic band of septum secundum is often deficient or virtually absent. Note that the septum primum is somewhat deficient and fenestrated. A prominent left hepatic vein connects with the RA close to the ostium of the coronary sinus. Note how broad, large, and anterior the right sided RAA and its pectinate muscles are. The right-sided tricuspid valve is normally formed, and the AV canal is normally divided (not in common).

Fig. 29.11B is a posterior view of the same heart and liver. Note that the liver looks *bilaterally symmetrical,* with the right-sided lobe (to the viewer's right) and the left-sided lobe (to the viewer's left) both being approximately equal in size. An abnormal degree of bilateral symmetry of the liver is characteristic of the heterotaxy syndromes, both with asplenia and with polysplenia. This is often amusingly called a "midline liver." Can you imagine a truly midline liver? If present, it would have to protrude anteriorly like the bow of the Queen Elizabeth. A more or less bilaterally symmetrical liver is what is meant. Note also that the left-sided atrial appendage is relatively small, posterior, and finger-shaped, just as the LAA typically is in atrial situs solitus. LAA isomerism is not present. The left hepatic vein flows into the floor of the coronary sinus (just below the LAA) and then draining into RA along with the coronary sinus. However, if the coronary sinus septum and the atrial septum were both absent, the large left hepatic vein would then seem to connect directly with the LA. We think that the hepatic veins and the IVC always connect with the sinus venosus—with the right horn, the left horn, or both. If the coronary sinus (which is the left horn of the sinus venosus in atrial situs solitus) is unroofed, and if the atrial septum is very deficient, both of which often occur with the heterotaxy syndromes, some of the hepatic veins can *drain* directly into the LA, even though the hepatic veins are normally *connected* with the sinus venosus. In this patient, the coronary sinus was not unroofed and the atrial septum was quite well formed. Hence, both the left hepatic veins and the IVC drained normally into the RA.

Fig. 29.11 endeavors to answer the question: **What is the sinus venosus, and how does it normally develop in the human embryo and fetus?** These diagrams show the sinus venosus and the atria from a posterior or dorsal perspective. Fig. 29.11A shows the undivided atrium and the bilaterally symmetrical sinus venosus of a normal human embryo with a crown rump length of 3 mm, which corresponds to the Streeter horizon XI, which in turn corresponds to an embryonic age of 22 to 24 days. On both sides, the anterior (or superior) cardinal vein and the posterior (or inferior) cardinal vein join together to form the common cardinal vein (or duct of Cuvier). Inferiorly, the right-sided and left-sided umbilical veins flow into the common cardinal veins, marking the lateral limits of the right sided and left-sided sinus horns. More medially, the right-sided vitelline veins from the yolk sac flow into the inferior aspect of the sinus venosus, serving as the medial margins of the right and left sinus horns and the lateral margins of the central or transverse portion of the sinus venosus (between the right and left sinus horns). These conventional designations are for the purposes of description; they do not indicate any physical demarcations or delimitations within the sinus venosus.

Fig. 29.11B represents the 5-mm stage, corresponding to horizon XIII, that is, to 26 to 28 days of age. Note that the right sinus horn normally is starting to become larger than the left sinus horn. The common pulmonary vein has appeared inferiorly and posteriorly, just above the transverse portion of the sinus venosus. Note that only the right horn of the sinus venosus is confluent with and opens into the RA *(broken lines)*. By contrast, the left horn of the sinus venosus normally does not open into the LA but rather remains a separate structure that will become the coronary sinus. Note also that the umbilical and vitelline veins have fused bilaterally, forming the omphalomesenteric veins. The "omphalo" part is the umbilical venous contribution, and the "mesenteric" part is the vitelline vein contribution. The right omphalomesenteric vein is getting larger, whereas the left omphalomesenteric vein is getting smaller. The earliest stage at which we were able to identify the common pulmonary vein in normal human embryos of the Minot Collection at Harvard Medical School was in an embryo with an estimated age of 27 days,[24] just as Fig. 29.4B indicates.

Fig. 29.4C represents a 12-mm human embryo, which corresponds to horizon XVII, that is, 34 to 36 days of age. The common pulmonary vein is becoming incorporated into the dorsal left atrial wall. The left sinus horn is slowly involuting, whereas the right sinus horn is enlarging. The left omphalomesenteric vein has involuted completely and no longer flows into the left sinus horn.

Fig. 29.4 represents the state found in the normal newborn infant. The left sinus horn has become reduced to the coronary sinus. The left anterior (superior) cardinal vein, also known as the vein of Marshall or the LSVC, normally has undergone involution and become the ligament of Marshall. If this process of involution fails to occur, the result is a persistent LSVC connecting with the coronary sinus and flowing into the RA. If the coronary sinus is unroofed, that is, if a coronary sinus septal defect is present, venous blood from the coronary sinus, with or without venous blood from the persistent LSVC, flows into the LA. Note that the ligament of Marshall, or the persistent LSVC, runs just behind the LAA (not shown) and just in front of the left pulmonary veins (shown). The right horn of the sinus venosus is now much larger than the left horn (normally), and the right sinus horn—the smooth, nontrabeculated, venous component of the morphologically RA—is well incorporated into this chamber. The right sinus horn is limited superiorly by the RSVC, inferiorly by the right IVC, right laterally by the remnant of the right venous valve and the crista terminalis, and right medially by the remnants of the left venous valve and the atrial septum. The pulmonary veins are now well incorporated into the dorsal wall of the LA, up to beyond the primary divisions of the right and left pulmonary venous branches. This is why it normally looks as though there are two (or three) right pulmonary veins and two left pulmonary veins, because the common pulmonary vein has undergone incorporation up to and beyond the primary divisions of both right and left pulmonary venous branches. In fact, there is only one pulmonary vein, as Fig. 29.4B accurately shows. The pulmonary vein and its primary branches (one for each lobe of both lungs, hence four or five) are surrounded on three sides by the sinus venosus: to the left by the left sinus horn; inferiorly by the left sinus horn and by a little of the right sinus horn; and on the right by the right sinus horn. Hence, the pulmonary veins are normally surrounded on three sides by a "horseshoe" of sinus venosus tissue (see Fig. 29.4D).

Fig. 29.12 shows the heart and lungs of a 13-week-old girl with the heterotaxy syndrome and right-sided polysplenia {A(S),D,S}. Fig. 29.12A presents the interior of the right-sided morphologically RA. Note the large, triangular, right sided and anterior RAA with abundant pectinate muscles. However, the tip of this appendage was somewhat finger-like, reminiscent of a LAA. There was interruption of the IVC, characteristic of the polysplenia syndrome. The suprahepatic segment of the IVC and the hepatic veins connected with the RA as did the RSVC. Note that the right pulmonary veins drain into the morphologically RA; ipsilateral pulmonary veins are present. The right pulmonary veins drain into the right-sided RA, resulting in partially anomalous pulmonary venous drainage, whereas only the left pulmonary veins drain into the left-sided LA. *The septum primum is malpositioned to the left of the right pulmonary veins,* resulting in partially anomalous pulmonary venous *drainage,* despite what we think is a normal pulmonary venous *connection.*

Note the *white arrowhead* through the restrictively small *septum primum malposition defect in the interatrial septum.* This interatrial communication resembles a patent foramen ovale or a secundum type of ASD, except that it occurs in a very malpositioned septum primum, far removed from the septum secundum, which is either very deficient or absent. Hence, this interatrial communication is anatomically different from a normal patent foramen ovale and from the usual secundum type of ASD. The septum primum, just beneath the white arrowhead, is well seen, but only from the right atrial view, not from the left atrial view. Easy visualization of septum primum from the right

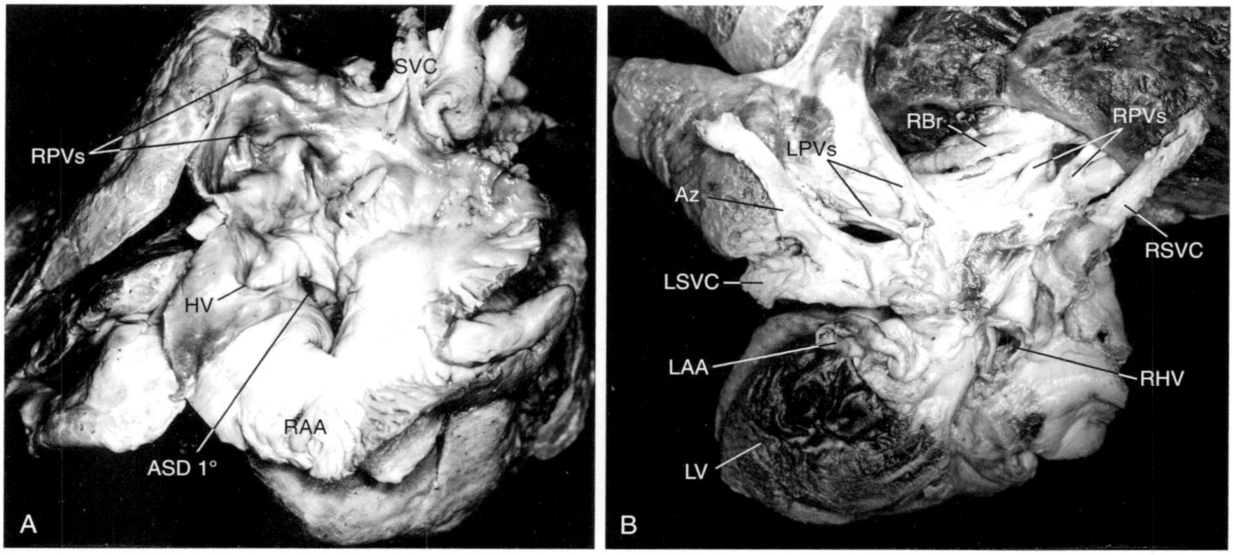

Fig. 29.12 Heterotaxy syndrome with right-sided polysplenia, interrupted inferior vena cava (IVC), and ipsilateral pulmonary veins in a 13-week-old girl. The segmental anatomy is {S,D,S}, that is, situs solitus of the atria, concordant D-loop ventricles, and solitus normally related great arteries. (A) Interior of the right-sided morphologically right atrium *(RA)*. Note the large, well-pectinated right atrial appendage *(RAA)*, only the tip of which resembles a left atrial appendage *(LAA)*. The RA receives the suprahepatic segment of the interrupted IVC and the hepatic veins *(HV)*, the right superior vena cava *(SVC)*, and the right pulmonary veins *(RPVs)*. The septum primum (to the right of the shaft of the *white arrow*) is malpositioned to the left of the RPVs, resulting in ipsilateral pulmonary venous drainage. The septum primum malposition atrial septal defect (ASD) is restrictively small and is filled by the white arrow. An ostium primum type of ASD *(ASD 1°)* indicates a partially common atrioventricular canal. (B) Posterior view of the heart. The left pulmonary veins (LPVs) and the RPVs connect with the atrial portion of the heart as in normal hearts, that is, between the left superior vena cava *(LSVC)* and the right superior vena cava (RSVC) and above the left sinus horn (see Fig. 29.4). Hence, ipsilateral pulmonary venous drainage is considered to be due to leftward malposition of the septum primum, not to anomalous connection of the RPVs. The left atrial appendage (LAA) is posterior, finger-like, and much smaller than the RAA. Interruption of the IVC is associated with connection of the right hepatic veins *(RHVs)* and the suprahepatic segment of the IVC with the RA, and a prominent left azygos vein *(Az)* connecting with the LSVC. *LV*, Left ventricle; *R Br*, right bronchus. (Reproduced with permission from Van Praagh S, Santini F, Sanders SP. Cardiac malpositions with special emphasis on visceral heterotaxy (asplenia and polysplenia syndromes). In: Fyler DC, ed. *Nadas' Pediatric Cardiology*. Philadelphia, PA: Hanley & Belfus; 1992:589.13.[15])

atrial view, and difficulty seeing the septum primum from the left atrial view, both are anatomically very abnormal, but characteristic of the polysplenia syndrome because of deficiency or absence of the superior limbic band of septum secundum. An ostium primum type of ASD can also be seen (see Fig. 29.12A), indicating the coexistence of common AV canal (partial type).

Fig. 29.12B is a posterior and somewhat left-sided view of this heart. Note that the LAA is left-sided, posterior, small, and finger-like, typical of the morphologically LA. The left and right pulmonary veins connect with the posterior atrial wall between the LSVC and the RSVC, this being a normal pulmonary venous connection, as is shown in Fig. 29.4. Consequently, we think that the pulmonary veins are normally connected, but drain in part anomalously (ipsilateral pulmonary veins) because of leftward malposition of the septum primum. The septum primum could not be well visualized from the left atrial aspect, a very unusual and abnormal phenomenon. A large left-sided azygos vein connected with the LSVC, which was unroofed by a large coronary sinus septal defect and hence drained into the morphologically LA.

To summarize, this patient (see Fig. 29.12A–B) with the heterotaxy syndrome and right-sided polysplenia had situs solitus of the atria (right-sided suprahepatic segment of the IVC, and the morphology of the atrial appendages), partially anomalous pulmonary venous drainage (ipsilateral pulmonary veins), and partially anomalous systemic venous drainage (unroofing of the left-sided coronary sinus receiving the persistent LSVC and the enlarged left azygos vein associated with interruption of the IVC).

Our conclusions are as follows:

1. When pulmonary veins connect with the posterior atrial wall between the RSVC and LSVC and above the coronary sinus, such pulmonary veins are normally connected (see Fig. 29.4).
2. Normally connected pulmonary veins may drain partly or totally anomalously if the septum primum is malpositioned between the pulmonary veins, or entirely to the left of the pulmonary veins, respectively (see Figs. 29.1, 29.2, 29.12).
3. Normally connected systemic veins can drain anomalously, for example, when the coronary sinus is unroofed into the LA.
4. In this patient (see Fig. 29.12A–B), we think that both the pulmonary and the systemic veins were normally connected, but that both drained anomalously, for the reasons described.

Hence, it is important to distinguish between anomalous venous drainage and anomalous venous connections.

Conclusions 1 and 2 concerning normal pulmonary venous connections with anomalous pulmonary venous drainage produced by malposition of the septum primum and associated with a newly recognized type of interatrial communication, that is, a septum primum malposition defect, represents relatively new understanding.[9,12-15,46,131] Although this was a new understanding for us in Boston, as a result of the work of one of us (SVP),[9,12-15] we subsequently found that very similar conclusions had been reached by Edwards[131] in 1953 and by Moller et al[46] in 1967. This important understanding, which was documented echocardiographically for the first time in Figs. 29.1 and 29.2, is relevant not only to the comprehension of the heterotaxy syndromes of asplenia and polysplenia but also to the comprehension and general classification of pulmonary venous anomalies, systemic venous anomalies, and interatrial communications.

Fig. 29.13 presents the heart of a 12 7/12-year-old boy (A67- 2) with the heterotaxy syndrome and right-sided polysplenia with DORV {I,L,L}; that is, there were situs inversus of the atria, concordant L-loop ventricles, and L malposition of the great arteries. CCAVC (type A of Rastelli) and a subpulmonary conus only with aortic-AV valvar fibrous continuity were also present.

Fig. 29.13A shows the interior of the left-sided morphologically RA. Anterior is toward the viewer's left hand, and posterior is toward the viewer's right hand. Note the large, broad, triangular and heavily pectinated RAA that was left-sided. The suprahepatic segment of the interrupted left-sided IVC and the hepatic veins connect with the left-sided RA, as do the coronary sinus and the left-sided SVC. Both the left and right pulmonary veins also drain into the left-sided RA. The septum primum is readily seen from within the left-sided RA. The septum primum is malpositioned to the right of all of the pulmonary veins. A small septum primum malposition type of ASD is seen above the malposed septum primum. A large primum type of ASD and a common AV valve are present beneath the malpositioned septum primum; CCAVC is found, there being a VSD of the AV canal type.

Fig. 29.13B shows the opened right-sided morphologically LA. Anterior is toward the viewer's right hand, and posterior is toward the viewer's left hand, and posterior is toward the viewer's left hand. The small, long, thin, and finger like LAA is reflected posteriorly. (Left isomerism of the left-sided and right-sided atrial appendages is not present.) The large primum type of ASD, the common AV valve, and the right-sided morphologically LV are seen. Note that the septum primum is difficult to identify from this left atrial viewpoint. No caval or pulmonary vein enters this right-sided LA. Consequently, it would be easy to make this misdiagnosis of the left-sided RA (Fig. 29.13A) as a common atrium because it receives all of the systemic and pulmonary veins. It would be similarly easy to miss the presence of the small right sided LA because it receives none of the systemic or pulmonary veins. This relatively small right-sided LA leads by a relatively small mitral component of the common AV valve into the right-sided LV, from which no great artery originates because DORV coexists.

Nonetheless, *from a diagnostic standpoint,* it is helpful to understand that marked malposition of septum primum in the direction of the morphologically LAA can simulate common atrium by facilitating drainage of all the normally connected pulmonary veins into the morphologically RA. Hence, the understanding of septum primum malposition is of very practical diagnostic assistance. This understanding can be lifesaving if a normally arising aorta emerges from the right-sided LV. *Surgically,* what needs to be done, among other things, is resection of the rightwardly malpositioned atrial septum and creation of a correctly positioned atrial septum to the left of these inverted but otherwise normally connected pulmonary veins.

Fig. 29.13C shows this same heart and the right lung from the posterior aspect. The patient's left side is toward the viewer's left hand and the patient's right side is toward the viewer's right hand. Note that the LSVC and the left sided suprahepatic segment of the interrupted IVC that receives the hepatic veins both lie to the left of the connections of the left pulmonary veins, just as one would expect in otherwise unremarkable atrial situs inversus. Both the left and the right pulmonary veins connect with the dorsal atrial wall in an inverted normal way. The fact that all of these inverted normally connected pulmonary veins drain into the left-sided right atrium is not due to anomalous connection of the pulmonary veins, but to rightward malposition of the atrial septum—to the right of the right pulmonary veins. Malposition of the atrial septum may be more clearly seen and understood echocardiographically (see Figs. 29.1 and 29.2) than anatomically (see Fig. 29.13A–B). Note also that the left-sided bronchus is seen passing beneath the large left pulmonary artery. In situs inversus totalis but without visceral heterotaxy, the left-sided bronchus is eparterial: the bronchus to the left upper lobe passes above the left pulmonary artery and hence is upon or above (Greek, *epi*) the left pulmonary artery (epiarterial being contracted to eparterial). However, in this patient with polysplenia, both bronchi were hyparterial (Greek, *hypo,* "below" or "beneath"), as is seen in Fig. 29.13C. Bilaterally hyparterial bronchi is characteristic of the heterotaxy syndrome with polysplenia.

Fig. 29.14 presents the heart and lungs of a 7-year-old girl with the heterotaxy syndrome with right-sided polysplenia, solitus atria, D-loop ventricles, and solitus normally related great arteries, that is, {S,D,S} (A68-66).

Fig. 29.14A shows the interior of the right-sided morphologically RA. The appendage was broad and triangular but has been partially amputated. The IVC, coronary sinus, and RSVC all connect with this RA. The septum primum is well seen from within the RA, although the superior limbic band of septum secundum is virtually absent (perhaps explaining, at least in part, why the septum primum is so well visualized from the right atrial view). The septum primum is malpositioned, lying to the left of the entry of the left pulmonary veins (the lower pulmonary veins in this photograph) and to the left of the right pulmonary veins (the upper pulmonary veins in this photograph). Hence, TAPVD is associated with markedly leftward malposition of the atrial septum. The septum primum malposition type of ASD is seen above the superior rim of the septum primum. Note also the divided AV canal, the unremarkable appearing

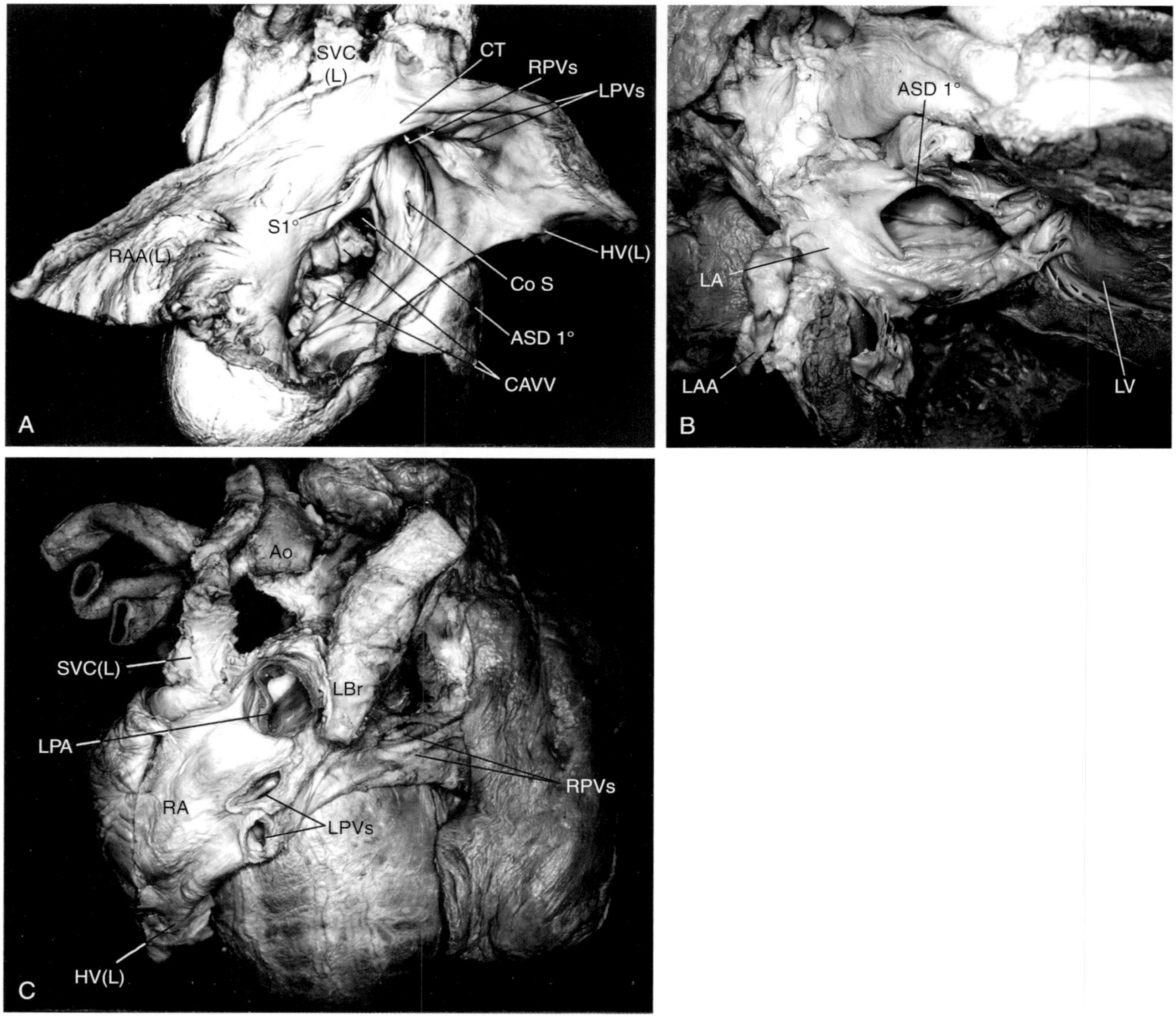

Fig. 29.13 The heterotaxy syndrome with right-sided polysplenia and double-outlet right ventricle {I,L,L} in a 12 7/12-year-old boy. (A) Interior of morphologically right atrium *(RA)* with broad triangular right atrial appendage that is left-sided *(RAA[L])*. Anterior is to the viewer's left. There was interruption of the inferior vena cava (IVC). This left-sided *RA* receives the left-sided suprahepatic segment of the inferior vena cava (IVC) and the hepatic veins, left-sided *(HV[L])*, the left-sided superior vena cava *(SVC[L])*, the coronary sinus *(CoS)*, the right pulmonary veins *(RPVs)* and the left pulmonary veins *(LPVs)*. Septum primum *(S1°)* is displaced into the right-sided morphologically left atrium *(LA)*, to the right of all the pulmonary veins. The septum primum malposition type of atrial septal defect (above S1°) is small and restrictive. S1° is visible only from RA side (not from LA side, as normally is the case). Completely common atrioventricular canal type A of Rastelli is present; note the ostium primum type of atrial septal defect (ASD 1°) and the common atrioventricular valve *(CAVV)*. The left-sided crista terminalis *(CT)* is seen between the venous component of the RA associated with the SVC(L) and the RAA(L). (B) Interior of the right-sided morphologically LA. The long, thin, narrow, left atrial appendage *(LAA)* has been reflected posteroinferiorly. Note that no pulmonary veins enter the LA, and that the septum primum is difficult to identify from the left atrial view. The ASD 1° component of the atrioventricular septal defect, the right portion of the CAVV (unlabeled), and the right sided morphologically left ventricle (LV) are also seen. (C) In this posterior view, note that the LPVs and RPVs both connect to the right of the left-sided SVC, and the left-sided suprahepatic segment of the IVC and the HV(L)s. These relations are normal in visceroatrial situs inversus; that is, the pulmonary veins are not anomalously connected with the left-sided RA. Note that the left mainstem bronchus *(LBr)* is hyparterial, passing beneath the left pulmonary artery *(LPA)*. *Ao*, Aorta. (Reproduced with permission from Van Praagh S, Santini F, Sanders SP. Cardiac malpositions with special emphasis on visceral heterotaxy (asplenia and polysplenia syndromes). In: Fyler DC, ed. *Nadas' Pediatric Cardiology*. Philadelphia, PA: Hanley & Belfus; 1992:589.13.[15])

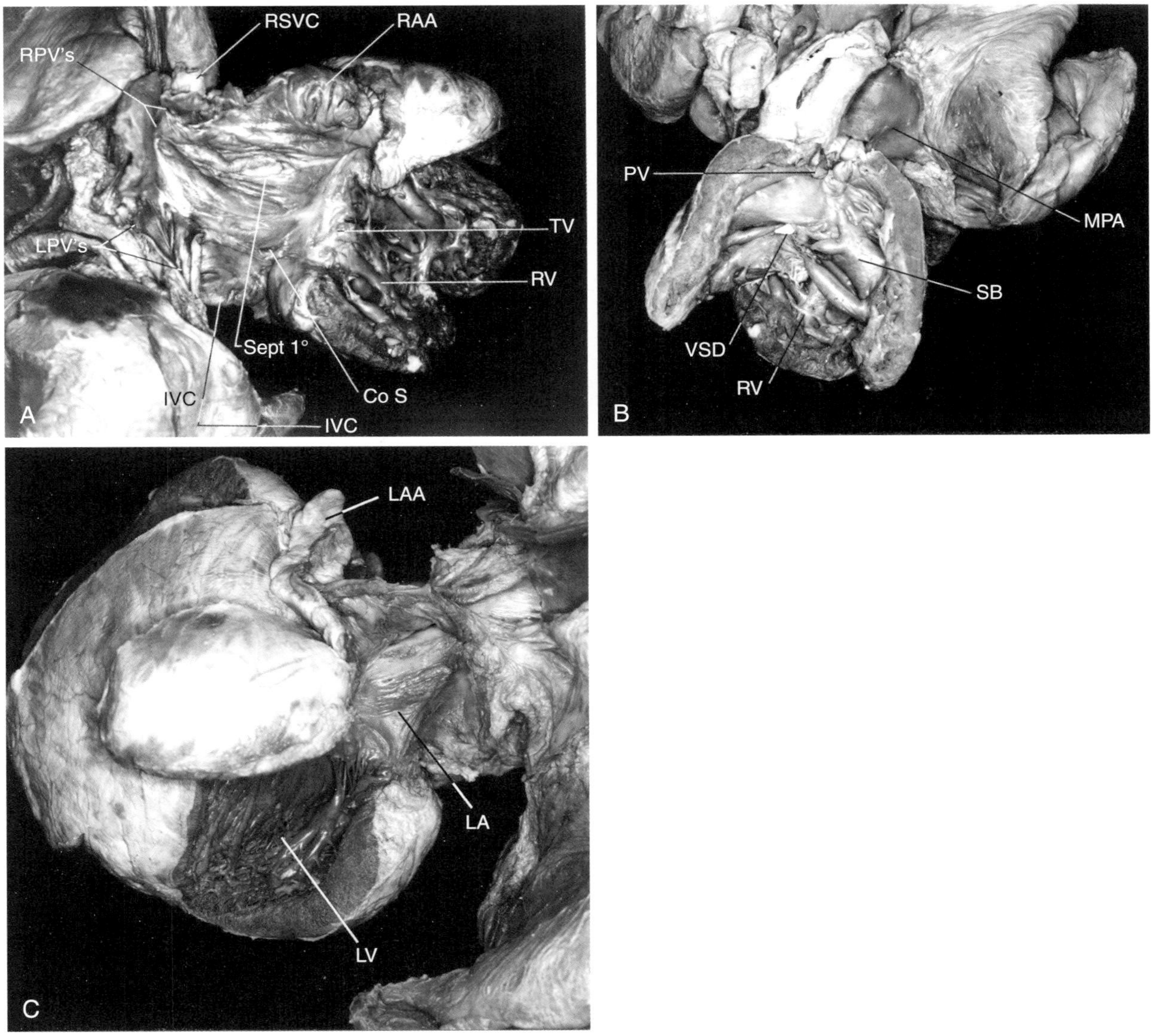

Fig. 29.14 Heterotaxy syndrome with right-sided polysplenia in a 7-year-old girl (A68-66) with normal segmental anatomy, that is, {S,D,S} and totally anomalous pulmonary venous drainage into the right atrium secondary to leftward malposition of the septum primum. (A) Interior view of right-sided morphologically right atrium, same view as shown in Fig. 29.3, except that restrictive septum primum malposition defect is filled with cotton wool (*white,* above *Sept 1°*) for greater clarity. (B) Interior of the markedly hypertrophied right ventricle *(RV)*. The *white arrowhead* is through a very small membranous ventricular septal defect *(VSD)*. The pulmonary valve *(PV)* and main pulmonary artery *(MPA)* are widely patent. The septal band *(SB)* and the papillary muscles are notably hypertrophied. (C) Interior of small left atrium *(LA)* and the inflow tract of the left ventricle *(LV)*. Note that the left atrial appendage *(LAA)* is long, thin, finger-like, and posterior. No pulmonary veins drain into the LA, and the septum primum is difficult to identify from the LA view. *Co S,* Coronary sinus; *IVC,* inferior vena cava; *LPVs,* left pulmonary veins; *RAA,* right atrial appendage; *RPVs,* right pulmonary veins; *RSVC,* right superior vena cava; *TV,* tricuspid valve. (Reproduced with permission from Van Praagh S, Santini F, Sanders SP. Cardiac malpositions with special emphasis on visceral heterotaxy (asplenia and polysplenia syndromes). In: Fyler DC, ed. *Nadas' Pediatric Cardiology*. Philadelphia, PA: Hanley & Belfus; 1992:589.13.[15])

tricuspid valve, and the hypertrophied right ventricular sinus (body, or inflow tract).

Fig. 29.14B shows the interior of the hypertrophied RV. The subpulmonary infundibulum is well developed and nonobstructive, and a small membranous VSD is seen.

Fig. 29.14C shows the interior of the markedly hypoplastic left atrium, mitral valve, and left ventricle, from which a hypoplastic ascending aorta (not seen) originates. Note that the malpositioned septum primum is not readily identified from the left atrial perspective. The atrial septal defect above the malpositioned septum primum was restrictively small, resulting in hypoplasia of the left heart. Note the long, thin, posterior, finger-like LAA. (Left isomerism of the atria or of the atrial appendages was not present.) *Diagnostically,* in cases such as this, it is

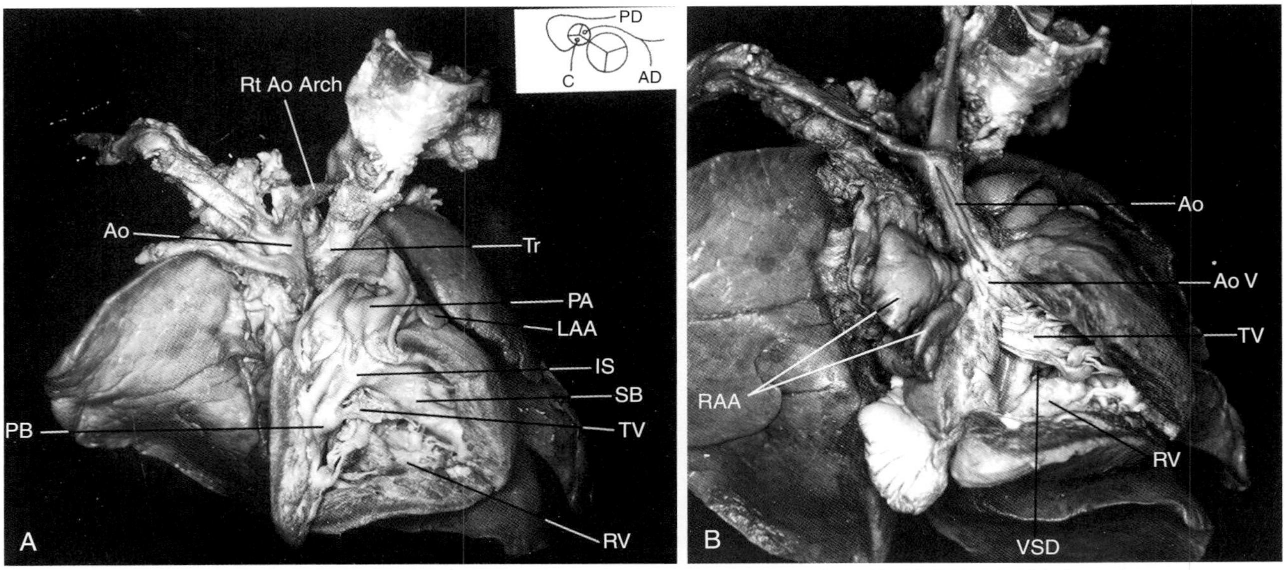

Fig. 29.15 The heterotaxy syndrome with right-sided polysplenia in a 3-day-old girl (C83-98). This heart has double-outlet right ventricle (DORV) {S,D,D}, interruption of the inferior vena cava (IVC), prominent left azygos vein connecting with left superior vena cava that drained into the left atrium because of unroofing of the coronary sinus, suprahepatic segment of the IVC and right superior vena cava connecting with the right atrium (RA), totally anomalous pulmonary venous drainage to RA because of leftward malposition of the septum primum, completely common atrioventricular canal, subpulmonary conus, severe subaortic stenosis, hypoplasia of aortic valve and ascending aorta *(Ao)* and right aortic arch *(Rt Ao Arch)*, left patent ductus arteriosus, and aberrant left subclavian artery. (A) Opened right ventricle *(RV)* with well-developed subpulmonary conus opening into widely patent pulmonary artery *(PA)*. Note the well-developed infundibular septum *(IS)*, parietal band *(PB)*, and septal band *(SB)*. The tricuspid valvar component *(TV)* of the common atrioventricular (AV) valve appears normally situated relative to the IS. Where is the aortic outflow tract? Note the hypoplasia of the aortic valve *(diagrammatic inset)*, of the ascending aorta, and of the right aortic arch. Such hypoplasia indicates severe subaortic stenosis. But where is it? (B) To show the subaortic stenosis, it was necessary to cut through the conal septum, as in a Konno procedure. The subaortic outflow tract was squeezed between the well-developed and normally located IS (best seen in A) and the tricuspid valvar component of the common AV valve, well seen here *(TV)*. Note the direct fibrous continuity between the hypoplastic aortic valve *(AoV)* and the superior leaflet of the common AV valve (TV). DORV with a unilateral conus, in this case with a subpulmonary conus only, resulted in severe aortic outflow tract stenosis apparently because of failure of expansile growth and development of the subaortic part of the conus, which is typical with polysplenia, but rare with asplenia. When DORV has a unilateral conus—subpulmonary (as here), or subaortic—the undeveloped conus often is associated with a stenotic outflow tract. The ventricular septal defect *(VSD)* component of the AV septal defect can also be seen. Note the large and anterior right atrial appendage *(RAA)*, which is much larger than the left atrial appendage *(LAA)*, seen here and in A. *AD*, anterior descending coronary artery; *C*, coronary artery, right; *PD*, posterior descending coronary artery; *Tr*, trachea. (Reproduced with permission from Van Praagh S, Santini F, Sanders SP. Cardiac malpositions with special emphasis on visceral heterotaxy (asplenia and polysplenia syndromes). In: Fyler DC, ed. *Nadas' Pediatric Cardiology*. Philadelphia, PA: Hanley & Belfus; 1992:589.13.[15])

vital to recognize that the RA (see Fig. 29.14A) is indeed the morphologically RA, and not a common atrium, despite the fact that this chamber receives all the systemic and all the pulmonary veins. This diagnostic realization is aided by the understanding that the septum primum can be displaced between the pulmonary veins (resulting in ipsilateral pulmonary venous drainage) or to the left of all the pulmonary veins (resulting in TAPVD, as in this patient). Understanding of septum primum or atrial septal malposition then spurs the diagnostic search for the diminutive LA into which little blood is flowing because the malpositioned atrial septum has a restrictively small ASD. Septum primum malposition ASDs often are restrictively small, this being one of the reasons why the displaced septum primum is difficult to identify from the left atrial perspective (see Fig. 29.14C). Surgically, these cases need to have the malpositioned atrial septum resected, with reconstruction of the atrial septum to the right of the pulmonary veins, thereby creating normal left- and right-heart hemodynamics.

Fig. 29.15 presents the heart and lungs of a 3-day-old girl with the heterotaxy syndrome and a right-sided polysplenia (C83-98). She had DORV {S,D,"S"}, with a subpulmonary conus, aortic outflow tract stenosis, right aortic arch, left ductus arteriosus, and an aberrant left subclavian artery. The suprahepatic segment of the interrupted IVC connected with the RA, as did the RSVC. A left-sided enlarged azygos vein connected with a LSVC that drained into the morphologically LA because the coronary sinus was unroofed by a large coronary sinus septal defect. All of the pulmonary veins drained into the morphologically RA because of leftward malposition of the septum primum, as in Figs. 29.12 and 29.14.

Fig. 29.15A presents the opened RV, pulmonary valve, and MPA of this patient. Note the small LAA to the left of the MPA. The subpulmonary infundibular septum is well developed and normally positioned. The ascending aorta is hypoplastic, as is the right aortic arch. In the diagrammatic *inset,* note that the aortic valve was tricuspid and tricommissural, but decidedly hypoplastic compared with the unobstructed pulmonary valve. The origins, courses, and distributions of the coronary arteries were unremarkable. Note that the semilunar interrelationship looks like that of solitus normally related great arteries, not like that of DORV. But remember, DORV is indeed present. Note also that the tricuspid component of this CCAVC presents a usual appearance. But the question is: Where is the aortic outflow tract? The answer is not at all obvious (see Fig. 29.15A). And that is the point. As the diagrammatic inset shows, the aortic valve is located approximately normally, being posterior, rightward, and inferior relative to the pulmonary valve. Blood had to slip between the conal septum anteriorly and the anterior leaflet of the tricuspid valvar component of the common AV valve posteriorly to reach the hypoplastic aortic valve.

Fig. 29.15B shows the highly stenotic aortic outflow tract, which is located between an essentially normally located conal septum anteriorly and the anterior leaflet of the common AV valve posteriorly. There is direct fibrous continuity between the aortic valve and the anterosuperior leaflet of the common AV valve.

The VA alignments, segmental set, and conal anatomy of this heart are DORV {S,D,D} with subpulmonary conus. The semilunar interrelation is very like that of solitus normally related great arteries (diagrammatic *inset,* Fig. 29.15A). However, the VA alignments were those of DORV, not solitus normally related great arteries. (Hence, we could not make the diagnosis of DORV {S,D,S} because the third element of the segmental set {-,-,S} is wrong. Also, DORV {S,D,S} would be a contradiction in terms: DORV cannot be entirely solitus normally related.) This is why quotation marks were placed around the third element of the segmental situs set: **DORV {S,D,"S"}.** "S" indicates that the infundibuloarterial part of the heart was very similar to the solitus normal conotruncus, but that the VA alignments were not solitus normal, but those of DORV. "S" means very similar to solitus normally related great arteries (i.e., with subpulmonary conus and aortic-AV fibrous continuity).

It should be understood what DORV {S,D,D} with a subpulmonary conus really means. Because there is a subpulmonary conus (only), consequently there is aortic-AV fibrous continuity because of the absence of subaortic conal free wall musculature.

Why was there severe subaortic stenosis? Because, when a well-expanded subaortic conus is not present, the aortic outflow tract in DORV can get squeezed between an approximately normally located conal septum anteriorly and the AV valve posteriorly. A well-developed, well-expanded conus prevents subsemilunar outflow tract obstruction—stenosis or atresia. This is precisely what was not present in this case: a well-developed and well-expanded subaortic conus. The larger point is that a well-developed and well-expanded subaortic conus is not characteristic of the polysplenia syndrome, even when DORV is present.

The VSD associated with this common AV canal can be seen (see Fig. 29.15B). Note also the large triangular RAA to the right of the hypoplastic ascending aorta. (Again, left isomerism of the atria or of the atrial appendages was not found.)

Visceral Heterotaxy With Normally Formed Spleen

We have seen only 5 postmortem cases of visceral heterotaxy with a normally formed spleen, which constitutes only 3% of our 168 patients with visceral heterotaxy (see Table 29.1). In all 5 cases, the spleen was right-sided.

Sex: Male-to-female, 3/2 (1.5/1).

Age at Death: Mean, 39 ± 79 days; range, 18 hours to 6 months; and median, 4 days. Lung Lobation: bilaterally trilobed, 3 (60%); normal (situs solitus), 1 (20%); and hypoplastic right lung with scimitar syndrome, 1 patient (20%).

Segmental Sets: Every case was different, but then our experience with this rare entity is very small: {S,D,S}, TGA {S,D,D}, DORV {S,1,D}, {I, D,I }, and DORV {I,D,D}.

Visceral Situs: Situs ambiguus in all.

Atrial Situs: Solitus in 3, inversus in 2.

Ventricular Loop: D-loop ventricles in 4, 1-loop ventricles in 1.

Atrioventricular Alignments: AV concordance in 2, that is, {S,D,-}; and AV discordance in 3, that is, {S,L,-} in 1, and {I,D,-} in 2.

Ventriculoarterial Alignments: Normal in 2, that is, solitus normal (S) in 1 and inversus normal (I) in 1; 0-TGA in 1; and DORV with 0-malposition of the great arteries in 2.

However, as the segmental sets make clear, the patient with inverted normally related great arteries had the segmental combination of **{I,D,I}.** In words this may be called **isolated ventricular noninversion,** meaning that everything except the ventricles is inverted. This is another anatomic type of AV discordance with VA concordance. Therapeutically, an atrial switch procedure is indicated, if otherwise feasible. Hence, in this patient, the VA alignments are as normal as is possible between noninverted (0-loop) ventricles and inverted great arteries.

Ventriculoarterial Situs: Although {I,D,I} has VA alignment concordance (the LV ejects into the aorta, and the RV into the pulmonary artery), it is also noteworthy that VA situs discordance coexists (the ventricles are noninverted or 0-loop, whereas the great arteries are inverted normally related). This case clearly illustrates the difference between alignment concordance or discordance and situs concordance or discordance. Similarly, in DORV {S,L,D}, there is VA *situs* discordance: L-loop or inverted ventricles, with D-malposition or noninverted malposed great arteries.

Conus: Subpulmonary in 2, bilateral in 2, and bilaterally deficient in 1.

Superior Vena Cava: Unilateral, to RA, in 4; and bilateral, to RA and to the coronary sinus, in 1.

Inferior Vena Cava: Uninterrupted, to RA, in 5.

Pulmonary Veins: There was TAPVC in 3 of 5 cases: to the RA in 1; to the left innominate vein in 1; and to the RSVC in 1. Partially anomalous pulmonary venous connection in the form of the scimitar syndrome was found in 1. The pulmonary veins connected normally with the LA in 1 patient.

Atrial Septum: Common atrium in 3 of 5, secundum atrial septal defect in 1, and patent foramen ovale in 1.

Atrioventricular Valves: Common AV canal was present in 3 of 5 patients: 2 had a VSD of the AV canal type (typical complete form); but 1 case had a single RV (with absence of the LV), and consequently no interventricular septal defect could be present. Hence, whether the latter case had a complete or a partial form of common AV canal is unresolved. Normal AV valves were present in 2 of 5 patients.

Right Ventricle: Hypoplastic in 2, absent in 1 (single LV), normal in 1, and single RV because of absent LV in 1.

Left Ventricle: Hypertrophy and enlargement in 3 of 5; normal in 1; and absent (single RV) in 1.

Ventricular Septum: VSD of AV canal type in 2 of 5; conoventricular type of VSD in 1; and intact in 2.

Pulmonary Outflow Tract: Atretic in 3 of 5; stenotic in 1; and not obstructed in 1.

Aortic Outflow Tract: No obstruction in all 5.

Is visceral heterotaxy with a normally formed spleen more like the asplenia syndrome, or more like the polysplenia syndrome? Although only 5 cases is a very small series on which to base any generalizations, our impression is that heterotaxy with a normally formed spleen more closely resembles the asplenia syndrome than the polysplenia syndrome. For example, all 5 patients had continuous (noninterrupted) IVC, as in asplenia. However, more experience with heterotaxy and a normally formed spleen is needed before it will be possible to answer this question with confidence.

Comparison of Asplenia and Polysplenia

Are we dealing with the heterotaxy syndrome (singular), or are there really multiple heterotaxy syndromes (plural)? Is the polysplenia syndrome a *forme fruste* of the asplenia syndrome, or are the asplenia and the polysplenia syndromes really two significantly different syndromes? Is there really only one heterotaxy syndrome, or are there two or perhaps even three different heterotaxy syndromes? In an effort to answer these questions, let us compare the asplenia and the polysplenia syndromes both anatomically and statistically.

RELATIONS BETWEEN THE GREAT ARTERIES

The relations between the great arteries, that is, the VA alignments, in the heterotaxy syndrome with asplenia and in the heterotaxy syndrome with polysplenia are summarized in Table 29.43. As will be seen, the VA alignments in these two syndromes are significantly different.

Normally related great arteries was the least frequent type of VA alignment with asplenia (9%), but was the most frequent type with polysplenia (69%) ($p < .0001$). DORV was the most frequent type of VA alignment with asplenia (67%) but was much less common with polysplenia (24%) ($p < .0001$). *TGA* occurred in 22% of the cases with the asplenia syndrome but in only 6% of patients with the polysplenia syndrome ($p < .005$). Hence, abnormally related great arteries (i.e., conotruncal anomalies, either DORV or TGA) were characteristic of patients with asplenia (85/94, 90%), whereas normally related great arteries were typical of patients with polysplenia (47/67, 69%) ($p < .0001$).

TABLE 29.43 Relations Between the Great Arteries

Type of VA Alignment	Asplenia (n = 94)	Polysplenia (n = 67)	*p* Value
Normally related great arteries	9 (9%)	47 (69%)	<.0001
Double-outlet right ventricle	64 (67%)	16 (24%)	<.0001
Transposition of the great arteries	21 (22%)	4 (6%)	<.005

VA, Ventriculoarterial.

TABLE 29.44 The Superior Vena(e) Cava(e)

Status of the SVC(s)	Asplenia (n = 72)	Polysplenia (n = 67)	*p* Value
	17 (20%)	30 (45%)	<.005
RSVC only	8 (9%)	8 (12%)	NS
LSVC only	47 (55%)	29 (43%)	NS

LSVC, Left superior vena cava; *NS,* statistically not significant; *RSVC,* right superior vena cava; *SVC(s),* superior vena cava or superior venae cavae.

The Superior Vena Cava

The anatomic status of the SVC (or of the SVCs) in the heterotaxy syndrome with asplenia and in the heterotaxy syndrome with polysplenia is summarized in Table 29.44.

The only significant difference in the anatomic status of the SVC between the asplenia and the polysplenia syndromes was that a RSVC (only) was more likely to occur in the polysplenia syndrome (45%) than in the asplenia syndrome (20%) ($p < .005$). The prevalences of an LSVC (only) and of bilateral SVCs were not statistically significantly different between the asplenia and the polysplenia syndromes.

The Inferior Vena Cava

The anatomic status of the IVC in the heterotaxy syndromes of asplenia and polysplenia are summarized in Table 29.45.

Interruption of the IVC (between the renal veins below and the hepatic veins above, with an enlarged azygos vein to an SVC) was much more common with the polysplenia syndrome (56%) than with the asplenia syndrome (3%) ($p < .0001$). Thus interruption of the IVC can occur in the asplenia syndrome, but it is rare.

A left-sided LVC was much more common with asplenia (37%) than with polysplenia (10%) ($p < .001$). A right-sided IVC was equally common with asplenia and with polysplenia (32% with both; see Table 29.4).

The Atrial Appendages

The morphologic anatomic findings concerning the atrial appendages in the heterotaxy syndromes with asplenia and with polysplenia are summarized in Table 29.46. *Solitus appearing*

TABLE 29.45 The Inferior Vena Cava

Status of the IVC	Asplenia (n = 54)	Polysplenia (n = 67)	*p* Value
Right-sided IVC	24 (32%)	22 (32%)	NS
Left-sided IVC	28 (37%)	7 (10%)	<.001
Interrupted IVC	2 (3%)	38 (56%)	<.0001

IVC, Inferior vena cava; *NS*, statistically not significant.

TABLE 29.46 The Atrial Appendages

Findings	Asplenia (n = 43)	Polysplenia (n = 16)	*p* Value
Solitus appendages	22 (51%)	8 (50%)	NS
Inversus appendages	12 (28%)	3 (19%)	NS
Both rightish	9 (21%)	0 (0%)	.04[a]
Both leftish	0 (0%)	5 (31%)	.0009[a]

[a]Fisher exact test.
NS, Statistically not significant.

atrial appendages (morphologically RAA right-sided and morphologically LAA left-sided) was the commonest pattern both with asplenia (51%) and with polysplenia (50%) (p = not significant). *Inverted appearing atrial appendages* (morphologically RAA left-sided and morphologically LAA right-sided) was the second most common pattern in the asplenia syndrome (28%), and third most prevalent in the polysplenia syndrome (19%) (p = not significant). Both atrial appendages appearing rightish (large, broad, triangular atrial appendages bilaterally) was the least frequent pattern in these 43 postmortem cases of visceral heterotaxy with asplenia (21%), this appendage pattern being found in no case with polysplenia (0%) ($p = .04$).

Both atrial appendages appearing leftish (long, thin, fingerlike atrial appendages bilaterally) was the second most common pattern with polysplenia (31%) but did not occur with asplenia (0%) ($p = .0009$) (see Table 29.5). In an effort to avoid observer bias, the foregoing conclusions are what multiple different observers thought at the time of autopsy. None of our original observations has been altered to support any point of view. If no conclusion was recorded at the time of necropsy, such cases are not included here.

TYPES OF ATRIAL SITUS

Realizing that it is usually possible to diagnose the basic type of atrial situs despite the presence of visceral heterotaxy,[9,10,12-15] we summarize these findings in Table 29.47.

The type of atrial situs was *situs solitus* much more often in the polysplenia syndrome (72%) than in the asplenia syndrome (42%) ($p < .001$).

Conversely, the type of atrial situs was judged to be *situs inversus* more often with asplenia (31%) than with polysplenia (22%), but this difference was not statistically significant (see Table 29.47). *Visceroatrial situs discordance* occurred both with asplenia and with polysplenia. It was always of the same anatomic type: situs inversus of the abdominal viscera, with situs

TABLE 29.47 Types of Atrial Situs

Types of Situs	Asplenia (n = 95)	Polysplenia (n = 67)	*p* Value
Situs solitus situs	40 (42%)	48 (72%)	<.001
Inversus	29 (31%)	15 (22%)	NS
Inversus viscera with solitus atria	1 (1%)	3 (4%)	—
Situs ambiguous (undiagnosed)	25 (26%)	1 (1%)	<.0001

NS, Statistically not significant.

TABLE 29.48 Types of AV Alignment

Type of AV Alignment	Asplenia (n = 95)	Polysplenia (n = 67)	*p* Value
AV Concordance	29 (31%)	53 (79%)	<.0001
AV Discordance	28 (29%)	11 (16%)	NS (.056)
Common-Inlet RV	17 (18%)	0 (0%)	<.001
Common-Inlet LV	4 (4%)	2 (3%)	—
Indeterminate	17 (18%)	1 (1%)	<.01

AV, Atrioventricular; *LV*, morphologically left ventricle; *NS*, statistically not significant; *RV*, morphologically right ventricle.

solitus of the atria (never vice versa). (It will be recalled that almost always, visceroatrial situs concordance (not discordance) is present: both viscera and atria in situs solitus, or both viscera and atria in situs inversus. These cases are the exceptions.)

The rare situation of inverted viscera with solitus atria (thinking in sequential or blood-flow order) was somewhat more common with polysplenia (4%) than with asplenia (1%).

Visceroatrial situs ambiguus, that is, undiagnosed type(s) of visceral and atrial situs was much more common with asplenia (26%) than with polysplenia (1%) ($p < .0001$) (see Table 29.6).

Atrioventricular Alignments

The types of AV alignments (which many call connections) are presented and compared in Table 29.48.

AV concordance was much more common with polysplenia (79%) than with asplenia (31%) ($p < .0001$). Conversely, AV discordance was more common with asplenia (29%) than with polysplenia (16%), but this difference was statistically not significant, although it was very close to statistical significance ($p = .056$).

Common-inlet RV, that is, a common AV valve opening entirely or predominantly into the morphologically RV, occurred in 18% of these 95 postmortem cases with asplenia, but in none of these 67 patients with polysplenia (0%) ($p < .001$). *Common-inlet LV*, that is, a common AV valve opening entirely or predominantly into the morphologically LV, occurred with an approximately equally low prevalence in both the asplenia syndrome (4%) and in the polysplenia syndrome (3%).

An indeterminate AV alignment was much more common with asplenia (18%) than with polysplenia (1%) ($p < .01$) (see Table 29.7). The reason for an indeterminate AV alignment is the presence of undiagnosed atrial situs (situs ambiguus), which was far more common with asplenia than with polysplenia.

TABLE 29.49 Types of Ventricular Loop

Type of Loop	Asplenia (n = 95)	Polysplenia (n = 67)	*p* Value
D-Loop ventricles	62 (65%)	50 (75%)	NS
L-Loop ventricles	33 (35%)	17 (25%)	NS

NS, Statistically not significant.

TABLE 29.50 Types of Aortic Arch

Types of Aortic Arch	Asplenia (n = 93)	Polysplenia (n = 61)	*p* Value
Left	37 (40%)	43 (70%)	<.001
Right	56 (60%)	18 (30%)	<.001

Ventricular Loop

The types of ventricular loop are summarized in Table 29.49. *D-loop ventricles* were more common with polysplenia (75%) than with asplenia (65%). Conversely, *L-loop ventricles* were more frequent with asplenia (35%) than with polysplenia (25%). However, neither of these differences reached statistical significance (see Table 29.49).

Aortic Arch

The types of aortic arch are summarized and compared in Table 29.50. A *left aortic arch* was much more common with polysplenia (70%) than with asplenia (40%) ($p < .001$). Conversely, a *right aortic arch* was twice as frequent with asplenia (60%) as with polysplenia (30%) ($p < .001$). Note that a double aortic arch was not encountered.

Ductus Arteriosus

The findings concerning the ductus arteriosus are presented and compared in Table 29.51. Although the prevalences of patent ductus arteriosus and of closed ductus arteriosus were not significantly different with asplenia and polysplenia, the prevalence of congenital absence of the ductus arteriosus was much higher with asplenia (27%) than with polysplenia (12%) ($p < .05$).

The Atrioventricular Valves

The findings concerning the AV valves are presented and compared in Table 29.52. *Common AV canal* was more than twice as common with asplenia (96%) as with polysplenia (45%) ($p < .0001$). *The complete form* of common AV canal was much more common with asplenia than with polysplenia (33%) ($p < .001$). However, *the partial form* of common AV canal was statistically not significantly different with asplenia (15%) than with polysplenia (12%).

Normal AV valves were quite common with polysplenia (55%), but rare with asplenia (4%) ($p < .0001$). The foregoing statistical analysis of the anatomic data led us to suggest several conclusions:

1. **Two different syndromes.** In view of the many statistically highly significant differences between the asplenia and the polysplenia syndromes documented earlier, we regard them as two different syndromes.

TABLE 29.51 The Ductus Arteriosus

Findings	Asplenia (n = 90)	Polysplenia (n = 60)	*p* Value
Patent Ductus Arteriosus	44 (49%)	33 (55%)	NS
Closed Ductus Arteriosus	22 (24%)	20 (33%)	NS
Absent Ductus Arteriosus	24 (27%)	7 (12%)	<.05

TABLE 29.52 The Atrioventricular Valves

Findings	Asplenia (n = 95)	Polysplenia (n = 67)	*p* Value
Common AV Canal	91 (96%)	30 (45%)	<.0001
Complete	77 (81%)	22 (33%)	<.001
Partial	14 (15%)	8 (12%)	NS
Normal AV Valves	4 (4%)	37 (55%)	<.0001

AV, Atrioventricular; *NS*, statistically not significant.

2. **Visceral heterotaxy with a normally formed spleen.** A definitive conclusion concerning whether this is a third and different heterotaxy syndrome requires more data.
3. **Etiologic implications.** The anatomic differences between the asplenia and the polysplenia syndromes suggest that the causes of these two syndromes, presumably genetic, may well prove to be nonidentical. Molecular genetics and time will tell (see later).
4. **Lung lobation.** Bilaterally trilobed lungs were much more common with asplenia (84%) than with polysplenia (3%) ($p < .0001$). Bilaterally bilobed lungs were much more common with polysplenia (57%) than with asplenia (1%) ($p < .0001$). Bilaterally unilobed lungs were infrequent with both asplenia (1%) and with polysplenia (5%). Normal lobation of the lungs was not observed with asplenia but occurred in 22% of patients with polysplenia. Inverted lobation was infrequent with asplenia (3%) and with polysplenia (10%). Other patterns of lobation were found with asplenia (11%) and with polysplenia (2%).
5. **Liver.** The liver was more often bilaterally symmetrical with asplenia (82%) than with polysplenia (61%) ($p < .05$). A solitus liver was more common with polysplenia (29%) than with asplenia (9%) ($p = .017$). An inversus liver was approximately equally frequent with asplenia (9%) and with polysplenia (11%) (p = not significant).
6. **Gallbladder.** The only statistically significant difference was that the gallbladder was more likely to be absent with polysplenia (12%) than with asplenia (6%) ($p <. 01$).
7. **Stomach.** No significant differences were found between the asplenia and the polysplenia syndromes.
8. **Atrial Situs.** The type of atrial situs was more likely to be situs solitus with polysplenia (72%) than with asplenia (42%) ($p < .001$). Undiagnosed atrial situs (situs ambiguus) was more frequent with asplenia (26%) than with polysplenia (1%) ($p <.0001$). No other statistically significant differences were found.
9. **Inferior Vena Cava.** A right-sided IVC was equally common both with asplenia and with polysplenia (32%). A

left-sided IVC was more frequent with asplenia (37%) than with polysplenia (10%) ($p < .001$). An interrupted IVC was much more common with polysplenia (56%) than with asplenia (3%) ($p < .0001$).

10. **Superior Vena Cava.** An RSVC only was more common with polysplenia (45%) than with asplenia (20%) ($p < .005$). Bilateral SVCs were somewhat more frequent with asplenia (55%) than with polysplenia (43%) (p = not significant). An LSVC (only) was infrequent both with asplenia (9%) and polysplenia (12%) (p = not significant).
11. **Pulmonary Veins.** TAPVD was more common with asplenia (69%) than with polysplenia (22%) ($p < .0001$). Partially anomalous pulmonary venous drainage was more frequent with polysplenia (15%) than with asplenia (5%) ($p < .05$). Normally connected pulmonary veins were much more common with polysplenia (63%) than with asplenia (26%) ($p < .0001$).
12. **Atrial Appendages.** Solitus atrial appendages occurred with asplenia in 51% and with polysplenia in 50% (p = not significant). Inverted atrial appendages were found in 28% with asplenia and 19% with polysplenia (p = not significant). Both atrial appendages resembled RAAs in 21% with asplenia and in none with polysplenia ($p = .04$). Both atrial appendages resembled LAAs in none with asplenia and in 31% with polysplenia ($p = .0009$).
13. **Atrial Septum.** Common atrium was much more frequent with asplenia (72%) than with polysplenia (32%) ($p < .001$). An ostium primum type of ASD only was commoner with asplenia (23%) than with polysplenia (10%) ($p < .05$). An ostium secundum type of ASD was somewhat more common with polysplenia (31%) than with asplenia (20%) (p = not significant). A patent foramen ovale or an intact atrial septum was more frequent with polysplenia (22%) than with asplenia (2%) ($p < .001$).
14. **Atrioventricular Valves.** Common AV canal was more frequent with asplenia (96%) than with polysplenia (45%) ($p < .0001$). The complete form of AV canal was more prevalent with asplenia (81%) than with polysplenia (33%) ($p < .0001$). The partial form of common AV canal was about equally infrequent with asplenia (15%) and with polysplenia (12%) (p = not significant). Normal AV valves occurred in more than half of the patients with polysplenia (55%) but were very infrequent with asplenia (4%) ($p < .0001$).
15. **Right Ventricle.** Single morphologically RV (because of absence of the morphologically LV) and functionally single RV (with a diminutive LV) were much more frequent with asplenia (38%) than with polysplenia (2%) ($p < .0001$). Right ventricular hypertrophy and enlargement with a well-developed LV was much more common with polysplenia (71%) than with asplenia (28%) ($p < .0001$). A normal RV was more frequent with polysplenia (16%) than with asplenia (4%) ($p < .025$). Hypoplasia of the right ventricular sinus was somewhat more common with asplenia (19%) than with polysplenia (9%) (p = not significant). Absence of the right ventricular sinus resulting in single LV with an infundibular outlet chamber was approximately equally infrequent both with asplenia (5%) and with polysplenia (3%) (p = not significant).
16. **Left Ventricle.** An absent or rudimentary LV, resulting in an anatomically or functionally single RV was more frequent with asplenia (38%) than with polysplenia (2%) ($p < .0001$). However, mild to moderate left ventricular hypoplasia was more common with polysplenia (38%) than with asplenia (11%) ($p < .0001$). Left ventricular hypertrophy and enlargement was approximately equally prevalent with asplenia (28%) and with polysplenia (22%) (p = not significant). Single LV with infundibular outlet chamber, as a result of absence of the right ventricular sinus, occurred infrequently both with asplenia (5%) and with polysplenia (2%) (p = not significant).
17. **Ventricular Loop.** D-loop ventricles were more common than L-loop ventricles both with asplenia (65%) and with polysplenia (75%) (p = not significant). Conversely, L-loop ventricles were less frequent than D-loop ventricles both with asplenia (35%) and with polysplenia (25%) (p = not significant).
18. **Conus.** Bilateral conus (subaortic and subpulmonary) was much more frequent with asplenia (60%) than with polysplenia (9%) ($p < .0001$). Subaortic conus (only) occurred exclusively with asplenia (27%), never with polysplenia ($p < .0001$). A subpulmonary conus (only) was much more frequent with polysplenia (89%) than with asplenia (14%) ($p < .0001$). A bilaterally deficient conus (permitting aortic-AV valvar and pulmonary AV valvar fibrous continuity) occurred, rarely, with polysplenia (2%) and never with asplenia.
19. **Pulmonary Outflow Tract.** Absence of pulmonary outflow tract obstruction was much more common with polysplenia (63%) than with asplenia (11%) ($p < .0001$). Conversely, pulmonary outflow tract stenosis was more frequent with asplenia (47%) than with polysplenia (31%) ($p < .05$). Similarly, pulmonary outflow tract atresia was much more common with asplenia (42%) than with polysplenia (6%) ($p > .0001$).
20. **Aortic Outflow Tract.** Absence of aortic outflow tract obstruction was the rule both with asplenia (93%) and with polysplenia (89%) (p = not significant). Aortic outflow tract stenosis was rare both with asplenia (3%) and with polysplenia (8%) (p = not significant). Similarly, aortic outflow tract atresia was rare both with asplenia and polysplenia (3% in both) (p = not significant).
21. **Great Arteries.** Normally related great arteries were much more common with polysplenia (69%) than with asplenia (9%) ($p < .0001$). DORV was more frequent with asplenia (67%) than with polysplenia (24%) ($p < .0001$). TGA was also more common with asplenia (22%) than with polysplenia (6%) ($p < .005$).
22. **Aortic Arch.** A left aortic arch was much more frequent with polysplenia (70%) than with asplenia (40%) ($p < .001$). Conversely, a right aortic arch was more common with asplenia (60%) than with polysplenia (30%) ($p < .001$).
23. **Ductus Arteriosus.** The only statistically significant difference was that absence of the ductus arteriosus was more frequent with asplenia (27%) than with polysplenia (12%) ($p < .05$).

In the foregoing anatomic and statistical comparison of the asplenia and polysplenia syndromes, 20 anatomic features were compared and contrasted (items 4 to 23, inclusive). Of these 20 anatomic features, statistically significant differences between the asplenia and polysplenia syndromes were found in 17 (85%). Concerning only 3 anatomic considerations (15%) were statistically significant differences not found: (1) the stomach (item 7); (2) D-loop ventricles and L-loop ventricles (item 17); and (3) the aortic outflow tract (item 20).

We think that the previously mentioned findings support the conclusion that the constellations of findings associated with asplenia and polysplenia have many significant differences, but that these syndromes also share some findings that do not differ significantly: 85% difference, 15% overlap, as documented above.

Appendage Shapes. Why are atrial appendages shaped as they are? Why is the normal RAA broad, large, and triangular, with the appendage well incorporated into the right atrial chamber? Conversely, why is the normal LAA long, thin, and finger-like, with the appendage poorly incorporated into the left atrial chamber? In the heterotaxy syndrome with asplenia, why may both atrial appendages appear "rightish," as in 21% of our cases? In the heterotaxy syndrome with polysplenia, why may both atrial appendages appear "leftish," as in 31% of our cases?

Although there may well be some still unknown genetic factors controlling the shapes of atrial appendages, we think that hemodynamic factors probably also play an important role. The following may be regarded as the hemodynamic hypothesis concerning the shapes of the atrial appendages. Blood from the placenta and lower body flows up the IVC and into the RA. This IVC blood stream flows directly into the RAA, distending it and incorporating it into the cavity of the RA. Some of this IVC blood stream also flows over the top of the septum primum into the LA, where it passes down behind the LAA, through the mitral valve, and into the LV. It is noteworthy that this via sinistra of the embryonic and fetal circulation does not flow directly into the LAA but passes *behind* this appendage. Consequently, the LAA is not distended by hemodynamic forces (as the RAA is). Hence, the LAA remains an undistended appendix to the left atrial cavity. This, we think, may well help to explain the normal differences between the shapes of the RAA and LAA. *But what happens in the heterotaxy syndrome with asplenia?* The IVC is almost never interrupted (97% of our asplenia patients had a noninterrupted IVC). Consequently, as in the normal heart, the blood flows from the placenta and lower body up the IVC and enters the RA. But in asplenia, the atrial septum is often poorly formed (the atrial septum was abnormally formed in 98% of our cases). Consequently, the IVC blood stream often can flow directly into both atrial appendages, distending both, and making both atrial appendages look rightish (as in 21% of our asplenia patients). Also, hepatic veins frequently drain into the LA in the asplenia syndrome.

What happens with the heterotaxy syndrome with polysplenia? The IVC is often interrupted (as in 56% of these polysplenic patients and as in 80% of other series[13]).

Consequently, the blood from the placenta and lower body returns to the heart by an enlarged azygos vein that connects with the SVC. Then, most of the systemic venous blood (except for the hepatic venous return by the suprahepatic segment of the IVC) flows down the SVC into the atrial level, where it passes behind the atrial appendages, through the AV valve, and into the ventricular level. Thus, in the polysplenia syndrome, the systemic venous blood flows behind the atrial appendages, leaving their tips undistended and hence "leftish" in appearance (as in 31% of our polysplenic patients).

When the atrial appendages appear bilaterally rightish, diagnostically this should certainly suggest asplenia. Conversely, when the atrial appendages appear bilaterally leftish, diagnostically this should certainly suggest polysplenia. These atrial appendage appearances are diagnostically very helpful, even though they were found in only a minority of our asplenic patients (21%) and in only a minority of our polysplenic patients (31%).

These atrial appendage shapes are appearances that are hemodynamically understandable. These atrial appendage shapes do not indicate anatomic identity. The RAA is not present bilaterally in a literally accurate sense in some cases of asplenia; this is an appearance, not an anatomic reality.

Similarly, the LAA is not present bilaterally in a literally accurate sense in some cases of polysplenia; again, this is an appearance, not an anatomic reality. These, at least in part, hemodynamically based appearances of the atrial appendages did not prevent the diagnosis of the atrial situs in the majority of our patients with asplenia (74%) and in virtually all of our patients with polysplenia (99%).

Thus the foregoing is our best present understanding of the shapes of the atrial appendages both normally and in the heterotaxy syndromes with asplenia and polysplenia.

Midline-Associated Extracardiac Anomalies

Ticho, Goldstein, and one of us (RVP)[25] completed a study of postmortem cases of the heterotaxy syndromes examined either at Children's Hospital, Boston, or at the Massachusetts General Hospital, Boston, focusing on midline-associated anomalies: asplenia, 90 patients; polysplenia, 60; and right-sided single spleen present, 11 patients (total n = 161). In the heterotaxy syndromes as a whole: levocardia in 84 of 132 (64%), dextrocardia in 42 of 132 (32%), mesocardia in 6 of 132 (4%), D-loop ventricles in 91 of 132 (69%), and loop ventricles in 41 of 132 (32%).

There is a significant correlation between the type of ventricular loop and cardiac sidedness[25]:

1. When D-loop ventricles were present, the heart was left-sided (levocardia) in 74 of 91 patients (81%), right-sided (dextrocardia) in 13 (14%), and midline (mesocardia) in 4 (4%).
2. However, when L-loop ventricles were present, the heart was left-sided in only 10 of 41 patients (24%), right-sided in 29 (71%), and midline in 2 (5%).

These differences between levocardia and dextrocardia with D-loop ventricles and L-loop ventricles are statistically highly significant ($p < .0001$). In other words, with D-loop ventricles, levocardia "should" be present, as in 81% of these heterotaxic patients; whereas, when L-loop ventricles are present, dextrocardia "should" be present, as in 71% of these cases.

Hence, there is a highly significant correlation between the type of ventricular loop (D- or L-) and the sidedness of the heart in the chest (left-sided or right-sided). There is also a significant correlation between the ·atrial situs and the location of the stomach[25]:

1. When the atria were in situs solitus, the stomach was left-sided in 45 of 74 (61%) and right-sided in 29 (39%).
2. However, when the atria were inverted, the stomach was left-sided in only 15 of 46 cases (33%) and right-sided in 31 patients (67%).

The location of the stomach (left-sided or right-sided) was statistically significantly different, depending on the type of atrial situs that coexisted ($p < .01$). In other words, when the atria were in situs solitus, the stomach usually was left-sided, as in 61% of these cases. However, when the atria were in situs inversus, the stomach usually was right-sided, as in 67% of these patients. This is why we speak of the visceroatrial situs, because there is a strong positive correlation between the visceral situs and atrial situs, even in the presence of visceral heterotaxy. In the heterotaxy syndromes, however, the visceroatrial correlations are not nearly as strong as they normally are in visceroatrial situs solitus or visceroatrial situs inversus.

The severity of congenital heart disease was less with left-sided polysplenia than with right-sided polysplenia. For example, the complete form of common AV canal with *left-sided polysplenia* occurred in 7 of 23 patients (30%); whereas with *right-sided polysplenia*, the complete form of common AV canal was found in 12 of 27 patients (44%) ($p < .01$). *Solitary right-sided spleen with visceral heterotaxy* was even more severe, with *CCAVC* in 7 of 11 patients (64%). Asplenia was the most severe, with CCAVC occurring in 72 of 90 patients (80%).

Hence, as far as the status of the AV canal was concerned, a gradient from a lower frequency to a higher frequency of the complete form of common AV canal was found to be as follows: left-sided polysplenia, 30%; right-sided polysplenia, 44%; right-sided spleen with heterotaxy, 64%; and asplenia, 80%.[25] **Lung morphology** was abnormal in 90% of this series as a whole.

In the 90 patients with asplenia, bilaterally trilobed lungs with eparterial bronchi were present in 74 (83%). Among the 60 patients with polysplenia, bilaterally bilobed lungs with hyparterial bronchi were found in 34 (61%). In the remaining polysplenic patients, solitus lobation occurred in 11 (20%), inversus lobation in 6 (11%), bilaterally trilobed in 4 (7%), and bilaterally unilobed in 2 (3.5%).[25] **Gastrointestinal anomalies** were present in all.

A right-sided stomach was found in 40% of asplenics (36 of 90), in 45% of polysplenics (27 of 60), and in 100% of patients with a right-sided spleen and heterotaxy.

Malrotation of the bowel was present in 52 of the 161 (33%): with asplenia, 33 of 90 (37%); with polysplenia, 16 of 60 (27%); and with right-sided spleen, 3 of 11 (27%). Typically, so-called malrotation of the bowel involves the presence of a common GI mesentery; absence of the ligament of Treitz; a nonretroperitoneal pancreas, cecum, and appendix not in the right lower quadrant; and occasionally most of the small bowel in half of the peritoneal cavity; and most of the large bowel in the other half of the peritoneal cavity.

A midline GI defect was present in 10 of 161 patients (6%). Tracheoesophageal fistula was found in 6 (4%): asplenia, 3; and left-sided polysplenia, 3. Omphalocele occurred in 4 patients (2.5%): asplenia, 2; left polysplenia, 1; and right polysplenia, 1. Anal stenosis or atresia occurred in 4 patients (2.5%), only with asplenia ($p = .07$). Genitourinary anomalies were found in 22 of 161 heterotaxic patients (14%). Hypoplastic kidney was present in 7 patients (4%): asplenia, 5; and left polysplenia, 2. Hypospadias was found in 6 cases (4%): asplenia, 1; left polysplenia, 2; right polysplenia, 2; and right spleen with heterotaxy, 1. Absence of a kidney occurred in 3 patients (2%): asplenia, 2; and right polysplenia, 1. Horseshoe kidney occurred in 2 (1%): asplenia, 1; and left polysplenia, 1. A urethral anomaly was present in 2 patients (1%): left polysplenia, 1; and right polysplenia, 1. Duplication of the vagina was present in 3 patients (2%): asplenia, 1; and left polysplenia, 2. A duplicated uterus occurred in 2 patients (1%): asplenia, 1; and left polysplenia, 1. A bicornuate uterus was present in 1 asplenic (1%). A unicornuate uterus occurred in 1 right polysplenic (1%). Vaginal atresia was observed in 1 asplenic (1%).

Musculoskeletal abnormalities involving midline structures were present in 21 of 161 heterotaxic patients (13%).

Most common was severe kyphosis or scoliosis in 9 patients (5.5%): asplenia, 4; left polysplenia, 2; and right polysplenia, 3. Hemivertebrae were second in frequency, occurring in 5 patients (3%): asplenia, 2; left polysplenia, 1; right polysplenia, 1; and right spleen with heterotaxy, 1. The caudal regression syndrome was found in 4 patients (2.5%): asplenia, 1; left polysplenia, 2; and right polysplenia, 1. Fused vertebrae were present in 2 patients (1%): asplenia, 1; and left polysplenia, 1. Pectus deformity was present in 2 patients (1%): asplenia, 1; and right polysplenia, 1.

Vertebral anomalies were found in 2 patients (1%): asplenia, 1; and left polysplenia, 1. A bifid sacrum occurred in 1 left polysplenic patient (1%). Sacral agenesis was observed in 1 other left polysplenic case (1%). Craniofacial defects were present in 14 of 161 patients (9%). Each patient had one or more of the following midline associated defects: Cleft lip and palate were found in 10 cases (6%): asplenia, 7; left polysplenia, 2; and right polysplenia, 1.

Agnathia or micrognathia was observed in 7 patients (4%): asplenia, 4; left polysplenia, 1; and right polysplenia, 2. There was 1 case each (1%) of: choanal atresia (left polysplenia); high-arched palate (asplenia); laryngeal cleft (right polysplenia); and cyclopia (left polysplenia). **Central nervous system anomalies** involving midline defects were found in 12 of 161 patients (7%). Meningomyelocele occurred in 2 patients (1%): asplenia, 1; and right polysplenia, 1. Agenesis of the corpus callosum was observed in 2 cases (1%): left polysplenia, 2. Porencephalic cyst was found in 2 patients (1%): asplenia, 1; and right polysplenia, 1. Cerebellar agenesis occurred in 2 right polysplenic patients (1%). One case each (1%) had the following: encephalocele (asplenia); Dandy-Walker syndrome (left polysplenia); holoprosencephaly (left polysplenia); arhinencephaly (right polysplenia); diplomyelia (asplenia); and hydromyelia (left polysplenia).

Endocrine anomalies took only one form: fusion of the adrenal glands across the midline. Although rare in the general population, this defect occurred in 8 of 90 patients with asplenia (9%) and was not observed in other forms of heterotaxy ($p = .01$).

To summarize, a total of 111 midline-associated anomalies was found in these 161 heterotaxic patients. The most commonly affected systems were the genitourinary (28/111 anomalies, 25%) and the musculoskeletal (26, 23%), followed by craniofacial structures (21, 19%), the nervous and GI systems (both 14/111 anomalies, 13%), and endocrine (8, 7%).

The type of autopsy significantly influenced the discovery of midline-associated defects. When a complete autopsy was performed, a midline-associated defect was found in 43% of patients (56/131); whereas when the autopsy was incomplete (for example, heart and lungs only), a midline-associated defect was described in only 20% (6/30) ($p = .02$).

Single or multiple midline-associated defects were found in the 62 patients with a complete autopsy. Asplenic patients had a single midline-associated defect in 56% (18/32) and multiple defects in 44% (14/32). By contrast, polysplenic patients had a single midline-associated defect in only 22% (5/22), whereas polysplenic patients had multiple defects in 78% (17/22).

Thus, polysplenic patients had significantly more multiple midline-associated anomalies (78%) than did asplenic patients (44%) ($p = .01$). Additional syndromes coexisted in the 31 heterotaxic patients with multiple midline-associated anomalies: Goldenhaar syndrome in 1 (3%), and Meckel-Gruber syndrome in 1 (3%).

The frequency of midline-associated defects in this heterotaxy population is 10 to 60 times greater than that described in the general population,[26] suggesting that midline associated defects occur in the heterotaxic syndromes much more often than would be expected by chance alone. A single midline-associated defect occurred in 95% of nonsyndromic infants with such malformations in a recent population study,[26] whereas multiple midline-associated defects were found in 44% of our asplenia syndrome patients and in 78% of our polysplenia syndrome cases. These data point to the need for further clarification of the association between midline associated defects and laterality defects, with special emphasis on cause (molecular genetics) and pathogenesis (embryology). An association between lateralization defects and midline anomalies has been reported.[27,28] So too has an association between an X-linked heterotaxy and midline malformations of brain, sacrum, and anus.[29,30]

Developmental Implications. The relatively high incidence of midline-associated defects in patients with heterotaxy supports the theory that the midline plays a critical role in establishing normal left-right asymmetry.[31,33] Cells in the midline, such as notochord cells, may act as sources of signals that direct left-right asymmetry and may act as a barrier to maintain a gradient of left-right signaling molecules.[34]

Leftward flow of extraembryonic fluid at the Hensen node has been shown to be essential for normal left-right determination.[35] These findings then lead to the hypothesis that disruption of the midline barrier separating left from right may permit mixing of molecules that are normally distributed asymmetrically in the early embryo, subsequently leading in later development to abnormalities of left-right organ sidedness.[25]

The midline developmental field concept[28] may explain the occurrence of apparently unrelated malformations in the same individual. Deficiencies in the midline field are likely to arise from single gene defects, as observed in mouse models of lateralization defects.[36]

The phenotype of mice lacking the activin receptor II B *is* **similar to the human asplenia syndrome.**[25] Of the several mouse models that have been investigated,[36] Ticho et al[25] have demonstrated a marked similarity between the phenotypes of human patients with the heterotaxy syndrome with asplenia and mice with selective disruption of the activin receptor type II gene.[31] These mice frequently have pulmonary right isomerism, asplenia, midline defects, and CCAVC. These observations lead to the hypothesis that the molecule activin, or nodal, or others in the same transforming growth factor beta (TGFP) pathway, may be mutated in human patients with asplenia.[25] The investigation continues.

LITERATURE

In 1826, G. Martin,[132] a medical student from L'Ecole Pratique and the Hopitaux Civils of Paris, described the first known case of asplenia with visceral heterotaxy and congenital heart disease in humans. In 1901, Lawrence and Nabarro[37] first reported the association of congenital heart disease, asplenia, and interruption of the IVC—a truly rare constellation of anomalies because, as we now know, asplenia almost never has interruption of the IVC. It was not until 1952 that Polhemus and Schafer[1] appreciated that the association between common AV canal and congenital asplenia constitute a syndrome. Then in 1955, working at the Children's Hospital in Boston, Ivemark[2] described the asplenia syndrome so well that for many years this entity was known as the **Ivemark syndrome.** In 1967, Moller et al[46] first noted the association between polysplenia and interruption of the IVC. To our knowledge, this chapter is the first statistically analyzed comparison of the heterotaxy syndrome with asplenia and the heterotaxy syndrome with polysplenia.

Diagnosis of the Heterotaxy Syndromes

The diagnosis of visceral heterotaxy with asplenia can be established during life on the basis of (1) Howell-Jolly bodies in the blood smear; (2) bilateral eparterial bronchi in the air bronchogram of the chest radiograph; (3) juxtaposition of the IVC and the descending aorta; (4) absence of normal uptake on splenic scan using heat-damaged red blood cells; and (5) the constellation of congenital heart defects described earlier that can be demonstrated by two- and three-dimensional echocardiography, angiocardiography, and magnetic resonance imaging (MRI).

The diagnosis of visceral heterotaxy with polysplenia can be established during life on the basis of (1) interruption of the IVC with prominent unilateral or bilateral azygos vein(s) to ipsilateral SVC(s); (2) bilateral hyparterial bronchi in the air bronchogram of the chest radiograph; (3) ectopic atrial pacemakers in the electrogram with coronary sinus rhythms (inferior to superior atrial depolarization); (4) the presence of multiple splenuli or a multilobed spleen on splenic scan; and (5) the presence of many of the previously characteristic forms of congenital heart disease, demonstrated by echocardiography, angiocardiography, or MRI. A chest radiograph showing an abnormally symmetrical liver, a right-sided stomach bubble, or dextrocardia is often the first clue that visceral heterotaxy is present.

MANAGEMENT

When the diagnosis of asplenia is established, as earlier, antibiotic prophylaxis should be given.[133] The recommended regimen for infants and young children was amoxicillin, 125 mg twice daily. For older children and adults, the usual prophylaxis is penicillin G, 200,000 units twice daily (in patients not allergic to penicillin). Penicillin (or other) prophylaxis should continue for life because fatal fulminating septicemia can occur rapidly after the onset of an apparently mild upper respiratory tract infection.

This is another Children's Hospital story. We had a patient with asplenia who was well palliated for pulmonary outflow tract stenosis with a Blalock-Taussig shunt. The patient was doing well until he developed a fulminating septicemia secondary to pneumococcus infection. The patient rapidly became hypothermic and leukopenic and died in less than 24 hours from the onset. One of us (RVP) was asked by an outside hospital in the western part of the Commonwealth of Massachusetts to come and help with the autopsy because they knew that the patient had complex congenital heart disease.

The most impressive thing about the autopsy was not the congenital heart disease, with which we were familiar, but the overwhelming septicemia. As a pediatrician, I put two and two together: asplenia is an open invitation to septicemia. When I returned to Children's Hospital, I was surprised to learn that our infectious disease experts and immunologists did not agree. Fortunately, Drs. Dean Waldman and Amnon Rosenthal then did a comparative study of asplenics versus normal-spleen patients, both groups with similar forms of congenital heart disease. Waldman et al[133] found that asplenic patients were much more prone to sepsis than were otherwise similar patients with normal spleens. This then is the background story of their very important paper advocating prophylaxis.

But another word should be added. Acquired asplenia—resulting from splenectomy for any reason—is just as dangerous as congenital asplenia. Prophylaxis is similarly mandatory.

The patient may be an adult, even a brilliant medical scientist. He may feel sure that he would recognize the symptoms and signs of incipient septicemia. But he may not. Pneumococcal meningitis produces confusion and may lessen one's mental acuity. So all asplenics—congenital and acquired—should receive lifetime prophylaxis.

Medical and surgical treatment of congenital heart disease associated with the heterotaxy syndromes should, insofar as possible, be just the same as for patients without heterotaxy. Please see the relevant chapters (for DORV, TGA, etc). The heterotaxy difference is not only the greater risk for sepsis but also the grater complexity of the congenital heart disease. This is why it is essential for cardiologists and surgeons to really understand the heterotaxy syndromes.

SUMMARY

1. The heterotaxy syndromes are anomalies of visceroatrial situs characterized by malformations of right-left asymmetry by defects of midline-associated structures, and by anomalies of the spleen, which may be absent (asplenia), hypoplastic (polysplenia), or abnormally located (right-sided).
2. The phenotypes of the cardiovascular and other anomalies of heterotaxy with asplenia and of heterotaxy with polysplenia have many statistically significant differences (85%) and some areas of overlap without significant differences (15%) (Tables 29.1 to 29.52). We therefore conclude that they are two different but related syndromes.
3. Whether visceral heterotaxy with right-sided spleen is a third and different heterotaxy syndrome awaits further data. We have studied only 5 such postmortem cases. We conclude that such a small series ($n = 5$) is too small to permit reliable generalizations.
4. Right atrial isomerism and left atrial isomerism have never been documented anatomically, accurately speaking.
5. Partial atrial isomerism (appendage isomerism or pectinate isomerism) is not isomerism. Accurately, isomerism involves all parts of two different composite structures that must be mirror-images to be isomers as, for example, the two molecules D-glucose and L-glucose are.
6. The realization that the concepts of right atrial isomerism and left atrial isomerism are anatomically inaccurate and conceptually flawed opens the door to the diagnosis of the atrial situs in the heterotaxy syndromes.
7. In 95 postmortem cases of visceral heterotaxy with asplenia and in 67 cases of visceral heterotaxy with polysplenia, situs solitus of the atria was present in 42% of the asplenic patients and in 72% of the polysplenic patients ($p < .001$). Situs inversus of the atria was found in 31% of the asplenic cases and in 22% of the polysplenic cases (p = not significant). Undiagnosed atrial situs (situs ambiguus) was significantly more frequent in patients with asplenia (26%) than in those with polysplenia (1%) ($p < .0001$).
8. Diagnosing the atrial situs in the heterotaxy syndromes, when it is possible to do so with confidence, also makes it possible to diagnose the presence of AV concordance and AV discordance in such cases. For example, AV concordance was found to be much more frequent in visceral heterotaxy with polysplenia (79%) than in visceral heterotaxy with asplenia (31%) ($p < .0001$).
9. The heterotaxy syndromes with asplenia, or polyspenia, or with a normally formed but right-sided spleen are anomalies of bilateral asymmetry, not anomalies of bilateral symmetry. Patients with visceral heterotaxy do not have bilateral right-sidedness, or bilateral left-sidedness. Instead, there is a lot of crossover of findings between the two main heterotaxy syndromes with asplenia or polysplenia.
10. The principal advantages of the concept of the heterotaxy syndromes, as opposed to the concept of right or left isomerism, are the following:
    a. The concept of the heterotaxy syndromes is anatomically accurate.
    b. The concept of the heterotaxy syndromes facilitates, in many cases, the diagnosis of the basic type of visceral situs and atrial situs in these patients, and the presence of AV concordance or discordance.

REFERENCES

1. Polhemus D, Schafer WB. Congenital absence of the spleen: syndrome with atrioventricularis and situs inversus; case reports and review of the literature. *Pediatrics.* 1952;9:696.
2. Ivemark BI. Implications of agenesis of the spleen on the pathogenesis of conotruncus anomalies in childhood. *Acta Pediatr Scand.* 1955;44(suppl 104):1.
3. Putschar WGJ, Manion WC. Congenital absence of the spleen and associated anomalies. *Am J Clin Pathol.* 1956;26:429.
4. Freedom RM. Aortic valve and arch anomalies in the congenital asplenia syndrome. Case report, literature review and re-examination of the embryology of the congenital asplenia syndrome. *Johns Hopkins Med J.* 1974;135:124.
5. Rose V, Izukawa T, Moes CAF. Syndromes of asplenia and polysplenia. *Br Heart J.* 1975;37:840.
6. Van Mierop LHS, Wiglesworth FW. Isomerism of the cardiac atria in the asplenia syndrome. *Lab Invest.* 1962;11:1303.
7. Moller JH, Hakib A, Anderson RC. Congenital cardiac disease associated with polysplenia. *Circulation.* 1967;36:789.
8. Freedom RM, Culham JAG, Moes CA. Asplenia and polysplenia (a consideration of syndromes characterized by right or left atrial isomerism). In: *Angiocardiography of Congenital Heart Disease.* New York: Macmillan; 1984:643.
9. Van Praagh S, Kakou-Guikahue M, Kim H-S, Becker J, Alday L, Van Praagh R. Atrial situs in patients with visceral heterotaxy and congenital heart disease: conclusions based on findings in 104 postmortem cases. *Coeur.* 1988;19:484.
10. Van Praagh R, Van Praagh S. Atrial isomerism in the heterotaxy syndromes with asplenia, or polysplenia, or normally formed spleen: an erroneous concept. *Am J Cardiol.* 1990;66:1504.
11. Waldman JD, Rosenthal A, Smith AL, Shurin S, Nadas AS. Sepsis and congenital asplenia. *J Pediat.* 1977;90:555.
12. Van Praagh S, Kreutzer J, Alday L, Van Praagh R. Systemic and pulmonary venous connections in visceral heterotaxy, with emphasis on the diagnosis of the atrial situs: a study of 109 postmortem cases. In: *Developmental Cardiology: Morphogenesis and Function.* Mount Kisco, NY: Futura Publishing Co, Inc; 1990:671.
13. Van Praagh S, Santini F, Sanders SP. Cardiac malpositions with special emphasis on visceral heterotaxy (asplenia and polysplenia syndromes). In: Fyler DC, ed. *Nadas' Pediatric Cardiology.* Philadelphia: Hanley & Belfus; 1992:589.
14. Rubino M, Van Praagh S, Kadoba K, Pessotto R, Van Praagh R. Systemic and pulmonary venous connections in visceral heterotaxy with asplenia, diagnostic and surgical considerations based on seventy-two autopsied cases. *J Thorac Cardiovasc Surg.* 1995;110:641.
15. Van Praagh S, Carrera ME, Sanders S, Mayer JE, Van Praagh R. Partial or total direct pulmonary venous drainage to right atrium due to malposition of septum primum, anatomic and echocardiographic findings and surgical treatment: a study based on 36 cases. *Chest.* 1995;107:1488.
16. David I, Castaneda AR, Van Praagh R. Potentially parachute mitral valve in common atrioventricular canal: pathologic anatomy and surgical importance. *J Thorac Cardiovasc Surg.* 1982;84:178.
17. Van Praagh R, Plett JA, Van Praagh S. Single ventricle: pathology, embryology, terminology, and classification. *Herz.* 1979;4:113.
18. Van Praagh R, Van Praagh S. Isolated ventricular inversion, a consideration of the morphogenesis, definition, and diagnosis of nontransposed and transposed great arteries. *Am J Cardiol.* 1966;17:395.
19. Van Praagh R, Van Praagh S. Anatomically corrected transposition of the great arteries. *Br Heart J.* 1967;29:112.
20. Van Praagh R, Durnin RE, Jockin H, et al. Anatomically corrected malposition of the great arteries {S,D,L}. *Circulation.* 1975;51:20.
21. Delisle G, Ando M, Calder AL, et al. Total anomalous pulmonary venous connection: report of 93 autopsied cases with emphasis on diagnostic and surgical considerations. *Am Heart J.* 1976;91:99.
22. Pasquini L, Sanders SP, Parness I, et al. Echocardiographic and anatomic findings in atrioventricular discordance with ventriculoarterial concordance. *Am J Cardiol.* 1988;62:1256.
23. Van Praagh S, LaCorte M, Fellows KE, et al. Supero-inferior ventricles, anatomic and angiocardiographic findings in 10 postmortem cases. In: Van Praagh R, Takao A, eds. *Etiology and Morphogenesis of Congenital Heart Disease.* Mount Kisco, NY: Futura Publishing Co, Inc; 1980:379.
24. Van Praagh R, Corsini I. Cor triatriatum: pathologic anatomy and a consideration of morphogenesis based on 13 postmortem cases and a study of normal development of the pulmonary vein and atrial septum in 83 human embryos. *Am Heart J.* 1969;78:379.
25. Ticho BS, Goldstein AM, Van Praagh R. Extracardiac anomalies in the heterotaxy syndromes with focus on anomalies of midline-associated structures. *Am J Cardiol.* 2000;85:729.
26. Khoury MJ, Cordero JF, Mulinare J, Opitz JM. Selected midline defect associations: a population study. *Pediatrics.* 1989;84:266.
27. de Meeus A, Sarda P, Tenconi R, Ferriere M, Bouvagnet P. Blastogenesis dominant 1: a sequence with midline anomalies and heterotaxy. *Am J Med Genet.* 1997;68:405.
28. Martinez-Frias ML, Urioste M, Bermejo E, et al. Primary midline developmental field: II. Clinical/epidemiological analysis of alteration of laterality (normal body symmetry and asymmetry). *Amer J Med Gen.* 1995;56:382.
29. Casey B, Devoto M, Jones KL, Ballabio A. Mapping a gene for familial situs abnormalities to human chromosome Xq24-q27.1. *Nature Genetics.* 1993;5:403.
30. Ferrero GB, Gebbia M, Pilia G, et al. A submicroscopic deletion in Xq26 associated with familial situs ambiguus. *Am J Hum Genet.* 1997;61:395.
31. Oh SP, Li E. The signaling pathway mediated by the type IIB activin receptor controls axial patterning and lateral asymmetry in the mouse. *Genes Dev.* 1997;11:1812.
32. Danos MC, Yost HJ. Role of notochord in specification of cardiac left-right orientation in zebrafish and Xenopus. *Dev Biol.* 1996;177:96.
33. Lohr JL, Danos MC, Yost HJ. Left-right asymmetry of a nodal related gene is regulated by dorsoanterior midline structures during Xenopus development. *Dev.* 1997;124:1465.
34. Yost HJ. Left-right development in Xenopus and zebrafish. *Semin Cell Dev Biol.* 1998;9:61.
35. Nonaka S, Tanaka Y, Okada Y, et al. Randomization of left-right asymmetry due to loss of nodal cilia generating leftward flow of extraembryonic fluid in mice lacking KIF3B motor protein. *Cell.* 1998;95:829.
36. Supp DM, Brueckner M, Potter SS. Handed asymmetry in the mouse: understanding how things go right (or left) by studying how they go wrong. *Semin Cell Dev Biol.* 1998;9:77.
37. Lawrence TMP, Nabarro D. A case of congenital malformation of the heart, with abnormalities of abdominal viscera: absence of spleen, absence of hepatic section of inferior cava. *J Anat and Physiol.* 1901;36:63.

38. Blattner RJ. Agenesis of the spleen. *J Pediat*. 1957;51:350.
39. Schonfeld EA, Frischman B. Syndrome of spleen agenesis, defect of the heart and vessels and situs inversus. *Helvetica Pediatrica Acta*. 1958;13:636.
40. Lucas Jr RV, Neufeld HN, Lester RG, Edwards JE. The symmetrical liver as a roentgen sign of asplenia. *Circulation*. 1962;25:973.
41. Roberts WE, Berry WB, Morrow G. The significance of asplenia in the recognition of inoperable congenital heart disease. *Circulation*. 1962;26:1251.
42. Ruttenberg HD, Neufeld HN, Lucas Jr RV, et al. Syndrome of congenital cardiac disease with asplenia: distinction from other forms of congenital heart disease. *Am Heart J*. 1964;13:387.
43. Ongley PA, Titus JL, Khoury GH, Rahimtoola SH, Marshall HJ, Edwards JE. Anomalous connection of pulmonary veins to right atrium associated with anomalous inferior vena cava, situs inversus and multiple spleens: a developmental complex. *Mayo Clin Proc*. 1965;40:609.
44. Campbell M, Deuchar DC. Absent inferior vena cava, symmetrical liver, splenic agenesis, and situs inversus, and their embryology. *Brit Heart J*. 1967;29:268.
45. Layman TE, Levine M, Amplatz K, Edwards JE. Asplenia syndrome in association with rudimentary spleen. *Am J Cardiol*. 1967;20:136.
46. Moller JH, Nakib A, Anderson RC, Edwards JE. Congenital cardiac disease associated with polysplenia. A developmental complex of bilateral "left-sidedness". *Circulation*. 1967;36:789.
47. Niibori S, Ando M, Takao A, Sakakibara S. Visceroatrial heterotaxic syndrome. *Bull Heart Inst Japan*. 1971;13:72.
48. Van Mierop LHS, Gessner I, Schiebler G. Asplenia and polysplenia syndromes - Birth defects. *Original article series*. 1972;8:36.
49. Silver W, Steier M, Chandra N. Asplenia syndrome with congenital heart disease and tetralogy of Fallot in siblings. *Am Heart J*. 1972;30:91.
50. Freedom RM. The asplenia syndrome: a review of significant extracardiac structural abnormalities in 29 necropsied patients. *J Pediat*. 1972;81:1130.
51. Blieden LC, Moller JH. Analysis of the P wave in congenital cardiac malformations associated with splenic anomalies. *Amer Heart J*. 1973;85:439.
52. Padmabhan J, Risenberg HM, Rowe RD. Howell-Jolly bodies in the peripheral blood of full-term and premature neonates. *Hopkins Med J*. 1973;132:146.
53. Freedom RM, Ellison RC. Coronary sinus rhythm in the polysplenia syndrome. *Chest*. 1973;63:952.
54. Freedom RM. Aortic valve and arch anomalies in the congenital asplenia syndrome. Case report, literature review and re-examination of the embryology of the congenital asplenia syndrome. *Johns Hopkins Med J*. 1974;135:124.
55. Chandra RS. Biliary atresia and other structural anomalies in the congenital polysplenia syndrome. *J Pediat*. 1974;85:649.
56. Winkelstein JA, Lambert GH. Pneumococcal serum opsonizing activity in splenectomized children. *J Pediat*. 1975;87:430.
57. Patridge JB, Scott O, Deverall PB, Macartney FJ. Visualization and measurement of the main bronchi by tomography as an objective indicator of thoracic situs in congenital heart disease. *Circulation*. 1975;51:188.
58. Hyslop NE, McCluskey RT. Fever and circulatory collapse in an asplenic man. *New Engl J Med*. 1975;293:547.
59. Ando F, Shirotani H, Kawai J, et al. Successful total repair of complicated cardiac anomalies with asplenia syndrome. *J Thorac & Cardiovasc Surg*. 1976;33.
60. Lamberti JJ, Thilenius 0, de la Fuente D, Lin CY, Arcilla R, Replogle RL. Right atrial partition and right ventricular exclusion. Another surgical approach for complex cyanotic congenital heart disease. *J Thorac & Cardiovasc Surg*. 1976;71:386.
61. Ammann AJ, Addiego J, Wara DW, Lubin B, Smith WB, Mentzer WC. Polyvalent pneumococcal-polysaccharide immunization of patients with sickle cell anemia and patients with splenectomy. *New Engl J Med*. 1977;297:897.
62. Freedom RM, Olley PM, Coceani F, Rowe RD. The prostaglandin challenge test to unmask obstructed total anomalous pulmonary venous connections in a splenia syndrome. *Brit Heart J*. 1978;40:91.
63. Caruso G, Becker AE. How to determine atrial situs? Considerations initiated by 3 cases of absent spleen with a discordant anatomy between bronchi and atria. *Brit Heart J*. 1979;41:559.
64. Pohamka I, Vitek B. The conducting system of the heart in the syndrome of visceral symmetry. *Folia Morph*. 1978;26:379.
65. Dickinson DF, Wilkinson JL, Anderson KR, Smith A, Ho SY, Anderson RH. The cardiac conduction system in situs ambiguus. *Circulation*. 1979;59:879.
66. Katcher AL. Familial asplenia, other malformations, and sudden death. *Pediatrics*. 1980;65:633.
67. Macartney FJ, Zuberbuhler JR, Anderson RH. Morphological considerations pertaining to recognition of atrial isomerism. Consequences for sequential chamber localization. *Br Heart J*. 1980;44:657.
68. Garcia OL, Mehta AV, Pickoff AS, et al. Left isomerism and complete atrioventricular block: a report of six cases. *Am J Cardiol*. 1981;48:1103.
69. Wick MR, Rife CC. Paratesticular accessory spleen. *Mayo Clin Proc*. 1981;56:455.
70. Turley K, Tarnoff H, Snider R, Ebert PA. Repair of combined total anomalous pulmonary venous connection and anomalous systemic connection in early infancy. *Ann Thorac Surg*. 1981;31:70.
71. Biggar WD, Ramirez RA, Rose V. Congenital asplenia: immunologic assessment and clinical review of eight surviving patients. *Pediatrics*. 1981;67:548.
72. Huhta JC, Smallhorn F, Macartney FJ. Two dimensional echocardiographic diagnosis of situs. *Br Heart J*. 1982;48:97.
73. Berman W, Yabek SM, Burnstein J, Dillon T. Asplenia syndrome with atypical cardiac anomalies. *Ped Cardiol*. 1982;3:35.
74. Marcelletti C, Di Donato R, Nojveld A, et al. Right and left isomerism: the cardiac surgeon's view. *Ann Thor Surg*. 1983;35:400.
75. Peoples WM, Moller JH, Edwards JE. Polysplenia: a review of 146 cases. *Ped Cardiol*. 1983;4:129.
76. Monie IW. The asplenia syndrome: an explanation for absence of the spleen. *Teratology*. 1982;25:215.
77. Stewart PA, Becker AE, Wladimiroff JW, Essed CE. Left atrial isomerism associated with asplenia: prenatal echo cardiographic detection of complex congenital cardiac malformations. *JACC*. 1984;4:1015.
78. Kine K-M, Ueda T. Asplenia syndrome complicated by purulent pericarditis. *Pediatr Cardiol*. 1985;6:114.
79. Sharma S, Devine W, Anderson RH, Zuberbuhler JR. Identification and analysis of left atrial isomerism. *Am J Cardiol*. 1987;60:1157.
80. Calder L. *Morphological Features in Situs Ambiguus*. Bergamo: First World Congress of Pediatric Cardiac Surgery; 1988:134. Abstracts.
81. Sharma S, Devine W, Anderson RH, Zuberbuhler JR. The determination of atrial arrangement examination of appendage morphology in 1842 hearts specimens. *Br Heart J*. 1988;60:227.

82. Wren C, Macartney FJ, Deanfield JE. Cardiac rhythm in atrial isomerism. *Am J Cardiol.* 1987;59:1156.
83. Sapire DW, Ho SY, Anderson RH, Rigby ML. Diagnosis and significance of atrial isomerism. *Am J Cardiol.* 1986;58:342.
84. Waldman JD, Lamberti JJ. Anastomosis of systemic veins to pulmonary arteries for physiologic repair of asplenia syndrome. *Pediatr Cardiol.* 1986;6:327.
85. Chiu I-S, How S-W, Wang JK, et al. Clinical implications of atrial isomerism. *Br Heart J.* 1988;60:72.
86. DiDonato R, di Carlo D, Squitieri C, et al. Palliation of cardiac malformations associated with right isomerism (asplenia syndrome) in infancy. *Ann Thorac Surg.* 1987;44:35.
87. Humes RA, Feldt RH, Porter CJ, Julsrud PR, Puga FJ, Danielson GK. The modified Fontan operation for asplenia and polysplenia syndromes. *J Thorac Cardiovasc Surg.* 1988;96:212.
88. Brueckner M, D'Eustachio P, Horwich AL. Linkage mapping of mouse gene, iv, that controls left-right symmetry of the heart and viscera. *Proc Natl Acad Sci USA.* 1989;86:5035.
89. Escarous A. Left pulmonary isomerism with normal arrangement of the heart and abdominal organs. Computed tomography of two adults. *Internat J Cardiol.* 1989;24:118.
90. Momma K, Takao A, Shibata T. Characteristics and natural history of abnormal atrial rhythms in left isomerism. *Am J Cardiel.* 1990;65:231.
91. Anderson C, Devine WA, Anderson RH, Debich DE, Zuberbuhler JR. Abnormalities of the spleen in relation to congenital malformations of the heart: a survey of necropsy findings in children. *Br Heart J.* 1990;63:122.
92. Debich DE, Devine WA, Anderson RH. Polysplenia with normally structured hearts. *Am J Cardiol.* 1990;65:1274.
93. Arisawa J, Morimoto S, Ikezoe J, et al. Cross-sectional echocardiographic anatomy of common atrioventricular valve in atrial isomerism. *Br Heart J.* 1989;62:291.
94. Murdoch IA, Dos Anjos R, Mitchell A. Fatal pneumococcal septicaemia associated with asplenia and isomerism of the right atrial appendages. *Br Heart J.* 1991;65:102.
95. Mauser I, Deutinger J, Bernaschek G. Prenatal diagnosis of a complex fetal cardiac malformation associated with asplenia. *Br Heart J.* 1991;65:293.
96. Seo J-W, Brown AN, Ho SY, Anderson RH. Abnormal laterality and congenital cardiac anomalies: relations of visceral and cardiac morphologies in the IV/IV mouse. *Circulation.* 1992;86:642.
97. Lee HJ, Ko JK, Kim SH, Park YK, Lee YK. Atrioventricular and ventriculoarterial morphology in isomeric patient with double outlet right ventricle. *Cardiol Young.* 1993;3:1–69 (Abstract207).
98. Sauer U, Maier M, Kolb S, Heimisch W, Btihlmeyer K, Sebening F. Sixty-three children with congenital cardiovascular anomalies and heterotaxy - follow-up and suitability for staged or definitive cavopulmonary connection. *Cardiol Young.* 1993;3:1–151.
99. Webber SA, Boyle GJ, Ettedgui JA, Sandor GGS. Can pulmonary venous obstruction be reliably diagnosed in the newborn with atrial isomerism. *Cardiol Young.* 1993;3:1–146.
100. Gillis S, Dann EJ, Berkman N, Koganox Y, Kramer MR. Fatal haemophilus influenzae septicemia following bronchoscopy in a splenectomized patient. *Chest.* 1993;104:1607.
101. Kawashima Y, Matsuda H, Naito Y, Yagihara T, Kadoba K, Matsuki O. Biventricular repair of cardiac isomerism with common atrioventricular canal with the aid of an endocardial cushion prosthesis. *J Thorac Cardiovasc Surg.* 1993;106:248.
102. O'Leary PW, Seward JB, Hagler DL, Tajik AJ. Echocardiographic documentation of splenic anatomy in complex congenital heart disease. *Am J Cardiol.* 1991;68:1536.
103. Phoon CK, Neill CA. Asplenia syndrome: insight into embryology through an analysis of cardiac and extracardiac anomalies. *Am J Cardiol.* 1994;73:581.
104. Niwa K, Uchishiba M, Aotsuka H, et al. Magnetic resonance imaging of heterotaxia in infancy. *J Am Coll Cardiol.* 1994;23:177.
105. Oku H, Iemura J, Kitayama H, Saga T, Shirotani H. Bivalvation with briding for common atrioventricular valve regurgitation in right isomerism. *Ann Thorac Surg.* 1994;57:1324.
106. Geva T, Vick GW, Wendt RE, Rokey R. Role of spin echo and cine magnetic resonance imaging in presurgical planning of heterotaxy syndrome, comparison with echocardiography and catheterization. *Circulation.* 1994;90:348.
107. Ho SY, Fagg N, Anderson RH, Cook A, Allan I. Disposition of the atrioventricular conduction tissues in the heart with isomerism of the atrial appendages: its relation to congenital complete heart block. *J Am Coll Cardiol.* 1992;20:904.
108. Anderson RH, Devine WA, Uemura H. Diagnosis of heterotaxy syndrome. *Circulation.* 1995;91:906.
109. Geva T, Vick GW, Wendt RE, Rokey R. Diagnosis of heterotaxy syndrome. Reply. *Circulation.* 1995;91:907.
110. Vitiello R, Moller JH, Marino B, Vairo U, Edwards JE, Titus JL. Pulmonary circulation in pulmonary atresia associated with the asplenia cardiac syndrome. *JAm Coll Cardiol.* 1992;20:363.
111. Hirooka K, Yagihara T, Kishimoto H, et al. Biventricular repair in cardiac isomerism, report of seventeen cases. *J Thorac Cardiovasc Surg.* 1995;109:530.
112. Wang J-K, Li Y-W, Chiu I-S, et al. Usefulness of magnetic resonance imaging in the assessment of venoatrial connections, atrial morphology, bronchial situs, and other anomalies in right atrial isomerism. *Am J Cardiol.* 1994;74:701.
113. Uemura H, Anderson RH, Ho SY, et al. Left ventricular structures in atrioventricular septal defect associated with isomerism of atrial appendages compared with similar features with usual atrial arrangement. *J Thorac Cardiovasc Surg.* 1995;110:445.
114. Uemura H, Ho SY, Anderson RH, et al. The surgical anatomy of coronary venous return in hearts with isomeric atrial appendages. *J Thorac Cardiovasc Surg.* 1995;110:436.
115. Uemura H, Ho SY, Devine WA, Kilpatrick LL, Anderson RH. Atrial appendages and venoatrial connections in hearts from patients with visceral heterotaxy. *Ann Thorac Surg.* 1995;60:561.
116. Uemura H, Yagihara T, Kawashima Y, Okada K, Anderson RH. The earliest site of atrial activation in patients with isomeric appendages. *Br Heart J.* 1995;74:305.
117. Uemura H, Ho SY, Devine WA, Anderson RH. Analysis of visceral heterotaxy according to splenic status, appendage morphology, or both. *Am Heart J.* 1995;76:846.
118. Ho SY, Seo J-W, Brown NA, Cook AC, Fagg NLK, Anderson RH. Morphology of the sinus node in human and mouse hearts with isomerism of the atrial appendages. *Br Heart J.* 1995;74:437.
119. Wu M-H, Lin J-L, Wange J-K, Chiu I-S, Young M-L. Electrophysiological properties of dual atrioventricular nodes in patients with right atrial isomerism. *Br Heart J.* 1995;74:553.
120. Sadiq M, Stümper O, De Giovanni JV, et al. Management and outcome of infants and children with right atrial isomerism. *Heart.* 1996;75:314.
121. Marino B, Pasquini L. Systemic and venous connection in asplenia syndrome, letter to the editor. *J Thorac Cardiovasc Surg.* 1996;111:1109.
122. Rubino M, Van Praagh S, Kadoba K, Pessotto R, Van Praagh R. Venoarterial connections in visceral heterotaxy. *J Thorac Cardiovasc Surg.* 1996;111:1107.

123. Phoon CK, Villegas MD, Ursell PC, Silverman NH. Left atrial isomerism detected in fetal life. *Am J Cardiol.* 1996;77:1083.
124. Uemura H, Yagihara T, Kawashima Y. Surgical approach for right heart bypass in patients with isomeric atrial appendages. *Rev Argent Cardiol.* 1996;64:391.
125. Gebbia M, Towbin JA, Casey B. Failure to detect connexin 43 mutations in 38 cases of sporadic and familial heterotaxy. *Circulation.* 1996;94:1909.
126. Van Praagh S, Geva T, Friedberg DZ, et al. Aortic outflow obstruction in visceral heterotaxy: a study based on twenty postmortem cases. *Am Heart J.* 1997;133:558.
127. Cesko I, Hajdu J, Tóth T, Marton T, Papp C, Papp Z. Ivemark syndrome with asplenia in siblings. *J Pediatr.* 1997;130:822.
128. Yates RWM, Raymond FL, Cook A, Sharland GK. Isomerism of the atrial appendages associated with 22q11 deletion in a fetus. *Heart.* 1996;76:548.
129. Bowers PN, Nelson-Williams CJ, Casey B, Lifton RP, Brueckner M. Identification, chromosomal localization and mutational analysis of human left-right dynein in human heterotaxia. *Circulation.* 1998;98:1–57.
130. Ruscazio M, Van Praagh S, Marrass AR, Catani G, Iliceto S, Van Praagh R. Interrupted inferior vena cava in asplenia syndrome and a review of the hereditary patterns of visceral situs abnormalities. *Am J Cardiol.* 1998;81:111.
131. Edwards JE. Pathologic and developmental considerations in anomalous pulmonary venous connection. *Mayo Clin Proc.* 1953;28:441.
132. Martin G. Observations d'une deviation organique de l'estomac, d'une anomalie dans la situation, dans la configuration du coeur et des vaisseaux qui en partent au qui s'y rendent. *Bulletin de la Societe Anatomique de Paris.* 1826;3:39.
133. Waldman JD, Rosenthal A, Smith AL, Shurin S, Nadas AS. Sepsis and congenital asplenia. *J Pediatr.* 1977;90:555.

30

Conclusions

The new information,[1] also presented in Chapters 15, 26, and 27, raises questions about how best to name and define various types of congenital heart disease.

Consider, for example, transposition of the great arteries (TGA). At the present time, TGA is defined and named *with reference to the anatomy of the normal heart.* Compared with the normal human heart, in TGA the aorta is placed across the ventricular septum (Latin, *trans,* "across," and *positio,* "a placing"), and consequently the aorta arises above the anatomically inappropriate ventricle, the morphologically right ventricle. Similarly, the transposed pulmonary artery has been "placed across" the ventricular septum and thus originates above the anatomically inappropriate ventricle, the morphologically left ventricle.

Complete TGA meant transposition of *both* great arteries, usually typical D-TGA. *Partial* TGA meant transposition of only one great artery, typically the aorta. We now call this *double-outlet right ventricle (DORV).* Rarely, only the pulmonary artery is transposed, resulting in *double-outlet left ventricle (DOLV).* Thus, *partial TGA* includes both *DORV* and *DOLV.*

By the late 1920s, any spatial anomaly between the great arteries themselves, and/or between the great arteries and the underlying ventricles, was regarded as some form of TGA—complete or partial. So "transposition" of the great arteries included "everything."[2]

But gradually, more accurate and specific terminology emerged. People who are interested in languages and meanings started using *transposition* of the great arteries with literal accuracy, that is, only for cases in which it looked as though both great arteries had been placed across the ventricular septum (Latin, *trans* + *positio,* or English, transposed) and thus both great arteries arose above the morphologically wrong ventricles. This change caught on because it was based on accuracy in terminology.

When you do this, the names of a lot of other anomalies have to change because transposition of *both* great arteries is not present, accurately speaking. Anomalies that had to have their names changed include:

1. double-outlet right ventricle (DORV)[3];
2. double-outlet left ventricle (DOLV)[4];
3. anatomically corrected malposition of the great arteries (ACMGA)[5]; and
4. absence of subpulmonary infundibulum (AOSPI), erroneously known as truncus arteriosus communis.[6]

Now, our diagnoses are *anatomically* accurate, that is, relative to normal cardiac *anatomy.* However, *developmentally,* our anatomic diagnoses are often erroneous. Consider D-TGA (Table 30.1):

$$\text{TGA }\{S,D,D\} = 4R + 0L$$

This is the defining equation of D-TGA. It shows that the subarterial component of D-TGA (to the right of the equal sign) is inverted, that is, the same as in the equation for inverted normally related great arteries with situs inversus totalis.

Consequently, the subarterial infundibular free wall apoptosis is inverted, that is, left-sided and subpulmonary, instead of right-sided and subaortic. Hence, the wrong great artery (the pulmonary artery [PA]) gets switched from the right ventricle (RV) to the left ventricle (LV).

In D-TGA the well-developed, right-sided subaortic infundibulum prevents a switch of the aorta to the LV.

According to current *developmental* understanding, our *anatomic* understanding of D-TGA may be regarded as approximately 50% correct. The PA does get switched or transposed from the RV into the LV. But the aorta does not get switched or transposed from the LV into the RV because the RV is the beginning, or starting, location of the aorta. The anatomic understanding of D-TGA usually does not include the concepts of infundibular inversion, inverted apoptosis, and inverted great arterial migration of only the PA.

Just as typical D-TGA, that is, TGA {S,D,D}, is isolated infundibular inversion (4R + 0L), typical L-TGA, that is, TGA {S,L,L} is isolated infundibular noninversion (0R + 4L) (see Table 30.1). The *anatomic* understanding of typical L-TGA correctly holds that the right-sided PA is switched from the left-sided RV into the right-sided LV. But this *anatomic* hypothesis also predicts, erroneously, that the left-sided aorta is switched from the right-sided LV into the left-sided RV. This prediction of aortic transposition from the LV into the RV is erroneous because the RV is the starting position of both great arteries. *Thus, accurately speaking, in TGA (D- and L-), transposition is never "complete."*

Only the PA is transposed from the RV to the LV. The aorta is not switched. The anomaly that befalls the aorta is not being switched from the RV (the normal starting position) into the LV (the normal destination).

Tetralogy of Fallot, accurately speaking, is just one malformation—variable hypoplasia of the subpulmonary infundibulum[7]—that is now thought to cause the classic tetrad of (1) pulmonary outflow tract obstruction (stenosis or atresia), (2) subaortic ventricular septal defect, (3) aortic overriding, and (4) right ventricular hypertrophy postnatally.

TABLE 30.1 Equations That Define Normally and Abnormally Related Great Arteries

1.	SNRGA {S,D,S} = 0R + 4L
2.	INRGA {I,L,I} = 4R + 0L
3.	TOF {S,D,S} = 0R + 3L + VSD
4.	TOF {S,D,S} = 0R + 2L + VSD
5.	TOF {S,D,S} = 0R + 1L + VSD
6.	AOSPI {S,D,-} = 0R + (-L) + APSD
7.	AOSPI {S,D,-}= 0R + (-L) + VSD – PV – MPA
8.	AOAPS {S,D,S} = 0R + 4L – APS
9.	TGA {S,D,D} = 4R + 0L
10.	TGA {S,L,L} = 0R + 4L
11.	DORV {S,D,D} = 4R + 4L
12.	DOLV {S,D,D} = 0R + 0L
13.	ACMGA {S,D,L} = 0R + 4L
14.	ACMGA {S,L,D} = 4R + 4L
15.	IVI {S,L,S} = 0R + 4L + VSD

ACMGA, Anatomically corrected malposition of the great arteries; *AOAPS,* absence of aortopulmonary septum; *AOSPI,* absence of subpulmonary infundibulum; *APS,* aorta pulmonary septum; *DOLV,* double-outlet left ventricle; *DORV,* double-outlet right ventricle; *INRGA,* inverted normally related great arteries; *IVI,* isolated ventricular inversion; *LV,* left ventricle; *MPA,* main pulmonary artery; *PA,* pulmonary artery; *RV,* right ventricle; *SNRGA,* solitus normally related great arteries; *TGA,* transposition of the great arteries; *TOF,* tetralogy of Fallot; *VSD,* ventricular septal defect.
Equation 30.1, solitus normally related great arteries.
Equation 30.2, inverted normally related great arteries.
Equation 30.3, TOF, with mild/moderate PS, that is, 3L.
Equation 30.4, TOF with severe PS, i.e., 2L.
Equation 30.5, TOF with pulmonary atresia, that is, 1L.
Equation 30.6, absence of subpulmonary infundibulum, conventionally called truncus arteriosus communis type A1.
Equation 30.7, AOSPI with absence of the PV and absence of the MPA, our "TAC" type A2. Absence of the MPA makes the diagnosis of a huge PA window (TAC) impossible. This is a solitary aorta, not both great arteries in common.
Equation 30.8, absence of aortopulmonary septum, which I have never examined personally.
Equation 30.9, typical D-TGA.
Equation 30.10, TGA {S,L,L}.
Equation 30.11, DORV of the Taussig-Bing type.[7]
Equation 30.12, DOLV of the Paul type.[4]
Equation 30.13, ACGMA that is also potentially physiologically corrected.
Equation 30.14, ACMGA that is potentially physiologically uncorrected.
Equation 30.15, isolated ventricular inversion.

Truncus arteriosus communis (TAC) persistens, or persistent common arterial trunk, or its interpretation, can be anatomically erroneous, for example, our type of TAC type A2 in which the main pulmonary artery (MPA) is absent.[6] One cannot make the diagnosis of a huge AP window when the MPA is absent, as it is our TAC type A2.

However, it must be added that I think that TAC as described by Abbott in 1927 does exist, because I have seen a photograph, from a reputable source, of isolated absence of the aortopulmonary septum.[6] I have never examined such a case myself.

The evolutionary significance[7,8] of AOSPI {S,D,-} = 0R + (-L) + VSD – PV – MPA is huge. Absence of the subpulmonary infundibulum, absence of the pulmonary valve, and absence of the MPA represents absence of the main cardiovascular evolutionary adaptations that made possible permanent air-breathing and permanent land-living.

The full range of development of the pulmonary outflow tract is expressed in the equations in Table 30.1[7]:
Equation 30.7, absence;
Equation 30.6, pulmonary artery is present;
Equation 30.5, extreme infundibular hypoplasia;
Equation 30.4, severe infundibular hypoplasia;
Equation 30.3, mild to moderate infundibular hypoplasia; and
Equation 30.1, normal development.

Development of the right ventricular sinus (body, or inflow tract)—the lung pump—is not helpful physiologically if there is no pulmonary outflow tract, or if the pulmonary outflow tract is hypoplastic and highly obstructive hemodynamically.

Thus, absence or hypoplasia of the pulmonary outflow tract is one form of interrelated congenital heart disease.

What is really going on with transposition of the great arteries? Equations 30.9 and 30.10[6] suggest an answer (see Table 30.1):

$$\text{TGA }\{S,D,D\} = 4R + 0L \qquad \textbf{Equation 30.9}$$

$$\text{TGA }\{S,L,L\} = 0R + 4L \qquad \textbf{Equation 30.10}$$

In Equation 30.9 of D-TGA, the subarterial infundibular situs is inverted (4R + 0L), the same as in Equation 30.2 of situs inversus (4R + 0L). Thus, D-TGA is isolated infundibular inversion:

only the subarterial infundibulum is inverted, but nothing else is. Apoptosis is related to infundibular situs. Consequently, apoptosis is left-sided and subpulmonary, not right-sided and subaortic, which is normal. Hence the pulmonary artery is switched from the RV into the LV, not the aorta.

In Equation 30.10, congenitally physiologically corrected L-TGA has isolated infundibular nonnversion (or situs solitus): 0R + 4L is the same as in Equation 30.1.

For the human heart to be normally formed, there must be total segmental situs uniformity (all solitus or all inversus, not a mixture) and every segment must be normally formed, as in Equation 30.1 and as in its mirror-image, Equation 30.2.

Every other equation in Table 30.1 has either segmental situs nonuniformity (Equations 30.9 to 30.15), or segmental hypoplasia or absence (Equations 30.3 to 30.8).

Segmental situs is important not only structurally, but also because of the role situs plays in great arterial switches and non-switches, rotation, and synergy.

All of the equations are repeated in Table 30.1, all together, for the reader's convenience. Many additional equations could and should be written, to accurately reflect other variations in the pathologic anatomy.

SIDEDNESS OF THE SEMILUNAR VALVES

1. When the semilunar valves are solitus normally or abnormally related (e.g., SNRGA or D-TGA), the aortic valve (AoV) typically is right-sided relative to the PV, that is, AoV (R) and PV (L).
2. When the semilunar valves are inversus normally or abnormally related (e.g., INRGA or L-TGA), the AoV typically is left-sided relative to the PV, that is, AoV (L) and PV (R).
3. If the semilunar valvar relationship is atypical, note the relationship carefully. This is important both algebraically (for the equations) and geometrically (for measuring rotations of the atrial septum, ventricular septum, and semilunar valves).

THE IMPORTANCE OF SEGMENTAL SITUS

Segmental situs is a fundamental concept. The pattern of anatomic organization (or situs) may be solitus (normal), inversus (a mirror-image of solitus), or heterotaxy (uncertain, or unknown). Congenital heart disease often is characterized by a segmental situs "salad" (mixture). What are these equations really (see Table 30.1)?

Well, these certainly are *diagnostic equations*. These equations describe each type of congenital heart disease in a specific and different way. Each equation is accurately diagnostic. These equations are also *situs equations*. Consider Equation 30.1:

$$\text{SNRGA }\{S,D,S\} = 0R + 4L$$

This is an equation concerning *solitus* normally related great arteries with a segmental *situs* set of solitus atria, *D-loop* or *solitus* ventricles, and *solitus* normally related arteries. These are situs-based equations (see Table 30.1).

Summary

Segmental situs is important not only structurally, but also because of the role situs plays in great arterial switches and non-switches, apoptosis, rotations, and synergy. There is no better summary than the equations (see Table 30.1).

REFERENCES

1. Van Praagh R. What determines whether the great arteries are normally or abnormally related? *Am J Cardiol.* 2016;118: 1390.
2. Abbott ME. Transposition or reversed torsion of the arterial trunks. In: Osler W, McCree T, eds. *Modern Medicine: Its Theory and Practice.* Vol. 4. Philadelphia: Lea & Febiger; 1927: 716.
3. Van Praagh S, Davidoff A, Chin A, Shiel FS, Reynolds J, Van Praagh R. Double outlet right ventricle: anatomic types and developmental implications based on a study of 101 autopsied cases. *Coeur.* 1982;13:389.
4. Paul MH, Muster AJ, Sinha SN, Cole RB, Van Praagh R. Double-outlet left ventricle with an intact ventricular septum: clinical and autopsy diagnosis and developmental implications. *Circulation.* 1970;41:129.
5. Van Praagh R. The story of anatomically corrected malposition of the great arteries. *Chest.* 1976;69:2.
6. Van Praagh R, Van Praagh S. The anatomy of common aorticopulmonary trunk (truncus arteriosus communis) and its embryologic implications, a study of 59 necropsied cases. *Am J Cardiol.* 1965;16:406.
7. Taussig HB, Bing RJ. Complete transposition of the aorta and a levoposition of the pulmonary artery. Clinical, physiological, and pathological findings. *Am Heart J.* 1949;37:551.
8. Van Praagh R. The evolution of the human heart and its relevance to congenital heart disease. *Kardiochirurgia i Torakochirurgia Polska.* 2011;8:427.

Understanding Normally and Abnormally Related Great Arteries

Equations, Apoptosis, Switches, Rotations, and Synergy

BASIC PRINCIPLES

1. When the situs (pattern of anatomic organization) of the subarterial infundibulum and the situs of the great arteries are the same (concordant), the great arteries are normally related—solitus normally related, or inversus normally related.
2. When the situs of the infundibulum and the situs of the great arteries are different (discordant), the great arteries are abnormally related.

GREAT ARTERIAL EQUATIONS*

Normally Related Great Arteries With or Without Associated Malformations

1. SNRGA {S,D,**S**} = **0R + 4L**

$$\uparrow \qquad \uparrow$$

GA **Inf**

Situs of infundibulum (Inf) + Situs of great arteries (GA) = Solitus + Solitus, that is, concordant, **solitus normal**

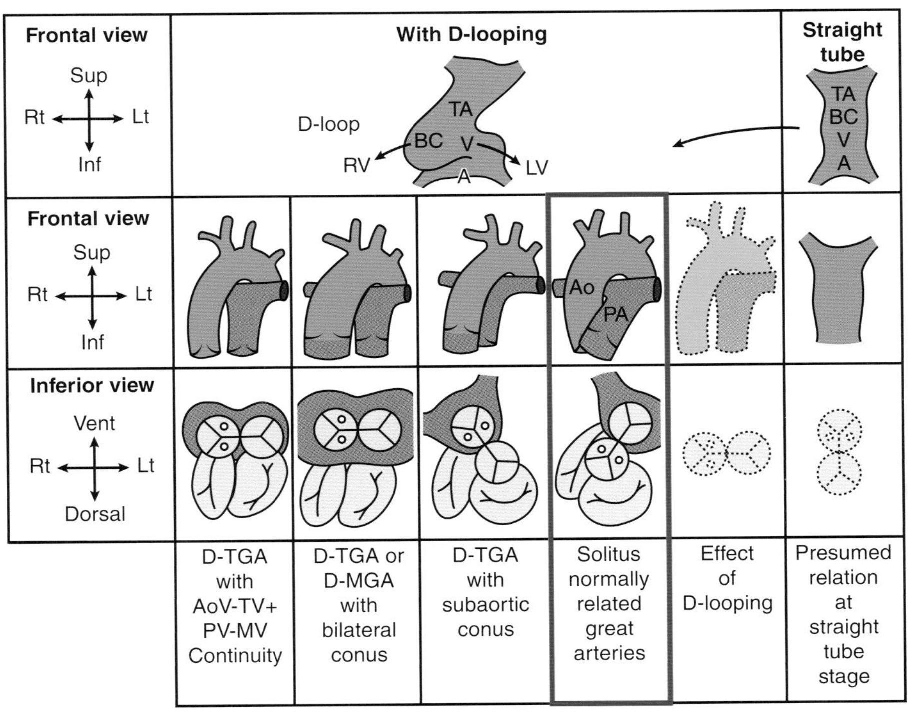

A.1 Solitus or D-Loop Hearts. (Reproduced with permission from Van Praagh R, Van Praagh S. Isolated ventricular inversion: A consideration of the morphogenesis, definition, and diagnosis of nontransposed and transposed great arteries. *Am J Cardiol.* 1966;17:395-406.)

*Equal sign is intended for clarity of understanding. However, morphogenetic movements are typically a range of values not equal to simply one mean or median value.

2. INRGA {I,L,**I**} = **4R + 0L**

↑ ↑

GA **Inf**

Situs of inf + Situs of GA = Inversus + Inversus, that is, concordant, **inversus normal**

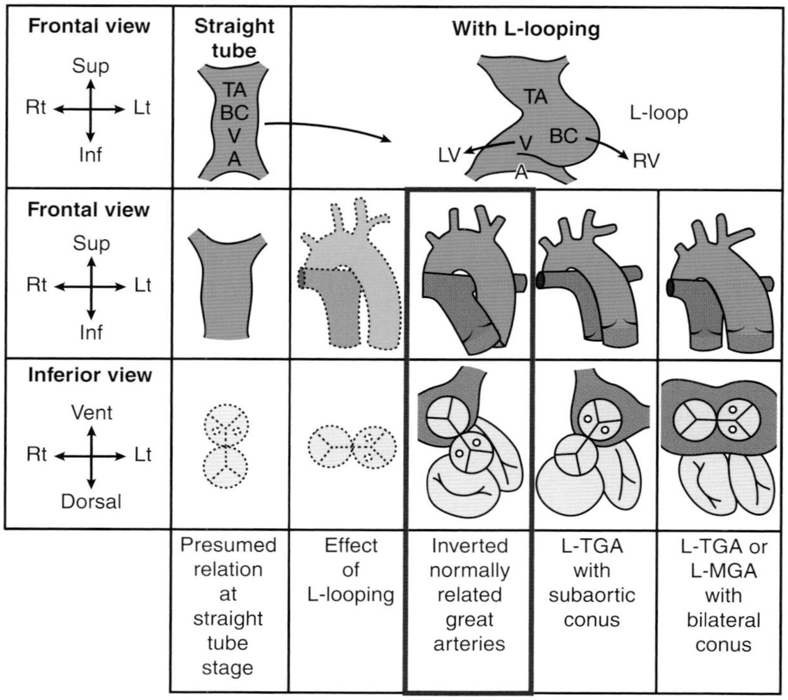

A.2 Inverted or L-Loop Hearts. (Reproduced with permission from Van Praagh R, Van Praagh S. Isolated ventricular inversion: A consideration of the morphogenesis, definition, and diagnosis of nontransposed and transposed great arteries. *Am J Cardiol.* 1966;17:395-406.)

Tetralogy of Fallot

3. TOF {S,D,**S**} = 0R + **3L** (TOF, mild/moderate PS)
4. TOF {S,D,**S**} = 0R + **2L** (TOF, severe PS)
5. TOF {S,D,**S**} = 0R + **1L** (TOF, P Atresia)

↑ ↑
GA **Inf**

Situs of inf + GA

Situs of the infundibulum is of the solitus normal type, except that the subpulmonary infundibulum is hypoplastic: mildly (3L), moderately (2L), or severely (1L). The situs of the great arteries is solitus normal. Hence, the sum of the infundibular situs and the great arterial situs is Solitus + Solitus, that is, concordant, and therefore **solitus normal**.

Tetralogy of Fallot may also be regarded as the Monology of Stensen. First described by Niels Stensen, the Dane of parotid duct fame, in 1671, all four of these anomalies are now thought to be sequelae of subpulmonary infundibular hypoplasia: pulmonary outflow tract obstruction, subaortic ventricular septal defect (VSD), aortic overriding (subnormal semilunar dextral rotation), and postnatal right ventricular hypertrophy.

Inverted or L-Loop Hearts

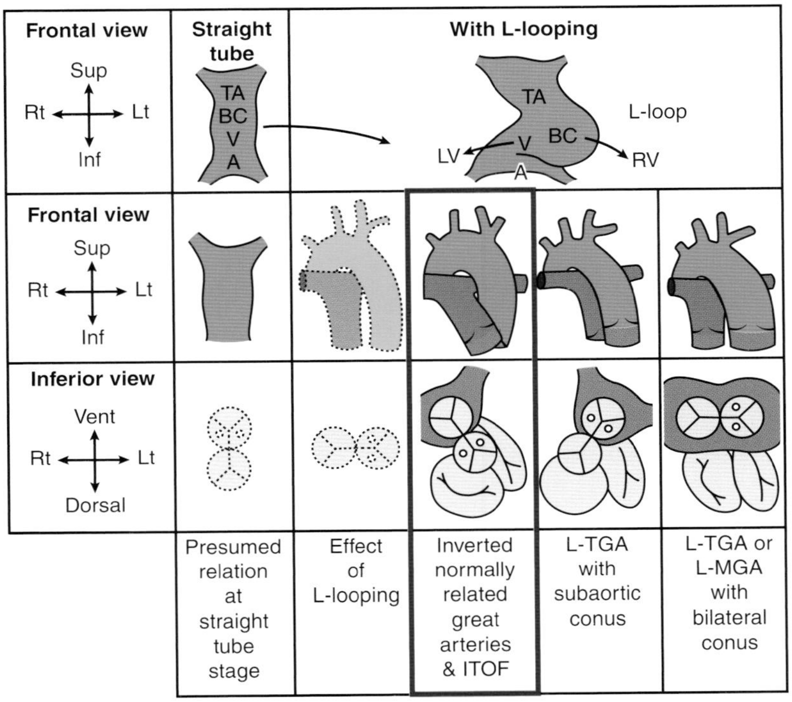

A.3 Inverted Tetralogy of Fallot. (Reproduced with permission from Van Praagh R, Van Praagh S. Isolated ventricular inversion: A consideration of the morphogenesis, definition, and diagnosis of nontransposed and transposed great arteries. *Am J Cardiol.* 1966;17:395-406.)

Absence of Subpulmonary Infundibulum (Formerly Called "Truncus Arteriosus Communis")

6. AOSPI {S,D,–} = 0R + (**–L**) + APW ("TAC" type A1)
7. AOSPI {S,D,–} = 0R + (**–L**) – PV – MPA ("TAC" type A2)

TOF does not have absence of subpulmonary infundibulum. AOSPI + TOF are closely associated anomalies.

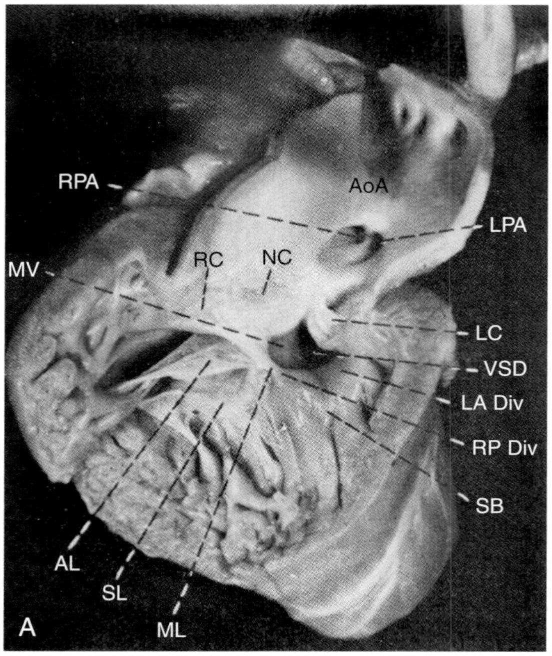

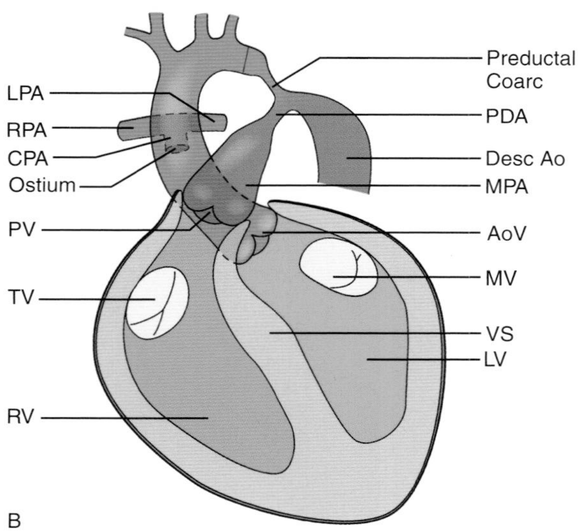

A.4 A, B: Absence of Subpulmonary Infundibulum (Formerly Called "Truncus Arteriosus Communis"). **B:** Absence of the right and left sixth aortic arches results in non-migration of the right pulmonary artery (RPA) branch and the left pulmonary artery (LPA) branch from the aortic sac or common pulmonary artery (CPA), and also results in the main pulmonary artery (MPA) in having no branches. (Reproduced with permission from Vizcaino A, Campbell J, Litovsky S, Van Praagh R. Single origin of right and left pulmonary artery branches from ascending aorta with nonbranching main pulmonary artery: Relevance to a new understanding of truncus arteriosus. *Pediatr Cardiol.* 2002;23:230.)

CORRECT

Understanding of Truncus Arteriosus Communis

In "truncus arteriosus communis" type A2 – with right pulmonary artery (RPA) and left pulmonary artery (LPA) from the aortic sac, the main pulmonary artery (MPA) is absent (Fig. A.4a). Without an MPA, "TAC" is impossible.

However, rarely it is possible to have isolated absence of the Ao – PA septum (Fig. A.5).

8. AOAPS {S,D,S} = 0R + 4L – **APS**

Absence of the aortopulmonary septum (AOAPS), as an isolated anomaly, appears to be very rare.

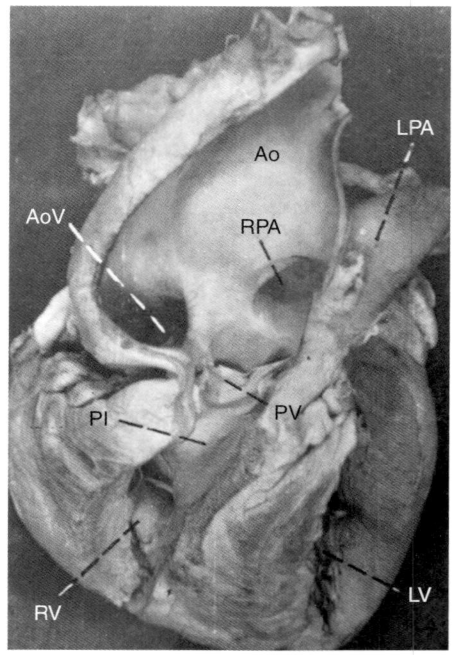

A.5 Isolated absence of the aortopulmonary septum is a true example of common aortopulmonary trunk (truncus arteriosus communis). Therefore, truncus arteriosus communis or absence of the common aortopulmonary trunk rarely does exist as an isolated anomaly. (Reproduced with permission from Vizcaino A, Campbell J, Litovsky S, Van Praagh R. Single origin of right and left pulmonary artery branches from ascending aorta with nonbranching main pulmonary artery: Relevance to a new understanding of truncus arteriosus. *Pediatr Cardiol.* 2002;23:230.)

ABNORMALLY RELATED GREAT ARTERIES

D-Transposition of the Great Arteries

9. TGA {S,D,**D**} = **4R + 0L**

↑ ↑

GA **Inf**

Infundibular situs is situs inversus, the same as in Equation 2 of situs inversus totalis.

Infundibular situs = Inversus
Great arterial situs = solitus, abnormal
Infundibuloarterial situs analysis = inversus + solitus, discordant, abnormal

Typical D-TGA is isolated infundibular inversion.

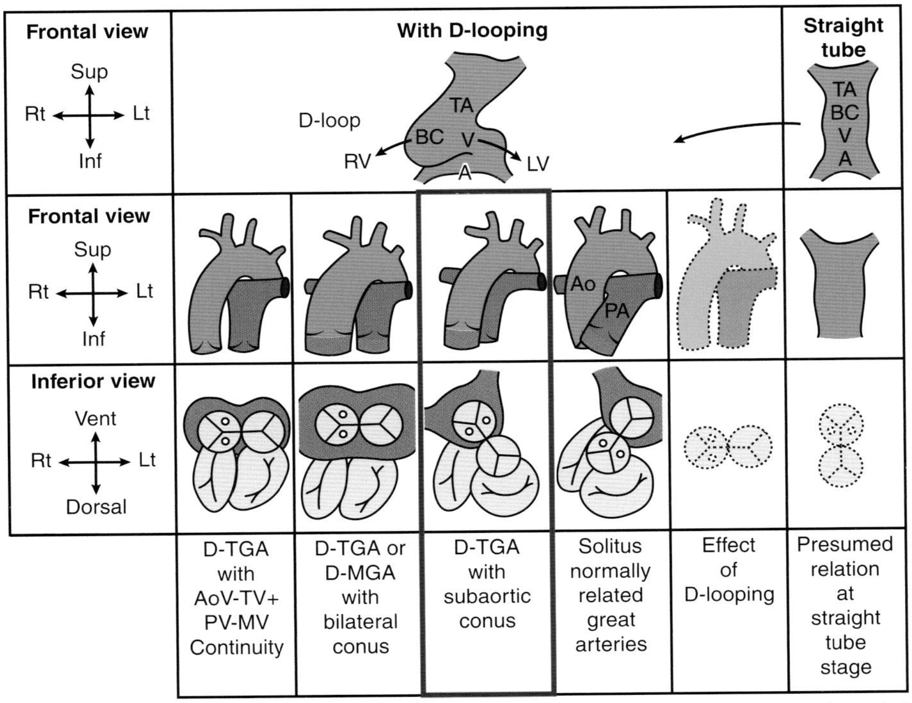

A.6 D-Transposition of the Great Arteries. (Reproduced with permission from Van Praagh R, Van Praagh S. Isolated ventricular inversion: A consideration of the morphogenesis, definition, and diagnosis of nontransposed and transposed great arteries. *Am J Cardiol.* 1966;17:395-406.)

L-Transposition of the Great Arteries

10. TGA {S,L,**L**} = **0R** + **4L**

↑ ↑

GA **Inf**

Infundibular situs = Solitus normal, the same as in Equation 1.

The great arterial situs = inverted.

I-A situs analysis = Solitus + Inversus.

Conclusion: Discordant, that is, abnormal

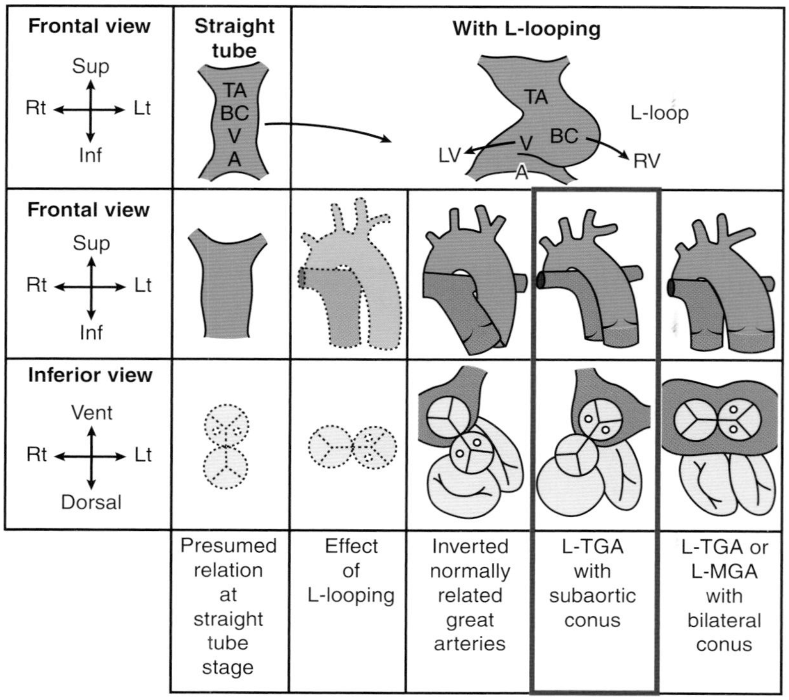

A.7 Congenitally, Physiologically Corrected L-TGA Is Isolated Infundibular Noninversion. (Reproduced with permission from Van Praagh R, Van Praagh S. Isolated ventricular inversion: A consideration of the morphogenesis, definition, and diagnosis of nontransposed and transposed great arteries. *Am J Cardiol.* 1966;17:395-406.)

Double-Outlet Right Ventricle

11. DORV {S,D,**D**} = **4R + 4L (Taussig-Bing type)**

↑ ↑

GA Inf

I-A situs analysis:

Inf situs = situs ambiguus

GA situs = solitus, abnormal

I-A situs = Ambiguus + Solitus

Conclusion: discordant, therefore abnormal. DORV with bilateral infundibular free walls results from no apoptosis.[1]

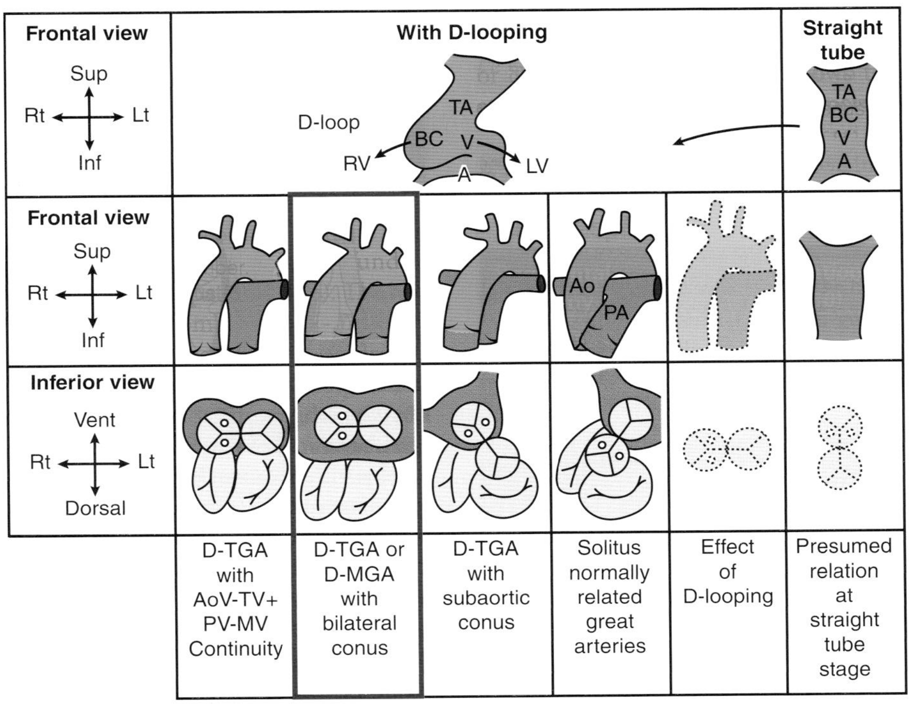

A.8 D malposition of the great artery (D-MGA). (Reproduced with permission from Van Praagh R, Van Praagh S. Isolated ventricular inversion: A consideration of the morphogenesis, definition, and diagnosis of nontransposed and transposed great arteries. *Am J Cardiol*. 1966;17:395-406.)

Double-Outlet Left Ventricle, Paul Type

12. DOLV {S,D,**D**} = 0R + 0L

↑ ↑

GA **Inf**

I-A situs combination:

Inf situs = situs ambiguus

GA situs = situs solitus, abnormal

I-A situs combination = Ambiguus + Solitus, that is, discordant, abnormal

DOLV with bilateral absence of the subarterial infundibular free walls results in a double great arterial switch and DOLV.[2]

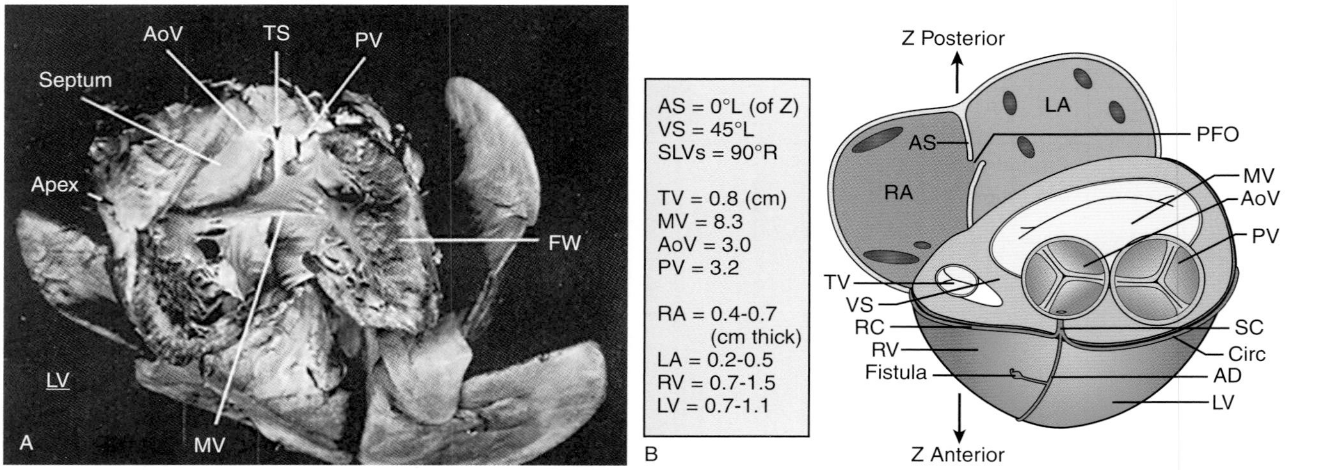

A.9 (Reproduced with permission from Paul MH, Muster AJ, Sinha SN, Cole RB, Van Praagh R. Double-outlet left ventricle with an intact ventricular septum: Clinical and autopsy diagnosis and developmental implications. *Circulation.* 1970;41:129.)

Anatomically Corrected Malposition of the Great Arteries

13. ACMGA {S,D,**L**} = **0R** + **4L**

↑ ↑

GA **Inf**

I-A situs combination = Solitus normal + Inverted, that is, discordant, abnormal.

In ACMGA, abnormally related great arteries emerge from morphologically appropriate ventricles because the ventricles loop in one direction and the infundibulum and great arteries twist in the opposite direction.

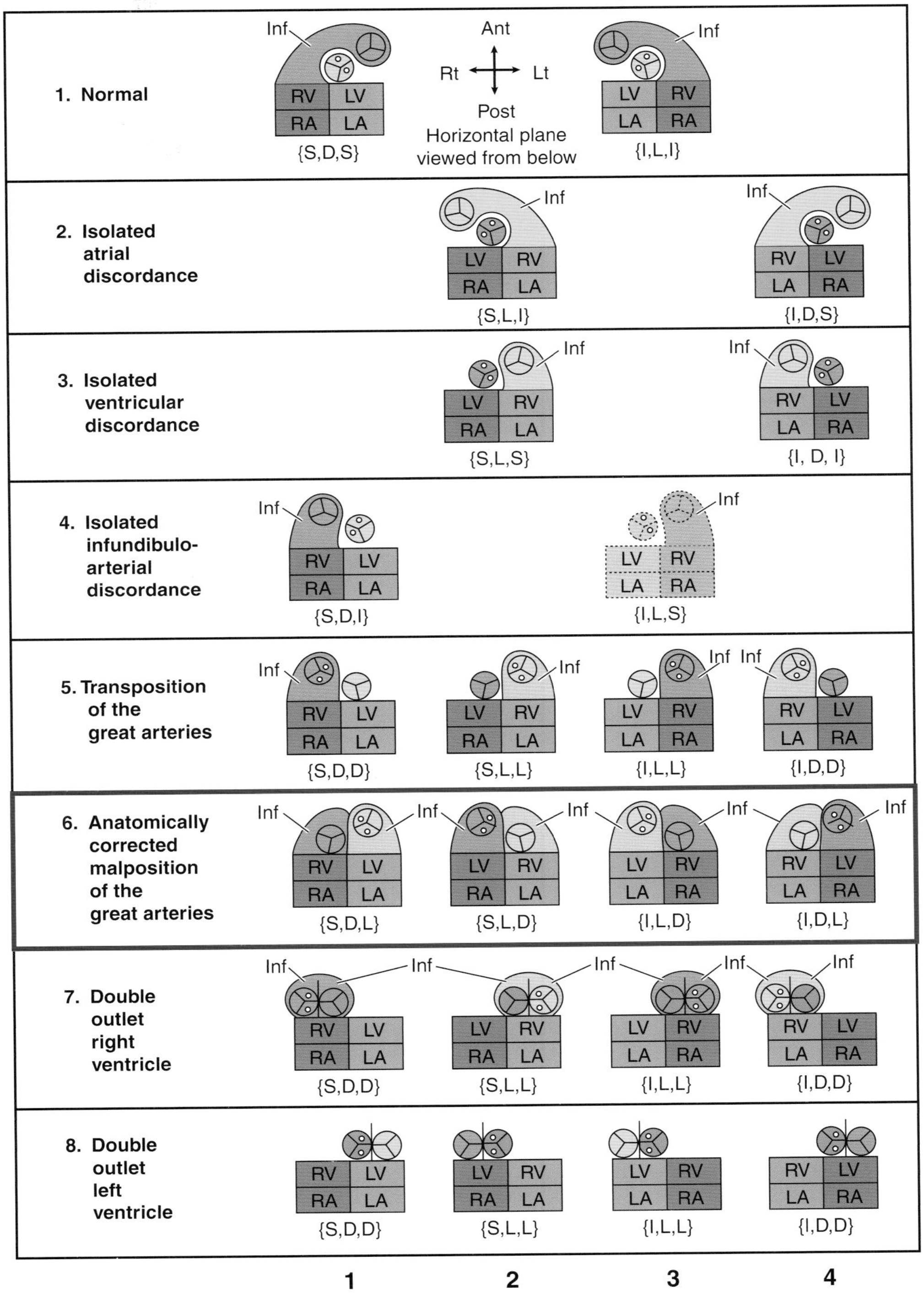

A.10 (From Foran RB, Belcourt C, Nanton MA, Murphy DA, Weinberg AG, Liebman J, Castaneda AR, Van Praagh R. Isolated infundibuloarterial inversion {S,D,I}: A newly recognized form of congenital heart disease. *Am Heart J.* 1988;116:1337, with permission.)

14. ACMGA {S,L,**D**} = **4R** + **4L**

↑ ↑

GA **Inf**

Situs of inf + Situs of GA = Ambiguus + Solitus abnormal, that is, **discordant**

Isolated Ventricular Inversion

15. IVI {S,**L**,S} = 0R + 4L + VSD + Ventricular L-loop

This is a rare malformation of the ventricles that are inverted (ventricular L-loop), not of the infundibulum that is solitus normal. Because there is one segmental alignment discordance at the atrioventricular level, the systemic venous and pulmonary venous circulations are physiologically uncorrected, similar to typical D-TGA.

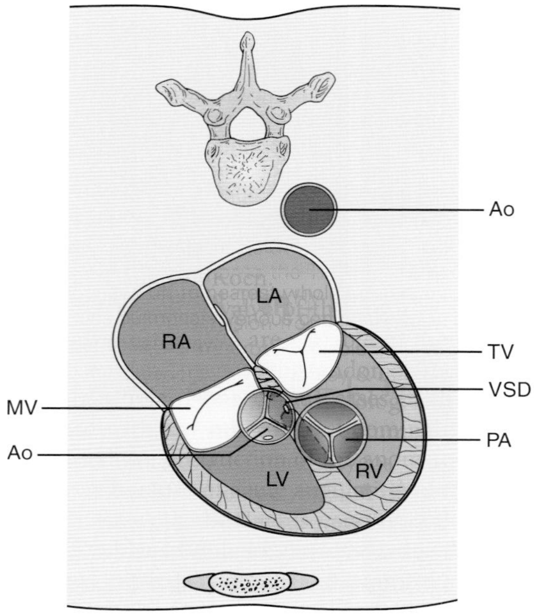

A.11 IVI {S,**L**,S} = 0R + 4L + **L-loop** + VSD. (Reprinted with permission from Van Praagh R, Van Praagh S. Isolated ventricular inversion. *Am J Cardiol.* 1966;17:395.)

BASIC PRINCIPLES (ADDRESSED THUS FAR)

Thus far, this presentation has been mostly concerned with the effects of two basic principles:

1. When the situs of the subarterial infundibulum and the situs of the great arteries are the same (concordant), the great arteries are normally related.
2. When the situs of the subarterial infundibulum and the situs of the great arteries are different (discordant), the great arteries are abnormally related.
3. The developmental effect of infundibular muscle beneath a great artery typically prevents an embryonic switch of that great artery from the RV to the LV.
4. The developmental effect of the absence of infundibular muscle beneath a great artery typically is facilitation of an embryonic switch of that great artery from the RV to the LV.

Look at the equations: every 0 is a switch, every 1, 2, 3, or 4 is a nonswitch:

1. SNRGA {S,D,S} = 0R + 4L
2. INRGA {I,L,I} = 4R + 0L
3. TOF {S,D,S} = 0R + 3L + VSD
4. TOF {S,D,S} = 0R + 2L + VSD
5. TOF {S,D,S} = 0R + 1L + VSD
6. AOSPI {S,D,–} = 0R + (–L) + APSD
7. AOSPI {S,D,–} = 0R + (–L) + VSD – PV – MPA
8. AOAPS {S,D,S} = 0R + 4L – APS
9. TGA {S,D,D} = 4R + 0L
10. TGA {S,L,L} = 0R + 4L
11. DORV {S,D,D} = 4R + 4L
12. DOLV {S,D,D} = 0R + 0L
13. ACMGA {S,D,L} = 0R + 4L
14. ACMGA {S,L,D} = 4R + 4L
15. IVI {S,L,S} = 0R + 4L + VSD + L-loop

THE EMBRYONIC ARTERIAL SWITCH

How Does It Happen Normally?

Normally, the subaortic infundibular free wall is killed and removed by **apoptosis,** that is, programmed cell death. Then the aorta, which is above the RV, can migrate inferiorly, posteriorly, and leftward. The aortic valve then passes through the interventricular foramen (the normal ventral septal defect [VSD]) into the LV and then gets into fibrous continuity with the mitral valve via the intervalvar fibrosa.

How Does It Happen in D-TGA?

D-TGA results from infundibular inversion, that is, R-L switching of infundibular development:

SNRGA {S,D,S} = 0R + 4L

TGA {S,D,D} = 4R + 0L

In D-TGA, apoptosis occurs beneath the left-sided pulmonary artery (0L), not normally beneath the right-sided aorta (0R). Left-sided subpulmonary apoptosis results in switching the left-sided pulmonary artery into the LV. The right-sided aorta sits unswitched atop a well-developed subaortic infundibulum, in turn above the right-sided RV.

How Does It Happen in DORV?

DORV of the Taussig-Bing type results from bilateral absence of apoptosis, SubAo + SubPA.

DORV {S,D,D} = 4R + 4L.

Absence of apoptosis results in a well-developed subaortic infundibulum (4R) and in a well-developed subpulmonary infundibulum (4L).

Bilaterally well-developed subarterial infundibula prevent aortic and pulmonary artery switches, resulting in DORV.

IA situs analysis: Inf situs	=	4R + 4L = Ambiguus
Arterial situs = {S,D,D}	=	Solitus abnormal
IA situs combination	=	Ambiguus + Solitus, that is, discordant, abnormal

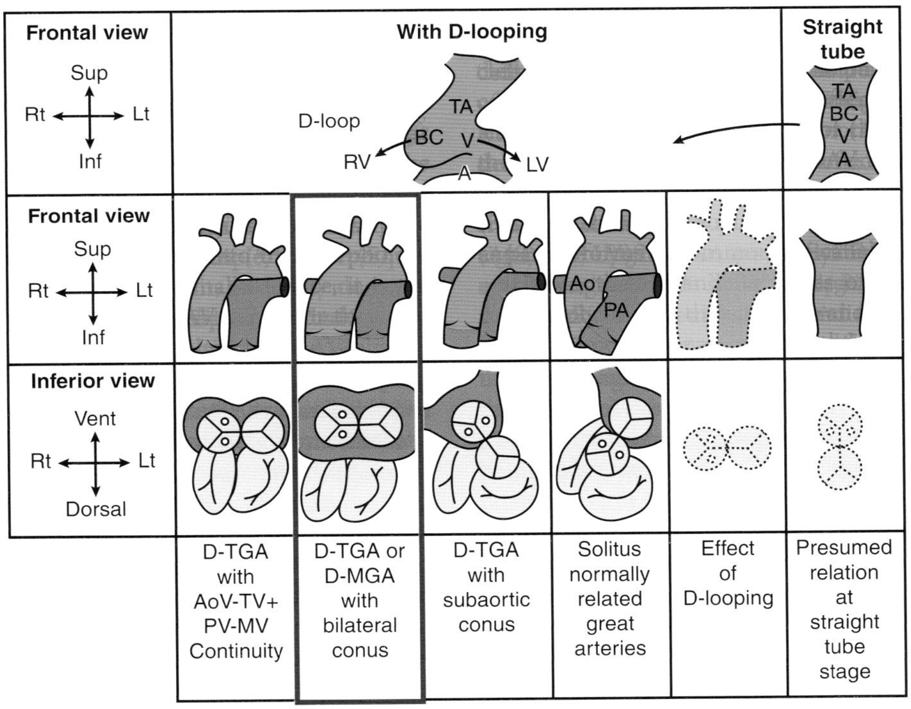

A.12 (Reproduced with permission from Van Praagh R, Van Praagh S. Isolated ventricular inversion: A consideration of the morphogenesis, definition, and diagnosis of nontransposed and transposed great arteries. *Am J Cardiol.* 1966;17:395-406.)

DOLV {S,**D**,D} = **0R + 0L**

DOLV of the Paul type results from absence of the right-sided subaortic muscular infundibulum (0R) and absence of the left-sided subpulmonary muscular infundibulum (0L).

Bilateral infundibular absence is thought to be due to bilateral apoptosis (programmed cell death) of the subarterial infundibula.

The infundibuloarterial situs combination is (0R + 0L) + {-,-,D}, that is, Ambiguus + Solitus, discordant, or abnormal.

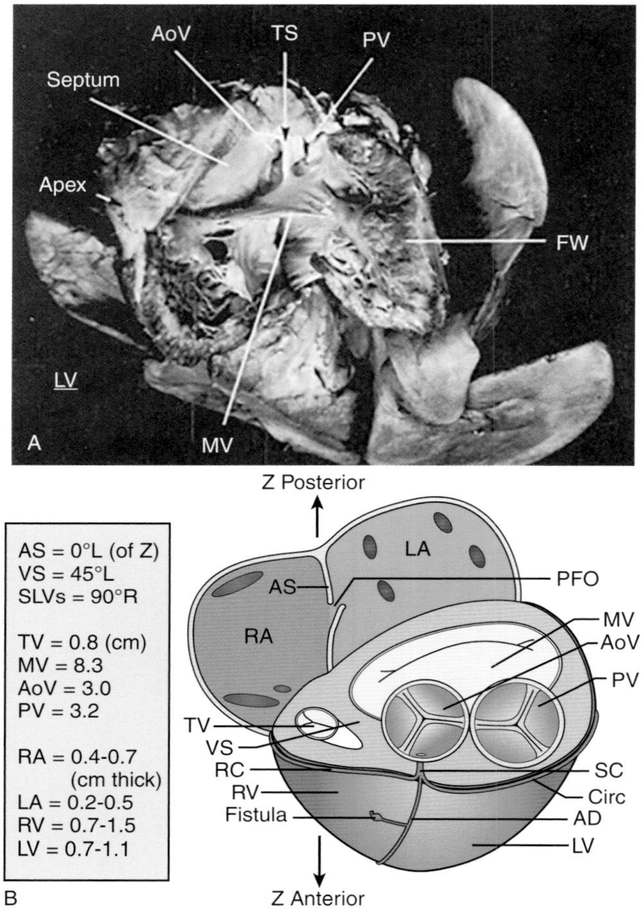

A.13 (Reproduced with permission from Paul MH, Muster AJ, Sinha SN, Cole RB, Van Praagh R. Double-outlet left ventricle with an intact ventricular septum: Clinical and autopsy diagnosis and developmental implications. *Circulation.* 1970:41:129.)

Central Role of the Subarterial Infundibulum

We have finally figured out what the subarterial infundibulum is doing!

1. The subarterial infundibulum prevents the embryonic great arterial switch from RV to LV and mitral valve.
2. The absence of a subarterial infundibulum permits or facilitates an embryonic great arterial switch from RV to LV.
3. Apoptosis, or programmed cell death, determines where absences of subarterial infundibular muscle occur and therefore which great arteries get switched and which do not get switched.

ANATOMICALLY CORRECTED MALPOSITION OF THE GREAT ARTERIES

ACMGA {S,D,**L**} = **0R + 4L**
ACMGA {S,L,**D**} = **4R + 4L**

In ACMGA, the malposed great arteries nonetheless arise from the appropriate ventricles, aorta (Ao) above the LV, and pulmonary artery (PA) above the RV. This apparent impossibility is related to the fact that the ventricles loop in one direction but infundibulum and great arteries twist in the opposite direction: {-,D,L} and {-,L,D}.

Infundibuloarterial situs analysis is discordant in both equations:

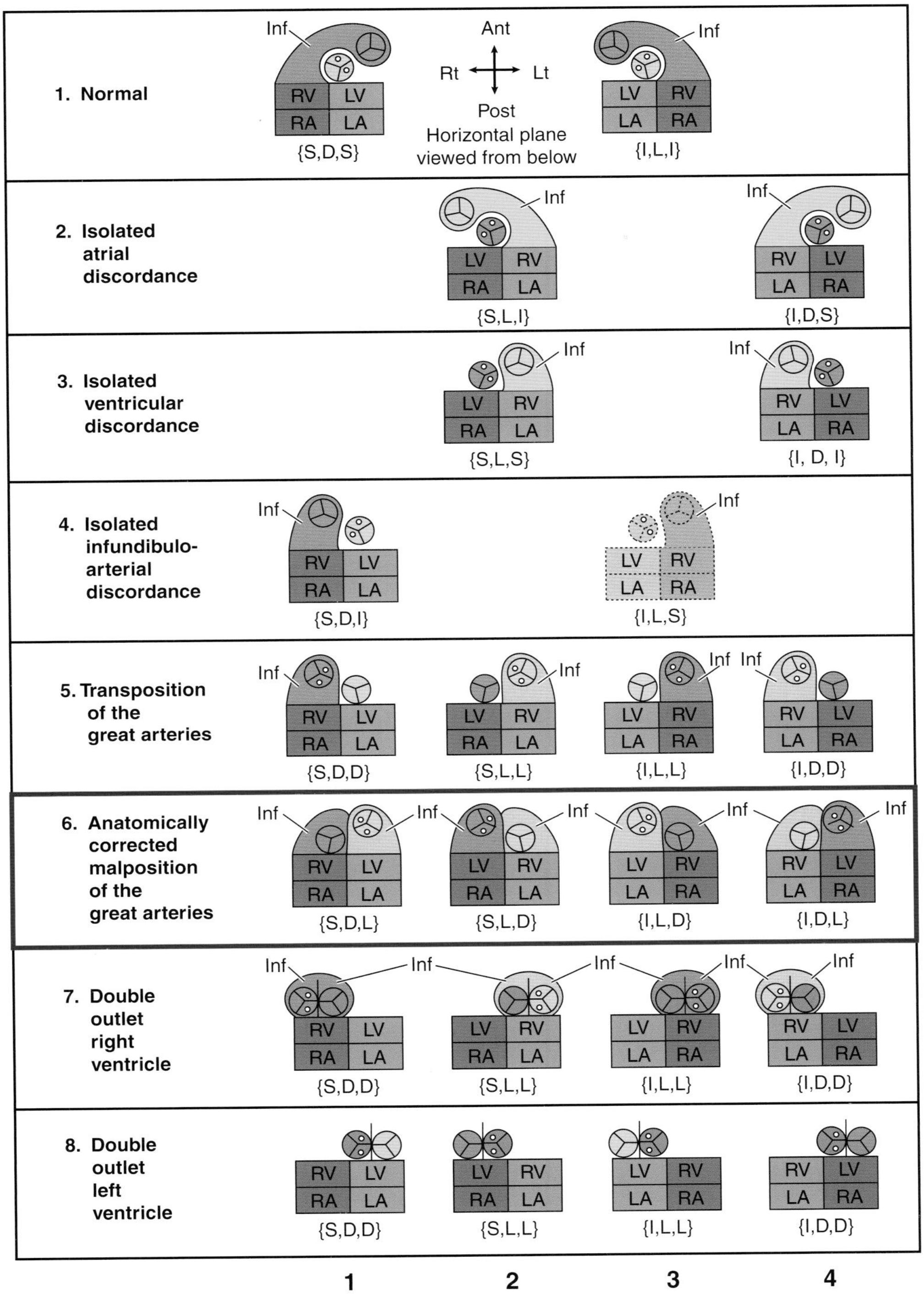

A.14 Anatomically corrected malposition of the great arteries (ACMGA): S,D,L and S,L,D. In ACMGA {S,D,L}, the ventricles loop to the right and the infundibulum and great arteries twist to the left. In ACMGA {S,L,D}, the ventricles loop to the left and the infundibulum and great arteries twist to the right. (From Foran RB, Belcourt C, Nanton MA, Murphy DA, Weinberg AG, Liebman J, Castaneda AR, Van Praagh R. Isolated infundibuloarterial inversion {S,D,I}: A newly recognized form of congenital heart disease. *Am Heart J.* 1988;116:1337, with permission.)

Rotation

In the cardiovascular system:

1. Solitus structures rotate to the right, as in D-loops, that is, dextral rotation.
2. Inversus structures rotate to the left, as in L-loops, that is, levorotation.

Rotations, D- and L-

Equation 1:

1. SNRGA {S,D,**S**} = **0R** + **4L**

   ↑ Situs solitus of the great arteries (**S**); ↑ Situs of the infundibulum (**0R + 4L**)

   What happens?

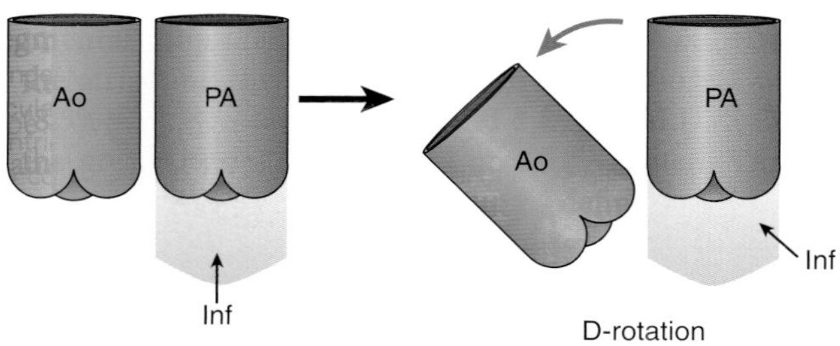

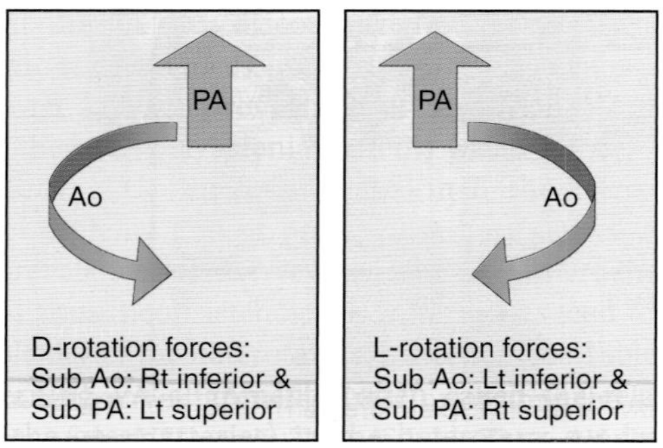

Normal:

- Normally, the subaortic force appears to be *negative*, because of apoptosis (programmed cell death) of the subaortic infundibular free wall.
- Normally, the subpulmonary force appears to be *positive*, due to growth and development of the subpulmonary muscular infundibulum.

Thus there are ***two opposite forces acting*** to produce dextrorotation at the semilunar valves.

Equation 2 (inversus heart):

2. INRGA {I,L,**I**} = **4R** + **0L**

   ↑ Situs inversus of the great arteries (**I**); ↑ Well-developed right-sided subpulmonary infundibulum and zero infundibulum under the left-sided aorta (**4R + 0L**)

   What happens?

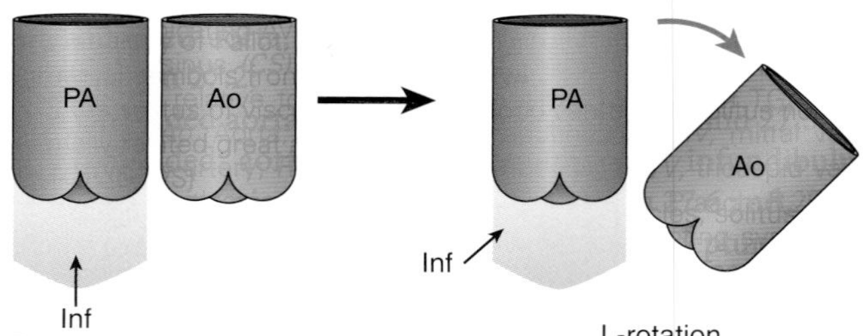

B

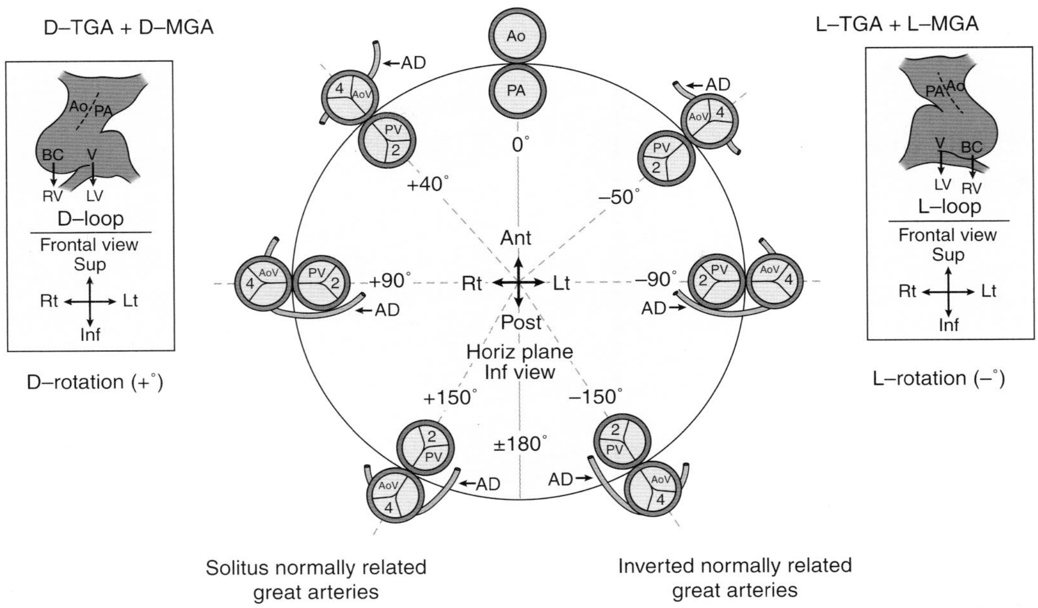

A.15 Normal and abnormal geometric relations between the great arteries at the semilunar valves. (From Van Praagh R. Approccio segmentario alla diagnosi delle cardiopatie congenite. In Squarcia U, ed. *Progressi in Cardiologia Pediatrica.* Milan: Casa Editrice Ambrosiana; 1978:7.)

Synergy

Syn (together) + ergon (to work), Greek

Normal:

Ventricular force = 90 degrees D-rotation at valves, as in the Taussig-Bing type of DORV

Infundibular force = 60 degrees D-rotation at valves

Normal total D-rotation at semilunar valves = 90 degrees + 60 degrees = 150 degrees

Inverted normal heart = –90 degrees + (–60 degrees) = –150 degrees of levorotation, expressed in negative degrees

WHAT IS GOING ON IN TRANSPOSITION OF THE GREAT ARTERIES?

The absence of synergy and the presence of L-rotation or negative forces related to infundibular situs inversus.

D-TGA is basically isolated infundibular inversion:

TGA {S,D,D} = **4R + 0L**

SNRGA {S,D,S} = **0R + 4L**

Infundibular inversion ≈ 60 degrees L-rotation

In D-TGA, rotation at the semilunar valves:

Ventricular force = 90 degrees D-rotation

Infundibular force = 60 degrees

In D-TGA, rotation at semilunar valves

≈ (equals the sum of) + (90 degrees D-rotation) + (– 60 degrees L-rotation) = 30 degrees D-rotation

SUMMARY

This appendix is about normally and abnormally related great arteries, presented in terms of:

- defining equations,
- apoptosis,
- switches and nonswitches,
- D- and L- rotations, and
- synergy and its absence and the presence of antagonistic situs-based force(s)

This work is a contribution to the algebra and the geometry of congenital heart disease in humans.

ACKNOWLEDGMENTS

This work was greatly facilitated by the assistance of:

- Prof. Janusz Skalski
- Michael Goderre
- Susan Boissonneault
- Andrew D.G. Van Praagh, PhD

REFERENCES

1. Taussig HB, Bing RJ. Complete transposition of the aorta and a levoposition of the pulmonary artery. Clinical, physiological, and pathological findings. *Am Heart J*. 1949;37:551.
2. Paul MH, Sinha SN, Muster AJ, Cole RB, Van Praagh R. Double-outlet left ventricle. Report of an autopsy case with an intact ventricular septum and consideration of its developmental implications. *Circulation.* 1970;41:129.

POST SCRIPTUM

CONGENITAL HEART DISEASES AS FAILURES OF EVOLUTIONARY ADAPTATIONS

Fish hearts are single-pump systems with a single atrium, a single ventricle, and a single great artery. Land-living vertebrates such as humans typically have a double-pump cardiovascular system with two atria, two ventricles, and two great arteries.

Fish started coming ashore about 500 million years ago and gradually evolved into many different kinds of vertebrates. Those that functioned normally we decided had normal anatomy. Those that did not function normally we decided had congenital heart disease. This book is concerned with both the normal and the abnormal.

CONGENITAL HEART DISEASES ASSOCIATED WITH EVOLUTIONARY FAILURE

Single left ventricle (LV) with absence of the right ventricle (RV) and with double-inlet or common-inlet LV is an anomaly that reduces what normally should be a biventricular heart (LV and RV) to a univentricular heart (LV only). Absence of the RV is a major evolutionary failure.

TETRALOGY OF FALLOT

Obstructive hypoplasia of the normal subpulmonary infundibulum decreases pulmonary blood flow (<QP), and this anomaly increases the systemic blood flow (>QS) and typically also increases systemic cyanosis.

There is only one formula for a normal human heart and its inverted or mirror-image form.

The solitus normal heart: SNRGA {S,D,S} = 0R + 4L

The inverted normal heart: INRGA {I,L,I} = 4R + 0L

All other formulas result in abnormal hearts. For example:

Abnormal cardiovascular formulas

1. Single LV: SNRGA {S,D,S} = 0R + 4L-RV
2. TOF {S,D,S} = 0R + 3L + VSD
   TOF {S,D,S} = 0R + 2L + VSD
   TOF {S,D,S} = 0R + 1L + VSD
3. TGA {S,D,D} = 4R + 0L
4. TGA {S,L,L} = 0R + 4L + VSD
5. DORV {S,D,D} = 4R + 4L + VSD
6. DOLV {S,D,D} = 0R + 0L
7. ACM {S,D,L} = 0R + 4L

INDEX

S

U